DUKES' PHYSIOLOGY OF DOMESTIC ANIMALS | ELEVENTH EDITION

Melvin J. Swenson,
Editor
William O. Reece,
Editor
Milton J. Allison
Bengt E. Andersson
Robert A. Argenzio
Harpal S. Bal
Gary K. Beauchamp
Donald C. Beitz
Emmett N. Bergman
James E. Breazile
William H. Burke
Dwight B. Coulter
David K. Detweiler
William M. Dickson
Harry G. Downie
Gary E. Duke
Lars-Eric Edqvist
Howard H. Erickson
Richard C. Ewan
M. Roger Fedde
Patricia A. Gentry
Virgil W. Hays
T. Richard Houpt
Ainsley Iggo
Norman L. Jacobson
Hallgrímur Jónasson
F. A. Kallfelz
Morley R. Kare
W. R. Klemm
David H. Knight
Barry F. Leek
George Lust
Roger R. Marsh
Julius Melbin
Michael S. Miller
Chung S. Park
Dean H. Riedesel
David Robertshaw
Gretchen M. Schmidt
George H. Stabenfeldt
Larry Patrick Tilley
R. H. Wasserman

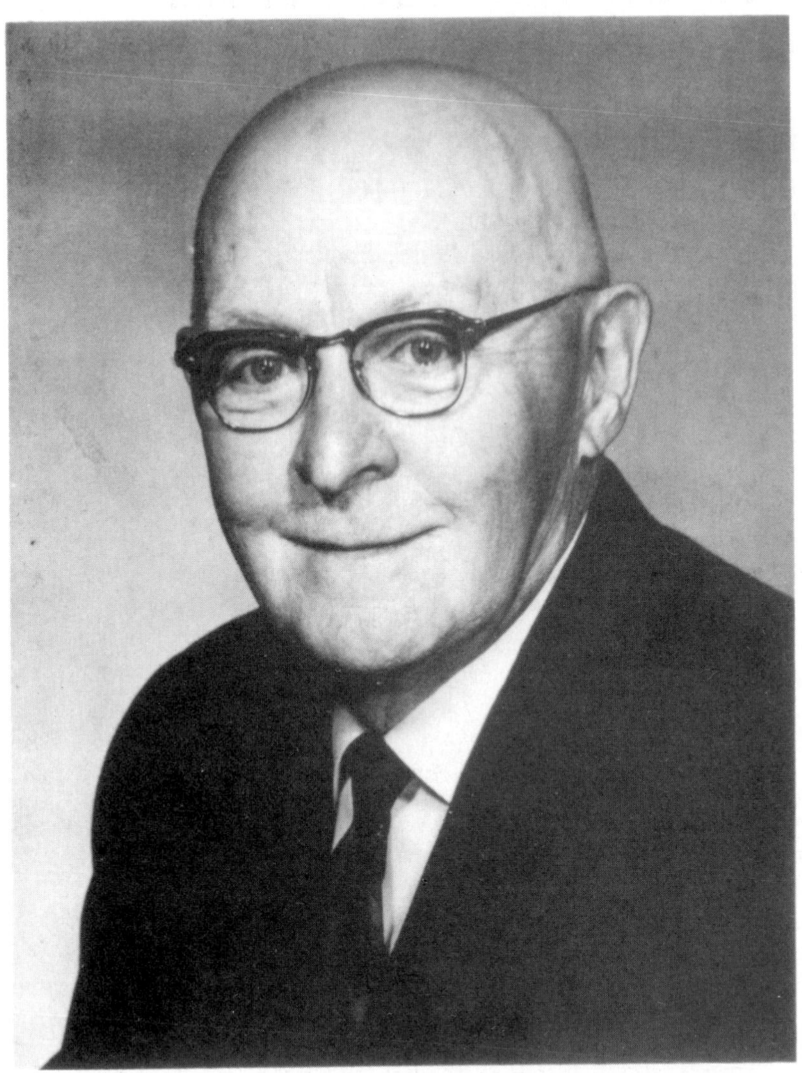

H. Hugh Dukes, teacher extraordinary and benefactor to veterinarians throughout the world.

DUKES' PHYSIOLOGY OF DOMESTIC ANIMALS | ELEVENTH EDITION

EDITED BY

MELVIN J. SWENSON D.V.M., M.S., Ph.D.

WILLIAM O. REECE D.V.M., Ph.D.

COMSTOCK PUBLISHING ASSOCIATES a division of

CORNELL UNIVERSITY PRESS | Ithaca and London

The Physiology of Domestic Animals, by H. H. Dukes
First edition, 1933
Second edition, 1934
Third edition, 1935
Fourth edition, 1937
Fifth edition, 1942
Sixth edition, 1947
Seventh edition, 1955

Dukes' Physiology of Domestic Animals, edited by Melvin J. Swenson
Eighth edition, 1970
Ninth edition, 1977
Tenth edition, 1984
Eleventh edition, 1993 (coeditor William O. Reece)

Library of Congress Cataloging-in-Publication Data
Dukes, H. H. (Henry Hugh), 1895–1987
[Physiology of domestic animals]
Dukes' Physiology of domestic animals/edited by Melvin J. Swenson, William O. Reece—11th ed.
p. cm.
Includes bibliographical references and index.
ISBN 0-8014-2804-1
1. Veterinary physiology. I. Swenson, Melvin J., 1917– . II. Reece, William O. III. Title. IV. Title: Physiology of domestic animals.
SF768.D77 1993
636.089'2—dc20 92-56781

Printed in the United States of America

This edition is dedicated to my son, Myron, who has been called home to be with our Lord since the last edition was published. He was always an inspiring and encouraging son and companion to me through the years I worked on the book.

M. J. S.

Contents

Preface

Since 1933, H. Hugh Dukes' *Physiology of Domestic Animals* has been an inspiring and indispensable textbook for undergraduate students of veterinary medicine and animal science. Moreover, because of its comprehensive treatment, it is used extensively by graduate students, research workers, and practitioners.

The purpose of the eleventh edition continues in the same tradition as that expressed by Dr. Dukes in the Preface to the first: "This book, based on years of experience in the field of animal physiology, represents an attempt to provide students of veterinary medicine with a suitable textbook for their courses in physiology. I believe also, on the basis of experience, that much of the book will be useful to students of animal science. Furthermore, I venture the opinion that practitioners of veterinary medicine who wish to keep up with the trend in physiology will find the book helpful."

This edition has been thoroughly revised and updated. Three chapters have been added, and seven chapters have been either incorporated into other chapters or deleted to make room for new material. Chapter outlines are provided once again to assist instructors in making specific assignments to students, and in turn, students should be able to find reading assignments quickly. References at the end of each chapter will lead researchers to recent work in many areas.

Years ago, Hippocrates, the father of medicine, laid down certain principles of science upon which modern medicine is built. These principles are (1) there is no authority except facts, (2) facts are obtained by accurate observations, and (3) deductions are to be made only from facts. The scientific method of today still consists of correct observations, the absence of prejudices, and proper conclusions. These principles have guided us in editing this book.

We are indebted to several people who have helped in the preparation of this book. Dr. Dukes was always a constant source of encouragement, and W. R. Klemm of Texas A & M University offered helpful recommendations in the organization of the book, for which we are grateful. We obtained constructive suggestions for each chapter from faculty members at various colleges of veterinary medicine who used the tenth edition. We sent these suggestions to each contributor, and many of them have been incorporated into the eleventh edition. The advice of these reviewers has been a valued service.

The cooperation of several faculty members in the Department of Veterinary Physiology and Pharmacology and in other departments of the College of Veterinary Medicine at Iowa State University is acknowledged. Among them are Franklin A. Ahrens, Harpal S. Bal, Richard L. Engen, Frederick B. Hembrough, Walter H. Hsu, Kenneth B. Platt, and Dean H. Riedesel. Computer assistance and secretarial service from Arthur R. Anderson and Linda Erickson, respectively, are also acknowledged.

The staff of Cornell University Press has been very helpful in the preparation of this edition. The cooperation and patience of Joy Moore, Cracom Corporation, are deeply appreciated by the editors.

MELVIN J. SWENSON
WILLIAM O. REECE

Above all I thank God for His guidance and inspiration; my deceased wife, Mildred, for her support, loyalty, and devotion; our children, Myron, Pamela, and Brita, their spouses, and our grandchildren for their encouragement and the joy and happiness they share with me; and my mother and father for their divine wisdom, discipline, and counsel.

M. J. S.

The Authors

Milton J. Allison, Ph.D. Lead Scientist, Physiopathology Research Unit, National Animal Disease Center, USDA, ARS, Ames, Iowa (Author of Chapter 22)

Bengt E. Andersson, D.V.M. Professor Emeritus, Department of Physiology, Faculty of Veterinary Medicine, Swedish University of Agricultural Sciences (Senior author of Chapter 47)

Robert A. Argenzio, Ph.D. Professor of Physiology, College of Veterinary Medicine, North Carolina State University (Author of Chapters 16–20)

Harpal S. Bal, B.V.Sc., M.S., Ph.D. Professor of Veterinary Anatomy, College of Veterinary Medicine, Iowa State University (Author of Chapter 33)

Gary K. Beauchamp, Ph.D. Director, Monell Chemical Senses Center, Philadelphia (Coauthor of Chapter 43)

Donald C. Beitz, Ph.D. Distinguished Professor, Departments of Animal Science and Biochemistry-Biophysics, Iowa State University (Author of Chapters 24–26)

Emmett N. Bergman, D.V.M, M.S., Ph.D. (deceased) Professor, Department of Physiology, College of Veterinary Medicine, Cornell University (Author of Chapter 27)

James E. Breazile, D.V.M., M.A., Ph.D. Professor of Physiology and Director of Laboratory Animal Resources, College of Veterinary Medicine, Oklahoma State University (Author of Chapters 44 and 45)

William H. Burke, M.S., Ph.D. Professor, Department of Poultry Science, College of Agricultural and Environmental Sciences, University of Georgia (Author of Chapter 38)

Dwight B. Coulter, D.V.M., M.S., Ph.D. Professor of Physiology and Pharmacology, and Associate Dean for Academic Affairs, College of Veterinary Medicine, University of Georgia (Senior author of Chapter 42)

David K. Detweiler, V.M.D., D.Sc. (h.c.), M.V.D. (h.c.), D.M.V. (h.c.) Diplomate, American College of Veterinary Internal Medicine (Cardiology); Professor of Physiology, Emeritus, School of Veterinary Medicine, Graduate Faculty of Arts and Sciences, University of Pennsylvania (Coauthor of Chapters 5 and 7; senior author of Chapters 6, 8, and 11; author of Chapters 9, 10, and 12)

William M. Dickson, D.V.M., M.S., Ph.D. Professor Emeritus, College of Veterinary Medicine, Washington State University (Author of Chapter 34)

Harry G. Downie, D.V.M., M.S., M.V.Sc., Ph.D. Professor (retired), Department of Biomedical Sciences, Ontario Veterinary College, University of Guelph (Coauthor of Chapter 4)

Gary E. Duke, M.S., Ph.D. Professor, Department of PathoBiology, College of Veterinary Medicine, University of Minnesota (Author of Chapter 23)

Lars-Eric Edqvist, D.V.M., Ph.D. Professor, Department of Clinical Chemistry, College of Veterinary Medicine, Swedish University of Agricultural Sciences (Coauthor of Chapters 35 and 36)

Howard H. Erickson, D.V.M., Ph.D. Professor, Department of Anatomy and Physiology, College of Veterinary Medicine, Kansas State University (Author of Chapter 15)

Richard C. Ewan, Ph.D. Professor, Department of Animal Science, College of Agriculture, Iowa State University (Author of Chapter 28)

M. Roger Fedde, Ph.D. Professor, Department of Anatomy and Physiology, College of Veterinary Medicine, Kansas State University (Author of Chapter 14)

Patricia A. Gentry, Ph.D. Professor, Department of Biomedical Sciences, Ontario Veterinary College, University of Guelph (Senior author of Chapter 4)

Virgil W. Hays, Ph.D. Professor, Department of Animal Sciences, University of Kentucky (Senior author of Chapter 29)

T. Richard Houpt, V.M.D., Ph.D. Professor of Veterinary Physiology, Department of Physiology, College of Veterinary Medicine, Cornell University (Author of Chapters 2 and 32)

Ainsley Iggo, M.Agr.Sc., D.Sc., F.R.S. Professor, Department of Veterinary Preclinical Sciences, University of Edinburgh (Senior author of Chapters 40 and 41)

Norman L. Jacobson, B.S., M.S., Ph.D. Emeritus Professor, Department of Animal Science, College of Agriculture, Iowa State University (Coauthor of Chapter 37)

Hallgrímur Jónasson, Dr.Med.Sc. Associate Professor, Department of Physiology, Faculty of Veterinary Medicine, Swedish University of Agricultural Sciences (Coauthor of Chapter 47)

F. A. Kallfelz, D.V.M., Ph.D. Diplomate, American College of Veterinary Nutrition; Director, Veterinary Medical Teaching Hospital, and Professor, Departments of Physiology and Clinical Sciences, College of Veterinary Medicine, Cornell University (Coauthor of Chapter 30)

Morley R. Kare, Ph.D. (deceased) Founding Director, Monell Chemical Senses Center, Philadelphia (Senior author of Chapter 43)

W. R. Klemm, D.V.M., Ph.D. Professor of Neuroscience, Cellular and Molecular Biology, and Toxicology, Department of Veterinary Anatomy and Public Health, Texas A & M University (Author of Chapters 39, 48, and 49; coauthor of Chapters 40 and 41)

David H. Knight, D.V.M. Professor of Cardiology and Chief, Section of Cardiology, School of Veterinary Medicine, University of Pennsylvania (Coauthor of Chapter 8)

Barry F. Leek, B.V.M.&S., B.Sc., Ph.D., M.R.C.V.S. Professor and Head, Department of Veterinary Physiology and Biochemistry, University College, Dublin (Author of Chapter 21)

George Lust, Ph.D. Professor of Physiological Chemistry, Department of Veterinary Microbiology, Immunology, and Parasitology, Baker Institute of Animal Health, College of Veterinary Medicine, Cornell University (Coauthor of Chapter 30)

Roger R. Marsh, Ph.D. Director, Otolaryngology Research, Department of Pediatric Otolaryngology, Children's Hospital of Philadelphia (Coauthor of Chapter 43)

Julius Melbin, B.Sc., V.M.D., D.Sc., Ph.D. Professor of Physiology and Bioengineering (retired), University of Pennsylvania (Senior author of Chapter 5)

Michael S. Miller, M.S., V.M.D. Diplomate, American Board of Veterinary Practitioners; Vice President and Staff Consultant, Department of Cardiology, Cardiopet Inc., Floral Park, New York; Staff Clinician and Cardiologist, A & A Veterinary Hospital, Franklin Square, New York (Senior author of Chapter 7)

Chung S. Park, M.S., Ph.D. Professor, Department of Animal Sciences, College of Agriculture, North Dakota State University (Senior author of Chapter 37)

William O. Reece, D.V.M., Ph.D. Professor, Department of Veterinary Physiology and Pharmacology, College of Veterinary Medicine, Iowa State University (Author of Chapters 1, 13, and 31; editor)

Dean H. Riedesel, D.V.M., Ph.D. Professor, Department of Veterinary Clinical Sciences, College of Veterinary Medicine, Iowa State University (Coauthor of Chapters 6, 8, and 11)

David Robertshaw, Ph.D., B.V.M.S., M.R.C.V.S. Professor and Chairman, Department/Section of Physiology, College of Veterinary Medicine, Cornell University (Author of Chapter 46)

Gretchen M. Schmidt, D.V.M. Animal Eye Associates, Wheeling, Illinois (Coauthor of Chapter 42)

George H. Stabenfeldt, D.V.M., Ph.D. (deceased) Professor, Department of Reproduction, School of Veterinary Medicine, University of California, Davis (Senior author of Chapters 35 and 36)

Melvin J. Swenson, D.V.M., M.S., Ph.D. Emeritus Professor, Department of Veterinary Physiology and Pharmacology, College of Veterinary Medicine, Iowa State University (Author of Chapter 3; coauthor of Chapter 29; editor)

Larry Patrick Tilley, D.V.M. Diplomate, American College of Veterinary Internal Medicine (Internal Medicine); President and Chief Medical Officer, Department of Cardiology, Cardiopet Inc., Floral Park, New York (Coauthor of Chapter 7)

R. H. Wasserman, Ph.D. James Law Professor of Physiology, Department of Physiology, College of Veterinary Medicine, Cornell University (Senior author of Chapter 30)

DUKES' PHYSIOLOGY OF DOMESTIC ANIMALS | ELEVENTH EDITION

PART I BLOOD, CIRCULATION, AND THE CARDIOVASCULAR SYSTEM

CHAPTER 1

PHYSICOCHEMICAL PROPERTIES OF SOLUTIONS | by William O. Reece

The animal body contains 60 to 70 percent water in the form of aqueous solutions. Basic to most physiological phenomena, functions of aqueous solutions include glomerular filtration in the kidney, production of a solute concentration gradient in the renal medulla, maintenance of cell size, excitability of cell membranes, and, in particular, generation of a nerve impulse, among others. In the practice of veterinary medicine, knowledge about solutions is used in planning treatment regimens for fluid replacement and electrolyte loss. Therefore, it is important that the physicochemical properties of solutions be considered early in physiology education. When H.F. Weisberg approached this topic, he seemed to have a feel for its basic importance when he quoted the following biblical verse (Proverbs 4:7): "Wisdom is the principal thing; therefore get wisdom: and with all thy getting get understanding." It is in this context that the physicochemical properties of solutions are presented, beginning with the definition of terms fundamental to the topic.

TERMINOLOGY

Solution. Applied to any homogeneous mixture. Solutions most frequently encountered are in the liquid state.

Solvent. The substance whose physical state is preserved when a solution is formed.

Solute. The substance whose physical state is changed when the solution is formed. Examples: (1) NaCl in water (water = solvent; NaCl = solute). (2) Alcohol in water (substance present in larger amount arbitrarily taken as the solvent).

Percent solution. The concentration of solute in grams per 100 ml of aqueous solution. A 5% aqueous solution of dextrose would contain 5 g of dextrose and sufficient water to make 100 ml of solution.

Specific gravity of solutions. Specific gravity is the number of times heavier an object is than an equal volume of water at the same temperature. Specific gravity is simply a number and has no dimensions. As applied to blood and urine, it is the ratio of the weight of a volume of blood or urine to the weight of the same volume of water.

Mole (gram molecule). The weight, in grams, of 6×10^{23} (Avogadro's number) molecules of a substance and referred to as the *gram molecular weight* (the same numerically as the molecular weight of the substance but expressed in grams). Similarly, the *gram atomic weight* refers to the weight, in grams, of 6×10^{23} atoms of an element (the same numerically as the atomic weight of an element but expressed in grams).

Molar and molal. Concentration measurements for solutes in a solution. A *molar* solution defines the number of moles in a liter of solution, whereas a *molal* solution defines the number of moles in a kilogram of solvent (1 L if water).

Example: There is 58.5 g of NaCl/mole.

1. A 1 molar aqueous solution would contain 58.5 g NaCl plus sufficient water for 1 L of solution.
2. A 1 molal aqueous solution would contain 58.5 g NaCl plus 1 kg of water (1 L).

Semipermeable membrane. A membrane that permits the passage of solvent but not of solute.

Selectively permeable membrane. A membrane that permits the passage not only of solvent but also of selected solutes (most cell membranes in the body are of this type).

Osmosis. Variably defined as follows: (1) The process of diffusion of solvent through a semipermeable membrane from a solution of higher solvent concentration to a solution of lower solvent concentration. (2) Net movement of water caused by a concentration difference for water developing across a membrane. (3) Movement of solvent molecules across a membrane into an area in which there is a higher concentration of solute for which the membrane is not permeable.

Colligative properties. The properties of a solution that are determined by the number of particles (ions, molecules) rather than by kind (size, charge). These include (1) vapor pressure lowering, (2) freezing point depression, (3) boiling point elevation, and (4) osmotic pressure. A measurement of any one colligative property of a solution permits calculation of the others. For this reason, osmotic pressure can be determined by freezing point depression or by vapor pressure lowering (frequently used methods).

Osmotic pressure. A quantitative measure of the tendency for water to osmose. For two aqueous solutions separated by a semipermeable membrane, the osmotic pressure refers to the pressure that would be needed to prevent the diffusion of water to the solution that has the highest solute concentration (greater number of particles). Water diffuses to the greater osmotic pressure. Osmotic pressure is measured in millimeters of mercury.

Effective osmotic pressure. Measurement used in referring to the tendency for water to osmose through a selectively permeable membrane. Only those particles that are unable to pass through the membrane contribute to the effective osmotic pressure. Water diffuses to the greater effective osmotic pressure.

Osmole. A measurement of solute concentration in terms of the number of dissolved particles and not their mass, which is in contrast to the mole. One osmole is the number of particles in 1 mole of undissociated (not ionized) solute. When a substance ionizes into two particles, $\frac{1}{2}$ mole would equal 1 osmole and 1 mole would equal 2 osmoles. When a substance ionizes into three particles, $\frac{1}{3}$ mole would equal 1 osmole and 1 mole would equal 3 osmoles. Osmole is abbreviated osm, and milliosmole (0.001 osm) is abbreviated mOsm.

Osmolarity and osmolality. Measurements of total solute concentrations based on the number of particles in a solution. A one *osmolar* solution contains 1 osm in 1 L of solution. A one osmolal solution contains 1 osm in 1 kg of solvent (1 L if water). For dilute solutions (as in the body), the quantitative difference between osmolality and osmolarity is less than 1%. These measurements are proportional to the osmotic pressure of solutes in solution because they are based on particle numbers. A one osmolal solution has an osmotic pressure of 22.4 atmospheres at 0°C or 17,024 mm Hg (one atmosphere equals 760 mm Hg). Therefore, each milliosmole per kilogram of water has an osmotic pressure of 17.024 mm Hg. When extrapolated to bovine (body temperature about 39°C) serum and corrected for body temperature [(273°K + 39°C)/273°K], each milliosmole per kilogram of serum (the aqueous solution) has an osmotic pressure of approximately 19.5 mm Hg.

Tone (tonicity). The effective osmotic pressure with respect to a selectively permeable membrane. Tone is not a colligative property because it is not determined by the total number of particles in the solution. Only those particles that cannot diffuse through the membrane contribute to tone. Solutions are judged to be hypotonic, isotonic, or hypertonic depending on the definition of the membrane that separates them and the nature of the solution with which they are being compared. They are hypotonic, isotonic, or hypertonic if they have less, the same, or greater effective osmotic pressure, respectively.

Equivalent weight. Substances react with each other in proportion to their equivalent weights rather than on a weight basis. One equivalent weight is that weight of a substance which will displace or otherwise react with 1.008 g of hydrogen (gram atomic weight of hydrogen), 35.5 g of chlorine (gram atomic weight of chlorine), or 8.0 g of oxygen ($\frac{1}{2}$ gram atomic weight of oxygen). Examples: (1) In 1 gram molecular weight of NaCl there is 1 gram atomic weight of sodium and 1 gram atomic weight of chlorine; thus, there is one equivalent of sodium and one equivalent of chlorine. (2) In 1 gram molecular weight of magnesium chloride ($MgCl_2$) there is 1 gram atomic weight of magnesium and 2 gram atomic weights of chlorine; thus, there are two equivalents of magnesium and two equivalents of chlorine (according to the above definition).

Electrolytes. Materials that dissolve to yield a conducting solution. In a solution of an electrolyte there are charged particles known as *ions*, positive (cations) and negative (anions), which are formed directly from the solute or result from its interaction with the solvent. The ions formed are measured in equivalents, and since electrolyte concentrations are small in biologic fluids, it is more convenient to use the milliequivalent. A milliequivalent (mEq) is one-thousandth (0.001) of an equivalent. Because substances react with each other on an equivalent basis rather than on a weight basis, 1 mEq of Na^+ (23 mg) will react with 1 mEq of Cl^- (35.5 mg).

DIFFUSION

The water in blood is circulated throughout the body because of the hydrostatic pressure created by the heart. Its distribution to the interstitial and intracellular fluid from the blood depends on diffusion in response to gradients. Simple diffusion is the random movement of molecules, ions, and suspended colloid particles under the influence of brownian (thermal) motion. Where a concentration gradient exists, the movement provided for the molecules, ions, and colloidal particles is from an area of higher concentration to an area of lower concentration. The movement is specific for each substance (i.e., Na^+ or water molecules will diffuse from an area of higher concentration to an area of lower concentration regardless of the presence and concentrations of other substances). When the ions and molecules are equally dispersed, the random motion continues but does not accomplish net movement and there is a state of equilibrium.

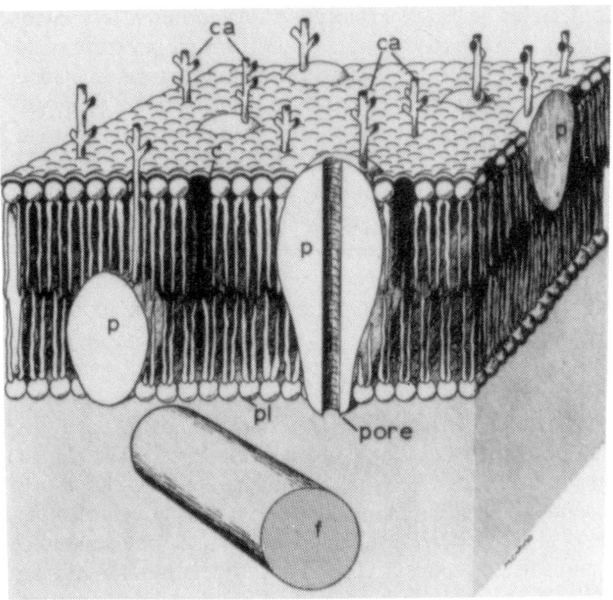

Figure 1.1. Structures of the plasma membrane surrounding cells. The plasma membrane contains phospholipids (pl), cholesterol (c), and proteins (p). Portions of carbohydrates (ca) extend from the external surface, where some are attached to protein and some to lipid. Many of the proteins extend from outside the membrane to the interior, where some serve as pores (aqueous channels) and others are involved with facilitated transport. Filaments (f) from the cytoplasm permit membrane interactions. Because of the fluid nature of the plasma membrane, proteins in the membrane move about, changing the sites of surface-active areas. (From Kelly, Wood, and Enders 1984, *Bailey's Textbook of Microscopic Anatomy*, 18th ed. Williams & Wilkins, Baltimore.)

Membranes of the cells can present barriers to diffusion. The cell membranes consist of a lipid bilayer, which is a thin film of lipid only two molecules thick through which fat-soluble substances (notable examples are carbon dioxide and oxygen) may diffuse readily (Fig. 1.1). Very small molecules can diffuse through postulated pores (protein channels), while larger molecules are transported through the membrane by facilitated diffusion, for which a carrier (transport protein) is required (Fig. 1.2). Because cell membranes are predominantly lipid, they are relatively hydrophobic (water repelling) and the diffusion of water through those portions is impeded. There are, however, protein channels through which water can diffuse. The protein channels are protein molecules that extend through the lipid bilayer from exposure on one side to exposure on the other. Some are thought to form aqueous channels (pores), and some are involved with facilitated transport. The aqueous channels permit diffusion not only of water but also of water-soluble substances. Some substances may be excluded from diffusion through the pores because of their large size, and others may be helped because of their relatively smaller size or because of other characteristics of the pore, such as its electrical charge (negative pore charge assists Na^+ diffusion). The number of protein channels is not considered sufficient to account for the volume and rapidity of water exchange between the inner and outer aspects of cells; therefore it is believed that the random motion of the water molecules causes them to bombard and penetrate the lipid bilayer before the hydrophobic character of the lipids can prevent their diffusion.

OSMOSIS

The most abundant substance in the body to diffuse is water, and this diffusion occurs throughout the body with relative ease. The amount diffusing into cells is usually balanced by an equal amount that is diffusing out. When two aqueous solutions differ in their concentration of water and are separated by a membrane that is permeable to water but not to its solutes (semipermeable membrane), there will be a net diffusion of water from the side with the greatest water concentration to the side with the least water concentration. This phenomenon is referred to as osmosis. When water concentrations of solutions are compared, it is

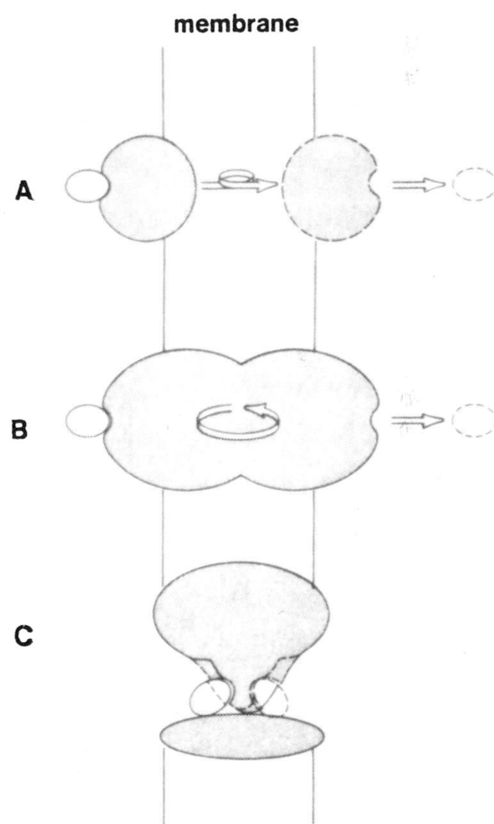

Figure 1.2. Membrane transport by proteins. (*A*) Rotation of the protein while it moves through the lipid core to expose the binding site on the opposite face. (*B*) Simple rotation of a protein that extends the entire distance through the membrane, moves the binding site from one side to the other. (*C*) Protein conformational change that exposes the binding site to the opposite side of the membrane. (From McGilvery 1983, *Biochemistry: A Functional Approach*. 3d ed. WB Saunders, Philadelphia.)

implied that a solution with the highest water concentration has the lowest solute concentration. A situation in which osmosis occurs is shown in Fig. 1.3. Net diffusion has occurred from the compartment that has the highest water concentration to the compartment that has the lowest water concentration.

OSMOTIC PRESSURE

Osmotic pressure is the pressure that would have to be applied to the compartment in Fig. 1.3 with the lowest water concentration to prevent net diffusion of water from the compartment with the highest water concentration. It is a colligative property in that the total number of particles in a solution (ions, molecules) determines its osmotic pressure. The greater the number of particles, the greater the osmotic pressure. In this regard, 1 L of an aqueous solution that contains 1 g of a protein with a molecular mass of 50,000 Da (molecular weight of 50,000) would contain more molecules than 1 L of solution that contains 1 g of a protein with a molecular mass of 400,000 Da (molecular weight of 400,000). Accordingly, the osmotic pressure of the former solution would be greater than that of the latter solution. For two aqueous solutions of NaCl separated by a membrane that permits diffusion of water but not NaCl, the greatest osmotic pressure would be measured for the solution with the highest concentration of NaCl (lowest concentration of water). Water would diffuse to the greatest osmotic pressure. Actually, it is a potential pressure in that it is the pressure that would have to be applied to prevent osmosis (i.e., in the body, osmosis is not prevented when water imbalances exist).

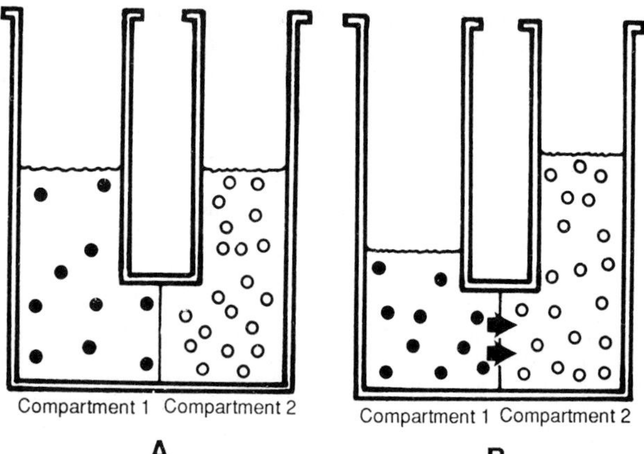

Figure 1.3. Osmosis. (*A*) Before osmosis. (*B*) During osmosis. Equal volumes of aqueous solutions (solutes represented by black circles and open circles) are placed in compartments that are separated by membranes that are permeable to water but not to solutes (semipermeable membrane). The aqueous solution in compartment 1 has the highest concentration of water (lowest concentration of solute). Osmosis (diffusion of water) occurs from compartment 1 to compartment 2 (highest water concentration to lowest water concentration), and the water level rises in compartment 2. (From Reece 1991, *Physiology of Domestic Animals*, Lea & Febiger, Philadelphia.)

Osmolar or osmolal concentrations are used to prepare solutions that will exert a specific osmotic pressure or to express the osmotic strength of solutions (urine, plasma, NaCl). A solution of glucose with an osmolality of 300 mOsm would exert the same osmotic pressure as a solution of NaCl with an osmolality of 300 mOsm. Because urine is a mixture of solutes in an aqueous medium and analysis of the exact composition is impractical, osmolality is a convenient measurement for comparative purposes. A urine specimen with an osmolality of 300 mOsm would therefore exert the same osmotic pressure as the above solutions of glucose and NaCl.

TONE OF SOLUTIONS

A selectively permeable membrane can restrict the diffusion of some solutes and permit diffusion of others. Most membranes of the body are of this nature. If a membrane separating two solutions permitted the diffusion through its pores of all the solutes in either solution, the solutes would establish equal concentrations for themselves on either side of the membrane. There would be no change in the water concentration on either side of the membrane or in the subsequent tendency for water to osmose. Therefore, the measured osmotic pressure for a solution that has solutes that can diffuse through membranes would not be an index of its tendency to cause osmosis. There is defined instead the tone of a solution, which is the effective osmotic pressure. Only those particles (molecules, ions) for which the membrane prevents diffusion contribute to tone. The principles of osmosis continue to prevail, except that it must now be stated that water will diffuse to the greatest effective osmotic pressure. Figure 1.4 illustrates tone of solutions. Two solutions of equal volumes and particle numbers are shown to be separated by a membrane that permits passage through it by diffusion of water and the particles in compartment 2. Before osmosis, each of the solutions would have the same measured osmotic pressure (same concentration of particles). Because compartment 1 has particles that cannot diffuse through the membrane, these particles are the ones that contribute to an effective osmotic pressure. Since the solution in compartment 2 has no effective osmotic pressure, water diffuses to the greatest effective osmotic pressure or from compartment 2 to compartment 1.

Physiological significance

From a practical standpoint, the tone of a solution that can be infused into the blood of animals is usually compared with plasma because plasma is in osmotic equilibrium with the suspended erythrocytes, or red blood cells (RBCs). A solution with the same effective osmotic pressure as plasma is isotonic. When RBCs are placed in this solution, they will not increase or decrease in size. A solution that is hypotonic when compared with plasma has a less effective osmotic pressure, and RBCs placed in this solution will increase in size. If the solution is sufficiently hypo-

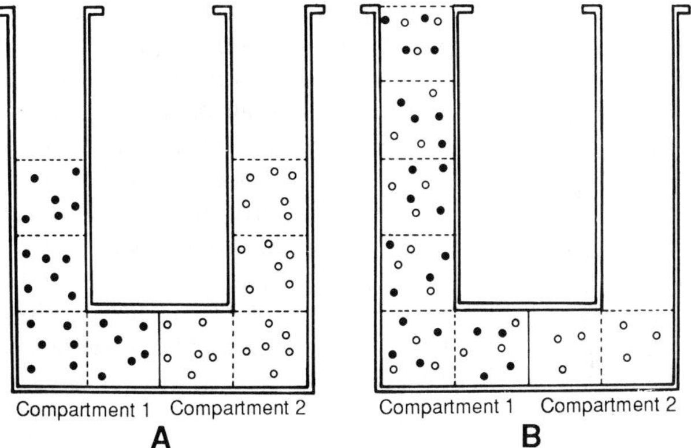

Figure 1.4. Hypothetic example of tone of solutions. (*A*) Before osmosis. (*B*) After osmosis. Two aqueous solutions (solutes represented by black circles and open circles) of equal osmotic pressure are separated by a membrane that is permeable to water and open circle solutes. Effective osmotic pressure is exerted only by black circle solute, and water diffuses to compartment 1. At equilibrium, open circle solute has a new, lower concentration that is equal throughout compartments 1 and 2. (Dashed lines represent divisions of equal volumes.) (From Reece 1991, *Physiology of Domestic Animals*, Lea & Febiger, Philadelphia.)

tonic, the RBCs will increase in size until they rupture (hemolyze) and liberate their contents into the solution. Plasma from an animal in which hemolysis has occurred will have some degree of redness, depending on the amount of hemolysis. The condition that results when this occurs is known as hemoglobinemia because the redness is due to the liberated hemoglobin. There may be enough hemolysis that hemoglobin enters the kidney tubules and appears in the urine. A red color is imparted to the urine, and the condition is called hemoglobinuria. A solution that is hypertonic when compared with plasma has a greater effective osmotic pressure, and when RBCs are suspended in this solution they decrease in size. Loss of sufficient water can cause the RBC's to appear wrinkled, and they are said to be crenated. The effect of solutions with different tone on erythrocytes is illustrated in Fig. 1.5.

Because freezing point and osmolality are determined by the number of particles in a solution, the osmolality of

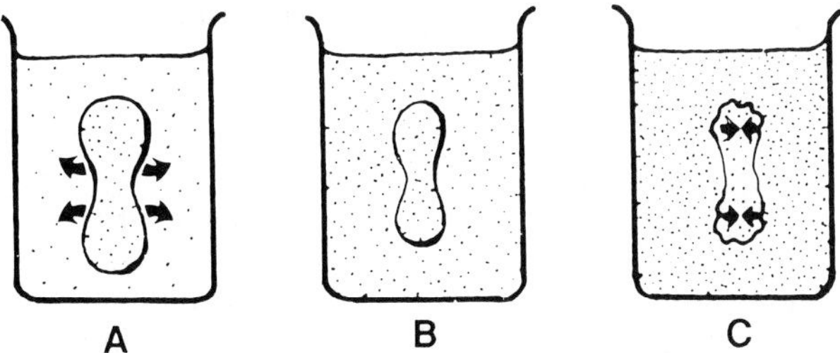

Figure 1.5. Effect of tone of solution on erythrocytes. (*A*) The solution is hypotonic and the erythrocyte expands. (*B*) The solution is isotonic and no change occurs in erythrocyte size. (*C*) The solution is hypertonic and the erythrocyte decreases in size. (From Reece 1991, *Physiology of Domestic Animals*, Lea & Febiger, Philadelphia.)

plasma can be estimated by measurement of its freezing point (freezing point depression, a colligative property, depends on the number of particles). A one osmolal solution has a freezing point that is 1.858°C lower than solute-free water. Isotonic plasma has a freezing point depression of 0.56°C. According to these values, isotonic plasma has an osmolality of about 0.30 osm (0.56°C/1.858°C) or, as more commonly stated, 300 mOsm.

Isotonic saline solutions are prepared according to the freezing point relationship. Because NaCl ionizes in aqueous solutions to form Na^+ and Cl^-, the osmolar quantity is obtained with the use of one-half the molar amount. Accordingly, a 0.15 molar solution of NaCl is equivalent to a 0.30 osmolar solution. Incomplete dissociation and interionic attractions cause a 0.15M solution of NaCl to be only 0.93 as osmotically active as that which is calculated. Because of this, a 0.161 M (0.15/0.93) solution of NaCl more closely approximates an isotonic solution. From this relationship, a more convenient concentration of 1/6 M (0.167 M) became more commonplace. A 0.167 M NaCl solution is the same as a 0.977% solution (58.5 g × 0.167 = 9.77 g/dL = 0.977 g/dl = 0.977%), whereas a 0.15 M solution of NaCl is equal to a 0.875% solution. On that basis, the 0.15 M NaCl solution would be considered slightly hypotonic. The physiological difference between the 0.15 M and 0.167 M solutions is not significant and quite often a physiological NaCl (saline) solution is prepared as a 0.9% NaCl solution.

OSMOTIC FRAGILITY OF ERYTHROCYTES

Erythrocytes of most domestic animal species usually appear as biconcave, circular disks. Those closest to being round or spherical have a limited capacity to expand and will burst on intake of small amounts of water. The osmotic fragility of these erythrocytes is increased and their osmotic resistance is decreased. Thin or flat erythrocytes can take in considerable amounts of water before they expand to the point of rupture. Their osmotic fragility is decreased, and their osmotic resistance is increased. As an example of decreased osmotic fragility, consider the condition of iron deficiency anemia in calves. In iron deficiency, hemoglobin synthesis is more deficient than erythrocyte production; thus the red cell count is not as markedly reduced as the hemoglobin concentration. This occurs because a maturation arrest takes place in the late rubricyte stage so that while these cells are awaiting hemoglobin synthesis, further cell division may take place with the production of some cells that are smaller than normal and deficient in hemoglobin (microcytic, hypochromic anemia). When stained and viewed microscopically, the resultant erythrocyte has a narrow rim of highly stained hemoglobin with a variable but greater than normal area of central pallor. (The cell would be more biconcave and have a greater potential for volume expansion.)

The results of osmotic fragility tests that compare blood

Table 1.1. A comparison of osmotic fragility of erythrocytes from a normal calf and a calf with iron deficiency anemia

Tube no.	% NaCl	Normal calf % hemolysis	Anemic calf % hemolysis
1	0.95	0.0	0.0
2	0.85	0.0	0.0
3	0.75	0.0	0.0
4	0.65	3.4	0.0
5	0.60	51.2	27.8
6	0.55	80.3	40.9
7	0.50	100.0	62.9
8	0.45	100.0	73.4
9	0.40	100.0	81.9
10	0.35	100.0	96.6
11	0.30	100.0	100.0

from normal calves and calves with iron-deficiency anemia are presented in Table 1.1. The packed cell volumes of normal and anemic calves are 34 and 16 percent, respectively. Exactly 0.05 ml of blood was delivered to each of 11 tubes containing 5 ml of NaCl solutions that were reduced in concentration beginning at 0.95%. A spectrophotometer was used to determine the degree of hemolysis. It is noted that hemolysis is complete for the blood from the normal calf in the 0.50% NaCl solution. The blood from the anemic calf is not completely hemolyzed until the NaCl solution concentration reaches 0.30%. It is also noted that there is no hemolysis for the blood from the normal calf and the anemic calf until the NaCl concentration was reduced to 0.65% and 0.60%, respectively. It is apparent that there is a relative degree of tolerance to hemolysis when hypotonic solutions are infused.

INTERCONVERSION OF UNITS OF MEASUREMENT

Various circumstances can require the preparation of solutions with exacting compositions and can also require the conversion of solute concentrations given in one unit of measurement (i.e., equivalents) to another (i.e., osmoles). Interconversion must proceed according to the pathways shown in Fig. 1.6.

When solutions have the amounts of the various components listed in grams and one wishes to know the composition in milliosmoles and milliequivalents, it is necessary to (1) calculate the millimolar amount and (2) comply with the definitions of osmoles and equivalents and convert to the milliosmolar and milliequivalent amounts.

Example:
One liter of solution contains:
6 g (6000 mg) NaCl (MW 58.5)
210 mg $MgCl_2$ (MW 95.24)

Step 1 (millimolar amount):
a. NaCl = 6000/58.5 = 102.56 mM
b. $MgCl_2$ = 210/95.24 = 2.20 mM

Step 2 (milliosmolar amount):
a. NaCl = 102.56 mM × 2 ions/molecule = 205.12 mOsm
b. $MgCl_2$ = 2.20 mM × 3 ions/molecule = 6.60 mOsm

Step 3 (milliequivalent amount):
a. 102.56 mM NaCl = 102.56 mEq Na^+ and 102.56 mEq Cl^-
b. 2.20 mM $MgCl_2$ = 4.40 mEq Mg^{2+} and 4.40 mEq Cl^-

For the solution (concentration in milliosmoles per liter):
a. Contribution of NaCl = 102.56 × 2 = 205.12 mOsm
b. Contribution of $MgCl_2$ = 2.20 × 3 = 6.60 mOsm
c. Calculated milliosmolarity = 205.12 mOsm + 6.60 mOsm = 211.72 mOsm

For the solution (concentration in milliequivalents):
a. Na^+ = 102.56 mEq/L
b. Mg^{2+} = 4.40 mEq/L
c. Cl^- = 102.56 + 4.40 = 106.96 mEq/L

When the concentrations of a solution's ionic components are listed in milliequivalents per liter and one wishes to know how many grams of each electrolyte are needed to prepare the solution, the following steps are taken:

1. It is decided which molecular compounds were used.
2. The milliequivalent concentrations are converted to the millimolar concentrations.
3. The millimolar (or molar) concentration is multiplied by molecular weight to yield the weight in milligrams (or grams) of the electrolytes used.

Example
A liter of solution has the following composition:

Component	Concentration (mEq/L)
Na^+	121
K^+	5
Ca^{2+}	32
Cl^-	132
Acetate	26

Step 1:
Electrolytes used are NaCl, Na acetate, $CaCl_2$, and KCl.

Step 2 (millimolar concentration):
KCl = 5 mM (same as mEq concentration)

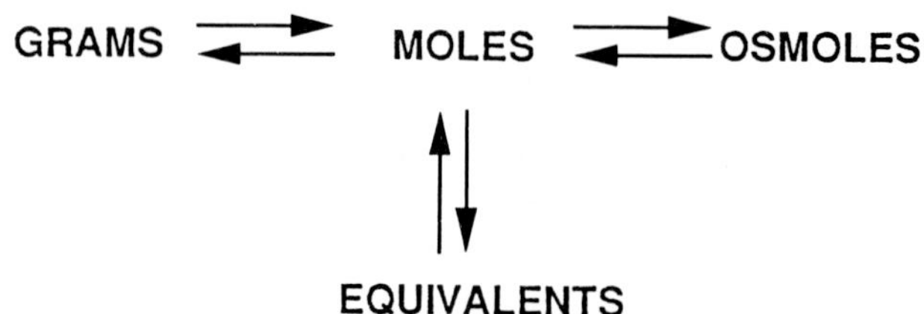

Figure 1.6. Pathways for the interconversion of grams, moles, osmoles, and equivalents.

$CaCl_2$ = 16 mM ($\frac{1}{2}$ mEq concentration)
Na acetate = 26 mM (same as mEq concentration)
NaCl = 95 mM (amount of Na^+ and Cl^- remaining after subtraction of the amount needed for KCl, NaCl, and Na acetate from the listed values; for Na^+ = 121 mEq − 26 mEq (from Na acetate) = 95 mEq; for Cl^- = 132 mEq − 32 mEq (from $CaCl_2$) − 5 mEq (from KCl) = 95 mEq.

Step 3 (milligrams of electrolyte needed for 1 L solution):
Grams KCl = 0.005 M × 74.5 g/M = 0.373 g = 373 mg
Grams $CaCl_2$ = 0.016 M × 111 g/M = 1.776 g = 1776 mg
Grams Na acetate = 0.026 M × 82 g/M = 2.132 g = 2132 mg
Grams NaCl = 0.095 M × 58.5 g/M = 5.558 g = 5558 mg

Calculation of osmolarity for this solution would show the contribution from NaCl, Na acetate, $CaCl_2$, and KCl to be 190, 52, 48, and 10, respectively, for a total of 300 mOsm/L. The actual osmotic activity would be less by a factor of about 0.93 (0.93 × 300 = 279).

PROBLEM SOLVING

The following exercises represent hypothetical situations and provide an additional opportunity to understand the physicochemical properties of solutions:

1. The plasma urea concentration has been increased from 40 mg/dl to 220 mg/dl in a cow with nephritis (an increase of 180 mg/dl). Urea is freely diffusible through the cell membranes of most cells of the body. Urea molecular weight is 60, and it does not dissociate in solution. In this cow:
   a. What is the increase in plasma osmolarity?
   b. Is the plasma isotonic or hypertonic with erythrocytes?
   c. Is the osmotic pressure of plasma higher, lower, or the same as the osmotic pressure of the erythrocyte intracellular fluid?
2. A one osmolal solution of $MgCl_2$ has a freezing point depressed 1.858°C. What is the osmolality of a NaCl solution that depresses the freezing point 1.858°C?
3. A solution contains 60 mEq of Ca^{2+} and 60 mEq of Cl^- in each liter. How many grams of $CaCl_2$ would be needed to make 1 L of this solution (MW $CaCl_2$ = 111)?
4. Equal volumes of aqueous solution A and aqueous solution B are placed on opposite sides of a membrane. Solution A contains particles x and y. Solution B contains particles y and z. The membrane is permeable to water and particles y and z. At equilibrium which side will have the greatest volume?
   a. The side that originally contained solution A
   b. The side that originally contained solution B
   c. Equal volumes remain on both sides
5. Which one of the following statements about $CaCl_2$ is *true* (when placed in water each molecule ionizes into 1 Ca^{2+} and 2 Cl^-)?
   a. One-half gram molecular weight dissolved in 1 L of solution would be equal to one osmole
   b. One-third gram molecular weight would be equal to 1 mole
   c. One gram molecular weight would be equal to two equivalents of calcium and two equivalents of chloride
6. Which one of the following solutions would lower the freezing point the most:
   a. 1 pound of glucose (MW 180) dissolved in 4 L of water
   b. 1 pound of urea (MW 60) dissolved in 4 L of water
7. Two solutions are separated by a membrane that permits the diffusion of water and particles X and Y. Both are aqueous solutions containing X, Y, and Z. The concentration of Z is higher in solution A than it is in solution B. Which one of the following statements about the tone of the solutions is correct?
   a. The solutions are isotonic to each other
   b. Solution A is hypertonic to solution B
   c. Solution A is hypotonic to solution B
8. Aqueous solutions of 0.167M NH_4Cl, NaCl, and Na acetate and 0.334M urea are considered to have osmotic pressures approximately equal to plasma. Erythrocyte membranes are permeable to urea, chloride ion, acetate ion, and ammonium ion but not to sodium ion. Indicate whether the tone of each of the following solutions is isotonic, hypotonic, or hypertonic when compared with plasma.
   a. 0.334 M urea + 0.167 M NH_4Cl
   b. 0.334 M urea + 0.167 NaCl
   c. 0.167 M NaCl + 0.167 M Na acetate
   d. 0.0835 M NaCl + 0.0835 M Na acetate
9. How many grams of Na lactate are needed to prepare 1 L of Na lactate solution (Na^+ and lactate $^-$) with an osmolarity of 300 mOsm/L (MW Na lactate = 112)?
10. One liter of a solution contains
    155 mEq Na^+
    5 mEq K^+
    10 mEq Ca^{++}
    145 mEq Cl^-
    25 mEq lactate$^-$
    How many millimoles (mM) are there of NaCl, KCl, $CaCl_2$, and Na lactate?
11. If it was desired to increase the osmolarity of a solution by 60 mOsm with $CaCl_2$, what weight of $CaCl_2$ would be needed (MW $CaCl_2$ = 111)?
12. A veterinary clinic prepares a solution for large volume use known as "ECF (extracellular fluid) solution."
    A concentrate is prepared as follows:
    116 g NaCl (MW = 58.5)
    44 g Na acetate (MW = 82.0)
    7 g KCl (MW = 74.5)
    Distilled water (quantity sufficient for 1 L)
    Before use, 1 L of concentrate is added to 17 L of distilled water and the resulting solution is approximately isotonic with plasma.
    In the 18 L of solution that are finally used:
    a. How many milliequivalents per liter are there for Na^+, K^+, Cl^-, and acetate?
    b. What is the osmolarity?
13. A person wishes to prepare 1 L of an isotonic solution containing NaCl and glucose wherein each constituent would contribute $\frac{1}{2}$ of the tone. The molecular weight of NaCl is 58.5 and that of glucose is 180. What weight of each compound (NaCl and glucose) would be present in 1 L of the solution? (Consider the erythrocyte membrane not permeable to Na^+ and glucose).

14. A solution is 0.075M NaCl and 0.05M $CaCl_2$. What are the concentrations of Na^+, Ca^{2+}, and Cl^- in milliequivalents per liter?
15. Which one of the following is the best indicator of water equilibrium between the interstitial and intracellular compartments?
    a. Equal molar concentrations
    b. Equal osmolar concentrations
    c. Equal equivalent concentrations

Answers

1. a. 30 mOsm b. isotonic c. same as
2. one osmolal
3. 3.33
4. a
5. c
6. b
7. b
8. Hypotonic, isotonic, hypertonic, and isotonic, for a, b, c, and d, respectively
9. 16.8
10. 130, 5, 5, and 25, respectively.
11. 2.22 g
12. a. 140, 5.2, 115, and 29.8, respectively
    b. 290 mOsm/L
13. 4.3875 g NaCl, 27.0 g glucose
14. 75, 100, and 175, respectively
15. b

REFERENCES

Brey, W.S., Jr. 1958. *Principles of Physical Chemistry,* Appleton-Century-Crofts, New York.

Davidsohn, I., and Henry, J.B. 1969. *Todd-Sanford Clinical Diagnosis by Laboratory Methods.* 14th ed. W.B. Saunders, Philadelphia.

Kelly, D.E., Wood, R.L., and Enders, A.C. 1984. *Bailey's Textbook of Microscopic Anatomy.* 18th ed. William & Wilkins, Baltimore.

McGilvery, R.W. 1983. *Biochemistry: A Functional Approach.* 3d ed. W.B. Saunders, Philadelphia.

Reece, W.O. 1991. *Physiology of Domestic Animals,* Lea & Febiger, Philadelphia.

Weisberg, H. F. 1962. *Water, Electrolyte, and Acid-Base Balance.* 2d ed. Baltimore, Williams & Wilkins, 1962.

CHAPTER 2

Water and Electrolytes | by T. Richard Houpt

Normal tissue function and development of the higher forms of animal life depend on the maintenance and control of the composition of the body fluids that bathe all tissue cells. Claude Bernard pointed out more than 100 years ago that this extracellular fluid constitutes an internal environment, and early in this century W.B. Cannon coined the word *homeostasis* to express the existence and maintenance of stability within this environment.

WATER

All life is intimately associated with water. Most of the ions and molecules that make up living matter have chemical and physical relationships with water, and the number of chemical compounds that can be put into aqueous solution is exceptionally large. Water not only supplies the matrix in which all living processes occur, but it also participates significantly in those processes.

Distribution of body water

Total body water and fluid compartments

There is considerable variation in total body water content among different species, ages, sexes, nutritional states, and other conditions. Generally, the lean adult nonherbivore has a total body water content of about 70 percent of its body weight. Water content is highest in the newborn animal, declines rapidly at first, and then declines slowly (Fig. 2.1). Fat tissue is exceptional in its low water content (10 percent or less); thus the total water content of a fat animal will be lower than that of a lean one. In very lean cattle about 70 percent of body weight is water, while in very fat animals, total body water accounts for only about 40 percent.

Water contained within cells is called *intracellular fluid*. All fluid lying outside cells is called *extracellular fluid* (ECF). The ECF is, in turn, divided by the walls of the vascular system into the *interstitial fluid* and the *plasma*. Roughly, in the lean animal, an amount of water equal to 50 percent of the body weight lies within the cells, 15 percent in the interstitial spaces, and 5 percent in blood plasma. Water in the alimentary canal, although strictly speaking outside the body tissues proper, is usually included as extracellular water. The cerebrospinal fluid, aqueous humor of the eye, synovial fluids, urine, and bile also are subdivisions of ECF that may exhibit special characteristics. These fluids, which are somewhat separated from the main body of ECF, as well as the water in the alimentary canal, are called *transcellular fluids*.

Note that the terms *water* and *fluid* are almost, but not

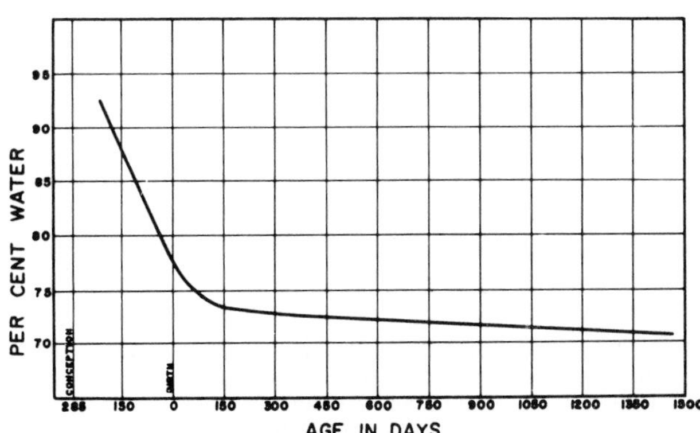

Figure 2.1. Relation between water content and age in cattle. (From Armsby and Moulton 1925, *The Animal as a Converter of Matter and Energy*, Chemical Catalog Co., New York.)

quite, interchangeable. A fluid such as blood plasma includes various solutes, and actual plasma water volume is slightly smaller than total plasma volume. Most methods measure the entire space occupied by blood, plasma, or extracellular fluid, including solutes; hence, such volumes are usually called fluid volumes. Measurement of total body water, if done with heavy water, radioactive water, or dehydration, gives an estimate of that water volume.

Water movement between fluid compartments

Water molecules can rapidly penetrate most cell membranes. If an osmotic or hydrostatic pressure gradient exists between body fluid compartments, a shift of water will occur. If there is no appreciable hydrostatic pressure involved, the result of the water movement will be to equalize the osmoconcentrations of the fluids. The hypothetical response to an intravenous injection of water is illustrated in Fig. 2.2. If, for any reason, a very large amount of water were added to the ECF, the water movement into cells might disrupt normal metabolic function and might even cause death. This condition of cellular overhydration is known as *water intoxication*.

Water shifts similar to those described above will occur after the addition of any hypotonic NaCl solution to the ECF. If an isotonic NaCl solution were injected, it would become evenly distributed throughout the extracellular compartment but would have little effect on cellular water. If a hypertonic NaCl solution were administered intravenously, water would begin to shift into the plasma. Since the capillaries are freely permeable to both water and electrolytes, however, the osmotic gradient would disappear as solvent and solute were distributed throughout the extra-

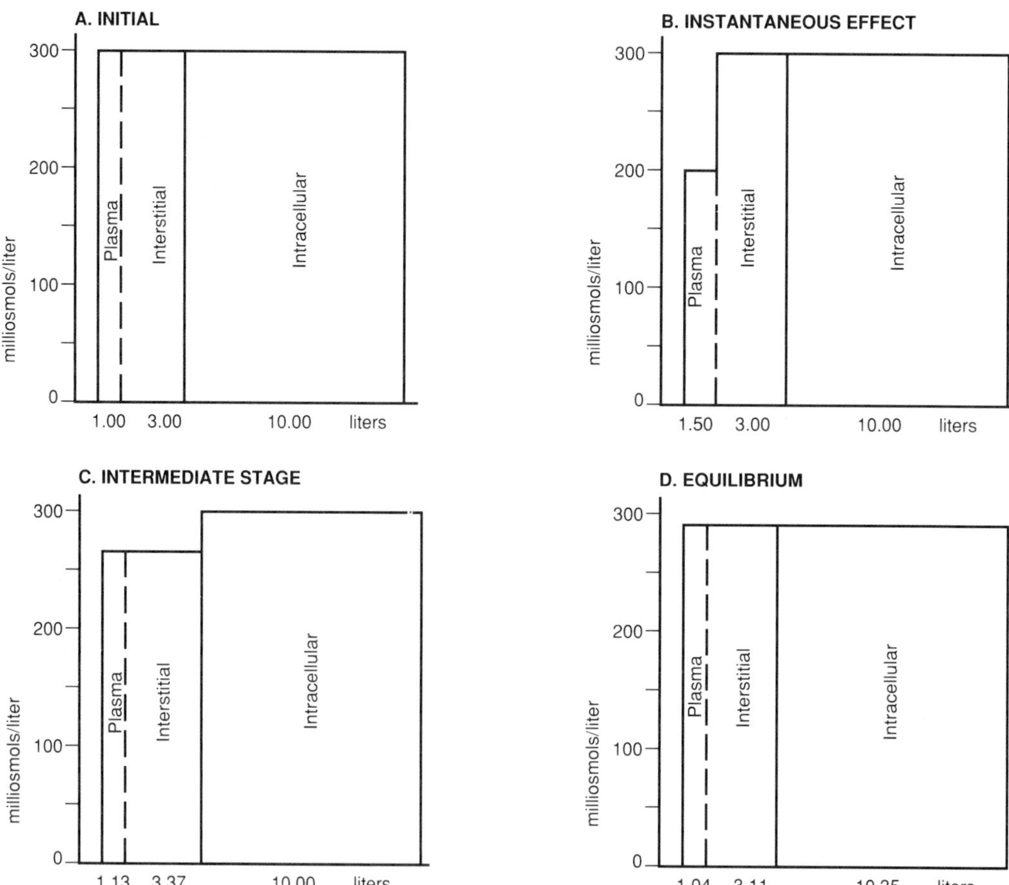

Figure 2.2. Hypothetical water shifts among fluid compartments as a result of injection of 500 ml water intravenously into a 20-kg dog. Height of each compartment represents osmoconcentration in milliosmoles per liter; width represents volume in liters. Initially osmoconcentration is identical in all compartments (*A*), but there is a rapid dilution of plasma osmoconcentration as the injection is being made. (*B*) The extent of plasma dilution that would occur if the distribution of the injected water was instantaneous and limited to the plasma. Actually the osmotic gradient between plasma and interstitial fluid, plus a rise of blood pressure due to the increased volume of fluid, causes water to begin its shift out of the vascular system, even while the injection is occurring. This prevents the extreme dilution of plasma shown in (*B*), and instead osmoconcentrations shortly after the injection are approximately as shown in (*C*). Of course, as soon as the interstitial fluid osmoconcentration begins to drop, water begins to move into the cells. Within a few minutes equality of osmoconcentration has been reestablished for all fluid compartments at a slightly subnormal level (*D*).

cellular compartment. However, the cell membrane, unlike the capillary wall, does not permit the free movement of Na^+, and thus the increased osmoconcentration of the ECF would cause a cellular dehydration.

Measurement of body fluid volumes

One can determine total body water directly by drying the whole animal and measuring the loss of weight. Blood volume has been estimated directly, but inaccurately, by measurements of the volume of blood that can be bled from the circulatory system. These methods are inconvenient, however, and necessitate the death of the animal. Instead, the method commonly used to estimate these and other fluid volumes is the dilution technique. A compound is injected and becomes distributed throughout the fluid volume in question. The compound must be restricted to that particular fluid volume. After distribution of the compound is complete, a sample of the fluid is obtained and the concentration of the compound is determined. The volume of that fluid compartment then equals the weight of the compound injected divided by its concentration after distribution. Unfortunately, while the compound is being distributed throughout the fluid compartment, it may also be excreted or metabolized, and corrections must be made for these losses that occur during the distribution time. Furthermore, it is difficult to find suitable substances that will be distributed only within the fluid volume under study.

An example will illustrate the measurement of a body fluid compartment by this dilution technique. A schematic representation of this method of determining plasma volume is shown in Fig. 2.3A, along with a log plot of the data from the animal against time (Fig. 2.3B). This was done in a nonpregnant, nonlactating cow with the use of Evans blue dye. This dye is rapidly bound to plasma proteins after injection. As a result, its distribution in the body is the same as that of the plasma proteins; that is, it is limited to the plasma volume. In this case, 120 mg of the dye was injected intravenously. A series of blood samples was taken, and the concentration of the dye was plotted on a log scale against time (Fig. 2.3B). This plot permitted extrapolation of dye concentration back to the time it had been injected, as though it had been instantaneously mixed throughout the plasma at zero time. This procedure corrects for the slow loss of dye during the 60 minutes. In this case the "instantaneous" dye concentration was 1 mg/dl. The amount of plasma needed to dilute the injected dye is then calculated: 120 mg divided by 1 mg/dl = 12,000 ml, the plasma volume. This plasma volume can also be expressed on a body weight basis:

$$12{,}000 \text{ ml} \div 320 \text{ kg} = 37.5 \text{ ml/kg},$$
$$\text{or } 3.75\% \text{ of body weight.}$$

The best compounds for measurement of total body water are heavy water (deuterium oxide) and radioactive water (tritium oxide). Isotopically labeled water distributes itself in the same way as the normal water of the body. Other compounds used include antipyrine, sulfanilamide, thiourea, and urea. Estimation of ECF volume requires a sub-

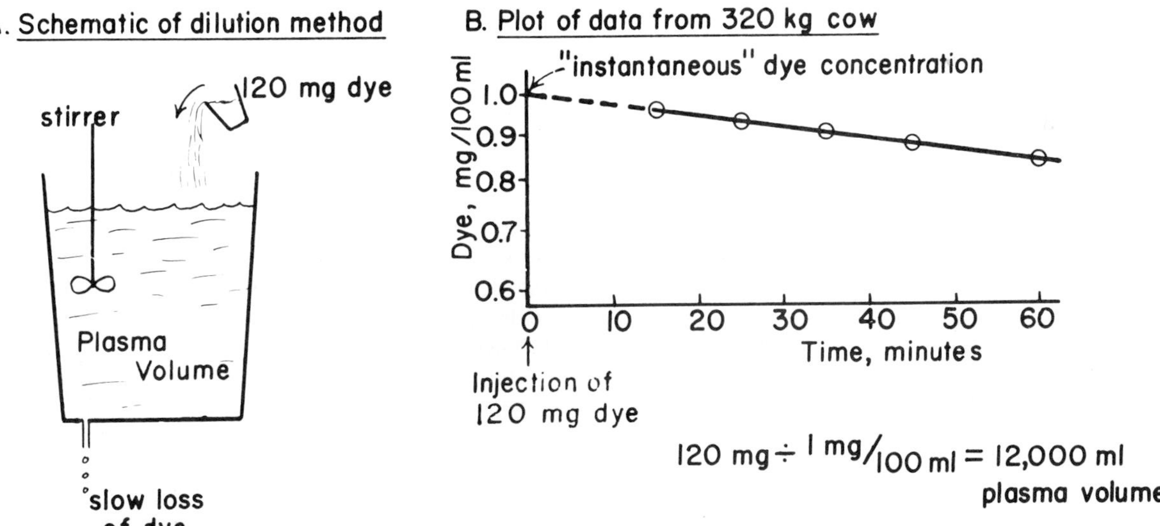

Figure 2.3. Dye dilution method of determining blood plasma volume. (*A*). Model of method. At zero time 120 mg dye was added to a container of water. When there was no loss of dye from the container, the concentration was found to be 1 mg/100 ml after mixing. If, as shown, dye was slowly lost from the container, the zero time concentration of the dye could be found by taking a series of samples, plotting the declining concentrations on a log scale against time, and extrapolating back to zero time. This would also have given 1 mg/100 ml, and the calculated volume of the water in the container would be 12,000 ml. (*B*). The method applied to a cow. The dye was injected at zero time and mixed by the circulation in the first few minutes; and then its concentration slowly declined. A plot of concentration values on a log scale against time permitted extrapolation back to zero time to give the "instantaneously mixed" concentration of 1 mg/100 ml. Calculated plasma volume was 12,000 ml.

stance that does not enter cells. Inulin, a large dextran molecule, is frequently used for this purpose, but sucrose, thiocyanate, sulfate, radioactive sodium, and others are also used. Intracellular fluid volume cannot be estimated directly but must be calculated as the difference between total and ECF volumes. Plasma volume can be measured by injection of a substance, such as Evans blue dye (also known as T-1824), that is adsorbed to plasma proteins. An alternative way to measure plasma volume is to measure blood volume with erythrocytes labeled with radioactive phosphorus or chromium. Plasma volume can be easily calculated from blood volume if the fractional volume of erythrocytes (i.e., the packed cell volume) is also determined. The measurement of the various body fluid compartments is not precise; repetition of measurements or use of different substances often gives variations of several percent in the same animal.

Water balance

The total amount of water in the body remains relatively constant from day to day. Water is gained by ingestion or as an end product of cellular metabolism; water loss occurs in urine, from the skin, with expired gases, and in the feces. The lactating animal also loses large amounts of water in milk. Typical values for lactating and nonlactating cows under moderate environmental conditions are given in Table 2.1. Most of these routes of water loss or gain are not controlled with respect to body water content. Only ingestion of water and urinary water excretion are controlled in order to regulate body water volume.

Table 2.1. Daily water balance of Holstein cows eating legume hay

Balance	Nonlactating (L)	Lactating (L)
Intake		
Drinking water	26	51
Food water	1	2
Metabolic water	2	3
Total	29	56
Output		
Feces	12	19
Urine	7	11
Vaporized	10	14
Milk	0	12
Total	29	56

Modified from Leitch and Thomson 1944, *Nutr. Abstr. Rev.* 14:197–223.

Thirst and ingestion of water

Much of the loss of water from the body is continuous, and in time a deficit in body water develops. This is then corrected periodically by the ingestion of water. The ingestion of water may be partly due to habit or to a daily rhythm of eating and drinking without overt thirst. When any appreciable water deficit in the body fluids develops, however, specific controls of water intake act to correct that deficit. Water deprivation causes both the sensation of thirst and an associated behavioral drive to drink water.

There appear to be several mechanisms that control the amount of water ingested so that it equals the body water deficit. Most obviously, thirst is characterized by a dryness of the throat and mouth due to a decrease in salivary secretion. This sensation of dryness may become so intense in the human as to be acutely painful, but thirst can be relieved only partially and temporarily by wetting the mouth and throat. Temporary inhibition of drinking can also be caused by other stimuli in the alimentary canal in addition to oral dryness. If a dog equipped with an esophageal fistula is deprived of water and is then permitted to drink, it will drink about double the amount needed but will then stop, even though none of the water has reached the stomach. Apparently the amount of water passing through the mouth and pharynx is measured, but imprecisely. After about 20 minutes the inhibition to drinking disappears, and the animal will drink more water. Similar temporary inhibition of drinking can be induced by placement in the stomach of a balloon containing an amount of water equal to the water deficit or by infusion of a small amount of water into the duodenum. Clearly, signals arising from the alimentary tract inform the central nervous system of the approximate amount of water being ingested. These immediate feedback signals from the digestive tract are essential for preventing overingestion of water before longer-lasting inhibition can be achieved by absorption of the water and actual correction of the deficit in the body fluids.

The neuronal system that controls thirst and drinking behavior is located in the hypothalamic region of the brain. This locus of control has been demonstrated dramatically in the goat by implantation of electrodes in the hypothalamus and application of electrical stimuli. The goats immediately went to water and drank, even though no deficit in body water existed. The goats continued drinking as long as the stimulus continued but not beyond the consumption of an excess of water equal to 40 percent of their body weight. During water deprivation the osmotic concentration of body fluids rises by a few percent, and it has been found that injections of minute amounts of hypertonic NaCl solutions into the same regions of the hypothalamus cause the animal to drink water. Such experimental results indicate that certain cells of the hypothalamus, and probably cells in nearby tissues close to the cerebral ventricles, are sensitive to changes in osmoconcentration that cause cellular dehydration, thirst, and drinking behavior. The site of stimulus may be cells that are exposed to blood circulation, that is, where the blood-brain barrier is deficient. It should be noted that as a water deficit develops, both osmotic and sodium concentrations rise in the ECF. The rise in sodium and associated anion concentration is usually the cause of the increase in osmolality. Because sodium is relatively retained in the ECF, it contributes to an effective osmotic pressure that causes diffusion of water from cells. An increase in osmolality caused by urea (freely diffusible) does not contribute to effective osmotic pressure, and thirst is not stimulated.

Changes in composition of body fluids bathing the cells of the hypothalamic control systems are not the only source of information to the central nervous system about body water content. A water deficit produces a fall in fluid volume as well as a rise in ECF concentration. Although initially blood volume is defended at the expense of interstitial and intracellular fluid, the general fall of ECF volume will be reflected by some fall in blood volume and pressure. There appear to be two detection mechanisms associated with the vascular system: stretch receptors in the large veins and atria of the heart and the renin-releasing cells of the kidney which are sensitive to a fall in vascular pressure. A fall in venous return resulting in a lessening of stretch of the walls of the veins, atria, and possibly the arterial baroreceptors in the carotid sinus and aortic arch acts as a stimulus by way of vagal afferents to the hypothalamic centers. Thirst and increased drinking result, as well as release of the antidiuretic hormone (ADH), which causes a decrease in urine volume. A fall in arterial blood pressure will also directly cause the release of renin from the juxtaglomerular cells of the afferent arterioles of the kidney glomeruli. Renin acts on plasma angiotensinogen to form angiotensin I, which is, in turn, converted to angiotensin II by converting enzyme. In a variety of animals angiotensin II has been shown to cause an increase in water drinking. However, the exact mode of angiotensin II action on the hypothalamic region is not clear. It is believed that compounds that cannot pass the blood-brain barrier stimulate receptors in periventricular highly vascular structures that are exposed to both cerebral circulation and cerebrospinal fluid (for example, the subfornical organ). The problem of how blood-borne angiotensin influences hypothalamic activity is further complicated by the presence of an isorenin-angiotensin complex located within brain tissue. Whether and how this cerebral isorenin-angiotensin combination interacts with blood angiotensin or acts independently to cause thirst is not known.

When a dehydrated animal drinks, thirst is temporarily inhibited after ingestion of an amount approximately equal to the water deficit. Prolonged satisfaction, however, is not attained until absorption and dilution of the body fluids remove the osmotic and volume stimuli to the hypothalamic control systems. The main features of the water intake control systems are summarized schematically in Fig. 2.4.

Urinary excretion of water and its hormonal control

If an animal is deprived of water, the rate of water excretion in the urine decreases, the converse is also true, but there are limitations. On the one hand, a minimum urine volume is determined by the quantity of solutes to be excreted and by the ability of the kidney to concentrate urine. The maximum urine concentration possible varies greatly among animals. Some approximate values (osm/L) are as follows: human, 1.5; dog, 2.3; cat, 3.3; sheep, 3.2; rabbit, 1.9; kangaroo, rat 5.5; beaver, 0.6. On the other hand, maximum urine volume is also limited, but the limit is very high and ordinarily excess water will be excreted rapidly. The excretion of water by the kidney is controlled primarily by the ADH of the posterior pituitary gland (see Chaps. 31 and 34). ADH (also known as vasopressin) acts on the nephron to permit increased reabsorption of water and hence decreased excretion in the urine. During water deprivation the concentration of ADH in the blood rises and urine volume falls. If the animal is overhydrated, less ADH will be present in the blood, urine flow will rise, and the concentration of the urine may decrease until it approaches that of the plasma.

The release of ADH from the posterior pituitary gland is believed to be caused primarily by changes in the osmoconcentration of the plasma. If a hypertonic saline solution is injected into the carotid artery, a decrease in urine flow results. Other evidence indicates that the hypertonic solution acts on structures in the ventral diencephalon and suggests that the supraoptic nuclei of the hypothalamus contain cells that are sensitive to changes in osmoconcentration of plasma. These nuclei exert their control by way of the hypothalamic-hypophyseal nerve tracts to cause release of ADH. This hypothesis states that when the osmotic concentration of plasma rises, it stimulates a greater release of ADH; when osmoconcentration falls, less ADH is released. There is also evidence that an osmoreceptive mechanism is located in the hepatic portal vein, or in the liver itself, and that the mechanism similarly signals an increased osmoconcentration there with resultant ADH release. Whether this hepatic control of ADH release operates normally is uncertain.

The hypothalamic osmoreceptor system is involved with the regulation of the ECF osmoconcentration through variation in water excretion, but ADH also functions as a control for regulation of ECF volume (Fig. 2.4). A fall in ECF volume generally involves a fall in circulating blood volume. However, there appear to be no true volume receptors. Instead, the degree of distention of the left atrium and large arteries is monitored by stretch receptors located at those sites. This afferent limb of the pathway is the same as that for thirst. The resultant change in afferent nerve discharge frequently causes, by way of the hypothalamus, an increase in ADH release from the posterior pituitary. The consequent conservation of water by the kidneys aids restoration of ECF volume. Another consequence of this hypothalamic response is the increased retention of sodium that is necessary to maintain normal osmoconcentration as water retention occurs. The release of ADH can also be stimulated by pain, exercise, and many other stresses.

Variations in glomerular filtration rate (GFR) may also have an important influence on water conservation in some domestic animals. For example, a 50 percent fall in GFR

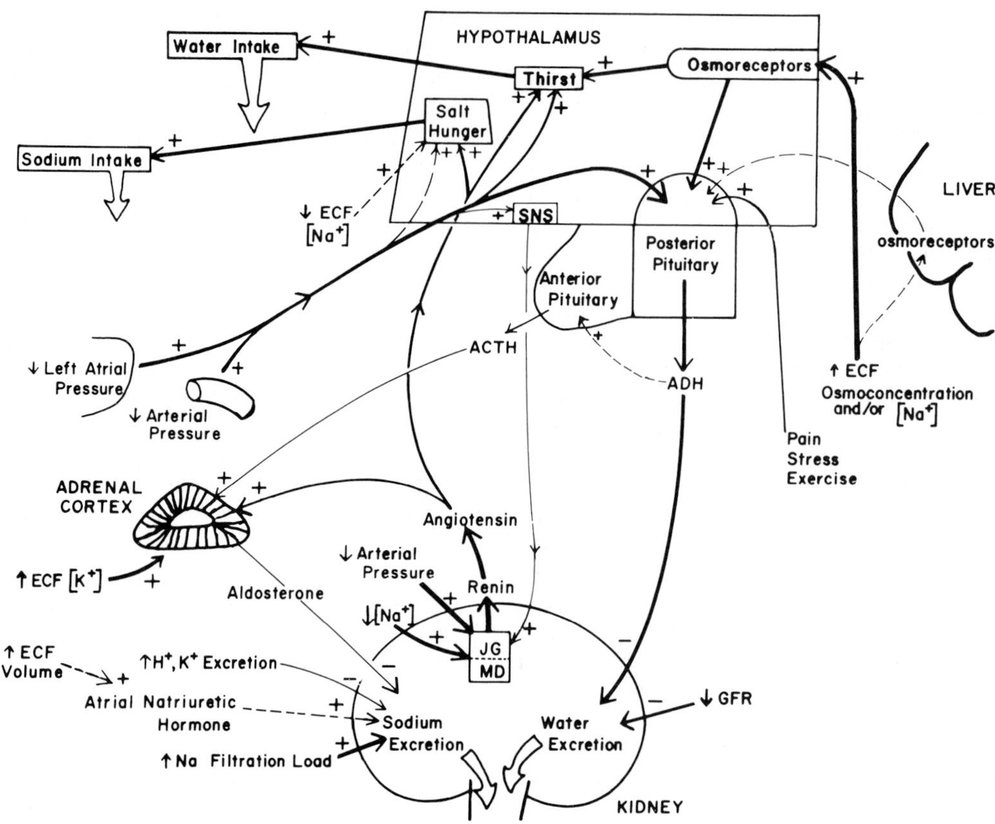

Figure 2.4. Controls of water and sodium intake and excretion. Well-established pathways are shown with solid lines; others with dashed lines. Each pathway is initiated by a deviation of an ECF variable from normal; typical deviations are indicated by an arrow before the variable. The effect of the deviation on the next structure or process in the pathway is shown as + for increase or − for decrease in its action. JG, juxtaglomerular cells; MD, macula densa. Control mechanisms indicated in the hypothalamus are not meant to represent cellular nuclei or centers; rather, systems may actually include structures in other parts of the brain. SNS, sympathetic nervous system.

has been reported in sheep deprived of drinking water for 5 days.

Water in food and metabolic water

Although the bulk of the water obtained by the animal is ingested as drinking water, under certain circumstances much water may be obtained in food. Most foodstuffs contain at least a small amount of water, and lush green vegetation may contain 75 to 90 percent water. Nonlactating ruminants, when on succulent pasture, may ingest little or no drinking water. In fact, cattle on such pasture may appear to be somewhat overhydrated and, as a result, excrete copious amounts of urine. The oxidation of foodstuffs also yields some water. The oxidation of each gram of carbohydrate yields about 0.6 ml of water; the corresponding amounts for fats and protein are 1.1 and 0.4 ml, respectively, per gram metabolized. For most domestic animals this oxidative or metabolic water represents only 5 to 10 percent of the total water intake and remains constant, provided metabolic rate is constant.

Metabolic water, however, can be of great importance in the water balance of many small desert rodents and may constitute 100 percent of their water intake. Best known of this group are the kangaroo rats, which may live indefinitely on dried food with no drinking water. These animals are able to maintain water balance, first, by avoiding the greatest daily heat load and hence the necessity to expend water for heat dissipation and, second, by minimizing water loss to an unusual degree. These rodents remain in their relatively cool burrows during the heat of the day and emerge only during the night. Loss of water is minimized by a nearly water-impermeable skin, low respiratory water loss due to a low temperature of the expired air (cooled as it passes through the nasal passages), a highly concentrated urine of small volume, and exceptionally dry feces. Under these circumstances, the metabolic water gained exceeds or equals water lost from the body.

Water loss by other routes

Besides excretion in the urine, water is lost from the body in feces, with respiratory gases, and from the surface of the body. These routes of water loss are not generally regulated with respect to the water content of the body. The amount of fecal water varies with the species of animal; for example, it is small in sheep but considerable in cattle. In all animals water loss during gastrointestinal disturbances may be substantial and rapid. The air inspired by an animal ordinarily has a lower water content than the air that is expired. This is because the incoming air is warmed and saturated with water before expiration. Loss by this route under moderate conditions is constant, but when an animal is exposed to a hot environment, evaporation of water from the respiratory tract increases as the respiratory minute volume rises. Water loss from animals that show a marked thermal polypnea, such as the dog and the sheep, may become considerable under these circumstances (except for the camel, see below).

Water loss from the surface of the skin occurs in two ways. Water may simply diffuse to the surface from the blood vessels and body fluids in the skin and evaporate from the surface. This diffusion of water will vary according to the temperature of the skin and circulation. Diffusion water loss through the skin and evaporation of water from the respiratory tract together are known as *insensible water loss*. Sweating, which is varied with respect to body temperature, is another process by which water is lost from the body surface. Under moderate environmental conditions, water loss in sweat is insignificant. Under heat stress, however, sweating losses may be tremendous in freely sweating animals, such as humans and horses. Finally, some animals, such as cats, rats, and kangaroos, produce large amounts of saliva when they are under heat stress and then spread the saliva over the body surface.

Dehydration

Since the intake of water is intermittent and loss of water is continuous, the animal is always faced with the problem of slow dehydration. Any serious dehydration involves the loss of both water and electrolytes. The process of dehydration will vary somewhat according to whether the loss of water and electrolytes is rapid or slow and according to the relative rates of water and electrolyte loss. Only simple dehydration due to a lack of drinking water under moderate environmental conditions is considered here.

The first sign of dehydration is a tendency to seek and drink water. Concomitantly, there is a decrease in urine volume. These changes can be observed when only 1 to 2 percent of the body weight has been lost as water. Dehydration to the extent of 10 percent of the body weight is considered severe. A dog deprived of water under moderate conditions will lose about 10 percent of its body weight in 5 days. Most animals will not eat during moderate or severe dehydration; hence part of the body weight loss is loss of tissue substance used for energy metabolism. Notable exceptions are donkeys, which will eat before drinking, and the camel, which blithely continues to eat in a normal fashion despite what for other animals would be severe dehydration. The immediate source of water lost from the body is the ECF; if the rate of loss is very rapid, ECF volume may be severely reduced. In slow dehydration, however, there will be a shift of water from the cells into the ECF. After 5 days of water deprivation in a dog, 67 percent of the water loss is from the ECF volume and 33 percent is from the cells.

During water deprivation the slow loss of water from the body results in a rise of ECF osmoconcentration and a fall of ECF volume which stimulate both drinking behavior and decreased urine flow. Electrolyte concentration does not, however, continue to rise during dehydration. Instead, electrolytes are also excreted from the body roughly in proportion to water loss, and this prevents a further rise of osmoconcentration until dehydration has proceeded nearly to the point of death. In early dehydration increased quantities of sodium chloride appear in the urine as ECF is reduced. Then, as cellular water shifts to the extracellular compartment, cellular potassium also is excreted in the urine. Thus after a long period of dehydration the animal will be depleted of both water and the primary electrolytes. The proportion of body weight that can be lost as water before death occurs varies widely according to dietary and environmental conditions. In humans, for example, this limit may range from 15 to 25 percent.

Adaptation to water lack

Among domestic animals there is a wide range of adaptation to water lack. Some species (e.g., cattle, dogs, cats, and swine) exhibit little special adaptation; generally neither they nor their wild progenitors have inhabited arid regions. On the other hand, some common domestic animals indigenous to arid regions, such as the camel and the donkey, have acquired adaptations that enable them to withstand severe water lack. Almost without exception, the problem of water lack is compounded by exposure to high temperatures. During the cool season of most arid areas the small amount of rainfall is sufficient to increase the water content of the vegetation appreciably, and some herbivores are able to maintain water balance on plant water for long periods (for example, camels in the Sahara). High summer temperatures, however, necessitate expenditures of increased amounts of water to control body temperature, and during the hot season the natural vegetation contains far less water. Under these circumstances even the camel must drink water periodically.

Cattle appear to have no special water conservation mechanisms, but there is an important difference between European cattle (*Bos taurus*) and Brahman cattle (*Bos indicus*). Brahman cattle are better able to regulate their body temperatures when exposed to heat stress; they can dissipate larger quantities of heat by evaporation of larger quantities of water from their body surface. Furthermore, Brahman cattle have more and larger sweat glands over most of their body surface. This heat resistance, however, depends on an ample supply of water.

The legendary ability of the dromedary camel to withstand heat and water lack has been substantiated by experimental studies. It is necessary to point out that, contrary to legend, the camel can neither store water nor derive important additional amounts of water from metabolism of the fat in its hump. When severely dehydrated camels are permitted to drink, they do not store water by overhydration. Only if an excessive amount of salt is ingested will the animal, in effect, overhydrate. Peculiar small sacs located in the wall of the rumen have given rise to the legend that the camel stores water in its rumen. Although rumen fluid may act as a source of water when the animal is deprived of water, there is no evidence that more water is present in the camel rumen than in the rumen of other ruminants. The small rumen sacs, on the contrary, contain comparatively dry ingesta when examined after the animal's death and may have absorptive functions. The camel stores water only in the sense that it can withstand a greater degree of dehydration (i.e., loss of body water) than can many other mammals.

It has been suggested that since the metabolism of each gram of fat yields 1.1 ml of water, the fatty hump of the camel should represent an important store of water. The camel, like other animals, does derive a certain amount of water from oxidation of nutrients. Presumably, the special value of the hump fat would be due to a shift from the metabolism of starch and protein to that of fat, total metabolic rate remaining relatively constant. However, this additional metabolic water can be of little value. First, although the camel has a remarkable ability to conserve water, its daily needs in absolute terms are sizable. Even when conserving water maximally, a medium-sized camel will expend more than 10 L of water daily during summer months. Obviously, only an enormous hump could supply enough water to meet needs for more than 2 or 3 days. Second, in the desert a fat animal is a rarity; most camel humps there contain relatively little fat. Finally, whether energy needs are satisfied by the oxidation of fat or by the oxidation of starch and protein, about the same total amount of metabolic water will be produced. This is because, although more water will be produced per gram of fat oxidized, less than one-half as much fat will be required to replace the starch and proteins. The actual amounts of water formed per kilocalorie derived from the oxidation of the nutrients are as follows: for fat, 0.12 g/kcal; for carbohydrate, 0.14 g/kcal; and for protein, 0.10 g/kcal. Further, the oxidation of the smaller amount of fat will require more than twice as much oxygen. Hence the animal's oxygen consumption will be nearly the same regardless of the nutrients metabolized. It follows that respiratory water loss is also nearly the same, whether fat or other nutrients are oxidized. Little or no net gain of water is accrued from fat metabolism under these circumstances. Needless to say, the hump fat does constitute an energy reserve of great importance.

Under conditions of heat stress in which a human could survive only a single day without drinking water, camels can easily survive for a week and, in fact, show little discomfort. At the end of that first day, a human will have lost about 12 percent of body weight as water, while by the end of the week the camel will have lost more than 25 percent. In addition to being able to withstand greater degrees of dehydration, the camel has several means of conserving water. During the day, when the heat stress is greatest, the camel's body temperature rises, thereby storing heat and saving the water that would have been required to dissipate this heat. During the cooler desert night this stored heat is dissipated and body temperature is normal or even slightly subnormal by dawn. In addition, the camel's summer fur, which is most prominent on the dorsal surfaces, is very effective in reducing solar heat gain. Although the camel has considerable ability to concentrate its urine and to form very dry feces, the amounts of water conserved by these means are less significant in maintaining water balance. The animal does, of course, dissipate heat through the evaporation of water. Sweating may be the most important route of evaporative heat dissipation, for a marked thermal polypnea is not observed. In fact, respiratory water loss can be very low in the camel because of an ability to reduce the relative humidity of expired air to below 100 percent. This is possible because of the hygroscopic nature of nasal secretions. A final remarkable attribute of the camel is its ability to rehydrate rapidly. It is not unusual for a camel to ingest more than one-fourth of its body weight as water in a few minutes. In other ruminants such rapid ingestion of water often depresses plasma osmoconcentration to the point where hemolysis of red cells occurs. The oval biconcave erythrocytes of the camel are highly resistant to such osmotic hemolysis.

There have been relatively few investigations of resistance to water lack by equids; most of these investigations concern the donkey, which is the domestic member of this group most frequently seen in arid areas. Even deep in the Sahara, the donkey is found in regions where its equine relatives are rarely seen. The donkey matches the camel with respect to the degree of dehydration it will withstand and the rapidity with which it can rehydrate. Although the donkey can survive up to a 30 percent loss of body weight as water under heat stress, it uses water for cooling (sweating) at a rate three times that of a camel, with a corresponding reduction in the donkey's survival time. On rehydrating, a small donkey has been observed to drink 20.5 L of water in 2.5 minutes.

Sheep also have an outstanding ability to withstand high environmental temperatures and lack of water. The principal adaptations are an ability to endure a degree of dehydration equal to about 30 percent of their body weight and to minimize absorption of solar heat. When exposed to intense solar radiation, the temperature of the wool surface may rise to 87°C. Apparently the insulative capacity of the wool prevents a rapid transfer of heat from the wool surface to the skin, while at the same time the high surface temperature will cause radiation of heat to the cooler environment. The sheep also conserves water by excreting dry feces and a relatively concentrated urine. Dissipation of heat by evaporation of water is effected primarily by panting. Sweating does occur, but the rate is considerably lower than, for example, that of the cow. Finally, the sheep is similar to the camel and donkey in being able to consume nearly one-fourth of its body weight in water at one drinking without harmful effects.

ELECTROLYTES

The ionic composition of the body fluids typical of mammals is illustrated in Fig. 2.5. The height of each pair of columns represents the concentration of electrolytes in terms of chemical equivalents. The necessity for electrical neutrality dictates that the height of each column representing the cations must exactly equal the height of its adjacent column representing the anions. All of the ECF is similar, consisting primarily of sodium, chloride, and bicarbonate ions. In addition, the blood plasma component has an appreciable amount of protein, the plasma proteins. Furthermore, there is a slightly unequal distribution of all diffusible ions across the capillary wall, in compliance with the Gibbs-Donnan phenomenon. The small block representing nonelectrolytes refers to glucose, urea, and so forth. The major cations of the fluid of the cells, on the other hand, are potassium and magnesium with only small amounts of sodium. These cellular cations are balanced by organic phosphates, proteinate, sulfate, and a small amount of bicarbonate. The ionic composition of the cells depicted in this figure is typical of many body cells, but there are important exceptions. For example, although little chloride ion is found in muscle cells, significant quantities are found in certain other cells, such as erythrocytes and those of the gastric mucosa. Variations of electrolyte concentration in plasma and red blood cells are given in Chapter 29.

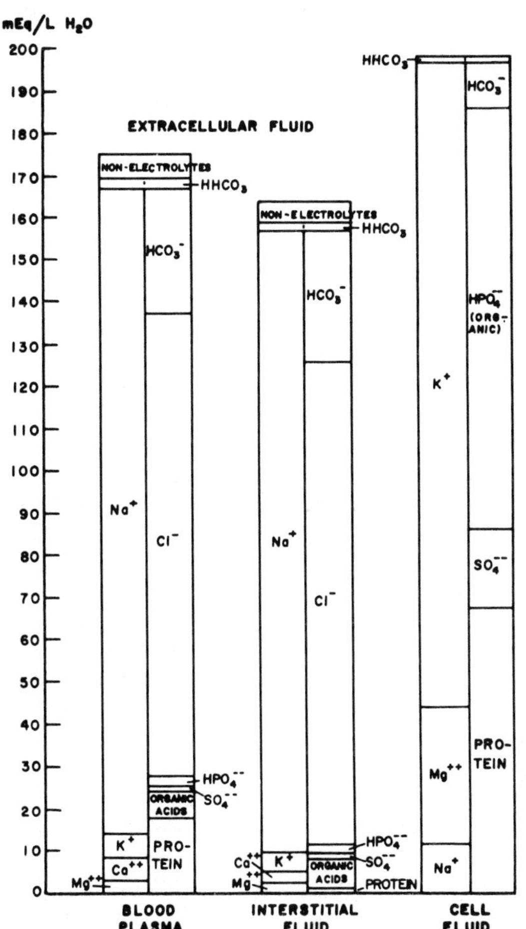

Figure 2.5. Composition of human body fluids. (From Gamble 1954, *Chemical Anatomy, Physiology, and Pathology of Extracellular Fluid*, Harvard Univ. Press, Cambridge.)

Table 2.2. Osmotically active substances in human body fluids (in milliosmoles per kilogram of water)

Substances	Plasma	Interstitial	Intracellular
Na^+	146	142	14
K^+	4.2	4.0	140
Ca^{2+}	2.5	2.4	0
Mg^{2+}	1.5	1.4	31
Cl^-	105	108	4
HCO_3^-	27	28.3	10
HPO_4^{2-}, $H_2PO_4^-$	2	2	11
SO_4^{2-}	0.5	0.5	1
Glucose	5.6	5.6	
Proteins	1.2	0.2	4
Urea	4	4	4
Other organic substances	3.4	3.4	83.2
Total	302.9	301.8	302.2
Total osmotic pressure at 37°C (mm Hg)	5453	5430	5430

Modified from Guyton 1981, *Textbook of Medical Physiology,* 6th ed., W.B. Saunders, Philadelphia.

If the composition of the body fluids is expressed in terms of osmoconcentration instead of chemical equivalents, a somewhat similar pattern is found, except that the multivalent ions have less osmotic effect (Table 2.2). Variations from this exist in domestic animals (see Chapter 29). Nearly all of the osmoconcentration of the ECF is due to sodium, chloride, and bicarbonate ions, while that of the intracellular fluid is mostly due to potassium, magnesium, and organic substances. Because of intermolecular and interionic attractive forces, the actual osmotic effect of the solutes in body fluids is only about 93 percent of that which would be calculated from their chemical composition. Total osmotic pressure values given on the bottom line of the table have been corrected for this depression of osmotic effect. The osmotic activity of all body fluids is nearly equal except for the small difference between plasma and interstitial fluid. The plasma proteins create this osmotic pressure difference across the capillary wall, and, although it is small in comparison with the total osmotic pressure of the extracellular fluids, it is of great importance for maintenance of blood volume and pressure.

Sodium

Sodium is the major cation of ECF and an important component of the skeleton. About 45 percent of the body store of sodium is found in ECF, 45 percent in bone, and the remainder is intracellular. Although most body sodium is in a readily exchangeable form, nearly one-half of that in bone does not exchange with sodium ions in the fluid compartments. The nonexchangeable sodium is adsorbed on the surfaces of hydroxyapatite crystals deep in long bones. None of the bone sodium is osmotically active, although part of it may become available to ameliorate the osmotic effects of ECF dilution.

Regulation of sodium concentration

A relatively constant [Na^+] of the ECF is attained over the long term by control of both ingestion and urinary excretion of sodium so as to maintain a salt balance, keeping [Na^+] within about 2 percent of its average value. In the short term, however, adjustments of disturbed [Na^+] are brought about quickly by the ADH-thirst–control system causing changes in water content of the ECF. If ECF [Na^+] rises above normal, the inevitable accompanying rise of osmolality stimulates release of ADH and usually thirst. The water gained by this action of the ADH-thirst system dilutes ECF, restoring [Na^+] to its normal level. This will increase ECF volume for the moment, but this is not life threatening. The rise of ECF volume includes a rise of blood volume, which results in a slight increase of blood pressure. This pressure increase causes an increase in glomerular filtration rate, and excess sodium and water are both excreted over a period of hours, restoring ECF volume to its normal level. In addition, if the increase of [Na^+] in blood plasma were to develop rapidly, changes in rate of sodium excretion in urine would also occur rapidly.

Excretion of sodium by the kidney involves first the filtration at the glomerulus of plasma sodium and then reabsorption from the tubule of most of the filtered sodium. The difference between the amount of sodium filtered and the amount reabsorbed is the amount excreted in the urine. Changes in sodium excretion can be effected in two ways. First, if the plasma [Na^+] or glomerular filtration rate suddenly increases, the amount of sodium filtered per unit of time into the tubule will also increase. However, sodium reabsorption from the tubule will not increase proportionately in such a short period of time. The difference between sodium filtered and sodium reabsorbed therefore will be greater, and more sodium will be excreted in the urine.

A deficit of sodium in the ECF leads to a rapid excretion of excess water because the depressed osmolality inhibits the release of ADH and urinary volume rises. Thirst usually will not be evident in the early stages of salt-deficient states. If blood volume is also depressed, the glomerular filtration rate will decline, with consequent increase in reabsorption of sodium and water. In addition, many sodium-deficient animals have a strong behavioral drive to ingest salt and show a remarkable ability to control ingestion of sodium chloride so that they just replace a body deficit of sodium. This salt hunger is most vigorous in ruminants and other herbivores. Although a fall in plasma sodium is associated with a salt-deficient state, the connection between plasma sodium concentration and the behavior is not clear. An injection of sodium chloride to correct a depressed [Na^+] will not immediately abolish the salt appetite, but raising the cerebrospinal fluid sodium level will. A decrease in blood volume can also result in an increase in salt intake, but only after a long time lag. Both a fall in arterial blood pressure and in [Na^+] will stimulate the release of renin from the kidney, and the consequent increase of angiotensin II can stimulate salt hunger. Further, there is evidence that aldosterone has a permissive role (e.g., it must be present for angiotensin to be effective in causing a salt appetite or hunger). These findings suggest that salt hunger is controlled by stimuli acting in the hypothalamus or close by in periventricular tissue. When more than very small amounts of salt are ingested with the ration, however, as is usually the case, salt appetite will not be evident, and excess salt will be excreted.

The urinary excretion rate of sodium will also decline because of renal events. If plasma [Na^+] and blood pressure fall as a consequence of salt deficiency, the glomerular filtration rate of sodium will also fall. Less sodium is then presented to the renal tubules and a larger fraction will be reabsorbed. A fall of plasma [Na^+] will also stimulate, via the renin-angiotensin system, release of aldosterone from the adrenal cortex. One action of aldosterone is to increase sodium reabsorption from the renal tubules; as noted below, however, aldosterone's effect on sodium excretion is minimal in the short term. Only in states of prolonged salt deficiency is aldosterone a significant factor in sodium conservation. The combination of all these mechanisms that cause a decrease in sodium excretion can result in a virtually sodium-free urine during prolonged salt deficiency (see Chap. 31).

As discussed below, aldosterone not only enhances sodium reabsorption from the renal tubule, but it also has an important action in enhancing secretion of potassium ions from tubular cells into the lumen. An increase in plasma [$K+$] directly causes increased aldosterone release from the adrenal cortex. In fact, the central role of aldosterone is believed to be the regulation of plasma [K^+], not of plasma [Na^+]. Angiotensin is relatively weak in causing aldosterone release and thus is of less importance in varying sodium excretion in urine. Instead, it has been suggested that the ADH-thirst system plays the major role of maintaining plasma [Na^+] at its normal level by varying ECF water content.

Distention of the atria of the heart, particularly the right atrium, causes the release of a hormone known as atrial natriuretic factor or hormone. This substance causes an increase in excretion of sodium salts with water by the kidney lowering the blood volume. Although of great interest in relation to such cardiac diseases as congestive heart failure in which distention of the atria occurs, this hormone may not be important under normal circumstances. Because the exact role of atrial natriuretic factor in a physiologic setting is not proven it is represented in Fig. 2.4 with a light dashed line.

Adrenocorticotropic hormone (ACTH) from the anterior pituitary has a positive influence on the release of aldosterone by maintaining the tropic state of cortical cells. ACTH is released after many general stresses and also by increased plasma ADH.

The multiple-control systems that regulate ECF osmolality volume through control of water and sodium intake and excretion are summarized in Fig. 2.4. In this figure the relative importance of each pathway is suggested by the thickness of its line.

Potassium

Potassium is the major cation of the intracellular fluid, and 89 percent of the total body content of potassium is located within the cells. Nearly all of the intracellular potassium is readily exchangeable with potassium in the ECF. The $[K+]$ in ECF is well regulated, and deviations of more than a few percent from normal values are uncommon. Dietary intake is usually in excess of needs because most foodstuffs contain considerable potassium, and the kidneys are more capable of excreting this excess than of conserving it. Dogs fed a potassium-deficient diet for several days, however, gradually decrease the amount of potassium excreted in the urine to a very low level and are able to reestablish potassium balance. Ruminants can also vary their urinary excretion rate of potassium to meet wide and rapid changes in intake.

Renal handling of potassium is complex. Nearly all filtered potassium is reabsorbed by the proximal convoluted tubules. Consequently, the potassium that appears in the urine is the result of secretion by the distal convoluted tubules and collecting ducts. There are two important mechanisms of potassium transport from plasma across the renal tubular cells and on into the tubular fluid.

First, secretion of potassium is very sensitive to ECF $[K^+]$, the secretion rate rising and falling in proportion to blood plasma concentrations. At the basolateral surfaces of the tubular cells, potassium is actively transported into the cells by the ubiquitous sodium/potassium adenosinetriphosphatase (Na/K ATPase) system: sodium is pumped out of the cells in exchange for potassium entering. In addition the transport of sodium is electrogenic, creating a potential that favors the movement of potassium into the cell and toward the tubular lumen. Intracellular $[K^+]$ becomes elevated, and potassium diffuses down its electrochemical gradient from the cells across the luminal border into the tubular lumen. This pathway is very sensitive to ECF potassium concentrations: a rise in the K^+ level of a few tenths of a milliequivalent per liter causes urinary excretion to increase several fold. This automatically results in appropriate changes in excretion rate as body potassium rises or falls (see Chap. 31).

The second major control of potassium concentration in the ECF involves aldosterone. Secretion of aldosterone from the adrenal cortex is sensitive to the ECF $[K^+]$, that is, a small rise of $[K^+]$ causes a great increase in aldosterone secretion. The regulatory sequence is as follows: An increase in plasma $[K^+]$ results in aldosterone release, which increases potassium excretion in urine, and plasma potassium declines to its normal level. If aldosterone is absent because of dysfunction of the adrenal cortex, as in Addison's disease, a severe hyperkalemia develops and can cause cardiac arrest and death. Conversely, excessive aldosterone can result in a serious hypokalemia. Normally, smaller variations of aldosterone concentration in blood cause corresponding variations in renal tubular secretion of potassium. This enhancement of potassium secretion into the tubular fluid is secondary to the stimulation of sodium reabsorption by aldosterone. Sodium channels in the luminal border of the tubular cells are activated, and the Na/K ATPase system at the basolateral border is stimulated by aldosterone. The result is an increase of intracellular potassium, an increase in the potential between blood and lumen (negative in lumen), and an increase in potassium permeability of the luminal membrane; consequently the rate of potassium secretion into the urine increases greatly.

There are two additional, but minor, influences on urinary excretion of potassium: rate of H^+ secretion and rate of Na^+ reabsorption. Because both H^+ secretion and K^+ secretion involve exchanges for Na^+ at the luminal border of the tubular cells, H^+ secretion will compete with K^+ for Na^+ with which to exchange. Consequently, increased H^+ secretion will depress K^+ secretion. Likewise, an appreciable increase in $Na+$ reabsorption will facilitate K^+ secretion. The dietary level of sodium intake, plasma $[Na^+]$, and filtered Na load can in this way influence potassium excretion rates.

Chloride and bicarbonate

Sodium ions of ECF are balanced electrically for the most part by chloride ions and bicarbonate ions. Osmotically, the effect of these ions equals that of sodium ions, but the variations of osmoconcentration are usually a consequence of changes in cation concentration (or water content) rather than that of anions. The $[Cl^-]$ tends to be regulated secondarily to regulation of $[Na^+]$ and $[HCO_3^-]$. If excess sodium is excreted by the kidney, chloride usually accompanies it. If, because of an alkalotic condition, the plasma level of bicarbonate ion rises, an equivalent amount of chloride ion is excreted in order that electroneutrality may be maintained in the ECF.

The bicarbonate ion is unique in that it can be formed in or removed by the body with great rapidity. It is formed in solution from its anhydride:

$$CO_2 + H_2O \rightleftarrows H_2CO_3 \rightleftarrows H^+ + HCO_3^-$$

There is a ready supply of carbon dioxide from cellular metabolism and a rapid means for its removal by the respiratory tract.

REFERENCES

Adolph, E.F., Barker, J.P., and Hoy, P.A. 1954. Multiple factors in thirst. *Am. J. Physiol.* 178:538–62.

Andersson, B. 1978. Regulation of water intake. *Physiol. Rev.* 58:582–603.

Andersson, B., and McCann, S.M. 1955. A further study of polydipsia evoked by hypothalamic stimulation in the goat. *Acta Physiol. Scand.* 33:333–46.

Baertschi, A.J., and Vallet, P.G. 1981. Osmosensitivity of the hepatic portal vein area and vasopressin release in rats. *J. Physiol.* 315:217–30.

Bell, F.R., Drury, P.L., and Sly, J. 1981. The effect on salt appetite and the renin-aldosterone system on replacing the depleted ions to sodium-deficient cattle. *J. Physiol.* 313:263–74.

Bellows, R.T. 1939. Time factors in water drinking in dogs. *Am. J. Physiol.* 125:87–97.

Cizek, L.J. 1959. Long-term observations on relationship between food and water ingestion in the dog. *Am. J. Physiol.* 197:342–46.

Coghlan, J.P., Considine, P.J., Denton, D.A., Fei, D.T.W., Leksell, L.G., McKinley, J.J., Muller, A.F., Tarjan, E., Weisinger, R.S., and Bradshaw, R.A. 1981. Sodium appetite in sheep induced by cerebral ventricular infusion of angiotensin: Comparison with sodium deficiency. *Science* 214:195–97.

de Caro, G., Epstein, A.N., and Massi, M, eds. 1986. *The Physiology of Thirst and Sodium Appetite.* Plenum Press, New York.

Denton, D. 1982. *The Hunger for Salt.* Springer-Verlag, Berlin.

Dill, D.B. 1938. *Life, Heat, and Altitude.* Harvard Univ. Press, Cambridge.

Dill, D.B., Yousef, M.K., Cox, C.R., and Barton, R.G. 1980. Hunger vs. thirst in the burro (*Equus asinus*). *Physiol. Behav.* 24:975–78.

Edelman, I.S., and Leibman, J. 1959. Anatomy of body water and electrolytes. *Am. J. Med.* 27:256–77.

Elkinton, J.R., and Taffel, M. 1942. Prolonged water deprivation in the dog. *J. Clin. Invest.* 21:787–94.

Epstein, A.N. 1976. The physiology of thirst. *Can. J. Physiol. Pharmacol.* 54:639–49.

Fitzsimons, J.T. 1980a. Thirst and sodium appetite. *Endeavor* 4:97–101.

Fitzsimons, J.T. 1980b. Angiotensin and other peptides in the control of water and sodium intake. *Proc. Roy. Soc.*, ser. B, 210:165–82.

Golob, P., O'Connor, W.J., and Potts, D.J. 1977. Post-prandial drinking by dogs. *Q. J. Exp. Physiol.* 62:275–85.

Hansard, S.L. 1964. Total body water in farm animals. *Am. J. Physiol.* 206:1369–72.

Hix, E.L., Underbjerg, G.K.L., and Hughes, J.S. 1959. The body fluids of ruminants and their simultaneous determination. *Am. J. Vet. Res.* 20:184–91.

Honstein, R.N., and Monty, D.E.,Jr. 1977. Physiologic responses of the horse to a hot, arid environment. *Am. J. Vet. Res.* 38:1041–48.

Hosutt, J.A., and Stricker, E.M. 1981. Hypotension and thirst in rats after phentolamine treatment. *Physiol. Behav.* 27:463–68.

Jackson, T.E., Guyton, A.C., and Hall, J.E. 1977. Transient response of glomerular filtration rate and renal blood flow to step changes in arterial pressure. *Am. J. Physiol.* 233:F396–F402.

Johnson, A.K., Mann, J.F.E., Rascher, W., Johnson, J.K., and Ganten, D. 1981. Plasma angiotensin II concentrations and experimentally induced thirst. *Am. J. Physiol.* 240:R229–R234.

Johnson, J.A., Zehr, J.E., and Moore, W.W. 1970. Effects of separate and concurrent osmotic and volume stimuli on plasma ADH in sheep. *Am. J. Physiol.* 218:1273–80.

Kraybill, H.F., Hankins, O.G., and Bitter, H.L. 1951. Body composition of cattle. I. Estimation of body fat from measurement in vivo of body water by the use of antipyrine. *J. Appl. Physiol.* 3:681–89.

Lee, D.H.K., and Robinson, K. 1941. Reactions of the sheep to hot atmospheres. *Proc. R. Soc. Queensl.* 53:189–200.

Lemieux, G., Warren, Y., and Gervais, M. 1964. Characteristics of potassium conservation by the dog kidney. *Am. J. Physiol.* 206:743–79.

Macallum, A.B. 1926. The paleochemistry of the body fluids and tissues. *Physiol. Rev.* 6:316–57.

Macfarlane, W.V. 1964. Terrestrial animals in dry heat: Ungulates. In D.B. Dill et al., eds., *Handbook of Physiology*. Sec. 4, *Adaptation to the Environment*. Am. Physiol. Soc., Washington. Pp. 509–39.

Maloiy, G.M.O. 1970. Water economy of the Somali donkey. *Am. J. Physiol.* 219:1522–27.

Mayland, H.F., and Grunes, D.L. 1974. Shade-induced grass-tetany-prone chemical changes in *Agropyron desertorum* and *Elymus cinereus*. *J. Range Mgmt.* 27:198–201.

McLean, J.A. 1963. The partition of insensible losses of body weight and heat from cattle under various climatic conditions. *J. Physiol.* 167:427–47.

Nay, T., and Hayman, R.H. 1956. Sweat glands in Zebu (*Bos indicus* L.) and European (*B. taurus* L.) cattle. *Aust. J. Agric. Res.* 7:482–94.

Needham, A.D., Dawson, T.J., and Hales, J.R.S. 1974. Forelimb blood flow and saliva spreading in the thermoregulation of the red kangaroo *Megaleia rufa*. *Comp. Biochem. Physiol.*, ser. A. 49:555–65.

Painter, E.E., Holmes, J.H., and Gregersen, M.I. 1948. Exchange and distribution of fluid in dehydration in the dog. *Am. J. Physiol.* 152:66–76.

Pickering, E.C. 1965. The role of the kidney in sodium and potassium balance in the cow. *Proc. Nutr. Soc.* 24:73–80.

Prentiss, P.G., Wolf, A.V., and Eddy, H.A. 1959. Hydropenia in cat and dog: Ability of the cat to meet its water requirements solely from a diet of fish or meat. *Am. J. Physiol.* 196:626–32.

Ramsay, D.J., Rolls, B.J., and Wood, R.J. 1977. Thirst following water deprivation in dogs. *Am. J. Physiol.* 232:R93–R100.

Reynolds, M. 1953. Plasma and blood volume in the cow using the T-1824 hematocrit method. *Am. J. Physiol.* 173:421–27.

Rolls, B.J., and Rolls, E.T. 1982. *Thirst.* Cambridge Univ. Press, Cambridge.

Schmidt-Nielsen, B., Schmidt-Nielsen, K., Houpt, T.R., and Jarnum, S.A. 1956. Water balance of the camel. *Am. J. Physiol.* 185:185–94

Schmidt-Nielsen, K. 1964. *Desert Animals: Physiological Problems of Heat and Water.* Oxford Univ. Press, London.

Schmidt-Nielsen, K., Schmidt-Nielsen, B., Jarnum, S.A., and Houpt, T.R. 1957. Body temperature of the camel and its relation to water economy. *Am. J. Physiol.* 188:103–12.

Schmidt-Nielsen, K., Schroter, R.C., and Shkolnik, A. 1981. Desaturation of exhaled air in camels. *Proc. R. Soc. Lond. Ser B. Biol. Sci.* 211:305–19.

Sellers, A.F., Gitis, T.L., and Roepke, M.H. 1951. Studies of electrolytes in body fluids of dairy cattle. III. Effects of potassium on electrolyte levels in body fluids in midlactation. *Am. J. Vet. Res.* 12: 296–301.

Stricker, E.M., and Verbalis, J.G. 1988. Hormones and behavior: The biology of thirst and sodium appetite. *Am. Sci.* 76:261–68.

Thrasher, T.N., Brown, C.J., Keil, L.C., and Ramsay, D.J. 1980. Thirst and vasopressin release in the dog: An osmoreceptor or sodium receptor mechanism? *Am. J. Physiol.* 238:R333–R339.

Towbin, E.J. 1949. Gastric distention as a factor in satiation of thirst in esophagostomized dogs. *Am. J. Physiol.* 159:533–41.

Wardener, H.E. de. 1973. The control of sodium excretion. In J. Orloff and R.W. Berliner, eds., *Handbook of Physiology.* Sec. 8, *Renal Physiology*. Am. Physiol. Soc., Washington. Pp. 677–720.
Widdowson, E.M., and McCance, R.A. 1956. The effect of development on the composition of the serum and extracellular fluids. *Clin. Sci.* 56:361–65.
Wolf, A.V. 1958. *Thirst: Physiology of the Urge to Drink and Problems of Water Lack*. Charles C Thomas, Springfield, Ill.
Young, D.B., McCaa, R.E., Pan, Y-J., and Guyton, A.C. 1976. Effectiveness of the aldosterone-sodium and -potassium feedback control system. *Am. J. Physiol.* 231:945–53.
Yousef, M.K., Dill, D.B., and Mayes, M.G. 1970. Shifts in body fluids during dehydration in the burro, *Equus asinus*. *J. Appl. Physiol.* 29:345–49.
Zimmerman, M.B., Blaine, E.H., and Stricker, E.M. 1981. Water intake in hypovolemic sheep: Effects of crushing the left atrial appendage. *Science* 211:489–91.

CHAPTER 3

Physiological Properties and Cellular and Chemical Constituents of Blood | by Melvin J. Swenson

Blood serves as a transport medium. It carries nutrients from the digestive tract to the tissues, the end products of metabolism from the cells to the organs of excretion, oxygen from the lungs to the tissues, carbon dioxide from the tissues to the lungs, and the secretions of the endocrine glands throughout the body. Blood also helps regulate body temperature, maintain a constant concentration of water and electrolytes in the cells, regulate the body's hydrogen ion concentration, and defend against microorganisms.

The cells of the blood and fluid compartments of the body assist in these functions. Leukocytes defend the body; erythrocytes contain hemoglobin, which transports oxygen and carbon dioxide. The extracellular constituents include water, electrolytes, proteins, glucose, enzymes, and hormones. Maintenance of uniformity and stability in this extracellular fluid is called homeostasis. In this environment cells function at their optimum. Homeostasis is maintained by physiological processes, such as diffusion, pressure gradients, concentration gradients, and active transport, and by regulatory mechanisms in the lungs and kidneys controlled by the nervous and endocrine systems (see Chaps. 13 and 31).

Blood Cells, Plasma, And Serum

Three classes of blood cells (corpuscles) are recognized: erythrocytes (red cells), leukocytes (white cells), and thrombocytes (platelets). The red color of blood is caused by the hemoglobin in the erythrocytes. All these cells are suspended in the fluid called *plasma*.

Plasma itself is yellow to colorless, depending on the quantity, the species of the animal, and the animal's diet. When examined as a thin film, plasma is almost colorless. In some species, such as cats, dogs, sheep, and goats, it is colorless or only slightly yellow in larger quantities; in cows and especially in horses it is usually darker. The color results chiefly from varying concentrations of a pigment called bilirubin, although carotene and other pigments are contributing factors.

In coagulation, blood lost from the body becomes a gelatinous mass (see Chap. 4). After coagulation, the blood clot retracts, thereby forcing from the clot a clear, watery fluid called *serum*. Serum is similar to plasma except that fibrinogen and other clotting factors have been removed.

One may obtain plasma by adding an anticoagulant to whole blood to prevent clotting and by letting the cells settle out, since they are heavier than plasma. Centrifuging the blood hastens the settling of the cells so that plasma may be obtained more readily.

In the adult animal, plasma contains 91 to 92 percent water and 8 to 9 percent solids. More than 7 percent of the plasma consists of proteins such as albumin, globulins, and fibrinogen. Other proteins in microquantities are antibodies, enzymes, and some of the hormones. The balance of the organic constituents includes the nonprotein nitrogen

(NPN) compounds (urea, uric acid, creatine, creatinine, amino acids, glutathione, xanthine, hypoxanthine), glucose, neutral fats, phospholipids, cholesterol, and others. The inorganic constituents make up about 1 percent of the plasma. They include the minerals (electrolytes) calcium, phosphorus, magnesium, potasium, sodium, chloride, sulfur, iodine, iron, copper, cobalt, manganese, zinc, selenium, and molybdenum. Some of these minerals are used for bone formation; some are constituents of proteins and lipids in muscles, organs, blood cells, and other tissues and of various enzymes. Minerals are involved in the maintenance of osmotic pressures, acid-base equilibria, and the irritability of muscles and nerves. (See Chap. 29 for details on minerals.)

At the time of conception the fertilized egg is about 90 to 95 percent water. From conception until maturity there is a constant decrease in the percentage of body water in mammals. As the percentage of body water decreases, the concentration of red blood cells increases in the bloodstream, and adult values for blood cells, plasma, and their constituents are eventually established. In addition to this gerontological change, there is an even greater decrease in body water when large amounts of fat are deposited in the adult. Thus the percentage of body water is related not only to age but also to the mass of the lean tissues. Obese animals such as swine will therefore have a much lower percentage of water on a body-weight basis than lean animals, and yet the adult blood picture will remain normal.

Anticoagulants

Many anticoagulants can be used to obtain blood samples that are free of clots for transfusion and for analytical work. Heparin, a conjugated polysaccharide, is a natural anticoagulant, produced by basophils (leukocytes of a particular kind) in the blood and by mast cells throughout the body. Mast cells are part of the connective tissue surrounding capillaries in the lungs and other organs. From this tissue, heparin is released and passes into the capillaries. A concentration of 0.2 mg (20 units) of heparin per milliliter of blood is used as an anticoagulant. However, 1 mg of heparin will prevent the coagulation of 100 to 500 ml of blood at 0°C and 10 to 20 ml at room temperature. One unit of heparin is approximately 0.01 mg of heparin sodium.

An anticoagulant commonly used for blood transfusions in animals is sodium citrate. The citrate combines with calcium ions of the plasma, forming an insoluble calcium salt. One must be careful not to give too much citrate because citrate can combine with sufficient calcium ions to produce a hypocalcemia, which may interfere with the functioning of nerves and of skeletal and cardiac muscles and lead to tetany, hypotension, and cardiac arrest. Sodium citrate and similar salts are used in concentrations of 0.2 to 0.4 percent of blood to prevent coagulation. Sodium citrate is the anticoagulant of choice for studies of blood coagulation. Potassium salts are not used in transfusions because of the possibility of producing hyperkalemia, which might alter cardiac electrical activity (tall peaked T waves, bradycardia, atrial standstill, heart block, or cardiac arrest).

Other useful anticoagulants are sodium, potassium, and ammonium salts of oxalates and fluorides. Chelating compounds, such as salts of ethylenediaminetetraacetic acid (EDTA), are also used for hematologic studies. Ammonium salts are not recommended when compounds that contain nitrogen are being determined quantitatively, because of nitrogen in the anticoagulant.

In the calculation of mean corpuscular volume (MCV), mean corpuscular hemoglobin (MCH), and mean corpuscular hemoglobin concentration (MCHC) as diagnostic aids, it is essential to maintain the cell size as it existed in the circulating blood when the packed cell volume (PCV) was determined.

Heparin or EDTA keeps the size of erythrocytes constant when recommended concentrations are used in hematologic procedures. A combination of 6 mg of ammonium oxalate and 4 mg of potassium oxalate inhibits the coagulation of 5 ml of blood and keeps the cell size constant. EDTA is the preferred anticoagulant for studies of blood morphology, quantitative methods involving cells, and the blood indices.

ERYTHROCYTES

Erythrocytes in the circulating blood of mammals are nonnucleated, nonmotile cells. They usually appear as biconcave circular disks with a central pale spot. The biconcavity increases the surface area, thus facilitating the exchange of oxygen and carbon dioxide carried by the red blood cells. To facilitate the transport of carbon dioxide, the red blood cells contain the enzyme *carbonic anhydrase*, which catalyzes the reversible reaction of carbon dioxide to form bicarbonate ions, thereby readily eliminating carbon dioxide from the body by the lungs (see Chap. 13 for more details).

Erythrocytes vary in diameter and thickness according to species and nutritional status of the animal, but they are capable of undergoing changes in shape while passing through capillary beds. The dog erythrocyte is markedly biconcave; cat and horse erythrocytes are slightly biconcave. The small red blood cell of the goat shows little biconcavity. Figure 3.1 shows erythrocytes from blood of normal animals. There is considerable variation in shape and size of erythrocytes within species and among species. Goats have the largest number of red cells per unit of volume (page 27) and the smallest cells in diameter and cubic volume (Table 3.1). Figure 3.1H shows fusiform and spindle-shaped erythrocytes from a normal Angora goat. Figure 3.1G shows elliptical red cells from a camel. Animals of the ruminant family Camellidae, including the alpaca, camel, llama, and vicuna, have elliptical erythrocytes without nuclei. The red cells of cold-blooded animals are

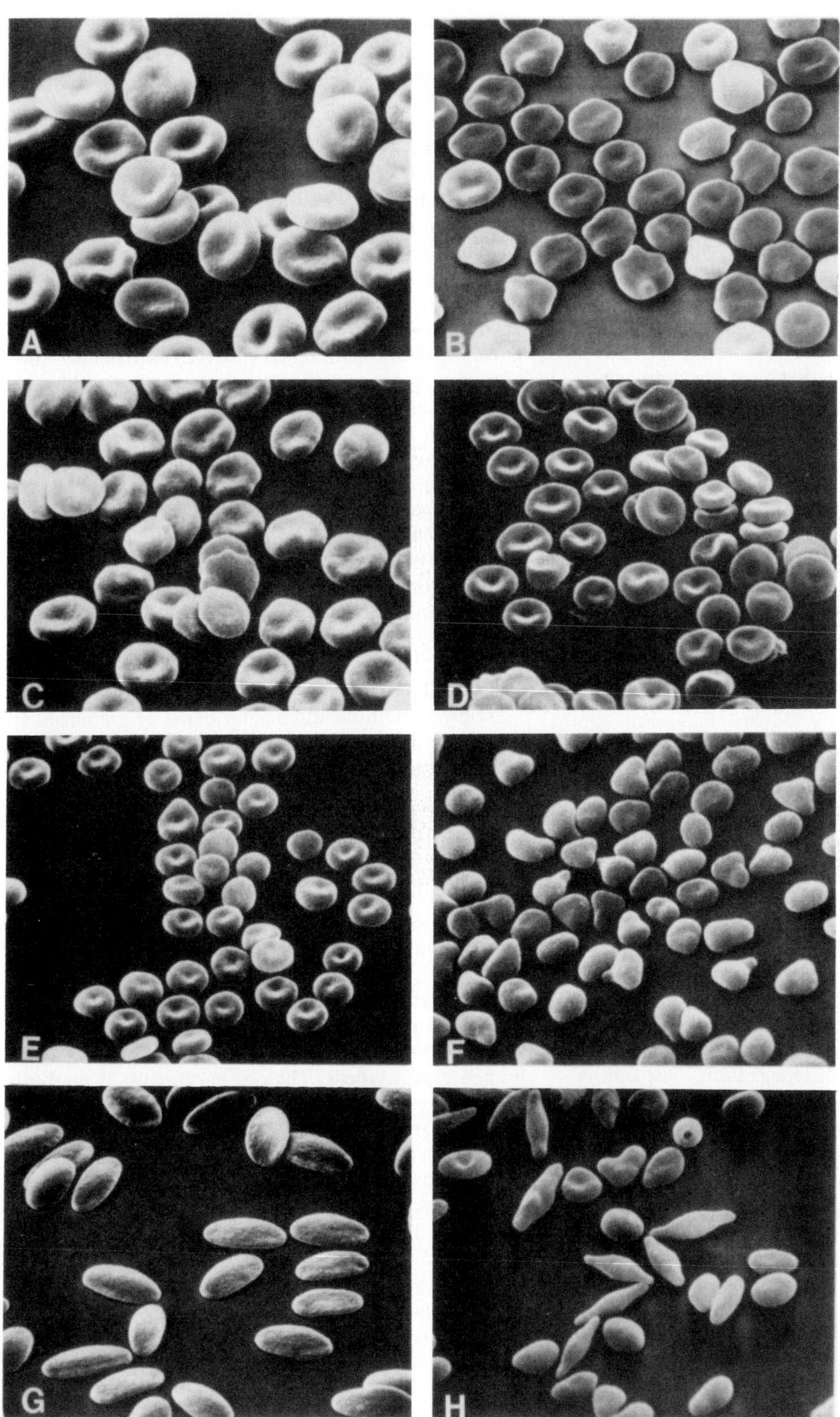

Figure 3.1. Scanning electron photomicrographs of erythrocytes. (*A*) Dog, ×2300. (*B*) Cat, ×2040. (*C*) Horse, ×2100. (*D*) Cow, ×1800. (*E*) Sheep, ×1620. (*F*) Goat, ×2100. (*G*) Camel, ×1440. (*H*) Goat with fusiform and spindle-shaped erythrocytes, ×1890. (*A* through *F* supplied by Dr. N.C. Jain, Department of Clinical Pathology, School of Veterinary Medicine, University of California, Davis; *G* from Jain and Keeton 1974, *Br. Vet. J.* 130:288–91; and *H* from Schalm, Jain, and Carroll 1975, *Veterinary Hematology*, 3d ed., Lea & Febiger, Philadelphia.)

Table 3.1. Erythrocyte size and hemoglobin content in adult domestic animals

Animal	MCV (μm^3)	MCH (pg)	MCHC (g/dl)	References
Cat	51–63	13–17	32–34	Coffin 1953
Cattle	52	19	32	Drastisch 1928
	58	20	34	Wintrobe 1933
	46–54	15–20	32–39	Swenson et al. 1962
Chicken	115–125	25–27	21–23	Calculated from Swenson 1951
Dog	59–69	20–24	30–35	Ranges from 7 references cited by Wintrobe 1961
Goat	16	8	32	Drastisch 1928
	19	7	35	Wintrobe 1933
Horse	52	18	34	Drastisch 1928
	42	13	33	Macleod and Ponder 1946
Pig	58	19	33	Wintrobe 1961
At birth	64–96	21–31	32–34	Swenson et al. 1958
1 week	71–78	22–25	30–33	Swenson et al. 1958
3 weeks	61–75	20–23	29–33	Swenson et al. 1958
4–8	53–66	16–20	28–35	Swenson et al. 1958
weeks	35	11	31	Drastisch 1928
Sheep	35	13	35	Wintrobe 1933
	30–44	10–14	27–36	Carlson et al. 1961

elliptical in shape and have nuclei. Avian erythrocytes in the circulating blood are elliptical, and they have nuclei.

Origin

In early fetal development nucleated red blood cells are produced in the yolk sac. Later in embryonic development, the liver, spleen, and lymph nodes are involved. During the latter part of gestation and after birth, the formation of red cells (erythropoiesis) takes place in the bone marrow. In adulthood the marrow of long bones, which was active in erythropoiesis in the young animal, is replaced with fat. The marrow of the membranous bones (bodies of the vertebrae, pelvis, ribs, and sternum) remains active in older animals, and there is a gradual tendency for the marrow to decrease in activity with age. The potential for erythropoietic activity of all embryonic sites (except the yolk sac), including the bone marrow, is present in the adult. One may see these sites with regenerative capacity reverting to the production of red cells. For example, the liver, spleen, and lymph nodes may produce red cells in adult animals that have severe, prolonged anemia. The same applies to inactive bone marrow locations such as the long bones and the spines of the vertebrae.

From the mesenchymal cells of the splanchnic mesoderm of the yolk sac there is formed a primitive stem cell called a colony-forming unit (CFU), which forms several pluripotent stem cells or CFUs. These pluripotent cells seed the sinusoids of the liver and the spleen by hormonal influence. The liver seeds the thymus and the bone marrow. The thymus seeds the lymph nodes and the spleen. The lymph nodes produce the T and B lymphocytes (discussed later).

In regard to the precise origin of the erythrocyte, the pluripotent stem cells in the bone marrow are capable of self-renewal and the production of unipotent cells of several hematopoietic lines. With appropriate stimulation, pluripotent stem cells differentiate into unipotent CFUs or committed progenitor cells, which have the ability to proliferate and differentiate into cells of only one hematopoietic line. They form the erythroid, myeloid, B lymphocyte, or megakaryocytic series. Thus, erythrocytes, granulocytes, monocytes, B lymphocytes, and platelets are produced. The lymphoid stem cell from the thymus is responsible for T lymphocytes to be produced in the lymph nodes.

Rubriblasts proliferate from the erythrocytic unipotent CFU. Table 3.2 shows that, as rubriblasts proliferate, they develop into prorubricytes; as prorubricytes mature, they form rubricytes, which eventually form the erythrocyte.

As one views the development of red blood cells, one may draw these conclusions:

1. The younger the cell, the larger it is. As cells develop, they become smaller.

2. The younger the cell, the larger the nucleus. This decreases in size with development and is finally lost from the red cells of domestic animals (mammals).

3. In the nucleus the chromatin containing deoxyribonucleic acid (DNA) becomes more compact or dense (pyknotic) as development proceeds and stains a deeper blue (Wright's stain).

4. The cytoplasm of rubriblasts contains ribonucleic acid (RNA) and stains blue. As cells develop into the various types, the cytoplasm takes on a reddish hue (first in the rubricyte) because of the presence of hemoglobin.

In the adult, erythropoiesis goes on continuously in the bone marrow, and corpuscles are poured into the bloodstream at a rate to balance the destruction of red cells. The total number in the blood therefore does not fluctuate greatly. It usually takes 4 to 5 days for a rubriblast to develop into an erythrocyte.

The metarubricyte, the bone marrow cell that is a fore-

Table 3.2. Developmental stages of various blood cells

Series	Cells
Erythrocytic	Rubriblast Prorubricyte Rubricyte Metarubricyte Basophilic erythrocyte (reticulocyte) Erythrocyte
Granulocytic	Myeloblast Progranulocyte Myelocyte Metamyelocyte Band cell Neutrophil, eosinophil, basophil
Lymphocytic	Lymphoblast Prolymphocyte Lymphocyte
Monocytic	Monoblast Promonocyte Monocyte
Thrombocytic	Megakaryoblast Promegakaryocyte Megakaryocyte Thrombocyte or platelet

runner of the erythrocyte, is nucleated whereas the mammalian erythrocyte is not (Table 3.2). The nucleus of the latter is lost by extrusion or by absorption before the corpuscle enters the bloodstream. Normally 1 to 3 percent of the erythrocytes are basophilic cells without a nucleus. With a supravital stain (new methylene blue) the RNA is precipitated, giving a network or reticulum of blue fibers, hence the name *reticulocyte*. Basically, reticulocytes are young red cells that contain the remains of a fragmented nucleus, with the ribosomes and polyribosomes in the cytoplasm being partially precipitated by staining.

Most animals respond with a release of young, nucleated red cells and reticulocytes from the bone marrow into the circulating blood in time of need, such as during hemorrhage, hemolytic diseases, and parasitism. The horse, however, does not usually respond in this manner. Reticulocytes and nucleated red cells are seldom seen in the peripheral blood of horses.

Composition

Erythrocytes in adult animals contain 62 to 72 percent water; the remaining approximately 35 percent consists of solids. Of the solids, hemoglobin constitutes about 95 percent. The major solids of the other 5 percent are proteins in the stroma and cell membrane; lipids such as phospholipids (lecithin, cephalin, sphingomyelin), free cholesterol, cholesterol esters, and neutral fat; vitamins functioning as coenzymes; glucose for energy; enzymes such as cholinesterase, phosphatases, carbonic anhydrase, peptidases, and those concerned with glycolysis; and minerals (electrolytes) such as phosphorus, sulfur, chlorine (principal intracellular anion), magnesium, potassium, and sodium.

Sodium is the principal cation in extracellular fluid. Serum or plasma sodium and potassium values of most domestic animals vary from 140 to 150 and 4.0 to 5.0 mEq/L, respectively. Cations and anions within and outside the cell help in the establishment and maintenance of electrical gradients across cell membranes by the sodium pump, by active transport of cations and anions, and by diffusion. These physiological processes help maintain a steady state of electrolytes within cells (see Chap. 32).

Potassium is the principal cation of erythrocytes of some species. In other animals sodium predominates (Table 3.3). It is well documented that domestic animals exhibit genetic differences in the potassium content of erythrocytes. There are both low-potassium (LK) and high-potassium (HK) erythrocytes in dogs, cats, cattle, goats, and sheep. Red blood cells in LK sheep are higher in potassium at birth than in adulthood. Potassium gradually decreases to adult values in 1 to 2 months after birth, when fetal hemoglobin is no longer present.

In animals with LK red cells all other tissues are indistinguishable between HK and LK animals. Table 3.3 gives potassium and sodium values for various domestic animals.

Table 3.3. Mean potassium and sodium values of erythrocytes

Species	Potassium (mM/kg)	Sodium (mM/kg)
Cat	5.9	103.7
Cow	21.8	79.8
Dog	8.7	107.0
Goat	18.4	93.2
Pig	99.5	10.8
Sheep	18.4	83.5
	64.2	15.6
	58.1	46.0
Chicken	97.3	7.1
Turkey	99.5	9.7

Data from Kerr 1937, *J. Biol. Chem.* 117:227–35.

Genetic differences are evident, especially for sheep with HK and LK red cells. The reported potassium values of red cells in horses average 88 mM/L. The serum values of potassium and sodium for horses are 2.4 to 4.7 and 132 to 146 mEq/L, respectively.

Animals with HK erythrocytes, such as the horse, pig, and some ruminants, have an active sodium pump that exchanges intracellular sodium for extracellular potassium with the hydrolysis of adenosine triphosphate (ATP). On the other hand, some sheep, goats, and cattle have relatively low potassium values and consequently higher sodium values in the red cells. LK red blood cells have low sodium pump activity and high passive potassium permeability.

Size and hemoglobin content

The diameter of erythrocytes has been measured frequently. For most domestic mammals, the mean diameters from dry smears vary from 4 μm for the goat to 7 μm for the dog (Table 3.4). There are shortcomings in this measurement: (1) the cells in a dry smear (or in a moist state but losing water) are smaller, (2) very few cells are measured from the blood sample taken, and (3) the depth or third dimension of the cell cannot be taken into account. For these reasons, diameters of erythrocytes are less important than their cubic volume, which should be used to measure cells.

The following formulas (indices) provide mean corpuscular volume (MCV), mean corpuscular hemoglobin (MCH), and mean corpuscular hemoglobin concentration (MCHC) values for erythrocytes (see below for abbreviations used):

MCV in μm^3 or fl

$$= \frac{\text{PCV} \times 10}{\text{No. of erythrocytes per } \mu\text{l blood} \times 10^{-6}}$$

MCH in μμg or pg

$$= \frac{\text{Hemoglobin in g/dl} \times 10}{\text{No. of erythrocytes per } \mu\text{l blood} \times 10^{-6}}$$

MCHC in g/dl or g%

$$= \frac{\text{Hemoglobin in g/dl} \times 100}{\text{PCV in ml/dl}}$$

Prefixes commonly used in physiology with gram (g), meters (m), and liter (L or l) are as follows:

Prefix	Abbreviation	Quantity
deci	d	one tenth (10^{-1})
centi	c	one hundredth (10^{-2})
milli	m	one thousandth (10^{-3})
micro	μ	one millionth (10^{-6})
nano	n	one billionth (10^{-9})
pico	p	one trillionth (10^{-12})
femto	f	one quadrillionth (10^{-15})

Thus mμm = nm; μμm = pm; mμμm = fm; pg = μμg; μl = cu mm or mm^3; dl = 100 ml; g/dl (or %) = g/100 ml; fl = cu μ or μm^3; μm is often written as μ (micron).

These indices are an aid in the diagnosis of various anemias. Iron deficiency in all mammals, including humans characterizes a microcytic type of anemia (very small cells). The MCV expresses the average cell size in cubic micrometers. Most mammals are born with large erythrocytes. Pigs are usually born with large erythrocytes measuring 80 to 90 μm^3, which then decrease to 55 to 65 μm^3 in 8 weeks. MCH expresses the average weight of hemoglobin present in erythrocytes, while MCHC gives the average percentage of the MCV that the hemoglobin occupies. These values vary among species (Table 3.1). Pernicious anemia in humans is macrocytic, but this kind of anemia does not occur in domestic animals. The variation in these values is considerable in domestic animals. Error in counting erythrocytes contributes to variations in MCV and MCH.

Number

The number of red blood cells varies greatly among species. The number varies also within species and within individuals of a species (because the cells are not uniformly distributed in the blood vascular system). Since plasma is constantly being shifted across capillary walls, cell counts vary as well between arterial and venous blood samples. The following figures show the range of erythrocytes in blood of domestic animals and humans:

Animal	Millions per mm^3 or μl
Cat	6–8
Cattle	6–8
Chicken	2.5–3.2
Dog	6–8
Goat	13–14
Horse (light or hot-blooded)	9–12
Horse (draft or cold-blooded)	7–10
Pig	6–8
Pigeon	3.5–4.5
Rabbit	5.5–6.5
Sheep	10–13
Man	5–6
Woman	4–5

Other factors affect not only erythrocytic counts but also hemoglobin concentration of other blood constituents: these factors are chiefly age, sex, exercise, nutritional status, lactation, pregnancy, egg production, excitement (release of epinephrine), blood volume (hemodilution or hemoconcentration), stage of estrous cycle, breed, time of day, environmental temperature, altitude, and other climatic factors.

Blood from light horses such as Thoroughbreds frequently has more red cells per unit of volume than blood from draft horses. This finding is partially explained on the basis of excitement causing a release of epinephrine, which makes the spleen contract and increases the number of red cells in the circulating blood. In addition, the erythrocytes of Thoroughbreds are smaller in size. Thus there is a greater erythrocyte surface area, which facilitates the transport of oxygen from the lungs to the tissues. The erythrocyte count per unit of volume for mules is practically the same as that for draft horses.

Table 3.4. Estimated values for calculating total erythrocyte surface area

Species	Human	Cattle	Goat	Sheep	Pig	Horse	Dog	Cat	Chicken
Weight (kg)	70	500	30	40	100	500	20	3	2
Blood volume (ml, calculated as 8% body weight)	5,600	40,000	2,400	3,200	8,000	40,000	1,600	240	160
Total RBC/μl blood × 10^6	5	7	14	11	7	10	7	7	3
Diameter of RBC (μm, dry films)	7.5	5.9	4	4.8	6	5.5	7	6	11.2 × 6.8
Total mm^3 of blood × 10^6	5.6	40	2.4	3.2	8.0	40	1.6	0.24	0.16
Total number of RBC × 10^{13}	2.8	28	3.4	3.5	5.6	40	1.1	0.17	0.048
Estimated surface area/RBC (μm^2) based on diameter and thickness (wet films)	162	110	50	66	113	84	121	113	183
μm^2 in 1 m^2 × 10^{12}	1	1	1	1	1	1	1	1	1
Estimated total erythrocyte surface area (m^2)	4,536	30,800	1,700	2,310	6,328	33,600	1,330	192	88
Ratio of erythrocyte surface area to body weight (m^2/kg body weight)	65	62	57	58	63	67	67	64	44

Surface area

Total erythrocyte surface area can be estimated when blood volume, erythrocyte count, diameter, and thickness are known. The surface areas are amazingly large (Table 3.4). This surface area is of great importance to the respiratory or gas-transport function of the blood. A relatively constant value of erythrocyte surface area to body weight is maintained. For mammals it varies from 57 to 67 m^2/kg. The value for the chickens, 44 m^2/kg, is quite low compared with the value for mammals. The estimated mean surface area per erythrocyte was calculated first from the dimensions reported on dry films. This value was increased by 20 percent to arrive at the estimated wet erythrocyte surface area. The average thickness was calculated as 2 μm. Although considerable error may be introduced with this and other values, these measurements do provide some comparative values to help one understand gas-transport mechanisms.

Life span

The life span of erythrocytes varies with species, and the reported values vary with the method used in measuring the life span. The erythrocytes are tagged with isotopes of iron, chromium, phosphorus, and carbon (^{51}Cr, ^{59}Fe, ^{55}Fe, ^{32}P, and ^{14}C); then their half-life is measured, and the life span is calculated.

In the dog the life span varies from 100 to 130 days, with an average of 118. Reported values for the cat are 70 to 80 days, and for horses they are 140 to 150 days. In adult ruminants (cattle, sheep, and goats) the erythrocyte life span varies from 125 to 150 days. In lambs and calves the life span is shorter, ranging from 50 to 100 days.

Reticulocytes are usually present in the blood of animals when the life span of erythrocytes is less than 100 days. The dog is an exception. Cattle and especially horses with longer life spans do not have reticulocytes in the circulating blood.

In the pig, reported life span of erythrocytes is 51 to 79 days, which appears too short for adult swine. When red cells were tagged with an isotope and infused back into the same animal, the half-life for autologous cells was 28 ± 4 days and for homologous cells (cells infused into a different animal) it was 13.8 ± 5.7 days. Thus erythrocytes from one animal infused into another animal of the same species do not live as long. With the autologous cells, the life span for erythrocytes in swine approaches that reported for humans (100 to 120 days). In practice, it is evident that the life span of red cells is less when the cells are transferred from a donor to the recipient in a blood transfusion.

The life span of erythrocytes of chickens is 20 to 30 days, and for the duck it is 30 to 40 days. It is possible that the short life span of erythrocytes in birds may be due to their high body temperature and rapid metabolic rate.

Erythrocytes are destroyed in great numbers daily. The total number of erythrocytes in the body of a 450-kg animal with a blood volume of 8 percent of body weight is 300 trillion. If the average life of individual erythrocytes is 100 days, then 3 trillion must be destroyed (and formed) in the body every day, or about 35 million every second.

Since erythrocytes become smaller as they develop, one might think that in iron-deficiency anemia the life span of red cells is prolonged because the cells are abnormally small. This is not the case. In iron-deficiency anemia there is a maturation arrest of erythrocytes in the late rubricyte stage. As these cells wait for iron needed in the synthesis of hemoglobin, there is further cell division producing smaller than normal red cells that are deficient in hemoglobin. This is characteristic of the microcytic-hypochromic anemia in iron deficiency.

Fate of erythrocytes

Erythrocytes have the remarkable ability to change shape as they pass through capillaries. Red cells with a diameter of 7 to 10 μm may pass through capillaries with a diameter of 3 to 5 μm. As these cells reach the end of their life span, they become less deformable. At this time approximately 10 percent of the older red cells may undergo lysis as they pass through capillary beds as a consequence of membrane permeability changes and osmotic swelling. When this happens, the hemoglobin is released, combines with haptoglobin (a plasma protein), and is subsequently engulfed by the cells of the mononuclear phagocytic system (MPS). This mode of destruction is known as *intravascular hemolysis*. Cellular fragments and the majority (90 percent) of aging red blood cells may be directly phagocytized by the MPS cells. This mode of destruction of red cells is known as *extravascular hemolysis*. The cells of the MPS are derived from monocytes, and they include the stellate, or Küpffer, cells found in the walls of the blood sinuses of the liver, similar cells in the spleen, and certain cells of the bone marrow and lymph nodes. Figure 3.2 shows that iron is released from the hemoglobin and is either (1) transported in the bloodstream by transferrin (a beta-globulin) to the erythropoietic organs to produce more red cells or (2) stored in the liver, spleen, bone marrow, and intestinal mucosa as ferritin or as hemosiderin (see Chap. 29). In pathological conditions, iron is stored in all tissues of the body. Both storage compounds (ferritin and hemosiderin) may be used in the synthesis of hemoglobin as needed. The pigmentary part of hemoglobin (heme) is converted in the liver into bile pigments such as bilirubin, which is secreted into the bile as an excretory product (see Chap. 17).

The MPS cells in different organs are important in the destruction of erythrocytes. In most domestic animals the red bone marrow is the principal place of erythrocyte destruction. In humans the spleen is probably of great importance; in the rabbit and guinea pig it is less so; in birds the liver is the main site. In some species of animals the liver is also an important site. The protein portion (globin) of the hemoglobin molecule may be broken down to amino

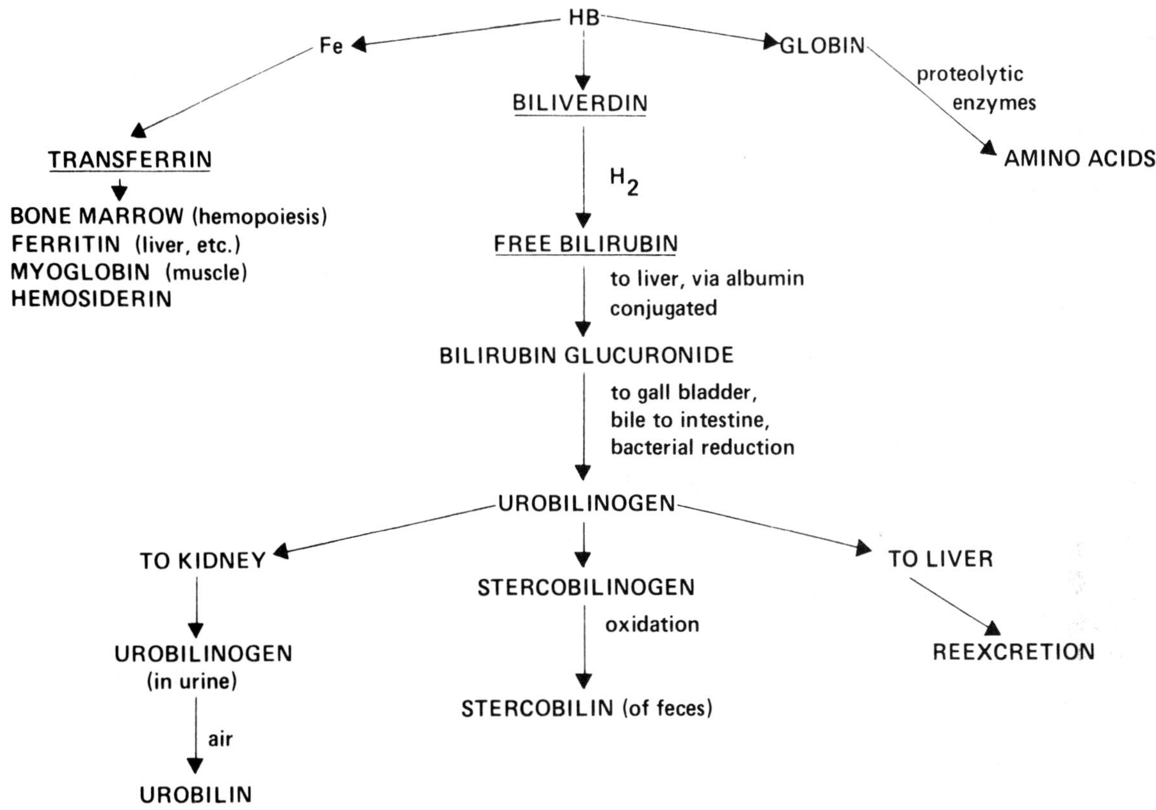

Figure 3.2. Fate of hemoglobin showing disposition of the iron (Fe), pigment (HB), and protein (globin) portion. (Redrawn from Frandson 1981, *Anatomy and Physiology of Farm Animals*, 3d ed., Lea & Febiger, Philadelphia.)

acids and used in the formation of new hemoglobin or other proteins.

Erythropoiesis

Erythropoiesis (the formation of red blood cells) is a continuous process. Many nutrients are essential for this process. Vitamin B_{12} (cyanocobalamin) contains one atom of cobalt in each molecule. It functions in the maturation of erythrocytes. It is required (as is folic acid) for the synthesis of DNA in all cells of the body, including erythrocytes. These vitamins function in different metabolic pathways in the red cell for DNA synthesis. Folic acid (pteroylglutamic acid) is also necessary for RNA synthesis in red cells. Both vitamins act as coenzymes in the synthesis of nucleic acids or their constituents, the purine and pyrimidine bases. Vitamin B_{12} deficiency in humans causes a macrocytic, hyperchromic anemia. In domestic animals the deficiency of vitamin B_{12} produces an anemia, but the size of the red cell is not altered as much as in humans.

Cobalt is a dietary essential for ruminants and is needed in the bacterial synthesis of vitamin B_{12} in the rumen. Cobalt given in excess will cause polycythemia. Animals placed at a high altitude may also show polycythemia because of decreased oxygen pressure (PO_2).

Other vitamins that aid erythropoiesis are pyridoxine, riboflavin, nicotinic acid, pantothenic acid, thiamine, biotin, and ascorbic acid. When these vitamins are deficient, growth and development of erythrocytes are impaired. Pyridoxine deficiency in swine produces a microcytic, hypochromic anemia.

In addition to vitamins, nutrients such as minerals and amino acids, as well as water and energy, are needed for the synthesis of blood proteins. The minerals most commonly needed are iron, copper, and cobalt. Iron is built into the hemoglobin molecule, and copper is essential as a coenzyme or catalyst in hemoglobin synthesis. Copper is part of the enzyme ferroxidase (ceruloplasmin), which is necessary for the oxidation of ferrous iron to the ferric form and the incorporation of iron into hemoglobin. Many enzymes in the body contain iron, copper, zinc, manganese, and molybdenum. For example, catalase, peroxidase, cytochrome oxidase, succinic dehydrogenase, aconitase, and xanthine oxidase contain iron.

With all the nutrients available for the maturation of erythrocytes, there still remain various governing mechanisms for the production and release of these cells from the bone marrow. Normally about 1 percent of the red cells are replaced daily; this figure is based on the fact that red cells live approximately 120 days. The body has a reserve capacity for replenishing or producing many times this quantity as the need arises.

Nonregenerative anemias such as trichostrongylosis in cattle, anemia associated with chronic infection, leukemia, aplastic bone marrow, lack of erythropoietin, and other cachectic diseases do not elicit greater red cell production. On the other hand, hemorrhage, hemolytic diseases, chronic blood loss, blood-sucking parasites, and nutritional deficiencies do elicit the response of greater red cell production. In these conditions the anemia is regenerative.

In hypoxic conditions caused by an inadequate number (anemia) or improper functioning of erythrocytes, the tissues are not supplied with enough oxygen. As a result, a humoral factor is released from the tissues and stimulates erythropoiesis. The substance is called erythropoietin (EPO). It is neither vitamin B_{12} nor the intrinsic factor of Castle. The kidney is the principal site of EPO production in the adults of most species (the sole source in the dog). Extrarenal EPO production in certain animals and humans helps to maintain erythropoiesis during anemia caused by severe kidney diseases. It is during these times that hypoxic tissue cells in general may produce EPO. When EPO is released, it stimulates erythrocyte formation in the bone marrow.

It has been demonstrated that acute hypoxia, whether due to anemia or to decreased oxygen pressure of the inspired air, will cause production and subsequent release of EPO into the blood plasma. This compound has been found in the blood plasma of rats, mice, rabbits, dogs, cattle, sheep, swine, and humans.

EPO stimulates committed stem cells, including rubriblasts, prorubricytes, and young rubricytes, to increase their mitotic activity for more rapid production and release of erythrocytes. As a result, reticulocytosis can be observed in hypoxic animals or when EPO is injected into animals.

The concentration of blood EPO does not increase above normal when the arterial PO_2 is 50 mm Hg or more and the O_2 saturation is 80 percent or greater (Fig. 13.16). When these values are decreased, the EPO levels are increased.

Since hydrochloric acid from the parietal cells of the stomach increases absorption of iron from food and also converts ferric to ferrous iron to facilitate absorption, an achlorhydria markedly reduces iron absorption. High doses of antacids also impair iron absorption and subsequent development of the red cell.

PACKED CELL VOLUME

The volume of cells in the circulating blood is usually less than the plasma volume. Data for this relationship are readily obtained from blood samples with the appropriate kind and quantity of anticoagulant (see Anticoagulants, above). The microhematocrit centrifuge and tubes are used to obtain PCV values very quickly (within 5 minutes). A layer of packed leukocytes occurs just above the packed erythrocytes. This layer is referred to as the *buffy coat*.

The PCV is expressed as a percent volume of packed cells in whole blood after centrifugation. Most species of domestic animals have PCV values of 38 to 45 percent with a mean of 40. Cold-blooded (draft) horses usually have PCV values of 35 to 38 percent; lactating dairy cows, 32 to 35 percent; and chickens, 30 to 33 percent. In adult male chickens the PCV value may reach 35 to 40 percent. Hemoconcentration due to dehydration, asphyxia, or excitement causing release of erythrocytes concentrated in the spleen can result in abnormally high PCV values. Excitement in dogs may cause the PCV values to change from 42 to 53 percent. In excitement the epinephrine causes splenic contraction, which forces the stored red cells into the circulating blood and increases the PCV. Normally, the PCV is approximately three times the hemoglobin concentration in grams/deciliter.

HEMOGLOBIN

Hemoglobin, the pigment of erythrocytes, is a complex, iron-containing, conjugated protein composed of a pigment and a simple protein. The protein is globin, a histone. The red color of hemoglobin is due to heme, a metallic compound containing an iron atom (Fig. 3.3). Hemoglobin has four polypeptide chains—alpha, beta, gamma, and delta. Each of the four chains unites with a heme group, resulting in the hemoglobin molecule.

Biosynthesis of hemoglobin starts in the rubricyte (polychromatophil erythroblast) and continues in the subsequent stages of cell development. As long as nuclear material is present in the cell, whether the cells are in the bone marrow or in the circulating blood, formation of hemoglobin may

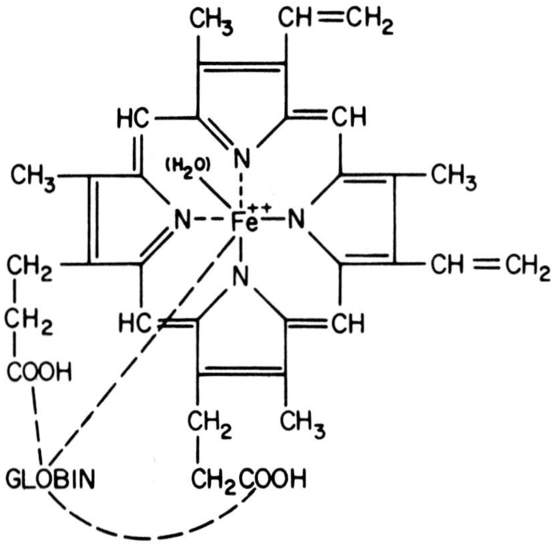

Figure 3.3. Structural formula of heme and its combination with globin. Globin consists of four polypeptides, each of which is united to a heme group to form hemoglobin.

Mitochondrion

Glycine
+
Succinyl-CoA
ALA(δ -aminolevulinic Acid)
ALA
ALA Dehydrase
Porphobilinogen
Uroporphyrinogen III
Coproporphyrinogen III
Protoporphyrin IX + Iron
Ferrochelatase
Heme
4 Heme Molecules + Protein
Mitochondrial Cytochromes
Hemoprotein
[e.g. hemoglobin,
myoglobin,
catalase, peroxidase,
cytochromes, etc.]

Figure 3.4. Biosynthetic pathway of heme in the formation of hemoproteins. (Modified from Tephly, Webb, Trussler, Kniffen, Hasegawa, and Piper 1973, *Drug Metab. Dispos.* 1:259–66.)

continue. Reticulocytes containing RNA and a portion of the nucleus have the ability to synthesize hemoglobin.

In hemoglobin synthesis (Fig. 3.4) the amino acid glycine coming from the amino acid pool and succinyl coenzyme A from the citric acid cycle form δ-aminolevulinic acid (ALA) with the help of ALA synthetase. In the presence of ALA dehydrase, porphobilinogen is then formed. Four of the pyrrole

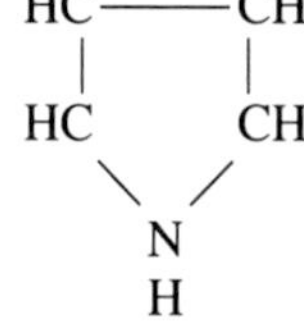

structures are present in the porphyrin molecule (Fig. 3.3). Four porpho-bilinogens unite to form uroporphyrinogen. The enzymes, uroporphyrinogen III cosynthetase and uroporphyrinogen I synthetase, form the type III isomer necessary for heme synthesis. Protoporphyrin IX plus iron in the presence of copper and ferrochelatase (synthetase) produce the heme structure. Then four heme molecules unite with four polypeptides to form the hemoglobin molecule (Fig. 3.3). As shown in Fig. 3.4, heme combines with specific proteins to form several proteins, such as hemoglobin, myoglobin, and various enzymes.

The molecular weights of hemoglobin from most species are reported to vary from 66,000 to 69,000. With the iron content of hemoglobin being 0.334 percent and the atomic weight of iron being 55.84, a value of 16,718 is derived as the minimal molecular weight of one heme and one polypeptide. Since hemoglobin comprises four of these units, the molecular weight ($16{,}718 \times 4 = 66{,}872$) is in the range given above. Differences in the globin molecules among species probably account for the slight differences in their molecular weights.

When erythrocytes are hemolyzed in the bloodstream by protozoa, toxins, or chemical agents, thereby releasing hemoglobin into the plasma, a hemoglobinuria may result. Hemoglobinuria will occur only when the plasma α_2-globulin, haptoglobin, is saturated with free hemoglobin in the plasma. The hemoglobin-haptoglobin complex cannot pass the glomerular filter, whereas free hemoglobin can. The pores or fenestrae in the capillary endothelium in the glomerular tufts of the kidneys place the blood plasma in direct contact with the underlying basement membrane, which permits passage of small proteins such as hemoglobin.

Fetal and adult hemoglobin

The hemoglobins of the fetus and the adult differ in many species. These differences have been noted when the amino acid compositions, oxygen dissociation curves, electrophoretic mobilities, solubilities, and ultraviolet absorption spectra were studied. The oxygen dissociation curve of fetal hemoglobin is steeper than that of adult hemoglobin (Fig. 3.5). At a given oxygen tension, fetal hemoglobin will take up more oxygen than adult hemoglobin. On the other hand, oxygen is passed from the mother to the fetus by

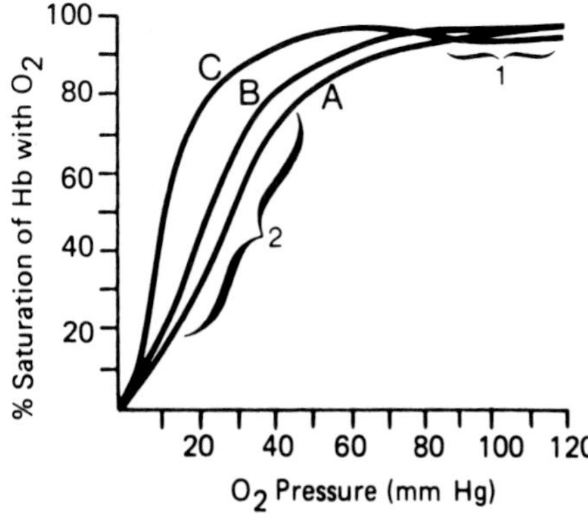

Figure 3.5. Oxygen-hemoglobin dissociation curves of (*A*) adult blood [(1) oxygenated blood from lungs and (2) reduced blood from tissues loaded with carbon dioxide], (*B*) fetal blood, and (*C*) myoglobin.

diffusion, and the tension of oxygen in the blood of the umbilical vein is the same as the arterial blood on the maternal side of the placenta. In the airless lungs of the fetus the blood vessels are bypassed, for the most part, and blood returns to the left atrium of the heart. A high percentage of the blood is thus shunted to the arterial side through vessels that normally become closed at birth or shortly after.

In calves fetal hemoglobin (F) makes up 41 to 100 percent of the total hemoglobin at birth. It diminishes rapidly after birth and is usually replaced with hemoglobin A (the more common adult type) at 2 to 3 months of age. In some calves hemoglobin B (a less common adult type) appears in early life and has the same electrophoretic mobility as fetal hemoglobin. Figure 3.6 shows the variation in the rate of disappearance of fetal hemoglobin in the blood of calves.

The production of fetal hemoglobin is dependent on the presence and availability of amino acids at the site of formation and on the anatomical origin of the erythrocytes. Other factors are probably involved. At birth in infants one-half to three-fourths of the hemoglobin may be of the fetal type. By the end of the first year, fetal-type hemoglobin may reach 1 percent. The animal retains the ability to make fetal hemoglobin in adult life.

Hemoglobin is present in the blood of all mammals and of other animals. In addition to variations in the hemoglobins within individuals (fetal and adult types), there are variations among species. The differences are in the globin part of the hemoglobin molecule, for heme does not vary in composition either in vertebrate animals or in the plant kingdom.

Amount

The amount of hemoglobin in the blood is expressed as grams per deciliter of blood. The quantity may vary within

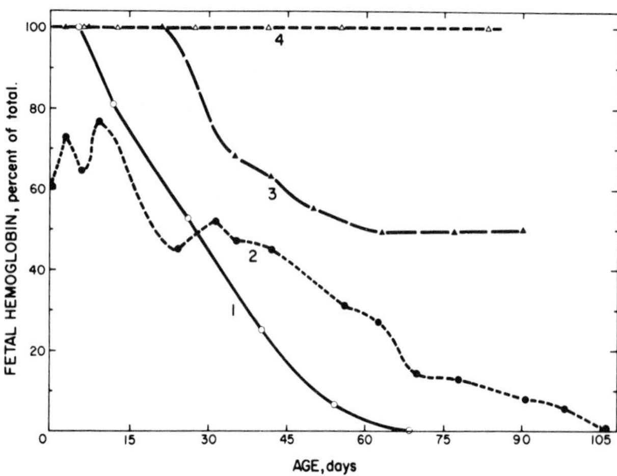

Figure 3.6. Variation in the rate of disappearance of fetal hemoglobin in the blood of calves. Curve 1, Holstein bull; curve 2, Holstein heifer; curves 3 and 4, Guernsey bulls. (From Grimes, Duncan, and Lassiter 1958, *J. Dairy Sci.*, 41:1529–33.)

certain normal limits. As a rule, in most mammals normal blood hemoglobin values are between 13 and 15 g/dl. Exceptions may be found in the lactating cow (11 to 12 g/dl). The hemoglobin values in cold-blooded horses are usually lower—12 to 13 g/dl. It is common to obtain values greater than 15 g/dl in some animals. Excitement may increase not only the hemoglobin concentration but also the PCV and erythrocyte numbers per unit of volume. These changes are due to the release of catecholamines (epinephrine and norepinephrine), causing an increase in blood pressure and contraction of the spleen, which mobilizes erythrocytes into the circulatory system. The changes can easily be demonstrated in an anesthetized dog. The values for PCV may increase from 40 to 45 percent or from 50 to 54 percent after a release or injection of epinephrine.

The hemoglobin concentration in avian blood is more difficult to determine. Various correction factors have been used in the past to adjust for the nucleated erythrocytes, which cause false high readings when conventional methods are used. A method has been devised to determine hemoglobin in the blood of chickens; the values obtained are similar to those determined with the iron method. The normal hemoglobin concentration in chicken blood ranges from 6.5 to 9 g/dl with this method.

In conditions that lower PO_2 in the blood (e.g., decreasing barometric pressure at increasing altitude), there is an increase in the number of erythrocytes and in the production of hemoglobin to help offset the deficiency of oxygen to the tissues. At high altitudes of 14,000 to 16,000 feet, the red cell count may increase (*polycythemia*) as much as 40 to 50 percent.

Oxyhemoglobin

Hemoglobin has important physiological relationships with oxygen. During the passage of the red corpuscles through the pulmonary capillaries, hemoglobin combines with oxygen to form oxyhemoglobin, which, as it traverses the systemic capillaries, loses its oxygen to the tissues and again becomes hemoglobin. Under appropriate conditions these reactions take place readily. Hemoglobin functions as the respiratory pigment of the blood. The red cells, the hemoglobin carriers, spend only about 1 second traversing a capillary. The relation between hemoglobin and oxygen may be expressed in its simplest form as follows: $Hb + O_2 \rightleftarrows HbO_2$. Hemoglobin owes its oxygen-carrying capacity to the pigment it contains, and this in turn owes its oxygen-combining capacity to its iron content. The amount of iron in the blood is small—about 0.334 percent of the hemoglobin molecule or 0.04 to 0.05 percent of the blood itself. The plasma iron concentration is normally 100 to 300 μg/dl, while in iron-deficient animals it may be as low as 40 to 50 μg/dl.

The body carefully conserves the iron resulting from hemoglobin destruction, with only a small amount being lost daily. The dietary iron needed for hemoglobin formation is therefore small.

When saturated with oxygen, 1 g of hemoglobin carries about 1.34 ml of oxygen. As a result, 15 g of hemoglobin in 100 ml of blood may carry approximately 20 ml of oxygen (see Chap. 13 for more details).

Oxyhemoglobin, its aqueous solutions, and arterial blood are bright red in color, whereas reduced (deoxygenated) hemoglobin, its aqueous solutions, and venous blood are purplish red.

Myoglobin (myohemoglobin, muscle hemoglobin)

Myoglobin, or muscle hemoglobin, is a true hemoglobin, being composed of heme and one polypeptide chain. The heme is identical to that in blood hemoglobin. The globins of different species, like the globins of blood hemoglobins, differ somewhat because of variations in their amino acid content. Muscle hemoglobin contains only one heme group and hence only one iron atom per molecule. The iron content is 0.32 percent. Its molecular weight is approximately 16,700. The oxygen-hemoglobin dissociation curve of muscle hemoglobin is hyperbolic (very steep), as shown in Fig. 3.5, whereas the curve for blood hemoglobin is S shaped.

Myoglobin resembles blood hemoglobin in function. It serves as a brief oxygen store within the muscle fiber from one contraction to another. Myoglobin has a greater affinity for oxygen than blood hemoglobin. Consistent with its steeper oxygen-dissociation curve, however, oxygen is rapidly released when the PO_2 level is sufficiently lowered during muscle contraction. Myoglobin is replenished with oxygen during the resting state.

Carboxyhemoglobin

Hemoglobin has the power of combining not only with oxygen but also with certain other gases (e.g., carbon monoxide). The resulting compound is carboxyhemoglobin, or carbonmonoxyhemoglobin. When carbon monoxide is present in the inspired air, it enters the blood and combines with hemoglobin to the exclusion of oxygen, for the affinity of hemoglobin for carbon monoxide is more than 200 times greater than for oxygen. Carbon monoxide attaches to the iron of heme in the same manner as oxygen. Carbon monoxide prevents hemoglobin from being a carrier of oxygen; thus it interferes with hemoglobin supplying oxygen to the tissues. The breathing of air containing 0.1 percent of carbon monoxide will cause severe effects in 30 to 60 minutes; under these conditions some 20 percent of the hemoglobin will be converted to carboxyhemoglobin (HbCO). The carbon monoxide in combination with hemoglobin will be replaced with oxygen if the partial pressure of the latter is great enough. The replacement follows the law of mass action. The reaction $HbCO + O_2 \rightleftharpoons HbO_2 + CO$ will also be displaced to the right by an increase of carbon dioxide pressure by stimulation of the respiratory center.

Carboxyhemoglobin is a bright cherry red. Blood samples and tissues from an animal poisoned with carbon monoxide may mislead one into thinking that the animal has had an abundant supply of oxygen.

Methemoglobin

Methemoglobin, a derivative of hemoglobin, is formed by the oxidation of the ferrous iron of hemoglobin to the ferric state. Methemoglobin is thus the true oxide of hemoglobin, whereas oxyhemoglobin is an oxygenated derivative. Methemoglobin is a nontoxic compound but it cannot combine with oxygen in the sense that hemoglobin does. It is therefore useless as a respiratory pigment in the blood. Methemoglobin is formed in small amounts in the circulating blood, but reducing systems or compounds in the erythrocytes (ascorbic acid, glutathione) prevent its accumulation. Under some conditions, however, as after the administration of certain drugs (nitrites, aminophenols, acetanilid, sulfonamides, etc.), it may occur in the bloodstream in larger amounts. Methemoglobin produces a dark-colored (chocolate brown) blood, and it may cause an animal to be cyanotic. Methemoglobin will form spontaneously in blood or in hemoglobin solutions kept in vitro. Partial deoxygenation of the samples favors its formation. Many chemical substances, including certain oxidizing agents, promote the conversion of hemoglobin to methemoglobin in vitro.

Under field conditions the veterinarian is often called to treat animals poisoned with nitrites and chlorates. These compounds cause methemoglobin to form (see below). Chlorates are sometimes present in herbicides that might be ingested by livestock. Fertilizers may contain a high percentage of nitrate. Foliage of plants grown on highly fertilized soils and water drained from these soils may contain high levels of nitrate and can poison livestock. When nitrates are ingested by ruminants, they are converted to nitrites in the rumen (farther on in the digestive tract of pigs), causing methemoglobin to form; methemoglobin does not transport oxygen to the tissues.

Cattle sometimes eat stunted grain sorghums during periods of drought or after a frost. Under these circumstances, hydrocyanic acid (prussic acid) is usually present in the plants. Cattle that eat these plants are often poisoned with cyanide. Asphyxia occurs because the utilization of oxygen at the tissue level is greatly impaired. To expedite detoxification, veterinarians give various compounds intravenously to form methemoglobin, which unites with cyanide to form cyanmethemoglobin. This compound is then broken down and detoxified by the body. For example, sodium thiosulfate ($Na_2S_2O_3$) unites with the cyanide to form thiocyanate (SCN), which does not have cyanide action and is practically nontoxic. Sodium nitrite and other compounds may be given to form methemoglobin in the poisoned animal. A solution of methylene blue aids in the reduction of methemoglobin to hemoglobin.

LEUKOCYTES

Leukocytes, the white blood cells, are much less numerous than erythrocytes in the circulating blood. Erythrocytes

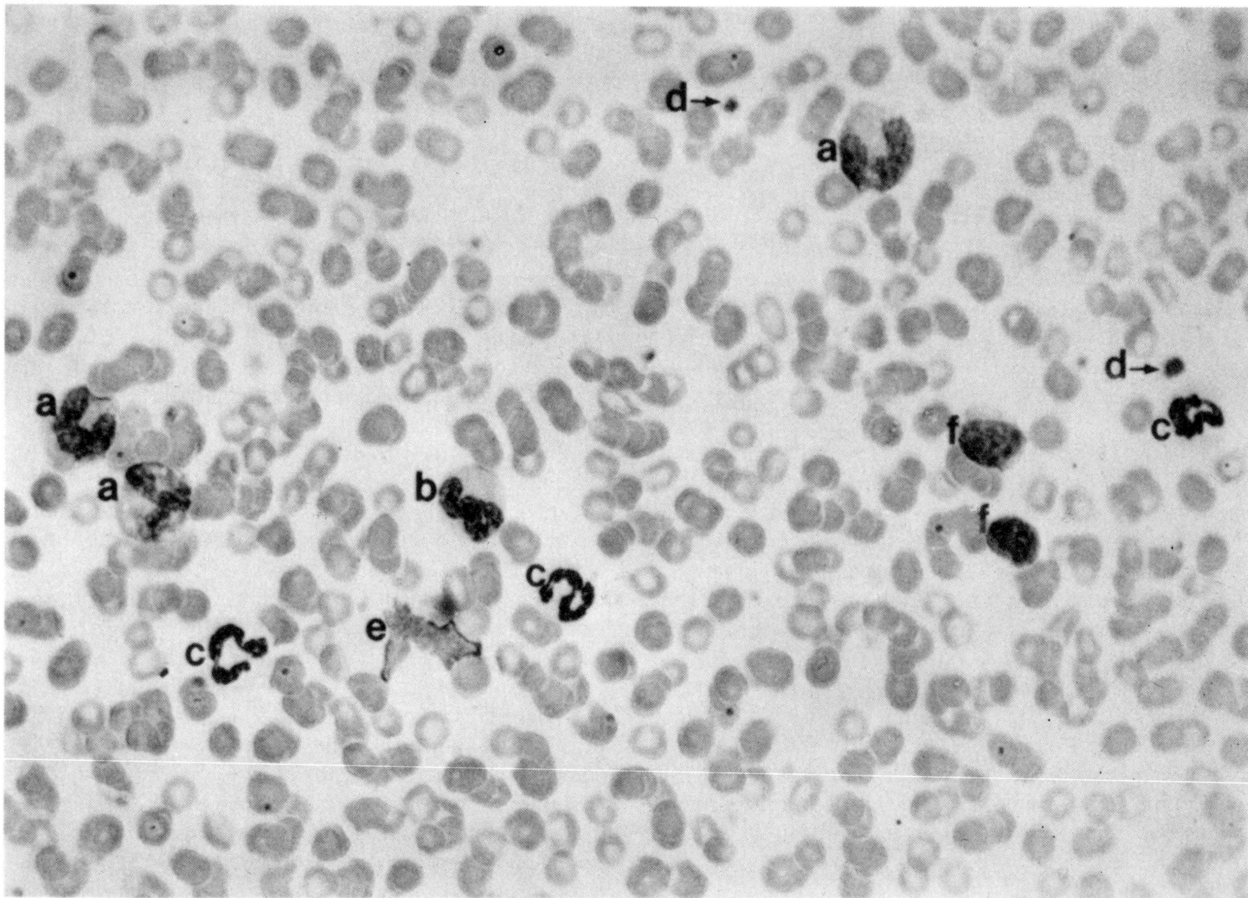

Figure 3.7. Blood smear from a dog (Gram's stain) showing (a) monocyte, (b) immature neutrophil (band cell), (c) neutrophil, (d) platelet, (e) ruptured leukocyte, and (f) lymphocyte. ×1415. (Provided by Dr. Harpal S. Bal, Department of Veterinary Anatomy, College of Veterinary Medicine, Iowa State University, Ames, Iowa.)

function in the bloodstream whereas leukocytes carry on their functions predominantly in the tissues. There are approximately 1300 erythrocytes to every leukocyte in the bloodstream of goats; 1200 to 1 in sheep; 1000 to 1 in horses; 800 to 1 in cattle; 700 to 1 in humans; 600 to 1 in dogs and cats; 400 to 1 in swine; and 100 to 1 in chickens. In anemia the number of erythrocytes may be reduced considerably. In bacterial infections the leukocytes, especially neutrophils, may be increased greatly (leukocytosis). In viral diseases the number of leukocytes, especially neutrophils, may be reduced (leukopenia). Leukopenia is also encountered with bacterial endotoxins, septicemia, and toxemia. In tumors (neoplasms) involving the lymphatic system the number of lymphocytes in the bloodstream may show a marked increase, which changes the usual ratios of erythrocytes to leukocytes.

Leukocytes normally found in the blood are classified as granulocytes and agranulocytes. The granulocytes are characterized by specific granules in their cytoplasm. According to their staining reactions, they are neutrophils, eosinophils, or basophils. The agranulocytes are lymphocytes and monocytes. Figures 3.7 and 3.8 show various white blood cells and platelets among the erythrocytes in a blood smear. Each kind of cell has its own characteristics.

Granulocytes

Neutrophils

Neutrophils are comparatively numerous in the blood of most animals (Table 3.5). They are formed in the bone marrow from extravascular neutrophilic myelocytes (see Table 3.2). They have abundant, finely granular cytoplasm, and the granules stain with neutral dyes. The nucleus of each mature cell is generally divided into lobes or segments connected by filaments; such cells are called *segmented*. Those cells with nuclei that appear as curved or coiled bands, rodlike, or even deeply indented but without segmentation, are known as *band cells*; they are younger or immature forms. Neutrophils show ameboid activity and are active in phagocytosis to defend the body against infection or foreign matter, as they engulf bacteria, viruses, and

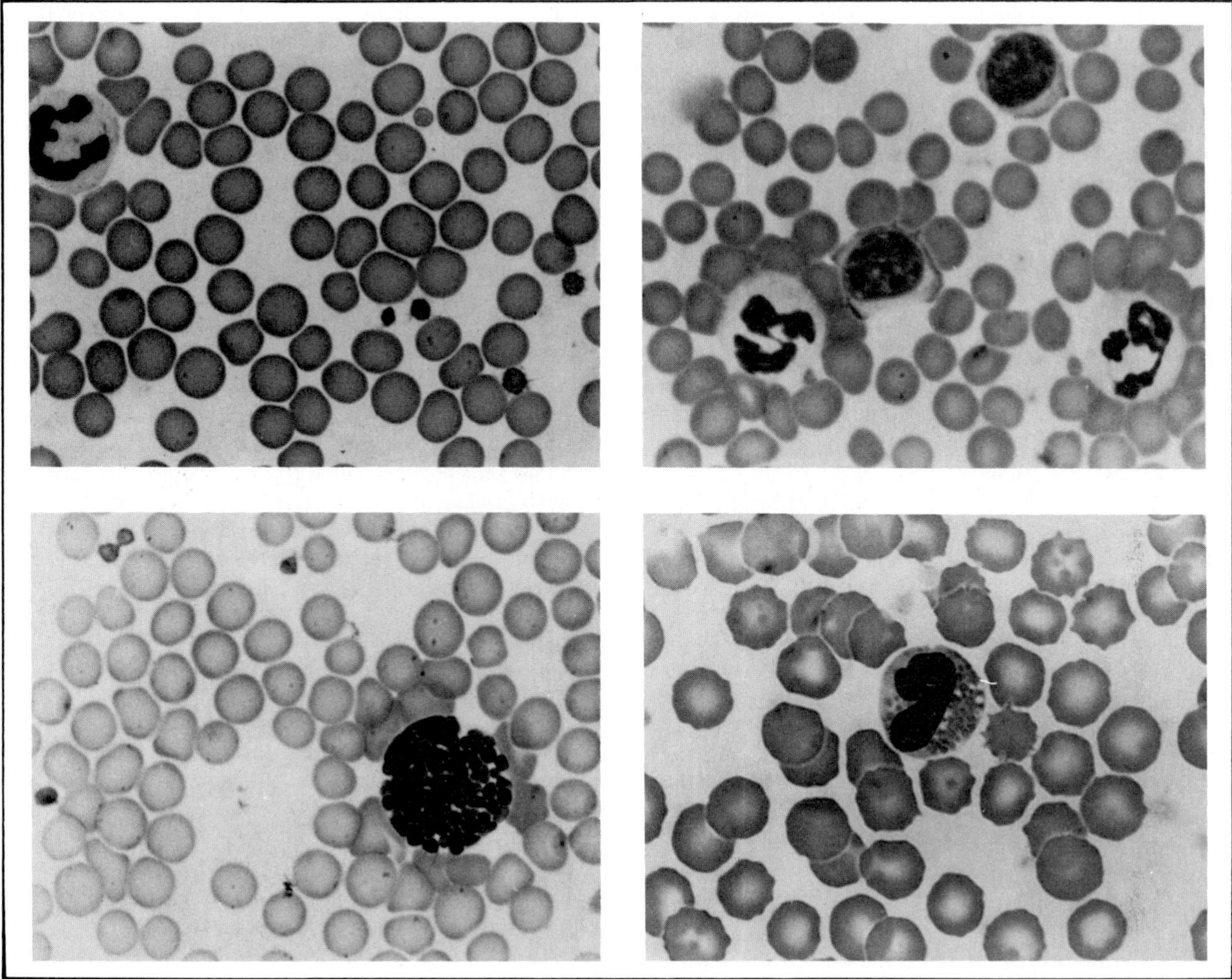

Figure 3.8. Blood smears (Wright's stain) showing erythrocytes, leukocytes, and platelets. (*Upper left*) Five platelets and a band cell (immature neutrophil) from a dog. (*Upper right*) Two large lymphocytes and two neutrophils from a dog. (*Lower left*) One eosinophil and five platelets from a horse. (*Lower right*) One basophil from a dog. ×2300. (Provided by Dr. Harpal S. Bal, Department of Veterinary Anatomy, College of Veterinary Medicine, Iowa State University, Ames, Iowa.)

other small particles. They appear in large numbers at sites of inflammation.

The granules of neutrophils contain lysosomes, which supply enzymes to digest the engulfed material such as bacteria, viruses, and cellular remnants. The lysosomes are antibacterial agents that contain hydrolytic and oxidative enzymes, which attack the bacterial cell wall. The proteolytic enzymes and lipases are especially active on the cell wall. Neutrophils produce hydrogen peroxide; this and the aldehydes are bactericidal.

As bacteria are killed by neutrophils, fewer granules are present in them. A single neutrophil may contain 10 to 20 dead or dying bacteria at the area of inflammation in the tissues. In the process of degranulation of the lysosomes in the neutrophils, enzymes and histamine are released before the death of the neutrophil. In a bacteremia one may observe engulfed bacteria in neutrophils.

Leukocytes may be found in the circulating blood or attached to or passing slowly along the endothelial lining of capillaries and small vessels. The latter comprise a marginal pool of leukocytes, which may account for 50 percent or more of the leukocytes. The total white cell counts given in Table 3.5 usually do not include the marginal cells. Epinephrine (released in response to excitement) will mobilize cells from the marginal pool into the circulation, which accounts for the increase in the total count of white blood cells after epinephrine is given to an animal or when the animal is excited. Exercise acts as a counterforce to margination and distributes the white cells in the circulatory blood.

As trauma, toxins, hemorrhage, ischemia, thermal or radiant injury, or invasion by bacteria, viruses, or parasites occur in tissues, neutrophils are mobilized to these sites by diapedesis and ameboid action. Neutrophils are attracted to these locations by chemotactic compounds from the damaged cells to phagocytize the bacteria and other foreign particles. Inflammation is produced to help fight the infection.

At the onset of infection neutrophils produce pyrogens, which cause the temperature-regulating center in the brain to raise the temperature of the body (fever). A rise in temperature helps the white cells combat an infection and slow the reproduction of bacteria and viruses. In the healthy animal neutrophils are constantly passing from the marginal pool to the tissues to remove antigenic substances, which are potentially harmful to the animal.

In avian blood the cell comparable to the neutrophil is the heterophil. It contains large, rod- or spindle-shaped granules that stain brilliant red to pink with eosin. These granules are acid in reaction, in contrast to the neutral-staining granules of the neutrophil.

Eosinophils

Eosinophils are large cells containing numerous large cytoplasmic granules that stain with acid dyes. They appear in small numbers in the circulating blood (Table 3.5). Their nuclei are less lobulated than those of neutrophils. Eosinophils originate in bone marrow, are very motile, and are slightly phagocytic. They may increase greatly in allergic conditions, anaphylactic shock, and certain parasitisms, such as trichinosis caused by eating uncooked, *Trichina*-infested pork. Eosinophils participate in detoxifying proteins, especially of parasites. They are attracted to the sites of antigen-antibody reactions, and after an animal has been sensitized to an antigen, injection of that antigen will cause eosinophils to appear in large numbers at the injection site, where they may phagocytize antigen-antibody complexes. Eosinopenia follows stress conditions in which the hypothalamic-adenohypophyseal-adrenocortical response occurs or when exogenous adrenocorticotropic hormone (ACTH) is given. ACTH stimulates the production of cortisol from the adrenal cortex, which causes the eosinopenia. The eosinopenia is so consistent that it is used as a means of assaying the potency of adrenocortical hormones and ACTH. Epinephrine also produces an eosinopenia by causing a release of ACTH.

Basophils

Basophils occur in normal blood in very low numbers (Table 3.5) and have water-soluble cytoplasmic granules that stain with alkaline dyes. Phagocytic power is slight or absent. They originate in bone marrow and are closely related to tissue mast cells, which are found around capillaries. Basophils resemble mast cells histologically. In areas of inflammation, both cells produce heparin, histamine, bradykinin, serotonin, and lysosomal enzymes. Basophils and mast cells have receptors for immunoglobulin E (IgE), which is produced in allergic reactions. Thus in hypersensitive reactions the released compounds help initiate and promote the inflammatory changes to combat the invading etiological agent.

Agranulocytes

Lymphocytes

Lymphocytes are relatively numerous in the blood of most species of domestic animals—most numerous in cattle, sheep, goats, swine (6 weeks and older), and chickens (see Table 3.5). They are formed in lymphoid tissue (e.g., lymph nodes, Peyer's patches, spleen, tonsils, and thymus) and are the main constituent of this tissue. The chromatin material of the nucleus of a lymphocyte stains dense and darker than that of monocytes. It has the appearance of being in blocks or aggregates, and this appearance helps in the identification of lymphocytes (Figs. 3.7, 3.8). The nucleus is large and round, and the cell has little cytoplasm. Lymphocytes play a very important role in immunity. They

Table 3.5. Total leukocytes per microliter of blood and percentage of each leukocyte

Species	Total leukocyte count (range)	Percentage of each leukocyte				
		Neutrophil	Lymphocyte	Monocyte	Eosinophil	Basophil
Pig: 1 day	10,000–12,000	70	20	5–6	2–5	<1
1 week	10,000–12,000	50	40	5–6	2–5	<1
2 weeks	10,000–12,000	40	50	5–6	2–5	<1
6 weeks and older	15,000–22,000	30–35	55–60	5–6	2–5	<1
Horse	8000–11,000	50–60	30–40	5–6	2–5	<1
Cow	7000–10,000	25–30	60–65	5	2–5	<1
Sheep	7000–10,000	25–30	60–65	5	2–5	<1
Goat	8000–12,000	35–40	50–55	5	2–5	<1
Dog	9000–13,000	65–70	20–25	5	2–5	<1
Cat	10,000–15,000	55–60	30–35	5	2–5	<1
Chicken	20,000–30,000	25–30	55–60	10	3–8	1–4

produce antibodies, mainly IgG. There are two types; T and B lymphocytes (Fig. 3.9). Lymphocytes are lost in large numbers by migration to the intestinal, uterine, and respiratory mucous membranes. They are actively motile and show ameboid activity, but they are not phagocytic.

There are four types of T lymphocyte: the cytotoxic T cells, helper T cells, suppressor T cells, and the memory T cells. The cytotoxic T cells are also called "killer" cells because they kill foreign invaders by producing H_2O_2 from their lysosomal enzymes (peroxidases, phosphatases, and oxygenases), as the macrophages do. Hydrogen peroxide is lethal to microorganisms. The cytotoxic T cells also attack cells of transplanted organs or other cells foreign to the body. They eliminate antigen-bearing cells that invade the body. Cancer cells are derived from the body's own tissues. They start to generate unique antigens when they become cancerous. The body's immune system recognizes when a cell changes from its normal self to a neoplastic (cancerous) cell that is foreign to the body. Then the cytotoxic T cells attack the cancer cells with their defense mechanism.

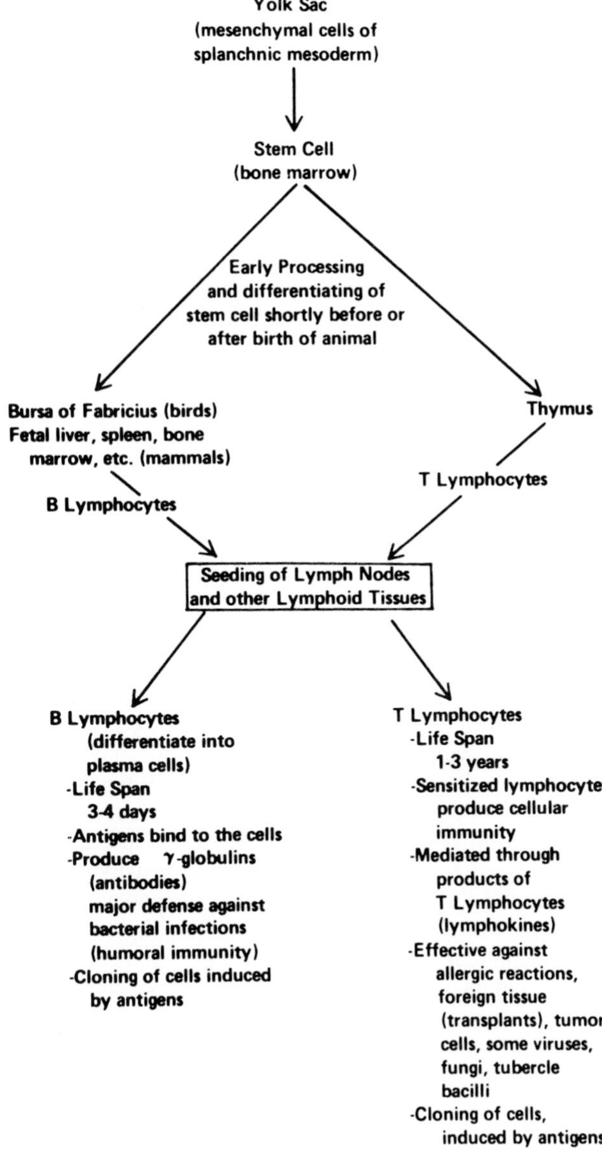

Figure 3.9. Origin, development, and functions of B and T lymphocytes.

Cloning of B and T lymphocytes is a process of responding to many different antigens with specific antibodies that are being produced by specialized cells. It is through this means that animals can build up immunity to various diseases. After each exposure to the same antigen, previous clones are reactivated to produce more antibodies. Thus a greater immunity is produced. The responses by the body may vary with each antigen, some being more antigenic than others.

T lymphocytes play a role in humoral-antibody response as well as in cell-mediated immunity. Although B cells can produce antibodies in the absence of T cells, there is usually cooperation with T cells. Helper T cells are involved in the recognition of antigens and in the stimulation of B lymphocytes to produce antibodies. Helper T cells are not capable of secreting antibodies by themselves. Counterparts of the helper T cells are suppressor T cells. They are called suppressor T cells because they suppress both humoral and cellular-immune responses. They regulate the activity of helper T cells and also regulate the production of antibodies by B cells. Memory T and B cells help in retaining the capacity of T and B cells to respond to the same antigen in producing antibodies when exposed at a later date. Interleukin-2 is produced by helper T cells. It serves as a lymphocytic growth factor and modulates immune responses. It may also promote the production of lymphokines and cytotoxic T cells.

In Fig. 3.9 a flow chart shows the origin, development, and functions of lymphocytes, including their life spans. The T and B lymphocytes have their origin in a common stem cell in the bone marrow. For mammals shortly before or after birth, the site of early processing and differentiation of the stem cells for T lymphocytes is the thymus gland; for B lymphocytes, the sites are the fetal liver, spleen, and bone marrow. The bursa of Fabricius in birds performs a function similar to that the bone marrow in mammals for processing and differentiating B lymphocytes.

The origin of the B lymphocytes is mainly in the lymphocytic follicles around the germinal centers of lymph nodes, spleen, bone marrow, and other places where they are formed. They account for about 15 percent of the circulating lymphocytes in the blood vessels. In contrast, the T lymphocytes are produced in the interfollicular areas of these organs. They account for about 85 percent of the circulating lymphocytes in the bloodstream. As the lymphocytes are produced, they pass to the bloodstream by way of the lymphatics. They stay in the blood a few hours, pass into the tissues by diapedesis, return to the bloodstream via the lymphatics, and recirculate. In this respect, lymphocytes are unique in that granulocytes and monocytes do not recirculate from the tissues.

B lymphocytes are concerned with humoral immunity, and they produce antibodies against extracellular bacteria and viruses. T lymphocytes respond to antigens such as fungi, transplants, neoplastic cells, and intracellular pathogenic organisms. Receptors for the antigens are on the surface of B lymphocytes. As antigen and B cell unite, the cell is activated to form a clone of plasma cells producing antibodies (IgA) that are specific for that antigen for release into the circulating blood. Also, antigens sensitize T lymphocytes to produce cellular immunity. As the T cells come into contact with antigens in the lymphoid tissue, the cells divide and form clones as the B cells do. The T cells also produce lymphokines, which may inhibit or stimulate the movement of macrophages and neutrophils according to the needs of the body.

Adrenocortical steroids (glucocorticoids) under the influence of ACTH cause an increase in antibody concentration in the blood through dissolution of lymphocytes in lymphoid tissue. Thus lymphopenia results from the administration of ACTH or cortisol, as it may occur after prolonged stress.

Interferon is an antiviral compound produced by lymphocytes. As body cells come into contact with a virus, they produce an interferon, which may prevent the virus from reproducing. The viral RNA and DNA replication is inhibited, thus making the virus less effective in the extension and seriousness of the disease. As a virus elicits the lymphocytic response, interferon is produced and circulated throughout the body, protecting other body cells from the virus.

Interferons are glycoproteins of 20,000 to 160,000 molecular weight produced by B cells after viral infections. These are the α and β interferons. T cells, after antigenic stimulation, produce γ interferon. Interferons that have antiviral activity may also inhibit tumor growth. They may regulate cellular and humoral immune responses and macrophage function.

Monocytes

Monocytes originate in cells of the mononuclear phagocytic system (MPS) in the spleen and bone marrow. They occur in normal blood to only a limited extent. They are relatively large, with a single nucleus and a fairly abundant, faintly granular cytoplasm (Fig. 3.7). They are motile and phagocytic. Monocytes have enzyme systems that are designed to engulf tissue debris from chronic inflammatory reactions.

When monocytes leave the blood and are attracted to the tissues by chemotaxis and lymphokines, they become macrophages. Lymphokines are products of lymphocyte activation. When T lymphocytes are stimulated by antigens, they undergo metabolic changes and become activated to produce many factors with various biological activities. Some lymphokines inhibit the migration of macrophages, while others are chemotactic and thus mobilize and activate macrophages. Macrophages are pinocytotic and phagocytic; they kill ingested microbes by their pH, bacteriostatic proteins, and degradative enzymes. Mononuclear phagocytes such as monocytes produce H_2O_2, as cytotoxic T cells do, in even greater quantity than the neutrophils. Hydrogen peroxide is lethal to microorganisms and is produced by these cells to combat various organisms that cause diseases in animals.

Macrophages also kill tumor cells extracellularly by proteases. Macrophages may ingest numerous bacteria (up to 100 or more in each cell) and can increase in diameter two or three times, thus giving the cell a much larger volume for ingesting bacteria, viruses, cellular debris, and even red blood cells.

Differential leukocyte counts

Differential leukocyte counts are made by classifying at least 100 leukocytes, according to their kind, from a single stained blood smear. Normal values are known for each species of animal (Table 3.5). Differential counts are made to determine whether the health of the animal on which the count is being made is normal or abnormal. The values for each kind of leukocyte should be expressed as the number per microliter of blood when differential leukocyte counts are made, rather than on a percentage basis. The percentage is needed with the total leukocyte count to arrive at the number of each kind of cell per microliter of blood. From Table 3.5 one can obtain the actual number of each kind of leukocyte per microliter of blood by multiplying the total count by the known percentage of each cell. If this is not done, one may be misled by relative values and make serious errors in conclusions.

For example, animals given therapeutic antimetabolites (purine and pyrimidine analogues) or chloramphenicol, an antibiotic, may have severe bone marrow depression. In such cases very few granulocytes are in the circulating blood, and there is a marked reduction in the red cells (anemia). If one should rely on the percentage figures of a differential leukocyte count in animals with bone marrow depression, a lymphocytosis and a neutropenia may appear to be present. Cattle poisoned with compounds that cause a bone marrow depression may have 96–98 percent lymphocytes in the differential count. One might conclude that the animal has a marked lymphocytosis and a marked neutropenia. The latter is correct, but the lymphocyte count may be normal (5000–6000/μl in cattle blood). Also, cattle with traumatic reticulitis may have 70 percent neutrophils (mature and immature) and 20 percent lymphocytes. From these data one might erroneously conclude that neutrophilia and lymphopenia are present. Actually, the total leukocyte count may be 25,000; therefore the lymphocyte count is normal, but there are seven times as many neutrophils in the circulating blood as normal, whereas the percentages would show approximately three times as many as normal.

Shift to the left is a term used to describe an increase in the number of immature neutrophils (band cells) in the circulating blood. This status is characteristic of bacterial infections. The body is mobilizing more neutrophils to fight the infection. *Shift to the right* may denote more maturity of the cells, with a greater number of neutrophils showing hypersegmentation or lobulation of the nucleus. It is reported that hypersegmentation of the nuclei of neutrophils may be an inherited anomaly with failure of cytoplasmic division following nuclear division.

Total leukocyte counts

Various factors may contribute to physiological leukocytosis, such as time of day, a meal, exercise, epinephrine (endogenous or exogenous), ether anesthesia, and other stress conditions. Neutrophilia occurs following exercise. As a rule, epinephrine causes an increase in the number of neutrophils in the circulating blood and, in some species, an increase in the number of lymphocytes. With ether anesthesia, animals undergo an excitement period that causes epinephrine release, which contributes to a leukocytosis. Digestive leukocytosis occurs in some animals; with grazing and eating habits rather continuous in some animals, however, it is probably of less importance. Shifts of body water and secretions into the digestive tract during and after meals may provide a partial explanation for this phenomenon.

In the postnatal period marked changes take place in the number of circulating leukocytes. Some species of animals may be born with an increased number, but frequently the counts are comparable with those of adults or even less. In the newborn calf the number is similar to that found in the adult. In the newborn pig (see Table 3.5) the number per microliter of blood is approximately one-half that of adult swine. During this 5- to 6-week period, counts made at weekly intervals may show a transitory rise at 1 to 2 weeks of age. The reported rise is due to an increase in nucleated erythrocytes that are counted as leukocytes. This error is introduced if the mathematical correction for the percentage of nucleated erythrocytes is not made.

As presented earlier, a leukocytosis showing principally a neutrophilia usually signifies a bacterial infection. In viral diseases a neutropenia may be evident. A lymphocytosis is usually present in neoplasms of lymphoid tissue. It is very important to know which leukocyte is increased or decreased before a diagnosis of a disease is made.

Life span

The life span of leukocytes is not so easily measured as that of erythrocytes. The circulating blood transports the leukocytes to sites of action, where they function in an extravascular capacity.

The mean life span of granulocytes, including the time of development in the bone marrow, is approximately 9 days. When granulocytes enter the bloodstream, they are about 6 days old. They spend only a few (6 to 20) hours in the circulating blood. They are constantly leaving the bloodstream by diapedesis to tissues at sites of inflammation, where they may live 2 to 3 days. They also leave the bloodstream by way of the gastrointestinal, urinary, and reproductive tracts and other areas. As they line the membranes of these organs, they help prevent entry of organisms into the body. The number of granulocytes in the circulating blood may decrease because of diminished production or because of their increased passage to tissues by diapedesis. Inflammatory processes hasten the passage of these cells to the site of infection. A decrease in bone marrow myeloid proliferation or impaired release of granulocytes from the marrow may cause a decrease in circulating granulocytes.

Monocytes enter the circulation from the bone marrow. They remain in the circulating blood only 24 hours or less. At this time they enter the tissues, where they become tissue macrophages (e.g., the alveolar macrophages in the lungs and the Küpffer cells of the liver). As tissue macrophages, they may live for many months and even longer, or they may die earlier as a result of combat experience. The mononuclear phagocytic system, previously called the reticuloendothelial system, is a remarkable defense system of the body in conjunction with the neutrophils and other defense mechanisms.

The life span of B lymphocytes is very short, 3 to 4 days on average with some living only a few hours; others, which migrate through the postcapillary venules, enter the lymphatics, and reside in the peripheral lymphatic tissue, may live a week to a month. The T lymphocytes may live 1 to 3 years in the tissues and recirculate many times. One cannot differentiate the two kinds of lymphocytes in a blood smear. Special staining procedures help to identify these cells.

PLATELETS

Platelets (thrombocytes) are small, colorless, round or rod-shaped bodies in the circulating blood of mammals. They average about 3 μm in diameter, but in some cases they are considerably larger. In chickens and other submammalian species they are nucleated cells, usually oval in shape. In the chicken they range from 3 to 5 μm in width and 7 to 10 μm in length and have a round nucleus in the center. Platelets are formed in fetal liver, spleen, and bone marrow. In adult mammals the principal source is bone marrow, where the platelets originate from the megakaryocyte (see Table 3.2). The lung also has been cited as a source of platelets. In birds megakaryocytes are not present, but it is thought that their thrombocytes originate in the bone marrow from large mononucleated cells.

Platelets are extremely numerous in the circulating blood, with considerable species variation. Venous and arterial platelet counts of the same individual also vary. In addition, variations have been found within the arterial or venous systems, depending on the blood vessel from which the sample is taken.

Many domestic mammals have blood platelet counts around 450,000 ± 150,000/μl of blood. The count for chickens usually ranges from 25,000 to 40,000/μl. Draft horses usually have around 300,000 ± 150,000/μl while light horses have approximately one-half this number. Platelets in pigs usually number 350,000 ± 150,000/μl.

There seems to be a variation between young and adult animals in some species. Lambs and calves have more platelets than adult sheep and cows. The young dog has fewer than an adult dog. Infants have fewer platelets than human adults. During the first 48 hours of life the number is considerably less than in adults. Usually at 3 months the infant has the number normally reported for adults. (For specific platelet counts, see Jain 1986.)

The survival time of platelets is relatively short. They survive 8 to 11 days in the circulating blood. The half-life of platelets is 2 to 3 days. The principal role of platelets is to assist in the prevention of hemorrhage when blood vessels are injured (see Chap. 4).

Table 3.6. F_{cells} factors of various animals

Animal	F_{cells} factors	References
Cat		
Normal	0.88–1.06	Farnsworth et al. 1960
After splenectomy	0.76–0.80	Farnsworth et al. 1960
Dog		
Normal	0.89	Clark and Woodley 1959
	1.02	Baker and Remington 1960
After splenectomy	0.84	Baker and Remington 1960
	0.87–0.90	Reeve et al. 1953
	0.88	Rawson et al. 1959
Goat	0.90	O'Brien et al. 1957
Human	0.91	Gray and Frank 1953
Infant	0.87	Chaplin et al. 1953
	0.73–0.95	Mollison et al. 1950
Monkey	0.83	Gregersen et al. 1959
Pig		
At birth	0.72	Talbot and Swenson 1963b
6 weeks	0.71	Talbot and Swenson 1963b
Rabbit	0.89	Zizza and Reeve 1958
Rat	0.74	Wang 1959

SPLEEN

The spleen is the largest lymphoid organ in the animal body. More complex than other lymphoid tissue, it has been compared histologically with a large hemolymph node, as found in ruminants. The spleen is abundantly supplied with blood. The splenic pulp consists primarily of lymphoid cells, but MPS cells line the venous sinuses. Granulocytes and erythrocytes are also present. In the postnatal period the spleen usually produces lymphocytes and monocytes but may produce erythrocytes, granulocytes, and megakaryocytes.

The more common functions of the spleen are as follows:

1. In the fetus the spleen is concerned with red blood cell formation, and in the adult it forms lymphocytes, monocytes, and possibly other cells. The fetal activity of erythropoiesis can be resumed under certain pathologic conditions. The spleen may produce erythropoietin in some species.

2. The spleen is an important reservoir of blood, to be called upon when the body has a greater need for oxygen in the tissues. This may occur during exercise, after hemorrhage, in carbon monoxide poisoning, during the administration of certain anesthetics (chloroform, ether), and in emotional states. When an animal is excited, there is a release of catecholamines such as epinephrine and norepinephrine. Under these conditions there are increased values for erythrocyte counts, PCV, and hemoglobin. The ability of the spleen to contract is reflected in the larger F_{cells} factor. Table 3.6 gives F_{cells} factors for various animals.

The F_{cells} factor provides a correction for the disparity of lower PCV (more blood plasma) in smaller vessels than in larger veins and arteries in order to obtain the overall or body PCV. The blood values for red cell counts, hemoglobin, and PCV obtained after the release of catecholamines may be similar as during hemoconcentration. In birds the spleen is too small to serve as a blood reservoir.

3. The spleen is concerned with the destruction of erythrocytes; it removes aged and abnormal ones from the circulating blood. The numerous MPS cells lining the venous sinuses and in the red pulp are active in this process.

4. The spleen helps the body to resist pathogenic organisms because its T and B lymphocytes produce antibodies and because its MPS cells engulf bacteria, viruses, and foreign particles.

5. The spleen is of importance in the formation of bile pigment, in the storage of iron, and possibly in other phases of metabolism.

Hemal (hemolymph) nodes, found only in ruminants, are similar in structure and probably in function to the spleen. Erythropoiesis usually occurs in these nodes during the fetal period; granulopoiesis is more prevalent in the postnatal period.

SPECIFIC GRAVITY OF BLOOD

The specific gravities (with ranges) of whole blood of several species of domestic animals are as follows: horse, 1.053 (1.046 to 1.059); cattle, 1.052 (1.046 to 1.061); sheep, 1.051 (1.041 to 1.061); goat, 1.042 (1.036 to 1.051); pig, 1.045 (1.035 to 1.055); and dog, 1.045 to 1.052; cat, 1.050 (1.045 to 1.057). The specific gravity of the corpuscles, especially the erythrocytes, is greater than that of the plasma. In cattle and sheep the erythrocytes have a specific gravity of 1.084 (1.079 to 1.090), and the serum has a specific gravity of 1.027 (1.021 to 1.029). The plasma protein concentration is largely responsible for the specific gravity of plasma or serum.

Because of the higher specific gravities of the cellular elements, the corpuscles of a sample of blood in which coagulation has been prevented will tend to settle out. The red blood cells gravitate to the bottom, the white blood cells occupy a thin intermediate zone, and the plasma rises to the top. This is commonly seen when blood containing an anticoagulant is permitted to stand for a period of time. Other factors, such as rouleaux formation of the erythrocytes, also influence the settling of blood cells.

ERYTHROCYTE SEDIMENTATION RATE

The erythrocyte sedimentation rate (ESR) is a test performed on blood to help determine the health status of an animal. An anticoagulant such as heparin or EDTA is used to keep the cell volume constant. ESR varies greatly among different species of animals (Table 3.7). It also increases with certain diseases. Microcirculatory changes that occur in disease are often manifested by "sludged blood" (partial or complete stasis of blood in capillaries).

It is not known specifically whether sludged blood and an increased ESR are directly related, but an increased ESR is frequently found when microcirculatory changes such as sludged blood are present in morbid animals.

It is difficult to explain the marked variation of ESR among some species of animals. Erythrocytes of horse blood settle quickly, whereas those of ruminants settle very slowly. The ESR is measured in standard tubes by the distance in millimeters through which the uppermost layers of erythrocytes pass in a certain length of time.

Frequently a rapid ESR may be observed in newborn pigs; when not present at birth, it usually develops quickly if the pigs are not provided with adequate iron. The rapid ESR develops simultaneously with the anemia; but an intramuscular injection of iron (iron-dextran) will usually correct the rapid ESR before the anemia is corrected.

The ESR is usually determined in standard tubes placed in a vertical position. Tubes held at a 45-degree angle will produce the maximum sedimentation rate of erythrocytes. This is advantageous when the ESR is needed quickly or the rate is slow. It is helpful with ruminant blood.

Changes in the viscosity of the plasma, the specific gravities of the corpuscles or plasma, or the size of the erythrocytes have practically nothing to do with the sedimentation rate. The only factor of importance is the degree of agglutination of erythrocytes (size of sedimenting particles or rouleaux formation), and it is certain that the plasma proteins markedly influence this factor. According to some workers, it is an increase in the fibrinogen content of the plasma that hastens agglutination and settling, whereas others believe it is an increase in the globulin.

Horse erythrocytes will sediment rapidly, even in ox and sheep plasma, and ox and sheep erythrocytes will sediment slowly in horse plasma. These findings indicate that the plasma is not the only factor that determines the rapid ESR of horses.

Changes in the ESR are nonspecific reactions and do not indicate a pathological condition. The ESR is not pathognomonic for the diagnosis of a specific disease; it merely helps in the evaluation of the health status of the animal. At times a rapid ESR may be present and yet one is unable to make a diagnosis or observe symptoms of a disease. A rapid ESR may occur with normal hemoglobin and PCV values.

Usually the rate is increased in acute general infections, in the presence of malignant tumors, in inflammatory conditions, in hypothyroidism, and also in pregnancy.

Table 3.7. Erythrocyte sedimentation rates (vertical tubes)

Species	mm	Time	PCV	References
Cat	53	1 h	27	Didisheim et al. 1959
	15.4 (7–27)	1 h	37.3 (34.5–41.0)	Schalm et al. 1975
	22.7 (0.5–51)	1 h	38.7 (30–48.5)	Swenson 1966
Cattle	2.4	7 h		Ferguson 1937
Chicken	0.5 (0–1)	30 min	30.6 (29.8–31.6)	Swenson 1951
	1.5 (1–3)	1 h		
	6.7 (3–10)	3 h		
	14.4 (10–18)	6 h		
Dog	1–5	30 min		Coffin 1953
	6–10	1 h		
Horse	2–12	10 min		Coffin 1953
	15–38	20 min		
Pig	0–6	30 min		Coffin 1953
	1–14	60 min		

COMPOSITION OF BLOOD PLASMA

Plasma, which forms 55 to 70 percent of the blood, may be obtained from blood in which coagulation has been prevented. Chemical and physical analyses reveal that the composition of blood plasma, serum, and whole blood is extremely complex. This is to be expected because blood has so many functions. Table 3.8 provides blood data from domestic animals, which the student may use while studying each physiologic element or compound. Species differences are present. Also, age and activity of the animal are important factors that may alter these blood values.

Plasma proteins

The plasma proteins have been identified as albumin, α_1-, α_2-, β_1-, β_2-, and γ-, globulins, and fibrinogen. The γ-globulins produced by lymphocytes and plasma cells contain antibodies commonly called immunoglobulins. The immunoglobulins are classified as IgM, IgG, IgA, IgD, and IgE. IgG is the most abundant immunoglobulin of normal animals. It is present in the blood and is found in the tissues. It also crosses the placental barrier. IgE is produced by animals with various allergies. It causes the release of histamine from the basophils and mast cells. IgA is a glycoprotein found in external secretions such as saliva, tears, and colostrum. It is present in blood plasma and does not cross the placental barrier but collects in the colostrum for use by newborn animals. It is effective against microorganisms present in the mouth and gastrointestinal tract. IgM is the naturally occurring antibody against red blood cells in certain incompatible blood types. This is why blood

Table 3.8. Ranges of some chemical constituents of blood from mature domestic animals

Constituents	Unit of measurement	Source	Horse	Cow	Sheep	Goat	Pig	Dog	Cat	Chicken
Glucose	mg/dl	P, S, WB	60–110	40–80 80–120 (calf)	40–80 80–120 (lamb)	40–75 80–120 (kid)	80–120	70–120	70–120	130–270
Nonprotein nitrogen	mg/dl	P, S, WB	20–40	20–40	20–38	30–44	20–45	17–38		20–35
Urea nitrogen (BUN)	mg/dl	P, S, WB	10–24	10–30	8–20	10–28	8–24	10–30	10–30	0.4–1.0
Uric acid	mg/dl	WB	0.5–1	0.1–2	0.1–2	0.3–1	0.1–2	0.1–1.5	0.2–2.5	1–2 1–7 (laying hen)
Creatinine	mg/dl	P, S, WB	1–2	1–2	1–2	1–2	1–2.5	1–2	0.8–2	1–2
Amino acid nitrogen	mg/dl	WB	5–7	4–8	5–8		6–8	7–8		4–10
Lactic acid	mg/dl	WB	10–16	5–20	9–12			8–20		47–56 20–98 (laying hen)
Cholesterol	mg/dl	P, S, WB	75–150	80–180	60–150	80–160	60–200	120–250	80–180	125–200
Bilirubin										
Direct	mg/dl	P, S, WB	0–0.4	0–0.3	0–0.3		0–0.3	0.06–0.1	0.05–0.1	
Indirect	mg/dl	P, S, WB	0.2–5	0.1–0.5	0–0.1		0–0.3	0.01–0.5	0.15–0.3	
Total	mg/dl	P, S, WB	0.2–6	0.2–1.5	0.1–0.4		0–0.6	0.1–0.6	0.2–0.6	
Sodium	mEq/L	P, S	132–152	132–152	139–152	142–155	135–150	141–155	142–158	151–161
Potassium	mEq/L	P, S	2.5–5.0	3.9–5.8	3.9–5.4	3.5–6.7	4.4–6.7	3.7–5.8	3.4–5.4	4.6–4.7
Calcium	mEq/L	P, S	4.5–6.5	4.5–6.0	4.5–6.0	4.5–6.0	4.5–6.5	4.5–6.0	4.5–6.0	4.5–6.0 8.5–19.5 (laying hen)
Phosphorus	mEq/L	P, S	2–6	2–7	2–7	2–6	3–6	2–6	4–7	3–6
Magnesium	mEq/L	P, S	1.5–2.5	1.5–2.5	1.8–2.3	2–3	2–3	1.5–2.0	1.6–2.5	
Chlorine	mEq/L	P, S	99–109	97–111	95–105	99–110	94–106	100–115	117–123	119–130

P, plasma; S, serum; WB, whole blood.

Data compiled from previous editions of *Dukes' Physiology of Domestic Animals*; Clinical Pathology Laboratory, College of Veterinary Medicine, Iowa State University, Ames, Iowa; Department of Clinical Pathology, School of Veterinary Medicine, University of California, Davis, California; Schalm, Jain, and Carroll 1975, *Veterinary Hematology,* 3d ed., Lea & Febiger, Philadelphia; and from unpublished data of author.

has to be typed or cross-matched to assure that red cells will not agglutinate in blood transfusions between donor and recipient. IgD is related in some way to the recognition of B lymphocytes to some antigens and the inducement of these B cells to proliferate and form clones.

In humans, sheep, goats, and dogs, albumin predominates over the globulins; in horses, pigs, cows, and cats the relative proportions of albumin and globulins are nearly equal (Table 3.9).

In most newborn animals (except rodents and primates) plasma γ-globulin is either lacking or present in minute amounts since the placenta is impermeable to these protein molecules. The fetus is not capable of synthesizing them. To counteract this deficiency, large quantities of γ-globulin are concentrated in the dam's colostrum. When the newborn ingests colostrum, the γ-globulin easily crosses the intestinal barrier and provides passive immunity in the form of antibodies.

The serum of laying hens contains 5.40 ± 0.71 g of protein per deciliter. Serum of cockerels and nonlaying hens contains somewhat less (3.6 g/dl) and that of chicks still less. Simultaneous with the increase in plasma proteins in the laying hen is a marked increase in serum calcium. The nonlaying chicken has 4.5 to 6 mEq of calcium per liter of serum (9 to 12 mg/dl), while the laying hen has 8.5 to 19.5 mEq/L. The increase is attributed to the rise in estrogens from the follicles of the active ovary.

Origin

Plasma albumin, fibrinogen, some of the globulins, and prothrombin are formed in the liver. The balance of the globulins, including γ-globulins, are formed in the lymph nodes and in other MPS of the spleen and bone marrow.

Plasma protein synthesis is markedly reduced in severe

Table 3.9. Proteins of blood plasma (g/dl)

Animal	Albumin	Globulin	Fibrinogen	Total
Horse	2.8–3.8	2.8–3.8	0.2–0.4	6.0–8.0
Cow	3.0–3.8	3.6–4.4	0.2–0.5	7.0–8.5
Sheep	3.5–4.5	2.5–3.5	0.2–0.4	6.0–8.0
Goat	3.7–4.5	2.4–3.2	0.2–0.5	6.5–7.5
Pig	3.2–4.0	3.4–4.0	0.2–0.4	6.5–8.5
Dog	3.4–4.4	2.2–3.2	0.1–0.4	6.0–7.8
Cat	3.0–3.8	2.5–3.5	0.1–0.4	6.0–7.5
Chicken	1.6–2.0	2.3–3.3		4.0–5.2
Human	4.0–5.8	1.5–3.3	0.20–0.39	6.2–7.9

Data from Altman and Dittmer 1961, *Blood and Other Body Fluids,* Fed. Am. Soc. Exp. Biol., Washington; Department of Clinical Pathology, School of Veterinary Medicine, University of California, Davis, California; Clinical Pathology Laboratory, College of Veterinary Medicine, Iowa State University, Ames, Iowa; and Sturkle 1976, *Avian Physiology,* 3d ed., Springer-Verlag, New York.

liver damage or prolonged dietary protein deficiency. This can reduce the plasma fibrinogen, resulting in increased prothrombin time and prolonged blood coagulation time (see Chap. 4 and below). The prothrombin time is a liver function test. The normal plasma prothrombin time of most domestic animals, determined by the one-stage method of Quick, varies between 9 and 12 seconds; for cattle, sheep, and chickens it ranges between 20 and 25 seconds.

The prothrombin time of newborn pups is prolonged during the first 48 hours of life, that of newborn lambs during the first 72 hours, and that of calves during the first week. Low values of fibrinogen are found during this time. Adult values are reached after 1 day in the dog and 3 days in the lamb.

The time it takes blood to coagulate varies among and within species. The capillary tube method requires less blood and is used most frequently. The normal blood coagulation times of most animals, as determined with the capillary tube method, are between 1 and 5 minutes; with cows and horses, however, the coagulation times may be 10 to 12 minutes. With the method of Lee and White when a larger quantity of blood is used (1 to 5 ml), the coagulation times are 2 to 5 minutes longer than with the capillary tube method.

Functions

The plasma proteins, amino acids, and tissue proteins are in a state of equilibrium. When the amino acid concentration in tissue cells decreases below that in plasma, amino acids enter the cells and are used for synthesis of essential plasma and tissue proteins. The plasma proteins, formed chiefly by hepatic cells, may also be broken down into amino acids by MPS cells and made available for the formation of cellular proteins, especially when the amino acid supply from the digestive processes is not adequate.

The plasma proteins help to maintain the colloid osmotic pressure of blood. The colloid osmotic pressure, not to be confused with the crystalloid osmotic pressure of blood, amounts to 25 to 30 mm Hg (see Chap. 32). The proteins are colloidal and nondiffusible. The osmotic pressure produced by them opposes the hydrostatic blood pressure in the capillaries and thus prevents excess passage of fluid into the tissues, which might cause edema. The water-holding capacity of the blood depends on the concentration of plasma proteins. A hypoproteinemia usually leads to edema. The albumins account for nearly 80 percent of the colloid osmotic pressure of the plasma because of their abundance and smaller molecular weight. The osmotic pressure that each protein fraction contributes is inversely related to the molecular weight and directly related to its concentration in terms of the number of particles in the plasma. The molecular weights of fibrinogen, albumin, and globulins are approximately 300,000, 70,000, and 180,000, respectively. Since the concentration of fibrinogen is low, the osmotic pressure exerted by this protein is likewise low. When the concentrations of α-globulin and albumin are nearly the same, the albumin will contribute two to three times as much osmotic pressure as globulins.

Other functions of plasma proteins are (1) to help maintain normal blood pressure by contributing to the viscosity of the blood; (2) to influence the suspension stability of the erythrocytes; (3) to help regulate the acid-base balance of the blood; (4) to affect the solubility of carbohydrates, lipids, and other substances held in solution in the plasma; and (5) to transport substances bound by plasma proteins, such as nutrients (calcium, phosphorus, iron, copper, lipids, fat-soluble vitamins, amino acids), hormones (thyroxine, steroids), cholesterol, bilirubin, heme, enzymes, and many others. Foreign substances such as T-1824 dye (used in measuring blood volume) and various therapeutic agents (sulfonamides, streptomycin, barbiturates, digitoxin) are united with the plasma proteins in the circulating blood.

REACTION OF BLOOD

The term *reaction of blood* usually refers to the pH of blood plasma in the intact animal. The balance of all cations against all anions is reflected in the hydrogen ion concentration. The negative logarithm of the hydrogen ion concentration is pH. For accurate measurements of pH, blood must be examined under conditions that prevent loss of its gases, particularly carbon dioxide. The reaction under these conditions is on the alkaline side of neutrality. The average reaction is about pH 7.4. The pH fluctuates only within narrow limits. The mean blood pH values and ranges for several species are given in Table 3.10. Arterial blood is slightly more alkaline than venous blood because of the greater abundance of carbon dioxide in the venous blood. The plasma is more alkaline than the corpuscles. The limits of pH range of blood compatible with life are approximately 7.0 and 7.8.

A large amount of acid or alkali may be added to blood, in vitro or in vivo, without any considerable change in reaction. Some of the acids that are added to the blood in vivo as a result of normal metabolism are carbonic, lactic, pyruvic, phosphoric, sulfuric, and uric acids. Blood can maintain a constant reaction, even with this acid metabolism, primarily because of its buffer systems and secondarily because of its respiratory and renal mechanisms in

Table 3.10. Mean blood pH values and ranges for several species

Animal	Blood sample	Mean blood pH (range)
Cattle	Arterial	7.38 (7.27–7.49)
Sheep	Venous	7.44 (7.32–7.54)
Horse	Venous	N.A. (7.20–7.55)
Dog	Arterial	7.36 (7.31–7.42)
Cat	Mixed	7.35 (7.24–7.40)
Chicken	Venous	7.54 (7.45–7.63)
Human	Arterial	7.39 (7.33–7.45)

eliminating carbon dioxide, ammonia, and hydrogen ions (see Chap. 3 and 31).

In maintenance of the normal acid-base balance, and thus the alkali reserve, of the body it is essential that adequate electrolytes be ingested by the animal. The pH of the urine is affected by the constituents of the ration. Meat products that contain chlorides, phosphates, and sulfates contribute to an acid urine in both ruminants and nonruminants. High-protein diets typical of carnivores and some omnivores usually produce an acid urine. Citrus fruits and plant products containing abundant sodium and potassium make the body more alkaline and produce an alkaline urine. Sodium and potassium salts of strong bases and weak acids exist in citrus fruits. The anions of organic acids are metabolized, leaving the sodium and potassium for use by the body.

Frequently the pH of the urine in a sick animal may have to be changed. For example, normal cow urine is usually alkaline, while urine from a cow with ketosis is usually acid in reaction. Various salts can be used to change the reaction of urine. Salts of a strong base and a weak acid (sodium propionate, lactate, or acetate) will have an alkaline effect on the body and produce an alkaline urine. The sodium is retained by the body if needed and the organic anions are metabolized into carbon dioxide and water. Salts of a weak base and a strong acid (e.g., ammonium chloride) will produce an acid urine.

BLOOD VOLUME

The blood volume of an animal is an important consideration in the understanding and interpretation of PCV, hemoglobin, red cell counts, plasma protein concentration, and other hematologic values. These values are altered when blood volume changes; they can even be misleading if hemoconcentration or hemodilution occurs. The status of blood volume in an animal is especially important when a blood transfusion is being considered, in the diagnosis of anemia, or in the differentiation of various kinds of anemia. Changes in the volumes of red cells and blood plasma in the circulating blood will alter the PCV when increases or decreases in red cells and plasma are not proportional.

It is impossible to determine the volume of blood in the body merely by bleeding an animal to death. A considerable amount of blood is left in the vessels, even after the animal dies of hemorrhage. Clotting and vasoconstrictor mechanisms retain a large amount of blood in the vessels. Attempts to wash out the blood retained in the vessels after bleeding have been made in the past, but the animal must be killed. Blood volume data obtained in this manner are not accurate and precise. In analytical work, accuracy refers to closeness to actual value, while precision concerns the repeatability of values obtained from a specific sample. Thus, one can have precision without accuracy.

Methods based on dilution procedures have greater accuracy and precision and can be repeated on the same conscious animal.

There are numerous indirect methods of estimating blood volume in the living animal. With these, one may determine the plasma volume by injecting into the blood a foreign substance such as Evans blue dye (T-1824) or radioactive iodine, which combines with plasma proteins. Then one calculates the dilution that the foreign substance has undergone in the plasma over a period of time by using the formula

$$\frac{\text{Amount injected}}{\text{Concentration per milliliter of plasma}}$$

The erythrocyte volume may be determined in a similar manner by injection of radioactive phosphorus (^{32}P), iron (^{59}Fe), or chromium (^{51}Cr), which combines with erythrocytes, or by injection of red cells previously labeled with ^{32}P, ^{59}Fe, ^{51}Cr either in vitro or in a donor animal, followed by measurement of the dilution the tagged erythrocytes have undergone with time. After the plasma and red cell volumes are obtained, the blood volume can be calculated from the formula

$$\text{Plasma volume} \times \frac{100}{100 - \text{PCV}}$$

or

$$\text{Red cell volume} \times \frac{100}{\text{PCV}}$$

Blood is not homogenous. To calculate blood volumes accurately, therefore, one must determine plasma volume and red cell volume and then use correction factors for true PCV and body PCV according to the following formulas:

$$\text{Blood volume} = \text{Plasma volume} \times \frac{100}{100 - (\text{Venous PCV})(\text{correction factor for true PCV and body PCV})}$$

$$\text{Red cell volume} = \text{Plasma volume} \times \frac{(\text{Venous PCV})(\text{correction factor for true PCV and body PCV})}{100 - (\text{Venous PCV})(\text{correction factor for true PCV and body PCV})}$$

$$\text{Plasma volume} = \text{Red cell volume} \times \frac{100 - (\text{Venous PCV})(\text{correction factor for true PCV and body PCV})}{(\text{Venous PCV})(\text{correction factor for true PCV and body PCV})}$$

In calculating blood volume, one multiplies the correction factor for true PCV by that for body PCV to obtain the appropriate correction factor to be multiplied by the venous PCV. For example, when the correction factor for trapped plasma in arriving at the true PCV is 0.96 and the F_{cells} factor in arriving at the body PCV is 0.90, one obtains the overall correction factor (0.864) by multiplying 0.96 by 0.90.

The *true PCV* of venous blood is the venous PCV minus the trapped plasma. It is impossible to centrifuge blood so that no plasma remains in the packed cells. In blood volume determinations, therefore, a correction must be made. The amount of plasma left in the packed cells varies with the time and force of centrifugation. PCV values obtained with a microhematocrit centrifuge usually contain less trapped plasma than those obtained with larger quantities of blood centrifuged for 30 minutes at 3000 rpm. A great variation is obtained among blood samples from anemic animals, normal animals, and animals that have hemoconcentration. As a rule, the smaller PCV values contain less trapped plasma on a percentage basis. Microhematocrit PCV values ranging from 13 to 20 percent contain 1.5 to 2.5 percent trapped plasma in the packed cells; values of 40 to 45 percent contain 4.5 to 5.5 percent; and those of 60 to 65 percent contain 7 to 8 percent.

An additional factor that regulates the amount of trapped plasma in the PCV is the size of the erythrocytes. As a rule, the larger mean corpuscular volumes of erythrocytes have less trapped plasma in the PCV than the smaller cells. For example, the correction factors reported for trapped plasma in the PCV of elephants, humans, dogs, sheep, and goats were 0.96, 0.99, 0.97, 0.96, and 0.91, respectively, as

Table 3.11. Reportd blood volumes (ml/kg body weight)

Animal	Plasma volume	Red cell volume	Total blood volume	References
Cat	47.7 (34–56)			Gregersen and Stewart 1939
	46.5 (34.3–65.8)			Conley 1941
	46.8		66.7	Spink et al. 1966
Cattle				
Beef			57	Hansard et al. 1953
Dairy	38.8 (36.3–40.6)		57.4 (52.4–60.6)	Reynolds 1953
	36.6		62	Dale et al. 1957
Chicken	55		83	Pappenheimer et al. 1939
Male		21		Rodnan et al. 1957
Female		10		Rodnan et al. 1957
2–5 wk	65.6		95.5	Hegsted et al. 1951
1 wk	87		120	Medway and Kare 1959
32 wk	46		65	Medway and Kare 1959
Dog	(42–58)	38–43	83–101	Ranges from 17 references cited by Altman and Dittmer 1961
	52.8	34.1		Baker and Remington 1960
	48.3	26.4		Baker 1963
	41.6			Baker 1963
			81	Clark and Woodley 1959
	51.4	43	94.4	Parkinson and Dougherty 1959
	50.2	33.5		Deavers et al. 1960
	54		79	Courtice 1943
Goat	53		70	Courtice 1943
	55.9	14.7	70.6	Klement et al. 1955
Horse	51		72	Courtice 1943
Draft	43.2	28.5	71.7	Julian et al. 1956
	43.5	18.2	61.4	Marcilese et al. 1964
Thoroughbred	61.9	47.1	109.6	Julian et al. 1956
	63.3	39.8	103.1	Marcilese et al. 1964
Saddle	52.5	25.3	77.5	Marcilese et al. 1964
Pig				
0–2 mo	48–81	13–33	74–100	Ranges from 8 references cited by Swenson 1975
2–12 ml	35–59	21–27	52–69	
1–3 yr			35–46	
Sheep			58	Schambye 1952
			57	Hansard et al. 1953
	61.9			MacFarlane et al. 1959
	44.6			Hodgetts 1961
	46.7	19.7	66.4	Hodgetts 1961

determined by the microhematocrit method. The mean corpuscular volumes for these same animals were 112, 91, 72, 37, and 18 μm^3. As a rule, the smaller the cell, the greater the amount of trapped plasma, a fact that may be explained by the greater amount of erythrocyte surface area per equal volume of packed cells. To arrive at the true PCV from the venous PCV, one must multiply the venous PCV by a correction factor such as 0.96, assuming 4 percent trapped plasma.

The overall cell volume percentage or body PVC is the true PCV multiplied by the F_{cells} factor (obtained by dividing the body PCV by the venous PCV). The F_{cells} factor is used to correct the venous PCV and is based on a discrepancy between the true blood volume as actually measured and the total blood volume calculated from the venous PCV. The venous PCV gives a higher value than actually exists as an overall or body PCV because most blood samples are taken from large veins and arteries, which have higher PCV readings than samples from capillaries, arterioles, and other minute vessels. The ratio of the endothelial surface area to the blood volume in small blood vessels is considerably larger than in large arteries and veins. When blood circulates, plasma passes near the endothelial lining more rapidly than erythrocytes do, granting that there may be "no slip" or passage of plasma in intimate contact with the endothelium. As a result, erythrocytes are more to the center of the blood vessels and plasma more to the periphery; this hastens circulation. Thus, in the process of blood flow, capillaries and other small vessels with a greater ratio of endothelial lining to blood volume will have more plasma at the periphery and a lower PCV reading. The F_{cells} factor corrects this disparity.

Considerable variation exists in the F_{cells} factor among species of animals (see Table 3.6). The F_{cells} factor is influenced by the spleen, as shown by the fact that it is stable in cats and dogs after splenectomy. The spleen does not function as a large blood reservoir in humans; however, the F_{cells} factor is rather constant when it is compared in persons whose spleens are intact with those who have undergone splenectomy.

It is generally thought that the venous circulation contains approximately 50 percent of the blood volume and that the capillaries contain 5 percent. While an animal rests, only 10 percent of the capillaries may be patent in skeletal muscle. The volumes of the capillary beds in various tissues and organs are subject to change, depending on the needs of the cells for oxygen and nutrients. The status of the animal with regard to age, size, activity, health, excitement, and quantity of hemoglobin may affect the F_{cells} factor. Considerable variation in blood volume values can be expected as a result of the methods used, species variation, and variations within species, such as age, nutrition, health of the animal, degree of physical activity, lactation, sex, and environmental factors such as temperature and altitude. Larger blood volumes are present in light-weight horses (hot-blooded) than in draft horses (cold-blooded) (Table 3.11). Animals that are more excitable and active usually have greater blood volumes.

The plasma, erythrocyte, and total blood volumes vary greatly with age in swine. The plasma volume of newborn pigs is 53 to 55 ml per kilogram body weight and increases to 81 after nursing. There is a progressive decrease in these percentage values as pigs and other animals grow and become fat. The percentage of total body water is similarly decreased as the body fat increases.

REFERENCES

Albert, S.N. 1964. Blood volume. *Scintillator* 8:1–6.

Altman, P.L., and Dittmer, D.S. 1961. *Blood and Other Body Fluids*. Fed. Am. Soc. Exp. Biol., Washington.

Altura, B.M. 1980. Reticuloendothelial cells and host defense. In B.M. Altura, E. Davis, and H. Harders, eds., *Advances in Microcirculation*. Vol. 9, *Vascular Endothelium and Basement Membranes*. S. Karger, Basel. Pp. 252–94.

Baker, C.H. 1963. Cr^{51} labeled red cell, I^{131}-fibrinogen, and T-1824 dilution spaces. *Am. J. Physiol.* 204:176–80.

Baker, C.H., and Remington, J.W. 1960. Role of the spleen in determining total body hematocrit. *Am. J. Physiol.* 198:906–10.

Bauer, C., and Kurtz, A. 1989. Oxygen sensing in the kidney and its relation to erythropoietin production. *Annu. Rev. Physiol.* 51:845–46.

Brown, B.A. 1984. *Hematology: Principles and Procedures*. 4th ed. Lea & Febiger, Philadelphia.

Burwell, E.L., Brickley, B.A., and Finch, C.A. 1953. Erythrocyte life span in small animals. *Am. J. Physiol.* 172:718–24.

Bush, J.A., Berlin, N.I., Jensen, W.N., Brill, A.B., Cartwright, G.E., and Wintrobe, M.M. 1955. Erythrocyte life span in growing swine-determined by glycine-2-C^{14}. *J. Exp. Med.* 101:451–59.

Bush, J.A., Jensen, W.N., Athens, J.W., Ashenbrucker, H., Cartwright, G.E., and Wintrobe, M.M. 1956. Studies on copper metabolism. XIX. The kinetics of iron metabolism and erythrocyte life span in copper-deficient swine. *J. Exp. Med.* 103:701–12.

Carlson, R.H., Swenson, M.J., Ward, G.M., and Booth, N.H. 1961. Effects of intramuscular injections of iron-dextran in newborn lambs and calves. *J. Am. Vet. Med. Ass.* 139:457–61.

Chaplin, H., Jr., Mollison, P.L., and Vetter, H. 1953. The body-venous hematocrit ratio: Its constancy over a wide hematocrit range. *J. Clin. Invest.* 32:1309–16.

Clark, C.H., and Woodley, C.H. 1959. A comparison of blood volumes as measured by rose bengal, T-1824 (Evans blue), radio-chromium-tagged erythrocytes, and a combination of the latter two. *Am. J. Vet. Res.* 20:1067–68.

Coffin, D.L. 1953. *Manual of Veterinary Clinical Pathology*. 3d ed. Cornell Univ. Press, Ithaca, N.Y.

Conley, C.L. 1941. The effect of ether anesthesia on the plasma volume of cats. *Am. J. Physiol.* 32:796–800.

Cormack, D.C. 1987. *Ham's Histology*. 9th ed., J.B. Lippincott, Philadelphia.

Courtice, F.C. 1943. The blood volume of normal animals. *J. Physiol.* 102:290–305.

Dale, H.E., Brody, S., and Burge, G.J. 1957. The effect of environmental temperature on blood volume and the antipyrine space in dairy cattle. *Am. J. Vet. Res.* 18:97–100.

Davson, H. 1958. Cellular aspects of the electrolytes and water in body fluids. In G.E.W. Wolstenholme and M. O'Connor, eds., *Water and Electrolyte Metabolism in Relation to Age and Sex*. Ciba Foundation Colloquia on Ageing, vol. 4. Churchill, London. Pp. 15–35.

Deavers, S., Smith, E.L., and Huggins, R.A. 1960. Control circulatory values of morphine-pentobarbitalized dogs. *Am. J. Physiol.* 199:797–99.

Didisheim, P., Hattori, K., and Lewis, J.H. 1959. Hematologic and coagulation studies in various animal species. *J. Lab. Clin. Med.* 53:866–75.

Dixon, E. 1990. Monensin-induced cation movements in bovine erythrocytes. *Life Sci.* 47:37–50.

Drastisch, L. 1928. Ist die Konzentration des Blutfarbstoffes im Blutkörperchen bei allen Tieren Konstant? *Arch. f. g. ges. Physiol.* 219:227–32.

Evans, J.V. 1954. Electrolyte concentrations in red blood cells of British breeds of sheep. *Nature* 174:931–32.

Evans, J.V., and Phillipson, A.T. 1957. Electrolyte concentrations in the erythrocytes of the goat and ox. *J. Physiol.* 139:87–96.

Fåhraeus, R. 1929. The suspension stability of the blood. *Physiol. Rev.* 9:241–74.

Farnsworth, P.N., Paulino-Gonzalez, C.M., and Gregersen, M.I. 1960. F_{cells} values in the normal and splenectomized cat: Relation of F_{cells} to body size. *Proc. Soc. Exp. Biol. Med.* 104:729–33.

Fegler, G. 1948. Haemoglobin concentration, hematocrit value, and sedimentation rate of horse blood. *Q. J. Exp. Physiol.* 35:129–39.

Ferguson, L.C. 1937. Studies on bovine blood. I. The sedimentation rate and percentage volume of erythrocytes in normal blood. *J. Am. Vet. Med. Assoc.* 91:163–75.

Field, J.B., Spero, L., and Link, K.P. 1951. Prothrombin and fibrinogen deficiency in new-born pups and lambs. *Am. J. Physiol.* 165:188–94.

Frandson, R.D. 1986. *Anatomy and Physiology of Farm Animals.* 4th ed. Lea & Febiger, Philadelphia.

Fudenberg, H., Baldini, H., Mahoney, J.P., and Dameshek, W. 1961. The body hematocrit/venous hematocrit ratio and the splenic reservoir. *Blood* 17:71–82.

Gasson, J.C. 1991. Molecular physiology of granulocyte-macrophage colony-stimulating factor. *Blood* 77:1131–45.

Gray, S.J., and Frank, H. 1953. The simultaneous determination of red cell mass and plasma volume in man with radioactive sodium chromate and chromic chloride. *J. Clin. Invest.* 32:1000–1004.

Gregersen, M.I., Sear, H., Rawson, R.A., Chien, S., and Saiger, G.I. 1959. Cell volume, plasma volume, total blood volume, and F_{cells} factor in the Rhesus monkey. *Am. J. Physiol.* 196:184–87.

Gregersen, M.I., and Stewart, J.D. 1939. Simultaneous determination of the plasma volume with T-1824, and the available fluid volume with sodium thiocyanate. *Am. J. Physiol.* 125:142–52.

Grimes, R.M., Duncan, C.W., and Lassiter, C.A. 1958. Bovine fetal hemoglobin. I. Postnatal persistence and relation to adult hemoglobins. *J. Dairy Sci.* 41:1527–33.

Guyton, A.C. 1986. *Textbook of Medical Physiology.* 7th ed. W.B. Saunders, Philadelphia.

Hansard, S.L., Butler, W.O., Comar, C.L., and Hobbs, C.S. 1953. Blood volume of farm animals. *J. Anim. Sci.* 12:402–13.

Hansard, S.L., and Kincaid, E. 1956. Red cell life span of farm animals. *J. Anim. Sci.* 15:1300.

Hawkins, W.B., and Whipple, G.H. 1938. The life cycle of the red blood cell in the dog. *Am. J. Physiol.* 122:418–27.

Hegsted, D.M., Wilson, D., Milner, J.P., and Ginna, P.H. 1951. Blood and plasma volume and thiocyanate space of normal chicks. *Proc. Soc. Exp. Biol. Med.* 78:114–15.

Heller, V.G., and Paul, H. 1934. Changes in cell volume produced by varying concentrations of different anticoagulants. *J. Lab. Clin. Med.* 19:777–80.

Hevesy, G., and Ottesen, J. 1945. Life-cycle of the red corpuscles of the hen. *Nature* 156:534.

Hodgetts, V.E. 1961. The dynamic red cell storage function of the spleen in sheep. III. Relationship to determination of blood volume, total red cell volume, and plasma volume. *Aust. J. Exp. Biol.* 39:187–96.

Jain, N.C. 1986. *Schalm's Veterinary Hematology.* 4th ed. Lea & Febiger, Philadelphia.

Jensen, W.N., Bush, J.A., Ashenbrucker, H., Cartwright, G.E., and Wintrobe, M.M. 1956. The kinetics of iron metabolism in normal growing swine. *J. Exp. Med.* 103:145–59.

Jones, W.G., Hughes, C.D., Swenson, M.J., and Underbjerg, G.K.L. 1956. Plasma prothrombin time and hematocrit values of blood of dairy cattle. *Proc. Soc. Exp. Biol. Med.* 91:14–18.

Julian, L.M., Lawrence, J.H., Berlin, N.I., and Hyde, G.M. 1956. Blood volume, body water, and body fat of the horse. *J. Appl. Physiol.* 8:651–53.

Kaneko, J.J., and Cornelius, C.E. 1970. *Clinical Biochemistry of Domestic Animals.* 2d ed. Vols. 1, 2. Academic Press, New York.

Kerr, S.E. 1937. Studies on the inorganic composition of blood. IV. The relationship of potassium to the acid-soluble phosphorus fractions. *J. Biol. Chem.* 117:227–35.

Klement, A.W., Jr., Ayer, D.E., and Rogers, E.B. 1955. Simultaneous use of Cr^{51} and T-1824 dye in blood volume studies in the goat. *Am. J. Physiol.* 181:15–18.

Krantz, S.B. 1991. Erythropoietin. *Blood* 77:419–34.

MacFarlane, W.V., Morris, R.J.H., Howard, B., and Budtz-Olsen, O.E. 1959. Extracellular fluid distribution in tropical Merino sheep. *Aust. J. Agric. Res.* 10:269–86.

Macleod, J., and Ponder, E. 1946. An observation on the red cell content of the blood of the Thoroughbred horse. *Science* 103:73–75.

Mann, F.D., Shonyo, E.S., and Mann, F.C. 1951. Effect of removal of the liver on blood coagulation. *Am. J. Physiol.* 164:111–16.

Marcilese, N.A., Valsecchi, R.M., Figueiras, H.D., Camberos, H.R., and Varela, J.E. 1964. Normal blood volumes in the horse. *Am. J. Physiol.* 207:223–27.

McCance, R.A., and Widdowson, E.M. 1959. The effect of colostrum on the composition and volume of the plasma of newborn piglets. *J. Physiol.* 145:547–50.

Medway, W., and Kare, M.R. 1959. Blood and plasma volume, hematocrit, blood specific gravity, and serum protein electrophoresis of the chicken. *Poult. Sci.* 38:624–31.

Mollison, P.L., Veall, N., and Cutbush, M. 1950. Red cell and plasma volume in newborn infants. *Arch. Dis. Childhood* 25:242–53.

O'Brien, W.A., Howie, D.L., and Crosby, W.H. 1957. Blood volume studies in wounded animals. *J. Appl. Physiol.* 11:110-14.

Pappenheimer, A.M., Goettsch, M., and Jungherr, E. 1939. *Nutritional Encephalomalacia in Chicks and Certain Related Disorders of Domestic Birds.* Conn. Ag. Exp. Sta. Bull. 229. Storrs.

Parkinson, J.E., and Dougherty, J.H. 1958. Effect of internal emitters on red cell plasma volumes of beagle dogs. *Proc. Soc. Exp. Biol. Med.* 97:722–25.

Perk, K., Frei, Y.F., and Herz, A. 1964. Osmotic fragility of red blood cells of young and mature domestic and laboratory animals. *Am. J. Vet. Res.* 25:1241–48.

Porter, K.R., and Bonneville, M.A. 1964. *An Introduction to Fine Structure of Cells and Tissues.* Lea & Febiger, Philadelphia.

Rawson, R.A., Chien, S., Peng, M.T., and Dellenback, R.J. 1959. Determination of residual blood volume required for survival in rapidly hemorrhaged splenectomized dogs. *Am. J. Physiol.* 196:179–83.

Reece, W.O. 1991. *Physiology of Domestic Animals.* Lea & Febiger, Philadelphia.

Reece, W.O., and Wahlstrom, J.D. 1970. Effect of feeding and excitement on the packed cell volume of dogs. *Lab. Anim. Care* 20:1114–17.

Reeve, E.B., Gregersen, M.I., Allen, T.H., Sear, H., and Walcott, W.W. 1953. Effects of alteration in blood volume and venous hematocrit in splenectomized dogs on estimates of total blood volume with P^{32} and T-1824. *Am. J. Physiol.* 175:204–10.

Reynolds, M. 1953. Plasma and blood volume in the cow using the T-1824 hematocrit method. *Am. J. Physiol.* 173:421–27.

Rodnan, G.P., Ebaugh, E.G., Jr., and Fox, M.R.S. 1957. Red cell turnover rate in the mammal, bird, and reptile. *Blood* 12:355–66.

Rowsell, H.C., Downie, H.G., and Mustard, J.F. 1960. Comparison of the effect of egg yolk or butter on the development of atherosclerosis in swine. *Can. Med. Assoc. J.* 83:1175–86.

Rowsell, H.C., and Mustard, J.F. 1963. Blood coagulation in some common laboratory animals. *Lab. Anim. Care* 13:752–62.

Schalm, O.W., Jain, N.C., and Carroll, E.J. 1975. *Veterinary Hematology*. 3d ed. Lea & Febiger, Philadelphia.
Schambye, A.P. 1952. Det cirkulerende Blodvolumen hos får bestemt med P^{32}-maerkede Erytrocyter og T-1824. *Nord. Veterinaermed.* 4:929–61.
Spink, R.R., Malvin, R.L., and Cohen, B.J. 1966. Determination of erythrocyte half life and blood volume in cats. *Am. J. Vet. Res.* 27:1041–43.
Swenson, M.J. 1951. Effect of a vitamin B_{12} concentrate and liver meal on the hematology of chicks fed on all-plant protein ration. *Am. J. Vet. Res.* 12:147–51.
Swenson, M.J. 1966. Erythrocyte sedimentation rates of cats. Unpublished data.
Swenson, M.J. 1975. Composition of body fluids. In H.W. Dunne and A.D. Leman, eds., *Diseases of Swine*, 4th ed. Iowa State Univ. Press, Ames. Pp. 95–124.
Swenson, M.J., Goetsch, D.D., and Underbjerg, G.K.L. 1955. The effect of the sow's ration on the hematology of the newborn pig. *Proc. Book*. Am. Vet. Med. Assoc., 92d Ann. Mtg., Minneapolis. Pp. 159–62.
Swenson, M.J., Goetsch, D.D., and Underbjerg, G.K.L. 1962. Effects of dietary trace minerals, excess calcium, and various roughages on the hemogram, tissues, and estrous cycles of Hereford heifers. *Am. J. Vet. Res.* 23:803–8.
Swenson, M.J., Underbjerg, G.K.L., Bartley, E.E., and Jones, W.G. 1957. Effects of trace minerals, aureomycin, and other supplements on certain hematologic values and organ weights of dairy calves. *J. Dairy Sci.* 40:1525–33.
Swenson, M.J., Underbjerg, G.K.L., Goetsch, D.D., and Aubel, C.E. 1958. Blood values and growth of newborn pigs following subcutaneous implantation of bacitracin pellets. *Am. J. Vet. Res.* 19:554–59.
Talbot, R.B., and Swenson, M.J. 1963a. Survival of Cr^{51} labeled erythrocytes in swine. *Proc. Soc. Exp. Biol. Med.* 112:573–76.
Talbot, R.G., and Swenson, M.J. 1963b. Plasma volume, erythrocyte volume, total blood volume, and F_{cells} factor in the suckling pig. *Fed. Proc.* 22 (pt. I):682.
Tosteson, D.C. 1963. Active transport, genetics, and cellular evolution. *Fed. Proc.* 22 (pt. I):19–26.
Wang, L. 1959. Plasma volume, cell volume, total blood volume, and F_{cells} factor in the normal and splenectomized Sherman rat. *Am. J. Physiol.* 196:188–92.
White, P. 1972. Degradation of hemoglobin. In W.J. Williams, E. Beutler, A.J. Ersley, and R.W. Rundles, eds, *Hematology*. McGraw-Hill, New York.
Wintrobe, M.M. 1933. Variations in the size and hemoglobin content of erythrocytes in the blood of various vertebrates. *Folia Haematol.* 51:32–49.
Wintrobe, M.M. 1961. *Clinical Hematology,* 5th Ed. Lea & Febiger, Philadelphia.
Zizza, F., and Reeve, E.B. 1958. Erroneous measurement of plasma volume in the rabbit by T-1824. *Am. J. Physiol.* 194:522–26.

CHAPTER 4

Blood Coagulation and Hemostasis

by Patricia A. Gentry and Harry G. Downie

Blood coagulation, the system for preventing blood loss from a damaged vessel, is a major component of the mammalian homeostatic mechanism. Not only does blood coagulation function in conjunction with cellular and fibrinolytic processes to maintain vascular integrity, but some components of the coagulation mechanism also contribute to the inflammatory and immunological systems.

Hemostasis involves a complex system of interrelated processes (Fig. 4.1). The hemostatic process includes (1) contraction of the blood vessel wall and adhesion of platelets to the damaged subendothelium; (2) the primary hemostatic process, which consists of the formation of platelet aggregates and the activation of the coagulation mechanism; (3) the secondary hemostatic process, which encompasses the consolidation of the platelet aggregates with the formation of thrombin and an insoluble fibrin mesh or clot; (4) regeneration of the damaged endothelium, reduction in size of the platelet-fibrin complex, and initiation of the fibrinolytic process; and (5) degradation of the platelet-fibrin complex and removal of the protein and cellular debris from the circulation, once endothelial repair is complete.

The appropriate balance of blood clot formation and clot dissolution is maintained by the intricate balance of molecular reactions involving endothelial cells, blood platelets, and adhesive, procoagulant, and fibrinolytic proteins. In addition, the hemostatic process is elegantly controlled by a counterbalance of activation and inhibitory mechanisms.

Most of the plasma proteins, or factors, involved in the coagulation system were first identified in human patients who were congenitally deficient in a specific protein. A standard nomenclature has been devised for these proteins. The major components of the coagulation and fibrinolytic systems are listed in Table 4.1, along with the role of each component.

VASCULAR ENDOTHELIUM

The integrity of the endothelium is essential for the normal functioning of blood vessels and also for the maintenance of a nonthrombogenic state, which ensures that as blood circulates neither the blood platelets nor the procoagulant proteins are activated. Part of this thromboresistance is due to several properties of the normal vasculature. These include (1) the negative charge on the endothelial cell surface, which can repel the negatively charged platelets; (2) the ability of the metabolically active endothelial cells to synthesize inhibitors of both platelet function (e.g., prostacyclin) and fibrin formation (e.g., thrombomodulin); and (3) generation of activators of fibrin degradation (e.g., tissue plasminogen activator [t-PA]).

Whenever the integrity of the vascular endothelium is compromised, the endothelial cells can contribute actively to the processes of platelet aggregation, coagulation, and fibrinolysis. The subendothelium, which is exposed after vascular damage, contains collagen (types III and IV), a potent platelet activator. Also present in the subendothelial

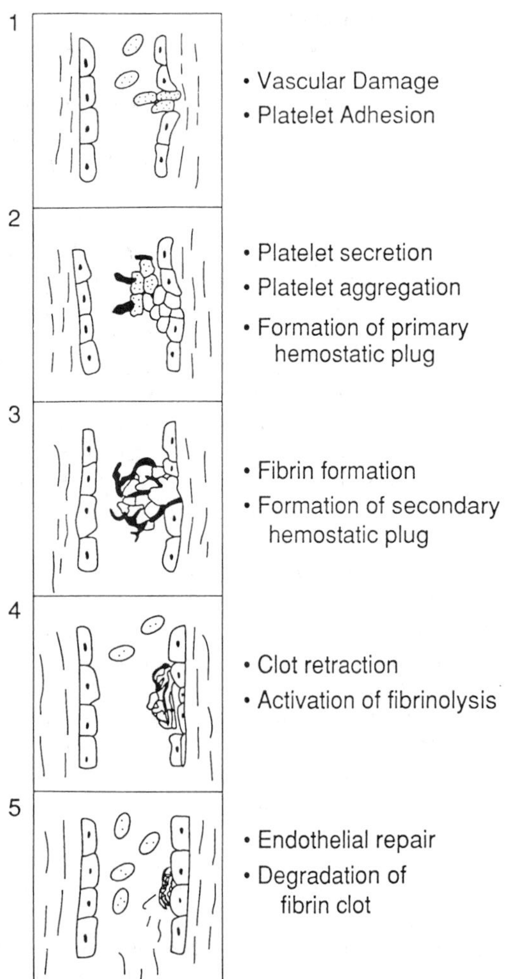

Figure 4.1. A schematic diagram representing the formation and dissolution of a blood clot, or thrombus, around the site of vascular injury. Panel *1* represents the initial adhesion of blood platelets to a site of vascular damage; *2* represents the formation of a platelet aggregate; *3* represents the formation of the insoluble fibrin network resulting in the impermeable blood clot; *4* represents the resolution of the blood clot by the processes of clot retraction and fibrinolysis; *5* represents the final degradation of the fibrin clot and the repair of vascular endothelium.

layer are proteins such as von Willebrand factor (vWF) and fibronectin, which have adhesive properties that can serve to enhance the formation of platelet aggregates.

PLATELET FUNCTION

Blood platelets are highly reactive cellular components that are equally as important as the coagulation proteins in the hemostatic process.

Platelet structure

Mammalian platelets are nonnucleated disk-shaped structures, 2 to 4 μm in diameter (Fig. 4.2). The major source of blood platelets is the megakaryocyte of the bone marrow. As the megakaryocyte matures, pseudopods form and, as the extremities bud off, platelets are released.

There is a close correlation between several of the characteristic ultrastructural features and the functional activity of the platelet. The circumferential band of microtubules, which can be observed just under the cell wall in the nonstimulated cell, is essential for maintenance of the discoid shape as platelets circulate and is also involved in the shape change and contractility that the platelets undergo on activation. Two morphologically distinguishable types of storage granules—the alpha granules and the dense granules—are apparent in the platelet cytoplasm. Alpha granules are protein-storage sites that contain (1) platelet-specific proteins, such as β-thromboglobulin and platelet factor 4; (2) coagulation factors, such as fibrinogen, factor V, and von Willebrand factor (vWF); and (3) other proteins, including albumin, fibronectin, and platelet-derived growth factor (PDGF). The dense granules are the storage sites for calcium, serotonin and adenine nucleotides, such as adenosine triphosphate (ATP) and adenosine diphosphate (ADP). The release of the contents of both the alpha granules and the dense granules is an energy-dependent process that requires ionized calcium. The energy is supplied by the platelet mitochondria and glycogen granules, whereas calcium is made available by the dense tubular system, a component of the membranous system of the platelet. The platelets of most mammalian species also exhibit a characteristic open canalicular system (OCS) that generally is closely associated with the outer membrane and serves as a conduit for the extrusion of the granular contents. The porcine platelet illustrated in Fig. 4.2 is typical of this type of platelet. In contrast, in the bovine platelet, the OCS appears to be poorly developed and is frequently not visible in intact cells (Fig. 4.2).

Platelet adhesion

Platelets may be activated by any contact with a "foreign surface," such as damaged endothelium or an atherosclerotic plaque on the vessel wall, or by a variety of agonists released from damaged cells, such as ADP, platelet-activating factor (PAF), thromboxane A_2 (TXA_2), and serotonin. Irrespective of the stimulus to activation, platelet adhesion (the attachment of platelets to surfaces) and change in platelet shape are the initial physiological responses. Any pathophysiological vascular injury that causes the exposure of subendothelial tissue will result in the adhesion of a monolayer of single platelets to the endothelial surface. The platelets lose their discoid shape and form pseudopods. The pseudopods allow the platelets to spread over the surface and facilitate interplatelet contact between unstimulated platelets flowing past the site of damage and those already adhering to the subendothelium. The adhesion of platelets to the subendothelium requires the cofactors, vWF and fibronectin, which may initially be supplied from endothelial cells but can also be released

Table 4.1. Proteins involved in coagulation and fibrinolysis

Factor	Synonym	Molecular weight	Site of synthesis	Biological activity	Pathway*
Fibrinogen	Factor I	320–340	Liver	Substrate	I E
Prothrombin	Factor II	68–72	Liver	Serine protease	I E
Tissue factor	Thromboplastin, factor III	43–46	Tissues	Activator	E
Factor V	Proaccelerin	290–350	Platelets	Cofactor	I E
Factor VII	Proconvertin	45–53	Liver	Serine protease	E
Factor VIII	Factor VIII:C, antihemophilic factor	265–300	Vascular endothelium	Cofactor	I
Factor IX	Christmas factor	55–60	Liver	Serine protease	I
Factor X	Stuart factor	54–56	Liver	Serine protease	I E
Factor XI	Plasma thromboplastin antecedent	140–175	Liver	Serine protease	I
Factor XII	Hageman factor	80–90	Liver	Serine protease	I F
Factor XIII	Fibrin stabilizing factor	310–320	Liver	Transaminase	I E
von Willebrand factor	VWF	800–2000	Megakaryocytes, endothelial cells	Platelet adhesion	I E
Prekallikrein	Fletcher factor	85–100	Liver	Serine protease	I
High-molecular-weight kininogen	HMWK	110–120	Liver	Cofactor	I F
Fibronectin	Cold-insoluble globulin	440–550	Liver	Platelet adhesion	I E
Tissue plasminogen activator	t-PA	68–70	Tissues	Activator	F
Urokinase	—	32–55	Tissues	Serine protease	F
Plasminogen	—	83–88	Liver	Serine protease	F

*I represents the intrinsic pathway, E the extrinsic pathway, and F the fibrinolytic pathway.

from the activated platelets as the coagulation process develops. Adhesion of platelets and subsequent aggregation (the attachment of platelets to each other) also require the unmasking of fibrinogen receptors on the platelet membrane as the platelets are activated in the presence of fibrinogen. Multiple bonds are formed between the protein molecules and the platelets, resulting in the formation of the *primary hemostatic plug*.

Platelet release reaction

The formation of large irreversible platelet aggregates and the formation of an insoluble fibrin network require the secretion of the contents of the platelet granules. The secretion of proteins from the alpha granules provides high, localized concentrations of fibrinogen, fibronectin, factor V, and vWF at the platelet surface. This release reaction is mediated by ADP and calcium secreted from the dense granules along with arachidonic acid metabolites formed by the platelets in response to stimulation. The granular secretions can occur by two morphologically distinct mechanisms. In platelets with a well-developed OCS, stimulation causes the granules to migrate centrally. The granules fuse with the channels of the OCS, and the granular contents are extruded through the channel pores on the platelet surface. After stimulation of platelets with a poorly developed OCS, the granules move to the periphery of the cell where they fuse with the platelet membrane, and the granular contents are extruded directly into the surrounding medium.

Mechanisms of platelet activation

The platelet, like all reactive cells, is activated by the binding of an agonist to a specific receptor on the cell surface with the formation of an activated agonist-receptor complex, which then initiates the transmission of a signal through the membrane with the subsequent activation of intracellular messengers that, in turn, initiate the biological response. There appear to be at least three intracellular mechanisms by which the platelet response may be modulated. A common pathway, shared by the platelet responses to most agonists, is the increase in the cytoplasmic concentration of ionized calcium, which is an essential prerequisite for irreversible platelet aggregation (Fig. 4.3).

One of the major pathways of platelet stimulation is the liberation of arachidonic acid (AA) from membrane phospholipids, either by the direct action of phospholipase A_2 or by the indirect action of phospholipase C. The released AA is subsequently metabolized by the cyclooxygenase enzyme system to endoperoxides and TXA_2. TXA_2 has ionophoric activity that enables it to facilitate the transport of calcium across intracellular membranes and thus redistribute calcium from dense granule stores to the cell cytoplasm. In some mammalian platelets (e.g., rabbit and human platelets), TXA_2 can also function as a potent platelet agonist that accelerates the formation of platelet aggregates around the primary site of platelet adhesion. For these species, the TXA_2 pathway is generally considered to be of major importance. However, there are other species, (e.g., bovine and elephant) in which platelet aggregation appears to proceed normally even in the presence of drugs, such as aspirin, that inhibit the cyclooxygenase enzyme system and prevent the formation of TXA_2, indicating that other biochemical pathways are also important.

One alternative pathway involves the formation of PAF (1-O-alkyl-2-O-acetyl glyceryl phosphoryl choline) from membrane phospholipids. PAF may, in turn, modulate calcium mobilization by the phosphatidyl inositol-diacylglycerol second messenger system.

As with other cells in which calcium mobilization plays a key role, the adenylate cyclase–cyclic AMP (cAMP) system has an important regulatory function in the platelet.

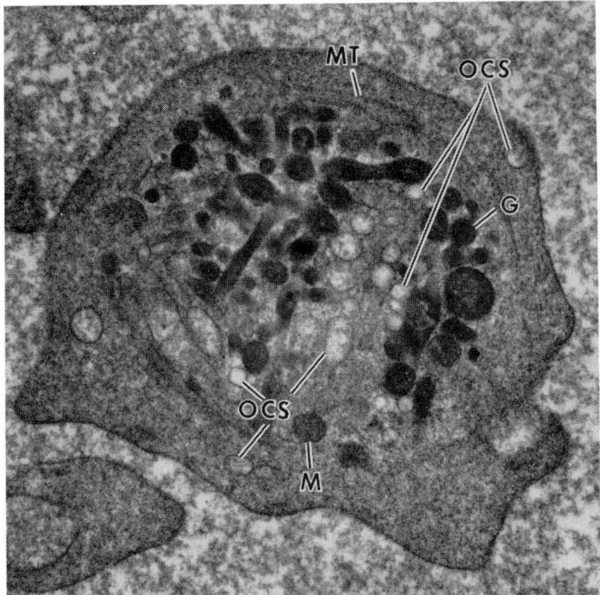

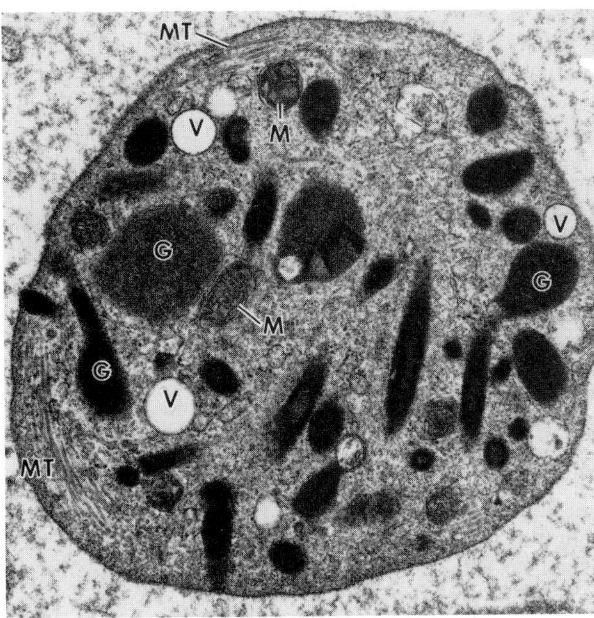

Figure 4.2. Electron micrographs of porcine (*upper plate*) and bovine (*lower plate*) platelets. The electron micrographs illustrate bands of microtubules (MT), mitochondria (M), the open canalicular system (OCS), vacuoles (V), and granules of various configurations and size (G). Note the extensive OCS system in the porcine platelet, which is absent in the bovine platelet. Note also the difference in the distribution of granules in the platelet cytoplasm. The granules are centrally located in the porcine platelet, whereas those of the bovine platelet are randomly distributed. Vacuoles are present in the bovine platelet but absent in the porcine cell. ×10,200. (Courtesy P.K. Basrur, University of Guelph.)

Platelet agonists, such as ADP, can bind to a regulatory portion of the membrane adenylate cyclase complex and cause a reduction of intracellular cAMP levels which, in turn, facilitates calcium mobilization. In contrast, inhibitory agents such as prostacyclin, which can be generated from AA in the damaged vascular endothelium, cause an elevation of intracellular cAMP levels as a result of forming a complex with the membrane adenylate cyclase receptor. In this way prostacyclin acts as an inhibitor of platelet aggregation by inhibiting calcium mobilization.

Platelet aggregation

The mobilization of calcium and the extrusion of the platelet granular contents lead to the growth and consolidation of the primary hemostatic plug. After the release reaction has occurred, the platelets begin to lose their individual integrity and the subsequent fusion of lipoprotein membranes, and the concomitant exposure of specific membrane receptors for coagulation proteins provides a highly reactive surface for the molecular reactions involved in thrombin and fibrin formation. Thrombin, formed in the penultimate stage of the blood coagulation pathway, is a potent agonist of platelet stimulation and granule release, and it serves as a positive effector of additional platelet aggregation at the site of vascular damage (Fig. 4.3). The platelet plug is stabilized by the formation of insoluble fibrin, first around the periphery of the platelet aggregates and then throughout the platelet plug. With the formation of the *secondary hemostatic plug* or thrombus, blood loss through the damaged endothelial surface is completely stopped and the tissue repair processes can proceed, mediated in part by such components as PDGF released from the platelet alpha granules.

THE COAGULATION MECHANISM

The biochemical mechanism of blood clot formation involves a regulated sequence of protein-protein interactions along with the molecular assembly of enzyme-cofactor-substrate complexes. These reactions are designed to confer maximum efficiency and speed to the molecular reactions, which culminate in the formation of macromolecular complexes of fibrin around the platelet aggregates associated with damaged endothelial tissue. The majority of proteins that participate in the hemostatic process circulate in plasma as inactive proenzymes, and each undergoes sequential activation as coagulation proceeds (Fig. 4.4).

It is convenient to consider the sequence of enzymatic reactions that produce the fibrin clot in several steps: (1) the surface or contact activation phase, (2) the activation of factor X, (3) the formation of thrombin, and (4) the formation of insoluble fibrin.

There are two closely related mechanisms that, when stimulated, can generate fibrin (Fig. 4.4). The *intrinsic mechanism* is the sequence of enzymatic reactions that are

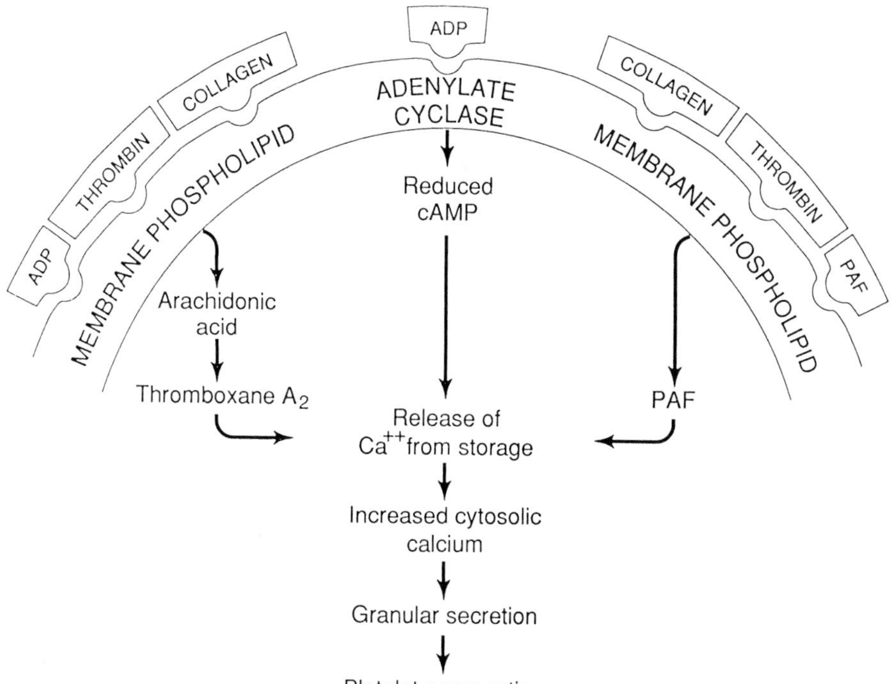

Figure 4.3. A diagrammatic representation of the major biochemical pathways of platelet activation. Agonists interact with receptors on the platelet membrane and initiate a biochemical messenger, which in turn initiates calcium release from storage pools, secretion of granular contents, and platelet aggregation. PAF, platelet activating factor.

initiated when blood comes into contact with a "foreign surface." Any surface, other than the intact endothelial lining of the blood vessel wall, can activate the coagulation process. The *extrinsic mechanism* is the sequence of reactions that occur when the damage to a blood vessel is sufficiently traumatic to involve not only the vascular wall but also the surrounding tissues. Until recently, it was considered that these two mechanisms were independent pathways that converged into a final common pathway with the activation of factor X. It is now recognized that these two pathways are interrelated by a number of enzymatic reactions that function to enhance fibrin formation (Fig. 4.4).

Contact-activation phase

The so-called contact system involves four proteins: factor XII, prekallikrein, factor XI, and high-molecular-weight kininogen (HMWK). Factors XI and XII are proenzymes, while prekallikrein is the precursor of plasma kallikrein. Both factor XI and prekallikrein circulate in plasma bound to HMWK, a glycoprotein that serves both as a cofactor in the coagulation mechanism and as a precursor of bradykinin in the inflammatory response (Fig. 4.5).

The sequence of reactions involved in thrombin generation is sometimes referred to as a "waterfall" or "cascade," since a small stimulus can rapidly result in a disproportionately large response. Factor XII, the first protein in the sequence of reactions, can be activated either by contact with a negatively charged surface or by enzymatic cleavage by a protease. A wide range of insoluble particles, such as glass, celite, and kaolin, will activate factor XII, as will a variety of biological components, including fatty acids, sodium urate crystals, and endotoxin. The physiological activator is thought to be subendothelial vascular basement membrane.

When plasma factor XII binds to a negatively charged surface, the protein undergoes autoactivation to the active serine protease form, factor XIIa. The formation of a small amount of factor XIIa is sufficient to initiate the activation of its substrates, prekallikrein, factor XI, and HMWK (Fig. 4.5). Once kallikrein and activated HMWK (HMWKa) are formed, the molecular interactions accelerate both the rate of additional factor XIIa formation and the extent of factor XIa formation. The HMWKa serves as a cofactor for formation of both factors XIIa and XIa by binding to the negatively charged surface alongside factor XIIa and by enhancing the local surface binding of prekallikrein and factor XI. The HMWKa, in effect, provides an anchor for factor XIIa and its substrates and thus increases the local concentration of the substrates for factor XIIa, which facilitates the rate of the enzymatic reactions. Kallikrein can convert factor XII to factor XIIa at a faster rate than the initial factor XII autocatalytic reaction, thereby serving as a positive feedback mechanism to further enhance the activation rate. Kallikrein also liberates the nonapeptide, bradykinin, from HMWK with the formation of HMWKa. The extent of the surface-bound activation of the coagulation mechanism is

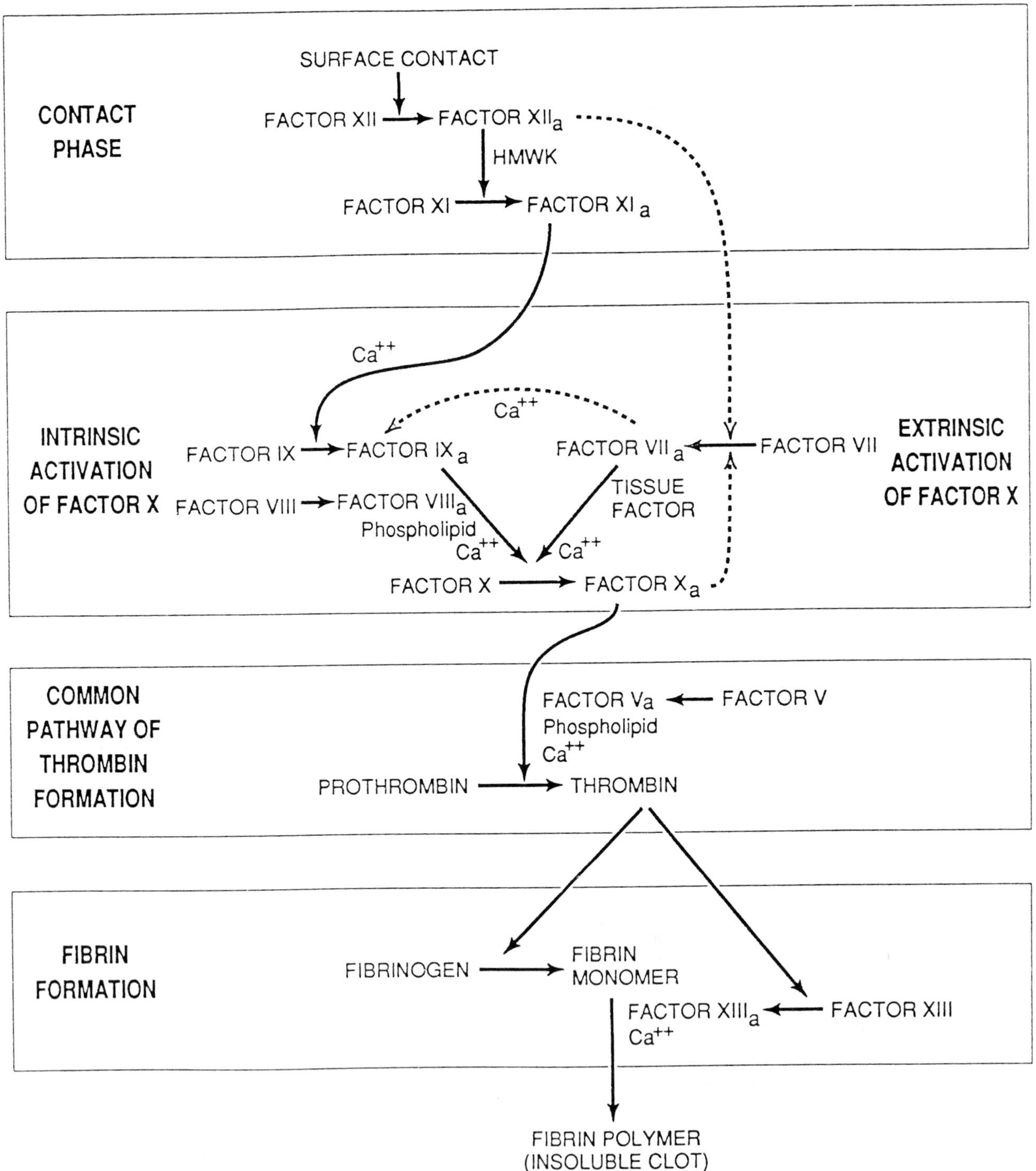

Figure 4.4. A schematic view of molecular interactions beginning with the interaction of factor XII with an abnormal surface and culminating in the formation of insoluble fibrin. The broken lines represent the interactions that link the intrinsic and extrinsic pathways of factor X activation. HMWK, high-molecular-weight kininogen.

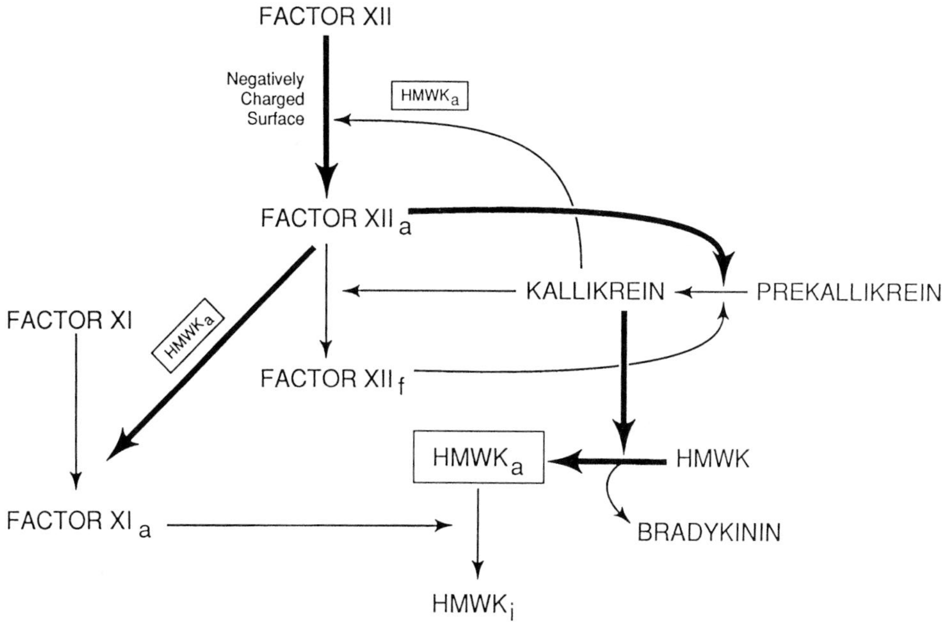

Figure 4.5. A schematic diagram illustrating the interactions of the various components of the contact-activation phase of blood coagulation. The heavy solid lines represent the major reactions; the light solid lines represent feedback reactions that assist in modulating the process. HMWK, high-molecular-weight kininogen; HMWKa, activated HMWK; HMWKi, inactive HMWK; factor XIIf, factor XII fragment.

controlled or limited by (1) the conversion of factor XIIa to a factor XII fragment (factor XIIf), which retains the property of activating prekallikrein while losing its procoagulant activity; and (2) the proteolytic cleavage of HMWKa by factor XIa to an inactive product (HMWKi) that lacks cofactor activity. This local modulation of proteolytic activity by complex molecular interactions is characteristic of each phase of the coagulation process.

Intrinsic activation of factor X

Factor XIa, in the presence of calcium ions, exerts a proteolytic effect on the glycoprotein, factor IX, to convert it to factor IXa, a serine protease. For factor IXa to activate factor X at a rate adequate to support hemostasis, two cofactors, in addition to calcium, are required: (1) a phospholipid component supplied by platelets and (2) a large protein cofactor, factor VIII.

The term *factor VIII* is used to designate the protein that corrects the clotting defect in hemophilia A plasma. The term *factor VIII* denotes the protein, and the term *factor VIII:C* denotes the functional activity. Factor VIII circulates in plasma bound to vWF. Since vWF constitutes the major component of this protein complex, much of the literature before the early 1980s describes vWF rather than factor VIII:C. It is now recognized that factor VIII and vWF are distinct proteins and are products of different genes.

Factor IXa, factor VIII, and calcium form a complex on the phospholipid surface that converts factor X to an active proteolytic product, factor Xa. The rate of this reaction is enhanced by the proteolytic modification of the factor VIII molecule to a more active cofactor form (factor VIIIa) either by the product of the reaction, factor Xa, or by the final protease formed in the coagulation pathway—thrombin (Fig. 4.4). Phospholipid also plays a critical role in the factor X activator complex. The binding of factor VIII to the phospholipid vesicle releases it from the complex with vWF, facilitates the activation of the factor VIII molecule, and stabilizes the factor VIIIa form of the cofactor. When either thrombin or factor Xa interacts with factor VIII unbound to phospholipid, the factor VIII molecule undergoes successive proteolytic cleavages that produce protein fragments with no procoagulant activity.

Extrinsic activation of factor X

The extrinsic or tissue factor pathway of factor Xa formation is unique because it is initiated by the release of a lipoprotein cofactor, tissue factor, into the circulation. Some types of tissue, such as brain, lung, and placenta, have a higher tissue factor content than others (e.g., kidney and spleen), whereas muscle tissue and platelets are thought to be devoid of tissue factor.

In the presence of calcium, the procoagulant protein, factor VII, forms a complex with tissue factor (TF), which will slowly activate factors IX and X. The activation products, factors IXa and Xa, respectively, proteolytically activate factor VII to produce a TF–factor VIIa complex that is approximately 100 times more active than the initial TF–factor VII complex. The factor Xa formed by this TF–factor VIIa complex is identical to the product formed by the factor IXa–factor VIIIa complex of the intrinsic system.

Although factor VII can be activated by the first proteolytic enzyme of the intrinsic pathway (i.e., factor XIIa), this activation alone is not sufficient to promote the activation of factor X by way of the extrinsic pathway. For factor VIIa to produce factor Xa, the obligatory cofactor, tissue factor, must also be present.

Formation of thrombin

Factor Xa, like factor IXa, is a proteolytic enzyme that can, in the presence of calcium ions, slowly convert prothrombin to the active enzyme form, thrombin. For the reaction to proceed at a hemostatically adequate rate, however, two additional cofactors are required: a phospholipid component and a protein, factor V (Fig. 4.4). It has been shown that factor V is released from the alpha granules of platelets during the platelet release reaction and that factor V then becomes bound to the platelet plasma membrane, where it serves as a receptor for factor Xa, which then also becomes bound to the platelet membrane. In a reaction analogous to the factor IXa–factor VIII–phospholipid complex activation of factor X, the thrombin generated by the factor Xa–factor V–phospholipid complex can proteolytically modify the factor V molecule to a more reactive cofactor form, factor Va, which results in significant enhancement of the rate of thrombin formation.

The arrangement of the prothrombin activator complex on the surface of the activated platelet serves to ensure that large amounts of thrombin, perhaps the most critical enzyme of the coagulation pathway, are formed at the site of the primary hemostatic platelet plug (Fig. 4.1). Consequently, the fibrin mesh formed by the proteolytic action of thrombin is also localized around the platelet aggregates.

Formation of fibrin

Once thrombin has been generated, the final steps of fibrin formation can proceed. The first step is the proteolytic cleavage by thrombin of two small peptide chains from each end of the fibrinogen molecule. This activity alters the surface charge on the fibrinogen molecule and permits fibrin monomers to form a loosely knit mesh of fibrin polymers (Fig. 4.4). This fibrin polymer structure, which is still permeable to the flow of blood, is referred to as soluble fibrin. The transformation or "stabilization" of the soluble fibrin to an insoluble fibrin clot requires the formation of stable peptide bonds to complete fibrin polymerization. This transamination, or peptide bond–forming reaction, is catalyzed by activated factor XIII in the presence of calcium ions. Factor XIII normally circulates in plasma in the form of an inactive proenzyme (also released from platelets) and is converted to its active form by thrombin.

The fibrin mesh, by interacting with other adhesive proteins such as fibronectin and platelet fibrinogen, which are released from the activated platelets, not only binds the platelets together but also contributes to the attachment of the platelets to the blood vessel wall. This adhesion of the blood clot (at this stage, usually referred to as a thrombus) to the vessel wall is not only important for the subsequent stages of wound healing and dissolution of the fibrin clot but also prevents the thrombus from becoming dislodged from the vessel wall by the shear force of the flowing blood. If the blood clot does break off from its attachment to the vessel wall, it can circulate in the blood stream as an embolus, which has the potential of becoming lodged in small capillary vessels distant from the original site of formation. The trapped embolus can thus disrupt normal blood circulation at a site removed from the original vascular injury.

DISSOLUTION OF THE FIBRIN CLOT

Equally as important as formation of the fibrin clot, which stops the loss of blood and allows cellular regeneration to repair the blood vessel wall, is removal of the thrombus to allow normal blood circulation to proceed. Removal of the thrombus depends on two processes: reduction in size of the clot (clot retraction) and degradation of the insoluble fibrin (fibrinolysis). As with formation of the thrombus, these processes depend on interaction of the vascular endothelium, platelets, and plasma proteins.

Clot retraction

Adequate numbers of normal, functional platelets are essential to support shrinkage of the fibrin-platelet mass. Shrinkage of the clot depends on interaction of the pseudopods formed in the initial adhesion reaction of the platelets and the fibrin strands. This process is dependent on both energy and calcium and involves the specific platelet contractile protein, thrombosthenin, which functions in a fashion analogous to muscle actinomyosin. The physiological function of this process is (1) to bring the lips of the wound closer together, (2) to stabilize the fibrin clot, (3) to improve the conditions for tissue repair with minimal scarring, and (4) to activate the process of clot lysis.

Platelet-derived growth factors

At least three growth factors can be released from activated platelets when they undergo the release reaction. These proteins have been identified as platelet-derived growth factor (PDGF), epidermal growth factor (EGF), and transforming growth factor (TGF-beta). The growth factors, once released from the platelet, can bind with specific receptors on arterial endothelial cells. The activated growth factor–receptor complex generates an intracellular signal that initiates the early phases of cell division, resulting in endothelial cell proliferation. The importance of these growth promoters is reflected in the experimental observation that a normal, blood vascular, smooth muscle repair response does not occur in thrombocytopenic animals after intra-arterial injury.

THE FIBRINOLYTIC MECHANISM

The fibrinolytic mechanism is the counterpart of the coagulation mechanism, consisting of an ordered sequence of interactions of an enzyme and cofactor on a specific substrate. The major components of the fibrinolytic system include (1) the glycoprotein plasminogen; (2) tissue plasminogen activator (t-PA), a serine protease released from endothelial cells; (3) urokinase (UK), also a protease that is released in a precursor form from tissues such as kidney, macrophages, and fetal organs; and (4) kallikrein.

Activators of plasminogen

Endogenous activators

The principal endogenous activator of plasminogen in blood is t-PA, which is released from endothelial cells "on demand" by such stimuli as thrombin and venous stasis (Fig. 4.6). This plasminogen activator binds avidly to fibrin and exhibits greater enzymatic activity in the fibrin-bound form than in the free form. These characteristics ensure that t-PA activity is localized and its fibrinolytic potential is enhanced at sites of fibrin deposition.

Urokinase (UK) is a tissue-type plasminogen activator that was originally identified as responsible for the fibrinolytic activity of urine. It is structurally and immunologically distinct from t-PA. In plasma, UK exists in a proenzyme form (proUK), which has minimal enzymatic activity and which can be activated either by kallikrein or by the product of plasminogen activation—plasmin (Fig. 4.6). Unlike t-PA, UK has very little affinity for fibrin.

In addition to the activation of the intrinsic coagulation mechanism, the contact-activation process can also result in the generation of plasmin, provided that factor XIIa, prekallikrein, and HMWK are all present. This factor XII–mediated pathway is thought to function via the kallikrein-mediated conversion of proUK to UK. Although the physiological significance of this pathway is uncertain, it may serve to amplify the fibrinolytic process in the location of the fibrin clot since plasmin itself can cause activation of factor XII.

Exogenous activators

Streptokinase (SK), a protein produced by certain strains of streptococci, can combine with human plasminogen in a stoichiometric 1:1 complex that has the capacity to convert human plasminogen to plasmin. Although SK is widely used in the treatment of human thrombotic disorders, its use in veterinary medicine is likely to be limited. For example, SK is only a weak activator of the fibrinolytic system in both the equine and the bovine species.

Formation of plasmin

During formation of the thrombus, some of the circulating plasminogen binds to the fibrin and is incorporated throughout the fibrin clot. Additional plasminogen binding to the fibrin mesh is induced by the locally released t-PA. This enhancement of plasminogen binding ensures a continuous supply of plasminogen substrate for the proteolytic action of t-PA.

Cleavage of a single peptide bond by any of the plasminogen activators converts plasminogen to the trypsinlike protease, plasmin. Although fibrin is the preferred sub-

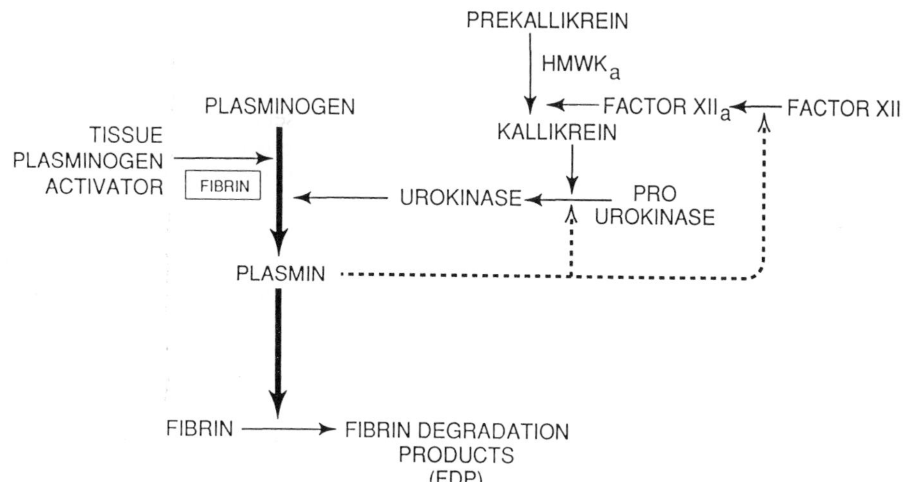

Figure 4.6. A schematic diagram representing the reactions that are involved in the activation of plasminogen and that initiate the fibrinolytic mechanism. The heavy solid line represents the major steps leading to the proteolytic cleavage of fibrin. The broken line represents feedback activation reactions. HMWKa, activated high-molecular-weight kininogen.

strate for plasmin, this enzyme is capable of hydrolyzing other plasma proteins, including fibrinogen, factors XII, VIII, and V, and proteins of the complement system.

Degradation of fibrin

Plasmin successively degrades the fibrin molecule into distinct protein derivatives, known as fibrin degradation products. Although the proteolytic action of plasmin on fibrinogen and fibrin is similar, the protein derivatives produced during fibrin degradation are unique because of the intermolecular peptide bonds formed during the process of fibrin polymerization by factor XIIIa. The significance of this is that circulating FDPs serve as diagnostic markers that reflect prior clot formation and ongoing fibrinolysis.

When the surface of the fibrin clot is removed, fresh surfaces are exposed; these are progressively hydrolyzed until the process of clot lysis is complete. The fibrin fragments and the cellular debris are removed from the circulation by the mononuclear phagocytic system.

REGULATION OF THE HEMOSTATIC PROCESS

Since the stimulation of platelets and proteins results in thrombin formation and a positive feedback system that, in turn, enhances platelet aggregation and additional thrombin formation, it is pertinent to consider the limiting factors that prevent the hemostatic mechanism from proceeding unchecked until all the available platelets and fibrinogen have been used. Some of the factors that exert restraint on the coagulation process include (1) the production of inhibitors of platelet aggregation by vascular endothelium, (2) the localization of the proteolytic reactions of the coagulation mechanism on the phospholipid surfaces associated with the activated platelets, (3) the short half-life in the circulation of activated coagulation factors compared with the nonactivated forms, and, perhaps most important, (4) the presence in plasma of inhibitors of both procoagulant and fibrinolytic reactions.

Under normal circumstances, blood clots are not formed at random in the circulation but only at sites of damage to vascular endothelium. This limitation of blood clot formation is the result of the biochemical constraints on the reactions of the coagulation mechanism, namely, the bonding of factors XII and XI to damaged endothelium, the phospholipid-protein complexes required to ensure that the reactions proceed at functionally adequate rates, and the close interaction among platelet aggregates, fibrin formation, and fibrinolysis. Any of the activated clotting factors that escape from the microenvironment of the clot are either rapidly inactivated by circulating inhibitors or removed from the circulation by the mononuclear phagocytic system.

Inhibitors of the hemostatic process

The similarity of the amino acid sequences of the various protease inhibitors of both the coagulation and fibrinolytic mechanisms indicates that they belong to a family of *ser*ine *pr*otease *in*hibitors, known collectively as "serpins" (Table 4.2).

Table 4.2. Major inhibitors of hemostasis

Inhibitor	Molecular weight	Major proteins inhibited
C1 inhibitor	105	Factor XIIa, kallikrein
α_1-Antitrypsin	55	Factor XIa, elastase
Antithrombin III	58	Factors IXa and Xa, thrombin
α_2-Macroglobulin	725	Kallikrein, thrombin, plasmin
Antiplasmin	67	Plasmin
Plasminogen activator inhibitor	57	Plasminogen activators

The major inhibitor of the intrinsic contact activation system is C1 inhibitor, which accounts for 95 percent of the plasma inhibitory capacity for factor XIIa and more than 50 percent of the kallikrein inhibitory capacity. The name for this inhibitor is derived from its ability to inhibit both the proteolytic and the esterolytic activities of C1, the activated first component of human complement. C1 inhibitor may also function as an inhibitor of factor XIa and plasmin.

Although alpha$_1$-antitrypsin (α_1AT) is found in plasma in the highest concentration of any of the protease inhibitors, its role as a regulator of the coagulation mechanism appears to be confined to its ability to inhibit factor XIa. The major substrate for the inhibitory action of α_1AT appears to be the neutrophil elastase enzyme.

Antithrombin (ATIII), also known as antithrombin III or antithrombin-heparin cofactor, is one of the major inhibitors of the coagulation process since it inhibits a wide range of the coagulant proteases, including thrombin, and the activated factors XIIa, XIa, IXa, and Xa. Although ATIII can also inhibit plasmin and kallikrein, the physiological significance of these reactions is unclear. One molecule of ATIII binds to one molecule of enzyme to form an inactive complex. The rate of formation of the ATIII-enzyme complex is accelerated by the presence of heparin, a highly negatively charged sulfated polysaccharide related to the heparan that exists on the endothelial cell surface.

Alpha$_2$-macroglobulin is a plasma protein that exhibits a wide range of protease inhibitory activity. Not only can it inhibit plasma coagulant and fibrinolytic enzymes such as kallikrein, thrombin, and plasmin, but it can also inhibit protein-cleaving enzymes derived from white blood cells, bacteria, and snake venoms. The physiological role of alpha$_2$-macroglobulin has not been fully elucidated, but, with respect to the hemostatic mechanism, it is sometimes considered a "backup" inhibitor or a modulator of proteolytic activity. The hemostatic enzymes that form a complex with this large protein can still exhibit some residual enzymatic activity. Once the enzyme is bound to or "trapped" in the cagelike structure of the alpha$_2$-macroglobulin molecule, it is protected from attack by other inhibitors.

Antiplasmin, also referred to as alpha$_2$-antiplasmin, is physiologically the most important inhibitor of plasmin mediated fibrinolysis (Table 4.2). The reaction between plasmin and antiplasmin occurs rapidly, with one molecule of the enzyme and one molecule of the inhibitor combining to form an inactive complex. Antiplasmin can function as an inhibitor of plasmin while the proteins are free in the circulation and also when they are bound to fibrin. Antiplasmin can be released from the alpha granules during the platelet release reaction, and during the subsequent coagulation process it can be covalently bound to fibrin strands by the activity of factor XIIIa. Not only does the bound antiplasmin retain full inhibitory activity, but it can also interfere with the binding of plasminogen to the fibrin network. Although these activities appear to be the major physiological function for antiplasmin, this protein can also inhibit other fibrinolytic components, including UK and t-PA, as well as some procoagulant enzymes, including thrombin and the activated forms of factors XI and X.

Plasminogen activator inhibitor (PA inhibitor) can function to inactivate both t-PA and UK (Table 4.2). This inhibitor may play an important role in the regulation of hemostasis despite the fact that in healthy animals it is present in the circulating blood at a markedly lower concentration than are the other protease inhibitors and that it is also rapidly cleared from the circulation. During the coagulation process, PA inhibitor can be released both by endothelial cells and from the platelet alpha granules at the site of formation of the fibrin clot. This release of PA inhibitor can potentially serve to protect the fibrin clot from premature lysis.

Protein C

The protein C anticoagulant pathway is now recognized to be an important regulatory mechanism for both the coagulant and fibrinolytic systems (Fig. 4.7). The major components of this pathway are (1) protein C (PC), a vitamin K–dependent protein synthesized in the liver, which circulates in plasma in an inactive form; (2) protein S, also a vitamin K–dependent protein, which circulates in plasma both in a free form and reversibly bound to C4bBP, a regulatory component of the complement system; (3) thrombomodulin, an endothelial cell surface receptor; and (4) thrombin, which is generated during the coagulation process. The protein C inhibitory pathway is distinct from the serpin effects in that it initiates selective inactivation of the activated cofactors, factors Va and VIIIa. In a reaction sequence analogous to those described for the coagulation and fibrinolytic pathways, the protein C pathway involves, first, the activation of PC, followed by the assembly of factor Va/factor VIIIa inactivation complexes.

Thrombin by itself is an extremely weak activator of PC, but when thrombin becomes bound to the specific endothelial cell surface receptor, thrombomodulin (TM), the thrombin molecule undergoes a change in substrate specificity and becomes an effective PC activator. In contrast to many other proteins that bind to cell surface receptors, thrombin is not internalized by the endothelial cell but remains bound to the cell surface from which it only slowly dissociates. The thrombin-thrombomodulin (thrombin-TM) complex converts PC into an active serine protease (APC) which, like the other procoagulant vitamin K–dependent proteins, exhibits limited substrate specificity and also has specific cofactor requirements for full enzymatic activity (Fig. 4.7). Protein S, the cofactor for APC, binds both calcium and phospholipid and functions to facilitate the interaction of the APC with the factor Va complex formed on the activated platelet surface as part of the factor Xa receptor during the coagulation process. A similar inhibitory complex forms with factor VIIIa. This APC complex inactivates both factors Va and VIIIa by limited proteolytic cleavage of the protein molecule. The progressive inactivation of these cofactors effectively inhibits the formation of factor Xa and thrombin.

The protein C anticoagulant pathway is yet another example of the close knit interactions that occur among the

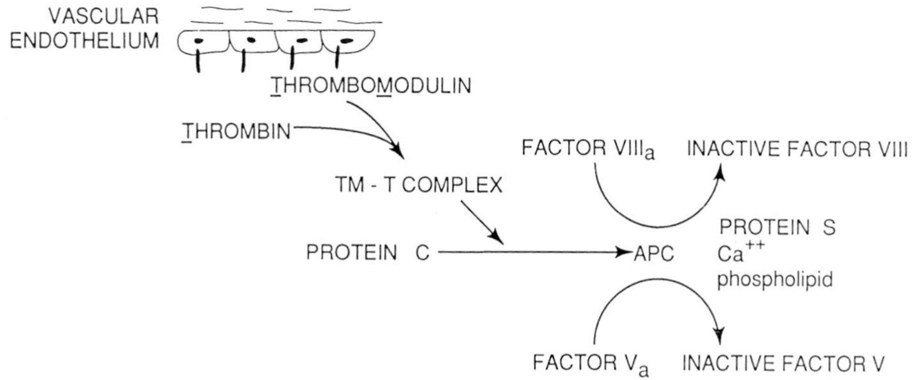

Figure 4.7. A schematic diagram illustrating activation of the protein C anticoagulant pathway by the thrombin-thrombomodulin complex with the subsequent inactivation of factors V and VIII. TM-T complex, thrombomodulin-thrombin complex; APC, activated protein C.

vascular endothelial cells, platelets, and plasma proteins in the hemostatic process.

HEMOSTATIC MECHANISM IN DIFFERENT SPECIES

Striking similarities are observed when the overall coagulation profiles for different species are compared. The circulating biological activity of individual coagulation factors has been found to vary between species when compared with human reference standards. There appears to be considerable homology between species in the amino acid sequences of each of the procoagulant and fibrinolytic proteins. In some instances, however, the differences in the amino acid sequences are sufficient that species specificity is observed, especially when the hemostatic mechanism is examined in the laboratory. For example, homologous tissue factor is a more effective cofactor in the activation of factor X than is tissue factor derived from an unrelated species. The current interest in biotechnology and the expanding use of gene cloning may aid in elucidation of the functional significance of the differences in the amino acid sequences and the species specificity exhibited by protein associated with the hemostatic mechanism.

Although circulating platelet numbers, platelet morphology, and the response to both platelet agonists and antagonists varies not only between birds and mammals but also between mammalian species, it appears that the interaction of activated platelets with damaged endothelium and coagulation proteins is a universal requirement for a normal hemostatic mechanism. In animals other than humans the fibrinolytic system has been less well studied than the coagulation system, but it has been demonstrated that fibrinolysis occurs in amphibians, birds, and mammals.

One of the most striking differences in the hemostatic mechanism is observed when the coagulation profiles of marine mammals, birds, and reptiles are compared with those of terrestrial mammals. In marine mammals the in vitro clotting time of blood is prolonged, apparently as a result of the absence of factor XII. A similar situation has been documented in poultry, except that in birds the entire contact phase is absent. Factor XII is also absent from the blood of most reptiles. Since none of these species exhibit unusual hemorrhagic problems, it appears that factor XII is not essential for the maintenance of adequate hemostasis and that factor VII may play a more prominent role in both the intrinsic and extrinsic pathways in these species.

The quantitative differences in the coagulation profiles not only exist between species but can also be found within a given species. The coagulation profiles of newborn calves, kittens, pups, foals, guinea pigs, rabbits, and pigs exhibit marked differences from those of the comparable adult animals. It should be noted, however, that in most species the coagulation profile resembles that of the adult, at least by the end of the first week of life. In the dog, horse, and pig such factors as exercise, stress, trauma, and hormonal changes are known to influence the hemostatic process. Cattle appear to be less sensitive than other species to these influences.

HEMORRHAGIC DISORDERS

Congenital coagulation defects

Hemophilia A (factor VIII:C deficiency) is one of the most common coagulation defects recognized in domestic animals. The problem is most frequently found in dogs, having been reported in almost every breed, but it also occurs in cats and to a more limited extent in horses and cattle. In dogs the spectrum of mild, moderate, and severe forms of hemophilia A has been recognized. Although the clinical severity of the disorder in some instances is correlated with the reduction in plasma factor VIII:C activity, bleeding episodes in the larger breeds of dogs are reported more frequently and tend to be more severe than in the small breeds. This observation may correlate with the finding that hemophilia A is generally severe in horses and mild in cats. In all species the defect is transmitted on the X chromosome as a recessive trait. In the laboratory the plasma clotting time is prolonged, and the factor VIII:C coagulant activity is reduced. Animals with hemophilia A generally have normal bleeding times since they are able to form the primary hemostatic platelet plug.

Another relatively common coagulation disorder is hemophilia B, which is characterized by a reduction of functional factor IX levels in the circulation. This defect has been identified in many breeds of dogs and in several breeds of cats. The genetic inheritance, clinical symptoms, and variation in severity resemble those of hemophilia A.

Von Willebrand's disease (vWD) has been reported frequently in numerous breeds of dogs, occurs in swine and cats, and has even been reported in the laboratory rabbit. It is one of the most common inherited hemorrhagic problems encountered in dogs. The hemorrhagic condition is generally less severe than that found in the hemophilias and tends to be characterized by mucosal, gastrointestinal, and urogenital bleeding and epistaxis. Since platelet vWF activity is reduced, platelet function is impaired; this, in turn, impedes the formation of the primary hemostatic platelet plug and results in prolonged bleeding times. Immunological assays are generally used to quantitate the antigenic level of vWF in plasma, which is reduced in vWD. This disease can be inherited as an autosomal recessive trait or as an autosomal incompletely dominant trait with variable penetrance and expression. Unlike the hemophilias, in which only homozygotes exhibit a bleeding tendency, in vWD, hemorrhagic problems can occur in both homozygotes and heterozygotes. The clinical severity of vWD decreases with age in males and with both age and successive pregnancies in females.

Other congenital defects that have been identified in dogs include factor VII deficiency and factor X deficiency. Hereditary factor VII deficiency has been reported in a number of families and colonies of beagles in North America and Great Britain. This autosomally transmitted disorder is expressed in dogs as a mild clinical condition that requires no therapy. Factor X deficiency in the dog is manifest as a severe bleeding diathesis in newborn and young adult dogs, although in dogs that survive to maturity the disorder seems to be clinically mild unless the dogs undergo surgery. This disorder is transmitted as an autosomal recessive trait.

Factor XI deficiency is the only congenital coagulation disorder that has been reported in cattle. In some affected animals excessive bleeding has been noted after dehorning, and frank bleeding into the milk has also been reported occasionally. The disorder is transmitted as an autosomal recessive trait. Factor XI deficiency has also been identified in springer spaniel dogs. In this breed the disorder is also transmitted as an autosomal trait, and affected animals exhibit mild bleeding. Factor XII deficiency has been reported infrequently in both cats and dogs. It appears that the disorder is clinically asymptomatic and is transmitted as an autosomal recessive trait.

Bleeding problems associated with defective platelets have also been reported in domestic animals. In one type of dysfunction, referred to as thrombasthenia, which has been identified in a family of otter hounds, the platelets exhibit normal morphology but fail to respond normally to standard aggregating agents and do not sustain normal clot retraction. Affected animals have prolonged bleeding times, and epistaxis is common. A canine thrombopathia has been identified as an autosomally inherited disorder in the basset hound. The platelets appear morphologically normal, and although they may aggregate in response to thrombin, they do not respond to other physiological stimuli or support normal platelet adhesion and clot retraction. Other thrombopathies that have been identified include an ultrastructural defect in cattle in which the dense granules are absent and a storage pool deficiency in fawn-hooded rats in which a reduction in platelet serotonin and release occurs.

Acquired coagulation defects

Acquired bleeding disorders are much more common than are the inherited coagulation disorders and can be induced by a wide variety of factors, including trauma, septicemia, liver disease, malignant tumors, and drug intoxication.

Platelet defects

Acquired platelet defects generally fall into one of two categories: (1) quantitative defects that are usually associated with a reduced platelet count, or thrombocytopenia; or (2) qualitative defects, or thrombopathies, in which circulating platelet numbers may be normal but platelet function is impaired. Immune-mediated thrombocytopenia is the most common type of quantitative disorder. When the cause of the reduction in platelet number is not known, the disorder is referred to as idiopathic thrombocytopenic purpura. The majority of thrombopathies are the result of drug ingestion, especially the nonsteroidal anti-inflammatory drugs such as phenylbutazone, aspirin, and indomethacin. It is relevant to note that there are marked species differences in the platelet response to these drugs; hence caution should be exercised in the extrapolation of data between species. For example, canine and feline platelets are sensitive to such drugs as aspirin and indomethacin, to which bovine and elephant platelets are insensitive. In all species, these drugs inhibit platelet function by interfering with prostaglandin and thromboxane synthesis in the activated platelet. The most common disorders associated with thrombopathies are uremia and liver disease.

Liver disease

The liver is not only the major source of nonimmunological plasma proteins, it is also the primary site of synthesis of most of the plasma coagulation factors in addition to plasminogen and the inhibitors alpha$_1$-antitrypsin, alpha$_2$-macroglobulin, and ATIII (Table 4.1). The hepatic synthesis of functionally normal forms of factors IX, X, VII, prothrombin, protein C, and protein S is dependent on the availability of adequate amounts of vitamin K. Oral anticoagulants, belonging to the coumarin group, antagonize the action of vitamin K and induce the synthesis of nonfunctional forms of the vitamin K–dependent proteins. Since the nonfunctional factors cannot bind to phospholipids, as required for the formation of the protein-phospholipid-calcium complexes (Fig. 4.4), thrombin formation is impaired. This type of hemorrhagic problem can be differentiated from clinical problems associated with liver dysfunction, since the results of liver function tests will generally be normal in coumarin-related bleeding disorders.

Disseminated intravascular coagulation

A rather complex hemorrhagic problem known as disseminated intravascular coagulation (DIC, consumption coagulopathy, defibrination syndrome) can occur secondary to many disease processes, including liver dysfunction, cancer, and infections. This disorder has been reported in dogs, cats, horses, and cattle. DIC is defined as the pathological activation of the coagulation mechanism in the microvasculature with the simultaneous activation of the fibrinolytic system. On the one hand, generation of thrombin during the coagulation process can lead to platelet aggregation and fibrin formation, which may result in the thrombosis of small blood vessels. On the other hand, uncontrolled activation of the fibrinolytic system leads to the degradation of both fibrin and fibrinogen, with the release of both fibrin and fibrinogen degradation products into the circulation. Since both circulating platelets and procoagulant proteins are used in the coagulation process, and since the circulating fibrin(ogen) degradation products can interfere with the normal processes of fibrin formation, there arises a paradoxical situation in which a hemorrhagic condition is produced. DIC is one of the most common coagulopathies encountered in small animal medicine.

EVALUATION OF HEMOSTASIS

Since there are a number of excellent reference sources that describe laboratory diagnosis in detail, only a brief description of the most commonly used routine procedures is given here.

Bleeding time

In dogs, the buccal mucosal bleeding time, which is defined as the duration of hemorrhage from standardized cuts made with a spring-loaded disposable device in the mucosal surface of the upper lip, has been shown to be a reliable method for evaluating disorders that involve the primary hemostatic process. Hence, a prolonged buccal mucosal bleeding time is generally indicative of vascular and/or platelet dysfunction.

Laboratory evaluation

Anticoagulants must be added to blood taken for hemostatic tests. The preferred anticoagulants are the chelating agents trisodium citrate and EDTA (ethylenediaminetetraacetic acid disodium salt), both of which bind the calcium ions present in blood and prevent any of the calcium-dependent reactions from proceeding. To prevent contact activation of the blood, samples collected for coagulation screening should not be exposed to glass surfaces. Heparin is not an appropriate anticoagulant for hemostatic testing, since it functions to accelerate the complex formation between ATIII and factor Xa and thrombin. Thus the presence of heparin interferes with coagulation testing by slowing the rate of thrombin formation.

General screening tests

The two most commonly used laboratory screening tests of the coagulation mechanism are the activated partial thromboplastin time (APTT), which provides an assessment of the intrinsic coagulation pathway, and the one-stage prothrombin time (OSPT, PT), which assesses the extrinsic pathway. For the APTT test, plasma is contact-activated with an inert substance, such as kaolin or celite, in the presence of phospholipid, and fibrin formation is initiated by the addition of calcium. This test will detect abnormalities of factors XII, XI, IX, VIII, X, prothrombin, and fibrinogen. Unfortunately, a prolonged APTT may not be found when there is a mild deficiency of a single factor, since the test is sensitive only to specific factor levels in the 20 to 25 percent of normal range. For the OSPT assay, plasma is activated with tissue thromboplastin, a mixture of tissue factor and phospholipids, before the mixture is recalcified. This assay will detect abnormalities in factors V, VII, X, prothrombin, and fibrinogen and is subject to the same sensitivity constraints as the APTT assay.

Specific tests

Plasma fibrinogen concentrations can be quantitated by several methods, including biological and immunological assays. Fibrin degradation products, a measure of excessive fibrinolysis, can be evaluated by one of several commercially available agglutination or immunological methods. The biological activity of specific coagulation factors is usually evaluated by a modification of the APTT or OSPT assays with specific congenitally deficient plasma.

REFERENCES

Bachmann, F., and Kruithof, I.E.K.O. 1984. Tissue plasminogen activator: chemical and physiological aspects. *Semin. Thromb. Hemostasis.* 10:6–17.

Badylak, S.F. 1988. Coagulation disorders and liver disease. *Vet. Clin. North Am.: Small Anim. Pract.* 18:87–93.

Bevers, E.M., Rosing, J., and Zwaal, R.F.A. 1987. Platelets and coagulation. In D.E. MacIntyre and J.L. Gordon, eds., *Platelets in Biology and Pathology. III*. Elsevier Science Publishers, New York.

Bondy, G.S., and Gentry, P.A. 1989. Characterization of the normal bovine platelet aggregation response. *Comp. Biochem. Physiol.* 92C:67–72.

Catalfamo, J.L., and Dodds, W.J. 1988. Hereditary and acquired thrombopathias. *Vet. Clin. North Amer.: Small Anim. Pract.* 18:185–93.

Colman, R.W., Marder, V.J., Salzman, E.W., and Hirsh, J. 1987. Overview of hemostasis. In R.W. Colman, J. Hirsh, Marder, V.J., and E.W. Salzman, eds., *Hemostasis and Thrombosis: Basic Principles and Clinical Practice*. 2d ed. J.B. Lippincott, Philadelphia.

Dodds, W.J. 1989. Hemostasis. In J.J. Kaneko, ed., *Clinical Biochemistry of Domestic Animals*. Academic Press, New York.

Esmon, C.T. 1989. The roles of protein C and thrombomodulin in the regulation of blood coagulation. *J. Biol. Chem.* 264:4743–46.

Fogh, J.M., and Fogh, I.T. 1988. Inherited coagulation disorders. *Vet. Clin. North Am.: Small. Anim. Pract.* 18:231–43.

Francis, C.W., and Marder, V.J. 1986. Concepts of clot lysis. *Ann. Rev. Med.* 37:187–204.

Gentry, P.A., and Black, W.D. 1980. Prevalence and inheritance of factor XI (plasma thromboplastin antecedent) deficiency in cattle. *J. Dairy Sci.* 63:616–20.

Gentry, P.A., and Liptrap, R.M. 1988. Comparative hemostatic protein alterations accompanying pregnancy and parturition. *Can. J. Physiol. Pharmacol.* 66:671–678.

Gentry, P.A., Niemuller, C., Ross, M.L., and Liptrap, R.M. 1989. Platelet aggregation in the Asian elephant is not dependent on thromboxane B_2 production. *Comp. Biochem. Physiol.* 94A:47–51.

Johnstone, G.S., Turrentine, M.A., Kraus, K.H. 1988. Canine von Willebrand's disease: A heterogeneous group of bleeding disorders. *Vet. Clin. North Am.: Small Anim. Pract.* 18:195–229.

Johnstone, I.B. 1988. Clinical and laboratory diagnosis of bleeding disorders. *Vet. Clin. North. Am.: Small Anim. Pract.* 18:21–23.

Kane, W.H., and Davie, E.W. 1988. Blood coagulation factors V and VIII: structural and functional similarities and their relationship to hemorrhagic and thrombotic disorders. *Blood* 71:539–55.

Kaplan, A.P., and Silverberg, M. 1987. The coagulation-kinin pathway of human plasma. *Blood* 70:1–15.

Littlewood, J.D., Herrtage, M.E., Gorman, N.T., and McGlennon, N.J. 1987. Von Willebrand's disease in dogs in the United Kingdom. *Vet. Rec.* 121:463–68.

Marder, V.J., and Francis, C.W. 1987. Physiological balance of haemostasis and bleeding. *Drugs* 33:13–21.

Meyers, K.M. 1986. Species differences. In H. Holmsen, ed., *Platelet Responses and Metabolism*. Vol. 1. CRC Press, Boca Raton, Fla.

Meyers, K.M., Katz, J.B., Clemmons, R.M., Smith, J.B., and Holmsen, H. 1980. An evaluation of the arachidonate pathway of platelets from companion animals and food-producing animals, mink, and man. *Thromb. Res.* 20:13–24.

Meyers, K.M., Menard, M., and Wardrop, K.J. 1987. Equine hemostasis. *Vet. Clin. North. Am.: Equine Pract.* 3:485–505.

Morris, D.D. 1988. Recognition and management of disseminated intravascular coagulation in horses. *Vet. Clin. North. Am: Equine Pract.* 4:115–43.

Nemerson, Y. 1988. Tissue factor and hemostasis. *Blood* 71:1–8.

Packham, M.A. 1988. The behaviour of platelets at foreign surfaces. *Proc. Soc. Exp. Biol.* 189:261–74.

Rao, A.K., and Holmsen, H. 1986. Congenital disorders of platelet function. *Semin. Haematol.* 23:102–18.

Rosenberg, R.D. 1987. The biochemistry and pathophysiology of the prethrombotic state. *Ann. Rev. Med.* 38:493–508.

Schafer, A.I. 1987. Focussing of the clot: Normal and pathological mechanisms. *Ann. Rev. Med.* 38:211–20.

Siess, W. 1989. Molecular mechanisms of platelet activation. *Physiol. Rev.* 69: 58–178.

Slappendel, R.J. 1988. Disseminated intravascular coagulation. *Vet. Clin. North Am.: Small Anim. Pract.* 18:169–84.

Sprengers, E.D., and Kluft, C. 1987. Plasminogen activator inhibitors. *Blood* 69:381–87.

Troy, G.C. 1988. An overview of hemostasis. *Vet. Clin. North Am.: Small Anim. Pract.* 18:5–20.

White, J.G. 1987. The secretory pathway of bovine platelets. *Blood* 69:878–85.

Zucker-Franklin, D., Benson, K.A., and Meyers, K.M. 1985. Absence of a surface-connected canalicular system in bovine platelets. *Blood* 65:241–44.

CHAPTER 5

The Cardiovascular System and Blood Flow | by Julius Melbin and David K. Detweiler

GENERAL FEATURES OF THE VASCULAR SYSTEM

Leonardo da Vinci is credited with conceiving of the heart as a pump, but it was William Harvey (1628) who described the anatomic and physiologic principles of the circulation and is considered to be the "discoverer" of the circulation. The cardiovascular system of the normal adult mammal is shown in a schematic drawing in Fig. 5.1. The mammalian heart consists of four chambers—two atria and two ventricles—that pump blood. The right ventricle supplies blood to the pulmonic or lung circulation, from which it returns to the left atrium. Blood in this chamber passes to the left ventricle. The left ventricle supplies blood to the remainder of the body via the systemic circulation, which includes all other organ systems. Blood from this latter circulation returns to the right atrium and passes to the right ventricle to complete the cycle. Although the pulmonic and systemic circulations are in series, in the systemic circulation the vascular supply to the various organs exists primarily in a parallel arrangement. Functionally, the two ventricles are also connected in series except for a small bronchial shunt and thus, except for transients, their steady-state outputs or flows (volume/time) must equilibrate. Normally this equilibration is preserved, even with wide variation in output as, for example, during strenuous exercise. If this balance is upset because of cardiac dysfunction, clinical signs of respiratory distress become evident because of fluid accumulation in the lungs. Because of low pressures in the atria (Fig. 5.2D, Fig. 5.4), even moderate increases in intrapericardial pressure (which can result from inflammatory effusions or hemorrhage) can compromise or interrupt ventricular filling (cardiac tamponade) and either seriously reduce or terminate cardiac output.

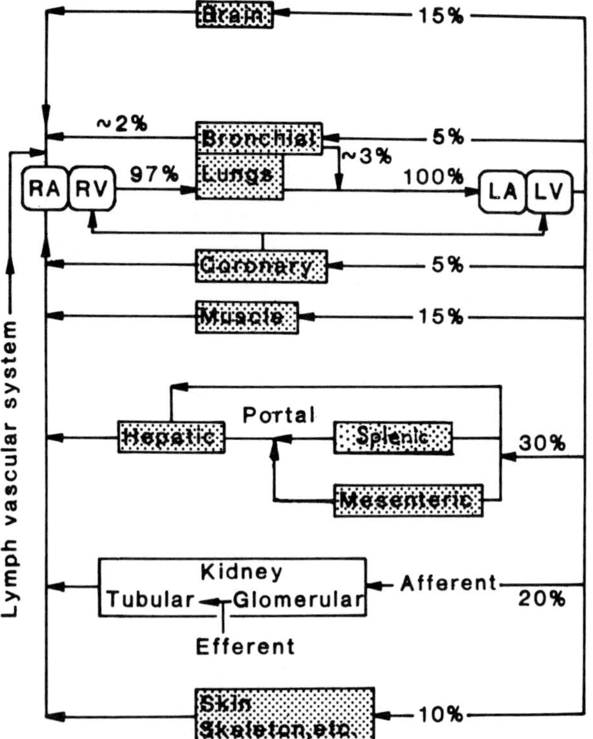

Figure 5.1. Diagram of a mammalian circulatory system. Lines depict arteries and veins, arrowheads show the direction of flow, and boxed and shaded regions indicate the microcirculation (arteries, capillaries, venules). Approximate percentages of cardiac output to the different circulatory beds are indicated. Although these values are representative of many mammals, there can be marked species differences. RA, Right atrium; LA, left atrium, RV, right ventricle; LV, left ventricle. (Modified from Detweiler 1979, in Brobeck 1979, *Best and Taylor's Physiological Basis of Medical Practice,* 10th ed., Williams & Wilkins Co., Baltimore.)

The blood vascular system can be subcategorized into three groups, each with different functions: (1) arteries, the conduit system that distributes blood to organs and tissues; (2) the microcirculation (arterioles, capillaries), the system concerned with blood distribution and with filtration and diffusion within organs and tissues; and (3) veins, the conduit system that collects blood from the organs and tissues for return to the heart. All of these vessels share some geometric and structural features but have some features that differ greatly; individual design is suited to specific function and existing blood pressure (Fig. 5.2D, Fig. 5.3). For example, arteries of the pulmonic circulation operate at a mean arterial pressure about one-seventh that of systemic arteries. Pressures are highest in arteries, fall to very low values in the microcirculation, and remain low in the veins (Fig. 5.2D, Fig. 5.4). This gradient of mean pressure indicates that pressure energy is gradually converted to thermal form by viscosity or friction during blood flow through the circuit (i.e., dissipated as heat). The relatively abrupt and substantial drop in pressure that occurs in the microcirculation implies high frictional properties associated with these vascular beds.

Vascular patterns at the microcirculatory level vary, depending on the organ. In the hepatic circulation (Fig. 5.1) arterial blood flowing to liver stroma and sinusoids combines with venous blood that enters liver sinusoids from the splenic and mesenteric circulations (via the portal vein) before leaving the liver in the hepatic vein. In the pulmonary system, arterial blood of the bronchial circulation combines in the lung capillaries with venous blood from the right ventricle. In the case of congenital absence of the pulmonary artery, unoxygenated blood can bypass the lung circulation by entering the left atrium through a patent foramen ovale. A portion of left ventricular output will perfuse lung capillaries through an enlarged bronchial artery, and the blood thus oxygenated may be sufficient for marginal support of postnatal life (see p. 217, Bronchial Circulation).

Different animal species may have different characteristic levels of arterial blood pressure that correlate with form and activity. For example, in the erect posture the resting mean systemic arterial pressures at heart level in giraffes, oxen, and humans are 219, 135, and 90 mm Hg, respectively. At brain level the values are 100, 88, and 65 mm Hg, respectively (Fig. 5.5A). Thus the species with the longest distances between heart and brain (e.g., 160 cm in giraffes, 34 cm in humans) have the highest pressure at heart level. Pressures become more uniform at brain level because energy dissipated in flowing blood is proportional to the length over which this viscous fluid is moved (Fig. 5.5A and B). As a class, birds, which are subject to marked alteration in gravitational and other transient accelerations associated with flying, have higher arterial pressures than do mammals.

The total volume of blood is not uniformly distributed among different segments of the circulation. The volume in a given segment, although not rigidly fixed, is normally maintained within fairly narrow limits (Fig. 5.2E, Tables 5.1 and 5.2). The blood volume contained in the systemic arteries is the least, and it is also the least variable. This high-pressure system contains about 14 percent of the blood volume. The heart contains about 7 percent, and the remainder (about 79 percent) is in the low-pressure (pulmo-

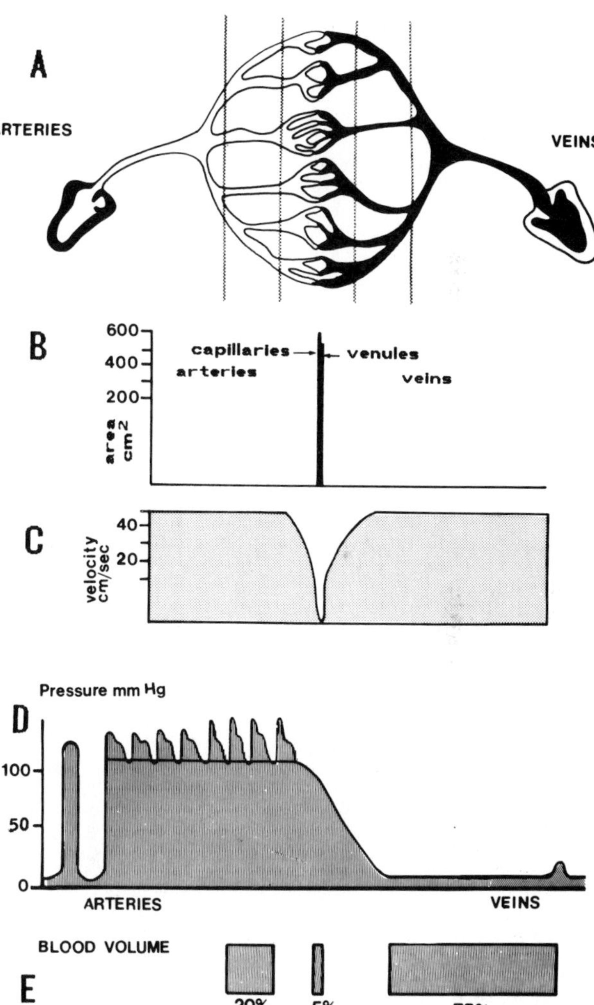

Figure 5.2. Schema correlating cross-sectional areas, flow velocities, pressures, and volumes in the mammalian circulation. (*A*) Illustration of the increasing and then decreasing total cross sections developed by the branching vasculature. Vertical lines separate segments of greatly differing total cross sections, but volume flow through one segment equals that of any other. (*B*) Cross-sectional areas of different segments of the circulation computed from a 13 kg dog. (*C*) Graph of blood flow velocity to demonstrate inverse relationship to cross-sectional area. Velocity of flow in the capillaries averages about 0.07 cm/s. (*D*) Approximate pressures throughout the circulation. Pressure is high and pulsatile in the arteries and falls rapidly in the microcirculation, and pulsations are damped in the capillaries and veins. (*E*) Distribution of blood volume in the vascular system. (Modified from Detweiler 1979, in Brobeck 1979, *Best and Taylor's Physiological Basis of Medical Practice*, 10th ed., Williams & Wilkins Co., Baltimore.)

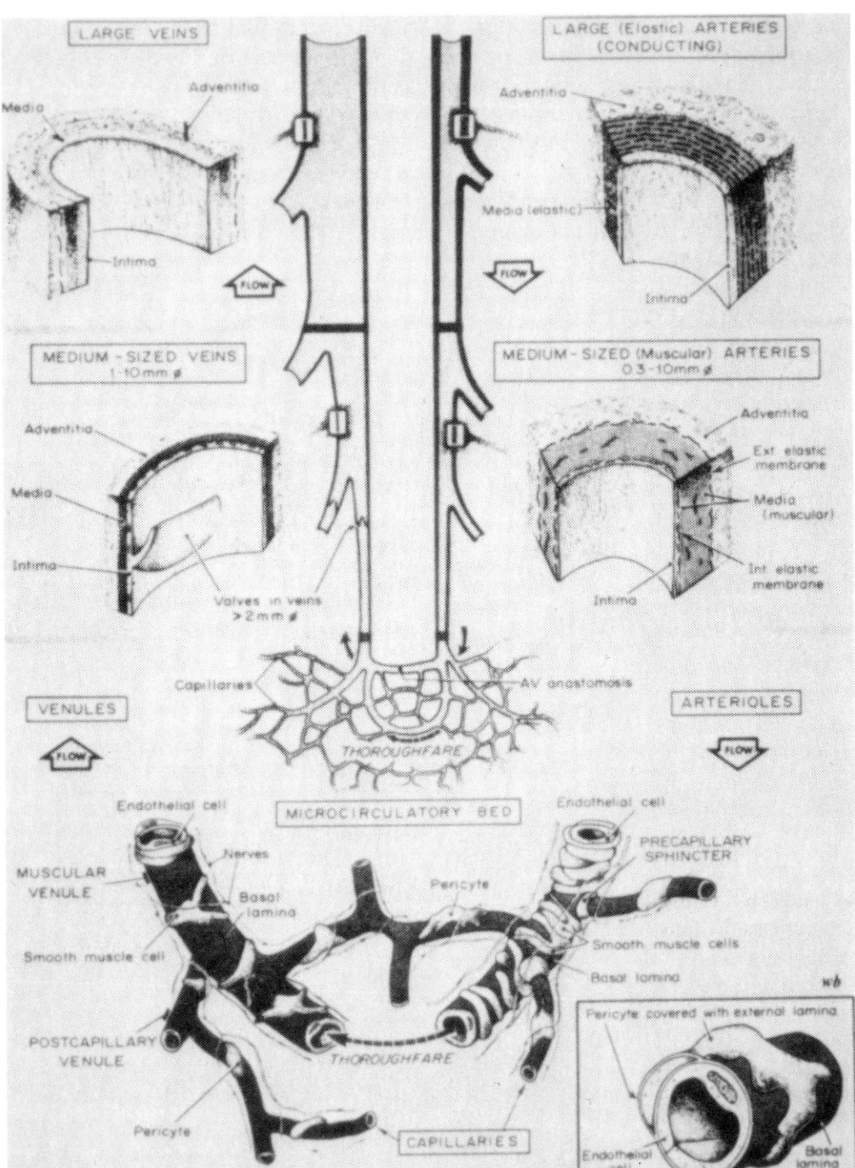

Figure 5.3. Schema depicting chief structural components of main segments of mammalian blood vessels. (From Rhodin 1980, in *Handbook of Physiology,* sect. 2, vol. 2., Bohr, Somlyo, and Sparks, eds., *The Cardiovascular System,* Am. Physiol. Soc., Baltimore.)

nary and venous) systems. Of this latter volume, about 9 percent is in the pulmonary system (Tables 5.1 and 5.2). The low-pressure system can also be readily distended. If blood volume is increased, as by transfusion, only about 1 percent of the added volume distributes to the high-pressure system. Thus the low-pressure system functions as a reservoir. Located in the low-pressure system are receptors that are sensitive to changes in fluid volume (i.e., responsive to the degree of stretch of these vessels). These receptors are thought to serve as sensors for the regulation of fluid volume by the central nervous system.

In addition to the blood vascular system, there exists a lymphatic system whose capillaries are closely associated with blood capillaries. These capillaries serve to collect fluids and macromolecules that accumulate in tissue spaces. Larger lymph vessels are formed by the confluence of lymph capillaries, and these return lymph to the right atrium.

SCALING AND CIRCULATORY VARIABLES

In biology, scaling deals with structural and functional relationships among organisms that differ in size but otherwise are similar. For a general concept of scaling of the cardiovascular system, it is useful to consider certain ratios that relate body and organ sizes. Although these ratios are informative, marked deviations that appear in particular species and individuals can be associated with characteristic differences in other variables, such as autonomic tone

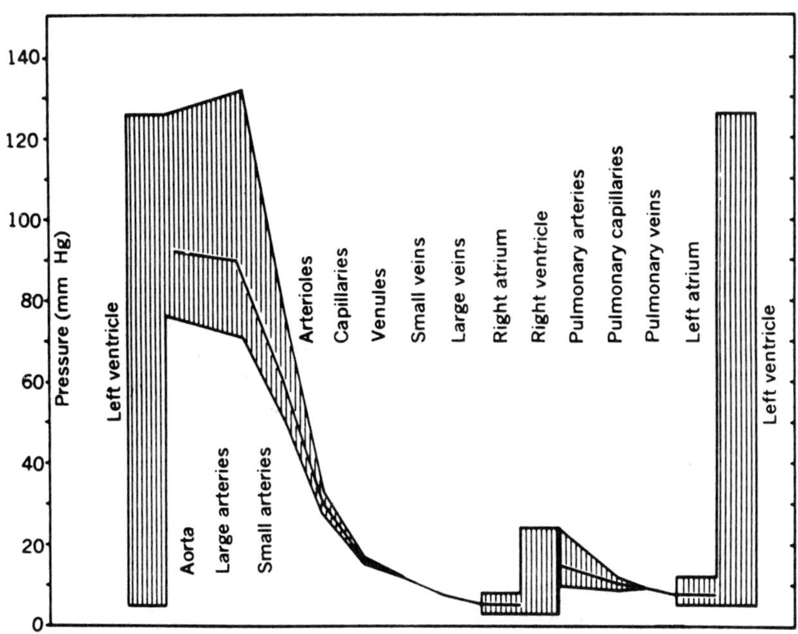

Figure 5.4. Pressure distribution in the human cardiovascular system. The shaded area extends between diastolic and systolic pressures and indicates the amplitude of pulse pressure. The central solid line represents mean pressure. (Redrawn from Milnor, in Mountcastle 1980, *Medical Physiology,* 14th ed. C.V. Mosby, St. Louis.)

(e.g., vagotonic animals such as the horse) and metabolic rate (e.g., milking cows vs. nonlactating animals of similar size) or with genetically controlled characteristics such as cardiac size (e.g., racing greyhound vs. mongrel dogs).

The mass of a mammalian heart (M_{heart}) is generally equal to about 0.6 percent of the body mass or weight (M_{body}). Blood volume or mass (M_{blood}), although it varies among species, is in the order of about 8 percent of the body weight, i.e.,

$$M_{heart}/M_{body} = 0.006$$

$$M_{blood}/M_{body} = 0.08$$

Thus, according to these values, blood and heart mass are related by

$$\frac{M_{blood}}{M_{heart}} = \frac{0.08}{0.006} = 13.3$$

That is, the blood mass (or volume) is about 13 times the heart mass (or volume) in mammals. Since the density of myocardium is close to that of blood, volume and mass are used interchangeably.

Several cardiovascular functions have been shown to be related to body mass. These include cardiac output, heart rate, and electrocardiographic time intervals. With body mass or weight as the independent variable, morphological and physiological variables (dependent variables) relative to body size have been scaled in accordance with allometric equations of the general form as

$$y = a \cdot x^b$$

where x = body weight. When these variables (x,y) are plotted on logarithmic coordinates, the result is a straight line, even when the relationship is nonlinear (i.e., when b $\neq$ 1). On logarithmic coordinates, the slope of the regression line representing log y versus log x is given by the

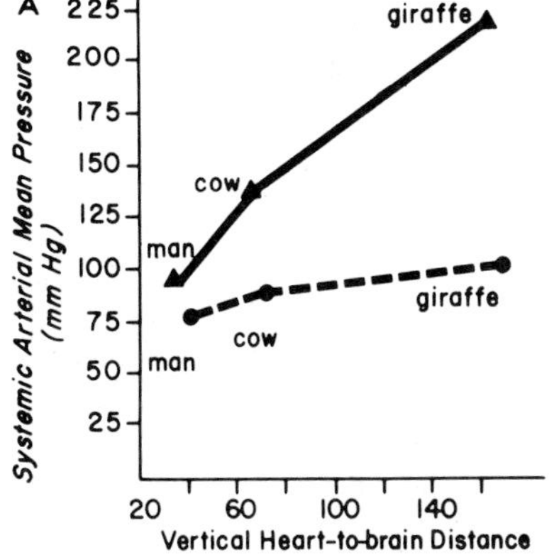

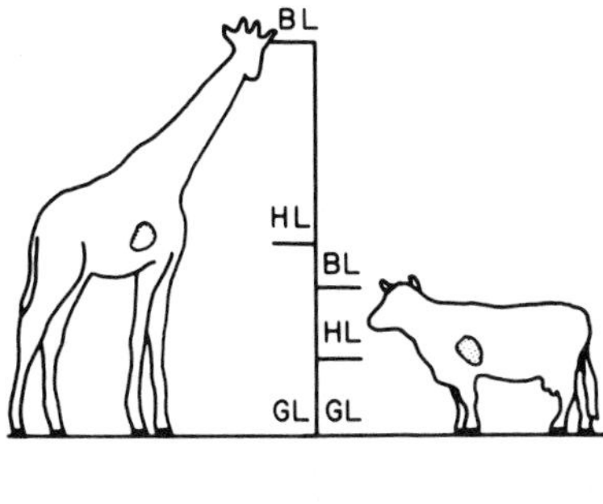

Figure 5.5. (*A*) Mean arterial pressures at the heart level (solid line) and brain level (dashed line) in human, cow, and giraffe. (*B*) Scale drawings of the giraffe and cow indicating relative levels of ground (GL), heart (HL), and brain (BL). (Redrawn from Patterson et al. 1965, *Ann. N.Y. Acad. Sci.* 127:393–413.)

Table 5.1. Estimates of relative blood volumes in segments of the circulatory system from data on the mesenteric vascular bed of the dog

Structure	Diameter (mm)	Number	Total cross-sectional area (cm^2)	Length (cm)	Total volume (ml)
Aorta	10.0	1	0.8	40.0	30
Large arteries	3.0	40	3.0	20.0	60
Main arterial branches	1.0	600	5.0	10.0	50
Terminal branches	0.6	1,800	5.0	1.0	5
Arterioles	0.02	40,000,000	125.0	0.2	25
Capillaries	0.008	1,200,000,000	600.0	0.1	60
Venules	0.03	80,000,000	570.0	0.2	110
Terminal veins	1.5	1,800	30.0	1.0	30
Main venous branches	2.4	600	27.0	10.0	270
Large veins	6.0	40	11.0	20.0	220
Vena cava	12.5	1	1.2	40.0	40
Total					910

Data of F. Mall, cited from Green 1944, in Glasser, ed., *Medical Physics,* vol. 2, Year Book, New York.

Table 5.2. Estimated distribution of blood in vascular system of hypothetical adult man*

Region	Volume (ml)		Volume percent	
Heart (diastole)	360		7.2	
Pulmonary				
Arteries	130	440	2.6	8.8
Capillaries	110		2.2	
Veins	200		4.0	
Systemic				
Aorta and large arteries	300	4,200	6.0	84.0
Small arteries	400		8.0	
Capillaries	300		6.0	
Small veins	2,300		46.0	
Large veins	900		18.0	
Total	5,000		100	

From Milnor 1968, in Mountcastle, ed., *Medical Physiology,* vol. 1, Mosby, St. Louis.

*Age, 40 years; weight, 75 kg; surface area, 1.85 m^2.

value of the exponent b. If the slope is unity (b = 1), the change of y with respect to x is in 1 to 1 proportion. A slope greater than 1 indicates that the dependent variable, y, increases in a greater than 1 to 1 proportion to the independent variable, x. If the slope is less than 1 but greater than 0, it indicates that y increases by less than a 1 to 1 proportion with respect to x. A slope of 0 indicates that y is independent of x, and a slope of less than 0 (i.e., negative) indicates that y decreases with increasing x. Several of these relationships are found in the cardiovascular systems of mammals. Figure 5.6 illustrates pictorially how heart size varies among mammals, and Fig. 5.7 includes a log-log plot of the relationship between heart and body weights.

Electrocardiographic intervals, like heart rates, can also be related to body mass. Important intervals or durations include the PR interval indicating atrioventricular conduction time, the QRS duration indicating ventricular depolarization to completion of repolarization. More detailed discussions of the electrocardiogram are given in Chapter 7. Figure 5.8 illustrates log-log plots of these intervals for a range of mammals. The relations of these variables to body weight have slopes considerably less than 1.0 on logarithmic coordinates.

In most mammals blood volume is a constant fraction of

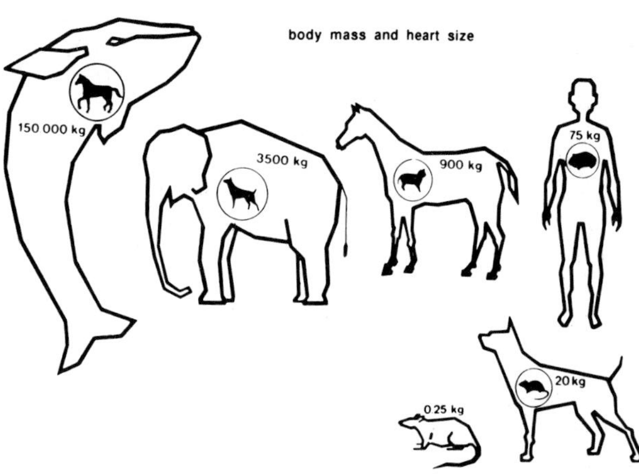

Figure 5.6. Pictorial illustration of body weight and heart weight. Heart size is represented by the image of a mammal of corresponding weight. (Modified from R.E. Rushmer, in collaboration with and published by F.L. Meijler, 1985, *Med. Tidschr. Geneesk.* 129:1329, with permission.)

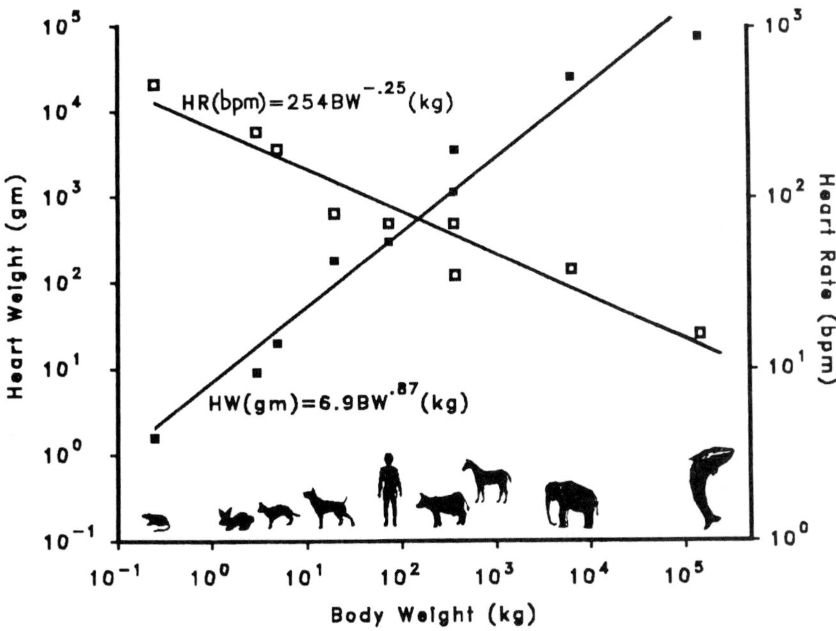

Figure 5.7. Log-log plots of heart weight (g) and heart rate (bpm) versus body weight for a range of mammals. Data are from various sources. Allometric relations are shown as inserts.

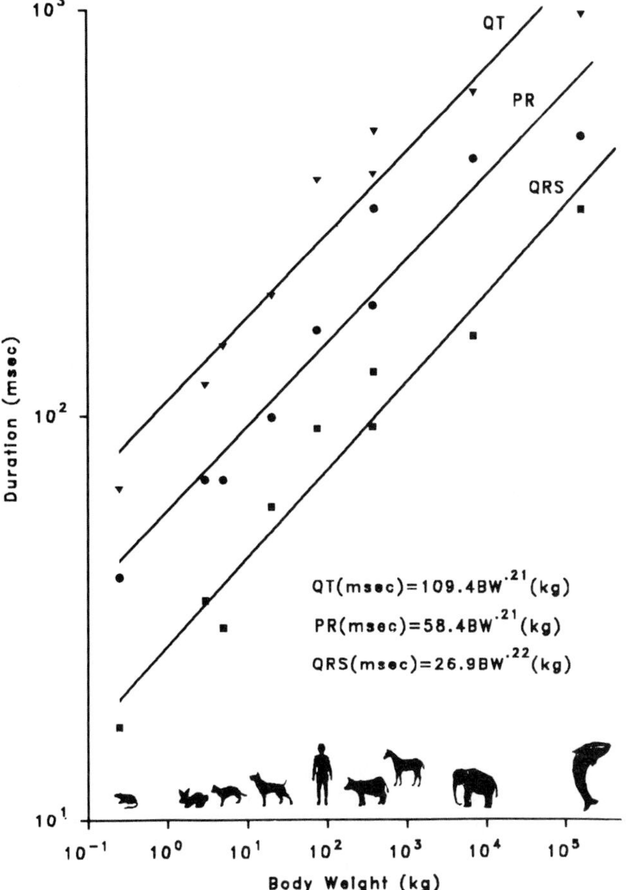

Figure 5.8. Log-log plots of relationships of electrocardiographic time durations (ms) versus body weight (kg) for a range of mammals. Data are from various sources. Allometric relations for PR interval, QRS duration, and QT interval are shown as inserts.

body weight (ranging between about 50 and 80 ml/kg of body weight) with the exponent on body weight close to 1.0; i.e., blood (L) = 0.0655·BW (kg). Some diving mammals, however, have higher blood volumes than this as an adaptation that serves their frequent need for a reservoir of oxygen during prolonged dives (see Chap. 12). Differences are also found within some species; for example, racing greyhounds have higher relative blood volumes than do mongrels (114/kg vs. 79 ml/kg). Early methods often overestimated the volume, and published values for various species that range from 5.5 to 10.9 percent of body weight may be found.

The total blood circulation time has also been scaled to body size. Circulation time is the time it takes a quantity of blood to travel a given distance over a part or all of the circulatory system. A marker, such as a dye or radioactive substance, is injected at one point in the circulation, and the time it takes for it to arrive at a sampling site is determined. The measured time interval provides an estimate of the flow rate over the shortest circuit between the injection and sampling sites. Since neither distance, blood velocity, nor volume flow is known, determinations of these factors do not accurately estimate the state of the circulation.

Total blood circulation time is the time required for the total blood volume to complete a round trip of the entire circulatory system. If the cardiac output (CO) and the blood volume (bl.v.) are known, the time for the heart to pump the entire blood volume can be determined by the following formula:

$$\text{Circulation time (s)} = \frac{\text{Bl.v. (ml)}}{\text{CO (ml) (s}^{-1})}$$

With the scaling equation for blood volume (in liters), i.e., 0.6555·BW(kg), and that for the cardiac output (in liters per second) taken as 20 times the per second rate of oxygen consumption ($20 \cdot 1.88 \cdot 10^{-4} \cdot BW^{0.75}$kg), the theoretical blood volume circulation time is approximately

Circulation time =

$$\frac{\text{Bl.v.}}{\text{CO}} = \frac{0.0655 \cdot \text{BW (kg)}}{3.76 \cdot 10^{-3} \cdot \text{BW}^{0.75} \text{ (kg)}} = 17.4 \cdot \text{BW}^{0.25} \text{ (kg)}$$

Accordingly, body weight and total blood volume circulation time for different mammals were determined to be as follows: elephant, 3000 to 4000 kg, about 140 seconds; horse, 700 to 900 kg, about 90 seconds; human 70 to 75 kg, about 50 seconds; rat, 0.2 to 0.25 kg, about 12 seconds; mouse, 0.03 kg, about 7 seconds; shrew, 0.003 kg, about 4 seconds. The dramatic difference between circulation times of large versus small mammals is a reflection of the relatively high metabolic rate and tissue oxygen requirements of the smaller species, since the oxygen-carrying capacity of the blood is about the same. In smaller mammals the blood must circulate through the lungs more often to adequately supply the tissues with oxygen.

Although there are interspecies and interstrain differences, several circulatory variables are not scaleable and change little with body size. These include blood viscosity, blood pressure, erythrocyte size, packed cell volume, and capillary diameter.

BLOOD AS A VISCOUS FLUID

Rheology is the study of fluid (liquid or gas) deformation and flow. Hemodynamics is the branch of physiology that deals with the forces and physical mechanisms concerned with the circulation of blood. Unlike solids, fluids deform continuously with continuous application of force. Molecular layers slide over each other (shear), and, since fluids are viscous to a varying extent, force application is necessary to maintain flow. If a fluid were inviscid, flow would be maintained, once it had commenced, without continual force application if no new forces acted to halt the flow. A quantitative measure of the degree of viscosity is expressed as a coefficient of viscosity (expressed in units called poises that, in the centimeter-gram-second or cgs system, is dyne-seconds/cm^3; the dyne is a unit for force). Viscosity relates the force required to develop a measured rate of shear over a surface area with the rate of shear itself. Different fluids have different viscous properties. A newtonian fluid is a homogeneous fluid whose viscosity remains constant at any flow velocity. A thixotropic fluid is a nonnewtonian fluid whose viscosity may alter with velocity (i.e., viscosity decreases with increased shear rate). A Bingham body is a semifluid material that will not flow unless a minimum or threshold unbalanced pressure (termed "yield stress" or "yield pressure") has been exceeded. Nonnewtonian fluids may exhibit more than one such complex property.

Blood plasma behaves much as a newtonian fluid, but the behavior of whole blood varies in different regions of the circulation and with the percentage of cellular components. Because of mixing in the large vessels close to the heart, blood appears largely as a newtonian fluid here. It appears more thixotropic in smaller vessels and acts as a Bingham body in the capillaries because, in these vessels whose diameters are smaller than those of blood cells, force is required to deform cells before flow develops. Factors that affect blood viscosity include the following:

1. Packed cell volume (PCV). This is the most important governor of blood viscosity. Figure 5.9 illustrates how viscosity depends on PCV. Because the geometry of erythrocytes contributes to the manner in which these cells affect viscosity and because this geometry varies among animals, distinctions among species can be seen.

2. Flow velocity. Apparent viscosity decreases with increase in velocity since cell distribution and alignment of formed elements within the vessels vary with velocity. The development of relatively cell-free zones next to the vessel wall affects overall viscosity and thus resistance to flow, as does a lower PCV (Fig. 5.10).

3. Temperature. Viscosity is inversely proportional to temperature.

4. Vessel diameter. This effect is observed in vessels that are less than 0.5 mm in diameter but larger than erythrocytes (approximately 8 μm in diameter) so that cellular elements occupy an appreciable fraction of the cross-section. Here a single coefficient of viscosity is not applicable, as would be the case for a homogeneous fluid. Cells are transported as intact units (without continual shearing as is the case with fluids), and a plasma layer forms near the walls. Since total shearing is reduced for a given mass of flowing plasma and cells, flow occurs with a smaller unbalanced force and the apparent viscosity is decreased substantially (Fig. 5.11). If hemoglobin were not packaged in erythrocytes, a substantially greater mean pressure would be required to perfuse the circulatory system, since this effect would not be present.

Because of these factors, the apparent viscosity of blood is dependent on circumstances and is not constant in the vascular system.

CIRCULATORY MECHANICS

Regardless of the system in question and of particular terminology with respect to physiologically related mechanics, all systems obey universal laws and behave as do all newtonian physical systems. All forms of energy (i.e., kinetic, thermal, and potential) participate. The relative

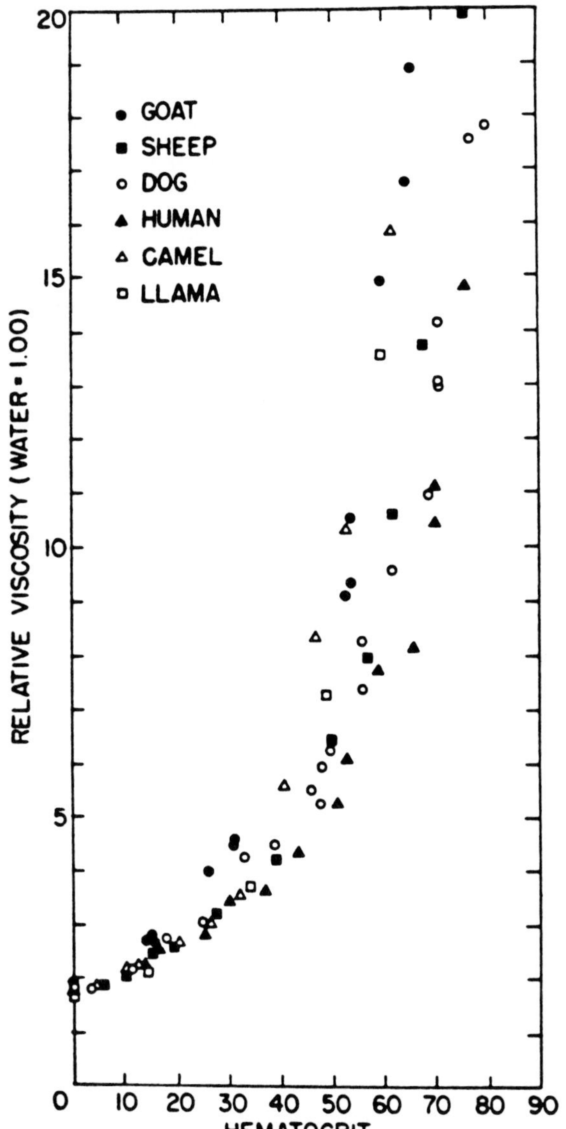

Figure 5.9. The effect of packed cell volume (hematocrit) on viscosity. Most domestic animals have resting PCVs between about 38 and 45 percent with a mean of 40 percent. Exercise, excitement, dehydration, hypoxia, etc. can raise this value. Lactating dairy cattle have hematocrit values of about 35 percent, and birds have even lower values. (From Stone, Thompson, and Schmidt-Nielsen 1968, *Am. J. Physiol.*, 214:913–18.)

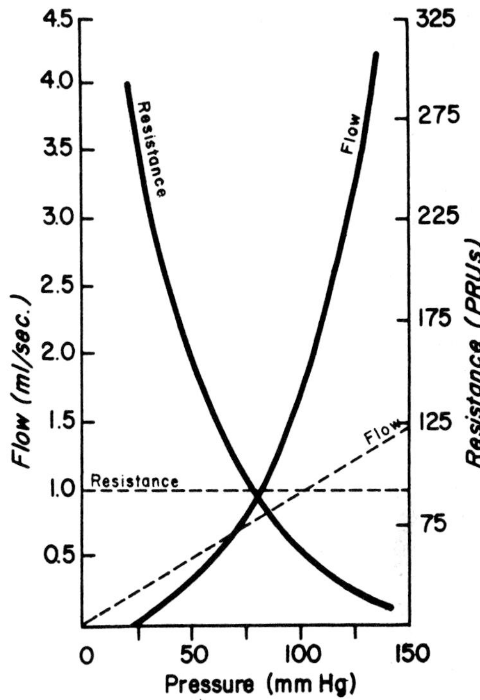

Figure 5.10. The relationships of flow, pressure, and resistances in non-distensible tubes at constant temperature (Poiseuille's equation). Broken lines: Newtonian fluids. Solid lines: Blood.

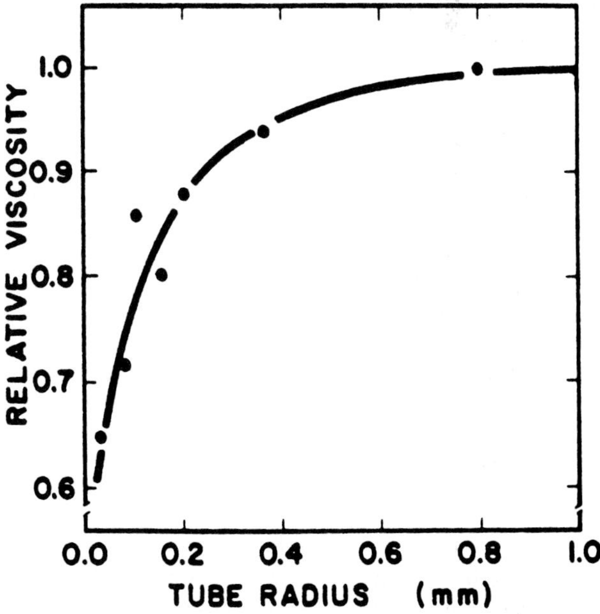

Figure 5.11. The relationship between the relative viscosity of a dog erythrocyte suspension and the radius of the viscometer tube. The smooth curve is a least-squares fit to the data. (From Snyder 1973, *Respiration Physiol.* 19:271–78.)

significance of each form can vary greatly, however, depending on the system. Since energy converts from one form to another but is never lost, the energy or work balance relation applies to all systems, i.e.

Total energy = Kinetic energy + Thermal energy + Potential energy

Kinetic energy relates to motion and inertial forces (i.e., mass and its accelerations and velocity of movement).

Thermal energy is related to the temperature and also to velocity of movement but as associated with viscosity and frictional resistance in the system. Potential energy is associated with the elastic nature of the system and displacements as well as with position in space. Potential energy may also imply chemical or nutrient storage that provides source energy for the mechanical forms. Energy, or the capacity to accomplish work, has the units of work (i.e., dyne-centimeters). Commonly only the more significant physical properties (mass, viscosity, elasticity) observed in a particular system are emphasized, and the energy balance relation is simplified accordingly. Examples are as follows:

Nutrient energy for heat balance =
Heat (body temperature) + Stored energy (e.g., fat)

Respiratory work =
Frictional losses (heat dissipation) + Lung distention and air compression

Cardiac work =
Accelerations (e.g., of blood) + Frictional losses + Vascular distentions and blood storage

Although the heart is the primary source of mechanical energy or forces (or pressures, i.e., force per unit area) that move blood, other features of the mammalian system also contribute to blood movement. These include (1) vascular elasticity, which permits transient blood storage; (2) skeletal muscles, which develop respiratory movements and imbalances of intrathoracic and extrathoracic pressure (respiratory pump) that cause abdominal movements and that compress veins; and (3) unidirectional venous valves in limbs (Fig. 5.3), which assist in return of blood to the heart when these veins are compressed. The alteration of body position also invokes gravitational contributions that affect blood volume distribution. Thus the mechanical potential energy component in the circulation consists of two forms—fluid pressure energy and that related to gravitational force. It is convenient to express the energy relationships for flow in the circulation in terms of a force balance equation, e.g.,

$$\Delta F = M\,a + R\,Q + \Delta vol/C + \rho g\,H\,A$$

where ΔF is the unbalanced force or force difference over a length of vessel in dynes, M is the mass of blood in grams, a is the imparted acceleration in centimeters/second squared, R is the frictional resistance in the vessel in dyne-seconds per cubic centimeter, $\dot{Q}$ is flow in cubic centimeters per second, Δ vol is the volume stored in the vessel segment in cubic centimeters, C is a form of the volumetric compliance of the vessel in cubic centimeters per dyne, ρ is the blood density in grams per cubic centimeter, g is the gravitational acceleration of 980 cm/s^2, A is the surface area of the vessel lumen in square centimeters, and H is the vertical distance between the distal and proximal ends of the vessel segment in centimeters. For example, H can be termed positive if the distal end is above or negative if it is below the proximal end. If every term in the above expression were divided by the cross-sectional area of the vessel (in square centimeters), it would become a pressure balance equation with units of dynes per square centimeter. Pressure in the circulation is also often expressed in millimeters of mercury or centimeters of water. Approximate relationships between these units are 1 mm Hg = 1.36 cm H_2O = 1333 dyne/cm^2.

The pulsatile nature of blood flow (pulsations) is concerned largely with accelerations and vascular distentions because of the elastic nature of blood vessels and thus with conversions of kinetic and potential energy. There is, however, some conversion to thermal form because blood and vascular tissues also have viscous properties. If flow is distributed by the pulsations, additional conversions can occur in the blood (see Laminar and Turbulent Flow below). Conversions between kinetic and potential energy forms conserve the energy that can develop imbalances of pressure that pump blood. Energy converted to heat, however, is dissipated or "lost" in the sense of this direct capability. Thermal energy can affect flow indirectly by altering viscosity. In the circulation, the major loss of pressure energy is due to the viscosity of flowing blood; in particular, it is related to the resistive component of the system and the mean flow. The mean flow is the average of the pulsatile flow over the time period of the heart cycle. For mean flow, only the resistive component is involved in force-balance relations. The term *cardiac output* defines the mean flow, and this is the primary aspect of the total pulsatile flow that delivers blood to organs and tissues. In the circulation, pressure–mean flow relations in different regions vary according to the flow resistance developed by different-sized vessels in different series and parallel arrangements.

LAMINAR AND TURBULENT FLOW

Shortly beyond the root of the aorta, the pumped blood tends to stabilize into a streamline or laminar flow pattern in which each molecular fluid layer remains intact and retains its relative position in the stream. Thus the moving cylinder of fluid consists of concentric, tubular laminae that slide or shear over each other in a defined fashion. If the conduit vessel were sufficiently long and straight before any geometric or other disturbance was imposed, the fluid velocity profile would approach a parabolic form (Fig. 5.12). This is termed *fully developed flow.* Although it is not achieved in the circulation, laminar flow with flatter velocity profiles is attained. Features of laminar blood flow include the following:

1. The greatest velocity occurs at the center of the tube, and the fluid layer adjacent to the wall is considered stationary. Maximal shearing (and thus maximal thermal energy conversions) occurs near the wall. Fluid toward the center contains greater kinetic energy.

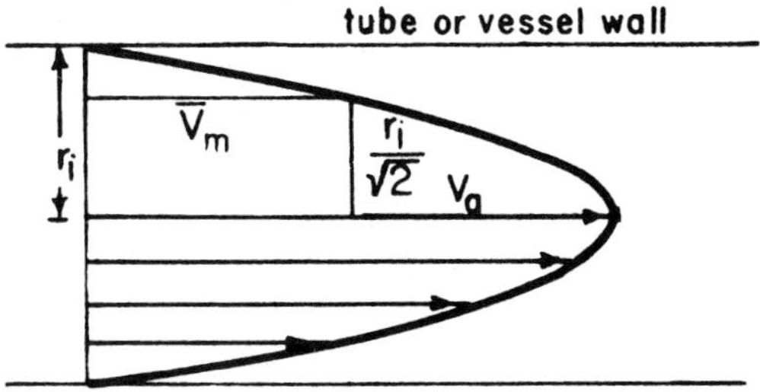

Figure 5.12. Plot of a parabolic velocity profile representing various flow velocities (v, represented by the lengths of the horizontal vectors) at different radial distances (r) measured from the center of the tube to the wall where flow is assumed to be stationary (v = O). Velocity at r (v_r) varies in accordance with $v_r = \Delta p(r_i^2 - r^2)/4L\mu$, where Δp = pressure head, L = length of tube over which this pressure difference occurs, μ = coefficient of viscosity, r_i = internal radius of tube, and r = radial distance from the center of the tube. Velocity is greatest at the central axis (v_a). At the radial distance $r_i/2^{1/2}$, $v = v_a/2$, which is also the mean velocity ($\bar{V}m$) in the tube.

2. A radial pressure gradient develops so that pressures are higher toward the wall than at the center of the tube.

3. Plasma skimming. The radial pressure gradient results in the suspended elements in blood (macromolecules, cells) moving toward the center of the vessel so that cell concentration decreases near the wall. Thus blood flowing into some branches may contain a reduced cell concentration compared with that in the main vessel (i.e., plasma is skimmed). In the abdominal aorta the relatively cell-free zone that develops near the wall results in blood with different PCVs flowing to different organs. This varies with location and function of the organs. For example, a primary function of the kidneys is to filter plasma. The kidneys receive about 20 percent of the cardiac output, which is well beyond that required to provide sufficient erythrocytes for their metabolic requirements. Thus efficiency of this organ system is increased when the renal blood consists of more plasma and fewer cells. Blood beyond the renal arteries has a larger PCV and thus the greater oxygen-carrying capacity required for the function of large leg muscles (Fig. 5.13).

When there are disturbances in a fluid system, such as are caused by the beating heart or by abrupt anatomical constriction (stenosis), dilatation (aneurysm), or vascular branching, the laminar flow pattern may be disrupted. Even in straight, long tubes if flow velocity is sufficiently high, a transient disturbance can disrupt a laminar flow pattern so that flow then persists in a disorganized manner with total, random mixing of fluid over the cross section. Such flows are termed turbulent. Transitional flow patterns that have features of both laminar and turbulent flows also occur (Fig. 5.14). Turbulent flows have flat velocity profiles and manifest a greater apparent viscosity than do identical fluids in laminar flow because of greater losses through thermal conversions in the blood.

In 1883 Reynolds recognized that the persistence of turbulent flow depends on a ratio that expresses the inertial properties to the viscous properties of the system. The ratio, known as Reynolds' number (N_R), is dimensionless and, for a cross-section of any shape, is given by

$$N_R = 4\ m\ v\ \rho/\mu$$

in which m is the "mean hydraulic depth," defined as the cross-sectional area divided by the perimeter. For a circular tube, m = *Lumen diameter.* Here v is the mean flow velocity, ρ is the fluid density, and μ is the coefficient 4 of viscosity. Reynolds' number achieves different values for different fluids. For water ($\rho = 1$, $\mu = 0.01$), turbulence is maintained when N_R exceeds 2000. For blood ($\rho = 1.05$, $\mu = 0.03 - 0.05$), the N_R does not exceed 2000 in most parts

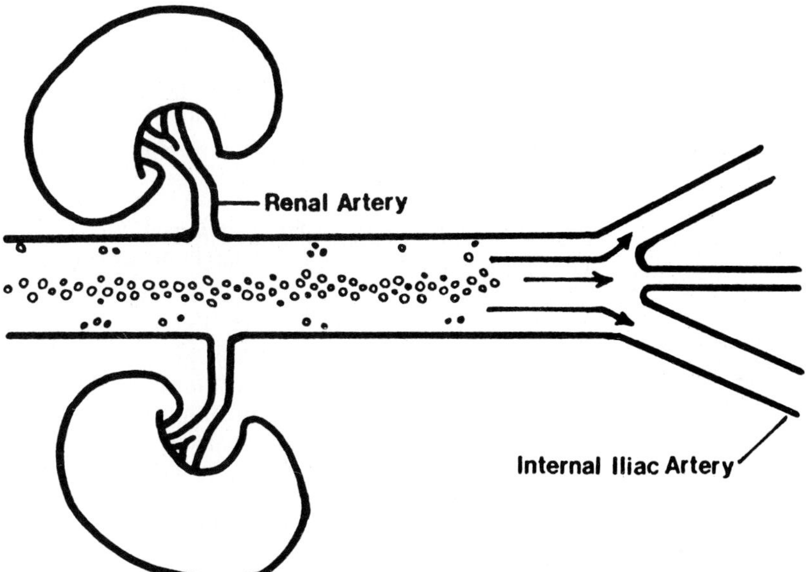

Figure 5.13. Diagram of a section of abdominal aorta to illustrate plasma skimming. The renal arteries, branching approximately orthogonal to the axis of the aorta, skim relatively cell-free plasma for filtration. Erythrocytes remaining in the aorta flow to muscles require a greater oxygen supply for their metabolic activity.

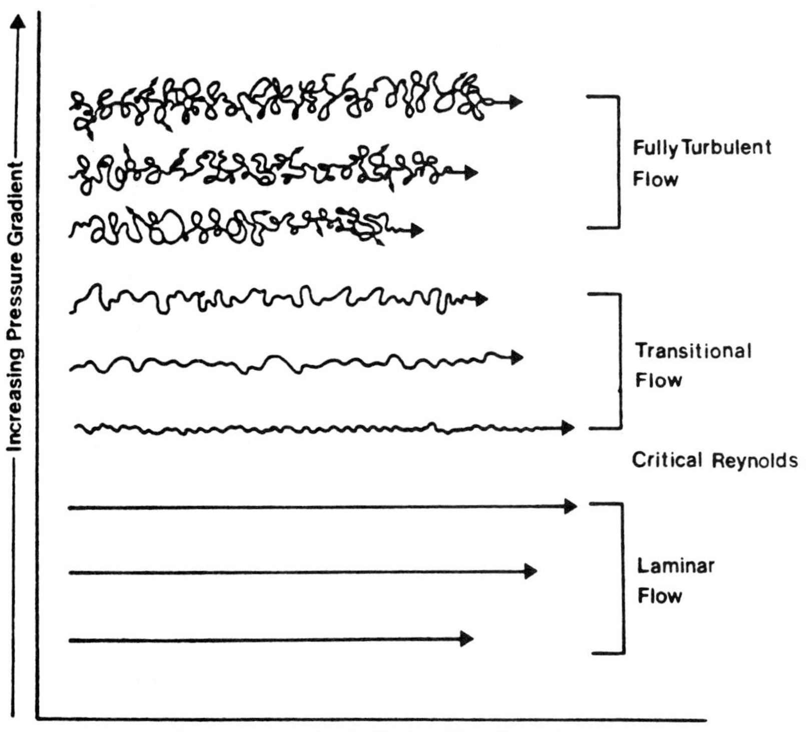

Figure 5.14. Diagram of different flow patterns. With increasing pressure gradient, flow velocity increases until the critical velocity is achieved, at which point laminar flow is disrupted. Transitional flows may exist before fully turbulent flow develops. Losses in turbulent flows reduce the flow velocity relative to that for laminar flow for a given pressure gradient.

of the circulation (Table 5.3). In large vessels such as the aorta, greater values of N_R may be achieved. In larger mammals high Reynolds numbers can extend farther into the circulation. In horses, for example, peak flow velocities of nearly 100 cm/s and an N_R on the order of 10,000 have been reported. Other factors that contribute to higher values include increased flow rates (as with exercise) and lowered viscosity (as in anemia).

Flows that are not steady or laminar can develop intermittent local circulations or vortices that may generate vibrations. If these vibrations occur at acoustic frequency and contain sufficient energy, they may produce audible sounds, such as murmurs. Conditions favorable for local disturbances with significant energy are those that increase Reynolds' number. These include increased flow velocity, large vessel diameter, stenoses or aneurysms, and decreased blood viscosity. Anemia is especially likely to alter conditions that tend toward turbulence because the PCV is an important determinant of blood viscosity. Also, the larger the species, the larger the aortic diameter and the potential for high peak flow velocity and the more likely that innocent (not related to disease) flow murmurs will be heard.

Table 5.3. Vessel diameter, blood velocity, and Reynolds' number for the systemic circulation of the dog

Vessel	Diameter (cm)	Blood velocity (cm/s)	Reynolds' number
Aorta			
Ascending	1.0	40 (mean systolic)	2360
Proximal thoracic	1.0	112 (peak)	3000–3500
Distal thoracic	0.77–0.82	114–128 (peak)	2450–2590
Abdominal	0.53–0.61	106–141 (peak)	1710–1970
Femoral	0.3	100 (peak)	1300
Saphenous	0.1	30 (peak)	80
Small mesenteric	0.005	2.1	0.28
Arteriole	0.0025	0.28	0.018
Capillary	0.0008	0.05	0.001
Abdominal vena cava	1.0	15.0 (peak)	930

From McDonald 1974, *Blood Flow in Arteries,* Williams & Wilkins, Baltimore.

THERMAL AND PRESSURE ENERGY CONVERSIONS AND RESISTANCE TO FLOW

In 1839 Hagen studied water flow in brass tubes and found that flow varied with about the fourth of the power radius and was inversely proportional to tube length. In 1846, Poiseuille, a physician known as the father of hemodynamics, studied more precisely the flow of water in narrow glass tubes (less than 1 mm in diameter) and confirmed these findings. He showed that the factors that influence the steady (nonpulsatile) laminar flow of newtonian fluids in long tubes are related to the tube length, unbalanced pressure between two points in the tube, and the fourth power of the radius. The mathematical development of the relationship for fully developed flow is usually termed the Poiseuille equation. It appears as

$$\dot{Q} = \Delta p\, \pi r^4/(8\ L\ \mu)$$

where $\dot{Q}$ is the mean flow, Δp is the pressure difference over a length of tube (L), r is the radius of the lumen, and μ is the coefficient of fluid viscosity in poises. The pressure gradient is defined as $\Delta p/L$. $\dot{Q}$ may always be written as the product of mean velocity in the tube (v) and cross-sectional area (A), regardless of the type of flow (i.e., $\dot{Q} = v\ A$).

For fully developed flow, the mean velocity is one-half of the center line velocity and occurs at a radius equal to the tube radius divided by $2^{\frac{1}{2}}$ (Fig. 5.11). Although the conditions underlying the Poiseuille expression are not fully met in the circulation, the relation applies in general if not exactly quantitatively. The most important feature of the relationship that concerns blood vessel function is that $\dot{Q}$ is proportional to r^4. Thus a change in the radius by a factor of 2 results in a change of flow by a factor of 16. This is a particularly important feature in the microcirculation, where substantial vasoconstriction can occur in arterioles. Also, since the resistance to flow manifested by a blood vessel is inversely proportional to the fourth power of its radius, the resistance of large blood vessels can become negligible, even though the blood is viscous.

The general relation between mean flow and pressure difference is: $\dot{Q} = \Delta p/R$.

Flow is seen to be directly proportional to Δp and inversely proportional to R. This is analogous to Ohm's law in electric circuits, where current flow (I) equals the potential difference (E) divided by the resistance (R)—$I = E/R$. For the Poiseuille expression, $R = 8\ L\ \mu/(\pi r^4)$, so that R is seen to be proportional to vessel length and fluid viscosity and inversely proportional to vessel radius. Since the use of R does not define details of the resistive contributors, $\dot{Q} = \Delta p/R$ applies to any laminar flow. In turbulent flow, however, random motion of the viscous fluid causes greater heat dissipation than develops in laminar flow so that, even with the same vessel and blood properties, fully turbulent flow relates more to $(\Delta p)^{1/2}$ (Fig. 5.14). In Poiseuille's experiments, resistance was constant since tube geometry and viscosity were not affected by variations in flow. As discussed above, however, blood is a complex fluid whose viscosity can depend on the particular flow circumstance, and flow is affected differently in distensible versus nondistensible tubes. Nevertheless, the nature of the flow is often unknown, and pressure and flow measurements for a particular circumstance would simply develop a value for R based on the relationship $R = \Delta p/\dot{Q}$. Thus it should be recognized that R determined in this manner may reflect not only the physical properties of the underlying system but also the flow pattern.

Conventionally, such a computation applied across the entire circulation is defined as total peripheral resistance (TPR). In the medical field, the unit of resistance is often computed in terms of pressure (1 mm Hg = 1333 dynes/cm^2) with flow in millimeters per second and expressed in peripheral resistance units (PRU), i.e.,

$$\text{PRU} = \Delta p(\text{mm Hg})/\dot{Q}[\text{ml/sec}])$$

Thus, for example, a dog with a cardiac output (mean flow) of 2 L/min and a mean systemic pressure difference between root aorta and right atrium of 100 mm Hg has a TPR = 3.0 PRU. Alternatively, for the pulmonary circulation, with a mean pressure difference of 10 mm Hg between the main pulmonary artery and the left atrium, the TPR is 0.3 PRU. Mean blood pressures vary much less with animal size than do cardiac outputs, so the relatively large number of small vessels in parallel in larger animals can be seen to develop less TPR than do the smaller number in smaller animals. For example, TPR ranges from 2000 to 9000 dyne-sec/cm^5 for the dog, whereas it ranges from 11,500 to 12,000 dyne-sec/cm^5 for the rabbit.

The number and arrangement of vessels affect total resistance of a vascular bed. In the circulation, blood vessels appear in both series and parallel arrangement with each serial segment comprising vessels in parallel. For example, in Fig. 5.2A, each serial segment defined by the vertical lines consists of vessels in parallel arrangement. The total resistance of vessels in series (R_{ts}) is simply the sum of their individual resistances, i.e., $R_{ts} = R_1 + R_2 + \ldots\ldots\ldots + R_n$.

For vessels arranged in parallel, the total flow across all the vessels equals the sum of the individual vessel flows. The total resistance of the parallel vessels (R_{tp}) equals the reciprocal of the sum of all reciprocal resistances of the individual vessels, i.e., $R_{tp} = 1/(1/R_1 + 1/R_2 + \ldots\ldots\ldots 1/R_n)$. Thus R_{tp} is always less than the R for any individual vessel.

The resistance across an organ system can be computed similarly to that for the entire circulation (i.e., with use of the pressure drop across the organ system and the flow through the system). In an ideal electrical system, circuits in parallel with other circuits divide total current (flow) between themselves in accordance with individual resistances, but all the parallel circuits have the same voltage drop if they begin and end at common junctions. Since the large conduit vessels themselves have relatively low resistance, this is roughly approximated in the circulation (see Fig. 5.1). Thus the mean systemic pressure drop approximates pressure drop across individual systemic organs. Table 5.4 lists the resistance in PRUs for the parallel circulations shown in Fig. 5.1 as computed with a mean systemic pressure drop of 100 mm Hg and a cardiac output of 2 L/min. From these data, one can also determine systemic TPR as done above (TPR = 100 mm Hg/33.3 ml/s = 3.0 PRU), i.e.

$$\text{TPR} = 1/(1/20 + 1/60 + 1/60 + 1/20 + 1/10 + 1/15 + 1/30) = 3.0\ \text{PRU}$$

Table 5.4. Regional flow, flow rates, and peripheral resistance units (PR of blood)

Region	Percent flow	Flow (ml/s)	PR
Brain	15	5.00	20
Bronchial	5	1.66	60
Coronary	5	1.66	60
Muscle (resting)	15	5.00	20
Splanchnic	30	10.00	10
Renal	20	6.66	15
Skin, skeletal	10	3.33	30
Total	100	33.3	

KINETIC AND POTENTIAL ENERGY CONVERSIONS

The kinetic energy (KE) of a fluid particle is equivalent to the work (force × distance) done on the particle by virtue of its motion or translation over a length of vessel in a time period (t). The velocity (v) of a particle with uniform acceleration (a) from rest is a function of that time, i.e., $v = a\,t$. Under such circumstances, the average velocity of the particle in that time period is v/2. The distance (L) traveled (translated) in this time is $L = (v/2)\,t$ or $L = (v/2)\,(v/a) = v^2/(2\,a)$. From the force balance relation it is noted that the force associated with the kinetic energy is M a. Thus $KE = M\,a\,L = M\,v^2/2$ or, on a per unit volume or energy density basis, $KE/vol = \rho v^2/2$.

The potential energy (PE) is equivalent to the work that is not related to the existing velocity; i.e., it is either work accomplished to attain a position or height (H) from a reference by overcoming gravitational force or work by forces other than those related to gravity. The total energy density (E_d) at a point in the vessel for the inviscid circumstance, therefore, is

$$E_d = KE/vol + PE/vol = \rho v^2/2 + p$$

Since, with flow of completely inviscid fluids, no thermal conversions (losses) occur, E_d remains unchanged. Note also that, in such a case, the velocity profile remains flat, even if flow is not turbulent, since viscous drag does not exist between molecular layers of the fluid. If the flow of incompressible fluid remains constant in a tube (i.e., no branches exist in that section), axial flow persists because of the kinetic component, even if adverse, *local* pressure gradients arise. For example, with an obstruction, stenosis, or dilatation in such a tube, fluid kinetic energy and fluid pressure energy continuously convert between themselves so as to maintain E_d constant on any given streamline. At an obstruction, where all local flow ceases, all kinetic energy at the region may convert to pressure, which can thus achieve a value higher than surrounding pressures. Such regions are termed "stagnation" regions. In the circulation, degrees of stagnation can exist for both physiological (e.g., relating to the sinuses of Valsalva) and pathological (e.g., relating to atheromatous plaques) reasons.

Figure 5.15 illustrates a vessel that has both a stenosis (constriction) and an aneurysm (dilatation) and is oriented so that any two points on a streamline are at the same H (the term ρgH is ignored). Regardless of axial location, E_d on the streamline is constant. If no branches exist, total flow must also be equal at all sites, regardless of cross-sectional areas (A). Thus, for the planes marked by a,b,c one has

$$p_a + \rho v_a^2 = p_b + \rho v_b^2 = p_c + \rho v_c^2$$

$$\dot{Q} = v_a\,A_a = v_b\,A_b = v_c\,A_c$$

Because of constant $\dot{Q}$ and since $A_c < A_a < A_b$, one must have $v_c > v_a > v_b$. Therefore, because of constant E_d, we also have $p_c < p_a < p_b$. These conversions of local pressure energy with kinetic energy express the Bernoulli principle, which also appears in many circumstances outside the circulation, where the velocity of a given mass of air or fluid is altered (e.g., Venturi tubes, airfoils, etc.). In an abnormal aneurysm the intraluminal pressures, and consequently the wall tension, can be increased and thus exacerbate the problem by progressive distention of the arterial wall. In such cases the wall structure may also be weakened by disease. Conversely, in the stenotic region, the lower pressure is less

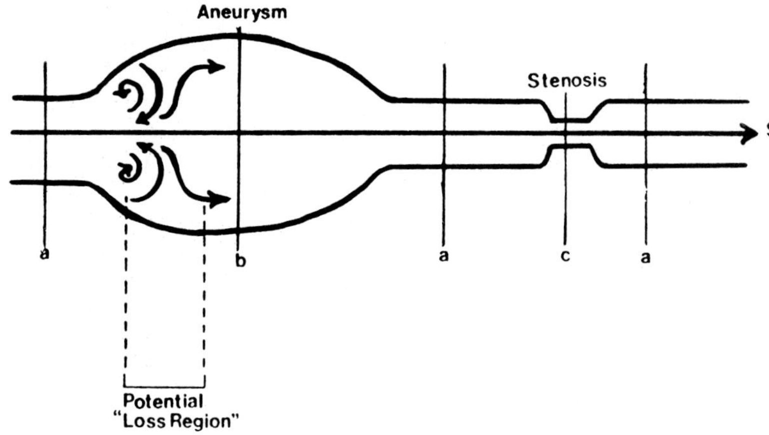

Figure 5.15. Tubular section containing a dilatation (aneurysm) and a constriction (stenosis). Under laminar flow conditions, flow velocity is less at *b* than at *a* which in turn is less than at *c*. Pressure at *b* is greater than at *a*, which in turn is greater than at *c*. An area where pressure energy is converted to thermal energy is called a "loss region." If a sufficient loss region develops, these pressure relations can change.

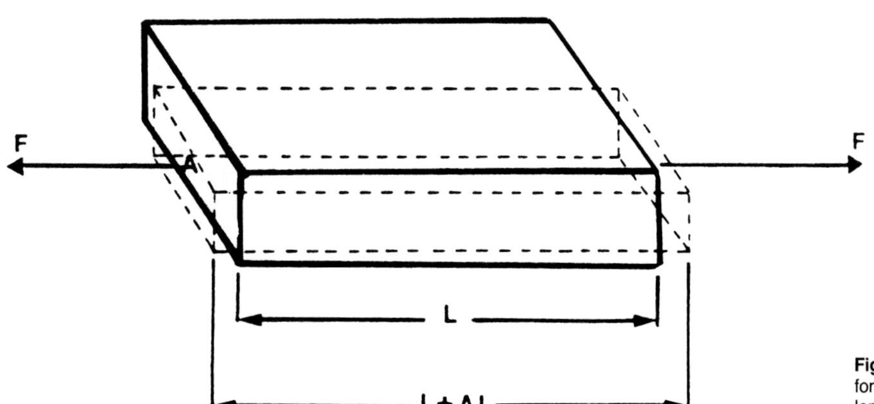

Figure 5.16. Section of material under a tensile force (F) applied over cross section (A). The initial length (L) is elongated to the new length L + ΔL.

effective in enlarging the lumen. With stenoses of an artery or of valves, such as the cardiac semilunar valves, if blood flow has not been decreased, the velocity of flow is increased. This can develop a jet with high kinetic energy that may be interrupted by a downstream region (effective stagnation site) where local high pressure develops because of energy conversion to the potential form. If the site is not designed to accommodate the high pressure, the consequence can be an abnormal enlargement of the region (poststenotic dilatation). In addition to the effect of pressure variations due to energy conversions, pressure can also have adverse effects in dilated regions because tensile stresses induced in the wall by the transmural pressure gradient vary in accordance with the size of the lumen. This is discussed in the next section.

The Bernoulli principle suggests the direction of site-dependent pressure alterations in Fig. 5.15. In reality, however, the situation may be complicated by other factors. In the circulation, for example, pressure in an aneurysm may not show an observable increase because of the viscous blood and losses due to thermal conversion. The degree of conversion is particularly subject to the entrance geometry of the aneurysm which, if abrupt, can cause a substantial "loss region," where the development of local fluid circulations or disruption of laminar flow and turbulence magnify conversion of pressure energy to the thermal form (Fig. 5.15, region upstream of plane b). As with Reynolds' number elsewhere, larger diameters and higher flow velocities favor the development of a loss region. Pulsatile flow can also enhance this phenomenon.

PROPERTIES OF BLOOD VESSELS

Many solid materials manifest elastic properties, but the degree can vary greatly. Elasticity is the property that restores the original shape to a deformed material after removal of the deforming force. Small deformations of vascular wall material are generally related to the deforming force, essentially by a constant or scale factor (termed elastic modulus) that quantifies the elastic property. Such linear behavior (constant modulus) of elastic materials is explained by Hooke's law. The modulus is usually expressed in terms of stress (i.e., the force per unit area of material to which the force is applied) and strain, which expresses the deformation in terms of a change in dimension with respect to the original dimension. Thus, for the case of a rectangular section of wall material with surface area A, initial length L, under tensile force F (Fig. 5.16),

$$F/A = E\,\Delta L/L$$

where F/A is the stress, and ΔL/L is the strain. E is the measure of elasticity or elastic modulus and takes on units of stress (dynes per square centimeter) since strain is dimensionless. The term *compliance* is often used to express the concept of the reciprocal of E or strain/stress.

Vascular wall material is not homogeneous but is composed of three principal types of tissue (smooth muscle, collagen, elastin) that support the transmural pressure, each with its own elastic property. Thus the manifestation of E for the wall material is a composite of all contributions. Approximate values of E for the different components are given in Table 5.5. Smooth muscle is so compliant with respect to collagen and elastin that it participates least in "load bearing" or wall stress equilibration with the intraluminal pressure (stress) in conduit vessels. The structure and arrangement of collagen and elastin are such that in the undistended vessel elastin bears much of the stress. As the vessel wall is distended, more of the load is transferred to collagen fibers. Since the E of collagen is greater than that of elastin, the wall material normally appears more com-

Table 5.5. Major components of arterial wall

	Young's modulus (static) $E = \frac{\text{stress}}{\text{strain}}$
Collagen	$30–100 \times 10^6$
Elastin	6×10^6
Smooth Muscle	$0.1–2 \times 10^6$

pliant when the wall is less distended. Thus the value of E for the wall material is not constant but depends on the state of distention of the vessel (i.e., on transmural pressure). Since the linear relation (constant E) as expressed by Hooke's law does not hold over the range of physiological pressures, the wall material is described as nonlinear (Fig. 5.17A). Additional complications are presented when one considers the compliance of the whole vessel (i.e., as a structure rather than just in terms of wall material). To encompass all features of the structure, it is useful to consider the volumetric compliance. A convenient convention is to consider length unchanging and to express volumetric compliance in terms of change in vessel cross-sectional area (ΔA) per transmural pressure difference (Δp_t). In this case the strain is developed as $\Delta A/A$ and volumetric compliance as $\Delta A/(A\ \Delta p_t)$.

As one moves more peripherally, vessel walls become relatively less compliant, especially at higher tensions, because the relative quantity of collagen to elastin in the wall increases. This feature of the circulation persists until the arterioles are reached, where walls are dominated by smooth muscle. Also, the ratio of wall thickness to lumen diameter increases, although both the diameter and the wall thickness themselves decrease (Fig. 5.17B). This ratio is important in the determination of the stresses developed in the wall and is another reason for reduced apparent volumetric compliance of peripheral conduit vessels relative to proximal vessels.

The relation, $T = pr/h$, is commonly called the law of Laplace although it dates back to Bernoulli in the seventeenth century. The expression shows that for any given transmural pressure (p), the wall tension (T) will be proportional to the radius (r) of the vessel and inversely proportional to the wall thickness (h). Thus the smaller, circular vessels can behave as though they were less compliant volumetrically solely on the basis of geometry. For this reason, small, very thin-walled vessels in the microcirculation, such as arterioles and capillaries, can withstand relatively substantial pressures (Figs. 5.3, 5.4).

In addition to the size of the vessel, which provides a

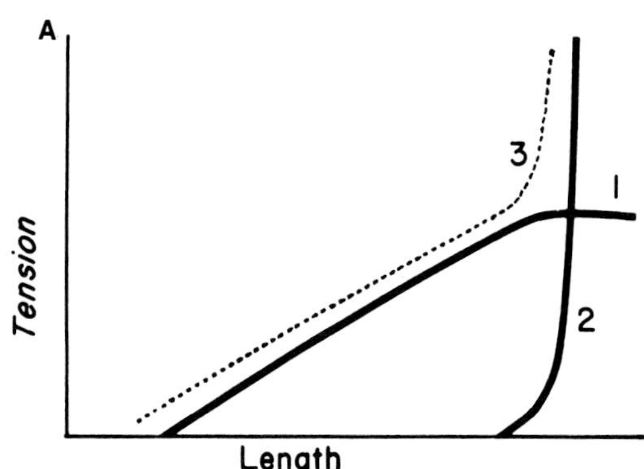

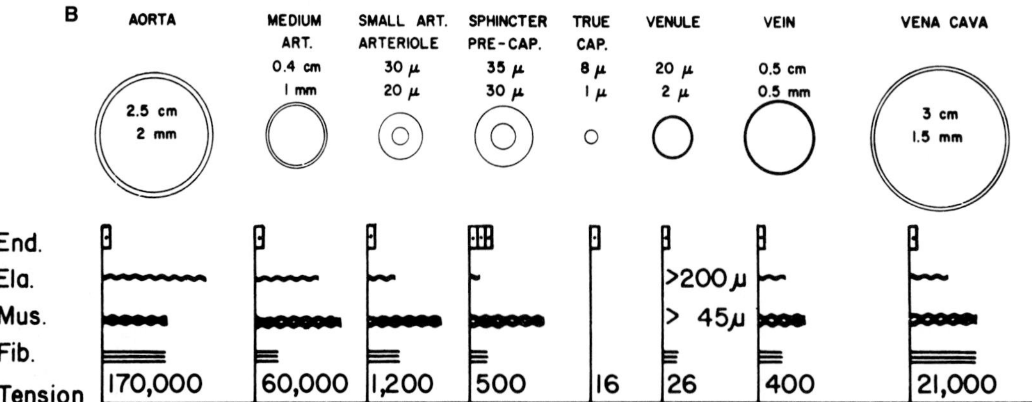

Figure 5.17. (*A*) Length-tension diagrams of (1) elastin, (2) collagen, and (3) elastin and collagen combined. (*B*) Lumen diameters, wall thickness, relative amounts of wall tissue constituents, and wall stress in various blood vessels. End, Endothelium; Ela, elastin; Mus, smooth muscle; Fib, collagen fibers; Tension, tensile stress (dynes/cm^2); Art, artery; Pre-Cap, precapillary. (From Wolf 1952, *Science*, 115:243–44, and Burton 1954, *Physiol. Rev.* 34:619–42.)

direct, geometric contribution to volumetric compliance, the cross-sectional shape is an important factor. Essentially three circumstances can be found in mammalian systems: (1) systemic arteries that remain circular even if unloaded ($p_t = 0$), (2) veins that can collapse when unloaded, and (3) major pulmonary arteries that assume oval but patent cross sections when unloaded. All other factors being equal, the more eccentric the cross section, the greater will be the volumetric compliance. This is because an eccentric cross-sectional area can increase in response to an increase in transmural pressure gradient by a primarily bending mode deformation rather than by wall stretch (i.e., the cross section increases with minimal change in perimeter length). Thin-walled vessels in an eccentric state can have such high geometric compliance that the wall material itself becomes insignificant in that (eccentric) operating range. As the cross-sectional area becomes more circular, wall material properties become more dominant in determining volumetric compliance. With continuing increase in cross section, geometry can again become a significant contributor because of Laplace law relations. Figure 5.18 illustrates these geometric relations for conditions of constant and increasing wall material moduli (E) with distention.

Veins offer examples of vessels with walls that have a high collagen/elastin ratio whose moduli may be greater than those of some arteries. Nevertheless, considerably greater volumetric compliance may be achieved at low transmural pressure. For normal transmural pressure cycles, the major pulmonary vessels manifest a volumetric compliance that is achieved in the systemic circulation by a length about 10 times greater. Thus these high-compliance vessels can accommodate substantial alterations in stroke volume with little change in pressure, which would not be the case if their construction were similar to that of systemic arteries. Since functioning lung tissue in mammals is much closer to the right side of the heart than are organs in the systemic circulation to the left side of the heart, the designs of both systems' conduit vessels serve to isolate or uncoupie the heart from the high resistances in the microcirculations.

PULSATILE PRESSURE AND FLOW

Although the steady pressure-flow relations discussed in previous sections carry important information about blood distribution in the mammal, they represent only a portion of the phenomena encountered in the circulatory system. The pulsatile nature of cardiac activity with accompanying pressures and flows is not represented. To also account for pulsatile features, Frank, in 1895 and 1927, proposed a model for the circulation that conceived of the heart as pumping into an elastic reservoir. This reservoir was called a *Windkessel,* the German word for air chamber or compression chamber. Instead of air providing the compliant medium, however, its equivalent was considered to be compliant vessels that included the aorta and its more proximal, larger branches. Beyond these, the vessels were considered to be essentially inelastic. Fig. 5.19 shows a schematic drawing of a Windkessel model. The provision of such a chamber explained how the heart could pump intermittent stroke volumes into the vasculature without having to accelerate the entire mass of incompressible blood that, if no compliance existed, would otherwise come to rest during each diastole. Since inertial force is the product of mass (represented by the blood density and volume accelerated) times acceleration, the Windkessel design limits the cardiac force required for cyclical pumping of blood. The high compliance embodied in the air chamber permits ejection of a relatively small volume of blood (stroke volume) at high acceleration during systole (by compression of the air) and

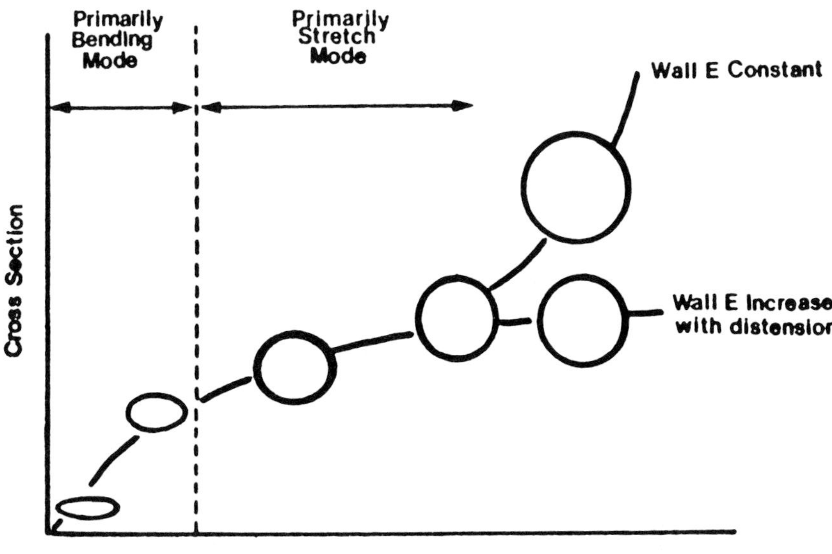

Figure 5.18. Plot illustrating the manner in which a collapsed vessel increases cross-sectional area with increasing transmural pressure gradient. In the bending mode, small increases in transmural pressure gradient result in large changes of cross-sectional area (high volumetric compliance) with minimal regard to wall material modulus. In the stretch mode, if the modulus is a constant, higher volumetric compliance develops with increasing cross section. If the wall modulus increases with wall stretch, a stable cross section of the vessel can be established after the bending mode.

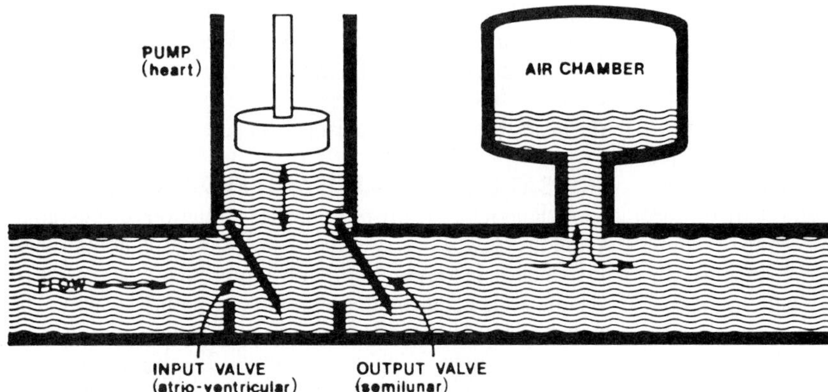

Figure 5.19. Schematic drawing of a Windkessel model of the circulation. During the slow upstroke of the piston in the pump, the input value opens and the output valve closes. Fluid is drawn into the pump cylinder. During the rapid downstroke, the input value closes and the output valve opens. The stroke volume is pumped preferentially into the air chamber because of the high compliance in this region and the large inertial property of the mass of fluid in the remaining vasculature. During the next slow upstroke, the slow expansion of the air in the chamber moves the fluid in the chamber downstream.

distribution of blood more slowly to the periphery during cardiac diastole (as the air expands). During diastole, semilunar valves are closed and the compliant vascular walls return to initial dimensions, thus forcing blood downstream. Low force is required during systole because the high acceleration is imparted to a relatively small mass. Low force is also adequate during diastole because a relatively low acceleration is imparted to the relatively large mass of blood in the vasculature.

A limitation of the Windkessel model is that it does not represent the manner in which pressure and flow pulses are propagated to the periphery. If vessels beyond the aorta were inelastic, the speed of pulse propagation beyond the aorta could, theoretically, approach infinity since blood is virtually incompressible. Thus the model represents compliance of the circulatory system in a lumped, rather than in its actually distributed, form.

In the natural environment transfer of energy occurs when equilibrium is perturbed. Periodic perturbations or oscillations of interest in the cardiovascular system include electrical (such as those that develop the electrocardiogram), acoustic (such as those that develop the heart sounds), and hemodynamic events (represented by pressure and flow pulses). Regardless of the nature of the oscillation, however, the shape of the oscillation wave form can be expressed conventionally in basic terms (i.e., as a mean value on which is superimposed a sum of sinusoidal oscillations). The shape of a pressure pulsation, for example, could be viewed as a compound wave form that consists simply of a mean value and the sum of different frequency oscillations or harmonics, much as one would view a musical note, the difference being that the frequencies differ. The lowest frequency or harmonic contained in a pulse is termed the fundamental frequency and in the circulation is, in fact, the heart rate. Note that although *heart rate* is conventional terminology, a more accurate descriptor would be *heart frequency*. Harmonics are integral multiples of the fundamental frequency. Frequency is expressed in terms of cycles per second, usually expressed as hertz. The time required to complete a cycle is called the period and is simply the reciprocal of the frequency. This manner of representing a pulse uniquely in terms of a mean value, fundamental frequency, and harmonics can be accomplished by a mathematical procedure known as Fourier analysis. An example of a pressure pulse wave form decomposed into its harmonics is shown in Fig. 5.20.

Each harmonic is a pure sine wave that oscillates about the mean value. Its maximum or minimum value is termed its modulus, and the position of a point on the wave with respect to some reference is given by a phase angle in degrees or radians (Fig. 5.21). A sine wave describes a complete cycle over 360 degrees. The relationship of the different harmonics to each other is fixed for each pulse and is expressed in terms of phase with respect to any convenient reference point. Figure 5.21 illustrates relationships

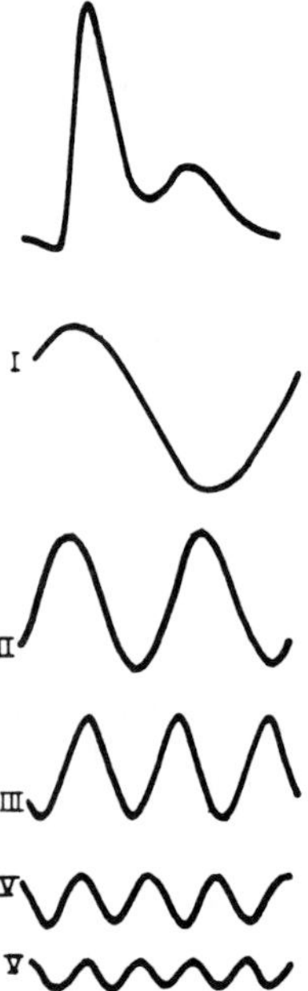

Figure 5.20. Pressure pulse from a peripheral artery and its first five harmonics. (From Taylor 1966, *Aust. Ann. Med.* 15:71–86.)

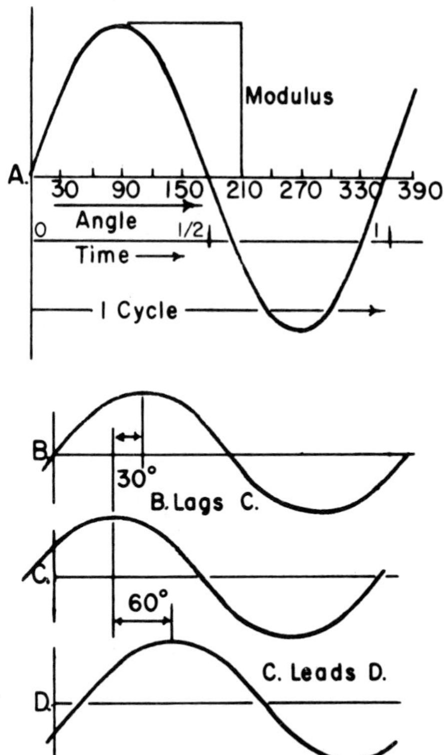

Figure 5.21. (*A*) Simple harmonic motion; a sine wave illustrating the definition of modulus. (*B, C, D*) Sine wave illustrating the definition of phase lag and phase lead. (From Taylor 1966, *Aust. Ann. Med.* 15:71–86.)

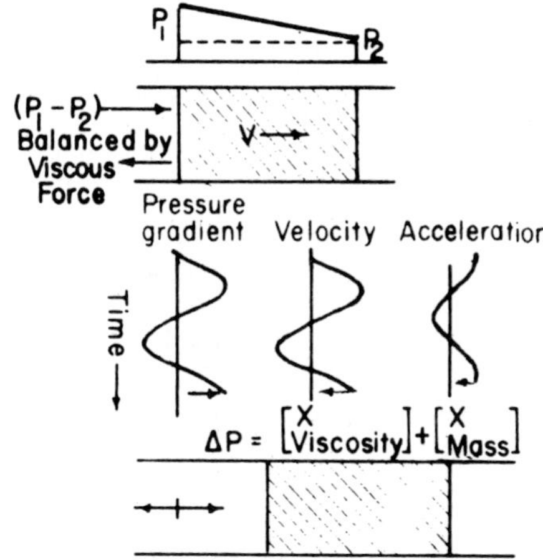

Figure 5.22. (*Top*) The relationship between a steady pressure difference ($p_1 - p_2$ or Δp) and flow velocity (v). In steady flow the pressure gradient that imparts movement of the fluid is entirely balanced by the frictional or viscous resistance (force) to flow. Inertial properties of the fluid are not involved, since flow is constant (i.e., no accelerations occur). (*Bottom*) The relationship between unbalanced pressure (Δp), flow velocity, and acceleration when Δp varies with time. Here Δp acts against both the viscous resistance and inertia as the fluid mass is accelerated. Since Δp is oscillatory, flow velocity and acceleration are also oscillatory but with a phase lag. If the oscillatory Δp passes through zero, flow direction may also reverse in an oscillatory fashion. This depends on the frequency of oscillation, viscosity, and inertial properties of the system. (From Taylor 1966, *Aust. Ann. Med.* 15:71–86.)

between three sine waves where the chosen reference is the zero value of sine wave B. The nature of a pulse, relationships between pulses, and propagation of pulses can be analyzed according to the characteristics of the harmonic components.

In steady flow, as defined by the Poiseuille equation, the pressure drop or difference ($p_1 - p_2$) or gradient *(p_l* (distance between p_1 and p_2)/, $- P_2$), is constant (Fig. 5.22 top) and balanced only by the viscous resistance to flow. In a pulsatile flow system it is the mean flow value that is the steady flow corollary for this resistance. With pulsatile flow, the pressure gradient varies with time and, in its most simple form, is a sinusoidal oscillation (Fig. 5.22 bottom). A more complex, cyclic gradient (compound wave form) is developed by the systolic-diastolic cardiac activity. A pressure gradient that varies with time in a stiff tube, such as seen in Fig. 5.22 bottom, not only acts against the viscous resistance but also accelerates the fluid mass, and thus both kinetic and thermal energy conversions occur. If, unlike that seen in Fig. 5.22, the pressure gradient were a transient occurring only once (i.e., rising to a peak value and falling to zero), fluid would be placed in motion, but in a viscous system it would eventually come to rest. Once in motion, fluid continues to move in the direction accelerated (even though the pressure gradient falls to zero) until resistive forces overcome the inertial forces developed by the momentum of the moving fluid. Thus blood flow follows Newton's laws of motion.

The pulsatile flow that is achieved in the circulation depends not only on frequency (f) but also on fluid density (ρ), viscosity (μ), and tube radius (r). Frequency and density become contributors because of inertial forces that develop in the pulsatile system. These four factors are related in the form of a dimensionless parameter (α) that characterizes the oscillatory flow system:

$$\alpha = r\,(2\,\pi\,f\,\rho/\mu)^{1/2}$$

Here α is used in a complex relationship to calculate oscillatory flow from an oscillating pressure gradient.

For steady flow (or mean flow in a pulsatile system), the pressure gradient (or mean pressure gradient in the pulsatile system) is related by the resistance due to viscosity. In the pulsatile system, where resistive, compliant, and inertial properties are all manifested, the compound wave form that is the pressure gradient is related to the compound flow wave form by all of these properties. *Impedance* is the term used for the relationship that encompasses all three properties. As resistance has its analogue in electrical systems for direct current (Ohm's law), impedance has its analogue in electrical circuits for alternating current. Since compound wave forms are constituted with different frequency harmonics, impedance is not single-valued but, rather, is dependent on frequency and includes for each frequency a value for magnitude (modulus) and phase. That is, the ratio of a particular frequency harmonic of pressure to the corresponding frequency harmonic of flow yields modulus and phase values of impedance that can differ from that derived with other frequency harmonics.

Since it is system properties that are manifested in the impedance, an overall assessment of the state of a system can be gleaned from the ratio of pressure and flow pulses (harmonic by harmonic) obtained at the input to a system. Impedance thus obtained is called input impedance. Figure 5.23 shows a plot of input impedance of the arterial system of a dog. The zero frequency value is derived from the mean pressure/flow ratio. Since the resistive properties of large vessels are minimal (primarily because of large radii), this value essentially represents peripheral resistance. The shape of pressure and flow wave forms and of impedance modulus and phase plots are generally similar in mammals of all species studied, which include large variation in body size (e.g., rabbit to horse). In all cases, the minimal modulus value is approached at the normal heart rate (or fundamental frequency) for the particular animal and remains low for higher frequencies. The lower the impedance values, the lower is the energy requirement for the heart to pump blood.

For the systemic circulation, the work required to develop the pulsatile component of flow at normal heart rate is about 5 to 15 percent of total left ventricular work. This relatively low value reflects the low impedance to oscillatory components of the pulse. The input impedance of the pulmonary circulation has, in general, a configuration similar to that of the systemic circulation, but the zero frequency value is much lower than that of the systemic circulation because the cyclic mean pressure is lower and cardiac output is essentially the same. Because of the low mean pressure–stroke volume product (work) in the pulmonary circulation, oscillatory work can be more than 50 percent of total right ventricular work.

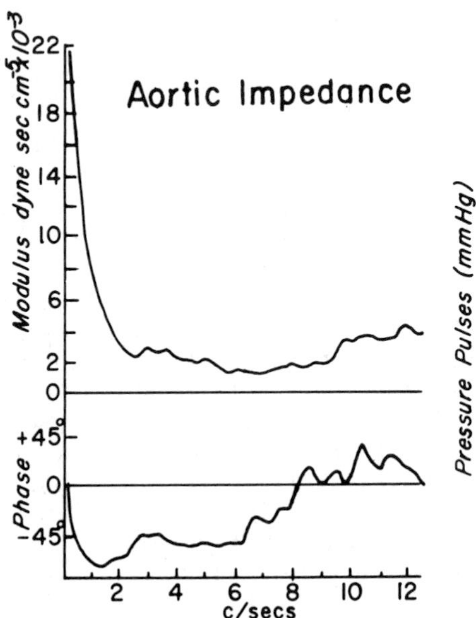

Figure 5.23. Modulus and phase of the input impedance of the arterial system of a dog measured at the ascending aorta. The peripheral resistance (modulus at 0 cps) falls steeply to an almost constant value above 1.5 to 2.0 cps. Phase represents the angle between the harmonics of flow and pressure (see Fig. 5.21). By convention, phase angle is negative when flow leads pressure. In the ascending aorta flow leads pressure for the lower-frequency harmonics. (From Taylor 1966, *Aust. Ann. Med.* 15:71–86.)

PULSE WAVE PROPAGATION

Oscillations introduced by the heart appear as wave forms that propagate (i.e., are transmitted) through the tissues in accordance with the nature of the oscillation (mechanical, electrical, magnetic) and respective properties of the tissues. Of particular interest in the circulation are the pulses of pressure that propagate in the walls of the blood vessels. Since the walls of blood vessels are elastic, the speed of propagation or pulse wave velocity is not infinite. Because the velocity of propagation in an elastic tube is finite, differences in pressure appear between two sites, even in close spatial proximity, at a point in time. This difference establishes an oscillating pressure gradient that develops an oscillating flow pulse. Figure 5.24 illustrates the generation of such a pressure gradient that derives from subtraction at each instant of the value of the downstream pulse from the upstream pulse. The general shape of the flow pulse can appear much like the shape of the pressure gradient.

In the conduit vessels of the circulation, pressure pulse waves propagate with a velocity about 10 times greater than the mean blood velocity. More specifically, the system is such that the propagation velocity of each harmonic of the pulse depends on its frequency, and velocities range from about 5 to 15 m/sec. Since the volumetric compliance of peripheral vessels is less than that of proximal vessels, the wave velocity in mammals can increase about threefold between the aortic arch and the periphery. The shape of a pressure pulse at any site in the circulation also differs from its shape at other sites. Wave shape develops from the summation of the constituent harmonics, each with its own modulus and phase relation. Thus alteration of shape occurs for a number of reasons, including (1) harmonic dispersion (frequency-dependent altering phase relations) as each harmonic propagates at its own velocity, (2) frequency-dependent conversions between pressure energy and kinetic energy that result in site-dependent amplitude alterations, (3) frequency-dependent attenuations—i.e., amplitude reduction because of energy conversions to thermal form (heat losses), (4) frequency-dependent reflections of the harmonics. This latter is a particularly important feature of mammalian circulations, but all factors are subject to the manner in which nonlinear, frequency-dependent system

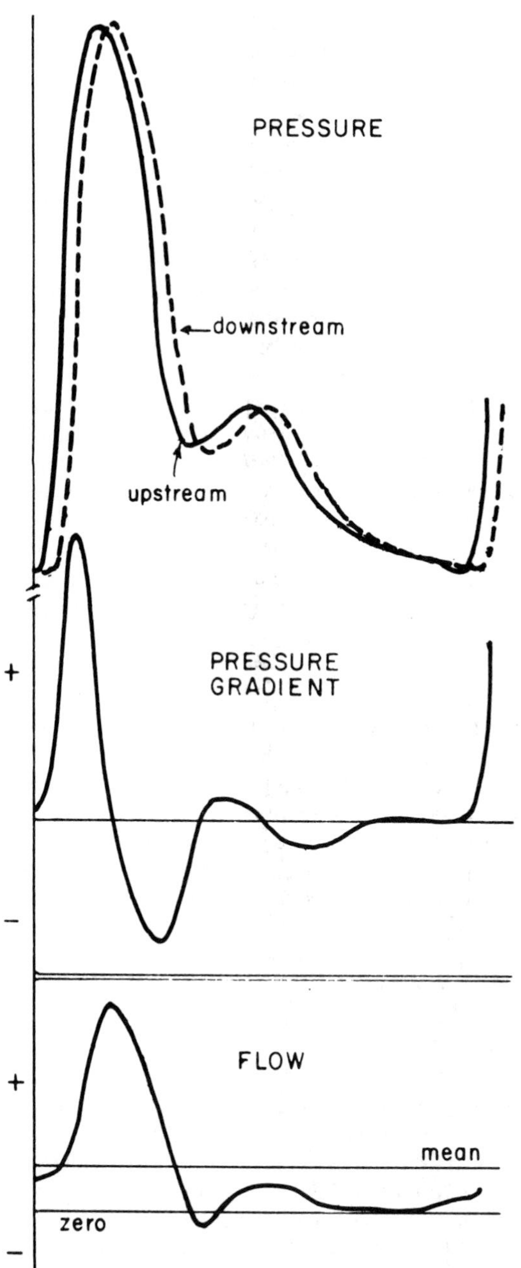

Figure 5.24. Generation of a pressure gradient by a propagating pulse wave and resultant flow pulse as appears in the femoral artery of a dog. Note small reversal of flow (below zero). (From Taylor 1966, *Aust. Ann. Med.* 15:71–86.)

components interact with the propagating pulses. In general, a pulse at any site should be considered to be the sum of all harmonics that propagate antegrade (toward the periphery) plus all harmonics that propagate retrograde (toward the heart) that are reflected from all peripheral sites.

In mammalian circulations an increasing pulse pressure is seen as one moves from the heart toward the periphery. Thus systolic peak blood pressure measured at a peripheral artery will be higher than more central pressures (e.g., root aorta) (Fig. 5.2D, Fig. 5.25). This is primarily due to reflections. An understanding of this phenomenon can be gained if one considers a simple system, such as a totally inviscid system that consists of a long elastic tube filled with incompressible fluid. There is no mean flow, but upstream one introduces a single, transient oscillation so that a pressure pulse is propagated antegrade (downstream) in the wall of the tube. At some point downstream the tube is terminated by a complete occlusion. As the pulse arrives at this site, it is completely reflected onto itself. Thus here the sum of the antegrade and retrograde components results in a doubling of the pulse amplitude. The reflected pulse continues to propagate retrograde with an amplitude equal to that of the original antegrade pulse because, without viscosity, there is no attenuation. The ratio of the reflected to the antegrade pulse is termed the reflection coefficient (C_R); therefore, in this example, $C_R = +1$. The opposite would be the case if the system terminated with the tube completely open to the atmosphere. Since atmospheric pressure can be taken as reference zero, pressure is always zero at the termination. Thus the sum of the arriving antegrade pressure pulse with its reflection at this termination must equal zero. Therefore the reflected pulse must be a negative pressure excursion whose amplitude is equal to that of the antegrade pulse. In fact, if the retrograde-propagating pulse were measured upstream of the termination this would be seen to be the case. For this circumstance, $C_R = -1$. In actuality, systems are more complex and C_R can vary between $+1$ and -1. In the circulation, it is dependent on the vasoconstrictive state. In the normal circulation in the resting mammal, C_R has been determined to be $+0.7$ to $+0.8$;

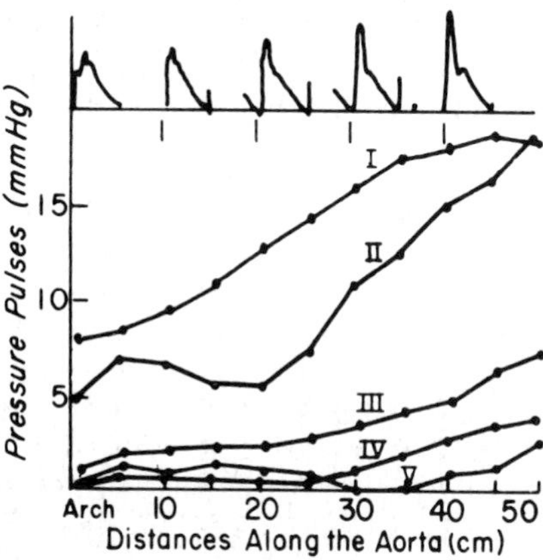

Figure 5.25. (*Top*) Pressure pulses recorded along the aorta of a dog from the arch to the femoral artery; distance given in centimeters. Pulse pressure increases with distance, and a secondary wave develops on the descending limb. (*Bottom*) Amplitudes of the first five harmonic components of these waves. Note that the relative energy content of more peripheral pulses is more concentrated in the lower-frequency harmonics (e.g., I, II). (From Taylor 1966, *Aust. Ann. Med.* 15:71–86.)

this implies that the periphery is established as more of a close termination that tends to maintain blood pressure.

An important design feature of the circulation is that reflective properties (arising because of system inhomogeneities, such as altering vessel compliances, branching sites, vasoactive sites, etc.) are less for antegrade-propagating pulses than for retrograde-propagating pulses. Consequently, pulse energy transmits preferentially toward the periphery. That is, reflected waves propagating retrograde toward the heart encounter substantial reflective properties that again reflect them toward the periphery. During all transmissions and reflections, attenuation occurs. Because viscous losses are greater for higher-frequency components of a pulse, the high-frequency content of more peripheral pulses is less than that of more proximal pulses, so that relatively more of their total pulse energy is contained in the low-frequency harmonics. Thus peripheral pulses appear smoother. Figure 5.25 illustrates pressure pulse amplifications, wave shapes, and relative energy distribution among pulse harmonics at different sites in the circulatory system. A consequence of the relatively low root aortic pressure seen in these figures is that the peak pressure required by the heart for ejection can be lower and is not directly dependent on the peripheral vasoactive state. The higher pulse pressure at the periphery, however, is advantageous for rapid flow responses (e.g., with arteriolar vasodilation) and blood flow distributions in the microcirculation.

Associated with the increase in peripheral pulse pressure is the appearance of a secondary wave in the descending portion of the wave form. This is not a transmission of the small incisura observed just after the peak in the root aortic pressure pulse. The high frequencies that are responsible for that manifestation are largely attenuated during transmission to the periphery. The secondary wave, which is also manifested in the aortic pulse, has been attributed to a second appearance of the high-energy, low-frequency components that have been reflected at the periphery and then again more centrally, making a complete round trip of the arterial system.

High-frequency harmonics in a compound pulse wave define, to a large extent, the initial rise of the pressure wave form from its baseline. This is known as the "foot" of the pulse. Since this portion of the pulse is not greatly affected by reflections from the periphery (high-frequency components having been attenuated during transmission to the periphery), it can be used to estimate pulse wave velocity. That is, the time required for antegrade transmission of this portion (foot) of the pulse from one site to another (foot-to-foot velocity) is an estimate of pulse velocity least affected by alteration of the wave form due to reflections. This measurement can provide a crude assessment of the compliant properties, and thus the degree of normalcy, of the system between the sites of measurements of the pulses.

Although the discussion in this section centers about the propagation of the pressure pulse, other oscillations or pulsations in the cardiovascular system follow similar physical laws. Each form of pulsation (mechanical, electrical) propagates in accordance with the tissue properties' effects on the specific pulse. Thus, for example, if a mechanical pulsation frequency were greater than 20 to 30 Hz, it could be perceived as sound by a stethoscope placed at different sites on the animal torso. The nature of the detected acoustic oscillations will differ, depending on the tissues intervening between the source of the sound and the detection site. Oscillations of much higher frequency (e.g., higher than 20,000 Hz) are beyond the frequency range of detection of the human ear and fall into a broad range termed ultrasound. Ultrasonic oscillations are useful in veterinary medicine but not because they are generated by the animal. Rather, they are used in diagnostic devices that transmit these oscillations into the animal system. By measuring and recording reflections and alterations of the ultrasound oscillations that are caused by the system, one gains information about the system itself. Ultrasound devices are used to measure boundaries and movements of structures that are defined, for example, by reflective properties of tissue interfaces and can also provide measurements of other variables such as flow. In this latter case, cellular elements in the blood define the blood velocity by an apparent velocity-dependent shift of the frequency of ultrasound. This is a Doppler shift caused when reflections of the ultrasound waves by these elements occur while these elements are moving. Applications of ultrasound are discussed in Chapter 8. Waves in the electromagnetic spectrum are also generated in mammals and are propagated throughout the system. There are instruments that use the electromagnetic spectrum to gain information about the animal. This information is presented in the form of, for example, electrocardiograms, radiographs, and magnetic resonance images.

CIRCULATORY CONTROL

Living systems maintain viability and stability by different negative-feedback control systems. Feedback implies that a system that is being controlled provides current-state information or signals to a controller that, in turn, alters its controlling signals accordingly. A negative-feedback system is one in which feedback information results in controlling signals that oppose a system alteration, so that the system is returned to the reference state. A positive-feedback system is one in which feedback information results in controlling signals that enhance a system alteration, so that the system moves consistently away from the reference state. Positive-feedback systems imply instability and, if unconstrained, can result in excessive alterations, such as are seen with fire storms or explosions. Negative-feedback systems are common to other than biological systems, as in thermostatic regulation of room temperature where the response to a decrease in temperature below an established reference is the provision of additional heat. Conversely, increases in temperature are followed by cooling until the reference state is reestablished.

Global Control

The components of biological control systems are not always understood. In such cases, it is useful to describe or quantify input and output relationships between given variables, such as blood pressure, cardiac output, and others. Such a relationship is termed a transfer function. The transfer function may appear equivalently as a mathematical expression, a table of observed values, a set of rules, or in graphic form (Fig. 5.26). The ratio of the change in output per unit change of input is called gain. An example of an important, controlled variable in mammals is blood pressure in large conduit arteries. An overview of the regulation of this pressure is shown in Fig. 5.27 in terms of transfer functions. Three subsystems are shown, each receiving the current state of pressure as input and each providing outputs in accordance with the particular subsystem. The input (pressure) is considered to be the independent variable and is plotted on the abscissas. Each transfer function is shown in the form of a plot whose value decreases with an increase in pressure, so that the output varies inversely with pressure. This expresses the negative-feedback concept. The contribution of each subsystem is temporally distinct from the others. The neural response occurs in the order of seconds or fractions thereof and has the shortest persistence (short-term regulation); the humoral response occurs in seconds to minutes and persists longer. Capillary fluid shifts occur over hours and days, and the effects persist the longest (long-term regulation). Neural responses act to directly regulate the heart and vasoactivity; the renal and adrenal responses introduce humoral agents into the circulation that also affect the heart and blood vessels; and capillary fluid shifts alter intravascular fluid volume. The effects of the systems on pressure are additive, as illustrated by the summating junction (Fig. 5.27). There also exist interactions among the systems that are not shown on this greatly simplified scheme.

Blood pressure can be affected by local vasodilations and

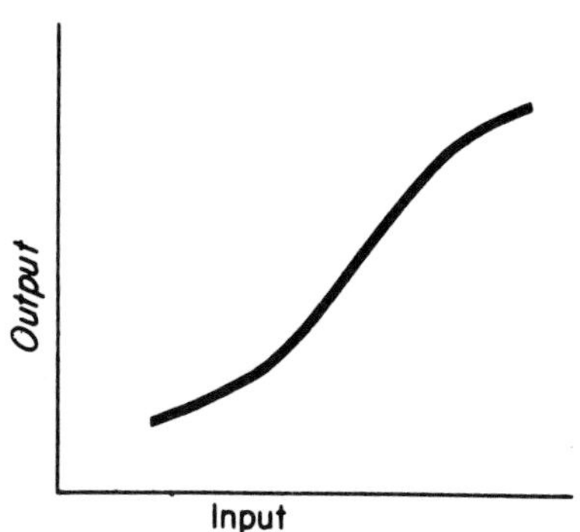

Figure 5.26. Illustration of a transfer function.

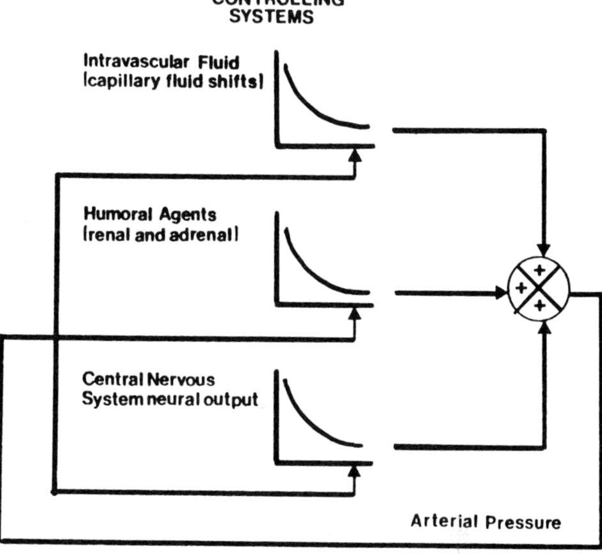

Figure 5.27. Illustration of controlling systems for arterial blood pressure in terms of transfer functions. Decreasing outputs (ordinates) that tend to decrease pressure with increasing pressure inputs (abscissas) imply negative feedback control. The system's effects are additive, as indicated by the summating junction.

vasoconstrictions of peripheral vascular beds that increase or decrease flow, respectively, in organs. Blood flow is maintained in organs according to priority of oxygen requirements, so that vasodilation in a high-priority organ may be accompanied by vasoconstriction in lower-priority organs. Thus increase of flow to one part of the circulatory system may be accompanied by a decrease in flow to another. High-priority organs include the brain and the heart, and low-priority organs include the splanchnic organs and the kidneys. Renal arteries in particular are richly invested with sympathetic nerves, and this may account for the renal function shutdown that occurs when mean arterial pressure falls below approximately 60 mm Hg. Despite flow variations, the dimensions of the conduit arteries will reflect their transmural pressure gradient, and this provides information to the central nervous system in the form of electrical signals arising from sensors located in the vessel walls. This leads to stabilization of pressure by a variety of mechanisms that include vasomotor activity and alterations in cardiac output. These sensors are known as pressoreceptors or baroreceptors, but they actually monitor stretch of the wall. Thus an abnormal (e.g., stiffer) wall may not reflect transmural pressure the same as would a normal wall. Flow (or true volume) receptors are not known to participate in such extrinsic circulatory control.

Important baroreceptors are located in the aortic arch and carotid sinus. These provide signals that reflect the state of pressure for the entire systemic circulation (aortic arch) and for pressures that are particularly important for blood flow

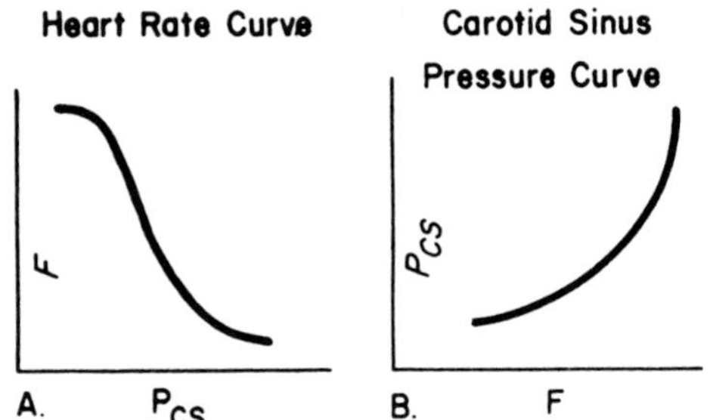

Figure 5.28. Illustration of two transfer functions. (*A*) Cardiac cyclic frequency or heart rate (F) response to carotid sinus pressure (p_{cs}). (*B*)P_{cs} response to F.

to the brain (carotid sinus). The central nervous system responds to baroreceptor information to maintain the reference state. For example, cardiac output may be increased by increasing cyclic frequency of heart contractions (heart rate), ejected volume per cycle (stroke volume), or both. An example of the form of rate changes that correlate with pressure alterations in a baroreceptor is shown in Fig. 5.28, left panel (A). Note that the curve relating carotid sinus pressure (P_{cs}) to heart rate (F) is sigmoid in shape. This is a characteristic of mammalian transfer functions in general. For such transfer functions, gain is minimal at very high or very low inputs and maximal at the central, more linear regions. This more responsive or sensitive region is usually the region of normal operation. Figure 5.28, right panel (B), indicates that heart rate (i.e., cyclic frequency, F) is also an independent variable that affects pressure in a predictable manner if all other variables (e.g., peripheral resistance) remain unchanged. Thus the variables are interdependent; such interdependence is common to biological systems.

The interaction of these two variables—carotid sinus pressure and heart rate (Fig. 5.29)—can be appreciated when the transfer functions of Fig. 5.28 are plotted on the same graph with the axis convention of the left panel of Fig. 5.28. The resulting intersection, S, of the two solid curves represents the steady-state heart rate and carotid sinus pressure in the undisturbed state. The dashed curves represent a different state, intersecting at T, that is achieved because of overall system alteration, such as by sustained exercise or disease. In each of these states pressure perturbation from the respective reference or operating point can be seen to become a transient event as heart rate and pressure track back to the reference point. Note the arrows on the transfer function pair.

Interaction becomes increasingly complex as additional variables are considered together. Figure 5.30 illustrates experimental findings in a dog with respect to the relationship of two independent variables (left atrial pressure, p_{LA}, and aortic pressure (p_{Ao}) with their regulation of left ventricular output ($\dot{Q}_{LV}$). If one of the independent variables is held constant and the other is altered, their individual roles can be determined. The three-dimensional plot shows that

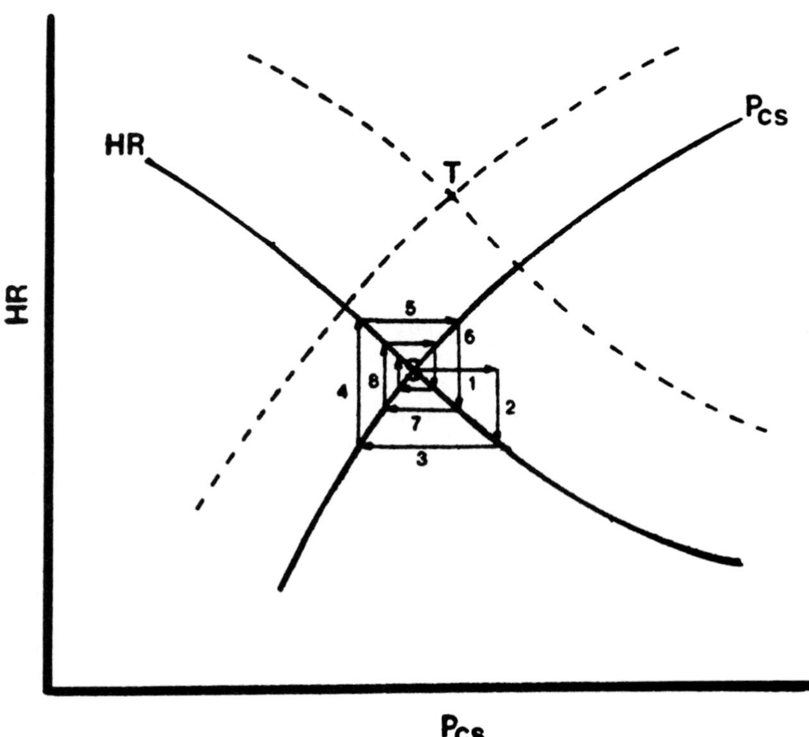

Figure 5.29. Relations and equilibrium points of heart rate (HR) and carotid sinus pressure (p_{cs}). A reference steady state is indicated by solid lines with equilibrium at S. Another "temporary" steady state can also exist (e.g., with sustained exercise); this alters the HR − p_{cs} relations so that the curves are displaced (broken lines) and a new steady-state equilibrium is established (T). At termination of this temporary steady state the curves return to their previous locations. A perturbation from equilibrium (e.g., of pressure as shown) by a transient event during the same steady state is controlled by HR − p_{cs} adjustments (sequentially numbered vectors) to reestablish the original (S).

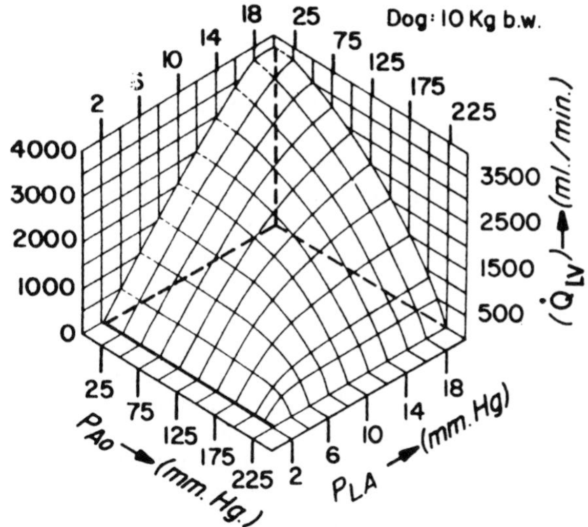

Figure 5.30. A three-dimensional plot of mean aortic pressure (p_{AO}), mean left atrial pressure (P_{LA}), and cardiac output ($\dot{Q}_{LV}$). (Modified from Milhorn 1966, *Application of Control Theory to Physiological Systems,* W.B. Saunders, Philadelphia.)

at low left atrial pressures, an increase in aortic pressure has little effect on left ventricular output until high aortic pressures are attained. At high left atrial pressures, the influence of increasing aortic pressure on output is greater across the entire range of aortic pressure. Similarly, at high aortic pressures, decreases in left atrial pressure have little effect on $\dot{Q}_{LV}$ until low values are reached. At low aortic pressures, however, the influence of increasing left atrial pressure on $\dot{Q}_{LV}$ is much greater.

Concomitant with the central control of cardiac activity is control of the resistance to flow out of the conduit arterial system by peripheral vasoactivity. Feedback loops that involve baroreceptors act through nerves and hormones to maintain pressures and adequate blood flow to tissues. Short-term regulation is augmented by long-term regulation. This latter governs intravascular and extravascular fluid volume, vascular tone, and vascular capacity. These, in turn, alter blood pressure, cardiac output, and vascular resistance that assists or opposes pressure and flow variations, which require days or weeks to develop. Short-term regulation maintains viable physiologic status in the presence of fluctuations that occur with activity or trauma and thus combats perturbations that could otherwise lead to shock or hypertension. Sustained departure, however, from normal physiologic values (e.g., chronic hypertension) requires long-term adjustments.

Local Control

Local control mechanisms are also present in the periphery of the circulatory system and have been shown to operate in the absence of central nervous system and peripheral autonomic innervation. Thus surgical or traumatic section of vasomotor nerves to many organs will not result in total loss of control of its blood supply. *Autoregulation* is the term applied to regulation of tissue and organ blood flow produced by such local mechanisms. The provision of adequate flows for diffusion and filtration processes at the capillary level is directly linked to metabolic needs and can take precedence over central control of the local perfusion pressure. Factors involved with local vascular responses include an intrinsic contractile response of vascular smooth muscle to increased tension, changes in tissue pressure, and consequences of metabolism such as accumulations of metabolites (lactate, pyruvate, adenosine diphosphate, adenosine monophosphate, etc.), increases in tissue K^+ concentration, and decreases in oxygen tension and pH, all of which are local vasodilators in the systemic circulation. The metabolically related factors can override neural influences that affect the arteriolar state. Conversely, in organs whose normal function involves blood flows that are in excess of metabolic needs (e.g., the skin or kidneys), reflex and hormonal control mechanisms can dominate over local control so that flow distribution is biased in favor of the higher-priority organs.

Autoregulation based on metabolic activity has been demonstrated in the circulations of the brain, heart, kidney, liver, intestine, and muscle. The renal bed, however, is encased in a tough capsule, and flow regulation is of a mechanical type whereby overall vascular resistance varies directly with blood pressure that develops extravascular pressure within the organ. Also, autoregulation is much less significant in the cutaneous and pulmonary circulations. In vascular beds in which flows are in excess of metabolic needs, there is little intrinsic tendency to maintain constancy of flow through metabolic responses when arterial pressure or metabolic rate is altered.

Autoregulatory responses normally occur in 1 to 3 minutes in individual organs. Figure 5.31 illustrates pressure-flow relations obtained from an isolated dog skeletal muscle preparation in the resting state. The immediate effect of an abrupt change in pressure is an alteration of flow (closed circles). After 30 to 60 seconds, however, flow returns, as shown by the direction of the arrows, to control levels (open circles). In experimental whole-dog preparations in which all nervous control has been ablated, the vascular system as a whole exhibits substantial, slowly developing autoregulatory responses over periods of 20 to 90 minutes; these responses may develop even further with time. This suggests that whole-body autoregulation exists, along with neural and humoral control of cardiac output and peripheral resistance, to regulate blood pressure.

MOLECULAR BIOLOGICAL ASPECTS

The mechanical functions of the cardiovascular system are accomplished chiefly by actions of proteins in the system. Thus cardiac output, vascular resistance and compliance, and mechanical deformation of blood cells and

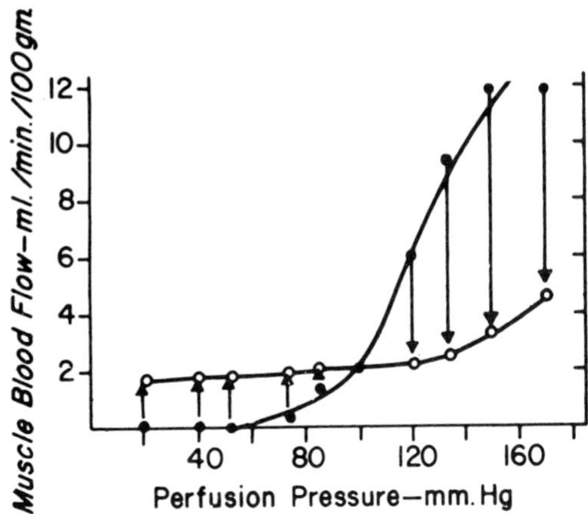

Figure 5.31. Pressure-flow relationships in the vascular bed of skeletal muscle in the dog. Closed circles represent flow rates measured when pressure was changed abruptly from the control perfusion pressure level of 100 mm Hg. Open circles are the steady-state flows eventually achieved at the new perfusion pressure. Vectors show the direction of flow changes. Intersection of the lines occurs at the control pressure. (From Berne and Levy, 1981, *Cardiovascular Physiology,* 4th ed., C.V. Mosby, St. Louis.)

vascular cells depend on active or passive properties of contractile proteins and cytoskeletal proteins in the blood, endothelial, and other cardiovascular cells. Active functions of effector cells and proteins are often mediated and regulated by the interaction of receptors on the cell surface with *ligands* from other sources. Ligands are specific chemicals that attach by forming weak noncovalent bonds with binding site regions of the cell surface proteins. The receptor and its ligand are called *mediator proteins*. The usual sequence of events in the control of cardiovascular function is that the specific interaction between the ligand and its receptor (forming the mediator proteins) causes a signal transmission via a *second intracellular messenger* to affect the function of the effector proteins. Examples of important second messengers in the cardiovascular system are cyclic AMP (cAMP) and calcium ions.

Cell-surface receptors generate intracellular signals in two general ways. One is by activation or inactivation of a plasma membrane–bound enzyme that catalyzes the production of a soluble intracellular messenger. For example, adenylate cyclase catalyzes the synthesis of cAMP from ATP located on the cytoplasmic side of the plasma membrane. When cAMP is increased in this manner in ventricular myocardial cells, the contractility of these cells is enhanced. cAMP has the opposite effect in vascular smooth muscle cells and causes relaxation. Inhibition of adenylate cyclase reduces intracellular cAMP, with resultant opposite effects.

Cell-surface receptors also act by opening or closing gated ion channels in the plasma membrane. In electrically active cells, such as neurons or muscle cells, this may cause a small and brief flux of ions, which produces a transient change in voltage across the membrane. In autonomic nerves, neurotransmitters regulate the membrane potential of the postsynaptic cell; a decrease in this membrane potential below a certain level triggers an action potential. When an action potential reaches the nerve terminal where voltage-gated Ca^{2+} channels exit, the lowering of the membrane potential (depolarization) opens these channels. Ca^{2+} ions enter the nerve terminal in accordance with their electrochemical gradient and act as second messengers to initiate neurotransmitter secretion.

Cell-surface receptors that regulate inward Ca^{2+} current channels are found in vascular smooth muscle. These interact with such agents as histamine, acetylcholine, and norepinephrine, causing relaxation or contraction unaccompanied by changes in the cell membrane potential. The receptor-operated channels presumably can increase the influx of calcium in response to the appropriate ligand. The process is called nonelectrical or pharmacomechanical activation and is assumed to depend on both an influx of Ca^{2+} and a release of Ca^{2+} from intracellular stores.

Further discussions of the molecular biology of cardiac and vascular muscle regulators are presented in Chapters 6 and 10.

REFERENCES

Binah, O. 1987. Tetanus in the mammalian heart: Studies in the shrew myocardium. *J. Mol. Cell Cardiol.* 19:1247–52.

Bramwell, J.C., and Hill, A.V. 1922. The velocity of the pulse wave in man. *Proc. R. Soc. Lond. (Biol.)* 93:298–306.

Droogman, G., and Casteels, R. 1989. Electromechanical and pharmacomechanical coupling in vascular smooth muscle. In N. Sperelakis, ed., *Physiology and Pathophysiology of the Heart.* 2d ed. Kluwer, Boston. pp. 813–24.

Fahraeus, R., and Linqvist, T. 1931. The viscosity of the blood in narrow capillary tubes. *Am. J. Physiol.* 96:562–8.

Frank, O. 1895. Zur Dynamik des Herzmuskels. *Z. Biol.* 32:370–437.

Frank, O. 1927. Die Theorie der Pulswellen, *Z. Biol.* 85:91–130.

Granger, H.S., and Guyton, A.C. 1969. Autoregulation of the total systemic circulation following destruction of the central nervous system in the dog. *Circ. Res.* 25:379–88.

Hagenbach, E. 1860. Über die Bestimming der Zähigkeit einer Flüssigkeit durch den Ausfluss aus Röhren. *Ann. der Physik.* 109:385–426 (cited in B. Folkow, and E. Neil, eds. *Circulation,* Oxford University Press, London.

Holt, J.P., Rhode, E.A., and Kines, H. 1968. Ventricular volumes and body weight in mammals. *Am. J. Physiol.* 215:704–15.

Korteweg, D.J. 1878. Cited in Lambossy P. (1950).

Lambossy, P. 1950. Apercu historique et critique sur le problème de la propagation des ondes dans un liquide compressible enfermé dans un tube elastique. *Helv. Physiol. Acta* 8:209–27 (cited in D. A. McDonald, ed., *Blood Flow in Arteries,* Williams & Wilkins, Baltimore).

Li, J.K.-J., Melbin, J., Riffle, R.A., and Noordegraaf, A. 1981. Pulse wave propagation. *Circ. Res.* 49:442–52.

Mainwood, G.W., and Lee, S.L. 1969. Rat heart papillary muscles: Action potentials and mechanical response to paired stimuli. *Science* 166:396–97.

Meijler, F.L. 1985. De functie van de atrivoventriuclaire knoop versus hartgroottee van muis tot walris. *Ned. Tijdschr. Geneeskd.* 129:1329–32.

McDonald, D.A. 1974. *Blood Flow in Arteries,* Williams & Wilkins, Baltimore.

McGuill, M.W., and Rowan, A.N. 1989. Biological effect of blood loss: Implications for sampling volumes and techniques. *ILAR News* 31:5–18.

Melbin, J., and Noordergraaf, A. 1983. Pressure gradient related to energy conversion in the aorta. *Circ. Res.* 52:143–50.

Milnor, W.R. 1979. Aortic wavelength as a determinant of the relation between heart rate and body size in mammals. *Am. J. Physiol.* 237(1):R3–R6.

Milnor, W. R., Bergel, W.H., and Bargainer, J.D. 1966. Hydraulic power associated with pulmonary blood flow and its relation to heart rate. *Circ. Res.* 19:467–80.

Moens, A.I. 1878. Die Pulskurve, Leiden (cited in D. A. McDonald, ed., *Blood Flow in Arteries,* Williams & Wilkins, Baltimore).

Nerem, R.M., Rumberger, J.A., Jr., Gross, D.R., Hamlin, R.L., and Geiger, G.L. 1974. Hot-film anemometer velocity measurements of arterial blood flow in horses. *Circ. Res.* 34:193–203.

Noordergraaf, A., Li, J.K.-J., and Campbell, K.B. 1979. Mammalian hemodynamics: A new similarity principle. *J. Theor. Biol.* 79:485–89.

O'Rourke, M.F., and Taylor, M.G. 1966. Vascular impedance of the femoral bed. *Circ. Res.* 18:126–39.

Patterson, J.L., Jr., Goetz, R.H., Doyle, J.T., Warren, J.V., Gauer, O.H., Detweiler, D.K., Said, S.I., Hoernicke, H., McGregor, M., Keen, E.N., Smith, M.H., Jr., Hardie, E.L., Reynolds, M., Flatt, W.P., and Waldo, D.R. 1965 Cardiorespiratory dynamics in the ox and giraffe, with comparative observations on man and other mammals. *Ann. N.Y. Acad. Sci.* 127:393–413.

Poiseuille, J.L.M. 1846. Recherches experimentales sur le mouvement des liquides dans les tubes de tres petits diametres. *Mem. Acad. Sci. Paris* 9:433–544.

Prothero, J. 1979. Heart weight as a function of body weight in mammals growth. 43:139–50.

Reynolds, O. 1883. An experimental investigation of the circumstances which determine whether the motion of water shall be direct or sinuous, and the law of resistance in parallel channels. *Philos. Trans. R. Soc.* (London) 174:935–82.

Schmidt-Nielsen, K. 1984. *Scaling: Why Is Animal Size So Important?* Cambridge University Press, Cambridge.

Shu, Chien, ed. 1990. *Molecular Biology of the Cardiovascular System.* Lea & Febiger, Philadelphia.

Stahl, W.R. 1967. Scaling of respiratory variables in mammals. *J. Appl. Physiol.* 22:453–60.

Taylor, M.G. 1966. An introduction to some recent developments in arterial hemodynamics. *Aust. Ann. Med.* 15:71–86.

Wiedemann, G. 1856. Ann. der Physik. 99:221 (quoted by E. Hatschek, 1928, in *The Viscosity of Liquids*. London: Bell. p. 239.

Womersly, J.R. 1957. Oscillatory flow in arteries: The constrained elastic tube as a model of arterial flow and pulse transmission. *Phys. Med. Biol.* 2:178–87.

CHAPTER 6

The Heart: Gross Structure, Myocardial Cells

by David K. Detweiler and Dean H. Riedesel

GROSS STRUCTURE

Some of the specialized structures and anatomical landmarks within the four-chambered mammalian heart are depicted in Fig. 6.1. A fibrous skeleton separates the muscular atria and ventricles. It forms the annuli fibrosi (fibrous rings) that surround the orifices of the aorta, pulmonary artery, and atrioventricular valves (Fig. 6.2.) These rings provide attachment sites for the cardiac valves, for the origin and insertion of the cardiac muscles, and for the electrical insulation or separation of the atria and ventricles. Table 6.1 gives historical highlights concerning the structure of the heart.

Atria

The thin-walled atria subserve three functions: (1) elastic reservoir and conduit from the venous bed to the ventricle; (2) booster pump action, enhancing ventricular filling and maintaining low mean atrial pressure; and (3) atrioventricular valve closure before ventricular systole. After atrial contraction, which increases ventricular pressure, pressure in the relaxing atria declines. The resultant ventriculoatrial pressure gradient aids or actually effects atrioventricular valve closure.

The pumping action of the atria is relatively unimportant at slow heart rates when the ventricles and atria fill as a common chamber during most of diastole. At the very end of this period the atria contract and increase cardiac output from 15 to 20 percent. At rapid heart rates and in certain heart diseases, atrial contraction becomes more important for ventricular filling and contributes perhaps 20 to 30 percent to cardiac output. If the atria cease to contract (e.g., in atrial fibrillation) and the atrial pump is lost, the ventricles continue to fill and function reasonably well under resting conditions.

Ventricles

The ventricular myocardial mass makes up most of the heart's weight. During contraction the volume of the left ventricle is reduced by a decrease in transverse diameter and some shortening of the base-apex diameter. The former is particularly effective, owing to the constrictor action of the midwall circumferential fibers (Fig. 6.3).

The right ventricle has much thinner walls and only about one-third the mass of the left ventricle. Its free wall is moved toward the interventricular septum by contraction of the spiral muscles. Systole in the left ventricle also functions to assist ejection from the right ventricle. As the constrictor muscles of the left ventricle contract, the curvature of the septum is increased, pulling the free right ventricular wall toward the septum (called *left ventricular aid*).

Pericardium

The pericardium is a double-walled sac that contains a few milliliters of serous fluid that gives a lubricated surface for the heart movements. The parietal or outer sac is slightly larger than the heart in diastole. It is relatively inelastic and thus protects against acute expansion of the heart. Because of this inelasticity, the acute accumulation of intrapericardial fluid under pressure will tend to collapse the veins that enter the atria and impede or halt cardiac filling (cardiac

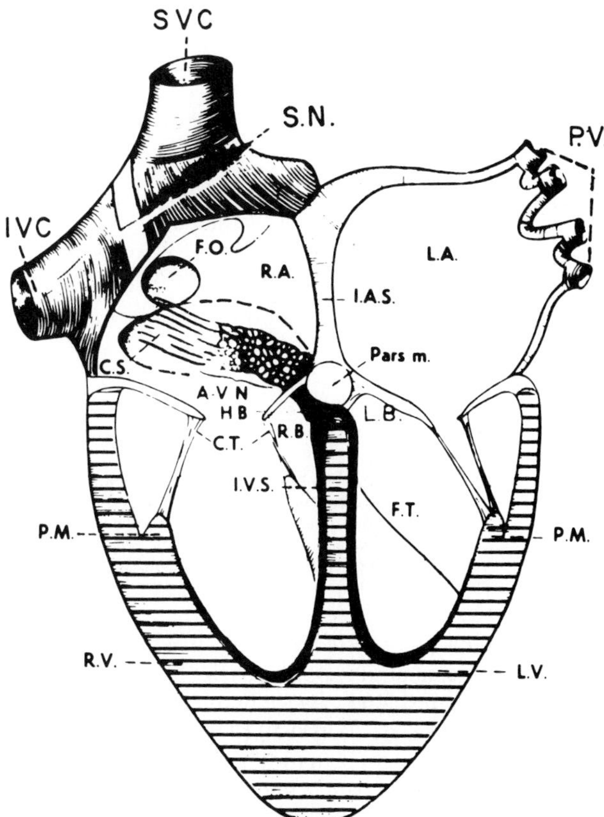

Figure 6.1. Specialized structures and anatomical landmarks within the mammalian heart. F.O., Foramen ovale (functional closure occurs at birth); S.N., sinoatrial node; P.V., pulmonary veins; R.A. and L.A., right and left atria; I.A.S., interatrial septum; C.S., coronary sinus; A-V.N., atrioventricular node; H.B., bundle of His; R.B. and L.B., right and left branches of the bundle of His; I.V.S., interventricular septum; P.M., papillary muscle; F.T., false tendon of the Purkinje network; R.V. and L.V., right and left ventricle; C.T., chordae tendinea; IVC, posterior vena cava; SVC, anterior vena cava; Pars M., Pars membranacea. (Redrawn from Schütz 1968, *Physiologie des Herzens,* Springer, Berlin.)

tamponade). When cardiac enlargement develops gradually, as in hypertrophy, or when there is chronic accumulation of fluid in pericardial effusion, the pericardium will enlarge to accommodate the increased contents. Large quantities (greater than the volume of the heart itself) of fluid may thus accumulate and cause only moderate cardiac tamponade compatible with life. Congenital absence or surgical removal of the pericardium ordinarily does not disturb cardiac function. Its restraining effect on the heart promotes mechanical interplay between the cardiac chambers, so that the volume and pressure effect of distention of one chamber will be transmitted more readily to the other chambers when the pericardium is intact. For example, enlargement of the right ventricle due to obstructed blood flow through the lungs will lead to displacement of the interventricular septum and reduce the volume of the left ventricular chamber.

Relative heart size in mammals correlates with differences in degree of physical activity characteristic of species or breed (Tables 6.2, 6.3, and Fig. 5.6). Adult greyhounds have relatively large hearts compared with mongrel dogs. Since newborn greyhounds also have relatively large hearts (i.e., the heart weight/body weight ratio is similar in both newborn and adult), relative heart weight appears to be a genetically determined characteristic.

MYOCARDIAL CELL MORPHOLOGY

Electron microscopic studies of the early 1950s demonstrated that myocardial cells are surrounded by an intact plasma membrane (sarcolemma) and do not form a syncytium. They do, however, form a functional syncytium because of the presence of tight or gap junctions (nexuses) that have low electrical resistance and allow passage of ions and perhaps small molecules.

Pacemaker and conducting cells

Three subtypes of cells are specialized for impulse formation: P cells, transitional cells, and Purkinje cells.

P cells are so named because (1) pacemaking seems to be their primary function, (2) their internal structure is more primitive than the highly differentiated contractile cells, and (3) they are pale staining. (Thus the *P* stands for pacemaking, primitive, and pale.) Located in the sinoatrial and atrioventricular nodes, these cells have no T tubules and little longitudinal sarcoplasmic reticulum.

Transitional cells are thinner than other myocardial cells, are intermediately differentiated between the P cells and contractile cells, and are thought to form the connection between P cells and surrounding tissue.

Purkinje cells are large (10–30 μm in diameter and 20–50 μm in length), and contain few contractile filaments. They make up the bundle of His, the bundle branches, and the Purkinje network.

Contractile or working myocardial cells

The heart is usually considered a mass of contractile tissue. However, the pacemaker, conducting, and working cells provide only 25 percent of the total number of cells in the heart. The remaining cells are fibroblasts, endocardial cells, endothelial cells, vascular smooth muscle cells, pericytes, neurons, and blood cellular elements (e.g., macrophages).

The working myocardial cells are specialized for contraction and conduction, but most cells do not initiate impulses. The contractile cells of smaller mammals (rat, guinea pig) are somewhat thinner (11–12 μm in diameter) than those of larger mammals (dog, ox) (16–17 μm diameter), but their size differs far less than the hearts themselves. Thus larger hearts contain many more cells than smaller hearts. Each myocardial cell has a centrally located nucleus, is packed with contractile myofibrils, and contains numerous mitochondria. Working myocardial cells are a specialized type of smooth muscle cell, like those in arteries,

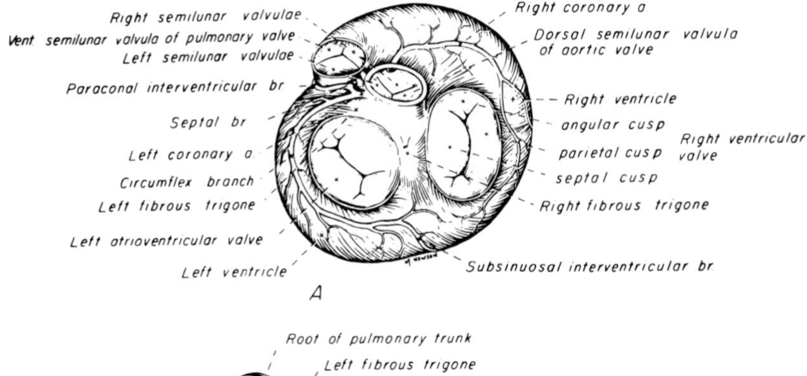

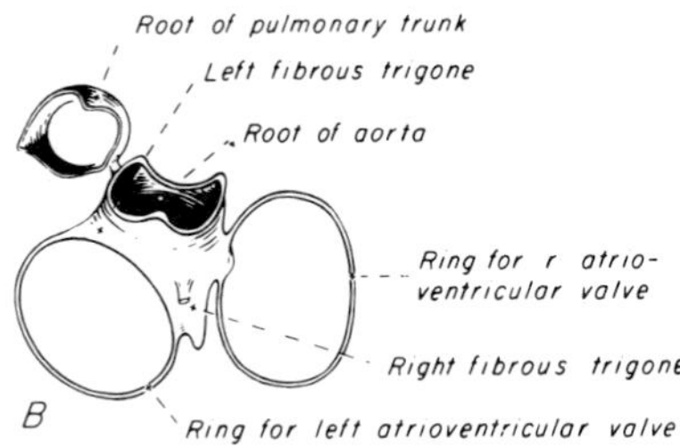

Figure 6.2. The base of the heart. (*A*) Atrioventricular, aortic, and pulmonary valves, craniodorsal aspect. (*B*) The fibrous base of the heart, craniodorsal aspect. (From Evans and Christensen, 1979, *Miller's Anatomy of the Dog*, W.B. Saunders, Philadelphia, p. 640.)

that have acquired features and properties resembling skeletal muscle.

Multiple cells are organized mainly in series and are connected end to end by the intercalated disks, forming the myocardial *fibers*. Parallel groups of fibers are separated into *bundles* that are invested by connective tissue sheaths. The heart wall contains layers of muscle fibers that characteristically show a smooth change in orientation across the wall. Dissection of the heart wall reveals that fiber paths take on a figure-of-eight pattern (Fig. 6.4). In the left ventricle, for example, the path may begin at the fibrous atrioventricular fibrous ring and spiral toward the apex and into the wall, course past midwall, and emerge on the endocardial surface. The fiber path then spirals up toward the base of the heart, again passing the midwall and returning to the epicardial surface. This completes the figure-of-eight.

Table 6.1. Historical highlights concerning heart structure

1664 Niels Stensen proved the heart consists of muscle fibers.
1669 Richard Lower observed the tamponade effect of pericardial effusion. Described the course and layering of the heart muscle.
1695 Antony van Leeuwenhoek described the syncytial arrangement of muscle fibers. Also discovered the cross-striations of muscle (1685).
1759–1769 Albrecht von Haller correctly described the myocardium, pericardium, and venous valves.
1839 Johannes Evangelista Purkinje described the subendocardial conduction system that bears his name, although he misunderstood its function.
1862 Albert von Kölliker rediscovered the "syncytial" structure of the heart that van Leeuwenhoek's studies had indicated.
1863 Christoph Theodor Aeby first observed the intercalated disks.
1866 Karl Joseph Eberth first described the intercalated disks in detail and interpreted them as a cementing material (*Kittstreiffen*) at the cell boundaries.
1892 A.F. Stanley Kent described accessory atrioventricular bundles of myocardial fibers.
1893 Wilhelm His, Jr., described the bundle of specialized (Purkinje) fibers connecting the atria and ventricles (bundle of His).
1902 Emilio Veratti published the key paper on the sarcoplasmic reticulum of skeletal muscle.
1906 Sunao Tawara described the atrioventricular node (Tawara's node) and was the first to conceive of the system consisting of the atrioventicular node, bundle of His, bundle branches, and Purkinje fiber network as a functional unit, specialized for rapid intraventicular conduction.
1907 Arthur Keith and Martin William Flack described the sinoatrial node and postulated that it initiated the heartbeat.
1900–1920 With the work of Victor von Ebner and Rudolf Peter Heinrich Heidenhain the syncytial continuity of the myocardium became generally accepted until electron microscopic studies in the early 1950s exploded this concept.
1954 F.S. Sjöstrand and Ebba Andersson showed with electron micrographs that the intercalated disks are cell boundaries and that the myocardial cells do not forms a syncytium.

Fibers, fibrils, and filaments

The term *fiber* is applied to individual cells as well as to chains of cells. Within each cell or fiber, *fibrils* (myofibrils) are densely packed in a linear arrangement that forms parallel groups. Each myofibril extends the full length of the cell and inserts into the cytoplasmic surface of the intercalated disk. These groups are cross-banded and appear as a series of repeating units or cross-striations. The sarcomere is the fundamental contractile unit between two cross-striations (Fig. 6.5). The sarcomeres of parallel myofibrils are aligned in transverse register across the cell, giving the cross-banded appearance.

The sarcomeres, in turn, are composed of still finer structures, the *filaments* (myofilaments). These are strands of contractile proteins; the two that are best defined and fundamental to contraction are *myosin* and *actin*. Their pattern of organization is summarized in Figs. 6.5 and 6.6. Dark transverse bands called Z lines form the boundaries of each contractile unit or sarcomere. Light (I band) and dark (A band) zones exist within the sarcomere because of the arrangement of actin and myosin. At least two other proteins,

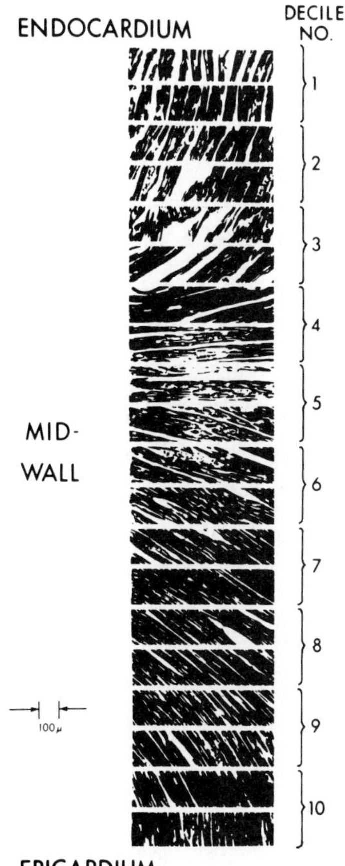

Figure 6.3. Myocardial fiber directions across the wall of the dog's left ventricle from endocardium (inner wall, decile 1) to epicardium (the outer wall, decile 10). The fibers are viewed as if facing the front of the heart, and it can be seen that the bulk of the fibers in the midwall tend to run in a circumferential (horizontal) direction, whereas fibers in the inner (endocardial) and outer (epicardial) layers tend to run more vertically, along the long axis of the heart. (From Streeter et al. 1969, *Circ Res* 24:339–47.)

Table 6.2. Heart weight (grams per kilogram of body weight) in various mammals arranged in order of increasing physical activity

Animal	Heart weight
Hedgehog	3.8
Guinea pig	4.2
Pig	4.5
Cat	4.6
Calf	5.4
Human	5.9
Goat	6.2
Horse	6.8
Hare	7.7
Dog	8.0
Fox	9.2
Wolf	10.2
Stag	11.5

From Grande and Taylor 1965, in Hamilton, ed., *Handbook of Physiology*, Am. Physiol. Soc., Washington.

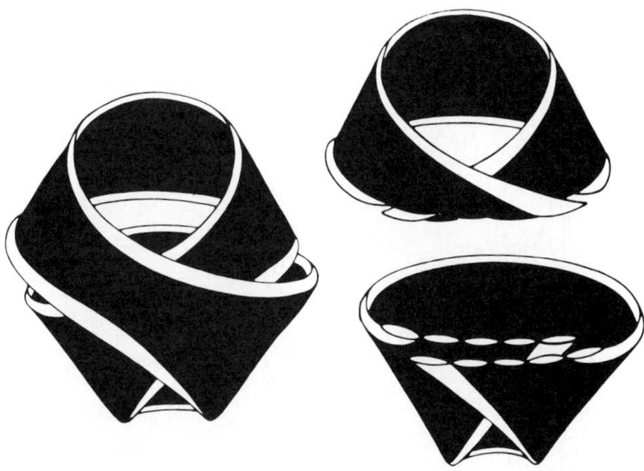

Figure 6.4. Representation of a number of fiber paths in a figure-of-eight construction for apical and basal portions as a single left ventricular unit. Note how sense of imbrication reverses at equatorial cut; unrolling procedure goes to the right in apical half, to the left in basal half. (From Torrent-Guasp 1973, *The Cardiac Muscle,* Juan March, Barcelona.)

tropomyosin and *troponin,* modulate the contractile process (see Chap. 45 for detail on skeletal muscle).

Intercalated disks

Intercalated disks are specialized paired membrane junctions that connect the ends of adjacent cells in series. The transverse portions of these disks are at right angles to the fibers. They are always located at the level of a terminal Z line. Neighboring transverse segments are often connected by a longitudinal segment that runs the length of a sarcomere to the next Z line, forming zigzag steps. Low electrical impedance at the nexus sites of the intercalated disks and firmness of their connection between pairs of cells cause the groups of discrete myocardial cells to function as a mechanical and electrical syncytium.

The intercalated disks have three types of functional specializations:

1. The *macula adherens* or desmosomes. These electron-dense round bodies appear to weld the sarcolemma of adjacent fibers together.

2. The *fascia adherens* or *intermediate junction.* This structure is generally larger than the macula adherens and

Table 6.3. Heart weight (grams per kilogram of body weight) differences within species or family

Animal	Heart weight
Dog	
Mongrels	7.98
Greyhound	13.40
Leporids	
Hutch rabbit	2.40
Wild rabbit	2.76
Hare	7.75

From Grande and Taylor 1965, in Hamilton, ed., *Handbook of Physiology,* Am. Physiol. Soc., Washington.

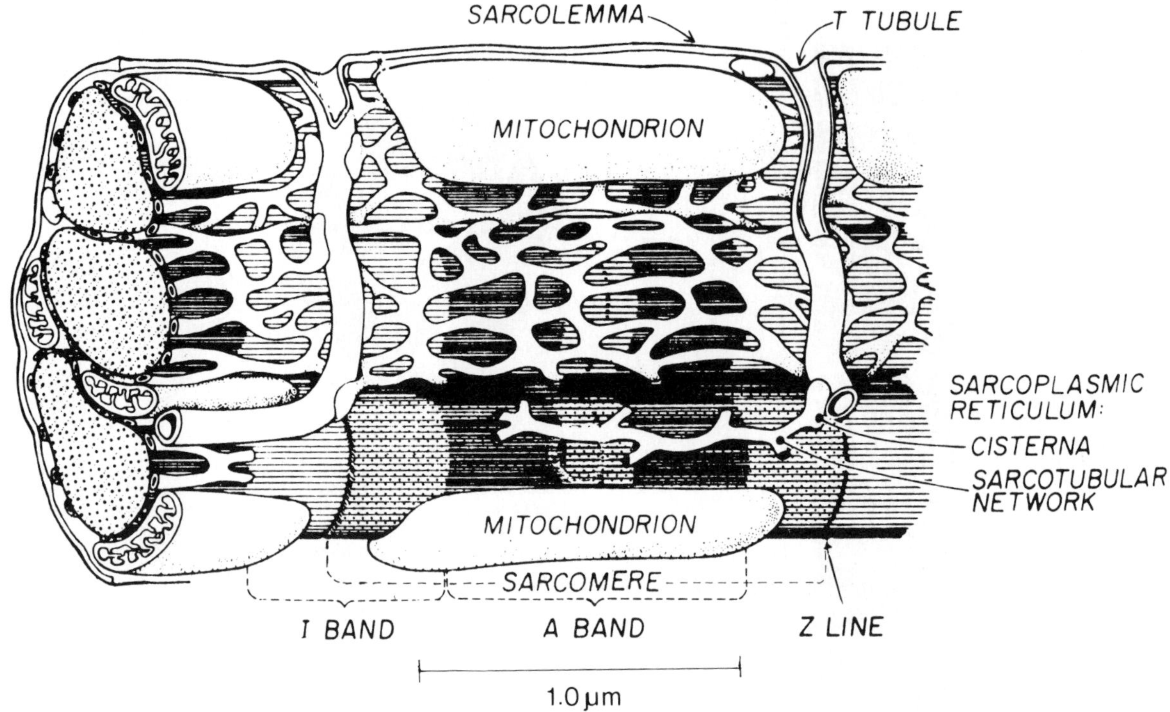

Figure 6.5. The working myocardial cell. The A band is the region occupied by the thick filaments (myosin) and thin filaments (actin) that extend between them from either side; the I band is the region occupied by thin filaments only. These thin filaments attach at the Z line (the line bisecting each I band) and extend toward the center of the sarcomere, which is the shaded area between two Z lines and is the functional contractile unit. The sarcoplasmic reticulum (SR) is a tubular structure that surrounds the contractile proteins forming the sacrotubular network at the center of the sarcomere and the cistermae that contact the T tubules and sarcolemma, which is a thin, enveloping sheath. The transverse tubules are continuous with the sarcolemma and thus extend the cell surface into the depths of the cell. (Modified from Katz 1975, *New Eng. J. Med.* 293:1184.)

occupies the major part of the transverse segments of the intercalated disk. The fascia adherens appears to provide adhesion between adjacent cells and a locus for insertion of myofilaments on either side of the intercalated disk. Thus, together with the maculae adherents, these structures provide for mechanical attachment of adjacent cells, allowing the transmission of contractile force from cell to cell.

3. *Nexus.* Nexuses (gap or tight junctions) are generally found in the lateral portions of the disk (Fig. 6.7). No filaments insert into them, and they seem to be out of the direct line of tension exerted by myofilaments. The plasma membrane of one cell comes into contact with that of an adjoining cell at the nexus. Nexuses appear to serve as efficient low-resistance pathways for electrical conduction between the cells. Nexuses are sparse and small in sinoatrial and atrioventricular nodal cells, where conduction is slow, and plentiful and elongated in Purkinje cells, where conduction is rapid.

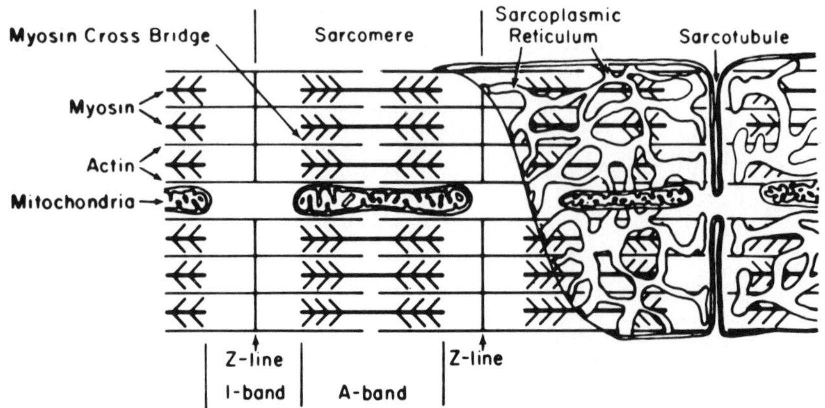

Figure 6.6. Drawing of myocardial fiber. (*Left*) Ultrastructural division into interdigitating actin and myosin filaments. The organization of one sarcomere is shown containing overlapping thick (myosin) and thin (actin) filaments with cross-bridges on the ends of myosin filaments. (*Right*) Abundant sarcoplasmic reticulum and prominent sarcotubules in the region of the Z line are shown. (From Little and Little 1989, *Physiology of the Heart and Circulation,* 4th ed., Yearbook Medical Publishers, Chicago, p. 73.)

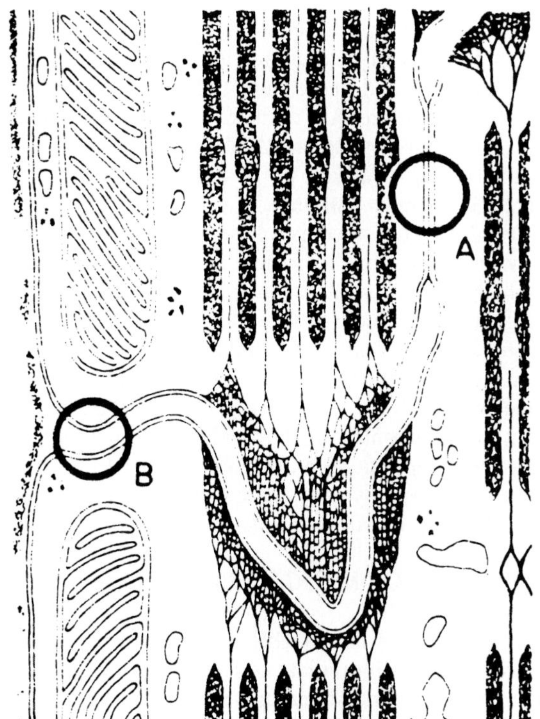

Figure 6.7. Region of the intercalated disk. The limiting membranes of two discrete cells are separated by a distinct extracellular space (*circle B*); the membranes fuse forming a nexus or tight junction (*circle A*). (Modified by Weidmann 1967, Harvey Lectures 61:1–15, from Sjöstrand et al. 1958, *Ultrastruct. Res.* 1:271–87.)

Mitochondria

The mitochondria or sarcosomes are remarkably numerous, making up 25 to 30 percent of the myocardium. In some myocardial cells the mass of the mitochondria equals that of the myofibrils. They are the major sites of oxidative phosphorylation, in which energy provided from substrate oxidation is converted to adenosine triphosphate, the source of energy for cell function.

Glycogen granules and lipid droplets

Glycogen granules are found in large numbers and are evenly dispersed in cardiac muscle. Lipid droplets are frequently encountered and are commonly located adjacent to mitochondria.

Transverse tubular system or interior sarcolemma

The transverse tubular or T system consists of relatively thick-walled transverse tubules formed by invaginations of the sarcolemma, which extend into the myocardial fiber. Although the T tubules are usually found at the level of the Z lines, T tubules may be disoriented to run longitudinally in the fibers. Nevertheless, the membrane forming the T tubule is continuous with the sarcolemma, and the lumen of the tubule is in direct connection with the extracellular space. These tubules are believed to (1) transmit the action potential from the outside surface of the sarcolemma to the interior of the fiber, (2) distribute substrates to and remove metabolites from the cell interior, and (3) accumulate calcium (see below).

Sarcoplasmic reticulum

The sarcoplasmic reticulum is also known as the *longitudinal* or *L system*. It consists of a series of anastomosing thin-walled tubules that invest the sarcomere. These tubules form a complex reticulum of anastomosing intracellular channels that have no direct contact with the cell exterior (Figs. 6.5 and 6.6). The longitudinal system is thought to function in the storage, release, and uptake of calcium ions, which are responsible for initiating myofibril contraction and relaxation. The juxtaposition of the T system with the L system has suggested the hypothesis that the depolarizing impulse travels along the transverse tubule from the outer-cell membrane, triggering release of calcium from stores within the longitudinal tubular system. The calcium then diffuses into the myofibril, activating contraction. Sarcoplasmic reticulum fragments are known to accumulate calcium in vitro. It is thought that they do this during contraction, thus lowering the ionic calcium available to act on myosin filaments, hence leading to relaxation.

Contractile proteins

The four major proteins that have been mentioned above (actin, myosin, tropomyosin, and troponin) have been extracted from myofibrils of cardiac muscle.

Actin and myosin of the heart convert the chemical energy of substrate metabolism into mechanical energy of contraction. The amount of energy so converted and the resulting force of contraction depend mainly on two factors: (1) the resting length of sarcomeres (the Frank-Starling mechanism) and (2) the chemical environment of the proteins before and during the activation-contraction reaction. The relationship of force developed by a muscle and the sarcomere length has been described in both skeletal and cardiac muscle (Fig. 6.8). The cross-bridge hypothesis suggests that in *striated* muscle the reduction in force as the sarcomere is lengthened is related to a reduction in the overlap of thin and thick filaments and that force approaches zero when this overlap is eliminated. This fits well with the hypothesis that force is related to the number of cross-bridges that can be formed. Likewise, at short sarcomere lengths, the actin filaments begin to overlap in the center of the sarcomere. This interferes with cross-bridge attachment and again the force is decreased.

Additional mechanisms, however, appear to be involved. In cardiac muscle the force developed at longer lengths seems to be greater than that dictated by overlap of crossbridges alone.

There is experimental evidence that stretch of the fiber increases the concentration of intracellular calcium and also increases the myofilament binding of calcium ions. Thus a

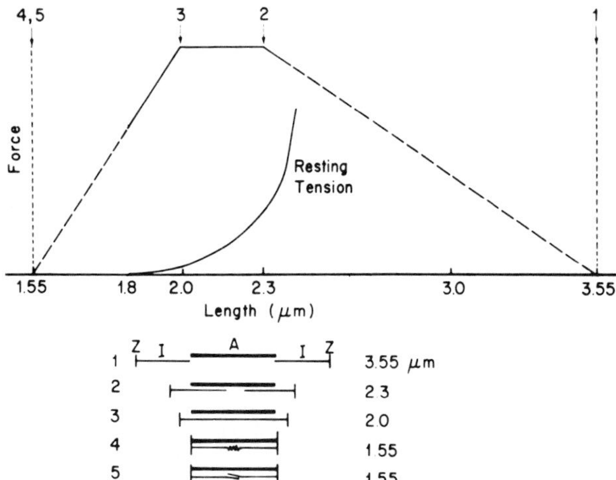

Figure 6.8. Sarcomere force-length relations and myofilament overlap in muscle. *Upper curve* represents active and resting force-length relations. Force is in arbitrary units. *Lower schematic* represents thick (A) and thin (I) filament overlap at varied sarcomere lengths. Z indicates Z lines of sarcomere. Number sequence at left corresponds to number at varied sarcomere lengths as indicated at top of force-length curve. Myofilament positions: 1, no overlap; 2, complete overlap except in regions of no thick filament cross-bridges; 3, thick filaments abut; 4, shortening with compression of thin filaments; 5, shortening with overlap of thin filaments. (From Brady, 1979, in Berne, Sperelakis, and Giger, eds., *Handbook of Physiology,* Am. Physiol. Soc., Bethesda, Md., p. 462.)

change in cross-bridge number or sarcomere geometry alone does not account for force-length relations, especially at short sarcomere lengths. The chemical environment includes the concentration of a positive inotropic agent such as calcium ions or a catecholamine (e.g., norepinephrine), which can alter tension development in the absence of changes in sarcomere length.

Myosin and actin form an organized lattice within the myocardial cells, which interact cyclically, generating contractile force. The thin actin filaments extend from the Z line into the sarcomere. The thick myosin filaments have a tail and an angled globular head attached at one end (Fig. 6.9). Tropomyosin is a long, thick regulatory protein that is wrapped around the actin filament and covers the active binding sites during the time between contractions. Attached to the tropomyosin are molecules of troponin. When the cell depolarizes, calcium diffuses into the sarcoplasma from outside the cell and is released from storage within the sarcomplasmic reticulum. The calcium combines with troponin, and a conformation change in the molecule causes tropomyosin to move away from the myosin-binding sites on actin (Fig. 6.9).

The hydrolysis of ATP provides the energy for muscle contraction. The sequence of events is as follows: (1) The myosin molecule, when bound to ATP, is only weakly bound to actin; (2) hydrolysis of ATP to ADP + Pi energizes the myosin headpiece, which still binds the hydrolysis products ADP and Pi; (3) with the increase in calcium ions caused by electrical excitation of the cell membrane, the myosin head binds to the adjacent actin filament; and (4) the actin-bound myosin head changes its conformation, causing it to move from a 90-degree angle with respect to the actin filament to a 45-degree angle. This motion moves the actin filament with respect to the myosin filament (contraction). During this step Pi and ADP are released, providing the free energy needed to power the conformational change. Subsequent binding of ATP to the myosin head releases or weakens the bond of the myosin head from actin (the situation in step 1). If there is a lack of high-energy phosphate (ATP or creatine phosphate) to replace the ADP and Pi, the muscle locks at step 4 and becomes stiff because the actin-myosin cross-bridge linkage is firm. This state is known as *rigor* and is seen as the stiffening of striated muscles shortly after death (*rigor mortis*). On repolarization of the cell membrane, the calcium is reaccumulated in the sarcoplasmic reticulum, troponin returns to its original shape, and tropomyosin again inhibits or covers the myosin-binding locations on the actin filament.

PROPERTIES OF MYOCARDIAL CELLS

Conductivity

Myocardial cells are capable of transmitting action potentials. Although individual cells are separated by plasma membranes, the impulse can pass from cell to cell, presumably through the specialized tight junctions known as nexuses.

Contraction

Contraction of the myocardium differs from that of skeletal muscle in several respects: (1) the individual myocardial

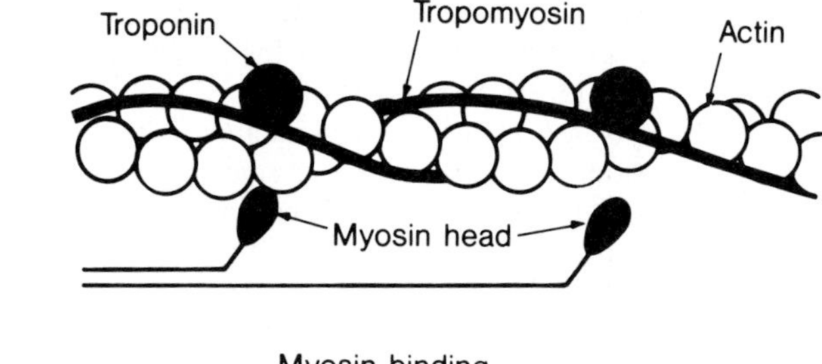

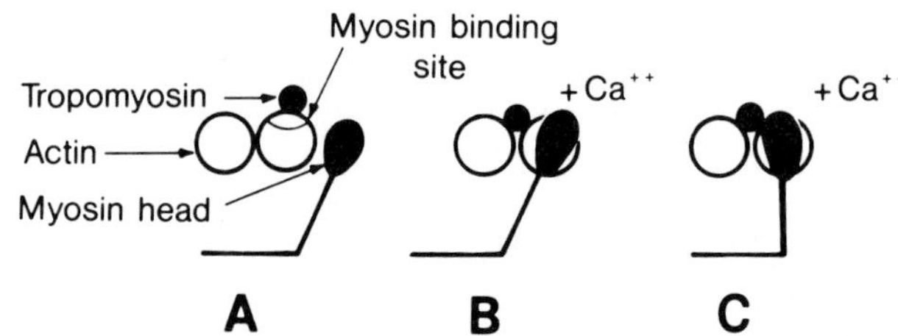

Figure 6.9. Schematic diagram showing actin monomers (*above*) arranged into a double helix with tropomyosin filaments running near the groove between the two chains and globular troponin molecules located about 40 nm apart. Two globular heavy meromyosin heads are shown. (*Below*): (*A*) Cross-section of actin helix showing the relaxed muscle with myosin-binding site on actin blocked by the tropomyosin filament. (*B*) Binding of calcium ions by troponin causes movement of the tropomyosin filament into the groove and permits binding of the myosin head to actin. (*C*) Movement of the actin-myosin cross-bridge causes sliding of the actin filament and muscle contraction. (From Little and Little, 1989, *Physiology of the Heart and Circulation,* 4th ed., Yearbook Medical Publishers, Chicago, p. 75.)

cells, while anatomically discrete, transmit impulses across the cell boundaries and thus behave as a functional syncytium; (2) the duration of contraction is longer; (3) the refractory period is longer; (4) the rate of force development during contraction is slower and the velocity of shortening is slower; and (5) the maximum tension developed per unit of cross-section of muscle is only one-third to one-half that of skeletal muscle.

The physiological features that distinguish cardiac from red and white skeletal muscle are outlined in Table 6.4. Tension development in skeletal muscle is regulated by the frequency of motor nerve impulses (temporal summation, tetanus) and by variations in the number of muscle units activated during a single contraction. Cardiac muscle is not organized on a muscle unit basis (nor are individual muscle fibers directly innervated) and behaves as a physiological syncytium so that all myocardial cells are activated during each contraction in an all-or-none fashion. Further, under physiological conditions, myocardial cells cannot be summated temporally; nor can they develop tetanic contraction because of their long refractory period.

There are other differences between cardiac and skeletal muscle. First, cardiac muscle has more mitochondria than skeletal muscle, probably because of its continual need for oxidative phosphorylation to supply high-energy phosphates for contraction. Skeletal muscle does not need this capability because it can develop an oxygen debt with a far greater lowering of pH and high-energy phosphate levels during activity than can cardiac muscle since, unlike the myocardium, it can go through a recovery period during rest to restore metabolites and pH. Second, skeletal muscle fibers can run the length of the muscle whereas cardiac muscle cells are bounded by intercalated disks. Finally, skeletal muscle has multiple peripheral nuclei while cardiac muscle cells have a single centrally placed nucleus.

Compared with certain types of smooth muscle on the one hand and red and white skeletal muscle on the other, myocardial cells have structural and functional features that are more closely allied with those of smooth muscle and red skeletal muscle than with white skeletal muscle. Smooth muscle cells are relatively poor in myofibrils, are often arranged as a syncytium, and contract slowly. Similarly, red skeletal muscle is richer in sarcoplasm than white skeletal muscle. Cardiac muscle is arranged as a functional syncytium, like certain types of smooth muscle, and is rich in mitochondria, like red skeletal muscle. These various features that smooth muscle and red striated skeletal muscle share with cardiac muscle correlate with functional similarities (e.g., smooth muscle, red striated muscle, and cardiac muscle contract more slowly and engage in more sustained activity than white skeletal muscle.)

Table 6.4. Regulation of contraction in cardiac and skeletal muscles

Mechanism	Cardiac muscle	Red and white skeletal muscle
Ability to summate responses to rapidly delivered stimuli	None	Marked
Ability to vary the number of active muscle fibers	None	Marked
Ability to alter contractility	Marked	Little
Ability to alter contractile response by changing of initial fiber length	Present: functions at short sarcomere lengths	Present: functions at long and short sarcomere lengths

From Katz 1967, in Tanz, Kavaler, and Roberts, eds., *Factors Influencing Myocardial Contractility,* Academic Press, New York.

Excitation and the membrane system of cardiac cells

As in all excitable cells, excitation is mediated in myocardial cells by depolarization of cell membranes (sarcolemma). From the sarcolemma, the excitatory process is distributed via intercalated disks to adjacent cells and over the transverse tubular system throughout the entire thickness of the cell. The intercalated disks with their nexuses of low electrical resistance permit rapid transmission of depolarizing impulses from cell to adjacent cell. The transverse tubular network extend the extracellular compartment to all levels of the myocardial cell, shortening diffusion distance from cell exterior to structures in the cell interior. Its depolarization and repolarization can occur in intimate association with intracellular structures.

Excitation-contraction coupling

Ionic calcium is the link between excitation and contraction. Table 6.5 provides some highlights of the history of excitation-contraction coupling. Calcium is released from more than one intracellular site and also enters the cell from the extracellular solution during the plateau of the action potential (Chap. 7).

The sarcolemma membrane not only regulates inward diffusion of calcium but also acts as a calcium-accumulating system. The highest concentrations of calcium are found in the parts of the sarcolemma that are invaginated in the form of T tubules. From this location, calcium ions enter the myocardial fiber through the slowly conducting inward calcium channel (see Chap. 7) as soon as the excitation wave depolarizes the membrane sufficiently

Table 6.5. Historical highlights of excitation-contraction coupling

1882	Sidney Ringer showed that Ca^{2+} was required in the bathing medium to maintain beating and response to electrical stimulation of perfused myocardial cells isolated from heart.
1913	G.R. Mines demonstrated that omission of Ca^{2+} from Ringer's solution uncoupled excitation from contraction.
1940	L.V. Heilbrunn proposed that excitation released Ca^{2+} from the cortical layer of the cell to cause contraction. Heilbrunn compared the myosin contractile process to that of fibrin precipitation in blood clotting as similar Ca^{2+}-requiring mechanisms.
1947	L.V. Heilbrunn and F.J. Wiercenski showed that of all physiologicial salts, only calcium salts caused contraction when injected into the muscle fiber.
1959	C.P. Bianchi and A.M. Shanes demonstrated increased Ca^{2+} influx during electrical stimulation of frog skeletal muscle.

to open the channel. The production of cyclic AMP (cAMP) probably leads to this calcium accumulation by inducing phosphorylation of membrane proteins in and around the slow channels. By this reaction, the number of negative phosphate groups is increased and they accumulate calcium ions. The action of beta-adrenergic catecholamines increases cAMP, and this increases the membrane calcium pool, making more calcium available for influx at the next membrane depolarization.

From kinetic studies of calcium binding and uptake by cardiac microsomes in vitro, there is evidence of the existence of two different Ca^{2+} pools within the myocardial cell: (1) a *calcium-binding site* (possibly the longitudinal tubules of the subcellular sarcoplasmic reticulum) and (2) a *calcium-storage site* (possibly the terminal cisternae of the sarcoplasmic reticulum) presumed to accumulate, store, and release Ca^{2+} within the muscle cell. In response to the action potential, Ca^{2+} is released and diffuses into the fibrils for interaction with the contractile proteins, causing contraction. Systole is terminated when the sarcoplasmic reticulum reaccumulates the Ca^{2+}, removing it from its site of interaction with the contractile proteins.

Thus Ca^{2+} for excitation-contraction coupling has three potential sources: (1) influx of extracellular Ca^{2+} during systole, (2) release from binding sites, and (3) release from storage sites. The importance of sarcoplasmic reticulum release of calcium can be illustrated by stimulation of an isolated ventricular muscle after a prolonged rest period (Fig. 6.10). The resulting contraction is weak because, under these circumstances, the sarcoplasmic reticulum is depleted of calcium. The only calcium available for contraction is that which enters the cell transsarcolemmally, and it is inadequate for a normal contractile force. Contractile force of the isolated myocardial cell increases with an increase in the frequency of beating (positive staircase) (Fig. 6.10). The sensitivity of the myofilaments to calcium is not altered, but the amount of calcium released is increased. Its exact source is not known, but it may involve an increase in both transsarcolemmal and sarcoplasmic reticulum release of calcium. Paired-pulse stimulation or stimulation after a brief rest following high-frequency stimulation of isolated cardiac muscle results in a potentiated forceful state that again is not due to an alteration in the sensitivity of the myofilaments to calcium (Fig. 6.10). These potentiated states depend on calcium derived from sarcoplasmic reticulum.

As the contractile event depends on the presence of calcium ions, so relaxation depends on their removal. When calcium ions are removed from the area of myofilaments, cross-bridge formation between actin and myosin ceases and the sarcomere returns to its resting length. Thus the sarcoplasmic reticulum, with its ability to bind, transport, and resequester calcium in an inactive site (lateral sac), is considered the subcellular system, which produces contraction, regulates tension, and achieves relaxation. These various functions are summarized in Fig. 6.11A and B.

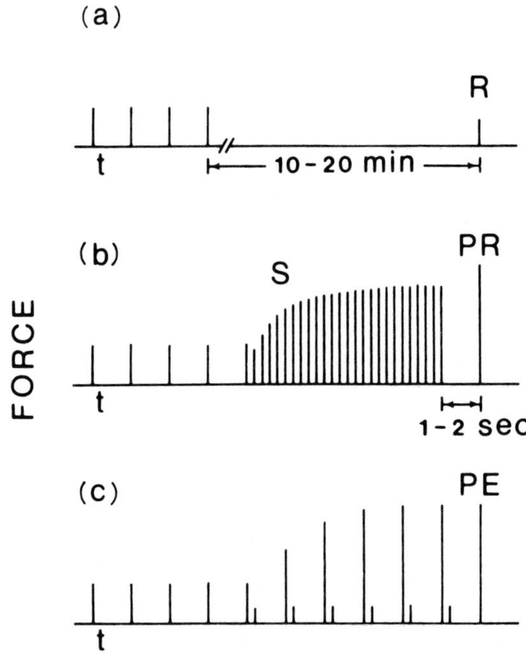

Figure 6.10. Effect of rate and pattern of stimulation on contractile state. (*a*) Rested-state contraction (R) is elicited by a stimulus that follows a long (10 to 20 minutes) rest period. During the rest, internal store of sarcoplasmic reticulum Ca^{2+} is depleted. Resting-state contraction is activated predominantly by Ca^{2+} supplied via transsarcolemmal influx. (b) Staircase (S) is also called positive staircase, Bowditch staircase, and Treppe. Force of contraction increases to a new steady state over several beats after an abrupt transition to a higher rate of stimulation. Postrest (PR) potentiated-state contraction is elicited by a stimulus delivered after 1 to 2 seconds of rest after a train of high-frequency stimuli. (c) Postextrasystolic potentiation (PE) is elicited in response to paired-pulse stimulation. The intrapair stimulus interval is approximately 300 ms. Ca^{2+} released internally from the SR assumes a major role in the activation of potentiated-state contractions. (From Rusy and Komai 1987, *Anesthesiology* 67:745–66.)

In summary, it is thought that the depolarizing impulse travels along the sarcolemma and is propagated throughout the cell via the T tubular network. Depolarization of the membranes of the lateral sacs associated with T tubules and those beneath the sarcolemma results in calcium ion release. Calcium ions induce interaction between actin and myosin, and contraction results. Relaxation is the result of sarcotubular removal of calcium from the area of the myofilaments.

Metabolism and energetics

Under normal circumstances, myocardial cells operate almost exclusively on an aerobic metabolic system that provides the constant supply of high-energy phosphate bonds for mechanical and chemical work. In Table 6.6 are listed various metabolic substrates together with their percentage contribution to myocardial oxygen use. Usually the major fuel for cardiac metabolism is free fatty acids. Glucose and lactate are also important contributors, whereas amino acids, ketones, and pyruvate make lesser contributions.

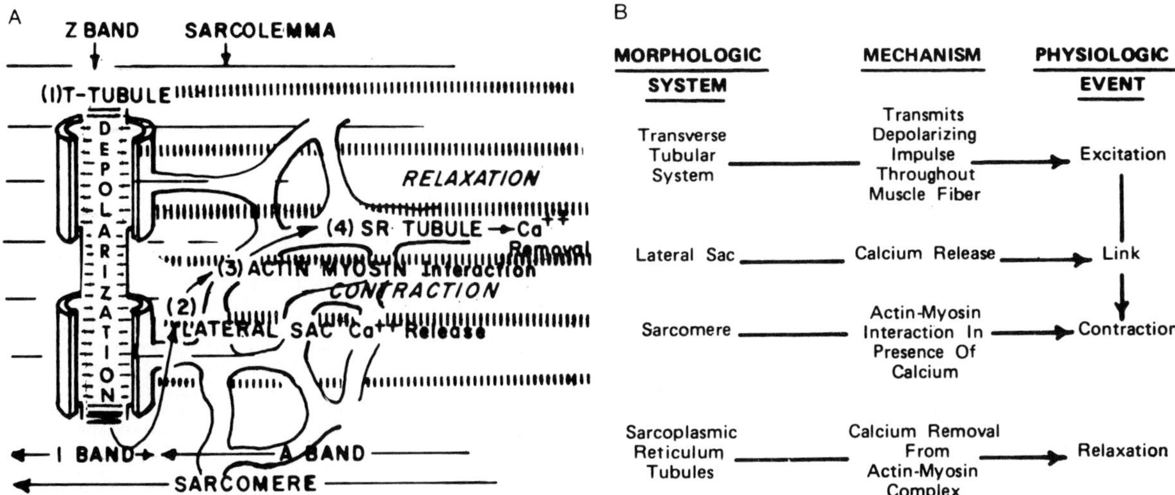

Figure 6.11. (*A*) Subcellular systems involved in excitation-contraction coupling and relaxation. (1) The depolarizing impulse travels over the sarcomeric membrane and along the T-tubule membrane into the depths of the cell. (2) Depolarization causes calcium ion release from storage depots of the lateral sacs. (3) Calcium ions bind with troponin of the tropomyosin-troponin complex and somehow abolish the inhibitory effect of these modulatory proteins on the interaction between actin and myosin, and contraction occurs. (4) Relaxation occurs when this freed calcium is removed by being taken up again by the lateral sacs. (*B*) The events of excitation-contraction coupling are summarized (Redrawn and modified from Legato 1969, *Prog. Cardiovasc. Dis.* 11:391–409, by permission.)

Myocardial metabolism has three phases (Fig. 6.12):

1. *Energy liberation* or production is the stage during which energy is released from the carbon-hydrogen bonds of substrates, including fatty acids, glucose, lactate, and other compounds used by the heart.
2. *Energy conservation* or storage is the transfer of the energy into synthesis of high-energy phosphate compounds, including ATP and creatine phosphate, as well as the mono- and diphosphates of adenosine (AMP, ADP).
3. *Energy utilization* is the release of this stored chemical energy into shortening or development of tension of the cardiac contraction.

The mitochondria (sarcosomes) are the sites of the major aerobic or oxidative processes on which the heart depends for its energy supply.

The relationships between the biochemical events, myocardial contraction, and cellular maintenance are diagrammed in Fig. 6.13. The physicochemical interaction of actin and myosin uses ATP. The latter is then replenished from high-energy phosphate bonds from creatine phosphate or from the electron transport chain. The increased amounts of ADP and inorganic phosphate (P_i) resulting from muscle contraction act to stimulate oxidative phosphorylation, the citric acid cycle, and glycolysis. This increases high-energy phosphate bond production. High levels of ATP depress these processes. Thus the relative levels of ADP and P_i on the one hand and ATP on the other serve as a regulatory feedback control governing aerobic mitochondrial processes leading to the production of high-energy compounds. Creatine phosphate functions as a small but immediately available source of high-energy phosphate bonds.

Table 6.6. Percentage contribution of various metabolic substrates to total myocardial oxygen usage

Carbohydrate		Noncarbohydrate	
Glucose	17.90%	Fatty acids	67.0%
Pyruvate	0.54%	Amino acids	5.6%
Lactate	16.46%	Ketones	4.3%
Total[a]	34.90%	Total[a]	76.9%

[a]The total is more than 100 percent because some of the substrates removed from the blood, in amounts measured by the arteriovenous differences, were stored by the heart or not completely metabolized.

From Bing 1955, *Circulation* 12:635–47.

To understand the dependence of cardiac muscle on the continual oxygen supply, it is useful to compare the patterns of energy production and use with those of red and white skeletal muscle. The heart, like red skeletal muscle, is organized to maintain its work over long periods of time without rest; both of these types of muscle rely on oxidative metabolism for ATP regeneration and have little ability to function anaerobically or to incur oxygen debt. This is in contrast to white skeletal muscle, which is organized for brief bursts of intense activity followed by periods of relaxation. The substrates, metabolites, pathways of intermediary metabolism, and intracellular energy reserves of the two types of muscle are strikingly different (Table 6.7). Cardiac muscle contains large numbers of mitochondria that are rich in the enzymes of the citric acid cycle and oxidative phosphorylation. The myoglobin content is large, favoring oxygen diffusion into the fiber. In white skeletal muscle the enzymes responsible for anaerobic glycolysis are more abundant, whereas cardiac muscle is richer in enzymes providing for oxidative metabolism of pyruvate, succinate, and acetoacetate. Un-

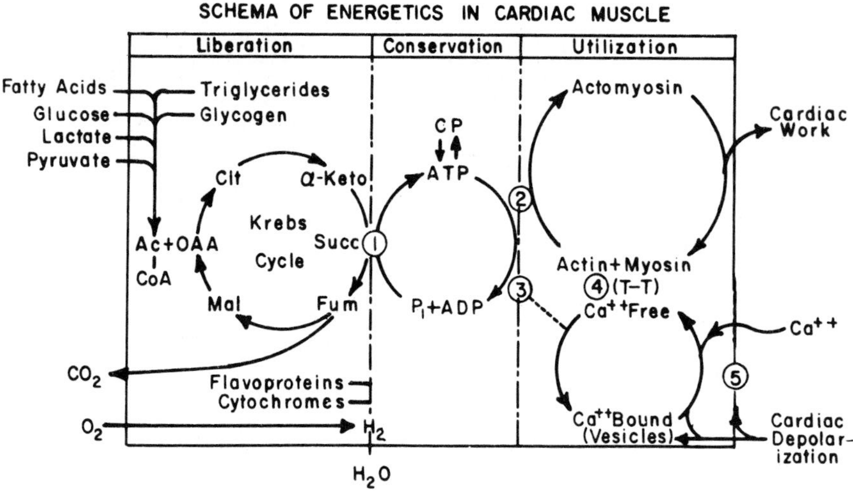

Figure 6.12. The three phases of myocardial energetics. Energy-coupling points affected by hypoxia include (1) oxidative phosphorylation, (2) actomyosin ATPase, (3) ATP-energized calcium pump of the reticulum, (4) troponin-tropomyosin-calcium system for regulating contractility, and (5) ion pumps in the cell membrane. Cit, citrate; α-Keto, alpha ketoglutarate; Succ, succinate; Fum, fumarate; Mal, malate; Ac CoA, acetyl CoA; OAA, oxaloacetate; CP, creatine phosphate; ATP, adenine triphosphate; ADP, adenosine diphosphate. (Slightly modified from Olson, Dhalla, and Sun 1971/1972, *Cardiology* 56:114–24.)

Table 6.7. Energy sources for contraction of red and white skeletal muscle and cardiac muscle

Energy source	White skeletal muscle	Red skeletal and cardiac muscle
Major substrates	Carbohydrate	Lipid
Major metabolic pathways	Anaerobic	Aerobic
Major products of metabolism	Lactic acid	CO_2 and H_2O
Oxygen debt on activity	Significant	Minor
Reserve of phosphate-bond energy (phosphocreatine)	Significant	Minor
Ability to function in the absence of oxygen	Good	Poor

From Katz 1967, *Physiol. Rev.* 50:63–168.

der anaerobic conditions the heart has a very limited capacity to use glycolysis for energy release, and its slender reserve of creatine phosphate is quickly depleted.

The energy-utilization phase of cardiac and red skeletal muscle also differs characteristically from that of white skeletal muscle. The ATPase of myosins from the former is less active than that of white skeletal myosin. The maximal shortening velocities of both red skeletal and cardiac muscles are slower than those of white skeletal muscle, presumably because shortening velocity may be determined by the rate of ATP hydrolysis by the contractile proteins. The relatively lower tensions developed by cardiac muscle, as contrasted with white skeletal muscle, may be attributed in part to the larger number of mitochondria in myocardial cells. These, by taking up considerable intracellular space, reduce the amount of contractile protein present per unit volume of myocardial tissue.

Regeneration

In the embryogenesis of skeletal muscle, once the cells have differentiated to the point where they are capable of contraction, there is no further cell division or increase in DNA content. In the developing heart, on the other hand, the cells multiply, that is, undergo *hyperplasia*. A similar division of myocardial cells occurs in tissue culture, involving both undifferentiated cells and those that have become contractile. At just what stage of development the heart

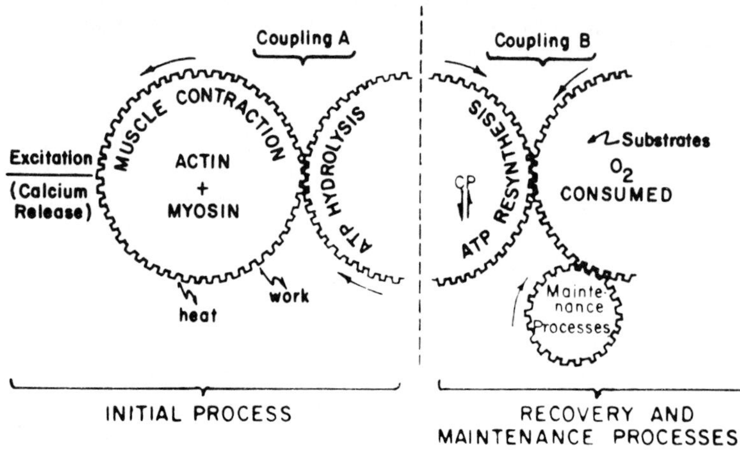

Figure 6.13. Diagram of mechanochemical coupling in cardiac muscle. The interaction of actin and myosin during contraction is initiated by Ca^{2+} release (initial process, *left*), and utilizes ATP through coupling A. Oxidative phosphorylation provides for the formation of creatine phosphate (CP) and adenosine triphosphate (ATP), CP serving as a reservoir for high-energy phosphate bonds available for ATP resynthesis. Oxygen utilization is related to CP and ATP synthesis through coupling B. Oxygen is also consumed in various cellular maintenance processes. (Redrawn from Braunwald, Ross, and Sonnenblick 1967, *Mechanisms of Contraction of the Normal and the Failing Heart,* Little, Brown, Boston, © 1967.)

loses its capacity for hyperplasia is not known for certain. The consensus is that an increase in myocardial mass, particularly in an adult, can be accomplished only through enlargement of *hypertrophy* of cardiac cells already differentiated. This means the enlargement and multiplication of intracellular structures such as myofilaments and mitochondria. This is in sharp contrast to skeletal muscle, which is capable of tissue repair involving both regeneration of individual fibers and reconstitution of the whole muscle.

Dilatation

The term *cardiac dilatation* refers to an increase in volumetric capacity of the heart chambers. Alterations in cardiac volume occur normally whenever there is a change in cardiac output, especially stroke volume. In various abnormal states, however, enlargement beyond usual physiological limits may occur, either acutely or as a chronic condition.

Three factors involved in acute dilatation are (1) sarcomere lengthening, (2) so-called fiber slippage, and (3) stratification change. Two of these factors are represented schematically in Fig. 6.14. In acute dilatation the sarcomeres become longer than 2.2 μm, and an H zone (due to the thin filaments withdrawing from the A band) that normally is absent in cardiac sarcomeres can be seen in electron micrographs. *Fiber slippage* means that individual fibers slide past one another longitudinally, and this can produce lengthening of the dimensions of the wall of the heart in any direction because there are fibers that run longitudinally in every direction. Different from this is the process of change in stratification of fibers where the wall lengthens at right angles to the direction of myocardial fibers. As the myocardium is stretched, the individual fibers become thinner and fibers from adjacent layers slip between one another. This increases the number of fibers within a single layer and decreases the number of layers of the myocardial wall. In this way, wall thickness is reduced and surface area is increased. The term *plastic dilatation* has been applied to longitudinal slippage and lateral rearrangement of myocardial fibers.

Dilatation, in that it involves an increase both in sarcomere length and in the internal diameter of cardiac chambers, has two functional implications: (1) Increasing sarcomere length, within limits, increases the contractile strength of myocardial fibers (Frank-Starling relationship, see Chap. 9); (2) increasing chamber diameter increases the wall tension for a given intracardiac pressure in accordance with the Laplace relation (tension = pressure × radius^2, see Chap. 8 and Fig. 8.10). Physiologically, increased stretch results in increased wall tension, but at the same time force of contraction is increased. If the sarcomeres are stretched too far, however, contractile strength decreases, even though for any given intraluminal pressure the tension within the wall is increased as a result of the dilatation.

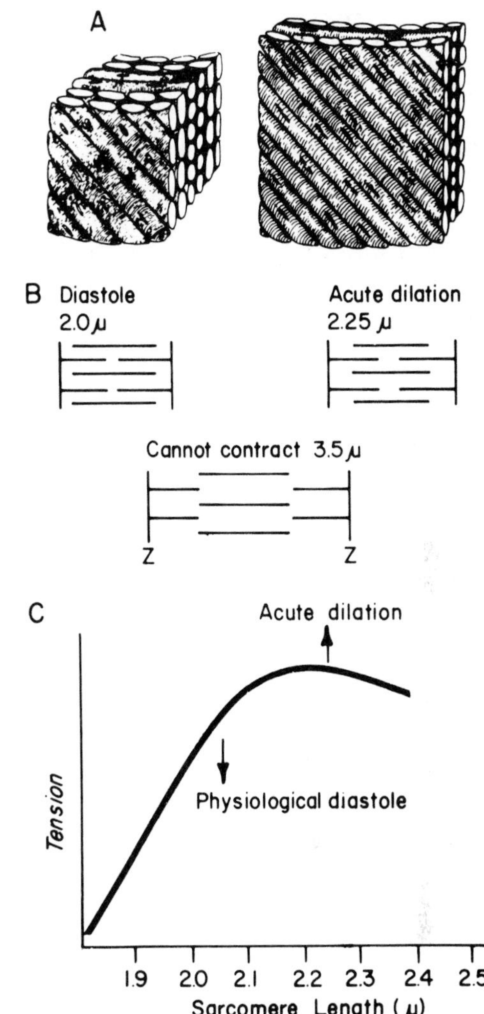

Figure 6.14. (*A*) Schemata of stratification change. The same part of the right ventricular wall is represented in normal state and with marked dilatation. (*B*) Schematic representation of sarcomeres in different states of stretch showing the relations of the thin and thick filaments. (*C*) Sarcomere length—active tension diagram of an isolated papillary muscle showing the sarcomere lengths for physiological diastole and acute dilatation. (Redrawn from Hort 1968, in Reindell, Keul, and Doll, eds., *Herzinsuffizienz,* Thieme, Stuttgart.)

Studies on experimental animals in which acute cardiac dilatation has been induced (e.g., acute asphyxia) indicate that sarcomere stretch beyond physiological limits does not ordinarily occur (Fig. 6.14). The increase in sarcomere length that does take place cannot fully account for the degree of observed dilatation, so that fiber slippage and stratification change must play a significant role. It does not appear that the sarcomeres become stretched to the point where this factor alone can account for contractile weakness or that individual sarcomeres are stretched to the point where they cannot contract at all. Sarcomere length is increased, however, to the point where there is little reserve for increase in contractile strength through the Frank-Starling mechanism.

In chronic dilatation it has been shown experimentally that fiber slippage and change in stratification, as well as a moderate increase in sarcomere length, occur as in acute dilatation.

In summary, acute and chronic dilatation results primarily from slippage and stratification change of fibers. Sarcomere length is increased moderately at most or, as some studies have shown, not at all. Because of the increased diameter, the heart must operate at increased wall tension for a given intracardiac pressure. Insofar as sarcomere lengthening does occur, the reserve for increased contractile force with increased sarcomere length is compromised.

Hypertrophy and atrophy

Myocardial hypertrophy is an increase in muscle mass beyond its usual limits. At present the molecular biology of myocardial hypertrophy is speculative. It is based on myocyte cell culture experiments. In most types of cell, the predominant extracellular signals for growth are soluble molecules called *growth factors*. For cardiac myocytes, the search of these factors is ongoing. Since mechanical stretch (as in cardiac dilatation) induces myocyte growth, this mechanism must be understood. Current work suggests that the receptor for the stimulation of stretch or growth may be a surface ion channel, while that for humoral induction of growth may be the alpha$_1$-adrenergic receptor. The latter is supported by the finding that norepinephrine increases cultured cardiac myocyte size 1.5 to 2-times and provides evidence of the long-held view that catecholamines may be a major growth factor for cardiac hypertrophy. *Physiological hypertrophy,* as seen in exercise training, is accompanied by a normal or enhanced contractile state, proportional growth of cellular constituents, and normal myosin ATPase activity. *Pathological hypertrophy,* seen in diseased hearts, is accompanied by a decrease in contractile state, decreased myosin ATPase activity, diminished cyclic AMP, and disproportionate biosynthesis of subcellular structures (e.g., mitochondria). There is no convincing evidence of hyperplasia in myocardial hypertrophy. Rather, the myocardial fibers increase in diameter by the addition of more myofibrils and in length by the addition of more sarcomeres. The sarcomeres may be added only at the intercalated disks. Possibly the Z substance serves as a source or template for the new sarcomeres. Proliferation of mitochondria also contributes to the increased diameter. Connective tissue and vasculature increase by hyperplasia; capillaries increase in length but not in numbers (i.e., the normal 1 : 1 ratio of capillaries to fibers is maintained).

Concentric hypertrophy consists of an increased thickness of the ventricular wall without an increase in size of the ventricular chamber. This adaptation occurs in response to a long-standing pressure overload (e.g., aortic valve or aortic outflow tract obstruction). Eccentric hypertrophy consists of an enlarged ventricular chamber with a relatively small increase in wall thickness. This adaptation is due to a long-standing volume overload (e.g., patent ductus arteriosus or atrioventricular valve insufficiency). The hypertrophied myocardium in cardiac disease frequently exhibits abnormal systolic or diastolic function and electrical instability leading to arrhythmias of various kinds.

Control mechanisms

Myocardial cells adjust their size to their workload: mechanical overload induces hypertrophy, the cells return to control size when the workload returns to normal, and reduction in workload below normal causes atrophy. Example of the latter are the reduction of left ventricular mass when right ventricular output is reduced in pulmonary hypertension, the small subepicardial myocardial cells seen in long-standing pericardial effusion that decreases cardiac output, and the reduction in heart and fiber size in Addison's disease and in starvation. Mechanical unloading of a single papillary muscle by section of the chordae tendinae results in atrophy of the involved cells to 66 percent of their control diameter within 3 days. Living cells maintain a state of dynamic equilibrium between synthesis and breakdown of cellular elements. This process is under control of the genetic apparatus in the nucleus (also in part in the mitochondria) and involves nuclear DNA and the sarcoplasmic RNA system. In hypertrophy there is an increase in synthesis over destruction of contractile proteins especially, as well as other cellular elements. The link between increased contractile activity and stimulation of the DNA-RNA system is obscure.

The mechanical stimulus for hypertrophy requires an increased energy expenditure per unit mass of myocardium. This may be caused by an increase in cardiac output, such as results from an increase in flow-work (as in valvular insufficiency, arteriovenous fistulas, or severe anemia) or from an increase in pressure-work (as in valvular stenosis or hypertension). In cardiomyopathies there is no increase in external workload, but the heart dilates and, in accordance with the Laplace relationship, wall tension increases for a given pressure and provides the stimulus for hypertrophy. The sequence of events for hypertrophy is outlined in Fig. 6.15. Normalization of the abnormal myocardial wall stress is considered feedback signal that governs the rate and degree of ventricular hypertrophy.

The following list gives some clinical applications about myocardial cells:

1. Atrial contraction is lost in atrial fibrillation, but this in itself is of little consequence in the maintenance of cardiac output except at rapid heart rates.
2. Systole in the left ventricle alone will cause some pumping of the right ventricle because of left ventricular aid.
3. Rapid fluid accumulation under pressure in the inelastic pericardial sac limits or halts cardiac output because of

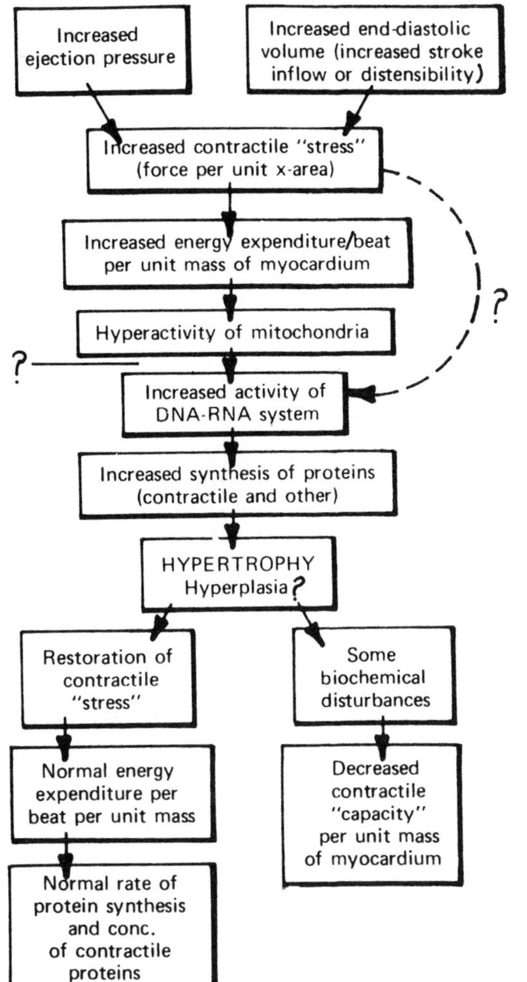

Figure 6.15. The pathogenesis of cardiac hypertrophy. (Redrawn from Badeer 1968, *Prog. Cardiovasc. Dis.* 11:52–63, by permission.)

cardiac tamponade. The pericardial sac can enlarge gradually in cardiac hypertrophy and can accommodate large volumes of slowly forming pericardial effusions.

4. Hypocalcemia, as in parturient paresis, has a negative inotropic effect and can cause death from cardiac failure. Hypercalcemia, especially when induced by infusions of Ca^{2+} solutions, has a positive inotropic effect but is dangerous because fatal arrhythmias may be produced.

5. The heart requires a continual supply of oxygen because it cannot function anaerobically or incur an oxygen debt.

6. The damaged myocardium cannot regenerate, and dead myocardial tissue is replaced by noncontractile connective tissue.

7. Cardiac dilatation occurs by longitudinal fiber slippage and lateral rearrangement of fibers, rather than by abnormal stretch of sarcomeres.

8. Physiological cardiac hypertrophy of exercise training does not disturb contractile function, whereas pathological hypertrophy is associated with diminished contractility and ultimate cardiac failure.

REFERENCES

Babu, A., Sonnenblick, E., Gulati, J. 1988. Molecular basis for the influence of muscle length on myocardial performance. *Science* 240:74–76.

Badeer, H.S. 1968. Metabolic basis of cardiac hypertrophy. *Prog. Cardiovasc. Dis.* 11:52–63.

Beznak, M.J. (1969. Regression of cardiac hypertrophy of various origins. *Can. J. Physiol. Pharmacol.* 47:579–86.

Bing, J.R. 1955. Myocardial metabolism. *Circulation* 12:635–47.

Brady, A.J. 1979. Mechanical properties of cardiac fibers. In R.M. Berne, N. Sperelakis, and S.R. Geiger, eds., *Handbook of Physiology.* Sec. 2, The Cardiovascular System. Vol. 1, *The Heart.* Am. Physiol. Soc., Bethesda, Md. Pp. 461–74.

Braunwald, E., Ross, J., Jr., and Sonnenblick, E.H. 1967. *Mechanisms of Contraction of the Normal and Failing Heart.* Little, Brown, Boston.

Bugaisky, L., and Zak, R. 1979. Cellular growth of cardiac muscle after birth. *Tex. Rep. Biol. Med.* 39:123–38.

Chacko, S. 1973. DNA synthesis, mitosis and differentiation in cardiac myogenesis. *Dev. Biol.* 35:1–18.

Cheung, W.Y. 1980. Calmodulin plays a pivotal role in cellular regulation. *Science* 207:19–27.

Cooper, S., IV, and Tomanek, R.J. 1982. Load regulation of the structure, composition, and function of mammalian myocardium. *Circ. Res.* 50:788–98.

Detweiler, D.K. 1981. The use of electrocardiography in toxicological studies with rats. In R. Budden, D.K. Detweiler, and G. Zbinden, eds., *The Rat Electrogardiogram in Pharmacology and Toxicology.* Pergamon, Oxford. Pp. 83–115.

Detweiler, D.K., Cox, R.H., Alonso, F.R., and Patterson, D.F. 1975. Characteristics of the greyhound cardiovascular system. *Fed. Proc.* 34:399.

Dhalla, N.S., Pierce, G.N., Panagra, V., Singal, P.K., and Beamish, R.E. 1982. Calcium movements in relation to heart function. *Basic Res. Cardiol.* 77:117–39.

Evans, H.E., and Christensen, G.C. 1979. The heart and arteries. In H.E. Evans and G.C. Christensen, eds., *Miller's Anatomy of the Dog.* 2d ed. W.B. Saunders, Philadelphia. Pp. 632–756.

Fleckenstein, A.H., Tritthart, H., Döring, H.-J., and Byon, K.Y. 1972. Bay a 1040-ein hochaktiver ($Ca^{(++)}$-angatonistischer Inhibitor der elektro-mechanischen Koppelungsprozesse im Warmblüter-Myokard. *Arzneim. Forsch.* 22:22–23.

Fleckenstein. A., and Fleckenstein-Grun. G. 1989. Effects of and the mechanism of action of calcium antagonists and other antianginal agents. In N. Sperelakis, ed., *Physiology and Pathophysiology of the Heart.* 2d ed. Klulver, Boston, Pp. 471–91.

Ford, L.E. 1991. Mechanical manifestations of activation in cardiac muscle. *Circ. Res.* 68:621–37.

Ford, L.E., and Forman, R. 1974. Tetanized cardiac muscle. In Ciba Foundation Symposium No. 27. *The Physiological Basis of Starling's Law of the Heart.* Elsevier, Amsterdam. Pp. 137–50.

Grande, F., and Taylor, H.L. 1965. Adaptive changes in the heart, vessels, and patterns of control under chronically high loads. *Handbook of Physiology.* Sec. 2, W.F. Hamilton, ed., *Circulation.* Am. Physiol. Soc., Washington. Vol. 3, 2615–77.

Hill, A.V. 1939. Heat of shortening and dynamic constants of muscle. *Proc. R. Soc.* (London) (Biol.), ser. B. 126:136–95.

Hort, W. 1968. Strukturelle Analyse akut insuffizienter Hertzen. In H. Reindell, J. Keul, and E. Doll, eds., *Herzinsuffizienz.* Thieme, Stuttgart. Pp. 6–11.

Jewell, B.R., and Wilkie, D.R. 1960. The mechanical properties of relaxing muscle. *J. Physiol.* (London) 152:30–47.

Katz, A.M. 1967. Patterns of energy production and energy utilization in cardiac and skeletal muscle. In R.D. Tanz, F. Kavaler, and J. Roberts, eds., *Factors Influencing Myocardial Contractility.* Academic Press, New York. Pp. 401–15.

Knight, D.H. 1967. Pulmonary hypertension and left ventricular atrophy in dogs with spontaneous cor pulmonale. *Physiologist* 10:223.

Knight, D.H. 1970. Sarcomergenesis in the human myocardium. *J. Mol. Cell Cardiol.* 1:425–37.

Linzbach, J., and Kyrieleis, C. 1968. Strukturelle Analyse chronisch insuffizienter menschlicher Herzen. In H. Reindell, H. Keul, and E. Doll, eds., *Herzinsuffizienz.* Thieme, Stuttgart. Pp. 11–19.

Little, R.C., and Little, W.C. 1989. *Physiology of the Heart and Circulation.* 4th ed. Yearbook Medical Publishers, Chicago.

McNutt, N.S. 1970. Ultrastructure of intercellular junctions in adult and developing cardiac muscle. *Am. J. Cardiol.* 25:169–83.

Maruyamia, T., Ashekawa, K., Isoyama, S., Kanatsuka, H., Ino-Oka, E., and Takishima. T. 1982. Mechanical interactions between four heart chambers with and without the pericardium in canine hearts. *Circ. Res.* 50:86–100.

Meerson, F.Z. 1969. The myocardium in hyperfunction, hypertrophy, and heart failure. *Circ. Res.* (suppl.) 2:1–163.

Olson, R.E., Dhalla, N.S., and Sun, C.N. 1971/72. Changes in energy stores in the hypoxic heart. *Cardiology* 56:114–24.

Olson, R.E., and Piatnek, D.A. 1959. Conservation of energy in cardiac muscle. *Ann. N.Y. Acad. Sci.* 72:466, 478.

Parmley, W.W., and Wikman-Coffelt, J. 1988. In W.W. Parmley and K. Chatterjee, eds., *Cardiology,* vol. 1. J. B. Lippincott, Philadelphia. Pp. 1–26.

Rusy, B.F., and Komai, H. 1987. Anesthetic depression of myocardial contractility: a review of possible mechanisms. *Anesthesiology* 67:745–66.

Schütz, E. 1958. *Physiologie des Herzens.* Springer, Berlin.

Simpson, P.C., Karns, L.R., and Long, C.S. 1990. An approach to the molecular regulation of cardiac myocyte hypertrophy. In S. Chien, ed., *Molecular Biology of the Cardiovascular System.* Lea & Febiger, Philadelphia. Pp. 53–81.

Sommer, J.R., and Johnson, E.A. 1970. Comparative ultrastructure of cardiac cell membrane specialization. A review. *Am. J. Cardiol.* 25:278–84.

Sommer, J.R., and Johnson, E.A. 1979. Ultrastructure of cardiac muscle. In R. M. Berne, N. Sperelakis, and S.R. Geiger, eds., *Handbook of Physiology.* Sec. 2, The Cardiovascular System. Vol. 1, *The Heart.* Am. Physiol. Soc., Bethesda, Md. Pp. 113–86.

Streeter, D.D., Jr. 1979. Gross morphology and fiber geometry of the heart. In R.M. Berne, N. Sperelakis, and S.R. Geiger, eds., *Handbook of Physiology.* Sec. 2, The Cardiovascular System. Vol. 1, *The Heart.* Am. Physiol. Soc., Bethesda, Md. Pp. 61–112.

Streeter, D.D., Jr., Spotnitz, H.M., Patel, D.P., Ross, J., Jr., and Sonnenblick, E.H. 1969. Fiber orientation in the canine left ventricle during diastole and systole. *Circ. Res.* 24:339–47.

Tomanek, R.J. 1979. Quantitative ultrastructural aspects of cardiac hypertrophy. *Tex. Rep. Biol. Med.* 9:111–21.

Urthaler, F., Kawamura, K., and James, T.N. 1978. The anatomical basis for cardiac rhythm and conduction. In T.E. Andreoli, J.F. Hoffman, and D.D. Fanstel, eds., *Physiology of Membrane Disorders.* Plenum, New York. Pp. 831–75.

Weidmann, S. 1965. Cardiac electrophysiology in the light of recent morphological findings. *Harvey Lectures* 61:1–15.

Weidmann, S. 1966. Diffusion of radio-potassium across intercalated discs of mammalian cardiac muscle. *J. Physiol.* (London) 187:323–42.

Wiegner, A.W., Beng, O.H.L., Borg, T.K., and Caulfield, J.B. 1981. Mechanical and structural correlates of canine pericardium. *Circ. Res.* 49:807–14.

Wikman-Coffelt, J., Laks, M.M., Riemenschneider, T., and Mason, D. 1980. Physiological versus pathological myocardial hypertrophy. In M. Tajudden, P.K. Das, M. Tariq, and N.S. Dhalla, eds., *Advances in Myocardiology.* Vol. 1. University Park Press, Baltimore. Pp. 469–76.

Woodworth, R.S. 1902. Maximal contraction, "staircase" contraction, refractory period and compensatory pause of the heart. *Am. J. Physiol.* 8:231–49.

Yin, F.C.P. 1981. Ventricular wall stress. *Circ. Res.* 49:829–42.

Zak, R. 1973. Cell proliferation during cardiac growth. *Am. J. Cardiol.* 31:211–19.

CHAPTER 7

Electrophysiology of the Heart | by Michael S. Miller, Larry Patrick Tilley, and David K. Detweiler

PACEMAKER AND CONDUCTION SYSTEM

The specialized pacemaking and conduction tissues of the heart consist of the sinus (sinoatrial) node, the atrioventricular (AV) node, the bundle of His, the right bundle branch and the left bundle branch of the bundle of His, and the peripheral Purkinje network (Fig. 7.1).

Normally, pacemaker cells located within the sinoatrial (SA) node serve to initiate the heartbeat. Although special anatomical tracts connecting the SA and AV nodes and atrial cells that are electrophysiologically specialized for conduction have been described, conduction in the atria is primarily through ordinary atrial myocardial cells. Conduction is more rapid along the long axis of these cells than transversely. This fiber orientation probably accounts for rapid conduction along preferential pathways to the AV node rather than bundlelike tracts of specialized cells. The crista terminalis and the anterior limbus of the fossa ovalis are the main routes for such preferential conduction between the SA and AV nodes in both dog and rabbit atria and allow early activation of the AV node.

Normally the cardiac impulses that reach the ventricle must traverse the AV node, a region of relatively slow conduction. The AV node is the normal pathway between the atrial myocardium and the bundle of His. Emerging from the AV node, the impulse reaches the rapidly conducting Purkinje fibers of the bundle of His and travels along the bundle branches to the Purkinje fiber network of the ventricles.

This complex system accounts for cardiac impulse origination and its distribution throughout the heart for each heartbeat. It provides for sequential contraction of the atria and ventricles and brings the entire myocardial mass of both ventricles rapidly into coordinated contraction. The diameters and conduction velocities of the mammalian heart fibers are provided in Table 7.1.

Sinus node

The sinus node is embedded in the right atrial wall at the junction of the anterior vena cava and the right atrium. This junction appears on the epicardial surface as the *sulcus terminalis* and on the endocardial surface as the *crista terminalis*. The SA node is ellipsoid in shape in dogs, humans, and several other species, but it is horseshoe-shaped with long tapering crura in the horse and is similarly shaped in other ungulates. Its ultrastructure is similar in several different species. Long thin myocardial cells, sparse in myofibrils, interlace with an abundant collagen network and make up this compact structure.

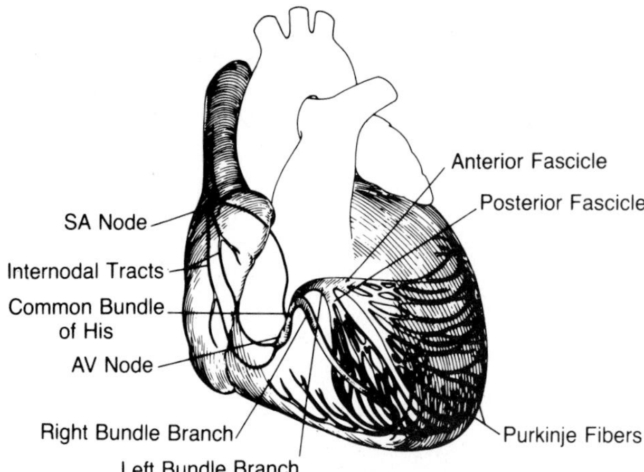

Figure 7.1. The mammalian cardiac conduction system of the heart. (From DeSanctis 1982, Disturbances of cardiac rhythm and conduction. In E. Rubenstein, ed. *Scientific American Medicine,* New York, Scientific American, 1982. *Scientific American Medicine,* Section 1, Subsection VI. © 1991 Scientific American, Inc. All rights reserved.)

Atrioventricular node

The AV node is located beneath the right atrial endocardium at the base of the interatrial septum just anterior to the ostium of the coronary sinus. On the atrial side, it receives branches from the atrial musculature and is continuous with the bundle of His on the ventricular side. Its fibers, which are smaller than those of atrial muscle, form a pattern of branching and interlacing strands in a connective tissue framework. The various cell types in this specialized cardiac tissue have different electrophysiological characteristics (see text below).

Bundle of His

At the transition region between the AV node and the bundle of His, the cells gather into more regular fascicles and take on the characteristics of Purkinje fibers. These collected Purkinje fibers are known as the bundle of His. The bundle of His passes from the right atrial endocardial location of the AV node medially and along the lower margin of the interventricular septum and then gives rise to a single right bundle branch and multiple left bundle branches.

Table 7.1. Fiber diameter and conduction velocity in mammalian heart cells

Cell type	Diameter (μm)	Conduction velocity (m/s)*
SA and AV nodes	5	0.02–0.1
Atrial and ventricular working cells	8–12	0.3–1.0
Purkinje cells	40–50	3–5

*The difference in conduction velocity between Purkinje cells and working myocardial cells can be partly explained by their different diameters. The difference between the conduction velocity of SA and AV nodal cells and that of the other cells cannot be explained by diameter difference but, rather, by differences in the rate of inward current during phase 0 of the action potential (rapid upstroke, see text), which is relatively slow in these cells (see definition of *slow response* in text).

From Fozzard 1979, in Berne, Sperelakis, and Geiger, eds., Cardiovascular System, *Handbook of Physiology,* Am. Physiol. Soc., Bethesda, Md.

Bundle branches

The right bundle is given off first and is the smaller of the two branches. The left bundle branch continues from the bundle of His as a broad fascicle that runs subendocardially down the left side of the interventricular septum and divides into major anterior and posterior fascicles before reaching the peripheral Purkinje network (Fig. 7.2).

The electron microscopic morphology of the fibers within the peripheral Purkinje network arborization varies with heart size in mammalian species. In small mammals (e.g., cat, rabbit, guinea pig, mouse) these cells are indistinguishable from those of the working myocardium, except that the Purkinje network cells lack a T system. In large mammals (e.g., ungulates, whales) these Purkinje cells are large and pale staining, and they contain little contractile protein. Also, the Purkinje network penetrates extensively into the depths of the ventricular myocardium in the large mammals and birds but is limited to the subendocardium in small mammals. No conduction system is present in the small, slow-beating hearts of lower vertebrates. Conduction is more rapid in the larger cells (Fig. 7.3). These morphological adaptations permit more rapid spread of excitation in the larger hearts (e.g., ungulates and whales) and fast conduction velocities for the rapid heart rates of birds.

A variable number of fibers of intermediate size (transitional fibers) are found intermingled with the Purkinje fibers of the bundle branches. These transitional fibers gradually diminish in size and become continuous with working myocardial fibers. In addition to their smaller diameter, they are characterized by an absence of T tubules and sarcoplasmic reticulum. They have a lower resting membrane potential (see text below), a slower rate of rise of phase 0, and a slower conduction velocity than Purkinje fibers.

Anatomical tracts that bypass the AV node

There are several anatomical pathways through which conduction from atria to ventricles can occur, bypassing the AV node. *James fibers* are fibers from the atria that pass around the AV node and reenter its inferior margin or penetrate as far as the interventricular septum. *Mahaim fibers* (paraspecific fibers) are short, direct connections between the AV node, the bundle of His, or bundle branches, and the interventricular septum. The *accessory bundle of Kent* is the right- and left-sided myocardial or specialized conduction tissue bridge between the atria and the ventricles. Although this bundle is most frequently found in fetal and infantile hearts, it may be identified in some adult hearts. Purkinje cells are not found in these accessory bundles.

All of these tracts are considered possible conduction routes that, when active, can account for anomalous AV

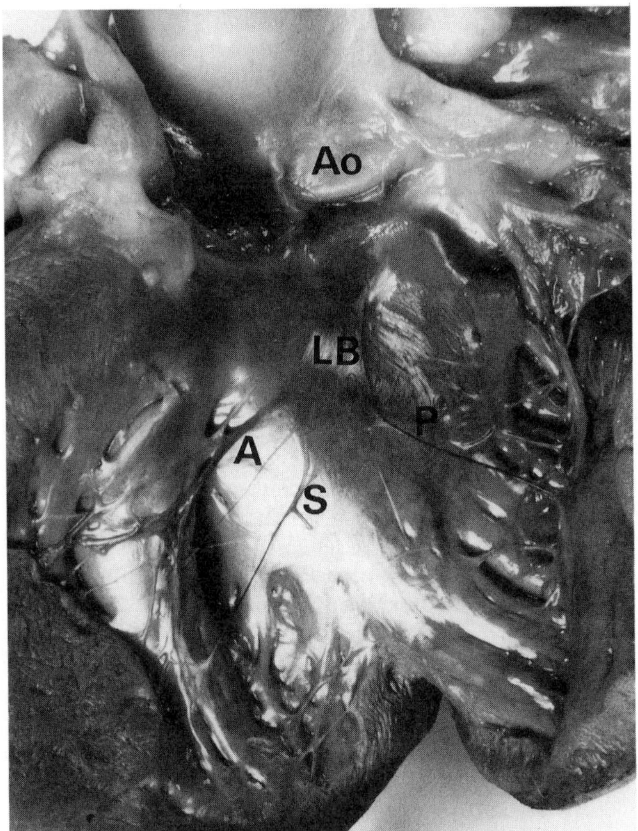

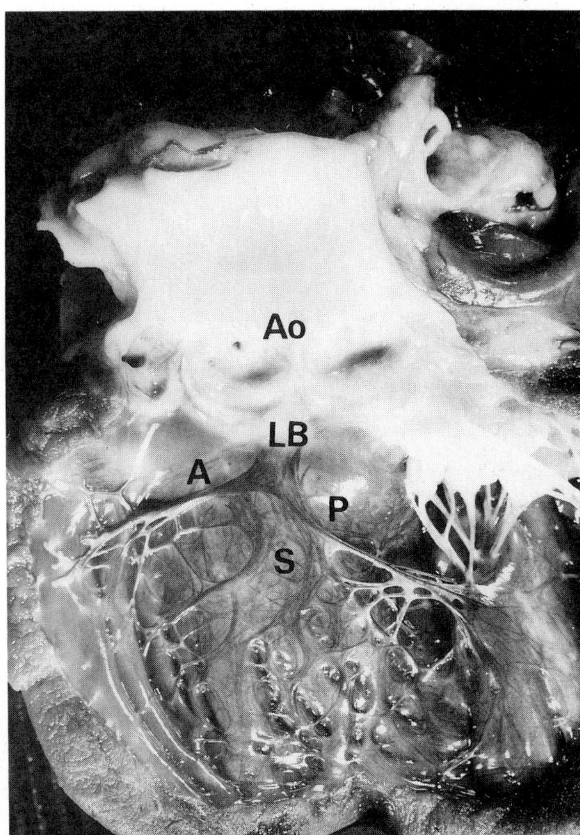

Figure 7.2. Left ventricular conduction system in two canine hearts. The endocardial surfaces have been stained with iodine. The left bundle branch (LB) emerges as a bandlike structure below the aortic root in both cases. The LB bifurcates into anterior (A) and posterior (P) fascicles, which are attached to the apical portions of the papillary muscles. A network of midseptal Purkinje fibers is distributed throughout the septal surface bordered by the two major fascicles. There is some variation between the Purkinje fibers of the two hearts. The aorta (Ao) and the interventricular septum (s) are also labeled. (From Tilley 1992, *Essentials of Canine and Feline Electrocardiography*, 3d ed., Lea & Febiger, Philadelphia.)

conduction, which bypasses the AV node and permits rapid conduction of the cardiac impulse from atria to ventricles (i.e., ventricular preexcitation). The anomolous paths that bypass the slow-conducting AV node completely (e.g., James fibers, Kent bundle) may permit rapid conduction of the cardiac impulse from atria to ventricles, causing a shorter than normal delay between atrial and ventricular excitation (i.e., ventricular preexcitation). The resultant electrocardiographic pattern (short PR and long QRS intervals) is part of the Wolff-Parkinson-White syndrome, which may be complicated by bouts of rapid arrhythmias (tachyarrhythmias) because of reentry involving circuits.

In summary, the sequence of normal electrical activation is as follows: The cardiac impulse originates in the sinus node. Depolarization (activation) spreads through the atrial myocardial cells in the direction of the AV node. The impulse then slows dramatically while traversing the specialized conduction tissue in the AV node. The impulse increases in velocity through the bundle of His, the bundle branches, and the Purkinje system. The AV nodal delay allows the atria to complete their contraction before flow into the ventricles is interrupted by ventricular contraction. Terminal Purkinje fibers connect with the ends of the bundle branches to form interweaving networks on the subendocardial surface of both ventricles that transmit the cardiac impulse almost simultaneously to the right and left ventricular myocardium. Purkinje fibers tend to be less concentrated at the base of the ventricle and at the papillary muscle tips. They penetrate the myocardium for varying distances, depending on the animal species; in the human and in the dog, they penetrate only the inner third of the myocardium, while in the ungulates they can almost reach the epicardium. The cardiac impulse then spreads through the ventricular myocardial cells by cell-to-cell conduction.

BASIC ELECTROPHYSIOLOGICAL PRINCIPLES

Each type of cardiac cell has a characteristic transmembrane action potential (Table 7.2 and Fig. 7.4) that is responsible for passing the cardiac impulse from one cell to the next. These moving transmembrane action potentials produce a traveling change in the external charges on the myocardial cell surfaces. The sequential potential dif-

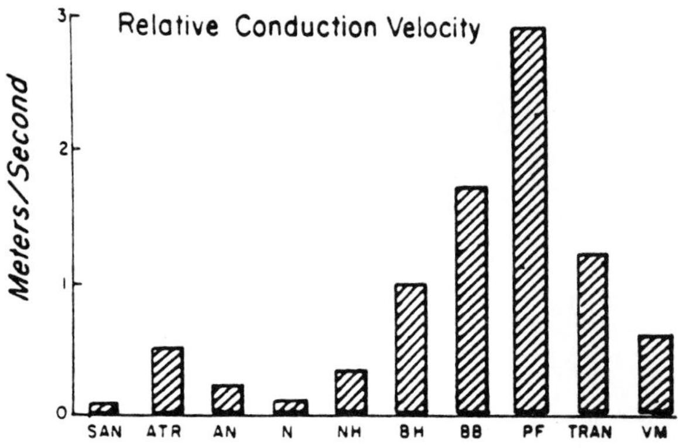

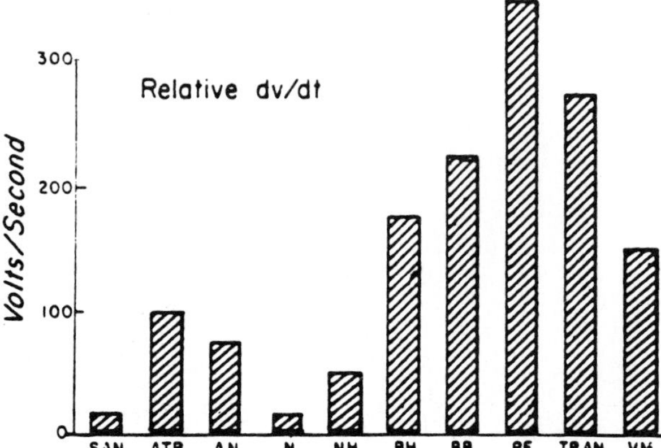

Figure 7.3. Relative conduction velocity (top) and maximum rate of depolarization (bottom) in cells of the sinoatrial node (SAN); atrium (ATR); nodal regions—atrionodal (AN), nodal (N), nodal-His (NH); bundle of His (BH); bundle branches (BB); Purkinje fibers (PF); transitional fibers (TRAN); and ventricular muscle (VM) of the dog. (Prepared by J.F. Spear, 1976. From Detweiler 1979, in Brobeck, ed., *Best and Taylor's Physiological Basis of Medical Practice,* 10th ed., the Williams & Wilkins Co., Baltimore.)

ferences thus produced in the myocardium create a varying electrical field that, when recorded at the body surface, is called the electrocardiogram (ECG) (Fig. 7.5). Intracellular properties of automaticity, excitability, conductivity, and refractoriness will be discussed; they are important when one is analyzing cardiac arrhythmias and considering antiarrhythmic drugs.

Transmembrane action potential

The myocardial cell transmembrane action potential (Figs. 7.6 to 7.8) consists of five phases: phase 0—rapid depolarization; phase 1—early, rapid repolarization; phase 2—plateau; phase 3—final, rapid repolarization; phase 4—resting membrane potential and diastolic depolarization. These phases are the result of ion fluxes that are passive. Ions move down electrochemical gradients established by the sodium pump and exchange mechanisms. Each ion moves primarily through its own ion-specific channel. Impulses spread from one cell to the next without requiring neural input (functional syncytium) via cell areas of low electrical resistance, the nexuses or gap junctions of the intercalated disks. Intracellular electrical activity can be measured by insertion of a glass microelectrode with a tip diameter of less than 0.5μm into a single cell. The microelectrode produces minimal cell membrane damage, its entry point being rapidly sealed. The five phases of the myocardial cell action potential comprise a rapid sequence of changes in electrical potential across the cell membrane during depolarization and repolarization.

Phase 4 is electrical diastole, and phases 0 to 3 represent electrical systole. At the end of phase 3 and the beginning of phase 4, the cell has been completely repolarized and has achieved its maximal resting potential. Nonpacemaker cells maintain this resting membrane potential until they are driven to threshold potential by the current from adjacent depolarizing tissue. In pacemaker cells, phase 4 slowly decreases (becomes less negative) on its own. Phase 4 depolarization is also termed slow diastolic depolarization or "automaticity." It is a normal process in pacemaker cells, although it may occur pathologically in other cardiac cells. In pacemaker cells, the resting membrane potential becomes less negative during phase 4 until the threshold potential is reached or until the cell is driven to threshold potential by an outside current (e.g., by another cardiac pacemaker). The threshold potential is the voltage to which the cell must be reduced before complete cell depolarization occurs. Except for the pacemaker cells, which reach threshold on their own, other cardiac cells remain at their resting potential during phase 4 and are driven to threshold potential by a conducted impulse spread from adjacent depolarizing tissue. Electrophysiologic studies show that di-

Table 7.2. Properties of transmembrane potentials in mammalian hearts

	Sinus nodal cell	Atrial muscle cell	AV nodal cell	Purkinje fiber	Ventricular muscle cell
Resting potential (mV)	−50 to −60	−80 to −90	−60 to −70	−90 to −95	−80 to −90
Action potential					
Amplitude (mV)	60 to 70	110 to 120	70 to 80	120	110 to 120
Overshoot (mV)	0 to 10	30	5 to 15	30	30
Duration (ms)	100 to 300	100 to 300	100 to 300	300 to 500	200 to 300
V_{max} (V/S)	1 to 10	100 to 200	5 to 15	500 to 700	100 to 200
Propagation velocity (m/s)	less than 0.05	0.3 to 0.4	0.1	2 to 3	0.3 to 0.4
Fiber diameter (μm)	5 to 10	10 to 15	5 to 10	100	10 to 16

Modified from Sperelakis, 1979. Origin of the cardiac resting potential, in Berne, Sperelakis, and Geiger, eds., Cardiovascular System, *Handbook of Physiology,* Am. Physiol. Soc., Bethesda, Md.

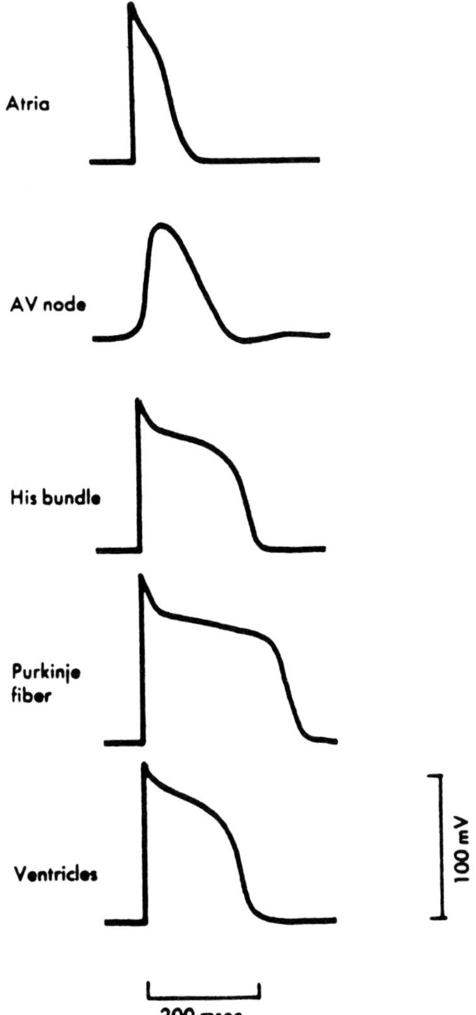

Figure 7.4. Action potential configuration from different areas of the heart. Note that action potential gets longer and longer in duration until it reaches its maximal duration in Purkinje fibers and decreases in duration in ventricular myocardium. The result is a mechanism called "gating." (From Marriot and Conover 1989, *Advanced Concepts in Arrhythmias*, 2d ed, C.V. Mosby, St. Louis.)

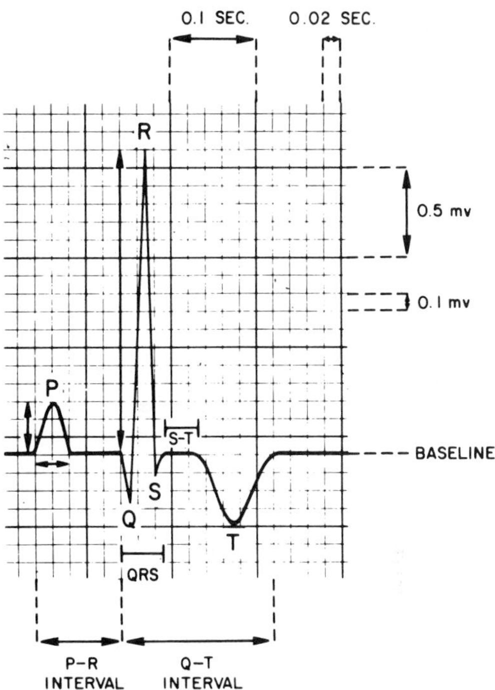

Figure 7.5. Close-up of normal canine lead II P-QRS-T complex with labels and intervals. Measurements for amplitude (in millivolts) are indicated by positive and negative movement; time intervals (in hundredths of a second) are indicated from left to right. Paper speed, 50 mm/s; 1 cm = 1 mV. (From Tilley 1992, *Essentials of Canine and Feline Electrocardiography*, 3d ed., Lea & Febiger, Philadelphia.)

astolic depolarization is due to a slow diastolic influx of sodium ions (Fig. 7.9). Recent electrophysiological studies in Purkinje fibers indicate that the pacemaker current is an inward I_{Na} inactivated at -50 mV and slowly activated by hyperpolarization. Potassium conductance (gK^+) falls as a consequence of depolarization because of increased inward rectification. When the membrane depolarizes, it passes inward current more easily than outward current. The decreasing gK^+helps to produce the depolarization.

Phase 0 is the initial and total upstroke of the action potential, and it is the phase of rapid depolarization that occurs when the cardiac cell is brought to threshold potential when the fast sodium channels are activated. The rate of

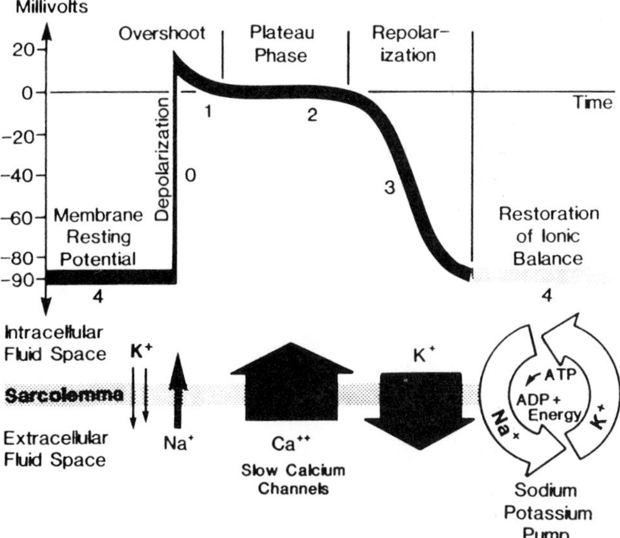

Figure 7.6. Phases and ionic gradients of the cardiac cell transmembrane action potential. (From Lipman, Dynn, and Massie 1984, *Clinical Electrocardiography*, 7th ed, Year Book Medical Publishers, Chicago.)

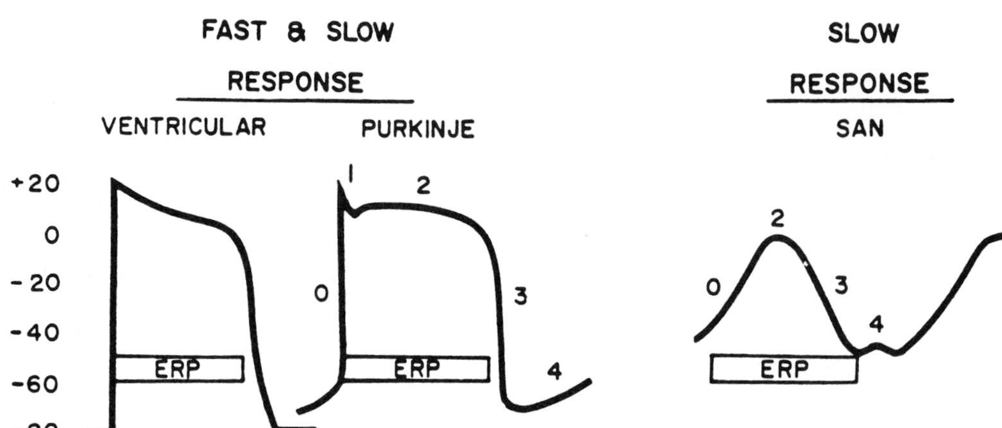

Figure 7.7. Diagrams of types of transmembrane action potentials. Ordinate: potential in millivolts. ERP, Effective refractory period; SAN, sinoatrial node. The two action potentials on the left are from a ventricular myocardial cell and a Purkinje cell, respectively. These action potentials have two components—the brief rapid spike potential (fast response) and a slower plateau phase (slow response). The fast response cells have an initial rapid depolarization (phase 0), followed by a rapid early repolarization (phase 1, most pronounced in the Purkinje cell), a plateau (phase 2), a final repolarization (phase 3) to the diastolic potential level, and a diastolic potential (phase 4). Phase 4 is a constant or resting membrane potential in myocardial cells, but in cells of the pacemaker (Purkinje) type gradual diastolic (phase 4) depolarization occurs until threshold is reached and another action potential is generated. In both fast-response cells, ERP terminates sometime during phase 3. The action potential on the right shows the slow response transmembrane potential of the SA node. Phase 0 is slow, phase 1 is lacking, phase 3 is gradual, there may or may not be an oscillatory afterpotential during phase 4, and phase 4 depolarization continues until phase 0 is triggered again. The effective refractory potential of the SA node may exceed the action potential in duration.

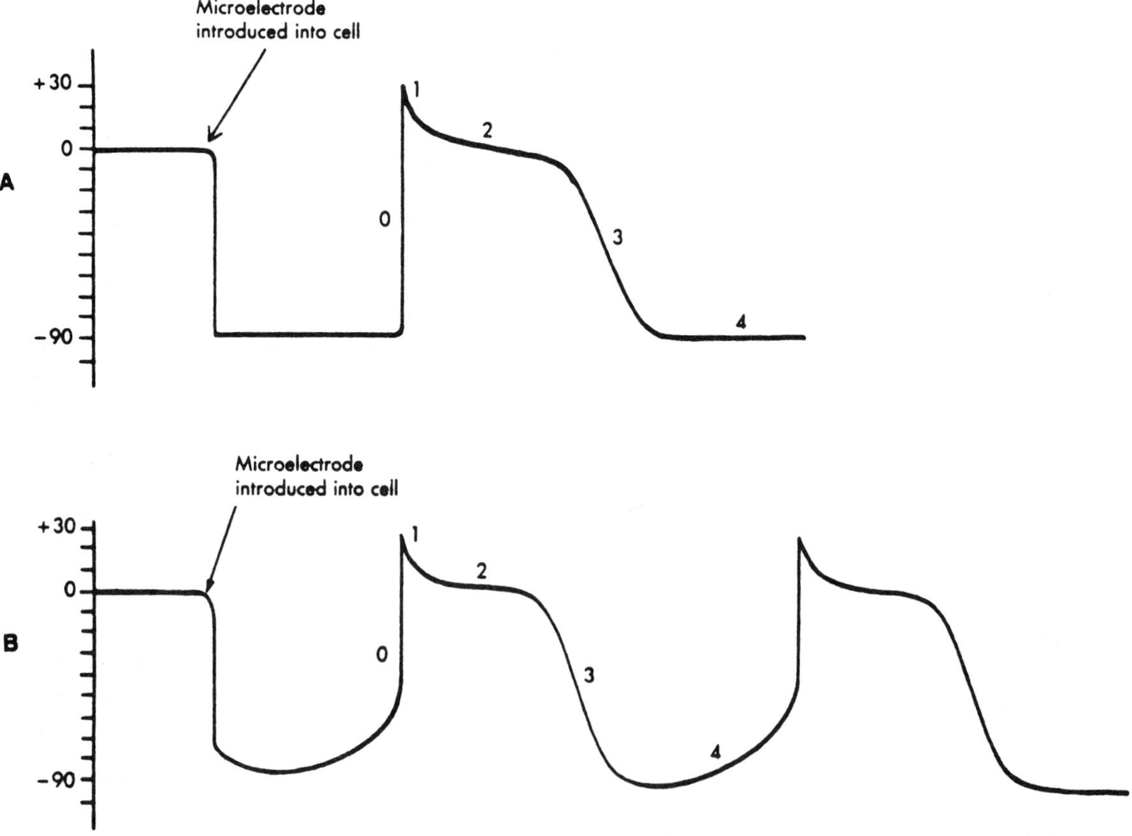

Figure 7.8. Action potentials of (*A*) a myocardial fiber and (*B*) a Purkinje fiber. Arrow indicates point at which microelectrode was introduced into cell. Note that graph suddenly dips to −90 mV as it records resting membrane potential. Diastolic (phase 4) depolarization occurs in Purkinje fiber but not in the myocardial fiber. Myocardial fibers await stimulation from adjoining cell action potential. (From Marriot and Conover 1989, *Advanced Concepts in Arrhythmias*, 2d ed, C.V. Mosby, St. Louis.)

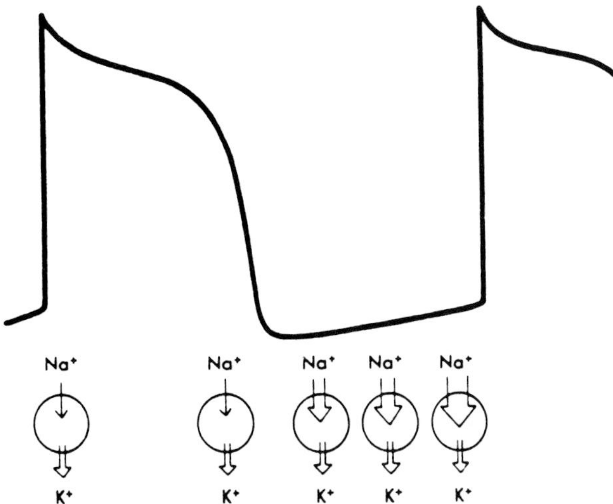

Figure 7.9. Pacemaker current. During phase 4 in pacemaker cells, a slow buildup of intracellular positive ions occurs (slow diastolic depolarization) as a result of an increasing amount of Na^+ entering the cell until the cell reaches threshold potential and depolarizes rapidly. Efflux of potassium (gK^+) varies during this period. (From Conover 1988, *Understanding Electrocardiography*, 5th ed., C.V. Mosby, St. Louis.)

rise of phase 0 (i.e., V_{max} or maximum voltage change per second) is determined by the number of available sodium ions and by the number of opened fast sodium channels, which is in turn related to the cell membrane potential in its resting state (Figs. 7.10 and 7.11). During phase 0 of the fast response action potential, a second inward current is initiated at a lower membrane potential. This second current is carried by calcium and sodium, and its upstroke velocity (V_{max}) and the velocity at which it propagates to other cells are much slower than that produced by the fast sodium current. This slow current is responsible for phase 0 depolarization in cells that do not have fast sodium channels (e.g., the sinus node cells and the AV node cells) and that have only slow calcium channels.

Phase 1 is the rapid, brief beginning of repolarization immediately after phase 0. It is caused by the abrupt closure of the fast sodium channels and occurs because of a transient outward potassium current. Phase 1 ends in the plateau of the action potential.

Phase 2 (the plateau) is maintained by the influx of positive ions (calcium and sodium) into the cell through the slow calcium channels (Figs. 7.6 and 7.11). It is the plateau phase of the action potential that accounts for the relatively long refractory period in myocardial cells as compared with skeletal muscle cells (Fig. 7.12). This slow inward calcium current maintains the cell in a prolonged depolarized state, allowing time for muscle contraction to occur before another impulse is started. Phase 2 is important for cardiac muscle contraction because the entering calcium helps to raise the myoplasmic calcium concentration required for excitation-contraction coupling. This increase in intracellular calcium also brings about a further release of additional calcium from the sarcoplasmic reticulum. The slow inward sodium and calcium currents, as well as an outward chloride current, maintain the positive plateau phase of the membrane potential.

Phase 3 is the final rapid repolarization of the action potential. It results from inactivation of the slow inward calcium channels, reversal or inward rectification (see below), and activation of the outward potassium channel. The sodium-potassium pump activity (see below) is increased by the higher concentration of intracellular sodium and functions to restore sodium and potassium concentrations to their resting levels. This pump is electrogenic and makes a small (about 10 mV) contribution to the resting transmembrane potential.

At least two voltage-dependent potassium channels are involved. One allows potassium ions to pass inward against the electrochemical gradient for potassium (the so-called inward rectifier or anomalous rectification). This channel is responsible for the rapid decrease in potassium conductance on depolarization (during phase 2) and the increase in conductance with repolarization. The second potassium channel allows the ion to pass outward (down the electrochemical gradient for potassium). Its activation produces the increase in total potassium conductance that terminates the phase 2 plateau.

Sodium-potassium pump

The sodium-potassium (Na^+–K^+) pump is an ATP-dependent enzyme, ATPase. This enzyme system apparently spans the entire thickness of the cell membrane. At the inner surface of the cell membrane it binds Na^+ and transports it to the external surface for release. At the external surface it binds K^+ and releases it at the inner surface of the membrane. Thus these ions are moved against their electrochemical gradients. This pump is electrogenic in that three Na^+ ions are transported for only two K^+ ions. Thus it carries a net positive charge out of the cell and can contribute up to 10 mV to the resting membrane potential. At each cardiac cycle the enzyme undergoes conformational changes and is phosphorylated from ATP, which is hydrolyzed to ADP and phosphate, the free energy being used for the cation transport. The pump is activated by increased intracellular Na^+ concentration ($[Na^+]_i$) or increased extracellular K^+ concentration ($[K^+]_o$).

The primary function of the Na^+–K^+ pump is to extrude the small amount of Na^+ that enters the cell during systole and to restore the small amount of K^+ lost from the cell at the end of systole (i.e., it acts to maintain constant intracellular $[Na^+]$ and $[K^+]$). Its activity is increased by elevation of $[Na^+]_i$ or $[K^+]_o$ and depressed by decreases in these specific ion concentrations inside (Na^+) or outside (K^+) the cell membrane.

This enzyme is also the receptor for the positive inotropic effect of digitalis and related glycosides. Cardiac glycosides bind to the external side of the enzyme, where K^+ is

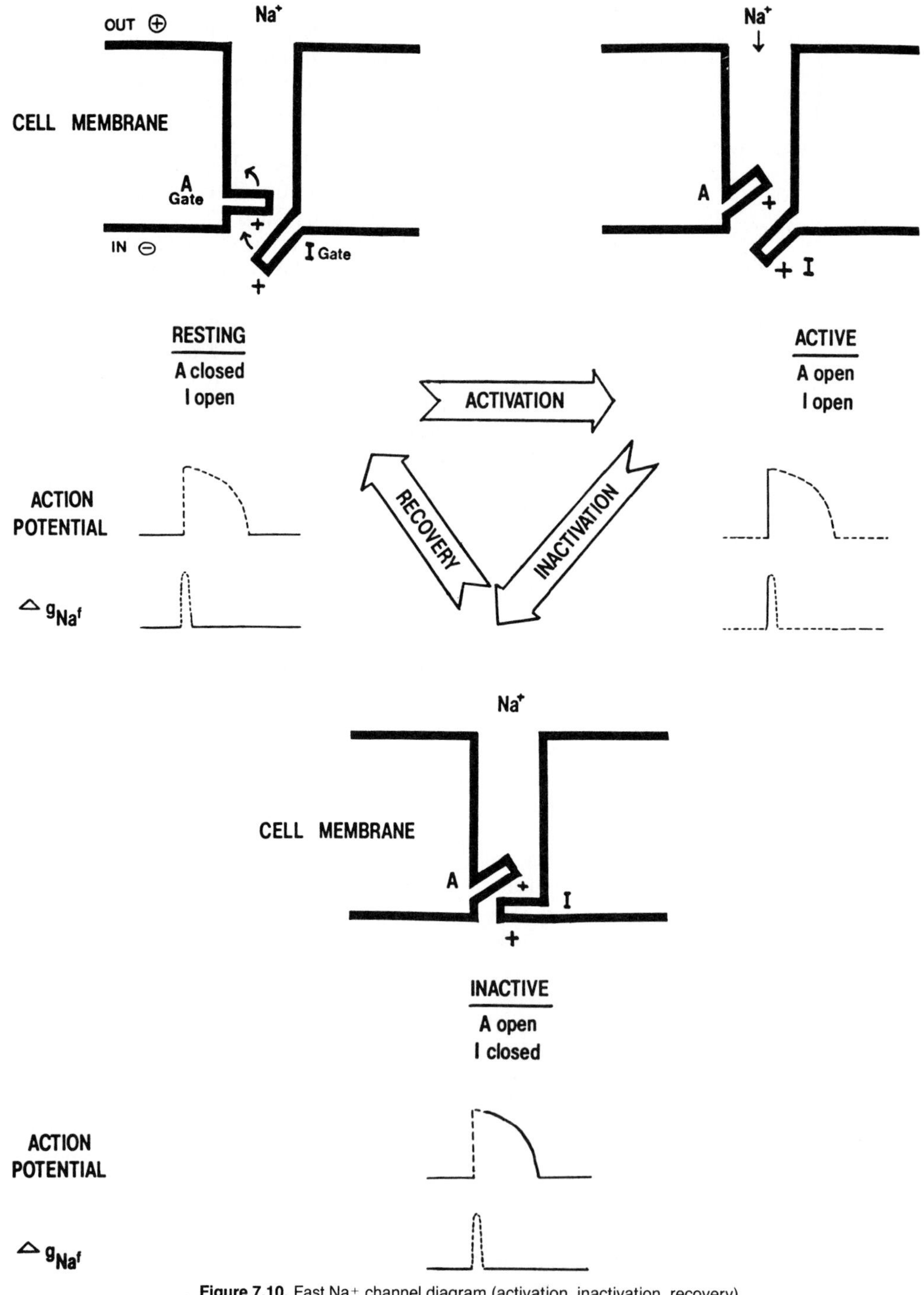

Figure 7.10. Fast Na+ channel diagram (activation, inactivation, recovery).

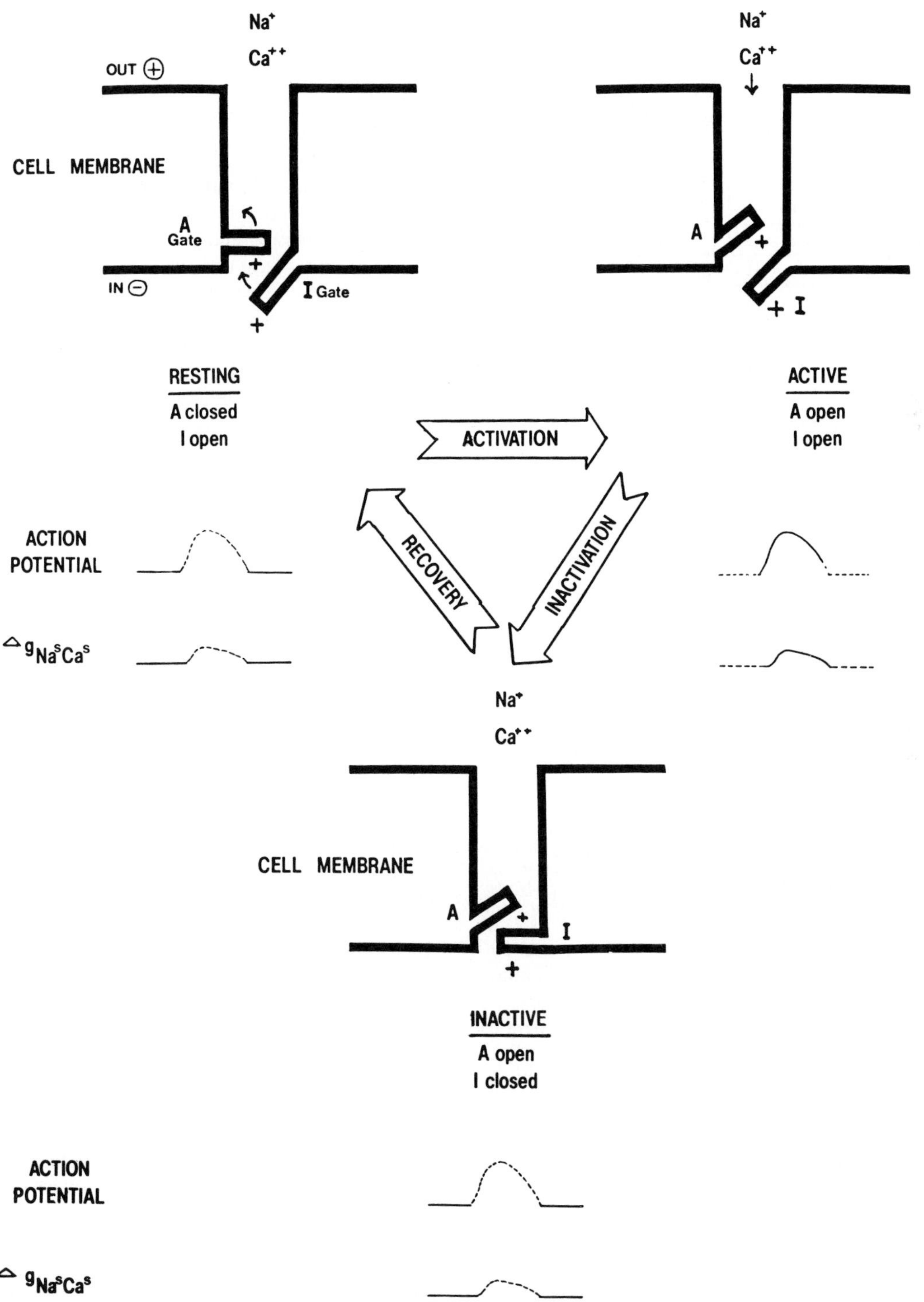

Figure 7.11. Slow Na^+–Ca^{2+} channel diagram (activation, inactivation, recovery).

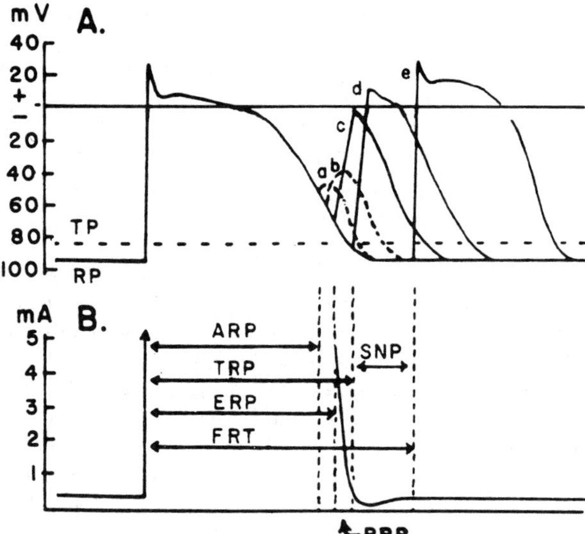

Figure 7.12. (*A*) Amplitude and upstroke velocity (V_{max}) are related to the membrane potential from which they arise. Earliest responses (a and b) are slow-response action potentials that arise from a relatively positive membrane potential; they do not propagate. Response c is the earliest propagated action potential (depressed fast response), but it propagates slowly because of its low upstroke velocity (V_{max}) and low amplitude. Response d is elicited before complete repolarization, and it has a greater V_{max} and amplitude than c because it arises from a more negative potential; it still propagates more slowly than normal. Response e is evoked after complete repolarization, which has the most negative-resting potential, has a normal dv/dt and amplitude, and propagates rapidly. TP, Threshold potential; RP, resting potential. (From Singer and Ten Eick 1969, *Prog Cardiovasc Dis* 11:488.) (*B*) Approximate duration of absolute refractory period (ARP), total refractory period (TRP), effective refractory period (ERP), full recovery time (FRT), supernormal period (SNP), and relative refractory period (RRP). Responses shown as dotted lines a and b in (*A*) are graded responses that do not propagate. Response c is the earliest propagated response and defines the end of the effective refractory period. Response is elicited after the end of repolarization and is normal in terms of rising velocity and amplitude, defining the end of full recovery time. Changes in threshold shown in (*B*) are related to an arbitrary scale of current strength. Curve shows onset of inexcitability coincident with phase 0 of transmembrane action potential, gradual decrease in threshold during phase 3 of repolarization, and restoration of full excitability after the end of phase 3 of transmembrane action potential (phases defined in Fig. 7.10). (Redrawn from Hoffman 1969, in Fisch and Surawicz, eds., *Digitalis: Mechanisms of the Inotropic Effect of Digitalis*, Grune & Stratton, New York.)

also bound. Hypokalemia enhances the glycoside binding, and hyperkalemia delays it.

The main function of the Na^+–K^+ pump is to generate large sodium and potassium gradients across the cardiac cell membrane by transporting sodium out of the cell in exchange for potassium (Fig. 7.6). The Na^+–K^+ pump moves sodium out of the cell against its electrochemical gradient and simultaneously pumps potassium into the cell against its chemical gradient. Intracellular potassium concentration remains high, and intracellular sodium concentration remains low. This pump is fueled by the Na^+–K^+ ATPase that hydrolyzes ATP for energy and is bound to the membrane. It requires both sodium and potassium to function and can transport three sodium ions outward for two potassium ions inward; therefore the pump can be electrogenic, generating a net outward movement of positive charges. As the heart rate increases, the Na^+–K^+ pump must increase its efforts to maintain the same ionic gradients since the cell gains a slight amount of sodium and loses a slight amount of potassium with each depolarization.

Sodium cannot freely diffuse into the cell, despite its concentration gradient to do so, because at the resting membrane potential the cell membrane is relatively impermeable to sodium. Potassium, however, can diffuse freely out of the cell down its concentration gradient at the resting membrane potential. The loss of this positive charge leaves the inside of the cell more negative. Negative intracellular charges due to large polyvalent ions such as proteins do not cross the membrane and thus help maintain intracellular negativity. Potassium continues to leave the cell until the forces driving it down its concentration gradient are balanced by the negative intracellular electrical charges that attract potassium back into the cell. The transmembrane voltage at which the electrical gradient is equal and opposite to the concentration gradient is the K electrochemical equilibrium potential (E_K) and is approximately described by the Nernst equation

$$E_K = (RT/F)\text{Ln}\,\frac{[K^+]_o}{[K^+]_i}.$$

In this equation R is the gas constant, T is the absolute temperature F is the Faraday number, Ln is the logarithm to the base E, is the extracellular K^+ concentration, and $[K^+]_i$, is the intracellular K^+ concentration. A resting transmembrane voltage of −96 mV is predicted from the Goldman equation (an expansion of the Nernst equation to include all permeable ions), which is close to the actual recorded voltage.

Membrane channels

In normal atrial and ventricular muscle and in the fibers of the His-Purkinje system, the action potentials are called fast responses and have very rapid upstrokes (V_{max}) mediated by the fast sodium membrane channels (Fig. 7.10). Action potentials in the normal sinus node and AV node are called slow responses and have very slow upstrokes (V_{max}) mediated by the slow calcium channels (Figs. 7.7 and 7.11). Upstrokes of slow responses are mediated by a slow inward predominantly calcium current rather than by the fast inward sodium current. The potentials are called *slow responses* because the time required for activation and inactivation of the slow inward current is much slower than that for the fast inward sodium current (Table 7.3).

As shown in Figs. 7.10 and 7.11, the fast Na^+ channels and the slow Na^+–Ca^{2+} channels at a given membrane site pass through three functional states—resting, active, and inactive—as a conducted impulse approaches, occupies, and departs the region. The sequence is shown in Fig. 7.10 for the fast Na^+ channel. This channel is guarded by two gates. Gates that open on depolarization are called activation (A) gates. Gates that close on depolarization are called inactivation (I) gates. In the resting state, the A gate is

Table 7.3. Characteristics of fast and slow inward currents in cardiac tissue

	Fast	Slow
Primary charge carrier	Na	Ca(Na)
Activation threshold	−70 to −55 mV	−55 to −30 mV
Magnitude	1 to 30 μA	0.1 to 0.3 μA
Time constant of		
Activation	Less than 1 ms	10 to 20 ms
Inactivation	Less than 1 ms	50 to 500 ms
Inhibitors	Tetrodotoxin, local anesthetics, sustained depolarization at less than 40 mV	Verapamil, D-600, nifedipine, diltiazem, Mn, Co, Ni, La
Resting membrane potential	−80 to −95 mV	−40 to −70 mV
Conduction velocity	0.3 to 3.0 M/s	0.01 to 0.10 M/s
Rate of rise (V_{max}) of action potential upstroke	200 to 1000 V/s	1 to 10 V/s
Action potential amplitude	100 to 130 mV	35 to 75 mV
Response to stimuli	All or none	Affected by characteristics of stimulus
Recovery of excitability	Prompt, ends with repolarization	Delayed, outlasts full repolarization
Safety factor for conduction	High	Low
Major current action potential upstroke in the following:		
SA node	−	+
Atrial myocardium	+	−
AV node (N region)	−	+
His-Purkinje system	+	−
Ventricular myocardium	+	−
Neurotransmitter influence		
Beta-adrenergic	−	↑ ↑
Alpha-adrenergic	−	↑ (?)
Muscarinic cholinergic	−	↓ In atrium ↓ (?) In ventricle

From Zipes 1988, Genesis of cardiac arrhythmias: Electrophysiological considerations, in Braunwald, ed., *Heart Disease,* W.B. Saunders Co., Philadelphia.

closed and the I gate is open. In the active state both gates are open. In the inactive state the A gate is open but the I gate is closed. This channel must go through a recovery process after it has been activated and then inactivated before it can pass into a state (resting) in which it can be reactivated. The recovery process requires repolarization of the membrane to −50 mV or so before it can begin, and it takes a few milliseconds to complete.

For the slow Na^+–Ca^{2+} channels, the recovery process requires tens of milliseconds (30 to 200 ms.). The kinetics of all these processes (activation, inactivation, and recovery) can be altered by drugs.

The K^+ channel, an outward going channel that is largely responsible for the resting potential, is thought not to inactivate and therefore is believed to have only an A gate.

Membrane channels are specific for certain ions and functions, and they open only at a certain transmembrane potential voltage, their threshold potential. Membrane channels are composed of a channel protein, a selectivity filter, and gating proteins. The selectivity filter guards the channel and is ion specific. The gating proteins provide resting, open, and inactivated states. The gating proteins will move to an open position when the threshold potential (i.e., −70 mV for the fast channels and −30 mV for the slow channels) is reached. Sodium enters through the fast channels, and both calcium and sodium enter through the slow channels. The movement of these gating proteins to open and closed positions is determined by transmembrane voltage and the length of time that the cell maintains that voltage. The slow calcium channels operate in the same way as the fast sodium channels except for different threshold potentials. The slow channels stay open longer, and recovery from inactivation also takes longer than in the fast channels. It is because of this slow current of positive ions (calcium and sodium) into the cell through the slow calcium channels that the plateau (phase 2) occurs and the rapid repolarization (phase 3) of the transmembrane potential is delayed. Cells with only slow calcium channels (e.g., nodal cells) have a resting membrane potential of −60 mV. The slow calcium current can be activated and play a prominent role in diseased, partially depolarized myocardial cells in which the fast channels have been inactivated. The fast sodium channel is voltage dependent and a particular membrane voltage must be reached before the recovery of excitability, whereas the slow calcium channel is time dependent and a certain amount of time must elapse before excitability is regained.

Voltage dependency

Voltage dependency of a specific ion channel signifies that it functions maximally (i.e., is highly permeable to the ion species) at a certain transmembrane potential range. For example, the V_{max} of phase 0 is largely determined by voltage-dependent opening of the fast sodium channel. In the resting cell the fast sodium channel is nearly closed and the potassium channel is open (sodium conductance is low and potassium conductance is high). When the membrane potential is decreased from the resting level, the degree of opening of the sodium channel increases and that of the potassium decreases. Once the membrane is depolarized, the fast sodium channels close, largely terminating the fast inward current. The level of resting potential before stimulation also influences V_{max}. When the resting potential is high the sodium channels open rapidly and widely, and when the resting potential is lower (but more negative than threshold) the sodium channels open less widely and V_{max} is lower. The slow calcium-sodium channels, for example, operate over lower (less negative) activation and inactivation voltage ranges than the fast sodium channel.

Time dependency

Time dependency of an ionic channel signifies that after activation (or inactivation) its continuation in an active (or inactive) status will follow a certain time course. Thus the permeability of ion channels is also dependent on several factors, including elapsed time after a polarity change. For example, the ability of fast sodium channels to reopen after being closed by depolarization of the membrane can take some time after resting potential levels are reached. In the case of the slow calcium-sodium channels, the current has a slow time-dependent inactivation period after its activation.

Fast and slow channels can be differentiated on the basis of their pharmacological sensitivity. Drugs that block the slow channels with some specificity include verapamil, nifedipine, diltiazem, and compounds that contain manganese and cobalt. Antiarrhythmic agents such as lidocaine, quinidine, and procainamide affect the fast sodium channels and not the slow calcium channels. Tetrodotoxin (puffer fish poison), which is too toxic to be used clinically, blocks the fast sodium channels with strong specificity. Although fast action potentials are characteristic of normal atrial and ventricular myocardial cells and His-Purkinje cells, the slow response action potentials are found in the normal sinus node, the normal AV node, and with certain diseased cardiac cells of any type.

The fast and slow channels may be affected by disease. Disease may change the resting transmembrane potential, which alters the percentage of fast and slow ion channels that can be activated. The lower the number of fast sodium channels that are activated, the slower the V_{max} (phase 0) and cardiac fiber conduction to the next cell. Slower cardiac conduction may contribute to the reentry mechanism for cardiac arrhythmias. Drugs that act on the fast sodium channels will normally affect only the atrial and ventricular myocardial cells and Purkinje fibers. Drugs that act on the slow calcium channels will affect primarily the pacemaker cells of the sinus and AV nodes. An example is lidocaine or procainamide, which can work only on cells that have activated fast sodium channels. Pacemaker cells are primarily depolarized by slow calcium channels and thus respond best to calcium channel blockers (e.g., verapamil).

During phase 3, rapid repolarization occurs. This phase starts with the closure of the slow calcium channels. During phase 3, potassium extrusion from the cell increases and the sodium pump restores the cell to its resting membrane potential (Fig. 7.6).

In summary, although the transmembrane action potentials of atrial and ventricular fibers are similar, they differ from pacemaker cell transmembrane potentials. Pacemaker cells have automaticity. They are characterized by a low resting membrane potential, slow channel activation during phase 0, short action potential duration, no overshoot, and spontaneous depolarization during phase 4 until the threshold potential is reached.

Automaticity

Automaticity (slow diastolic depolarization) is the ability of the cell to depolarize spontaneously, reach threshold potential, and initiate a propagated transmembrane action potential. Automaticity occurs during phase 4 by a slow buildup of positive ions inside the cell. In healthy hearts only the cells of the sinus node reach threshold potential without an outside stimulus, although cells in other areas of the heart are capable of automaticity and are referred to as *subsidiary* or *latent pacemakers*. Cells of the His-Purkinje system are potential pacemakers. The rate of automaticity decreases from the sinus node down to the Purkinje fibers, so that the sinus node depolarizes fastest during phase 4 and reaches threshold before the latent pacemaker cells have time to do so. From the sinus node the cardiac impulse travels to the rest of the heart, driving all the latent pacemaker cells to threshold before they can reach that point themselves. Abnormal automaticity can occur at low membrane potential levels in myocardial cells. This abnormal situation is caused by functional cell pathosis that lowers resting membrane potential to the point where there is a loss of fast sodium channels. Then the cells are left with slow calcium channels and slow response action potentials that are capable of automaticity. Arrhythmias caused by this type of pathological change are extremely resistant to drugs, such as lidocaine and procainamide, that act on the fast sodium channels.

Automaticity versus excitability

All normal myocardial cells are excitable; that is, they are capable of giving rise to an action potential when driven by an adequate stimulus. Normally only pacemaker cells can reach threshold potential without an adequate stimulus by the mechanism of automaticity.

Overdrive suppression

Overdrive suppression is the inhibitory effect of a fast pacemaker on a slower pacemaker. Stimulating a pacemaker cell at rates above its intrinsic frequency increases sodium influx and elevates $[Na^+]_i$, thereby markedly increasing the activity of the Na^+–K^+ pump. This, in turn, lowers $[K^+]_o$. The maximum diastolic potential is hyperpolarized, and there is a slowing or abolition of spontaneous firing. This effect on the intrinsic rate of firing is called *overdrive suppression*. Note that the major cause of this phenomenon is stimulation of the Na^+–K^+ pump by the elevated intracellular sodium.

Thus impulses from a faster pacemaker propagated to a slower pacemaker will inhibit the latter. The SA node exerts such inhibition on subsidiary pacemaker cells in the heart. Rapidly firing abnormal pacemakers can inhibit the normal SA node in certain atrial arrhythmias, and abnormal ectopic pacemakers can be inhibited if the heart is driven at still more rapid rates with an external pacemaker.

Resting membrane potential

The resting membrane potential is the electrical potential gradient that exists across cell membranes during electrical diastole (phase 4 of the action potential). The normal functioning cardiac cell is dependent on an intact resting membrane potential, which in turn is dependent on the electrical potential produced by sodium, potassium, and calcium concentration gradients across the cell membrane.

The normal resting potential recorded by a microelectrode is approximately −90 mV in normal atrial and ventricular myocardial cells and Purkinje fibers. Sinoatrial node and AV node cells have a less negative resting potential of approximately −60 mV. The normal resting potential of −90 mV is maintained by the electrogenic negativity produced by the Na^+–K^+ exchange pump and the flow of potassium out of the cell down its concentration gradient. The activity of the fast sodium channels increases as the transmembrane potential increases, so that the V_{max} of phase 0 increases with the negative voltage at which it starts. Thus, the magnitude of the resting membrane potential influences conduction velocity.

Threshold potential

The critical level of cell membrane depolarization (about −55 to −60 mV) at which an action potential is initiated is the *threshold potential*. Once this level of depolarizaion is reached, no greater stimulus is required for the upstroke of the action potential to become self-sustaining. Subthreshold stimuli produce only local nonpropagated responses.

The resting potential level and the form, duration, and amplitude of the action potential are characteristic of the different myocardial cell types (Figs. 7.4 and 7.7). The SA node pacemaker cells have a relatively low resting potential, a slower phase 0, no phase 1, an indistinct phase 2, a distinct phase 3, and slow depolarization during phase 4. Atrial muscle cells lack a distinct phase 2 (plateau), and phase 3 is prolonged. AV nodal cells may exhibit hyperpolarization at the end of phase 3, and phase 1 is not distinct. Purkinje fibers have a distinct phase 1, a relatively long phase 2, and a distinct phase 3, and phase 4 may exhibit spontaneous depolarization. In species with short QT intervals, phase 2 of the action potential is essentially absent in both atrial and ventricular cells.

Most atrial and ventricular cells maintain a relatively stable resting membrane potential throughout phase 4 and are termed *nonpacemaker cells*. Normally they cannot initiate impulses spontaneously. Pacemaker cells can spontaneously depolarize to the threshold potential.

Refractory period

Refractoriness is the inability of a cell to respond to a stimulus because it has been recently activated by a previous stimulus. The refractory period is the time interval during which the cell remains unresponsive (effective refractory period) or responds poorly (relative refractory period) to a second stimulus (Figs. 7.7 and 7.12). The refractory period is determined by the level of transmembrane potential. For instance, after phase 0 of the action potential, the fast ion channels are inactivated and cannot be reactivated until the membrane potential has achieved a higher (i.e., more negative) level during phase 3 of the action potential. When the higher membrane potential is reached, the fast sodium channels become partially activated (relative refractory period), and during this time a strong stimulus may cause another propagated response.

Refractory states

Under physiological conditions, cardiac cells are refractory to further stimulation during most of the action potential period. Excitability returns during the repolarization phase and goes through a period of supernormality (Fig. 7.12).

The absolute refractory period (ARP) extends from the onset of the action potential until repolarization has progressed to a potential of about −55 mV. The cell cannot be excited during this period. As repolarization continues there is a period during which a stimulus may produce a graded cellular response of membrane potential but no propagated action potential follows. The effective refractory period (ERP) (Fig. 7.7) is this interval plus the ARP. With further repolarization of the membrane, there is a progressive decrease in the stimulus strength required to excite the fiber, and stimulation begins to be followed by propagated action potentials that have a slow rate of rise of phase 0 and a submaximal amplitude. This is the relative refractory period (RRP). The total refractory period includes both stages of the ERP plus the RRP.

The supernormal period is an interval beginning at about the time the action potential reaches the resting threshold level. During this period the stimulus required for response is less than for a resting cell, but the amplitude and the rate of rise of the action potential are submaximal. Full recovery time includes all of the defined periods up to the time when the resting potential is stable and the rise time, action potential amplitude, and duration of the response and excitability are fully restored. The term *partial recovery period* is sometimes used in describing cardiac tissue or the entire heart to designate the interval during which some cells have recovered fully while others remain in some stage of refractoriness.

Conduction velocity

The rapidity with which the impulse is conducted in a given fiber is a function of the rate of rise and amplitude of the action potential and of the fiber diameter (Table 7.2). The lower (i.e., less negative) the resting potential, the lower is the speed of conduction velocity (see Fig. 7.10). Sinus and AV nodal fibers have lower resting potentials and are smaller in diameter than atrial and ventricular cells. These fibers conduct more slowly. Although conduction in sinus and AV nodal tissue is slow, it is qualitatively similar to conduction elsewhere. In normal AV conduction much of the slowing occurs in the upper or atrial zone of the AV node (the AN zone). When impulses reach the AV node at very rapid rates, conduction time increases until it finally fails. The site of conduction slowing and block now appears to be in the AV nodal cells. Because of this propensity to decrease or block conduction with rapid rates of stimulation, the AV node is said to have the lowest safety factor in the atrioventricular conduction system. When complete block occurs, with each successive beat, phase 0 in these AV nodal cells becomes slower and amplitude diminishes until finally a nonpropagated local response is present. This is called *decremental conduction*.

Gating function of Purkinje cells

In the dog the duration of the effective refractory period of Purkinje cells in the bundle of His, bundle branches, and peripheral network increases from the bundle of His onward to a point where there is an intermingling of transitional cells that gradually diminish in size and conduction velocity until they become continuous with working ventricular fibers. The longer refractory period of the cells toward the end of the bundle branches (Fig. 7.4) exceeds that of the ventricular myocardial cells as well as the more proximal conduction system cells. This region of long refractoriness is called a *gate* in that it can block premature depolarizations that arise from higher in the conduction system from leaving or those from beyond the conduction system in working ventricular muscle cells from entering the conduction system. This feature protects the ventricles from premature activations during their relative refractory period and the conduction system from premature retrograde conduction of impulses arising in the ventricles. The terms *gate* and *gating* are also used for conduction changes in membrane channels of myocardial cells.

Table 7.4. Historical highlights in electrocardiography

1786	Aloysio Luigi Galvani: Concept of animal electricity
1842	Carlo Matteucci: Rheoscopic muscle (muscle contracts when its nerve is in contact with another muscle)
1843	Emil Dubois-Reymond: Action potentials in nerve and muscle
1856	Albert von Kolliker and Johannes Muller: Muscle contracts if its nerve is laid across a contracting heart
1875	Gabriel Lippmann: Development of capillary electrometer
1876	Etienne-Jules Marey: Refractory period of the heart; ECG of frog and turtle heart with capillary electrometer (1881)
1878	T.W. Engelmann: Electrical excitation of frog heart
1879–1880	John Scott Burden-Sanderson and F.J.M. Page: ECG from intact animal (frog)
1887	August Desire Waller: Capillary electrometer ECGs (humans, horses, dogs)
1901–1903	Willem Einthoven: String galvanometer electrocardiograph (Nobel prize 1924)
1909–1920	Thomas Lewis: ECG and cardiac arrhythmias: Visual proof that fibrillating atria produce f waves in ECG of horses with spontaneous disease (1912); excitation wave in the dog heart (with M.A. Rothschild 1915).
1912	Willem Einthoven: Equilateral triangle hypothesis of ECG introduced
1913	Johannes Norr: Pioneer veterinary electrocardiographer's first publication on ECG of the horse
1914	W.E. Garrey: "Circus" movement mechanism of atrial flutter and fibrillation
1925	Thomas Lewis: Definition third edition of his classical: *The Mechanism and Graphic Registration of the Heart Beat*
1926	C.J. Rothberger: "Arrhythmias," in *Handbuch der normalen und pathologischen Physiologie*
1927	K.D. Wenckebach and H. Winterberg: Standard work on arrhythmias; Die unregeimassige Herztatigkeit
1930	F.N. Wilson: Modern theory of ECG; the central terminal V (now known as Wilson's central terminal); distribution of potentials in a volume conductor
1939	A.L. Hodgkin and A.F. Huxley: Transmembrane action potential in squid axon
1949	Gilbert Ling and R.W. Gerard: Transmembrane potentials in skeletal muscle
1951	Silvio Weidmann, M.H. Draper, E. Coraboeuf, J.W. Woodbury, H.H. Hecht, and W. Trautwein: Cardiac transmembrane potentials
1953	A.M. Scher: Ventricular activation.

THE ELECTROCARDIOGRAM

The electrocardiogram (ECG) is a record of the average electrical potential generated in the heart muscle and graphed in terms of voltage and time during the different phases of the cardiac cycle. The ECG is measured at the body surface. Table 7.4 lists some historical landmarks in electrocardiography.

Normally, each segment of the ECG arises from a specific area of the heart in sequential fashion. The P wave, QRS complex, and T wave are the recognizable deflections of the ECG tracing and indicate atrial depolarization (P), ventricular depolarization (QRS), and ventricular repolarization (T) (Fig. 7.5). The surface electrocardiogram wave forms represent the electrical activity of the atrial and ventricular myocardium but not the conduction system. Activity in the conduction system can sometimes be deduced from its effect on subsequent wave form amplitudes and intervals and is termed *concealed conduction* (Fig. 7.13).

Relation of action potential to surface electrocardiogram

Figures 7.14 and 7.15 relate the action potential to the surface ECG. Whenever there is a difference in electrical potential between fibers within the heart, electrical current will flow as is seen during the QRS and T-wave. The time difference between the first and last ventricular phase 0 depolarizations causes the QRS complex (Fig. 7.15). During phase 2 of the action potential, there is little difference in potential between the first and last fibers that depolarize (isoelectric S-T segment). Then, during rapid repolarization (phase 3), the differences in potential again become apparent: current flows and is reflected in the T wave. Abnormalities of depolarization are seen in the QRS complex and repolarization abnormalities are seen in the S-T segment, T wave, and Q-T interval.

In electrocardiography both scalar and vector values are used to describe the electrical potentials recorded. A single-magnitude value of a recorded electrical potential is called a *scalar* and is expressed in millivolts. When both magnitude (millivoltage) and direction of the physical quantity are needed, then magnitude in millivoltage, the direction in space, and polarity (or sense) of the potential are recorded. Vectors are represented by straight-line segments or arrows in which the length represents magnitude, the arrowhead

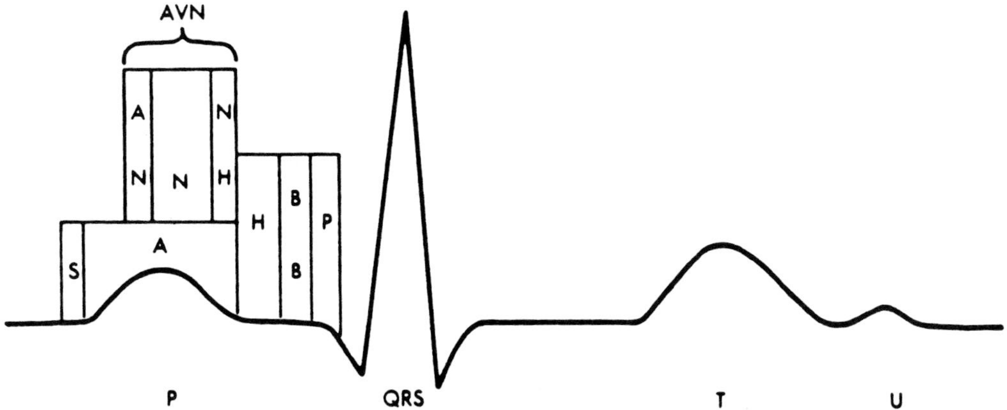

Figure 7.13. Sequence of activation through conduction system related to surface ECG. Note that QRS begins only after most of the conduction system has already been activated. The U wave seen following the T wave is related to Purkinje cell repolarization and is commonly seen in the human electrogram. S, SA conduction; A, atria; AVN, atrioventricular node; AN, atrionodal; N, nodal (central); NH, nodal-His; H, His bundle; BB, bundle branches; P, Purkinje fibers. (From Marriot and Conover 1989, *Advanced Concepts in Arrhythmias*, 2d ed., C.V. Mosby, St. Louis.)

represents the positive pole (or sense), and the orientation in space represents the direction.

Relation of excitation and specialized conduction system and ventricular myocardial action potentials to the electrocardiogram

Figure 7.14 shows the sequence of activation through the atria and conduction system and its relation to the electrocardiogram. Note that activation of the sinoatrial node (SAN), the atrioventricular node (AVN), the bundle of His (H), the bundle branches (BB), and the Purkinje network (P) does not result in measurable electrical potentials at the body surface and, therefore, no waves signaling these events appear in the electrocardiogram.

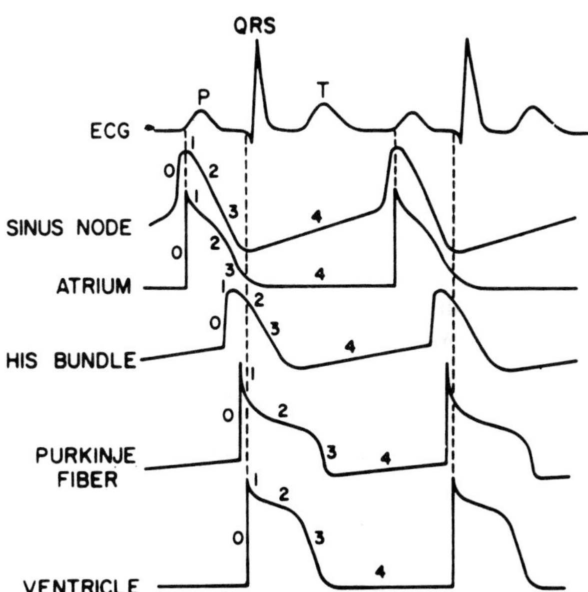

Figure 7.14. Action potentials for the sinus node, atrium, bundle of His, Purkinje fibers, and ventricular myocardium are shown relative to the production of the surface ECG. The corresponding phases of each action potential are labeled, representing electrolyte shifts across the cell membrane (see text). Note the difference in action potential shape, particularly the slope of phase 4 of the normal cardiac pacemaker (sinus node). (From Edwards 1987, *Bolton's Handbook of Canine and Feline Electrocardiography*, 2d ed., W.B. Saunders, Philadelphia.)

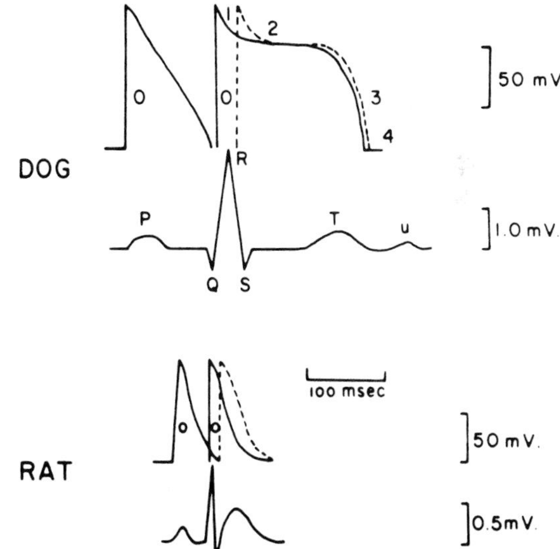

Figure 7.15. Schema of atrial and ventricular transmembrane action potentials (TMAP) and the electrocardiogram (ECG) drawn on the same time scale. The five phases of the dog TMAP are labeled: 0, initial rapid depolarization or spike; 1. initial rapid repolarization; 2, slow repolarization or plateau; 3, final rapid repolarization; 4, resting or diastolic transmembrane potential. Note that the rat and dog atrial and the rat ventricular TMAPs have no plateau. The TMAPs drawn with a solid line represent excitation of ventricular cells early during the QRS interval; those drawn with a dashed line represent excitation of ventricular cells later during the QRS interval. Note that in the dog the plateaus of the TMAPs overlap so that there is little difference in charge between groups of cells. This period of overlap coincides with the isopotential ST segment of the ECG. The T wave of the dog ECG is generated during final rapid repolarization, phase 3, when at any given instant in time the charges of different masses of cells are not the same. In the rat, the ventricular TMAPs do not have a plateau and there is no period during repolarization when most cells are isopotential. Thus no ST segment appears in the ECG.

In Fig. 7.15, the time relations between single-cell transmembrane action potentials and the electrocardiogram are depicted for mammalian species with long action potentials and those with short action potentials. In the latter the ST segment of the electrocardiogram is essentially absent. In animals such as carnivores, primates, lagomorphs, etc., the ventricular action potentials are nearly as long as the QT interval, a plateau (phase 2) is present, and an ST segment is present in the electrocardiogram. In animals such as many insectivores, rodents, and kangaroos the plateau is absent in the action potential and there is no distinct ST segment on the electrocardiogram. The ST segment of the electrocardiogram in species that have one corresponds to the period of time when the action potentials of the mass of ventricular myocardial cells are at phase 2 (plateau) and there is little difference in charge between groups of cells.

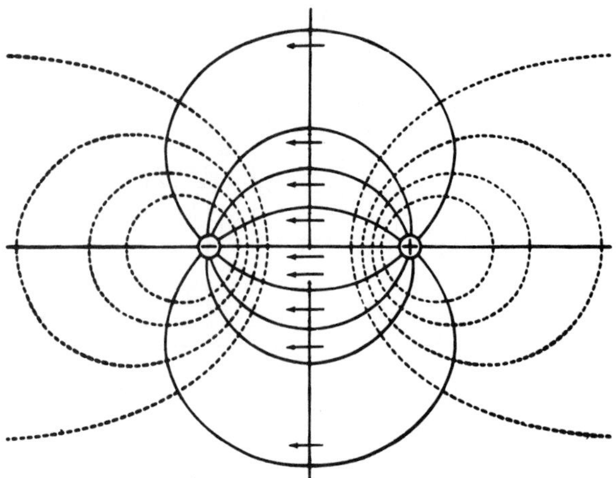

Figure 7.16. Electric field of a dipole in a volume conductor. This is a planar section through the "center" of a three-dimensional field. Solid lines represent current flow. Dotted lines represent isopotential lines.

Equivalent dipole theory

A review of the dipolar hypothesis can provide a theoretical basis for clinical ECG interpretation. A single pair of equal and opposite charges that are in close proximity to each other constitutes an electrical generator, termed a dipole. If the dipole is immersed in a conducting medium (e.g., animal thorax), the dipole will generate an electric field throughout the conducting medium. The electric potential measured at any position in the electric field depends on the position of the recording electrode with respect to the positive and negative charges of the dipole. If any two points (electrodes) with a different potential in the electric field are connected by a superior electric conductor (e.g., the ECG lead wires), the potential difference between the electrodes will result in a flow of current through the wires. This electromotive force or voltage is the quantity measured by the surface ECG.

Numerous surface dipoles are formed by the individual myocardial cells and muscle bundles and move during the depolarization-repolarization process (Fig. 7.16). They create an electric field in the surrounding body tissues and fluids. Conventionally, these electrical quantities or forces are represented by arrows (called vectors) in two- or three-dimensional space, so that the length of the arrow indicates the magnitude of the voltage, the arrowhead indicates the positive sense, the arrow tail indicates the negative sense of the potential difference, and the direction of the arrow indicates the orientation of the force in space. Dipoles differ in orientation and polarity because of their varied spatial relationships in the multidimensional heart. At any given instant during ventricular depolarization or repolarization, all the dipoles can be integrated and a resultant dipole or vector can be obtained by the ECG.

The equivalent dipole theory assumes that electric potentials at the body surface can be represented at any instant by a single resultant dipole vector. Although this concept is oversimplified, it is applicable to the surface ECG. The resultant electric field force registered in any given bipolar lead is in direct proportion to the projection of the instantaneous vector on the axis of the lead and is proportional to the square of the distance multiplied by the reciprocal of the conductance between the dipole and each of the lead electrodes. This vector concept was used by Einthoven to determine the mean electrical axis of the extremity leads (I, II, and III). The dipole theory has been criticized because heart muscle is anisotropic (i.e., does not conduct homogeneously in all directions). Another analogue of body surface potentials uses the electric field produced from epicardial potentials. Maps showing the potential distribution of the body surface (isopotential lines) can be constructed (Fig. 7.17).

Recording the electrocardiogram

Electrocardiographic recording paper is usually inscribed with horizontal and vertical lines spaced 1 mm apart (Fig. 7.5). They represent time and amplitude, respectively. The typical ECG examination is performed with electrodes attached at specific body sites (electrode positions). When two electrodes are connected to the positive and negative poles, the potential difference between the electrodes will be measured in appropriate units (e.g., millivolts). The electrodes are connected through wires (lead lines) to the positive and negative poles of the electrocardiograph amplifier-galvanometer system. Potential differences are thus measured between various combinations of electrode pairs or between the so-called central or V terminal and an exploring electrode. The ECG is a moving record of the deflections generated by the electrocardiograph stylus calibrated in voltage (vertical axis) and time (horizontal axis) and recorded on standardized graph paper.

Electrocardiographic electrodes (leads) sample cardiac potentials at the body surface. The electrocardiograph can combine the electrodes on the body (right and left arms, left leg, and exploring electrode) into the specific combinations or leads (Table 7.5). They include bipolar standard limb

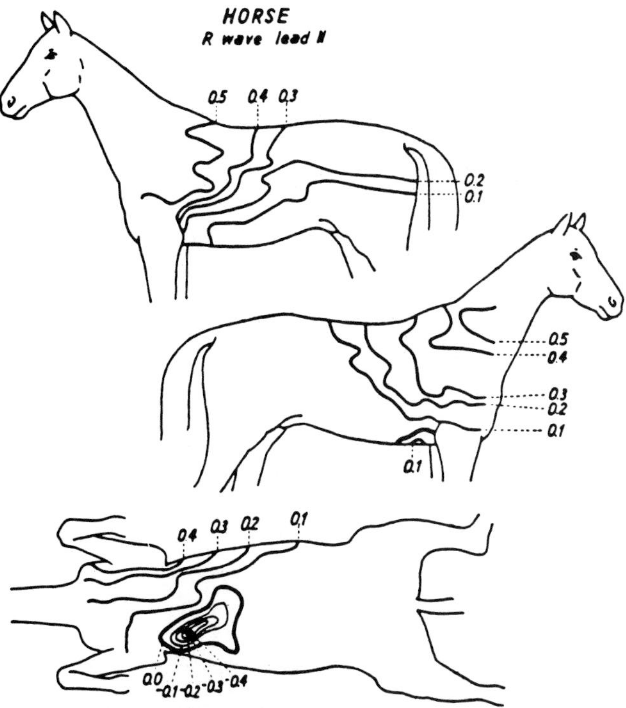

Figure 7.17. Equine isopotential lines mapped on the body of a horse during the peak of R wave in lead II. The values are in millivolts and represent the potentials recorded against the Wilson central terminal. The area of greatest negativity (−0.4 mV) was located on the ventral thorax to the right of the sternum, and the area of greatest positivity (+0.5 mV) toward the head. (From Detweiler and Patterson 1972, in Catcott and Smithcors eds, *The Cardiovascular System in Equine Medicine and Surgery,* 2d ed. Courtesy of American Veterinary Publications, Goleta, Calif.)

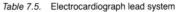

Table 7.5. Electrocardiograph lead system

Bipolar standard leads
Lead I: Right arm (−) compared with left arm (+)
Lead II: Right arm (−) compared with left leg (+)
Lead III: Left arm (−) compared with left leg (+)
Augmented unipolar limb leads
Lead aVR: Right arm (+) compared with left arm and left leg (−)
Lead aVL: Left arm (+) compared with right arm and left leg (−)
Lead aVF: Left leg (+) compared with right and left arms (−)
Special leads
Unipolar precordial chest leads
Lead CV_5RL (rV_2): Fifth right intercostal space near edge of sternum
Lead CV_6LL (V_2): Sixth left intercostal space near edge of sternum
Lead CV_6LU (V_4): Sixth left intercostal space at costochondral junction
Lead V_{10}: Over dorsal spinous process of seventh thoracic vertebra
Modified orthogonal lead systems
Lead X: Lead I; right (−) to left (+)
Lead Y: Lead aVF; cranial (−) to caudal (+)
Lead Z: Lead V_{10}: ventral (−) to dorsal (+)

From Tilley 1992, *Essentials of Canine and Feline Electrocardiography. Interpretation and Management,* 3d ed., Lea & Febiger, Philadelphia.

leads I, II, and III (Fig. 7.18), augmented unipolar limb leads aVR, aVL, and aVF (Fig. 7.19), and unipolar precordial (thoracic) leads V_2 (CV_6LL) (V_4) (CV_6LU) (rV_2) (CV_5RL), and V_{10} (Fig. 7.20). Right lateral recumbency is the standard body position for recording ECGs in the dog and cat. Foreleg positioning must be standardized and consistent to avoid QRS axis changes. Right lateral recumbency with the forelegs parallel and vertical to the long axis of the body is the standard body position for dogs and cats. If the positions of the forelimb and shoulder blades (or neck and shoulders) vary, spurious axis changes occur in serial records. If respiratory distress is evident, the ECG should

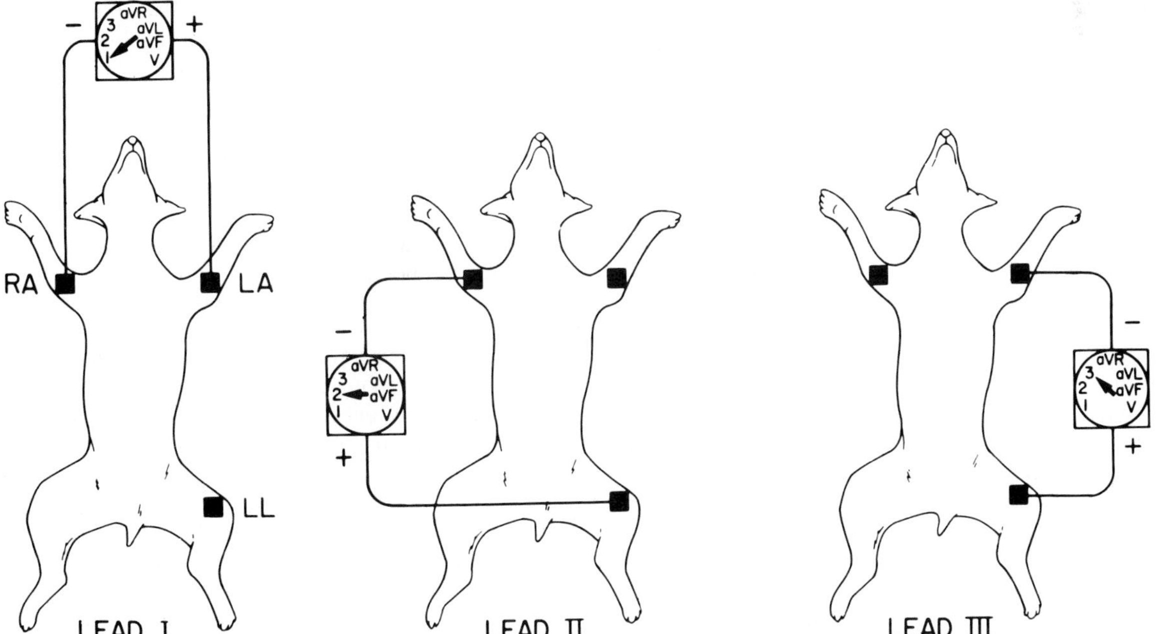

Figure 7.18. Three bipolar standard leads. By means of a switch incorporated in the instrument, the galvanometer can be connected across any pair of several electrodes. Each pair of electrodes is called a lead. The leads illustrated here are identified as I, II, and III. (From Tilley 1992, *Essentials of Canine and Feline Electrocardiography*, 3d ed., Lea & Febiger, Philadelphia.)

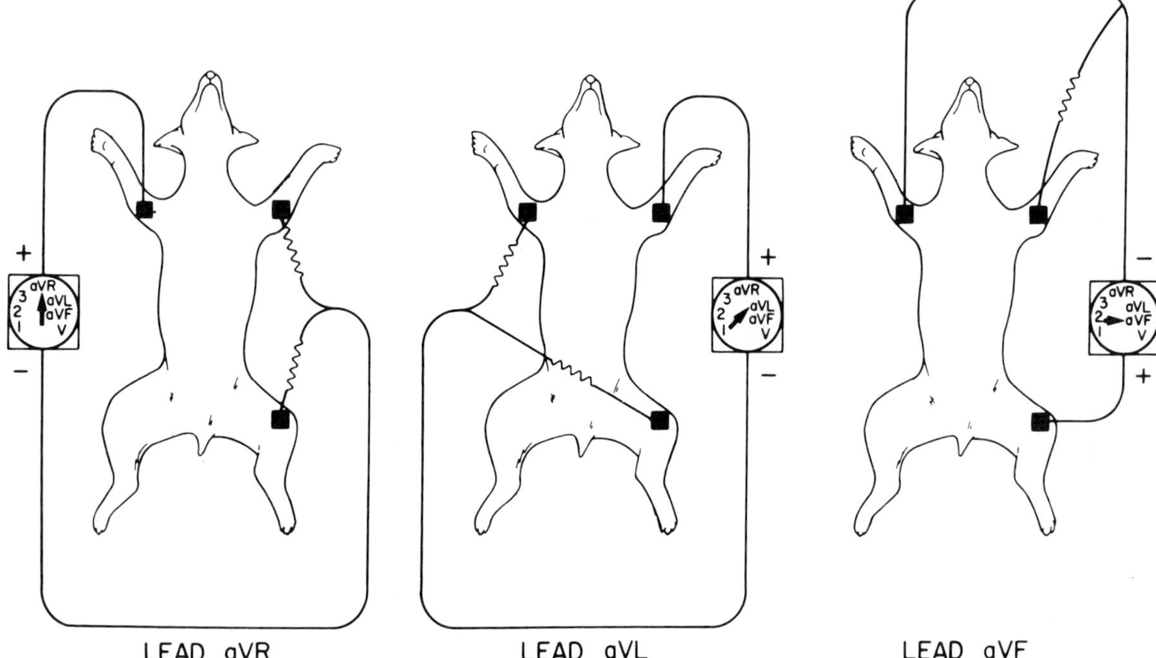

Figure 7.19. Augmented unipolar limb leads aVR, aVL, and aVF. (From Tilley 1992, *Essentials of Canine and Feline Electrocardiography*, 3d ed., Lea & Febiger, Philadelphia.)

be recorded with the animal standing or in a sternal position. Electrodes should be placed below the olecranons and over the patellar ligaments for bipolar standard and augmented unipolar limb leads. Precordial leads may be helpful in confirming areas of cardiac enlargement, emphasizing the deflections of the standard limb leads (this may be important if P waves are not clearly visible). Also, rV_2 and V_{10} have the only T waves with stable polarity in serial records and are used to detect myocardial injury. When the ECG lead selector is set to the V position, the exploring electrode potential is measured against the zero reference equivalent formed by the connected three limb electrodes.

The base-apex monitor lead is frequently recorded in the horse with the right forelimb electrode positioned in the right jugular furrow and the left forelimb electrode positioned over the heart or the left thorax. The electrocardiograph lead selector is turned to lead I to record the base-apex lead.

Orthogonal leads are oriented perpendicular to each other and view the heart in three different planes (leads X, Y, and Z). The X lead measures the frontal plane directed from right to left and is approximated by lead I. The Y lead axis indicates a midsagittal plane oriented craniocaudally and is approximated by lead aVF. The Z lead represents the transverse plane directed in a ventral to dorsal direction and is approximated by lead V_{10}. These uncorrected orthogonal leads can be used to generate a vectorcardiogram. Accurate orthogonal lead systems have been introduced (McFee, Schmidt, and Frank lead systems) and require the use of multiple electrodes at precise locations on the body.

Technical or mechanical problems that are superimposed on or distort the normal P-QRS-T complexes are known as artifacts. For accurate ECG interpretation, it is essential to recognize artifact and eliminate the source. Electrical 60-cycle artifact may be due to poor electric grounding of the ECG machine, the animal, or the table on which the animal is positioned. It is recognized on the ECG strip as a regular sequence of fine, sharp, vertical oscillations. Muscle tremor or body movement may also cause artifact, and efforts should be made to calm the animal.

Vectorcardiography

The vectorcardiogram (VCG) is another means of graphically displaying the heart's electrical activity (Figs. 7.21 and 7.22). The vectorcardiogram is produced when two simultaneously recorded perpendicular ECG leads are connected to the horizontal and vertical plates of a cathode ray tube. The magnitude (voltage) and spatial direction of the cardiac vector are visualized. Uncorrected orthogonal leads I and aVF (XY), I and V_{10} (XZ), aVF, and V_{10} (YZ) can be used to depict the magnitude and direction of the cardiac vector in the frontal, horizontal, and sagittal planes, respectively. The ECG differs in that magnitude and time are graphically depicted in each lead, and the values from more than one lead are required for spatial information such as the determination of mean electrical axis. Cardiac disease

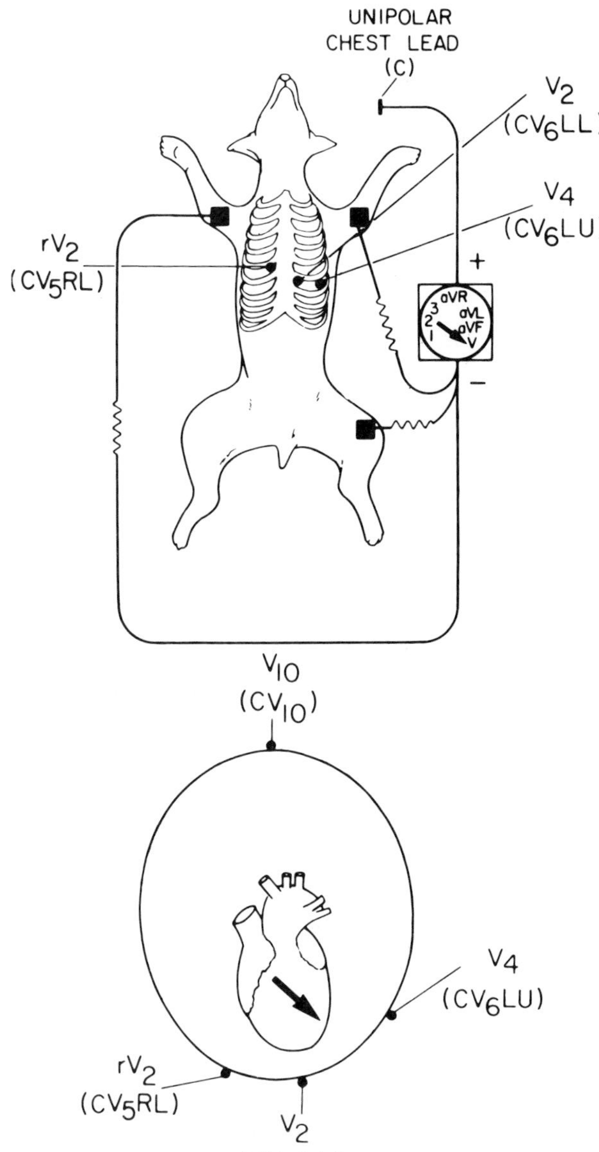

Figure 7.20. Unipolar precordial chest leads. The various positions of the chest electrodes on the thoracic cavity are viewed from the ventral aspect and in cross section. V_{10} is located over the seventh dorsal spinous process, CV_5RL on the right edge of the sternum at the fifth intercostal space, both CV_6LL and CV_6LU over the sixth intercostal space. Note that CV_6LL is near the sternum and CV_6LU is at the costochondral junction. (From Tilley 1992, *Essentials of Canine and Feline Electrocardiography*, 3d ed., Lea & Febiger, Philadelphia.)

that results in enlargement of the left or right heart chamber will change the vector loops of the P wave, QRS complex, and T wave. Because of the special equipment needed for the vectorcardiogram and the lack of emphasis on this technique when compared with the electrocardiogram, the vectorcardiogram has not had widespread use in human or veterinary clinical practice.

Transcription of the electrocardiogram

Atrial and ventricular contractions are preceded by electrical activity that initiates excitation-contraction coupling of myocardial cells. The sequence of normal electrical activation of the heart is illustrated in Fig. 7.23. The cardiac impulse originates in the pacemaking cells of the sinus node located at the junction of the cranial vena cava and right atrium and giving rise to the P wave. A depolarization (activation) wave spreads through the atria activating first the right and then the left atrium and giving rise to the P wave. The cardiac impulse then slows dramatically while traversing the specialized conduction tissue of the AV node and AV junctional tissue. This delay allows time for completion of atrial contraction before the onset of ventricular contraction. When the impulse emerges from the AV junctional tissue, its velocity increases through the bundle of His, the right bundle branch, the common left bundle branch, the anterior and posterior divisions of the common left bundle branch, and the Purkinje network. The cardiac impulse emerges from the Purkinje network and then spreads by cell-to-cell conduction through ventricular myocardial cells.

By convention, the Q wave is termed the first negative wave in the ventricular depolarization complex (Fig. 7.24). The R wave is the first positive wave, and the S wave is the first negative wave following the R wave. Collectively, these waves are called the QRS complex. Ventricular recovery (repolarization) is represented as the T wave on the ECG. The Q-T interval is the ventricular depolarization-repolarization time. It has clinical significance in specific disease processes. The sequential depolarization of atrial and ventricular myocardial fibers gives rise to the changing dipoles that result in the P wave and the QRS complex, respectively.

Analyzing the electrocardiogram

Before evaluation of the actual ECG strip, familiarization with the ECG machine, proper animal positioning restraint, electrode placement, and minimizing of electrical or mechanical artifacts are essential to ensure accurate analysis of the ECG.

A methodical approach to ECG interpretation is mandatory to avoid overlooking of vital information. Although many schemes have been advocated, a reasonable approach is described. The heart rate should be calculated from the lead II rhythm strip (Fig. 7.25). Both atrial and ventricular rates should be computed, since they may vary in some arrhythmias. When the basic rhythm is irregular, one can calculate the ventricular rate by counting the number of cycles (R-R intervals) within 3 seconds (paper speed of 50 mm/s) and multiplying by 20. When the rhythm is regular, the method explained in the legend of Fig. 7.25 may be used to calculate the heart rate. Paper speeds of 25 mm/s, or 50 mm/s are routinely employed.

After calculation of the heart rate, the heart rhythm

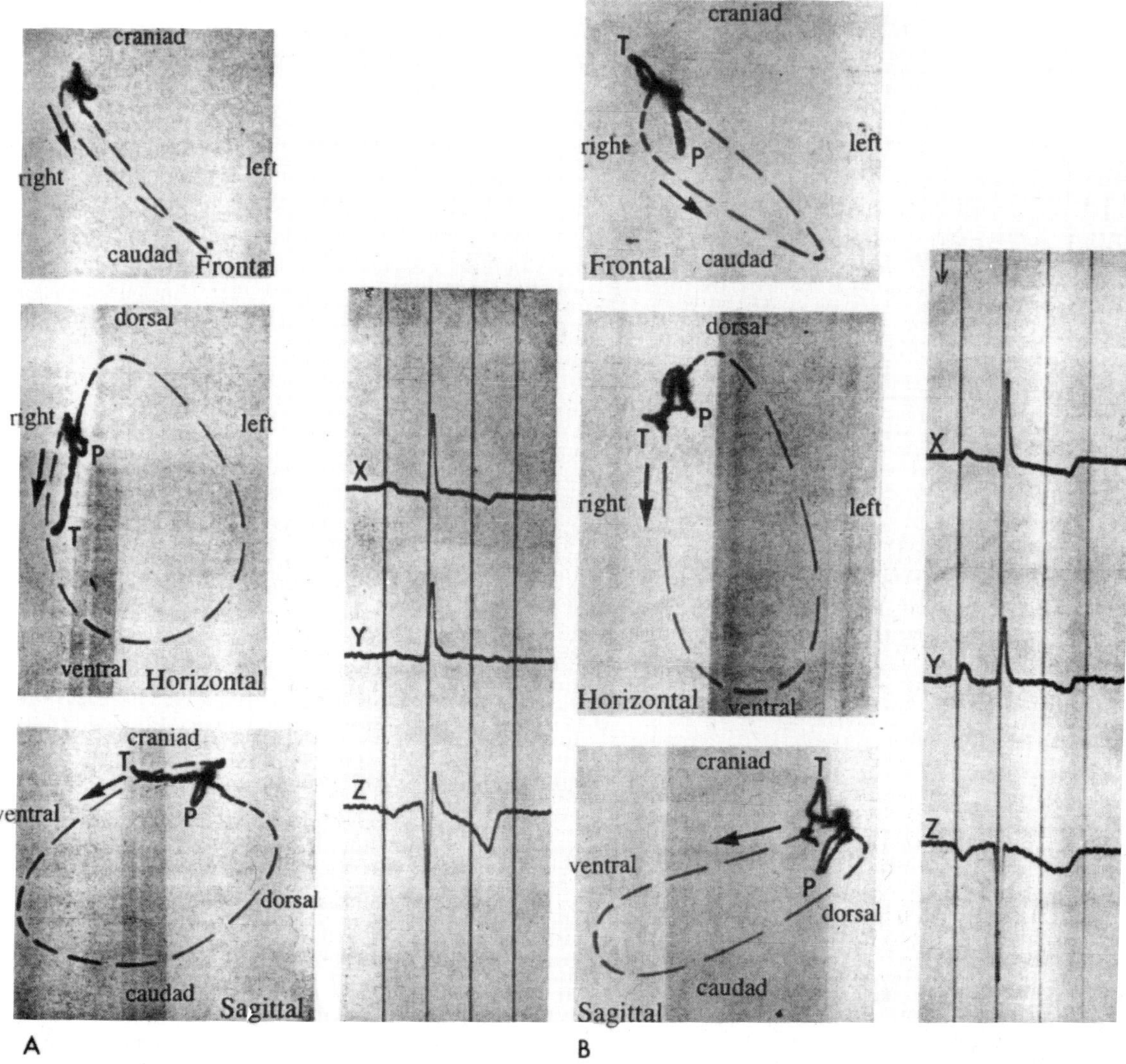

Figure 7.21. Normal vectorcardiogram. Scalar time lines = 0.1 second; teardrops = 0.002 second. (*A*) Vectorcardiogram, normal dog. The scalar X, Y, and Z leads are recorded, and the resultants of the X and Y leads (frontal plane), X and Z leads (horizontal plane), and Z and Y leads (sagittal plane) are then photographed. In the frontal plane the direction of the teardrops is counterclockwise (arrow). The forces are initially directed rightward and caudad and then turn leftward and caudad. In the horizontal plane the direction is counterclockwise, and the terminal forces are directed dorsally and leftward. The P (small) and T (large) loops are clearly recorded in the horizontal and sagittal planes of this vectorcardiogram. (*B*) The vectorcardiogram of a normal dog, similar to the vectorcardiogram in (*A*). A major difference in the two vectorcardiograms is the orientation of the T loop, which is more cranially directed in this case (frontal and sagittal planes). The P loop, normally directed leftward, caudad, and ventrad, is well produced. (From Ettinger and Suter 1970, *Canine Cardiology,* W.B. Saunders, Philadelphia.)

should then be evaluated. Calipers are helpful for making measurements. It is important to examine all recorded leads for arrhythmias. The following steps are important in the general evaluation of the cardiac rhythm:

1. General inspection will show whether the rhythm is characteristic of an arrhythmia or of a normal sinus rhythm. If an arrhythmia is present, it should be determined whether it is occasional, frequent, repetitive, regular, or irregular.
2. Identification of P waves plays a crucial role in the ECG examination. If P waves cannot be found, it is impossible to determine the relationship to QRS complexes. Doubling the sensitivity of the ECG may be helpful in magnifying the P waves. Precordial chest or esophageal leads may demonstrate P waves that are unrecognizable in other leads. When P waves are present it is important to determine whether they are uniform, multiform, regular, or irregular.
3. Recognition of QRS complexes and characterization of their configuration, uniformity, and regularity should then be done.
4. Analysis of the P-QRS relationship is the final step. Recognition of P waves is crucial in determining this relationship. Is the P-R interval consistent or is there no consistent relationship between the P wave and the QRS complexes?

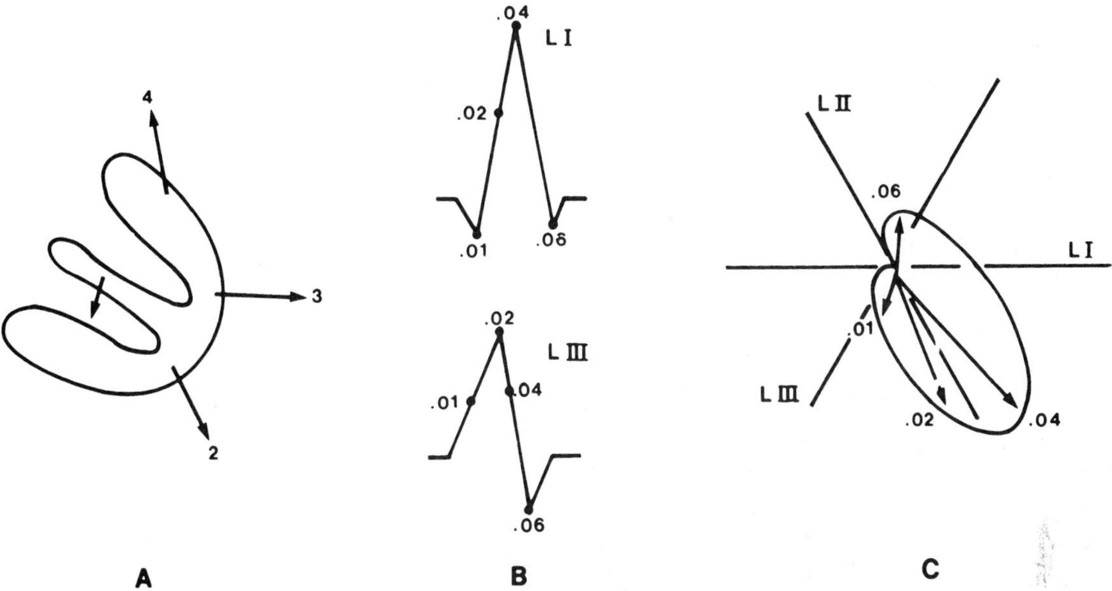

Figure 7.22. Correlation between the order of ventricular activation (*A*), scalar ECG (*B*), and vectorcardiogram (*C*). (*A*) The sequence of ventricular activation is represented by four instantaneous frontal plane vectors. (*B*) The four vectors plotted on leads I and III at the appropriate time during inscription of the QRS. (*C*) Using the method of construction of vectors described in Fig. 7.29, one can derive each of the four vectors in the frontal plane. A line joining the ends of the vectors results in a frontal plane QRS loop. The same method can be used to derive the orthogonal X, Y, and Z leads from the frontal, transverse, or sagittal planes. (Times given are in seconds.) (From Fisch 1988, Electrocardiography and vectorcardiography, in Braunwald, ed., *Heart Disease,* W.B. Saunders, Philadelphia.)

After the calculation of heart rate and analysis of rhythm, all amplitudes, durations, and intervals of P-QRS-T complexes can be determined on the lead II rhythm strip.

Measuring the normal P-QRS-T complex

Duration of the P wave is measured from its beginning to the end, and its amplitude is measured from the isoelectric line to the maximum height of the P wave (see Fig. 7.5). The P-R interval is measured from the beginning of the P wave to the beginning of the QRS complex. Duration of the QRS complex is measured from the beginning of the Q wave (if present) or the R wave if no Q wave is present to the end of the S wave (if present) or, if the S wave is absent, to where the R wave deflection reaches the baseline. The amplitude of the QRS complex is the sum of the excursions of the positive R wave and the negative Q or S wave (whichever is more negative). The Q-, R-, and S-wave amplitudes are measured from the baseline to the point of their maximal excursion. The interval between the end of the QRS complex and the beginning of the T wave is the S-T segment. The measurement between the beginning of the Q wave and the end of the T wave is referred to as the Q-T interval. The Q-T interval as well as the P-R interval may vary with many factors such as heart rate, cardiac disease, and electrolyte disorders. The T-wave amplitude and duration are variable and depend on a multitude of factors. Examples of normal canine and feline ECGs are shown in Fig. 7.26. Normal values for ECG complex amplitudes and intervals will vary depending on the species.

Mean electrical axis

Einthoven introduced the equilateral triangle concept to help analyze the ECG. This concept is based on the attachment of the three limb extremities that form the apexes of an equilateral triangle with the heart situated in the center. It is based on the assumption that the arms (or forelimbs in quadrupeds) and the left leg plus the lower (or caudal in quadrupeds) torso can be considered linear conductors attached at the apexes of an equilateral triangle. The apexes of the triangle are located at the shoulder attachment of the forelimbs or arms and approximately at the level of the diaphragm. In this simplified interpretation, the dipoles created by the heart are assumed to lie in the center of the equilateral triangle. The sides of the triangle are analogous to the standard limb leads. During ventricular depolarization-repolarization, many dipoles contribute to the electric field and may be represented by a single dipole or vector at any given instant. The average of all vectors is termed the *mean electrical axis*, which can be projected onto the three sides of Einthoven's triangle. When the three sides of the triangle (leads I, II, and III) are transposed so that their centers are superimposed on one another, the triaxial reference system is formed (Fig. 7.27). The hexaxial reference system is formed by addition of the unipolar limb lead axes to the triaxial system (Fig. 7.28).

The mean electrical axis (MEA) is the average direction of the electrical potential generated by the heart during the entire cardiac cycle. It is useful for suggesting chamber enlargement or intraventricular conduction defects. The MEA may be applied to atrial depolarization (P wave) or

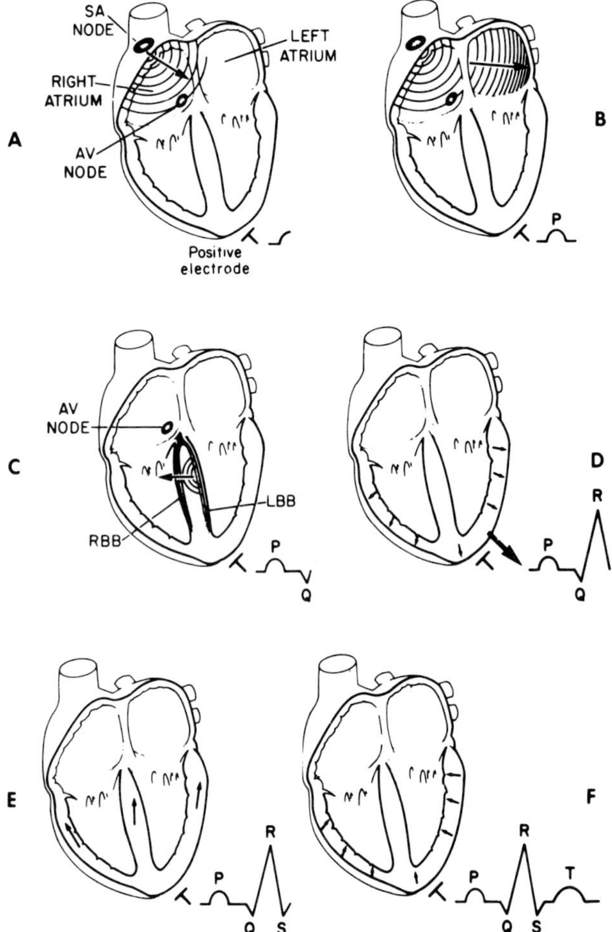

Figure 7.23. Electrocardiogram and the dog cardiac conduction system as an electrical impulse travels from the sinus node to the ventricular Purkinje network. (From Tilley 1992, *Essentials of Canine and Feline Electrocardiography,* 3d ed., Lea & Febiger, Philadelphia.)

ventricular repolarization (T wave), but traditionally it has been applied to ventricular depolarization (QRS complex). The MEA in the frontal plane can be calculated by means of the six limb leads and the hexaxial reference system. In the canine heart (Fig. 7.29) the axis most often falls between +40 and +100 degrees, and in the feline heart it most often falls between 0 and +160 degrees when the animals are placed in the right lateral recumbent position with forelimbs parallel and at right angles to the long axis of the body. In 27 of 36 70-day-old cats positioned in right lateral recumbency with forelimbs at a right angle to the long axis of the body, the frontal plane model electrical axis fell between 45 and 100 degrees.

There are several methods to determine the MEA. One method involves measurement of the net amplitudes in lead I and lead III and plotting of these vectors on the triaxial reference system (marked off from the zero point) (Fig. 7.30). Perpendicular lines are then drawn from these points to their intersection. A line drawn from the center of the axial reference system to this intersection represents the angle (in degrees) of the QRS axis. A more simple (and less accurate) method involves examination of all standard and augmented limb leads and identification of the one that is isoelectric (algebraic sum of the QRS deflections is zero) (Fig. 7.31). The MEA is directed approximately perpendicular to this isoelectric lead in the direction of its net (positive or negative) value of the perpendicular lead (Figs. 7.32 and 7.33).

Vector analysis

In analyzing the various leads of conventional scalar ECGs, it is common practice first to visualize the electromotive vector forces responsible for the deflections in the frontal plane from the limb lead deflections. and then to determine their orientation in three-dimensional space from the unipolar precordial leads. As with single-plane vectordiagrams, schematizing the information in the scalar ECG in this way simplifies interpretation of abnormalities and promotes understanding of their causes.

Types of adult mammalian electrocardiograms

Mammalian ECGs from different species (Table 7.6) can be classified in accordance with the following general characteristics: (1) relative duration of QT interval and ST segment; (2) QRS-vector direction and sense; and (3) constancy of T-wave polarity (T-wave lability). These differences, in turn, are determined by three elec-

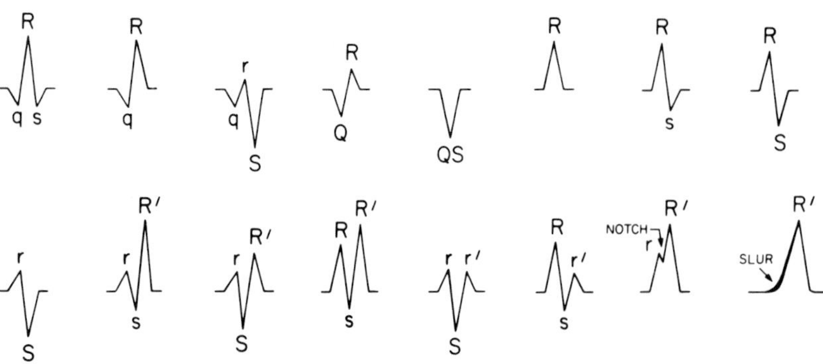

Figure 7.24. Components of QRS complex nomenclature of the various QRS complexes. The first positive wave is the r or R wave; the first negative complex is q or Q wave, and negative wave following the r or R wave is the s or S wave. By convention, capital letters are used if the Q, R, and S complexes are of large amplitude, and lowercase letters are used if the q, r, and s complexes are of low amplitude. The prime symbols (i.e., r′ and R′) are used for the second wave in any QRS complex. This also applies to Q and S waves. (From Tilley 1992, *Essentials of Canine and Feline Electrocardiography*, 3d ed., Lea & Febiger, Philadelphia.)

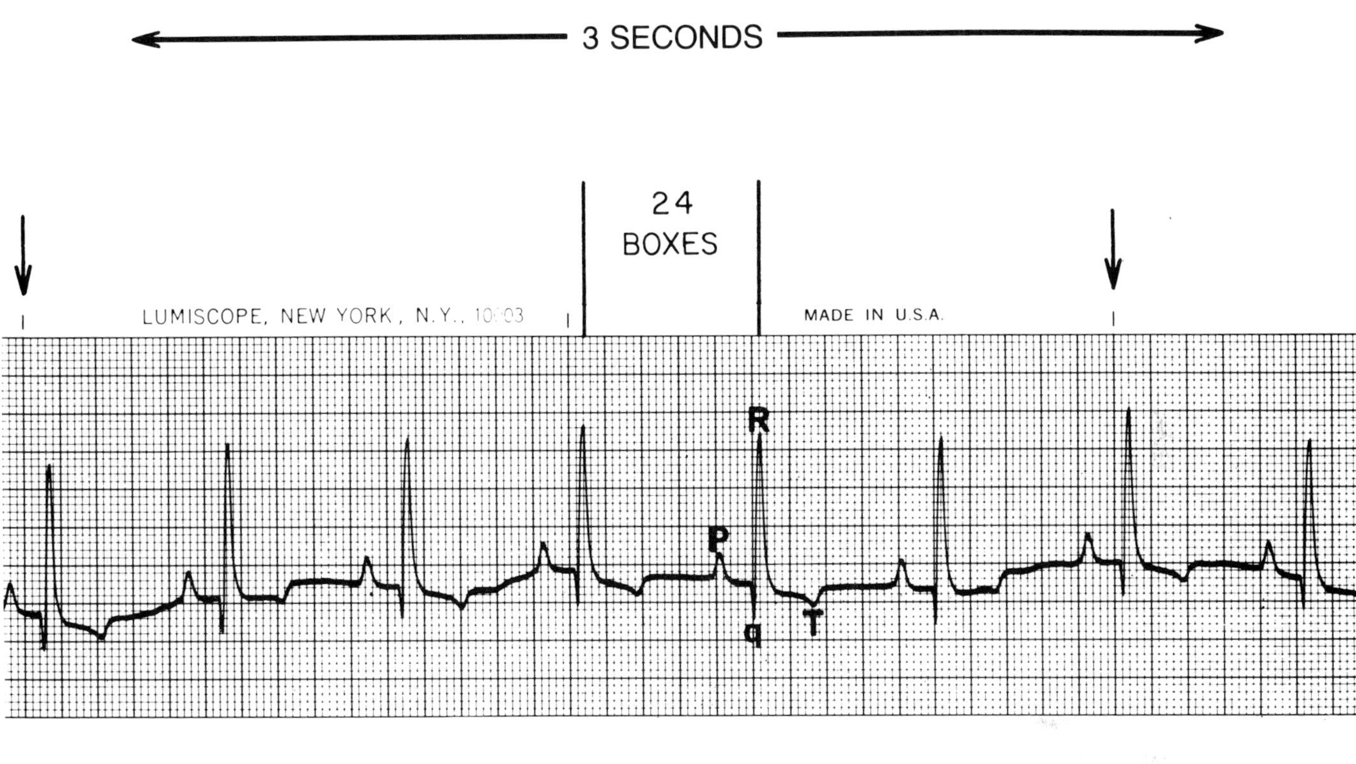

Figure 7.25. Calculation of the heart rate from a normal canine ECG. When the ventricular rate is regular, 3000 (number of small boxes per minute) divided by the number of small 0.02 second boxes per beat equals the heart rate (3000 ÷ 24 = 125). When the rhythm is irregular, the approximate number of cycles (R-R intervals) between two sets of marks (arrows) multiplied by 20 (60 seconds divided by 30 seconds) equals the heart rate (6 × 20 = 120). Paper speed, 50 mm/s. At a paper speed of 25 mm/s, each small box equals 0.04 second, and 12 such boxes would separate two consecutive beats; when 1500 is divided by the number, the heart rate is 125. At this paper speed, 15 cm equals 6 seconds, and the number of cycles counted is multiplied by 10 to get the heart rate. A heart rate calculator can also be used for rapid determination of the rate. These rulers may be calibrated for the paper speed of 25 mm/s. (From Tilley 1992, *Essentials of Canine and Feline Electrocardiography*, 3d ed., Lea & Febiger, Philadelphia.)

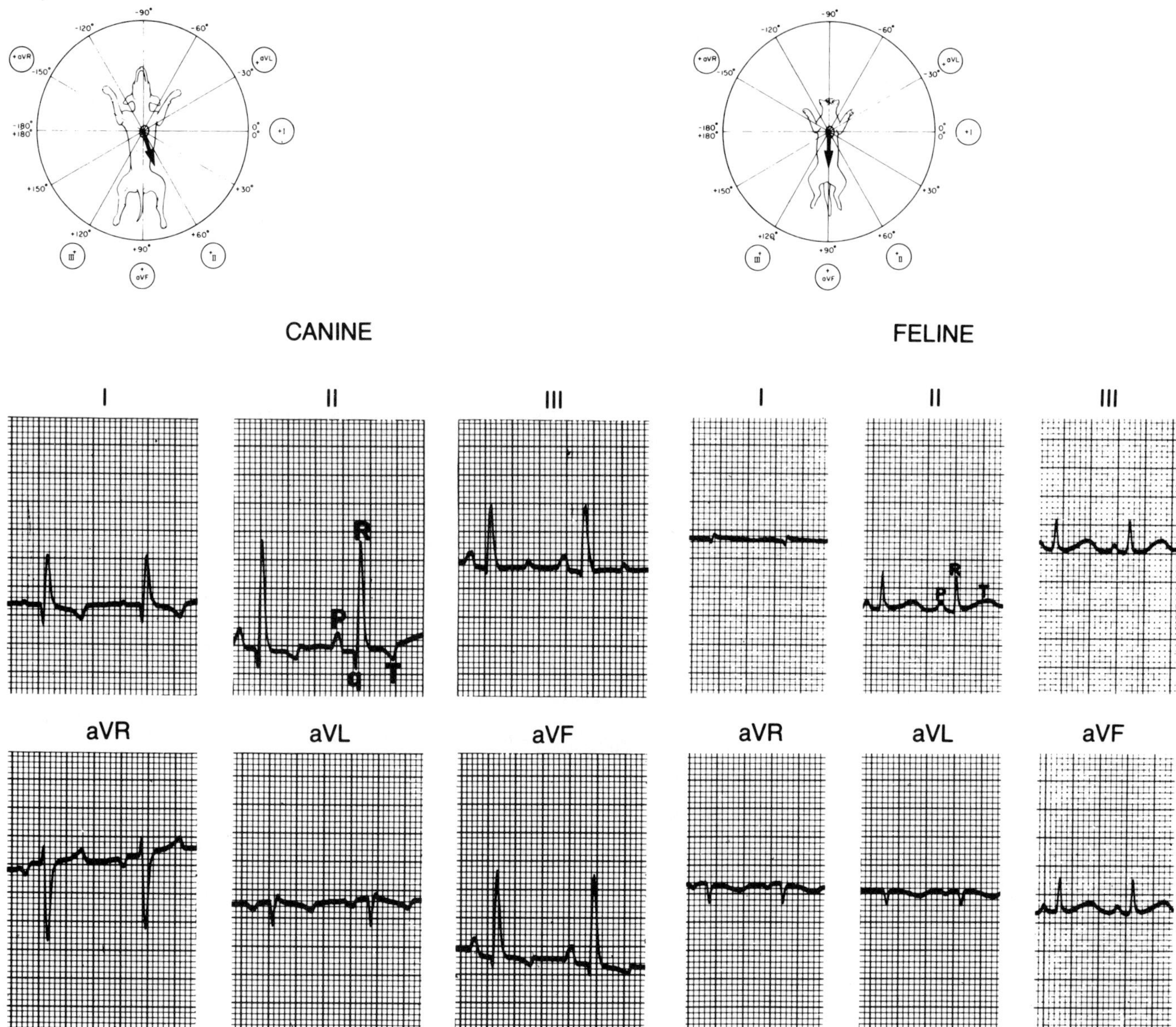

Figure 7.26. For the systematic analysis of the direction and magnitude of the electrical axis of the heart, the six basic limb leads (I, II, III, aVR, aVL, and aVF) are arranged in a circular field according to the direction of each lead and the location of the positive electrodes. The mean electrical axis is +70 degrees for this dog and +90 degrees for this cat. (From Tilley 1992, *Essentials of Canine and Feline Electrocardiography*, 3d ed., Lea & Febiger, Philadelphia.)

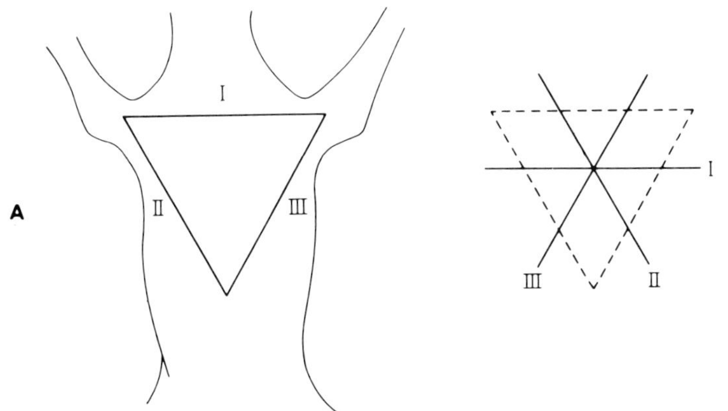

Figure 7.27. (*A*) The equilateral triangle of Einthoven, formed by leads I, II, and III. (*B*) The triaxial lead reference system is produced by transposition of the three sides of the triangle (leads I, II, and III) to a common central point of zero potential. This triaxial lead system will later be used to formulate the hexaxial lead system. (From Tilley 1992, *Essentials of Canine and Feline Electrocardiography*, 3d ed., Lea & Febiger, Philadelphia.)

trophysiological properties that are genetically governed: (1) the relative duration of the ventricular cell action potential as determined by the presence or absence of phase 2 (plateau);
(2) the pattern of spread of excitation throughout the ventricles; and (3) constancy of the pattern of repolarization, (i.e., the constancy of the ventricular gradient).

QT duration and ST segment

Many species (rodents, insectivores, bats, and kangaroos) have short QT intervals relative to the duration of mechanical systole. The ST segment is essentially absent. The QRS-T complex consists of rapid QRS deflections that merge with the slower T wave, and its duration is about one-half that of mechanical systole. The transmembrane action potentials of these species do not have a distinct plateau, which explains the absence of the ST segment. This is in contrast to the QRS-T complex of other mammalians that have an ST segment, a QT interval equivalent to mechanical systole, and an action potential with a distinct plateau.

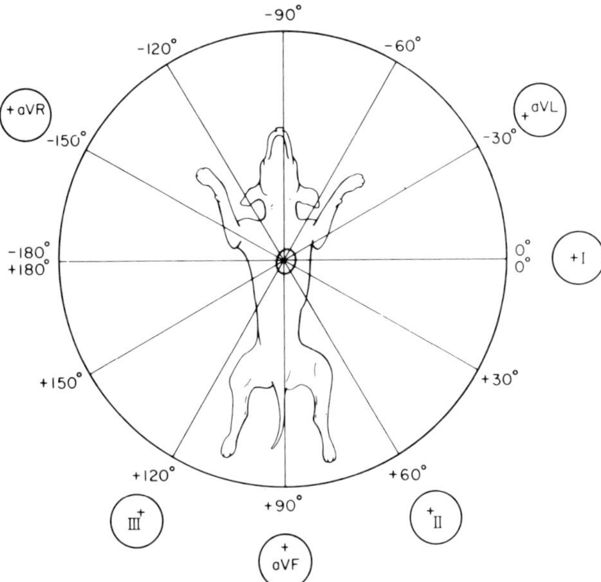

Figure 7.28. The hexaxial lead system for both the dog and the cat can be enclosed in a circle. The positive pole of each lead is indicated by a circle. (From Tilley 1992, *Essentials of Canine and Feline Electrocardiography*, 3d ed., Lea & Febiger, Philadelphia.)

Ventricular activation patterns

The ventricular activation patterns of various species fall into two general types:

1. Group A. Dogs, humans, monkeys, cats, and rats, for example, have QRS vectors that, generally, are directed along the long axis of the body, caudally and ventrally, and produce a largely negative deflection in lead V_{10} and a positive deflection in lead aVF.
2. Group B. Hoofed mammals and dolphins, for example, have QRS vectors, that, generally, are directed from the sternum toward the spine, and they produce largely positive deflections in lead V_{10} and negative deflections in lead aVF.

These differences are associated with the distributive characteristics of the Purkinje network. In group A animals, it is primarily a subendocardial network. In group B animals, the Purkinje network is more elaborate and penetrates deeply into the ventricular myocardium.

T-wave lability

In humans, primates, and many hoofed mammals, T-wave amplitude and polarity tend to be fairly constant in serial records. In dogs, and especially in horses, T-wave vectors are quite labile and the T waves vary in polarity and amplitude in limb leads and some thoracic leads in serial records and sometimes change during the course of recording of a given lead. In the dog there are two conventional thoracic leads in which the T-wave polarity is remarkably consistent: the T wave is normally positive in lead rV_2 (CV_5RL) and negative in V_{10} in about 90 percent of the animals.

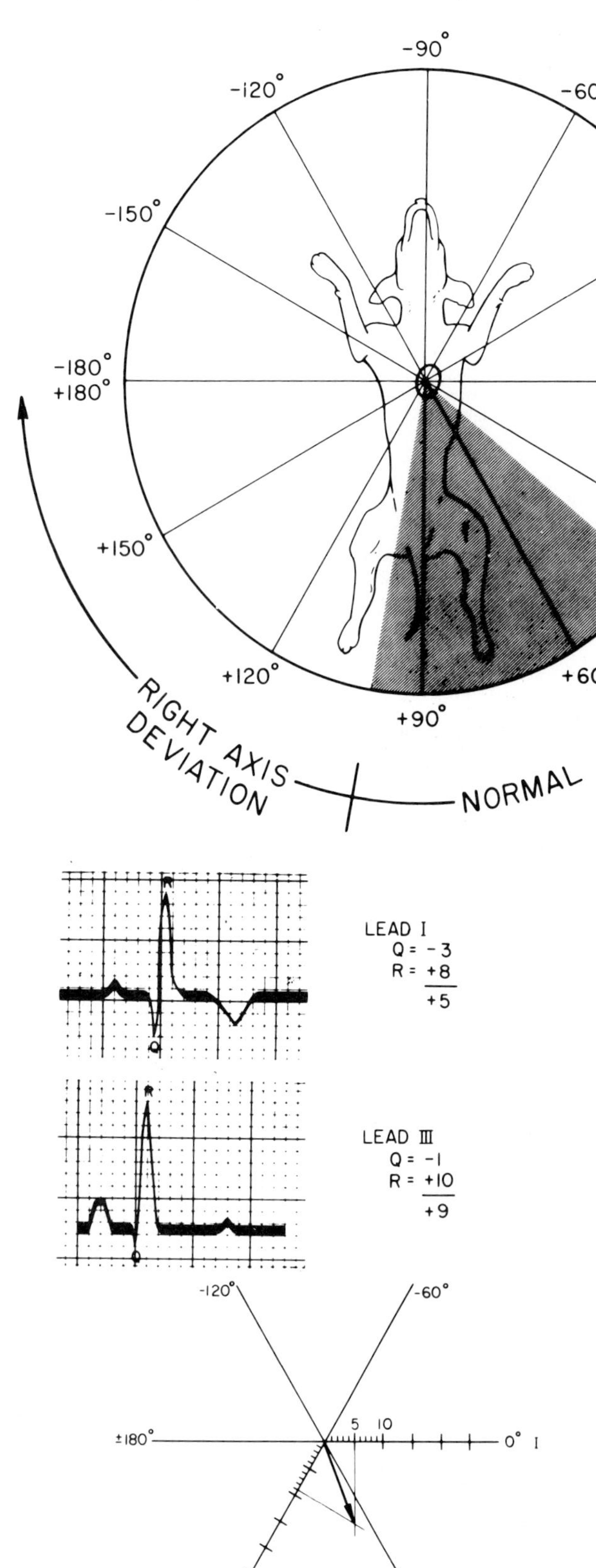

Figure 7.29. In the dog, the usual mean electrical axis in the frontal plane is from +40 to +100 degrees. If the axis departs substantially beyond these approximate limits, the term *axis deviation* is used. Right axis deviation means that the calculated axis angle is considerably greater than +100 degrees and left axis deviation means that the angle is substantially smaller than 40 degrees in either case when the axes reach the upper half of the circle in which, by convention, the degrees are expressed as negative values from 0 to 180 degrees. (From Tilley 1992, *Essentials of Canine and Feline Electrocardiography*, 3d ed., Lea & Febiger, Philadelphia.)

Figure 7.30. Plotting of the lead I and lead III values for calculation of the mean electrical axis. The positive and negative deflections for each lead are added (I = +5; III = +9). Perpendicular lines are then followed from the positive or negative point determined for each lead on the triaxial system. A line drawn from the center of the triaxial system to the point of the intersected perpendicular lines gives the direction and relative magnitude of the mean QRS vector (approximately +70 degrees). (From Tilley 1992, *Essentials of Canine and Feline Electrocardiography*, 3d ed., Lea & Febiger, Philadelphia.)

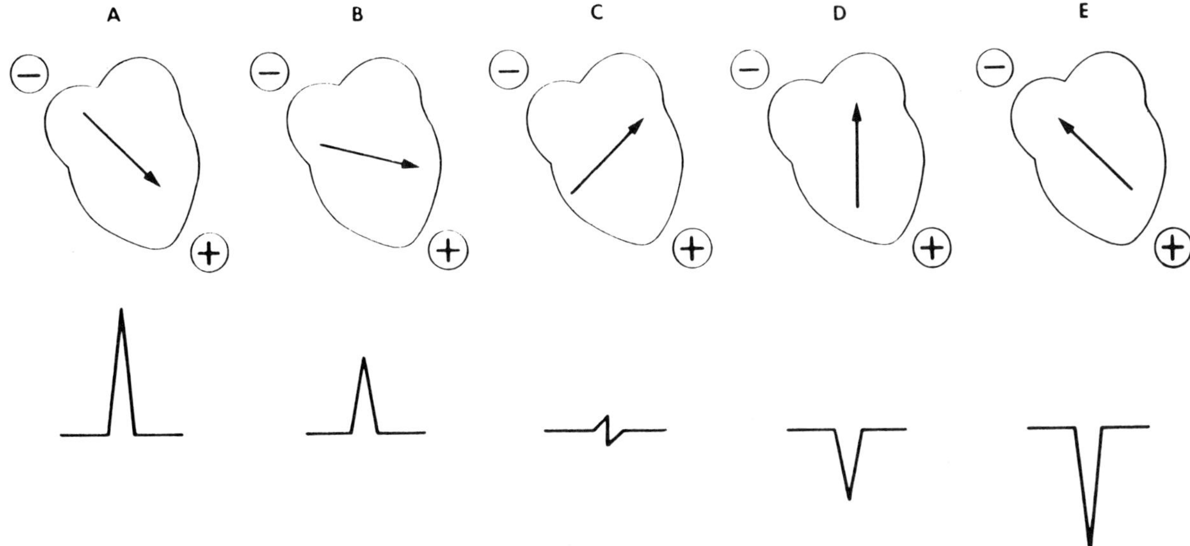

Figure 7.31. Effect of the depolarization wave on the deflections of the electrocardiogram, determined by wave direction. Each lead has a positive and a negative pole. By tradition, the electrocardiogram is generated in such a way that it shows a positive wave when the depolarization wave is flowing *toward* the positive electrode (*A* and *B*). A negative deflection is recorded when the depolarization wave moves *away* from the positive electrode (*D* and *E*). The deflection is *isoelectric* when depolarization is perpendicular to an imaginary line connecting the two electrodes (*C*). (From Tilley 1992, *Essentials of Canine and Feline Electrocardiography*, 3d ed., Lea & Febiger, Philadelphia.)

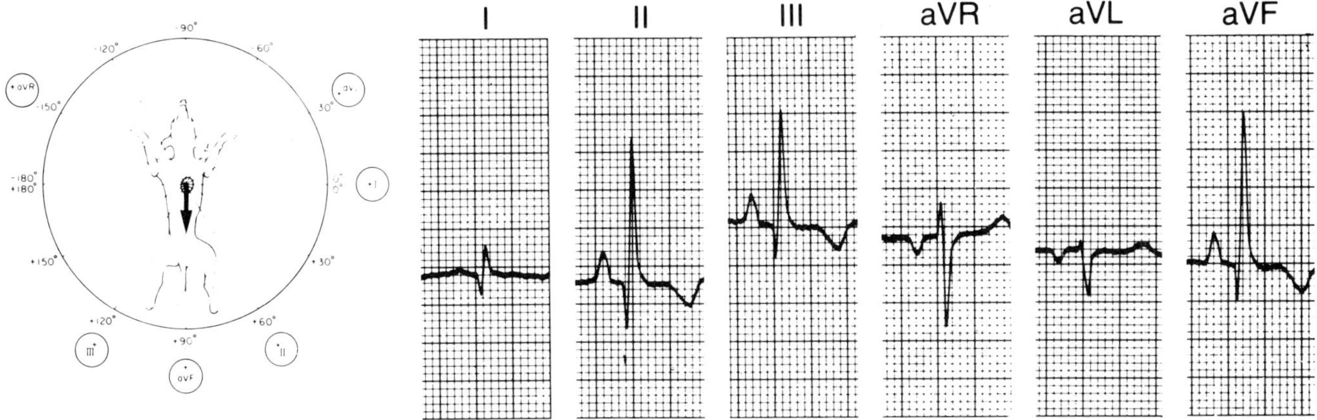

Figure 7.32. The mean electrical axis in this canine ECG is +90 degrees. Lead I is isoelectric. The lead perpendicular to lead I is aVF (see axis chart). Since lead aVF is positive, the axis is calculated to be +90 degrees (a normal axis). (From Tilley 1992, *Essentials of Canine and Feline Electrocardiography*, 3d ed., Lea & Febiger, Philadelphia.)

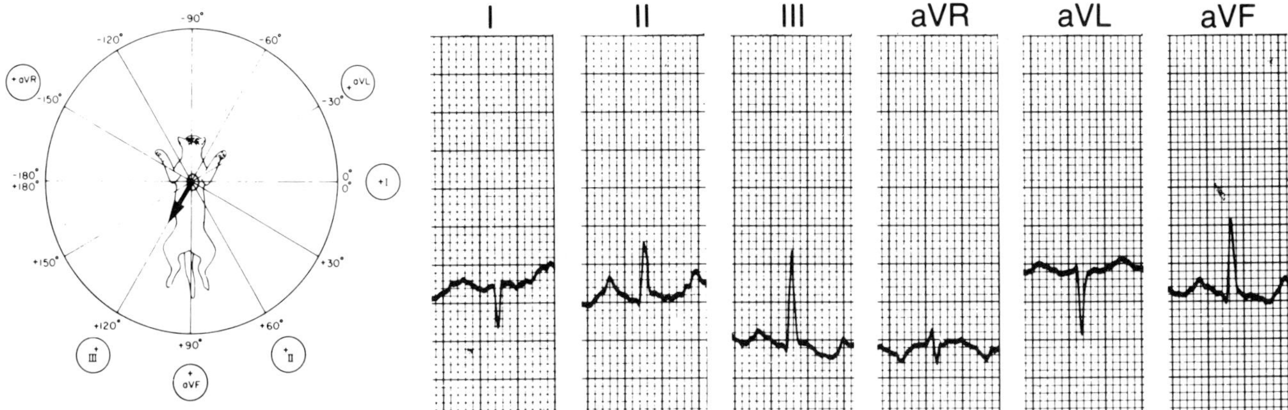

Figure 7.33. The isoelectric lead in this feline ECG is aVR. On the axis charge, lead aVR is perpendicular to lead III. Since lead III is positive on this tracing, the axis is directed toward the positive pole of lead III (or +120 degrees). An axis of +120 degrees is normal in the cat. (From Tilley 1992, *Essentials of Canine and Feline Electrocardiography*, 3d ed., Lea & Febiger, Philadelphia.)

Table 7.6. Representative values for electrocardiographic intervals in various species

Species	Average heart rate per minute	PR (s)	QRS (s)	QT (s)
Elephant	30	0.35	0.15	0.60
Horse	35	0.30	0.11	0.52
Ox	70	0.18	0.09	0.39
Swine	100	0.13	0.06	0.32
Sheep/goat	100	0.13	0.04	0.28
Dog	100	0.10	0.06	0.20
Cat	140	0.07	0.04	0.17
Rabbit	260	0.06	0.03	0.12
Guinea pig	250	0.06	0.03	0.12
White rat	350	0.04	0.015	0.07
Mouse	550	0.03	0.01	0.035

Importance of forelimb and body position in recording limb lead electrocardiograms in quadrupeds

The attachment of the forelimbs at the shoulder girdle and the shape of the thorax relative to the position of the heart in the chest differ in quadrupeds from those in humans and many other primates. In quadrupeds, the transverse diameter of the thorax is generally less than the dorsoventral diameter. Also, the forelimb muscular attachment is on either side of the thorax. When the forelimbs are moved, limb attachment location shifts relative to heart position, and the direction in space of electrocardiographic vectors appears to change, although there has been no change in spread of excitation or heart position. Accordingly, it is necessary to standardize limb position in quadrupeds to obtain consistent limb lead ECGs. In certain primates, because the shoulder girdle attachment is more posterior, on approximately the same plane behind the heart, variations in limb position have less effect on electrocardiographic vectors.

THE ABNORMAL ELECTROCARDIOGRAM

Electrocardiography is useful in clinical veterinary practice (1) in the definitive diagnosis of cardiac arrhythmias, (2) as an adjunct to determine cardiac enlargement (dilation or hypertrophy), and (3) as an indicator of certain electrolyte, acid-base, systemic, or metabolic disorders. The use of electrocardiography in the diagnosis of cardiac arrhythmias is based on well-understood electrophysiological principles. Vectorcardiographic and electrocardiographic diagnoses of other cardiac abnormalities, while supported by experimental work, are much more empirical.

The first and most important step in ECG interpretation is differentiation between normal and abnormal wave forms. The second step is differentiation between the various abnormal ECG patterns and correlation with known cardiac abnormalities. ECG abnormalities that suggest cardiac enlargement require further definition with thoracic radiography, echocardiography, or angiocardiography. A simple checklist for this process is provided in Table 7.7.

Table 7.7 Evaluation of the ECG for arrhythmias: a checklist

1. Are P waves present?
   a. If not, is there other evidence of atrial activity (flutter or fibrillatory waves)?
2. What is the relationship between atrial activity and QRS complexes?
   a. What are the atrial and ventricular rates?
   b. Is a P wave related to each QRS complex?
   c. Does a P wave precede or follow the QRS complex?
   d. Is the P-R or R-R interval constant?
   e. Are the P-R and R-R intervals regular or irregular?
3. Are the P waves and QRS complexes normal and of similar morphology?
4. Are the QRS complexes wide (greater than 0.05 s) or normal?
5. Is the ventricular rhythm regular or irregular?
6. Are durations and amplitudes of P, P-R, QRS, and Q-T intervals normal?
7. Are there pauses or premature complexes that require explanation?
8. What is the significance of the arrhythmias in context with the clinical setting?
   a. Is there a danger posed by the arrhythmia?
   b. Should attempts be made to directly terminate the arrhythmia?
   c. Can an underlying disorder be corrected, thereby abolishing the arrhythmia?

From Fox, Kaplan 1987, Feline arrhythmias, in Bonagura, ed., *Contemporary Issues Small Animal Medicine,* vol. 7, *Cardiology,* Churchill Livingstone, New York.

Ladder diagrams

The ladder (Lewis) diagram is a graphic illustration (Figs. 7.34 and 7.35) of cardiac impulse formation and conduction that enhances the understanding of arrhythmias and conduction disorders and allows deduction of complex mechanisms. These diagrams help explain and illustrate simple and complex rhythm disorders. The technique is easy to use and should be constructed routinely under the actual ECG strip being analyzed.

Cardiac arrhythmias

Cardiac arrhythmias (disorders of cardiac rhythm) are generally divided into categories of disorders of impulse formation, disorders of impulse conduction, or combinations of both (Table 7.8). The current view of the mechanisms for cardiac arrhythmias includes isolated or concurrent abnormalities in impulse initiation (automaticity), conduction (including reentry), and triggered activity (early and delayed after depolarizations).

Reentry mechanism for arrhythmias

Reentry is an established and proven mechanism underlying many supraventricular (atrial) and ventricular arrhythmias. Reentry occurs when a propagating cardiac impulse does not terminate after normal cardiac cell activation but persists to reexcite proximal cardiac tissue after expiration of the refractory period. Usually the reentrant impulse returns in a different pathway to reactivate cardiac tissue; this may occur in terminal Purkinje fibers, ischemic myocardial tissue, bundle branches, the bundle of His, AV nodal tissue, and anomalous accessory AV pathways (Figs. 7.36 and 7.37). Slowed conduction in one pathway and unidirectional block in the other pathway are typical requirements for reentry to occur.

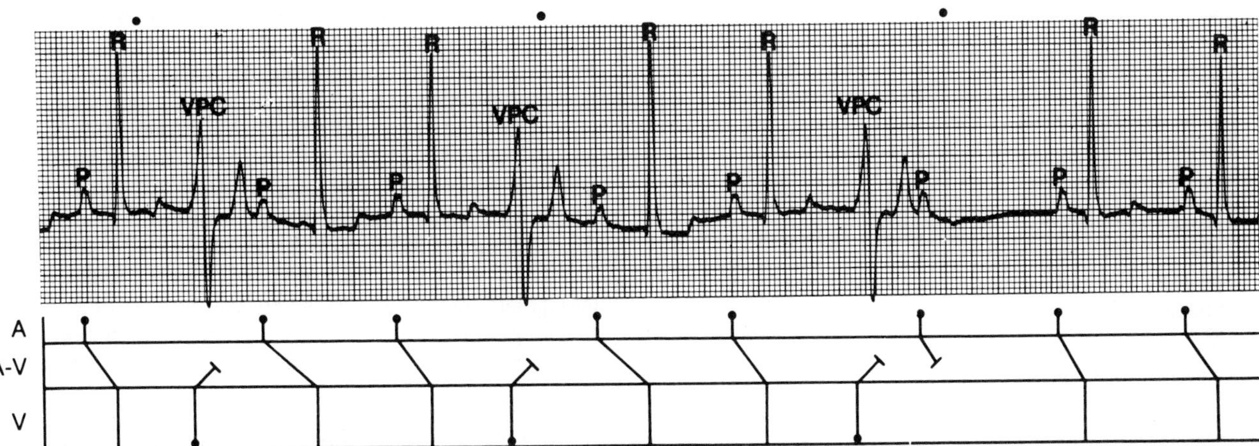

Figure 7.34. How to use the AV ladder diagram. First draw the lines for the P waves (A level) and QRS complexes (V level); the lines should coincide with the beginning of the P wave and the QRS complex, respectively. Then draw a line between the AV levels to indicate AV conduction. The site of impulse formation can be represented by a dot. The ladder diagram easily explains the prolonged P-R interval after the first two VPCs as well as the blocked P wave after the third VPC. The first two interpolated VPCs have penetrated the AV junction and caused the subsequent P-R interval to be prolonged. The third VPC has rendered the AV junction completely refractory, preventing conduction of the subsequent sinus P wave. A compensatory pause occurs after the third VPC. (From Tilley 1992, *Essentials of Canine and Feline Electrocardiography*, 3d ed., Lea & Febiger, Philadelphia.)

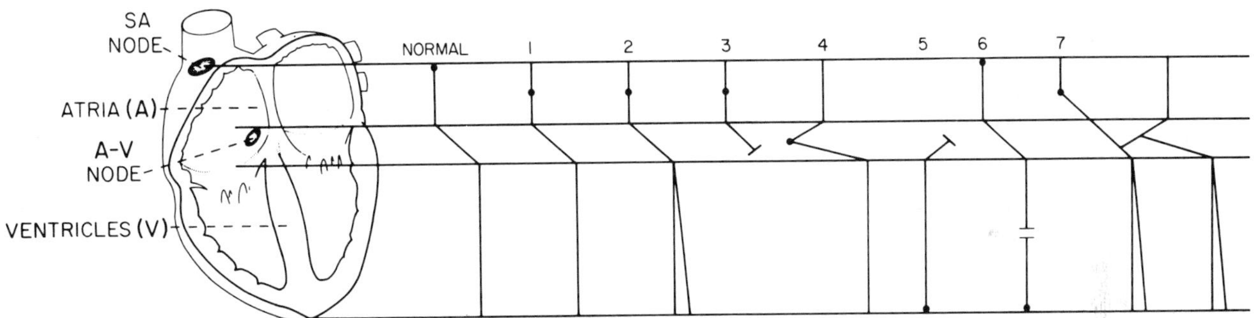

Figure 7.35. Representative examples of the AV ladder diagram: 1, atrial premature complex (APC) with normal conduction; 2, APC with aberrant ventricular conduction (also used to illustrate left and right bundle branches); 3, APC not conducted; 4, AV junctional premature complex with anterograde ventricular and retrograde atrial conduction; 5, ventricular premature complex (VPC) with partial penetration of the AV junction; 6, ventricular fusion complex between a sinus impulse and an ectopic ventricular impulse; 7, APC and one reciprocal complex (reentry) with aberrant ventricular conduction. (From Tilley 1992, *Essentials of Canine and Feline Electrocardiography,* 3d ed., Lea & Febiger, Philadelphia.)

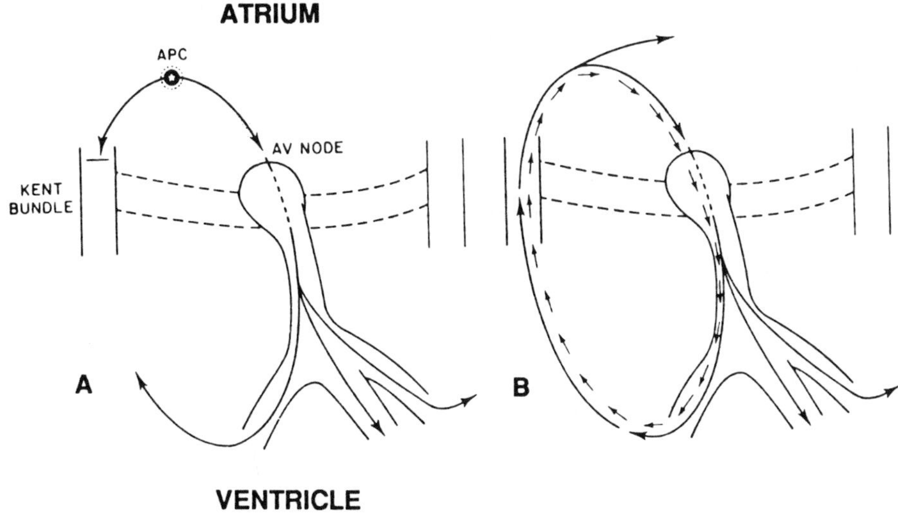

Figure 7.36. Reciprocal rhythm. Mechanisms of paroxysmal supraventricular tachycardia associated with ventricular preexcitation. The Wolff-Parkinson-White syndrome provides a classic example of macro-reentry (reentrant pathways that are used are long). The APC is conducted down the AV node and the His-Purkinje network but not the accessory bundle of Kent (*A*). After reaching the ventricles, the impulse reenters the atria by passing up through the bypass tract (Kent bundle shown here). This sequence is repeated, causing a reciprocal tachycardia (*B*). (From Tilley 1992, *Essentials of Canine and Feline Electrocardiography*, 3d ed., Lea & Febiger, Philadelphia.)

Table 7.8. Classification of cardiac arrhythmias

Normal sinus impulse formation
Normal sinus rhythm
Sinus arrhythmia
Disturbances of sinus impulse formation
Sinoatrial arrest
Atrial premature complexes
Atrial tachycardia
Atrial flutter
Atrial fibrillation
Atrioventricular junctional rhythm
Disturbances of ventricular impulse formation
Ventricular premature complexes
Ventricular tachycardia
Ventricular asystole
Ventricular fibrillation
Disturbances of impulse conduction
Sinoatrial block
Atrial standstill
First-degree AV block
Second-degree AV block
Disturbances of both impulse formation and impulse conduction
Sick sinus syndrome
Ventricular preexcitation

From Miller 1985, Treatment of cardiac arrhythmias and conduction disturbances, in Tilley and Owens, eds., *Manual of Small Animal Cardiology,* Churchill Livingstone, New York.

Triggered activity

Triggered activity is a depolarization that results from a preceding impulse or series of impulses. Triggered activity is initiated by afterdepolarizations (Fig. 7.38). *Afterpotentials* are oscillations in cell membrane potentials other than conventional phase 4 depolarization, that occur during or after repolarization of a conducted impulse. There are two kinds; afterdepolarizations and afterhyperpolarizations. *Afterdepolarizations* may occur during repolarization of the preceding impulse (*early afterdepolarizations*), or they may occur after repolarization of the preceding impulse (*delayed afterdepolarizations*). Both the early and delayed types can reach threshold and induce conducted impulses, resulting in ectopic heartbeats. *Afterhyperpolarizations* do not induce conducted impulses. The term *triggered extrasystoles* designates cardiac ectopic beats induced by afterdepolarizations. The action potential preceding the afterdepolarizations is considered the "trigger" and the afterdepolarization the "triggered activity" of the fiber. Afterdepolarizations are oscillations in the membrane potential that are induced by the preceding cardiac impulse.

Causes of arrhythmias

Cardiac arrhythmias may occur in the presence or absence of cardiac disease. Numerous systemic disorders may cause secondary cardiac arrhythmias, as there is a complex interaction among the cardiac cells, the autonomic nervous system, and the fluid that bathes and nourishes the heart. Arrhythmias are more likely to occur in hearts with diseases such as cardiomyopathy (e.g., atrial fibrillation) or AV valvular insufficiency (e.g., atrial arrhythmias) than in nondiseased hearts. Many cardiac arrhythmias are benign, clinically insignificant, and require no therapy. Arrhythmias may also cause severe clinical signs, such as dyspnea, coughing, weakness, and syncope, or degenerate into malignant arrhythmias, such as ventricular tachycardia or ventricular fibrillation. In the latter case, immediate therapeutic intervention may be lifesaving.

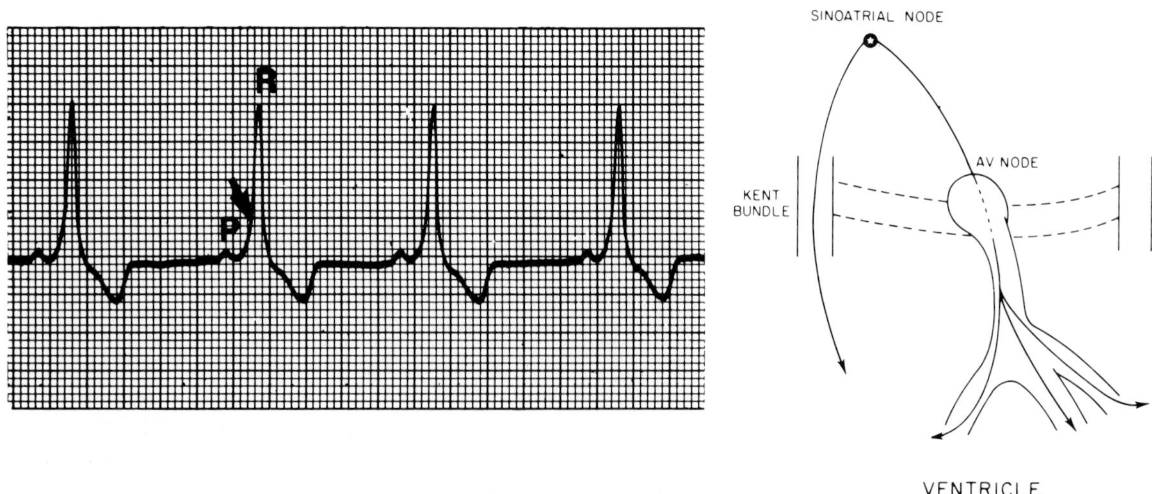

Figure 7.37. Ventricular preexcitation. The sinus impulse is conducted through the bundle of Kent without delay but is delayed physiologically in the AV node. The portion of the ventricle adjacent to the bundle of Kent is prematurely activated and causes a delta wave (arrow) on the electrocardiogram. The remainder of the ventricle is then activated from both the normal and the accessory pathways. The existence of an accessory pathway is not always evident on the ECG. The location of the accessory pathway, the intra-atrial conduction time, and the times required to traverse the AV node–His bundle branch pathway (James fibers) and the accessory pathway determine the configuration of the electrocardiogram in the Wolff-Parkinson-White syndrome. (From Tilley 1992, *Essentials of Canine and Feline Electrocardiography*, 3d ed., Lea & Febiger, Philadelphia.)

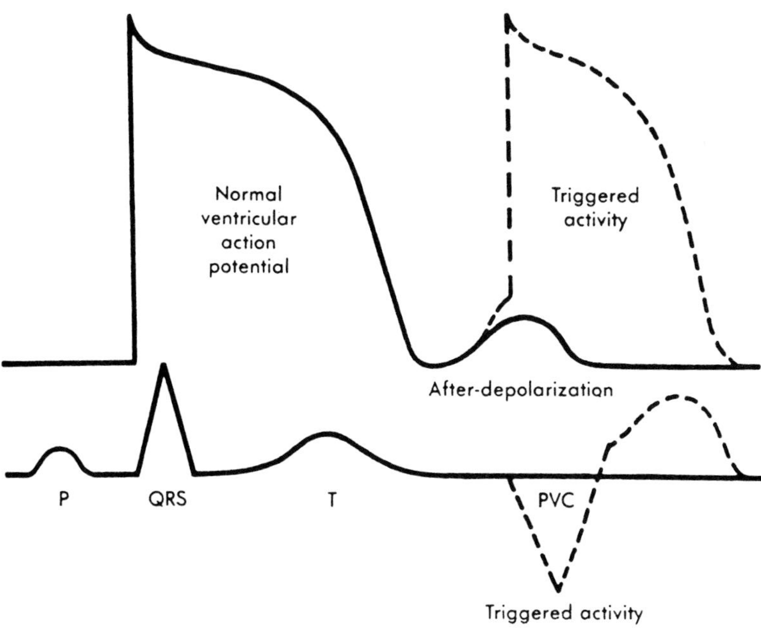

Figure 7.38. Myocardial action potential and delayed afterdepolarization as it relates to the surface ECG. Dashed lines represent the sequence of events that result when an afterdepolarization reaches threshold potential. (From Conover 1988, *Understanding Electrocardiography*, 5th ed., C.V. Mosby, St. Louis.)

Supraventricular arrhythmias

The term *supraventricular impulse* or *rhythm* was initially applied to any cardiac excitation arising "above" the ventricles in any part of the atria, atrioventricular junction, or sinoatrial node or even within the bundle of His before its bifurcation into the bundle branches. Essentially, it was used to describe arrhythmias that were not of ventricular origin although the precise location of their origin could not be established.

Electrophysiological studies have now shown that many rapid supraventricular rhythms are the result of closed anatomical conduction circuits involving such structures as the sinoatrial node, the atrioventricular (AV) node, and the AV nodal bypass tracts. Thus the term *supraventricular tachycardia* now means a tachycardia that requires participation of tissues above the bifurcation of the bundle of His. In some types part of a reentrant loop may traverse ventricular muscle. The basic mechanisms vary and include abnormal automaticity, triggered rhythms, and reentry via the aforementioned closed circuits. If the anatomical site of the supraventricular pacemaker is clear from the electrocardiographic criteria, then terms designating the anatomical site are used (e.g., *sinus rhythm* when the sinoatrial node is the pacemaker site, *atrial rhythm* when an ectopic location in the atria can be implicated from changes in P-wave morphology, and *AV junctional rhythms* when the pacemaker appears to be located in or around the atrioventricular node). Further details are given under "Abnormal Cardiac Rhythms". The pause after an atrial premature complex (APC) is often a noncompensatory (less than compensatory) R wave before and after the R wave of the APC. It is equal to two normal R-R intervals due to premature depolarization and resetting of the sinus node. Although the QRS complex is usually normal, an early APC may find the ventricular conduction system, especially the right bundle branch, in a refractory period and result in an abnormally shaped QRS complex (aberrant ventricular conduction). The aberrant QRS complex is often confused with a ventricular premature complex (VPC), and the aberrant APCs are repetitive and can be confused with ventricular tachycardia.

Ventricular arrhythmias

Ventricular arrhythmias are characterized by ectopic impulses that originate from a focus below the bifurcation of the bundle of His. If the ectopic impulse is in the AV node, the AV junction, or the bundle of His, spread of excitation in the ventricles is normal and the QRST complexes are normal. Ectopic impulses below these structures result in QRS complexes that are wide and bizarre, as ventricular conduction occurs mostly from cell to cell rather than through the conduction system. The P waves are not related to the wide and bizarre QRS complexes.

Normal cardiac rhythms

1. Sinus rhythm. The rhythm is regular; there is a normal P wave for each QRS complex with a consistent PR interval. A rapid sinus rhythm (the rate depends on the species) is termed sinus tachycardia, and a slow sinus rhythm (again the rate depends on the species) is referred to as sinus bradycardia. The parasympathetic and sympathetic divisions of the autonomic nervous system often determine whether there is a sinus bradycardia or sinus tachycardia.

2. Sinus arrhythmia (Fig. 7.39). The rhythm is irregular

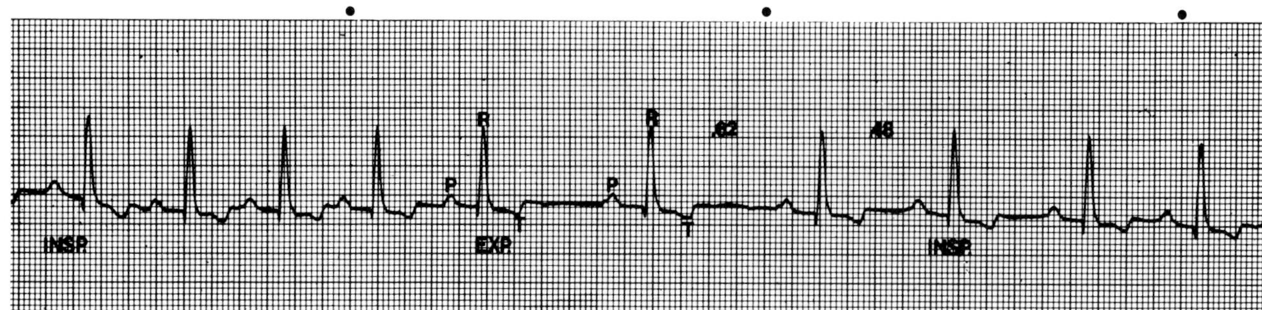

Figure 7.39. Respiratory sinus arrhythmia with an average rate of 120 beats per minute. The R-R intervals vary more than 0.12 second as the rate changes with inspiration (INSP) and expiration (EXP). (From Tilley 1992, *Essentials of Canine and Feline Electrocardiography*, 3d ed., Lea & Febiger, Philadelphia.)

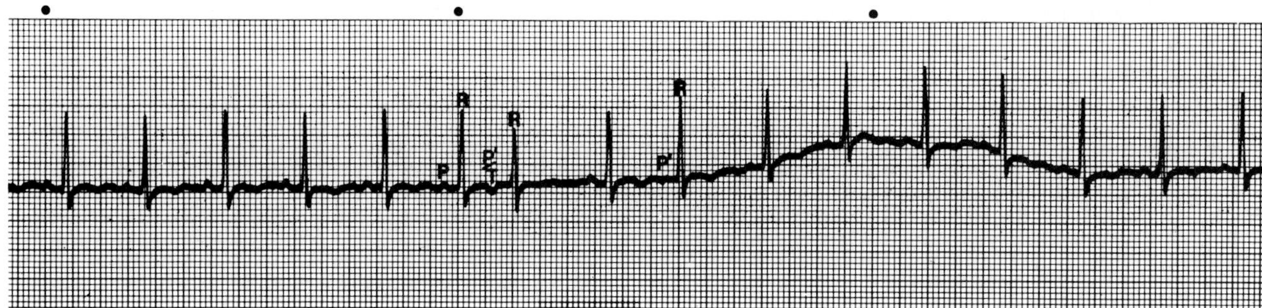

Figure 7.40. Two APCs, the seventh and ninth complexes, in a 15-year-old cat with chronic mitral insufficiency. The premature P waves vary in configuration and are superimposed on the T waves of the preceding QRS complexes. The pause after each APC is noncompensatory. (From Tilley 1992, *Essentials of Canine and Feline Electrocardiography*, 3d ed., Lea & Febiger, Philadelphia.)

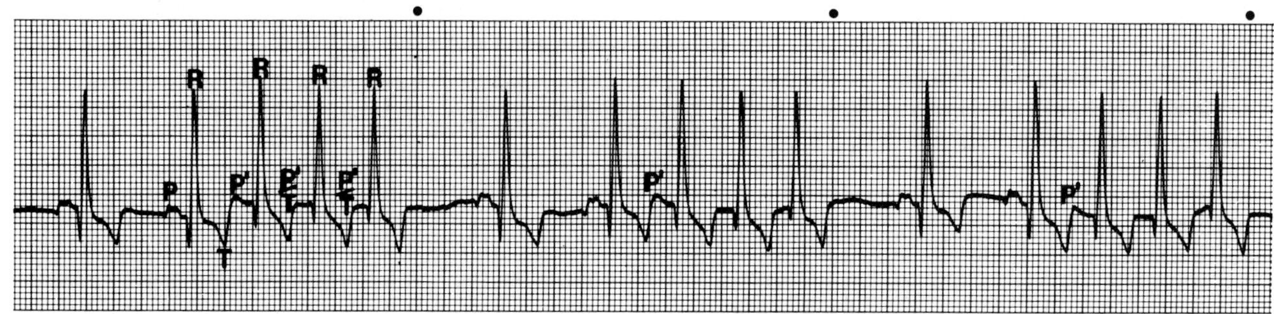

Figure 7.41. Paroxysms of atrial tachycardia in a dog with severe left atrial enlargement from mitral valvular insufficiency. A hint of a P′ wave can be seen in the previous T wave at the start of each brief period of tachycardia. The other premature P′ waves (*P′/T*) are hidden in the previous T waves. (From Tilley 1992, *Essentials of Canine and Feline Electrocardiography*, 3d ed., Lea & Febiger, Philadelphia.)

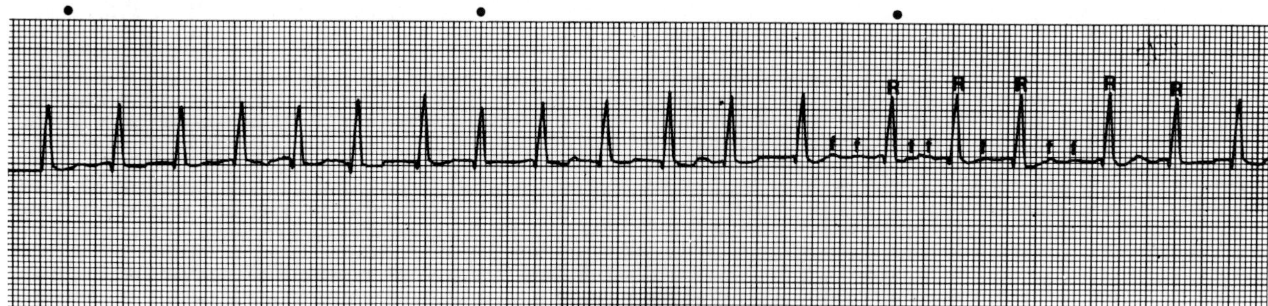

Figure 7.42. Atrial fibrillation with an average ventricular rate of 240 to 260 beats per minute. The ventricular rhythm is markedly irregular. The QRS complexes vary in amplitude, since numerous supraventricular impulses arrive when only part of the ventricle is completely recovered. (From Tilley 1992, *Essentials of Canine and Feline Electrocardiography*, 3d ed., Lea & Febiger, Philadelphia.)

with greater than a 10 percent variation in the P-P interval; there is a normal P wave for each QRS complex with a relatively constant P-R interval. Sinus arrhythmia is associated with the varying levels of parasympathetic (vagal) tone that influences the sinus node during the respiratory cycle. A wandering pacemaker (P waves vary in shape) caused by changes in intra-atrial conduction or pacemaker location often occurs with sinus arrhythmia.

3. There are two types of sinus arrhythmia—respiratory and nonrespiratory—and their presence or absence varies with species. The P-wave modification is characteristic of dogs but not necessarily of other species.

Abnormal cardiac rhythms

A. Supraventricular

1. Atrial premature complexes (APCs) (Fig. 7.40). The rhythm is irregular; there is usually an abnormal P′ wave (premature P wave) followed by a normally shaped QRS complex; the P′ wave may have various forms or may be fused with the T wave of the preceding beat.

2. Atrial tachycardia (Fig. 7.41). The impulses originate from an atrial site other than the sinus node; the rate is rapid; the rhythm is usually regular; there is a P′ wave for each QRS complex although the P wave may not be visualized; the P′ wave may be fused with the T wave or occur simultaneously with the preceding QRS complex. The QRS complex may also be of a different shape as a result of aberrant ventricular conduction.

3. Atrial fibrillation (Fig. 7.42). Atrial fibrillation is due to a large number of disorganized atrial impulses bombarding the AV node; many of these impulses find the AV node in a refractory period and are not conducted to the ventricles; the ventricular rate is usually rapid, although in the resting horse it is slow; the rhythm is irregular and is correlated with an arterial pulse deficit. No P waves are seen with atrial fibrillation, and the QRS complexes are of normal shape. Instead of P waves, small or large oscillations (f waves) are often seen. There may be variation with a widening of the QRS complexes because of aberrant ventricular conduction or concurrent enlargement.

4. AV junctional rhythm (Fig. 7.43). Impulses are generated in the AV junctional tissue and spread backward (retrograde) through the atrium and forward (antegrade) through the ventricles. The heart rate is variable, and the rhythm is usually regular; the negative P′ waves may occur before, during, or after the normal QRS complex, depending on the relative speed of retrograde conduction through the atrium compared with the speed of antegrade conduction through the AV node, the bundle of His, and the ventricular conduction system.

B. Ventricular

1. Ventricular premature complexes (Fig. 7.44A). Ectopic impulses are generated from a focus below the AV node and AV junction; the heart rate is variable, and the heart rhythm is irregular. Usually a full compensatory pause follows the VPCs, as the ectopic beat does not usually conduct back to the atrium and affect the spontaneous sinus node rate. The P waves that are seen are normal in shape and are not associated with the QRS complex of the VPCs. The QRS complex is often wide and bizarre because of an abnormal conduction pathway through the ventricles.

2. Ventricular tachycardia (Fig. 7.44B). Impulses repetitively (more than three VPCs in a row) originate from one or more ventricular foci and may be paroxysmal or sustained. The heart rate is rapid (depending on the species), and the rhythm is regular unless the arrhythmia is paroxysmal. The P waves that are seen are normal in shape but have no fixed relationship to the usually wide and bizarre QRS complexes.

Conduction Disturbances

1. First-degree AV block (Fig. 7.45). The cardiac impulse is delayed in the region of the AV node or the AV junction; the heart rate is variable, and the heart rhythm is regular or irregular with sinus arrhythmia. The ECG shows a prolonged, constant P-R interval.

2. Second-degree AV block (Fig. 7.46). The cardiac impulse is delayed or intermittently blocked in the region of the AV node or the AV junction; the heart rate is variable, and the heart rhythm is usually irregular. First-degree AV block shows a prolonged, constant P-R interval, and second-degree AV block has a normal P wave and QRS complex with intermittent P waves that are not followed by QRS complexes. The P-R interval either gradually prolongs or shortens (Mobitz type I or Wenckebach AV block) or has a consistent P-R interval (Mobitz type II AV block) prior to a dropped ventricular beat. Mobitz type I second-degree AV block is considered a normal rhythm in the resting horse.

3. Complete (third-degree) AV block (Fig. 7.47). The cardiac impulse is completely blocked in the region of the AV junction, the bundle of His or both. The atrial rate (P-P interval) is within normal limits, and there is a slow idioventricular escape rhythm. The rhythm is usually regular, the P wave is completely dissociated from the QRS complex, and the shape of the QRS complex varies, depending on the location of the ventricular escape pacemaker.

4. Atrial standstill. Impulses are generated in the sinus node but are not conducted through the atrial myocardial tissues, so no P waves are seen. The heart rate is slow, and the rhythm is regular; the QRS complexes are normal or bizarre, depending on the intraventricular conduction. Atrial standstill is a life-threatening abnormality that is usually associated with hyperkalemia, although it is also seen with a muscular dystrophy disorder that has been reported in English Springer Spaniel dogs and in some cats with severe heart disease.

5. Bundle branch block. The most common forms of intraventricular conduction disturbance are right (Figs. 7.48 and 7.49) and left bundle branch block (Figs. 7.50 and 7.51). These abnormalities exist when the cardiac impulse is blocked in the right bundle or the common left bundle,

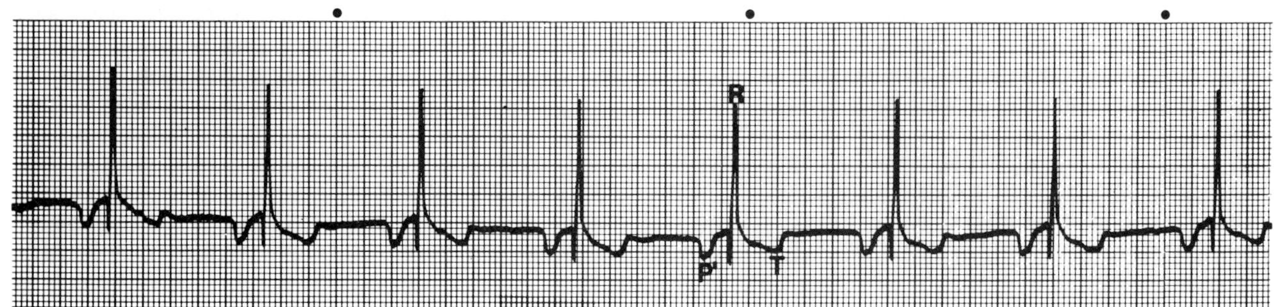

Figure 7.43. AV junctional tachycardia at a rate of 100 beats per minute in a dog with digitalis toxicity. (From Tilley 1992, *Essentials of Canine and Feline Electrocardiography*, 3d ed., Lea & Febiger, Philadelphia.)

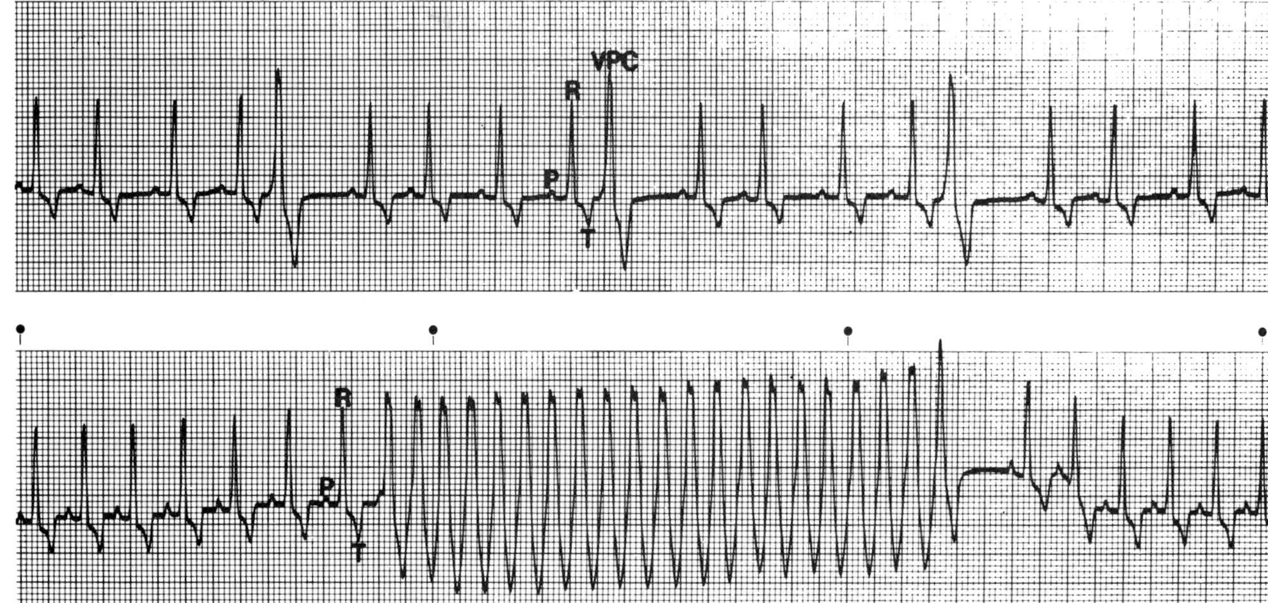

Figure 7.44. Two separate strips, made 1 hour apart, from ECGs of a dog with episodes of fainting. The upper strip reveals VPCs that represent the R-on-T phenomenon. The R wave of the VPC is near the peak of the preceding T wave, the vulnerable period. VPC during the vulnerable period may result in ventricular tachycardia (as observed later on the lower strip) or ventricular fibrillation. Paper speed, 25 mm/s. (From Tilley 1992, *Essentials of Canine and Feline Electrocardiography*, 3d ed., Lea & Febiger, Philadelphia.)

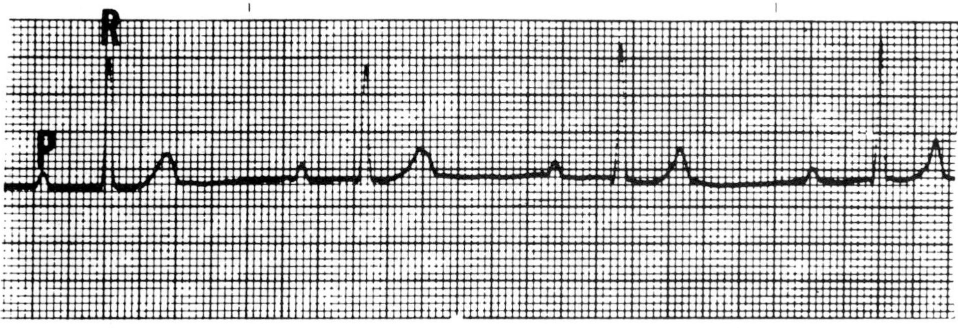

Figure 7.45. Tracing from a dog with digitalis toxicity. First-degree atrioventricular heart block is present because the P-R interval exceeds 0.13 second. In this case, it measures 0.18 second. (From Edwards 1987, *Bolton's Handbook of Canine and Feline Electrocardiography*, 2d ed., W.B. Saunders, Philadelphia.)

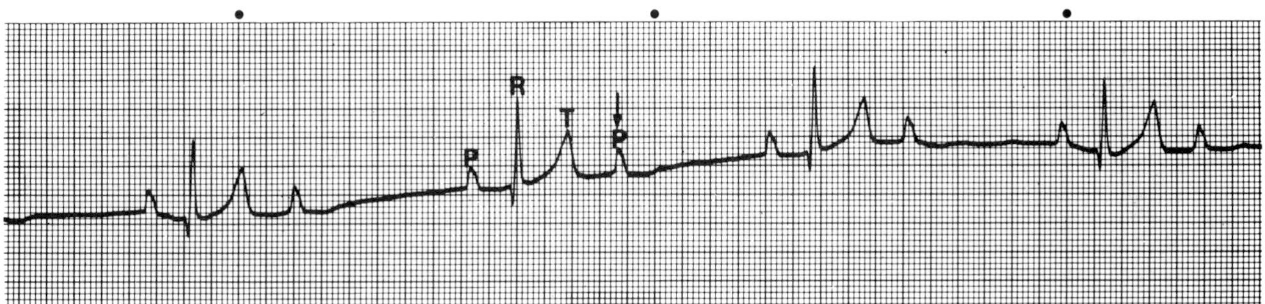

Figure 7.46. Second-degree 2:1 AV block (arrow) as well as first-degree AV block (PR interval 0.15 second). In most cases of advanced second-degree AV block with a 2:1 ratio, a distinctive pattern of the P-P interval often exists. The P-P interval that includes a QRS complex is shorter in duration than the P-P interval that does not contain a QRS complex. One explanation is that the shorter P-P cycle is associated with improved coronary perfusion subsequent to ventricular systole. The sinus node responds to the increased perfusion by a more rapid discharge. Another explanation is a baroreceptor response in association with a reduction of vagal tone in response to ventricular systole. (From Tilley 1992, *Essentials of Canine and Feline Electrocardiography* 3d ed., Lea & Febiger, Philadelphia.)

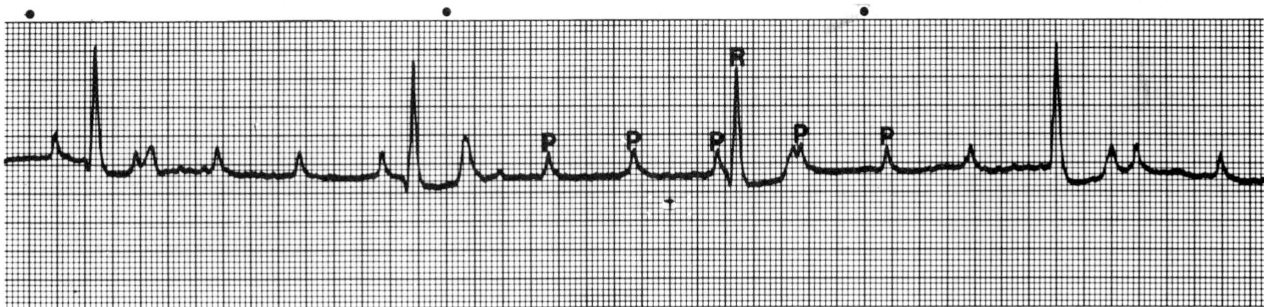

Figure 7.47. Complete heart block in a dog with congenital AV block. The P waves occur regularly at a rate of 200/min, totally independent of the ventricular rate of 50. Because the QRS complex is of normal configuration, the ventricular pacemaker is probably above the bifurcation of the bundle of His. (From Tilley 1992, *Essentials of Canine and Feline Electrocardiography*, 3d ed., Lea & Febiger, Philadelphia.)

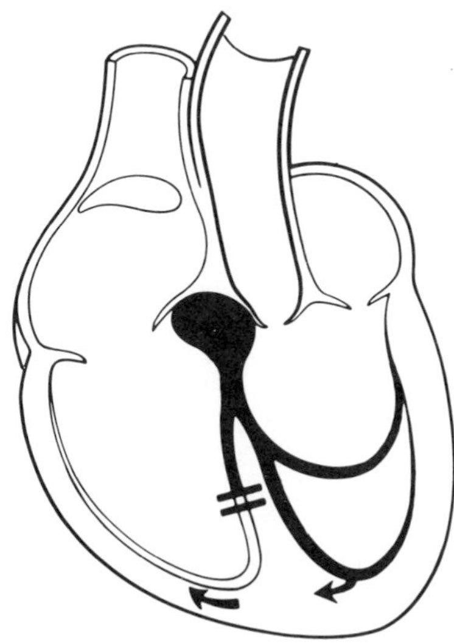

Figure 7.48. Right bundle branch block. The right ventricle is stimulated by the impulse, which passes from the left bundle branch to the right side of the septum below the block. It is then activated with delay, causing the QRS complex to become wide and bizarre. (From Phillips and Feeney 1980, *The Cardiac Rhythms*, W.B. Saunders, Philadelphia.)

respectively, and is conducted via the intact bundle branch so that the ventricle with the blocked bundle branch is activated later than the ventricle with the intact bundle branch by myocyte-to-myocyte conduction. A prolonged QRS complex interval is the key to recognition of bundle branch block. Right bundle branch block is recognized by a prolongation of the QRS complex interval, a relatively consistent P-R interval, and a right axis deviation due to deep and wide S waves in leads I, II, and aVF and the left precordial chest leads. Left bundle branch block is recognized by a normal or leftward axis orientation, a prolongation of the QRS complex interval, a relatively consistent P-R interval, absence of septal Q waves, or deep S waves in lead I, lead II or lead aVF.

CLINICAL APPLICATION OF ELECTROCARDIOGRAPHY

The ECG is useful clinically as a noninvasive method of evaluating cardiac electrical function (Table 7.9). When recorded from the body surface, the electrical signals generated by the heart give information on pacemaker location and on the rate and course of depolarization throughout the heart. Through laboratory investigation, the electrocar-

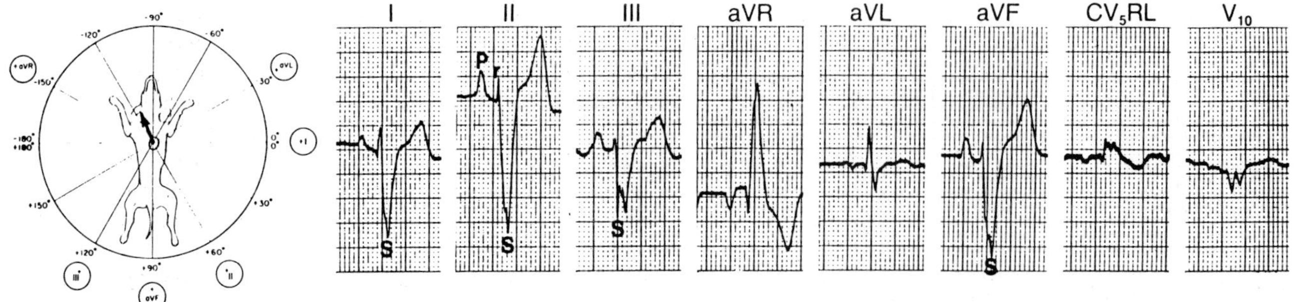

Figure 7.49. Right bundle branch block in a dog. The QRS duration is 0.09 second (4½ boxes). There are large, wide S waves in leads I, II, III, and aVF. The QRS in CV_5RL has a wide rsR′ pattern (M-shaped). A w pattern is seen in lead V_{10}. There is a right axis deviation (−110 degrees). (From Tilley 1992, *Essentials of Canine and Feline Electrocardiography,* 3d ed., Lea & Febiger, Philadelphia.)

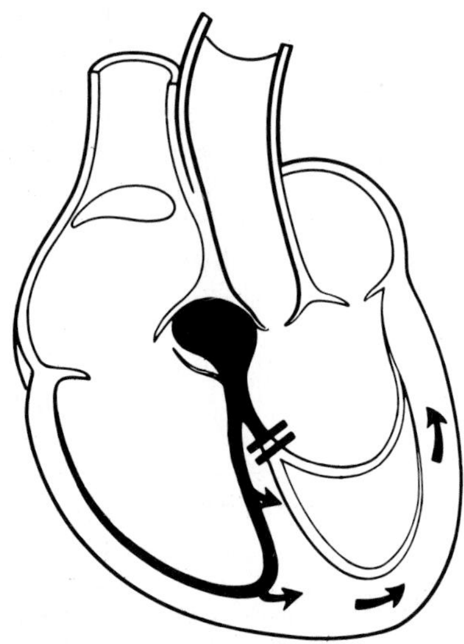

Figure 7.50. Left bundle branch block in the main left bundle branch. Block can also occur at the level of the anterior and posterior fascicles. The impulse cannot enter the left bundle system and activate the left septal fibers. Therefore, the septum is initially depolarized from fibers arising from the distal portion of the right bundle branch, resulting in an initial vector oriented to the left. The left ventricle is then activated late, causing the QRS complex to become wide and bizarre. (From Phillips and Feeney 1980, *The Cardiac Rhythm*, W.B. Saunders, Philadelphia.)

diographic events have been correlated with experimentally induced changes in action potentials, pacemaker location, and conduction disturbances. These correlations, in turn, have been related to clinical and necropsy observations to provide an empirical basis for diagnosis of cardiac conditions, such as enlargement of individual ventricles (Fig. 7.52), specific conduction-system blocks, myocardial infarction, pulmonary thromboembolus (blood clot blocking a pulmonary artery) (Fig. 7.53), and electrolyte disturbances, such as hyperkalemia, drug effects, and cardiotoxicity. The ECG is the established means of recording and analyzing the heart's electrical activity. The primary use for the ECG is to recognize clinically significant disorders of the heartbeat (arrhythmias) that result in congestive heart failure, dyspnea, weakness, syncope, and sudden death. The ECG is sensitive and specific for the recognition of cardiac arrhythmias. No other diagnostic tool, including auscultation, radiography, and ultrasonography (echocardiography), can be substituted for this purpose. All of the commonly diagnosed rhythm abnormalities, including atrial premature complexes, atrial tachycardia, atrial fibrillation, ventricular premature complexes, ventricular tachycardia, and the various degrees of AV block, have been defined and verified by means of the surface elec-

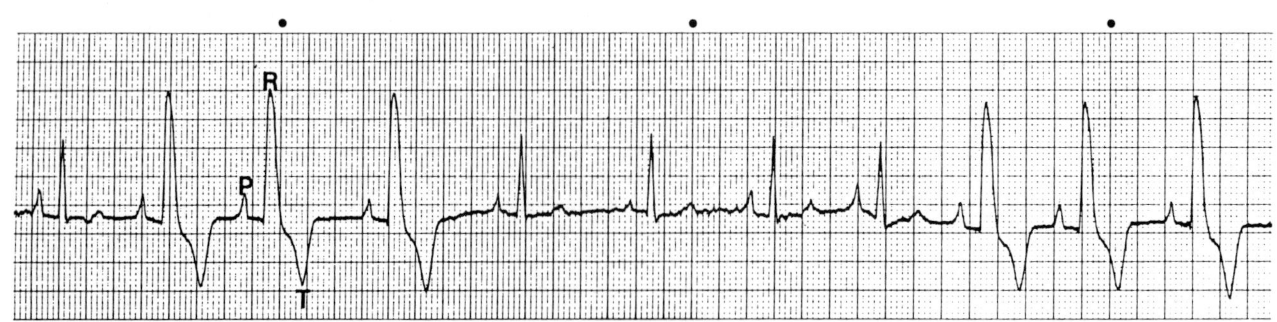

Figure 7.51. Intermittent left bundle branch block in a Chihuahua. The QRS complexes are wider (0.07 to 0.08 second) in the second, third, and fourth complexes and in the last three complexes. The consistent P-R interval of these complexes supports left bundle branch block rather than ventricular premature complexes. (From Tilley 1992, *Essentials of Canine and Feline Electrocardiography*, 3d ed., Lea & Febiger, Philadelphia.)

Table 7.9. Clinical indications for electrocardiography

Arrhythmias
Cardiac monitoring (anesthesia; critical care)
Pacemaker dysfunction
Heart chamber enlargement
Drug effects or toxicities
Myocardial disease
Congenital heart disease
Acquired valvular heart disease
Pericardial disease
Heart failure
Endocrine disorders (e.g., thyrotoxicosis)
Electrolyte imbalance (potassium, calcium)
Acid-base abnormalities
Shock
Dyspnea
Syncope or seizures
Heart murmurs
Gallop rhythms
Cyanosis
Geriatric or presurgical work-up
Systemic diseases

trocardiogram. An accurate diagnosis of arrythmia is essential before antiarrhythmic therapy, as many drugs may cause or worsen arrhythmias (proarrhythmia) with clinical deterioration rather than improvement.

The ECG also has numerous other applications, including detection of heart chamber enlargement and myocardial infarction (primarily in humans), and it is useful as an aid in detecting other medical problems, such as endocrinopathies (e.g., Addison's disease, hypothyroidism, and hyperthyroidism) and electrolyte disorders (e.g., hyperkalemia, hypocalcemia), and it may be useful in stimulating a further medical workup in an animal with nonspecific signs of illness and S-T segment or T-wave changes on the ECG. Changes in the S-T segment or T wave do not have the same sensitivity or specificity as when an ECG is used for detection of cardiac arrhythmias.

The essentials of electrocardiography include assessment of heart rate and heart rhythm and analysis of P-QRS-T complexes. The ECG reflects only the electrical potential of the heart, and it may be impossible to identify the actual cause of an ECG abnormality. Therefore a thorough physical examination, a thoracic radiograph, a laboratory blood profile, and, when applicable, an echocardiogram remain essential to a complete diagnosis. Recognizable ECG changes such as S-T segment shifts and T-wave changes are important, even though these changes are nonspecific and may have numerous causes.

The occurrence of arrhythmias is influenced by a combination of the transmembrane potentials of the individual cardiac muscle cells, the autonomic nervous system, and the electrolytes in the fluid of the pericardial sac. A disorder or dyssynergy in any of these components may account for arrhythmias.

Histopathologic findings of cardiac inflammation, fibrosis, or neoplasia do not correlate with cellular electrochemical changes or ECG abnormalities. Conversely, a heart that is normal radiographically and histopathologically may develop life-threatening arrhythmias after such clinical syndromes as gastrodilatation shock, ischemia, or cardiac arrest.

The following list gives selected clinical applications of cardiac electrophysiology:

1. The millions of cardiac cells relate to each other electrically as dipoles (areas of plus and minus charges) and create a changing electrical field that surrounds the heart. When electrode clips are attached to the limbs and these electrodes are connected to a galvanometer (electrocardiograph), this changing electric field is displayed on moving ECG graph paper as P-QRS-T complexes. The electrocardiograph combines the electrodes into specific combinations (leads), which sample electrical activity of the heart from different angles or aspects of the body. A complete ECG includes multiple leads, although the lead II rhythm strip is used for rhythm analysis.

2. The characteristics of the heart are essentially similar in all domestic mammals. The chief differences among species are in cardiac size, extent of penetration of the ven-

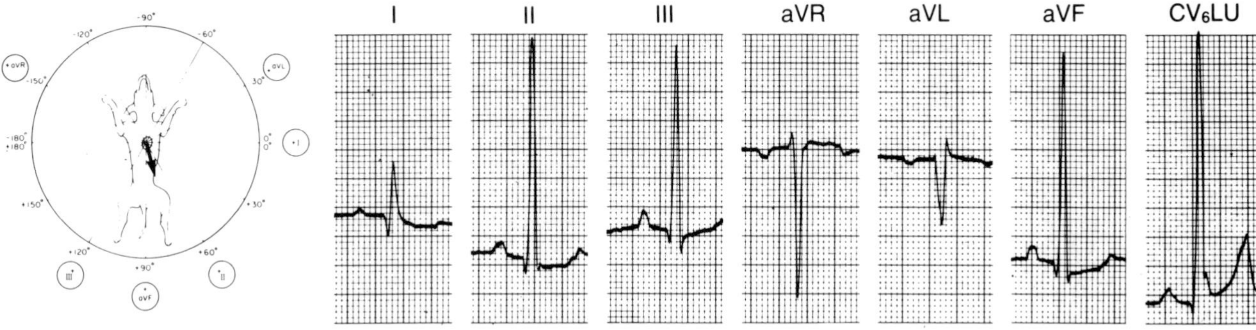

Figure 7.52. Left ventricular enlargement in an 8-year-old poodle with mitral valvular insufficiency. There are tall R waves in leads II, III, aVF, and CV_6LU. The QRS duration is wide (0.06 second, or 3 boxes). The electrical axis is normal (+75 degrees). (From Tilley 1992, *Essentials of Canine and Feline Electrocardiography*, 3d ed., Lea & Febiger, Philadelphia.)

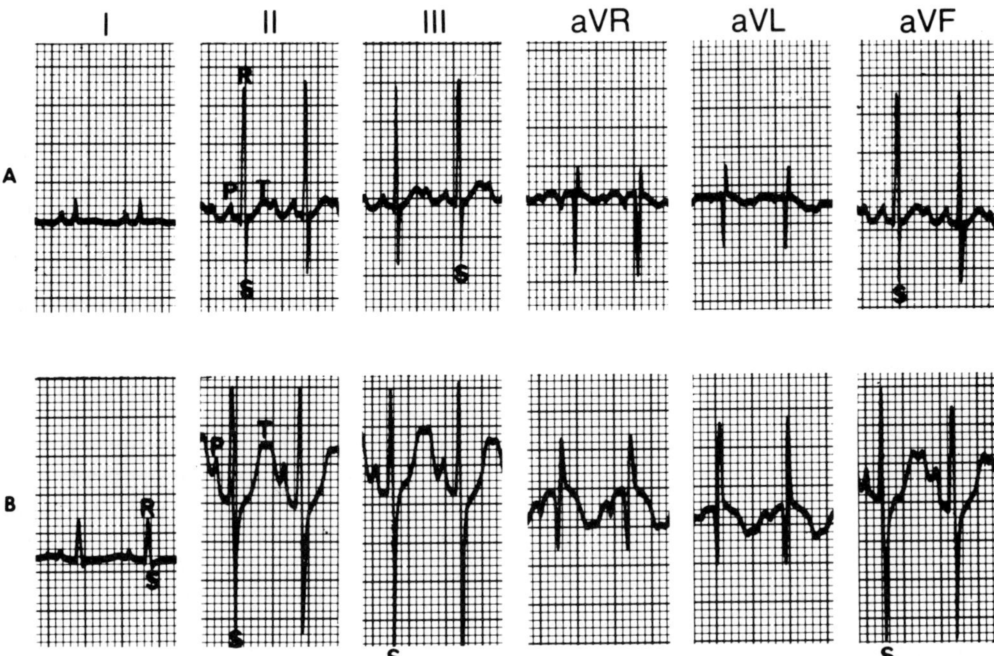

Figure 7.53. Acute cor pulmonale in a dog with heartworm disease. Paper speed, 25 mm/s. (*A*) Before chemotherapy for the adult heartworms. Right ventricular enlargement is present (large S waves in leads II, III, and aVF). The mean electrical axis is +75 degrees. (*B*) Three days after chemotherapy coughing was present as a result of pulmonary embolism. The sudden pulmonary hypertension results in right ventricular dilatation. An S wave has formed in lead I, and S waves are now larger in leads II, III, and aVF. Note also the increased height of the P waves and the T waves. The electrical axis is markedly deviated. (From Tilley 1992, *Essentials of Canine and Feline Electrocardiography*, 3d ed., Lea & Febiger, Philadelphia.)

tricular Purkinje network into the ventricular myocardium, and duration of ventricular action potentials.

3. The heart is especially vulnerable to changes in serum Ca^{2+} and K^+ concentration because of their profound effects on the action potential and excitation-contraction coupling. The negative inotropic effects that lead to acute cardiac failure of hypocalcemia or hyperkalemia are well-known clinical examples. Severe electrolyte disorders, acid-base disturbances, or metabolic diseases will affect the electrochemical gradients of the myocardial cells and result in an abnormal ECG.

4. Arrhythmias caused by conduction disturbances occur normally in some species. These include second-degree AV block in horses (common) and dogs (rare, except in telemetry records from undisturbed animals) and right bundle branch block in dogs (rare except in some purebred animals).

5. Respiratory sinus arrhythmia is the normal rhythm in resting dogs.

6. The AV node, because of its refractoriness, acts as an impulse filter to protect the ventricles from excessive rates when atrial tachyarrhythmias occur. It prevents atrial fibrillation from consistently spreading to the ventricles and causing them to beat at too rapid a rate.

7. Atrial fibrillation is more likely to occur in animals with larger atria (greater number of cells) and higher vagal tone. Horses and cattle are the most vulnerable of all domestic species, and large breeds of dogs are more susceptible than small breeds.

8. Electrical shock is likely to cause death by induction of ventricular fibrillation. An electric shock during the vulnerable period of the ECG (near the peak of the T wave) is dangerous, as fiber depolarization heterogeneity (many cardiac muscle cells are depolarized while others are in different stages of repolarization) causes the heart to be more susceptible to ventricular fibrillation. Electric shock (cardioversion) to terminate ventricular arrhythmias requires the electrical impulse to be triggered by the R wave of the ECG so as to avoid the vulnerable period for ventricular fibrillation.

9. Multiple ECG leads are required for recognition of such conditions as specific T-wave changes (e.g., in leads V_{10} or CV_6RL in dogs) and for diagnosis of bundle branch blocks, right ventricular hypertrophy, localized myocardial infarcts, and cardiomyopathies.

10. The ECG should be a consistent part of the cardiac data base as a way to recognize clinically significant arrhythmias, conduction disorders, cardiac enlargement patterns, and systemic disorders and as an aid in individualizing therapy in animals with cardiac disease.

11. The electrocardiogram recorded from the body surface reveals only the electrical activity on the atrial and

ventricular myocardial cells but does not provide direct information on the conduction system (e.g., AV node, bundle of His, and Purkinje system during the P-R interval of the ECG). Small electrodes positioned on the inner (endocardial) or outer (epicardial) surface of the heart record electrical activity, and the resulting graph is called a cardiac electrogram. When depolarization of the bundle of His is visible on the electrogram recording, it is termed a His bundle electrogram (Fig. 7.54). The His bundle electrogram is useful for measuring conduction time between atrial depolarization and His bundle depolarization and between His bundle depolarization and ventricular depolarization. These measurements "fine tune" our ability to determine whether AV block occurs above or below the bundle of His and clinically aids us in determining which animals with conduction disorders and a slow heart rate will respond to drug therapy or will require a permanent cardiac pacemaker. Electrograms are also useful in diagnosis of complex arrhythmias with rapid heart rates where the P-waves can be fused with the preceding T waves.

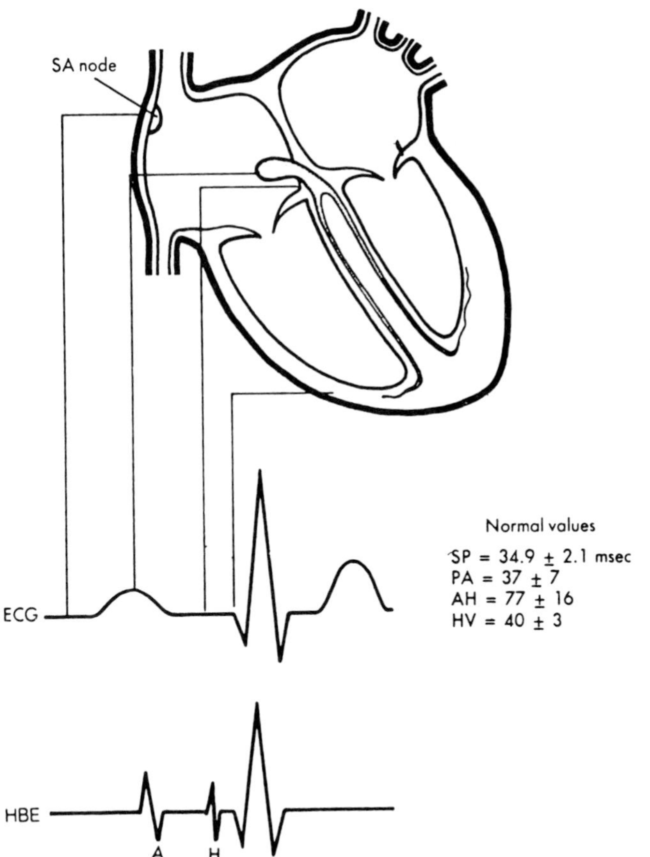

Figure 7.54. His bundle electrogram (HBE) recorded from the inner (endocardial) surface of the heart by means of an electrode attached to the tip of an intravascular catheter (tube) positioned within the heart. A, Atrial electrogram; H, His bundle electrogram; V, ventricular electrogram. Approximate relationship of the electrograms is also temporally related to surface ECG. (From Marriot and Conover 1989, *Advanced Concepts in Arrhythmias*, 2d ed., C.V. Mosby, St. Louis.)

REFERENCES

Akera, T. and Brody, T.M. 1989. Pharmacology of cardiac glycosides. In, N. Sperelakis, ed. *Physiology and Pathophysiology of the Heart*. 2d ed. Kluwer Acad. Publ., Boston. Pp. 453–69.

Bayley, R.H., Ashman, R., And Byer, E. 1943. The normal human ventricular gradient. I. Factors which affect its direction and its relation to the mean QRS axis, with an appendix on notation by R.H. Bayley. *Am. Heart J.* 25:16–35.

Baumgarten, C.M., and Fozzard, H.A. 1986. The resting and pacemaker potentials. In H.A. Fozzard et al., eds. *The Heart and Cardiovascular System*, vol. 1. Raven Press, New York. Pp. 601–26.

Bellet, S. 1972. *Essentials of Cardiac Arrhythmias*. W.B. Saunders, Philadelphia.

Bishop, S.P., and Cole, C.R. 1967. Morphology of the specialized conducting tissue in the atria of the equine heart. *Anat. Rec.* 158:401–15.

Burch, G.E., and Winsor, T. 1966. *A Primer of Electrocardiography*. Lea & Febiger, Philadelphia.

Carmeliet, E., and Vereecke, J. 1979. Electrogenesis of the action potential and automaticity. In R.M. Berne, N. Sperelakis, and S.R. Geiger, eds., *Handbook of Physiology*. Sec. 2, The Cardiovascular System. Vol. 1, *The Heart*. Am. Physiol. Soc., Bethesda, Md. Pp. 177–87.

Coraboeuf, E., Deroubaix, E., and Hoerter, J. 1976. Control of ionic permeabilities in normal and ischemic heart. *Circ. Res.* 38 (Suppl.): 1–92.

Cranefield, P.F. 1975. *The Conduction of the Cardiac Impulse*. Futura, Mt. Kisco, N.Y.

Detweiler, D.K. 1981. The use of electrocardiography in toxicological studies with rats. In R. Budden, D.K. Detweiler, and G. Zbinden, eds., *The Rat Electrocardiogram in Pharmacology and Toxicology*. Pergamon, Oxford. Pp. 83–115.

Detweiler, D.K., Buchanan, J.W., Fregin, G.F., and Hill, J.D. 1970. Heart. In A.C. Anderson, ed., *The Beagle as an Experimental Dog*. Iowa State University Press, Ames. Pp. 232–45.

Einthoven, W., Fahr, G., and de Waart, A. 1913. Über die Richtung and die manifeste Grosse der Potentialschwankungen im menschlichen Herzen und über den Einfluss der herzlage auf die Form des elektrokardiogrammes. *Pflugers Arch.* 150:275–315.

Ettinger, S.J., and Suter, P.F. 1970. *Canine Cardiology*. W.B. Saunders, Philadelphia. Pp. 158–68.

Fish, C. 1988. Electrocardiography and vectorcardiography. In E. Braunwald, ed., *Heart Disease*. W.B. Saunders, Philadelphia. Pp. 180–222.

Fozzard, H.A. 1979. Conduction of the action potential. In R.M. Berne, N. Sperelakis, and S.R. Geiger, eds., *Handbook of Physiology*. Sec. 2, The Cardiovascular System. Vol. 1, *The Heart*. Am. Physiol. Soc., Bethesda, Md. Pp. 335–56.

Fozzard, H.A., and Gibbons, W.V. 1973. Action potential and contraction of heart muscle. *Am. J. Cardiol.* 31:182–92.

Golderberger, E. 1947. *Unipolar Lead Electrocardiography*. Lea & Febiger, Philadelphia.

Hamlin, R.L., and Smith, C.R. 1965. Categorization of common domestic mammals based on their ventricular activation process. *Ann. N.Y. Acad. Sci.* 127:195–203.

Herre, J.M., and Scheinman, M.M. 1989. Supraventricular tachycardia. In W.N. Parmley and K. Chatterjee, eds. *Cardiology*. Vol. 1. J.B. Lippincott, Philadelphia, Pp. 11–18.

Hill, J.D. 1968a. The electrocardiogram in dogs with standardized body and limb positions. *J. Electrocardiol.* 1:175–82.

Hill, J.D. 1968b. The significance of foreleg position in the interpretation of electrocardiograms and vectorcardiograms from research animals. *Am. Heart J.* 75:518–27.

Hodgkin, A.L., and Huxley, A.F. 1952. A quantitative description of membrane current and its application to conduction and excitation in nerve. *J. Physiol.* (Lond.) 117:500–44.

Hoffman, B.F., Cranefield, P.F., and Wallace, A.G. 1966. Physiologic basis of cardiac arrhythmias. *Mod. Concepts Cardiovasc. Dis.* 35: 103–8.

Holsinger, J.W., Jr., Wallace, A.G., Sealy, W.C. 1968. The identification and surgical significance of the atrial internodal conduction. *Ann. Surg.* 167:447–53.

Katz, A.M. 1977. *Physiology of the Heart*. Raven Press, New York.

Keith, A., and Flack, M.W. 1907. The form and nature of the muscular connections between the primary divisions of the vertebrate heart. *J. Anat. Physiol.* 51:172–89.

Kishida, H., Cole, J.S., and Surawicz, B. 1982. Negative U wave: A highly specific but poorly understood sign of heart disease. *Am. J. Cardiol.* 49:2030–36.

Ling, G., and Gerard, R.W. 1949. The normal membrane potential of frog sartorious fibers. *J. Cell. Comp. Physiol.* 34:383–96.

Marriot, H.J.L., Conover, M.B. 1989. *Advanced Concepts in Arrhythmias*. C.V. Mosby, St. Louis.

Miller, M.S. 1985. Treatment of arrhythmias and conduction disturbances. In L.P. Tilley and J.M. Owends, eds., *Manual of Small Animal Cardiology.* Churchill Livingstone, New York. Pp. 333–86.

Miller, M.S. 1986. Electrocardiography. In G. Harrison and L. Harrison, eds., *Avian Medicine and Surgery*. W.B. Saunders, Philadelphia. Pp. 286–92.

Miller, M.S. 1988. Equine electrocardiography: Usage in clinical practice. In Proceedings of the American Association of Equine Practitioners. Annual meeting, San Diego. Pp. 577–586.

Miller, M.S., and Tilley, L.P. 1988. Electrocardiography. In P.R. Fox, ed., *Canine and Feline Cardiology*. Churchill Livingstone, New York. Pp. 43–89.

Myerburg, R.J. 1971. The gating mechanism in the distal AV conducting system. *Circulation* 43:955–60.

Myerburg, R.J., Stewart, J.W., and Hoffman, B.F. 1970. Electrophysiological properties of the canine peripheral AV conduction system. *Circ. Res.* 26:361–78.

Pagel, B.E., and Trautvetter, E. 1989. Elektrokardiographische und Kardio- morphologische Veranderungen bei Katzen in den ersten 70 Lebenstagen. *Waltham Rep.* No. 29:13–25.

Scheidt, S. 1983. Basic electrocardiography: Leads, axes, arrhythmias. *CIBA's Clinical Symposia* 35:1–32.

Scher, A.M., and Spach, M.J. 1979. Cardiac depolarization and repolarization and the electrocardiogram. In R.M. Berne, N. Sperelakis, and S.R. Geiger, eds., *Handbook of Physiology*. Sec. 2, The Cardiovascular System. Vol. 1, *The Heart*. Am. Physiol. Soc., Bethesda, Md. Pp. 357–92.

Sommer, J.R., and Johnson, E.A. 1979. Ultrastructure of cardiac muscle. In R.M. Berne, N. Sperelakis, and S.R. Geiger, eds., *Handbook of Physiology*. Sec. 2, The Cardiovascular System. Vol. 1. *The Heart*. Am. Physiol. Soc., Bethesda, Md. Pp. 113–86.

Sperelakis, N. 1989. Basis of the resting potential. In N. Sperelakis, ed. *Physiology and Pathophysiology of the Heart*. 2d ed. Kluwer Acad. Publ., Boston, pp. 59–80.

TenEick, R.E., Baumgarten, C.M., and Singer, D.H. 1981. Ventricular dysrhythmia: Membrane basis of currents, channels, gates, and cables. *Prog. Cardiovasc. Dis*. 24:157–88.

Thorel, Ch. 1910. Über den Aufbau des Sinusknotens und seine Verbindung mit der cava superior und den Wenckenbachischen Bundeln. *Munchen Med. Wochenschr*. 57:183–86.

Tilley, L.P. 1992. *Essentials of Canine and Feline Electrocardiography*. 3d ed. Lea & Febiger, Philadelphia.

Trautwein, W. 1973. Membrane currents in cardiac fibers. *Physiol. Rev*. 53:793–835.

Truex, R.C. 1973. Anatomy of the specialized tissues of the heart. In L.S. Dreifus and W. Likoff, eds., *Cardiac Arrhythmias*. Grune & Stratton, New York. Pp. 1–12.

Tisen, R.W., and Siegelbaum, S. 1978. Excitable tissues: The heart. In T.E. Andreoli, J.F. Hoffman, and D.D. Fanestil, eds., *Physiology of Membrane Disorders*. Plenum, New York. Pp. 517–38.

Urthaler, F., Kawamura, K., and James, T.M. 1978. The anatomical basis for cardiac rhythm and conduction. In T.E. Andreoli, J.F. Hoffman, and D.D. Fanestil, eds., *Physiology of Membrane Disorders*. Plenum, New York. Pp. 831–75.

Van Dam, R.Th., and Janse, M.J. 1989. Activation of the heart. In P.W. Macfarlane and T.D.V. Lawrie, eds. *Comprehensive Electrocardiology*. Vol. 1. Pergamon Press, New York, 101–217.

Wenckebach, K.F. 1907. Beitrage zur Kenntnis der menschlicher Herztatigkeit. *Arch. Anat. Physiol.* 1–2:1–24.

Wilson, F.N. 1954. F.D. Johnston and E. Lepeschkin, eds., *Selected Papers*. Heart Station, University Hospital, Ann Arbor, Mich.

Wilson, F.N., Johnston, F.D., MacLeod, A.G., and Baker, P.S. 1934. Electrocardiograms that represent the potential variations of a single electrode. *Am. Heart J.* 9:447–58.

Zipes, D.P. 1988. Genesis of cardiac arrhythmias: electrophysiological considerations. In E. Braunwald, ed., *Heart Disease*. W.B. Saunders, Philadelphia. Pp. 581–620.

CHAPTER 8

Mechanical Activity of the Heart | by David K. Detweiler, Dean H. Riedesel, and David H. Knight

MUSCLE MECHANICS

Studying an isolated piece of cardiac muscle may help one understand the response of the whole heart to changes in blood pressure (afterload), return of venous blood (preload), and myocardial contractility (inotropic state). The concepts and techniques are those of A.V. Hill, which were developed to analyze skeletal muscle. Two types of muscle contraction are used: isometric (*iso,* constant or equal; *metric,* length) and isotonic (at constant force or load). The force of contraction and the velocity of shortening are measured under variable loading conditions of the isolated muscle. Force and velocity are inversely related; thus, with no load, force is negligible and velocity is maximal. At the other extreme, an isometric contraction is characterized by maximal force and zero velocity of contraction.

Three-component model of muscle

The original skeletal muscle model proposed by Hill (Fig. 8.1) consists of a contractile element (CE), a series elastic element (SE), and a parallel elastic element (PE). The elastic elements have no anatomical counterpart. The muscle functions as if the elastic elements existed as shown in the model. Since the PE has no role in muscle contraction, it will not be considered further in this discussion.

Figure 8.2 shows the arrangement employed for studying muscle mechanics in the isolated papillary muscle from the right ventricle of a cat. One end of the muscle is fixed to a tension or force transducer, the other end to a movable isotonic lever; thus both tension and movement can be recorded simultaneously.

Preload (Fig. 8.2) is the term given to the weight attached to stretch the muscle to its normal resting length and tension. The mechanical energy produced by the contraction of cardiac or skeletal muscle is a function of its sarcomere length just before contraction. Preload is the force required to stretch the muscle to its precontraction length. In the intact ventricle, preload is analogous to factors that

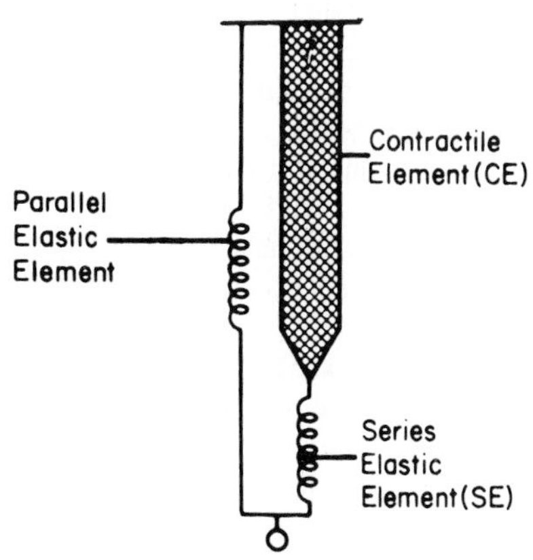

Figure 8.1. Three-component model for muscle proposed by A.V. Hill (1939). (Redrawn from Sonnenblick 1966, in Briller and Conn, eds., *The Myocardial Cell.* University of Pennsylvania Press, Philadelphia.)

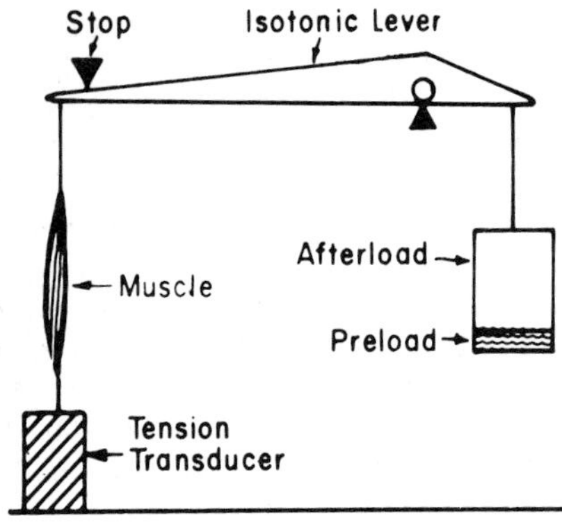

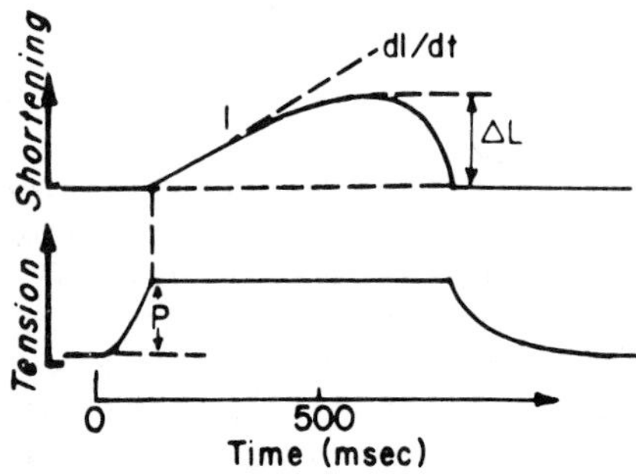

Figure 8.2. (*Top*) Arrangement for study of mechanics in isolated papillary muscle. (*Bottom*) Records of shortening and tension of afterloaded isotonic contraction. P, Afterload; *dl/dt*, initial shortening velocity; ΔL, change in length; I, isotonic. (Redrawn from Sonnenblick, Parmley, Urschel, and Brutsaert 1970, *Prog. Cardiovasc. Dis.* 12:449–66, by permission.)

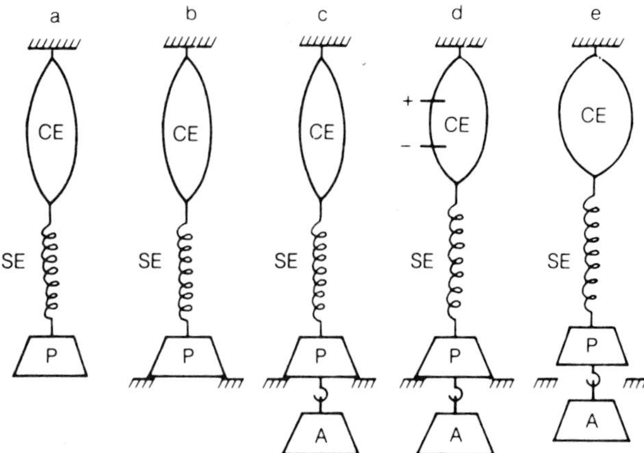

Figure 8.3. Schematic representation of an afterloaded isotonic contraction of a muscle. In (*a*) a preload (P) is attached to the muscle, which stretches the series elastic element (SE) to a certain degree. This creates a certain resting or initial length and tension in the muscle, depending on the magnitude of P. In (*b*) a stop or support is provided so that when an afterload (A) is added, as in (*c*), resting length or tension will not change. In (*d*) the muscle is stimulated electrically and the shortening of the contractile element (CE) will first stretch the series elastic element (SE) without causing external shortening of the muscle. In (*e*), the external length of the muscle shortens, lifting both the P and A. P + A is called the total load of the muscle. (Modified from Pollack, 1970, *Circ. Res.* 26:111–27.)

determine end-diastolic pressure. After the preload has been applied, a stop or support is placed (see Fig. 8.3) to prevent further stretching of the muscle. Additional weight then is added to the preload; in the system as diagrammed, this added weight, the *afterload,* has no effect on the muscle until it has been stimulated and begins to shorten. In the heart this afterload is approximated by the aortic pressure against which the ventricle contracts to raise pressure and eject blood. Together the preload and the afterload make up the *total load* or total weight against which the muscle contracts when stimulated.

The sequence of events during contraction is as follows (Fig. 8.3): When the muscle is stimulated, excitation-contraction coupling takes place, and the CE becomes capable of shortening and developing force. In Fig. 8.3 the SE element is given properties of a spring against which CE contracts. Consequently, the active state of CE is translated into mechanical force development or shortening only after some delay. The time course of the contraction depends on the contractile properties of CE, the duration of the active state, and the elastic properties of the SE element. As seen in Fig. 8.4, during the isometric phase of contraction when the muscle cannot shorten, force develops along a delayed time course relative to CE contraction, owing to the time required for stretching of the SE element. The model in Fig. 8.4 illustrates an afterloaded isotonic contraction. The load (afterload) rests on a surface and is not exerting tension. With stimulation, CE starts to contract and shortens, thus stretching one SE element. When contractile force stretches the SE element so that its elastic tension equals the load, the muscle begins to shorten and lifts the load.

Length-tension diagram

In both cardiac and skeletal muscle the force of contraction depends on initial muscle length (Fig. 8.5). Length-tension diagrams are similar for the two types of muscle, but there are certain significant differences. First, the maximum force of contraction per unit mass of heart muscle is less than for skeletal muscle because in cardiac muscle there is a relatively larger amount of noncontractile material, including mitochondria, per cross-sectional area than in skeletal muscle. When this difference is corrected for and heart muscle is induced to contract maximally, the force-generating capacity of the two varieties of muscle is similar. This means that their contractile elements have similar properties. Second, there is a considerable difference in the resting tension curves of the two muscles. If one compares the curves through (1) their ascending phase, (2) their maximal actively developed tension at the length designated as L_{max}, and (3) their descending limb, one notes that the resting tension at L_{max} is different for the two. In skeletal muscle the resting tension is small at L_{max} and increases significantly only during the descending limb of the active tension curve. In contrast, in heart muscle the resting ten-

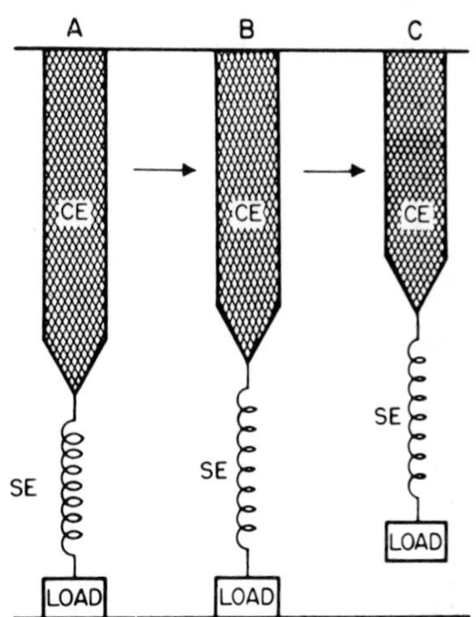

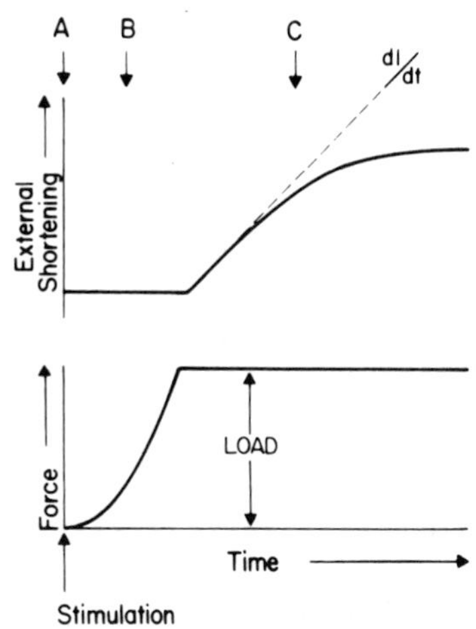

Figure 8.4. Model for an afterloaded isotonic contraction of a papillary muscle. (*A*) At rest; (*B*) partial contraction of the contractile element (CE) with stretch of the series elastic element (SE) but without external shortening (the isometric phase of the contraction); (*C*) further contraction of the CE with external shortening and lifting of the afterload. The tangent (*dl/dt*) to the initial slope of the shortening curve on the right is the velocity of initial shortening. (Redrawn from "The Mechanics of Myocardial Contraction," by Edmund H. Sonnenblick, M.D., in *The Myocardial Cell: Structure, Function, and Modification by Cardiac Drugs*, ed. Stanley A. Briller and Hadley L. Conn, Jr. Copyright 1966 by the Trustees of the University of Pennsylvania.)

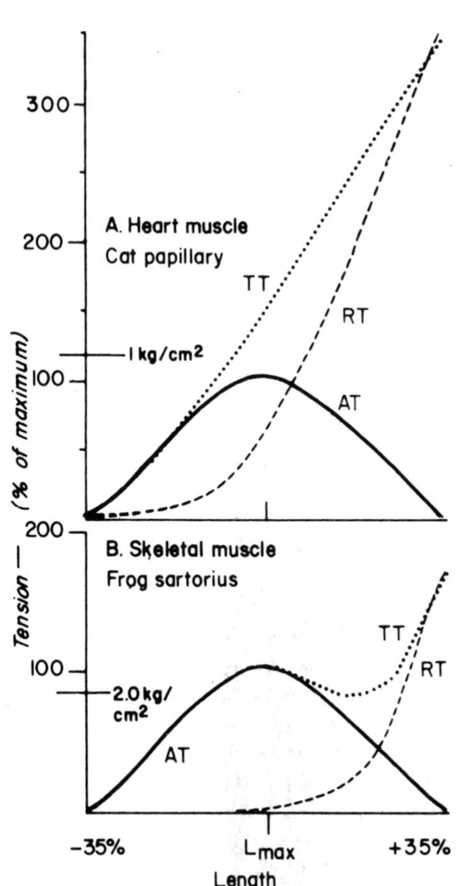

Figure 8.5. Length-tension diagrams for heart (*A*) and skeletal (*B*) muscle compared. RT, Resting tension; AT, actively developed tension; TT, total tension (AT + RT). (Redrawn from Spero and Sonnenblick 1964, *Circ. Res.* 15(Suppl. 2):14–37.)

sion is relatively high at L_{max}. The structures responsible for this difference in resting tension at L_{max} are not certainly known. Whatever the cause, in the intact heart the length-tension relationship of heart muscle is of great importance for adjusting the volume of blood pumped out by each ventricle as related to the degree of filling of the ventricle between contractions (initial length). Normally, the ventricles operate on the ascending limb of the length-tension curve so that any increase in the filling of the ventricle increases the force of contraction and thus the volume of the blood pumped out per beat. This relationship in the heart was first described by Otto Frank in 1895 and later elaborated by Ernest Starling in 1918; hence it is known as the Frank-Starling relationship or mechanism.

The sarcomere length-tension curve for papillary muscle is shown in Fig. 8.6, with the abscissa calibrated in micrometers. Active tension is minimal at a sarcomere length of 1.9 μm and then rises to its apex at lengths between 2.10 and 2.25 μm. When stretched beyond this L_{max}, tension decreases, but in this descending limb the relationship between sarcomere length and length of the muscle as a whole no longer applies strictly because changes occur in organization of the muscle. Resting tension increases markedly, but sarcomeres longer than 2.60 μm are seldom produced. Lengthening of the whole muscle, therefore, cannot be due to elongation of sarcomeres and must be the result of fiber slippage as explained in a preceding chapter.

According to the classic "sliding filament" theory of muscle contraction (Fig. 8.7), maximal tension depends on optimal overlap of actin and myosin filaments, so that all reactive sites between the two contractile protein filaments may be engaged. When the sarcomere is stretched, this overlapping is decreased and reduction in force development follows. If stretched sufficiently, so that no overlap occurs, the muscle becomes incapable of contraction. At the other end of the curve, where muscle length is less than L_{max}, the actin filaments slide into the center of the sar-

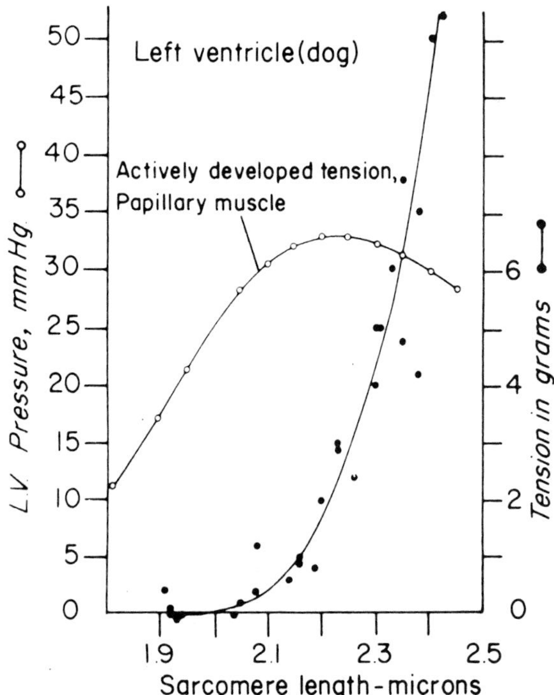

Figure 8.6. Sarcomere length plotted against left ventricular (LV) filling pressure (data from dog heart) and sarcomere length-tension diagram (from cat papillary muscle). Curves are displayed on the same coordinates to indicate the probable relation between sarcomere length and actively developed tension. (Redrawn from Spotnitz, Sonnenblick, and Spero 1966, *Circ. Res.* 18:49–66.)

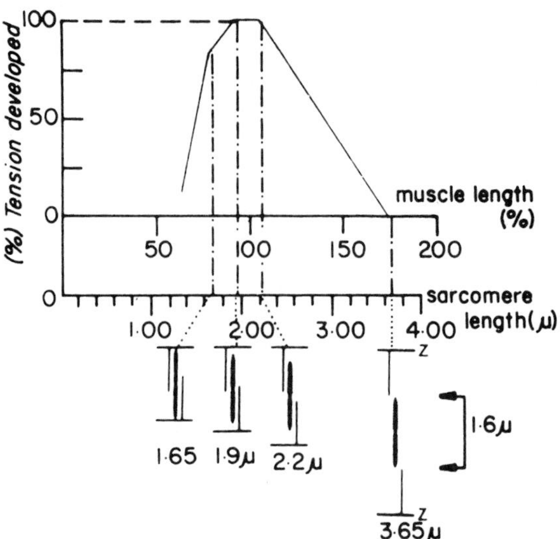

Figure 8.7. Sarcomere length in relation to tension development for skeletal muscle. (Redrawn from Hanson and Lowy 1965, *Br. Med. Bull.* 21:264–71.)

comere. This sliding is accompanied by a reduction in force development, which may be the result of disruption of bond formation in the opposite half of the sarcomere by the actin filaments or possibly the result of actual repelling forces between the filaments. The relationship between sarcomere length and contractile force, however, is not this simple. For example, the relation may depend on length-dependent changes in ionized calcium release for excitation-contraction coupling or sensitivity of the myofilaments to calcium, rather than on the degree of overlap of actin and myosin filaments.

Force-velocity curve

If an isolated muscle is allowed to contract isotonically against various total loads (preload and afterload), the relation between force and velocity may be determined (Fig. 8.8) (see below also). When preload and, therefore, initial muscle length are kept constant, an inverse relation is found between velocity and tension if the beginning or initial velocity is plotted as a function of load (p) (Fig. 8.9). The load at which the muscle cannot shorten and where its velocity is zero is denoted as p_0 on the abscissa; this represents maximum isometric force. If the curve is extrapolated to

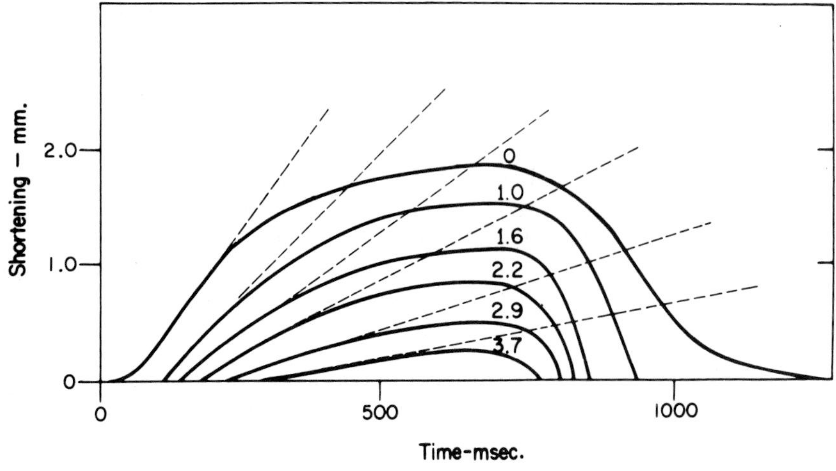

Figure 8.8. Series of superimposed afterloaded contractions of a papillary muscle at a constant initial length. The numbers refer to the magnitude of the afterload in grams, and the dashed lines represent the initial velocity of shortening. (Redrawn from "The Mechanics of Myocardial Contraction," by Edmund H. Sonnenblick, M.D., in *The Myocardial Cell: Structure, Function, and Modification by Cardiac Drugs,* ed. Stanley A. Briller and Hadley L. Conn, Jr. Copyright 1966 by the Trustees of the University of Pennsylvania.)

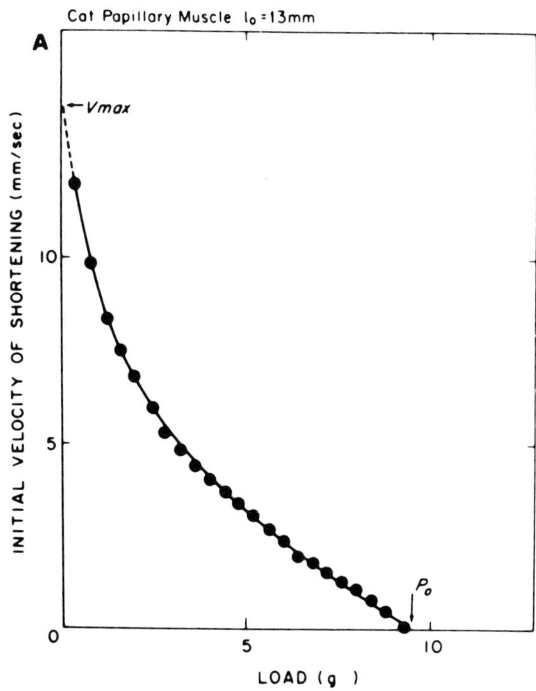

Figure 8.9. The force-velocity relationship in the cat papillary muscle. P_o is the force developed when the muscle is unable to lift the total load (i.e., isometric contraction). (From Sonnenblick 1962, *Fed. Proc.* 21:975.)

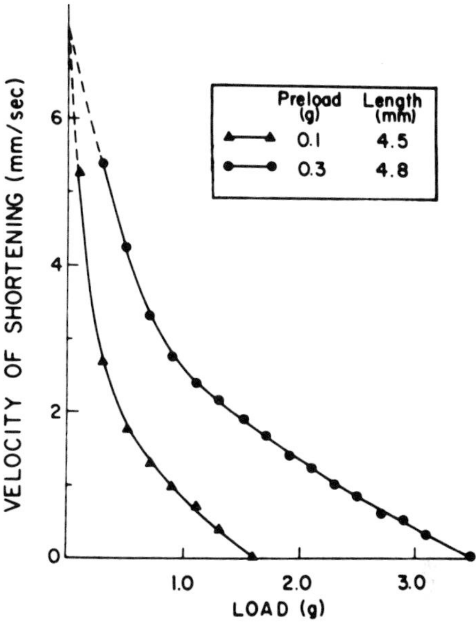

Figure 8.10. Effect of increasing initial muscle length on force-velocity relationship of cat papillary muscle. The initial velocity of shortening is plotted against the afterload for each curve. Preload and initial muscle length for each curve are shown in the inset. Increasing initial muscle length increases maximum force of contraction (P_o) with no change in maximum velocity of shortening (V_{max}). (From Sonnenblick 1965, *Fed. Proc.* 24:1396.)

intersection of the ordinate, the velocity at zero load, which is theoretically the maximum velocity of shortening (V_{max}), is obtained. The force (i.e., load) and velocity relationship of cardiac muscle varies with changes inherent in the contractile mechanism, including the property known as contractility, the contractile state, or the *inotropic state*. The relationship also changes when preload and initial muscle length are altered. When initial muscle length is increased, there is a change in maximal force developed (p_o) without any change in maximal velocity of shortening (see Fig. 8.10). In the intact heart this changing relationship has its counterpart in the Frank-Starling phenomenon in which the stroke volume and force of contraction are found to increase with increasing ventricular diastolic volume.

Inotropic agents increase contractility of the heart. They include norepinephrine, calcium, digitalis, and certain glycosides. They cause heart muscle to shorten faster for any given load and to contract more strongly for an isometric load. In view of the fact that V_{max} does not change when force is increased by stretching the muscle but does change during inotropism, the measurement of V_{max} can be used as an index of contractility.

The effect of initial muscle length on force of contraction is related to the length of the sarcomeres (Fig. 8.7), the degree of overlapping of the contractile filaments, and a length-dependent activation of the contractile unit. The relationship of contractile force to myofilament overlap is poorly understood. The basis of the Frank-Starling mechanism remains obscure.

The force-velocity relationship and the usefulness of V_{max} as an index of contractility have been strongly attacked and defended. It is considered by some to be devoid of fundamental significance, no more useful than other measures of contractility (e.g., maximum rate of isometric or isovolumetric contraction), and of limited empirical value.

Ventricular wall tension and the Laplace relationship

In the intact ventricle, the force of an isolated papillary muscle becomes analogous to ventricular myocardial wall tension, which is a function of the intraventricular pressure per unit area of ventricular surface and also of the total area of the ventricular endocardium. Thus the larger the surface, the greater will be the total pressure for any given unitary pressure. This relationship may be stated quantitatively according to the law of Laplace, which applies to any distensible membrane with a spherical or cylindrical shape. On the assumption that the ventricle has a spherical cavity, its contractile tension has been specified by the Laplace law (Fig. 8.11):

$$T = (P \cdot r)/2h$$

where T is mean stress (i.e., mean force per unit cross-sectional area of the wall during systole), which, for practi-

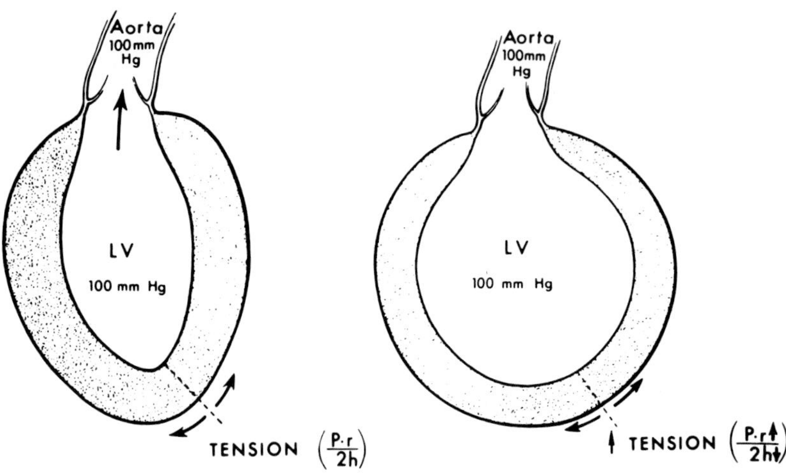

Figure 8.11. Afterload = wall tension (stress). Diagram showing how the systolic wall tension or wall stress (which represents the afterload in the myocardial fibers during left ventricular ejection) is affected by the geometry of the left ventricle (LV). A simplified Laplace relation relating pressure (P) to ventricular radius (r) and wall thickness (h) is shown. The acutely dilated ventricle on the right is developing the same systolic aortic and left ventricular pressure as the normal chamber on the left (100 mm Hg). However, since the radius of the chamber on the right is increased and its wall thickness is decreased, the wall tension is elevated compared with the chamber on the left. (From Ross 1985, in West, ed., *Best and Taylor's Physiological Basis of Medical Practice,* 11th ed., Williams & Wilkins, Baltimore, p. 206.)

cal purposes, is tension circumferentially directed: p is mean transmural pressure per unit endocardial area (again during systole), which, practically, is radially directed; r is mean radius of the chamber; h is mean thickness of the wall. One can see that if intraluminal pressure is increased, or the mean radius becomes greater, the ventricle will have to develop a greater circumferential tension in its wall if it is to shorten during systole. (The relation also applies, of course, to an atrium.)

The Laplace relationship results in a disadvantage when the ventricle is excessively dilated. In the normal ventricle the radius of the chamber during systole decreases as the blood is ejected. Thus the wall tension begins to decrease after the beginning of ejection and at the time of peak systolic pressure, may actually be less than at the onset of systole. When the ventricle is markedly dilated (Fig. 8.11), however, the wall tension is greater than normal and the magnitude of fiber shortening may be so compromised that reduction in chamber radius is minimal. In such instances, the tension produced by myocardial fibers may continue to increase from the beginning of ejection to the peak of systolic pressure. A further theoretical disadvantage of dilatation is that the sarcomeres may be stretched somewhat (although there is little anatomical evidence of this); and, if they are, the ventricle will be functioning on the descending limb of the length-tension curve. Further, the Laplace relation means that, at the same pressure, a dilated heart must generate greater force than normal and, in accordance with the force-velocity relationship, the rate of myocardial fiber shortening will be decreased. These factors diminish the ability of the ventricles to eject blood. It is this increased tension in dilated hearts that is believed to be the adequate stimulus for myocardial hypertrophy. Similarly, it may account for hypertrophy in conditions in which there is a volume overload, even though intraluminal pressure is not increased (e.g., right ventricular hypertrophy in atrial septal defects).

Tension-time index

The term time-tension index was introduced to reflect the total tension developed by the left ventricular myocardium. It is calculated as the product of the mean systolic pressure times duration of systole times heart rate and is expressed as millimeters of mercury seconds per minute. Thus at a mean systolic pressure (P) of 120 mm Hg, a systolic duration (S_d) of 0.2 second, and a heart rate (HR) of 120 beats per minute, the tension-time index (TTI) is

$$\begin{aligned} TTI &= P \times S_d \times HR = \text{mm Hg s/min} \\ &= 120 \times 0.2 \times 120 = 2880 \end{aligned}$$

Under certain experimental conditions, the TTI correlates well with myocardial oxygen utilization, although under other circumstances (e.g., exercise or sympathetic nerve stimulation in the dog or after isoproterenol administration in humans) the correlation is poor. This is because, in addition to tension developed and heart rate, the contractile state of the heart (as reflected by V_{max}) is also a major determinant of myocardial oxygen consumption (see Chap. 11). For clinical purposes, the rate-pressure product can be used to approximate myocardial oxygen consumption. The mean arterial pressure in millimeters of mercury is multiplied by the heart rate in beats per minute.

HEART AS A PUMP

Definitions and general considerations

The *atrial blood volume* is slightly greater than that of the corresponding ventricle, thus providing a reservoir of blood sufficient to fill the ventricle completely for each beat.

The output of each ventricle per beat is approximately equal and is termed the *stroke volume.* The stroke volume from either ventricle multiplied by the pulse rate gives the *cardiac output.* The quantity of blood ejected by each beat of the left ventricle in a 20 kg mongrel dog is about 27 ml, giving a cardiac output of 2.7 L/min when the heart rate is 100 beats per minute. An equal volume of blood is ejected at the same time by the right ventricle, giving a total ejected volume for the whole heart of 54 ml per beat. The stroke volumes and cardiac output, however, are always expressed in terms of one ventricle and thus represent the quantity of blood flowing consecutively through the lungs and into the systemic vessels during the same period. If the heart rate in our hypothetical dog averaged 100 beats per minute over 24 hours, the amount of blood circulated during that period would be 3888 L.

To compare the cardiac output in animals of different size, the values are generally expressed in terms of body surface area (m^2) or metabolic weight ($kg^{0.75}$) and referred to as indexes. Thus the cardiac index and the stroke volume index are obtained by dividing cardiac output or stroke volume by surface area of the body. In the dog, for example:

$$\text{Surface area} = k \times \text{weight}^{0.75}$$
$$m^2 = 0.112 \times kg^{0.75}$$

It follows that cardiac output and metabolism are similarly related to body surface area or to a power function of body weight and are therefore directly correlated. In fact, the total oxygen requirement of the tissues, which reflects the overall metabolism or energy exchange, is the primary determinant of cardiac output in all animals. There is some disagreement on which power function is more appropriate for normalizing cardiac output as a function of body mass. It has been shown that for dogs, horses, cows, humans, and other species the cardiac output is linearly related to body weight:

$$\text{Cardiac output (L/min)} = 0.1017 \times \text{body weight in } kg^{0.99}$$

In this regard, the relations between body mass and cardiovascular function in birds differ from those of mammals in that birds have relatively larger hearts, lower heart rates, higher blood pressure, and greater cardiac output (Grubb 1983). The cardiac output in birds is related to body mass as follows:

$$\text{Cardiac output (L/min)} = 0.2907 \times \text{body weight in } kg^{0.69}$$

It is now well established that the ventricle is not completely emptied of blood during systole. In experimental dogs, for example, under controlled conditions and with the animals under anesthesia, the fraction of the end-diastolic volume actually ejected by the left ventricle was only 47 percent. When outflow resistance (i.e., afterload) was decreased, however, the ejection rate rose to 73 percent.

Stroke volume (SV), the output per beat, is also the difference between end-diastolic volume (EDV) and end-systolic volume (ESV). The ratio SV/EDV (ejection fraction) has been shown to be quite constant in mammals varying in size from rat to horse and to vary linearly with body weight. This constancy in hearts of vastly different sizes is explained on the basis of sarcomere characteristics. In Fig. 8.12, percentage change in ventricular midwall circumference or in sarcomere length is plotted against ejection fraction (SV/EDV). The dashed lines represent ejection fractions within the reported range of 50 to 65 percent. This would require sarcomere shortening of 12 to 17 percent, which corresponds well with that predicted from afterloaded sarcomere shortening. Thus the characteristics of sarcomeres, which are uniform in different-sized hearts, would explain ventricular ejection and apply to hearts of any size.

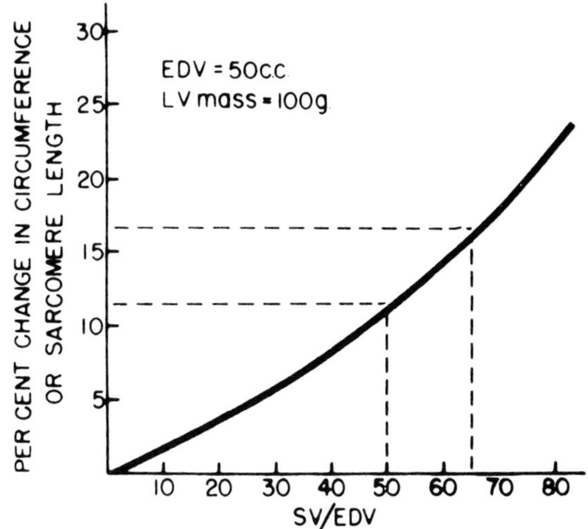

Figure 8.12. The percentage change in midwall circumference or sarcomere length to ventricular ejection fraction (SV/EDV, stroke volume/end-diastolic volume). LV, left ventricle. (Redrawn from Sonnenblick 1968, *Circulation* 38:29–44.)

Since the oxygen requirement of the tissues is the basic determinant of cardiac output, the volume of O_2 carried per unit of blood and the percentage extraction of O_2 by the tissues (arteriovenous O_2 difference) governs the actual cardiac output required to meet the tissue need. The former depends on the concentration of hemoglobin and its efficiency in transporting O_2; the latter depends on the gradient in partial pressure of O_2 between plasma and tissue, the capillary surface area available for exchange, and the time the blood is exposed to this surface. In species other than mammals, these factors become increasingly significant in determining cardiac output. Thus in fish or crustacea that have blood with low O_2-carrying capacity, a higher flow rate must be maintained. Similarly, in mammals, when the O_2-carrying capacity is reduced (as in severe anemia), cardiac output must increase. In humans and other mammals the ratio of cardiac output ($\dot{Q}$) to O_2 uptake ($\dot{V}_{O_2}$) approximates 20:1 (e.g., for a 20-kg dog, $\dot{Q}/\dot{V}_{O_2}$ = 3000 ml/150 ml). In anemia this ratio increases as blood flow (cardiac output) is elevated to carry the required amount of O_2. The general trend of change is similar to that observed when mammals, fish, and crustacea are compared. This further displays the importance of oxygen requirement as a fundamental determinant of circulatory volume flow.

Patterns of ventricular emptying

Direct measurements of changing ventricle dimensions in unanesthetized dogs indicate that the left ventricle resembles a cylinder with a conoid apical segment. Left ventricular systole involves primarily a reduction in transverse diameter. This action accounts for most of the power and volume of the ejection since the contained volume decreases with the square of the radius in a cylinder. There is relatively little rotation or shortening of the longitudinal axis. All this would be expected since the bulk of the fibers is circularly arranged.

By contrast, right ventricular ejection of blood can be effected by three means. (1) Longitudinal shortening of the chamber (i.e., base moving toward apex) is the most obvious movement. This might be expected since the inner and outer layers of spiral muscle making up most of the right ventricle are oriented at about 90 degrees from each other. Hence, simultaneous contraction of the two layers of spiral muscle produces shortening along the longitudinal axis. (2) The right ventricular chamber (Fig. 8.13) is roughly triangular in shape, being bounded by a convex septal wall and a concave free or lateral wall that enclose a crescent-shaped area between them. The free wall of the right ventricle moves toward the convex surface of the septum. This movement, although slight, should be extremely effective in moving blood. It would operate like a bellows; since the sides of the ventricle or bellows are large compared to the enclosed space, slight movement toward each other should cause displacement of a large volume of blood. (3) Contraction of the left ventricle must produce a greater curvature of the septum; thus, since this is attached to the right ventricular lateral wall, traction on it will add to the bellows' action. That this can be a potent mechanism is borne out by the observation that right ventricular ejection can be maintained when the free wall of the right ventricle has been almost completely destroyed by cautery in the dog or by coronary occlusion in humans.

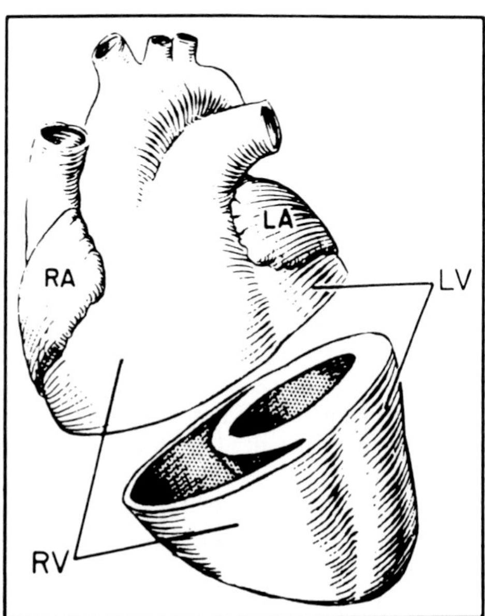

Figure 8.13. Diagram showing the shape and relationship of the two ventricles to each other. The left is ellipsoidal, and the right is crescent shaped, being wrapped around the left ventricle. (From Guyton 1976, *Textbook of Medical Physiology,* 5th ed., W.B. Saunders, Philadelphia.)

Pressure and volume events of a cardiac cycle

For describing the events of the cardiac cycle, terminology and symbols according to Wiggers (see Table 8.1) and the schema and time intervals shown in Fig. 8.14 are used.

Sequence of events

The upper set of pressure pulse curves in Fig. 8.14 is for the left side of the heart and the aorta and the lower set for the right side of the heart and the pulmonary artery. Events in these chambers are correlated with periods with semilunar and atrioventricular (AV) valves are opened or closed, with heart sounds, and with the electrocardiogram (ECG) (Fig. 8.14).

1. *Isovolumetric contraction.* At the time of the peak of the R wave in the ECG, ventricular contraction begins. The pressure curve starts to ascend, and at the moment it exceeds the atrial pressure curve, the AV valves close. The C wave in the atrial curves begins at this time, caused by bulging of the closed AV valves into the atria as ventricular pressure increases. The C waves are variable and may be absent. Both AV and semilunar valves are now closed, and the ventricles are contracting on the contained blood, which is incompressible. Therefore the volume of the ventricles does not change and pressure increases rapidly. This period terminates, and the next period begins at the moment ventricular pressures exceed aortic or pulmonic pressures. The semilunar valves open, and the blood is accelerated into the great arteries.

2. *Maximum ejection.* The period of maximum ejection begins with the opening of the semilunar valves. Most of the blood ejected during systole flows during this period, as can be seen by the rapid descent of the left ventricular volume curve. It lasts until the peak of the arterial pressure curve. For part of the period of systole, aortic pressure is exceeded by left ventricular pressure during this interval of greatest acceleration of aortic flow.

3. *Reduced ejection.* During rapid ejection blood flow into the aorta (and pulmonary artery) exceeds runoff into the peripheral arteries, and pressure continues to rise. As runoff reaches equilibrium with flow into the great arteries, the pressure curve reaches a maximum. This is the beginning of the reduced ejection period. Runoff now exceeds cardiac output, and the pressures begin to fall. The pressure in the left ventricle falls slightly below that in the root of the aorta, although forward flow continues as indicated by progressive decrease in ventricular volume.

4. *Protodiastole.* This marks the beginning of ventricular relaxation and is a point on the ventricular pressure curves

Table 8.1. Events of the cardiac cycle

Phase	Interval	Events at onset of phase	Main events during phase	Events at close of phase
Isovolumetric contraction	1	Onset of ventricular contraction	Closure of atrioventricular (AV) valves, rapid rise of intraventricular pressure	Opening of semilunar valves
Maximum ejection	2	Opening of semilunar valves	Rapid outflow of blood from ventricles	Peak of intraventricular pressure
Reduced ejection	3	Peak of intraventricular pressure	Declining outflow of blood from ventricles	Onset of ventricular relaxation
Protodiastole	4	Onset of ventricular relaxation	Rapid drop in intraventricular pressure	Closure of semilunar valves
Isovolumetric relaxation	5	Closure of semilunar valves	Continued ventricular relaxation with no volume change	Opening of AV valves
Rapid flow	6	Opening of AV valves	Rapid flow of blood from atria to ventricles	Slowing of inflow rate
Diastasis	7	Slowing of inflow from atria to ventricles	Continued slower flow from atria to ventricles	Onset of atrial contraction
Atrial systole	8	Onset of atrial contraction	Increased flow from atria to ventricles	Termination of atrial, and onset of ventricular, contraction

From Ditmer and Grebe, eds. 1963, *Handbook of Circulation,* Saunders, Philadelphia, modified from Wiggers 1952, *Circulatory Dynamics,* Grune and Stratton, New York.

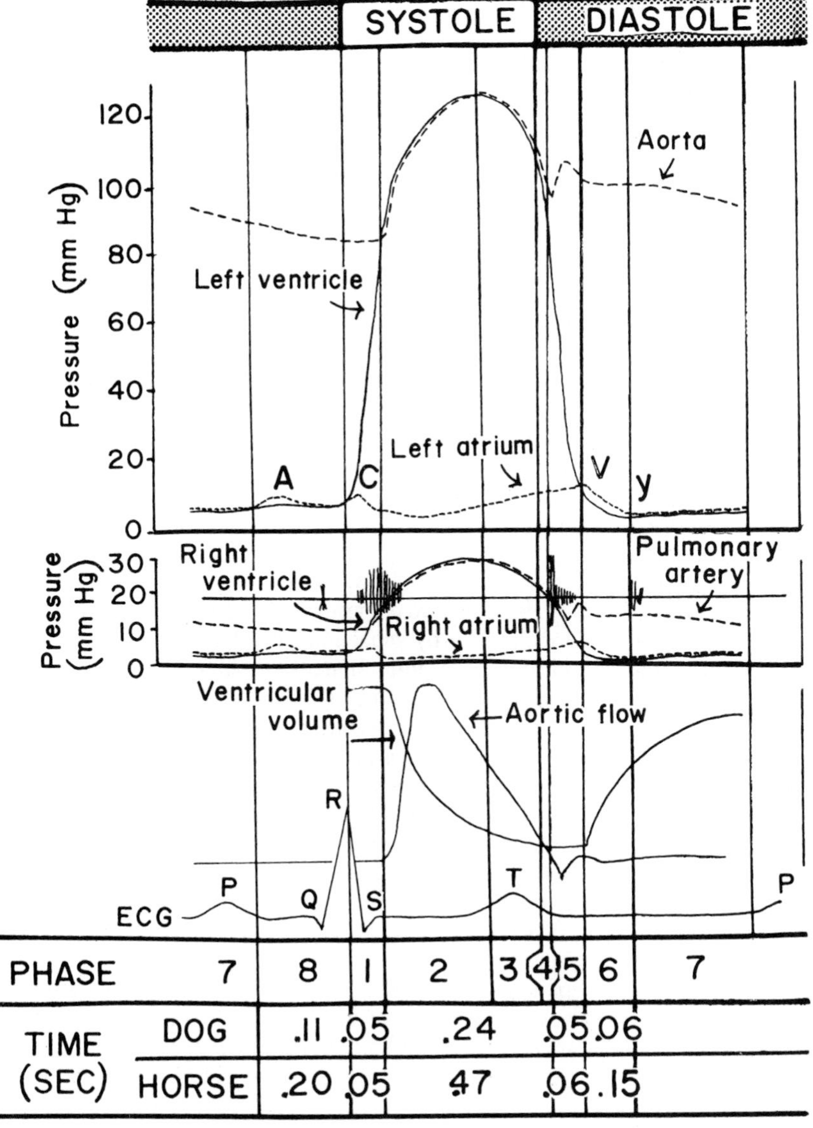

Figure 8.14. Events of the cardiac cycle. (*Top*) Pressure pulses of the left side of the heart. A, Atrial contraction wave; C, atrial pressure wave caused by bulging of AV valves into atria during phase 1; V, increasing pressure in atrium to end of phase 5; y, decline in atrial pressure curve as blood flows into ventricles (phase 6). (*Middle*) Pressure pulses of the right side of the heart; phonocardiogram displaying, from left to right, fourth (S_4), first (S_1), second (S_2), and third (S_3) heart sounds. S_4 appears during phase 8; S_1 starts during phase 1 and extends into phase 2; S_2 appears in phase 5; S_3 starts at the end of phase 6. (*Bottom*) Ventricular volume curve; aortic flow curve; ECG. P, Q, R, S, T, electrocardiographic waves. Phase indicates the eight phases of the cardiac cycle after Wiggers. Time indicates time intervals of the cardiac cycle for the horse and dog.

that is often difficult to identify. The pressures in the ventricles continue to fall below those in the aorta and pulmonary artery. A brief retrograde flow occurs, closing the semilunar valves. This marks the end of protodiastole and the beginning of the next phase.

5. *Isovolumetric relaxation.* With closure of the semilunar valves, an incisura in the arterial pressure curves is seen, marking the beginning of this phase. Once again, the ventricles are closed chambers; myocardial relaxation continues, causing a steep fall in intraventricular pressures but little alteration in ventricular volume. When the intraventricular pressures fall below those in the atria, the AV valves open, marking the end of this period. During this phase, the ventricles remain partially filled with blood, because they previously ejected only 50 to 65 percent of their diastolic volumes.

6. *Rapid filling.* Beginning with the opening of the AV valves, ventricular volumes increase rapidly as blood that has accumulated in the atria under increasing pressure flows quickly into the relaxed ventricles. During this phase the ventricular volume curve ascends steeply at first and then begins to level off. The end of this phase is not clear-cut as it merges with the next phase. At the transition between this and the following phase the usually inaudible third heart sound (S_3) may be recorded in the phonocardiogram. (See Heart Sounds, below, for description of other sounds.)

7. *Reduced filling (diastasis).* This is a period of slower filling during which blood continues to flow into both atria and ventricles as into a common chamber. It is terminated by onset of atrial systole.

8. *Atrial systole.* This period is marked by the onset of the atrial contraction (A) wave, which is reflected in the ventricle since the two chambers are now continuous. This atrial systolic pressure wave peaks and begins to decline, finally being interrupted by the onset of ventricular isovolumetric contraction, completing the cardiac cycle.

During each ventricular contraction, the C wave of atrial pressure is followed by a temporary abrupt decline as a result of an artifact imposed by cardiac movement. As blood pours into the cavity of the left atrium from the veins, however, the atrial pressure rises continuously to the end of the isometric relaxation period, forming the V wave. Then, when the intraventricular pressure drops below the intra-atrial pressure and the AV valves open, this accumulated blood flows rapidly into the ventricle. The period of rapid ventricular filling (i.e., the early diastolic inflow period) is marked by a continuous decline in ventricular pressure and in the V wave of the atrial pressure curve (the so-called *y* descent).

Filling of atria and ventricles

Inflow into the ventricular cavity always depends on the pressure gradient between atrium and ventricle, and one of the most important factors affecting this gradient is atrial filling. It is important, therefore, to know how the atria fill. There is no technique available for measuring flow into an atrium, but since the right atrium is continuous with the venae cavae without intervening valves, flow in the venae cavae may be taken as the equivalent of atrial filling. This flow shows the following three phases: (1) During ventricular diastole there is a considerable flow. (2) During atrial systole the flow is reduced nearly to zero because of the back pressure into the great veins. (3) During ventricular systole, when the AV valves are closed so that blood cannot enter the ventricle, the larger part of atrial filling takes place. This period of filling is particularly effective in the presence of tachycardia, in which the time available for diastolic inflow is shortened.

Ventricular systole aids atrial filling because there is a pistonlike downward movement of the AV junction that enlarges the atria and venae cavae and attracts blood into them. Their filling then depends on the quantity and pressure of blood available in the venous reservoir, and the vigor of the ventricle-induced movement of the AV junction. In this manner the contraction of the ventricle indirectly determines its own filling during its diastole, inasmuch as it is the filling of the atrium that later permits filling of the ventricle, particularly during the sixth phase.

Finally, in the sixth phase shown in Fig. 8.14, there is an alternate course for intraventricular pressure. When this curve attains a pressure that is more negative than intrathoracic pressure, it is said to represent a vis a fronte (force from in front; see Chap. 10), returning blood to the heart. For many years such a dip in the pressure curve of the ventricular relaxation was regarded as an artifact. Now, however, it is given more credence since (1) it can be recorded with an intraventricular micromanometer, which is supposedly free of artifacts, and (2) recent evidence suggests that the relaxing ventricle can, in fact, develop suction.

Atrial contraction

The dynamic importance of atrial contraction on ventricular filling has been much debated. The older view that the chief function of the atria is filling the ventricles is not now acceptable, since it is known that such filling occurs chiefly during the earlier portion of diastole when the difference between atrial and ventricular pressure is maximal. However, in a heart slowed by vagal stimulation to separate atrial and ventricular contraction or in a heart with 2:1 atrioventricular block, atrial contraction has a small but significant effect on the ventricular volume curve obtained with a cardiometer. Also in open-chest dogs with surgically induced complete AV block and a fixed, slow ventricular rate, there is an increase in left ventricular end-diastolic pressure, stroke volume, stroke work, and aortic systolic pressure when atrial systole precedes ventricular systole by an interval of 0.085 to 0.125 second, indicating enhanced ventricular filling through atrial contraction. Finally, atrial contraction and relaxation are instrumental in bringing about closure of the AV valves (see below).

Pressure pulse values

Aortic pressure throughout the cardiac cycle is uniformly higher than in the pulmonary artery. For dogs, the peak systolic pressure in the aorta is about 120 mm Hg, approximately 5 times higher than the corresponding pressure of 25 mm Hg in the pulmonary artery. The relative end-diastolic pressures are 80 mm Hg versus 10 mm Hg; the relative pulse pressures are 40 mm Hg versus 15 mm Hg. The diastolic pressure in both cavities is quite low, with a small pressure gradient from the left ventricle (0 to 5 mm Hg mean diastolic, 5 to 12 mm Hg end diastolic) to the right ventricle (0 to 3 mm Hg mean diastolic, 0 to 5 mm Hg end diastolic). The atrial pressure values are only a few millimeters of mercury and are uniformly somewhat higher in the left atrial (mean 0 to 5 mm Hg) curve.

Asynchronisms of pressure pulses. Although dynamic events on the two sides of the heart are generally similar, there is considerable asynchronism and some difference in duration of parts of the cardiac cycle. The onset of contraction of the right atrium precedes that of the left atrium, whereas the onset of contraction of the right ventricle follows that of the left ventricle. Nevertheless right ventricular ejection begins earlier and is completed later than left ventricular ejection.

Electrocardiogram versus onset of pressure events

In the dog the interval between the onset of electrical and mechanical activity in the left atrium (rise of P wave versus onset of rise of atrial A wave) is on the order of 0.04 second. For the left ventricle, the interval between the onset of ventricular depolarization (Q wave) and the onset of left ventricular contraction (onset of pressure rise) approximates 0.02 second. The T wave has a variable relation to the end of systole but terminates usually before the incisura of the aortic pressure curve.

Aortic flow

The relationship between left ventricular pressure pulse and aortic flow in a dog is seen in Fig. 8.14. The flow rate at the root of the aorta increases rapidly during the phase of rapid ejection when most of the systolic output of the heart is expelled; then flow falls off during the phase of reduced ejection and reverses at the end of ejection. During diastole the aortic flow remains at about zero, but forward flow continues in the more peripheral arteries under the impetus of its initial momentum and the elastic recoil of the larger arteries.

Ventricular pressure-volume diagram

For a complete representation of mechanical activity of the heart, the coordinates of pressure, volume, and time must be employed. In Fig. 8.14 this is done by plotting pressure and volume against time.

The cardiac cycle can also be diagrammed by plotting the changes in pressure and volume (Fig. 8.15). If the ventricle is prevented from ejecting and the peak isovolumetric pressure is determined for several different ventricular volumes, a linear relationship is found to exist. This line represents the end-systolic pressure-volume relationship and the upper left-hand corner at point 3 of the pressure-volume (P-V) loop of the ejecting beat (Fig. 8.16).

The normal P-V loop of an ejecting ventricle can begin at point 1 (Fig. 8.16), which is the end of diastole, mitral valve closure, and the onset of isovolumetric contraction. The ventricular pressure rises without ejection to point 2, where the aortic valve opens and ventricular ejection begins. The ventricular volume then decreases as the myocardial fibers shorten and blood is ejected into the aorta. At point 3 systole ends and the aortic valve closes. From point 3 to point 4 the ventricle relaxes isovolumically, and from point 4 to point 1 it fills again, with the mitral valve opening at point 4.

A ventricle that does not change its contractility will maintain an end-systolic point on a straight line, even though alterations in preload and afterload change the shape of the P-V loop.

Increasing the preload while holding the afterload and contractility constant produces a larger end-diastolic volume (Fig. 8.17). The ventricle will empty, however, to the

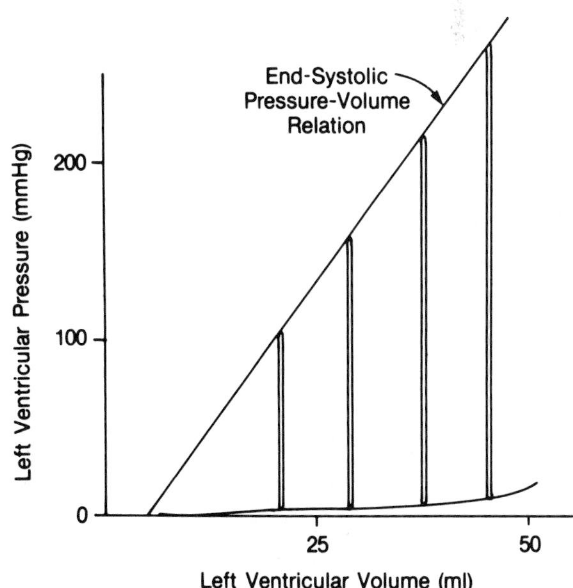

Figure 8.15. Left ventricular pressure-volume loops generated by isovolumetric (i.e., nonejecting) beats at various volumes. The peak pressure generated by each beat falls along a straight line, the end-systolic pressure-volume relation. (From Little and Little 1989, *Physiology of the Heart and Circulation,* 4th ed, Yearbook Medical Publishing, Chicago, p. 182.)

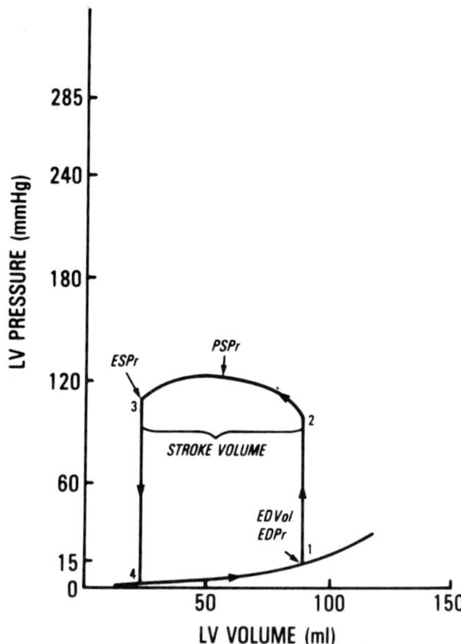

Figure 8.16. Left ventricular (LV) pressure-volume loop and the diastolic pressure-volume curve. During a normal contraction, point 1 shows end-diastolic (ED) pressure (Pr) and volume (Vol), point 2 the onset of left ventricular ejection, which continues to point 3 (the distance on the volume axis representing the stroke volume). This is followed by isovolumetric relaxation (point 3 to point 4) and then by filling of the ventricle along its diastolic pressure-volume curve (point 4 to point 1). The end-systolic (ES) pressure-volume point is indicated, as is the peak systolic pressure (PSPr). (From Ross 1985, in West, ed., *Best and Taylor's Physiological Basis of Medical Practice,* 11th ed, Williams & Wilkins, Baltimore, p. 210.)

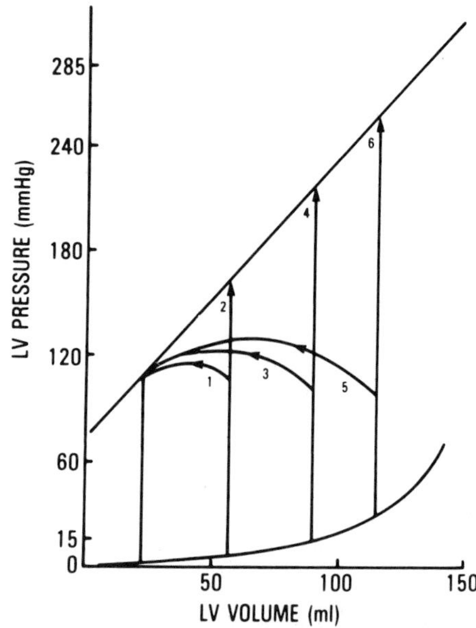

Figure 8.17. Left ventricular (LV) pressure-volume diagram showing effects of progressively increasing end-diastolic volume. In isovolumetric contractions (beats 2, 4, and 6), the peak pressure is increased at larger end-diastolic volumes, and at nearly the same left ventricular pressure during ejection the stroke volume progressively increases (beats 1, 3, and 5). (From Ross 1985, in West, ed., *Best and Taylor's Physiological Basis of Medical Practice,* 11th ed, Williams & Wilkins, Baltimore, p. 213.)

same end-systolic volume, thus increasing the stroke volume.

An increase in afterload with a constant preload and contractility results in a taller P-V loop with reduced stroke volume. The end-systolic point will be on the straight line developed from isovolumetric contractions.

If contractility is altered, there will be a change in the slope of the line representing the end-systolic pressure volume relationship (Fig. 8.18). If contractility were increased and the line were to shift from beat 1 to beat 3 with preload and afterload unchanged, the stroke volume would increase. Likewise, if contractility were decreased and the line changed from beat 1 to beat 5, the stroke volume would decrease.

The end-systolic relationship line has a slope with units of pressure per volume and denotes stiffness or elastance of the ventricle during systole. End-systolic elastance is unchanged by alterations in preload or afterload, but it increases and decreases with like changes in myocardial contractility.

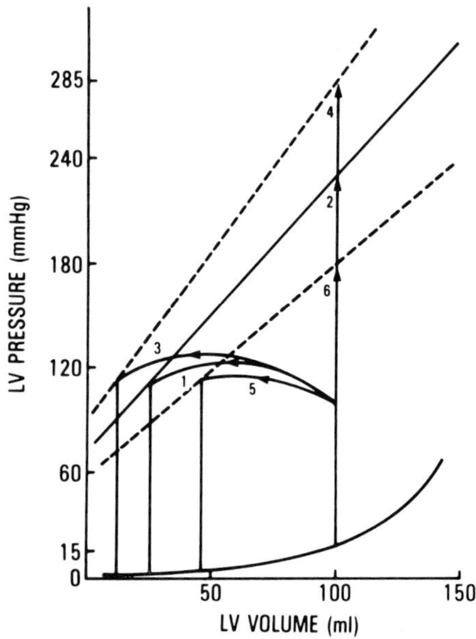

Figure 8.18. Pressure-volume diagram showing the effects of positive (upper dashed line) and negative inotropic stimuli (lower dashed line) compared with control (solid line); peak pressure in isovolumetric contractions is increased and decreased, respectively (beats 4 and 6, compared with beat 2), and the stroke volume is augmented with the positive inotropic stimulus (beat 3) and reduced with the negative inotropic intervention (beat 5). (From Ross 1985, in West, ed., *Best and Taylor's Physiological Basis of Medical Practice,* 11th ed, Williams & Wilkins, Baltimore, p. 216.)

Ventricular function curves

The "Starling curve" resulted from experiments on isolated dog heart-lung preparations. This curve, shown in

Fig. 8.19, describes the relationship between energy output (cardiac output) and ventricular diastolic size (mean venous pressure). In essence, the energy output is related to the presystolic length of individual fibers. Heterometric (*hetero,* different; *metric,* length) autoregulation is the name given to the heart's ability to alter its output in response to altered myocardial fiber length (Fig. 8.20).

Since these early experiments, ventricular function curves have been developed which plot some index of ventricular performance along the ordinate and some index of fiber length along the abscissa (Fig. 8.21). A ventricle may move from one curve to another, depending on the level and balance of autonomic input into the heart. Homeometric (*homeo,* same; *metric,* length) autoregulation refers to the ability of the ventricle to alter its vigor of contraction without altering the initial myocardial length.

Four major factors that influence ventricular performance

1. Preload (Frank-Starling mechanism)

Preload in the isolated muscle stretches the muscle and determines the resting fiber length. Increasing the preload of an isolated muscle causes an increased tension on contraction ("Starling's law of the heart"). In the whole heart, preload occurs by diastolic filling of the ventricle. The resting muscle fiber length is determined for practical purposes by ventricular end-diastolic pressure or volume. On the pressure-volume diagram, increasing the preload results in an increased stroke volume as well as the potential for a higher peak isovolumetric pressure (Fig. 8.17).

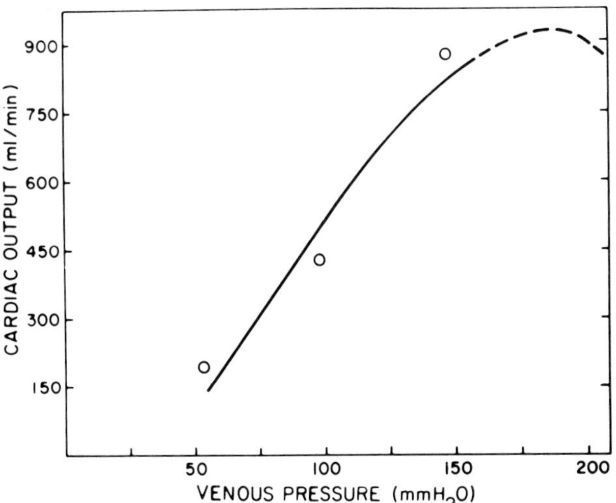

Figure 8.19. Schematic representation of a "Starling curve" showing energy output of the heart-lung preparation measured as cardiac output, plotted against ventricular diastolic size as reflected by the venous pressure level. (Modified from Patterson, Piper, and Starling 1914, *J. Physiol.* 48:465.)

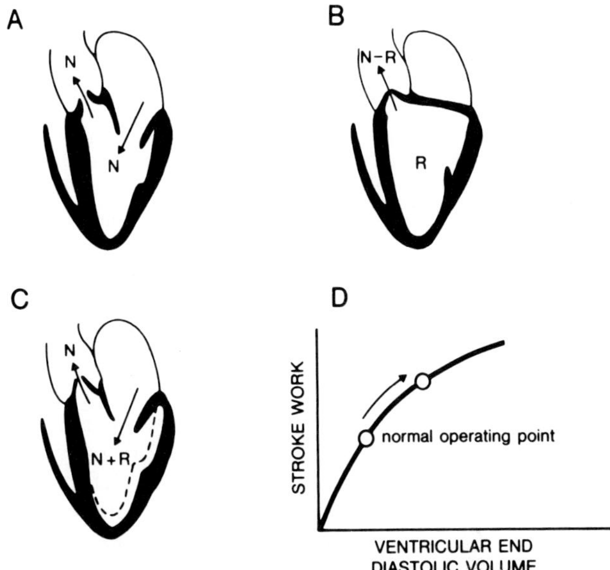

Figure 8.20. Schematic diagram illustrating the mechanism of heterometric regulation. (*A*) Control. The normal return (N) to the ventricle during diastole results in the same volume being ejected during systole. (*B*) A sudden increase in output resistance at the end of diastole results in the stroke volume being less than N; N − R is ejected, and R (remainder of the stroke volume) remains in the ventricle. (*C*) During the next beat, the normal venous return (N) is added to the volume remaining from the last beat (R). This increased diastolic volume (N + R) causes the next ventricular contraction to be more forceful. This returns stroke volume equal to venous return. (*D*) The above sequence of events causes the cardiac operating point to move on the cardiac function curve (Starling curve) from its normal operating point to a larger end-diastolic volume and increased stroke work. (From Little and Little 1989, *Physiology of the Heart and Circulation,* 4th ed, Yearbook Medical Publishers, Chicago, p. 176.)

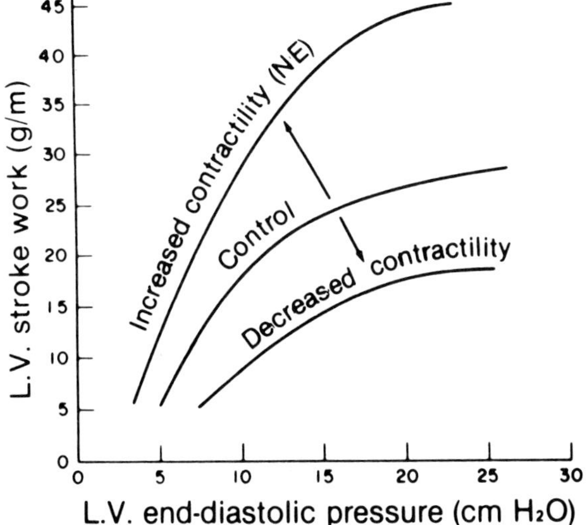

Figure 8.21. Left ventricular function curves. The administration of a positive inotropic agent (e.g., norepinephrine) characteristically increases the stroke work at a given left ventricular end-diastolic pressure (or volume) and is said to increase contractility. If the ventricle performs less stroke work at a given end-diastolic pressure (or volume), contractility is said to be decreased (negative inotropic state). (From Braunwald, Ross, and Sonnenblick 1967, *Mechanism of Contraction of the Normal and Failing Heart,* Little Brown & Co., Boston.)

2. Afterload

The major component of afterload for the left ventricle is systolic aortic pressure; for the right ventricle, it is the systolic pulmonary artery pressure. This pressure and aortic impedence together determine the tension that must be developed by the ventricular wall. If aortic pressure is decreased, the ensuing contractions of the ventricle will encounter less afterload and the ejected stoke volume will increase (Fig. 8.22), just as the isolated muscle experiments showed, decreasing the afterload increases the extent of wall shortening (Fig. 8.8) and the maximum rate of velocity of shortening.

3. Inotropic state

The inotropic state affects muscle performance independent of preload and afterload. The isometric length-tension curve (Fig. 8.23) is useful in illustrating how a change in inotropic state will affect muscle shortening and tension development. Increasing the inotropic state increases the peak (isometric) tension developed at each preload and the extent of fiber shortening. The whole heart, again, exhibits the same characteristics. The pressure-volume diagram (Fig. 8.18) illustrates that altering the inotropic state leads to changes in stroke volume (fiber shortening) and peak isometric tension. The sympathetic nervous system is an important determinant of inotropic state.

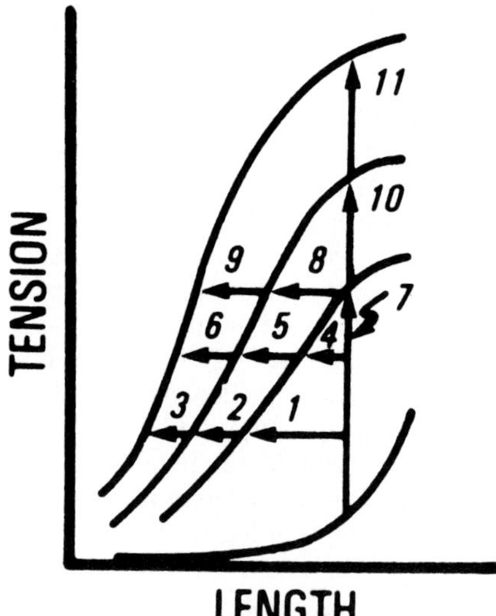

Figure 8.23. Effects of alterations of inotropic state on isometric and isotonic contractions from the same resting muscle length. Beat 10 represents an isometric contraction at the normal level of contractility, which forms a point on the isometric active length-tension relation. Beat 7 is an isometric contraction at a depressed level of inotropic state, which reaches the depressed isometric length-tension relation, and beat 11 is an isometric contraction in the presence of increased inotropic state, which reaches an elevated isometric length-active tension curve. At the same level of afterload beats 1 and 3 exhibit less and more active shortening, respectively, than beat 2 (the control beat), and this is the case at any given level of afterload. Notice that beat 9 shortens more than beat 8, while the depressed muscle is unable to shorten at that afterload. (From Ross 1985, in West, ed., *Best and Taylor's Physiological Basis of Medical Practice,* 11th ed, Williams & Wilkins, Baltimore, p. 204.)

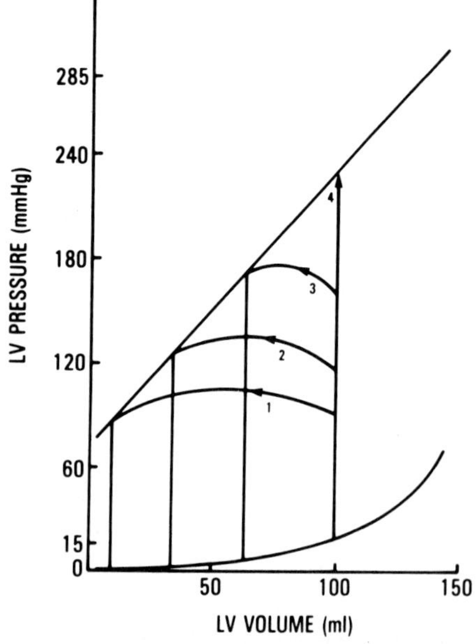

Figure 8.22. Pressure-volume diagram showing the effects of progressively increasing left ventricular systolic pressure from a constant left ventricular end-diastolic volume. There is progressive reduction of the stroke volume in beats 1, 2 and 3. Beat 4 represents an isovolumetric contraction. (From Ross 1985, in West, ed., *Best And Taylor's Physiologic Basis of Medical Practice,* 11th ed, Williams & Wilkins, Baltimore, p. 215.)

4. Heart rate

In the isolated muscle, an increase in stimulation frequency leads to an increase in developed tension. This effect is known as the staircase, or Treppe, phenomenon. Although the inotropic state is increased by an increase in heart rate (Fig. 8.24), the overall effect that overshadows all others is the increased cardiac output (performance) per minute. Since cardiac output is the product of heart rate times stroke volume, the cardiac output of a slowly beating heart can be doubled by doubling the heart rate.

CARDIAC OUTPUT MEASUREMENT

Three ways of measuring cardiac output (CO) are in general use: the *direct Fick,* the *indicator dilution,* and the *magnetic flowmeter* methods.

The *Fick principle* states that the amount of substance taken up by the circulation per unit of time equals the arterial level of the substance minus the venous level times the blood flow. The CO (left ventricle) can be determined by measuring the O_2 consumption per minute and the arteriovenous O_2 difference:

$$\text{CO/min} = \frac{O_2 \text{ consumption (ml/min)}}{\text{Arterial } O_2 \text{ concentration} - \text{venous } O_2 \text{ concentration}}$$

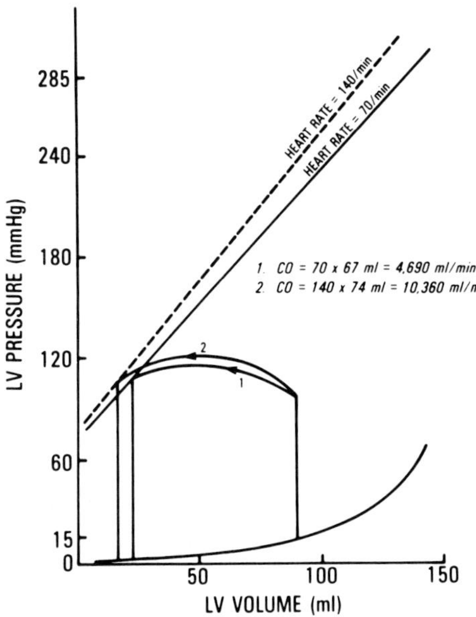

Figure 8.24. Pressure-volume diagram showing the effects of increasing heart rate while maintaining the end-diastolic pressure and volume of the ventricle constant with a pump or by transfusion. The end-systolic or isovolumetric pressure-volume relation is shifted upward and to the left by the force-frequency effect (dashed line), and beat 2 at the faster heart rate therefore delivers a slightly larger stroke volume. The effect of doubling the contraction frequency from 70 to 140/min at a constant end-diastolic volume is to more than double the cardiac output. (From Ross 1985, in West, ed., *Best and Taylor's Physiological Basis of Medical Practice,* 11th ed, Williams & Wilkins, Baltimore, p. 216.)

For a dog

$$CO = \frac{80 \text{ ml/min}}{190 - 140 \text{ ml/L}} = \frac{80 \text{ ml/min}}{50 \text{ ml/L}} = 1.6 \text{ L/min}$$

The *indicator dilution* method is based on the principle that if a known quantity of a substance is mixed with an unknown volume of fluid, the volume can be determined from the concentration of the substance in the fluid; volume equals amount of substance (in milligrams) divided by concentration of substance (in milligrams per liter).

In practice a known amount of some substance (e.g., radioactive isotope) that will not rapidly escape from the blood is injected into a vein, and the average concentration of this substance in the arterial blood is determined over a period of time from continuous or serial samples. The cardiac output is equal to the amount of indicator (I) substance injected, divided by its average concentration ($\int_0^\infty C\,dt$) in arterial blood after a single circulation through the heart. Thus

$$CO = \frac{I}{\int_0^\infty C\,dt}$$

In Fig. 8.25 a dye-dilution curve is shown. The mean concentration is 2.08 mg/L over the duration of the concentration curve when extrapolated to the baseline (21 seconds). The amount of indicator injected was 1.5 mg. Thus

$$CO = \frac{1.5 \text{ mg injected}}{2.08 \text{ mg/L}} = 0.72 \text{ L} \times \frac{60 \text{ s}}{21 \text{ s}} = 2.06 \text{ L/min}$$

A modification of this method is the *thermodilution* technique, in which a small quantity of chilled physiological saline solution is injected into a cardiac chamber and the temperature change in the blood is recorded over time as the temperature returns to the control level.

The *electromagnetic flowmeter* measures the electromotive force (EMF) generated when the blood flowing within a vessel of known diameter passes through a magnetic field at right angles to the magnetic lines of force. The induced EMF is detected by two electrodes positioned against the vessel wall perpendicular to both the lines of force and the direction of flow. Cardiac output is determined by placing the flowmeter probe around the root of the aorta. Such flowmeters can be used to measure regional flow in any artery.

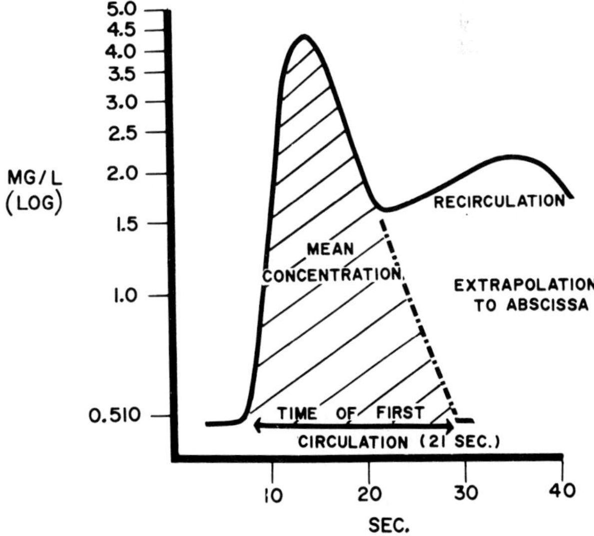

Figure 8.25. Dye-dilution curve for measuring cardiac output. An indicator was injected into the saphenous vein of a dog and its concentration measured in blood withdrawn from the opposite femoral artery. The resultant dye curve lasted about 21 s before recirculation of the indicator caused the second increase in the concentration curve. On log paper the total duration of the initial concentration curve can be estimated by extending its descending slope to the abscissa as a straight line. The mean concentration is the area under this curve.

MOVEMENTS OF HEART VALVES

Atrioventricular valves (tricuspid and mitral)

The valve leaflets or cusps, three in number on the right side and two on the left side, are attached by their bases to the fibrous rings surrounding the AV openings. Their free margins are connected through delicate tendons (chordae tendineae) to the papillary muscles, which prevent inversion of the valves into the atrium during ventricular systole. The chordae tendineae are tightened at the commencement of systole by the contraction of the papillary muscles.

The mechanism of valve closure

During systole the atrioventricular valves are closed by the intraventricular pressure. Early in diastole the valves open wide because of rapid ventricular filling. Within milliseconds the rate of diastolic filling slows and the leaflets partially close to occupy a midposition as a result of two opposing currents; the inflowing blood pressing upon their atrial surfaces keeps them open, while eddies reflected in the reverse direction from the ventricular walls strike their ventricular surfaces and tend to close them. Thus they float in a position of delicate balance. Atrial systole occurs late in diastole, and the additional ventricular filling causes the AV valves to reopen temporarily. When, as a result of the fall in intra-atrial pressure at the end of atrial systole, the incoming jet is diminished in force and finally ceases, the back eddies persisting for a brief space and being unopposed, approximate the valves. Firm closure of the valves is produced when the intraventricular pressure exceeds that in the corresponding atrium.

Semilunar valves

The dynamics of aortic and pulmonary closure are essentially the same in principle as those described for the AV valves. The valves and sinuses of Valsalva form three small pockets open toward the arterial lumen. During diastole the semilunar valves are closed by the aortic and pulmonary artery pressure. With the onset of systole, the valves open when the intraventricular pressure exceeds the arterial pressure on the other side of the valve. Back eddies set up during the ejection phase of systole prevent contact of the valves with the arterial wall. When ejection ceases, the centripetal currents carry the valves into apposition and firm closure is effected when the higher aortic or pulmonic pressure acts upon their arterial surfaces.

Heart sounds

Certain vibrations associated with the pulsatile events of the cardiac cycle produce sounds. Table 8.2 provides some historical highlights concerning heart sounds. These are divided into two groups, in accordance with their duration: (1) *transients*, sounds of relatively short duration, such as the four normal heart sounds and certain abnormal sounds of short duration (clicks and gallop sounds), and (2) *murmurs*, sounds of longer duration that are often associated with abnormal conditions such as valvular stenosis or insufficiency.

Table 8.2. Historical highlights concerning heart sounds

1819	Rene Theophile Hyacinthe Laennec, the father of clinical auscultation, erroneously attributed the first and second heart sounds to ventricular and atrial contraction, respectively.
1835	James Hope used stunned donkeys in open-chest experiments to identify the timing in the cardiac cycle and, in part, the source of the first and second heart sounds (assisted by veterinary surgeon John Fields of London).
1835	Charles J.B. Williams, from an experiment on a beating heart of a donkey from which the blood had been removed and the first sound was still audible, reasoned that it was produced by muscular contraction since he assumed that the value leaflets did not move.
1832 and 1844	Joseph Rouanet by pumping liquid intermittently through isolated hearts established valve closure (or tensing at the time of closure) as the cause of both heart sounds.
1855	August Chauveau and Jean Vaivre confirmed James Hope's initial observations on the production of heart sounds, by palpating the AV valves through the atrium (in horses).
1861	August Chauveau, in collaboration with Etienne-Jules Marey, recorded pressure pulses from horses with intraventricular balloon catheters and manually marked the time of the first and second heart sounds.
1893	Karl Huerthle led the output of a microphone to an inductorium that excited a frog nerve-muscle preparation which marked the "sounds" on a smoked drum producing a primitive phonocardiogram.
1894	Willem Einthoven and M.A.J. Geluk recorded the first phonocardiograms using a capillary electrometer.
1904	Otto Frank recorded precordial sound vibrations with optical amplification from a Frank segment capsule.
1907	Willem Einthoven recorded heart sounds with his string galvanometer.
1909	O. Weiss published the first monograph on phonocardiography.

The *phonocardiogram* (PCG) is a graphic recording of the heart sounds transduced to an electrical signal with a microphone. The PCG is usually recorded simultaneously with the ECG to identify phases of the cardiac cycle. A PCG of all four heart sounds and their temporal relationships is shown in Fig. 8.26.

The four heart sounds depicted in Figs. 8.14, 8.26, and 8.27 are induced by accelerations or decelerations of columns of blood that cause the cardiohemic system to vibrate. They are associated with the following hemodynamic events:

First heart sound (S_1): Closure and tensing of the AV valves with sudden deceleration of the blood being pushed against the valves.

Second heart sound (S_2): Closure of the semilunar valves and rapid deceleration of the blood flowing in a retrograde fashion toward the heart.

Third heart sound (S_3): Occurs early in diastole at the end of rapid ventricular filling, sudden tensing of the chordae tendineae, and deceleration of the filling wave of blood.

Fourth heart sound (S_4): Atrial contraction, acceleration of blood into the ventricles, and tensing of the AV valves when there is a transient reversal of the AV pressure gradient at the end of atrial systole.

The first and second heart sounds are auscultated normally in all domestic animals. The third and fourth sounds are normal in horses but a pathologic finding in dogs and cats. The presence of S_1 and S_2 plus a third or fourth heart

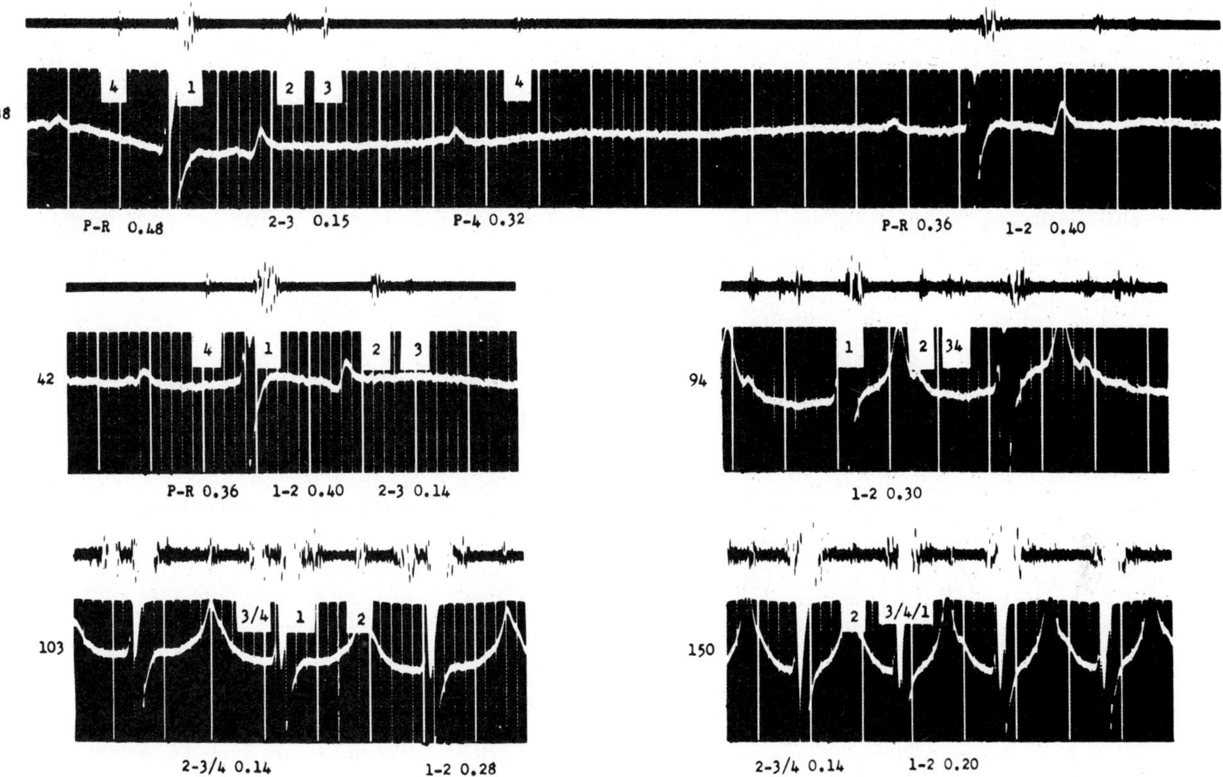

Figure 8.26. Effects of heart-rate changes on the heart sounds. Base-apex electrocardiogram and phonocardiogram from the mitral area of a 6-year-old thoroughbred mare. Heart rate per minute is given to the left of each record. Time intervals in seconds are given below each record for the PR, $S_1 - S_2$, $S_2 - S_3$, P $- S_4$ intervals. Fusion of two or three heart sounds into a single continuous sound is indicated by a slash separating the number of the sound: $\frac{3}{4}$ = fusion of S_3 and S_4; $\frac{3}{4}/1$ = fusion of S_3, S_4, and S_1. (*Top*) Heart rate: 38 beats per minute. Four heart sounds recorded. First-degree AV block with late S_4 recorded at the time of AV block. (*Middle left*) Heart rate: 42 beats per minute. (*Middle right*) Heart rate: 94 beats per minute. The PR interval has not shortened appreciably. S_3 follows the P wave and occurs just before S_4. (*Bottom left*) Heart rate: 103 beats per minute. P wave is buried in the preceding T wave. S_3 and S_4 summate ($\frac{3}{4}$) (summation gallop) producing a single sound that equals S_1 in amplitude. (*Bottom right*) Heart rate: 150 beats per minute. The summation sound ($\frac{3}{4}$) approaches and fuses with S_1 ($\frac{3}{4}/1$) producing a high-amplitude sound that begins before and ends after the QRS complex. S_2 is of lower amplitude.

sound gives an auscultated triple cadence much like the sound of a galloping horse; hence the name of *gallop rhythm*.

The first and second heart sounds may become split into two components when the right and left ventricles contract asynchronously. The most common split sound occurs in the dog with pulmonary hypertension secondary to heartworm disease. The elevated pulomonary vascular re-

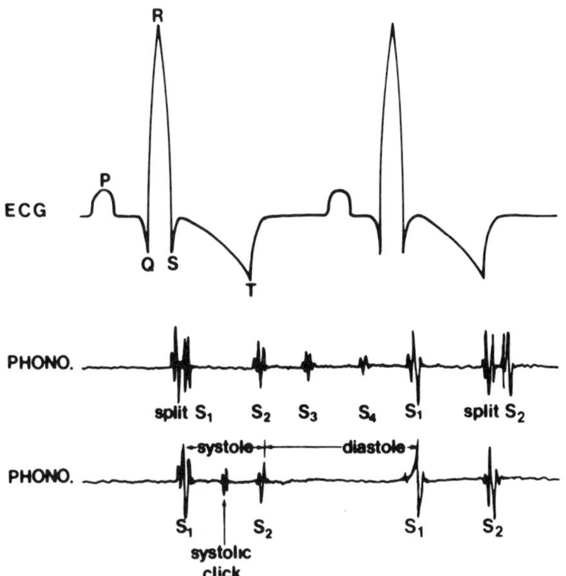

Figure 8.27. Illustration of relationships between the electrocardiogram (ECG) and timing of heart sounds. Electrical activity depicted on the ECG precedes cardiac mechanical activity shown by the phonocardiogram (PHONO). The QRS complex represents ventricular activation. The atrioventricular valves close as the ventricles eject blood through the semilunar valves and the first heart sound (S_1) occurs at the R-wave downstroke. The second heart sound (S_2) occurs at the end of ventricular contraction (i.e., ventricular systole) when the semilunar valves close, approximately at the time when ventricular repolarization is at its peak (e.g., peak of the T wave). The third heart sound (S_3) occurs during the first half of diastole, during passive ventricular filling (e.g., between the T wave and the ensuing P wave). The fourth heart sound (S_4) occurs late in diastole after atrial activation (P wave) and contraction. (From Gompf 1988, in Fox, ed., *Canine and Feline Cardiology,* Churchill, Livingstone, New York, p. 36.)

sistance, pulmonary arterial pressure, and right ventricular hypertrophy result in delayed relaxation of the right ventricle. Thus the aortic semilunar valve closes before the pulmonic semilunar valve.

In Figs. 8.28 and 8.29 the normal heart sounds and abnormal murmurs and transients are depicted schematically.

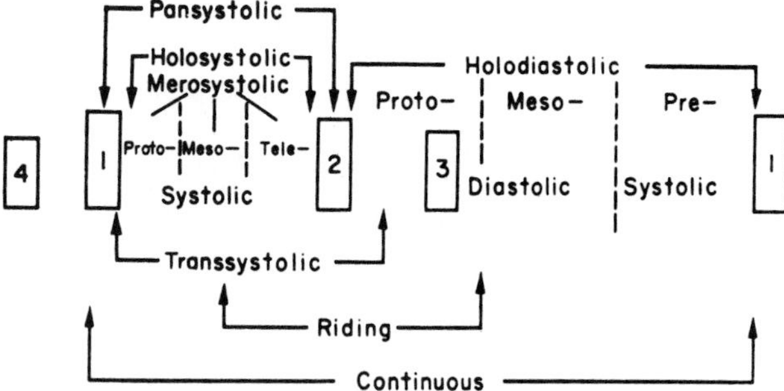

Figure 8.28. Various terms employed in describing cardiac murmurs. A pansystolic murmur begins before the end of S_1 (first heart sound) and ends after the onset of S_2 (second heart sound). A holosystolic murmur fills the systolic period but does not encroach on S_1 and S_2. Merosystolic murmurs occupy only a part of systole; protosystolic the first third, mesosystolic the middle third, and telesystolic the final third. A holodiastolic murmur fills the diastolic period: a protodiastolic the first third, mesodiastolic the middle third, and presystolic the last third. A transsystolic murmur is a holosystolic murmur that continues into diastole. A riding murmur begins before and ends after S_2. A continuous murmur lasts throughout the cardiac cycle from one heartbeat to the next.

The following list gives some clinical applications for cardiac muscle mechanisms and heart sounds:

1. The length-tension relationship of cardiac muscle is a crucial intrinsic factor in equalizing the right and left ventricular stroke volumes.
2. The Laplace relationship explains why the dilated heart functions at a mechanical disadvantage. Decreasing diastolic volume in acute cardiac failure is vital for resuscitation.
3. The basis of diagnostic cardiology is perfect knowledge of the pulsatile, acoustic, and electrical events of the cardiac cycle.
4. Appearance of S_3 (or its intensification in horses) is evidence of congestive heart failure.
5. Appearance of S_4 in species other than horses indicates some degree of AV block or that the atria are contracting against stiff, thick ventricles.
6. The timing of murmurs within the cardiac cycle aids in clinical diagnosis: systolic murmurs are associated with AV valve insufficiency or semilunar valve stenosis; continuous or "machinery" murmurs indicate *patent ductus arteriosus* (see Fig. 8.29).

ECHOCARDIOGRAPHY

Echocardiography is a noninvasive technique for evaluating cardiac dimensions, structure, and motion. It is a

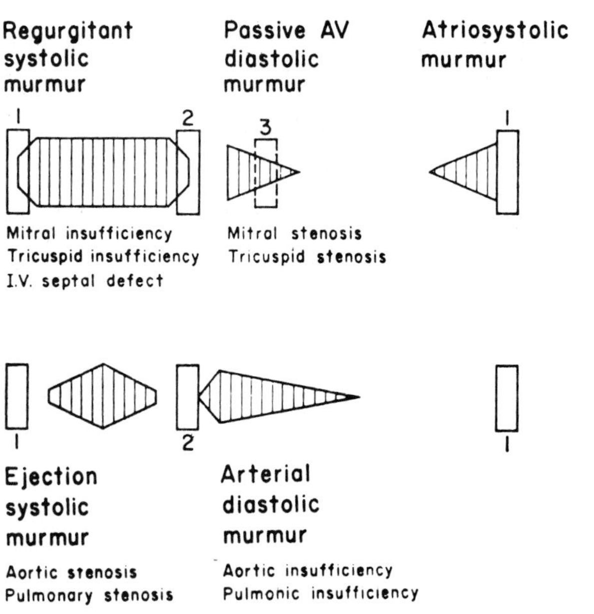

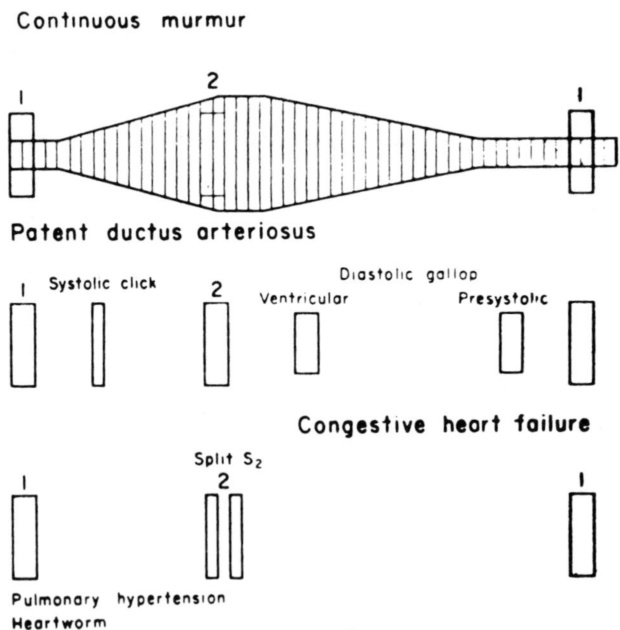

Figure 8.29. Some common abnormal murmurs. 1, 2, 3, First, second, and third heart sounds. Murmurs are shown in relation to heart sounds by figures with vertical lines. Widening of these figures indicates crescendo and narrowing decrescendo of sound intensity. Cardiac lesions or clinical syndromes associated with each murmur are listed below each diagram. (*Left*) The regurgitant murmur of mitral or tricuspid insufficiency is of constant intensity, the others shown vary in intensity. (*Right*) The *continuous murmur* of patent ductus arteriosus is often called a *machinery murmur.* It is caused by the waxing and waning of the intensity of sound vibrations set up by the continuous but pulsatile flow of blood from the aorta through the ductus arteriosus to the pulmonary artery. Splitting of the second heart sound occurs when the contraction of the two ventricles is asynchronous (as in bundle branch block) or when closure of the pulmonic valve is delayed because of pulmonic hypertension.

relatively recent addition to the armamentarium of the clinician, and interpretation of the results requires the mastery of basic cardiac physiology.

Genesis of an echocardiogram

Sound at frequencies in the millions of cycles per second (megahertz, MHz) resembles light in that it can be focused in a narrow beam and obeys the laws of reflection and refraction as it passes through tissue or some other dense medium. Diagnostic ultrasound is produced when a ceramic crystal with piezoelectric (pressure-electric) properties is induced to expand and contract, at frequencies between 2 and 10 MHz, in response to an electric current. Conversely, the pressure exerted on the piezoelectric element by the impact of a reflected sound wave (in the case of a sonogram) produces an electrical impulse. An ultrasound transducer contains a piezoelectric element that is rapidly pulsed to emit a brief burst of ultrasound and then switches into the receiving mode for collection of the reflected sound waves (echoes).

Imaging the heart with ultrasound

Ultrasound is reflected from the interface between tissues of dissimilar acoustic impedance, such as blood and muscle. The velocity of sound differs little as it passes through different tissues. Consequently, the distance separating sites of acoustic mismatch can be calculated from the time lapse between the sending of the primary packet of sound waves and the collection of returning echoes. Since the sound packets are pulsed at more than 1000 times per second, the spatial relationships between moving cardiac structures can be tracked at very short intervals of time. When the ultrasound beam is swept back and forth through the heart in a single plane, a sector scan is produced which creates a real-time, moving two-dimensional (2D) image. This format is complemented by the M-mode echogram in which reflections from moving structures intersected by a single stationary beam are displayed along a horizontal time axis (Fig. 8.30). The M-mode echogram is particularly useful for measuring cardiac dimensions and the velocity of moving structures.

Blood flow velocity and the Doppler echogram

Some hemodynamic information can be inferred from analysis of 2D and M-mode recordings. A more direct assessment of cardiac function can be obtained, however, by evaluation of the magnitude and timing of blood flow velocity during the cardiac cycle at specific locations within

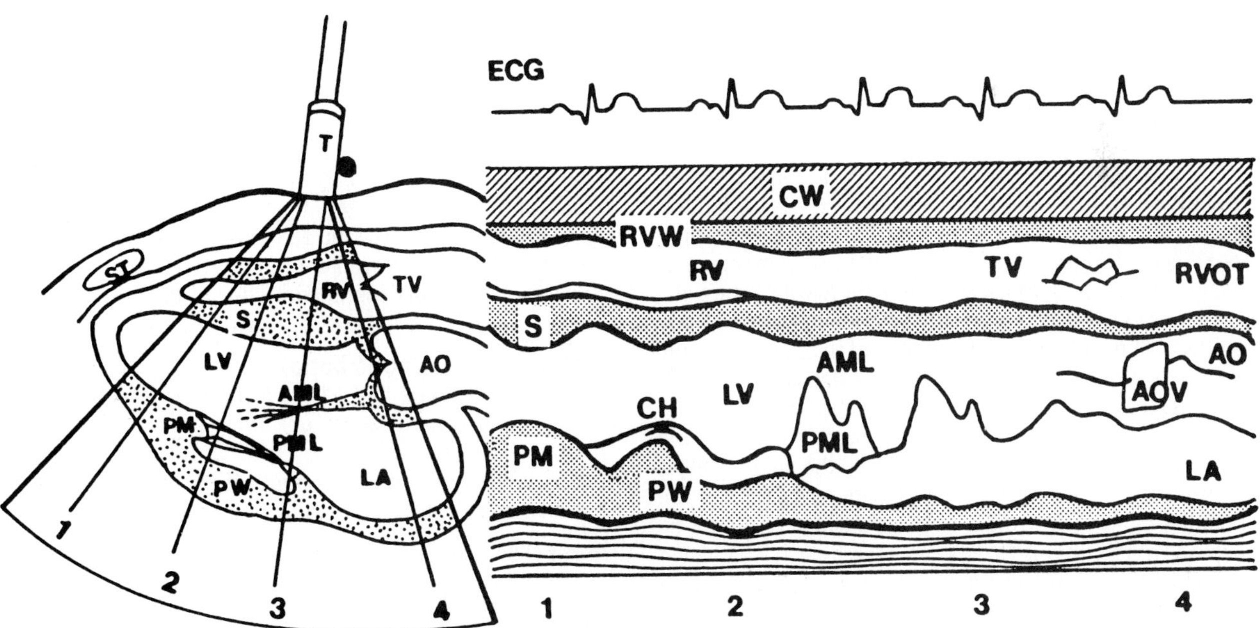

8.30. Schematic two-dimensional (2D) image of the dog heart (*left*) and corresponding M-mode echogram (*right*). The 2D image depicts the long-axis (heart base to apex) view that one can obtain by placing the transducer (T) on the right chest wall (CW). The boundaries of the sector scan and the orientation of the M-mode beam at four different positions are shown. The M-mode is illustrated as structures would appear in a continuous sweep of the echo beam, beginning at position 1 near the apex and finishing at the base of the heart in position 4. At least one full cardiac cycle is represented at each position. An M-mode echogram is always accompanied by an ECG for timing purposes. Notice the continuity between the interventricular septum (S) and the edge of the aortic root (Ao) nearest the transducer. Also, the chordae tendineae (CH) and anterior leaflet of the mitral valve (AML) are continuous with the posterior edge of the aortic root. ST, sternum; CW, chest wall artifact; RVW, right ventricular free wall; RV, right ventricular chamber; TV, tricuspid valve; RVOT, RV outflow tract; PM, papillary muscle; LV, left ventricular chamber; PW, LV posterior wall; PML, posterior mitral leaflet; AOV, aortic valve; LA, left atrium. The heavy echo bordering the posterior edge of the heart arises from the pericardium. Lung and echo reverberations appear in the far field behind the pericardium.

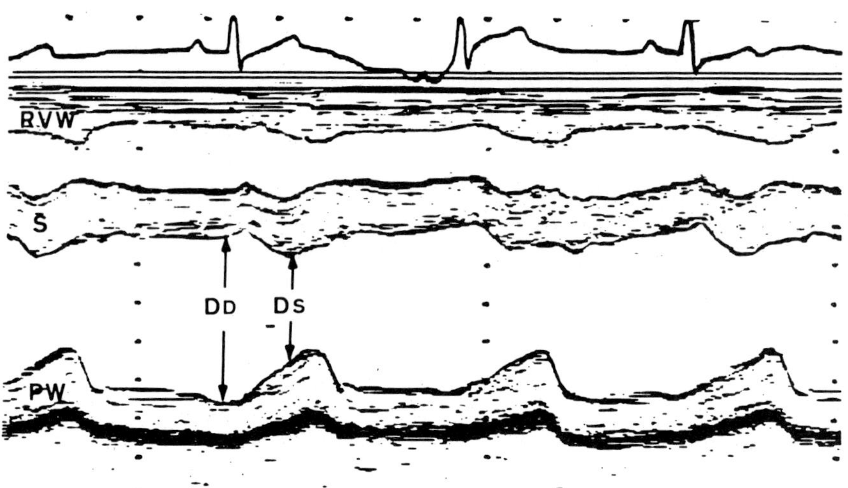

Figure 8.31. Vertical depth markers, 1 cm; horizontal time markers, 200 ms. M-mode echocardiogram at the midventricular level (position 2 in Fig. 8.30) of a normal 25 kg dog with a heart rate of approximately 100/min. The pericardium provides a highly reflective surface that is visible as the dense band of echoes behind the left ventricular posterior wall (PW). The pericardium over the right ventricular free wall (RVW) contributes to the chest wall artifact in the near field and is not visible as a distinct structure. Systolic thickening of the ventricular free wall and interventricular septum (S) with a corresponding reduction in chamber diameter is evident. The path of the echo beam approximates the true anatomic short axis of the left ventricular chamber. The diastolic (DD) and systolic (DS) short-axis dimensions of the left ventricle chamber are measured at the onset of the QRS complex and the nadir of the septal motion, respectively. If septal motion is ambiguous, the systolic dimension (DS) may be measured at the peak of the forward movement of the left ventricular posterior wall. Note that the septum and posterior wall move somewhat asynchronously. The short-axis dimension of the left ventricular chamber is reduced by 33 percent (shortening fraction). Early in diastole the left ventricular chamber opens up rapidly, as indicated by the steep slope of the posterior movement by the left ventricular endocardial surface. This coincides with the rapid, early passive filling phase, which at resting heart rates accounts for most of the stroke volume (stroke output) by the next beat. The chamber diameter then remains essentially unchanged until atrial systole produces a small additional posterior displacement of the left ventricular wall, adding slightly to the expansion of the chamber immediately preceding the QRS of the next ventricular contraction. The dynamics of the wall motion and changes in chamber dimension reflect the changes in the ventricular volume curve (see events of the cardiac cycle, Fig. 8.14).

the heart and great vessels. This can be accomplished by application of the Doppler principle to the analysis of ultrasound reflected from moving blood cells. When the ultrasound beam is directed at a column of blood moving away from the transducer, the echoes from these cells return at a frequency lower than that at which the sound was originally emitted.* If the blood is flowing toward the transducer, the frequency of the reflected ultrasound will exceed the emitted frequency. The difference between the emitted and reflected frequencies (Doppler shift) is directly related to the velocity of blood flow and the cosine of the angle (Theta) between the intersection of the ultrasound beam and the direction of flow. Since the angle of incidence cannot be determined reliably, flow velocity is ordinarily calculated by assumption of perfect alignment between the echo beam and the flow vector (i.e., $\cos \theta = 1$). As this angle widens ($\cos \theta < 1$) velocity will be increasingly underestimated.

*Doppler equation: $f_d = \frac{V \times \text{Cos } \theta \times 2f_0}{C}$, where F_d = Doppler shift frequency, V = flow velocity, $\cos \theta$ = angle of intersection between the interrogating beam of ultrasound and the flow velocity vector, fo = frequency of ultrasound emited by the transducer, and C = the velocity of ultrasound in tissue.

The velocity of blood cells moving away from the transducer produces a negative Doppler shift and, by convention, is displayed below the zero baseline. Conversely, the flow velocity is displayed above the zero baseline when a column of blood cells is moving toward the transducer.

Left ventricular contraction

Two-dimensional and M-mode echocardiography provides a convenient means of observing left ventricular wall motion. The most commonly used but highly imprecise index of left ventricular function is the reduction in chamber diameter (DD-DS) normalized to the end-diastolic diameter (DD) expressed in percent: $\left(\frac{\text{DD-DS}}{\text{DD}} \times 100\right)$ (Fig 8.31). Known as the "shortening fraction" (or fractional shortening), this index is the counterpart of the ejection fraction, which is based on the systolic reduction in ventricular volume. The shortening fraction is easily derived from an M-mode recording of the short-axis dimension (septum to posterior wall) of the left ventricle. Since the left ventricular volume is primarily reduced by circumferential fiber shortening, changes in the short-axis diameter are closely related to the state of myocardial contractility. Ventricular loading conditions, however, must also be taken into consideration when one is interpreting the functional significance of the shortening fraction since the ability of muscle fibers to shorten is inversely related to afterload and directly related to preload. Although individual variability is large, 35 to 40 percent is representative of the normal shortening fraction in medium-sized dogs. The value tends to be lower in giant breeds and higher in the miniature breeds.

Ventricular filling

Ventricular filling is a relatively complex phase of the cardiac cycle, during which work is performed on rather than by these two chambers. Information about filling mechanics can be obtained in a variety of ways from the echocardiogram by observation of the motion of the atrioventricular valves (Fig. 8.32), the velocity of blood flow into the ventricles (Fig. 8.33), and reciprocal changes in ventricular (Fig. 8.31) and atrial (Fig. 8.34) dimensions. Filling during diastole is passive and is affected primarily by the atrioventricular pressure gradient and ventricular compliance. Passive filling is compromised by a reduction in either of these two variables. At slow heart rates, there is adequate time for the ventricles to fill passively. As heart rate accelerates and diastole shortens, however, the atrial systolic contribution to ventricular filling becomes increasingly important and may ultimately account for 25 percent of the ventricular stroke volume.

The E point in the excursion of the anterior mitral leaflet (Fig. 8.32) represents the widest opening during the early passive phase of left ventricular filling. When the volume of flow through the mitral valve is low or the left ventricle becomes pathologically dilated, the distance between the E point of the anterior mitral leaflet and the interventricular septum increases. The timing and motion of the mitral and tricuspid valves are similar. The E point of an atrioventricular valve corresponds to the E wave of the Doppler recorded atrioventricular flow velocity profile (Fig. 8.33).

At slow heart rates following the period of ventricular diastasis, atrial systole reopens the partially closed atrioventricular valve, producing the A deflection in the M-mode recording of the valve's motion (Fig. 8.32). The A deflection of the valve corresponds to the A waves in the atrial pressure pulse (Fig. 8.14) and the Doppler-derived flow velocity profile recorded during atrial systole (8.33). Additional details about ventricular filling are provided in the legends for Figs. 8.32 to 8.34.

When they are audible, the third and fourth heart sounds

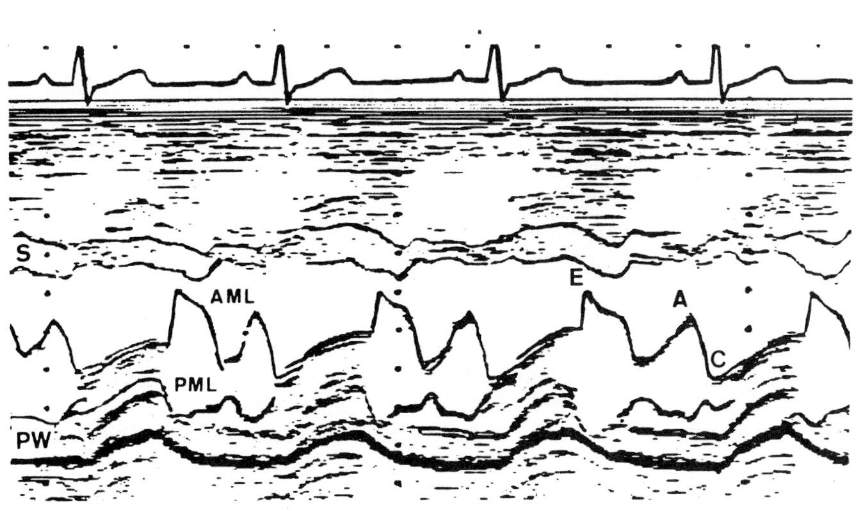

Figure 8.32. Vertical depth markers 1 cm; horizontal time markers, 200 ms. M-mode echocardiogram recorded from the dog heart illustrated in Fig. 8.31, but closer to the heart base through the mitral valve, corresponding to cursor No. 3 in Fig. 8.30. The M-mode beam is optimally positioned to produce echoes from the anterior (AML) and smaller posterior (PML) mitral leaflets but not the septum (S) and left ventricular posterior wall (PW). At the onset of diastole following the T wave of the electrocardiogram and coinciding with the beginning of rapid posterior movement of the left ventricular wall (Fig. 8.31), the valve opens rapidly. This is illustrated best by the AML, which swings toward the septum and, after reaching its most wide-open point (E), at first begins to close gradually and then quickly moves back toward the PML as the early passive filling phase ends abruptly. The rapid deceleration and cessation of blood flow into the left ventricle produce a slight pressure reversal across the valve and move it momentarily into a semiclosed position. After the P wave and subsequent atrial contraction, the valve reopens partially (A) during the atrial systolic phase of ventricular filling. Again, a transient pressure reversal closes the valve at the onset of ventricular systole (C). The first heart sound commences with tensing of the atrioventricular valves as ventricular pressure rises rapidly at the beginning of the isovolumetric contraction period. At this relatively slow heart rate (100/min), the two-part filling cycle of the left ventricle is evident from the M-shaped pattern of the mitral valve movement. As heart rate accelerates, the interval between the E and A excursions of the atrioventricular valves shortens. At rapid rates, passive and atrial systolic ventricular fillings occur at approximately the same time and the valve opens only once per cardiac cycle. This commonly occurs at heart rates exceeding 160/min.

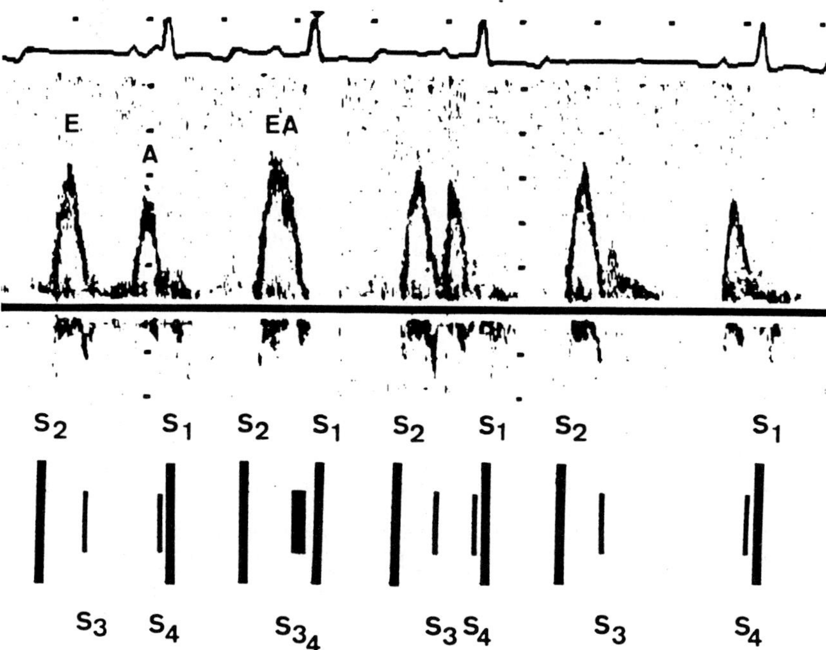

Figure 8.33. Vertical velocity markers, 20 cm/s; horizontal time markers, 200 ms. Pulsed-wave Doppler recording of the velocity of blood entering the left ventricle through the mitral valve in a normal 3.9 kg dog with sinus arrhythmia. The transducer is positioned near the left ventricular apex so that the echo beam can be directed into the orifice of the mitral valve. Since blood flows toward the transducer as it fills the left ventricle, the velocity is inscribed above the zero baseline. The interval between early passive (E) and late atrial systolic (A) phases of ventricular filling is determined by the length of diastole. The Doppler E and A waves correspond to the mitral valve E and A deflections (Fig. 8.32). Notice that during the longer cycles there is a period of diastasis during which ventricular inflow slows to an immeasurable rate or ceases, consistent with the static left ventricular chamber dimensions during the corresponding period (Fig. 8.31). During the shortest cycle, however, the two inflow phases overlap (EA). When the area beneath the E and A flow velocity profiles (mitral valve flow velocity integral) is used as an estimate of relative inflow volume, it can be seen that there is little difference in filling efficiency between the shortest and longest cycles. At heart rates in excess of 160/min passive filling is abbreviated and the atrial systolic contribution to ventricular filling becomes increasingly important. The shortest cycle in this illustration computes to a heart rate of 155/min. This Doppler illustration of ventricular filling dynamics also helps explain the genesis of the third (S_3) and fourth (S_4) heart sounds and summation gallop ($S_{3/4}$) in such species as the horse (Fig. 8.26) in which they are frequently audible even in normal animals. The events contributing to the genesis of these diastolic sounds are universal, but the audible threshold is reached only in large hearts where the hydraulic forces are sufficiently powerful to produce audible vibrations. The timing of the four heart sounds is diagrammed. The third and fourth heart sounds coincide with the end of the early passive and late atrial systolic phases of ventricular filling, respectively. The first (S_1) and second (S_2) heart sounds are synchronous with closure of the left and right atrioventricular valves at the onset of ventricular contraction and end-systolic closure of the aortic and pulmonary semilunar valves, respectively.

are associated with the rapid deceleration of blood at the end of the early passive and late atrial systolic phases of ventricular filling, respectively (Fig. 8.33). At rapid heart rates, an accentuated, single diastolic sound (summation gallop) may result from the simultaneous occurrence of the third and fourth sounds.

Systolic time intervals

The systolic time intervals of the ventricular pre-ejection period (PEP) and ejection time (ET) can be easily measured from the Doppler-derived flow velocity at the root of the aorta and pulmonary artery (Figs. 8.35 and 8.36). They are important conceptually for an understanding of ventricular performance. In a powerful, normally loaded ventricle, the intraventricular pressure rises rapidly during isovolumetric contraction. Consequently, the interval between the beginning of ventricular excitation (QRS complex of the electrocardiogram) and the onset of ejection (PEP) is short. An increase in inotropy or a decrease in afterload will further shorten the PEP, whereas a reduction in contractility or an elevation in afterload will have the opposite effect. Generally, a reciprocal relationship exists between changes in PEP and ET. For example, physiologic increases in preload will shorten PEP and lengthen ET by augmenting the total force of contraction according to the length-tension relationships of the Frank-Starling mechanism (heterometric autoregulation). Because the systolic time intervals are affected by loading conditions and heart rate, these variables must be taken into consideration in the interpretation of these indices of ventricular contraction. A comparison of the PEP and ET for the normal left and right ventricles is made in Figs. 8.35 and 8.36.

Echocardiography provides an easy way to evaluate the hemodynamic consequences of cardiac disease. Disturbances in heart rate and rhythm can significantly affect beat-to-beat performance of the heart and frequently com-

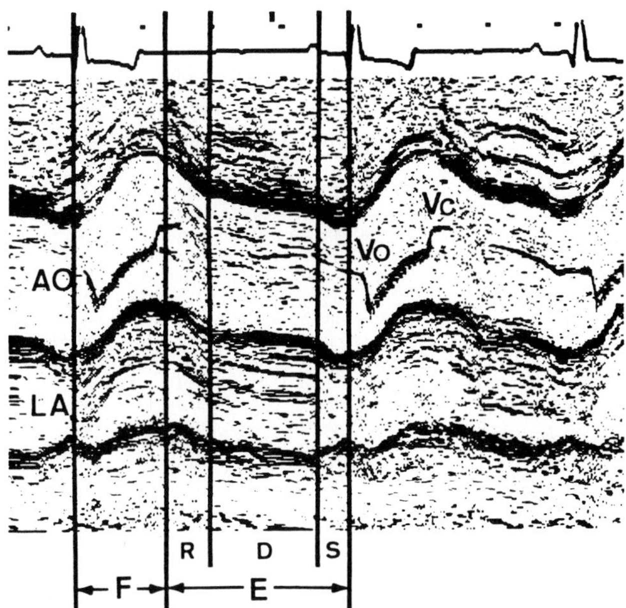

Figure 8.34. Vertical depth markers, 1 cm; horizontal time markers, 200 ms. M-mode echocardiogram of the aortic root (AO) and left atrium (LA) of a normal 30 kg dog. The ultrasound beam enters from the right chest wall corresponding to position 4 in Fig. 8.30. The aorta moves forward during ventricular systole as the left atrium fills (F) with blood returning from the pulmonary veins. At this relatively slow heart rate, left atrial emptying (E) occurs in three phases: rapid, passive ventricular inflow (R), a period of diastasis during which little or no flow occurs (D), and atrial systole (S). The slope of the adjacent aortic–left atrial walls corresponds to the rate at which atrial volume is changing during each phase. The motion of the left coronary cusp of the aortic valve is recorded. A high-frequency, low-amplitude flutter of the cusp occurs as blood is ejected rapidly through the open valve and lateral pressure across the cusp oscillates. The left ventricular ejection time can be measured from the interval between opening (Vo) and closing (Vc) of the aortic valve. The aortic component of the second heart sound (not shown) coincides with closure of the valve. The interval between the beginning of the QRS complex of the electrocardiogram and the opening of the aortic valve is the pre-ejection period of the left ventricle, which is composed of the electromechanical coupling interval and isovolumetric contraction period. Left ventricular isovolumetric relaxation occurs between closure of the aortic valve and the beginning of phase R of left atrial emptying, which also coincides with opening of the mitral valve (see Fig. 8.32).

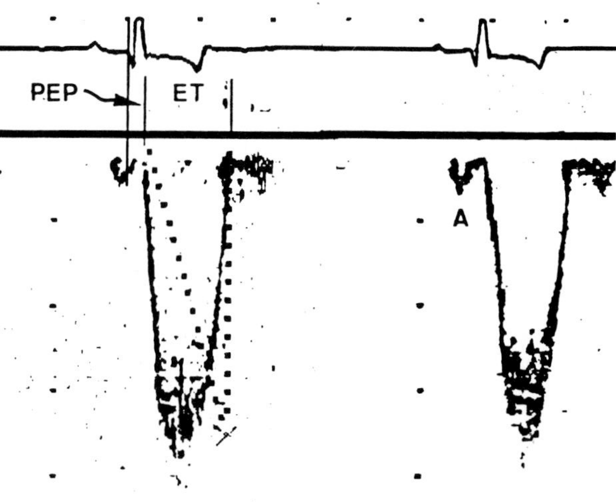

Figure 8.36. Vertical velocity markers, 20 cm/s; horizontal time markers, 200 ms. PEP, 40 ms; ET, 235 ms; modal velocity, 70 cm/s; peak flow velocity, 78 cm/s. Pulsed-wave Doppler echocardiogram of blood flow velocity at the pulmonic valve, recorded from the normal dog used to demonstrate aortic flow velocity in Fig. 8.35. Normally the systolic pressure in the right ventricle and main pulmonary artery is only about 20 percent as great as in the left ventricle and aorta. Consequently, the isovolumetric contraction period of the right ventricle is shorter than that of the left ventricle and blood flow into the low-pressure, more compliant pulmonary artery precedes flow into the aorta. A comparison of the pre-ejection periods (PEP) of the left (Fig. 8.35) and right (Fig. 8.36) ventricles confirms this sequence of events. Furthermore, because the end-diastolic pressure in the pulmonary artery may be only 5 to 10 mm Hg, atrial systole may generate enough pressure in the right ventricle to open the pulmonic valve briefly and produce a small ejection (A) before the ventricle actually begins to contract. Because the main pulmonary artery is wider and more distensible than the aorta, the right ventricle is able to empty more easily than the left ventricle. As a result, flow into the pulmonary artery does not accelerate as rapidly to a peak or reach as high a velocity as flow in the aorta. Also, since the afterload opposing shortening of muscle fibers in the right ventricular free wall is less than that faced by the left ventricle, the right ventricle normally has a longer ejection time (see Fig. 8.8.) A close comparison of Figs. 8.35 and 8.36 will illustrate these temporal differences. Because the ejection time (ET) of the right ventricle ordinarily exceeds that of the left, the pulmonary valve usually closes after the aortic valve. In normal animals separation of the two components of the second heart sound is sometimes wide enough during inspiratory augmentation of right ventricular filling to produce audible, "physiologic" splitting.

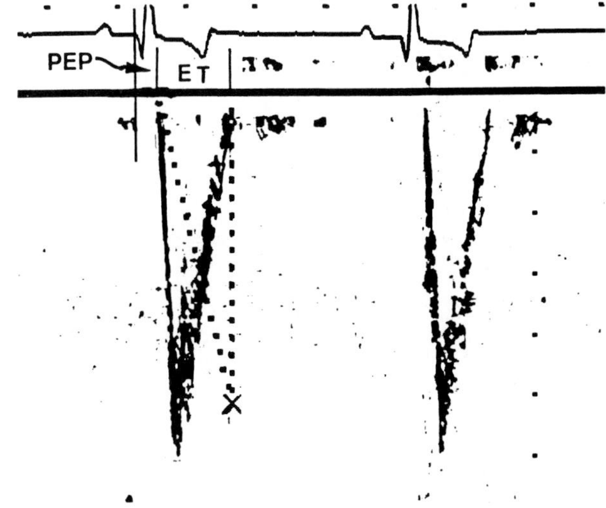

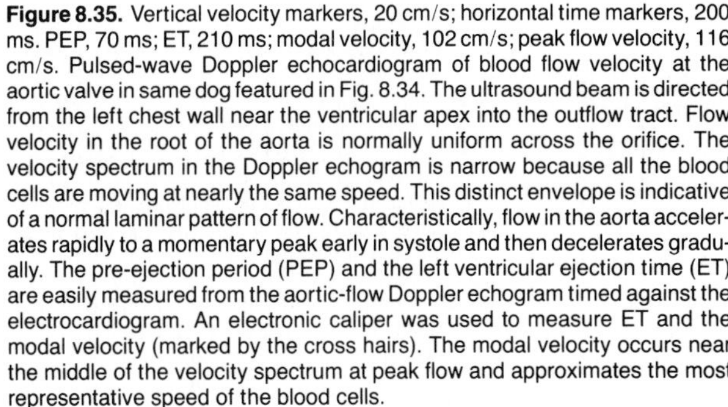

Figure 8.35. Vertical velocity markers, 20 cm/s; horizontal time markers, 200 ms. PEP, 70 ms; ET, 210 ms; modal velocity, 102 cm/s; peak flow velocity, 116 cm/s. Pulsed-wave Doppler echocardiogram of blood flow velocity at the aortic valve in same dog featured in Fig. 8.34. The ultrasound beam is directed from the left chest wall near the ventricular apex into the outflow tract. Flow velocity in the root of the aorta is normally uniform across the orifice. The velocity spectrum in the Doppler echogram is narrow because all the blood cells are moving at nearly the same speed. This distinct envelope is indicative of a normal laminar pattern of flow. Characteristically, flow in the aorta accelerates rapidly to a momentary peak early in systole and then decelerates gradually. The pre-ejection period (PEP) and the left ventricular ejection time (ET) are easily measured from the aortic-flow Doppler echogram timed against the electrocardiogram. An electronic caliper was used to measure ET and the modal velocity (marked by the cross hairs). The modal velocity occurs near the middle of the velocity spectrum at peak flow and approximates the most representative speed of the blood cells.

pound the deleterious effects of depressed contractility, malfunctioning valves or intracardiac and extracardiac shunting of blood. The importance of adequate ventricular end-diastolic volume on stroke output is illustrated by the great variability in cycle length (R-R electrocardiogram interval) and the absence of a coordinated atrial contraction immediately preceding ventricular systole in two dogs with atrial fibrillation (Figs. 8.37 and 8.38). In both dogs, myocardial contractility was depressed as a result of idiopathic dilated cardiomyopathy. A direct correlation between the

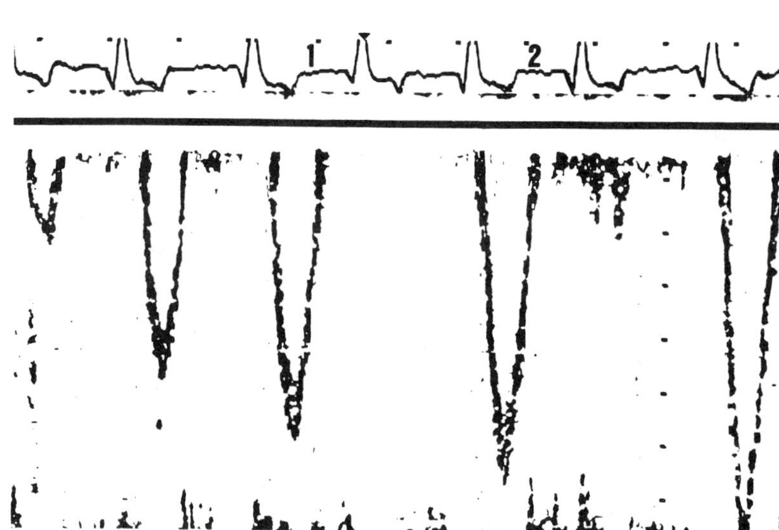

Figure 8.37. Vertical velocity markers, 20 cm/s; horizontal time markers, 200 ms. Pulsed-wave Doppler echocardiogram of blood flow velocity at the aortic valve of a 65 kg Great Dane in atrial fibrillation. The heart rate is approximately 180/min, and the rhythm is characteristically erratic. The areas within the flow-velocity inscriptions (flow velocity integrals) are proportional to the volume of blood (stroke volume) ejected by the left ventricle with each beat. The size of each stroke volume is influenced by the strength of ventricular contraction and the duration of the preceding filling cycle. The two shortest cardiac cycles (1 and 2) failed to produce ejections. During both, passive filling time was inadequate to distend the ventricle and thus stretch sarcomeres to a length from which they could generate sufficient force in accordance with Starling's law of the heart, to eject blood into the aorta. Ventricular filling in this dog was further compromised by the absence of a coordinated atrial contraction. However, partial distention of the ventricle preceding the two totally ineffective contractions, coupled with the next diastolic period, filled the ventricle sufficiently to produce the two beats with the highest peak flow velocity and longest ejection times. Notice that the larger of these two flow velocity integrals was preceded by a longer filling cycle. The discrepancy between heart rate and pulse rate (pulse deficit) that may exist when the heart rate is rapid and grossly irregular is illustrated by this Doppler echocardiogram. The variability of the pulse strength in this dog was palpable.

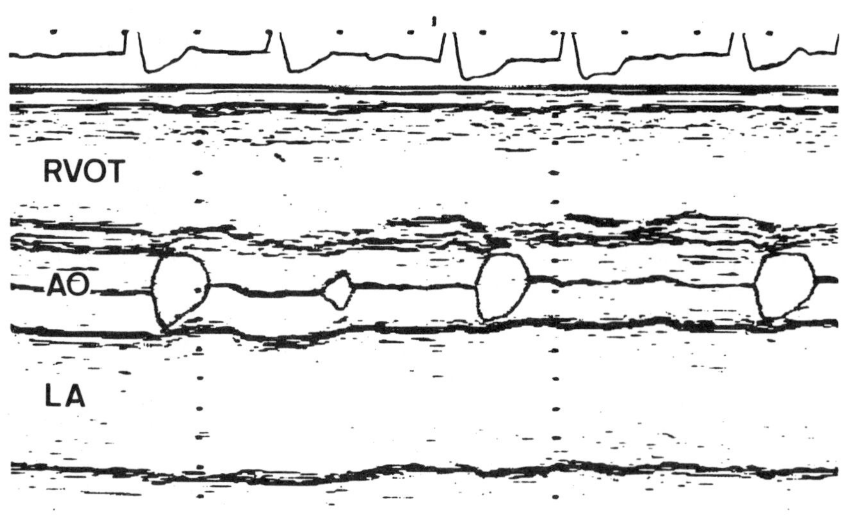

Figure 8.38. Vertical depth markers, 1 cm; horizontal time markers, 200 ms. M-mode echogram from a 25 kg dog with idiopathic dilated cardiomyopathy and atrial fibrillation. The heart rate is approximately 150/min and is characteristically erratic. The right ventricular outflow tract (RVOT) and left atrium (LA) are abnormally large. The absence of atrial systole is evident from the nonpulsatile movement of the aorta (AO) and left atrium. Echoes from the left and noncoronary cusps of the aortic valve in their open positions have been enhanced to facilitate visualization. The variability of left ventricular stroke volume illustrated by aortic flow velocity in Fig. 8.37 can also be inferred from the extent and duration of aortic valve opening in this dog. The longest left ventricular ejection times were measured from the first and last aortic valve echoes. In each instance, the preceding filling period was relatively long, accounting for the more effective ejection. The ventricular contraction preceding the last effective heartbeat had such a short filling cycle that no ejection occurred. The diastolic period preceding the second ventricular contraction from the left was slightly longer but still inadequate to generate much of an ejection, as can be seen by the delayed, gradual, and only partial opening of the valve cusps. Because of severe myocardial failure, left ventricular ejections were poorly sustained on each beat, resulting in gradual, premature closure of the aortic valve late in systole. From this illustration, it should be apparent why a second heart sound may not be generated when a ventricular contraction is very closely coupled to the preceding beat, as frequently happens in atrial fibrillation or premature ventricular ectopic beats.

duration of diastole or end-diastolic volume and ventricular stroke output can be recognized by comparison of the relative size of the flow velocity (velocity-time) integral of aortic blood flow velocity and the motion of the aortic valve (for details, see legends for Figs. 8.37 and 8.38).

REFERENCES

Badeer, H.S. 1963. Contractile tension in the myocardium. *Am. Heart J.* 66:432–34.

Badeer, H.S. 1984. *Cardiovascular Physiology.* Karger, New York.

Berne, R.M., and Levy, M.N. 1977. *Cardiovascular Physiology.* 3d ed. C.V. Mosby, St. Louis.

Brady, A.J. 1979. Mechanical properties of cardiac fibers. In R.M. Berne, N. Spereiakis, and S.R. Geiger, eds., *Handbook of Physiology.* Sec. 2, The Cardiovascular System. Vol. 1, *The Heart.* Am. Physiol. Soc., Bethesda Md., Pp. 461–74.

Braunwald, E. 1971. Control of myocardial oxygen consumption. *Am. J. Cardiol.* 27:416–32.

Braunwald, E., Ross, J., Jr., and Sonnenblick, E.H. 1967, 1968. *Mechanisms of Contraction of the Normal and Failing Heart.* Little, Brown. Boston.

Burns, J.W., Covell, J.W., and Ross, J., Jr. 1973. Mechanics of isotonic left ventricular contractions. *Am. J. Physiol.* 224:725–32.

Covell, J.W., Fuhrer, J.S., Boerth, R.C., and Ross, J., Jr. 1969. Production of isotonic contractions in the intact canine left ventricle. *J. Appl. Physiol.* 25:577–81.

Dejours, P., Garey, W., and Rahn, H. 1970. Comparison of ventilatory and circulatory flow between animals in various physiological conditions. *Respir. Physiol.* 9:108–17.

Detweiler, D.K., and Patterson, D.F. 1965. Heart sounds of the dog. *Ann. N.Y. Acad. Sci.* 127:322–40.

Ditmer, D.S., and Grebe, R.M., eds. 1963. *Handbook of Circulation.* W.B. Saunders, Philadelphia.

Dubois, E.F. 1936. *Basal Metabolism in Health and Disease.* Lea & Febiger, Philadelphia.

Fiegenbaum, H. 1986. *Echocardiography.* 4th ed., Lea & Febiger, Philadelphia.

Gompf, R.E. 1988. The clinical approach to heart disease: History and physical examination. In P.R. Fox, *Canine and Feline Cardiology.* Churchill, Livingstone, New York. Pp. 29–42.

Grubb, B.R. 1983. Allometric relations of cardiovascular function in birds. *Am. J. Physiol.*, 245:H567–72.

Guyton, A.C., Jones, C.E., and Coleman, T.G. 1973. *Circulatory Physiology: Cardiac Output and Its Regulation.* W.B. Saunders, Philadelphia.

Hatle, L., and Angelsen, B. 1985. *Doppler Ultrasound in Cardiology: Physical Principles and Clinical Applications.* 2nd ed., Lea & Febiger, Philadelphia.

Hill, A.V. 1939. Heat of shortening and dynamic constants of muscle. *Proc. R. Soc.* (London) (Biol.), ser. B 126:136–95.

Hoff, H.E., Geddes, L.A., and McCrady, J.E. 1966, 1965. The contributions of the horse to knowledge of the heart and circulation. I. Stephen Hales and the measurement of blood pressure. II. Cardiac catheterization and ventricular dynamics. III. James Mackenzie, Thomas Lewis, and the nature of atrial fibrillation. IV. James Hope and the heart sounds. *Conn. Med.* 29:795–801, 30:43–48, 126–32.

Holt, J.P., Rhode, E.A., and Kines, H. 1968. Ventricular volumes and body weight in mammals. *Am. J. Physiol.* 215:704–15.

Hope, J. 1835. *A Treatise on the Diseases of the Heart and Great Vessels.* W. Kidd, London.

Hori, M., Yelin, E.L., and Sonnenblick, E.H. 1982. Left ventricular diastolic suction as a mechanism of ventricular filling. *Jpn. Circ. J.* 46:125–29.

Jacobs, G., and Knight, D.H. 1985. M-mode echocardiographic measurements in nonanesthetized healthy cats: Effects of body weight, heart rate, and other variables. *Am. J. Vet. Res.* 46:1705–11.

Jewell, B.R., and Wilkie, D.R. 1958. An analysis of the mechanical components in frog's striated muscle. *J. Physiol.* (London) 143:515–40.

Jewell, B.R., and Wilkie, D.R. 1960. The mechanical properties of relaxing muscle. *J. Physiol.* (London) 152:30–47.

Knight, D.H. 1989. Pathophysiology of heart failure. In S.J. Ettinger, *Textbook of Veterinary Internal Medicine.* 3d ed. W.B. Saunders, Philadelphia. Pp. 899–922.

Laennec, R.T.H. 1962. *A Treatise on the Diseases of the Chest.* A translation of *Traite de l'Auscultation medicale.* 1819. Facsimile of London 1821 ed. Hafner, New York.

Little, R.C., and Little, W.C. 1989. *Physiology of the Heart and Circulation.* 4th ed. Yearbook Medical, Chicago.

Lombard, C.W. 1984. Normal values of the canine M-mode echocardiogram. *Am. J. Vet. Res.* 45:2015–18.

McKusick, V.A. 1958. *Cardiovascular Sound in Health and Disease.* Williams & Wilkins, Baltimore.

Milnor, W.R. 1982. *Hemodynamics.* Williams & Wilkins, Baltimore.

Patterson, D.F., Detweiler, D.K., and Glendenning, S.A. 1965. Heart-sounds and murmurs of the normal horse. *Ann. N.Y. Acad. Sci.* 127:242–305.

Pollack, G.H. 1970. Maximum velocity as an index of contractility in cardiac muscle: A critical evaluation. *Circ. Res.* 26:111–27.

Pollack, G.H. 1971. Is V max a valid contractile index? *Am. Heart J.* 81:572–73.

Pool, P.E., and Sonnenblick, E.H. 1967. The mechanochemistry of cardiac muscle. *J. Gen. Physiol.* 50:951–65.

Ross, J., Jr. 1985. Cardiovascular system. In J.B. West, *Best and Taylor's Physiological Basis of Medical Practice.* 11th ed. Williams & Wilkins, Baltimore. Pp. 184–222.

Sagawa, J. 1978. The ventricular pressure-volume diagram revisited. *Circ. Res.* 43:677–87.

Sagawa, K. 1981. The end-systolic pressure-volume relation of the ventricle: Definition, modifications, and clinical use. *Circulation* 63:1223–27.

Sarnoff, S.J., and Braunwald, E. 1959. Hemodynamic determinants of myocardial oxygen consumption. In A.A. Luisada, ed., *Cardiology.* McGraw-Hill, New York. Vol. 1, 2-24–2-30.

Skelton, C.L., and Sonnenblick, E.H. 1974. Myocardial energetics. In I. Mirsky, D.N. Ghista, and H. Sandler, eds., *Cardiac Mechanics.* Wiley, New York. Pp. 113–37.

Smetzer, D.L., Hamlin, R.L., and Smith, C.R. 1977. Cardiovascular sounds. In M.J. Swenson, *Dukes' Physiology of Domestic Animals.* 9th ed. Cornell University Press. Ithaca, N.Y. Pp. 95–101.

Smetzer, D.L., Smith, G.R., and Hamlin, R.L. 1965. The fourth heart sounds in the equine. *Ann. N.Y. Acad. Sci.* 127:306–21.

Snellen, H.A. 1980. *E.J. Marey and Cardiology.* Kooyker Scien. Publ., Rotterdam.

Sonnenblick, E.H. 1966. The mechanics of myocardial contraction. In S.A. Briller and H.L. Conn, Jr., eds., *The Myocardial Cell.* University of Pennsylvania Press, Philadelphia. Pp. 173–250.

Sonnenblick, E.H. 1968. Correlation of myocardial ultrastructure and function. *Circulation* 38:29–44.

Sonnenblick, E.H. 1970. Contractility of cardiac muscle (letter to editor). *Circ. Res.* 27:479–81.

Sonnenblick, E.H., Parmley, W.W., Urschel, C.W., and Brutsaert, D.L. 1970. Ventricular functions: Evaluations of myocardial contractility in health and disease. *Prog. Cardiovasc. Dis.* 12:449–66.

Spero, D., and Sonnenblick, E.H. 1964. Comparison of contractile process in heart and skeletal muscle. *Circ. Res.* 15(Suppl. 2):14–37.

Spotnitz, H.M., Sonnenblick, E.H., and Spero, D. 1966. Relationship of ultrastructure to function in intact heart: Sarcomere structure relative to pressure volume curves or intact left ventricles of dog and cat. *Circ. Res.* 18:49–66.

Thomas, W.P. 1984. Two-dimensional, real time echocardiography in the dog—technique and anatomic validation. *Vet. Radiol.* 25:50–64.

Tsakiris, A.G., Vandenberg, R.A., Banchero, N., Sturm, R.E., and Wood, E.H. 1968. Variation of left ventricular and diastolic pressure, volume, and ejection traction with changes in outflow resistance in anesthetized dogs. *Circ. Res.* 23:213–22.

Wiggers, C.J. 1952. *Circulatory Dynamics.* Grune & Stratton, New York.

CHAPTER 9

Regulation of the Heart | by David K. Detweiler

Regulation of cardiac output is effected through mechanisms that operate within the myocardium itself (*intrinsic* or *autoregulation*) and factors outside the heart (*extrinsic regulation*). These mechanisms adjust cardiac frequency and stroke volume by changing the force, velocity, duration, and extent of contraction. Conductivity is adjusted to maintain proper timing of atrial and ventricular systole and the temporal sequence of ventricular activation. Finally, the outputs of the left and right sides of the heart are coordinated so that they remain equal.

INTRINSIC REGULATION OF VENTRICULAR FUNCTION

Control mechanisms within the myocardium itself make it possible for isolated myocardial preparations to adapt to changes in work load. For example, in dogs with denervated hearts, cardiac output adjusts appropriately during exercise and rest. The best known of these intrinsic adaptive responses is the response to changes in resting myocardial fiber length, the Frank-Starling mechanism. It has been termed *heterometric autoregulation*. The term *homeometric autoregulation* is used to designate other intrinsic adaptive mechanisms that do not involve myocardial fiber length.

Heterometric autoregulation

As described for isolated papillary muscle and the entire isolated heart (Chap. 8), increasing fiber length or diastolic volume of the heart, within physiological limits, increases contractile force and ventricular stroke work. Thus the denervated heart can respond appropriately to alterations in filling pressure, duration of diastole (filling time), and its own distensibility.

Preload

The counterpart of the preload of an in vitro muscle strip described in Chapter 8 is the distending force in the ventricle at the end of diastolic filling (end-diastolic pressure). Assuming that ventricular compliance remains unchanged, it can be used as a measure of the volume change or stretch of the myocardial fibers.

Afterload

The intact ventricle also engages a counterpart of the afterload described for isolated ventricular muscle in Chapter 8. This is not a simple constant weight like that attached to an isolated muscle strip, because it is made up of changing forces that oppose ejection of blood into the aorta. These include aortic pressure (which rises and falls during ejection), blood viscosity, viscoelastic properties of the arterial system, and vascular resistance. Input impedance is the most complete measure of afterload, but it is complicated to analyze (Chap. 5). Thus in representing afterload as aortic pressure it must be recognized that this can only be a partial component of the real afterload.

These two terms, preload and afterload, have become part of the vocabulary of cardiac physiology, and their meaning and limitations require understanding.

Homeometric autoregulation

Frequency of contraction and temperature influence contractile strength for any given fiber length. Myocardial tension was thought to have a similar effect, but its importance is now in doubt.

Myocardial tension

When aortic resistance (and therefore aortic pressure) is elevated in a heart-lung preparation, ventricular volume at first increases. Then it returns toward its control value, indicating a positive inotropic effect that is not entirely dependent on a change in myocardial fiber length. This effect, first demonstrated by Anrep (1912) and sometimes called the *Anrep phenomenon,* implies that increased myocardial tension can, in some mysterious way, increase contractile strength. An alternate explanation is provided via evidence that in the intact heart an abrupt increase in intraventricular pressure causes a transient subendocardial ischemia. This results in a decrease in contractile strength, which accounts in part for the initial increase in ventricular volume. Subsequently, the subendocardial ischemia is relieved through vascular autoregulation, and the decrease in contractile strength is corrected. As ventricular contractility improves, the ventricular volume returns toward its control value. This effect has been demonstrated in intact, unanesthetized dogs and may have significance under either physiological or pathological states.

On isolated papillary muscle an increased load without increased stretch (i.e., afterload) may produce increased, decreased, or unchanged contractility, depending on temperature and contraction frequency. Little effect could be expected at physiological heart rates and body temperature. Accordingly, the effect of myocardial tension on contractility seems to be an elusive laboratory phenomenon that has little importance under physiological circumstances.

Rate and rhythm effects

The strength of myocardial contraction is markedly influenced by the time interval between beats. This was first described by Bowditch (1871) as the *staircase,* or *treppe, phenomenon* in the frog ventricle: after a period of rest, subsequent contractions increase stepwise in strength until a plateau is reached.

In mammalian ventricular muscle a premature contraction is weaker than the preceding beats, but then for several regular beats following the premature beat the contractions are greater than normal. This phenomenon has been called *postextrasystolic potentiation, premature activation potentiation,* or *prematurity potentiation.* Either of the last two terms seems to be more apt than the first. Another phenomenon exhibited by ventricular muscle of most mammals is that the rate of tension development, the peak tension developed, and the maximum shortening increase with frequency over the physiological range. This is known as *frequency potentiation.* It requires many beats to attain a steady state, whereas prematurity potentiation seems to be almost complete in the first potentiated contraction. (One must note, however, that if premature contractions are repeated in a series, the magnitude of prematurity potentiation increases; see below.)

These observations have been explained by an analysis which suggests that two interval-dependent processes influence myocardial contractility in opposite directions as follows: (1) *Negative inotropic effect of activation* (NIEA) is a temporary effect that tends to decrease the strength of contraction in subsequent beats. Each beat induces a relatively large NIEA, but it disappears rapidly a few seconds after any given contraction. (2) *Positive inotropic effect of activation* (PIEA) is a temporary effect that tends to increase the strength of contraction of subsequent beats. It disappears slowly, with a halftime of decay on the order of 0.5 to 1.0 minute.

Inasmuch as both NIEA and PIEA are cumulative, the strength of a given contraction in a series is equal to that of a rested, isolated, or standard contraction plus whatever PIEA and minus whatever NIEA may have accumulated and persisted. Under steady-state conditions at a regular frequency, the PIEA and NIEA increase and decrease by constant amounts during the interval between each two beats. Each beat produces more NIEA than PIEA, but the negative effect decays much more rapidly than the positive. Premature beats occur at an instant when there is more of both PIEA and NIEA than at the time of a regular beat, but the NIEA predominates and the premature beat therefore is weaker than a regular beat. At the instant when a regular beat begins in a normal series, the longer-lasting PIEA is predominant over the NIEA.

In Fig. 9.1 the various effects of interval changes on tension development of a mammalian papillary muscle are shown. The papillary muscle system clearly responds differently, depending on the preceding rate and rhythm of contractions. It exhibits information retention or "memory." At least three mechanisms appear to account for these interval-strength phenomena: (1) calcium-, (2) sodium-, and 3 regulatory protein phosphorylation–related effects of activation (Ca-REA, Na-REA, and PP-REA, respectively).

1. Ca-REA are discussed in Chapter 6 under excitation-contraction coupling. At excitation, sarcoplasmic reticulum (SR) Ca^{2+} is released from the functional cisternae of the SR to cause contraction. Relaxation is caused by pumping this Ca^{2+} back into the longitudinal SR. The SR release sites are then replenished with a time constant of less than 1.0 second (delayed restitution). The amount of available Ca^{2+} present at the release site will thus depend on the interval between contractions. Since Ca^{2+} enters the cell during each contraction, the availability of Ca^{2+} to replenish storage sites within the cell will also increase with the frequency of contraction.

2. In Na-REA, an electrogenic, potential-dependent sarcolemmal exchange of three Na^+ for one Ca^{2+} promotes influx of extracellular Ca^{2+} in exchange for intracellular Na^+. Na^+ influx through fast and slow channels produces a frequency-dependent increase in intracellular Na^+. This enhances Ca^{2+} influx during each activation in exchange for Na^+ and thus increases the availability of Ca^{2+} for excitation-contraction coupling.

3. In PP-REA, phosphorylation of slow channels by a cyclic adenosine monophosphate (AMP)-dependent protein kinase occurring at each activation may result in im-

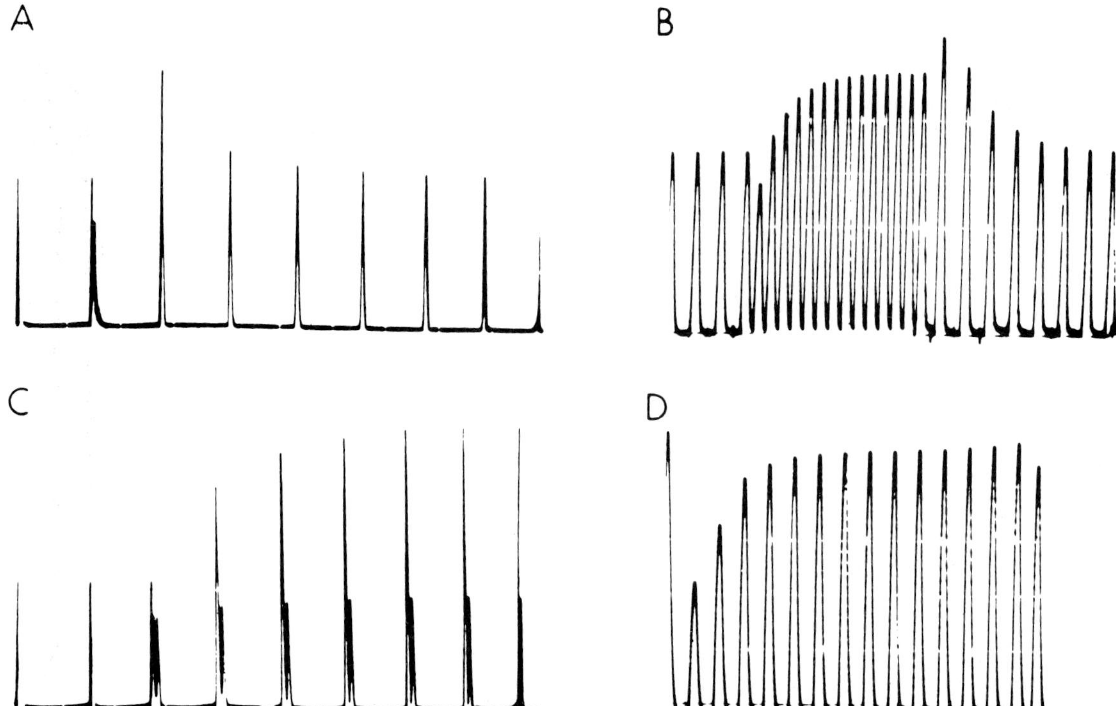

Figure 9.1. The effect of interval changes on rabbit papillary muscle. (*A*) In this example of *premature activation potentiation,* a markedly premature and weak contraction immediately follows the second contraction. It is inhibited by NIEA and therefore of lower amplitude than the two preceding contractions. The following (fourth) contraction is strongly potentiated by PIEA. This potentiation falls off, first abruptly then gradually, in the ensuing contractions. (*B*) Ascending (positive, Bowditch) and descending (negative, Woodworth) *staircase* (treppe) responses to sudden increase and then decrease in rate of stimulation. (*C*) The response to *paired pacing* in which the muscle is driven by paired stimuli. The second stimulus produces a small mechanical effect, but the following beat is potentiated (PIEA) progressively increasing the response to the first of the paired stimuli until a plateau is reached. (*D*) Response to a train of stimuli at constant intervals followed by a test stimulus at an interval shorter than the interval between stimuli in the train. The response is reduced. Had the interval preceding the test stimulus been greater than that between stimuli in the train, the test response would have been potentiated (as in *B*). (From Johnson 1979 in Berne, Sperelakis, and Geiger, eds., *Handbook of Physiol.,* sec. 2, vol. 1, *The Heart,* Am. Physiol. Soc., Washington.)

proved influx of Ca^{2+} during contraction. This mechanism may be active in the atria, but there is no evidence of its operation in the ventricles.

The force-interval relationships may differ in detail among mammals (e.g., rat vs. other mammals); they are present in heart muscle of birds, reptiles, and fish but are absent in amphibia.

From the foregoing, it can be seen that the three intrinsic factors that affect the inotropic state of the myocardium and thus cardiac performance are (1) *preload,* (2) *afterload,* and (3) *heart rate and rhythm.* In the following discussion various extrinsic factors that govern regulation of the inotropic state as well as heart rate will be elaborated.

Temperature

In isolated preparations of mammalian hearts, hypothermia augments contractile strength. In contrast, in intact dogs either moderate hypothermia (body temperature of 25 to 30°C) or pyrexia (body temperature of 41 to 43°C) decreases ventricular contractile capacity. A possible explanation of this apparent discrepancy is that in the intact heart the cooling depresses cardiac sympathetic tone; it is known that prior blockade of adrenergic receptor sites tends to counteract the inhibitory effect of cooling. The thermal limits of both human and dog hearts are between 26 and 44°C; as the heart approaches either of these limits, myocardial conduction and contractility are both depressed.

EXTRINSIC REGULATION

Nervous control of the heart

Innervation of the heart

The cardiac nerves arise bilaterally from sympathetic and parasympathetic (vagal) trunks. In all mammals the general anatomic plan is similar but differs in detail in the various species. Efferent sympathetic cardiac branches arise from the cranial, middle, and caudal cervical ganglia and from the first four or five thoracic ganglia. Their preganglionic fibers originate from the intermediolateral column of the spinal cord, usually from the second to the sixth thoracic segments. They synapse either in the cervical or vertebral ganglia or in the ganglia of the cardiac plexus. In addition, a substantial proportion of afferent fibers, probably mediating pain sensation, course in the sympathetic nerves. The parasympathetic fibers arise from the vagal trunks at the cranial cervical, caudal cervical, and thoracic levels with supplementation from the right and left recurrent laryngeal nerves. In addition to a considerable proportion of afferent fibers, the vagal branches are chiefly composed of preganglionic cholinergic axons that synapse in ganglia on or near the heart. The extrinsic autonomic nerves merge to form cardiac nerves and plexuses. These pass to the heart along the great veins and arteries. Within these plexuses, vagal components synapse on ganglion cells while sympathetic and afferent components pass through without relay. The term *plexus* may be misleading since careful study reveals continuity of individual cardiac nerves as they approach the heart.

The atria are extensively innervated by noradrenergic, cholinergic, and afferent fibers, and cholinergic ganglion cells are present, especially on their posterior surfaces. The sinoatrial (SA) and atrioventricular (AV) nodes are richly innervated; the SA node receives fibers primarily from the right side of the body and the AV node from both sides. Ventricular innervation, with the exception of the bundle of His, is much less profuse than atrial innervation (in mammals, not birds), and most species have only moderate cholinergic innervation, primarily following the course of the coronary arteries. Diving mammals may be exceptions since they can slow their hearts well below the AV rate as part of the diving reflex. In ungulates the AV bundle of His is richly supplied with nerves. The ventricular myocardium receives its modest innervation from the coronary plexuses that follow these arteries. They are predominantly composed of noradrenergic fibers.

In many species, the vagus and cervical sympathetic nerve fibers are enclosed in the same epineural sheath, the vagosympathetic trunk. The two nerves can sometimes be separated by blunt dissection (Figs. 9.2 and 9.3).

The aortic or depressor nerve, which carries impulses from the baroreceptor regions of the aortic arch and the brachiocephalic and common carotid arteries, is a separate nerve in the neck in rabbits (Fig. 9.2). This may be the case in some rats, and a separate nerve bound together with the vagus can be identified in cats and monkeys. In the dog and several other species the aortic nerve is rarely separate in the neck from the remainder of the vagal fibers. It has been called the depressor nerve ever since Cyon and Ludwig (1866) first described the fall in blood pressure and cardiac slowing caused by stimulation of its central end.

The stellate ganglia or cervicothoracic ganglia, right and left, result from fusion of certain vertebral sympathetic ganglia in the anterior thoracic and caudal cervical regions. The anatomical details vary in different species and to some extent within the same species. For example, the caudal cervical ganglion of the human is part of the stellate ganglion in the dog, and the caudal cervical ganglion of the dog corresponds to the middle cervical ganglion of the human.

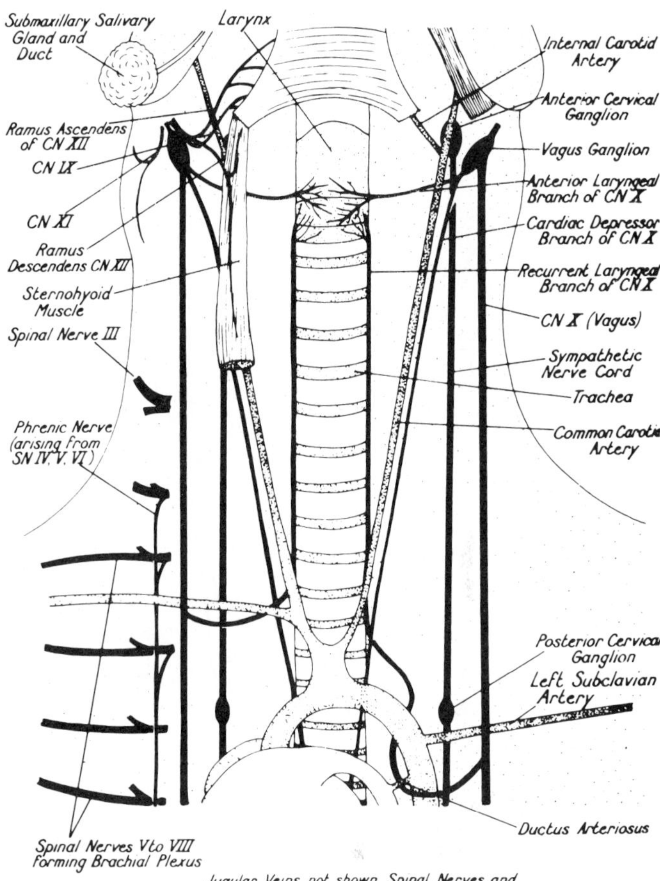

Figure 9.2. Diagram of the separate course of the cervical sympathetic nerve, cardiac depressor nerve, and vagus in the neck of the rabbit. CN, cranial nerve; SN, spinal nerve. (From Wells 1964, *The Rabbit: A Practical Guide,* Heinemann, London.)

In many species (including the dog, which has been most extensively studied) the sympathetic trunk cranioventral to the stellate ganglion splits to pass around the subclavian artery as two branches, the ansae subclavia. The majority of sympathetic nerve impulses reach the heart through the stellate ganglia; stimulation of the right stellate ganglion has a relatively greater effect on the heart rate, and stimulation of the left stellate has a relatively greater effect on the left ventricular contractility.

The sympathetic nerves have positive and the vagal fibers have negative chronotropic and inotropic actions on the heart. Vagal stimulation slows the discharge rate of the SA node, slows or blocks AV conduction, and decreases atrial and to a small extent ventricular contractility. Sympathetic stimulation has the opposite effect, and its positive inotropic action on the ventricles and atria is powerful.

Stimulation of the right vagus ordinarily has a greater effect on the SA node (negative chronotropy) than does

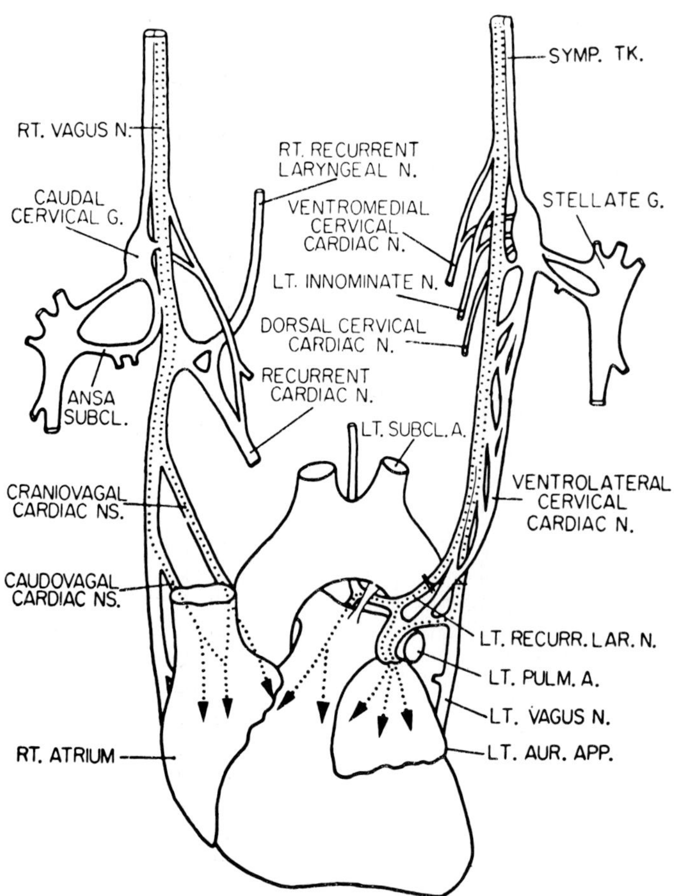

Figure 9.3. Diagram of the vagosympathetic trunks and their relations to the stellate ganglia, ansa subclavia, and caudal cervical ganglia in the dog. A., artery; AUR. APP., auricular appendage; G., ganglion; LT., left; N., nerve; NS., nerves; PULM. A., pulmonary artery; RECURR. LAR. N., recurrent laryngeal nerve; RT., right; SUBCL., subclavia; SYMP. TK., sympathetic trunk. (From Mizeres 1957, *Anat. Rec.* 127:109–15.)

stimulation of the left vagus. Most evidence indicates that the left vagus and left sympathetic nerves dominate over the right-sided innervation of the AV node, at least with maximal stimulation intensities. Stimulation of the right stellate ganglion in the dog has a marked cardioacceleratory (SA node) effect and a moderate inotropic effect on the left ventricle, while stimulation of the left stellate ganglion reverses these relations. The negative inotropic effects of the vagus are primarily exerted on the atria (where the vagal innervation is rich), but negative inotropic effects can also be demonstrated on the ventricles. This negative inotropic vagal effect becomes more potent as the level of cardiac sympathetic activity becomes greater. This is true because acetylcholine released from vagal endings reacts with presynaptic acetylcholine (muscarinic) receptors on sympathetic nerve endings that reduce the amount of norepinephrine released.

Heart rate

The resting heart rate is related to body size, metabolic rate, and autonomic balance characteristic of the species. Data on heart rates in the scientific literature are often disparate because of differing environmental conditions. For domestic animals, values found in the clinical literature appear to be more representative. Table 9.1 lists representative heart rates for various species.

Broadly considered, heart rate and body mass in different species are related. A logarithmic equation has been proposed to represent the relation between heart rate (HR) and body weight (in kg): $HR = 241 \cdot kg^{-0.25}$ (see Scaling, Chap. 5). Obviously, certain species depart from this relationship. The heart rate of the domestic rabbit ranges from 180 to 350 beats per minute, and that of the hare is much slower at 60 to 70 beats per minute. The heart rate range for dairy cattle is 48 to 84 beats per minute, and that for horses is lower at 28 to 40 beats per minute. Thus coursing animals like the hare and horse have higher vagal tone and lower resting heart rates than more sedentary species of similar size.

Heart rates in avians vary greatly, depending on age of subject and conditions of recording. In general, restraint tends to induce marked tachycardia. Some reported rates per minute for adult birds are as follows: chicken, 191 to 354; turkey, 160 to 219; duck, 175 to 194; and geese, 80 to 144.

Heart rate and cardiac output. At lower physiological heart rates and up to some maximum, cardiac output increases with increased heart rate. Depending on the physiological state of the circulatory system, as rate accelerates a point is reached where increasing the heart rate further results in a progressive decrease in cardiac output. For a physiological rate range, the relation is such that the larger the stroke volume is at the lowest rate, the higher are the heart rates at which peak outputs occur. Thus if the stroke

Table 9.1. Representative heart rate ranges in beats per minute

Animal	Rest*	Exercise	Newborn/young
Elephant	25–40		
Horse	28–40	180–240	
Ox	36–60		
Dairy cow	48–84		140–160
Swine	70–120		230
Human	60–80	100–200	100–160
Sheep, goat	70–80		
Dog	70–120	220–325	140–275
Cat	120–140		170–300
Rhesus monkey	160–330		
Rabbit	180–350		120–240
Hare	60–70		
Guinea pig	200–300		
Rat	250–400		
Mouse	450–750		

*More rapid resting rates are often reported for all nonhuman species owing to excitement tachycardia during restraint.

From various sources (see Grauwiler 1965; *Herz und Kreislauf der Säugetiere,* Berkhauser, Basel; Boyett and Jewell 1980, *Prog. Biophys. Mol. Biol.* 36:1–52).

volume is small at the resting or control heart rate, rate acceleration will increase output very little initially and output will begin to decline at relatively low frequencies. The smaller the initial stroke volume, the greater the fractional decrease of stroke volume as rate increases. Excessive rates result in lowered cardiac output; in dogs, for example, pacing the heart at 280 beats per minute for 11 to 29 days results in low-output congestive heart failure.

Denervated heart

Elimination of the extrinsic cardiac nervous supply by sectioning or destruction of the nerves or by excision and reimplantation (autotransplantation) of the heart permits evaluation of their role in regulation. In experimental dogs after surgery the resting heart rate stabilizes at 90 to 120 beats per minute, which appears to be the intrinsic rate of the denervated SA node. Respiratory sinus arrhythmia is abolished. The prompt acceleration of heart rate associated with a startle reaction or onset of exercise does not occur, but a slower increase in rate to values about one-third lower than those in control dogs occurs. Thus the innervated heart satisfies the need for increased cardiac output largely by increasing heart rate while the denervated heart responds with a lesser rate increase but a large increase in stroke volume through the Frank-Starling mechanism. The denervated heart is supersensitive to circulating catecholamines, which support the needed augmentation of ventricular performance and heart rate in exercise. Cardiac-denervated racing greyhounds ordinarily perform nearly as well as controls, but administration of a beta-adrenergic blocking agent results in a sharp reduction in exercise performance and heart rate.

There is depletion of catecholamine stores, but apparently there are no major alterations in myocardial metabolism in denervated hearts.

Parasympathectomy alone results in persistent sinus tachycardia at rest with rates of 140 to 160 beats per minute; this reveals the high vagal resting tone characteristic of normal dogs and the effect of unopposed sympathetic tone on heart rate.

Reinnervation becomes evident 1 to 2 months after denervation and is functionally complete in the dog in about 9 months. This does not occur in human cardiac transplantation.

Tonic action of nerves

Classically, the following qualitative terms have been applied to the effect on the heart of extrinsic nerve impulses, chemical mediators, hormones, drugs, and other compounds: *chronotropic action (chronotropy),* influence on heart rate; *inotropic action (inotropy),* influence on contractile strength, rate of pressure development (*dP/dt*), and ejection velocity; *dromotropic action (dromotropy),* influence on conduction velocity; and *bathmotropic action (bathmotropy),* influence on excitability or irritability (stimulation threshold). An increase in any action is termed *positive;* a decrease, *negative.* Thus a *positive inotropic* effect is one that increases strength of contraction; a *negative chronotropic* effect is one that slows heart rate.

The sympathetic fibers stimulate the heart and thus affect the aforementioned properties in a positive sense; the parasympathetic fibers inhibit the heart and affect these properties in a negative sense. The postganglionic chemical mediators of these autonomic effects—norepinephrine (sympathetic) and acetylcholine (parasympathetic)—act on the specific adrenergic (sympathetic) and cholinergic (parasympathetic) receptor sites in effector cells. Of the two types of adrenergic receptor sites recognized, alpha and beta, the heart contains chiefly beta receptors. Activation of the beta receptors causes vasodilatation and positive chronotropic and inotropic cardiac effects (see also Chap. 10). Beta receptors have been further separated into two subgroups: $beta_1$-adrenergic receptors, responsible for inotropic and chronotropic myocardial responses, lipolysis of fat cells, and inhibition of intestinal motility, and $beta_2$-adrenergic receptors, which mediate bronchodilatation, glycogenolysis, vasodilatation, and myometrial relaxation.

Initially it was generally accepted that myocardial adrenergic receptors were $beta_1$ and vascular smooth muscle receptors were $beta_2$. There are, however, exceptions to this generalization in various species. In most mammals tested the ventricular myocardium contains chiefly $beta_1$ receptors. $Beta_2$ receptors abound in the frog heart, however, and in the human ventricle the $beta_1$:$beta_2$ ratio is approximately 80:20 and an even higher percentage of $beta_2$ receptors is found in the atria. Unlike the foregoing functional properties of $beta_1$ and $beta_2$ receptors, in the hearts of many mammals $beta_1$ receptors apparently mediate glycogenolysis. It had been assumed that $beta_2$ receptors mediated coronary vasodilation, but in the coronary artery of the pig the majority of receptors have been found to be $beta_1$ subtype. In any case, beta-adrenergic receptors enhance myocardial contractility, dilate coronary arteries, mediate positive chronotropic effects, speed atrioventricular conduction, and increase automaticity (pacemaking, see Chap. 7).

Alpha-adrenergic receptors are also separated into two subgroups: $alpha_1$ and $alpha_2$. $Alpha_1$-adrenergic receptors are present in the myocardium, but their density is low in the ventricles, where their role appears to be unimportant. $Alpha_1$-adrenergic receptors have a higher concentration in atrial tissue, where they may participate to a greater extent in the production of positive inotropic effects.

$Alpha_2$-adrenergic receptors are present on presynaptic nerve terminals in the brain and can inhibit adrenergic discharge. Postsynaptic receptors mediate vasoconstriction in vascular smooth muscle in several locations, but their role in coronary artery regulation is unclear. There is older evidence that receptors of some type can mediate coronary vasoconstriction and negative chronotropy at the sinoatrial node and in ventricular pacemaker cells. (For a description of receptor functions, see Chap. 10.)

Sympathetic-parasympathetic interactions

Since the postganglionic sympathetic and parasympathetic nerve terminals intermingle, their respective mediators affect the other division of the autonomic nervous system. Thus vagal terminals inhibit the release of norepinephrine from sympathetic nerve terminals, and neuropeptide Y (see Chap. 10) released along with norepinephrine from sympathetic nerve terminals inhibits the release of acetylcholine from vagal nerve endings. Further, at the level of the effector muscle cells, the two antagonistic transmitters oppose one another's effects.

Accentuated antagonism. The term *accentuated antagonism* has been given to the inhibitory effect of a given level of vagal stimulation that becomes more pronounced as the level of sympathetic activity increases. The inhibiting effect of vagal activity in the ventricles, where vagal fibers are sparse, appears to be achieved chiefly by opposing the existing level of sympathetic activity. These interactions are dependent on both the prejunctional (nerve terminal mediator release) and postjunctional (effector cell) levels. The postjunctional effect has been shown by infusion of adrenergic and cholinergic agonists rather than by autonomic nerve stimulation. The opposing agonists interact postjunctionally at the level of the effector cell.

Tone of the vagus

At rest, the vagus nerves exert a continuous restraint on the action of the heart, which can be demonstrated in animals by cutting or freezing of the nerves. The heart's action then immediately becomes greatly accelerated. This increase occurs even though the stellate ganglia have been previously excised; the result, therefore, cannot be due to an increased action of the accelerator nerves. Various conditions, physiological and pathological, may alter the intensity of the vagal tone. It is naturally higher in some species (e.g., the horse) than in others (e.g., the domestic rabbit).

Vagal tone is apparently reflexive in nature, depending on afferent impulses flowing to the vagus center, especially along the sinus and aortic nerves. Sectioning of these afferent nerves causes an increase in heart rate so that little further acceleration occurs when the vagi themselves are subsequently severed.

Sympathetic tone

A tonic action of the sympathetic nerves has been postulated on the basis of experiments showing that after excision of the stellate ganglia the heart rate was slowed. A criticism of these experiments is that the control observations were not made under truly basal conditions. If not, then the control values would be higher than they should be for this comparison. This criticism was obviated by recording the heart rate of dogs after they were trained to lie quietly during the period of observation with all types of external stimulation (i.e., visual, auditory, and others) reduced to a minimum. The average "resting" heart rate before training was 90 to 112 beats per minute. After several weeks of training, the resting rate slowed and stabilized at 47 to 57 beats per minute. Cardiac sympathectomy was then performed. After the animals recovered from this procedure, the basal rate was 50 to 58 beats per minute (i.e., not different from control values). It was concluded that in the truly resting state the accelerator nerves are not in tonic activity but that the accelerator mechanism is more or less constantly involved in adapting the heart rate to the changing bodily conditions.

Sympathetic versus vagal stimulation

The heart rate responses to sympathetic versus vagal nerve stimulation follow different latent and decay periods. During sympathetic nerve stimulation the response is sluggish, with heart rate acceleration beginning in 1 to 2 seconds and reaching a plateau after 30 to 60 seconds. The reason for the delay is that the effects are mediated by adrenergic receptors coupled with the adenylate cyclase system that responds slowly. This positive chronotropic effect gradually decays as reuptake and diffusion dissipate the released norepinephrine.

With vagal stimulation, the latent period is short (0.15 to 0.2 second), a plateau is reached within a few heartbeats, and after cessation of stimulation cardiac acceleration occurs promptly, also within a few heartbeats, although the heart rate may oscillate somewhat for a few seconds. This rapid response allows beat-by-beat regulation of cardiac cycle length or heart period (i.e., the interval between two consecutive beats). The reasons for rapid response are twofold: (1) The sinoatrial nodal cells' automaticity is slowed primarily by hyperpolarization owing to the effect of released acetylcholine (ACh) on the potassium channel (and the muscarinic receptors are coupled directly to the potassium channels). (2) ACh is rapidly hydrolyzed. Accordingly, it is the sudden release and reinstatement of vagal tone that account for the brief acceleration and deceleration of the heart rate in a vagotonic animal, such as the horse, that is subject to a brief startle reaction (e.g., response to a loud noise). When such a rapid change in heart rate occurs in a startled horse, although the tachycardia is short-lived, the sympathetic effects on the myocardium as measured by the duration of the electrocardiographic QT interval and the interval between the first and second heart sounds (indicators of the duration of systole) are shortened for a substantial period after the heart has slowed.

Cardiac reflexes

A variety of reflexes affect both cardiac activity and vascular tone simultaneously. They are therefore discussed together in Chapter 10.

Under natural conditions, the rate of the heartbeat and

physiological variations in this rate are controlled by the interaction of the cardioinhibitory and cardioaccelerator centers in the medulla oblongata. These centers, in turn, are under the influence of other parts of the central nervous system, including the hypothalamus and the limbic system. They also receive impulses that stream into the brain stem from all parts of the body, including the heart itself. Under these influences, the level of activity of either center may be exalted or depressed, with corresponding changes in heart rate. If the cardiac vagus on one side is cut and its central end (i.e., the end conducting afferent impulses to the brain) is stimulated, a reflex through the cardioinhibitory center and the opposite vagus usually slows the heart rate. If the second vagus is then cut, stimulation of the central end of either vagus usually produces cardioacceleration. The results of this experiment, however, are unpredictable, because the vagus contains several kinds of afferent fiber, some making connection with the cardioinhibitory center, others with the cardioaccelerator. In fact, this is true of other nerves also, so that in student laboratories the stimulation of the central end of any mixed nerve may yield variable results, depending on intensity and frequency of the stimulating current. Stimulation of the central end of the cut sciatic nerve usually accelerates the heart.

There are certain reflex changes in heart rate that are of interest. For example, pressure on the eyeball at the outer canthus usually slows the heart (oculocardiac reflex), as does pressure on the carotid sinus. Stimulation of afferent fibers in the respiratory passages by the inhalation of irritating vapors (e.g., anesthetics) is particularly likely to cause reflex inhibition of the heart. Extrasystoles and bradycardia have been demonstrated electrocardiographically during abdominal operations, the irregularities apparently being the consequence of visceral stimulation. Changes in heart rate that accompany emotions or those that precede muscular exercise are believed to result from the influence of higher cerebral centers on the medullary cardiomotor mechanisms.

The pulse rate is generally inversely related to the arterial blood pressure, a rise or fall in pressure causing, respectively, a decrease or increase in heart rate. These adjustments are subserved by (1) a reflex whose afferent limb is the afferent vagal fibers (aortic nerve) originating from the aortic arch and heart and (2) a reflex in which the sinus nerve forms the afferent limb. These mechanisms are considered in Chapter 10. Presumably, such changes in heart rate are brought about not simply by an increase or a decrease in activity of one cardiac center or the other but by reciprocal variations in the tone of both. For example, the slowing of the heart that results from a rise in arterial pressure is much less pronounced if impulses from the cardioinhibitory center have been prevented from reaching the heart by sectioning of the vagi. After removal of the stellate ganglia, on the other hand, the cardiac response to a fall in blood pressure is reduced to a lesser extent. Other mechanisms are concerned, since a fall in blood pressure causes an increase in the rate of the heart even after it has been completely denervated.

Chemical control of the heart

Catecholamines, whether released from the adrenal medulla or from postganglionic adrenergic nerve endings, exert positive inotropic, chronotropic, dromotropic, and bathmotropic actions on the myocardium. Acting through the 3′,5′-adenosine monophosphate (cyclic AMP) system, they also induce biochemical changes in cardiac muscle cells, including glycogenolysis. All of these are beta-adrenergic receptor effects. The details of the action of beta-adrenergic receptors on cAMP are given in Chapter 10 under "Cardiovascular Receptors." The action of catecholamines on the cAMP system may be summarized as follows: Norepinephrine as a typical catecholamine activates the enzyme, adenyl cyclase, to catalyze the production of cAMP from adenosine triphosphate (ATP). The cAMP then promotes the conversion of inactive phosphorylase *b* to the active form, phosphorylase *a,* which brings about glycogenolysis to supply glucose phosphates (and thereby energy) to the working muscle.

Another and possibly related action of catecholamines on the heart involves calcium ions. Ca^{2+} is required for activation of phosphorylase and, through its action in excitation-contraction coupling, probably is responsible for the inotropic action of catecholamines. When applied to cardiac muscle, the catecholamines both increase the permeability of the cell membrane to extracellular Ca^{2+} and mobilize calcium ions from intracellular stores in the sarcoplasmic reticulum. Cyclic AMP is the intermediary of this latter calcium mobilization. These processes, therefore, involve two series of interrelated reactions. In the first the catecholamine, acting via adenyl cyclase, cAMP, and phosphorylase *b* and *a,* promotes glycogenolysis and simultaneously mobilizes intracellular calcium stores. In the second the catecholamine meanwhile has increased cell membrane permeability to extracellular Ca^{2+}. The overall results are provision of energy from carbohydrates, mobilization of calcium ions from both extracellular and intracellular sites, and positive inotropic actions on the heart. Similar mechanisms of activation are believed to operate also in other cells, with cAMP and Ca^{2+} serving in an integrated fashion as intracellular "messengers" in control of both contractile and secretory cells. The way this system may operate in heart muscle is illustrated in Fig. 9.4.

The role of 3′,5′-guanosine monophosphate (cyclic GMP) and its enzyme guanylate cyclase in the heart is much less clear. Early studies indicated that an increase in cGMP had a negative chronotropic effect and that acetylcholine increased tissue concentration of cGMP in isolated cardiac tissue. This led to the idea that there is a dual cyclic nucleotide system with opposing effects (e.g., cAMP with positive and cGMP with negative inotropic actions). Increases in cGMP, however, are not always associated with

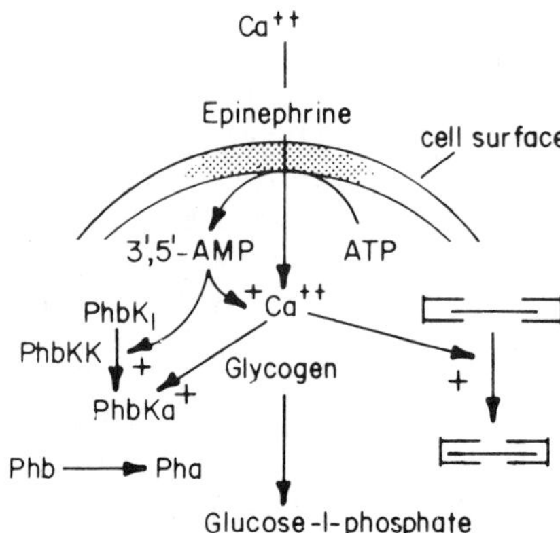

Figure 9.4. Hypothetical mechanism of epinephrine inotropic and glycogenolytic effects in heart muscle. Epinephrine stimulates 3′, 5′-adenosine monophosphate (cyclic AMP) production and calcium mobilization. These sequentially activate phosphorylase *b* kinase kinase (PhbKK) and inactive phosphorylase *b* kinase ($PHbK_1$) to active phosphorylase *b* kinase (PhbKa). Inactive phorphorylase *b* (Phb) is then converted to active phosphorylase *a* (Pha) and glycogenolysis is increased. The positive inotropic effect results from greater availability of Ca^{2+} made possible by increased Ca^{2+} uptake by the cell. This is induced by epinephrine and by more efficient Ca^{2+} mobilization from the sarcoplasmic reticulum stimulated by cyclic AMP. (Modified from Rasmussen 1970, *Science* 170:404–12.)

negative inotropy. The role of cGMP- and cAMP-dependent protein kinases, which in turn phosphorylate certain cellular proteins, has also not been resolved. This topic is explained further in Chapter 10, under "Cardiovascular Receptors."

Autonomic effects on contractility

Sympathetic effects, as indicated above, markedly increase both atrial and ventricular contractility. Parasympathetic effects profoundly inhibit the atria, decreasing heart rate and atrial contractility and, paradoxically, shortening the action potential and refractory period of atrial cells. The inhibitory effects on the ventricles are negligible compared with those on the atria, although a definite depression of ventricular contractility occurs with vagal stimulation, especially in the presence of high concurrent sympathetic activity. The reason for this latter characteristic is that the acetylcholine liberated by vagal stimulation acts to inhibit norepinephrine release from the postganglionic sympathetic nerve terminals. This dependency of the vagal effect on contractility on the background sympathetic activity has been termed *accentuated antagonism,* described in the foregoing. A related phenomenon is that neuropeptide Y (NPY), which is liberated from sympathetic nerve endings together with norepinephrine (NE), inhibits the release of acetylcholine (ACh) from vagal nerve endings. Thus ACh inhibits NE release while NPY inhibits ACh release in this interactive system.

Atrioventricular conduction

Atrioventricular (AV) conduction is also regulated by the autonomic nervous system and its transmitters. Sympathetic neural activity and catecholamines decrease AV conduction time, acting especially in the upper (i.e., atrionodal and nodal) regions of the AV junctional area. Conduction in the lower (i.e., nodal–His) region is little affected. Beta-adrenergic blockade decreases the sinoatrial node rate of discharge, prolongs AV conduction, and prolongs the refractory period of the AV junction.

Vagal stimulation and cholinergic drugs slow conduction through the AV junction and increase the refractory period, acting primarily at the atrionodal and nodal regions rather than at the nodal–His region.

The effects of various humoral agents on cardiac functions are tabulated in Table 9.2.

Glucagon causes a similar activation of glycogenolysis and a positive inotropic effect, possibly by a similar mechanism. It does not act as a beta receptor but appears to stimulate cardiac adenyl cyclase at a different receptor site. This suggests that there are at least two receptor sites affecting catalytic activity of the cyclase—one responding to adrenergic beta stimulation and one to glucagon.

Although a physiological role for *histamine* in cardiac regulation has not been established, a histamine receptor system analogous to the adrenergic receptor system is in place in the heart. Like $beta_1$-adrenergic receptors, $histamine_2$ receptors mediate positive chronotropy and inotropy, stimulate adenyl cyclase, and cause coronary vasodilatation. $Histamine_1$ receptors, like alpha-adrenergic receptors, mediate coronary vasoconstriction. Better known are the pathological effects of massive histamine release in anaphylactic shock, which causes hypotension, venodilatation, tachycardia, increased myocardial oxygen demand, and, ultimately, cardiovascular collapse. Although histamine may play a role in local vascular autoregulation, it does not appear to be a likely candidate as a physiologic regulator of cardiac function under ordinary circumstances.

The receptor sites and the physiological roles for the other agents listed in Table 9.2 are not well established.

Hypoxemia, hypercapnia, and *acidosis* of sufficient degree depress myocardial contractility.

COORDINATION OF ACTIVITY OF RIGHT AND LEFT SIDES OF THE HEART

As noted previously, and as shown in Fig. 9.5, the outputs of the left and right ventricles must be maintained in equilibrium if the blood volume and hemodynamic relations between the pulmonary and systemic circulations are to be preserved. There are five cardiac factors that serve to interrelate right and left ventricular activity:

1. *Frank-Starling mechanism.* This serves to adjust each ventricular output to its inflow.

2. *Ventricular end-diastolic volume.* Temporarily a discrepancy between output of the right and left ventricles can be buffered by changes in their end-diastolic volume. This is possible because neither one empties completely with each beat and because the degree of emptying seems to be

Table 9.2. Cardiac effects of humoral agents and adrenergic receptors stimulated

Hormone	Inotropic effect	Chronotropic effect	Coronary vasoactive effect	Remarks
Epinephrine	Positive, β_1	Positive, β_1	Constriction, α Dilation, β_1	Increased myocardial metabolism with β_1 stimulation causes coronary dilatation by autoregulation
Norepinephrine	Positive, β_1	Positive, β_1	Constriction, α Dilation, β_2	
Acetylcholine	Negative	Negative	Dilation	
Glucagon	Positive	Positive	Dilation	No β receptor effect; stimulates cyclase at another receptor site
Insulin	Positive	None	Dilation	
Somatostatin	None	Unknown	None	
Mineralocorticoids	Positive	None	None	
Glucocorticoids	None	None	None	
Adrenocorticotropic hormone	Little or none	Positive	None	May release corticosteroids
Melanocyte-stimulating hormone	Positive, weak	Positive, weak	Constriction	
Somatotropic growth hormone	None	None	None	
Vasopressin	Negative	Positive	Constriction, marked	Inotropic effect secondary to coronary constriction
Oxytocin	Little or none	Positive	Constriction, slight	
Renin	None	None	None	
Angiotensin I	Positive, moderate	Positive, moderate	Constriction, weak	
Angiotensin II	Positive	Variable	Constriction	Strong inotropic and vasoconstrictor effect
Angiotensin III	Positive	Unknown	Constriction	Strong vasoconstrictor effect
Thyroxin	Positive	Positive	Increased flow	Inotropic effect chiefly on V_{max}; coronary effect chiefly secondary to increased myocardial O_2 consumption
Prostaglandins	Positive	Variable	Dilation	Reflex tachycardia; central nervous system stimulation tachycardia

Data from Bourne, ed. 1980, *Hearts and Heart-like Organs,* vols. 1, 2, 3, Academic Press, New York; Berne, Sperelakis, and Geiger, eds. 1979, *Handbook of Physiology,* sec. 2, vol. 1, *The Heart,* Am. Physiol. Soc., Bethesda, Md.; and other sources.

under control of the sympathetic nervous system. In dogs, an abrupt onset of exercise causes a simultaneous increase in both right and left ventricular stroke volumes that is attributed to almost immediate increases in contractility brought about by increased sympathetic tone. This means that the two outputs do not have to be identical for every beat; small inequalities of volume output can be accommodated within the ventricles themselves or can be expelled when sympathetic tone is increased.

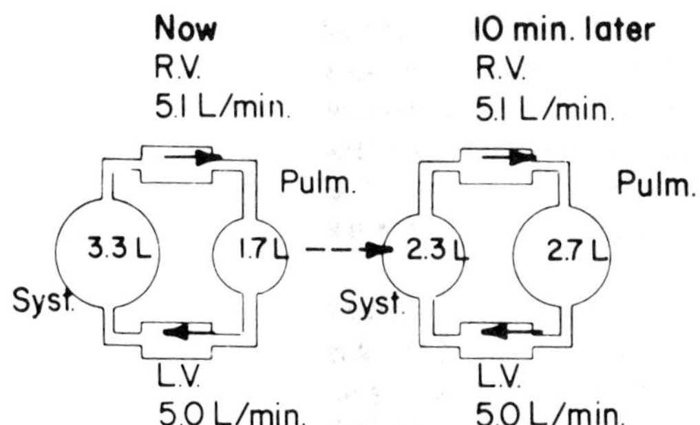

Figure 9.5. Diagram illustrating the consequences of a 2 percent difference in right ventricular (RV) over left ventricular (LV) outputs, if mechanisms did not come into play to keep the mean outputs of the two ventricles the same. Actually, death would supervene before a shift of blood volume of the magnitude depicted could occur. Syst., systemic blood volume; Pulm., pulmonic blood volume. (Reproduced with permission from Burton, A.C., *Physiology and Biophysics of the Circulation,* 2nd ed. Copyright © 1972 by Year Book Medical Publishers, Inc., Chicago.)

3. *Storage function of the pulmonary circulation.* This is another mechanism that permits moderate differences in output of the two ventricles for limited periods of time. For example, if saline solution is infused intravenously quickly, the right ventricular output increases almost at once. The left ventricular output similarly rises but only after a lag time of at least three cardiac cycles. In this interval the saline solution administered must have been added to the blood volume in pulmonary vessels.

4. *Flow transmission through the pulmonary vasculature.* In spite of the storage function of pulmonary vessels, there is a rather direct transmission of the pulse of systolic blood flow from right ventricle to left atrium; consequently, the wave of the pulmonary flow pulse is transmitted into the period of rapid filling of the left ventricle, with a delay of only 0.1 second between right ventricular contraction and left ventricular filling. Left ventricular end-diastolic volume, therefore, can be directly altered by right ventricular stroke output, with the result that what the right ventricle expels in any given beat to a degree determines what the left ventricle will expel in the following beat. The transmission of this stroke flow is related to the stiffness (compliance) of the pulmonary vasculature. Increased stiffness (sympathetic activity) increases flow-wave transmission, thus aiding in ventricular coordination.

5. *Bronchial circulation.* There is free communication between the capillaries of the pulmonary vascular bed and the bronchial circulation. The bronchial flow (part of left

ventricular output) returns in part to the left atrium through the pulmonary veins; a smaller fraction returns to the right atrium through the azygos vein and the superior vena cava. Thus a shunt is provided which could serve to equalize pressure and flow between the two circulatory systems. The possible importance of this mechanism in health and disease has not been established.

COORDINATION OF ATRIAL AND VENTRICULAR ACTIVITY

Correlation between activity of atria and ventricles during acceleration of the heart rate is maintained by the following: (1) AV conduction time decreases, (2) conduction time over ventricular muscle is shortened, and (3) the duration of depolarization) is reduced. Thus the whole cycle is shortened and the sequence of activation is maintained.

HEART AND VESSELS AS A COORDINATED SYSTEM

In coordination of the circulatory system, two types of coupling are significant. One is the mechanical interaction of the several parts on the basis of the closed nature of the system and the finite volume of blood it contains. Thus systolic output is bound to affect venous return; what the right side of the heart does determines what the left side of the heart can do. The volume of blood ejected from the heart has direct effects on peripheral blood flow, while the latter also acts to influence what the heart does. In this type of interdependence the important variables are heart rate, venous return, cardiac output, end-diastolic volume, stroke volume, peripheral resistance, blood pressure, blood volume, and blood flow. The venous side of the circulation is always coupled hemodynamically with the heart through the atria. The arterial side, however, is coupled with the ventricles only when the valves are open during systole; for the remainder of the cardiac cycle, its hemodynamic connection with the heart is downstream through arteries, arterioles, capillaries, and the venous system. The second type of coupling is extrinsic to the circulatory system and is represented by neural and humoral mechanisms of control. Usually they, too, represent circuits or closed loops, in that information from detectors within the circulatory system initiates reflexes through the central nervous system, which, in turn, bring into play the effector components that modify performance of the heart and blood vessels.

Cardiac function curves (so-called Starling curves) relate factors governed in part by venous return (e.g., mean right atrial pressure, end-diastolic ventricular volume, end-diastolic pressure) to cardiac output or some function of the ventricle that is a determinant of cardiac output (e.g., stroke volume, ventricular pressure, rate of pressure development: dP/dt, power, work). A group of curves relating left ventricular output to right atrial pressure is reproduced in Fig. 9.6, together with a simplified model of the circulation. As can be seen from the normal curve (curve b) of Fig. 9.6B, when right atrial pressure increases, cardiac output increases. When right atrial pressure falls sufficiently below zero (e.g., to −2.0 mm Hg), cardiac output is zero. At an atrial pressure of 0 mm Hg the output is 5 L/min, and at 5.0 mm Hg it is 12.5 L/min. Curves a and c are for hyperdynamic (a) and hypodynamic (c) hearts. The former represents the direction of change with, for example, sympathetic nerve stimulation or cardiac hypertrophy of lengthy physical training; the latter represents the direction of change associated with inhibition of sympathetic tone, vagal stimulation, or myocardial disease.

These curves permit an evaluation of the functional state of the heart based on the measurement of two factors (e.g., right atrial pressure and left ventricular output). Any influence of the right ventricle, pulmonary circulation, or left atrium that would alter the relationship between these two variables would not be distinguished from changes in left ventricular function by this analysis.

Venous return or systemic function curves (Fig. 9.6C and D) relate venous return to right atrial pressure. The relationship is between pressure and flow, but it is the inverse of the Starling relationship of Fig. 9.6B. An increase in atrial pressure decreases venous return. In these curves the right atrial pressure is the dependent variable plotted as a function of venous flow, the independent variable. Contrary to convention, however, the dependent variable is plotted here along the abscissa so that these curves can be compared with the Starling plot of Fig. 9.6B, with right atrial pressure on the same axis in both types of plot. The fact that the relationship between pressure and flow is reversed in the two types of curve is not contradictory. It simply means that the variables are interdependent and both relationships operate simultaneously in the system (see Chap. 5). When flow is considered first as the dependent variable (Starling curve) and then as the independent variable (systemic function curve), the individual roles of factors determining right atrial pressure, venous return, and cardiac output are emphasized. Starling curves deal with circulation through the heart and lungs; systemic function curves deal with circulation through the systemic vessels. In the former, the output of the heart is treated as the dependent variable that responds functionally to controlled alterations in pressure, flow, and resistance of the systemic vascular system that affect atrial pressure (independent variable). In the latter, the heart and lungs are replaced by a pump oxygenator, and, return flow in the systemic vascular system becomes the independent variable that determines right atrial pressure. Fig. 9.6C depicts a series of systemic function curves. Note that in the normal curve, blood flow into the right atrium reaches zero at an atrial pressure of 7 mm Hg. This is the expected pressure in all parts of the systemic circulation when equilibrium occurs after cessation of flow. Theoretically, it is the mean pressure in all parts of the systemic circulation when filled with nonmoving blood, and is termed *mean systemic pressure* (P_{MS}). The value 7 mm Hg

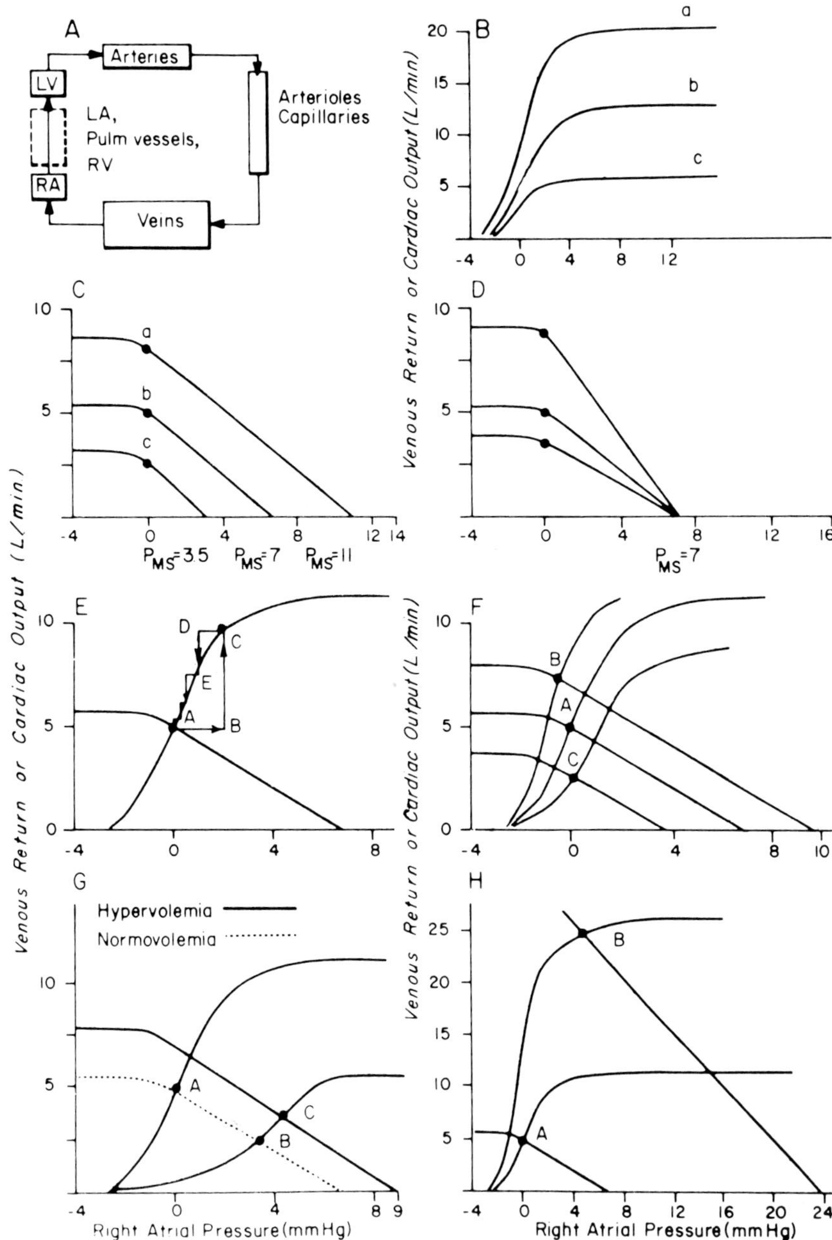

Figure 9.6. (*A*) Simplified model of the circulation. Cardiac function curves may be plotted from determinations of right atrial (RA) pressure and left ventricular (LV) output. The resultant curves characterize steady-state flow through the heart and lungs. When the only parameters measured are LV output and RA pressure, the possible effects of hemodynamic influences of the right ventricle, pulmonary vessels, and left atrium (*dotted square*) are ignored. (*B*) Cardiac function curves (Starling curves) for the heart: (a) hyperdynamic, (b) normal, and (c) hypodynamic cardiac states. (*C*) Systemic function curves and the effect of changing mean systemic pressure (P_{MS}): a, 11; b, 7; c, 3.5 mm Hg. (*D*) Systemic function curves and the effect of changing resistance to venous return. (*E*) Cardiac function (cardiac output) and systemic function (venous return) curves plotted on the same axes. Point A is the equilibrium point with coordinates of 5 L/min cardiac output and venous return (ordinate) and zero mm Hg. right atrial pressure (abscissa). These coordinates represent stable values at which the system is operating. When a perturbation occurs (such as a sudden shift of right atrial pressure from point A to B), the coordinates for cardiac output reach a new point (C). In a stable system, a series of changes is initiated (points D, E, etc.) and the original equilibrium value (point A) is regained. (*F*) The effect of altering sympathetic tone on the equilibrium point of cardiac function and systemic function curves. Point B is the equilibrium with sympathetic nerve stimulation, point C is the equilibrium with sympathetic nerve inhibition (e.g., with spinal anesthesia), and point A is the control. (*G*) Shifts in cardiac and systemic function curves in congestive heart failure. Point A is the equilibrium point of control curves; point B is the new equilibrium point when the heart fails (decrease in cardiac output and increase in right atrial pressure); and point C is the equilibrium point established when the increase in blood volume (which is expected in heart failure) occurs. Cardiac output is substantially increased owing to this shift in the equilibrium point. (*H*) The effect of exercise on cardiac and systemic function curves. Point A is the control equilibrium point; point B is the new equilibrium point when cardiac output and right atrial pressure are increased during strenuous exercise. (From Detweiler 1979, in Brobeck, ed., *Best & Taylor's Physiological Basis of Medical Practice* 10th ed., © 1979, the Williams & Wilkins Co., Baltimore.)

has been determined in dogs when the heart is stopped and, within 2 to 3 seconds, blood is pumped from the arterial to the venous side until the pressure is equalized. The P_{MS} is determined by the volume capacity of the vascular system and its degree of filling (blood volume). In the systemic function curves an increase of venous return is seen as atrial pressure falls (Figs. 9.6C and D) until a plateau is reached. This is the maximum venous return, which is not exceeded as atrial pressure continues to fall. The plateau is caused by progressive collapse of the veins (at the thoracic entrance), which increases resistance to flow. This automatically limits the rise in venous return with further fall in atrial pressure. When the P_{MS} is increased (increased blood volume, decreased vascular capacitance), the curve is shifted upward and to the right, and with a fall in P_{MS} it shifts to the left and downward (Fig. 9.6C). If the P_{MS} remains constant when vasodilatation occurs, venous return increases as resistance to flow decreases and the function curves rotate about the point of right atrial pressure which equals P_{MS} (Fig. 9.6D).

Figure 9.6E illustrates the normal relationship between right atrial pressure, venous return, and cardiac output.

These two function curves cross at point A, the *equilibrium point*. The coordinates of this point represent the cardiac output and mean right atrial pressure, which characterize the state of the heart and circulatory system at the time the curves are derived.

As long as the system is operating along these cardiac output and systemic function curves, it will tend to stabilize at this equilibrium point. For example, a sudden increase in right atrial pressure from point A to B, all other factors remaining unchanged, would result in increased cardiac output (point C). This could be induced experimentally by withdrawal of a given volume of blood from the arterial side and its injection during ventricular systole into the venous side. The increase in right atrial pressure would increase cardiac output (point C) while decreasing venous return. The cardiac output would then exceed venous return, and during the next four or five heartbeats blood from the heart and pulmonary circulation would be transferred into the systemic circulation. Thus artrial pressure would be reduced (points D, E, etc.) as cardiac output likewise decreased. The process would continue until the stable equilibrium point for the two function curves was reestablished.

With alteration in sympathetic tone, shifts occur as depicted in Fig. 9.6F: increased sympathetic tone shifts the ventricular function curve to the left and the systemic function curve upward and to the right. New coordinates are then established for the equilibrium (point B), representing an increase in cardiac output and venous return and a decrease in mean atrial pressure. Decreasing sympathetic tone has the opposite effect, and the new equilibrium (point C) shows that flow into and out of the heart is less for a given right atrial pressure. Marked reduction in cardiac output, as occurs in heart failure, shifts the cardiac output curve to the right and the equilibrium point lower on the systemic function curve (from point A to B, Fig. 9.6G). Even if cardiac function does not improve, fluid retention with hypervolemia increases P_{MS}, establishing a new equilibrium (point C).

With exercise, marked shifts in the function curves occur. In Fig. 9.6H, point A represents the equilibrium point at a resting cardiac output of 5 L/min and mean right atrial pressure of 0 mm Hg. Point B is the equilibrium point attained with a fivefold increase in cardiac output and elevation of right atrial pressure to about 5 mm Hg. Mean systemic pressure has increased to 24 mm Hg, the result of sympathetic contraction of capacitance vessels. The slope of the systemic function curve is steeper than that of the resting curve because vasodilatation in the active muscles reduces resistance to flow through part of the systemic circuit. The cardiac output curve is shifted to the left as the result of inotropic cardiac effects of sympathetic nerve activity. The two curves equilibrate at point B, a point near the maximum cardiac output.

The foregoing analysis is based on simplified assumptions regarding the vascular system and on reasonable presumptions regarding the course of the cardiac output curves. It serves to illustrate, however, the complex interactions between cardiac output, arterial pressure, right atrial pressure, and venous return in cardiac regulation. In this way the analyses have predictive value and agree with experimental observations.

CARDIAC RESERVE

The potential reserves available to the heart for coping with various stresses are heart rate, systolic and diastolic volumes, cardiac blood flow, oxygen content of the body mixed-venous blood, cardiac work, changing efficiency of the heart, and possibly the stores of catecholamines. Increases in these various functions with exercise are discussed in Chapter 15.

The following list provides some clinical applications on the regulation of the heart:

1. To permit rapid heart rates (e.g., 3 [dog] to 6 [horse] times greater than resting rates), the systolic ejection time, the refractory period of cardiac muscle, and the AV conduction interval must decrease. As heart rate increases, frequency potentiation increases contractile force, spread of excitation accelerates (QRS is shortened), and action potential duration and refractory period shorten (QT interval is shortened). AV conduction is accelerated (PR interval is shortened). These changes abbreviate systole and maintain the proper sequence of atrial and ventricular contraction. Diastole shortens more than systole and the atrial contraction component of ventricular filling becomes progressively more important.
2. Cardiac denervation studies demonstrate that adequate cardiac regulation during exercise in the absence of extrinsic nerves is achieved through heterometric autoregulation (increase in stroke volume and contractility) and the action of circulating catecholamines (increased heart rate and contractility).
3. The hypervolemia of congestive heart failure increases ventricular filling and thus increases cardiac output toward normal.
4. With exercise, cardiac output can increase fivefold, right atrial filling pressure increases to the same degree, and the venous return curve shifts to the right and becomes steeper.
5. The output of the two ventricles must be exquisitely coordinated to prevent shifts of blood volume from the systemic to the pulmonic circulations (or vice versa). Equalization of left and right ventricular stroke volumes is a primary function of the Frank-Starling mechanism. Storage functions of the ventricles and pulmonary circulation, rapid flow transmission through the pulmonary vasculature, and possibly the shunting mechanism of the bronchial circulation all serve to prevent volume overload of the pulmonary circulation with consequent fatal pulmonary edema.

REFERENCES

Anrep, G. 1912. On part played by suprarenals in normal vascular reactions of body. *J. Physiol.* (London) 45:307–17.

Berne, R.M., Sperelakis, N., and Geiger, S.R., eds. 1979. *Handbook of Physiology.* Sec. 2. Vol. 1, *The Heart.* Am. Physiol. Soc., Bethesda.

Blinks, J.R., and Koch-Weser, J. 1961. Analysis of the effect of changes in rate and rhythm upon myocardial contractility. *J. Pharmacol. Exp. Ther.* 134:373–89.

Bourne, G.H., ed. 1980. *Hearts and Heart-Like Organs,* vols. 1, 2, 3. Academic Press, New York.

Bowditch, H.P. 1871. Über die Eigenthümlichkeiten der Reizbarkeit, welche die Muskelfasern des Herzens zeigen. *Ber. Math. Phys. Sachs, Gesellsch. Wissensch.* (Leipzig) 23:652.

Boyett, M.R., and Jewell, B.R. 1980. Analysis of the effects of changes in rate and rhythm upon electrical activity in the heart. *Prog. Biophys. Mol. Biol.* 36:1–52.

Braunwald, E., Ross, J., Jr., and Sonnenblick, E.J. 1968. *Mechanisms of Contraction of the Normal and Failing Heart.* Little, Brown, Boston.

Bristow, M.R., Ginsburg, R., and Harrison, D.C. 1982. Histamine and the human heart: The other receptor system. *Am. J. Cardiol.* 49:249–51.

Bristow, M.R., and Port, J.D. 1990. Receptor pharmacology in the human heart. In O.B. Garfein (ed.), *Current Concepts in Cardiovascular Physiology.* Academic Press, New York. Pp. 73–132.

Bugge-Asperheim, B., and Kiil, F. 1969. Cardiac response to increased aortic pressure. *Scand. J. Clin. Lab. Invest.* 24:345–60.

Burton, A.C. 1972. *Physiology and Biophysics of the Circulation.* 2d ed. Year Book, Chicago.

Cooper, T. 1965. Physiologic and pharmacologic effects of cardiac denervation. *Fed. Proc.* 24:1428–31.

Cyon, E. de, and Ludwig, C. 1866. Die Reflexe eines sensiblen Nerven des Herzens auf die motorischen der Blutgefässe. *Ber. sachs. Ges. (Acad.) Wiss.* 18:307–28.

Donald, D.E., Milburn, S.E., and Shepherd, J.T. 1964. Effect of cardiac denervation on the maximal capacity for exercise in the racing greyhound. *J. Appl. Physiol.* 19:849–52.

Donald, T.C., Peterson, D.M., Walker, A.A., and Hefner, L.L. 1976. Afterload-induced homeometric autoregulation in isolated cardiac muscle. *Am. J. Physiol.* 231:545–50.

Feigl, E.O. 1967. Sympathetic control of coronary circulation. *Circ. Res.* 20:262–71.

Feigl, E.O. 1968. Carotid sinus reflex control of coronary blood flow. *Circ. Res.* 23:223–37.

Franklin, D.L., Van Citters, R.L., and Rushmer, R.F. 1962. Balance between right and left ventricular output. *Circ. Res.* 10:17–26.

George, W.J., and Graeff, R.M. 1981. Cyclic nucleotides and cardiac function. In R.D. Wilkerson, ed., *Cardiac Pharmacology.* Academic Press, New York. Pp. 75–93.

Grauwiler, J. 1965. *Herz und Kreislauf der Säugetiere.* Berkhauser, Basel.

Guyton, A.C. 1955. Determination of cardiac output by equating venous return curves with cardiac response curves. *Physiol. Rev.* 35:123–29.

Guyton, A.C., Polizo, C., and Armstrong, G.G., Jr. 1954. Mean circulatory filling pressure measured immediately after cessation of heart pumping. *Am. J. Physiol.* 179:261–67.

Hordof, A.J., Rose, E., Danilo, P., Jr., and Rosen, M.R. 1982. α- and β-Adrenergic effects of epinephrine on ventricular pacemaker cells in dogs. *Am. J. Physiol.* 242:H677–H682.

James, T.N., Bean, E.S., Land, K.F., and Green, E.W. 1968. Evidence of alpha receptor depressant activity in the heart. *Am. J. Physiol.* 215:1366–75.

Johnson, E.A. 1979. Force-interval relationship of cardiac muscle. In R.M. Berne, N. Sperelakis, and S.R. Geiger, eds., *Handbook of Physiology.* Sec. 2. The Cardiovascular System. Vol. 1, *The Heart.* Am. Physiol. Soc., Bethesda, Md. Pp. 475–96.

Kaye, M.P. 1977. Denervation and reinnervation of the heart. In W.C. Randall, ed., *Neural Regulation of the Heart.* Oxford University Press, New York. Pp. 345–78.

Levy, M.N. 1990. Neural and reflex control of the circulation. In O.B. Garfein (ed.), *Current Concepts in Cardiovascular Physiology.* Academic Press, New York. Pp. 133–207.

Levy, M.N., and Martin, P.J. 1979. Neural control of the heart. In R.M. Berne, N. Sperelakis, and S.R. Geiger, eds., *Handbook of Physiology.* Sec. 2, The Cardiovascular System. Vol. 1, *The Heart.* Am. Physiol. Soc., Bethesda. Pp. 581–620.

Mayer, S.E. 1970. Adrenergic receptors for metabolic responses in the heart. *Fed. Proc.* 29:1367–72.

Melbin, J., Detweiler, D.K., Riffle, R.A., and Noordergraaf, A. 1982. Coherence of cardiac output with rate changes. *Am. J. Physiol.* 243:H499–H504.

Mensing, N.J., and Hilgemann, D.W. 1981. Inotropic effects of activation and pharmacological mechanisms. *Trends Pharmacol. Sci.* 2:303–7.

Mizeres, N.J. 1957. The course of the left cardioinhibitory fibers in the dog heart. *Anat. Rec.* 127:109–15.

Monroe, R.G., Gamble, W.J., LaFarge, C.G., and Vatner, S.F. 1974. Homeometric autoregulation. In Ciba Foundation Symposium No. 27. *The Physiological Basis of Starling's Law of the Heart.* Elsevier, Amsterdam. Pp. 257–77.

Morkin, E., Collins, J.A., Goldman, H.S., and Fishman, A.P. 1965. Pattern of blood flow in the pulmonary veins of the dog. *J. Appl. Physiol.* 10:1118–28.

Murphy, Q. 1942. The influence of the accelerator nerves on the basal heart rate of the dog. *Am. J. Physiol.* 137:727–30.

Navaratnam, V. 1980. Anatomy of the mammalian heart. In G.H. Bourne, ed., *Hearts and Heart-like Organs.* American Press, New York. Vol. 1. Pp. 349–74.

Noble, M.I.M. 1979. *The Cardiac Cycle.* Blackwell, Oxford.

Patterson, D.F., Detweiler, D.K., Glendenning, S.A. 1965. Heart sounds and murmurs of the normal horse, *Ann. N.Y. Acad. Sci.* 127:242–305.

Priola, D.V. 1969. Individual chamber sensitivity to noreprinephrine after unilateral cardiac denervation. *J. Physiol.* (London) 216:604–14.

Randall, W.C., ed. 1977. *Neural Regulation of the Heart.* Oxford University Press, New York.

Rasmussen, H. 1970. Cell communication, calcium ion, and cyclic adenosine monophosphate. *Science* 170:404–12.

Stahl, W.R. 1967. Scaling of respiratory variables in mammals. *J. Appl. Physiol.* 22:453–60.

Sturkie, D.D., ed. 1976. *Avian Physiology.* 3d ed. Springer, New York.

Vatner, S.F., Monroe, R.G., and McRitchie, R.J. 1974. Effects of anesthesia, tachycardia, and autonomic blockade on the Anrep effect in intact dogs. *Am. J. Physiol.* 266:1450–56.

Wells, T.A.G. 1964. *The Rabbit: A Practical Guide.* Heinemann, London.

Woodworth, R.S. 1902. Maximal contraction, "staircase" contraction, refractory period and compensatory pause of the heart. *Am. J. Physiol.* 8:213–49.

Zelis, R., Delea, C.S., Coleman, H.N., and Mason, D. 1970. Arterial sodium content in experimental congestive heart failure. *Circulation* 41:213–16.

CHAPTER 10

Control Mechanisms of the Circulatory System | by David K. Detweiler

SYSTEMIC PRESSURE AND FLOW

Arterial pressure

Arterial blood pressure is determined by (1) the pumping action of the heart, (2) the peripheral resistance, (3) the viscosity of the blood, (4) the quantity of blood in the arterial system, and (5) the elasticity of the arterial walls. These factors are controlled by a complex regulatory system that ordinarily maintains the arterial pressure within narrow limits. Normal values for various species are given in Table 10.1. Unlike heart rate, there is no between-species blood pressure difference related to body weight; most mammals fall within the same ranges. There is a determining relationship, at least in the giraffe, between blood pressure and the height of the head above the heart level (see Fig. 5.5). Thus the resting blood pressure at heart level increases with neck length from dog to cow to giraffe, while the differences at brain level are much less. Birds have blood pressure ranges higher than mammals, possibly to buffer gravitational forces in flying.

Blood pressure of newborn animals is significantly lower than that of adults in both birds and mammals. The enormous mean peak blood pressures within the corpus cavernosum penis (CCP) (7000 to 14,000 mm Hg in the goat, bull, and stallion) and the corpus spongiosum penis (CSP) (994 mm Hg in the stallion) are caused by contractions of the ischiocavernosus (for the CCP) and bulbospongiosus (for the CSP) muscles. The peak systolic arterial pressures recorded at the same time ranged from 179 to 245 mm Hg and obviously could not account for these high penile pressures.

For the characteristics of capillary and venous pressure and flow, see Chap. 5.

Arterial blood pressure measurement

Direct measurement of arterial blood pressure is accomplished by means of a fluid-filled hypodermic needle or catheter inserted into the vessel or heart chamber, and the pressure at the external end is measured with a pressure-sensitive transducer (saline or mercury column; induc-

Table 10.1. Representative adult arterial blood pressures

Species	Systiolic/diastolic (mm Hg)*	Mean (mm Hg)
Giraffe	260/160	219
Horse	130/95	115
Cow	140/95	120
Swine	140/80	110
Sheep	140/90	114
Humans	120/70	100
Dog	120/70	100
Cat	140/90	110
Rabbit	120/80	100
Guinea pig	100/60	80
Rat	110/70	90
Mouse	111/80	100
Turkey	250/170	190
Chicken	175/145	160
Canary	220/150	185

*Published values are extremely variable because of the lability of blood pressure in response to environmental factors. These values were selected from various sources as reasonable for resting animals.

tance, capacitance, or strain-gauge transducer). This is by far the most reliable method.

Indirect blood pressure measurement has the advantage of being noninvasive, but the results are less reliable than those obtained with direct methods. Most indirect methods depend on compression of an artery with an inflatable cuff placed around a limb or the tail. The pressure in the cuff is then measured to determine when blood flow is interrupted (*systolic pressure*) and when flow is unimpeded again (*diastolic pressure*). One of three methods is used for determining the points of interruption and unimpeded flow: the *palpatory, oscillatory,* or *auscultatory.* The first method uses palpation of the arterial pulse below the cuff and determines systolic pressure only; the second, the presence of oscillations in the manometer; and the third, a sequence of sounds heard with a stethoscope over the artery adjacent to the cuff.

Auscultatory method

The auscultatory procedure is the one generally employed clinically. It was introduced in 1905 by the Russian physician Korotkoff. Certain sounds heard during auscultation over the brachial artery distal to the cuff are taken as the criteria for the systolic and diastolic pressures. Under ordinary circumstances if a stethoscope is placed over the artery, no sound can be heard as the flow of blood through the vessels is inaudible. If, however, the artery is compressed by the manometer cuff to arrest completely the flow of blood, a sharp, light tapping sound, in rhythm with the heartbeat, will be heard when the pressure in the cuff is released and falls just sufficiently to permit the arterial lumen to open. As the pressure in the cuff is progressively lowered, the sound undergoes a series of changes in quality and intensity.

Four phases of the sound, each having its distinctive character, may be heard in succession in the normal animal as the pressure is gradually reduced from about 120 to 80 mm Hg or less. These are described below with the average pressures at which they are normally heard (Fig. 10.1).

Sounds of Korotkoff

Phase I. Sudden appearance of a clear, but often faint, tapping sound that grows louder during the succeeding 10 to 14 mm Hg fall in pressure.

Phase II. The sound takes on a murmuring quality during the next 15 to 20 mm Hg fall in pressure.

Phase III. The sound changes little in quality but becomes clearer and louder during the next 5 to 7 mm Hg fall in pressure.

Phase IV. A muffled quality lasts throughout the next 5 to 6 mm Hg fall. After this all sound disappears.

Phase V. This is the point at which sounds disappear.

The muffling and disappearance are commonly referred to as the fourth and fifth points. If there is a detectable difference between these, it is recommended that they be recorded as, for example, 142/82/78 mm Hg (142 = systolic; 82 = fourth phase; 78 = fifth phase). If the fourth and fifth points are identical, this should be recorded (e.g., 144/76/76 mm Hg). Muffling (phase IV) occurs at pressures 7 to 10 mm Hg higher than direct intra-arterial diastolic pressures. Disappearance of sounds (phase V) occurs close to intra-arterial diastolic pressures at resting heart rate. With an increase in flow, as with exercise, phase V does not occur until far below true diastolic pressure because of the greater opportunity for intra-arterial turbulence. Under such circumstances, phases IV and V may be separated by 40 mm Hg or more, with phase IV being closest to true diastolic pressure.

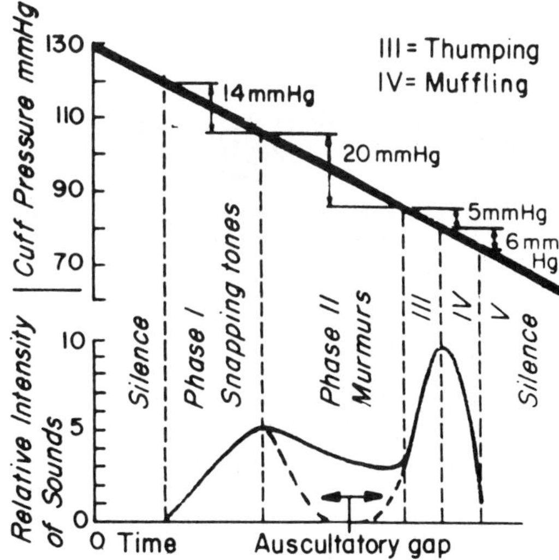

Figure 10.1. Characteristics of the auscultatory method of measuring blood pressure. (Redrawn from Geddes 1970. *The Direct and Indirect Measurement of Blood Pressure,* Year Book, Chicago, copyright © 1970 by Year Book Medical Publishers, Inc.)

Auscultatory gap

As shown by the sound intensity curve in Fig. 10.1, the Korotkoff sounds may temporarily disappear during the latter part of phase II. This gap may cover a range of 40 mm Hg and cause marked underestimation of systolic pressure if the cuff pressure is increased only to the level at which the sounds are first absent. This may be avoided by checking the systolic pressure first by palpation; when the palpatory systolic pressure is highest, it should be accepted as the reliable determination. Venous congestion associated with slow cuff deflation or rapidly repeated occlusions increases the occurrence of auscultatory gap. Thus, by rapidly deflating the cuff (2 to 3 mm Hg/s), allowing 2 to 3 minutes to elapse between determinations, and raising the limb to promote venous drainage, one can reduce or eliminate the auscultatory gap.

Other indirect methods

A variety of other methods based on the use of an occluding cuff employ various sensors for detecting sound, pulsation, or blood flow below the cuff.

Pulse detectors

Various types of pressure transducer have been applied below the cuff to detect the earliest arrival of pulsation as the indicator for systolic pressure. The size of the signal obtained varies as pulsation increases, and these characteristic variations have been used to estimate (in general, unreliably) mean or diastolic pressure.

Microphones

Korotkoff sounds may be amplified by means of piezoelectric microphones mounted within or below the cuff. The electrical signal obtained may be amplified to increase audibility or used to actuate a voltmeter or other visual signal such as a flashing light.

Ultrasound

Ultrasound may be used to detect arterial wall movements as pressure is decreased in the blood pressure cuff. Ultrasound transmitting and receiving crystals are placed over the artery beneath the cuff. The Doppler signal received identifies the opening and closing of the artery. At cuff pressure just below systolic level, opening of the artery occurs only at the peak of pressure, followed rapidly by closure. The time interval between these two signals increases as cuff pressure declines until it is low enough that the vessel remains open during the pulse.

Equipment and methods for radiotelemetry of blood pressure and flow have been developed and employed in free-ranging terrestrial and aquatic animals (Van Citters and Franklin 1969a, b).

FUNCTIONAL ORGANIZATION OF THE VASCULAR BED

As blood makes its circuit through the body, it passes in series through the parts of the circulatory system that have the functions designated in Fig. 10.2. Each part of the body receives its blood through a series of vessels of this kind. For the body as a whole, however, the circulation consists of multiple series like this arranged in parallel channels.

Classification by function

Vessels may be classified in accordance with their function as follows (Folkow 1960):

1. *Windkessel vessels* convert pulsatile inflow to a somewhat smoothed outflow.

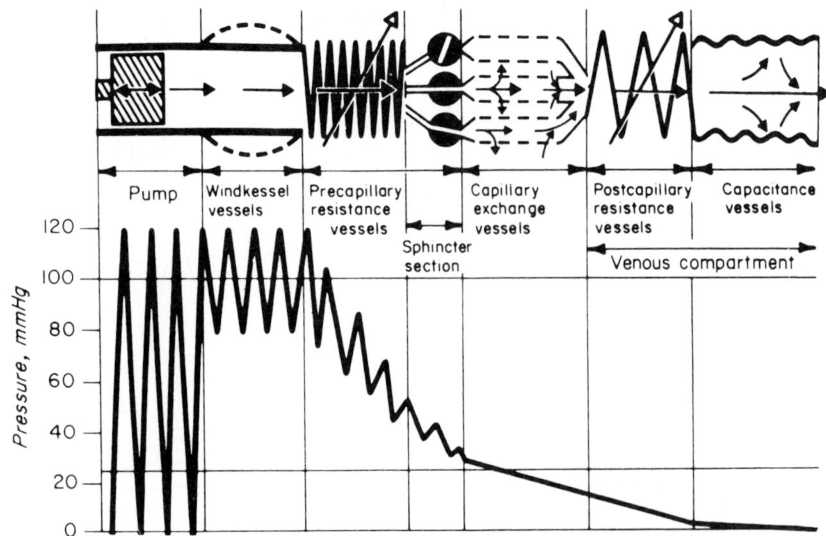

Figure 10.2. Functionally differentiated segments of the vascular bed. (From Mellander and Johansson 1968. *Pharmacol. Rev.* 20:117–96, © 1968, Am. Soc. for Pharmacology & Experimental Therapeutics.)

2. *Resistance vessels* are chiefly the small arteries, the arterioles, and to a lesser extent the capillaries and smallest veins.
   a. Precapillary resistance resides chiefly in the small arteries and arterioles; they are the major sites of resistance to flow.
   b. Postcapillary resistance is determined by the venules and veins. Capillary hydrostatic pressure and thus filtration-absorption exchange are determined by the ratio of pre-capillary to postcapillary resistance.
3. *Sphincter vessels* are terminal segments of precapillary arterioles that can constrict and restrict or shut off capillary flow. They determine the number of open capillaries and hence the area of capillary exchange surface.
4. *Exchange vessels* are the capillaries, which are not contractile but respond passively to changes in resistance and sphincter vessels.
5. *Capacitance vessels* are chiefly the veins that, through diameter changes that have little influence on resistance, can effect marked shifts of blood volume and thus dramatically affect cardiac venous return and volume flow. They contain about 80 percent of the regional blood volume.
6. *Shunt vessels* are arteriovenous anastomoses found in some tissues; these vessels allow the blood to bypass exchange vessels.

Resistance and capacitance vessels may react differently in accordance with their differing functions. Thus epinephrine dilates some resistance vessels while constricting capacitance vessels; norepinephrine constricts both but affects capacitance vessels more.

Musculoelastic thickenings, called *intimal cushions,* are found at branching sites of many small arteries; since according to some authorities they are often densely innervated, they are thought to be capable of differentially regulating distribution of blood flow within the tissues.

Microcirculation

The terminal vascular beds consisting of small arterioles, metarterioles, capillaries, and venules are included under the general term *microcirculation* (see Fig. 5.3).

Arterioles

The arterioles contain the smallest blood volume of the cardiovascular system, but the pressure and flow in the circulatory system are more sensitive to minute changes in diameter of the arterioles than to diameter changes in any other part of the circulatory system. The arterioles are the final or end branches of the distributing system and operate as stopcocks that control the runoff of blood from the arterial system into the capillaries. The caliber of arterioles is controlled by the state of contraction of their circularly disposed and strongly developed smooth muscle fibers as regulated by local metabolic processes and by blood-borne substances such as catecholamines. Arterioles are also supplied with vasomotor fibers controlled by centers in the spinal cord and medulla. Their distensibility depends on the state of the smooth muscle in their walls.

Capillaries

The blood content of the capillaries (5 percent of blood volume) is also very small, but the total filtering surface of the capillary endothelium is enormous.

The capillary wall is composed of a single layer of endothelial cells and does not exceed 0.5 μm in thickness (Fig. 10.3). Three general types of capillaries are distinguished on the basis of the completeness of their endothelial walls (Fig. 10.3). (1) *Continuous capillaries* with complete endothelial walls and basement membranes are found in adipose

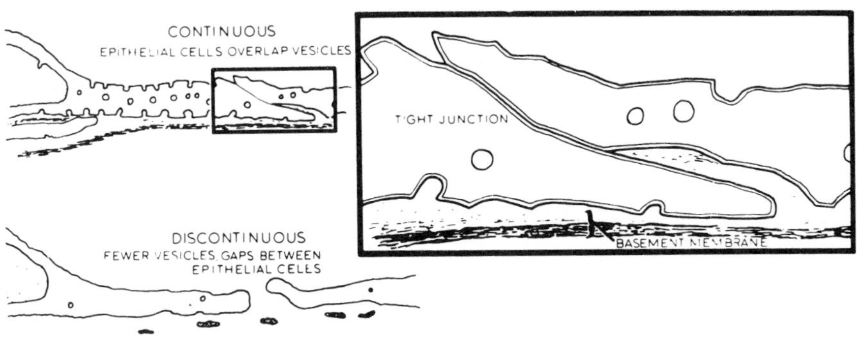

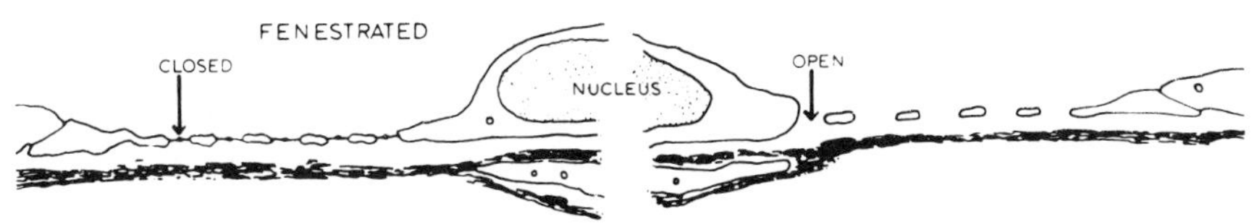

Figure 10.3. Three types of capillaries according to completeness of the endothelium. (Modified from Majno 1965, in Hamilton and Dow, eds. *Handbook of Physiology,* sec. 2, vol. 3, *Circulation,* Am. Physiol. Soc., Washington, pp. 2293–2375.)

tissue; smooth, skeletal, and cardiac muscle; placenta; lung; and central nervous system. They have pinocytic vesicles that are 60 to 70 nm in diameter along their luminal and basal borders, form tight junctions with adjacent cells, and have pores or intercellular clefts between cells that allow passage of water-soluble ions and molecules. (2) *Discontinuous capillaries* or sinusoids have gaps between the endothelial cells and incomplete or absent basement membranes. They are found in the liver, spleen, and bone marrow and allow passage of whole cells, macromolecules, and particles. (3) *Fenestrated capillaries* contain small openings, 0.1 μm or less in diameter, that are closed (except for glomerular capillaries) by a thin diaphragm. They allow rapid diffusion of solutes and water. Fenestrated capillaries are found in endocrine and exocrine glands, gallbladder, synovial membrane, ciliary body, and choroid plexus and in countercurrent flow systems such as those found in the renal medulla and the swim bladder.

The functional anatomy of the capillaries has been worked out for some cold-blooded animals and for the rat and dog mesentery through microscopic observations of the in vivo vessels and for the rat and dog myocardium by both anatomical and microscopic observations (Fig. 5.3). Briefly, blood flows generally from the arteriole directly into a metarteriole, which leads into capillaries as well as into capillarylike channels that connect rather directly with venules. The true capillaries that carry on most of the interchange between blood and tissues are arranged as interanastomosing side branches of the main channels through the bed. At the ostia of each capillary is a small precapillary sphincter of smooth muscle. Sympathetic vasoconstrictor fibers innervate the arterioles and occasionally extend as far as the metarterioles. The metarterioles and the precapillary sphincters, however, are not usually innervated and thus are chiefly under the control of local conditions in the tissues. Under natural conditions the metarterioles and their precapillary sphincters undergo periodic contractions at intervals of 15 seconds to 3 minutes. When the tissue is in a resting state, the constrictor phase of this rhythm predominates and the precapillary sphincters may be completely closed. When the tissue becomes active, the dilator phase of the metarterioles predominates and the precapillary sphincters are open. In contrast to this active vasomotion in metarterioles and precapillary sphincters is the passive opening or closing of the true capillaries. Whether they are open or closed depends on hydrostatic pressure relationships within and without; the intracapillary pressure is governed by the upstream sphincter mechanisms (e.g., the precapillary sphincters). The external capillary pressure depends on mechanical forces applied to the tissue in question. In skeletal muscle, the increase in blood flow with exercise comes in large measure from the opening up of large numbers of additional capillaries.

Although the capillary bed is traditionally considered a passive system, the recent finding of contractile protein in capillary walls and the presence of autonomic nerve endings indicate that the contractile protein and autonomic nerve endings may play a role in hemodynamic function (contraction and dilation).

Capillary exchanges

Diffusional flow, resulting from the spontaneous movement of molecules and particles from regions of higher to lower concentration, is the major mechanism for transcapillary exchanges. The volume of water diffusion through the total capillary surface is about 15,000 to 18,000 times that of filtration. Lipid-soluble substances, including oxygen and carbon dioxide, diffuse through the capillary membrane. Water molecules also diffuse through the capillary membrane as well as through intercellular clefts or pores. Water-soluble, lipid-insoluble substances (e.g., electrolytes, glucose, urea) cannot pass through the lipid membrane of endothelial cells but must diffuse through the capillary pores (see Fig. 1.1).

Bulk flow, in contrast to diffusional flow, is the movement of fluid and solutes in bulk through capillary pores in response to hydrostatic or osmotic pressure differences across the capillary wall. The direction of this flow, inward or outward, depends on the balance of hydrostatic and osmotic pressures within and outside the capillary. The relations of these governing forces were first formulated in 1896 by Starling (the *Starling hypothesis*), and later Landis verified the concept with specific pressure measurements. Typical values are given in Fig. 10.4. The effective outward *filtration pressure* depicted at the arterial end of the capillary is the difference between the sums of (1) blood pressure (25 mm Hg) plus the tissue colloid osmotic pressure (5 mm Hg) and (2) the plasma protein oncotic pressure (28 mm Hg) minus the tissue hydrostatic pressure (−6 mm Hg). This gives a net 8 mm Hg filtration pressure at the arterial end of the capillary. The blood hydrostatic pressure falls toward the venous end, while the other forces remain constant, resulting in an effective inward *absorption pressure* at the venous end of a −7 mm Hg. The net exchange is on the order of 40 ml/24 h/100 g of tissue. Such bulk flow explains fluid shifts between the plasma and interstitial compartments, which are important in the reflex vasomotor control of plasma volume. It contributes little to the actual rate of exchange of other materials across capillary membranes. Compared with bulk flow and total extracellular fluid volume, including plasma volume, the relatively enormous diffusional exchange mentioned above is the prime determinant of transcapillary exchanges, and for a given solute it may proceed along a concentration gradient in a direction opposite that of net bulk flow.

Pinocytosis, in which the endothelial cells ingest substances at their inner surface by forming vesicles around them for transport through the outer-cell surface, where they are discharged, accounts for absorption of large molecules (e.g., lipoproteins, polysaccharides).

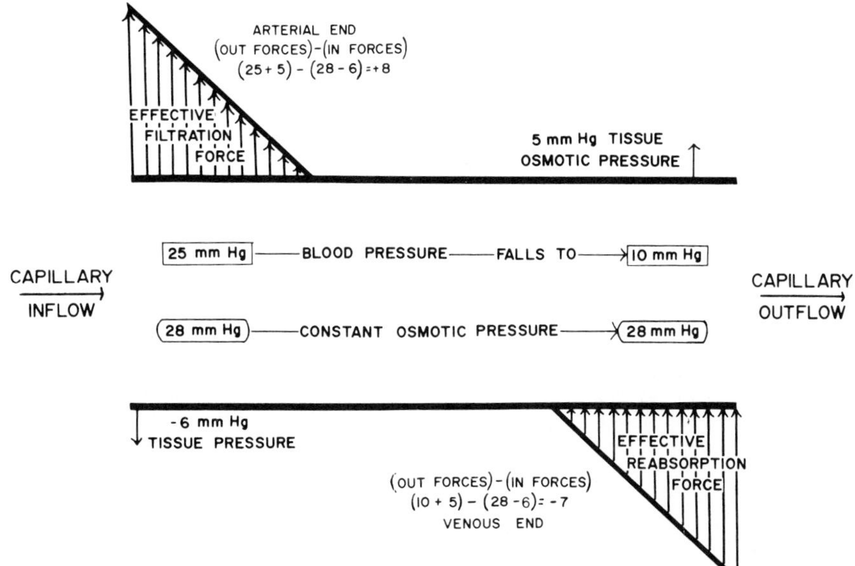

Figure 10.4. Forces accounting for capillary filtration and absorption.

Excess extracellular fluids and large molecules and particles that are not returned to the bloodstream through capillary absorption can return through the lymphatics.

Capillary hydrostatic pressures are not the same in all tissues. In the renal glomeruli, for example, the hydrostatic pressures are about double those elsewhere, favoring the large glomerular filtration required for renal function. In the lungs, by contrast, where it is crucial that fluid does not collect in the alveoli, the hydrostatic pressures are about one-half of those elsewhere, favoring absorption of fluid. Another site where capillary hydrostatic and other forces acting at the microvascular level are anomalous is in the vasculature of the fleshy lamina of the equine digit. The following values have been reported for healthy horses: capillary blood pressure, 37 mm Hg; plasma protein oncotic pressure 19 mm Hg; and tissue hydrostatic pressure, 25 mm Hg.

The importance of active contractility as a mechanism for altering permeability is still an open question, but it appears that permeability is not constant and may increase or decrease under both normal and pathological conditions.

CONTROL OF VASCULAR SMOOTH MUSCLE

Both single-unit and multiunit types of smooth muscle are found in vessel walls. Cells in the inner media of blood vessels are probably of the single-unit type, while outer medial cells probably have multiunit properties. Only these outer-ring cells are innervated. They are excited by neural activity, propagate the excitation poorly to adjoining cells, and are relatively unresponsive to stretch. The medial cells with single-unit properties are not innervated, have spontaneous pacemaker cells that generate action potentials that spread to adjacent cells, and respond actively to mechanical stretch. Sympathetic vasoconstrictor stimulation, catecholamines, and stretching of the vessel wall increase the frequency of discharge of these pacemaker cells, increasing the net tension developed in the vessel wall. There are two activation mechanisms in vascular smooth muscle: (1) excitation generated by action potentials and (2) excitation without action potentials. Thus some specific agonists can excite contraction without inducing membrane action potentials. Excitation-contraction coupling, whether or not associated with an action potential, is the result of increasing the cytoplasmic Ca^{2+} concentration from 10^{-7} mM to 10^{-5} mM or higher.

The role of vascular endothelium

Although the vascular endothelium is only a thin monolayer of squamous cells making up a small fraction of the vessel wall in larger arteries and veins, it lines the entire vascular system and, taken as a whole, has the bulk of such large organs as the liver. The study of endothelial function was vastly stimulated by the initial observation that acetylcholine (ACh) produces dilatation in the rabbit aorta, not by acting directly on ACh receptors in smooth muscle, but by acting on ACh receptors in the endothelium. The endothelial cells, in turn, produce and release a relaxing factor(s) that penetrates the smooth muscle cells and relaxes them (Fig. 10.5). This factor (or factors) has been named endothelium-derived relaxing factor (EDRF), and the principle of endothelium dependency of vascular responses (both constrictor and dilator) applies to vessels of all sizes, including arterioles (i.e., resistance vessels).

Recent research (especially during the last decade) has emphasized the functional role of vascular endothelium in circulation above and beyond its importance in capillary

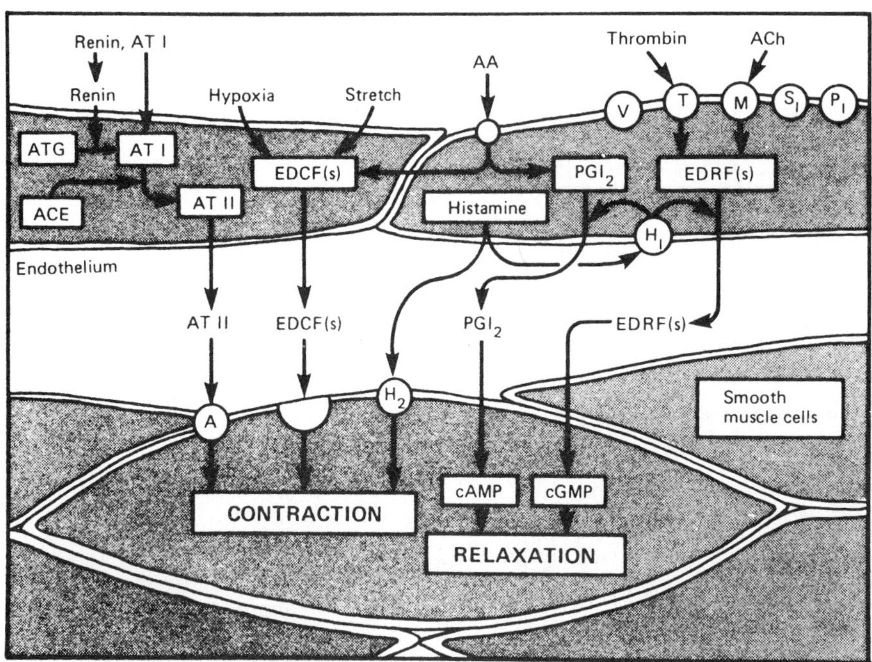

Figure 10.5. Vasoactive substances released from the vascular endothelium. AA, arachidonic acid; ACh, acetylcholine; V, vasopressinergic receptor; T, thrombin receptor; M, muscarinic receptor; S_1, serotonergic receptor; P_1, purinergic receptor; ATG, angiotensinogen; AT I, angiotensin I; AT II, angiotensin II; ACE, angiotensin-converting enzyme; EDCF(s), endothelium-derived constricting factors(s); PGI_2, prostacyclin; EDRF(s), endothelium-derived relaxing factor(s); H_1/H_2, histaminergic receptor; A, angiotensinergic receptor; cAMP, cyclic adenosine monophosphate; cGMP, cyclic guanosine monophosphate. (From Luescher 1988. *Endothelial Vasoactive Substances and Cardiovascular Disease.* Karger, Basel.)

transport and exchanges between blood and tissue. These functions include the following:

1. Prevention of the adherence of platelets, leukocytes and monocytes.
2. Production of blood clotting factors (e.g., von Willebrand factor VIII, plasminogen activators, and inhibitors).
3. Activation (e.g., angiotensin I) and inactivation (e.g., norepinephrine, serotonin, bradykinin, and adenosine 5′-diphosphate) of circulating hormones and other plasma constituents.
4. Synthesis and secretion of vasodilator (e.g., prostacyclin, EDRFs) and vasoconstrictor substances (e.g., endothelium-derived constrictor factors (EDCFs), prostanoids, angiotensin, and histamine).
5. Production of a heparinlike cell-growth inhibitor and growth factors that may regulate growth of vascular smooth muscle. (See "Metabolic Functions of Pulmonary Circulation," p. 222 of this chapter.)

Endothelium-derived vasoactive substances

The various vasoactive substances produced or released from the endothelium (Fig. 10.5) serve to regulate vascular smooth muscle tone or to modulate other regulatory influence. These substances include (1) prostacyclin and other prostanoids; (2) angiotensin II, either locally produced or carried in circulating blood; (3) EDRF or EDCF (or factors) that are released under certain conditions, such as hypoxia or stretch.

Endothelium-derived relaxing factor(s)

Among the several EDRFs are the following:

Nitrous oxide. Recent work indicates that release of nitrous oxide (NO) from the endothelium is one of the chief mediators of endothelium-dependent relaxation and that L-arginine is the physiologic substrate for its formulation.

The L-arginine–nitrous oxide pathway

The role of NO as a second messenger and its synthesis from L-arginine as a widespread pathway for cell regulation and communication have been demonstrated. In the vascular endothelium NO is released by such factors as acetylcholine and shear stress. Nitrous oxide activates guanylyl cyclase in the vascular smooth muscle cells, where it vasodilates, and in platelets, where it inhibits aggregation and adhesion. The mechanism whereby the cyclic guanosine monophosphate (cGMP), which is increased by the activation of guanylyl cyclase, mediates its effects on the smooth muscle cells is uncertain but may include protein phosphorylation.

Blockade of NO synthesis in experimental animals increases blood pressure. This suggests that a basal release of NO in arterial beds regulates arterial tone.

These findings that NO is an important determinant of blood vessel tone and platelet function indicate that the L-arginine–NO pathway may play a major role in such clinical states as hypertension, shock, and atherosclerosis (see Chap. 12).

Prostacyclin. Prostaglandins, derived primarily from arachidonic acid through the cyclooxygenase pathway, are the main source of prostacyclin, whose production from prostaglandins is catalyzed by the enzyme prostacyclin synthetase. In blood vessel walls it is the major product of the cyclooxygenase pathway and is largely produced by the endothelial cells. The endothelial cells can also produce prostacyclin from platelet-derived endoperoxides; this is a negative feedback mechanism that causes increased prostacyclin production where platelet aggregation occurs, since prostacyclin inhibits platelet aggregation.

Prostacyclin *release* can be caused by (1) shear stress, (2) hypoxia, or (3) receptor-operated mechanisms.

In most vascular beds prostacyclin causes relaxation of smooth muscle mediated by cyclic AMP (cAMP) and, infused intravenously, it causes a fall in blood pressure.

Endothelium-derived constricting factor(s)

Initially, a vasoconstrictor polypeptide was isolated from cultured endothelial cells. Later, a 21-residue vasoconstrictor peptide, termed *endothelin* (ET) was isolated from vascular endothelial cells. It is among the most potent of all known mammalian vasoconstricting substances. As yet its physiological role has not been established, although it is considered to have important as yet undetermined regulatory functions. ET is also produced by tracheal epithelial cells. Binding sites are not limited to the vasculature but are also found in kidneys, lungs, brain, gray matter of the spinal cord, nerves, liver, spleen, intestine, uterus, trachea, and placenta. ET density in the atria is double that in the ventricles, and there are clusters of high-affinity sites in the sinoatrial node. Sites have been identified in cardiac myocytes in which ET elicits a dose-dependent positive inotropic response accompanied by increased cytosolic Ca^{2+} concentration. Similarly, many smooth muscle cells contain binding sites and ET promotes dose-dependent sustained constriction accompanied by an increased cytosolic Ca^{2+} concentration.

Thus ET causes vasoconstriction, positive inotropy, and atrial natriuretic factor (ANF) release all at concentrations in the low nanomolar range.

The contractile apparatus of vascular smooth muscle

Unlike skeletal and cardiac muscle, smooth muscle actin and myosin filaments are not organized into sarcomeric units. Instead, these contractile proteins are scattered throughout the cytoplasm of the smooth muscle cell (SMC). SMC also differs from sarcomeric muscle in that the regulation of contraction is based on the thick (myosin) filament rather than on the thin (actin) filament. Actin serves as a structural element and activates myosin-associated Mg^{2+} ATPase. SMC myosin consists of a pair of heavy-molecular-weight chains and two pairs of light-molecular-weight chains. There are two types of myosin light chains (MLC). One is required for myosin ATPase activity and is called essential, or alkali, MLC. A second type regulates SMC activity and is called regulatory MLC. The SMC has a pair of each type of MLCs. In addition, the SMC contains tropomyosin. This protein interacts with actin and the group of proteins known as troponins to regulate the actin-myosin interaction in striated muscle. The role of tropomyosin in SMCs is uncertain.

The thick (myosin) filament regulation of SMC contraction depends on phosphorylation of a specific serine residue in the regulatory MLC. This is required for activation of the myosin Mg^{2+} ATPase by actin, which is needed to provide the energy for contraction. Phosphorylation occurs through a specific MLC kinase, which is regulated by calcium ions. The calcium ions are bound to the protein calmodulin (Ca^{2+}–calmodulin complex). The latter binds to inactive MLC kinase and activates it to cause regulatory MLC phosphorylation. This MLC kinase is also regulated by a cAMP-dependent protein kinase. Phosphorylation of the MLC kinase by this enzyme decreases the binding of the Ca^{2+}–calmodulin complex, favors the inactive form of MLC kinase, and promotes relaxation. Note that cAMP increases contractility in cardiac muscle and decreases it in vascular smooth muscle. (See Table 10.2.)

Thus contraction of the SMC is initiated by increasing Ca^{2+} that activates MLC kinase. The latter causes phosphorylation of regulatory MLC and the formation of cross-bridges between actin and myosin. Where these phosphorylated cross-bridges cycle rapidly, phasic vasoconstriction occurs as in response to vasocontrictor substances. Relaxation follows sufficient reduction in Ca^{2+} levels because of inactivation of MLC kinase. If Ca^{2+} levels are not reduced sufficiently to cause relaxation, a reduced cycling called the "latch" state will prevail and maintain a condition of steady vascular tone.

The myosin heavy chains (MHC) in SMCs are similar to those in striated muscle. They consist of an aminoterminal globular head, which binds two sets of MLC, and a long alpha helical tail, and they contain Mg^{2+} ATPase located in the head region, which is activated by interaction with actin.

Local control

Precapillary resistance vessels are in a constant state of partial constriction (i.e., tone) caused by inherent myogenic activity. This activity is particularly marked in the single-unit SMC present in these vessels. This tone persists in the absence of excitatory nervous or humoral effects. The venous capacitance vessels have little myogenic activity. Their tone depends on sympathetic vasoconstrictor action; their smooth muscle is of the multiunit type. The mechanism of this inherent vasomotion is unknown. Presumably, it arises from locally produced metabolites, which can have

Table 10.2. Adrenergic effects on the cardiovascular system

Receptor (R) subtype	Transduction pathway	Receptor location	Effect
Alpha$_1$	Increased phosphatidylinositol (PI) turnover: mediated by an undefined protein (G_x); hydrolysis of PI to phosphatidylinositol biphosphate (PIP_2) is stimulated with release of diacylglycerol (DG) and inositol triphosphate (IP_3). DG → C-kinase activation in membrane which may selectively limit or mimic alpha$_1$-mediated processes. IP_3 → Ca^{2+} release from sarcoplasmic reticulum.	Ventricular myocardium (VM) Atrial myocardium (AM) Purkinje fibers and sinoatrial node	Positive inotropy (prolonged action potential) Positive inotropy Negative chronotropy (reduced automaticity)
	Ca^{2+} binds to and activates calmodulin (CM). CM activates myosin light chain kinase (MLCK) → myosin light chain phosphate, which allows activation of myosin Mg^{2+} ATPase by actin → cross-bridge formation and vascular smooth muscle contraction	Arterioles and veins	Constriction
Alpha$_2$	Inhibition of adenylate cyclase: coupled to a guanine nucleotide-binding protein that is inhibitory (G_i) and linked to the catalytic subunit (C) of adenylate cyclase, this R − G_i − C complex inhibits C and cAMP synthesis is reduced.	Selected arterioles Presynaptic adrenergic terminals Platelets Inhibitory neurons, pontomedullary region	Constriction Inhibition of norepinephrine (NE) release Aggregation Decreased sympathetic tone, increased vagal tone → vasodilatation, negative chronotropy
Beta$_1$	Activation of adenylate cyclase: coupled to a guanine nucleotide binding protein that is stimulatory (G_s and linked to C; thus R-G_s-C complex stimulates C and cAMP synthesis is increased.	Sinoatrial node Atrial myocardium Atrioventricular node Ventricular myocardium	Positive chronotropy Positive inotropy, chronotropy Positive chronotropy, dromotropy Positive inotropy, dromotropy
	In cAMP relaxation cAMP activates protein kinase that phosphorylates a MLCK subunit, decreasing MLCK activity.	Renal arterioles	Relaxation
Beta$_2$	Activation of adenylate cyclase: coupled to G_s and linked to C causing increase in cAMP as with beta$_1$.	Sinoatrial node	Positive chronotropy
	cAMP activates a protein kinase that phosphorylates a MLCK subunit, decreasing MLCK activity. cGMP is also involved by mechanisms other than phosphorylation of MLCK (e.g., regulating Ca^{2+} uptake).	Coronary, skeletal muscle, abdominal, visceral, and pulmonary arterioles Systemic veins	Relaxation Relaxation

PI, phosphatidylinositol; DG, diacylglycerol; IP_3, inositol triphosphate; MLCK, myosin light chain kinase; VSM, vascular smooth muscle; G, nucleotide binding protein; G_s, stimulatory; G_i, inhibitory; G_x, undefined nucleotide binding protein; NE, norepinephrin; VM, ventricular myocardium; AM, atrial myocardium; R, receptor; C, catalytic subunit of adenylate cyclase.

Compiled from various sources: Bristow and Port, 1990; Green and Watanabe, 1989; Bennett et al., 1989; Graham and Lanier, 1986; Darnell et al., 1986.

complex effects. Locally about the arterioles, precapillaries, and capillaries there are released norepinephrine, acetylcholine, carbon dioxide, lactic acid, products of nuclear metabolism, and presumably many other substances, which can act in many different ways on these vessels. Other potent vasoactive substances such as histamine, prostaglandins, serotonin, and adenosine triphosphate and diphosphate are found in all metabolically active tissues, including the blood vessel walls themselves.

Although large quantitative differences are found in different parts of the vascular tree, in general the regions that have active intrinsic vasomotion have autonomic vasoconstriction that is not very powerful, whereas where the latter is prominent the myogenic contractions are less conspicuous. For example, the cutaneous arteriovenous anastomoses that are found in the paws of cats are strongly controlled from the hypothalamic heat-loss center and show maximal dilatation with little intrinsic tone after sympathectomy. However, elimination of vasomotor nerves that serve regions such as the brain and myocardium has scarcely any effect on local blood flow, and the small blood vessels retain their usual size. Similarly, in skeletal muscle, sectioning of vasomotor nerves leaves a very strong tone in the smooth muscle of small vessels (dogs and humans), which increases with time after the sympathectomy. Reactivity to local metabolic effects seems to be stronger in the metarterioles and precapillary sphincters, whereas constrictor nerve fibers affect predominantly the arterioles; this indicates that the two types of control may exist within the same vascular bed. It is the locally induced vasodilatation that protects a tissue against ischemia (1) when arterial pressure is decreased or (2) when constriction of arterioles tends to reduce blood flow unduly. (See Autoregulation, Chap. 5.)

Three mechanisms contributing to local control of blood flow account for autoregulation: myogenic response to stretch, vasomotor effects of local metabolites, and tissue pressure.

Myogenic response to stretch

The myogenic response to stretch has been termed the *Bayliss mechanism,* after the physiologist who first proposed that increased stretch might increase vascular tone.

The small precapillary vessels constrict actively when pressure is elevated and dilate when it is lowered. The response to a change in pressure requires 15 to 60 seconds after an initial passive phase. Two major objections to a regulatory myogenic mechanism have been offered on a priori grounds: (1) Increased vasoconstrictor response to increased wall tension constitutes a positive-feedback response leading to instability in the cardiovascular system. Thus increased blood pressure would elevate flow resistance, which would further raise the blood pressure and lead to additional vasoconstriction, and so on. (2) Smooth muscle contractile response to vascular distention would tend to abolish the stimulus of stretch. The vessel might thus oscillate around a diameter somewhat greater than that at the time of the stretch stimulus. These objections are not necessarily valid. Whether or not a system like this is unstable and oscillates depends on the time constants of the several components of the system. The possible instability caused by positive feedback could be limited by "metabolic vasodilators" and the maximum range of vasomotor response. It seems reasonable to conclude that the myogenic response to stretch is a major factor in determining autoregulatory pressure-flow relationships. Thus both local metabolic dilator factors and myogenic mechanisms may be envisioned as functioning together to produce autoregulation.

An increase in perfusion pressure can cause an increase in *tissue pressure* by increasing the capillary hydrostatic pressure and enhancing fluid movement into the extracellular tissue space. The increased tissue pressure then compresses capillaries, venules, and small veins and thus increases resistance to blood flow. This mechanism can be demonstrated, for example, in the isolated kidney. Since the kidney is encased in a nonelastic capsule, an increase in extracellular fluid volume will rapidly result in increased tissue pressure. In other tissues that do not have such a stiff capsule (e.g., intestine and muscle), this mechanism does not appear to play a role in autoregulation.

Hypertonic infusions produce vasodilatation through inhibition of visceral smooth muscle pacemaker activity and a negative inotropic effect. Thus changes in plasma *osmolarity* can influence blood flow. A decrease in *temperature* increases myogenic vascular tone, and vice versa.

Under resting conditions, the pressure range where autoregulation is effective varies in different vascular beds. The lower limit for autoregulation in different organs is approximately 20 to 30 mm Hg for brain, 60 to 70 mm Hg for kidney, and above 100 mm Hg for body skin.

In summary, the peripheral resistance caused by vascular smooth muscle tone is regulated in a variety of ways. It is influenced locally by chemical factors that can affect both multiunit outer medial cells and single-unit inner medial cells. The innervated outer cells are under direct autonomic neural regulation (see below). Maximal stimulation by stretch affects chiefly the inner-ring cells. Thus there is some spatial separation of the sites of action of these different regulatory factors. The effects of stretch on myogenic tone are modulated by the chemical environment, temperature, and alpha-adrenergic neural control.

Nervous control

All levels of the central nervous system participate in cardiovascular control. Stimulation of discrete central nervous system areas and ablation experiments have identified a hierarchical array of control levels in the spinal cord, medulla and pons (bulb), hypothalamus, thalamus, cerebellum, and cerebral hemispheres (Fig. 10.6). Although such experiments demonstrate a certain autonomy and dominance in blood pressure control for centers in the bulbar

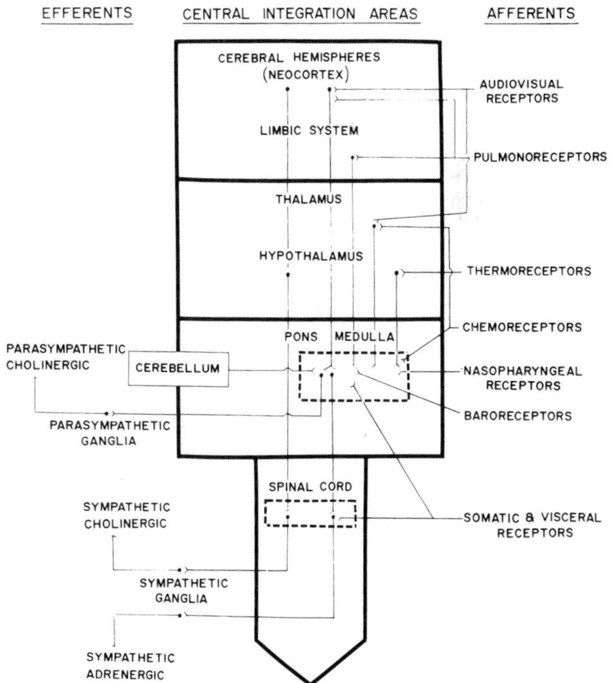

Figure 10.6. Summarizing schema of central nervous system cardiovascular control sites. This is a greatly simplified condensation of the large amount of experimental data on the location of control centers and their connections. The various centers, their cephalocaudal connections, and their afferents and efferents are actually bilateral. Specific vasomotor and cardioactive centers are not located; rather, the interplay of control areas at all levels of the central nervous system is emphasized. There has been no attempt to indicate the anatomical paths of the afferent input fibers.

region, they should not necessarily be considered the chief integrators for a given autonomic response when the various other control loops are not interrupted. The other areas all play an important complementary and modifying role in regulation in the intact animal, and selective destruction of one pathway or center may result in compensation by the remaining pathways.

The older idea that there are discrete centers for unitary control of spinal neurons has waned in favor of the concept that the inputs to the spinal nerves are organized at several levels, (e.g., pontomedullary region, midbrain, hypothalamus, and cerebral cortex). Thus complicated responses, such as the defense reaction, temperature control, and blood pressure control, are the result of integration longitudinally along the neuraxis.

The spinal cord

Neurons of nearby spinal cord segments, as well as descending axons from several cerebral centers, synapse with soma of preganglionic sympathetic neurons in the spinal cord. Therefore much of the integration of neural activity from various central nervous system levels occurs at these spinal synapses.

The preganglionic sympathetic neurons may, under some circumstances, exhibit spontaneous activity that is independent of an excitatory drive from afferent fibers or from higher levels of the nervous system. This phenomenon has been observed in spinal animals, where altered tensions of oxygen or carbon dioxide are believed to be responsible for the "spontaneous" activity.

Various types of afferent stimulation can call forth reflex vasoconstriction via the spinal cord. For example, pain or cold stimulation of the skin induces a segmentally arranged constriction of splanchnic vessels in spinal animals. Cutaneous vasodilatation occurs when the skin is moderately warmed.

Medulla oblongata. Neurons subserving vasomotor function from the spinal cord are under the control of higher-order neurons located particularly in the floor of the fourth ventricle of the medulla oblongata. Local electrical stimulation has revealed "pressor areas" and "depressor areas" that cause vasoconstriction and vasodilatation, respectively. The vasodilatation is caused by inhibition of vasoconstrictor tone, specific vasodilator fibers not being involved. Together these areas are known as the *vasomotor centers*. In the intact animal these centers, in turn, are controlled by still higher neurons from the hypothalamus and the cerebral cortex in response to a great variety of types of afferent stimulation and other neural inputs that become integrated into patterns of vasomotor activity. Special sympathetic cholinergic vasodilator pathways originating above the bulb also traverse the medulla (Fig. 10.6).

The state of activity of the medullary vasomotor centers similarly depends on afferent nerve impulses received from various organs and regions of the body, as well as from other nervous centers and respiratory centers, and on the chemical composition of the blood.

They exhibit inherent automaticity, in that they continue to discharge and maintain arterial blood pressure through vasoconstriction even after elimination of all incoming nerve influences. Sectioning of the brain stem above the medulla does not affect blood pressure; this indicates that upper levels do not dominate the medullary level, even though they can modify its state of activity.

The neurons of the nucleus tractus solitarius (NTS) in the medulla are the most important in the integration of sensory input from various afferents that affect cardiovascular and respiratory functions. Medial cells of the NTS, at the level of the obex, are involved in blood pressure regulation. The NTS has a close neural and vascular connection with the area postrema, which is devoid of a blood-brain barrier and is near the ventricular system. Afferents from arterial and cardiopulmonary baroreceptors, the trigeminal, facial, and vestibular nerves, and the hypothalamic nuclei all reach the NTS. The NTS, in turn, sends efferent fibers to hypothalamic nuclei, the amygdala, and to vagal and sympathetic preganglionic nuclei. Lesions of the NTS produce arterial hypertension.

The subretrofacial (SRF) nucleus located within the rostral ventrolateral medulla oblongata plays a pivotal role in the tonic and reflex control of the sympathetic nerves that innervate the heart and blood vessels. The SRF neurons are presympathetic nerve cells that are a major source of vasomotor tone.

This nucleus has distinctive histochemical and receptor binding properties, as follows. Bilateral application of neuroinhibitory compounds such as glycine directly to this nucleus in anesthetized cats causes collapse of the blood pressure to the level seen after complete severance of the spinal cord. This area has therefore been called the "glycine-sensitive area," and the cells here are considered responsible for maintaining resting arterial blood pressure through tonic sympathetic vasomotor activity. Since glycine does not affect nerve axons passing through this area, but affects only neuronal cell bodies, an effect on "axons of passage" that originate from cell bodies elsewhere is not involved. The glycine-blocking effect abolishes baroreceptor, other cardiovascular reflexes, and vasomotor responses from higher centers such as the cerebellum or the hypothalamus.

Unilateral microinjecton of neuroexcitatory amino acids such as L-glutamate (which excite cell bodies but not "axons of passage") into the SRF nucleus region causes large increases in sympathetic activity and blood pressure. The sympathetic activity thus induced is largely limited to sympathetic nerves innervating blood vessels, the heart, and the adrenal medulla but has little or no effect on noncardiovascular effectors (e.g., pupillary sphincters, sweat glands, etc.).

Further, the SRF nucleus contains subsets of neurons that control different regional beds. For example, chemical stimulation of the more rostral part of the nucleus preferentially increases vascular resistance in the kidney while stimulation of the caudal part preferentially increases vascular resistance in skeletal muscle of the hind limb. Similarly, differential effects on skin versus skeletal muscle arteries can be demonstrated by stimulation of different parts of the nucleus.

Afferent inputs to the SRF nucleus arise from several nuclei in the brain stem, the hypothalamus, and the NTS. A high proportion of efferent nerve fibers from the SRF projects to sympathetic preganglionic nuclei in the thoracic and lumbar spinal cord. Inputs through the NTS from baroreceptors inhibit the SRF cells, causing vasodilatation, and inputs from supramedullary regions of the brain can stimulate SRF cells to cause vasoconstriction and elevation of blood pressure as in the "defense reaction."

It is not certain what neurotransmitters are used by the SRF pressor cells in the control of the spinal preganglionic sympathetic nuclei. Neurotransmitters used by afferent nerves to the SRF include gamma-aminobutyric acid from inhibitory baroreceptor inputs, and there is a high density of angiotensin II receptor binding sites.

Sectioning of the spinal cord in the lower cervical region interrupts the stream of vasoconstrictor impulses passing from the medullary to the spinal mechanisms; the vessels dilate and arterial blood pressure falls. After a time, however, the blood pressure rises again. The spinal neurons thus exhibit their inherent power of autonomous action and, assuming the functions hitherto exercised by the medullary neurons, restore the vessels to their previous state of tonic constriction. The time required for the vessels to regain their tone after sectioning of the cord varies considerably in different species; for rats the time is measured in days, for cats it is measured in weeks.

After the animal with the sectioned spinal cord has recovered a nearly normal blood pressure, section of the splanchnic nerves once more leads to hypotension and vasodilatation, this time only in the splanchnic bed. In a normal animal sectioning of the splanchnic nerves doubles the flow of blood in the viscera they innervate (Burton-Opitz 1903). Once again, in the spinal animal with sectioning of the splanchnic nerves, a certain degree of tone ultimately returns to splanchnic blood vessels. It is intrinsic to the smooth muscle of the vessels and is known as *peripheral tone*. It develops still more slowly than the tone that originates in sympathetic neurons of the spinal cord.

Medullary vagal centers containing nuclei of cardiomotor fibers that regulate the heart differ in various species: in the dog these fibers arise from the dorsal motor nucleus of the vagus and the ambiguous nucleus; in the cat virtually all of these fibers arise from the ambiguous nucleus; in the monkey, rat, and pigeon the dorsal motor nucleus is the chief source.

Hypothalamus. Both increases and decreases in heart rate and arterial blood pressure may be elicited by stimulation of various areas in the hypothalamus. Pressor effects are subserved by sympathetic alpha-adrenergic fibers; depressor effects, by inhibition of sympathetic alpha-adrenergic fibers and stimulation of sympathetic cholinergic vasodilator fibers (cat and dog) and histaminergic vasodilator nerves.

An immediate and persistent lowering of blood pressure in both normotensive and renal hypertensive dogs occurs after large bilateral lesions that include the lateral hypothalamic areas. At least four possible explanations for this hypotension may be considered: (1) It may result from interruption of a tonic hypothalamic pressor action mediated by the autonomic vasoconstrictor nerves. (2) It may be a disturbance of the hypothalamicohypophyseal system that controls secretion of vasopressin (antidiuretic hormone, ADH) from the neurohypophysis; this seems unlikely because in diabetes insipidus, where ADH secretion does not occur, there is no characteristic change in blood pressure. (3) It may be related in some manner to adenohypophyseal dysfunction, inasmuch as total hypophysectomy does produce a lowering of blood pressure and the hypothalamus does control adenohypophyseal secretion. Against this possibility is the fact that a lowering of pressure follows hypothalamic injury immediately, whereas it develops more slowly and gradually after hypophysectomy. (4) Since renal hypertension depends initially on the renin-angiotensin-endocrine mechanism, there may be some as yet undisclosed relationship between it and the hypothalamus.

Centers in the perifornical regions of the hypothalamus and the central gray matter of the midbrain are involved in the vascular responses of the defense reaction. These include adrenergic arteriolar and venular constriction and cholinergically mediated arteriolar dilation in skeletal muscle. Electrical stimulation of the H_2 fields of Forel cause hemodynamic changes like those that occur during exercise.

The hypothalamus is involved in regulation of blood pressure and is essential for normal baroreceptor responses.

Another and principal function of the hypothalamus is control of body temperature. The rostral hypothalamus and preoptic area contain neurons that protect the body against overheating; they also control the discharge to the vasoconstrictor fibers of the cutaneous blood vessels and thus play an important role in adjusting blood pressure. Electrical stimulation or local cooling of this area brings about a rise in blood pressure (vasoconstriction), and direct warming of this region produces a fall in blood pressure (vasodilatation). The cutaneous arterioles and precapillary vessels, and especially the arteriovenous anastomoses (shunts), are the vessels most sensitively engaged in control of heat loss.

Cerebral cortex. Stimulation of the motor and premotor cerebral cortex results in marked elevation of blood pressure with constriction of the cutaneous, splanchnic, and renal vessels and, at the same time, a considerable vasodilatation in the skeletal muscle. A generalized depressor response accompanied by somatic inhibition ("playing dead" reaction) can be produced by stimulation of the cingulate gyrus. It is believed that these higher centers play significant roles in blood pressure response to pain and anxiety and also to exercise.

Cerebellum. Stimulation of various areas in the cerebellum can produce depressor and pressor effects and peripheral redistribution of blood supply (e.g., decrease renal blood flow and increase skin and muscle flow). In decerebrate cats, cerebellectomy facilitates baroreceptor reflexes and reverses somatosympathetic pressor reflexes. The actual role of the cerebellum in cardiovascular control is still unclear.

Central aminergic pathways. Numerous neurons containing catecholamines, dopamine, and serotonin are found in the brain. Their function in vasomotor control is uncertain. Some studies indicate that descending serotonergic fibers depress and descending adrenergic fibers excite sympathetic vasoconstrictor activity, but opposite effects have also been reported.

Sympathetic vasoconstrictor fibers

Distribution

Sympathetic vasoconstrictor fibers were discovered in 1852 by Claude Bernard, who stimulated the cervical sympathetic nerve in the rabbit and observed constriction of the vessels of the ear. These fibers belong to the thoracolumbar (sympathetic) division of the autonomic nervous system.

Adrenergic nerve endings have been identified in all types of blood vessels except the true capillaries. In general, precapillary resistance vessels (small arteries and arterioles) have a rich innervation, although in the smallest precapillary vessels the number of fibers is small. The venules have fewer adrenergic fibers than the larger veins, which themselves are less richly innervated than the precapillary vessels. It is solely through such sympathetic fibers traveling with somatic nerve trunks that constrictor impulses are conveyed to the minute vessels of the limbs. Unlike the larger vessels in the abdomen, the vessels in the extremities do not have ganglion cells in or on their walls. Sectioning of a peripheral nerve, therefore, causes complete degeneration of vasoconstrictor fibers in the area of its distribution.

Vasoconstrictor fibers to the head and neck are conveyed from the sympathetic chain through plexuses investing the blood vessels but also via peripheral nerve trunks (cervical and certain cranial nerves). The vessels of the abdomen and pelvis are supplied with fibers that pass along the vascular walls from plexuses surrounding the aorta and its branches. The sympathetic fibers to the heart arise chiefly in five upper dorsal segments of the cord, pass to the stellate ganglia and upper dorsal ganglia as white rami, and proceed to the heart by a complex plexus. Although the coronary vasomotor effect of sympathetic stimulation is overshadowed by metabolic, inotropic, and chronotropic effects associated with vasodilatation, stimulation of sympathetic C fibers has been shown to cause active vasodilatation directly when other factors are controlled (see Chap. 11).

Site and mode of action

The sympathetic nerve fibers constitute a group of powerful vasoconstrictor mechanisms. The physiological discharge rate of the vasoconstrictor fibers is 1 to 2 impulses per second to maintain normal vessel tone and reaches 10 impulses per second with maximal physiological excitation.

The chemical transmitter released at the smooth muscle cell is norepinephrine. Co-released with norepinephrine is the recently described neuropeptide Y (see below), and newer evidence indicates that ATP is also co-released with norepinephrine from some sympathetic fibers. When so released, ATP can apparently cause vasoconstriction by activating P_2 purinergic receptors of smooth muscle cells that open calcium channels. The vasodilatation produced by exogenous ATP or adenine occurs as the result of P_2 receptors' action on endothelial cells causing release of endothelium-derived relaxing factor. Because these constrictor fibers exert control over the resistance vessels, a marked increase in blood flow in a vasoconstricted limb immediately follows sympathetic blockade. During prolonged constriction, accumulation of "vasodilator metabolites" can oppose neurogenic influence, relaxing precapillary sphincters.

In addition, these fibers exert strong control over the heart size and the capacity of vessels, mainly the veins. These fibers can alter greatly the venous return to the heart and thus markedly influence cardiac output. The significance of vasomotor fibers in control of capacitance has been verified in functionally isolated parts of the superficial and deep venous system of the dog by records of pressure changes evoked by various types of reflex stimulation.

Excitation of sympathetic vasoconstrictor fibers to the aorta and largest arteries has only a moderate effect on these vessels. There is little or no rise in pressure as a direct effect of contraction of the vessels; presumably, the most significant change is in their distensibility. Even as far out along the arterial tree as the vessels that have a diameter of 1 mm, a marked vasoconstriction or vasodilatation does not alter diameter of the vessels by more than 5 percent.

The postganglionic sympathetic neurons to blood vessels usually form two plexuses in the vascular adventitia. The innermost plexus is made up of nonmedullated fibers located in the boundary between the adventitia and the media. Small varicosities (2 μm in diameter) along each axon contain storage granules that are released on depolarization. The chief neurotransmitter released is norepinephrine (NE), but other transmitters or modulators such as monamines, neuropeptides, and purines are also present.

Norepinephrine regulates its own release by a negative-feedback mechanism in which it activates alpha$_2$-adrenergic receptors on the membrane of the varicosity. These are called presynaptic receptors, and when NE concentration increases they act to decrease the release of NE and other transmitters. Thus drugs that block alpha$_2$-adrenergic receptors increase release of NE and other transmitters from the nerve endings. Biogenic substances also act on these receptors to affect NE release: acetylcholine and certain prostaglandins inhibit and angiotensin II enhances NE release.

The released NE attaches to the vascular smooth muscle alpha or beta-adrenergic receptors; much of it is taken up again by the nerve endings (NE "reuptake") to be recycled in the varicosities to storage granules. Some NE is degraded by monamine oxidase and catechol-O-methyltransferase in nerve and neighboring tissues. The neuronal reuptake mechanism, which is the most important for removal of NE from the smaller resistance vessels, can be blocked by a number of drugs. This is an active transport process requiring ATP, magnesium, and sodium. Drugs that block the reuptake process lead to depletion of NE stores on the one hand and, for a period of time, to potentiation and prolongation of the effects of sympathetic nerve stimulation or injected NE on the other hand. Among the familiar compounds that have this effect are cocaine, ouabain, amphetamine, chlorpromazine, and phenoxybenzamine.

Neuropeptide Y

In addition to NE, neuropeptide Y (NPY) (as well as other neurotransmitters or modulators) is released from the storage vesicles and, since it is a strong vasoconstrictor, probably contributes to the vascular response.

This 36-amino acid peptide (NPY) is widely distributed together with norepinephrine in the brain, adrenal medulla, and peripheral sympathetic nerve endings. The release of NE and NPY from sympathetic nerve endings is inhibited by beta$_2$-adrenergic presynaptic receptors. Neuropeptide Y is an independent vasoconstrictor to which the coronary vasculature is particularly sensitive. It also potentiates the vasoconstrictor actions of the adrenergic receptors, serotonin and K^+. On the other hand, it inhibits release of renin and stimulates the release of atrial natriuretic factor, actions that would tend to lower blood pressure. In the brain it is found in cardiovascular regulating tracts, and there is evidence that it may play a role in genetic hypertension in rats. Accordingly, it is apparent that this neurotransmitter plays at least a modulatory role in vascular regulation.)

Functional significance

Vasoconstrictor fibers are of major importance in homeostasis of blood pressure and blood flow, including those reflex adjustments that arise from baroreceptors and chemoreceptors. They also control blood flow through the skin and thus influence peripheral heat exchange. Vasodilatation, particularly when it is of a reflex nature, is predominantly merely an inhibition of vasoconstriction. In fulfilling its role as the main neural modulator of the peripheral circulation, the vasoconstrictor system may exhibit generalized, segmental, or regional function, depending on the type of stimulus.

Active dilation

With abolition of sympathetic vasoconstrictor effect, there remains in blood vessels a residual contractile state called basal tone. The term *active dilation* refers to a further reduction in vascular contractile tone below the basal level. Increased sympathetic activity can cause active dilation in three ways: (1) by increasing tissue metabolic rate (e.g., through autoregulation, coronary dilation occurs when cardiac work increases in response to sympathetic stimulation); (2) by action on beta$_2$-adrenergic receptors that cause vasodilation in certain vascular beds (e.g., skeletal muscle); and (3) through sympathetic cholinergic fibers (see below).

Vasodilator fibers

Vasodilator impulses emerge from the central nervous system by (1) the thoracolumbar outflow; (2) the cranial outflow of the parasympathetic division reaching the periphery by way of the chorda tympani, glossopharyngeal, and vagus nerves; (3) the sacral outflow of the pelvic nerve; and (4) the posterior spinal nerve roots–antidromic impulses.

Sympathetic cholinergic vasodilator fibers

In addition to the vasodilatation that follows inhibition of vasoconstriction, there exists also a system of efferent dilator nerves transmitting from the central nervous system, but they seem to be distributed only to skeletal muscle. Electrical stimulation of sympathetic fibers usually brings about vasoconstriction in the innervated area, since the vasoconstrictor influence usually predominates over that of vasodilatation. If the vasoconstrictor response is first blocked by alpha-adrenergic blockage, however, electrical stimulation will produce vasodilatation if the sympathetic outflow contains vasodilator fibers. The existence of a sympathetic vasodilator innervation to skeletal muscle of the dog and cat has been established by this technique, but it appears to be absent in rabbits and certain other mammals and has not been verified conclusively in humans. It appears that these vasodilator nerves can be activated by stimulation of the hypothalamus and also from the motor cortex. The pathway seems to originate in the cortex, synapses in the hypothalamus, and passes as a thin bundle through the ventrolateral portion of the brain stem to reach the intermediolateral cell column of the spinal cord where the fibers synapse upon preganglionic neurons. This pathway is anatomically and functionally distinct from the medullary vasomotor center, which mediates vasoconstrictor activity.

When this vasodilator system is stimulated in the hypothalamus, the venous outflow from skeletal muscle of the hind leg of a dog may increase so that the rate of flow approximates that of maximal dilatation achieved by other means, such as acetylcholine injection. It does not occur after atropine administration. Consequently, it is assumed to represent a vasodilatation brought about by vasodilator nerves that are cholinergic (as are the sympathetic nerves to sweat glands in many species). The dilator response seems to be limited to arterioles, since precapillary sphincters and the capacitance vessels of the venous side have no known cholinergic innervation.

The functional significance of the sympathetic cholinergic vasodilator fibers is not clear. It has been suggested that they are activated when the motor cortex becomes active, presumably in association with or in anticipation of skeletal muscle exercise. The dilation that accompanies physical exercise, however, is not entirely cholinergic or adrenergic because it is not completely blocked by atropine or sympathectomy. It is believed that these sympathetic cholinergic vasodilator fibers to skeletal muscle serve to cause an increase in blood flow just before exertion. These fibers are not universally present; they have been identified only in dogs and cats but not in the primates that have been studied.

Parasympathetic vasodilator fibers

Parasympathetic vasodilator fibers run to restricted cranial and sacral areas such as the cerebral vessels, tongue, salivary glands, external genitalia, and the bladder and rectum. These fibers are probably not concerned with baroreceptor and chemoreceptor control of blood vessels; nor are they tonically active. It is generally believed that they are cholinergic, but their vasodilator effect is notably resistant to atropine. The vasodilation caused by acetylcholine is caused by interaction with muscarinic receptors in three locations: (1) on vascular smooth muscle, (2) on vascular endothelial cells that then release the endothelium-derived relaxing factor, and (3) on sympathetic nerve terminals with inhibition of NE release.

In salivary glands and in the skin, the nerves that bring about cholinergic secretion of the exocrine glands somehow cause to be released into the circulation an enzyme that acts on plasma protein to produce the vasodilator polypeptide, bradykinin.

It has been suggested that the glandular kallikrein-kinin system, through the formation of lysyl-bradykinin (kallidin), mediates vasodilatation during glandular secretion, but the importance of this system remains controversial.

Histaminergic, purinergic, and other vasodilator fibers

Vasodilator fibers that apparently liberate histamine have been demonstrated to be present in the hind limb of the dog. The vasodilatation is not prevented by atropine or beta-adrenergic receptor blockade. It is abolished by antihistamines and is associated with release of histamine into the blood. Purinergic vasodilator fibers that liberate adenosine triphosphate (ATP) or adenosine have also been identified. The function of these fibers is not known. In this context, it can be mentioned again that it is now known that in many blood vessels the powerful dilator actions of extracellular ATP and ADP (unlike those of adenosine, which directly relaxes vascular smooth muscle) are mediated through the release of nitrous oxide by the endothelial cells (see p. 190). The receptors for adenosine actions have been designated P_1, and those for ATP and ADP have been designated P_2. ATP and ADP also release prostacyclin (a vasodilator in some blood vessels and the most potent platelet aggregation inhibitor known). The vasoconstrictor potential of neurally released ATP was explained in the discussion of sympathetic vasoconstrictor fibers above.

Antidromic vasodilator impulses

Stimulation of the peripheral segments of the cut dorsal roots of sacral nerves causes dilatation of vessels of the dog's paw. This observation appears to be at variance with the Bell-Magendie principle that the dorsal roots contain only afferent fibers; however, both the observation and the principle are correct. When they are stimulated artificially these afferent fibers conduct in the direction opposite their usual function (i.e., antidromically). They cannot be activated naturally by other neurons in the spinal cord, because afferent synapses do not conduct in an antidromic direction. It also implies that these fibers ordinarily serve some other function and that the antidromically induced vasodilatation is a laboratory curiosity; however, it is more than that. Peripheral parts of cutaneous afferent fibers are capable of producing what is known (inappropriately) as an "axon reflex." Such a response persists after sectioning of the main nerve trunk but not after degeneration of the afferent fibers. The stimulus applied to the skin travels up one branch of a fiber to a bifurcation, then out along another branch of the same afferent fiber to its terminal, where arrival of the impulse brings about a local vasodilatation. Inasmuch as these are afferent nerve terminals, conventional neurotransmitter arrangements may not apply here. Various substances have been proposed as the transmitter: a histamine-like compound, acetylcholine, or ATP. An axon reflex may be induced by any factor that injures the surface of the skin (e.g., trauma, cooling, heating, frostbite). It is believed to contribute to local defense and repair by increasing the blood flow in response to the injury.

Dorsal root vasodilatation, therefore, may represent a special case of activation of what is, in fact, an axon reflex, initiated in this instance by an unnatural type of antidromic stimulation of the roots rather than by the more natural kind of stimulation via sensory endings. It probably occurs only in tissues that have relatively rich innervation for pain, such as the skin and mucous membranes.

In summary, most vasomotor nerves that supply arteries are adrenergic. Parasympathetic and sympathetic cholinergic vasodilator nerves to special regions are present. Nonadrenergic and noncholinergic innervation has been demonstrated in many vessels. Many transmitters appear to be purinergic, but other possible vasodilator transmitters have also been identified: prostaglandin, serotonin, dopamine, angiotensin, bradykinin, vasoactive intestinal peptide, and ATP.

The largest elastic arteries that have relatively little smooth muscle are sparsely innervated. As smooth muscle content increases and arteries get smaller, innervation density increases; it is most dense in small arteries and in the larger arterioles. "Intimal cushions," ridgelike elevations of connective tissue and smooth muscle located at branching sites of coronary, renal, thyroid, and other arteries, are densely innervated, but the function of these structures is not known. Most precapillary sphincters are not innervated, but some are richly supplied with nerves. Veins are less densely innervated than arteries.

Neurohumoral regulating mechanisms

In addition to cardiovascular control by way of autonomic nerves and their chemical mediators, there are blood-borne *endocrine* secretions that act on the heart and blood vessels and *paracrine* substances made by cells in many tissues that diffuse in the extracellular spaces to affect nearby blood vessels. Some of these endocrine and paracrine substances are also neurally released, so that a clear distinction between endocrines, paracrines, and neurotransmitters cannot always be made (see norepinephrine, neuropeptide Y, and vasoactive intestinal peptide, substance P).

In nearly every instance the effect of a chemical regulator is transmitted to the cells regulated by a linkage of the regulator with a specific protein receptor in the cell membrane. (See also Chap. 5, "Molecular Biological Aspects.")

Vasoactive substances that are synthesized and released by nonneural cells have been variously classified as autacoids, local hormones, autopharmacological agents, autocrines, or paracrines. Among this array of terms, some confusion reigns. One classification is based on the distance over which these substances act: *Endocrines* are carried in the bloodstream and act on distant cells; *paracrines* act on target cells close to the releasing cell (in this sense, neurotransmitters and neurohormones would be classifed as paracrines); and *autocrines* act on the cells that release them (e.g., growth factors from tumor cells that stimulate their own growth).

Cardiovascular receptors

Receptors are discrete cellular structures that may be purification procedures. They are specific in the sense that, by combining with a restricted class of compounds, they initiate stimulation or inhibition of cellular function. They are usually located on the cell surface and mediate the cellular or subcellular action of biogenic compounds such as chemical mediators and hormones or extracorporeal drugs and chemicals. In addition to cell surface receptors, there surface receptors appear to be in dynamic equilibrium with the cell interior through endocytosis or internalization. For example, receptors may be newly formed by the endoplasmic reticulum, migrate to the surface, and return to be recycled or degraded. Receptors may also carry an agonist to the cell interior to initiate a specific event. (See also Chap. 5).

Receptor pathways. The receptor is linked to its physiological or biochemical response by a series of intermediate steps. Examples are the receptors for chemical mediators that act on myocardial cells. The receptor (R) is coupled with a guanine nucleotide–binding regulatory protein (G), which in turn is linked to the catalytic subunit (C) of adenylate cyclase: R — G — C complex. The G protein is so called because it binds guanosine triphosphate and diphosphate (GTP and GDP). G protein cycles between resting and active forms and may mediate stimulatory (G_s) or inhibitory (G_i) effects. G protein is composed of three peptide chains—alpha, beta, and gamma. The alpha subunit binds GTP and GDP. In the resting state GDP is bound to the alpha subunit of G (represented here in symbolic shorthand):

$$G_{\beta\gamma\alpha}(\mathrm{GDP})$$

and is inactive. When activated, R binds to G protein. This activates G protein so that it releases GDP and binds GTP, causing separation of the beta, gamma, and alpha subunits:

$$\mathrm{R}[G_{\beta\gamma} + G_{\alpha}(\mathrm{GTP})]$$

In the case of the stimulatory effects the $G_{s\alpha}$ (GTP) subunit binds to the catalytic subunit C of adenylate cyclase and activates it so that it catalyzes the synthesis of cAMP from ATP:

$$G_{s\alpha}(\mathrm{GTP})\mathrm{C}$$

When the GTP is hydrolyzed to GDP, the alpha subunit becomes inactive and reassociates with the beta and gamma subunits:

$$G_{s\beta\gamma\alpha}(\mathrm{GDP})$$

In the case of inhibitory effects, G_i may act directly on the catalytic subunit C through its alpha subunit in a coupling sequence that is analogous to stimulation (except that the effect is the opposite) or indirectly by allowing its beta and gamma subunits to combine with and inactivate any free stimulatory form of alpha from G_s.

In the heart, receptors coupled to G_s include beta$_1$-adrenergic, beta$_2$-adrenergic, and H_2-histaminic, all of which account for positive inotropic responses. Receptors coupled to G_i in the heart include muscarinic and A_1 adenosine, which mediate negative inotropic responses.

Although there is evidence that alpha$_2$-adrenergic receptors are present in the heart, they do not appear to be coupled to adenylate cyclase in the human myocardium.

When cAMP is activated, it in turn activates a cAMP-dependent protein kinase that phosphorylates the voltage-dependent Ca^{2+} channel, producing an increased influx of Ca^{2+} ions. This increased influx of Ca^{2+} replenishes intracellular stores (e.g., in the sarcoplasmic reticulum, SR) and also triggers the release of Ca^{2+} from the SR for excitation contraction coupling. The cAMP-mediated phosphorylation also affects phospholamban, a protein found in SR which, when phosphorylated, stimulates ATP-dependent Ca^{2+} uptake by the SR. This not only increases the Ca^{2+} available for release by the SR for the next contraction, but it also rapidly reduces intracytosolic Ca^{2+} favoring the subsequent relaxation.

A second receptor-coupled pathway is the stimulation of phosphatidylinositol (PI) hydrolysis to inositol triphosphate and diacylglycerol (DG), which increase cytoplasmic Ca^{2+}. The M_2 muscarinic and alpha$_1$-adrenergic receptors are coupled to this pathway. DG causes protein kinase activation in the myocardial cell membrane, and PI induces Ca^{2+} release from the SR. Table 10.2 summarizes adrenergic receptor pathways and effects on components of the cardiovascular system.

Muscarinic cholinergic receptors, of which three subtypes (M_1, M_2, M_3) have been identified, mediate a variety of inhibitory inotropic and electrophysiologic effects in the heart and vascular smooth muscle as well as the cerebral cortex and autonomic ganglia. The M_1 subtype is found in the cerebral cortex and autonomic ganglia; the M_2 subtype is present in the cerebellum, in cardiac muscle, and on presynaptic neurons of gastrointestinal smooth muscle; the M_3 subtype is located in exocrine glands and smooth muscle.

Most, or possibly all, muscarinic responses are also transduced through G proteins (see Table 10.3). Inhibition of adenylate cyclase is mediated by G_i protein and stimulation of PI hydrolysis by an undefined protein designated G_x. There is some evidence that stimulation of the myocardium by acetylcholine also elevates cGMP, although other studies failed to support this finding.

The interaction of the muscarinic receptor with the slow inward potassium (I_{ki}) channel in atrial muscle, sinoatrial and atrioventricular nodal cells, and Purkinje cells is clearly coupled with a G_i protein, but the effects are not mediated by a decrease in cAMP. In contrast, the inhibition of the slow inward channel (I_{si}) in the atrial and ventricular myocardium and in the sinoatrial and atrioventricular nodal cells is associated with decreases in cAMP.

The positive inotropic effect of high concentrations of acetylcholine may be caused by increased phosphoinositide turnover, but this remains unproven.

Activation of specific receptors

Autonomic receptors. The adrenergic and muscarinic receptors, their pathways, and effects of stimulation are given in Tables 10.2 and 10.3, and autonomic regulation is discussed further in subsequent chapters. These receptors respond to the specific autonomic chemical mediators, circulating epinephrine and norepinephrine and exogenous synthetic drugs with autonomic agonist or antagonist properties.

Histaminic receptors. Two general types of histamine receptor affect the cardiovascular system—H_1 and H_2. H_1 receptors can mediate vasoconstriction, probably by increasing phosphatidylinositol turnover. This does not lead to a positive inotropic effect on the heart, and there is experimental evidence that H_1 receptors are coupled with negative inotropic effects and histamine-mediated tissue damage. H_1 receptors can also mediate a vasodilator response that is mediated by endothelium-derived relaxing factor (EDRF), H_1 receptor stimulation can also prolong atrioventricular conduction time.

H_2 receptor actions generally resemble beta-adrenergic receptor effects, producing positive inotropic and chrono-

Table 10.3. Muscarinic effects on the cardiovascular system

Receptor (R) subtype	Transduction pathway	Receptor location	Effect
Muscarinic M_2	Inhibition of adenylate cyclase: coupled to G_i and linked with C, causing a decrease in cAMP.	Atrial myocardium	Negative inotropy (shortening of action potential duration, hyperpolarization, and shortened refractory period caused by increased inward K^+ current (I_{ki}) and reduced slow Ca^{2+} current (I_{si}) decreased cAMP)
		Sinoatrial node	Negative chronotropy (hyperpolarization of resting potential, reduction of diastolic depolarization rate caused by increased I_{ki})
		Atrioventricular node	Negative dromotropy (reduced rate of depolarization caused by increased I_{ki} and decreased I_{si})
		Purkinje fiber	Negative dromotropy (same as for AV node; decreases automaticity)
		Ventricular myocardium	Negative inotropy (inhibition of I_{si}, alpha$_1$-adrenergic effects reduced, decreased cAMP)
	Increased phosphatidylinositol (PI) turnover mediated by an undefined protein G_x	Myocardium	Positive inotropy (with higher concentrations of agonist possibly through increased PI turnover)
	G_x (?)	Arterioles	Relaxation (EDRF production, GC stimulation) Constriction (possibly through increased PI turnover)

G_i, inhibiting nucleotide-binding protein; G_x, undefined nucleotide-binding protein; C, catalytic subunit of adenylate cyclase; PI, phosphatidylinositol; I_{ki}, time-dependent inward potassium current; I_{si}, slow inward, largely calcium current; EDRF, endothelium-derived relaxing factor; GC, guanylate cyclase; (?), uncertain.
Compiled from various sources: Bristow and Port, 1990; Green and Watanabe, 1989; Bennett et al., 1989; Graham and Lanier, 1986; Darnell et al., 1986.

tropic responses and vasodilatation by adenylate cyclase stimulation. H_2 receptors are coupled with the catalytic subunit of adenylate cyclase through G_s as outlined earlier under "Receptor Pathways."

Adenosine receptors. Adenosine receptors are also called P_1 purinoreceptors. Two major subtypes are recognized: A_1, which inhibits adenylate cyclase, and A_2, which stimulates adenylate cyclase in some tissues. A_1, like the muscarine M_2 receptor (Table 10.3), is coupled with G_1 in the ventricular myocardium and inhibits cyclase; it also inhibits the hydrolysis of phosphatidylinositol. Through the A_2 receptors, adenosine is a powerful coronary vasodilator that has long been considered an integral factor in autoregulation of coronary blood flow. More recently, the importance of adenosine in coronary vascular control has been downgraded (see Chap. 11).

Vasoactive intestinal peptide (VIP), glucagon and secretin receptors. These three receptors can mediate a positive inotropic response through G_s coupling. VIP also causes vasodilation and stimulates the release of renin by an effect on juxtaglomerular cells although its physiological role in the regulation of renin release is unknown.

Atrial natriuretic factor receptors. Atrial natriuretic factor is a peptide, discussed below, that mediates vasodilation in some vascular beds by activating guanylate cyclase to form cGMP.

Serotonin receptors. Serotonin is an amine, 5-hydroxytryptamine, that acts as a neurotransmitter within the brain (excitatory in some sites and inhibitory in others), is liberated by platelets at sites of vascular injury where it will cause intense vasoconstriction (a hemostatic function), and inhibits gastric secretion. There are several recognized subtypes, of which S_1 mediates vasodilatation and S_2 mediates vasoconstriction. S_1 receptors are coupled through EDRF-guanylate cyclase and S_2 through PI hydrolysis. Serotonin can have a positive inotropic myocardial effect, presumably through the S_2 receptor.

Prostaglandin receptors. Several prostaglandins have powerful vasoactive properties (vasoconstrictor or vasodilator) and some exert positive inotropic effects on the myocardium. Vascular endothelium can produce prostacyclin, a vasodilator, and platelets can release a vasoconstrictor prostaglandin. Many of these effects are apparently caused by appropriate influences on adenylcyclase with subsequent increase or decrease of cAMP activity.

Angiotensin II receptors. The renin-angiotensin-aldosterone system is described below and in Chaps. 12 and 31. It plays a role in fluid balance and blood pressure regulation through effects on aldosterone production, thirst, sodium retention in the kidney, secretion of vasopressin (antidiuretic hormone), and vasoconstriction. Effector pathways are coupled through PI hydrolysis (type A receptor) and adenylate cyclase inhibition by G_i (type B receptor).

Miscellaneous receptors. Other receptors found in the cardiovascular system include those for myocardial calcium influx channels and potassium channels and a variety of hormone receptors. The physiological role of the latter (e.g., insulin, glucocorticoid, vasopressin) in cardiovascular regulation has not been determined.

Endocrine control

Adrenal medulla. One of the oldest known neurohumoral relationships is the secretion of epinephrine (with smaller quantities of norepinephrine) from the adrenal medulla after stimulation of (1) the splanchnic nerves, (2) the lateral columns of the spinal cord, (3) the vasomotor center in the medulla oblongata, or (4) the hypothalamus. These released catecholamines are thus true endocrines, although norepinephrine serves also as a neurotransmitter in the sympathetic nervous system. The alpha$_1$-, alpha$_2$-, beta$_1$-, and beta$_2$-adrenergic receptors and their functions are outlined in Table 10.2.

Epinephrine has a high affinity for both alpha- and beta-adrenergic receptors, and its effects in a particular vascular bed (and on the heart) are the result of the balance of each type of receptor in the tissue. Cutaneous and renal arterioles constrict, whereas striated muscle and splanchnic arterioles dilate and cardiac output is enhanced in response to epinephrine. Cardiac output is elevated, peripheral resistance decreases, and the blood pressure is raised. Ordinarily the baroreceptors moderate the rise in blood pressure and when large pharmacologic doses are given intravenously in the experimental laboratory, cardiac standstill can be induced for brief periods. When this occurs the blood pressure plummets and then rises abruptly when the heart beats again, causing wild gyrations of the blood pressure record.

Norepinephrine has about the same affinity for alpha-adrenergic receptors as epinephrine but much less affinity for beta-adrenergic receptors. With norepinephrine action, there is a greater vasoconstrictor action and less cardiac stimulation. Most arterioles constrict, peripheral resistance increases, and there is a greater rise in blood pressure.

The physiological role of adrenal medullary hormones in vasomotor control has long been debated. In experimental comparisons of these hormones and vasomotor fibers on peripheral vascular beds, most blood vessels have been found to be dominated by their vasomotor fibers. The exception is the peripheral resistance of skeletal muscle vessels, which are almost maximally dilated by epinephrine with a significant reduction in the ratio of precapillary to postcapillary resistance. Secreted epinephrine, therefore, is believed to produce vasodilatation in skeletal muscle in, for example, exercise. If the amount of secreted catecholamines is large, as after hemorrhage, alpha$_1$-adrenergic effects predominate and reinforce neurally mediated alpha$_1$-receptor vasoconstrictor effects, especially in the renal vascular bed.

Renin-angiotensin system

The renin-angiotensin system functions as a neurohumoral regulating mechanism in the control of normal blood pressure and is critically involved in the development of such clinical states as arterial hypertension and congestive heart failure (see Chap. 12).

Renin is a proteolytic enzyme that is synthesized, stored, and secreted by a variety of organs, including the kidney, brain, adrenal gland, arterial wall, uterus, placenta, fetal membranes, and amniotic fluid. Traditionally its role as a modulator of cardiovascular function has emphasized renal renin in the generation of angiotensin, but more recently it has become clear that angiotensin generated outside the kidney contributes to blood pressure control by local as well as systemic effects.

Renin cleaves the alpha$_2$-globulin, angiotensinogen (from the liver), to form a relatively vasoinactive decapeptide, *angiotensin I*. Angiotensin-converting enzyme, a dipeptidyl carboxypeptidase, then changes angiotensin I to an active vasopressor octapeptide, *angiotensin II*. This converting enzyme is derived mainly in the capillary endothelium of the lung but also is found in the circulating plasma, the kidney, and other organ beds. Next to vasopressin, angiotensin II is the second most potent vasoconstrictor produced in the body. It is rapidly destroyed in peripheral capillary beds by a number of enzymes called *angiotensinases*.

Angiotensin III is one of the metabolites produced by angiotensinase degradation of angiotensin II. Angiotensin III may be the mediator of aldosterone release in the adrenal cortex and is the most physiologically active component of the renin-angiotensin system in the brain.

The *juxtaglomerular apparatus* is the site of renin production in the kidney. Here renin production is increased by a decrease in renal arterial pressure, a decrease in extracellular fluid volume, stimulation of sympathetic nerves to the kidney, or alterations in the distal tubular sodium load. An elevated blood level of sodium ions, potassium ions, angiotensin II, or antidiuretic hormone each inhibits renin release. Thus the renin-angiotensin system is a closed-loop, negative-feedback system. Since angiotensin II stimulates the release of aldosterone from the adrenal cortex, the *renal-angiotensin-aldosterone* system plays a pivitol role in (1) body sodium and water content and (2) potassium balance. This feedback system, illustrated in Fig. 10.7., contributes to blood pressure control by regulating extracellular fluid balance and thus plasma volume.

In mammals the vasoconstrictor effect of angiotensin II is directly on receptors of the arterial smooth muscle. It also potentiates alpha-adrenergic effects. In nonmammalian vertebrates (e.g., chickens) its action is largely indirect, mediated by catecholamine release, and it may exert an initial vasodilator action by acting directly on smooth muscle. It has been suggested that the renin-angiotensin-aldosterone system contributes to the normal tonic control of blood pressure. In the normal animal, however, angiotensin II is not required for maintenance of blood pressure. When the extracellular fluid volume is depleted, however, angiotensin II blocking agents cause a fall in blood pressure and a rise in plasma renin activity. Small reductions in renal perfusion pressure between 100 and 65 mm Hg release enough renin to raise the blood pressure and cause, within 20 minutes, a 65 percent compensation of the fall in renal pressure. Thus the system has enough gain and operates with sufficient speed to function in moment-by-moment blood pressure control. It is probable that angiotensin II does play a significant role in blood pressure maintenance under certain stress conditions (e.g., salt deficiency, adrenalectomy, diuretic administration, reduction in renal perfusion pressure) through its vasoconstrictor and aldosterone-stimulating actions.

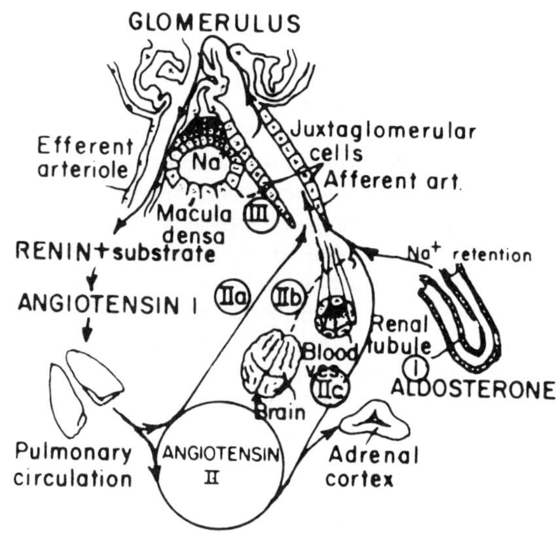

Figure 10.7. The juxtaglomerular apparatus and feedback regulation of renin release. Elevated angiotensin II concentration decreases renin secretion through several feedback loops: I, increased sodium retention causing increased extracellular fluid volume; IIa, direct negative feedback; IIb, increased blood pressure through the central nervous system; IIc, increased blood pressure through direct systemic vasoconstriction; III, direct sodium effects on the macula densa. (Redrawn from Oparil and Haber 1974, *New Eng. J. Med.* 291:389–401.)

Vascular wall renin. The renin-angiotensin system operates in blood vessel walls and is believed to control vascular tone by the local generation of angiotensin II. Since angiotensin II is a potent mitogen for vascular smooth muscle cells, it is thought that it may participate in the hypertrophy and hyperplasia of vascular smooth muscle seen in arterial hypertension.

Brain renin. All components of the renin-angiotensin system are found in the brain. Angiotensin II can increase arterial pressure acting on central neural structures that stimulate thirst, stimulate secretion of vasopressin (ADH) and ACTH, and increase sypathetic tone. This has led to the hypothesis that locally generated angiotensin II in the brain is involved in the pathogenesis of systemic hypertension and may have a functional role in cardiovascular regulation.

Activation of renal sympathetic nerves is an important stimulus for renin release, as are adrenergic agonists.

In summary, renin secretion is regulated by several humoral factors, including K^+, Na^+, Cl^-, angiotensin II, ADH (vasopressin), and vasoactive intestinal polypeptide, potassium and sodium chloride, by acting on the macula densa, reduce renin secretion. Chloride in the form of potassium and calcium salts also suppresses renin secretion, by acting on the macula densa. Chloride depletion is a potent stimulus for renin release. Antidiuretic hormone decreases renin secretion, presumably through an effect on the juxtaglomerular cells, and blocks renal nerve activity as part of its inhibitory action. Vasoactive intestinal polypeptide acts directly on juxtaglomerular cells to stimulate renin release, although its possible physiological role is not understood. The inhibitory effects of angiotensin are illustrated in Fig. 10.7. Finally, several lines of evidence indicate that prostaglandins may be the intracellular mediators of renin release; this would explain why the prostaglandin synthetase inhibitor, indomethacin, inhibits renin release.

The kidney itself, blood vessel walls, vascular smooth muscle, and brain tissue all contain the components of the renin-angiotensin system and the angiotensin-converting enzyme. There is increasing evidence that angiotensin II actions on vascular tone, secretion of ADH and ACTH, stimulation of thirst, and activation of the sympathetic nervous system can be brought about by locally produced as well as circulating angiotensin II.

Adrenal cortex

The mineralocorticoid hormones of the adrenal cortex regulate salt, water, and mineral metabolism. Aldosterone increases renal sodium reabsorption. This promotes expansion of body fluid volume, increasing blood volume and blood pressure. As an indirect result of the sodium retention and extracellular fluid volume expansion, the glomerular filtration rate and the renal plasma flow are increased and renin production is decreased. Under pathological conditions, its release, stimulated by angiotensin II, contributes to blood pressure elevation in hypertension and fluid retention in heart failure (see Chap. 12).

Other endocrines

Thyroid hormones stimulate protein synthesis (including the contractile proteins), increase heart rate, shorten the refractory period of myocytes, enhance myocardial contractility, and increase the heart's responsiveness to catecholamines. By increasing metabolic activity of most tissues, thyroid hormones increase demand for increased cardiac output and blood flow. Parathyroid hormone at physiological levels decreases the vasoconstrictor response to angiotensin II, but when injected in pharmacological doses it lowers arterial pressure. Paradoxically, *hyperparathyroidism* in humans is associated with clinical hypertension, although the pathogenesis of this relationship is uncertain. *Estrogens* increase cardiac output, stroke volume, and plasma volume. Progesterone has vasodilator and natriuretic properties. *Androgens* are associated with higher blood pressures in men than in premenopausal women and in male rats with hereditary hypertension and are therefore thought to influence blood pressure. Further, testosterone has recently been shown to increase the synthesis of extrarenal renins.

Vasopressin system

Vasopressin, or ADH, has two major actions that are important in blood pressure regulation: vasoconstriction and antidiuresis. While in vitro it is the most powerful vasoconstrictor known (even more potent than angiotensin II), the concentrations required for antidiuresis in the intact animal are 10 to 100 times less than those required to elevate the blood pressure. Its normal physiological role is primarily related to long-term regulation of blood pressure brought about by its influence on water reabsorption in the renal tubules. In hemorrhage, however, vasopressin is released in large quantities that are crucial to blood pressure maintenance. This is equal to the importance of the renin-angiotensin and baroreceptor compensatory responses in restoring blood pressure toward normal. Although plasma vasopressin levels are increased somewhat in experimental hypertension, its pathogenetic role is undecided.

Atrial natriuretic factor (ANF)

It has been thought that another hormone besides the renin-angiotensin-aldosterone system and ADH participates in the maintenance of sodium-water balance. Earlier investigations focused on a possible "natriuretic hormone" synthesized and released by the hypothalamus. Although the evidence of such a hypothalamic hormone continues to be reported, during the past decade atrial peptides with strong natriuretic properties have been isolated and characterized. These findings support and extend the postulate that the atria, because of their distensibility and independence of changes in systemic arterial blood pressure, are well situated and constructed to sense blood volume changes and initiate appropriate regulatory responses (see "Left Atrial Receptors" below.) Different laboratories have given this peptide different names (e.g., atriopeptin, auriculin, cardionatrin) based on differences in lengths of the peptide chains isolated, but the amino acid sequence is the same and chain length differences are presumably due to artifactual truncation during isolation.

Atrial natriuretic factor is synthesized in atrial cells and stored in membrane-bound secretory granules. Stretching the atria, as by an increase in blood volume, causes release of the hormone as a 24-28 amino acid peptide containing a 17-member disulfide-linked ring that is required for its biological activity. ANF acts on the intrarenal vascular resistance to increase glomerular filtration rate and possibly decreases tubular sodium chloride reabsorption, although the possible site of this action has not been established.

In addition to its natriuretic, diuretic, and vasodilator actions, ANF modulates other humoral effects on blood volume caused by renin, aldosterone, and vasopressin by inhibiting their secretion. Receptor site studies indicate that its cellular action is mediated by an increase in cGMP caused by activation of guanylate cyclase.

Paracrine control

As mentioned in the foregoing, these locally secreted agents may function purely as paracrine-control agents (e.g., bradykinin), may have paracrine and endocrine functions (e.g., renin and angiotensin II), or may serve as both paracrine and neurotransmitter substances (e.g., serotonin and various peptides that are thought to be also neurally released, such as VIP and substance P, among others).

Prostaglandins. Prostaglandins (PGs) are widely distributed in the body and have various cardiovascular effects. Prostaglandin synthesis begins with the liberation of the essential fatty acid arachidonic acid from tissue stores. It is converted into prostacyclin, PGs, thromboxanes, and leukotrienes. The first step in synthesis, catalyzed by the enzyme cyclooxygenase, is inhibited by anti-inflammatory drugs, including indomethacin. The enzymes that act on PG endoperoxide are tissue-specific so that the PG produced is characteristic of a tissue (e.g., thromboxane A_2 in platelets and prostacyclin [PGI_2] in blood vessels). Prostacyclin is a powerful vasodilator and inhibitor of platelet aggregation. It is synthesized mostly in the vascular endothelium, from endoperoxides. In platelets endoperoxides are converted to thromboxane A_2, which has the opposite effect, causing vasoconstriction and platelet aggregation. Other PG endoperoxides have opposing effects: PGE_2 dilates vascular and bronchial smooth muscle while PGF_{2a} constricts these smooth muscles. The functions of these various compounds in physiological control of the circulation has not been satisfactorily determined as yet, although some probably act in the regulation of renal blood flow and in this way contribute to blood pressure regulation. Their level in circulating blood is low because many of them are removed from the bloodstream by a single passage through the pulmonary circulation and are also taken up by the liver and kidney.

Vasodilator PGs are present, however, in the fetal plasma in relatively high concentrations. Since one of these, PGI_2 or prostacyclin, is little metabolized in the lungs, it probably acts as a circulatory hormone in the fetus, maintaining patency of the ductus arteriosus in utero. This has led to the use of indomethacin to aid closure of the patent ductus arteriosus in premature infants. (For further information on the ductus arteriosus see discussions of fetal circulation in Chap. 11 and congenital heart disease in Chap. 12.)

Leukotrienes are produced from arachidonic acid by the cyclooxygenase pathway and are not influenced by indomethacin or other anti-inflammatory drugs. The term *leukotriene* was used because these were first found in leukocytes and they contain three double bonds in the lipid portion of the molecules. It is now known that leukotrienes are produced not only by nucleated cells in bone marrow but by many other tissues, including skin, brain, liver, kidney, heart, and tracheal epithelium. They are powerful mediators of inflammation and smooth muscle contraction and are involved in immune-mediated disease. The slow-reacting substance of anaphylaxis is made up of three leukotrienes and produces marked hypotension, myocardial depression, and leakage of blood plasma into the tissues (see "Shock" Chap. 12.)

Thromboxane A_2 is released by activated platelets and by intestinal, pulmonary, and renal tissues in response to anaphylaxis, sepsis, and other inflammatory processes.

Tonin. The enzyme tonin, first discovered in rat submaxillary glands, is also found in many other tissues. It can generate both the vasoconstrictor angiotensin II and the vasodilator bradykinin from their precursors. There is evidence that it acts physiologically to sustain blood pressure, but at present its possible role in cardiovascular regulation has not been established.

Kallikrein-kinin system. Kinins are vasodilator peptides produced by proteases (kininogenases) from precursor proteins. Kallikrein is a potent kininogenase found in certain glands, in the brain, in plasma, and in many other tissues. Kallikrein can activate a number of prohormones, generate angiotensin, and stimulate renin release, besides having a contractile action on uterine and urethral smooth muscle.

Intrarenally released kinins cause natriuresis, diuresis, and the release of vasoactive prostaglandins. Glandular kallikrein-kinin systems appear to regulate local vasodilatation associated with secretion, and brain kinins such as bradykinin may play a role in central cardiovascular regulation.

Other paracrines, purine nucleotides, histamine, serotonin, and vasoactive intestinal peptide have been discussed under the heading "Cardiovascular Receptors."

Summary of neurohumoral circulatory control

The last decade has witnessed a remarkable and sometimes confusing expansion of observations on the local and general systemic cardiovascular effects of hormones, neurotransmitters, and autacoids. These have been reviewed in the foregoing section and elsewhere in this volume.

The autonomic nervous system neurotransmitters effect rapid regulatory changes, both local and general, through actions on the specific adrenergic and cholinergic receptors.

Neuropeptide Y (NPY) is released together with catecholamines from nerve endings in the brain, adrenal medulla, and peripheral sympathetic nervous system. Neuropeptide Y has direct vasoconstrictor properties, regulates the release of vasoactive autacoids (e.g., atrial natriuretic factor, angiotensin II), potentiates the effects of norepinephrine as well as the vasocontrictor actions of serotonin and K^+, and inhibits renin release.

In general, NPY effects, like those of norepinephrine and actylcholine, are short lived, permitting moment-by-moment regulation of blood pressure and blood flow.

The renin-angiotensin system can be activated rapidly by sympathetic stimulation, including such mechanisms as baroreceptor and chemoreceptor reflexes. The resultant support or increase in arterial blood pressure is sustained for minutes to hours because of aldosterone release, which has a long half-life in the circulation and increases plasma volume by renal sodium and associated water retention.

Atrial natriuretic factor release in response to increased blood volume–induced atrial stretch serves as the essential part of a negative feedback loop to regulate volume effects on blood pressure. Atrial natriuretic factor promotes natriuresis, diuresis, and vasodilatation, thus opposing the accumulation of increased fluid in the extracellular fluid compartment and its hypertensive effects.

Vasopressin, although a potent vasoconstrictor, is thought to function in blood pressure control primarily through its antidiuretic properties in the maintenance of optimal blood volume. Since it is also found in cardiovascular regulatory centers of the brain, there is speculation that it may play some role in central control.

The kallikrein-kinin system and tonin are enzymes that can generate both the vasoconstrictor peptide angiotensin II and the vasodilator peptide bradykinin. The kinins are considered primarily local vasodilators and tonin primarily a vasoconstrictor, but the individual roles and interactions of these factors remain to be established.

Other recently identified vasoactive substances include calcitonin gene–related peptides, potent vasodilator and positive inotropic/chronotropic agents that are widely distributed in periadventitial nerves of blood vessels (especially the coronary arteries) in sinoatrial and atrioventricular nodes, in sensory neurons, and in the central nervous system; endothelin, a strong vasoconstrictor produced by the vascular endothelium; endothelium-derived relaxing and constricting factors released from vascular endothelial cells; and various local growth factors with vasoconstrictor properties. Their functional relationships to the other regulatory systems remain to be established.

Circulatory ions, Na^+, K^+, Ca^{2+}, and Cl^-, modulate cardiovascular function through their effects on responses to autonomic nervous system transmitters and autacoids. Thyroid hormone tends to elevate blood pressure through its positive inotropic action, and parathyroid has a calcium level–dependent, vasodilatory hypotensive action. Estrogens stimulate synthesis and release of angiotensinogen and promote renal sodium retention, both hypertensive effects. Progestins are vasodilatory and natriuretic, both hypotensive actions. Androgens produce elevation of blood pressure, possibly through the release of mineralocorticoids. Although these various hormone effects can be demonstrated, they are relatively unimportant in the physiological regulation of blood pressure.

Various prostaglandins have diverse cardiovascular effects: Prostacyclin, a vasodilator and platelet aggregation inhibitor is synthesized in the vascular wall. Thromboxane A_2, produced in platelets, is a vasoconstrictor and promotes platelet aggregation. Other prostaglandins that have opposing effects on vascular tone appear to have a variety of localized effects on blood flow in various tissues, including the kidney.

Vascular tone

Vascular tone designates the state of contractile tension in vessel walls. *Basal tone* is defined as the degree of contractile tension remaining in vessels after complete elimination of known extrinsic excitatory influences. In the smaller precapillary vessels tone is maintained in the form of rhythmic contractions, the frequency, duration, and amplitude of which determine resistance to blood flow through those vessels. The underlying smooth muscle contractile activity may be established by different mechanisms. Myogenic automaticity and propagation, which may be modulated by vasomotor nerves and vasoactive agents, are characteristic of some vessels. Other vessels develop tone from asynchronous spike discharges in smooth muscle cells, which are dependent on the integrity of activity in vasomotor nerves. Nontetanic-graded contractures of smooth muscle may be another mechanism. These various types of contractile activity might operate in the same vessel, depending on changes in the local ionic and metabolic environment.

The consecutive segments of a given vascular bed have different degrees of basal tone; in precapillary resistance vessels tone is high, while it is less so in capacitance vessels. The degree of basal tone varies also in different tissues: it is high in resistance vessels of the brain, myocardium, skeletal muscle, and splanchnic organs but is practically absent in the arteriovenous anastomoses of the skin. Variations in vascular tone are determinants of vascular resistance, capillary exchange, arteriovenous shunting, vascular capacitance, and vascular compliance.

VASCULAR CIRCULATORY DIMENSIONS AND VESSEL TONE

As shown in Fig. 10.8, the parallel coupled vascular circuits to individual organs differ markedly in the ratio of resting to maximal flow rates. Three relations are distinguishable:

1. There are vascular beds in which dimensions are sufficient that, with maximal dilatation blood flow and capillary surface area, they will meet maximal metabolic needs (e.g., myocardium and central nervous system).

2. There are vascular beds that are too small to provide for maximal metabolic activity (e.g., during strenuous exercise skeletal muscle must go into "oxygen debt").

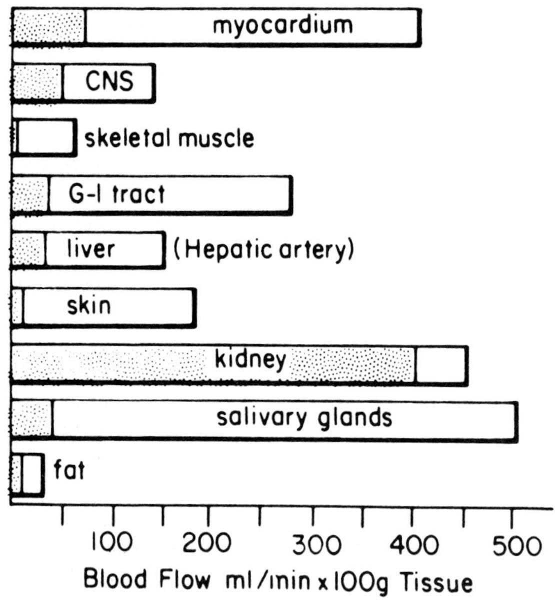

	Rest. blood flow (l/min.)	Max. blood flow (l/min.)	Organ weight (kg)
Myocardium	0.21	1.2	0.3
CNS	0.75	2.1	1.5
Skeletal muscle	0.75	18.0	30.0
G-I tract	0.7	5.5	2.0
Liver (hep. artery)	0.5	3.0	1.7
Skin	0.2	3.8	2.1
Kidney	1.2	1.4	0.3
Salivary glands	0.02	0.25	0.05
Fat	0.8	3.0	10.0
Total ≈	5.1	38.0	48.0

Figure 10.8. (*Top*) Bar graph representing approximate blood flows in various organs at maximal vasodilatation (total bar) and at "rest" (hatched areas in ml/min × 100 g of tissue at perfusion pressure of 100 mm Hg. (*Bottom*) Approximate values for regional blood flows in a 70 kg human at "rest" and at maximal dilatation, deduced from organ weights. The organs included comprise about 70 percent of total body weight. CNS, central nervous system; G-I, gastrointestinal. (Redrawn from Mellander and Johansson 1968. *Pharmacol. Rev.* 20:117–96, © 1968, Am. Soc. for Pharmacology & Experimental Therapeutics.)

3. There are vascular beds in which maximal vascular dimensions exceed maximal metabolic needs (e.g., kidney, skin, glands, and adipose tissue). Here regional circulation has functions in addition to provision of nutrients and removal of wastes (e.g., excretory function of the kidney, thermoregulatory function of the skin, glandular synthesis of secretory materials, and mobilization of energy stores from adipose tissue).

If all circulatory beds dilated maximally at once, cardiac output could not equal the total flow rate required and pressure would fall. Thus overall vascular resistance must be maintained at some minimal level by appropriate reciprocal adjustments when maximal flows prevail in some organs.

SUMMARY OF REMOTE AND LOCAL CONTROL MECHANISMS

Remote control systems (e.g., autonomic nervous system, adrenomedullary glands) bring about regional and general circulatory adjustments as required for thermoregulation, fluid balance, exercise, defense-alarm reactions, sexual responses, diving reflexes, and other conditions, including digestion of food.

Vasomotor regulation of plasma volume is called forth by arterial baroreceptors and chemoreceptors and by cardiac stretch receptors and is brought about through changes in peripheral resistance. Thus vasoconstrictor nerve stimulation with constant arterial and venous pressures can increase the precapillary/postcapillary resistance ratio in muscle from 4:1 to as high as 8:1 or 9:1. As a result, capillary hydrostatic pressure is lowered, interstitial fluid is returned to the plasma, and circulating blood volume rises. The atrial stretch receptors (see below) are the most important sensors governing precapillary to postcapillary resistance and respond to quite small changes in blood volume. A similar vasoconstrictor action on capacitance vessels may lead to expulsion of 30 percent of the blood previously contained in a given region of the circulation, with a proportional increase in venous return and cardiac output.

Vasoconstriction or dilatation in cutaneous vessels alters their resistance and capacitance; arteriovenous shunts play a leading role in these changes because they represent low-resistance channels in parallel with the capillary circulation. Reflex venoconstriction is, for the most part, transitory in the skin. The more important variable is the volume of blood flowing through the skin rather than the amount contained in the skin at any moment. As mentioned above, this is appropriate to the function of the skin in temperature regulation.

In the intestine, sympathetic adrenergic activation induces initial elevation of arteriolar resistance, which is later overcome by an autoregulatory escape from the vasoconstrictor influence. Changes in precapillary/postcapillary resistance ratio are similarly transient, so that capillary hydrostatic pressure returns to control levels. The decrease in vascular capacitance produced is sustained and can mobilize substantial volumes of blood from the splanchnic region. Thus the intestinal vascular response to increased sympathetic nerve activity is characterized by moderate alterations in arteriolar resistance and sustained decreases in blood volume with little change in capillary fluid absorption. In contrast to muscle, the intestine participates little in neurogenic plasma volume control. It does contribute effectively to blood pressure homeostasis through reflex arteriolar resistance and capacitance alterations.

The sympathetic cholinergic vasodilator system confined to skeletal muscle in those species in which it has been demonstrated has its predominant effect on arteriolar vessels, while precapillary sphincters and capacitance vessels have little or no cholinergic innervation. Stimulation of these fibers decreases the precapillary/postcapillary resistance ratio, thus increasing net transcapillary fluid filtration. The sympathetic cholinergic dilator system does not appear to be activated by homeostatic, chemoreceptor, or baroreceptor reflexes but may play a role in behavioral responses, such as alerting, flight, or attack in conscious animals.

The parasympathetic cholinergic vasodilator fibers function in vasodilatation associated with specific organ activity such as salivary secretion and penile erection. Dorsal root vasodilator fibers are not activated reflexly from the central nervous system and appear to be involved only in local vascular effects of the "axon reflex" type. In general, reflex vasodilatation such as that induced by baroreceptor stimulation results from diminished sympathetic vasoconstrictor discharge rather than parasympathetic cholinergic vasodilator effects.

The adrenomedullary hormones can produce alpha-adrenergic vasoconstriction similar to that of sympathetic vasoconstrictor fibers. The latter dominate during reflex pressor responses. The beta$_2$-adrenergic vasodilator effect is of unique significance since these receptors are not ordinarily activated by nerves. For example, skeletal muscle beta$_2$-receptor dilator response to epinephrine is unquestioned, even though it cannot be elicited by nerve action except under special experimental conditions (see above). The metabolic actions of epinephrine are also of importance in influencing local factors that govern blood flow.

Local mechanisms of vascular control affect so-called autoregulation and have as their chief targets precapillary resistance vessels and sphincters. Changes in the ionic and chemical metabolic milieu and vascular smooth muscle response to stretch cause vasomotor reactions appropriate to tissue metabolic needs, which can oppose or override the remote effects. This permits a degree of local autonomy that is important as a regional safeguard against the more generalized responses to homeostatic circulatory reflexes and adrenomedullary hormones. Thus "metabolic vasodilators" protect against excessive vasoconstriction, and myogenic control of precapillary resistance vessels and sphincters protects against capillary hydrostatic overload.

REFLEX CONTROL MECHANISMS

The vasomotor system of nerve fibers is the efferent side of the reflexes that bring about moment-by-moment adjustments in distribution of blood flow in response to variations in regional or organ function (Fig. 10.5). Stimulation of practically any afferent nerve will result in some kind of reflex vasomotor change.

Vascular reflexes from stimulation of somatic nerves

Historically reflexes from stimulation of somatic nerves are among the earliest vascular reflex mechanisms known, although their importance in overall circulatory regulation is relatively minor.

Stimulation of the central end of a nerve, such as the sciatic, the median, or a sensory cranial nerve, may result in either a rise or a fall in the arterial blood pressure, according to the frequency, strength, and type of the stimulus employed. The components of the reflex arc upon which the responses depend are (1) afferent fibers in the peripheral nerve; (2) reflex centers that usually lie in the spinal cord, but that may include the vasomotor center of the medulla, especially when the afferent fibers belong to a cranial nerve; and (3) the efferent vascular nerves (i.e., the vasoconstrictors or vasodilators). As a rule, to elicit a pressor reflex, a stimulus much stronger than that necessary to provoke a depressor response must be applied (i.e., one that would elicit pain in a conscious animal). In the elicitation of either reflex, the magnitude of the response is apparently dependent on the number of afferent fibers involved. For example, stimulation of various nerves of the brachial or lumbar plexus causes practically equivalent depressions or elevations in the blood pressure when the number of afferent fibers in the respective nerves is taken into account.

Arterial stretch receptors

A fundamental regulation of systemic blood pressure is reflex control by the action of the arterial pressure itself on *baroreceptors* located in the vascular walls, especially of the aortic arch and carotid sinus area.

Aortic or cardiac depressor nerve

The branch of the vagus that is known as the *aortic* or *cardiac depressor* nerve (Fig. 9.2) is purely afferent and depressor in function; when it is sectioned and its central (cerebral) end is stimulated, a pronounced fall in pressure occurs; excitation of the cardiac end, on the other hand, causes no effect. Two factors are involved in the depressor response after stimulation of the fibers; (1) *Slowing of the heart rate*. The efferent fibers of the vagus of the same side and of the opposite side constitute the efferent limb of the reflex arc through which this response is chiefly brought about; therefore, for its full elicitation one vagus must remain intact. (2) *Vasodilatation*. The vasomotor pathways constitute the efferent limb of this reflex. Vasoconstriction is inhibited and vasodilatation results.

The receptors of the reflex (the terminals of the aortic nerve) are situated in the aortic arch and the upper part of the thoracic aorta, in the ventricles, and possibly in the coronary and pulmonary vessels. Although they are called pressure receptors, their natural stimulus is stretching of the vessel wall. They can be stimulated artificially by mechanical or electrical manipulation of the wall.

The reflex fall in pressure is due mainly to dilation of splanchnic vessels. The dilation is not confined to these vessels, however, for it includes those of the skin and muscles. As a primary response, the pulmonary vascular bed may also show vasodilatation. Cardiac slowing plays some role in the fall in blood pressure, although after sectioning of both vagi to remove the cardiac component, the magnitude of the reflex hypotension may be almost unchanged.

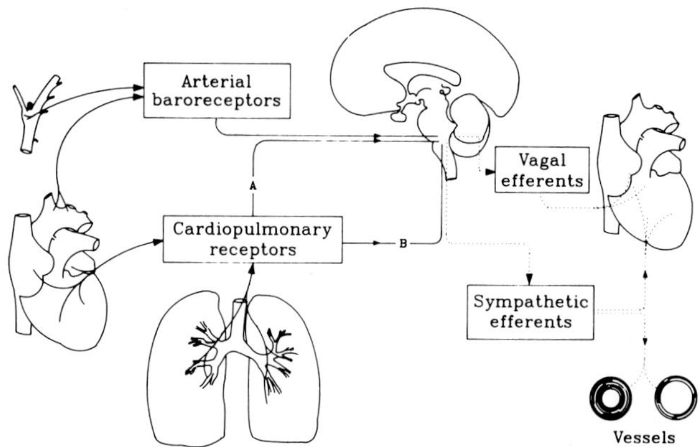

Figure 10.9. Schema of the afferent and efferent pathways of the cardiopulmonary and arterial baroreceptor reflexes. The carotid sinus and aortic arch baroreceptor sites send impulses to the nucleus tractus solitarius via the glossopharyngeal and vagal nerves, respectively. Vagal afferents from the heart and lungs (A) reach the cardiovascular centers, and cardiac sympathetic afferents (B) lead to spinal and supraspinal structures although their role in cardiopulmonary function is not clear at present. Dotted lines show the pathways of the vagal and sympathetic efferents to the heart and blood vessels. (From Persson et al. 1989. *News Physiol. Sci.* 4:56.)

Carotid sinus mechanism

The carotid sinus is the slight enlargement of the common carotid artery where it bifurcates into the internal and external carotids. The carotid sinus was shown by Hering in 1923 to play an important role in the regulation of the cardiac rate and arterial blood pressure. Compression of the common carotid at its bifurcation (so as to raise the common pressure within the sinus) causes a marked slowing of the heart rate, vasodilatation, and a fall in blood pressure. Electrical stimulation of the sinus wall produces similar effects. Pressure upon the common carotid some distance below the sinus (so as to reduce the blood pressure within the sinus itself) causes cardiac acceleration, vasoconstriction, and a rise in arterial pressure. The carotid sinus therefore constitutes a mechanism whereby both pressor and depressor effects are mediated. The effects are brought about through the following neural mechanism.

The sinus reflex arc. The afferent fibers of the reflex arc are contained in the *sinus nerve,* a branch of the glossopharyngeal. Nerve fibers of this delicate filament originate in sensory organs that are stretch receptors (proprioceptors) situated between the connective tissue fibers in the adventitia of the sinus wall. They ascend between the external and internal carotids to join the glossopharyngeal nerve. In the medulla they make connections with the cardioinhibitory and vasomotor centers. The efferent limb of the cardiac part of the reflex is the vagus. The efferent limbs of the vasodilator and vasoconstrictor reflexes are apparently sympathetic fibers, for these reflexes are abolished by complete removal of the sympathetic chains (Fig. 10.9).

The sinus and aortic nerves, the so-called buffer nerves, constitute a mechanism of the utmost importance in controlling the arterial blood pressure and in maintaining the circulation to the brain. The rise in diastolic pressure and the increase heart rate that occur when the body changes from the recumbent to the standing position are apparently brought about through these nerves; they therefore play an essential part in compensating for the effect of gravity on the circulation.

An underfilled state of the vessels, as may result from hemorrhage or shock, or any other condition that tends to cause a fall in blood pressure, will call these mechanisms into play so as to produce a generalized vasoconstriction. Excessive elevation of the blood pressure, on the other hand, is countered by a depressor reflex. The great importance of these reflex mechanisms in hemorrhage is shown by the fact that in an animal in which all four buffer nerves have been sectioned the rapid loss of only about one-tenth of the blood volume proves fatal, whereas usually a reduction in blood volume of from 35 to 45 percent is required to cause death.

A rise of pressure within the carotid sinus produces the behavioral signs of sleep and can induce cortical electroencephalographic synchronization and diminish or abolish drug-induced convulsions. The physiological significance of this effect in the regulation of sleep-wake patterns is somewhat uncertain. Studies in cats suggest that synchronous inflow from baroreceptors is in part responsible for synchronous sleep. Paradoxically, an acute rise in blood pressure due to inflation of an intra-aortic balloon causes arousal from sleep in lambs.

Mechanism of action. How the blood pressure stimulates the baroreceptors is complex and only partially understood. If deformation of the baroreceptive arterial wall is prevented so that no stretch occurs, the receptors no longer respond to pressure change. The reaction of baroreceptors to pulsatile pressure is asymmetrical in that the response, as measured by the impulse traffic in the afferent nerve, is less to falling than to rising pressure. Reflex blood pressure depression from carotid sinus stimulation is also less marked with steady stimulation than it is with pulsatile pressure stimulation. At moderate pressure, where the pulsatile change has a sinusoidal character, the greater the amplitude and the higher the frequency of the stimulating pressure change, the more intense is the blood pressure depression. This frequency effect, however, disappears at higher pressures within the carotid sinus; if stimulation pressure exceeds a range of 160 to 180 mm Hg in dogs, the blood pressure reaction is inverted.

Local application of epinephrine or norepinephrine or sympathetic nerve stimulation to an isolated carotid sinus preparation increases the smooth muscle tension in the arterial wall so that the wall becomes stiffer. This brings about a pronounced increase in impulse traffic along the baroreceptor fibers throughout the cardiac cycle and resets the baroreceptive mechanisms at a higher level of function. Norepinephrine administration has a similar effect on aortic baroreceptors. In the intact animal such a change would lower systemic arterial pressure. Sodium nitrite applied to the sinus relaxes the smooth muscle, reduces intramural tension, decreases impulse traffic, and resets the blood pressure regulation at a lower level. In the intact animals this would raise arterial pressure.

In experimental and clinical hypertension the pressure sensitivity of the carotid sinus receptor response is reduced. Thus baroreceptor response seems to be reset so as to maintain blood pressure at a higher level. When hypertension is relieved, the range of function can be reset downward. In dogs in which the carotid sinus is experimentally isolated and perfused separately while aortic blood pressure is being recorded, the point at which the mean aortic pressure and mean carotid pressure are equal is called the closed-loop operating point of the carotid sinus reflex. When carotid sinus pressure is above this point the reflex acts to lower systemic pressure, and vice versa. In greyhounds, which characteristically maintain higher blood pressure levels than control mongrel dogs under laboratory conditions, this closed-loop operating point is also higher.

Interaction of cardiopulmonary and arterial baroreceptors in the control of systemic arterial blood pressure

Unmyelinated cardiac vagal afferents and unmyelinated pulmonary afferents tonically inhibit the cardiovascular centers in a manner similar to that of the arterial baroreceptors. Vagal cold block of afferents from the atria, the ventricles, or the pulmonary arteries increases the systemic blood pressure substantially. It is assumed, therefore, that these cardiopulmonary receptors are important in maintenance of blood pressure at a level about which arterial baroreceptors operate. Figure 10.9 illustrates the convergence (labeled A) of unmyelinated cardiopulmonary afferents and arterial baroreceptor afferents on the same general pool of central neurons (i.e., the nucleus tractus solitarius of the medulla oblongata). Sympathetic afferents from the heart and lungs also converge (labeled B) on similar spinal and supraspinal structures. Their role in cardiopulmonary baroreceptor function is not clear at this time.

The stimulus-response behaviors of arterial baroreceptors and cardiopulmonary mechanoreceptors differ considerably: (1) The cardiopulmonary receptors cannot sense rapid fluctuations in arterial pressure as well as the arterial baroreceptors can and (2) the cardiopulmonary receptors affect neurons that supply renal resistance vessels to a greater extent and those that supply skeletal muscle resistance vessels to a lesser extent than do arterial baroreceptors.

When the arterial baroreceptors are denervated in dogs the lability of arterial blood pressure is greatly increased, but the mean blood pressure remains the same (Fig. 10.10). When both arterial and cardiopulmonary receptors are denervated, both mean arterial pressure and blood pressure lability are increased. Thus it appears that the cardio-

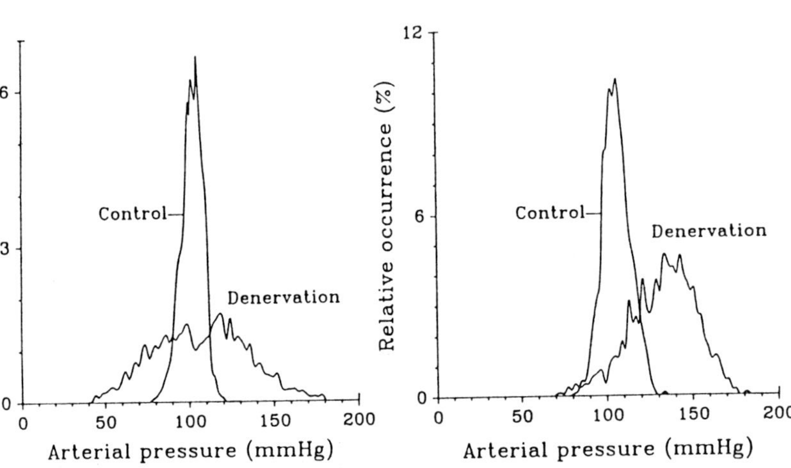

Figure 10.10. Frequency distributions of mean arterial pressures. These curves are frequency polygons in which the various blood pressure values determined for each group of dogs are plotted along the abscissa and the percentage of measurements falling in a given pressure range (e.g., pressure intervals of 5 to 10 mm/Hg) are plotted along the ordinate. The points plotted are then connected with a line to form a graph of the percentage distribution of the values formed. (*Left*) Response to arterial baroreceptor denervation. There was no increase in the mean arterial pressure, but the blood pressure fluctuations were much greater in denervated dogs than in the control animals. (*Right*) Both cardiopulmonary and arterial baroreceptors were denervated. In this case, both the blood pressure fluctuations and the mean arterial pressure increased. Thus the combined loss of baroreceptor input from arterial and cardiopulmonary receptor regions is required to produce sustained hypertension. Note that the scale of relative occurrence (%) of arterial pressures measured on the right is twice as high as that on the left because larger pressure intervals were used on the right. (From Persson et al. 1989, *News Physiol. Sci.* 4:56–59.)

pulmonary baroreceptors account for maintenance of normal mean blood pressure after arterial baroreceptor denervation but that they cannot limit blood pressure fluctuations, as the arterial baroreceptors can. This latter finding is attributed to the relative insensitivity of the cardiopulmonry baroreceptors to rapid pressure fluctuations mentioned in the foregoing discussion. (See also "Neurogenic Hypertension," Chap. 12, p. 248).

The foregoing is based on dog experiments; similar results have not always been obtained by other investigators or with application to other species. Cardiac reflexes are less pronounced in primates; carotid baroreceptor reflexes are less sensitive and have a lower set point in primates than in quadrupeds, and hypertension has been reported in a variety of species, even after only partial baroreceptor denervation.

Other arterial baroreceptors

Possible additional arterial baroreceptors have been studied in the common carotid artery and in the thoracic and mesenteric arteries. Experiments in which a sudden rise in intracranial pressure causes systemic hypertension (the *Cushing phenomenon* described in 1902) or in which a sudden reduction in intracranial pressure leads to systemic hypotension have been interpreted to mean that pressure-sensitive receptors are present within the cranial cavity. The hypertensive effect, however, is known to be largely or even entirely secondary to asphyxia of medullary centers. The mesenteric baroreceptors produce afferent impulses throughout the cardiac cycle; if pressure in the vessel is changed, or if the vessel is occluded, vasomotor reflexes are induced. These latter are capable of modifying systemic blood pressure after receptors in the aorta and carotid sinus have been denervated. They represent segmental spinal reflexes that have an influence on pressure and flow in a given region of the body. They are present in cats but have not been observed in dogs. Other reflexes have been obtained by varying pressure in the descending portion of the thoracic aorta or by administration of epinephrine to this vessel.

Another mechanism exists, at least in experimental animals, whereby afferent impulses arising from within an organ lead both to a generalized vasoconstriction that increases systemic arterial pressure and to a local vasodilatation with increased blood flow. This is sometimes called the *Lovén reflex,* after the investigator who first described it in 1866.

Cardiovascular reflexes of chemoreceptor origin

Adjacent to the carotid sinus and the root of the aorta are the carotid and aortic bodies that contain epithelioid cells and nerve endings sensitive to the chemical composition of the arterial blood. The fibers of the aortic body run in the vagus nerves, while the fibers of the carotid body are branches of the glossopharyngeal nerves. The blood supply of the aortic body is a branch of a fine artery arising from the aorta beyond its arch. The carotid body (glomus caroticum) is a small structure situated on a branch of the occipital artery or on a small vessel arising directly from the external carotid just above the bifurcation of the common carotid. It is composed of rounded clumps of polyhedral cells and has a rich network of capillaries of sinusoidal character. Microglomeruli that are located along the carotid artery and that have a chemosensory function have been described in the cat. Both the carotid and the aortic chemoreceptors sample the blood for its Po_2, Pco_2, pH, and possibly other chemical substances. Blood flow through the carotid body per gram of tissue appears to be by far the largest for any body tissue. Direct flow measurements indicate a flow of 2000 ml/100 g/min (left ventricle = 80 to 100 ml/100 g/min) while oxygen usage of 9 ml/100 g/min compares with that of the left ventricle. This flow can be cut to one-third by stimulation of the cervical sympathetic nerves. In general, the chemoreceptors are stimulated by hypoxia, hypercapnia, and acidosis. The mechanism by which changes in blood chemical composition effect a response in these two structures is not clearly understood; nor has the chemoreceptor intermediate that stimulates the nerve endings been identified. Nerve impulses can be recorded from the afferent nerves at CO_2 tensions above 30 mm Hg and at O_2 tensions of approximately 90 mm Hg or less, but the discharge with increasing CO_2 tension is rarely as great as that resulting from anoxia. Acute hypoxia (inhalation of low oxygen mixtures or of nitrogen) causes systemic hypertension and vasoconstriction in the limbs and intestine; responses are abolished if the chemoreceptor areas are blocked.

Cardiac response to chemoreceptor stimulation is complex. In experimental preparations arranged so as to prevent secondary influence of respiratory stimulation on cardiac activity, stimulation of the carotid bodies produces reflex bradycardia while stimulation of the aortic bodies produces reflex tachycardia. Where respiratory effects are allowed, cardiac response to carotid body stimulation is related to the intensity of the ventilatory augmentation. With mild ventilatory stimulation, the heart rate is usually decreased; with marked increase in ventilation, cardiac acceleration occurs. Carotid body reflex bradycardia appears to be part of the diving response (see Chap. 12).

The primary effect of chemoreceptor stimulation on the pulmonary circulation is vasoconstriction.

Reflexes from heart and lungs

From various intrathoracic vessels (including the chambers of the heart) arise other reflexes that affect vasomotor tone. Although their importance in the regulation of the circulation may possibly be comparable to that of previously mentioned reflexes, much less is known about their function since it is much more difficult to investigate cardiopulmonary reflexes than those related to the baroreceptors in the systemic circuit.

Reflexes of the right side of the heart

In the walls of the atria and great veins there are receptors that have fairly large afferent nerve fibers and that respond to changes of pressure in the atria by firing during atrial contraction (type A) or during the passive distention of atrial diastole (type B). Their afferent fibers are in the vagi.

Bainbridge reflex, McDowall reflex. In 1914 Bainbridge reported that intravenous injection of saline solution or blood to raise venous pressure induced tachycardia. Sectioning of the sympathetic nerves or administration of atropine reduced this response. Bilateral vagotomy abolished the effect. He concluded that receptors in the great veins and possibly the right atrium were responsible for this reflex. McDowall (1924) described a reflex that, in effect would have a hemodynamic action opposite to that of the Bainbridge reflex. Sectioning of the vagi in cats subjected to severe hemorrhage caused a decrease in blood pressure. He presumed that in hemorrhage atrial receptors were stimulated by the fall in pressure and caused reflex vasoconstriction.

Since these early reports, the findings have been both confirmed and refuted. Some workers have found that distention of the right atrium produces bradycardia and hypotension instead of the reverse. Others have reported that balloon distention of either the right or the left atrium causes tachycardia and that electrical stimulation of afferents from the heart produces tachycardia and vasoconstriction. The existing heart rate and hemodynamic state may determine the response, since in dogs when the initial heart rate is above 140 to 150 beats per minute a reflex cardiac slowing and vasodilatation follow stimulation of atrial receptors. At lower heart rates tachycardia and a decrease in blood pressure result. In any case, the circulatory effects of changes in heart rate elicited from these low-pressure atrial receptors are quantitatively small and their physiological significance undecided. The vasomotor effects may be concerned primarily with mobilization of blood volume (see "Left Atrial Receptors," below).

In anesthetized dogs, partial occlusion of the pulmonary artery leads to an increase in pulmonary blood flow. This reflex is dependent on an intact sympathetic innervation of the heart; the vagi and medullary centers are not involved. Presumably the increase in pulmonary blood flow is due to a reflex myocardial stimulation initiated by a rise in right ventricular systolic pressure.

The Bainbridge reflex versus the baroreceptor reflex. In unanesthetized dogs, infusion of blood that increases blood volume and arterial blood pressure also increases heart rate. In this case the Bainbridge reflex prevails over the baroreceptor reflex. Removal of blood volume by bleeding sufficient to reduce cardiac output and arterial blood pressure also increases the heart rate; here the baroreceptor reflex prevails over the Bainbridge reflex.

Pulmonary vessel reflexes

Most investigators now agree that the pulmonary blood vessels have tone and that possibly this tone can be altered. There is evidence in the anesthetized dog that the pulmonary vascular resistance is controlled by extrinsic vasomotor nerves. Both vasoconstrictor and vasodilator responses have been demonstrated. The primary effect of either baroreceptor (i.e., carotid sinus) or chemoreceptor (carotid body) stimulation is pulmonary vasoconstriction, although with chemoreceptor stimulation the reflex vasoconstrictor effect on the bronchial circulation, which occurs simultaneously, may actually produce a decrease in pulmonary vascular resistance (see above).

Pulmonary artery reflexes. Elevation of pressure in the main pulmonary artery and its bifurcation within physiological limits reflexly induces systemic hypotension and inconstant bradycardia. Vagotomy abolishes the response. Paradoxically, elevation of the pressure above physiological limits (e.g., 80 to 120 mm Hg) causes a rise in systemic arterial pressure.

Reflexes from the smaller pulmonary vessels. Despite a tremendous amount of investigation, it is questionable whether reflexes are initiated from the smaller vessels of the pulmonary circuit—arterioles, capillaries, and venules. In many experiments a pulmonary vasoconstriction has been observed in response to pulmonary venous congestion or after embolization by clots, starch grains, or glass or plastic beads. Whether the results have a mechanical or reflex explanation, however, or depend on a local response such as a pulmonary axon reflex has not been determined. It is known that the sympathetic innervation of pulmonary vessels is largely vasoconstrictor and that stimulation of the stellate ganglion may, at times, reduce lung blood flow by as much as 30 percent because of increased resistance.

Cardiac receptors

Atrial receptors. Two histological types of receptor are found in the heart: (1) free afferent nerve endings that often anastomose into "end nets" and (2) complex unencapsulated afferent endings. The end nets are more plentiful in the endocardium than in the epicardium. The complex unencapsulated endings are found throughout the atrial and ventricular epicardium but are less numerous in the endocardium. Both myelinated and unmyelinated C fiber afferents travel in the vagi to the medulla, and afferents from some of the ventricular receptors travel centrally as spinal cord afferents.

In the atria two types of receptor are distinguished functionally (but not histologically): type A receptors that initiate impulses with each atrial contraction and type B receptors that respond during the stretch of atrial filling when the atrioventricular valves are closed (see discussion of pressure and volume events of the cardiac cycle, Chap. 8). Presumably, type A receptors monitor strength of atrial contraction and type B receptors initiate responses to the stretch of atrial filling (i.e., act as "volume" receptors).

Ventricular receptors. Two physiological types of receptor are found in the ventricles. Ventricular pressure receptors, located in the endocardium, increase their discharge with increasing ventricular pressure. These impulses are carried in myelinated vagal afferent fibers. Epicardial fibers that discharge with no relationship to the phases of the cardiac cycle send impulses via unmyelinated afferent fibers centrally.

Reflexes of the left side of the heart

Left ventricle. Daly and Verney (1926) were the first to show that pressor receptors exist in the left side of the heart. In an innervated heart-lung preparation in which the aortic pressure was kept constant, an increased pressure in the left side of the heart caused cardiac slowing. Later it was shown that elevation of the pressure in a vascularly isolated left side of the heart results in reflex bradycardia, systemic hypotension, and vasodilatation of the leg vessels. Since left atrial pressure elevation alone was ineffective, it was concluded that the receptors are in the left ventricle. On vagal blockage, the effect disappeared. These effects may also arise from baroreceptors of the aortic arch, which are known to extend into the left side of the heart.

Coronary chemoreflex (Bezold-Jarisch reflex). Intravenous injection of veratridine and certain other agents (e.g., nicotine, some antihistaminics) produces reflex cardiac slowing, hypotension, and apnea (the *Bezold-Jarisch reflex*). The receptors for the reflex apnea are located in the lung and normally are responsible for the Hering-Breuer (lung-inflation) reflex. The receptors that evoke the reflex bradycardia and hypotension, however, are believed to lie within the heart, inasmuch as they can be stimulated by injection of veratridine into the coronary arteries or the pericardial sac. In the cat, injection into the right or left coronary artery elicits the response; in the dog, only injections into the left coronary arteries or pericardial sac are effective. The hypotension is independent of the bradycardia, as it is caused by reflex vasodilatation.

In the left ventricle there are numerous nonmedulated vagal afferent endings described as *epimyocardial* receptors. They are excited by increases in diastolic distention of the ventricle and also by various drugs (nicotine, veratridine, etc.). The response is of the Bezold-Jarisch type (bradycardia, vasodilatation). Because the ventricles during diastole are part of the low-pressure system, it has been suggested that they may have a blood volume–regulating function similar to that suggested for the atrial receptors (discussed below). In support of this is the finding that after cardiac autotransplantation carried out so that the atrial receptors have intact afferent connections but the ventricular receptor afferents are interrupted, there is an increase in blood volume and a decrease in renin release after hemorrhage.

Ventricular receptors with sympathetic afferents are also located in the ventricles. Many of these are mechanosensitive (pressure, distention) and also respond to drugs such as veratridine. The responses elicited are mainly pressor, producing vasoconstriction and acceleration of the heart. Thus, while these receptors respond to the same types of stimuli as the vagal epimyocardial receptors mentioned above, their reflex hemodynamic effects are opposite. Little is known about the functional role of these receptors or about their interaction with the depressor vagal afferents. The net effect when both are stimulated, as during obstruction of coronary artery flow, is often dominated by the depressor response characteristic of the vagal receptors.

Cardiogenic hypertensive chemoreflex. Injections of small doses of serotonin into the proximal left coronary artery of the dog elicits a brief systemic and pulmonic hypertension and positive inotropic effect on the heart. The afferent nerve is the vagus, and efferent effects are carried in both the vagus and the sympathetic nerves.

The region surrounding the left main coronary artery of the dog's heart contains the chemoreceptors for the cardiogenic hypertensive reflex (hypertension, tachycardia) and the afferents from the Bezold-Jarisch reflex receptors (hypotension, bradycardia).

Injection of the local anesthetic lidocaine (Xylocaine) into this region around the left main coronary artery eliminates both the cardiovascular Bezold-Jarisch reflex and the cardiogenic hypertensive chemoreflex.

Left atrial receptors

Receptors in the left atrium (and probably the pulmonary veins), which respond to stretch, have been implicated in the regulation of blood volume. Acute distention of the left atrium, as with inflation of an intra-atrial balloon, increases heart rate, in general decreases arterial pressure (although the reverse may occur), and causes diuresis. Similarly, procedures that produce a shift of blood into the intrathoracic circulation, thus elevating central blood volume and atrial pressure, produce diuresis and lead to reduction of plasma volume. This redistribution of blood can be produced, for example, by continuous *negative-pressure breathing,* by head-out body immersion in a thermoindifferent bath, or by human centrifuge simulated *gravitational effects* (so-called transverse G). The reduction in plasma volume observed in *bed rest* or during *weightlessness* of space pilots is presumed to have a similar basis. Procedures that decrease central blood volume (e.g., *hemorrhage, positive-pressure breathing*) have the opposite effect. The effects on fluid volume are mediated reflexly by changes in ADH and aldosterone release and in renal blood flow. Right atrial receptors and arterial baroreceptors similarly can be stimulated to evoke these responses. Vagal cooling or vagotomy blocks many of them. Fig 10.11 illustrates several of these

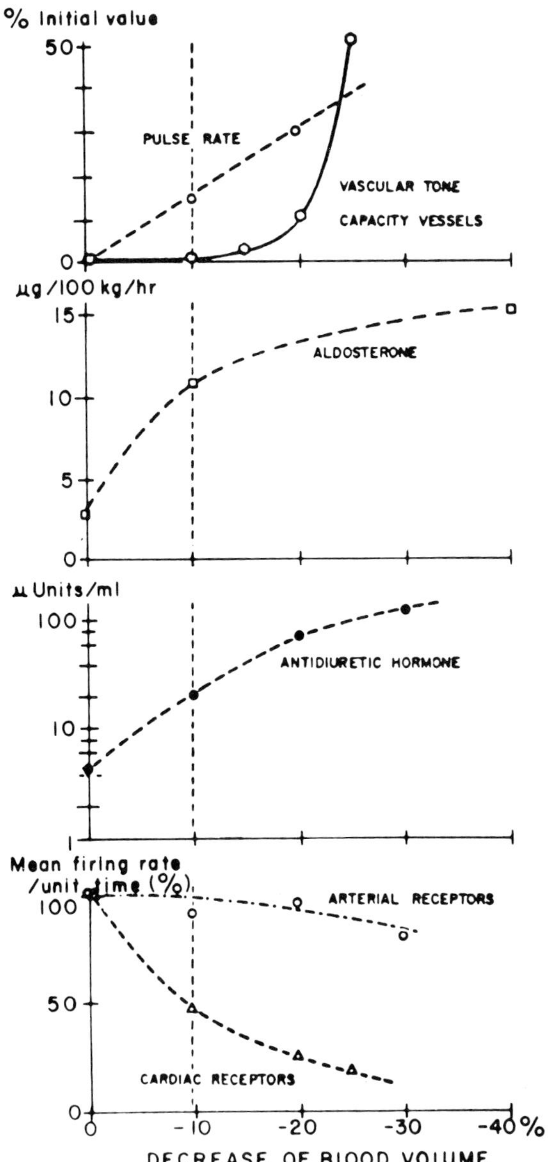

Figure 10.11. Responses to a graded hemorrhage. With loss of the first 10 percent of blood volume, the firing rate of atrial (cardiac) receptors falls to one-half. As the loss exceeds 20 percent there is a fall in firing rate of aortic (arterial) baroreceptors. The plasma aldosterone (micrograms released into the plasma) and antidiuretic hormone (microunits per milliliter) concentrations rise, causing sodium and water retention. The pulse rate increases steadily as blood volume falls. There is little change in tone of capacity vessels until collapse threatens, when it increases effectively to move blood to central regions. (Redrawn from Gauer, Henry, and Behn 1970, *Ann. Rev. Physiol.* 32:547–95, © 1970 by Annual Reviews Inc.)

effects in response to graded hemorrhage (see also Chap. 12).

The left atrial volume-receptor hypothesis for regulation of extracellular fluid volume described above is attractive because it seems logical. A cautionary note, however, should be voiced because the evidence of its physiological role is largely indirect. Actually, the atrial receptors may be of little importance in reflex regulation of renal function. Under physiological conditions, the secretion of ADH appears to be influenced primarily by hypothalamic osmoreceptors. As mentioned above, atrial receptors are the most important sensors reflexly altering precapillary to postcapillary resistance and can evoke sustained vasoconstriction in the intestinal vascular bed. Increased precapillary to postcapillary resistance increases plasma volume, and vasoconstriction of intestinal capacitance vessels can mobilize substantial amounts of blood for central circulation. These neurogenic vasomotor adjustments for producing rapid increases in blood volume appear to be important in the maintenance of cardiovascular homeostasis. Another view is that these atrial receptors are concerned in the control of heart volume and not blood volume per se. Thus the atrial receptor reflex could be a negative-feedback loop that prevents increased heart volume initially by causing tachycardia (Bainbridge reflex) when venous return increases and in the long run by causing diuresis when blood volume is increased. In cardiac-denervated dogs, however, the diuretic and natriuretic responses to atrial stretch are abolished, while those to fluid infusion remain unaltered. Thus the physiological role of these receptors in fluid volume regulation remains controversial.

After both renal denervation and destruction of the posterior pituitary, atrial distention still causes increased urine and sodium excretion through the release of atrial natriuretic factor. The cardiovascular reflexes are summarized in Table 10.3.

Arterial-cardiopulmonary interaction in blood pressure control

The carotid sinus and aortic arch baroreceptors buffer short-term pressure changes and when denervated blood pressure becomes labile (variable) but sustained, hypertension is not produced (see also discussion of neurogenic hypertension in Chap. 12, p. 248); their importance for long-term regulation of blood pressure appears to be minor. The cardiopulmonary baroreceptor reflexes reviewed in the foregoing (pulmonary artery and left ventricular reflexes), on the other hand, appear to be unimportant in the short term but active in long-term regulation of blood pressure. These cardiopulmonary mechanoreceptors tonically inhibit the vasomotor center, largely through unmyelinated vagal afferents that converge to the same central neuron pool as the arterial baroreceptor afferents (see Fig. 10.9) in the nucleus tractus solitarius of the medulla oblongata. If both arterial baroreceptor and cardiopulmonary baroreceptor regions are denervated together, the labile blood pressure characteristic of arterial baroreceptor denervation alone is present, but now there is also a sustained increase in blood pressure as well (i.e., neurogenic hypertension, see p. 248). Thus it appears that while arterial baroreceptor dener-

Table 10.4. Cardiovascular reflexes

Stimulus	Receptor	Afferent nerve	Reflex pattern	Responses: Heart	Responses: Arteries	Responses: Capacitance vessels
Pain, pressure, electrical	Somatic (pain, temperature, pressure, chemoreceptors)	Somatic nerves	(a) Hypotension (b) Hypertension	Bradycardia Tachycardia	Vasodilatation Vasoconstriction	Skeletal muscle exercise reflexly constricts splanchnic and limb veins and dilates cutaneous veins
Atrial mechanical						
1. Atriocaval or pulmonary vein junction	Stretch	Vagus	Diuresis	Tachycardia (?Bainbridge reflex)		No effect
2. Entire atrium	Stretch	Vagus	Hypotension	Bradycardia	Vasodilatation	
Ventricular						
1. Pressure	Stretch (left ventricular epicardium)	Vagus	Hypotension	Bradycardia	Vasodilatation	Increased capacitance (dilation) with high intraventricular pressures
2. Increase heart size	Low pressure (stretch)	Sympathetic	Hypertension	Tachycardia	Vasoconstriction	
3. Increase coronary artery and coronary sinus pressure	Stretch	Vagus	Hypotension	Bradycardia	Vasodilatation	
Stretch (increased arterial pressure)	Baroreceptors					
	Carotid sinus	Glossopharyngeal	Hypotension	Bradycardia	Vasodilatation	Decreased capacitance (constriction) of abdominal vessels (not limb vessels) with fall in arterial pressure
	Aortic arch	Vagus (aortic nerve)	Hypotension	Bradycardia, negative inotropy	Vasodilatation	
Hypoxia, hypercapnia, acidemia	Chemoreceptors					
	Carotid body	Glossopharyngeal	Hypertension	Primary bradycardia,* negative inotropy	Vasoconstriction	Hypoxia causes decrease in capacitance (constriction) Role of chemoreceptors uncertain
	Aortic body	Vagus (aortic nerve)	Hypertension	Primary tachycardia, positive inotropy	Vasoconstriction	

*See Diving, Chap. 12.

vation alone produces labile blood pressure and transient hypertension, the subsequent return to a normal blood pressure range is caused by the action of cardiopulmonary receptors.

These various cardiac reflex effects may be summarized as follows:

1. Both right and left atrial receptor stimulation by stretch increases urine flow via three mechanisms; (a) decreased vasopressin (ADH) release, (b) decreased sympathetic nerve activity to the kidney, which increases sodium excretion, and (c) release of ANF from atrial granules

2. Atrial stretch at slow heart rates can increase heart rate by means of the Bainbridge reflex, but sufficient atrial stretch can also elicit hypotension, bradycardia, and vasodilatation.

3. Reduction in atrial stretch, as by blood volume loss, increases precapillary to postcapillary resistance, allowing interstitial fluid return to the plasma and thus increasing blood volume and augmenting mobilization of blood for circulation from capacitance vessels.

4. Endocardial receptors in the left ventricle act like receptors in the arterial baroreceptors to lower blood pressure and heart rate in response to stretch.

5. Epicardial receptors in the ventricles can respond to chemical stimulants to evoke the Bezold-Jarisch reflex. Also, similar ventricular receptors can be shown to respond to increased stretch, causing the opposite effect, viz., vasoconstriction and tachycardia. Serotonin injection in the area of the left coronary artery can also induce systemic and pulmonary hypertension. The physiological roles of these reflexes are little understood, but it is thought they may account for various abnormal responses such as reflex bradycardia and hypotension with certain drugs, myocardial hypoxemia, and myocardial disease, as well as the induction of dangerous cardiac arrhythmias.

Respiratory reflexes: lung inflation

Stretch receptors in the lung parenchyma affect the respiratory cycle primarily (Hering-Breuer reflexes) but also induce cardiovascular changes. Lung inflation reflexly reduces sympathetic vasoconstrictor tone in the skin, splanchnic, and muscle vascular beds. The effect is greatest in skeletal muscle, and the chief redistribution of blood flow is to muscle. Presumably, the hyperventilation that accompanies strenuous exercise can contribute to increased blood flow to muscles through this reflex.

Respiratory sinus arrhythmia

An increase in heart rate during inspiration and a decrease during expiration is known as *respiratory sinus arrhythmia* (See Fig. 7.39). A number of different control systems appear to interact in producing the phasic variation in vagal tone that causes this type of sinus arrhythmia, which has no pathological implications. These include radiation of respiratory center activity to medullary cardiovascular centers, the cardiac component of the respiratory Hering-Breuer reflex, the Bainbridge reflex that produces cardiac acceleration (at least at slow heart rates and owing to increased filling of the right atrium and great veins during inspiration), and the baroreceptor reflex (which slows heart rate when blood pressure increases as a result of the acceleratory phase of sinus arrhythmia). In addition to the effect on heart rate, a positive inotropic action on left ventricular contraction during the acceleratory phase has been demonstrated. Why respiratory sinus arrhythmia should be so extraordinarily pronounced in the resting dog and minimal or absent in most other species is not clear.

CENTRALLY INTEGRATED PATTERNS OF CIRCULATORY RESPONSE

Stereotyped patterns of circulatory response characterized by changes in blood flow distribution and cardiac output occur in exercise, the defense reaction, diving, thermoregulation, and emotional responses. The integrating centers are in the hypothalamus. Influences from cortical and subcortical autonomic areas (especially the limbic system) and the premotor and motor cortex are superimposed on these hypothalamic integrating centers. Relay stations are found in mesencephalic structures and the medulla oblongata.

Patterned responses of exercise and emotional stress

Exercise response

At the onset of exercise there is sympathetic adrenergic discharge to the heart and many vascular beds that results in increased cardiac output and vasoconstriction in nonexercising parts of the body. Vasodilatation occurs in the vascular beds of the exercising muscles, and vasoconstriction occurs in nonexercising muscles and elsewhere. This results in alterations in regional peripheral resistance so that most of the increased blood flow goes to the exercising muscles. The cardiac and blood pressure adjustments that occur during exercise, in fact, begin before the exercise starts. In dogs these responses can be simulated by stimulation of the diencephalic H_2 fields of Forel (or area tegmentalis H_2, located below the thalamus in the region of the basal ganglia) in sites that are close to or identical with the so-called *defense area,* where stimulation in conscious cats produces alerting and aggressive behavior. The cardiovascular changes during such stimulation are like those in exercise: positive inotropic and chronotropic cardiac effects, generalized adrenergic vasoconstriction, and sympathetic cholinergic vasodilatation in skeletal muscle beds. Similar responses can be evoked by stimulation of selected areas in the motor cortex or in the amygdala.

Emotional stress

In humans, *emotional stress* produces the exercise pattern of cardiovascular change (increased cardiac output and blood pressure accompanied by increased muscle blood flow) in the absence of muscular exercise. It appears that the cortical motor area can turn on the hypothalamically integrated pattern of autonomic cardiovascular control that is characteristic of exercise. There is also evidence of vasoconstrictor and cardioaccelerating reflex effects from chemosensitive receptors that respond to accumulating metabolites in the contracting muscle. The baroreceptor responses that would limit these hemodynamic changes are suppressed to some extent at the medullary level, permitting continuation of the altered state during exercise and emotional stress.

Central nervous system role

The various cardiovascular afferents project to the pontomedullary circulatory centers and beyond to suprapontine centers in the hypothalamus, limbic region, and frontoorbital cortex (Fig. 10.6). The impulses arriving in the central nervous system signal changes in a large number of variables, including intravascular pressures (arterial and cardiac baroreceptors), lung inflation (lung stretch receptors), muscle activity (muscle afferents), temperature changes (central and peripheral thermoreceptors), and blood gas tension (chemoreceptors). Thus the central cardiovascular regulating centers receive a "profile" of afferent information. The distinctive patterns of change in autonomic vasomotor and cardioregulatory outflow are presumably preprogrammed in the neural circuits of the cardioregulatory centers. Which response is called forth depends on the interaction of the various inputs. Some of the major components of the cardiovascular control system are diagrammed in Figs. 10.6 and 10.12. It is important to note two features of this control system: (1) Various reflexes can be modulated or suppressed by other reflex effects (e.g., suppression of the arterial baroreceptor reflex at the medullary level during the defense reaction) and (2) local tissue flow regulators may be equally important or more important determinants of flow patterns between the various organ beds than are reflex autonomic effects.

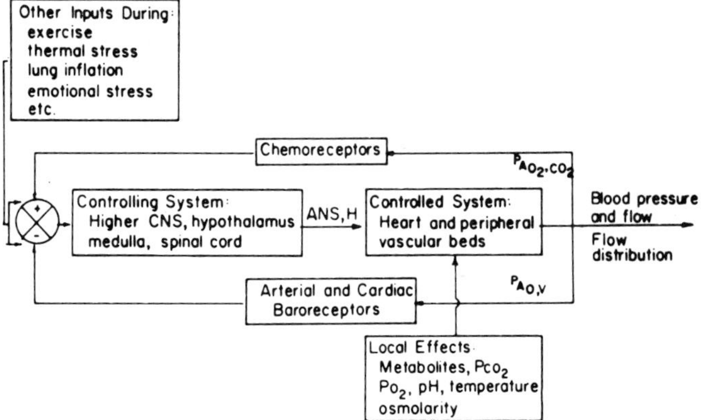

Figure 10.12. Block diagram showing several components of the circulatory control system in simplified form. Stimulation of baroreceptors by elevated arterial pressure reflexly lowers blood pressure, and stimulation of chemoreceptors by increased Pco_2 and decreased Po_2 has the opposite effect. These effects are modulated reflexly by inputs from lung stretch receptors, muscle chemoreceptors, central and peripheral thermoreceptors, and directly from the higher central nervous system (CNS) centers in exercise and in various emotional states. Peripherally, intrinsic local blood flow regulators in the various vascular beds are as important as reflex autonomic vascular effects on vascular smooth muscle and may oppose them. During various types of perturbation, the redistribution of blood flow to different organs results from a combination of nonuniform local effects and differential patterns of autonomic discharge from the CNS. ANS, autonomic nervous system; H, hormones; $P_{AO,V}$ aortic and intraventricular pressure; PA_{O_2,CO_2} arterial oxygen and carbon dioxide tension. The symbol at the left represents an algebraic "adder" of negative feedback effects on the controlling system that act to stabilize blood pressure and flow. A drop in blood pressure causes reflex effects on the controlling system to raise (+) the blood pressure; an increase in blood pressure reflexly tends to decrease (−) the blood pressure. (From Detweiler 1979, in Brobeck, ed., *Best & Taylor's Physiological Basis of Medical Practice,* 10th ed., © 1979, the Williams & Wilkins Co., Baltimore.)

As mentioned earlier, stimulation of certain areas of the cingulate gyrus in cats causes sympathetic inhibition with a vagal bradycardia and resultant hypotension. There is an increase in muscle blood flow despite the fall in blood pressure. These responses are like those observed in animals that "play dead" in the face of danger (e.g., the opossum) and in emotional fainting in humans.

In diving mammals and birds, reflex bradycardia and vasoconstriction occur when the nostrils are submerged. Blood flow to skeletal muscles and other tissues is thus restricted so that most of the blood flow is channeled to the heart and brain, conserving oxygen for these vital organs. Arteriovenous shunts in the skin remain patent, allowing a small venous return of blood that has lost no oxygen to the tissues. When the animal resurfaces, these changes are reversed; cardiac output promptly increases, as does muscle blood flow, the accumulated oxygen debt is repaid, and metabolites are removed from the muscles and other tissues that were poorly perfused.

Thermoregulatory responses

The thermoregulatory responses are under hypothalamic control. With increased heat load, these responses include cutaneous vasodilation and opening of arteriovenous anastomoses by reduced sympathetic vasoconstrictor discharge. The result is a redistribution of blood flow from other organs to increase cutaneous flow and favor heat loss. Local cooling of the hypothalamus or skin has the opposite effect.

SYSTEMIC ARTERIAL BLOOD FLOW

The principles of blood flow are presented in Chap. 5. The proximal aortic flow curve is depicted in Fig. 8.14. It is roughly triangular in shape and ends in a small negative flow (back flow) at the time of closure of the aortic valves. During most of diastole, this aortic flow curve is flat with almost zero velocity. A backflow component is present along the aorta and out into some of the larger aortic branches (e.g., femoral and common carotid arteries) for a variable distance. Flow continues to be pulsatile into the smaller arteries, but the pulsation is gradually damped. There is a pressure drop of about 40 mm Hg from small arteries to small veins, where flow is nonpulsatile.

Pulsus alternans, a change in pulse amplitude with every other beat, is usually a sign of severe depression of ventricular contractility. When the systolic pressure changes by more than 20 mm Hg, pulsus alternans can be detected by light palpation of a peripheral artery. When the arterial pulse is recorded with a transducer in anesthetized animals, the appearance of pulsus alternans usually indicates anesthetic overdose or hypoxia-induced ventricular depression.

Pulsus paradoxus designates a marked decrease in the amplitude of the arterial pulse during inspiration. Since the systolic arterial blood pressure normally decreases by a few millimeters of mercury during inspiration, pulsus paradoxus is simply an exaggeration of this effect of breathing on systolic blood pressure. Diastolic pressure may be little affected by respiration, even in the presence of pulsus paradoxus.

This exaggeration of the respiratory effect on the pulse occurs in such conditions as airway obstruction or stertorious breathing, which increase the fall in intrapleural pressure on inspiration, as well as in such conditions as hemorrhagic shock and cardiac tamponade (e.g., pericardial effusion in dogs and traumatic pericarditis in cattle).

SYSTEMIC VENOUS PRESSURE AND FLOW

Blood enters the venules from the capillaries with a small residuum of pressure (vis a tergo, see below) from the arterial side. Resistance to flow is present in the veins themselves and in the heart (vis a fronte). Various external or extramural factors (vis a latere), such as respiration, muscle compression, and gravity, together make up the pressure effect of surrounding tissues. Internal factors that affect venous pressure include the venous contractile tone, the venous capacity, and the volume of contained blood. These factors maintain the venous pressure at a level greater than that of the right atrium; when the latter rises, so does the peripheral venous pressure. The mean venous pressure of 9 to 10 mm Hg compared with the negligible right atrial pressure maintains the gradient responsible for venous flow. This small pressure gradient is sufficient to maintain flow equal to arterial flow because of the relatively large cross-sectional area and low flow resistance of the veins.

Vis a tergo (force from behind) is the pressure transmitted into the vascular system by ventricular systole. *Vis a fronte* (force from the front) designates any force that affects blood flow into the right atrium. Since both positive and negative pressures may participate, the uses of the term can be confusing. It has been variously used to designate (1) the back pressure from the right atrium, (2) the controversial suction effect of ventricular dilatation, (3) the "respiratory pump" effect of negative intrathoracic pressure that draws blood into thoracic veins, and (4) the impediment to venous return imposed by positive intrathoracic pressure (e.g., the Valsalva maneuver).

Two types of pressure change occur in the larger veins. Inspiration lowers and expiration raises the venous pressure, and the veins near the thoracic inlet can be seen to distend and collapse (the respiratory venous pulse). These great veins also act as a blood-filled manometer and reflect changes in right atrial pressure pattern (the cardiac *venous pressure pulse* or *jugular pulse*) so that A, C, and V waves (Fig. 8.14) can be recorded here as in the atria.

Contraction of skeletal muscle in the extremities and in the abdominal wall has a prominent effect on venous return. In the extremities the veins have valves so that massaging them by muscular activity pumps blood toward the heart; this pumping action is called *vis a latere*. There are no valves in the major abdominal and thoracic veins. Increasing intra-abdominal pressure relative to intrathoracic pressure favors flow toward the heart, and vice versa. Tonic contraction of abdominal muscles is suspended during inspiration and restored on its cessation. This abdominal muscle activity is increased if cardiac blood volume decreases. This compression of abdominal vessels may serve to enhance venous return.

REGULATION OF PULMONARY PRESSURE AND FLOW

Interposed between the right and left sides of the heart and entirely located within the negative pressure confines of the thorax, the functional characteristics of the pulmonary circulation are different from the systemic circulation. (1) It is an in-series system without parallel circuits. (2) It is the only circuit in the body to receive the total cardiac output. Consequently, blood flow is high. (3) It operates at a perfusion pressure one-seventh to one-eighth that of the systemic circulation. (4) It is a low-resistance system with a remarkable ability to lower resistance further as flow increases. In exercise, therefore, systemic blood flow can increase several times with little elevation of pulmonary artery pressure. (5) Because the distances from heart level are not as great as in the systemic circuit, the hydrostatic forces of gravity, acceleration, and deceleration have less effect. (6) Since it is situated within the rigid thoracic cage, it is largely protected from external pressure forces such as those that can compress systemic arteries and veins in, for example, the extremities. (7) It is, however, subject to intrathoracic pressure variations which, under certain circumstances, can exceed intravascular pressure and prevent flow. These various characteristics permit the pulmonary circuit to transport the same volume flow as the systemic circulation despite a much lower perfusion pressure. Normal data for the dog are given in Table 10.5.

Bronchial circulation

The blood supply to the bronchial connective tissue of the lung is part of the systemic circulation, but there is free communication between the capillaries of the pulmonary and bronchial systems. The bronchial capillary beds may drain either into the systemic venous system through the azygos vein or into the left atrium through the pulmonary veins. Thus oxygenated pulmonary venous blood is diluted to a small extent (perhaps 1 to 2 percent) by unoxygenated bronchial venous blood. The intermingling of the two circulations at the capillary level provides a potential shunt, which can serve to prevent elevation of capillary hydrostatic pressure if an increase should occur unilaterally in either right or left atrial pressure. Under such circumstances, capillary blood can drain through the venous system with the lower pressure.

The bronchial vessels can also provide collateral circulation to the lungs when the pulmonary arterial supply is inadequate. Thus, in pulmonary artery atresia the bronchial arteries enlarge, anastomoses with pulmonary arteries develop, and poorly oxygenated blood reaches alveolar capillaries from the aorta.

With the same volume perfusing both circuits, the pres-

Table 10.5. Representative pulmonary hemodynamic values under basal conditions in an unanesthetized 10 kg dog

	Systolic/diastolic	Mean
Pulmonary blood flow (L/min)		1.5
Radius, pulmonary artery lumen (cm)	± 0.07*	0.77
Average velocity of flow, pulmonary artery (cm/s)	47/0	13.4
Pressures (mm Hg)		
Right atrium		2
Right ventricle	27/2	
Pulmonary artery	27/9	14
Pulmonary capillaries		8
Left atrium		4
Pulmonary vascular resistance (dyne s cm^{-5})		534
Pulmonary blood volume (ml)		110
Pulmonary mean transit time (s)		4.4

*Maximal systolic/diastolic excursion around mean radius.

From Milnor 1968, in Mountcastle, ed., *Medical Physiology*, vol. 1, C.V. Mosby, St. Louis.

sure drop in the pulmonary circulation is only about one-fifth that in the systemic circulation. The tone of the terminal pulmonary vessels is relatively low, so that a rise in pulmonary venous pressure is readily transmitted to the arterial side, or vice versa. The pulmonary vascular bed is highly distensible, and blood added to perfusion of the pulmonary artery does not necessarily return at once via the pulmonary veins. It may be simply stored within the lung.

Pulmonary artery "wedge" pressure

If a small catheter is advanced along the pulmonary arterial tree until it wedges in a small branch artery, blood flow behind the catheter is blocked and fluid in the catheter perfuses the capillary bed beyond. Then the mean pressure in the catheter is believed to reflect that in the capillaries, so that the synonym *pulmonary capillary pressure* has been applied to such wedge pressures. Moreover, since the level of left atrial pressure influences that in the capillaries, arterial wedge pressure has been used as an indirect measure of the mean pressure in the left atrium. Large discrepancies between the two may prevail, however, and pulmonary arterial wedge pressure may not give a sufficiently accurate representation of the left atrial pressure for hemodynamic studies.

Pressure pulse in the pulmonary circuit

The pattern of the pulmonary arterial pressure is distinctive, showing a marked incisura low on the dicrotic limb. In late diastole, the pressure descent almost ceases and becomes horizontal (Fig. 10.13). Pulse contours of the peripheral and central portions of the pulmonary artery display differences somewhat like those of the systemic circuit. In open-chest dogs a 4 to 5 mm Hg pressure gradient was found between mean pulmonary venular (small pulmonary venous) and mean left atrial pressures.

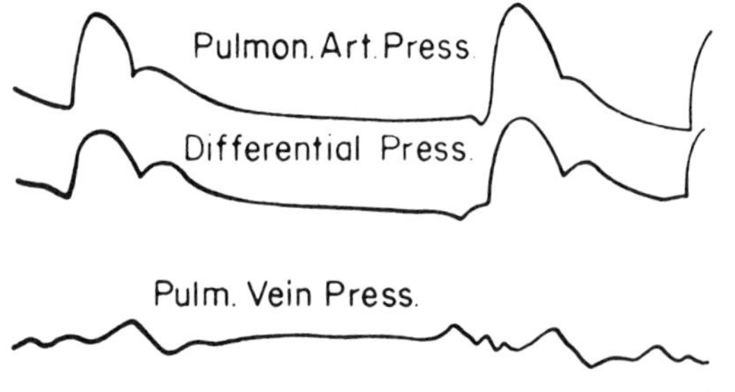

Figure 10.13. Record from an unanesthetized dog showing the pressure pulse contours in the pulmonary artery (*upper curve*), pulmonary vein (*lower curve*), and the differential pressure between the two (*middle curve*). Pulmonary artery pressure, 42/11 (systolic/diastolic) mm Hg; mean pulmonary vein pressure, 2–12 mm Hg; differential pressure had an average value of 30/1 mm Hg in six dogs. (From Hamilton et al. 1939, *Am. J. Physiol.* 125:130–41.)

Pulmonary blood volume

The pulmonary blood volume is the volume of blood contained in the vessels of the lungs and should not be confused with the *central blood volume,* which includes the pulmonary blood volume plus the blood volumes in the heart and great vessels. Only some one-third of the central blood volume is contained in the pulmonary blood vessels. Approximately 9 percent of the total blood volume in humans and dogs is contained in the pulmonary vessels. It is distributed about equally among the arteries, capillaries, and veins, although some earlier accounts placed up to 50 percent in the veins. Increases in pulmonary blood volume amounting to 25 or 50 percent may occur when the low-pressure system (systemic veins and pulmonary circulation, see Chap. 5) serves its reservoir function to accommodate increases in total blood volume or when extensive systemic arterial and venous constriction causes a shift of blood volume from the systemic to the pulmonary circuit.

PULMONARY BLOOD FLOW

Phasic flow

In the pulmonary artery the flow of blood rises and falls more slowly than in the aorta. A small backflow occurs at the end of systole, as in the aorta. Flow remains pulsatile throughout arteries and capillaries, and small oscillations persist into the left atrium. The distribution of flow within the lungs is affected by gravitational hydrostatic forces. In humans the capillaries in the lung apices more than 15 cm above the heart base are nearly or completely closed, whereas those at the bases are distended and regional blood flow is greater here. The net effect of low capillary pressure combined with normal plasma oncotic pressure is to favor fluid reabsorption from the lung interstitial tissue. Pulmonary edema appears first in the lower lobes because this is where hydrostatic pressure is highest.

Sheet-flow concept

It has been suggested on morphological grounds that the alveolar microcirculation is organized into a vascular sheet. That is, an arrangement in which two walls of endothelium held apart by connective tissue and cellular posts enclose a sheetlike space, rather than the conventional model of a network of cylindrical tubes. The interalveolar capillary bed would thus be visualized as an endothelium-lined, flat vascular sinus with variable reservoir capacity through which blood advances as a moving sheet. The validity of this concept as a basis for understanding microcirculatory flow and gas exchanges across the capillary alveolar barrier has not yet been realized.

Vascular waterfall concept

Some of the pressure-flow relationships in the pulmonary circulation suggest that, under certain conditions, the only significant resistance is found in the arterioles, rather than in capillaries and venules. Consequently, the flow rate through capillaries is influenced only by the hydrostatic pressure on the distal end of the arterioles and not by the pressure on the distal end of the arterioles and not by the pressure drop across the arterioles themselves. If the pulmonary artery is perfused with different volumes of flow at a constant pressure, the maximal flow will be found to coincide with a pressure in the pulmonary veins that just exceeds intra-alveolar pressure. If the pulmonary venous pressure is below the intra-alveolar level, changes in the former will not affect the rate of blood flow. Since capillary pressure must exceed alveolar pressure for flow to occur at all through collapsible capillaries, lowering venous pressure must create a larger pressure drop between end capillaries and pulmonary veins, even though the flow remains constant. Thus a *waterfall* can exist between capillaries and veins. Physiologically, this mechanism would operate only where arterial pressure is greater than and venous pressure is less than alveolar pressure (Fig. 10.15). *Waterfall* denotes a locus where flow rate is independent of pressure drop.

The influence of pulsatile arterial pressure on flow distribution in the lung appears to be dependent on frequency. Effective pulsatile pressure transmission to capillaries falls with increasing frequency of the arterial pressure pulse. Thus, in the vertical lung, the height above the heart level at which blood flow will be detected decreases with increasing pulse frequency. Factors that act to influence distribution of blood flow in vertical lungs are diagrammed in Fig. 10.14.

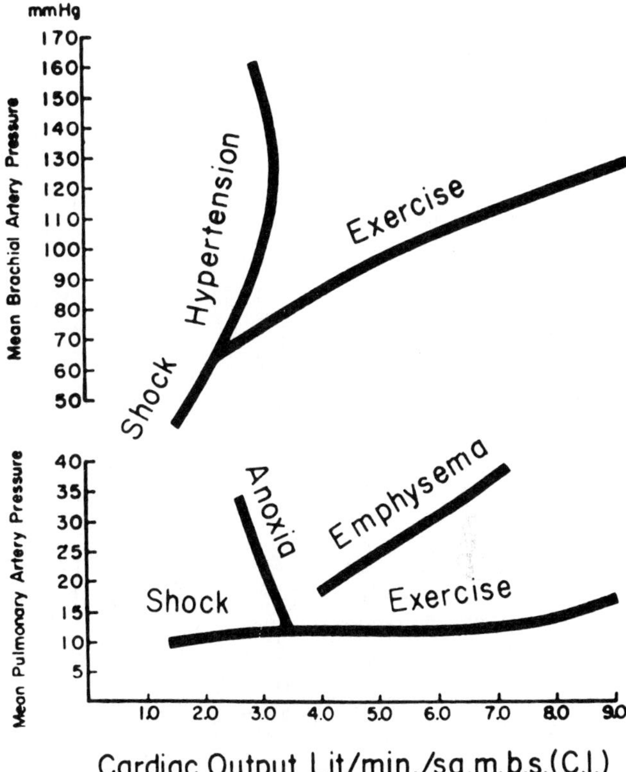

Figure 10.14. The relationship of pressure to flow in the systemic circulation and pulmonary circulation in normal and abnormal states in the dog. Note the difference in response of the two circulations to exercise. C.I., cardiac index; sq.m.b.s., square meters of body surface. (From Detweiler 1979, in Brobeck, ed., *Best & Taylor's Physiological Basis of Medical Practice,* 10th ed., © 1979, the Williams and Wilkins Co., Baltimore.)

Critical closing pressure in pulmonary vessels

There is experimental evidence that in both alveolar and extra-alveolar vessels of the pulmonary circulation, critical closing pressure exceeding intra-alveolar pressure can be caused by a low pH or a high CO_2 level.

Hydrostatic and osmotic pressures across the capillary membrane

Production and reabsorption of interstitial fluid in the lung ("lung water") in accordance with the Starling principle (see above) are somewhat controversial because of disagreements about the level of interstitial hydrostatic and oncotic pressures. Capillary pressures within the lung are low compared with those in the systemic circulation. Capillary hydrostatic pressure is determined in part by gravity, being low at the apex and high at the base; a mean value of 9 mm Hg has been suggested. Because of the prevailing negative intrathoracic pressures, it is generally assumed that lung interstitial fluid pressure is subatmospheric (perhaps −12 mm Hg). If colloid oncotic pressures of 26 mm Hg in the plasma and 5 mm Hg in the interstitial fluid are assumed, then these forces at equilibrium across the capillary membrane would balance as follows (Cumming 1974): The total *outward force* of 26 mm Hg is the sum of 9 mm Hg of capillary hydrostatic pressure, 5 mm Hg of interstitial colloid osmotic pressure, and 12 mm Hg of negative interstitial fluid pressure. The total *inward force* of the plasma colloid osmotic pressure is 26 mm Hg, and thus there is equilibrium.

Presumably, net outward forces slightly exceed the inward force, causing a very small excess of fluid to filter out of the capillaries. This is returned to the circulation through the lymphatics. In fact, it is the exceptionally rich lymphatic network that prevents pulmonary edema until capillary hydrostatic pressure exceeds 25 mm Hg. The negative interstitial fluid pressure favors passage of fluid across the alveolar membranes into the interstitial fluid spaces, thus preventing accumulation of fluid in the alveoli.

Effects of respiration on pulmonary and systemic blood pressures and flows

Representative pulmonary artery and right ventricular pressures are given in Table 10.6. The pulmonary arterial pressure falls during inspiration and rises during expiration. One might expect that, as a result of the increased flow of blood into the right ventricle during inspiration and the

Table 10.6. Pressures in the pulmonary circulation (mm Hg)

	Right ventricle pressures			Pulmonary artery pressures			
Species	Systolic	Diastolic	Source	Systolic	Diastolic	Mean	Source
Cow	45–56	0–1	Doyle et al. 1960	33–46	19–21	24–31	Doyle et al. 1960
Horse	49 ± 11 (35–72)	14 ± 6 (7–24)	Gall 1967	36 ± 9 (25–51)	21 ± 5 (14–28)	28	Gall 1967
Calf	55 (15–60)	0	McCrady et al. 1968	45 (36–52)	16 (12–18)	26 (20–35)	McCrady et al. 1968
Pig	51	0	Wachtel et al. 1963	40	16 (9–20)	22.5	Maaske et al. 1965
Dog	24	2	Moscovitz et al. 1956	21	10	15	Moscovitz et al. 1956
Human	25 (17–32)	4 (1–7)	Dittmer et al. 1959	22 (11–29)	9 (4–13)	15 (9–19)	Dittmer et al. 1959
Goat	24.5 (24–32)	−1.5 (−3 to 0)	Spörri 1962				
Sheep	26.3 (18–37)	−3.1 (−6 to 0)	Spörri 1962			9	Halmagi et al. 1961
Cat	26	0	Tashjian et al. 1965	26–36	15–17		Grauwiler 1965

greater systolic discharge, both the pulmonary pressure and pulmonary flow would rise during this phase of respiration; however, only the pulmonary flow rises. Because of the traction exerted on the circumference of the pulmonary vessels by the surrounding lung tissue, their capacity is increased. This more than counteracts the tendency for pressure to rise, and it accommodates the greater amount of blood entering the pulmonary circuit during the inspiratory phase. During expiration these effects are reversed. The right systolic discharge is less, but the capacity of the vascular bed of the lungs is at the same time reduced and an upward swing in pulmonary arterial pressure occurs. With maximal expansion of the lungs, or during a forced expiration with the glottis closed (Valsalva's experiment), the vessels are strongly compressed by the surrounding lung tissue and the pulmonary arterial pressure rises sharply.

The increased capacity of the pulmonary vessels during inspiration reduces, momentarily, the flow of blood into the left atrium; the consequent reduction in the systolic discharge of the left ventricle causes a fall in aortic pressure. After a few beats of the right ventricle, the greater capacity of the pulmonary vessels again becomes filled, the flow of blood into the left chambers of the heart increases, and the aortic pressure rises. The succeeding expiration, by reducing the capacity of the pulmonary vessels, drives blood to the left side and further increases the discharge into the aorta; the systemic pressure, in consequence, continues its rise until near the end of the expiratory phase. If the respiratory movements and the systemic blood pressure are recorded simultaneously, it is found that the blood pressure commences to fall at the beginning of inspiration and reaches its lowest point in the latter half of this phase; the blood pressure tracing then commences to rise and reaches its maximum toward the latter part of expiration. In addition to these mechanical effects of respiration on systemic flow and pressure, radiation of impulses to the vasomotor centers from the respiratory center during inspiration can increase arterial pressure. These are correctly called *Traube-Hering waves* after their discoverers. Also, reflex and chemoreceptor influences that accompany fluctuations in pressure and blood oxygen during the respiratory cycle can contribute to this effect.

Distinguished from the respiratory waves in systemic arterial blood pressure are slower fluctuations called *Mayer waves* (sometimes erroneously referred to as Traube-Hering waves), which occur at rates of one to three waves per minute. These represent oscillations in baroreceptor and chemoreceptor reflex control systems, which are exaggerated under conditions of hypotension and tissue hypoxia. For example, elevation of cerebrospinal fluid pressure elicits an increase in arterial blood pressure, the *medullary ischemic response of Cushing*. When the arterial blood pressure becomes high enough, ischemia is relieved and the pressure falls again until tissue hypoxia builds up once more and the cycle is repeated. Similar oscillations from cyclic carotid and aortic body chemoreceptor stimulation are seen, especially in hypotension after hemorrhage. The carotid sinus and aortic arch baroreceptors likewise participate in generation of these waves and may be the primary reflex influence under certain circumstances.

Spectral power analysis has been applied to these circulatory rhythms, and the current trend is to get away from classification of blood pressure oscillations according to the names of their discoverers and to order them by their frequency or period duration. In a recent study in normal and baroreceptor- and cardiopulmonary-deafferentated dogs (see above) three major oscillations in blood pressure peaks were identified: (1) those due to the heartbeat at the frequency of the heart rate; (2) those correlated with the respiratory rate; and (3) a very slow oscillation with a cycle length of about 20 minutes (or about three waves per hour). These patterns were of far greater magnitude in the denervated dogs than in the intact dogs since the baroreceptors tend to buffer the oscillations. The origin of these slow waves has not been determined.

In addition to the three categories of periodic blood pressure alterations cited above, others have been described in experimental dogs, such as an oscillatory blood pressure cycle with periods of about 1.5 hours. The primary cause of this blood pressure oscillation appears to be a similar oscillation in the heart rate and cardiac arrhythmia. The arterial baroreceptor system fails to buffer these oscillations. The cause of these oscillations is unknown, as is the question of whether it is an intrinsic cardiovascular periodicity or the result of entrainment by another system interacting via the central nervous system with the blood pressure–regulating system.

Effects of exercise on pulmonary circulation

The general form of the curves relating systemic and pulmonary artery pressure and blood flow in the dog as cardiac output changes in various normal and abnormal states is shown in Fig. 10.14. Pulmonary artery pressure is maintained below the upper limit of normal until the flow exceeds at least three times the base level, whereupon it increases progressively. This absence of pressure rise with increased flow implies an expansion of the vascular bed from opening of new channels, widening of those already perfused, or a combination of both. Thus the resistance decreases. It is believed (without proof) that this represents passive distention of the lung vasculature, especially since the same relationship holds when attempts are made to denervate the lungs, when isolated lung lobes are perfused, or when variation in the quantity of blood in the lungs is induced by different procedures.

In the exercising horse, unlike the dog, the pulmonary artery pressure rises about 30 percent during exercise (see Chap. 15).

Factors that passively affect pulmonary vascular pressure, volume, and flow include (1) cardiac output, (2) systemic arterial pressure, (3) bronchial blood flow, (4) ventilation, (5) bronchomotor activity, and (6) release of hormones (e.g., catecholamines) into the circulation. Active pulmonary vasomotion can be demonstrated by causing hypoxia, which produces vasoconstriction, or by infusing acetylcholine, which causes vasodilatation. Pulmonary blood volume changes, however, are primarily passive in response to alterations in vascular distending pressure. Thus pulmonary blood volume increases with exercise, systemic vasoconstriction, impaired left ventricular function, and infusion of fluid. It decreases with fall in systemic arterial pressure (vasodepressor reactions), improved left ventricular function, or a drop in total blood volume (hemorrhage).

Vasomotor control of pulmonary circulation

Evidence for and against the significance of vasomotor control of the pulmonary circulation may be summarized as follows.

The small pulmonary vessels have muscular coats and are equipped with a dual nerve supply: sympathetic and parasympathetic. Stimulation of the sympathetic pulmonary nerves increases the pulmonary vascular resistance; stimulation of the baroreceptors gives increased pulmonary flow and decreased pulmonary arterial pressure. Casts of the two sides of a lung are markedly different if one side is perfused with norepinephrine up to the time of plastic injection (the latter showing marked constriction in the vessels less than 25 μm in diameter). Narrowing and gnarling of the small, muscular pulmonary arteries can be demonstrated angiographically in response to hypoxia and to the intrapulmonary arterial injection of catecholamines and serotonin in the closed-chest dog. Although there is little doubt that wide variations in vascular resistance can normally occur in a purely passive way, active changes in sympathetic tone causing alterations in stiffness of large pulmonary arteries have been implicated in rapid circulatory adjustments (see Chap. 9).

Sympathetic fibers to pulmonary vessels are both vasoconstrictor through alpha$_1$-adrenergic receptors and vasodilator through beta$_2$-adrenergic receptors, respectively. Cholinergic vasodilator fibers have also been identified.

Unlike most other blood vessels, those of the lungs constrict in response to hypoxia. Alveolar hypoxia, but not pulmonary arterial hypoxemia, causes this response; the latter changes oxygen tension little and the smaller vessels receive oxygen from the alveoli. Hypoxia, induced by breathing 12 percent oxygen in nitrogen, considerably increases pulmonary arterial pressure, mildly increases cardiac output, and is without effect on left atrial pressure or central blood volume. This suggests that the vasoconstriction induced is on an active basis. Although generalized vasoconstriction of the pulmonary bed would seem to serve no useful purpose, a local hypoxia could be helpful in regulating the distribution of blood by causing vasoconstriction, which would divert blood from the anoxic region to vessels in better-aerated parts of the lung. In experiments on animals in which one lung was respired with a hypoxic mixture, that lung probably developed vasoconstriction, since the overall arterial saturation returned to normal. This response occurred as if the vessels in the hypoxic lung constricted and forced the blood normally flowing through them into well-oxygenated channels.

In addition to the neural effects on pulmonary circulation described in the foregoing under "Reflexes From Heart and Lungs," there is evidence that mechanically sensitive C fiber endings in the lung tissue (called *juxtacapillary* or *J receptors,* respond to the stretch caused by an increase in the volume of interstitial fluid. The reflex response to J receptor stimulation is bronchoconstriction and rapid, shallow breathing, but no responses that reduce pulmonary capillary hydrostatic pressure have been found.

Neurogenic pulmonary edema is the term given to acute pulmonary edema that may follow severe head injuries or experimental lesions of the medulla or hypothalmus. In some cases severe systemic hypertension leads to rising pulmonary capillary pressures that account for the pulmonary edema. In other instances increased pulmonary capillary pressure is not involved and an increase in capillary permeability apparently occurs. There is some vague speculation that the J receptors might be involved in some way in inducing vasomotor changes that cause the alteration in capillary exchange.

Epinephrine, norepinephrine, angiotensin, and serotonin (5-hydroxytryptamine) are pulmonary vasoconstrictors. Histamine causes pulmonary vasoconstriction in the dog, cat, and rat but vasodilatation in the calf.

Metabolic functions of pulmonary circulation

Because of the large area of the pulmonary vascular bed and the fact that practically the entire cardiac output passes through it during each circulatory cycle, uptake, inactivation, or production of circulating biologically active substances is maximized. Although similar metabolic processes may take place elsewhere, in other organ beds their access to the blood is only in proportion to the percentage of cardiac output they receive.

Up to 98 percent of serotonin, 30 percent of norepinephrine, 90 percent of certain prostaglandins (PGE_1, $PGE_{2\alpha}$), 80 percent of bradykinin and other substances such as leukotrienes (see p. 250) and adenosine tri- and monophosphate are taken up and inactivated in the lung vasculature. Other compounds that pass through the lungs are little affected. These include epinephrine, dopamine, tyramine and possibly histamine, prostaglandin A compounds, substance P, oxytocin, vasopressin, and angiotensin II. In addition to the important conversion of angiotensin I to angiotensin II, already discussed, certain other biologically active substances are generated in the lung (e.g., other vasoactive peptides, histamine, and certain prostaglandins). The detailed physiological role of many of these various functions in the regulation of the pulmonary vasculature, bronchial smooth muscle, and systemic circulation requires further investigation.

SUMMARY

The pulmonary vessels are capable of considerable passive dilatation as part of their function as a blood reservoir. Pulmonary blood volume and vascular resistance thus are adjusted so as to minimize pressure changes (e.g., as in exercise when blood flow can increase severalfold with little increase in pulmonary arterial pressure). Factors that increase systemic arterial pressure often have little effect on pulmonary arterial pressure (e.g., pressor reflexes and pressor drugs), and pulmonary hypertension ordinarily does not accompany essential hypertension. There is evidence, however, that variations in sympathetic tone may alter vascular compliance in the lungs and thus affect pulsatile flow and pressure transmission between the two ventricles. In this sense, the pulmonary vascular bed probably serves as more than a passive conduit and participates directly in maintaining equality of right and left ventricular output (Chap. 9). The local vasoconstrictor effect of hypoxia serves to shunt blood away from poorly ventilated lung areas to areas where oxygenation can take place. In the upright position, flow is minimal dorsal to the heart and increases at heart level and below until the most dependent areas are reached, where it declines again (Fig. 10.15). These differences in flow have to do with the effects of gravity on vascular filling and therefore resistance to flow rather than with the erroneous concept that the heart pumps against or with gravity to cause flow. The latter concept is not true because gravity affects all vessels (arteries, capillaries, and veins) equally and neither hinders nor increases flow; the flow through the vessels is an example of the siphon principle in hydraulics. The lower flow dorsal to the heart (region 1, Fig. 10.15) is a consequence of increased vascular resistance because the pressure of blood due to gravity is minimal here and the vessels collapse somewhat. In regions 2 and 3 of Fig. 10.15, vessels are distended by gravity, their resistance therefore decreases, and flow is greater than in region 1. In the deepest region, zone 4 in Fig. 10.15, vascular resistance is elevated owing to in-

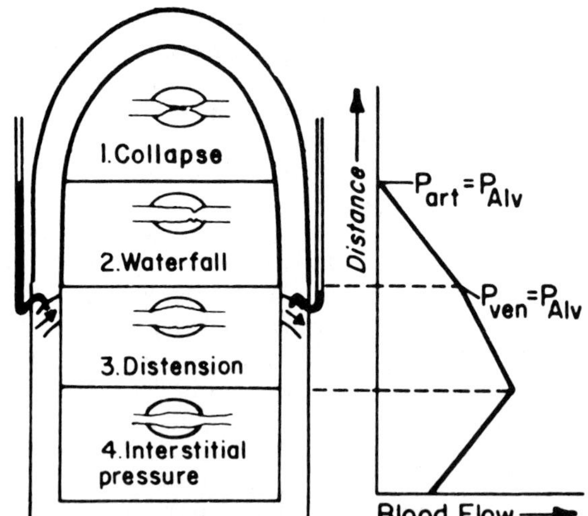

Figure 10.15. The resistance of vessels in different parts of the vertical lung. (*1*) In this region, the lung capillaries are collapsed if alveolar pressure exceeds arterial pressure and no flow occurs. (*2*) In this zone, arterial pressure exceeds alveolar pressure and alveolar pressure is greater than venous pressure. Flow is determined by the arterial-alveolar pressure difference (vascular waterfall). (*3*) Both arterial pressure (P_{art}) and venous pressure (P_{ven}) exceed alveolar pressure (P_{alv}) and flow depends on arterial-venous pressure difference. Flow increases down this zone owing to vessel distention by gravity and to recruitment of vessels. (*4*) In the deepest zone, flow decreases as the base is approached, probably owing to interstitial pressure narrowing the diameter of extra-alveolar pulmonary vessels. Distance (abscissa) is vertical height above ventral lung surface. (Redrawn from Hughes, Gracier, Maloney, and West 1968, *Resp. Physiol.* 4:58.)

creased interstitial pressure, which narrows the extra-alveolar pulmonary vessels.

INTERSTITIAL-LYMPHATIC FLOW SYSTEM

The blood vascular system transports compounds such as nutrients and metabolites to and from the blood-tissue exchange system at the capillary level. The interstitium is filled with a gel-like matrix (a water-filled network of fibers containing macromolecules) that can be considered "bounded" by two fluid compartments—the capillary network and the terminal lymphatics. The interstitium and the lymphatics constitute an extravascular flow system upon which the blood capillary-tissue exchanges depend. The steady state of the interstitium depends on the passage of materials in and out of the blood capillaries and passage of materials into the lymph system and then back to the bloodstream. The excess of capillary filtration over reabsorption is balanced by lymph flow. Large molecules, such as plasma proteins, cannot be reabsorbed into the capillaries against their concentration gradients. A primary function of the lymphatic system is to prevent accumulation of such large molecules in the interstitium.

The lymphatic system originates in a network of terminal sacs or spaces that converge to enter collecting channels. The tissue or interstitium pressure is subatmospheric, from −0.2 to −8.0 mm Hg. The blood capillary filtrate leaves the interstitium either by reabsorption by the Starling mechanism or via the lymphatic system. The latter is the only route for proteins and other macromolecules. This is aided by the pumping or suction action of the collecting lymphatic channels, which are spontaneously motile, have one-way valves, and are massaged by mechanical movement of the tissue. The transcapillary flux (Starling mechanism) is substantially higher than the lymph flow, perhaps 8 to 10 times higher.

Lymph transport mechanisms in lymphatics are vastly different from those in veins, as has been shown by work during the past decade. Intravenous and intralymphatic pressure records from the limbs of sheep show that the venous pressure is steady at about 15 to 20 mm Hg and fluctuates slightly with each heartbeat, whereas the intralymphatic pressure has a pressure pulse with an amplitude that reaches 25 mm Hg and a frequency of about 5 per minute. These lymphatic pressure pulses are generated by contractions of the lymphatics themselves. The lymphatics may be thought of as a series of contracting chambers, demarcated by the lymph valves, rather than as a continuous vessel like a vein. Thus it is better to describe their hydrodynamic function in terms used for the heart, such as systole, diastole, preload (filling pressure), afterload (outflow resistance), stroke volume, and rate of beating. The main determinants of lymph flow are filling pressure (preload) and outflow resistance (afterload). When afterload, preload, or both are increased, the lymph vessel is stretched; it responds by increasing the rate and strength of contraction, and vice versa. Empty lymph vessels, as when preload is reduced to zero, do not contract. Complete obstruction increases contraction amplitude and frequency to raise peak lymphatic pressures to about 60 mm Hg or even higher.

Hormones, vasoactive substances, and nerves affect lymph vessel rate and strength of contraction. Norepinephrine, epinephrine, and alpha-adrenergic sympathetic nerves stimulate motor activity and local lymph flow. There is no evidence, however, that such motor effects can cause negative pressure (or suction) at the lymph capillaries. Apparently, certain endotoxins can paralyze lymphatics.

Ordinarily, gravity has little effect on lymph flow because the column of fluid in the lymphatic is not continuous and a hydrostatic gradient (standpipe effect) is not present as in veins. If, however, lymphatics are markedly distended and their fluid column is continuous, then they behave like veins. Thus muscle or other massage can propel lymph in lymphatics as well as blood in veins centrally under conditions of lymph vessel distention. Also, movement of the limbs, manual massage, or both can induce lymphatic contractions as well as increase local production of lymph, causing an increase in lymph flow.

Thus the lymphatic system behaves more like the intestinal tract than the venous system in that it propels its contents by smooth-muscle activity. When no lymph is present, its smooth muscle becomes quiescent and lymph pressure fails to zero. Stretching of the vessels by the lymph causes rhythmical contractions that increase in rate and strength, depending on the degree of stretch.

Tissue edema

Tissue edema is an abnormal accumulation of interstitial fluid accompanied by swelling. It may occur in the extremities during prolonged standing or elsewhere as the result of cardiac decompensation (see Chap. 12), decreased plasma-protein concentration in starvation or glomerulonephritis, or mechanical obstruction of the lymph channels.

Overnight "stocking" ("ankle") edema of horses is caused by a deficiency of venous massage to aid in the return of venous blood from pendant blood capillaries and the inability of the lymphatic system to remove this excessive interstitital fluid. With exercise, muscle massage decreases venous pressure, and insofar as the lymphatics are distended exercise would aid lymph return. With exercise, "stocking" edema soon disappears. The lymphatics ordinarily handle minor increases in tissue flow, preventing edema formation. A cardinal reaction of tissue trauma is swelling caused by edema formation secondary to capillary damage. The edema that occurs in immunologically mediated tissue reactions (e.g., urticaria) and in various renal diseases apparently is caused by damage of capillary basement membrane. After severe hemorrhage, capillary hydrostatic pressure falls and the resulting capillary uptake of tissue fluid immediately begins to dilute plasma proteins and red cell concentration, depending on the intensity of the hypotension. Spontaneous vasomotion of the lymphatic collecting channels also occurs, further increasing fluid return to the bloodstream.

In the lungs, where edema is especially dangerous, the heightened rapid removal of capillary filtrate by the lymph system is especially important in preventing fluid accumulation in the alveoli when capillary hydrostatic pressure increases (e.g., in congestive heart failure) or when plasma protein concentration decreases.

REFERENCES

Abboud, F.M. 1982. The sympathetic system in hypertension. State-of-the-art review. *Hypertension* 4 (Suppl. II):II-208–II-225.

Allen, D., Jr., Clark, S., Moore, J.N., and Prasse, K.W. 1990. Evaluation of equine digital Starling forces and hemodynamics during early laminits. *Am. J. Vet. Res.* 51:1903–34.

Andersen, H.T. 1966. Physiological adaptations in diving vertebrates. *Physiol. Rev.* 46:212–43.

Badeer, H. 1982. Gravitational effect on the distribution of pulmonary blood flow: Hemodynamic misconceptions. *Respiration* 43:408–413.

Bainbridge, F.A. 1914. On some cardiac reflexes. *J. Physiol.* (London) 48:332–40.

Baust, W., and Heinemann, H. 1967. The role of the baroreceptors and of blood pressure in the regulation of sleep and wakefulness. *Exp. Brain Res.* 3:12–24.

Beckett, S.D., Hudson, R.S., Walker, D.F., Reynolds, T.M., and Vachon, R.I. 1972. Corpus cavernosum penis pressure and external penile muscle activity during erection in the goat. *Biol. Reprod.* 7:359–64.

Beckett, S.D., Walker, D.F., Hudson, R.S., Reynolds, T.M., and Vachon, R.I. 1973. Blood pressures and penile muscle activity in the stallion during coitus. *Am. J. Physiol.* 225:1072–75.

Beckett, S.D., Walker, D.F., Hudson, R.D., Reynolds, T.M., and Vachon, R.T. 1974. Corpus cavernosum penis pressure and penile muscle activity in the bull during coitus. *Am. J. Vet. Res.* 35:761–63.

Beckett, S.D., Walker, D.F., Hudson, R.S., Reynolds, T.M., and Purohit, R.C. 1975. Corpus spongiosum penis pressure and penile muscle activity in the stallion during coitus. *Am. J. Vet. Res.* 36:431–33.

Bennett, B.M., Molina, C.R., Waldman, S.A., and Murad, F. 1989. Cyclic nucleotides and protein phosphorylation in vascular smooth muscle relaxation. In N. Sperelakis, ed., *Physiology and Pathophysiology of the Heart.* Kluwer, Boston, Pp. 825–846.

Berne, R.M., and Levy, M.N. 1967. *Cardiovascular Physiology.* C.V. Mosby, St. Louis.

Blumenthal, H.T., and Cowdry, E.V. 1967. Functional anatomy of the vascular system. In H.T. Blumenthal, ed., *Cowdry's Arteriosclerosis.* Charles C Thomas, Springfield, Ill. Pp. 47–65.

Boeynaems, J-M., and Pearson, J.D. 1990. P_2 purinoceptors on vascular endothelial cells: Physiological significance and transduction mechanisms. *Trends. Pharmacol. Sci.* 11:34–37.

Bristow, M.R., and Port, J.P. 1990. Receptor pharmacology of the human heart. In O.B. Garfein, *Current Concepts in Cardiovascular Physiology.* Academic Press, San Diego. Pp. 73–132.

Brod, J., Fencl, V., Hejl, Z., and Jirka, J. 1959. Circulatory changes underlying blood pressure elevation during acute emotional stress (mental arithmetic) in normotensive and hypertensive subjects. *Clin. Sci.* 18:269–79.

Burnstock, G. 1980. Cholinergic and purinergic regulation of blood vessels. D.F. Bhor. A.P. Somlyo, and H.V. Sparks, Jr., eds. In *Handbook of Physiology.* Sec. 2, The Cardiovascular System. Vol. II, *Vascular Smooth Muscle.* Am. Physiol. Soc., Bethesda, Md. Pp. 577–612.

Burton-Opitz, R. 1903. Venous pressures. *Am. J. Physiol.* 9:198–206.

Coleridge, H.M., and Coleridge, S.C.G. 1986. Reflexes from the tracheobronchial tree. In N. Cherniak and S.D. Widdicombe, eds., *The Handbook of Physiology: The Respiratory System.* Vol. 2, *Control of Breathing,* Part I. Am. Physiol. Soc., Washington, D.C. Pp. 395–429.

Collier, J., and Vallance, P. 1989. Second messenger role for NO widens to nervous and immune systems. *Trends Pharmacol. Sci.* 10:428–31.

Cumming, G. 1974. The pulmonary circulation. In A.C. Guyton and D.E. Jones, eds., *Cardiovascular Physiology.* University Park Press, Baltimore, Pp. 93–122.

Cushing, H. 1902. Some experimental and clinical observations concerning states of increased intracranial tension. *Am. J. Med. Sci.* 124:375–400.

Daly, I.deB., and Hebb, C. 1966. *Pulmonary and Bronchial Vascular Systems.* Williams & Wilkins, Baltimore.

Daly, I.deB., and Verney, E.B. 1926. Cardiovascular reflexes. *J. Physiol.* (Paris) 61:268–74.

Dampney, R. 1990. The subretrofacial nucleus: Its pivotal role in cardiovascular regulation. *News Physiol. Sci.* 5:63–67.

Darnell, J., Lodish, H., and Baltimore, D. 1986. *Molecular cell biology.* Sci. Am. Books, New York.

Detweiler, D.K. 1981. The use of electrocardiography in toxicological studies with beagle dogs. In T. Balazs, ed., *Cardiac Toxicology.* vol. 3, CRC Press, Boca Raton, Fla. Pp. 33–82.

Detweiler, D.K., and Patterson, D.F. 1972. Diseases of the blood and cardiovascular system. In E.J. Catcott, ed., *Equine Medicine and Surgery.* Am. Vet. Public., Santa Barbara. Pp. 277–347.

de Wardener, H.E. 1987. Natriuretic and sodium-transport inhibitory factors associated with volume control and hypertension. In P.J. Mulrow and R. Schrier. *Atrial Hormones and Other Natriuretic Factors.* Am. Physiol. Soc., Bethesda, Md. Pp. 127–41.

Dittmer, D.S., and Grebe, R.M. 1959. *Handbook of Circulation.* WADA Technical Report 59–593. Wright Air Development Center, Wright-Patterson Air Force Base, Ohio.

Doyle, J.T., Patterson, J.L., Warren, J.V., and Detweiler, D.K. 1960. Observations on the circulation of domestic cattle. *Circ. Res.* 8:4–15.

Edis, A.J., Donald, D.E., and Shepherd, J.T. 1970. Cardiovascular reflexes from stretch of pulmonary vein-atrial junctions in the dog. *Circ. Res.* 27:1091–1100.

Fater, D.C., Schultz, H.D., Sundet, W.D., Mapes, J.S., and Goetz, K.L. 1982. Effects of left atrial stretch in cardiac-denervated and intact conscious dogs. *Am. J. Physiol.* 242:H1056–H1064.

Fewell, J.E., and Johnson, P. 1981. Acute increases in blood pressure cause arousal from sleep in lambs. *J. Physiol.* 320:127P.

Folkow, B. 1960. Range of control of the cardiovascular system by the central nervous system. *Physiol. Rev.* 40(Suppl. 4):93–100.

Folkow, B., and Neil, E. 1971. *Circulation.* Oxford University Press. New York.

Fregin, G.F., and Thomas, D.P. 1983. Cardiovascular response to exercise in the horse: A Review. In D.H. Snow, S.G.B. Persson, and R.J. Ross, eds., *Equine Exercise Physiology.* Burlington Press, Ltd., Cambridge. Pp. 76–90.

Furchgott, R.F., and Zawadzki, J.V. 1980. The obligatory role of endothelial cells in the relaxation of arterial smooth muscle by acetylcholine. *Nature* 299:373–76.

Gall, C.M. 1967. Intra-carotid and right heart pressures. M.S. thesis, Ohio State University, Columbus.

Gauer, O.N., Henry, J.P., and Behn, C. 1970. The regulation of extracellular fluid volume. *Annu. Rev. Physiol.* 32:547–95.

Geddes, L.A. 1970. The Direct and Indirect Measurement of Blood Pressure. Year Book, Chicago.

Goetz, K.L., Bond, G.C., and Bloxham, D.D. 1975. Atrial receptors and renal function. *Physiol. Rev.* 55:157–205.

Graham, R.M., and Lanier, S.M. 1986. Identification and characterization of alpha-adrenergic receptors. In H.A. Fozzard, E. Haber, R.B. Jennings, A. Katz, and H.B. Morgan, eds., *The Heart and Cardiovascular System.* Vol. 2. Raven Press, New York. Pp. 1059–95.

Graham, R.M., and Zisfein, J.B. 1986. Atrial natriuretic factor: Biosynthetic regulation and role in circulatory homeostasis. In H.A. Fozzard, E. Haber, R.B. Jennings, A. Katz, and H.E. Morgan, eds., *The Heart and Cardiovascular System.* Vol. 2. Raven Press, New York. Pp. 1559–69.

Green, F.J., and Watanabe, A.M. 1989. Cardiovascular adrenergic and cholinergic muscarinic receptors. In W.W. Parmley and K. Chatterjee, eds., *Cardiology.* Vol. 1. J.B. Lippincott, Philadelphia. Chap. 3. Pp. 1–21.

Guyton, A.C., Coleman, T.G., Cowley, A.W., Jr., Scheel, K.W., Manning, R.D., and Norman, R.A. 1974. Arterial pressure regulation. Overriding dominance of the kidneys in long-term regulation and in hypertension. In J.H. Laragh, ed., *Hypertension Manual.* Yorke Med., New York. Pp. 111–34.

Guyton, A.C., Jones, C.E., and Coleman, T.G. 1973. *Circulatory Physiology: Cardiac Output and Its Regulation.* 2d ed. W.B. Saunders, Philadelphia.

Halmagyi, D.F.J., and Colebatch, H.J.H. 1961. Ventilation and circulation after fluid aspiration. *J. Appl. Physiol.* 16:35–40.

Hamilton, W.F., Woodbury, R.A., and Vogt, E. 1939. Differential pressures in the lesser circulation of the unanesthetized dog. *Am. J. Physiol.* 125:560–68.

Hansen, B. 1989. Leukotrienes; biology and role in disease. *J. Vet. Intern. Med.* 3:59–72.

Hering, H.E. 1923. Der Karotisdruck-versuch. *Münch Med. Wochenschr.* 70:1287–90.

Heymans, C., and Neil, E. 1958. *Reflexogenic Areas of the Cardiovascular System.* Little, Brown, Boston.

Highsmith, R.F., and Fitzgerald, O.M. 1989. Endothelial cell regulation of vascular smooth muscle. In N. Sperelakis, ed., *Physiology and Pathophysiology of the Heart.* 2d ed. Kluwer Acad. Publ., Boston. Pp. 755–71.

Hughes, J.M.B., Gracier, J.B., Maloney, J.E., and West, J.B. 1968. Effect of lung volume on the distribution of pulmonary blood flow in man. *Resp. Physiol.* 4:58–69.

Ignarro, L.J., 1989. Endothelium-derived nitrous oxide: actions and properties. *FASEB J.* 3:31–6.

James, T.N. 1986. Degenerative lesions of a coronary chemoreceptor and nearby neural elements in the hearts of victims of sudden death. *J. Am. Col. Cardiol.* 8:12A–21A.

Johnson, P.C. 1964. Review of previous studies and current theories of autoregulation. *Circ. Res.* 15(Suppl 2):2–9.

Johnston, C.I., Newman, M., and Woods, R. 1981. Role of vasopressin in cardiovascular homeostasis and hypertension. *Clin. Sci.* 61:129s–139s.

Koch, E. 1932. Die Irradiation der pressoreceptorischen Kreislaufreflexe. *Klin. Wochenschr.* 11:225–27.

Korner, P.I. 1974. Control of blood flow to special vascular areas: Brain, kidney, muscle, skin, liver, and intestines. In A.C. Guyton and C.E. Jones, eds., *Cardiovascular Physiology.* University Park Press, Baltimore. Pp. 123–62.

Korner, P.I. 1979. Central nervous control of autonomic cardiovascular function. In R.M. Berne, N. Sperelakis, and S.R. Geiger, eds., *Handbook of Physiology.* Sec. 2, The Cardiovascular System. Vol. 1, *The Heart.* Am. Physiol. Soc., Bethesda, Md. Pp. 691–739.

Korotkov, N.S. 1905. K. Voprosu o metodach isledovaniya krovyanogo davleniya. *Izvestia Imperaratorskoi Voenno-Meditskoi Akademii* 11:365–67.

Laragh, J.H., Baer, L., Brunner, H.R., Buhler, F.R., Sealy, J.E., and Vaughan, E.D., Jr. 1972. Renin, angiotensin and aldosterone system in pathogenesis and management of hypertensive vascular disease. *Am. J. Med.* 52:633–52.

Levy, M.N. 1990. Neural and reflex control of circulation. In, O.B. Garfein (ed.), *Current concepts in Cardiovascular Physiology.* Academic Press, New York. Pp. 133–207.

Lewis, D.H. 1988. The effect of multiple organ failure on the regulation of circulation with special reference to the microcirculation. In H. Manabe, B.W. Zweifach, and K. Messmer, eds., *Microcirculation in Circulatory Disorders.* Springer, Tokyo, Pp. 103–108.

Linden, R.J. 1975. Reflexes from the heart. *Prog. Cardiovasc. Dis.* 18:201–21.

Lindermann, J.P., and Watanabe, A. 1989. Mechanisms of adrenergic and cholinergic regulation of myocardial contractility. In N. Sperelakis, ed., *Physiology and Pathophysiology of the Heart.* Kluwer, Boston, Pp. 423–52.

Loven, C. 1866. Über die Erweiterung von Arterien in Folge einer Nervenerregung. *Ber. Sachs. Ges. (Akad.) Wiss.* 18:85–100.

Luescher, T.F. 1988. *Endothelial Vasoactive Substances and Cardiovascular Disease.* S. Karger, Basel.

Maaske, C.A., Booth, N.H., and Nielson, T.W. 1965. Experimental right heart failure in swine. In L.K. Bustad, R.O. McClellan, and M.P. Burns, eds., *Swine in Biomedical Research.* Frayn, Seattle.

McCrady, J.D., Hallman, G.L., McNamara, D.G., and Vogel, J.H.K. 1968. Effects of increased flow of pulmonary blood on pulmonary vascular resistance and structure in calves. *Am. J. Vet. Res.* 29:1539–47.

McDowall, R.J.S. 1924. A vago-pressor reflex. *J. Physiol.* (London) 59:41–47.

Majno, G. 1965. Ultrastructure of the vascular membrane. In W.F. Hamilton and P. Dow, eds., *Handbook of Physiology.* Sec. 2., vol. 3, *Circulation.* Am. Physiol. Soc., Washington. Pp. 2293–2375.

Matsuura, S. 1973. Chemoreceptor properties of glomous tissue found in the carotid region of the cat. *J. Physiol.* 235:57–73.

Mellander, S. 1970. Systemic circulation: local control. *Ann. Rev. Physiol.* 32:313–44.

Mellander, S., and Johansson, B. 1968. Control of resistance, exchanges, and capacitance functions in the peripheral circulation. *Pharmacol. Rev.* 20:117–96.

Miller, A.S. 1982. *Lymphatics of the Heart.* Raven Press. New York.

Milnor, W.R. 1968. Pulmonary circulation. In V.B. Mountcastle, ed., *Medical Physiology.* vol. 1. C.V. Mosby, St. Louis. Pp. 24–34.

Milnor, W.R. 1990. *Cardiovascular Physiology.* Oxford Univ. Press, Oxford.

Moscovitz, H.L., and Wilder, R.J. 1956. Pressure events of the cardiac cycle in the dog: Normal right and left heart. *Circ. Res.* 4:574–78.

Mulrow, P.J., and Schrier, R. 1987. *Atrial Hormones and Other Natriuretic Factors.* Am. Physiol. Soc., Bethesda, Md.

Nayler, W.C. 1990. Endothelin: isoforms, binding sites, and possible implications in pathology. *Trends Pharmacol. Sci.* 11:96–99.

Nishimura, H., Nakamura, Y., Sumner, R.P., and Khosla, M.C. 1982. Vasopressor and depressor actions of angiotension in the anesthetized fowl. *Am. J. Physiol.* 242:H314–H324.

Öberg, B. 1976. Overall cardiovascular regulation. *Ann. Rev. Physiol. 38*:537–70.

Oparil, S., and Haber, E. 1974. The renin-angiotensin system. *New Engl. J. Med.* 291:389–401.

Oparil, S., and Katholi, R. 1990. Humoral control of the circulation. In O.B. Garfein, ed., *Current Concepts in Cardiovascular Physiology.* Academic Press, New York, Pp. 209–87.

Orstavik, T.B., Carretero, O.A., and Scici, A.G. 1982. Kallikrein-kinin system in regulation of submandibular gland blood flow. *Am. J. Physiol.* 242:H1010–H1014.

Owman, C. 1986. Neurogenic control of the vascular system: focus on cerebral circulation, p. 527. Neurogenic control of the vascular system. In V.B. Mountcastle, F.E. Bloom, and S.R. Geiger, eds., *Handbook of Physiology.* Sec. 1, vol. IV, Am. Physiol. Soc., Bethesda, Md. Chap. 10, pp. 525–80.

Patterson, J.L., Jr., et al. Cardiorespiratory dynamics in the ox and giraffe with comparative observations on man and other animals. *Ann. N.Y. Acad. Sci.* 127:393–413.

Permutt, S., and Riley, R.L. 1963. Hemodynamics of collapsible vessels with tone: The vascular waterfall. *J. Appl. Physiol.* 18:924–32.

Persson, P.B. 1990. Personal communication.

Persson, P.B., Ehmke, H., and Kirchheim, H.P. 1989. Cardiopulmonary-arterial baroreceptors interaction in control of blood pressure. *News Physiol. Sci.* 4:56–59.

Persson, P.B., Ehmke, H., Koeler, W.W., and Kirchheim, H.R. 1990. Identification of major slow blood pressure oscillations in conscious dogs. *Am. J. Physiol.* 259 (4 Pt 2):H1050–55.

Peñaz, J. 1978. Mayer waves: history and methodology. *Automedica* 2:135–41.

Quarton, G.C., Melnechuk, T., and Schmitt, F.O. 1967. *The Neurosciences.* Rockefeller University Press, New York.

Robinson, R.B. 1990. α-Adrenergic receptor-effector coupling. In M.R. Rosen, M.J. Janse, and A.L. Wit, eds. *Cardiac Electrophysiology: A Textbook.* Futura, Mount Kisco, N.Y. Pp. 819–29.

Roddie, I.C. 1990. Lymph transport mechanisms in peripheral lymphatics. *News Physiol. Sci.* 5:85–9.

Rosenblum, W.I. 1988. Endothelium-dependent relaxing factors in brain microvessels. In H. Manabe, B.W. Zweifach, and K. Messmer, eds., *Microcirculation in Circulatory Disorders.* Springer, Berlin, Pp. 267–70.

Rushmer, R.F. 1970. *Cardiovascular Dynamics.* 3d ed. W B Saunders, Philadelphia.

Sagawa, K., Kumada, M., and Schramm, L.P. 1974. Nervous control of the circulation. In A.C. Guyton and C.E. Jones, eds., *Cardiovascular Physiology.* University Park Press, Baltimore, Pp. 197–232.

Said, S.I. 1982. Metabolic functions of the pulmonary circulation. *Circ. Res.* 50:325–33.

Schmid, P.G., and Abboud, F.M. 1974. Neurohumoral control of vascular resistance. *Arch. Intern. Med.* 133:935–45.

Schweitzer, A. 1945. Rhythmical fluctuations of the arterial blood pressure. *J. Physiol.* (London) 104:25.

Shimada, S.G., and Marsh, D.J. 1979. Oscillations in mean arterial blood pressure in conscious dogs. *Circ. Res.* 44:692–700.

Sobin, S.S., Tremer, H.M., and Fung, Y.C. 1970. Morphometric basis of the sheet-flow concept of the pulmonary alveolar microcirculation. *Circ. Res.* 26:397–414.

Solez, K., and Heptinstall, R.H. 1980. The renal circulation: Physiology and hormonal control. In C.J. Schwartz, N.T. Werthessen, and S. Wolf, eds., *Structure and Function of the Circulation,* vol. 1. Plenum, New York. 661–727.

Sorota, S., and Pappano, A.J. 1990. Muscarinic receptor-effector coupling in the heart. In M.R. Rosen, M.J. Janse, and A.L. Wit, eds., *Cardiac Electrophysiology: A Textbook.* Futura, Mount Kisco, N.Y. Pp 803–17.

Sparks, H.V., Jr. 1980. Effect of local metabolic factors on vascular smooth muscle. In D.F. Bohr, A.P. Somlyo, and H.V. Sparks, Jr., eds., *Handbook of Physiology.* Sec. 2, *The Cardiovascular System.* Vol. 2, *Vascular Smooth Muscle.* Am. Physiol. Soc., Bethesda, Md. Pp. 475–513.

Spodick, D.H. 1988. Diseases of the pericardium. In W.W. Parmley and K. Chatterjee, eds., *Cardiology.* Vol. 2, J.B. Lippincott, Philadelphia. Chap. 43, pp. 1–33.

Spörri, H. 1962. The study of cardiac dynamics and its clinical significance. In C.A. Brandly and E.L. Jungherr, eds., *Advances in Veterinary Science* Vol. 7, Academic Press, New York. Pp. 1–41.

Stegemann, J., and Tibes, A. 1969. Sinusoidal stimulation of carotid sinus baroreceptors and peripheral blood pressure in dogs. *Ann. N.Y. Acad. Sci.* 156:787–95.

Tashjian, R.T., Das, K.M., Palich, W.E., Hamlin, R.L., and Yarns, E.E. 1965. Studies on cardiovascular disease in the cat. *Ann. N.Y. Acad. Sci.* 127:581–605.

Taubman, M.B. 1990. Molecular biology of the vascular smooth muscle contractile apparatus. In S. Chiens, ed., *Molecular Biology of the Cardiovascular System.* Lea & Febiger, Philadelphia, Pp. 91–113.

Urthaler, F., Hageman, G.R., and James, T.N. 1978. Hemodynamic components of a cardiogenic hypertensive chemoreflex in dogs. *Circ. Res.* 42:135–42.

Van Citters, R.L., and Franklin, D.L. 1969a. Cardiovascular research in wild animals: Telemetry technics and applications. *Acta. Zool. Pathol. Antverp.* 48:243–63.

Van Citters, R.L., and Franklin, D.L. 1969b. Cardiovascular responses in Alaska sled dogs during exercise. *Cir. Res.* 24:33–42.

Viveros, O.H., Garlick, D.C., and Renkin, E.M. 1968. Sympathetic beta adrenergic vasodilatation in skeletal muscle of the dog. *Am. J. Physiol.* 215:1218–25.

Webb, R.C., and Bohr, D.F. 1981. Regulation of vascular tone, molecular mechanisms. *Prog. Cardiovasc. Dis.* 24:213–42.

Yanagisawa, M., Kurihara, H., et al., 1988. A novel potent vasoconstrictor peptide produced by vascular endothelial cells. *Nature* 332: 411–15.

Zweifach, B.W., and Silberberg, A. 1979. The interstitial-lymphatic flow system. In A.C. Guyton and D.B. Young, eds., *Cardiovascular Physiology III,* vol. 18. University Park Press, Baltimore. Pp. 215–60.

CHAPTER 11

Regional and Fetal Circulations | by David K. Detweiler and Dean H. Riedesel

REGIONAL DISTRIBUTION OF CARDIAC OUTPUT

Values for blood flow to various organs in swine are given in Fig. 11.1A and B. Blood flow (in milliliters per minute per 100 g of tissue) for humans and swine is similar for various internal organs (e.g., brain, heart, kidney); however, the percentage of cardiac output going to certain organs (e.g., brain, kidney) is much lower in the swine because the organ weight/body weight ratios are smaller. The values for myocardial blood flow per 100 g of tissue and for the percentage of cardiac output reaching the heart in swine are similar to those values for calves, ponies, and humans but are markedly lower than the values for rats. Hepatic arterial flow and gastrointestinal flow are lower for swine than for rats and monkeys.

Coronary circulation

Compared with that of other organs, the coronary circulation is unique in several respects: (1) the heart is the only organ that perfuses itself; (2) flow is reduced during systole, especially in the left ventricle, because ventricular contractions compress the intramural vascular beds; (3) the myocardium, unlike skeletal muscle, depends largely on aerobic metabolism and cannot sustain a significant oxygen debt via anaerobic metabolism; (4) oxygen extraction from the blood is nearly maximal at rest, and therefore any increased oxygen demand must be met by an immediate increase in blood flow; (5) intrinsic mechanisms respond rapidly to adjust flow to oxygen used, hypoxia causes maximal vasodilatation, while the response to increased CO_2 or decreased pH is minimal; (6) metabolic factors exert primary control over vessel diameter and can override or mask extrinsic (i.e., neural and humoral) regulation; and (7) capillary density per square millimeter is enormous as compared with that of skeletal muscle.

Coronary arteries

Two coronary arteries, the right and the left, arise from the aortic sinuses of Valsalva and follow a branching course over the subepicardium. Interspecies and intraspecies differences abound in the (1) relative predominance of right versus left coronary arterial supply, (2) occurrence of intercoronary anastomoses, (3) number of collateral arteries, and (4) details of arterial branching. These differences affect the consequences of spontaneous or experimental coronary occlusion. Although once regarded as end arteries, the coronary arteries have collateral channels which are thin-walled vessels that connect coronary arteries without an intervening capillary bed. They can enlarge dramatically in

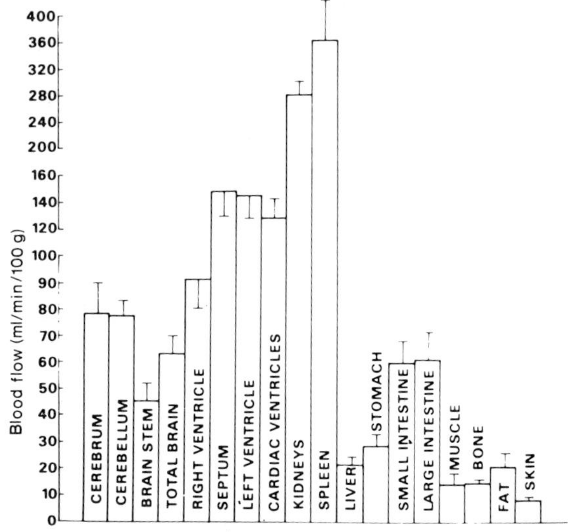

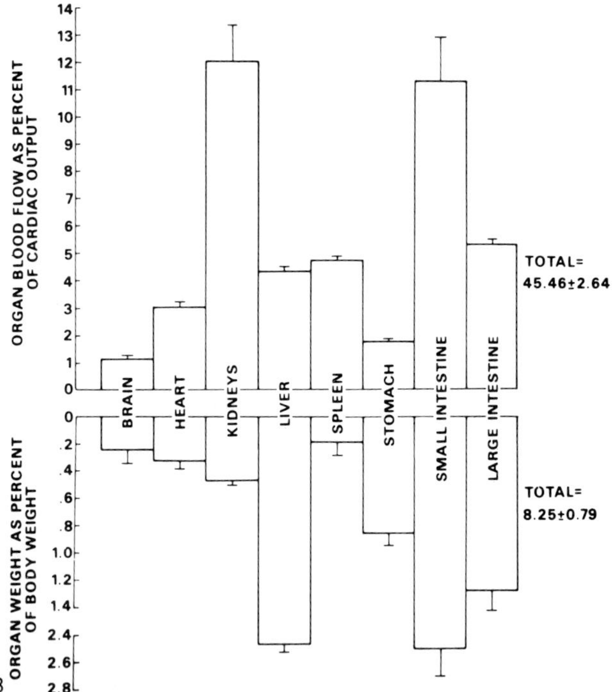

Figure 11.1. (*A*) Abscissa: values (mean ± standard error of the mean) for regional blood flow (ml/min/100 g) to various organs and tissues of unanesthetized swine (No. 9:28–55 kg). The liver value is for hepatic arterial flow only and does not include portal blood flow. (*B*) Values for blood flow to internal organs as percentage of cardiac output (CO) (i.e., distribution of CO) as related to organ weight as percentage of body weight. These internal organs make up only about 8 percent of the body mass but receive more than 45 percent of the resting CO. The CO fractions received by the various organs are 1.13 percent for the brain, 3.04 percent for the heart, 12.95 percent for the kidneys, 4.27 percent for the liver (hepatic artery only, portal flow not included), and 18.71 percent for the gastrointestinal tract. (Modified from Tranquilli, Parks, Thurmon, Benson, Koritz, Manohar, and Theodorakis 1982, *Am. J. Vet. Res.* 43:895–97.)

response to ischemia, but the extent and location of collateral circulation vary among species.

The relative predominance of the left and right coronary arterial supply to the myocardium differs within and among various mammalian species. Predominance is determined topographically by which coronary artery, right or left, crosses the crux (i.e., the point where posterior interventricular and atrioventricular sulci meet) or whether both arteries reach the crux and supply the posterior interventricular sulcus region. By this single criterion, most human hearts are classified as right coronary predominant; the remainder are classified as either left predominant or balanced. Right coronary predominance prevails in swine, horses, and certain primates; however, in dogs, cats, domestic ruminants, certain primates, and some whales, left coronary predominance is most frequent. It is not certain that this anatomical method of classification satisfactorily indicates which artery dominates in supplying the myocardium. For example, injection-corrosion preparations and arteriography show that 75 percent of human hearts have a balanced coronary arterial supply.

Veins

The great cardiac vein that, together with other tributaries, empties through the coronary sinus into the right atrium is the main drainage channel for the subepicardial veins of the left side of the heart. In the dog 80 to 90 percent of coronary sinus blood is from the left coronary artery and represents a large percentage of venous blood from the left ventricular myocardium. Changes in coronary sinus blood flow and composition can be used, therefore, to estimate metabolic changes in the left ventricle. Veins of the right side of the heart merge to form the right cardiac veins (venae cordis dextrae), which empty directly into the right atrium.

Small cardiac or thebesian veins

Thebesian veins are small vessels that connect small intramural veins and capillary beds with the cardiac chambers. In dogs the largest part of the interventricular septal arterial blood flow drains through these vessels directly into the right ventricle.

Capillaries

As noted above, the density of the myocardial capillary network and the corresponding capillary surface area are far greater per unit of cross-sectional area than in skeletal muscle. Although cardiac and skeletal muscle are alike in having about one capillary per muscle fiber, and although their capillaries are of the same diameter, the fiber diameter is 20 μm in myocardial muscle compared with about 50 μm in skeletal muscle. In the heart muscle there are 1400 to 5000 capillaries per square millimeter of cross-sectional area in various species (the variation is both biological and methodological)— with a reasonable average of about 3000 per square millimeter. In resting skeletal muscle about one-half of the capillaries are closed; experiments in rat hearts indicate that this is also true for the normally oxygenated and beating myocardium. Hypoxia increases the number of open capillaries.

Calculations based on capillary density or from coronary flow estimates indicate that the blood volume in the left ventricular free wall (dog) can vary from 10 to 20 percent of its myocardial mass and that most of it resides in the microvessels. The left ventricular coronary arterial inflow is primarily diastolic, whereas coronary venous outflow is almost entirely systolic. This means that coronary blood volume fluctuates with each heartbeat, increasing during each diastole and decreasing during systole. The blood volume change between diastole and systole is moderate and is estimated to be about 8 to 9 percent of the total coronary blood volume.

Collateral vessels

If a coronary artery is suddenly occluded, an infarction of the heart usually occurs; such a result is characteristic of end arteries without collateral vessels. A more gradual stenosis, however, leading to complete occlusion may result in progressive enlargement of small arterial collaterals and in development of new collateral channels from preexisting capillaries or from new capillaries growing in granulation tissue.

Collateral arteries have been demonstrated in normal hearts of most mammals, but their number, size, and distribution vary among species. In humans and pigs most collaterals are located subendocardially and intramurally. In dogs these vessels are found subepicardially, and they are larger but less numerous than in pigs and humans. Despite these species differences between dog and pig hearts, there are also marked individual differences among hearts of one species, so that some dog hearts will behave like pig hearts and vice versa in response to coronary ligation. Most collaterals have the dimension of arterioles until their size increases under the influence of tissue hypoxia (anemia, arterial stenosis). After coronary artery constriction (dog) active growth of collaterals begins within 36 hours and peaks at day 4. Flow to the ischemic area through the collateral vessels is only adequate in amount to maintain myocardial viability. Collateral flow does not allow the normal increase in coronary artery flow that is seen with skeletal muscle exercise.

Cardiac lymphatic vessels

The lymphatics are arranged in subepicardial, myocardial, and epicardial plexuses; of these, the epicardial plexuses have valves. Lymph flow in the dog is continuous (about 3 ml per hour in dogs weighing 15 to 24 kg), driven by intramural systolic pressure that forces lymph into the valved epicardial lymphatics and then through two or more main vessels into the mediastinal lymphatic network. Interruption of the cardiac lymphatic outflow produces acute cardiac edema with electrocardiographic changes characteristic of myocardial hypoxia or infarction; chronic interruption leads to fibrotic thickening of the atrioventricular valves, which contain lymphatics (the semilunar valves do not), and fibroelastic thickening of the endocardium.

REGULATION OF CORONARY FLOW

The control of coronary arterial resistance is exerted chiefly by intrinsic factors, namely, the local chemical milieu and mechanical compression secondary to myocardial contraction. Extrinsic regulation (neural and humoral) is of secondary importance. Rate of coronary blood flow parallels oxygen need and increases or decreases with changes in myocardial work.

Work and efficiency

In physics work is defined as force times distance or displacement. When applied to the heart, work is the transfer of energy from metabolic substrates to the development of pressure and the flow of blood. The external mechanical work of the heart results in the ejection of a stroke volume against the pressure of the aorta or pulmonary artery.

Stroke work is the area within a single cardiac pressure-volume cycle (Fig. 11.2) bounded by ABCDA. The shaded area at the bottom of Fig. 11.2 is the work performed by returning venous blood used to stretch the ventricular walls during diastole. Increased work demand can be in two forms: pressure or volume. If the ventricle needs to raise the pressure of the blood before ejection occurs, the area of the pressure-volume diagram increases. Likewise, if the ventricle needs to eject more volume than normal against the same arterial pressure, more work will be done. Pressure work is more costly in terms of oxygen consumption than

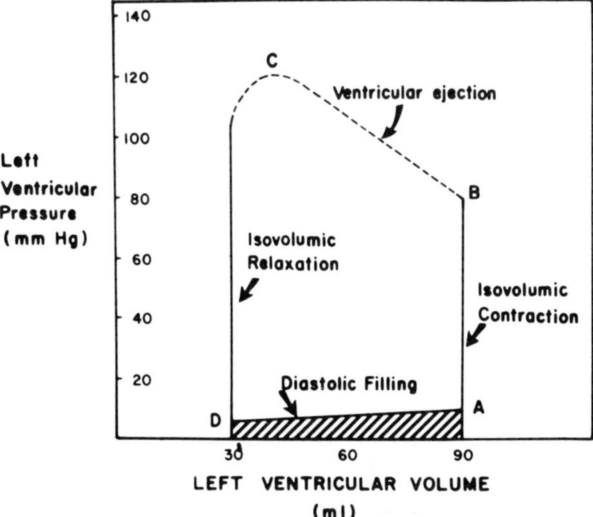

Figure 11.2. Schematic diagram of the relationship between left ventricular pressure and volume for one cardiac cycle. The area *ABCDA* represents net pressure-volume work. (From Little and Little 1989, *Physiology of the Heart and Circulation,* Yearbook Medical Publishers, Chicago, p. 210.)

volume work because of the increased amount of internal work necessary to develop the additional pressure. Other factors that affect the amount of oxygen consumption required to perform the same amount of work are the size of the heart (a dilated heart will require more oxygen), level of contractility (an increase in contractility by sympathetic nerve stimulation or drugs will increase oxygen consumption), and heart rate (an increase in heart rate leads to more oxygen consumption).

Various expressions of cardiac work are summarized in Fig. 11.3. *Effective cardiac work* is the production of forward movement of blood against arterial pressure (e.g., into the aorta or pulmonary artery in the natural direction). *Total cardiac work* includes all of the work accomplished during the contraction period, including any movement of blood in the wrong direction (regurgitation) in case the cardiac valves are incompetent. *Contractile element work* is not the same as the other two expressions, because it is applied to the development of tension in the contractile element (CE), even when the contraction is isometric and the muscle does not shorten. Strictly, it is the shortening of the CE against the series elastic component (SEC).

Efficiency (Eff), most simply defined, is the ratio of useful energy output (work) to total energy expenditure (work plus heat):

$$\text{Eff} = \frac{\text{Work}}{(\text{Work} + \text{Heat})} = \frac{\text{W}}{\text{W} + \text{h}}$$

Work plus heat is the equivalent of total chemical energy expended (E). Thus, efficiency can be represented as Eff = W/E, as in Fig. 11.3.

Since practically all energy exchange of the myocardium is linked to oxidative metabolism, myocardial oxygen consumption ($M\dot{V}O_2$) can be considered an equivalent of total chemical energy. Then the efficiency ratio becomes

$$\text{Eff} = \frac{\text{W}}{\text{Total } M\dot{V}O_2 - \text{Resting } M\dot{V}O_2}$$

W as represented here includes both contraction against pressure and kinetic energy imparted to the blood.

Values for cardiac efficiency calculated in this way have varied between 10 and 20 percent in experimental animals.

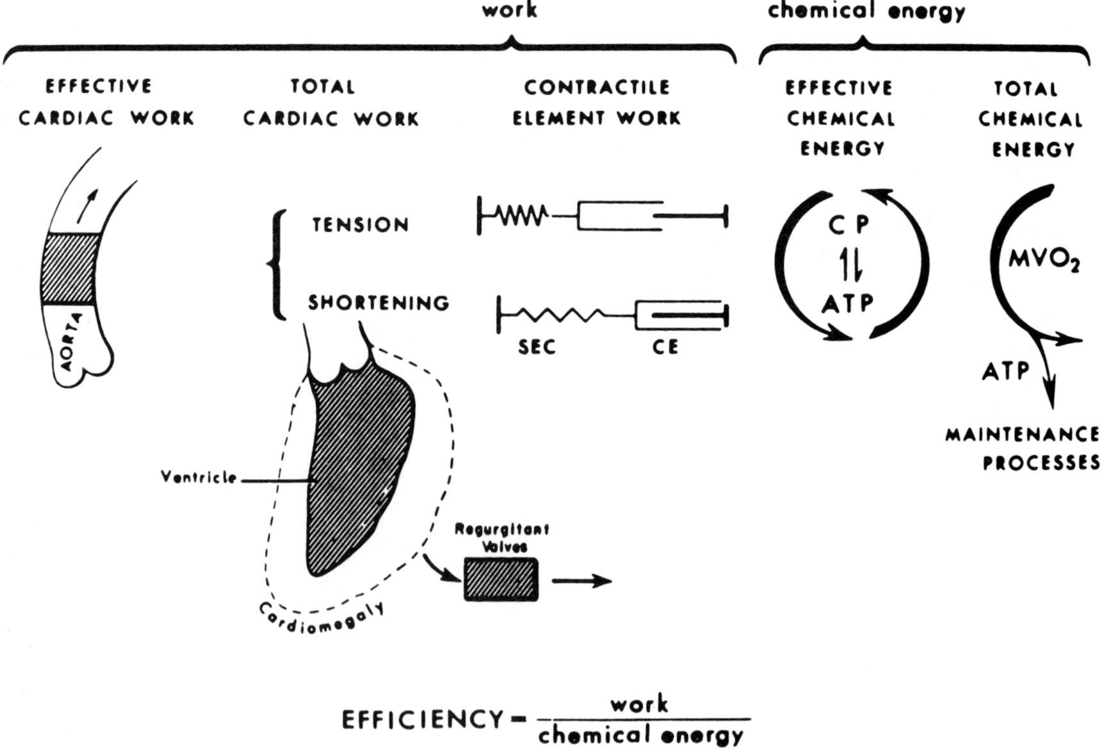

Figure 11.3. Various factors employed to calculate cardiac efficiency. Chemical energy can be taken as total myocardial consumption (MVO_2) or as effective energy used in the contractile process (adenosine triphosphate, ATP, utilization). Work can be considered as merely contractile element (CE) shortening against load or as the total cardiac work (which is a product of volume of blood ejected against pressure). The latter is affected by ventricular geometry, dimensions, and regurgitation of cardiac valves (see text). Effective cardiac work considers only what may be calculated from the stroke volume delivered forward into the great vessels (e.g., aorta) against a given pressure. (Redrawn from Braunwald, Ross, and Sonnenblick 1967, *Mechanisms of Contraction of the Normal and Failing Heart,* Little, Brown, Boston, © 1967.)

This expression of efficiency relates oxygen consumption only to effective cardiac work (Fig. 11.3) and neglects a number of factors linking the chemical and mechanical processes. A closer approximation to true cardiac efficiency, therefore, is the ratio of contractile element work (CEW) to the sum of chemical energy of activation (AE) and chemical energy of work (WE) less resting energy (RE).

$$\text{Eff} = \frac{\text{CEW}}{(\text{AE} + \text{WE}) - \text{RE}}$$

An efficiency of 33 percent was obtained for the anaerobic iodoacetate-treated papillary muscle with the use of this approach. When RE was not subtracted, the efficiency was 23 percent.

Pressure, flow, and resistance

Flow rates and patterns under resting conditions

In *unanesthetized* resting dogs, 37 to 58 ml/min of coronary flow and 4.4 to 8.6 ml/min of oxygen usage per 100 g of myocardium have been reported. Since an important determinant of coronary flow is myocardial work, flow per 100 g of myocardium is less in the right side of the heart (where pressure and, therefore, work are low) than in the left. Flow rates per unit mass to the right ventricle are roughly two-thirds and to the right atria roughly one-half those to the corresponding left chambers. The following values were found in *anesthetized* dogs: coronary flow, 94 ml/min/100 g; mean circulation time from left coronary artery to coronary sinus, 10 seconds; shortest circulation time, 2 seconds; intracoronary blood volume 16 ml/100 g. Increasing coronary flow by 200 percent with coronary dilator drugs increases intracoronary blood volume by 150 percent and decreases mean circulation time by 25 percent. Coronary blood flow rate is affected by five factors: (1) metabolic needs, (2) perfusion pressure, (3) systolic compression, (4) autonomic nervous system, and (5) exogenous drug administration.

Metabolic needs

The single most important factor is metabolic need or oxygen-consumption rate. There exists a linear relationship between myocardial oxygen consumption and coronary flow rate. Myocardial oxygen consumption consists of a basal requirement (20 percent of the total oxygen usage by the heart) for maintenance of chemical processes in the cell, a very small amount (less than 1 percent of the total) for activation of contraction, and the primary requirement (79 percent of the total) for performing work (pumping blood).

The exact mechanism by which myocardial oxygen consumption alters coronary blood flow is not known. Most current theories revolve around the buildup of cell metabolites that cause vasodilatation of precapillary arterioles. An increase in coronary flow will wash out the metabolites, and vasodilatation is limited at that level. The metabolite receiving the most attention is adenosine. Despite evidence that favors the central role of adenosine as one of the chief regulators of coronary blood flow, more recent findings indicate that its importance has been overrated and that it may not be necessary for normal coronary vasomotion. This conclusion was supported by the finding that during autoregulation the concentration of interstitial adenosine did not change and that decreasing interstitial adenosine by 90 percent of its control value by infusion of adenosine deaminase failed to alter autoregulation. Although adenosine's potent pharmacological vasodilator effects are undoubted, its physiological role in regulating coronary flow remains controversial.

The various humoral regulating mechanisms reviewed in Chapter 10 under the headings "Endocrine Control," "Cardiovascular Receptors" and "Neurohumoral Regulating Mechanisms" likewise apply to coronary arterial regulation. Thus the various biogenic vasodilators (e.g., prostaglandin E_2, prostacyclin, bradykinin, histamine, serotonin, atrial natriopeptide, vasoactive intestinal peptide, substance P, adenosine triphosphate, endothelium-derived relaxing factor) and vasoconstrictors (e.g., certain prostaglandins, thromboxane A_2, leukotriene D_4, angiotensin II, vasopressin, neuropeptide Y, endothelin) appear to have as yet incompletely defined actions as mediators or modulators of coronary vasomotion. Some of them are contained in the cytosol of autonomic nerves that run between the adventitia and media of arteries or occur in nerve endings. For example, postganglionic sympathetic nerve terminals contain neuropeptide Y as well as norepinephrine, and postganglionic parasympathetic fibers contain somatostatin and vasoactive intestinal polypeptide as well as acetylcholine. These agents are coreleased after nerve stimulation with the respective classic neurotransmitters (norepinephrine or acetylcholine). Presumably, their release may result in actions on specific receptors, or they may modulate the effects of their accompanying neurotransmitters.

Reactive hyperemia

After the release of a temporary occlusion of a coronary artery, there is an increase in blood flow and oxygen usage that exceeds the supposed deficit that occurred during the period when flow was stopped. This increase is known as reactive hyperemia. If the theoretical blood flow "debt" is estimated as the rate of control flow multiplied by duration of occlusion, the enhanced flow during the period of hyperemia is found to "overpay" greatly the supposed deficit. In contrast, in skeletal muscle the blood flow debt of vascular occlusion is sometimes underpaid and sometimes overpaid by reactive hyperemia (see below). It may be that metabolites accumulating locally while the oxygen tension is low continue to have a vasodilator influence beyond the period of oxygen deficiency.

Perfusion pressure—autoregulation

When coronary perfusion pressure is increased or decreased (Fig. 11.4), flow at first follows suit, but then the resistance changes and flow returns toward the control level. One plausible explanation of these changes in resistance after changes in perfusion pressure is that they are examples of the metabolic type of control just described. Coronary blood flow is kept fairly constant at mean arterial blood pressures between 50 and 130 mm Hg.

Systolic compression

Rhythmic variations in flow

Owing to systolic compression and diastolic release of the coronary vessels, arterial inflow and venous outflow vary rhythmically. Flow curves from an electromagnetic flowmeter are shown in Fig. 11.5. The characteristics of these flow patterns may vary greatly with changes in heart rate and myocardial oxygen demand and under the influence of perturbations such as exercise, excitement, hemorrhagic hypotension, or stellate ganglion stimulation.

Flow during a cardiac cycle

Flow in the *left* coronary artery is abruptly decreased or may be reversed (backflow) at the onset of left ventricular isometric contraction. Then as the aortic pressure rises during ventricular ejection, a forward flow peak occurs and is followed by a decline in flow during late systole. Actually, most of the systolic flow measured in extramural coronary arteries to the left ventricle distends these extramural arteries and is stored there. Beyond this storage area there is little coronary flow to the left ventricle during systole; perhaps only about 5 to 7 percent of the total left ventricular coronary flow reaches terminal intramural arteries during systole. With onset of isometric relaxation, the flow suddenly increases again, peaks during early diastole, and then declines progressively as diastole continues. A late diastolic transient fall in flow may be recorded at about the time of atrial systole, just before the isometric contraction period. Thus, of the total left coronary arterial flow in dogs during the cardiac cycle, 10 to 20 percent occurs in systole and 80 to 90 percent during diastole, but much of the systolic flow does not penetrate the intramural arteries and there is little intramyocardial flow until diastole. In the *right* coronary artery (dog) the flow curve pattern peaks during systole and again during diastole, with a late diastolic decline at the time of atrial systole. In contrast to what happens on the left side, the systolic flow component in the right coronary artery amounts to 30 to 50 percent of the total flow, and flow oscillations remain above the zero flow level. Thus systole inhibits flow less in the right than in the left coronary artery. The compliant extramural coronary arteries become distended during systole with stored blood. As blood pressure falls during diastole, the volume of extramural coronary arteries decreases because of the blood flowing downstream.

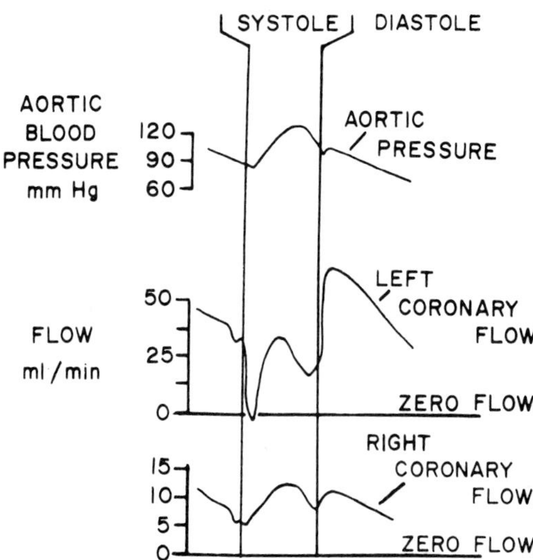

Figure 11.5. Aortic pressure and left and right coronary artery flow curves (dog). Note the relative systolic and diastolic flows in the left and right coronary artery and the flow reversal (i.e., less than zero flow) in the left coronary artery during left ventricular isometric contraction.

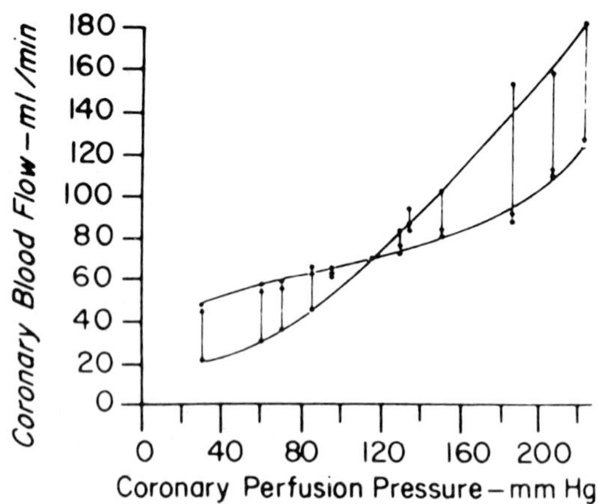

Figure 11.4. Pressure-flow relationships in the coronary vascular bed. The control level of coronary perfusion pressure and flow is at the point where the two lines cross. Abrupt decrease (left of control point) or increase (right of control point) in perfusion pressure changes flow immediately to a new level (any one of the closed circles). Flow returns toward the control level (a corresponding open circle) before becoming fixed at a new steady state (autoregulation of blood flow). (Redrawn from Berne and Levy 1981, *Cardiovascular Physiology,* 4th ed., C.V. Mosby, St. Louis.)

Extravascular pressure and resistance

The intramyocardial compression associated with systole is not uniform across the heart wall; rather, there is a gradient from higher pressures in subendocardium to lower pressures in subepicardium. In the left ventricle, cardiac contraction doubles the resistance in the subendocardial region, whereas it has virtually no effect at the subepicardium. Between these two extremes there is a gradient of resistance increasing from epicardium to endocardium during systole. The transmural distribution of blood flow (i.e., flow determined at four depths in the ventricular free wall from epicardium to endocardium), however, is uniform in the normal heart at rest and during exercise (dog). Despite this seeming equality of transmural distribution of blood flow under physiological conditions, the left ventricular subendocardium and papillary muscles are the most vulnerable sites for myocardial damage from various pathological and toxicological effects, such as coronary vascular disease, sustained tachycardia, hypotensive drugs, cyanotic heart disease, aortic stenosis, severe anemia, and hemorrhagic shock. Although generally accepted at first, the vulnerability of subendocardial tissues to various types of injury being blamed on greater extravascular resistance alone has become more controversial.

The current view regarding greater subendocardial vulnerability to ischemic damage is based on the observation that systole causes reversed coronary flow because the contracting myocardium squeezes blood out of the coronary vessels retrogradely. Because of the greater intramyocardial pressure in the deeper (i.e., subendocardial) muscles, it is thought that more blood is forced out of the deep vessels than out of the superficial vessels. Thus the vascular volume change would be greater in the subendocardial vessels than in the subepicardial vessels. Therefore at the onset of diastole the subendocardial vessels would have greater resistance and capacitance than the more superficial vessels and would require more time to reach adequate flow rates. Under conditions when diastolic pressure is low or diastole is short, the shorter time requirement for attainment of adequate flow in superficial vessels would favor subepicardial over subendocardial flow.

Autonomic nervous system

Both parasympathetic and beta-adrenergic receptor vasodilatation and alpha-adrenergic receptor vasoconstriction are the primary autonomic effects on the coronary arteries, which can be demonstrated under experimental conditions that allow separation of neural and metabolic autoregulatory control. A major part of large coronary artery adrenergic dilation is due to $beta_1$ and $beta_2$ receptor effects. Sympathetic cholinergic vasodilator nerves have not been demonstrated. Resting coronary blood flow is limited by alpha-adrenergic vasoconstrictor tone. This extrinsic neural control of coronary flow is clearly secondary to metabolic control. Neurally mediated reflex coronary vasomotor effects can also be elicited from the carotid sinus and the carotid body. For example, carotid sinus hypotension elicits generalized peripheral sympathetic nerve activation. The resulting coronary vasodilation could be explained by the metabolic needs of the myocardium being increased and by beta-receptor activation. However, beta-receptor blockade reveals that alpha-adrenergic vasoconstriction is also present and limiting the coronary artery's ability to dilate. These neurogenic effects are, at best, weak and evanescent. Vasoconstriction during postganglionic sympathetic nerve stimulation under beta-adrenergic receptor blockade increases coronary resistance only 30 percent (compared to 600 percent in skeletal muscle) and cannot be maintained. Presumably, the increased resistance is soon overcome by vasodilatation induced by tissue hypoxia. Parasympathetic vasodilatation from vagal stimulation also cannot be maintained. It seems that neural control is of little importance in the normal, unstressed heart, although under certain pathophysiological circumstances neural effects might become critical.

Thus the effects of coronary underperfusion on decreasing subendocardial/subepicardial flow ratio are greater when there is alpha-adrenergic blockade, and during exercise in dogs an intact alpha-adrenergic system helps to maintain equal transmural perfusion across the ventricular wall.

Exogenous drug administration

Drugs administered to a patient may affect coronary blood flow. Obviously, catecholamines such as epinephrine and norepinephrine will have predictable effects. Vasodilators (e.g., nitroglycerine) dilate the coronary arteries, and inhalant anesthetics (e.g., isoflurane and halothane) can also dilate the coronary arteries.

CEREBRAL CIRCULATION

The arterial blood supply to the brain reaches the anterior, middle, and posterior cerebral arteries of both sides through a common arterial pathway, the circle of Willis. The completeness of this circle, the arteries that supply it, and the direction of flow in its branches vary in different species. In several species the circle is supplied through the internal carotid arteries and the vertebral arteries via the basilar artery. In many other mammalian species (e.g., cat, sheep, dog, goat) the circle is supplied chiefly through a vascular net (a rete mirabile) that is interposed between the carotid system and the circle. This carotid rete appears to function in temperature regulation of the brain in species subject to high body-heat loads during exercise (e.g., sheep, Thomson's gazelle, eland, oryx).

Brain function is especially vulnerable to heat, and if the brain is kept cool then tolerance to elevated body core temperature is increased. Venous blood in the nasal cavities is cooled evaporatively by panting. When a carotid rete is present it lies in a lake of this venous blood, or if no rete is present the internal carotid artery traverses the cavernous sinus; the arterial blood in both cases is cooled by heat exchange, thus maintaining the brain temperature at 0.4 to 2.7°C below carotid temperature.

Through the circle of Willis there is free communication to the contralateral side of the brain from both the carotid and the vertebral arterial systems (and also between the circle and the extracranial arteries in humans). Thus arterial blood flow can continue to the brain despite occlusion at a single point in the system. Arteriovenous anastomoses are not found.

The capillary walls are of the nonporous type and are separated from direct contact with neuronal cells by neuroglia. This arrangement appears to be the anatomical basis for the diffusion barrier (blood-brain barrier), which allows passage of small molecules (ions, glucose) but prevents passage of many high-molecular-weight substances (e.g., dyes, proteins, organic molecules). Venous drainage is through interconnecting vascular sinuses, and veins are so arranged that blood can flow through the internal jugular venous system or can reach the vertebral venous plexus and external jugular system.

The cerebrospinal fluid (CSF), a thin watery filtrate of the blood plasma, fills the subarachnoid space, its perivascular extensions, the ventricles of the brain, and the central canal of the spinal cord. It serves as a fluid cushion for the central nervous system (CNS) and for fluid volume exchange with the cerebral blood. It is formed chiefly at the choroid plexus (brain tissues, ventricular walls, and subarachnoid pial surfaces also contribute) and flows out of the subarachnoid spaces into the sagittal sinus. Its confining membranes govern passage of certain materials between it and the brain (CSF-brain barrier) and between it and the blood (blood-CSF barrier), depending on the molecular size, charge, and lipid solubility of the materials. CSF pressure, ranging from 80 to 150 mm H_2O, is determined by its rate of formation and absorption. Trauma or space-occupying lesions that interfere with CSF or venous drainage from the brain can increase the CSF pressure, causing such signs as headache, vomiting, papilledema, arterial hypertension, and respiratory depression possibly leading to coma and death.

The presence of alternate vascular inflow and drainage pathways complicates *direct* determination of cerebral blood flow (CBF) with flowmeters. Techniques have been developed, however, for measurement of total venous outflow in dogs through a single contrived conduit. CBF may be estimated *indirectly* by the nitrous oxide method or by an indicator washout technique. The recent use of short-lived radioiostopes (oxygen or metabolic substrates) and positron emission tomography allows the measurement of regional CBF and cerebral metabolic rate (CMR). CBF in experimental mammals averages about 56 ml/min per 100 g of tissue, and cerebral metabolic rate for oxygen ($CMRO_2$) amounts to about 3.0 ml/min per 100 g. The ratio of CBF to CMR is usually maintained at 14 to 18:1 in the normal brain but is dependent on the partial pressure of arterial carbon dioxide (P_aco_2).

Responses to carbon dioxide and oxygen tension

The cerebral vasculature is markedly sensitive to changes in arterial carbon dioxide ($Paco_2$) and oxygen (Pao_2) tension. A normal P_aco_2 is approximately 40 mm Hg, and over the range of 20 to 80 mm Hg there is a linear fourfold increase in CBF (Fig. 11.6) with no change in $CMRO_2$. The mechanism for the altered vascular resistance is probably related to alterations in the hydrogen ion concentration in the extracellular fluid that occurs secondarily to hypercapnia or hypocapnia. The same mechanism may explain the consistent CBF/CMR ratio. The rate of oxygen metabolism affects the production and concentration of carbon dioxide which, in turn, affects vascular tone and blood flow. Under physiological conditions, arterial Pco_2 above 100 mm Hg increases CBF to a maximum of about 100 ml/min per 100 g; decreasing arterial Pco_2 to 20 mm Hg decreases CBF to about 20 ml/min per 100 g. The arterial partial pressure of oxygen (P_ao_2) has little effect on CBF except during extreme hypoxia (Fig. 11.6). The normal P_ao_2 of an animal breathing room air is approximately 100 mm Hg. With hypoxia, CBF changes little until an arterial Po_2 of 50 mm Hg is reached. Between 50 and 25 mm Hg arterial Po_2, the CBF increases markedly to a maximum of about 110 ml/min per 100 g.

Hydrogen, potassium, and bicarbonate ions

The vasodilator effect of increased arterial Pco_2 or decreased arterial Po_2 is mediated by an increase in hydrogen ion concentration. Potassium ions produce cerebral vasodilatation. Focal changes in K^+ concentration presumably act directly on neurons of the cerebral cortex that function to bring about vasodilatation by way of sympathetic nerves carrying impulses from the cortex to pial arteries. Increasing perivascular bicarbonate concentration produces vasoconstriction, which is opposed by elevating K^+ concentration. The interaction of these various ion effects is not

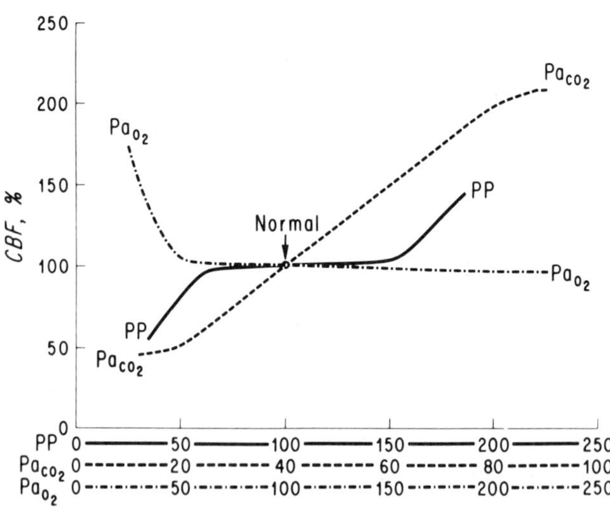

Figure 11.6. The relationship of cerebral blood flow to perfusion pressure (PP), $Paco_2$, and Pao_2. Units on the abscissa are in millimeters of Hg. (From Mitchenfelder 1988, *Anesthesia and the Brain,* Churchill Livingstone, New York, p. 6.)

completely understood. Chronic acidosis increases and chronic alkalosis decreases CBF.

Response to perfusion pressure

CBF is determined by two opposing sets of forces: effective perfusion pressure and cerebral vascular resistance (CVR). *Effective perfusion pressure* is the gradient between mean arterial pressure (MAP) and internal jugular venous pressure (IJP). MAP is affected by cardiac output and total peripheral resistance. CVR is the sum of all factors opposing the flow of blood through the brain, such as intracranial pressure, blood viscosity, and vascular diameter. The latter is affected by structural changes, neurogenic factors, and humoral agents. Cerebral blood flow is determined by the above variables according to the following equation:

$$\mathrm{CBF} = k\,\frac{\mathrm{MAP} - \mathrm{IJP}}{\mathrm{CVR}}$$

where k is a constant.

Elevation of arterial blood pressure or reduction to a mean level of 60 to 70 mm Hg has little effect on CBF, but this autoregulation of flow is abolished below an MAP of 50 mm Hg (Fig. 11.6). Reduction of MAP to 41 mm Hg reduces CBF, O_2 uptake. CO_2 production, and glucose utilization of the brain. Thus, when the MAP falls below about 40 mm Hg, oxidative metabolism of the brain is impaired. In anemia, on the other hand, CBF is increased in proportion to the decreased red cell mass; transfusion produces a return to normal flow.

Neural control

The cerebral vessels receive both sympathetic and parasympathetic fibers. There is little or no tonic *sympathetic* vasoconstriction present, since cerebral blood flow is little affected by sympathectomy or stellate ganglion blockade. Stimulation of the stellate ganglion in dogs, however, produces marked vasoconstriction and reduction in CBF, which are prevented by alpha-adrenergic receptor blockade. Catecholamines injected intra-arterially have little effect on CBF, but local application to pial vessels causes vasoconstriction. This difference between the effects of locally applied and circulating catecholamines suggests that the blood-brain barrier prevents the blood-borne agent from reaching vascular receptors.

Parasympathetic-induced increase in CBF has been demonstrated during stimulation of the distal end of the seventh cranial nerve, brain-stem stimulation, or local application of cholinergic drugs.

Although such autonomic vasoactive effects can be demonstrated experimentally, the role of neural control in CBF regulation has not been established.

Regulation of cerebral blood flow

Cerebral blood flow appears to be controlled principally by the mechanisms of autoregulation mediated mainly by local pH changes, as already mentioned. Neural regulation appears to play only a secondary and modulatory role. Total blood flow to the brain is little affected by general cardiovascular reflexes and hence is remarkably stable under a considerable variety of conditions, such as exercise, intellectual efforts, and anxiety; sleep induces a small increase in CBF. Measurement of regional blood flow in localized areas, however, disclosed a relationship between activity and CBF. When a portion of the brain increases activity, it is accompanied by an appropriate increase in blood flow. A close relationship has been found between local oxygen consumption and blood flow to that same area. The exact mechanism by which activity affects blood flow is not known for certain, but it may involve the production of metabolites, which act as vasodilators.

When, through trauma or disease, CSF pressure increases above about 33 mm Hg, brain ischemia results because of compression of the microvasculature. This creates a rise in tissue P_{CO_2} and a fall in pH, triggering intense stimulation of vasomotor centers. This causes systemic vasoconstriction and arterial hypertension (the Cushing reaction or CNS ischemic response) which, if high enough, will restore blood flow to the brain. Cerebral arterial stretch receptors (baroreceptors) cause reflex vasoconstriction when blood pressure falls. Compression of these arteries by increased intracranial pressure has the same effect on these receptors as a fall in blood pressure and thus may contribute to the Cushing effect.

CUTANEOUS CIRCULATION

Sympathetic adrenergic vasoconstrictor fibers, which are tonically active, innervate the cutaneous vessels. The vascular smooth muscles of cutaneous nutrient arterioles have both alpha- and beta-adrenergic receptors while the arteriovenous anastomoses have only alpha receptors. The physiological importance of cutaneous beta receptors is not known.

The vasodilator nonapeptide, *bradykinin,* was suggested as a mediator of cutaneous vasodilator effects associated with sweat gland activity, but the importance of this mechanism is now considered doubtful.

Body warming elicits a reflex active vasodilatation in addition to a release of vasoconstrictor tone (a decreased number of impulses traveling over the sympathetic nerve fibers). The reflex may originate either in cutaneous receptors or by CNS stimulation. The vessels themselves are also sensitive to warm temperature, for the dilation following blocking of vasomotor nerves can be augmented by local heating.

Arteriovenous anastomoses are communications between smaller arteries and arterioles and the corresponding venous channels, through which the blood may be shunted and capillary areas short-circuited. These arteriovenous anastomoses do not appear to be under metabolic control; rather, they appear to be governed chiefly by reflex influences from temperature receptors and from CNS centers.

Cutaneous veins

In dogs and cats the superficial large and small veins of the skin have a nerve supply, undergo rhythmic changes in diameter, and respond to pharmacological agents. The small veins may contract separately and independently from the large veins or arterial vessels during sympathetic nerve stimulation. When the veins constrict, an increase in pressure results. Thus there may be a reduced blood flow through the vascular bed without any obstruction or constriction of the arterial tree.

Dorsal root vasodilator fibers

The dorsal roots of the spinal cord contain fibers that, on electrical stimulation, produce cutaneous vasodilatation. They are believed to be sensory fibers that, at their peripheral ends, can release a substance that dilates small blood vessels. They do not convey impulses to or from the higher CNS centers for control of the cutaneous circulation. No true cutaneous vasomotor reflexes are seen after sympathectomy. Experiments have shown that the vasodilator fibers of the dorsal root do not engage in the baroreceptor or chemoreceptor control of vascular tone or in the regulation of heat loss from the skin. The transmitter substance of these fibers is not known. They probably act in an axon reflex arrangement to affect regional blood vessels. These are probably the fibers that, on damage to the superficial tissues, are involved in the vasodilator (flare) reaction of the skin. Any stimulus that causes damage to the skin, such as severe cooling and heating, activates these fibers.

Central neural control of cutaneous and muscle blood flow

The central neural control of blood flow is through the sympathetic fibers.

A variety of stimuli affecting peripheral receptors elicits spinal vasomotor reflexes; the efferent limbs are the cutaneous sympathetic vasoconstrictor fibers. These reflexes are usually segmentally or regionally arranged. Distinct from these reflexes, it has been observed that, in certain animal preparations, the preganglionic sympathetic neurons in the lateral horns of the spinal medulla may exhibit spontaneous activity independent of afferent stimuli.

The vasomotor center located in the medulla oblongata is believed to be the primary controlling factor of cutaneous and muscle vasoconstrictor tone. Experiments on dogs and cats have shown that stimulation of the midline of the medulla oblongata leads to vasodilatation in both skin and muscle. This vasodilatory response is not blocked by atropine and, therefore, is secondary to a release of vasoconstrictor tone. Stimulation lateral to this vasodilator area elicits vasoconstriction in the same regions. Both of these responses are absent in animals after sympathectomy. The vasodilator and vasoconstrictor areas may act as an integrated unit and, evidently, are primarily involved in vascular reflexes arising from the baroreceptors in the carotid sinus and aorta. A decrease in blood pressure causes reflex vasoconstriction in the dog hind limb via the carotid sinus baroreceptors, whereas stimulation of the carotid sinus nerve induces vasodilatation in skin and muscle.

Stimulation of an area still more lateral to the vasomotor center invokes a vasodilatation in skeletal muscle through the activity of the cholinergic (blocked by atropine) sympathetic fibers. The more medial vasodilatory area of the vasomotor center per se has no anatomical or apparent functional connection with these cholinergic fibers, which pass through but do not synapse in the medulla oblongata.

The rostral hypothalamus, often referred to as the *heat-loss center,* is thought predominantly to regulate the cutaneous vessels and perhaps the arteriovenous anastomoses. Sympathectomy abolishes these effects of the hypothalamus. Stimulation of certain areas in the hypothalamus may elicit a vasodilatation in muscle via the cholinergic fibers that synapse in this area. This muscle vasodilatation is often associated with a vasoconstriction of the skin.

Stimulation of the motor or premotor cortical areas results in cutaneous vasoconstriction. A muscle vasodilatation also occurs but is evidently secondary to a baroreceptor reflex from a rise in blood pressure.

SKELETAL MUSCLE CIRCULATION

Blood flow rate in resting mammalian skeletal muscle ranges from 2 to 5 ml/min per 100 g in humans to 10 to 20 ml/min per 100 g in cats and rabbits. One reason for this difference is the proportion of red and white fibers in the muscle groups studied, red muscle having about double the resting flow of white muscle. Skeletal muscle in general undergoes very active and widely ranging fluctuations in blood flow.

Neural control of muscle blood flow

Sympathetic vasoconstrictor fibers

Control of muscle blood flow over a wide range is affected by variations in alpha-adrenergic sympathetic tone acting on the resistance vessels. This forms the basis of most reflex regulation of vascular resistance in skeletal muscle. The transmitter substance is norepinephrine, which stimulates alpha receptors in vascular smooth muscle. Maximal stimulation of these fibers doubles vascular resistance in red muscle and increases it sevenfold in white muscle. These fibers also produce venoconstriction. After sympathectomy, muscle blood flow increases transiently and then returns to control values because of intrinsic regulation. During exercise, the effect of alpha-adrenergic stimulation on the arterioles is markedly reduced or abolished by the effects of intrinsic vasodilator mechanisms (see below). Venoconstriction, however, is well maintained. Sympathetic vasoconstrictor fibers are primarily concerned in postural and other reflex, homeostatic, hemodynamic adjustments, in regulation of precapillary to postcapillary resistance, and in changes in the caliber of capacitance vessels (veins). The vasoconstriction evoked by sympathetic fibers is reflexly influenced by arterial baroreceptors, chemoreceptors, and cardiac baroreceptors.

Sympathetic vasodilator fibers

Sympathetic nerve stimulation after alpha-adrenergic blockade produces in skeletal muscle a vasodilation that is blocked by atropine. The transmitter substance is thought to be acetylcholine acting on the gamma receptors. This sympathetic outflow is not activated by the baroreceptors and chemoreceptors mentioned above. It appears to originate in the cerebral cortex via fibers that have connections in the hypothalamus. Such sympathetic vasodilator activity increases in humans during stressful mental activity and vasovagal fainting. A similar sympathetic vasodilatation, blocked by atropine, can be demonstrated in the dog, cat, fox, sheep, and goat but not in primates or the rat. (A homologous vasodilator system, however, not blocked by atropine, has been described in monkeys). This response is transient, and resistance returns to control levels in about 1 minute, despite continued nerve stimulation. This type of active vasodilatation is thought to be part of a centrally integrated neural mechanism that controls cardiovascular adjustments (increased heart rate, blood pressure, and muscle blood flow) in preparation for exercise or the defense reaction.

A *histaminic vasodilator* neural system has been suggested for muscle. Histamine is found in the venous blood during nerve stimulation, and antihistamines block the vasodilatation. Its vasodilator effects, however, are evanescent, histaminergic nerves have not been identified, and histamine can be demonstrated only when adrenergic effects are blocked. The possible functional significance of this postulated system is not understood.

Beta-adrenergic receptors

The effects of circulating catecholamines on muscle blood flow are explained on the basis that both alpha and beta$_2$ receptors exist in vascular smooth muscle. Alpha receptors are innervated by the sympathetic vasoconstrictor nerves and respond to circulating norepinephrine, which has little beta-receptor stimulating activity. Beta$_2$ receptors cause vasodilatation. Epinephrine stimulates both alpha and beta receptors. Since the alpha receptors in muscle have the higher threshold of the two types, the usual effect of physiological amounts of epinephrine is to increase muscle blood flow. Sympathectomy does not abolish the increased flow; thus it is not neurogenic. Intra-arterial injections also cause vasodilatation, but flow rapidly returns to or below the control level. When alpha-adrenergic receptors are blocked pharmacologically, epinephrine produces a sustained increase in blood flow. Thus epinephrine stimulates alpha receptors to cause vasoconstriction and beta$_2$ receptors to cause vasodilatation, and the over-all effect of epinephrine is the sum of these opposing actions.

Intrinsic nerves

After surgical sectioning of nerves, the peripheral ends degenerate and disappear in a few days. Vasomotor responses in such "denervated" organs have been considered to be nonneural. Intact neuronal cell bodies, however, have been found to persist in the adventitia of small arteries and arterioles. By histochemical means, they have been shown to contain norepinephrine or acetylcholinesterase. Indirect evidence indicates that these nerves release peptide transmitters and are involved in local vasodilatation mechanisms. They presumably account in part for exercise vasodilatation.

Local control of resistance vessels in skeletal muscle

The extrinsic neurally mediated changes in muscle blood flow are small in contrast to those caused by local intrinsic mechanisms. The perfused muscle bed exhibits autoregulation, which minimizes changes in flow caused by alterations in perfusion pressure. Autoregulation is present in muscle both at rest and during exercise, and it is not affected by the level of metabolic activity. The hyperemia that accompanies muscle contractions is secondary to local physicochemical changes and intrinsic nerves.

In the dog, muscular activity induces a dilation of the femoral artery, which is mediated by an axon reflex that has cholinergic terminations. This mechanism, if it were shown to be present in the smaller arterial branches, could account for the vasodilatation of exercise. In the cat limb, postexercise muscle hyperemia is blocked by substances (cocaine, botulinum toxin) that are likely to abolish such axon reflexes. The vascular smooth muscle is not paralyzed by these agents, for the vessels continue to respond to epinephrine and acetylcholine. Since botulinum toxin specifically blocks cholinergic nerve endings, the fibers in this reflex may be cholinergic. A strong argument against this theory, however, is that the vasodilatation of exercise hyperemia is not blocked by atropine (although atropine does not block all cholinergic fibers in all areas).

Although the role that local metabolites might play in stimulating such axon reflexes is not known, anoxia, increased carbon dioxide tension, lactic acid, hydrogen ions, bradykinin, histamine, acetylcholine, adenosine triphosphate, adenylic acid, and potassium ions have been suggested as local determinants of exercise vasodilatation. Most of the metabolites have been tested by infusion into the vascular bed of skeletal muscle or by determination of their concentration in venous blood leaving the muscle after exercise hyperemia. Each one has received only a little support as the dilator agent, but a combination of two or more of these factors may provide the answer.

Both nerves and metabolites contribute to vasodilatation in the exercising muscle. (1) Extrinsic alpha-adrenergic vasoconstriction is reduced by local vasodilator effects; (2) sympathetic cholinergic vasodilatation can initiate vasodilatation in anticipation of exercise by carrying impulses from the motor cortex; (3) when muscle contraction starts, the intrinsic vasodilator nerves that are independent of the CNS rapidly cause and sustain vasodilatation; (4) circulating epinephrine stimulates beta-adrenergic vasodilator receptors; and (5) metabolites accumulate and maintain vasodilatation until the oxygen debt is repaid.

Reactive hyperemia

After a period of complete occlusion of the arterial supply to a limb, the blood flow at first increases markedly and then later returns to the control level. This phenomenon has been named *reactive hyperemia*. The response occurs in both skin and muscle and can be decreased in the skin by cooling, increased levels of epinephrine, or, in humans, tobacco smoking. The amount and duration of reactive hyperemia correlate with the previous length of arterial occlusion. This has been shown to be true for occlusion periods up to 10 minutes.

The blood flow or the oxygen debt incurred during the period of occlusion can be calculated when the control blood flow or the oxygen usage before circulatory arrest is multiplied by the duration of occlusion. In isolated gracilis muscle of the dog, as well as in the human forearm, the oxygen debt is approximately repaid for different periods of occlusion, but the blood-flow debt repayment ranges anywhere from 50 to 200 percent of that expected. This is what happened when the muscles are at rest. The phenomenon of reactive hyperemia has also been demonstrated in the dog hind limb during exercise. Flow debts then are underpaid or barely repaid. Oxygen debts are entirely or partially repaid, depending on the level of muscle performance and the duration of the ischemic period.

In resting muscle and during light exercise, both increased blood flow and oxygen extraction are involved in repayment of the oxygen debts, but during medium and strong exercise the increased blood flow is most important. Since during strong exercise oxygen debts are often not repaid in the presence of a *decreased* arteriovenous oxygen difference, oxygen extraction is the limiting factor.

It has been postulated the metabolites believed to cause exercise hyperemia also elicit reactive hyperemia. Since reactive hyperemia occurs in sympathectomized and denervated limbs, nervous system control is considered to be unimportant.

SPLANCHNIC CIRCULATION

The splanchnic circulation may be represented as consisting of three parts: (1) the mesenteric bed, supplying the gastrointestinal tract; (2) the splenic bed; and (3) the hepatic bed.

A unique feature of this circulatory system is that the combined outflow from two of the components (mesenteric and splenic) constitutes the major portion of the inflow of the third one (hepatic) through the portal vein. In its hemodynamic implications, this anatomical arrangement has been compared to the Wheatstone bridge in an electrical circuit because of the placement of the resistance vessels (Fig. 11.7). This serves mainly to emphasize the large number of variables that influence blood pressure and flow in any one point of the system and to illustrate the potential fallacy of conclusions based on measurements of a single variable, such as portal venous pressure.

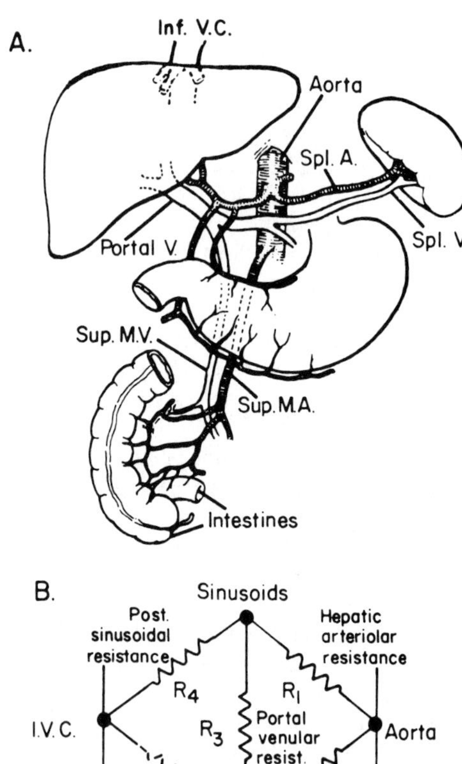

Figure 11.7. The splanchnic circuits. The vascular resistances in the splanchnic bed (*A*) are shown here in diagrammatic form (*B*). The resistances indicated are determinants of pressures in the portal vein and in the liver sinusoids and of flows through the portal vein and hepatic artery. R_1, hepatic arteriolar resistance; R_2, splanchnic (i.e., mesenteric, pancreatic, gastric, and splenic) arteriolar resistance; R_3, portal venular resistance; R_4, postsinusoidal or hepatic venular resistance. The dotted line represents a fifth resistance lying in the direct communications between the portal vein and inferior venae cavae. Inf. V.C., inferior venae cavae; Spl. A., splenic artery; Spl. V, splenic vein; Sup. M.V., superior mesenteric vein; Sup. M.A., superior mesenteric artery. (From Bradley 1958, in McMichael, ed., *Circulation,* Blackwell, Oxford.)

All of the splanchnic flow eventually reaches the liver. Perhaps 70 percent arrives there via the portal vein from the stomach, intestines, spleen, and pancreas; the remaining 30 percent comes via the hepatic artery. Together these fractions constitute the splanchnic flow, the hepatic blood flow, and the total flow through the hepatic veins.

Although autoregulation is not as pronounced in the gut as in other organs, three mechanisms operate to regulate blood flow at the local level: (1) enhanced metabolism of parenchymal cells of the villi lowers tissue Po_2 and increases vasodilator metabolites, relaxing arteriolar smooth muscle and precapillary sphincters to increase mucosal blood flow; (2) increased muscle activity, similarly, metabolically produces active hyperemia of the muscularis mucosae; and (3) intrinsic myogenic response to stretch (the Bayliss mechanism) (see Chap. 10) autoregulates blood flow when blood pressure fluctuates. Added to these effects, muscle contractions modify blood flow by causing extravascular compression. The absorptive process interacts with these local mechanisms through several phenomena, such as countercurrent exchange, washout of absorbed substances, and passive effects of Starling forces. Knowledge of the interplay of these various factors does not permit a simple description at present.

Neural control

The function of vasomotor nerves has been discussed in detail in Chapter 10. Electrical stimulation of the splanchnic nerves in anesthetized dogs produces sharp decline in blood flow in the mesenteric artery and increases both the arterial and the portal venous pressures, indicating that vasoconstriction has occurred. Intra-arterially injected norepinephrine reproduces the effect of splanchnic nerve stimulation, and sectioning of the nerves or administration of ganglionic blocking agents increases mesenteric flow. There is no evidence of the existence of vasodilator fibers in the splanchnic nerves. Stimulation of the vagi (parasympathetic supply) to the stomach and lower colon increases blood flow secondary to increased motility and glandular secretion. Colonic blood flow is not directly affected by vagal stimulation, but pelvic nerve stimulation produces transient intense hyperemia and prolonged increase in rhythmic flow.

Vasomotor reactions in the mesenteric circuit are of considerable importance in various circulatory adjustments. Not all of this vasomotor activity, however, is necessarily mediated by the nervous system. In the dog, experimental elevation of the portal venous pressure reduces the mesenteric blood flow to a degree that is greater than the decrease in mesenteric artery–portal vein pressure gradient. This indicates that mesenteric vascular resistance has increased. This change in resistance is shown to be independent from nervous activity and due to "myogenic" response of the arterioles to the pressure increase transmitted through the capillaries. It is not known what role, if any, this venous-arteriolar response plays in the intact animal.

Rumen blood flow

Feeding and the products of rumen digestion, carbon dioxide and volatile fatty acids, increase rumen blood flow. The effects of these chemical mediators appear to be independent of increases in rumen motility and content.

A major emergency function of the sympathetic vasoconstriction is a sustained decrease in the capacity of intestinal and mesenteric veins. This function facilitates mobilization of large amounts of blood into other more critical circulatory beds and thereby helps sustain blood pressure under stress conditions such as hyperthermia, exercise, and circulatory shock.

SPLENIC CIRCULATION

The nature of the intrasplenic circulation has long been controversial, especially the manner of connection between arterial and venous capillaries. It is uncertain whether their lumina are continuous with one another to form a *closed circulation,* or whether arterial blood is discharged into the meshwork of the splenic pulp per se, from which it later seeps back into the venous capillaries in an *open circulation.* The possibility of discontinuity between arterioles and venules is suggested by microscopic evidence that blood cells and intra-arterially injected foreign materials can be found within the splenic pulp. Advocates of the closed system, however, view these as artifacts of histological techniques. Microscopic transillumination studies in living animals indicated that both open and closed patterns of circulation may function simultaneously; this has been called a *combined circulatory pattern.* When studied with a scanning electron microscope, the cordal spaces in the splenic pulp seem to represent a special variety of enclosed vascular space through which blood moves from arterial vessel to venous sinus. However, no permanent physical connection comparable to capillaries or sinusoids has been found. Pressure-flow relationships in the dog spleen during artificial perfusion show a continuous drop in resistance with increasing pressure; there is no plateau even at high pressure and flow rates. This great distensibility is probably due to the opening of vascular sinuses.

In certain mammals (dog, cat, horse, guinea pig) the spleen serves as a reservoir of blood. Under ordinary circumstances, blood is stored in the distensible venous sinuses, to be released into the circulation when the need arises (as during exercise, anoxia, hemorrhage). This splenic emptying mechanism is under sympathetic regulation. Stimulation of splenic nerve fibers in the dog results in simultaneous decrease in arterial inflow, increase in venous outflow, and decrease in splenic weight. The inflow response can be reproduced by intra-arterial norepinephrine injection, and the outflow response can best be reproduced by injection of epinephrine. This suggests the existence of separate mechanisms for the control of splenic inflow and outflow: a norepinephrine-mediated arteriolar inflow constriction and an epinephrine-mediated emptying. This latter might be due either to venular relaxation causing passive elastic recoil of splenic tissues or to primary contraction of splenic smooth muscle fibers.

HEPATIC CIRCULATION

The dual hepatic blood supply from the hepatic artery and portal vein is governed by (1) hepatic arterial vascular resistance; (2) the arterial tone in the vascular beds of the gastrointestinal tract, pancreas, and the spleen; and (3) the intrahepatic portal venous vascular resistance. The total hepatic blood flow in humans, cats, and dogs averages 100 to 130 ml/min per 100 g, which represents about 25% of the cardiac output. The portal vein contributes about 70 to 75% of the total hepatic blood flow. Connections occur presinusoidally between the arterial and portal systems so that circulating vasoactive substances entering the portal vein will also reach the arterial system and vice versa. Sympathetic nerve stimulation increases hepatic arterial and portal venous tone. Since the liver, like the gut, is a major blood reservoir, sympathetic stimulation can rapidly mobilize substantial amounts of blood for redistribution to vital circulatory beds under stress conditions. Epinephrine infusions decrease hepatic artery flow and total hepatic blood volume. The hepatic vasculature contains both alpha- and beta-adrenergic receptors.

The hepatic arterial vascular bed exhibits relatively weak local control of its blood flow through both myogenic and metabolic types of autoregulation. The portal system lacks such intrinsic local control mechanisms. A partial reciprocity between the hepatic artery and the portal vein helps maintain total liver blood flow constant. Vasopressin has three effects on the liver circulation: (1) hepatic arterial constriction; (2) mesenteric vasoconstriction, and (3) dilator action on intrahepatic portal resistance vessels. Angiotensin II causes marked vasoconstriction of both hepatic arterial and portal beds. Neither of these effects ordinarily appears to be of physiological significance except possibly under conditions of extreme stress, such as circulatory shock.

Hepatic lymph and ascitic fluid

The liver produces large quantities of lymph with a high protein content. The principal site of formation is the liver sinusoids, where hydrostatic pressure is low but endothelial permeability to fluids and serum proteins is high. Increased resistance in postsinusoidal vessels, as occurs in congestive heart failure, increases the rate of lymph formation; the lymphatic drainage system is overwhelmed, and fluid escapes through the liver capsule into the peritoneal cavity. In quadrupeds this is the site most prone to the accumulation of excess fluid in congestive heart failure, and ascitic fluid often increases before edema in the limbs appears.

RENAL CIRCULATION

Renal circulation is discussed in Chapter 31.

FETAL AND NEONATAL CIRCULATION

In the fetus, the left and right halves of the heart act essentially as parallel pumps, discharging blood into the systemic and placental circuits (Fig. 11.8). Blood from the right side of the heart largely bypasses the lung circulation by flowing through the ductus arteriosus into the aorta. In contrast, the two sides of the heart in the adult pump chiefly in series; blood passes sequentially through the right side of the heart and the pulmonary circulation and then to the left side of the heart and the systemic circulation. It is only after birth that a large pressure differential develops between the pulmonary and systemic arterial systems. Consequent to this, the relative work load (pressure times volume) of the left side of the heart is increased greatly over that of the right. This difference is reflected in the relative masses of the adult left and right ventricles (about 2:1). The transition from fetal to adult circulatory patterns is accomplished by

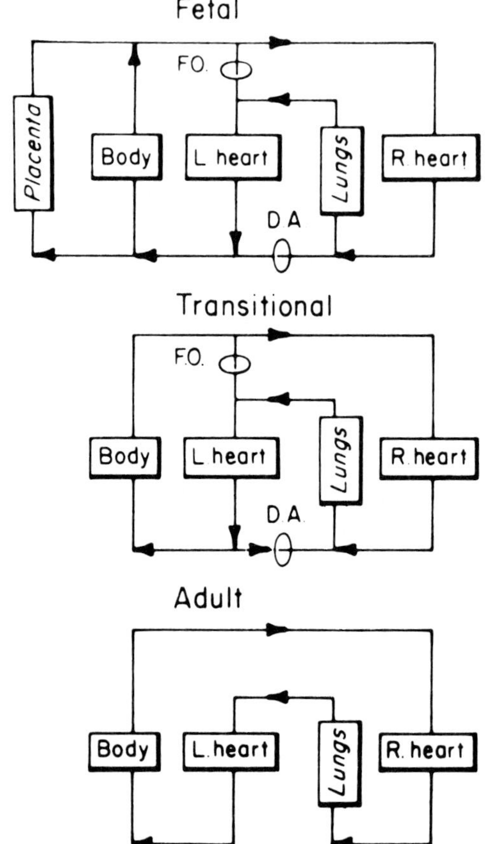

Figure 11.8. The fetal, transitional (neonatal), and adult types of circulation. F.O., foramen ovale; D.A., ductus arteriosus. (Redrawn from Dawes 1968, *Foetal and Neonatal Physiology,* Year Book, Chicago, copyright © 1968 by Year Book Medical Publishers, Inc., as modified from Born, Dawes, Mott, and Widdicombe 1954, *Symp. Quant. Biol.* 19:102–7.)

functional and anatomical closure of fetal flow paths (ductus arteriosus, foramen ovale, ductus venosus), expansion of the pulmonary circuit with expansion of the lungs, and interruption of the placental circulation. Failure of closure of ductus arteriosus or foramen ovale is a frequent congenital cardiac defect with hemodynamic consequences proportional to their degree of ultimate patency. A functional closure of these fetal bypass routes is almost complete in the early neonatal period, but anatomical closure requires weeks, months, or longer.

Circulation in the fetus

The placenta serves as the "fetal lung" and access port to the maternal circulation for uptake of nutritional substances and excretion of metabolic wastes. The major circulatory circuitry of the fetus is diagrammed in Fig. 11.8.

Most studies of the physiology of the fetal and neonatal circulation have been carried out on sheep and goats. Results and interpretations reported in the literature contain unresolved differences in certain details.

In the fetus, the combined output of the left and right ventricles is about equally divided between the placenta and fetal membranes and the body of the fetus itself. These two circulations are arranged in parallel (Fig. 11.8), and the following percentage distributions of flow have been calculated from data on lambs: placenta and fetal membranes, 57 percent; fetal lungs, 10 percent; foreparts of the body, 15 percent; hind parts of the body, 18 percent.

The blood circulating through the placenta enters with an oxygen saturation of about 58 percent and returns in the umbilical veins 80 percent saturated (contrasted with 98 percent oxygen saturation of maternal arterial blood). The fetal ductus venosus carries some of this blood, bypassing the liver, directly into the inferior vena cava, where it joins blood from the lower trunk and extremities (26 percent saturated) and from the liver.

Anatomically, the foramen ovale opens directly off the posterior vena cava so as to favor a flow of blood into the left atrium. There is evidence that the edge of the interarterial septum, the *crista dividens,* divides the posterior vena cava blood into two unequal streams. According to this view, the larger stream is composed mainly of umbilical vein blood and is shunted through the foramen ovale into the left atrium. The smaller stream mixes in the right atrium with anterior vena cava blood from the upper body and with blood from the heart. This less saturated blood largely passes into the right ventricle and is pumped out the pulmonary artery. Pulmonary arterial resistance is relatively high, the pressure being about 5 mm Hg above that in the aorta; consequently, more than two-thirds of the right ventricular output flows through the ductus arteriosus into the aorta. Entering the aorta at a point distal to the origins of the arteries to the head and upper limbs, this blood is thus directed to the posterior body and umbilical arteries. The larger stream of highly oxygenated blood from the foramen ovale and the blood entering the left atrium from the pulmonary veins mix and are pumped out of the left ventricle into the ascending aorta. About one-third of this blood reaches the arteries that supply the upper extremities and head. The more this separation of anterior and posterior caval flow takes place, the greater will be the oxygen saturation of the blood reaching the upper body and brain. Nevertheless, a difference in percentage of oxygen saturation of carotid and descending aortic blood is not always found experimentally, and fetuses with cardiac malformations that prevent such separation survive to term.

Fetal hemoglobin has a greater affinity for oxygen than adult hemoglobin, so that at equal oxygen tension fetal blood carries more oxygen than maternal blood. Also, fetal tissues are more resistant to hypoxia than are adult tissues. The fetal heart can function without oxygen for longer periods than the adult heart because these myocardial cells contain relatively large amounts of glycogen (an anaerobic energy source) throughout gestation. These two factors make possible an adequate oxygen supply to fetal tissues, despite a relatively low oxygen tension in blood leaving the placenta.

Changes at birth

With separation from the placental circulation, the peripheral resistance rises and asphyxia develops in the infant. The pressure in the aorta rises, and gasping respiratory movements expand the lungs. Constriction of the muscular umbilical veins squeezes up to 100 ml of blood into the fetal veins (so-called placental transfusion), and ventilatory movements aid venous return. With lung expansion, pulmonary blood flow increases as pulmonary vascular resistance falls below one-fifth of the in utero value. Pulmonary venous return to the left atrium increases left atrial pressure over right atrial pressure, and the valve of the foramen ovale is closed. In response to the increased oxygen tension in blood flowing through the ductus arteriosus, the smooth muscle constricts and the ductus is narrowed. Fetal Po_2 is about 20 mm Hg, and when the blood Po_2 reaches 50 to 60 mm Hg ductus blood flow continues to decrease. Aortic pressure now exceeds pulmonic artery pressure, and flow through the ductus arteriosus is reversed. This is the transitional (neonatal) state of the circulatory system. Functional closure of the ductus is complete within 1 or 2 days after birth. Prostaglandins can reopen the closing duct, and the prostaglandin synthetase inhibitor indomethacin contracts the duct. The murmur of patent ductus arteriosus can be heard in newborn animals varying in size from puppies to foals; in the normal lamb, calf, and foal it may be heard for several hours to several days after birth. Anatomical closure of the foramen ovale and ductus arteriosus may take several weeks. Normally, however, there is little flow through these channels after the first few days. With complete closure the adult separation of pulmonary and systemic vascular systems is accomplished (Fig. 11.8). The only shunt remaining in the adult is that through the bronchial artery and capillary system, from which a small amount of blood returns to the left side of the heart via pulmonary veins without having gone through the right side of the heart.

Summary

Fetal circulation is especially arranged to meet the needs of a rapidly growing organism living in a state of relative hypoxia. These requirements include high cardiac output, partial bypass of the lung circulation, and high placental blood flow. At birth, the fetus abruptly becomes an air breather, hypoxia disappears, blood-gas exchange occurs in the lungs, and the large placental flow is abolished. As a result, the cardiac output is reduced, pulmonary artery pressure drastically declines, and the two sides of the heart function serially rather than in parallel. Blood oxygen tension is the chief determinant of the pattern of fetal blood flow distribution and the changes in this distribution that occur at birth.

The ductus arteriosus permits up to 70 percent of the right ventricular output to enter the aorta and thus provides a major source of blood, which flows to the posterior fetal body and placenta. Because of the parallel arrangement of left and right ventricles in the fetus, both contribute to the high systemic flow required for the fetus and the placenta.

Blood flow to the lungs is minimal because of the differential effect of low oxygen tension on lung vessels and ductus arteriosus. Hypoxemia dilates the latter and constricts the former, thus favoring flow away from the collapsed fetal lungs where peripheral resistance is high and toward the aorta (and placenta) where peripheral resistance is low. At birth, the reciprocal effect of increased oxygen tension on ductus arteriosus and lung vessels results in constriction of the former and dilatation of the latter; pulmonary vascular resistance also decreases as a result of expansion of the lungs with the onset of breathing. Interruption of the placental circulation increases peripheral resistance in the systemic circuit. Thus pulmonary peripheral resistance and pulmonary arterial pressure decrease; systemic arterial peripheral resistance and pressure increase; shunting of blood from pulmonary artery to aorta through the ductus arteriosus is first curtailed, then reversed, and finally ceases; and cardiac output decreases.

The function of the foramen ovale is to shunt highly oxygenated blood to the left ventricle, aorta, and head and also to supply blood to the left ventricle, ensuring that it works mechanically and develops adequately to accommodate the abrupt increase in work load at birth.

The function of the ductus venosus is uncertain, and this structure is absent or disappears early in fetal life in certain species (horse, pig). The concept that it supplies a route for direct return of highly oxygenated umbilical venous blood, unmixed with fetal venous blood, is not supported by recent studies.

REFERENCES

Ahmed, S.H., El-Rakhawy, M.T., Abdalla, A., and Harrison, R.G. 1972. A new conception of coronary artery preponderance. *Acta Anat.* 83:87–94.

Assali, N.S., ed. 1968. *Biology of Gestation,* vol. 2. Academic Press, New York.

Assali, N.S., Bekey, G.A., and Morrison, L.W. 1968. Fetal and neonatal circulation. In N.S. Assali, ed., *Biology of Gestation,* vol. 2. Academic Press, New York, 51–142.

Baker, M.A. 1982. Brain cooling in endotherms in heat and exercise. *Ann. Rev. Physiol.* 44:85–96.

Barry, A., and Patten, B.M. 1968. The structure of the adult heart. In S.E. Gould, ed., *Pathology of the Heart,* 3d ed. Charles C. Thomas, Springfield, Ill. Pp. 91-130.

Beck, L., Pollard, A.A., Kayaaip, S.O., and Weiner, L.M. 1966. Sustained vasodilation elicited by sympathetic nerve stimulation. *Fed. Proc.* 25:1596–1606.

Berne, R.M., and Levy, M.N. 1967. *Cardiovascular Physiology.* C.V. Mosby, St. Louis.

Berne, R.M., and Rubio, R. 1979. Coronary circulation in R.M. Berne, N. Sperelakis, and I.R. Geiger, eds., *Handbook of Physiology.* Sec. 2, The Cardiovascular System. Vol. 1, *The Heart,* Am. Physiol. Soc., Bethesda, Md. Pp. 873-952.

Blum, R.L., Alpern, H., Jaffe, H., Lang, T.W., and Corday, E. 1970. Determination of interarterial coronary anastomosis by radioactive spherules: Effect on coronary occlusion and hypoxemia. *Am. Heart J.* 79:244–49.

Bourdeau-Martini, J., and Honig, C.R. 1973. Control of coronary intercapillary distance: Effect of arterial Pco_2 and pH. *Microvasc. Res.* 6:286–96.

Bradley, S.E. 1958. Methods for the evaluation of the splanchnic circulation. In J. McMichael, ed., *Circulation.* Proceedings of the Harvey Tercentenary Congress. Blackwell, Oxford. P. 355.

Braunwald. E. 1971. Control of myocardial oxygen consumption. *Am. J. Cardiol.* 27:416–32.

Brody, M.J. 1966. Neurohumoral mediation of active reflex vasodilation. *Fed. Proc.* 25:1483–1592.

Chou, C.C. 1972. Relationship between intestinal blood flow and motility. *Ann Rev. Physiol.* 44:29–42.

Chou, C.C., and Gallavan, R.H. 1982. Blood flow and intestinal motility. *Fed. Proc.* 41:2090–95.

Colborn, G.L. 1966. The gross morphology of the coronary arteries of the common squirrel monkey. *Anat. Rec.* 155:353–68.

D'Alecy, L.G. 1973. Sympathetic cerebral vasoconstriction blocked by adrenergic alpha receptor antagonists. *Stroke* 4:30–37.

D'Alecy, L.G., and Feigl, E.O. 1972. Sympathetic control of cerebral blood flow in dogs. *Circ. Res.* 31:267–83.

Dawes, G.S. 1968. *Foetal and Neonatal Physiology: A Comparative Study of the Changes at Birth.* Year Book. Chicago.

Deal, C.P., Jr., and Green, H.D. 1956. Comparison of changes in mesenteric resistance following splanchnic nerve stimulation with responses to epinephrine and norepinephrine. *Circ. Res.* 4:38–44.

Detweiler, D.K. 1989. Spontaneous and induced arterial disease in the dog: Pathology and pathogenesis. *Toxicol. Pathol.* 17:94–108.

Domenech, R.J., Hoffman, J.I.E., Noble, M.I.H.,. Saunders, D.B., Henson, J.R., and Sbijanto, S. 1969. Total and regional coronary blood flow measured by radioactive microspheres in conscious and unanesthetized dogs. *Circ. Res.* 25:581–96.

Downey, J.M. 1989. Extrasvascular coronary resistance. In N. Sperelakis, ed., *Physiology and Pathophysiology of the Heart,* 2d ed. Kluiver Publishing, Boston. Pp. 939–53.

Feigl, E.O. 1967. Sympathetic control of coronary circulation. *Circ. Res.* 20:262–71.

Feigl, E.O. 1969. Parasympathetic control of coronary blood flow in dogs. *Circ. Res.* 25:509–19.

Gregg, D.E. 1967. Introduction. In G. Marchette and B. Taccardi, eds., *Coronary Circulation and Energetics of the Myocardium.* Karger, New York. Pp. xiii–xv.

Gregg, D.E., Khouri, E.M., and Rayford, C.R. 1965. Systemic and coronary energetics in the resting unanesthetized dog. *Circ. Res.* 16:102–13.

Hadžiselimović, H., Šećerov, D., and Gmaz-Ni-Kulin, E. 1974. Comparative anatomical investigations on coronary arteries in wild and domestic animals. *Acta Anat.* 90:16–35.

Hammond, G.L., Juca, E.R., and Austen, W.G. 1969. The nature of intercoronary arterial flow. *Am. Heart J.* 78:559–68.

Heistad, D.P., and Kontos, H.A. 1983. Cerebral circulation. In J.T. Shepherd and F.M. Abboud, eds., *Handbook of Physiology.* Sec. 3, vol. 3, *Peripheral Circulation and Organ Blood Flow, Part 1.* Am. Physiol. Soc., Bethesda, Md.

Hoffman, S.I.E. 1990. Coronary physiology. In O.B. Garfein ed., *Current Concepts in Cardiovascular Physiology.* Academic Press, New York. Pp. 289–349.

Honig, C.R. 1981. *Modern Cardiovascular Physiology.* Little, Brown, Boston.

Jacobsen, E.D. 1982. Gastrointestinal physiology. *Ann. Rev. Physiol.* 44:1–2.

Janse, M.J., and Wilms-Schopman, F. 1982. Effect of changes in perfusion pressure on the position of the electrophysiologic border zone in acute regional ischemia in isolated perfused dog and pig hearts. *Am. J. Cardiol.* 50:74–82.

Johnson, P.C. 1959. Myogenic nature of increase in intestinal vascular resistance with venous pressure elevation. *Circ. Res.* 7:992–99.

Kaltenbach, M., and Spahn, F. 1975. Koronargraphische Nomenclatur und Typologie der Koronararterien des Menschen. *Z. Kardiol.* 64:193–202.

Kety, S.S. 1958. Physiology of the cerebral circulation in man. In J. McMichael, ed., *Circulation (Proc. Harvey Terc. Congress).* Blackwell, Oxford. Pp. 324–40.

Kety, S.S. 1963. Circulation and energy metabolism of the brain. *Clin. Neurosurg.* 9:56–66.

Kety, S.S., and Schmidt, C.F. 1948. The nitrous oxide method for the quantitative determination of cerebral blood flow in man: Theory, procedure and normal values. *J. Clin. Invest.* 27:476–83.

Kirk, E.S., Wischel, C.W., and Sonnenblick, E.H. 1974. Problems in cardiac performance: Regulation of coronary blood flow and the physiology of heart failure. In A.C. Guyton and C.E. Jones, eds., *Cardiovascular Physiology.* University Park Press, Baltimore. Pp. 299–334.

Klocke, F.J., Braunwald, E., and Ross, J., Jr. 1966. Oxygen cost of electrical activation of the heart. *Circ. Res.* 18:357–65.

Klocke, F.J., Kaiser, G.A., Ross, J., Jr., and Braunwald, E. 1965. Mechanism of increase of myocardial oxygen uptake produced by catecholamines. *Am. J. Physiol.* 209:913–18.

Korner, P.I. 1974. Control of blood flow to special vascular areas: Brain, kidney, muscle, skin, liver, and intestine. In A.C. Guyton and C.E. Jones, eds., *Cardiovascular Physiology.* University Park Press, Baltimore. Pp. 123–62.

Kvietys, P.R., and Granger, D.N. 1982. Regulation of colonic blood flow. *Fed. Proc.* 41:2106–10.

Langfitt, T.W., and Kassell, N.F. 1968. Cerebral vasodilatation produced by brain stem stimulation: Neurogenic control vs. autoregulation. *Am. J. Physiol.* 215:90–97.

Lochner, W. 1971. Herz. In E. Bauereisen, ed., *Physiologie des Kreislaufs,* vol. 1 Springer Verlag, New York. Pp. 184–228.

Mellander, S., and Johansson, B. 1968. Control of resistance, exchanges, and capacitance functions in the peripheral circulation. *Pharmacol. Rev.* 20:117–96.

Michenfelder, J.D. 1988. *Anesthesia and the Brain.* Churchill Livingstone, New York. Pp. 3–21.

Miller, A.J. 1982. *Lymphatics of the Heart.* Raven Press, New York.

Moir, T.W., Eckstein, W., and Driscol, T.E. 1963. Thebesian drainage of the septal artery. *Circ. Res.* 12:212–19.

Öberg, B. 1976. Overall cardiovascular regulation. *Ann. Rev. Physiol.* 38:537–70.

Pasyk, S., Schaper, W., Schaper, J., Pasyk, K., Miskiewicz, G., and Steinseifer, B. 1982. DNA synthesis in coronary collaterals after coronary artery occlusion in conscious dog. *Am. J. Physiol.* 242:H1031–H1037.

Pitt, A., Friesinger, G.C., and Ross, R.S. 1969. Measurement of blood flow in the right and left coronary artery beds in humans and dogs using the ^{133}xenon technique. *Cardiovasc. Res.* 3:100–106.

Renkin, E.M. 1967. Blood flow and transcapillary exchange in skeletal and cardiac muscle. In G. Marchetti and B. Taccardi, eds., *International Symposium on Coronary Circulation and Energetics of Myocardium.* Karger, Basel. Pp. 18–30.

Richardson, P.D.I., and Withrington, P.G. 1972. Physiological regulation of the hepatic circulation. *Ann. Rev. Physiol.* 44:57–69.

Rudolph, A.M. 1985. Distribution and regulation of blood flow in the fetal and neonatal lamb. *Circ. Res.* 57:811–21.

Salanga, V.D., and Waltz, A.G. 1973. Regional cerebral blood flow during stimulation of seventh cranial nerve. *Stroke* 4:213–17.

Schaper, W. 1970. The physiology of the collateral circulation in the normal and hypoxic myocardium. *Ergeb. Physiol.* 63:102–45.

Schaper, W. 1971. *The Collateral Circulation of the Heart.* Elsevier, New York. P. 176.

Schaper, W. 1982. Collateral anatomy and blood flow: Its potential role in sudden coronary death. *Ann. N.Y. Acad. Sci.* 382:69–74.

Schramm, L.P., Honig, C.R., and Bignall, K.E. 1971. Active muscle vasodilation in primates homologous with sympathetic vasodilation in carnivores. *Am. J. Physiol.* 221:768–77.

Selkurt, E.E., and Johnson, P.C. 1958. Effect of acute elevation of portal venous pressure on mesenteric blood volume, interstitial fluid volume and hemodynamics. *Circ. Res.* 6:592–99.

Sellers, A.F. 1965. Blood flow in rumen vessels. In R.W. Dougherty, R.S. Allen, W. Burroughs, N.L. Jacobson, and A.D. McGilliard, eds., *Physiology of Digestion in the Ruminant.* Butterworths, Washington. Pp. 171–84.

Shepherd, A.P. 1982. Local control of intestinal oxygenation and blood flow. *Ann. Rev. Physiol.* 44:13-27.

Shepherd, J.T. 1963. *Physiology of the Circulation in Human Limbs in Health and Disease.* W.B. Saunders, Philadelphia.

Solez, K., and Heptinstall, R.H. 1980. The anatomy of the renal circulation. The renal circulation: Physiology and hormonal control. In W. Schwartz, N.T., Werthessen, and S. Wolf, *Structure and Function of the Circulation,* vol. 1, Plenum, New York. 631-727.

Sparks, H.V., Jr. 1980. Effect of local metabolic factors on vascular smooth muscle. In D.F. Bohr, A.P. Somlyo, and H.V. Sparks, Jr., eds., *Handbook of Physiology.* Sec 2, The Cardiovascular System. Vol. 2, *Vascular Smooth Muscle.* Am. Physiol. Soc., Bethesda, Md. Pp. 475–513.

Tranquilli, W.J., Parks, C.M., Thurmon, J.C., Benson, G.J., Koritz, G.E., Manohar, M., and Theodorakis, M.C. 1982. Organ blood flow and distribution of cardiac output in nonanesthetized swine. *Am. J. Vet. Res.* 43:895–97.

Vatner, S.F., Hintze, T.H., and Macho, P. 1982. Regulation of large coronary arteries by (beta)-adrenergic mechanisms in the conscious dog. *Circ. Res.* 51:56-66.

Walsh, S.Z., and Lind, J. 1978. The fetal circulation and its alteration at birth. In R. Stave, ed., *Perinatal Physiology.* 2d ed. Plenum, New York. Pp. 129–79.

Weiss, L. 1974. A scanning electron microscopic study of the spleen. *Blood* 43:665–91.

CHAPTER 12

Normal and Pathological Circulatory Stresses | by David K. Detweiler

The central integration of short-term responses to circulatory demands of exercise, the defense reaction, thermoregulation, and emotional disturbances are reviewed in Chap. 10. The control mechanisms affecting blood pressure and flow are diagrammed in Fig. 10.12. These regulatory responses cause appropriate increases in cardiac output and shifts in blood flow distribution to accommodate increasing metabolic requirements of the heart and skeletal muscle while sustaining blood flow to vital organs and to the skin for thermoregulation.

The cardiovascular response to exercise is one of the most important examples of regulatory adjustment (see Chap. 15).

GRAVITY, WEIGHTLESSNESS, HEAD-OUT WATER IMMERSION

In humans, factors that increase intrathoracic blood volume produce natriuresis and water diuresis, and factors that decrease intrathoracic (central) blood volume have the reverse effect. Presumably, left (and possibly right) atrial stretch receptors sense increases in central blood volume leading to reflex reduction in release of antidiuretic hormone (ADH) and renal circulatory changes that decrease renin release, thus lowering aldosterone levels through the renin-angiotensin-aldosterone mechanism; decreases in central blood volume have the reverse effect. Prolonged head-out immersion in water and weightlessness, because of the lack of gravitational force in space, cause increases in central blood volume. Diuresis and dehydration with decreased blood volume result.

Head-out water immersion (WI) has somewhat different effects in experimental dogs than in humans. In this species, the heart rate is increased despite an increase in blood pressure, indicating a change in baroreceptor regulation of the heart rate. The mechanism is considered to be either a "resetting" of arterial baroreceptor sensitivity or increased central input from those cardiac mechanoreceptors that elicit acceleration of the heart rate (see Chap. 10). Although in humans there is suppression of ADH, renin, and aldosterone secretion, these secretions are not altered in the dog during water immersion. The modulation of baroreceptor control in the dog during WI resembles that during blood volume expansion. The rise in mean blood pressure occurs with no change in total peripheral resistance. This indicates that a volume of blood is translocated from the venous to the arterial side of the systemic circulation during WI.

DIVING

The cardiovascular-respiratory response to diving inhibits breathing and conserves oxygen after immersion of the nares. The mechanisms activated are represented broadly in the animal kingdom; for example, similar responses occur in fish and diving frogs when they are removed from water and in nondiving species when the nares are immersed. Aquatic species are found in most mammalian and in many avian orders. The duration of submersion and the depths reached by these mammalian divers vary from 3 to 15 minutes and from less than 20 m (e.g., mink, muskrats, and porpoises) to 40 to 120 minutes and 80 to more than 900 m (e.g., seals and whales). In addition to respiratory arrest and oxygen conservation, deep divers such as seals and whales must have adaptations that prevent bends (aeroembolism, or decompression sickness), the narcotic effect of gases, and the direct effects of high pressures (1 atm for each 10 m in depth). Mammalian and avian divers remain submerged up to four times longer than their oxygen reserves would last were it not for reduction in their prediving rate of oxidative metabolism.

Comparison with other responses

The stereotypic cardiovascular response to diving is essentially opposite that of the defense reaction. In the former there is bradycardia, decreased cardiac output, peripheral vasoconstriction in most organs including skeletal muscle, and either an increase (short dives) or a decrease (long dives) in blood pressure; in the latter there is tachycardia, increased cardiac output, vasodilatation in skeletal muscle, and an increase in blood pressure. The distribution of vasoconstrictor activity during diving is reminiscent of that during hemorrhage. Renal, splanchnic, and cutaneous vasoconstriction with maintenance of adequate cerebral and coronary circulation occur in both states; muscle blood flow is more profoundly restricted in diving than in hemorrhage.

Reflexes

Several cardiovascular and respiratory reflexes are activated during diving and cause (1) apnea, (2) bradycardia, and (3) peripheral vasoconstriction in arterial beds and capacitance vessels in all organs except those of the central nervous system and the heart. The receptors stimulated are located in the (1) external and internal nares, (2) the lung, (3) the carotid body chemoreceptors, (4) the arterial baroreceptors, and (5) mechanoreceptors in the left ventricle. The trigeminal and inferior and superior laryngeal nerves innervate the nasal receptors. This nasal reflex induces bradycardia and apnea in the expiratory position. Lung deflation also causes reflex bradycardia. The cardiac effects are mediated by an increase in vagal tone and a decrease in sympathetic tone. Bradycardia is accompanied by an intense peripheral constriction of the *muscular distributing arteries* (i.e., large arteries with a thick medial muscular layer) close to their origin at the aorta; blood flow to the muscles, skin, kidney, liver, and spleen is virtually cut off; the capacitance vessels also contract. There is a translocation of blood volume into the heart and central nervous system circuit (in deep divers, water pressure causes marked collapse of the lungs forcing the air into the dead space), and the central blood volume increases. This, together with the bradycardia, dilates the left ventricle, stimulating mechanoreceptors that further reinforce the bradycardia. About 20 seconds into the dive, the arterial Po_2 decreases (accompanied by an increased Pco_2 and a decreased pH) sufficiently to stimulate the carotid body chemoreceptors and intensify the bradycardia. Cardiac output falls and systemic blood pressure rises initially and then decreases. There is a decrease in cardiac work, an increase in coronary dilatation, a reduction in metabolic oxygen demand by the heart, and a decrease in oxidative metabolism in the nonperfused organs. The cardiac and vascular effects initiated by stimulation of the trigeminal and laryngeal nerve receptors are thus reinforced by the carotid body stimulation.

Since the bradycardia and vasoconstriction during diving occur at the same level of blood pressure as in the nondiving state, there must be a change in the relationships between blood pressure, heart rate, and vascular resistance in the diving state compared with the nondiving state. The baroreceptor-vasomotor reflex is reset toward decreased sensitivity to vasodilatation. The changes in sensitivity do not occur at the baroreceptors but, rather, result from the modulating effect of inputs from the nasal receptors and the carotid chemoreceptors, combined with the cessation of breathing. Although the neural mechanisms involved are not entirely clear, it is known that a reduction in lung ventilation or apnea potentiates the vasoconstrictor responses to trigeminal receptors and carotid chemoreceptors.

Deep divers avoid the bends by exhaling initially, and at great pressures the flexibility of the thorax permits collapse of the lungs, forcing the residual air into the dead space (bronchi, trachea, nasal cavity) where gases cannot enter the blood despite high external pressure. Diving animals are not subject to oxygen toxicity and nitrogen narcosis because they do not breathe a continuous supply of air when at great depths (i.e., when under several atmospheres of pressure).

The importance of the reflex responses to diving is seen dramatically in seals, which drown during voluntary dives exceeding 4 minutes if the bradycardia is prevented by pretreatment with atropine.

The long dives of some seals (e.g., 1 hour in Weddell seals, 25 minutes in harbor seals) are made possible in part by their oxygen-storage capacity, which is two to four times that of terrestrial mammals on a body weight basis. This is because they have higher blood volumes per kilogram of body weight and higher concentrations of blood hemoglobin and of skeletal and cardiac muscle myoglobin. Further, these species are adapted to tolerate a decline in blood oxygen tension to 8 to 10 torr. There is also evidence that at these low levels of oxygen tension both the brain tissue and the myocardium can convert to anaerobic metabolism to a greater extent than can those of terrestrial mammals.

The bradycardiac response in the fetus differs from that in the pregnant female Weddell seal in that the maternal heart rate decreases precipitously and recovers rapidly as in nonpregnant seals, while in the fetus both the onset and the offset of bradycardia after the mother's dive are gradual. Thus the bradycardiac mechanisms appear to differ in the fetus from those in the adult. Possibly the response in the fetus is governed by a special chemoreceptor influence of unknown origin.

HYPERTENSION

Blood pressure homeostasis

The interdependent systems that regulate blood flow and blood pressure, already discussed in some detail in Chapters 5, 9, 10, and 11, include (1) the baroreceptor mechanism, (2) the chemoreceptor system, (3) the central nervous system ischemic response (the Cushing effect), (4) the renin-angiotensin vasoconstrictor mechanism, (5) the capillary fluid-shift mechanism, (6) the renal regulation of body fluid, and (7) the renin-angiotensin-aldosterone system. Finally, (8) the stress-relaxation mechanism (not described previously) also tends to return pressure toward normal, because when arterial pressure rises markedly the arterial walls actually stretch.

In addition to the various tissue autoregulatory factors, there are other control mechanisms of lesser or questionable significance: (1) A fall in arterial pressure stimulates secretion of ADH, which brings about both vasoconstriction and water retention. (2) Release of vasodilator substances such as histamine and bradykinin follows tissue damage. (3) Prostaglandins influence renal function or peripheral resistance.

Effective pressure ranges for the different systems

The differing mean arterial pressure ranges over which these eight systems operate are shown in Fig. 12.1. For example, arterial stress-relaxation, capillary fluid shift, and renal-body fluid mechanisms are effective at all pressure ranges. The baroreceptor system, however, is most effective when pressures are within physiological ranges, and it becomes ineffective when pressures fall below 60 to 70 mm Hg. At pressures below 60 to 70 mm Hg and down to about 40 mm Hg, the chemoreceptors are stimulated intensely, produce strong pressor responses, and, in fact, respond maximally. When the pressure falls below 40 mm Hg, the ischemic response of the central nervous system is activated and results in vigorous sympathetic stimulation that opposes further decline in pressure. This final reaction is the "last resort" response in defense against extreme hypotension.

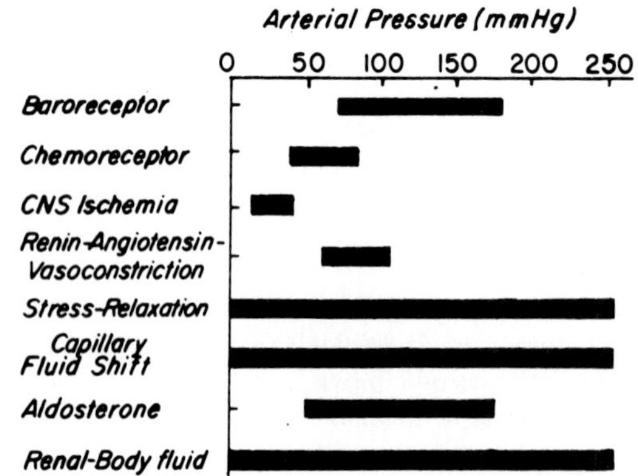

Figure 12.1. Approximate pressure ranges for function of different arterial pressure regulating mechanisms. CNS, central nervous system. (From Guyton, Coleman, Cowley, Scheel, Manning, and Norman 1974, in Laragh, ed., *Hypertension Manual,* Yorke Med., New York.)

Response times of the pressure control systems

These control systems also have different response times (Fig. 12.2). The three nervous reflex mechanisms (baroreceptor, chemoreceptor, and central nervous system ischemic response) respond within seconds. They are particularly effective in limiting excessive changes in pressure in the presence of acute perturbations, as in excitement, exercise, rapid hemorrhage, or positive or negative gravitational forces associated with postural changes or with acceleration or deceleration.

The stress-relaxation system, the renin-angiotensin-vasoconstrictor system, and the capillary fluid-shift system respond within a range of a few minutes to a few hours. Their role is more important in correction of pressure changes that would follow more deliberately acting disturbances such as slow hemorrhage or overtransfusion.

The renin-angiotensin-aldosterone system and the renal-body-fluid control mechanism do not produce significant effects on blood pressure for several hours after an alteration, but they continue to respond indefinitely.

Feedback gains of the pressure control systems

Feedback gain (see Chap. 5) may be expressed by division of the amount of correction of an aberration by the still-

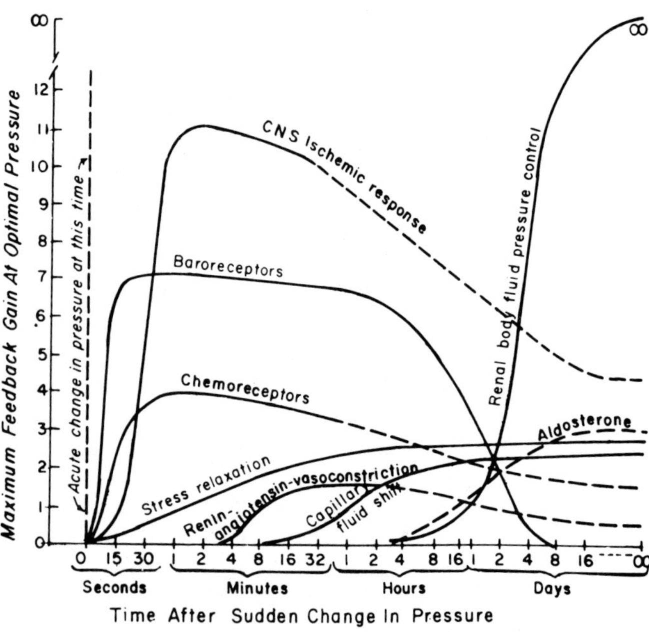

Figure 12.2. Response times and maximum feedback gains in the optimum pressure ranges for different arterial pressure regulating mechanisms. The dashed portions of the curves are not well determined. (From Guyton, Coleman, Cowley, Scheel, Manning, and Norman 1974, in Laragh, ed., *Hypertension Manual,* Yorke Med., New York.)

remaining degree of aberration. Thus, if there is no correction, the gain is zero; if the control system brings the pressure seven-eighths of the way back to normal, the gain is seven; if the control system corrects the aberration completely, its gain is infinite. Typical gains for the blood pressure control systems are diagrammed in Fig. 12.2. Of the three nervous reflex mechanisms, the central nervous system ischemic response has the highest gain, followed by the baroreceptor and chemoreceptor systems. The only system that can approach infinity is the slowly responding renal-body-fluid system, and the other systems have relatively low gains. Gains sum algebraically, however, so that the systems complement one another when acting in unison.

Clinical hypertension

The prevalence of hypertension in humans in the United States is about 15 percent. Hypertension of unknown etiology (*primary,* or *essential, hypertension*) accounts for 80 to 85 percent of these cases. *Benign* essential hypertension usually follows a chronic course over many years; *accelerated,* or *malignant,* hypertension is rapidly progressive and is commonly associated with renal insufficiency. Elevated blood pressure damages the blood vessels. Because the chief "target" organs affected are the brain, eyes, heart, and kidneys, this vascular damage leads to disability and even death from cerebral vascular accident, coronary occlusion, left ventricular failure, or renal disease (including uremia). The remaining types of human hypertension are called *secondary hypertension* and result from a variety of clinical conditions, such as renal disease (glomerulonephritis, pyelonephritis); pheochromocytomas; and coarctation of the aorta. The hypertension is limited to the systemic arterial system, and the pulmonary arterial pressure remains normal unless secondarily involved as the result of left ventricular failure induced by the primary hypertension.

Secondary hypertension occurs in domestic animals and is a recognized clinical entity in dogs. The usual cause is glomerular or nonglomerular renal disease and hyperadrenalcorticism (most often due to adrenocortical hyperplasia or carcinoma). A frequent presenting symptom in dogs with severe hypertension is blindness caused by retinopathy, including retinal detachment; with antihypertensive therapy, the detached retinas may reattach. In horses with acute laminitis, arterial hypertension associated with doubling of the cardiac output and unchanged peripheral resistance occurs during the period of lameness and pain.

Experimental hypertension

By manipulating components of the blood pressure control systems in a variety of ways, including selective breeding, experimentalists have created a number of animal models of hypertension.

Elevated cardiac output

It is generally agreed that in both humans and experimental animals cardiac output is elevated in early stages of most types of hypertension. The racing greyhound's physiological high blood pressure is associated with high cardiac output, and increasing the cardiac output experimentally will cause a transient elevation of the blood pressure. In sustained hypertension, however, the cardiac output is not elevated; rather, the hypertension depends on an increased peripheral resistance. This has led to the hypothesis that hypertension can arise from an initial increase in cardiac output that, through vascular autoregulation, leads to functional and morphological changes in the resistance vessels (chronic increase in vasoconstriction and hypertrophy of the muscular arterial walls). After these vascular changes the peripheral resistance is increased to a level sufficient to maintain hypertension despite a normal cardiac output. This hypothesis is supported by some studies but remains unproved experimentally because chronic elevations of cardiac output (e.g., stellate ganglion stimulation, atrial pacing) have failed to induce sustained hypertension after the cardiac output has returned to control values.

Renal hypertension

There is considerable evidence that the renal-body-fluid mechanism and the renin-angiotensin-aldosterone system are involved in the sustained blood pressure elevation that accompanies renal disease and also in essential hypertension in humans. A variety of experimental manipulations that reduce either renal blood flow, functional renal tissue, or sodium and water excretion relative to intake produce chronic hypertension. Interest in the role of the kidneys in hypertension was greatly stimulated by Goldblatt's finding in 1934 that in the dog a transient hypertension follows constriction of one renal artery and persistent hypertension develops if both renal arteries are constricted. The hypertension is not necessarily accompanied by a significant disturbance of renal excretory function. Subsequent studies led to elucidation of the renin-angiotensin-aldosterone system. In the dog, constriction of a single renal artery followed by removal of the opposite kidney (a "one-kidney Goldblatt preparation") produces a continuing hypertension, whereas in other species (rat, rabbit, goat, sheep) constriction of only one main renal artery is sufficient (a "two-kidney Goldblatt preparation"). Even in dogs, a unilateral constriction of the renal artery may result in a sustained hypertension, provided the reduction in renal blood flow is optimal. Hypertension is abolished by ipsilateral nephrectomy of the affected kidney performed as long as 16 months after constriction. Elevation of serum renin and angiotensin may be demonstrable in early stages but does not necessarily persist. Either active or passive immunization against renin counteracts experimental renal hypertension. During the early stages, the administration of competitive antagonists for angiotensin II similarly antagonizes the rapid hypertensive effects of acute renal artery constriction and lowers blood pressure but fails to reduce long-standing renal hypertension. Antibodies to angiotensin II do not prevent this hypertension, but it is reduced by peptide-blocking agents that prevent conversion of angiotensin I to angiotensin II. Thus it appears that interference only with the steps preceding angiotensin II formation reduces chronic renal hypertension. These findings suggest that it is short-term, acute renal hypertension that depends on an angiotensin II increase, while sustained renal hypertension requires renin but not angiotensin II. This could be explained by an action of renin other than angiotensin II formation or by the participation of other renal humoral factors. In the accelerated or malignant form of renal hypertension, the renin-angiotensin-aldosterone system appears to play a critical role, as it does in early acute hypertension.

The kidney also has antihypertensive properties. In the dog, Goldblatt hypertension from constriction of a single renal artery becomes more severe when the nonischemic kidney is removed, and removal of both kidneys in rats and dogs can lead to hypertension when the animal is well hydrated. Finally, subcutaneous implantation of renal medullary cells can lower Goldblatt hypertension, as can transplantation of a healthy kidney. Prostaglandin E_2 and a neutral lipid isolated from the renal medulla each has an antihypertensive effect when given to rats or rabbits with Goldblatt hypertension. It is of interest that analysis of the various regulatory systems in blood pressure control leads to the conclusion that the infinite gain of the renal-body-fluid mechanism requires that any long-term elevation of arterial pressure almost invariably involves the kidneys. This is because the kidney plays a pivotal role in most hypertensive states through its regulation of extracellular fluid volume, as well as through its production of both hypertensive and antihypertensive humoral agents. Neural afferent signals from the damaged kidney apparently potentiate the humoral effects on blood pressure through central nervous system excitation.

Neurogenic hypertension

Manipulation of the central nervous system and its afferent nerves is capable of inducing arterial hypertension varying in severity from labile bouts of high blood pressure to sustained hypertension and rapidly fatal fulminant hypertension.

Elevation of the cerebrospinal fluid pressure by injection of kaolin into the cisterna magna or by ligation of cerebral vessels produces hypertension via the central nervous system ischemic response. In the dog, bilateral destruction of the nucleus tractus solitarii or deafferentation of the carotid sinus and aortic arch baroreceptors induces mild, labile hypertension; when both of these procedures are performed simultaneously, or if the entire dorsal portion of the dog's brain stem is destroyed, fulminant hypertension, fatal within a few hours, results.

As mentioned in Chapter 10, p. 210, if both the arterial baroreceptors and the cardiopulmonary baroreceptor regions are denervated together, the labile blood pressure characteristic of arterial baroreceptor denervation alone is present, but now there is also a sustained increase in blood pressure as well.

In the rat, destruction of the nucleus tractus solitarii alone produces fatal fulminant hypertension. These procedures demonstrate that when the inhibitory feedback baroreceptor loop is completely opened, the unrestrained release of sympathetic outflow, causing extreme tachycardia and hypertension, results in acute heart failure and pulmonary edema.

Both sympathetic nervous system activity and vascular sensitivity to adrenergic effects are enhanced in practically all types of hypertension. This enhanced sympathetic activity contributes to the blood pressure elevation by causing or supporting increased vascular resistance, increased cardiac output, renal sodium retention and increased renin release, exaggeration of vasoconstrictor responses, and increased production of vascular contractile protein.

Other types of neurogenic hypertension include those produced in rats by repeated exposure to strong auditory stimuli or by provision of psychosocial conflict situations for caged animals.

Salt loading and renal mass

In rats, either reducing renal mass to one-sixth of normal or increasing salt intake by substituting 2 percent saline solution for drinking water will induce hypertension. The effect of excess salt is variable and under genetic control, since salt-sensitive strains of rats have been bred. The two conditions are interrelated in that a reduction in renal mass enhances the effect of salt loading. A combination of saline loading and reduction in renal mass produces hypertension also in dogs (a species largely immune to the hypertensive effect of either procedure alone). There is a transient increase in extracellular fluid volume, right atrial pressure, mean systemic pressure, and cardiac output. A secondary rise in peripheral resistance then occurs as a result of autoregulation in other tissues, and the cardiac output eventually returns toward normal. The elevated pressure is now maintained primarily by the increased peripheral resistance. During the initial stage when cardiac output is increased, the rise in arterial blood pressure also increases renal excretion of salt and water. Thus fluid volume and cardiac output both come to be reduced, but so long as the increased salt and water loading is continued, the increased peripheral resistance will sustain the hypertension. This sequence of events illustrates the long-term control of blood pressure by renal function and fluid volume.

In almost all forms of experimental chronic hypertension the concentration of sodium and potassium ions and the volume of intracellular water are increased in arterial smooth muscle. These changes could cause swelling of the vascular walls and encroachment on the lumen. They might also enhance the response of arterial smooth muscle to vasoconstrictor influences and thus contribute to the elevation of peripheral resistance.

An interesting hypothesis in this context is that a circulatory sodium transport inhibitor is increased when the kidney's ability to excrete sodium is comprised; this inhibitor adjusts sodium excretion toward normal but inhibits sodium transport in arteriolar smooth muscle, thereby raising both intracellular sodium and calcium and thus increasing vascular reactivity.

The proven antihypertensive effect of diuretic therapy or salt restriction probably results from reduction of extracellular fluid volume and of vascular ionic and water content.

Adrenal steroids

Many adrenal steroids can cause elevation of blood pressure and enhance the hypertensive effects of salt loading or renal ischemia. These effects are similar to those seen in Cushing's syndrome or in primary aldosteronism in humans. The mineralocorticoid hormones (aldosterone, corticosterone or compound B, and deoxycorticosterone) are most often identified as the primary cause of hypertension, although glucocorticoids may be involved because they also have some mineralocorticoid property. *Adrenal regeneration hypertension* can be induced in young rats by salt loading after removal of one adrenal gland and the medulla of the other, coupled with removal of one kidney. The hypertension is attributed to overproduction of adrenal steroids during adrenal regeneration.

Angiotensin II

In addition to its powerful direct vasoconstrictor properties, angiotensin II has been shown to have a number of other actions implicated in blood pressure elevation. These actions include enhancement of sympathetic activity by central activation of sympathetic vasoconstrictor nerves, by sensitization of vascular smooth muscle to catecholamines, by inhibition of norepinephrine inactivation and reuptake in sympathetic nerve endings, and by release of catecholamines from the adrenal medulla. Angiotensin II also stimulates aldosterone secretion, has direct antidiuretic and antinatriuretic actions on the kidney, induces thirst when injected into the diencephalic region or intravenously in high doses, and exerts a positive inotropic effect on the heart. Increased thirst has been noted in one-kidney Goldblatt preparations, as well as in hypertensive patients with chronic renal failure and high renin levels.

The response to injection of angiotensin II into the cerebral ventricles further distinguishes greyhound from mongrel cardiovascular control: the arterial pressure is increased in both; in greyhounds this result is due to increased cardiac output but in mongrels it is due to increased peripheral resistance.

Heredity

Breeding experiments in rats, rabbits, mice, chickens, and turkeys have shown that blood pressure is polygenically determined. In laboratory rats, however, hypertension is not a single entity, since the several hypertensive strains have differing physiological characteristics. In chickens, rats, and mice about 20 percent of the variation in blood pressure in a genetically heterogeneous population is inherited, while 80 percent results from environmental factors. This appears to be true in humans as well. The differing patterns of blood pressure elevation observed with age suggest that unknown environmental factors interact with the genetic substrate to produce the hypertensive pattern.

The form of hereditary hypertension in animals that has received the most attention is that of the spontaneously hypertensive rat. Of all the varieties thus far discovered, this seems to be most nearly the experimental counterpart of human essential hypertension. In these rats the hypertensive state is characterized hemodynamically by an early phase when the cardiac output is elevated, even though the peripheral resistance is normal. This hyperkinetic state is then transformed with aging to one in which there is a sustained increase in peripheral resistance and a normal cardiac output. This sequence fits in well with the speculation that an elevated cardiac output may initiate hypertension in humans. Nevertheless, it is unlikely that the elevated cardiac output plays a significant etiological role in hypertension in the spontaneously hypertensive rat since, if the increase in cardiac output is prevented by chronic administration of a beta-adrenergic blocking agent, the course of the development of hypertension is unaltered.

The greyhound breed of dogs (see "Exercise", Chap. 15) is another example of the effect of inheritance on hemodynamic variables and regulation.

Summary

Normal blood pressure is maintained by the complex interaction of short-term and long-term feedback control loops (Fig. 12.3). Acute perturbances in blood pressure levels are minimized by the rapidly acting short-term control mechanisms. Long-term control determines the mean blood pressure level in the steady state. Long-term control includes interrelations between arterial pressure, renal function, and body fluid volume. Renal function, in turn, is regulated by extrinsic influences, including the nervous system, the renin-angiotensin-aldosterone mechanism, ADH, and other factors that can produce brief or moderately prolonged effects. Such changes contribute to long-term control, during which the short-term regulators modulate blood pressure around the new pressure level. For example, the short-term mechanism that depends on the baroreceptors becomes "reset" in hypertension.

When blood pressure is elevated, the initial hemodynamic change is frequently an increase in cardiac output. Whether this is neurogenically engendered or results from a

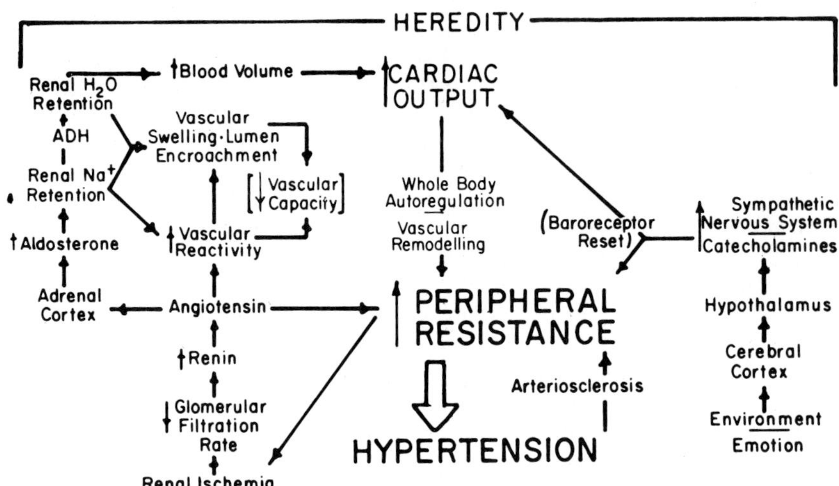

Figure 12.3. Schema depicting interrelationships of the chief factors identified as being involved in the development of hypertension. Increased peripheral resistance is placed centrally because this is the final dominant hemodynamic feature of most forms of established hypertension. (From Detweiler 1979, in Brobeck, ed., *Best & Taylor's Physiological Basis of Medical Practice,* 10th ed., © 1979, the Williams & Wilkins Co., Baltimore.)

renally induced increase in extracellular fluid volume, or both, cannot always be established. That a primary increase in cardiac output can, in itself, lead to hypertension remains to be proved. According to one view, when blood pressure is chronically elevated, the arterial vessels exhibit both structural and functional changes that lead to a persistent rise in peripheral resistance, even though the cardiac output and extracellular fluid volume eventually return toward normal. In time, a chronically elevated blood pressure induces degenerative arterial disease chiefly affecting the heart, brain, and kidneys.

Both blood pressure levels and susceptibility to arterial disease are genetically influenced so that the incidence of hypertension and its consequences vary among different species and breeds.

Therapeutic reduction of blood pressure in hypertensive patients has been shown to prolong life. Effective regimens include diuretics or salt restriction, which initially decrease plasma volume and later may alter the electrolyte and water content of vascular smooth muscle. Propranolol, a beta-adrenergic antagonist that decreases cardiac output, decreases renin secretion by the kidney, and it may reduce vasoconstriction by acting on the central nervous system. Drugs that relax arteriolar smooth muscle by direct action (e.g., hydralazine), peripheral sympatholytic effects (e.g., guanethidine), adrenergic ganglionic blockade (e.g., mecamylamine), or central nervous system effects are useful. Angiotensin II blockers and agents that block the enzyme that converts angiotensin I to angiotensin II are also effective.

CHRONIC CONGESTIVE HEART FAILURE

The clinical syndrome, chronic *congestive heart failure* (CHF), is characterized by complex alterations in cardiovascular control mechanisms that develop when the mechanical work capacity of the cardiac pump is diminished and cardiac output becomes insufficient to meet blood flow requirements of the body (Fig. 12.4). Ordinarily, failure develops gradually; in the early stages only cardiac responses to excessive demands, such as strenuous exercise, are compromised. Later the increase in cardiac work required for even moderate elevations in blood pressure and blood flow are curtailed, until a state is reached in which the cardiac output cannot be augmented above the resting level. Finally, when the cardiac output can no longer sustain a blood flow adequate even for the resting state, death supervenes.

These stages in the development of CHF do not necessarily form a progressive continuum. Rather, a given state of failure may remain fairly static for a varying period of time, depending on the effectiveness of adjustments in circulatory regulatory mechanisms and of limitations in demands placed on the heart (e.g., voluntary reduction in bodily activity).

Causes of chronic congestive heart failure

Primary diseases of the myocardium (e.g., myocardial infarction, myocarditis, cardiomyopathy) can sufficiently reduce the amount of normally active contractile tissue and result in CHF.

Abnormalities that increase the work of one or both ventricles and that lead to hypertrophy, if severe enough, may culminate in CHF. These include acquired or congenital lesions that cause valvular stenosis or insufficiency, systemic arterial hypertension, and pulmonary arterial hypertension.

Conditions that cause sustained increase in output of one or both ventricles in effect increase heart work, causing high-output failure. This occurs when peripheral resistance is markedly reduced, as in arteriovenous fistula or in congenital malformations that have large left-to-right shunts (e.g., patent ductus arteriosus). In anemia and hyperthroid-

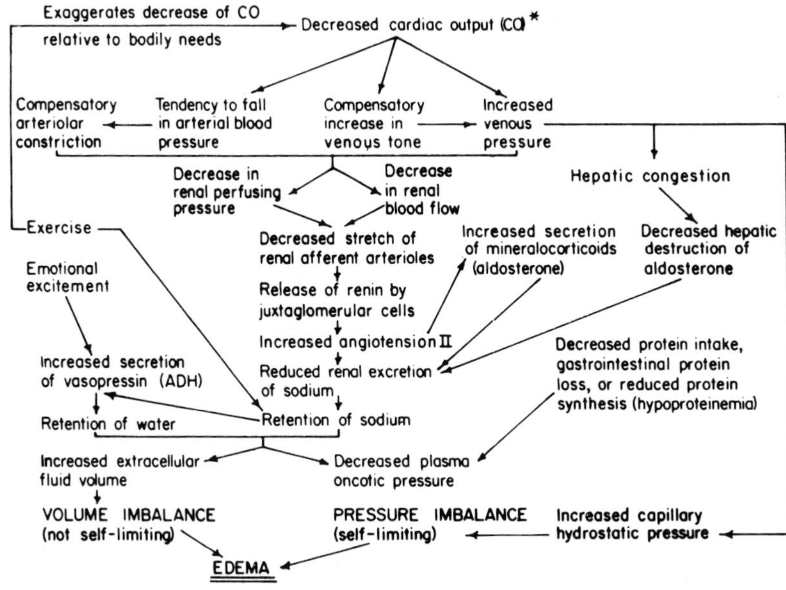

Figure 12.4. Schematic diagram of the principal mechanisms operating in congestive heart failure. (From Detweiler 1977, in Booth and McDonald, eds., *Veterinary Pharmacology,* Iowa State University Press, Ames.)

ism a high output is necessary to meet tissue metabolic needs.

Conditions that interfere with cardiac filling do not necessarily affect the myocardium directly but result in venous congestion with a low cardiac output. These include pericarditis with effusion (tamponade), constrictive pericarditis, and tricuspid stenosis.

The failing heart

Mechanical factors

Myocardial hypertrophy is one of the fundamental compensatory mechanisms of increased work load per unit of contractile tissue. When hypertrophy is severe enough, however, there is depression of contractile strength per unit mass of myocardium with a decrease in the velocity and extent of shortening of cardiac muscle and a lower value for the maximal developed tension. These changes progress in severity as CHF develops.

Ventricular dilation results in increased wall tension (T) per unit of intraventricular pressure (P), in accordance with the Laplace relation, $P = 2T/r$, where r is the radius that is being altered by the dilation. Thus, as the heart weakens and dilates, its work load per beat increases because wall tension needed to produce a given systolic pressure increases with diameter.

In the intact but diseased heart, in addition to the effect of ventricular dilation, there are other morphological factors (e.g., valvular stenosis or regurgitation), as well as cardiac arrhythmias or marked bradycardia or tachycardia, that decrease effective cardiac work.

Besides the changes in myocardial cells during the hypertrophy process that precedes cardiac failure, there are important accompanying abnormalities in the intramyocardial coronary arteries and cardiac fibroblasts. Myocytes represent only about 33 percent of all myocardial cells, but their volume amounts to two-thirds of the normal myocardium. In hypertrophy they increase either in diameter by parallel addition of sarcomeres or in length by series addition of sarcomeres (see also Chap. 6). Fibroblasts represent about 67 percent of all myocardial cells. The cardiac hypertrophy caused by pressure overload (e.g., aortic banding) causes an initial rise in collagen synthesis followed by fibroplasia. This does not occur in cardiac hypertrophy caused by volume overload (e.g., that secondary to arteriovenous fistula, anemia, or thyroxine administration). Collagen accumulation also occurs as the reactive (reparative) fibrosis to myocardial cell loss in the diseased myocardium. Such increases in collagen content lead to a marked rise in passive stiffness of the ventricle that interferes with diastolic filling and requires an increase in ventricular filling pressure. When the ventricular filling pressure of the left ventricle exceeds 25 mm Hg (the colloidal osmotic pressure of plasma), clinical signs of pulmonic congestion appear.

The intramural coronary artery disease that is a common feature of all cardiac failure states in animals has long been neglected in analyses of myocardial disease. It now appears that both impaired vasomotor reactivity and interstitial fibrosis play important roles in converting initial myocardial hypertrophy in response to increased work load to a pathological state.

Biochemical factors

Mitochondria isolated from failing hearts shows a decrease in *energy production,* which may account for myocardial depression, at least in advanced cardiac failure. By contrast, *energy stores* of creatine phosphate and adenosine triphosphate apparently are not significantly reduced. There is some evidence that myofibrillar adenosine triphosphatase activity is reduced in hypertrophy and failure and that this slows the rate of conversion of chemical energy (adenosine triphosphate) to mechanical energy (*energy utilization defect*).

Excitation-contraction coupling

The rate and total uptake of calcium by mitochondria and also by the sarcoplasmic reticulum in preparations from failing hearts are markedly decreased. Both calcium binding and calcium release are impaired in the reticular membranes. These findings indicate a defect in calcium transport for excitation-contraction coupling.

Supporting factors

In the failing myocardium, norepinephrine stores and biosynthesis are reduced and the response to sympathetic nerve stimulation is curtailed. Moreover, a beta-adrenergic blockade intensifies cardiac failure. Possibly the function of the failing myocardium is sustained by circulating catecholamines.

In any case, circulating levels of norepinephrine and epinephrine are inversely related to the degree of CHF, while at the same time the heart rate and blood pressure responses to these catecholamines are reduced.

Summary

The myocardial deficits that have been identified in CHF include (1) depression of contractile strength, (2) reduction in effective cardiac work owing to geometrical factors, (3) depression of mitochondrial energy production, (4) reduction in the rate of energy utilization, and (5) possibly a defect in excitation-contraction coupling.

Consequences of cardiac failure

Edema formation

The accumulation of an excessive volume of extracellular fluid in CHF results in increased blood volume, edema, ascites, and (sometimes) hydrothorax. These increases are brought about mainly by renal retention of salt and water, aggravated by increased thirst and possibly by an increased appetite for salt. With the increase in blood volume, the blood vessels are more completely filled, whereas the swollen interstitial fluid volume compresses the blood vessels externally. Both of these processes increase the mean systemic pressure (for definition, see Chap. 9). The mean systemic pressure is a measure of the cardiac filling pressure in the intact circulation, because the higher the mean systemic pressure, the higher the pressure inducing venous return. Another factor that raises cardiac filling pressure in CHF is the reflex venoconstriction that accompanies the reduction in cardiac output. Consequently, there is increased filling of the heart during diastole, and the end-diastolic volume is increased. Through operation of the intrinsic Starling mechanism, the change in end-diastolic volume will elevate cardiac output if the heart has any remaining intrinsic compensatory capacity. This mechanism is probably effective in early stages of chronic CHF, before clinical signs are obvious. By the time failure becomes evident, however, in the form of decreased exercise tolerance and edema, this mechanism usually has had its maximal effect, and a further retention of fluid can only exacerbate the condition of failure. Unfortunately, the processes that lead to accumulation of extracellular fluid are not turned off when they become ineffective. The result is that the kidney continues to function as though the body required additional extracellular fluid, even though vital organs are "waterlogged" and ascites and hydrothorax have become severe. At this stage, in the absence of therapeutic intervention, this vicious cycle of advancing cardiac failure and fluid retention inexorably leads to death.

Fluid retention mechanisms

There are at least two (and probably more) processes that account for renal reabsorption of sodium and water in CHF: (1) the direct effect of underperfusion on renal function and (2) a humoral sequence triggered by this hemodynamic insufficiency (Fig. 12.4). When the cardiac output is decreased, the renal blood flow is curtailed because of slightly decreased arterial pressure and reflexly engendered constriction of renal arterioles. Elevation of venous pressure accompanying CHF may also reduce renal blood flow. The result is a reduction in glomerular filtration rate and an increase in tubular reabsorption, the latter being mainly responsible for fluid retention.

The hormonal mechanism is the renin-angiotensin-aldosterone system. Underperfusion of the kidneys results in the release of *renin* from the juxtaglomerular cells with the consequent formation of angiotensin II (Fig. 12.5). The latter increases *aldosterone* secretion, and sodium retention follows. By raising the electrolyte concentration of extracellular fluid, this could bring about the release of ADH from the posterior pituitary gland. In dogs, for example, there is strong evidence that in experimental CHF there are marked increases in plasma ADH in animals that develop ascites and a positive sodium balance.

Experiments with dogs after adrenalectomy indicate that the renin-angiotensin-aldosterone mechanism is essential for the development of cardiac edema. Nevertheless, an elevation of plasma renin or aldosterone levels is not consistently found. This observation suggests that the renin-angiotensin-aldosterone system is activated only at certain times (e.g., during and after exercise) and that hyperaldosteronism is, therefore, not always present.

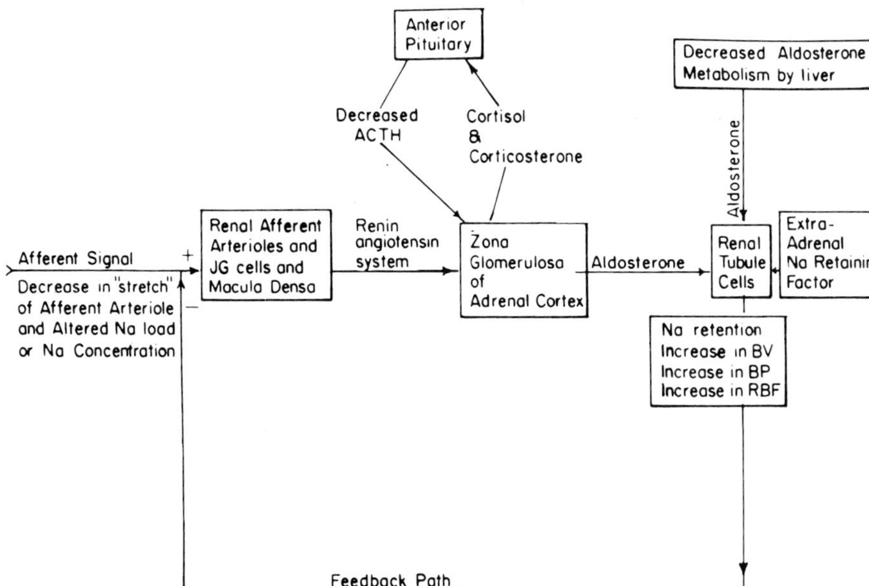

Figure 12.5. Negative-feedback diagram to explain the renin-angiotensin-aldosterone system. Two intrarenal receptors are postulated: (1) a stretch in the renal afferent arterioles and (2) the macula densa, which are sensitive to signals leading to renin release by juxtaglomerular apparatus cells. The vascular stretch receptor responds to changes in wall tension and the macula densa to changes in sodium load or transport. ACTH, adrenocorticotropic hormone; JG, juxtaglomerular; BP, blood pressure; BV, blood volume; RBF, renal blood flow. (From Davis 1974, in Page and Bumpus, eds., *Handbuch der experimentellen Pharmakologie,* Springer, Berlin.)

In dogs with experimental CHF there is also an increase in sympathetic tone that reduces renal blood flow. This may be part of a baroreceptor reflex associated with the tendency toward a decrease in arterial pressure. In normal dogs in which severe exercise results in an increase in renal vascular resistance, a concomitant rise in blood pressure prevents a sustained fall in renal blood flow. On the contrary, in the presence of experimental right-sided CHF, the renal vasoconstriction is greater and the pressor response is much less, resulting in a marked reduction in renal blood flow with exercise. A chief component of this renal vasoconstriction in CHF is prevented by renal denervation, whereas a smaller component is removed by alpha-adrenergic blockage (phentolamine). These findings indicate that in the dog with CHF a reduction of renal blood flow is mediated primarily by renal nerves and secondarily by circulating norepinephrine. These changes could account for exercise-induced retention of sodium, with or without participation of the renin-angiotensin-aldosterone system.

When hepatic congestion is severe enough, a decreased rate of metabolic destruction of aldosterone in the liver contributes to the elevation of its blood level.

Exercise and emotional stress increase the work of the heart and cause renal retention of sodium.

In experimental CHF the increase in venous pressure mentioned above becomes evident only after retention of sodium and water has been initiated. It is a major factor accounting for the extravascular accumulation of the fluid that has been retained by the kidneys, because it enhances the capillary hydrostatic pressure, creates a *pressure imbalance* across the capillary membrane, and causes water to move across the capillary walls at a faster rate. There is a concomitant reduction in plasma protein concentration that reduces the colloid osmotic pressure of the plasma; this also will promote a loss of fluid, especially into the interstitial spaces of dependent areas (limbs) and into the abdominal cavity. Such a reduction in plasma protein concentration has two chief origins: (1) dilution of the extracellular fluid (which includes the blood plasma) by the retained sodium and water and (2) loss of plasma protein into interstitial spaces and the ascitic fluid. Other factors that may operate to reduce plasma proteins include (3) reduced food intake, (4) poor gastrointestinal absorption, (5) gastrointestinal loss of protein, and (6) interference with hepatic protein synthesis owing to liver damage. Despite the decrease in plasma protein *concentration* in the blood, the total *quantity* of plasma protein, including that in the blood and extracellular fluids, may exceed the total blood protein in normal dogs.

To be considered, therefore, in the pathogenesis of edema are two processes: (1) a *volume imbalance* owing to the renal retention of sodium and water and (2) a *pressure imbalance* owing to increased hydrostatic pressure and decreased plasma oncotic pressure in the capillaries. Figure 12.5 summarizes the interrelated mechanisms.

As explained above, the pressure imbalance accounts for movement of fluid out of capillaries, but it cannot account for the relatively enormous quantity of edema fluid that may accumulate in CHF. If it were acting alone, either an increased hydrostatic pressure or a decreased plasma oncotic pressure would limit itself, because the blood concentration would increase, the capillary hydrostatic pressure would decrease, and tissue hydrostatic pressure would increase as a result of transudation of plasma fluid into the interstitial compartment. Consequently, the volume of the edema fluid could never exceed that of the plasma compartment. Actually, the volume of ascitic (abdominal) fluid alone may be much greater than that of the entire blood volume. It is the volume imbalance brought about by the retention of water and salt which causes the relatively unlimited accumulation of edema fluid found in CHF.

As described previously, the increase in interstitial and blood volumes increases mean systemic pressure, augments cardiac filling, and thus tends to increase cardiac output (see Fig. 9.5). Renal blood flow is thus increased, and if it becomes adequate the glomerular filtration rate will become sufficient, renin release will be reduced, the aldosterone level will return to normal, and fluid retention will cease.

One aspect of the humoral mechanism has not been explained. In normal dogs the sodium-retaining effects of aldosterone are transient, lasting only 1 or 2 days despite continued injection of the hormone. Yet in CHF the fluid retention continues indefinitely. It appears, therefore, that in CHF the retained fluid fails to restore renal arteriolar hemodynamics to normal, despite the increase in blood volume, and that this accounts for continued hypersecretion of renin and aldosterone. This same renal hemodynamic deficit might also cause, in some way, the continued sensitivity of the renal tubule to circulating aldosterone. Another, more controversial, explanation is that a salt-losing factor (natriuretic hormone) normally acts upon cells in the proximal tubule, independently of glomerular filtration rate and mineralocorticoid activity. Lack of production of this factor in CHF could account for the continued action of aldosterone.

Thirst

Increased thirst occurs at certain stages of the development of CHF in humans and dogs. It can be induced experimentally also by constriction of the thoracic posterior vena cava. The renin-angiotensin system is thought to be involved since such drinking responses can be blocked by the competitive angiotensin inhibitor, saralasin, and intracranial injection of angiotensin II induces thirst in practically all species tested. Whether angiotensin II is a natural dipsogen governing physiological thirst is more controversial.

Arterial pressure

Arterial pressure is usually maintained within normal limits despite the low cardiac output. Angiotensin II appears to be of primary importance in sustaining the arterial pressure since competitive angiotensin II blockers (e.g., saralasin) reduce the pressure. Increased neurogenic vasomotor tone and increased circulating norepinephrine contribute similarly to blood pressure maintenance.

Other humoral influences

The increase in plasma ADH (vasopressin) levels in CHF, already mentioned for its fluid-retention effect, raises the question of the importance of its vasoconstrictor effect. The current consensus is that its influence on vasoconstriction in CHF is less than that of circulating catecholamines or angiotensin II.

Atrial natriuretic factor. Atrial natriuretic factor (ANF) secretion is increased three- to fivefold in CHF, and it is thought to contribute perhaps 5 to 10 percent of the daily sodium excretion in chronic CHF, counterbalancing to some extent the effect of aldosterone. In addition, it promotes vasodilation, antagonizing angiotensin II, and causes a fall in renin activity. It has been shown, however, that the natriuretic response to ANF infusion is reduced in the presence of CHF and its effectiveness may be overridden when edema develops.

Paracrine and autocrine effects. The paracrine/autocrine substances that cause vasoconstrictor effects include thromboxane A_2, certain prostaglandins, serotonin, and endothelin (see Chap. 10). Conversely, prostaglandin E_2, prostacyclin, bradykinin, and endothelium-derived relaxation factor are vasodilators. Their various roles in CHF have not been determined. It is likely that their effects would be limited to regional vascular beds such as the coronary and renal circulations.

Clinical significance

While the array of mechanisms involved in the pathogenesis of CHF may seem confusing, the understanding of them has led to important changes in therapy, especially during the last decade. The traditional treatment for CHF has involved the use of digitalis glycosides for their positive inotropic and negative chronotropic actions, coupled with diuretics and low-sodium diets to reduce extracellular fluid (including plasma) volume. Recent years have witnessed the introduction of new positive inotropic drugs with mechanisms of action that differ from those of digitalis glycosides and the use of vasodilators to reduce afterload. Among the latter, the most interesting from a physiological standpoint are a series of drugs that inhibit angiotensin-converting enzyme (ACE) (see Chap. 10 and Fig. 12.4). These ACE inhibitors effectively lower peripheral resistance by reducing angiotensin II and are useful therapeutic agents in both CHF and hypertension. Available data indicate that the use of ACE inhibitors in humans has reduced the annual death rate from CHF by one-half.

SHOCK

Shock is an acute circulatory state in which the cardiac output is insufficient to maintain adequate blood flow to the tissues. Any condition that causes a sudden reduction in circulating blood volume or an enlargement of the vascular system can reduce mean circulatory pressure and cause shock. For example, shock may be induced by the following: (1) hemorrhage; (2) severe thirsting dehydration with reduction of extracellular fluid volume, including plasma volume; (3) extensive loss of plasma through capillaries damaged by mechanical, chemical, or thermal injury; (4) severe loss of body fluids through excessive sweating, vomiting, or diarrhea; (5) entrapment of blood in engorged capillaries, as in septic shock in fulminating gram-negative bacterial infections; (6) widespread vasodilatation caused by anaphylaxis; (7) abrupt enlargement of the vascular system after rapid removal of pressure around the vascular tree (e.g., after a quick withdrawal of ascitic fluid, removal of a large abdominal tumor, or sudden reduction in skeletal muscular tone); (8) sharp reduction in cardiac output from myocardial damage such as acute myocarditis; and (9) increased resistance to venous return as a result of cardiac tamponade, positive intrathoracic pressure, or compression of the inferior vena cava. Shock induced primarily by blood loss is called *hemorrhagic shock;* that following initial myocardial damage is termed *cardiogenic shock;* and that accompanying massive bacterial infections is designated *septic* or *endotoxic shock.*

Anaphylactic shock is an immunological reaction in which an antigen, when combining with an antibody, provokes a sudden release of harmful chemical substances: histamines, slow-reacting substance, and eosinophil leukocyte chemotactic factor are the chief mediators of the resultant cardiac failure and vascular fluid loss. Histamine increases capillary permeability (so that fluid and plasma proteins are lost) and causes contraction of visceral smooth muscle, including that of the bronchi (bronchospasm), an effect shared with certain prostaglandins. Slow-reacting substance also increases capillary transudation and stimulates visceral smooth muscle and is a far more potent bronchoconstrictor than histamine or prostaglandins. In addition, it has a negative inotropic action on the heart and causes coronary artery constriction. Slow-reacting substance has been recently identified chemically as a mixture of three leukotrienes, substances discovered in 1979 that are related to prostaglandins and thromboxanes.

The mortality rate from uncomplicated hemorrhagic shock is low, provided that adequate replacement of blood volume is effected early. Endotoxic or gram-negative septic shock and cardiogenic shock are usually fatal despite treatment with massive blood transfusions and vasopressor agents.

In shock the visible mucous membranes are pale, the extremities are cold and clammy, rectal temperature is subnormal, pulse and respiratory rates are elevated, blood pressure is decreased, and the central nervous system is depressed. The perception of pain is dulled, but the sensation of thirst is intense.

During fully developed shock as seen after hemorrhage, skeletal injury, or extensive muscle contusion in experiments on dogs, the circulating blood volume is reduced by 30 to 40 percent. For the treatment of shock after hemorrhage, the quantity of blood transfused should be in excess of the apparent blood loss to make up for the pooling of blood in dilated capillaries and for the loss of plasma into the interstitial space.

Stages of shock

Shock has been divided arbitrarily into three phases that define (1) degree of severity and (2) response to transfusion.

1. *Compensated or recovering shock.* Blood volume and blood pressure are reduced, but because compensatory mechanisms maintain adequate blood flow to vital organs the subject will recover without blood transfusion or other intervention.

2. *Progressive or degenerating shock.* The blood pressure slowly and progressively falls despite continuing compensatory changes such as reflex tachycardia and vasoconstriction of the skin, muscle, and splanchnic area and despite fluid shift from the interstitial fluid compartment into the plasma. As the mean arterial pressure falls to 60 mm Hg or below, the functions of the heart, kidneys, central nervous system, and other vital organs are impaired. This stage may be arrested by transfusion and other treatment, and the blood pressure may be restored to normal.

3. *Irreversible shock.* Cardiac output and blood pressure are very low; vital functions are depressed. Even though blood transfusion may restore cardiac output and blood pressure temporarily, the effect is transient. Blood pressure falls once again, and the subject dies of myocardial failure and cerebral depression. Unfortunately, the pathogenesis of the irreversible state is not yet well understood.

A *critical point* between compensated and progressive shock has been demonstrated in experiments on hemorrhagic shock in dogs. Animals bled to arterial pressures not lower than 47 mm Hg recover spontaneously, whereas animals bled to pressures only a few millimeters of mercury below this level develop progressive shock and die. Similarly, if animals are bled so that their cardiac output is below a critical level, they die; however, if hemorrhage is stopped so that the cardiac output, although reduced, remains even a few milliliters per minute above this level, the animals recover. Thus a difference of only a few milliliters per minute in cardiac output or of only a few millimeters of mercury in arterial blood pressure determines whether a dog will recover or die after blood loss.

Positive feedback in progressive shock

Progressive shock, if untreated, inexorably leads to irreversible shock—a vicious cycle in which each decrement in cardiac output and blood pressure induces further hemodynamic deterioration until death ensues. At least five types of positive feedback account for this advancing process: (1)

As shock proceeds, the cerebral blood flow is reduced progressively and the vasomotor and respiratory centers become increasingly depressed. (2) As the severity of shock increases, the blood vessels themselves are inadequately perfused, vascular tone is thereby reduced to the point that mean circulatory pressure falls and cardiac output is further compromised by a fall in venous return. (3) Reduced capillary perfusion causes a loss in capillary integrity, which is accompanied by a reduction in precapillary resistance and an increase in postcapillary resistance; hence, intravascular fluid is lost to extravascular spaces. (In the dog, marked congestion of the capillaries and venules of the small intestine occurs with substantial extravasation of fluid and frank hemorrhage into the intestinal lumen, but this mechanism is apparently of little importance in primates.) (4) Stasis of blood in some vascular beds is severe enough to result in blood clotting, which further impedes tissue nutrition. (5) Coronary blood flow is reduced to the point that impaired myocardial oxygenation causes a further fall in cardiac output. Further, a cardiodepressant factor may be formed in hypoxic tissues (see "Myocardial Depressant Factor," below) and produces a negative inotropic effect.

Negative-feedback resistance to shock

The circulatory regulatory systems reviewed in the section on hypertension and described in detail elsewhere are negative-feedback mechanisms that tend to return cardiac output and blood pressure toward normal after a perturbation. The effects of acute loss of blood volume on cardiac output and blood pressure are combatted almost immediately by those mechanisms that have the shortest response times (i.e., the baroreceptor, chemoreceptor, and central nervous ischemic systems). Within minutes to a few hours, the stress relaxation, the renin-angiotensin-vasoconstrictor, and the capillary fluid-shift systems also respond. The renin-angiotensin-aldosterone and the renal-body-fluid systems may begin to respond immediately, but their effects develop more gradually over a period of several hours.

The resultant of the respective gains (see section on hypertension) of these negative- and positive-feedback effects on blood pressure and cardiac output determines the outcome of the shock. At very low levels of arterial pressure, the negative gains of the pressoreceptor, chemoreceptor, and central nervous system ischemic reflex are reduced to zero, while the positive gain of cardiac deterioration increases to one or higher. This means that at mean arterial pressures of 50 mm Hg or less, the positive gain exceeds the sum of the negative gains, and progressive circulatory deterioration continues. Only at mean arterial pressure levels above 50 mm Hg do the negative-feedback mechanisms generally overcome the positive-feedback effects and break the vicious cycle so that spontaneous recovery follows.

The responses of the venous capacitance system to the stresses of hypertension, congestive heart failure, and shock have not been nearly as thoroughly studied as those of the heart and arterial system. The obvious importance of capacitance system responses to the stresses of hemorrhage and shock gave special impetus to studies in the area.

Much of the information comes from experiments in dogs. In a dog with a total blood volume of, say, 80 ml/kg, at 5 minutes after a rapid hemorrhage to reduce the mean arterial blood pressure below 50 mm Hg, about one-third of the blood lost is from passive elastic recoil of the vasculature, about one-third from transcapillary fluid shifts from the interstitial fluid compartment to the plasma compartment, and the remaining one-third is from reflexly induced capacitance vessel constriction. Capillary reabsorption of extravascular fluid owing to the decreased capillary hydrostatic pressure can add 30 ml/kg or more fluid to the blood volume during the first hour of blood loss. Reflex venoconstriction during the first few minutes after hemorrhage reduces venous capacitance, transferring about 10 ml/kg of blood toward the heart.

The arterial baroreceptors and chemoreceptors, acting in parallel with the atrial, pulmonary, and cardiac mechanoreceptors, account for reflex arterial and venous constriction that lowers the capillary pressure on the one hand and reduces venous capacity on the other.

The spleen of the dog is relatively larger than that of other species and, because its capsule contains large amounts of smooth muscle under sympathetic control, constricts after hemorrhage in response to the same reflexes that cause vascular constriction. It is capable of providing about 8 percent of the total blood volume into the active circulation after hemorrhage. The spleens of the horse and cat also have capsules rich in smooth muscle and can similarly increase blood volume and erythrocyte count when stimulated. The spleens of other domestic species (e.g., ruminants, swine, rabbits) and humans have little smooth muscle in their capsules and do not contract.

The liver is highly vascular, and about half of its blood volume can be mobilized for redistribution. In endotoxic shock in dogs, however, hepatic venoconstriction causes a large increase in portal venous pressure with hepatosplanchnic pooling of blood of up to 50 ml/kg. Such massive loss of circulating blood volume causes a rapid decrease in cardiac output, marked hypotension, and death. The spleen remains constricted in dogs with endotoxic shock. Hepatosplanchnic pooling is not an important component of endotoxic shock in monkeys, rabbits, or cats. In cats, on the other hand, pulmonary vascular constriction is prominent, leading to pulmonary edema and right heart overload. This reaction is also prominent in monkeys and rabbits. Histamine is a major mediator of these responses to endotoxic shock.

With respect to the effect of other stresses on venous compliance, it has been found that compliance is reduced in both hypertension and congestive heart failure. Because of the marked increase in extracellular fluid volume and the associated edema in congestive heart failure, it is thought that the decrease in compliance is probably of little primary importance in compensating for the failure state. In the early stages, however, before CHF is fully established, the early increase in blood volume coupled with venoconstriction may serve the function of increasing cardiac output as depicted in Fig. 9.6G. There appears to be no general consensus on the possible role of reduced venous compliance in hypertension except that a resultant reduction in venous volume might increase venous return, leading to increased cardiac output and a shift in blood volume favoring hypertension. This argument is weakened by the finding that cardiac output is normal and blood volume is reduced in established hypertension.

Antidiuretic hormone, aldosterone, adrenocorticotropic hormone, and epinephrine

Increases in plasma ADH and aldosterone concentrations after graded hemorrhage are depicted in Fig. 10.11. The release of ADH is attributed to a reflex mechanism in which a decrease in left atrial filling pressure leads to reduced input from stretch receptors in the wall of that chamber. (Ordinarily the input from these receptors inhibits ADH secretion.) The fall in atrial pressure also increases sympathetic activity in renal nerves and causes renal release of renin. Aldosterone levels increase after hemorrhage; there is also increased liberation of adrenocorticotropic hormone and epinephrine into the bloodstream. Receptor zones in the other atrium (right side) similarly contribute to the control of renin and corticosteroids. Through the combined effects of increased ADH, aldosterone, and sympathetic vasoconstriction of renal vessels, excretion of sodium and water is diminished and the fall in extracellular fluid volume is reduced.

Effects of shock on various organs

Heart

Reduction in cardiac output is one of the chief features of shock. An important initial cause is the reduction in cardiac filling that accompanies the reduction in blood volume. There is good evidence, however, that negative inotropic effects supervene during the course of shock. Thus primary myocardial failure has been said to be an integral and perhaps the principal factor responsible for irreversible shock. Prior digitalization of dogs before the hemorrhage tends to protect them against shock. The reduction in coronary blood flow at low blood pressures with consequent myocardial hypoxia (see "Positive Feedback in Progressive Shock" above) certainly has a negative inotropic action. This effect is reversible if transfusion restores myocardial oxygenation before cellular structural damage occurs. Postmortem examinations of hearts from animals that have died in shock, however, disclose subendocardial hemorrhage, focal areas of necrosis, and so-called zonal lesions. The latter consist of hypercontraction of the portion of myocytes adjacent to intercalated disks, fragmentation of the Z band, distortion of the myofilaments, and displacement of mitochondria from the region near the intercalated disks. These several lesions are like those seen after catecholamine overdosage and hypoxia.

Myocardial depressant factors (MDF). A variety of cardioinhibitory substances originating in the splanchnic region (i.e., pancreas, intestine, and perhaps liver) are liberated into the bloodstream during all types of circulatory shock. For the most part they appear to be small peptides in the range of 250 to 1000 Da. In addition to a negative inotropic effect, they exhibit other positive-feedback effects: (1) vasoconstriction, which increases splanchnic ischemia and further MDF formation, and (2) reticuloendothelial depression, which impairs clearance of MDF from the blood. They are probably produced by lysosomal and zymogenic proteolytic degradation of intracellular protein and are transported to the circulation via lymphatics and microcirculatory vessels.

Brain

At least a minimal blood flow to the brain is preserved in shock at the sacrifice of flow to the skin, splanchnic area, and kidneys. The latter experience vasoconstriction, whereas the cerebral circulation undergoes a compensatory vasodilatation. Despite this, brain function is compromised in severe shock as evidenced by depression of alertness and of the respiratory and vasomotor centers. In rats subjected to hemorrhage, the electrocorticographic activity is depressed and finally abolished, not to return even after restoration of blood pressure after transfusion.

Kidney

In progressive shock an intense renal arterial vasoconstriction causes ischemia of the kidney, with a reduction in glomerular filtration rate as well as in renal blood flow. Anuria may result, with retention of urea, creatinine, uric acid, and other metabolic products. Metabolic acidosis may ensue owing to failure of renal hydrogen ion excretion and the accumulation of serum phosphates and lactates. In shock following muscle contusion the released hemoglobin, myoglobin, and products of muscle autolysis may accumulate in the renal tubules and collecting ducts, blocking them (*lower nephron nephrosis*). In this instance, the renal failure may lead to death from uremia, even though transfusions have restored hemodynamic function.

The postshock kidney may fail to concentrate urine adequately. This is attributed to the loss of high osmolality in the papillary region, owing to a reduction of glomerular filtration while blood flow continues through the medulla. Thus, osmotically active substances are "washed out" of the normally hyperosmotic part of the medulla, and the concentrating mechanism of ADH is diminished or lost.

Prostaglandins of the renal medulla (PGE and PGE_2) may be involved in ADH antagonism and reduction of the electrolyte (Na^+, Ca^{2+}, and K^+) absorption in the postshock kidney. When released, these substances can relax vascular smooth muscle. This would increase medullary blood flow, favor the washout of electrolytes from the medullary interstitium, and thus oppose ADH action. Both catecholamines and angiotensin II, which are increased after hemorrhage, promote synthesis and release of these prostaglandins.

Liver

Liver function is disorganized in shock. A reduction in adenosine triphosphate and adenosine diphosphate concentrations accompanies impairment of urea formation, gluconeogenesis, and sodium-potassium transport across cell membranes. Intracellular sodium increases, water enters the cells, and cellular swelling results. Finally, liver cells lose their integrity and necrosis occurs.

Lung

A major determinant of survival after hemorrhagic or traumatic shock is the degree of associated pulmonary damage. In cats the most consistent finding is extensive interstitial edema around blood vessels that have a thick muscular tunica media. Apparently the precapillary arterioles and surrounding interstitium are the initial sites of injury, with the resulting edema, hemorrhage, and injury to the alveolar walls presumably contributing to the decreased oxygen saturation of blood that occurs in shock. Pulmonary edema is a consistent finding in the lungs of animals in shock, and intravascular coagulation in the microvasculature is a common terminal finding.

Irreversible shock and oxygen debt

In dogs with experimental irreversible shock, there is a positive correlation between the absolute amount of oxygen debt that the body builds up and the onset of shock. When the oxygen debt for the whole animal reaches about 120 ml of O_2 per kilogram of body weight, the irreversible stage of shock is reached. Prior digitalization raises the value of oxygen debt at which irreversible shock occurs, an example of the beneficial effect of digitalis mentioned previously. When an animal has incurred a lethal level of oxygen debt, transfusion may raise the cardiac output to control values temporarily, but ultimately cardiac output and blood pressure fall fatally.

Thirst

The insatiable thirst characteristic of shock is attributed to stimulation of hypothalamic drinking centers by angiotensin II, the formation of which is initiated by renin released from the kidney.

The cardinal treatment of shock is restoration of blood volume with transfusion of whole blood, blood plasma, or, if neither is available, plasma expanders such as dextran or polyvinylpyrrolidone. The use of vasopressor agents (e.g., norepinephrine, metaraminol) has been unsuccessful in hypovolemic shock because the high levels of sympathetic activity and circulating catecholamines have already effected maximal vasoconstriction. In fact, there is evidence that dogs previously rendered tolerant to the action of epinephrine are resistant to the induction of cardiogenic, hemorrhagic, or endotoxic shock. Presumably, excessive vasoconstriction in shock throttles regional blood supply and, in itself, has an untoward action. This may be another example of a positive feedback. It has led to the therapeutic use of vasodilator agents (e.g., methylprednisolone), provided that the blood pressure has first been restored by transfusion. Although transfusion appears to overcome the principal problem of peripheral vascular failure in shock, it does not counteract the primary myocardial depression. Glucocorticoids and the protease inhibitors (e.g., aprotinin) and certain prostaglandins are beneficial in preventing MDF formation. Positive inotropic agents (e.g., digitalis, glucagon, isoproterenol, dopamine, calcium ion) combat the myocardial depression but have not been notably successful in improving survival. In anaphylactic shock, catecholamines antagonize histamine therapeutically, and antihistaminic agents are useful prophylactically but have far less therapeutic value.

Summary

Figure 12.6 summarizes many of the interacting mechanisms involved in the development of circulatory shock.

Renin release

The renin-angiotensin-aldosterone system is involved in the several circulatory stress states just reviewed. Figure 12.7 summarizes factors that have been shown to stimulate or inhibit renin release.

PULMONARY HYPERTENSION

Three chief types of pulmonary hypertension (a vascular disease of the lung) are distinguished: (1) *passive,* caused by increased pulmonary venous pressure as seen in mitral valve insufficiency or left ventricular failure; (2) *hyperkinetic,* owing to marked increase in pulmonary blood flow as in large left-to-right shunts such as patent ductus arteriosus and ventricular septal defects; and (3) *vaso-occlusive,* resulting from a variety of causes that produce obliteration, obstruction, or increased vasoconstriction of pulmonary arteries (e.g., chronic pneumonia, emphysema, dirofilariasis, and brisket disease). It can overtax the right ventricle, causing right ventricular CHF. *Cor pulmonale* is the term given to the resultant dilatation and hypertrophy of the heart.

Reflex effects of pulmonary venous congestion

When left ventricular dysfunction is the cause of reduced venous return from the lungs (e.g., in mitral insuffiency), such clinical signs as restlessness at night, coughing, dyspnea with exercise, and respiratory wheezing ("cardiac

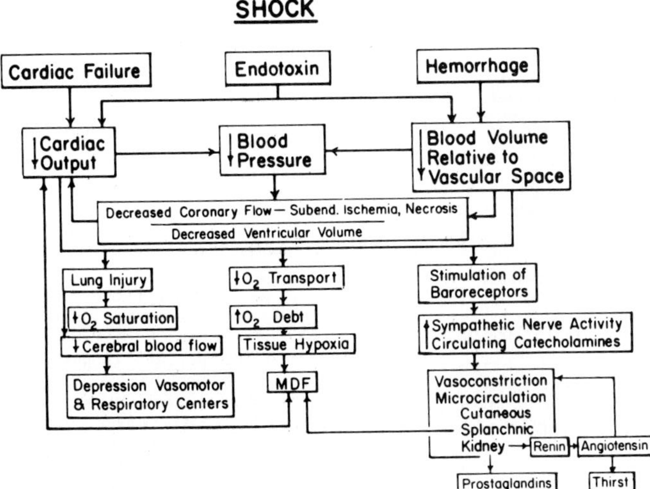

Figure 12.6. Schema representing interrelations of various factors contributing to the development of irreversible shock from various causes. Positive-feedback effects that further cardiovascular deterioration are emphasized. Arrows in boxes indicate increase (↑) or decrease (↓). The arrows connecting the boxes indicate the effects of the various changes depicted. MDF, myocardial depressant factors; Subend., subendocardial. The effects of endotoxin injected into healthy dogs (as well as cardiac failure and hemorrhage) are represented in this diagram. The mechanism in endotoxic shock is thought to result from peripheral pooling of blood, hemoconcentration owing to transudation of plasma water into the extravascular space, and consequent decreased venous return to the heart (Dedichen and Schenk 1967, Gilder et al. 1970). Endotoxin may also depress the myocardium (Bell and Thal 1970). In septic shock in humans, the hemodynamic picture varies with the underlying clinical state. Although reduction in cardiac output is often observed, it may be normal or elevated. In the latter cases there is evidence of precapillary arteriovenous shunting of blood (Bell and Thal 1970). (From Detweiler 1979, in Brobeck, ed., *Best & Taylor's Physiological Basis of Medical Practice,* 10th ed., © 1979, the Williams & Wilkins Co., Baltimore.)

asthma") occur. These signs result from accumulation of fluid in the peribronchial space. Such venous congestion can be induced in anesthetized dogs when the left atrial pressure is raised to 5 to 10 mm Hg by obstruction of the mitral valve with a balloon. Increasing the left atrial pressure to about 23 mm Hg leads to flooding of the alveoli to produce acute pulmonary edema.

The vagal rapidly adapting (stretch) receptors, located in the larger airways, respond to the increased microvascular pressures in pulmonary congestion and are markedly sensitive to increases in the quantity of fluid in the pulmonary extravascular space, apparently because this compresses the venous drainage of the bronchial mucosa. One of the reflex effects of stimulation of the rapidly adapting receptors is bronchoconstriction, which may account for the wheezing of "cardiac asthma" and the accelerated respiratory rate.

Three clinical syndromes associated with pulmonary hypertension in domestic animals are recognized: (1) brisket disease of cattle, (2) emphysema (heaves) in horses, and (3) heartworm heart disease in dogs. *Brisket disease* (named for the edema in the brisket region that develops in cattle with CHF) or *high mountain disease* results from a vasoconstrictive pulmonary hypertension that develops from alveolar hypoxia in cattle kept at altitudes above 7000 feet. Calves and pigs have relatively more vascular smooth muscle in both pulmonary arteries and veins and are highly responsive to hypoxia-induced pulmonary hypertension. In emphysema or heaves of horses, when alveolar hypoxia becomes severe enough pulmonary hypertension results, but cor pulmonale is found only infrequently. In heartworm heart disease in dogs, occlusive sclerosis of the smaller pulmonary arteries, resulting from the presence of adult worms in the heart and in the arterial lumina, causes pulmonary hypertension, cor pulmonale, and right-sided CHF.

CONGENITAL HEART DISEASE

Patent ductus arteriosus, pulmonic stenosis, subaortic stenosis, interventricular septal defect, and tetralogy of Fallot are common examples of congenital heart lesions in domestic animals (Fig. 12.8A and B). Review of the cardiac cycle events (Chap. 8) will permit an understanding of the physiological effects of these anomalies. In patent

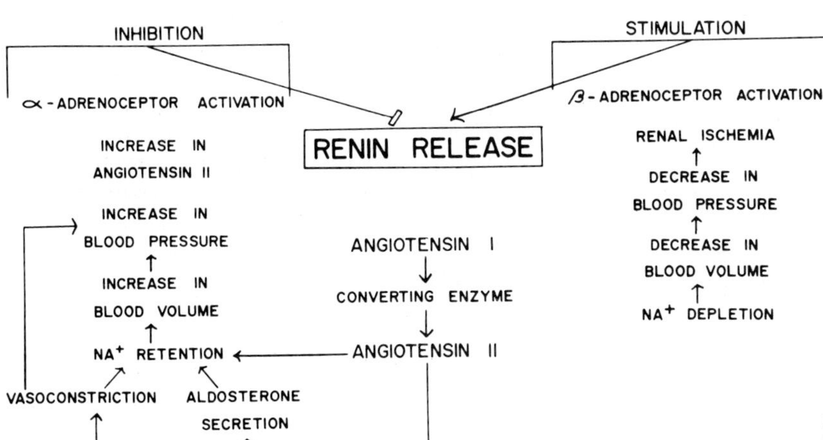

Figure 12.7. Summary of factors that regulate the release of renin. NA+, sodium ion.

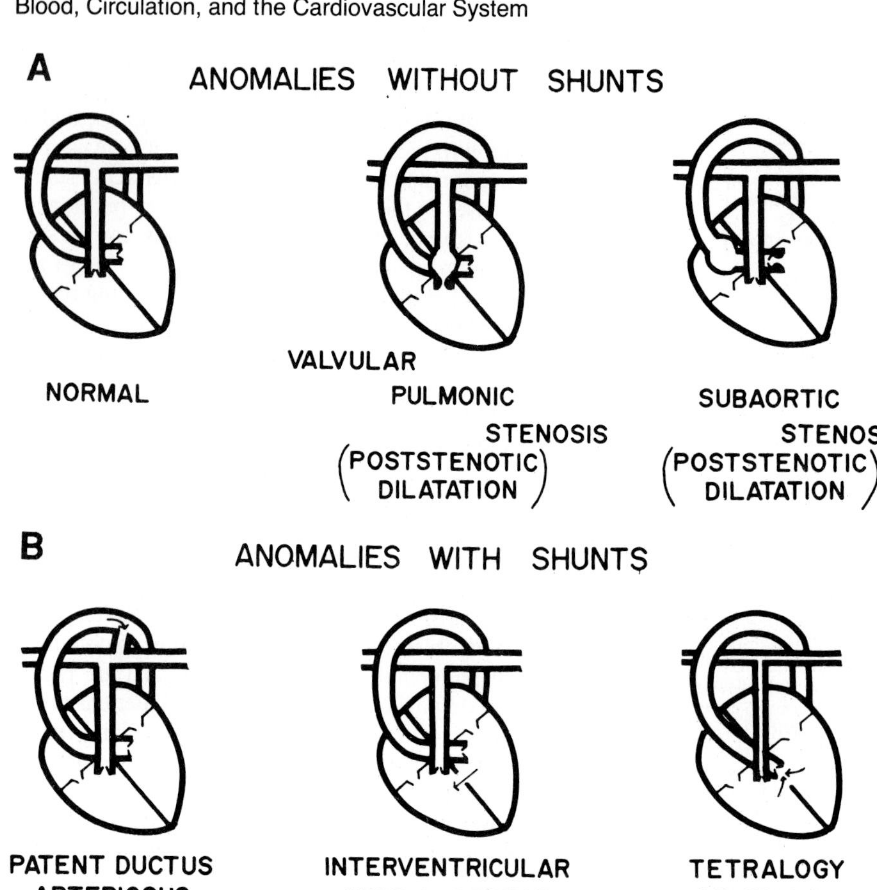

Figure 12.8. (*A*) Schemata of some common congenital cardiac anomalies without shunts. The basic scheme is seen in the normal sketch. The left cardiac chambers are depicted on the right (and vice versa), and the aorta arches over the T-shaped pulmonary artery and its major branches. The pulmonary artery arises from the right ventricle and crosses the aorta. Poststenotic dilatations are likely to occur downstream from stenoses and are shown here for pulmonic valvular stenosis in the pulmonary artery (middle diagram) and for subaortic stenosis in the aorta (right diagram). The stenoses are here represented by the thickened walls and narrowed orifices at the vessel origin. (*B*) Schemata of some common congenital cardiac anomalies with shunts. Shunts are abnormal communications between the right and left sides of the heart or between the pulmonic and systemic circulations. When the flow of blood through the shunt is from right to left, unoxygenated blood can bypass the lungs and reach the systemic arterial system, causing cyanosis of visible mucous membranes and reduced oxygen delivery to all tissues.

ductus arteriosus some of the blood is shunted from the aorta to the pulmonary artery, increasing pulmonary blood flow by the addition of already oxygenated blood and increasing left ventricular work. The flow of blood causes a continuous murmur that waxes and wanes with each pulse beat, the *machinery murmur.* Less commonly, the flow through the patent ductus is reversed (i.e., from right to left) because of pulmonary hypertension, and unoxygenated blood enters the aorta and causes peripheral cyanosis. In this case there is no machinery murmur, but affected dogs cannot run far because oxygen-poor blood is delivered to their hind legs, causing muscle exhaustion (their tongues and other cranial mucous membranes are not cyanotic because the patent ductus shunt enters the aorta after the cranial arteries are given off). In *aortic* or *pulmonic stenosis* (Fig. 12.8A) the affected ventricle must generate high systolic pressures to maintain normal arterial pressure and flow; this results in ventricular hypertrophy and turbulence during ejection of blood, causing a systolic murmur and poststenotic dilatation of the artery (Fig. 12.8B). In tetralogy of Fallot there is (1) pulmonary artery stenosis, (2) high ventricular septal defect, (3) dextroposition of the aorta over the ventricular septum, and (4) right ventricular hypertrophy. Blood flow to the lung is deficient, and unoxygenated blood enters the aorta, causing cyanosis; there are no distinctive murmurs.

VALVULAR HEART DISEASE

When the cardiac valves are sufficiently deformed by acquired disease changes, their openings may be narrowed or *stenosed* or proper closure may be prevented, and regurgitation or *insufficiency* occurs. These impediments to forward flow of blood result in increased myocardial work in one or more of the cardiac chambers; dilatation and hypertrophy result and may end in CHF. In addition to the congenital stenosis mentioned in the foregoing, mitral insufficiency is especially common in dogs and accounts for most acquired heart disease in this species.

REFERENCES

Abboud, F. 1982. The sympathetic system in hypertension. State-of-the-art review. *Hypertension* 4(Suppl. II):II-208–II-225.

Alonso, F.R.A. 1972. Distribution of the cardiac output in the greyhound dog. Thesis, University of Pennsylvania.

Andersen, H.T. 1967. Cardiovascular adaptations in diving mammals. *Am. Heart J.* 74:295–98.

Ayers, C.R., Davies, J.O., Lieberman, F., Carpenter, C.C.J., and Ber-man, M. 1962. The effects of chronic hepatic venous congestion on the metabolism of d, l-aldosterone and d-aldosterone. *J. Clin. Invest.* 41:884–95.

Barger, A.C., Muldowney, F.P., and Lubowitz, M.R. 1959. Role of the kidney in the pathogenesis of congestive heart failure. *Circulation* 20:273–85.

Barger, A.C., Yates, T.E., and Rudolph, A.M. 1961. Renal hemodynamics and sodium excretion in dogs with graded valvular damage. *Am. J. Physiol.* 200:601–8.

Bell, H., and Thal, A. 1970. The peculiar hemodynamics of septic shock. *Postgrad. Med.* 48:106–14.

Belleau, L., Mion, H., Simard, S., Granger, P., Bertranou, E., Nowaczynski, W., Boucher, R., and Genest, J. 1970. Studies on the mechanism of congestive heart failure in dogs. *Can. J. Physiol. Pharmacol.* 48:450–56.

Braunwald, E., Ross, J., Jr., and Sonnenblick, E.H. 1967, 1968. *Mechanisms of Contraction of the Normal and Failing Heart.* Little, Brown, Boston.

Brody, M.J. 1981. New developments in our knowledge of blood pressure regulation. *Fed. Proc.* 40:2257–61.

Bron, K.M., Murdaugh, H.V., Jr., Millen, J.E., Lenthall, R., Raskin, P., and Robin, E.D. 1966. Arterial constrictor response in a diving mammal. *Science* 152:540–43.

Buckley, J.P., Lokhandwala, M.F., Steenberg, M., Francis, J.S., and Tadepalli, A.S. 1981. Cardiovascular effects of chronic intraventricular administration of angiotensin II in dogs. *Clin. Exp. Hypertens.* 3:1001–18.

Buller, A.J., Mommaerts, W.F.H., and Seraydarian, K. 1969. Enzymatic properties of mysoin in fast and slow twitch muscles of the cat following cross-innervation. *J. Physiol.* 205:581–97.

Bumpus, F.M., Sen, S., Smeby, R.R., Sweet, C., Ferrario, C.M., and Koshla, M.C. 1973. Use of angiotensin II antagonists in experimental hypertension. *Circ. Res.* 32, 33(Suppl. I):150–58.

Cannon, P.J. 1989. Sodium retention in heart failure. *Cardiol. Clin.* 7:49–62.

Carew, T.E., and Covell, J.W. 1978. Left ventricular function in exercise-induced hypertrophy in dogs. *Am. J. Cardiol.* 42:82–88.

Clausen, J.P. 1969. The effects of physical conditioning: A hypothesis concerning circulatory adjustments to exercise. *Scand. J. Clin. Lab. Invest.* 24:305–13.

Cody, R.J. 1989. Neurohumoral influences in the pathogenesis of congestive heart failure. *Cardiol. Clin.* 7, 73–86.

Coleman, T.G., Cowley, A.W., Jr., and Guyton, A. 1974. Experimental hypertension and long-term control of arterial pressure. In A.C. Guyton and C.E. Jones, eds., *Cardiovascular Physiology.* University Park Press, Baltimore. Pp. 259–97.

Courtice, F.C. 1943. The blood volume of normal animals. *J. Physiol.* 102:290–305.

Cox, R.H., Peterson, L.H., and Detweiler, D.K. 1976. Hemodynamics in the mongrel dog and the racing greyhound. *Am. J. Physiol.* 230:211–18.

Davis, J.O. 1974. The renin angiotensin system in the control of aldosterone secretion. In I.H. Page and F.M. Bumpus, eds., *Handbuch der experimentellen Pharmakologie.* Springer, Berlin. P. 372.

Davis, J.O., and Freeman, R.H. 1982. Historical perspectives on the renin-angiotensin-aldosterone system and angiotensin blockade. *Am. J. Cardiol.* 49:1385–89.

Davis, J.O., Howell, D.S., and Hyatt, R.E. 1955. Sodium excretion in adrenalectomized dogs with chronic cardiac failure produced by pulmonary artery constriction. *Am. J. Physiol.* 183:263–68.

Dedichen, H., and Schenk, W.G., Jr. 1967. Hemodynamics of endotoxin shock in the dog. *Arch. Surg.* 95:1013–16.

Dequattro, V., and Miura, Y. 1974. Neurogenic factors in human hypertension: Mechanism or myth? In J.H. Laragh, ed., *Hypertension Manual.* Yorke Med., New York. Pp. 227–311.

Detweiler, D.K. 1964. Genetic aspects of cardiovascular diseases in animals. *Circulation* 30:114–27.

Detweiler, D.K., Cox, R.H., Alonso, R., Knight, D.H., Bagshaw, R., Jones, A., and Peterson, L.H. 1974. Hemodynamic characteristics of the young adult greyhound. *Fed. Proc.* 33:360.

Detweiler, D.K., Cox, R.H., Alonso, F.R., and Patterson, D.F. 1975. Characteristics of the greyhound cardiovascular system. *Fed. Proc.* 34:399.

Detweiler, D.K., and Patterson, D.F. 1972. Diseases of the blood and cardiovascular system. In E.J. Catcott, ed., *Equine Medicine and Surgery.* Am. Vet. Public., Santa Barbara, Calif. Pp. 277–347.

Detweiler, D.K., and Trautvetter, E. 1980. Bluthochdruck, Vorkommen und klinische Bedeutung. *Kleintier Praxis* 25:227–34.

Dietzman, R.H., Motsay, G.J., and Lillehei, R.C. 1971. Shock: Circulatory effects and treatment. In H.L. Conn, Jr., and O. Horowitz, eds., *Cardiac and Vascular Diseases.* Vol. 1. Lea & Febiger, Philadelphia. Pp. 577–89.

Donald, D.E., and Ferguson, D.A. 1966. Response of heart rate, oxygen consumption, and arterial blood pressure to graded exercise in dogs. *Proc. Soc. Exp. Bio. Med.* 121:626–29.

Drummond, P.C., and Jones, D.R. 1979. The initiation and maintenance of bradycardia in a diving mammal, the muskrat, *Ondatra zibethica. J. Physiol.* 290:253–71.

Dustan, H.P., Tarazi, R.C., and Bravo, E.L. 1974. Physiologic characteristics of hypertension. In J.H. Laragh, ed., *Hypertension Manual.* Yorke Med., New York. Pp. 227–56.

Dzua, V.J., and Creager, M.A. 1989. Progress in angiotensin-converting enzyme inhibition in heart failure. *Cardiol. Clin.* 7, 119–30.

Elsner, R., and Daly, M. de B. 1988. Coping with asphyxia: Lessons from seals. *News Physiol. Sci.* 3:65–69.

Epstein, A. 1978. Consensus, controversies, and curiosities (angiotensin II and thirst). *Fed. Proc.* 37:2711–16.

Ferrario, C.M., Barnes, K.L., and Bohonek, S. 1981. Neurogenic hypertension produced by lesions of the nucleus tractus solitarii alone or with sinoaortic denervation in the dog. *Hypertension* 3(Suppl. II.):II-112–II-118.

Fitzsimmons, J.T. 1978. Angiotensin, thirst and sodium appetite: Retrospect and prospect. *Fed. Proc.* 37:2669–75.

Garner, H.E., Hahn, A.W., Salena, C., Coffman, J.R., Hutcheson, D.P., and Johnson, J.H. 1977. Cardiac output, left ventricular ejection rate, plasma volume, and heart rate changes in equine laminitis-hypertension. *Am. J. Vet. Res.* 38:725–29.

Gauer, O.H. 1968. Zentrales Blutvolumen, Herzleistung und Flussigkeitshaushalt. In H. Reindell, J. Keul, and E. Doll, eds., *Herzinsuffiziens.* Thieme, Stuttgart. Pp. 523–29.

Gauer, O.H., and Henry, J.P. 1976. Neurohumoral control of plasma volume. In A.C. Guyton and A.W. Cowley, eds., *Cardiovascular Physiology,* vol. 2. University Park Press, Baltimore. 145–90.

Gilder, H., Cortese, A.F., Loehr, W.J., Moore, H.V., and De Leon, V. 1970. Dilution studies in experimental hemorrhagic and endotoxic shock. *Ann. Surg.* 171:42–50.

Goldblatt, H. 1958. Experimental renal hypertension: Mechanism of production and maintenance. *Circulation* 17(pt. 2):642–47.

Goldblatt, H., Lynch, J., Hanzal, R.F., and Summerville, W.W. 1934. Studies in experimental hypertension. I. The production of persistent elevation of systolic blood pressure by means of renal ischemia. *J. Exp. Med.* 59:347–79.

Gordon, M. 1972. *Animal Physiology: Principles and Adaptations.* 2d ed. Macmillan, New York.

Guth, L. 1968. Trophic influences of nerve on muscle. *Physiol. Rev.* 48:645–87.

Guyton, A.C. 1981. The relationship of cardiac output and arterial pressure control. *Circulation* 64:1079–88.

Guyton, A.C., Coleman, T.G., Cowley, A.W., Jr., Scheel, K.W., Manning, R.D., and Norman, R.A. 1974. Arterial pressure regulation: Overriding dominance of the kidneys in long-term regulation and in hypertension. In J.H. Laragh, ed., *Hypertension Manual.* Yorke Med., New York. Pp. 111–34.

Guyton, A.C., Jones, C.E., and Coleman, T.G. 1973. *Circulatory Physi-*

ology: Cardiac Output and Its Regulation. 2d ed. W.B. Saunders, Philadelphia.

Hackel, D.B., Ratliff, N.B., and Mikat, E. 1974. The heart in shock. *Circ. Res.* 35:805–11.

Hecht, H.H. 1956. Heart failure and lung disease. *Circulation* 14:265–290.

Henry, J.P., and Meehan, J.P. 1971. *The Circulation*. Year Book, Chicago.

Kallet, A., and Cowgill, L.D. 1982. Hypertensive states in the dog. *Proc. Ann. Mtg. Am. Coll. Vet. Int. Med.* P. 79.

Kovach, A.G.B. 1971. Metabolic changes in hemorrhagic shock. *Adv. Exp. Med. Biol.* 23:275–78.

Laird, S.F., Tarazi, R.C., Ferrario, C.M., and Manger, W. 1975. Hemodynamic and humoral characteristics of hypertension induced by prolonged stellate ganglion stimulation in conscious dogs. *Circ. Res.* 36:455–64.

Lefer, A.M. 1978. Properties of cardioinhibitory factors produced in shock. *Fed. Proc.* 37:2734–40.

Lupu, A.N., Maxwell, H., Kaufman, J.J., and White, F.N. 1972. Experimental unilateral renal artery constriction in the dog. *Circ. Res.* 30:567–74.

MacGregor, G.A., and de Wardener, H.E. 1981. Is a circulating sodium transport inhibitor involved in the pathogenesis of essential hypertension? *Clin. Exp. Hypertens.* 3:815–30.

Marx, J. 1982. The leukotrienes in allergy and inflammation. *Science* 215:1380–83.

Meixner, R., Hörnicke, H., and Ehrlein, H. 1981. Oxygen consumption, pulmonary ventilation, and heart rate of riding horses during walk, trot, and gallop. In W. Sanson, ed., *Biotelemetry VI*. Univ. of Arkansas Press, Fayetteville.

Michelassi, F., Landa, L., Hill, R.D., Lowenstein, E., Watkins, W.D., Petkau, A.J., and Zapol, W. 1982. Leukotriene D(4): A potent coronary artery vasoconstrictor associated with impaired ventricular contraction. *Science* 217:841–43.

Millard, R.W., Higgins, C.B., Franklin, D., and Vatner, S.F. 1972. Regulation of renal circulation during severe exercise in normal dogs and dogs with experimental heart failure. *Circ. Res.* 31:881–88.

Noble, D., and Gregerson, M.I. 1946. Blood volume in clinical shock. II. The extent and cause of blood volume reduction in traumatic hemorrhagic and burn shock. *J. Clin. Invest.* 25:172.

Nylander, E., Sigvardson, K., and Kilbom, A. 1982. Training-induced bradycardia and intrinsic heart rate in rats. *Eur. J. Appl. Physiol.* 48:189–99.

Okamoto, K., ed. 1972. *Spontaneous Hypertension: Its Pathogenesis and Complications*. Igaku Shoin, Tokyo.

Page, I.H., and McCubbin, J.W. 1968. *Renal Hypertension*. Year Book, Chicago.

Pfeffer, M.A., and Frohlich, E.D. 1973. Hemodynamic and myocardial function in young and old normotensive and spontaneously hypertensive rats. *Circ. Res.* 31,32(Suppl. I):I-29–I-38.

Pfeffer, M.A., Frohlich, E.D., Pfeffer, J.M., and Weiss, A.K. 1974. Pathophysiological implications of the increased cardiac output of young spontaneously hypertensive rats. *Circ. Res.* 34,35(Suppl. I):I-235–I-244.

Ratliff, N.B., Wilson, J.W., Hackel, D.B., and Martin, A.M., Jr. 1970. The lung in hemorrhagic shock II. Observations on alveolar and vascular ultrastructure. *Am. J. Pathol.* 58:353–73.

Ravi, K., and Kappagoda, C.T. 1990. Reflex effects of pulmonary venous congestion: Role of vagal afferents. *News Physiol. Sci.* 5:95–9.

Rhodin, J.A.G. 1980. Architecture of the vessel wall. In D.F. Bohr, A.P. Somlyo, and H.V. Sparks, Jr., eds., *Handbook of Physiology.* Sec. 2, The Cardiovascular System. Vol. 2, *Vascular Smooth Muscle*. Am. Physiol. Soc., Bethesda, Md. Pp. 1–31.

Rothe, C.F. 1983. Venous system: Physiology of the capacitance vessels. In J.T. Shepperd and F.M. Abboud, eds., *Handbook of Physiology.* Sec. 2, *The Cardiovascular System,* vol. III. *Peripheral Circulation and Organ Blood Flow.* Part 1. Am. Physiol. Soc., Bethesda, Md. Pp. 397–452.

Rushmer, R.F. 1970. *Cardiovascular Dynamics,* 3d ed. W.B. Saunders, Philadelphia.

Schalekemp, M.A., Beevers, D.G., Briggs, J.D., Brown, J.J., Davies, D.L., Fraser, R., Lebel, M., Lever, A.F., Medina, A., Morton, JJ., Robertson, J.O.S., and Tree, M. 1974. Hypertension in chronic renal failure: An abnormal relation between sodium and the renin-angiotensin system. In J.H. Laragh, ed., *Hypertension Manual.* Yorke Med., New York. Pp. 485–508.

Schlager, G. 1972. Spontaneous hypertension in laboratory animals: A review of the genetic implications. *J. Heredity* 63:35–38.

Schmidt-Nielsen, K. 1975. *Animal Physiology.* Cambridge University Press, Cambridge.

Schwartz, A.L., Sordahl, A., Entman, M.L., Allen, J.C., Reddy, Y.S., Goldstern, M.A., Luchi, R.J., and Wyborny, L.E. 1976. Abnormal biochemistry in myocardial failure. In D.T. Mason, ed., *Congestive Heart Failure*. Yorke Med., New York. Pp. 25–44.

Selkurt, E.E. 1969. Primate kidney function in hemorrhagic shock. *Am. J. Physiol.* 217:955–61.

Selkurt, E.E. 1976. Physiology of shock. In E.E. Selkurt, ed. *Physiology.* Little, Brown, Boston. Pp. 419–34.

Spangler, W.L., Gribble, D.H., and Weisser, M.G. 1977. Canine hypertension: A review. *J. Am. Vet. Med. Assoc.* 170:995–98.

Staaden, R. 1980. Cardiovascular system of the racing dog. In R.W. Kirk, ed., *Current Veterinary Therapy. VII. Small Animal Practice.* Yorke Med., New York. Pp. 347–51.

Thoren, P. 1979. Role of vagal C-fibers in cardiovascular control. *Rev. Physiol. Biochem. and Pharmacol.* 86:1–94.

Tobian, L., Jr. 1974. A viewpoint concerning the enigma of hypertension. In J.H. Laragh, ed., *Hypertension Manual.* Yorke Med., New York. Pp. 135–62.

Tonkin, M.J., Rosen, S.M., and Mason, D.T. 1976. Renal function and edema formation in congestive heart failure. In D.T. Mason, ed., *Congestive Heart Failure.* Yorke Med., New York. Pp. 169–79.

Urquhart, J., and Davis, J.O. 1963. Role of the kidney and the adrenal cortex in congestive heart failure. *Mod. Concepts Cardiovasc. Dis.* 32:787–92.

Van Citters, R.L., and Franklin, D.L. 1969a. Cardiovascular research in wild animals: Telemetry technics and applications. *Acta Zool. Pathol. Antwerp.* 48:243–63.

Van Citters, R.L., and Franklin, D.L. 1969b. Cardiovascular responses in Alaska sled dogs during exercise. *Circ. Res.* 24:33–42.

von Engelhardt, W. 1977. Cardiovascular effects of exercise and training in horses. In C.A. Brandly, C.E. Cornelius, and C.F. Simpson, eds., *Advances in Vet. Sci.* 21:173-204. Academic Press, New York.

von Engelhardt, W. 1979. Die Wirking von Arbeit im Training auf Herz und Kreislauf des Pferdes. *Deutsche Tierärztl. Wochenschr.* 86:2–7.

Webb, R.C., and Bohr, D.F. 1981. Recent advances in the pathogenesis of hypertension: Consideration of structural, functional and metabolic vascular abnormalities resulting in elevated arterial resistance. *Am. Heart J.* 102:251–64.

Weber, K.T., and Janicki, J.S. 1989. Pathogenesis of heart failure. *Cardiol. Clin.* 7:11–24.

Wiggers, C.J. 1950. *Physiology of Shock.* Commonwealth Fund, New York.

Wilmore, J.H., and Norton, A.C. 1974. *The Heart and Lungs at Work: A Primer of Exercise Physiology.* Beckman Instruments, Schiller Park, Ill.

Wilson, J.W., Ratliff, N.B., and Hackel, D.B. 1970. The lung in hemorrhagic shock. 1. In vivo observations of pulmonary microcirculation in cats. *Am. J. Pathol.* 58:337–51.

Yonce, R., and Folkow, B. 1970. The integration of the cardiovascular response to diving. *Am. Heart J.* 79:1–4.

Yoshino, H., Curran-Everett, D.C., Hong, S.K., and Krasney, J.A. 1988. Altered heart rate-arterial pressure relation during head-out water immersion in conscious dog. *Am. J. Physiol.* 254:R595–R601.

Zelis, R., and Flaim, S.F. 1982. Alterations in vasomotor tone in congestive heart failure. *Prog. Cardiovasc. Dis.* 24:437–59.

PART **II** RESPIRATION AND EXERCISE

CHAPTER 13

Respiration in Mammals

by William O. Reece

Respiratory phenomena that now appear elementary were, in fact, important discoveries of their day. Galen, in the second century A.D., observed that blood entered the lung and became charged with a "vital spirit." By experimentation, he showed that arteries contain only blood and that they are not pneumatic structures as previously believed. Marcello Malpighi, in the seventeenth century, observed that air passes through the trachea in and out of saccules in the lung and ruled out the theory that there is a direct passage for air from the lung to the left ventricle of the heart. He also observed that closed blood vessels were spread out over the surface of these saccules and that the blood was always separated from the air. It was also during this period that Richard Lower showed that the change in blood color from dark red to bright red occurred in the lung as a result of receiving something from the air. Also, John Mayow found that a decrease in air volume accompanied both respiration and combustion; this finding provided proof that something was absorbed from the air. A century later, Antoine Lavoisier explained the true nature of combustion and respiration, showing that they are similar processes that involve the uptake of what he named "oxygine" from the air and the production of "carbonic acid gas."

The question of how oxygen and carbon dioxide moved between blood and pulmonary alveoli was not answered until the early twentieth century when August and Marie Krogh obtained quantitative evidence that pulmonary diffusion, without secretion, accounted for this movement. It is apparent that many views about respiratory function were developed and discarded throughout this long period of time. It should not be disappointing, then, when our understanding of a particular physiological phenomenon must be abandoned because newer knowledge proves it to be wrong. It has been this way for centuries and quite likely will continue into the future. The following presentation of respiratory physiology will include those concepts of a basic nature that at present appear logical.

PHYSICAL PRINCIPLES OF GAS EXCHANGE

Physics of gases

Several physical laws are helpful in the study of gases. *Boyle's law* relates pressure to volume. If the mass and temperature of a gas in a chamber remain constant but the pressure is increased or decreased, the volume of the gas varies inversely with the pressure:

$$\text{Volume} = \frac{\text{Constant}}{\text{Pressure}}$$

Charles' law notes the effect of temperature on gas volume. If the pressure of a given quantity of gas remains constant but the temperature is varied, the volume of the gas increases directly in proportion to the increase in temperature:

$$\text{Volume} = \text{Constant} \times \text{Temperature}$$

Temperature adjustment is critical in the operation of blood-gas analyzers used for the determination of gas partial pressures in blood. The water bath temperature needs to be adjusted to the temperature of the animal body. In these instruments, the volume is not expandable; temperature increases would show increases in partial pressure, and temperature decreases would show decreases in partial pressure. Finally, a very important law to understand is *Henry's law*, which relates to the volumes of gases that dissolve in water. Specifically, the quantity of gas dissolved in water at equilibrium is affected by the pressure of the gas to which the water is exposed and also by the solubility coefficient of the gas and is directly proportional to each:

$$\text{Volume} = \text{Pressure} \times \text{Solubility coefficient}$$

The gases of concern for the body water of animals are carbon dioxide, oxygen, and nitrogen. Carbon dioxide is the most soluble of these gases, being about 24 times more soluble than oxygen. Nitrogen is the least soluble, being about one-half as soluble as oxygen.

The partial pressure of a gas is a common concept associated with respiratory physiology. It may be defined as the pressure exerted by a given gas in a mixture of gases. The sum of the partial pressures of each of the gases in a mixture is always equal to the total pressure. Specific partial pressures are identified by symbols appended to P, which is the physiological designation for partial pressure. For example, the designation of the partial pressure of oxygen would be PO_2. Further particularization is achieved with the use of additional symbols. Arterial, venous, and alveolar descriptions are commonly used and are referred to by the symbols a, v, and A, respectively. The partial pressure of CO_2 in arterial blood is designated as either $PaCO_2$ or arterial PCO_2. Other symbols will be defined when used. They will become familiar with use.

If oxygen comprises 20 percent of a gas mixture that has a total pressure of 760 mm Hg, then the partial pressure of oxygen is the product of its percentage composition and total pressure of the mixture ($PO_2 = 0.20 \times 760$ mm Hg = 152 mm Hg).

Gases exhibit net movement by simple diffusion in response to pressure differences. Net diffusion occurs from areas of high pressure to areas of lower pressure, and this applies to gases in a gas mixture, gases in a solution, and gases from the gas phase into the dissolved state (application of Henry's law).

There is a tendency for students to believe that high partial pressures of gases in a liquid are invariably related to large volumes of a gas in that liquid. That this is not correct may be explained by the solubility factor associated with Henry's law. At equal partial pressures, one could expect to find 24 times more CO_2 than O_2 in water because of the greater solubility of CO_2.

It is difficult to visualize a partial pressure for water. One must remember that water has a gas phase known as vapor. The vapor pressure of water is caused by the molecules of water at the surface tending to escape into the gas above the liquid. When the temperature of the water is increased, the tendency of the water molecules to escape is also increased. The symbol for water vapor pressure is PH_2O, and at a barometric pressure of 760 mm Hg, PH_2O is equal to 47 mm Hg at 37°C and 52 mm Hg at 39°C. The average deep body temperature in many of the domestic animals is 39°C.

Factors affecting gas diffusion

The physical proximity of pulmonary alveolar gas to blood is shown in Fig. 13.1. Diffusion occurs between these two media, which are separated by the respiratory membrane. In general, the respiratory membrane is composed of alveolar epithelium, alveolar epithelium basement membrane, interstitial space, capillary endothelium basement membrane, and capillary endothelium. This figure probably represents a minimum distance between the gas and the blood; the pulmonary separation certainly can become greater, depending on the interposition of cells and the amount of interstitial space. The diffusion rate (DR) of gas through the respiratory membrane is related to pressure difference (PD), surface area (A), diffusion distance (D), solubility of the gas (S), and molecular weight of the gas (MW). An algebraic relationship exists as follows:

$$DR = \frac{PD \times A \times S}{D \times \sqrt{MW}}$$

The diffusion coefficient for any gas is proportional to $S/\sqrt{MW}$ so that these terms could be replaced by diffusion coefficient in the numerator. The diffusion coefficient for CO_2 through the respiratory membrane is about 20 times more than that for O_2. Also, as the distance of diffusion increases, as in pulmonary interstitial edema, the diffusion rate decreases. Under this condition, one may notice greater ventilation efforts in an attempt to compensate for the hypoxemia (decreased O_2 concentration in arterial blood) that has developed because of the reduced rate of diffusion. Blood-gas analysis shows reduced partial pressures for O_2 and CO_2. Because of the decrease in diffusion rate due to distance, one might have expected an increase in CO_2 in view of its reduced elimination. Its diffusion coefficient is much greater than that for O_2, however, so that the increased ventilation overcompensates for diffusion decrease due to distance. Another feature of the algebraic relation-

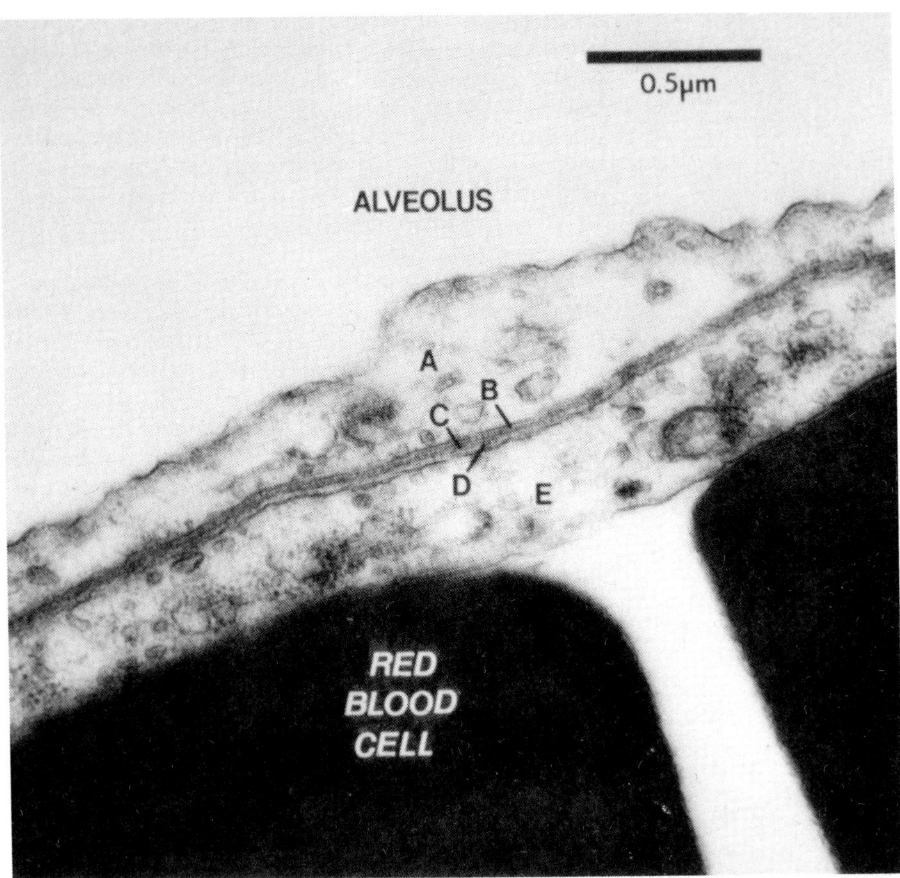

Figure 13.1. Electron micrograph of mouse lung showing attenuated portion of alveolar epithelium and its proximity to capillary endothelium. The respiratory membrane (without alveolar fluid layer) is composed of alveolar epithelium (A), alveolar epithelial basement membrane (B), interstitial space (C), capillary endothelial basement membrane (D), and capillary endothelium (E).

ship worth noting is the direct relationship of surface area to diffusion rate. Small mammals have very high oxygen requirements in comparison with large mammals because the basal oxygen requirement is more nearly proportional to body surface area than to body weight. Small mammals, however, have about the same proportion of lung volume to body weight as large mammals. They have greater lung efficiency for the given volume because of a greater number of smaller alveoli and thus an increased diffusion surface area. The efficiency of the lungs is decreased when alveolar walls are destroyed, thus reducing surface area and diffusion rate.

To this point, only diffusion between alveolar air and blood has been mentioned. It must be understood that the same principles apply for diffusion between the blood and the body tissues. The changes that occur in the blood, both at the lung and at the tissues, as a result of diffusion represent the difference between arterial blood and venous blood, respectively. Diffusion of gases in the body results from the generation of pressure differences according to the above diffusion-rate equation. With the exception of pressure difference, the other factors of the equation are somewhat fixed under normal conditions. Diffusion occurs because oxygen is consumed by the tissues, which lowers the Po_2, and CO_2 is produced by the tissues, which increases the Pco_2. As fresh air is brought into the lungs, a gradient is generated to replenish O_2 in the blood and to remove the CO_2 that has accumulated.

Partial pressures of gases in the lungs, blood, and tissues

The composition (and corresponding partial pressures) of dry, atmospheric air at sea level (760 mm Hg) is as follows: about 21.0 percent O_2 (Po_2, about 159 mm Hg); about 0.03 percent CO_2 (Pco_2, about 0.23 mm Hg); about 79.0 percent N_2 (PN_2, about 600 mm Hg). Values for the partial pressures of these gases in the tissues, blood, and pulmonary alveoli obtained from an animal at rest would be similar to those presented for humans in Table 13.1. Note that alveolar air Po_2 (104 mm Hg) is much reduced from the above value of 159 mm Hg for dry air that is inhaled. This reduction results from three factors: (1) O_2 is being consumed by the tissues and thus oxygen constantly leaves the alveoli and enters the blood; (2) the air is humidified, creating a PH_2O of 47 mm Hg at 37°C, which in turn dilutes the oxygen present; and (3) CO_2 constantly enters the alveoli, and thus also dilutes the oxygen present.

Increased ventilation could increase the alveolar Po_2 be-

Table 13.1. Total and partial pressures (in mm Hg) of respiratory gases in humans at rest (sea level)

Gases	Venous blood	Alveolar air	Arterial blood	Tissues
Oxygen	40	104	100	30 or less
Carbon dioxide	45	40	40	50 or more
Nitrogen	569	569	569	569
Water vapor	47	47	47	47
Total	701	760	756	696

Data from Comroe 1974, *Physiology of Respiration,* 2d ed., Year Book, Chicago.

cause the replacement with atmospheric air, which contains more O_2 than alveolar air, would be more rapid. Under these conditions, one observes that arterial Po_2 increases because of the greater pressure difference. Also worthy of note are the following, which are demonstrated in Table 13.1:

1. There may be a slight difference between arterial Po_2 and alveolar Po_2 because some of the blood leaving the lung is shunted (does not receive oxygen). A shunt is defined as any mechanism by which blood that has not been through ventilated areas of lung is added to the systemic arteries.

2. Alveolar Pco_2 and arterial Pco_2 are the same because of the greater diffusion coefficient for CO_2 and also because the small arterial-venous difference in Pco_2 results in an imperceptible change from shunted blood.

3. Nitrogen is in virtual equilibrium throughout the system because it is neither consumed nor produced.

4. Water vapor pressure is the same throughout the system because the gases remain at 100 percent humidification.

5. Whereas the sum of the partial pressures in the alveolar air and arterial columns total approximately that of the atmosphere (760 mm Hg), the venous and tissue columns do not. They are less by approximately the amount of O_2 that is consumed. Absorption of gas from closed spaces (peritoneal and pleural cavities) into venous blood occurs because of partial pressure differences in O_2 between venous blood and the closed spaces. This phenomenon is observed when the peritoneal cavity is surgically entered and a slight inrush of air occurs.

6. Each gas diffuses in response to its own partial pressure difference and is independent of the other gases. Thus a Pco_2 of 760 mm Hg and a Po_2 of 0 mm Hg in compartment A exposed to a Po_2 of 760 mm Hg and a Pco_2 of 0 mm Hg in compartment B would show diffusion of CO_2 from A to B and diffusion of O_2 from B to A, even though each has a total pressure of 760 mm Hg. This behavior exists because the *partial pressure differences* are represented by *concentration differences*. High and low pressures simply represent high and low concentrations, respectively. Simple diffusion occurs because of the random motion of molecules from an area of their higher concentration to an area of their lower concentration.

The direction of diffusion in response to differences in partial pressures is shown for oxygen and carbon dioxide in Fig. 13.2.

MECHANICS OF RESPIRATION

Respiratory cycle

Inspiration is an enlargement of the thorax and lungs with an accompanying inflow of air. The thorax is enlarged (1) by contraction of the diaphragm and (2) by a craniad and outward movement of the ribs. Expiration is a decrease in size of the thorax and lungs with air outflow. The previously

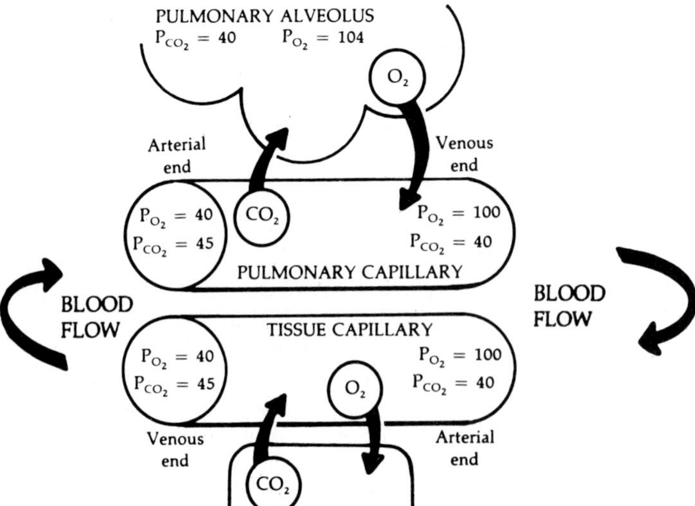

Figure 13.2. Direction of diffusion for oxygen (O_2) and carbon dioxide (CO_2) as shown by central arrows. Arrows on right and left show direction of blood flow. In the pulmonary alveolus the Pco_2 is 40 mm Hg and the Po_2 is 104 mm Hg; at the arterial end of the pulmonary capillary the Po_2 is 40 mm Hg and the Pco_2 is 45 mm Hg, while at the venous end the Po_2 is 100 mm Hg and the Pco_2 is 40 mm Hg; at the venous end of the tissue capillary the Po_2 is 40 mm Hg and the Pco_2 is 45 mm Hg, while at the arterial end the Po_2 is 100 mm Hg and the Pco_2 is 40 mm Hg; and in the tissue cell the Pco_2 is 50 mm Hg and the Po_2 is $<$ 30 mm Hg (recent evidence suggests Po_2 in resting skeletal muscle near 1.5 to 2.0 mm Hg throughout the cytoplasm). (From Reece 1991, *Physiology of Domestic Animals*, Lea & Febiger, Philadelphia.)

contracted muscles relax, and the enlarged thorax and distended abdomen rebound to their previous position with graded assistance from expiratory muscles, depending on the state of breathing. During times when the frequency must increase or when air outflow is impeded, abdominal muscles contract, press on abdominal viscera, and transmit the force to the caudal surface of the diaphragm. Also, intercostal muscles may contract and thus hasten the movement of the ribs to the expired position.

The respiratory pattern or wave form, when recorded, varies little among the mammalian species. The inspiratory and expiratory phases of the cycles are generally smooth and symmetrical. An exception to this general statement is the horse, in which there are two phases during inspiration and two phases during expiration (Fig. 13.3). This species difference may be due to a time delay in the firing of the late inspiratory neurons. These neurons will be described later, under "Regulation of Respiration."

Respiratory cycles are generally continuous. During anesthesia, however, there may be intervals between cycles, and the intervals may lengthen with increasing depth of anesthesia.

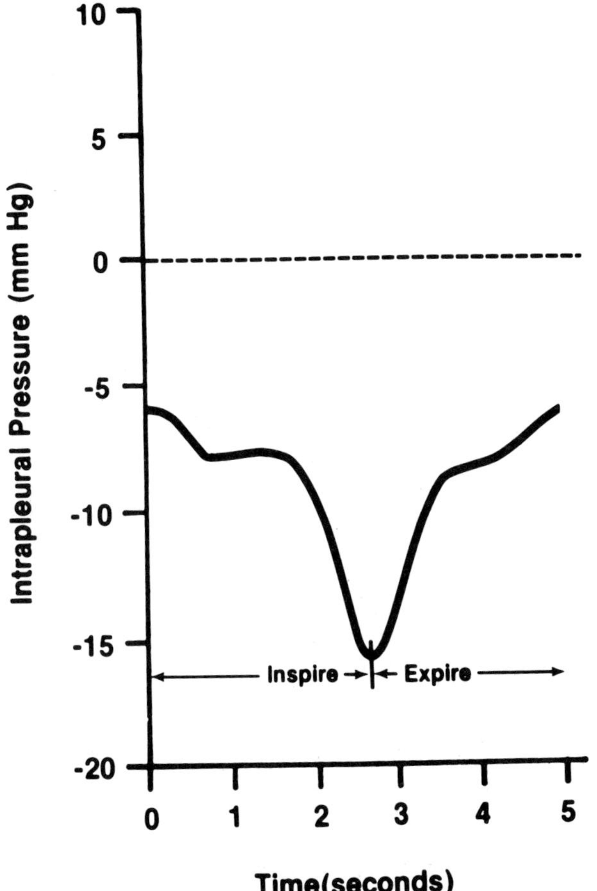

Figure 13.3. The respiratory cycle in the horse recorded by measuring intrapleural pressure. Note the two phases during inspiration and two phases during expiration. (Modified from McCutcheon 1951, *J. Cell. Comp. Physiol.* 37:455.)

Complementary breathing cycles are characterized by a deep, rapid inspiration followed by expiration of longer duration. They occur normally in many species but apparently not in the horse. This type of cycle has frequently been called a *sigh*. As it naturally occurs, it is probably a compensatory mechanism for poor ventilation. In laboratory exercises where ventilation is impaired by the addition of dead-space volume, not only do respiratory frequency and tidal volume increase but also the number of complementary breathing cycles increases. Anesthetists often create complementary cycles at regular intervals by manually compressing the rebreathing bag.

Types of breathing

Abdominal breathing predominates during normal, quiet respiration. This type of breathing is characterized by visible movements of the abdomen caused by visceral compression when the diaphragm contracts. During expiration the abdomen recoils.

Costal breathing is characterized by pronounced rib movements. When breathing becomes difficult, or during painful conditions of the abdomen, this type of breathing becomes pronounced.

Respiratory frequency

Respiratory frequency refers to the number of cycles or the number of breaths each minute. It is an excellent indicator of health status but must be properly interpreted because it is subject to numerous variations. In addition to variations observed among species, frequency may be affected by (1) body size, (2) age, (3) exercise, (4) excitement, (5) environmental temperature, (6) pregnancy, (7) degree of filling of the digestive tract, and (8) state of health. Pregnancy and digestive tract filling increase frequency because they limit the excursion of the diaphragm during inspiration. When expansion of the lungs is restricted, adequate ventilation is maintained by increased frequency. The same phenomenon may be observed when cattle lie down; the large rumen is pushed against the diaphragm and restricts its movement.

All domestic animals will increase frequency of breathing continuously as environmental temperature rises, thus aiding in thermoregulation. This often does not reach the stage of overt panting but can significantly increase alveolar ventilation and dead-space ventilation.

Respiratory frequency is usually increased and only rarely decreased during disease. This observation permits frequency to be a useful indicator of health status. Skill in its interpretation comes with experience and knowledge of the frequency for a species under various conditions. Values are meaningful only when obtained unobtrusively from animals at rest. A list of values for several species under different conditions is shown in Table 13.2.

Respiratory pressures

Air flows in and out of lungs in response to pressure differences created by enlargement or decrease of thoracic volume, respectively (Fig. 13.4). *Intrapulmonic pressure* refers to the air pressure in the lungs and the passages leading to them. The intrapulmonic pressure quickly equals the pressure of the atmosphere after the thoracic volume stabilizes because of free communication between the interior of the lungs and the outside. During inspiration the intrapulmonic pressure becomes slightly subatmospheric because the enlargement of the thorax and lungs is a little more rapid than the inrush of air. During expiration the intrapulmonic pressure becomes slightly greater than atmospheric pressure because the thorax decreases in size and allows the lungs to decrease in size (recoil tendency) and compress the air within them. The air moves out in response to this compression. It can thus be seen that pressure differences create the actual movement of air. Intrapulmonic pressure has also been referred to as alveolar or intra-alveolar pressure.

Intrapleural pressure refers to the pressure in the thorax outside the lungs (including the mediastinum). It has sometimes been called intrathoracic pressure. Ordinarily an intrapleural space does not exist and the lungs occupy all parts of the thoracic cavity not otherwise occupied. The intrapleural pressure is always less than the intrapulmonic pressure. This holds true not only during normal breathing but also under conditions of forceful expiration and under conditions of positive-pressure ventilation (forced-air inflation). Intrapleural pressure is less than intrapulmonic pressure because the lung is adhered to the thoracic wall by the liquid layer between the visceral and parietal pleura. Expansion of the thorax is followed by expansion of the lungs. However, the lungs always have a recoil tendency because

Table 13.2. Respiratory frequency for several animal species under different conditions

Animal	Condition	Cycles/minute Range	Mean
Horse	Standing (at rest)	10–14	12
Dairy cow	Standing (at rest)	26–35	29
	Sternal recumbency	24–50	35
Dairy calf	Standing (52 kg body weight, 3 weeks age)	18–22	20
	Lying down (52 kg body weight, 3 weeks age)	21–25	22
Swine	Lying down (23–27 kg body weight)	32–58	40
Dog	Sleeping (24°C)	18–25	21
	Standing (at rest)	20–34	24
Cat	Sleeping	16–25	22
	Lying down, awake	20–40	31
Sheep	Standing, ruminating, ½–1½ inch wool 18°C	20–34	25
	Same sheep and conditions except 10°C	16–22	19

Data from veterinary medical student laboratory assignments.

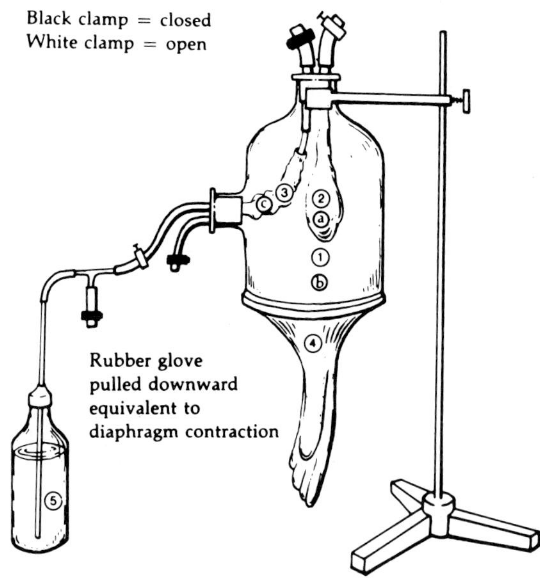

Figure 13.4. Laboratory model of the thorax. This illustrates the mechanics of breathing and the influence of breathing on venous blood return to the heart. Structures: 1, thorax; 2, lung; 3, vena cava (mediastinal structure); 4, diaphragm; 5, venous blood reservoir. Pressures: a, intrapulmonic; b, intrapleural; c, intravenous. During inspiration the diaphragm (4) contracts, resulting in an increase in thoracic volume (1) and a decrease in intrapleural pressure (b). This is followed by an increase in lung volume (2) and a decrease in intrapulmonic pressure (a). Air flows into the lung. Also, there is an increase in vena cava volume (3) and a decrease of its intravenous pressure (c). Blood (5) flow to the heart increases. During expiration the diaphragm (4) relaxes, resulting in a decrease in the volumes of the thorax (1), lung (2), and vena cava (3) and an increase in intrapleural (b), intrapulmonic (a), and intravenous (c) pressures. Air flows out of the lung. Valves prevent blood from flowing backward. Black clamp, closed; white clamp, open. (From Reece, 1991, *Physiology of Domestic Animals*, Lea & Febiger, Philadelphia.)

(1) the surface tension of the fluid lining the inside of the alveoli is always pulling the alveolar surface into the smallest possible size and (2) the elastic fibers that extend throughout the lungs tend to contract the lungs at all times. The inward recoil of the lung tissue pulls on the liquid layer causing a hydrostatic pressure that is subatmospheric. Normally, there is never gas in the liquid layer, and if gas is introduced the adhesion is broken and the lung collapses.

Under conditions of normal breathing, intrapulmonic pressure becomes only slightly negative (−1 mm Hg) during inspiration and only sightly positive (+1 mm Hg) during expiration. A simultaneous recording of intrapleural pressure would probably show a pressure of about −2 mm Hg at the end of expiration and a pressure of about −10 mm Hg at the end of inspiration (Fig. 13.5). All of these pressures are relative to atmospheric pressure.

In a condition called *pneumothorax*, air enters the space between the visceral and parietal pleurae, breaks the adhesion, and eliminates the potential for inflating the lungs. The lungs collapse because of the elastic and surface tension forces. Attempts by the animal to inhale will be unsuccessful, and death from asphyxia will result.

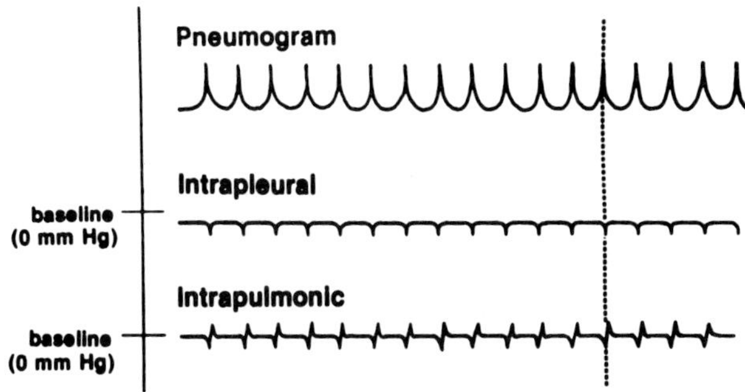

Figure 13.5. Simultaneous recording of intrapulmonic and intrapleural pressure during the respiratory cycle of an anesthetized dog. Each peak on the pneumogram indicates the end of inspiration (upsweep) and the beginning of expiration (downsweep). The transducers were not equally calibrated. Dashed line shows simultaneous position of pens at end of inspiration. Note that (1) intrapleural pressure remains subatmospheric at the end of expiration, (2) both pressure measurements have their greatest negativity at the end of inspiration, and (3) intrapulmonic pressure sharply becomes positive at the moment expiration begins. Drawn from actual recording.

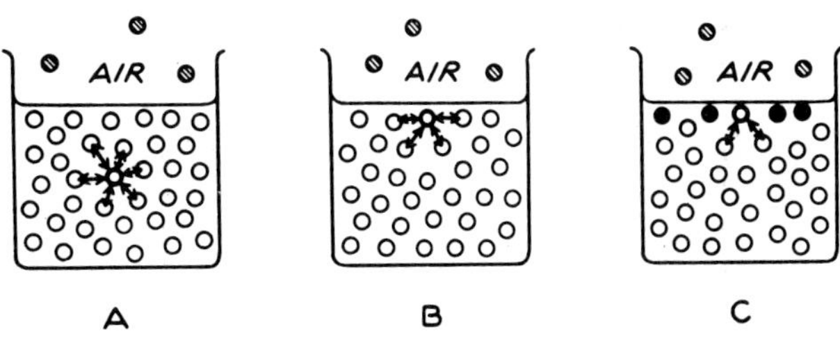

Figure 13.6. Surface tension. (*A*) Water molecules (*open circles*) below the surface of water standing in a beaker have equal attraction for each other in all directions. (*B*) Water molecules at the water-air interface do not have equal attracting forces. Note that the air molecules (*shaded circles*) are fewer in number and are less able to exert an upward force. Therefore the water molecules on the surface have more molecules pulling them down than up and they dive downward, creating a pull on the surface. Further, the attraction from molecules to the side causes a tightening of that surface. When translated to the inner aspect of a sphere (such as an alveolus), one can visualize that the sphere would be reduced in size by the tightening effect. (*C*) Accumulation of surfactant (*solid circles*) at the surface has the effect of reducing surface tension. (Reproduced with permission from Comroe, J.H., Jr.: *Physiology of Respiration*, 2d ed. Copyright © 1974 by Year Book Medical Publishers, Inc., Chicago.)

It is important to understand the relationship of the mediastinal structures to the intrapleural pressure. These structures are enveloped by mediastinal pleura. A subatmospheric intrapleural pressure is transmitted to the mediastinal structures, that is, the vena cava and the esophagus (see Fig. 13.4). This has important consequences of a helpful nature. During inspiration, when the intrapleural pressure becomes more negative to atmospheric pressure, the transmission of reduced pressure to the vena cava and the thoracic lymph duct assists the flow of blood and lymph to the heart. Because of valves in these vessels, the blood and lymph do not flow back when the pressure becomes less negative to atmospheric pressure during expiration. During the study of regurgitation in ruminants, it has been shown that entry of ruminal content into the esophagus is assisted when the animal inspires with a closed glottis. This creates a greater than normal subatmospheric intrapleural pressure, which is transmitted to the mediastinal structures. The intrapleural pressure is often measured by means of an appropriate transducer placed within the mediastinal esophagus.

Recoil tendency of lungs

There is a constant tendency for the lungs to collapse, and in doing so they recoil inward from the thoracic wall. This recoil tendency is mentioned in the above explanation of why intrapleural pressure is always less than intrapulmonic pressure. The recoil tendency is due to (1) stretching of elastic fibers by lung inflation and (2) surface tension of fluid lining the alveoli. The stretching of elastic fibers is easy to visualize as a force that contributes to recoil. *Surface tension*, which is less easily visualized, is a manifestation of attracting forces between atoms or molecules. Like atoms or molecules exert equal attractions for each other, whereas unlike atoms or molecules may have more attraction or less attraction for each other (Fig. 13.6).

To understand the effect of surface tension on pulmonary alveoli, it is helpful to compare the dynamics of alveoli and bubbles. Figure 13.7 shows a bubble under the influence of several forces. The tension (T) in the wall of the bubble tends to contract it, and the pressure (P) inside tends to expand it. When there is no movement of the bubble, there is an equilibrium between the forces of expansion and contraction so that

$$P = \frac{2T}{r}$$

where r equals the radius of the bubble. This is *Laplace's law*. If the surface tension in the bubble remains the same, regardless of the radius, then the pressure required to inflate increases as the radius decreases and decreases as the radius increases. Translating this to pulmonary alveoli, one would observe that a greater pressure would be required to begin inspiration (because the radius is smallest) and that small alveoli (with their greater pressure) would empty into larger alveoli. These untenable situations would occur if the surface tension remained the same, regardless of radius. This is not the case, however, because of pulmonary surfactant.

Surfactants are surface-active substances for which water molecules have a lesser attraction. Because of this property they accumulate at the surface (Fig. 13.6C), and a reduction in surface tension occurs. This results from the reduction in number of water molecules at the surface (displaced by surfactant molecules) and also because the surfactant molecules have a lesser attraction for each other as well as for water molecules and because the surface-tightening effect noted previously is reduced.

Pulmonary surfactant is a lipoprotein complex containing about 30 percent protein and 70 percent lipid. Most of the lipid fraction is composed of the phospholipid, di-

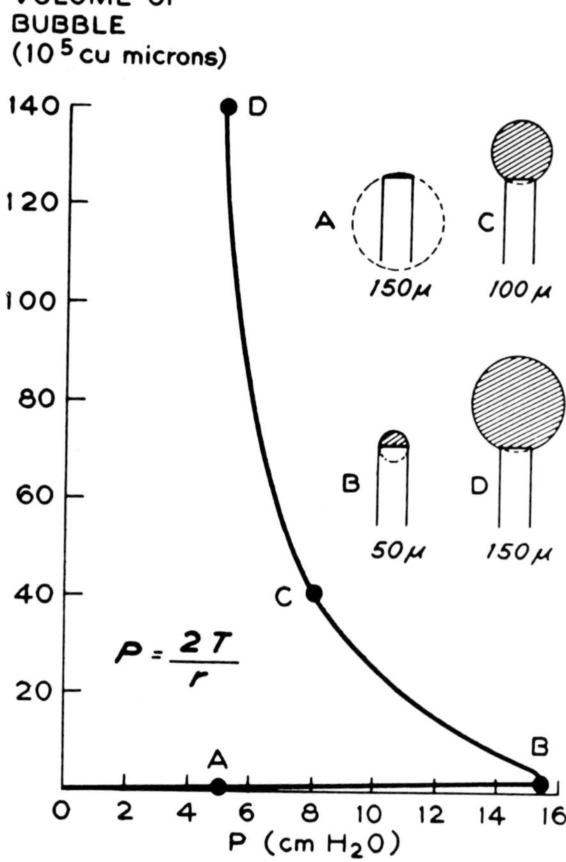

Figure 13.7. Pressure-volume curve of a bubble blown at the end of a glass tube and its conformance to Laplace's law. (A) The nascent bubble is just visible at the top of the tube, and the shaded sphere indicates the extrapolated continuation of the bubble boundary; it clearly has a large radius (note corresponding point A on graph). As the bubble is formed (*B*), its radius actually decreases and becomes minimal when it equals the radius of the tube. Therefore more and more pressure (see graph) is required for formation from *A* to *B*. Beyond this size, the radius begins to increase (*C* and *D*), and less pressure is required to enlarge the bubble. (Modified from Mead 1961, *Physiol. Rev.* 41:281. Reproduced with permission from Comroe, C.H., Jr.: *Physiology of Respiration*, 2d ed. Copyright © 1974 by Year Book Medical Publishers, Inc., Chicago.)

palmitoyl lecithin. Surfactant is synthesized by the type II alveolar epithelial cells (secretory cells). This fact places alveolar epithelium in the category of an active metabolic unit and not simply a passive membrane for the exchange of O_2 and CO_2. It is estimated that the lung may account for as much as 8 to 10 percent of the basal oxygen consumption of the body. Surfactant is formed relatively late in human fetal life and in some animal species. However, the time of its formation is not known for most of the domestic species. In the premature human infant, surfactant deficiency at birth leads to a respiratory distress syndrome characterized by dyspnea, cyanosis, and expiratory grunts. There are clinical, pathological, and biochemical resemblances to human respiratory distress syndrome among some animal species.

The syndrome in animals has been described most completely for horses and swine, in which it has been called barker syndrome. The name is derived from the noise that is associated with the expiratory grunts. The syndrome does not correlate with premature birth of foals and piglets. Although the primary cause may differ, development of the syndrome among human infants, foals, and piglets appears to involve a failure in the production of surfactant.

At the end of expiration, when the alveoli have assumed their smallest radius, it appears that increased pressure would be required to begin the next inspiration and thus inflate the alveoli. According to Laplace's law, this would be true if the surface tension factor remained the same at all stages of inflation. As the alveolar radius is reduced, however, the pulmonary surfactant becomes more compressed on the surface, is more active as a surface-active agent, and therefore reduces the surface tension. The reduction in surface tension tends to counteract the effect of reducing alveolar radius with regard to pressure needed to inflate the alveoli. It also stabilizes the alveoli so that small alveoli do not empty into larger alveoli. At the end of inspiration the alveoli will have expanded. For any beginning amount of surfactant, the surfactant is diluted at the surface and is thus less surface active. The surface tension at this point will have been increased. Physiologically, this provides an upper limiting factor to inspiration and assists the elastic fibers in providing recoil necessary for expiration.

Pulmonary compliance

Pulmonary *compliance* is a measurement of the distensibility of the lungs and thorax and is determined by measurement of the lung volume change for each unit of pressure change (Fig. 13.8). Compliance ($\Delta V/\Delta P$) equals the slope of the line that is made by joining the points when there is no air flow. These points are usually at the end-inspiratory and end-expiratory locations.

The standard units for pulmonary compliance are milliliters (or liters) per centimeter of water. If a compliance value in a particular animal has decreased over a period of time (less expansion volume for the same pressure), the tissues of the lung must be more rigid and less distensible or certain abnormalities may have further reduced the expansibility of the thorax. Factors that affect compliance are those conditions that destroy lung tissue or cause it to be fibrotic or edematous or that in any way impede lung expansion. It is also apparent that changes in surfactant (amount or composition) affect compliance values. Pressures associated with changes in lung volume are shown in Fig. 13.9 for both air-filled and saline-filled lungs.

The lung filled with saline solution has a greater compliance value than the one filled with air. Inasmuch as the gas-liquid interface has been eliminated by saline filling, surface tension as a retractive force has been eliminated. Expansion can be accomplished with less pressure. In the air-filled lung it is also noted that the inspiratory pressure-

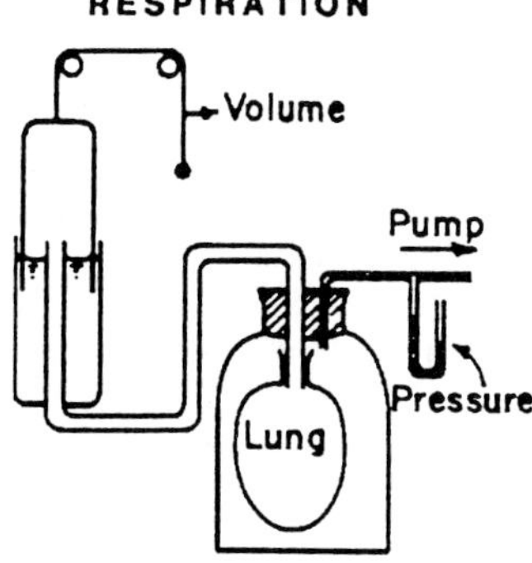

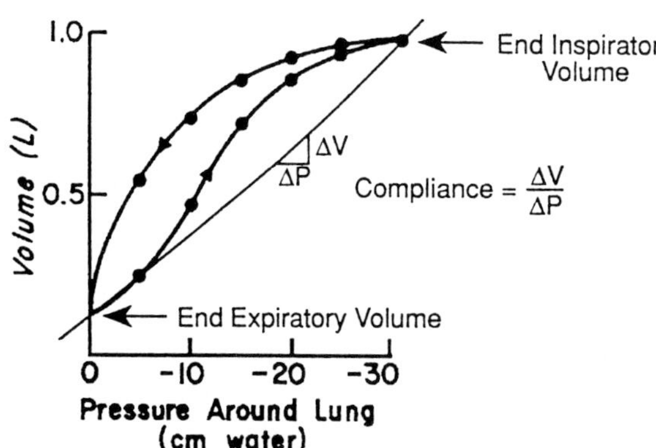

Figure 13.8. (*Bottom*) A pressure-volume curve for canine lung removed from the thorax and measured at various points by the method shown in the upper illustration. (*Top*) The pressure outside the lung is reduced by exhausting the gas in the jar with a pump. When the lung expands, it fills with air from a spirometer. The change in lung volume is measured with the spirometer. The pressure is reduced stepwise and held at the pressure for each step for a few seconds while the lung volume is measured. Compliance ($\Delta V/\Delta P$) for this lung equals the slope of the line that is made by joining the points at which there is no air flow. In the bottom illustration, the end-point of deflation is represented by end-expiratory volume. The end-point of inflation is represented by end-inspiratory volume. (Modified from West 1991, in West, ed., *Best and Taylor's Physiological Basis of Medical Practice*, 12th ed. © 1991, the Williams & Wilkins Co., Baltimore.)

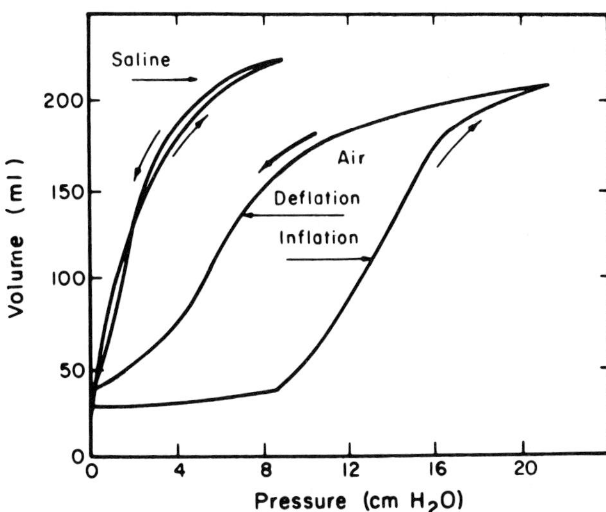

Figure 13.9. Pressure-volume curves of cat lung, showing results obtained when the lung is inflated with air and when it is filled with saline. In the latter case the surface-tension effect is eliminated. (Redrawn from Radford 1957, in Remington, ed., *Tissue Elasticity*, Am. Physiol. Soc., Washington.)

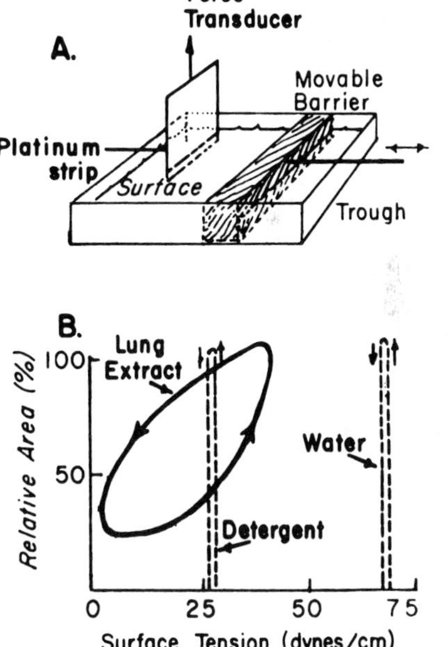

Figure 13.10. (*A*) Surface balance, an instrument used to measure surface tension of liquids. The surface area is increased or decreased with a movable barrier. The surface tension is simultaneously measured from the force exerted on a platinum strip dipped into the surface of the liquid being tested. (*B*) Plots of surface tension and area simultaneously obtained with a surface balance for water, detergent in water, and lung extract (washings from the alveoli that contain surfactant). Upward arrows denote surface area expansion, and downward arrows denote surface area reduction. If the trough contains pure water, the surface tension obtained is independent of the area of the surface. If detergent is added to the water, the surface tension falls considerably, but it is still independent of the area of the surface. For lung extract, note that the smaller the surface area, the lower the value for surface tension; also, for a given surface area, the surface tension during expansion is much greater than during compression. (From West 1991, in West, ed., *Best and Taylor's Physiological Basis of Medical Practice*, 12th ed. © 1991, the Williams & Wilkins Co., Baltimore.)

volume curve is different from the expiratory pressure-volume curve. This is related to the presence of surfactant in the lung. When the alveoli enlarge during inspiration, the distance between surfactant molecules is increased (separation). With reduction in alveolar size during expiration, the surfactant molecules return to their more compressed state (recombination). For surfactant, molecular separation is accomplished with greater difficulty than molecular recombination, so that a pressure measurement for a given lung volume during inspiration is greater than for the same lung volume during expiration. This is deduced from the observation that surface tension measurements of lung washings (which contain surfactant) show different values for the same relative area (volume), depending on whether the surface film is being compressed or expanded (Fig. 13.10).

Metabolic cost of breathing

An expenditure of energy is associated with breathing and is related to the muscle contractions necessary for expanding the lungs. During the expansion of the lungs there is muscle work associated with overcoming (1) the elastic and surface tension forces, (2) the nonelastic forces (rearrangement of tissues), and (3) airway resistance. All three of these may be increased during disease. Surfactant failures and fibrosis or stiffening of the tissues affect the first two factors, and airway obstruction affects the third. During chronic lung disease in livestock, more energy is required for breathing and a reduced feed efficiency can be measured.

Resistance to airflow

It has been pointed out that resistance to airflow is one of the factors associated with the work of breathing. Resistance is greater during expiration than it is during inspiration because the expansion of the lungs during inspiration pulls upon the airways in a manner that assists their greater opening. Accordingly, during many instances of pulmonary distress, the expiratory phase is more exaggerated than the inspiratory phase. The resistance to airflow is determined by the same factors that govern the flow of liquids in tubes. A modification of Poiseuille's law for laminar flow of liquids in rigid, smooth cylindrical tubes is

$$\text{Resistance} = \frac{8\ \text{nl}}{\pi r^4}$$

where n is the coefficient of viscosity, l is the length of the tube, and r is the radius of the tube. This equation renders some approximation of resistance, even though the respiratory tubes are not smooth, cylindrical, and rigid. If the length is increased 4 times, then the pressure must be increased 4 times to maintain constant airflow. If the radius of the tube is halved, however, then the pressure must be increased 16 times to maintain constant flow. For situations that require endotracheal intubation, this certainly points out the necessity of selecting an endotracheal tube that is of a maximum size compatible with the existing airway and an adapter that is similar in diameter to the endotracheal tube.

Pulmonary volumes and capacities

Although the lung for a particular animal may have its own limits for air volume, it is often helpful to designate certain arbitrary volumes related to fractions of the lung volume (Fig. 13.11). It is known that a certain volume of air, the *residual volume*, remains in the lungs even after the most forceful expiration. The amount of air breathed in or out during one respiratory cycle is called the *tidal volume*. This is probably the most used arbitrary volume. Table 13.3 lists average tidal volume values for several domestic animal species. The amount of air that may still be inspired after inhalation of the tidal volume is the *inspiratory reserve volume*. The amount that may still be expired after exhalation of the tidal volume is the *expiratory reserve volume*. It is also useful to define certain larger divisions. For example, two or more volumes may be said to constitute a *capac-*

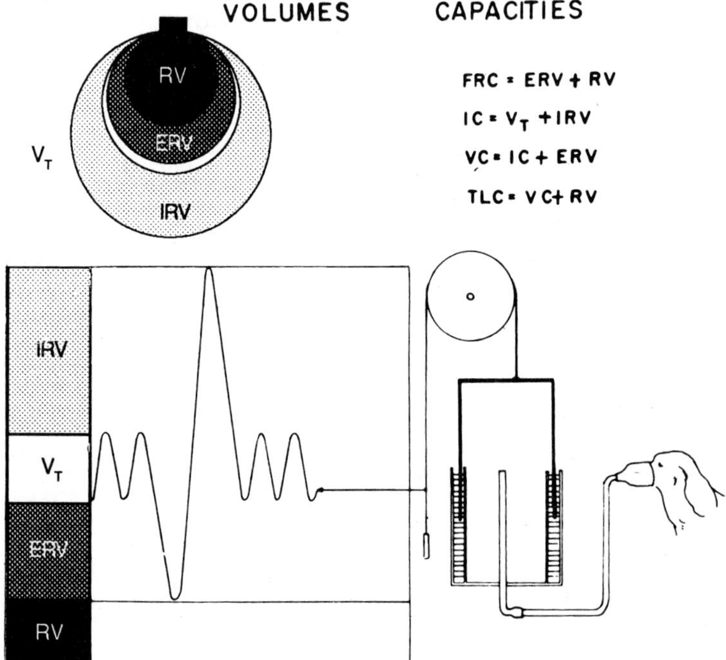

Figure 13.11. Subdivisions of the lung volume as illustrated on a spirometer record and a schematic spherical lung: RV, residual volume; ERV, expiratory reserve volume; V_T, tidal volume; IRV, inspiratory reserve volume; VC, vital capacity; FRC, functional residual capacity; IC, inspiratory capacity; TLC, total lung capacity. (Modified from Comroe, Forster, Dubois, Briscoe, and Carlsen 1962, *The Lung*, Year Book Medical Publishers, Inc., Chicago.)

Table 13.3. Average tidal volumes for several domestic animal species

Animal	Number	Average body weight (kg)	Condition	Respiratory frequency (breaths/min)	Tidal volume (ml/kg)	References
Cattle						
Holstein cows	11	516	Standing	26	8.20 S.D. 1.29	Hall & Brody (1933)
Jersey cows	13	405	Standing	27	8.44 S.D. 1.40	Hall & Brody (1933)
Clinical index*	—	—	Anesthetized	10–15	10–15	†
Horse						
Thoroughbred	15	486	Resting	10	15.4 S.D. 0.76	Gillespie et al. (1966)
Clinical index*	—	—	Anesthetized	10–15	10–15	†
Dog						
	77	19	Pentobarbital anesthesia	13.6	10.7 S.D. 5.3	Hamlin & Smith (1967)
	4	12.6	Pentobarbital anesthesia	21.0	11.4	Crosfil & Widdicombe (1961)
	20	13.8	Pentobarbital anesthesia	15.1	15.7 S.D. 5.8	‡
Beagles	20	—	25–26°C, sitting	23	16 S.D. 2.0	Park et al. (1970)
Clinical index*	—	—	Anesthetized	10–15	15–20	†
Cat						
	4	3.7	Pentobarbital anesthesia	30	9.2	Crosfil & Widdicombe (1961)
Clinical index*	—	—	Anesthetized	10–15	15–20	†

*Appropriate rate and volume for maintenance of pulmonary ventilation (blood gases analyzed) with mechanical intermittent positive pressure inflation anesthesia.

†Veterinary Teaching Hospital, College of Veterinary Medicine, Iowa State University.

‡Veterinary physiology student laboratory, College of Veterinary Medicine, Iowa State University.

ity. The sum of all volumes constitutes the *total lung capacity*. All of the volumes except the residual volume constitute the *vital capacity*. This represents the maximum amount of air that can be inhaled after the maximum amount has been exhaled. The tidal volume and the inspiratory reserve volume constitute the *inspiratory capacity*, which is the amount of air that can be inspired after expiration. The amount of air remaining in the lung after expiration is the *functional residual capacity*, and it is composed of the expiratory reserve volume and the residual volume. The functional residual capacity is the reservoir of air ventilated by the tidal volume that tends to provide constancy to the blood values for the respired gases.

PULMONARY VENTILATION

Respiratory dead space

There is virtually no diffusion of gases between the blood and the airways down to the level of the respiratory bronchioles, and this upper portion of the airways is termed a *respiratory dead space*. Its principal function is to conduct gas to and from those portions where diffusion occurs. Although there is no exchange of gas between air and blood in this conduction portion, some of its volume is exchanged with the environment in normal respiration, and it is a part of the tidal volume. Accordingly, not all of the tidal volume ventilates the alveoli, and it is recognized that tidal volume is composed of dead-space volume and alveolar volume ($V_D + V_A$).

The respiratory dead space may be defined as the volume of the conducting airways (*anatomical dead space*) or as the volume of gas that is inspired but takes no part in gas exchange in the airways and alveoli (*physiological dead space*). Anatomical dead space is a relatively fixed volume in a given animal, although it may change during a given respiratory cycle because of the lengthening and dilatation of bronchi and bronchioles during inspiration and their shortening and constriction during expiration. Physiological dead space is determined not only by the dimensions of the conducting airways but also by the volume of gas that may enter the alveoli and does not have diffusional interchange with the blood because of inadequate pulmonary capillary perfusion. Also, a physiological dead space takes into consideration differences in airflow characteristics. For the most part, the greatest air movement occurs in the central or axial portion of the airway. The gas adjacent to the wall of the airway may not be moving at all. Therefore it is apparent that the entire anatomical dead space is not moved during a respiratory cycle. Inasmuch as physiological dead space is the functional dead space, there is no constant comparison of its volume with anatomical dead space. It may be of lesser volume when only airways and the airflow characteristics thereof are considered; however, the volume of poorly perfused alveoli is variable and is additive to the airway volume.

Physiological dead-space volume for a respiratory cycle can be determined if the P_{CO_2} of alveolar and expired air is measured and if tidal volume is measured. Tidal volume can be measured by spirometry while P_{CO_2} is analyzed simultaneously in mixed expired air and in arterial blood. Since alveolar air is normally in equilibrium with arterial blood (especially for CO_2), the P_{CO_2} in arterial blood will be a reflection of the P_{CO_2} in the alveoli. Expired air is a mixture of atmospheric air from the airways and nonperfused alveoli together with air from perfused alveoli. Table 13.4 shows that the P_{CO_2} of expired air is lower than the P_{CO_2} of alveolar air. The lower value for P_{CO_2} occurs be-

Table 13.4. Total and partial pressures (in mm Hg) of respiratory gases in dogs at rest (sea level)

Gases	Atmospheric air*	Inspired gas†	Alveolar gas	Mixed expired gas
Oxygen	158	140	114	123
Carbon dioxide	0	0	45	29
Nitrogen	596	568	549	556
Water vapor	6	52	52	52
Total	760	760	760	760

*PH_2O arbitrarily assigned.

†Saturated with water vapor at body temperature (39°C) in region of bronchi.

Data from Tenney 1977, Respiration in mammals, in Swenson, ed., *Dukes' Physiology of Domestic Animals,* 9th ed, Cornell University Press, Ithaca, N.Y., and veterinary student laboratories.

cause of the dilution of the alveolar fraction (which is in equilibrium with arterial blood) by the dead-space fraction (which contains virtually no carbon dioxide). The equation for calculating the dead-space volume (known as the Bohr equation) is

$$V_D = \frac{P_ACO_2 - P_ECO_2}{P_ACO_2} \times V_T$$

where V_D is dead-space volume, V_T is tidal volume, P_ACO_2 is the partial pressure of carbon dioxide in alveolar air, and P_ECO_2 is the partial pressure of carbon dioxide in mixed expired air. The fraction on the right of the equation is the fraction of the tidal volume associated with physiological dead space. The numerical example below uses average values obtained from veterinary student physiology laboratory exercises. Dogs with an average body weight of 13 kg were used. They had been anesthetized with pentobarbital sodium and placed in a dorsal recumbent position for about 1 hour before measurement (partial pressures in millimeters of mercury).

$$V_D = \frac{P_ACO_2 - P_ECO_2}{P_ACO_2} \times V_T\ (\text{ml}) = \frac{54 - 27}{54} \times 170$$
$$= 85\ \text{ml}$$

Under these conditions, V_D was about 50 percent of the tidal volume.

In addition to providing a conduit for air on its way to the diffusional spaces, the dead space warms the inspired air, saturates it with water vapor at body temperature, and subjects it to clearance of particles.

Ventilation

Ventilation, as applied to the respiratory system, is the process of exchanging gas in the airways and alveoli with atmospheric air. Its purpose is to replenish oxygen and to remove carbon dioxide.

Total ventilation is the volume of gas moved into or out of the airways and alveoli over a certain period of time. *Minute ventilation* is the total volume of gas moved into or out of the airways and alveoli in 1 minute. It is determined by the relationship

$$\dot{V}_E = f\,V_T$$

where $\dot{V}_E$ is the minute ventilation (expired), f is respiratory frequency in cycles per minute, and V_T is the average tidal volume. Minute ventilation is also referred to as the *minute respiratory volume* (MRV).

Dead-space ventilation ($\dot{V}_D$) is the volume of air that does not take part in gas exchange over a certain period of time. *Alveolar ventilation* is determined by subtraction of dead-space ventilation from the total ventilation. Alveolar ventilation ($\dot{V}_A$) is the volume of gas that contributes to diffusional exchange each minute. A formula for its calculation is

$$\dot{V}_A = f(V_T - V_D) = f\,V_A$$

where f is the number of respiratory cycles each minute, V_T is tidal volume, V_D is dead-space volume, and V_A is alveolar volume. Substitution of values obtained from dogs in the same laboratory exercises as those in which dead-space volume was measured yields:

$$\dot{V}_A = 10(170 - 85)$$
$$= 850\ \text{ml/min}$$

In other words, 850 ml of gas in the alveoli of the lungs is replaced by air each minute. This represents only a portion of the total ventilation, which is obtained by substitution of data from our previous examples into the formula for minute ventilation ($\dot{V}_E = fV_T = 10$ cycles/min $\times$ 170 ml/cycle = 1700 ml/min).

Normoventilation refers to normal ventilation in which a P_ACO_2 of about 40 mm Hg is maintained. *Hyperventilation* refers to alveolar ventilation increased beyond the metabolic needs and a $P_ACO_2 < 40$ mm Hg. Hyperventilation is a characteristic of respiratory alkalosis. *Hypoventilation* is alveolar ventilation decreased below the metabolic needs and a $P_ACO_2 > 40$ mm Hg. Hypoventilation is a characteristic of respiratory acidosis. Respiratory alkalosis and respiratory acidosis are disturbances of acid-base equilibrium where the pH of blood is increased or decreased, respectively, from normal. An important regulator of alveolar ventilation is $Paco_2$ as determined by CO_2 production (see below under "Regulation of Respiration").

Physiological dead space may be increased under certain conditions, and it will be observed that tidal volume, respiratory frequency, or both increase in order to keep alveolar ventilation constant. It may also be observed that the frequency of complementary breaths increases as a compensation for added dead space. The limits of compensation must be recognized when dead space is added in the form of tubes and breathing devices. *Panting*, which is primarily dead-space ventilation, is an important temperature-regulating mechanism in many species. During panting the respiratory frequency is increased and the tidal volume is decreased so that alveolar ventilation remains relatively constant in order to provide protection from hyperventilation. Hyperventilation can occur in animals exposed to severe heat stress, however, and result in respiratory alkalosis.

Ventilation and perfusion relationships

The partial pressures of oxygen and carbon dioxide in the blood are related not only to alveolar ventilation but also to the amount of blood that perfuses the alveoli. The relationship of these two factors to each other is referred to as the ventilation/perfusion ratio and is abbreviated $\dot{V}_A/\dot{Q}$. The ratio can be calculated when appropriate measurements are obtained, and it may be useful in lung-function studies.

To understand the meaning of the ratios, one must consider relative ratios. For example, what do we mean when we say that a ratio is equal to zero or is equal to infinity? Further, what are the implications of deviations from normal toward zero or toward infinity? First, let us consider the ratio extremes of zero and infinity. For the ratio to become zero, the numerator must become zero. This would be the case when alveolar ventilation was nonexistent and perfusion of the alveoli continued (Fig. 13.12B). This condition does not allow for exchange of any gas between the atmosphere and the blood. For the ratio to become infinite, the denominator must become zero; this means that there is no perfusion of the alveoli, and they continue to be ventilated (Fig. 13.12C). This situation is also incompatible with the exchange of gas between the atmosphere and blood. A normal ventilation/perfusion ratio implies that there is a balance between ventilation and perfusion of the alveoli, so that exchange of oxygen and carbon dioxide between the alveoli and blood is optimal (Fig. 13.12A). Deviations from normal are known as mismatching of ventilation and blood flow within the lung.

Now let us consider the meaning of ratio deviations from the normal that lie between the extremes. A value less than normal (low $\dot{V}_A/\dot{Q}$) means that ventilation has declined but that perfusion remains adequate. A ventilation/perfusion ratio with a value greater than normal (high $\dot{V}_A/\dot{Q}$) means that ventilation is exceeding perfusion. Within the lung at any one time there may exist an uneven distribution of blood flow and ventilation so that areas of low $\dot{V}_A/\dot{Q}$, normal $\dot{V}_A/\dot{Q}$, and high $\dot{V}_A/\dot{Q}$ represent different lung units. For animals at rest and in the standing position, the dorsal aspects have a higher ventilation/perfusion ratio, resulting in high $\dot{V}_A/\dot{Q}$ lung units; the ventral aspects have a lower ventilation/perfusion ratio, resulting in low $\dot{V}_A/\dot{Q}$ lung units. It is likely that with greater activity a resumption of more equal matching of ventilation and perfusion occurs.

Blood leaving the lungs is a mixture from all lung units (low, normal, and high $\dot{V}_A/\dot{Q}$) as shown in Fig. 13.13. The high $\dot{V}_A/\dot{Q}$ units may have a greater oxygen content than blood from normal and low $\dot{V}_A/\dot{Q}$ units but, because of their restricted blood flow, a greater amount of blood is forced to perfuse low $\dot{V}_A/\dot{Q}$ units. Accordingly, the contribution of the high $\dot{V}_A/\dot{Q}$ units to oxygenation is not sufficient to compensate for the lesser contribution to oxygenation by low $\dot{V}_A/\dot{Q}$ units and the PaO_2 of systemic blood is less than blood from perfectly matched ventilation and perfusion (shunted blood).

Mismatches of ventilation and blood flow are probably the most common cause of hypoxemia. Chronic obstructive lung diseases, such as chronic bronchitis and alveolar pulmonary emphysema (alveoli unduly distended or with ruptured walls), are productive of mismatching of ventilation and blood flow throughout the lung. The initial restriction to air flow by chronic bronchitis produces low $\dot{V}_A/\dot{Q}$ lung units, and the emphysema that follows produces high $\dot{V}_A/\dot{Q}$ lung units. A diversity of lung units will be present along a ventilation/perfusion ratio line as shown in Fig. 13.14, and hypoxemia is a predominant feature. Mismatches can be accentuated under conditions of prolonged inactivity asso-

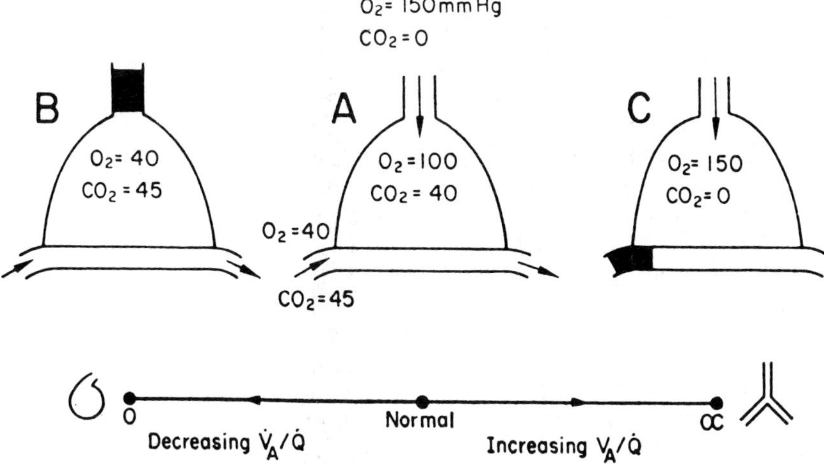

Figure 13.12. Ventilation/perfusion ratios ($\dot{V}_A/\dot{Q}$) that range from zero to infinity. In *(A)* ventilation and perfusion are normal and the $\dot{V}_A/\dot{Q}$ = about 1; in *(B)* perfusion is normal, but there is no ventilation and the $\dot{V}_A/\dot{Q} = 0$; in *(C)* ventilation is normal, but there is no perfusion and $\dot{V}_A/\dot{Q} = \alpha$. Symbol on the left shows the right ventricle; symbol on the right shows the trachea. (From West 1977, *Ventilation/Blood Flow and Gas Exchange*, 3d ed. Blackwell Scientific Publications, Oxford)

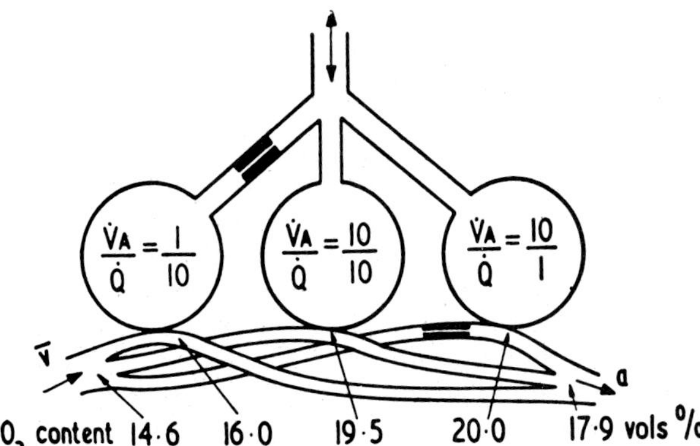

Figure 13.13. Three lung units represented by low $\dot{V}/\dot{Q}$ (ventilation/perfusion ratio) = 1/10, normal $\dot{V}/\dot{Q}$ = 10/10, and high $\dot{V}/\dot{Q}$ = 10/1. Mixed venous blood presented to the lungs is represented by v̄. Blood leaving the lungs is a mixture from all lung units and is represented by a. See text for explanation. (From West 1977, *Ventilation/Blood Flow and Gas Exchange*, 3d ed. Blackwell Scientific Publications, Oxford.)

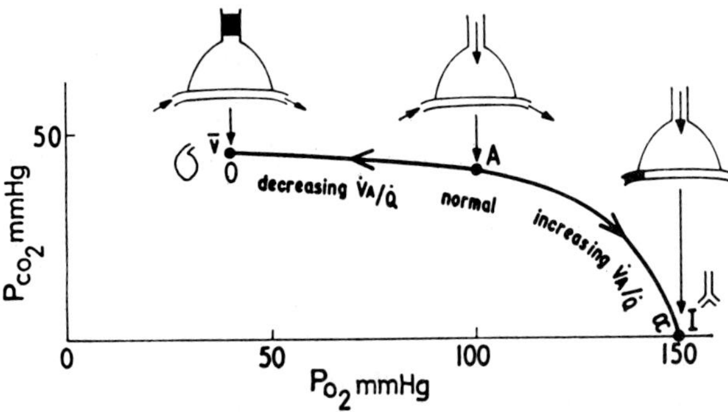

Figure 13.14. A ventilation/perfusion ratio ($\dot{V}_A/\dot{Q}$) line where v̄ represents the Po_2 and Pco_2 of mixed venous blood when ventilation is blocked ($\dot{V}/\dot{Q}$ = 0) and where I represents the Po_2 and Pco_2 of alveolar gas when perfusion is blocked ($\dot{V}/\dot{Q}$ = infinity). Mismatches of ventilation and perfusion within lung units at any point on the ratio line influence oxygenation of the blood accordingly. (From West 1977, *Ventilation/Blood Flow and Gas Exchange*, 3d ed. Blackwell Scientific Publications, Oxford.)

ciated with anesthesia. Deeper than normal inflation is regularly induced to reestablish patency in alveoli where their excursions have been limited. Also, if prolonged recovery periods are characteristic of the anesthetic, animals are regularly turned from one side to the other. The lower portions of the lung have a tendency to inadequate ventilation which, when coupled with adequate blood flow, results in low $\dot{V}_A/\dot{Q}$ lung units. Rotation provides for resumption of alveolar filling.

Hypoxic vasoconstriction

When the Po_2 of alveolar gas is reduced, the smooth muscle cells in the walls of the small arterioles contract in the hypoxic region. The vasoconstriction has the effect of directing blood flow away from hypoxic regions of lung to regions that have adequate oxygenation. The response is activated by the Po_2 of the alveolar gas, not the Po_2 of pulmonary arterial blood. The mediator of the vasoconstriction is not known, but it is thought that cells in the perivascular tissue release a vasoconstrictor substance in response to hypoxia.

Generalized pulmonary vasoconstriction occurs at altitudes above 2100 m where ambient Po_2 is less than 100 mm Hg. The generalized pulmonary vasoconstriction leads to a rise in pulmonary arterial pressure and a substantial increase in work for the right heart. Right ventricular failure may follow, with a subsequent increase in central venous pressure and a predisposition to edema. Pulmonary vascular smooth muscle responses vary with species, cattle and chickens being the most responsive domestic species and, therefore, potentially susceptible to generalized severe hypoxic pulmonary hypertension leading to right heart failure. Cattle raised at high altitudes have a condition referred to as *brisket disease* because of the accumulation of edematous fluid in the region of the brisket, the location in which overt edema is most likely to develop with right heart failure. Chickens are also susceptible to right ventricular failure at high altitude, and meat-type chickens, particularly growing males, which have a high oxygen requirement, are affected most severely. Overt edema in chickens is located in the peritoneal cavity, and the accumulation of fluid within that cavity is known as *ascites*. When caused by pulmonary hypertension, the condition is called *hypoxic ascites*.

OXYGEN TRANSPORT

General comments about hemoglobin

Hemoglobin is the red pigment of blood. When it is saturated with oxygen, it is bright red; as it loses oxygen, it becomes purplish. The hemoglobin molecule (Fig. 2.3), a chromoprotein, consists of a pigment component called heme and a protein. The protein component is composed of four polypeptide chains (globin subunits), each containing one heme. Each heme group contains an iron atom in the ferrous state, which combines loosely and reversibly with one oxygen molecule. Therefore one molecule of hemoglobin contains four iron atoms and can transport four molecules of oxygen. The exchange of oxygen does not involve a change in valence of iron. Electron shifts occur in groups close to iron during oxygen delivery and uptake, which influence oxygen binding and hydrogen ion balance.

General scheme of oxygen transport

When oxygen is consumed by the body cells, it is replenished by oxygen in solution from the internal environment (interstitial water) of the cell. In turn, the interstitial oxygen is replenished by the oxygen in solution from plasma, which is replenished by oxygen in solution from the erythrocytes. Finally, the oxygen in solution in the water of the erythrocytes is replenished by oxygen that is combined with hemoglobin. When the oxygen-depleted blood arrives at the lungs, there is a reversal of oxygen diffusion from the alveolus to the interstitial water, followed by oxygen diffusion to the water of the plasma and erythrocytes in the bloodstream, and finally diffusion to hemoglobin in the erythrocytes. It is important that this scheme for oxygen transport be understood (Fig. 13.15). The scheme considers the following points:

1. The amount (volume) of oxygen in solution (dissolved) is directly related to Po_2 and the solubility coefficient for oxygen (Henry's law).
2. Oxygen is relatively soluble in all membranes, so that diffusion is relatively uninhibited.
3. Oxygen is readily received and yielded by hemoglobin as influenced by the surrounding Po_2.
4. The surrounding Po_2 is determined by gradients generated by either cellular consumption or alveolar ventilation.
5. Because of oxygen-poor blood arriving at the lung, there is a diffusion gradient from the pulmonary alveolus to the interior of the red blood cell.

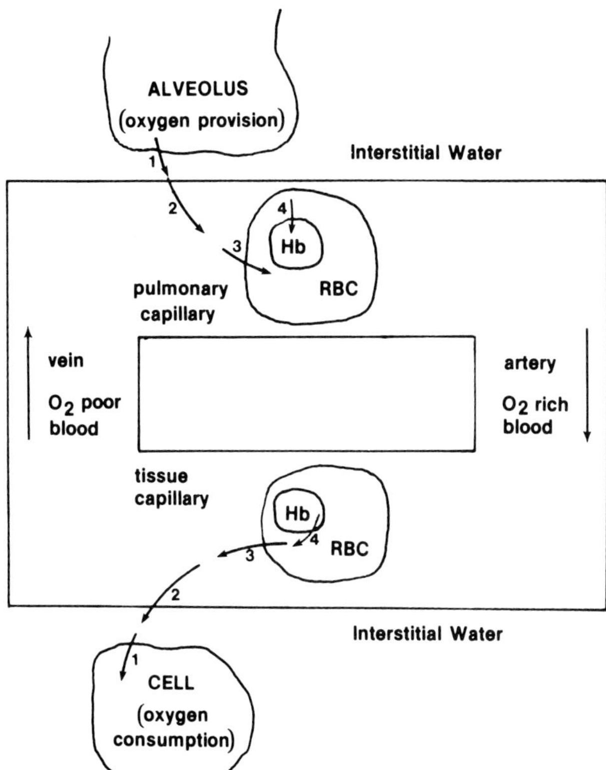

Figure 13.15. General scheme of oxygen transport showing oxygen procession. Procession occurs because of gradients. In this scheme, blood is oxygenated at top and deoxygenated at bottom; blood flow is clockwise. During oxygenation, oxygen diffuses from alveolus to interstitial water (1), followed by diffusion to plasma water (2), to RBC water (3) and to hemoglobin (4). For hemoglobin to be deoxygenated, oxygen in solution in interstitial water must diffuse first to cell water (1), followed by diffusion from plasma water (2), from RBC water (3), and finally from hemoglobin (4). Hb, hemoglobin; RBC, red blood cell.

6. Because consumption of oxygen at the body-cell level lowers Po_2, a diffusion gradient is established from the interior of the red blood cell to the consuming cell.

Relatively speaking, the last oxygen to enter solution from the alveolus is the first oxygen to be delivered to consuming cells. In other words, for oxygen uptake, there is a procession of oxygen from air in the alveolus to successive solution in interstitial water, in plasma, in erythrocyte water, and finally in hemoglobin. For oxygen yield, the procession of oxygen is from interstitial water, which is replenished by that which is in solution in plasma and erythrocyte water, which in turn is replenished by oxygen combined with hemoglobin.

Quantitative aspects

Most of the oxygen in blood is that which is combined with hemoglobin; relatively little is dissolved in water. The solubility coefficient of oxygen in water allows only 0.003 ml to be dissolved in each 100 ml of blood for each millimeter of mercury of partial pressure. For an arterial Po_2 of 100 mm Hg, this amounts to 0.3 ml of oxygen dissolved in each 100 ml of blood. The maximal volume of oxygen combined with hemoglobin is determined by the following:

1. One mole of hemoglobin can combine with 4 moles of oxygen (100% saturation).
2. One mole of any gas occupies 22,400 ml.
3. The gram molecular weight of hemoglobin is about 67,000 per mole.
4. The volume of oxygen combined with each gram of hemoglobin is about 1.34 ml (obtained by dividing the number of milliliters associated with 4 moles of gas [22,400 $\times$ 4 = 89,600] by the number of grams in each mole of hemoglobin [67,000]).
5. The volume of oxygen combined with hemoglobin in each deciliter of blood is the product of hemoglobin concentration (in grams per deciliter), volume of oxygen with each gram of hemoglobin (milliliters per gram), and oxygen saturation (decimal fraction) at the partial pressure of its measurement. For example, if the hemoglobin concentration in blood is 15 g/dl and hemoglobin is 97.5 percent saturated at 100 mm Hg, and 1.34 ml O_2 combines with each gram of hemoglobin when it is fully saturated, then 19.6 ml (15 g/dl $\times$ 1.34 ml/g $\times$ 0.975 = 19.6 ml/dl) of oxygen is combined with hemoglobin in each 100 ml of blood (19.6 volumes percent).

Of the total amount of oxygen transported by 100 ml of blood (0.3 ml in solution + 19.6 ml with hemoglobin = 19.9 ml), it can be seen that only 1.5 percent is carried in solution, whereas 98.5 percent is combined with hemoglobin. If hemoglobin were not present, it would take 66.3 times more blood to transport the same amount of oxygen.

The oxygen-hemoglobin dissociation curve

The loading and unloading of oxygen from hemoglobin are best described by the oxygen-hemoglobin dissociation

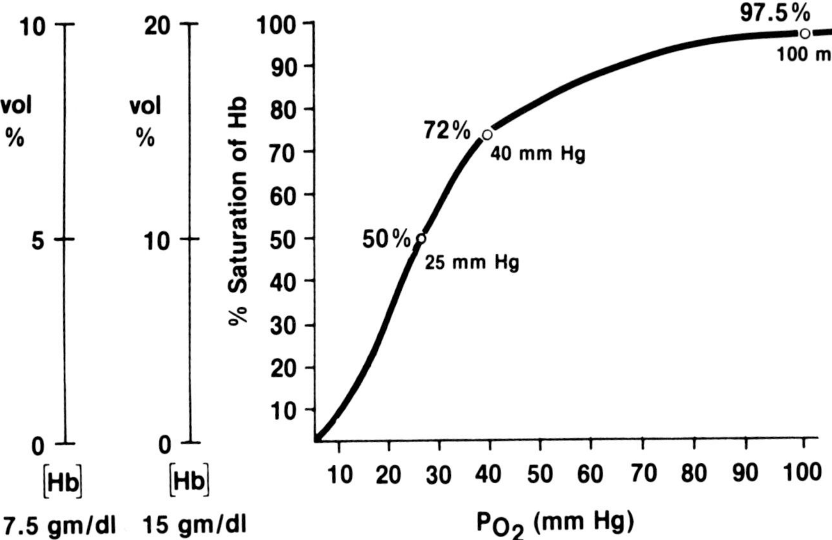

Figure 13.16. The oxygen-hemoglobin dissociation curve for human blood. Volumes percent of oxygen associated with normal (15 g/dl) and one-half of normal (7.5 g/dl) hemoglobin concentration (Hb) are shown relative to the hemoglobin saturation scale, so that the difference between hemoglobin saturation and volume of oxygen transported can be seen. The hemoglobin saturation scale refers to the percent of the total oxygen that hemoglobin is capable of binding.

curve (Fig. 13.16); the following points should be remembered:

1. The amount of oxygen associated with hemoglobin is related, but is not directly proportional (as was the amount in solution), to the pressure of dissolved oxygen in the water of the red blood cell and plasma.

2. Before the combination of oxygen with hemoglobin, there must be oxygen in solution; similarly, after its removal from hemoglobin, oxygen is again in solution so that it may diffuse to the consuming cells (the oxygen unloads because Po_2 in solution is lowered).

In addition to a scale for percent saturation of hemoglobin, Fig. 13.16 also has scales for volumes percent of oxygen (volumes [in milliliters] of oxygen per 100 ml of blood) associated with hemoglobin when the hemoglobin concentration of blood is normal (15 g/dl) or reduced (7.5 g/dl). In this way, the amount of oxygen transported by anemic blood might be compared with normal blood. A study of Fig. 13.16 will show the following:

1. At a Po_2 of 100 mm Hg (the approximate Po_2 of arterial blood), hemoglobin is about 97.5% saturated with oxygen. It will transport only about 19.6 volumes percent when the hemoglobin concentration is 15 g/dl. It will transport about 9.8 volumes percent when the hemoglobin concentration is 7.5 g/dl.

2. When the Po_2 is 40 mm Hg (approximately the Po_2 of venous blood), hemoglobin is still about 72 percent saturated with oxygen. It will transport about 14.5 volumes percent when the hemoglobin concentration is 15 g/dl but will transport only about 7.25 volumes percent when the hemoglobin concentration is lowered to 7.5 g/dl.

3. In going from a Po_2 of 100 mm Hg to one of 40 mm Hg, about 5 volumes percent of oxygen is yielded by 100 ml of blood when the hemoglobin concentration is 15 g/dl. However, only about 2.5 volumes percent is yielded when the hemoglobin concentration is 7.5 g/dl. The former value (5 volumes percent) reflects O_2 consumption under normal resting conditions.

4. For blood to yield 5 volumes percent of oxygen when an animal is anemic (7.5 g/dl of hemoglobin), it appears that the Po_2 of blood would have to be reduced to about 25 mm Hg. Reductions of this magnitude are unusual in the living animal, however, because cardiac output increases in order to transport more oxygen than would otherwise be available.

5. The P_{50} for this curve is about equal to 25 mm Hg. P_{50} is a notation for an associated Po_2 when hemoglobin is 50% saturated with oxygen. It is the same regardless of the concentration of hemoglobin. P_{50} changes when the dissociation constants for hemoglobin change (oxygen-hemoglobin dissociation curve shifts right or left).

The fraction of oxygen given up by blood as it passes through the tissue capillaries is known as the *utilization coefficient*. In the above example, where blood with a hemoglobin concentration of 15 g/dl carries about 20 volumes percent and yields about 5 volumes percent, the utilization coefficient is $\frac{1}{4}$. In the example of the anemic animal (hemoglobin concentration of 7.5 g/dl) this would become about $\frac{1}{2}$.

It can be seen that under normal conditions hemoglobin will set an upper limit on the Po_2 in the tissues at approximately 40 mm Hg, which is referred to as the *oxygen buffer function of hemoglobin*. The dissociation of oxygen from hemoglobin is such that the Po_2 of blood must fall to about 40 mm Hg in order to supply the minimal need of 5 volumes percent. Values below 40 mm Hg provide the desirable oxygen tension for optimum cell function. It is known that the prolonged provision of oxygen at high oxygen tension is detrimental to lung cells (cells that are intimately exposed to oxygen without the oxygen buffer function of hemoglobin). Also, the maintenance of capillary Po_2 close to 40 mm Hg assists the diffusion of O_2 into the tissue cells by providing a gradient for diffusion. Because the lower part of the dissociation curve is steep, large amounts of O_2 can be withdrawn from hemoglobin with little reduction in Po_2 from 40 mm Hg, and the diffusion gradient for O_2 will be maintained.

The association of oxygen with hemoglobin and its dissociation from hemoglobin are not stable under all conditions. Different conditions change the equilibrium of the reaction between hemoglobin and oxygen to form oxyhemoglobin. This equilibrium is represented by the oxygen-hemoglobin dissociation curve; when the equilibrium changes, shifts in the curve can be observed (Fig. 13.17). When the curve shifts to the right, it denotes a decreased affinity of hemoglobin for oxygen. Under these conditions more oxygen is yielded for each reduction in Po_2. Similarly, a shift to the left denotes an increased affinity of hemoglobin for oxygen, and less oxygen is yielded for each reduction in Po_2. Increases in hydrogen ion and carbon dioxide cause the curve to shift to the right; therefore a shift to the right would be expected at the level of the tissue capillaries where arterial blood becomes venous blood. This shift is appropriate because it provides for a greater yield of oxygen at the tissues where it should be unloaded. When the blood reaches the lungs and both the CO_2 and hydrogen ion concentrations are lowered, hemoglobin has a greater affinity for oxygen, and oxygen uptake is facilitated. The effect of CO_2 and hydrogen ions on the

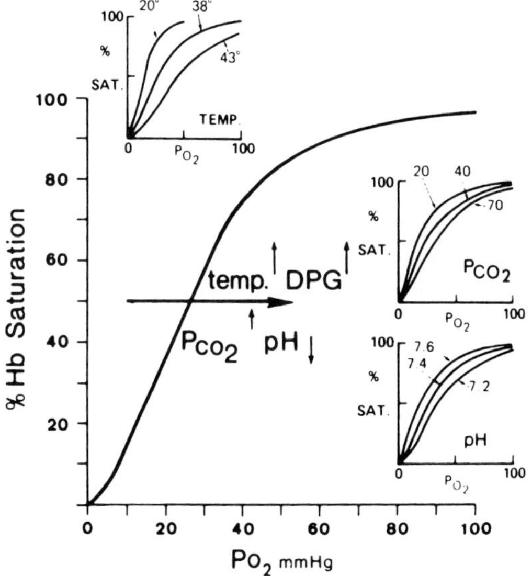

Figure 13.17. Shifts of the oxygen-hemoglobin dissociation curve for human blood as a result of changes in blood temperature, blood pH, blood Pco_2, and 2,3-diphosphoglycerate (DPG). A shift to the right, as shown by the large arrow, is caused by increases in temperature, DPG, and Pco_2 and decreases in pH. (From West, *Respiratory Physiology—the essentials*. 2d ed. © 1979, the Williams & Wilkins Co., Baltimore.)

ability of hemoglobin to yield or receive O_2 is referred to as the *Bohr effect*. Other factors noted to cause shifts in the curve are the temperature of the blood and the concentration of 2,3-diphosphoglycerate (DPG) within the red blood cell. There is a greater need for oxygen during hyperthermia, and, because increases in blood temperature cause the curve to shift to the right, greater yields of oxygen are provided to the tissues at these times. The normal utilization coefficient for avian blood is about $\frac{1}{2}$. The higher body temperature of these animals assists in the provision of easier oxygen yield. DPG is normally present in the blood, but its concentration varies under different conditions; DPG concentration is known to increase during conditions of hypoxia. During hypoxia the oxygen-hemoglobin dissociation curve is shifted to the right, and the dissociation of O_2 from hemoglobin is promoted. The magnitude of the shift caused by hypoxia is not as large at the Po_2 of oxygen loading as it is at the Po_2 of oxygen unloading, and an overall advantage is obtained.

CARBON DIOXIDE TRANSPORT

General scheme

A schematic illustration of carbon dioxide transport is shown in Fig. 13.18. This scheme considers the following aspects:

1. The amount (volume) of carbon dioxide that is dissolved (in solution) is consistent with Henry's law and is directly related to the Pco_2 and solubility coefficient. Carbon dioxide is about 24 times more soluble in water than O_2. Accordingly, one would expect greater volumes of carbon dioxide than of oxygen to be dissolved in water at a particular partial pressure.
2. Carbon dioxide is produced in body cells and readily diffuses through cell membranes. The diffusion coefficient for carbon dioxide is about 20 times greater than it is for oxygen.
3. Diffusion occurs because of partial pressure gradients; carbon dioxide will diffuse from its production site in cells to interstitial water, from interstitial water to plasma water, and from plasma water to erythrocyte water.
4. Ventilation will provide a lowered partial pressure gradient for carbon dioxide in the alveoli so that diffusion at this point will proceed to the alveoli from plasma water, followed by diffusion to plasma water from erythrocyte water.
5. Because the amount of carbon dioxide dissolved in water is not adequate for transporting the quantity produced, there are several reactions of importance in the plasma, and particularly in the erythrocytes that accommodate the remainder.

Carbon dioxide in plasma

Carbon dioxide that diffuses to the plasma from the cells not only will exist as dissolved carbon dioxide but also will combine with terminal amino groups of plasma proteins to

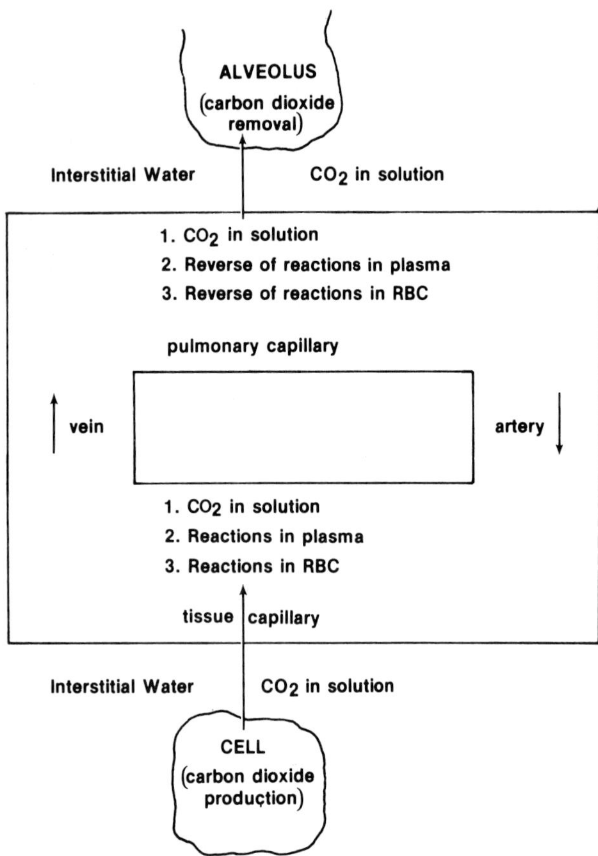

Figure 13.18. General scheme of carbon dioxide transport showing carbon dioxide procession. Procession occurs because of gradients. Blood flow is clockwise; carbon dioxide is taken up by blood from cells at bottom and removed from blood by the lungs at top. The items are numbered in the order of their occurrence. The reactions in plasma and the RBC are those associated with hydration of carbon dioxide, formation of carbamino compounds, and the buffering of hydrogen ion. These reactions are relatively minimal in plasma. The last carbon dioxide to go into plasma solution from the tissue cells is the first to leave at the alveolus. RBC, red blood cell.

form carbamino compounds and also will be hydrated to form ionization products of carbonic acid. The reaction with the amino groups is

$$R{-}NH_2 + CO_2 \rightleftharpoons R{-}N\begin{matrix} H \\ COOH \end{matrix} \rightleftharpoons R{-}N\begin{matrix} H \\ COO^- \end{matrix} + H^+$$

This reaction does not account for a significant amount of transport because there are relatively few free or terminal amino groups on plasma protein capable of combining with carbon dioxide.

The hydration of carbon dioxide proceeds as

$$CO_2 + H_2O \rightleftharpoons H_2CO_3$$

The equilibrium of the hydration reaction in plasma is far to the left. In fact, the concentration of carbon dioxide in plasma is about 1000 times greater than the concentration of carbonic acid. In summary, the reactions that occur in plasma with carbon dioxide are not significant when one considers the entirety of carbon dioxide transport.

Carbon dioxide in erythrocytes

Carbon dioxide readily diffuses into erythrocytes, and reactions with water and amino groups are more significant than in plasma. There are greater numbers of terminal amino groups on hemoglobin than there are on plasma proteins, so that this carriage form is more prominent. Also, the hydration reaction is facilitated by the presence of carbonic anhydrase, an enzyme found within erythrocytes. The carbonic acid that is formed ionizes to produce hydrogen and bicarbonate ions. Even though the equilibrium of the hydration reaction favors the formation of hydrogen and bicarbonate ions, it is rate-limited if the ionization products are not removed. The ionization products are removed, however, by the buffering of hydrogen ions by hemoglobin and by the diffusion of bicarbonate ions from the erythrocytes to the plasma.

Hydrogen ions are accommodated by hemoglobin as follows:

1. Combination with the basic carboxyl groups, suppressing their ionization and forming undissociated groups:

$$R{-}COO^- + H^+ \rightleftharpoons R{-}COOH$$

The electrical neutrality of the carboxyl groups was previously maintained by sodium and potassium ions.

2. Combination with imidazole groups of hemoglobin (see Fig. 13.19).

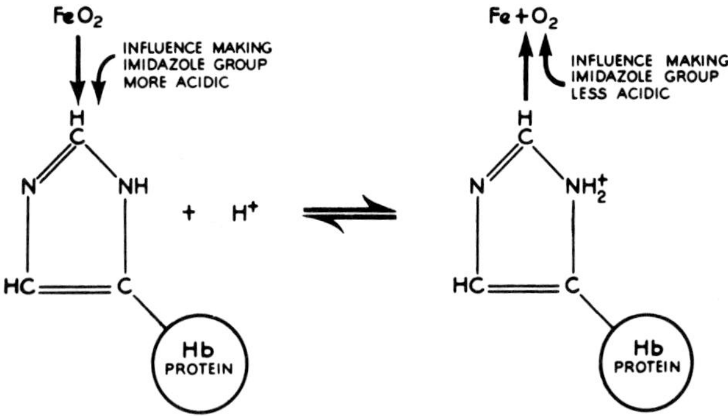

Figure 13.19. Schematic representation of the effect of oxygenation and deoxygenation on the chemical buffering action of the imidazole group ($C_3H_4N_2$) of hemoglobin. When oxygenated hemoglobin is deoxygenated (*right*), the beta chains of hemoglobin change their shape (not shown). In their new conformation, the C terminal histidines in the beta chains react with the aspartates at position 94 in the same chain. This interaction raises the apparent pK of the imidazole group of the histidines, and hydrogen ions are taken up from solution. When deoxygenated hemoglobin is again oxygenated (*left*), the C terminal histidines become free in solution once more; their pK falls, and they give off hydrogen ions. (Reprinted from *The ABC of Acid-Base Chemistry* by H.W. Davenport, by permission of the University of Chicago Press. © 1947, 1949, 1950, 1958, 1969, 1974 by the University of Chicago).

As noted above, electrical neutrality before buffering is maintained by sodium and potassium ions in balance with the carboxyl groups. After ionization of the carboxyl groups is suppressed by hydrogen ions, electrical neutrality of sodium and potassium ions is maintained by bicarbonate and chloride ions. As bicarbonate ions accumulate with continued hydration of carbon dioxide, they diffuse from the erythrocytes to the plasma because of a concentration gradient. Sodium and potassium ions do not readily diffuse, and electrical neutrality is then maintained because chloride ions diffuse from the plasma (where they are in relatively higher concentration) to the erythrocytes. This transfer of chloride ions is known as the *chloride shift* or, traditionally, as the *Hamburger shift*.

The reactions of carbon dioxide within erythrocytes are schematically represented by Fig. 13.20.

The chemical reactions within erythrocytes associated with carbon dioxide transport cause an increase in the effective osmotic pressure of the erythrocyte fluid, causing inward diffusion of water. An observation of slightly increased erythrocyte size in venous blood as compared with their size in arterial blood is explained by this phenomenon (see Fig. 13.21 for details).

When venous blood reaches the capillaries of the lung, the carbon dioxide in solution in plasma water begins to diffuse toward the alveoli. Ventilation of the alveoli lowers the P_{CO_2} and establishes the pressure gradient. The loss of carbon dioxide from the plasma water is followed by the loss of carbon dioxide that is in solution in the erythrocyte water. The equilibrium of the hydration reaction now favors formation of CO_2 and H_2O from H_2CO_3 because of the loss of carbon dioxide, and dehydration of carbonic acid proceeds. All of the reactions that had previously accommodated carbon dioxide transport are now reversed, so that carbon dioxide may be lost at the lung. The reverse reactions are facilitated because hemoglobin is becoming oxygenated. Oxygenated hemoglobin is more acidic and, accordingly, releases hydrogen ions. These hydrogen ions combine with bicarbonate ions to form carbonic acid, which in turn is dehydrated to carbon dioxide and water. The effect of oxygen on hydrogen ion and carbon dioxide loading and unloading from hemoglobin is known as the *Haldane effect*. The loss of O_2 from hemoglobin in the tissue capillaries makes hemoglobin more basic and hydrogen ions are received, facilitating the hydration reaction. The Haldane effect is an analogue of the Bohr effect. It was discovered by Christiansen, Douglas, and Haldane and is sometimes referred to as the *C-D-H effect*.

Carbon dioxide dissociation curve

By studying the oxygen-hemoglobin dissociation curve, it is possible to observe how the amount of O_2 carried by

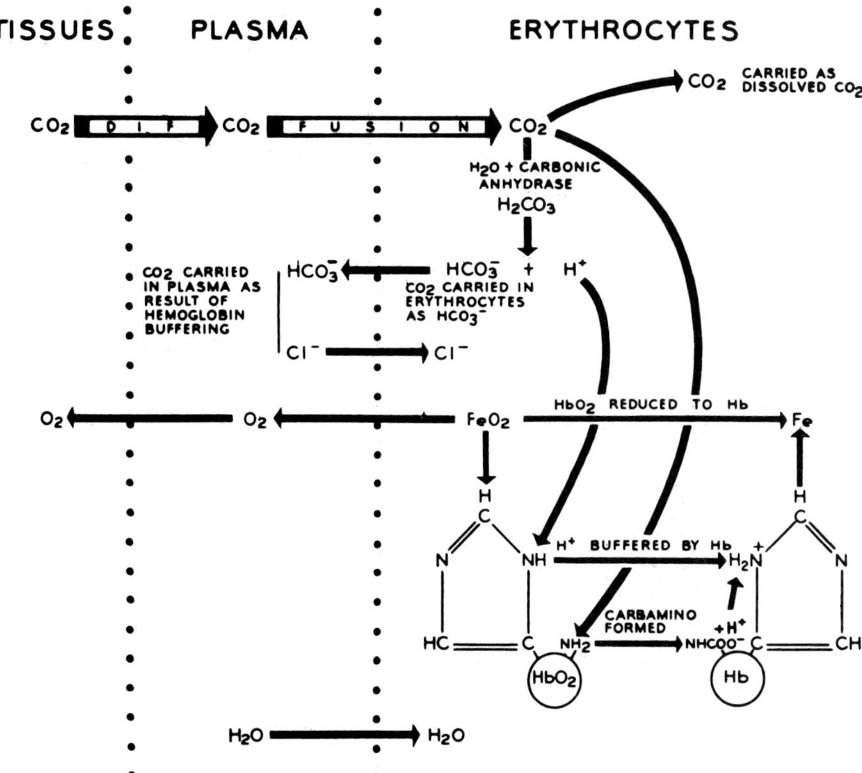

Figure 13.20. Schematic representation of the processes occurring when carbon dioxide diffuses from tissues into erythrocytes. The reactions shown as occurring in erythrocytes provide for the principal methods of transporting carbon dioxide from the cells to the lungs. (Reprinted from *The ABC of Acid-Base Chemistry* by H.W. Davenport, by permission of the University of Chicago Press. © 1947, 1949, 1950, 1958, 1969, 1974 by the University of Chicago).

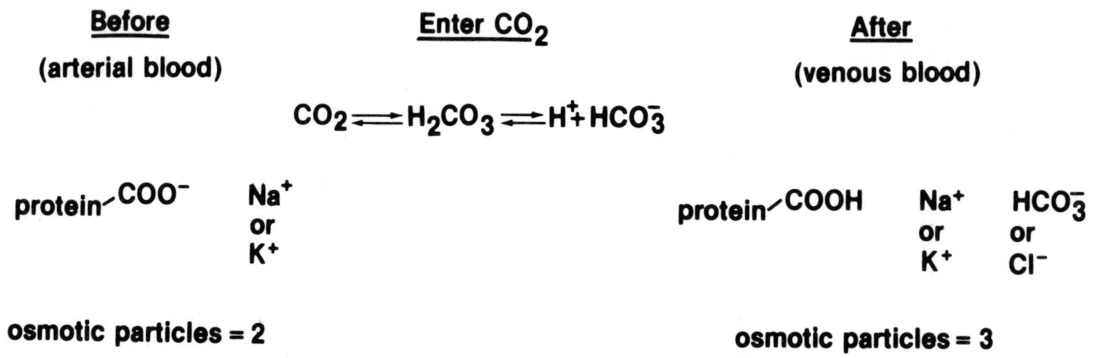

Before
(arterial blood)

Enter CO_2

$CO_2 \rightleftharpoons H_2CO_3 \rightleftharpoons H^+ + HCO_3^-$

After
(venous blood)

protein$\diagup$$COO^-$ Na^+ or K^+

protein$\diagup$COOH Na^+ or K^+ HCO_3^- or Cl^-

osmotic particles = 2

osmotic particles = 3

Figure 13.21. Effect of carbon dioxide transport on osmotic characteristics of erythrocytes. After the hydration of carbonic acid (H_2CO_3), both hydrogen (H^+) and bicarbonate (HCO_3^-) ions are formed. Carboxyl group anions (COO^-) associated with proteins and sodium or potassium ions (cations) represent two forms of osmotic particles that are present before the hydration of carbon dioxide (*left*). When a hydrogen ion is buffered, the carboxyl group becomes undissociated and still represents one osmotic particle form. The sodium or potassium ion, which maintained electrical neutrality with the carboxyl group, remains ionized and is in equilibrium with another anion (a bicarbonate ion formed from hydration or a chloride ion from the chloride shift) (*right*). Where there were previously two osmotic forms, there are now three; hence the increase in effective osmotic pressure. Particle numbers are relative to the amount of carbon dioxide transported.

hemoglobin changes with changes in the partial pressure of oxygen. Similarly, the amount of carbon dioxide transported in all of its forms (as CO_2, reactions with water, hemoglobin, and protein) varies with changes in partial pressure of carbon dioxide and is illustrated with a carbon dioxide dissociation curve (Fig. 13.22). Oxygen-hemoglobin dissociation curves are shifted to the right or left by several factors (Fig. 13.17) and because of the Bohr effect (influence of CO_2 on dissociation of O_2), a curve for venous blood is shifted to the right of that for arterial blood. In the upper carbon dioxide absorption curve it is seen that, for every increment of P_{CO_2}, a greater volume of CO_2 is transported. This happens because of the Haldane effect wherein loss of oxygen from arterial blood provides for greater accommodation of carbon dioxide. When arterial blood becomes venous blood, the partial pressure of carbon dioxide is about 5 mm Hg higher and contains about 4 volumes percent more carbon dioxide than arterial blood. If it were not for the Haldane effect, the partial pressure of carbon dioxide in venous blood would be about 12 mm Hg higher than that in arterial blood (rather than 5 mm Hg higher) in order to transport the added 4 volumes percent of carbon dioxide. This would seriously change acid-base balance and pulmonary ventilation.

It is instructive to relate volumes percent of oxygen consumed and volumes percent of carbon dioxide removed to the *respiratory quotient* (RQ), which is equated as

$$RQ = \frac{CO_2 \text{ production}}{O_2 \text{ consumption}}$$

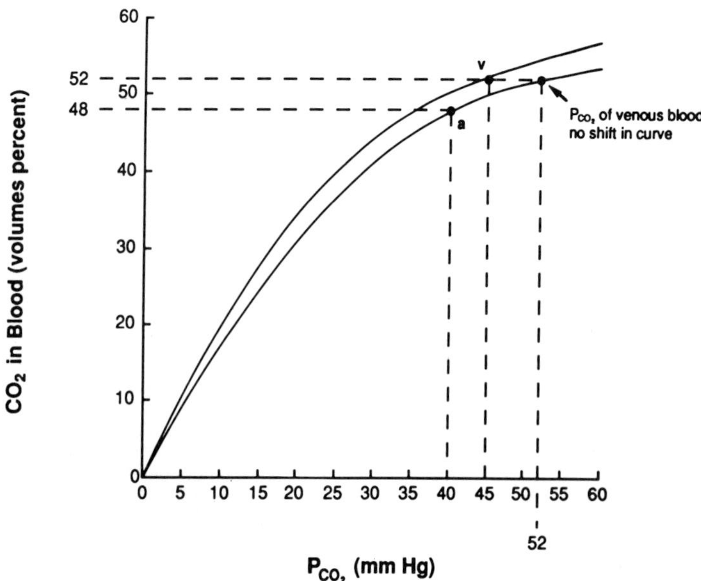

Figure 13.22. The carbon dioxide dissociation curves. The lower curve represents arterial blood, and the upper curve represents venous blood. Dashed lines are guides to the points indicated. Note that arterial blood with a P_{CO_2} of 40 mm Hg contains 48 volumes percent carbon dioxide and that venous blood with a P_{CO_2} of 45 mm Hg has 52 volumes percent, an increase of 4 volumes percent. The loss of oxygen from hemoglobin causes a greater accommodation for CO_2 by hemoglobin (Haldane effect whereby CO_2 dissociation curve shifts to the left). To transport the additional 4 volumes percent without the Haldane effect, the P_{CO_2} of venous blood would rise to 52 mm Hg.

Substituting the values used above, which represent normal values for inactivity, it is found that

$$RQ = \frac{4 \text{ vol } \%}{5 \text{ vol } \%} = 0.8$$

This represents a respiratory quotient that is common for intermediary metabolism, wherein the diet is balanced for carbohydrates, fats, and proteins.

REGULATION OF RESPIRATION

The respiratory center

The rhythmic pattern of breathing and the adjustments that occur therein are integrated within portions of the brain stem known as the respiratory center. Unlike many centers, it is not a collection of circumscribed nuclei but, rather, consists of regions within the medulla and pons associated with specific respiration-related functions. At the present time, four specific regions of the respiratory center have been identified: (1) the pneumotaxic center in the rostral portion of the pons, (2) the apneustic center in the caudal pons, (3) the dorsal respiratory group in the dorsal medulla, and (4) the ventral respiratory group in the ventral medulla.

Pneumotaxic center

The neurons within the pneumotaxic center receive their stimulation from the dorsal respiratory group (DRG) and exert their influence on the region of the ventral respiratory group (VRG). It is believed that the pneumotaxic center modulates the respiratory center sensitivity to inputs that activate the termination of inspiration and facilitate expiration.

Apneustic center

Of all the regions of the respiratory center, the apneustic center is the least understood; consequently, there is no consensus as to its role. Whereas the pneumotaxic center is concerned with the termination of inspiration, the apneustic center is believed to be associated with deep inspirations (apneusis). Perhaps complementary breaths are manifestations of apneustic center activity.

Dorsal respiratory group

Neurons of the DRG are predominantly associated with inspiratory activity. Two types of unit are recognized. One type projects mostly to phrenic motoneurons (diaphragm contraction) but also to the pneumotaxic center and the VRG (nucleus ambiguus only). The second type consists mainly of interneurons that are inhibitory to the first type and in this way are associated with inspiratory neurons. This second type is stimulated by afferents of lung receptors as the lung inflates. Therefore the DRG plays an important role in lung inflation–induced termination of inspiration.

Ventral respiratory group

Neurons of the VRG are composed of two separate nuclei—the nucleus ambiguus and the nucleus retroambigualis—each containing both inspiratory and expiratory cells. The nucleus ambiguus projects to the accessory muscles of respiration (mainly the larynx) via cranial nerves. The nucleus retroambigualis projects to phrenic and intercostal motoneurons. The nucleus retroambigualis inspiratory cells are of two types and are known as *early-burst* and *late-inspiratory* cells. The early-burst cells have an early peak of firing and then decline. These cells project to the late-inspiratory neurons, which they excite, and to nucleus retroambigualis expiratory neurons, which they inhibit. The late-inspiratory neurons have their peak firing late in the inspiratory phase. The nucleus retroambigualis expiratory neurons provide the excitatory drive to the expiratory intercostal and abdominal motoneurons. Excitation to the nucleus retroambigualis expiratory neurons is provided by receptors in the lung as it inflates.

Central pattern generator

The nature of the neural elements in the brain stem that produce rhythmicity is not known. The favored hypothesis is that there exists a neural network of interneurons known as the central pattern generator (CPG). It is believed that the CPG is paired, with one part existing in the region of the VRG and one in the region of the DRG; the pair has appropriate connections of coordinating fibers. The CPG is influenced by vagal inputs and chemoreceptors and has outputs to the dorsal and ventral respiratory groups.

Events of the respiratory cycle

A schematic representation of the respiratory center and its activity is shown in Fig. 13.23. This scheme will help the reader understand the explanation below of the events of the respiratory cycle. Commencing with the inspiratory phase of the cycle, the inspiratory neurons in the DRG and the VRG receive stimulation from the CPG. The neurons of the DRG stimulate simultaneously the motoneurons supplying the diaphragm, the neurons of the pneumotaxic center, and inspiratory neurons of the nucleus ambiguus in the VRG. The early-burst cells of the VRG's inspiratory group, having been stimulated by the CPG also, provide simultaneous stimuli to VRG late-inspiratory cells and to the VRG expiratory group. The VRG late-inspiratory cells (which project to phrenic and inspiratory intercostal motoneurons) are excited and the VRG expiratory group (which projects to expiratory intercostal and abdominal motoneurons and to inspiratory intercostal motoneurons) is inhibited. Inhibition to the VRG expiratory group provides for a release of inspiratory intercostal motoneuron inhibition inasmuch as they are inhibited when the VRG expiratory group is stimulated. As the lung inflates, afferents from lung receptors project to the inspiratory-inhibitory neurons of the DRG and to the expiratory neurons of the VRG,

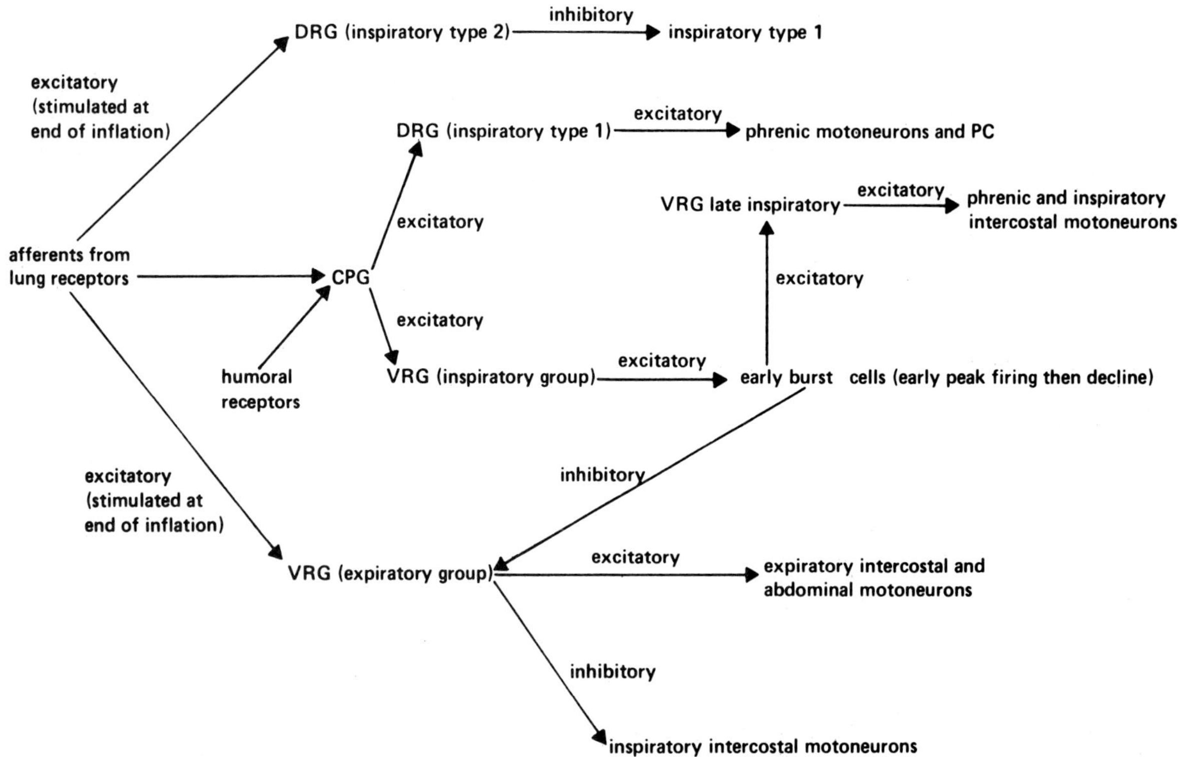

Figure 13.23. Schematic representation of the respiratory center and its activity. Only the nucleus retroambigualis projection is depicted for the VRG (ventral respiratory group). The nucleus ambiguus is not shown. Arrows designate projecting neurons. Excitatory and inhibitory notations on the arrows indicate the nature of the neurosecretion of the projecting neurons. CPG, central pattern generator; DRG, dorsal respiratory group; VRG, ventral respiratory group; PC, pneumotaxic center. See text for details of this model's function.

which assist in terminating inspiration and in beginning expiration. These afferents also project to the CPG to modify its output. The pneumotaxic center, which is stimulated when inspiration begins, influences the sensitivity of cells that provide for the termination of inspiration and the beginning of expiration. At the conclusion of expiration stimulation is again received from the CPG to initiate inspiration, and the cycle is repeated.

There are elements of this model that are not clearly understood, but it does provide a basis on which to visualize the many neural interconnections involved in rhythmic breathing. The model uses terminology consistent with the most recent findings, and further research will clarify its precise function.

Neural control of ventilation

The basic rhythm of respiration may be modified so that the breathing rate, depth, or both are changed. The reason for the modification is to change the rate of ventilation in response to body needs. Afferent impulses to the respiratory center from several receptor sources have been identified. The most noteworthy of these among many of the animals are the Hering-Breuer reflexes. The receptors for these reflexes are located in the lung and particularly in the bronchi and bronchioles. The nerve impulses that are generated by the receptors of the Hering-Breuer reflexes are transmitted by fibers in the vagus nerves to the respiratory center. The effect of inflation-receptor stimulation is to inhibit further inspiration (stimulation of neurons in the DRG) and to stimulate expiratory neurons in the VRG. Tidal volume can be increased, however, when stimuli from several sources exceed those that terminate inspiration.

Figure 13.24 is a pneumogram that shows respiratory cycles in a dog before and after anesthesia of first the right and then the left vagus nerves. Note the graded increase in tidal volume and decrease in frequency as the number of impulses from the lung receptors to the respiratory center is decreased by local anesthetic action.

A particular degree of deflation stimulates the deflation receptors, which in turn stimulate the respiratory center so that the next inspiration begins. It is not known whether these receptors are stimulated during eupnea. It appears that they may be most active when deflation is more complete. Receptor stimulation is elicited in anesthetized dogs by compression of the thorax. The inflation-receptor stimulation of the Hering-Breuer reflexes has been referred to as the inspiratory-inhibitory reflex (or inflation reflex), and

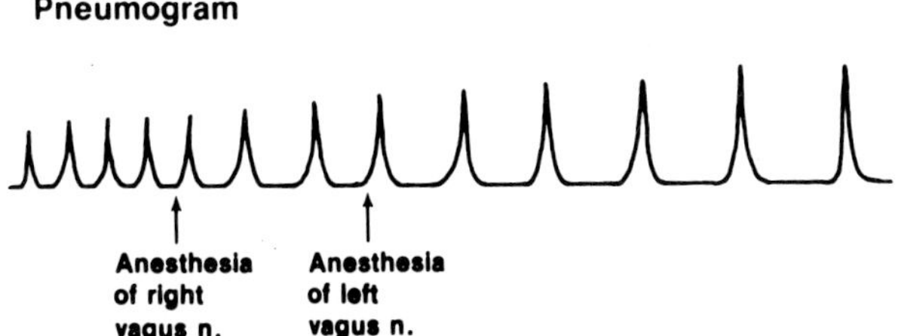

Figure 13.24. Changes in amplitude and frequency of respiratory cycles that occur after loss of vagus nerve afferent impulses by local infiltration of anesthetic. Higher peaks indicate increased tidal volume. Wider peaks indicate slower respiratory frequency. Drawn from actual recording.

the deflation-receptor stimulation has been referred to as the inspiratory reflex (or deflation reflex).

In addition to the receptors located in the lung, there are other peripherally located receptors that assist in modifying the basic rhythm. Stimulation of receptors in the skin is excitatory to the respiratory center, and deeper than usual inspiration may be noted. Perhaps their excitation to the inspiratory area is through the apneustic area, inasmuch as inspiratory gasps are occasionally seen. Advantage is taken of these receptors when stimulation of breathing is desired in newborn animals. Rubbing the skin with a rough cloth often starts the breathing cycles. An assist to ventilation needed during muscle activity is obtained from receptors located in tendons and joints. They will be stimulated when muscle contraction causes movement. It is also believed that when impulses go to skeletal muscles from the cerebral cortex, collateral impulses go to the brain stem and stimulate the respiratory center to increase alveolar ventilation. This mechanism might account for increases in ventilation that are not explainable by mere observation of changes in carbon dioxide, oxygen, and hydrogen ion concentration in the blood.

A number of respiratory reflexes take place from the upper air passages. Stimulation of the mucous membrane in these regions causes reflex inhibition of respiration. A striking example of this reflex is the inhibition of respiration that occurs during swallowing. Another example is seen in diving birds and mammals; submergence of the head causes reflex inhibition of breathing. Stimulation of the mucous membrane of the larynx in the unanesthetized animal causes not only inhibition of respiration but, usually, also powerful expiratory efforts (coughing). Similarly, stimulation of the nasal mucous membrane frequently leads to sneezing. Obviously, the function of all these latter reflexes is to protect the delicate respiratory passages and the depths of the lungs from harmful substances (irritating gases, dust, food particles) that otherwise might be inspired. To make the protection more certain, the glottis is closed and the bronchi may be constricted. Endotracheal intubation is often difficult in lightly anesthetized animals because of reflex closure of the glottis.

Ordinary respirations proceed quite involuntarily. It is, however, a matter of everyday experience that they may be altered voluntarily within wide limits; they may be hastened, slowed, or stopped altogether for a while. If respirations are entirely inhibited voluntarily, there soon comes a time when the animal must breathe again; the cells of the respiratory center escape from the inhibition. Phonation and related acts and the use of the abdominal press in the expulsive acts of defecation, urination, and parturition are examples of more or less complete voluntary control of the respiratory movements.

Afferent impulses from baroreceptors in the carotid and aortic sinuses have as their principal function a role in the regulation of the circulation. The same receptors are able to modify respiration. The receptors are constantly generating impulses that increase in frequency when the blood pressure increases and decrease in frequency when the blood pressure decreases. These impulses to the respiratory center are inhibitory in nature, and respiratory frequency decreases. It is believed that the function of this response is to modify the return of blood to the heart. For example, when blood pressure is reduced, respiration increases and the return of blood to the heart is facilitated. The effect of increased respiratory excursions, as evidenced by thoracic enlargement, is to provide a greater negativity of intrapleural pressure. Reduction in intrapleural pressure is transmitted to the mediastinal space, which aids in the expansion of the vena cava and reduction of the blood pressure within (see Fig. 13.4). The larger blood pressure difference created between the vena cava and the peripheral veins assists in the return of blood to the heart.

Humoral control of ventilation

In addition to the rather direct neural impingement on the respiratory center that has just been described, there are also blood chemicals that modify the basic rhythm. Inasmuch as these factors are present in the blood, this control mechanism may be referred to as *humoral control*. Specifically, the chemicals referred to are carbon dioxide, oxygen, and hydrogen ions. Their concentrations in arterial blood change alveolar ventilation as follows:

1. An increase in carbon dioxide partial pressure causes alveolar ventilation to increase; a decrease in carbon dioxide partial pressure causes alveolar ventilation to decrease.
2. An increase in hydrogen ion concentration causes alveolar ventilation to increase; a decrease in hydrogen ion concentration causes alveolar ventilation to decrease.
3. A decrease in oxygen partial pressure causes alveolar ventilation to increase; an increase in oxygen partial pressure causes alveolar ventilation to decrease.

Chemosensitive areas near the ventral surface of the medulla are highly sensitive to changes in hydrogen ion concentration of the interstitial fluid of the brain. The chemoreceptors in these areas are excitatory to the respiratory center, causing increases in tidal volume and in frequency. Whereas hydrogen ions diffuse poorly through the blood-cerebrospinal fluid barrier and the blood-brain barrier, carbon dioxide is freely diffusible and indirectly exerts its influence on ventilation through the intermediary of hydrogen ions after hydration ($CO_2 + H_2O \rightleftharpoons H_2CO_3 \rightleftharpoons H^+ + HCO_3^-$). Therefore, whenever the concentration of carbon dioxide in the blood increases, the P_{CO_2} of both the interstitial fluid of the medulla and of the cerebrospinal fluid increases, forming H^+ through hydration. It is believed that most of the respiratory center stimulation results from the H^+ changes in the interstitial fluid. Since the chemoreceptors are located near the surface of the medulla, however, diffusion of H^+ from the cerebrospinal fluid to the chemoreceptors is also considered a source of stimulation.

It is important to recognize that the accumulation of those substances (carbon dioxide and hydrogen ions) produced by the cells increases ventilation in order to eliminate them and that a reduction in the amount of the substance consumed (oxygen) increases ventilation so that the supply will be replenished. It is just as important to recognize also that reductions of carbon dioxide and hydrogen ions decrease ventilation. This decreased ventilation, in turn, prevents their extreme loss, which otherwise would cause drastic changes in body fluid pH. In other words, hyperventilation might lower the carbon dioxide concentration, and consequently the hydrogen ion concentration, to a point where the body fluids are too alkaline. This effect, whereby reduced concentrations of carbon dioxide and hydrogen ions decrease alveolar ventilation, is known as a *braking effect*. It can be observed to some extent with increased concentrations of oxygen, but the effect is far more subtle.

The interactions of carbon dioxide, oxygen, and hydrogen ion concentrations are quite apparent under certain conditions. It is possible for a lack of oxygen to increase ventilation to the point where carbon dioxide and hydrogen ion reduction by hyperventilation exert a braking effect. This prevents severe respiratory alkalosis, which might otherwise develop. This situation develops during ascent to high altitudes with reduced oxygen. The braking effects of carbon dioxide and hydrogen ions are most apparent for the first several days, but adaptation reduces their influence so that ventilation does increase to compensate for the reduced oxygen in the atmosphere. Part of the adaptation relates to a less responsive carbon dioxide and hydrogen ion braking effect.

Peripheral chemoreception

Up to this point, the chemical control of alveolar ventilation has been discussed only in terms of its direct effect on the medulla (the chemosensitive area). It should be noticed that oxygen did not exert its influence in that area. The anatomical entities known as the carotid and aortic bodies, found in the region of the bifurcation of the carotid arteries and the arch of the aorta, respectively, are chemoreceptors. They detect changes in the partial pressures of carbon dioxide and oxygen and hydrogen ion concentration and affect the respiratory center by transmission of impulses in afferent nerve fibers of the glossopharyngeal nerves (from the carotid bodies) and vagus nerves (from the aortic arch). Although the medulla is the principal location for detection of changes in CO_2 and H^+ concentrations, it has been shown that these peripheral chemoreceptors supply about 30 percent of the ventilatory drive in response to Pa_{CO_2} changes. Denervation of the carotid bodies in most of the domestic animals (dogs, cats, sheep, goats, ponies, cattle) causes chronic hypoventilation (Pa_{CO_2} increased by 5 to 10 mm Hg), indicating that the carotid bodies supply an important part of the tonic drive to resting ventilation in normoxic conditions. Carotid and aortic body chemoreceptors, however, are the only places where the partial pressure of oxygen is detected. These small organs are highly perfused with blood, and the O_2 needed for baseline activity is obtained from the oxygen in solution. The arteriovenous difference in O_2 content across the carotid body is too small for measurement. It should be emphasized that stimulation of the receptors is accomplished by the partial pressure of oxygen and carbon dioxide rather than by the amount of oxygen and carbon dioxide. Arterial blood with one-half as much hemoglobin may have a partial pressure of oxygen of 100 mm Hg, even though it has only half as much oxygen as normal blood. Any increased respiratory frequency in anemic animals would not be brought about because of the oxygen-lack mechanism. The carotid and aortic bodies are responding to the partial pressure of oxygen and not to the amount. Similarly, persons suffering from carbon monoxide poisoning (severe oxygen lack) do not experience a corresponding increase in respiratory frequency.

Nerve impulse transmission by the carotid and aortic bodies to the respiratory center varies with the partial pressure of oxygen perfusing them, as mentioned above. This is illustrated for the carotid bodies by Fig. 13.25. Note that the impulse discharge rate is increased most significantly in the P_{O_2} range of 30 to 60 mm Hg. The oxygen-hemoglobin dissociation curve (Fig. 13.16) shows that hemoglobin is still about 90 percent saturated with oxygen at a partial pressure of 60 mm Hg. No serious oxygen lack is present, and little change in ventilation occurs. Figure 13.25 also illustrates why the braking effect from oxygen excess is so subtle. It is virtually unnoticed in animals breathing atmospheric air because the partial pressure of oxygen in arterial blood seldom exceeds a pressure of 100 mm Hg. It is noticed only when the animal breathes gas mixtures that contain greater partial pressures of oxygen than atmospheric air. Figure 13.26 shows the respiratory frequency recorded in an anesthetized animal before and during the breathing of air enriched with oxygen. The partial pressure of oxygen of arterial blood in this instance was 350 mm Hg.

It is apparent that oxygen regulation is not normally needed. Hemoglobin is nearly saturated at an oxygen partial pressure of 100 mm Hg, and there would be no advantage to a higher partial pressure. Also, alveolar ventilation

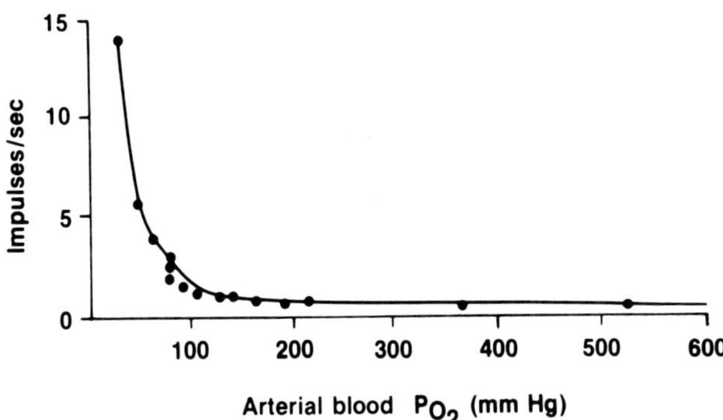

Figure 13.25. Effect of arterial oxygen partial pressure on the number of impulses per second from the carotid body to the respiratory center. The impulses are excitatory. (Redrawn and slightly modified from Biscoe, Purves, and Sampson 1970, *J. Physiol.* 208:121–31.)

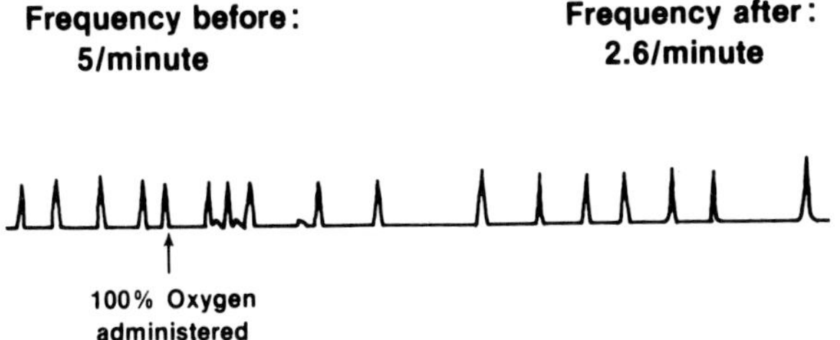

Figure 13.26. Pneumogram showing effect of oxygen enrichment on respiratory frequency. Oxygen was provided to a dog anesthetized with pentobarbital by means of an anesthesia machine. Note decreased frequency after administration of oxygen. Drawn from actual recording.

can be reduced to about one-half normal, and hemoglobin will retain considerable saturation. Accordingly, it is generally recognized that the leading chemical factor in normal regulation of ventilation resides with carbon dioxide. A ready response is obtained from relatively small changes in its partial pressure. Regulation by oxygen partial pressure, however, becomes more important in pneumonia, pulmonary edema, and the pneumoconioses, in which gases are not as readily diffusible through the respiratory membrane. Decreased diffusion is more readily noticed for oxygen than for carbon dioxide because of the smaller diffusion coefficient for oxygen. Accordingly, hyperventilation caused by oxygen lack may reduce carbon dioxide partial pressure and hydrogen ion concentration, whereby they become ineffective in stimulating increased ventilation. The oxygen-lack mechanism continues to function and provides the drive to increase ventilation. It should also be remembered that the oxygen-lack mechanism is useful in increasing ventilation at high altitudes after the adaptation period.

Periodic breathing

Breathing is considered abnormal when normal respiratory cycles and frequency patterns do not occur. The cycles sometimes occur in rapid succession (in pairs, triplets, or quadruplets) and are followed by varying intervals of apnea. This has been referred to as *grouped breathing* (Fig. 13.27). This may be common with head injuries and is frequently observed in animals anesthetized with pentobarbital.

Another form of periodic breathing is known as *Cheyne-Stokes breathing*. This is not frequently reported in veterinary medicine. Perhaps it is unrecognized. It is characterized by successive occurrence of the respiratory cycles in a waxing and waning pattern (Fig. 13.27). This breathing pattern is believed to be caused by a delay in the time from perfusion of the lungs with blood to the subsequent arrival of that blood at the brain. In other words, the chemoreceptors sense an increased Pa_{CO_2} and ventilation is increased. The perfused blood then equilibrates with the hyperventilated lungs, and the Pa_{CO_2} is lowered. When this blood reaches the brain, it exerts a braking effect on ventilation and the Pa_{CO_2} increases. The pattern of breathing is successively repeated because hyperventilation occurs again with the rise in Pa_{CO_2}. In normal breathing, circulation time between the lungs and the brain is relatively short; Pa_{CO_2} remains relatively constant, and respiratory cycles are of equal duration.

Another explanation for Cheyne-Stokes breathing postulates that some part of the respiratory control mechanism (possibly a chemoreceptor) has an increased gain so that the response to a stimulus causes an overly large ventilatory response, which in turn produces a larger than normal fall in Pa_{CO_2}. The braking effect is initiated and is followed by an oscillatory change in ventilation and blood gases.

RESPIRATORY CLEARANCE

Aerosols that arise from feedlot dusts or other livestock-confinement sources contain populations of particles that may be inhaled. Accordingly, bacteria and viruses may be aerosolized either by animal coughing and sneezing or by mechanical generation. An important function of the lung is to remove these particles (microorganisms or dusts) before they have an opportunity to invade cells or otherwise cause disease.

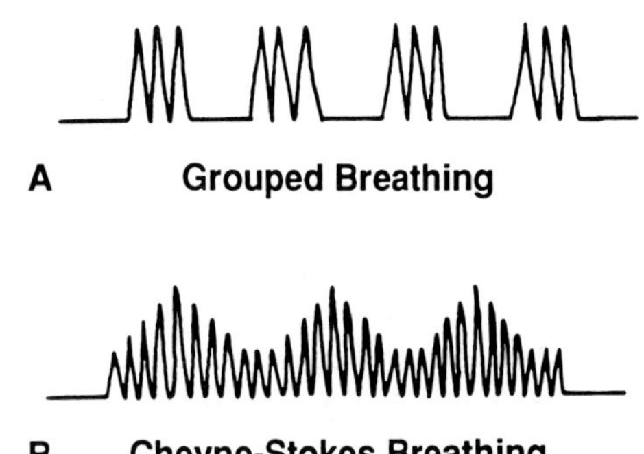

Figure 13.27. Drawings that illustrate pneumograms of periodic breathing. In grouped breathing, cycles appear in clusters of two or three. In Cheyne-Stoke's breathing, cycles alternately wax and wane.

Physical forces

Three different physical forces operate within the respiratory system to cause settlement of particles from the inhaled air just as they do to cause settlement of dust from the environmental air outside the body. The settlement of particles upon a mucous membrane is referred to as deposition. These physical forces are as follows:

1. Gravitational settling (sedimentation) causes deposition of particles simply because of the force of gravity and the mass of the particles. This provides for deposition in the nasal cavity and the tracheobronchial tree.

2. Inertial forces cause deposition in the nasal cavity, the pharynx, and the tracheobronchial tree. Since this deposition involves the factor of velocity, it probably promotes earlier deposition than gravitational settling. It becomes more of a factor at points of branching of the airways where the direction of flow changes. Inertial forces and gravitational settling are probably the most important deposition factors. Particle deposition increases, with increased particle size and increased density for both gravity and inertia.

3. Brownian motion accounts for deposition of submicron particles. These very small particles show a random motion that is imparted by air molecule bombardment. This factor becomes significant where there is a large area of intimate surface, as in the very small airways and alveoli.

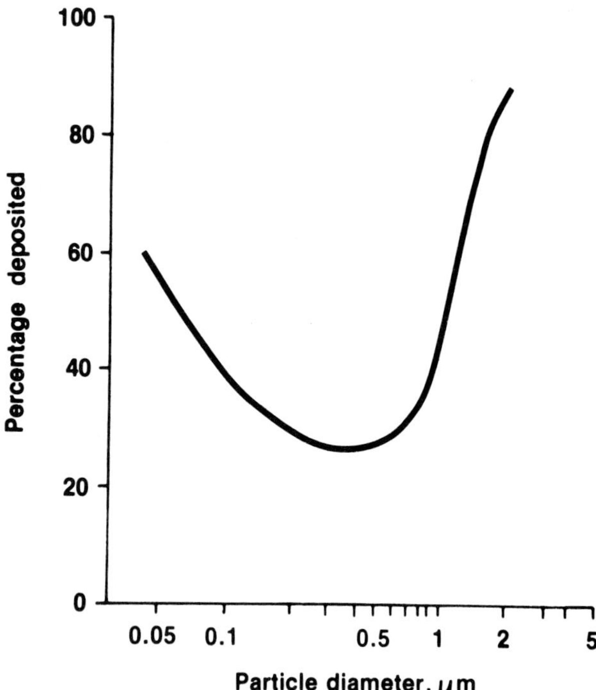

Figure 13.28. Percentage of inhaled particles (unit density) deposited in the lung according to their size. Particles in the range of 0.1 to 1.0 μm are those least affected by combined Brownian motion, sedimentation, and inertial impaction. (Redrawn, with permission, from *Health Physics* 2:372, P.E. Morrow. "Some Physical and Physiological Factors Controlling the Fate of Inhaled Substances—I." Copyright 1960, Pergamon Press, Ltd. Figure slightly modified.)

Particle size

The fraction of inhaled particles that is retained in the respiratory system and the depth to which the particles penetrate before deposition are closely related to particle size. Large particles settle onto the mucosa of the upper respiratory tract, and smaller particles penetrate more deeply into the lungs. For unit-density particles, those larger than 10 μm are essentially all removed in the nasal cavity. The deposition of particles proximal to the respiratory bronchioles decreases as particle size becomes smaller and is almost zero at diameters of 1 μm or less. Particles that penetrate to the pulmonary air spaces (including respiratory bronchioles and all distal structures) are generally smaller than 1 to 2 μm in diameter. Particle deposition is the least when the diameters are between 0.3 and 0.5 μm but begins to increase again when diameters are less than 0.3 μm (Fig. 13.28). Particles less than 0.3 μm diameter are more susceptible to Brownian movement.

Upper respiratory tract clearance

Once deposited, particles are cleared (removed) according to the location of their deposition. *Upper respiratory tract clearance* refers to the removal of particles that have been deposited at points proximal to the alveolar ducts. *Alveolar clearance* refers to the removal of particles that have been deposited within the alveoli. Upper respiratory tract clearance is dependent on the proximal movement of a blanket of mucinous fluid. The movement is provided by the ciliary activity of the columnar epithelium lining the tracheobronchial mucous membrane. The components of the mucous blanket are derived from three sources: (1) the film of fluid covering the alveolar membrane, (2) the apocrine, mucus-secreting cells that line the respiratory bronchioles, and (3) the goblet cells of the tracheobronchial mucosa proximal to the respiratory bronchioles. The rate of transport of the mucinous fluid is about 15 mm/min. When the mucous blanket and its contents reach the pharynx, it is ultimately swallowed. This is the means whereby inhaled materials appear in the feces.

Alveolar clearance

Several concepts of alveolar clearance have been developed, as follows:

1. There may be specialized absorptive sites near the alveolar ducts. It has been observed that visible deposits of particulate matter accumulate there. There are distal branches of the lymphatics at that location, and the accumulated particulates and fluid may be awaiting their entry into those lymphatics.

2. There may be a continuous flow of alveolar fluid to the bronchial epithelium, where it is then conveyed onward by the moving mucous blanket. It is believed that the fluid flow is facilitated by the mechanical action of breathing and

its associated changes in alveolar surface area. The result is that the cells and the particulate matter on the surface are moved out of the alveoli while the lower fluid layer accommodates changes in the surface area. This is similar to the accumulation of driftwood on the beach as water moves toward and recedes from the shore.

3. There is a general consensus that phagocyte activity is the most important process for clearance of inhaled insoluble particles and microorganisms. The current view is that alveolar phagocytes develop from monocytes that come to the alveolar wall from a capillary and migrate through the epithelial lining to enter the lumen of an alveolus. Once in the alveolus, they transform to macrophages and phagocytize large amounts of particulate material. These macrophages frequently have been referred to as "dust cells" because of particles noted within their cytoplasm. The process by which macrophages move from the alveoli to the moving mucous blanket is not clearly understood. It may be by random travel or by mechanical and directional assistance derived from alveolar fluid flow.

4. Although alveolar epithelial cells are not considered to be phagocytic, endocytosis does occur and particles may appear within the cytoplasm of these cells. Through normal cell turnover, desquamation occurs and they become "free cells" in the alveoli. Their subsequent movement to the moving mucous blanket would provide a clearance mechanism similar to that of macrophages, except that the quantity cleared is less. This mechanism is the important one in birds.

5. An inhaled particle may be solubilized by the alveolar fluid and be cleared from the alveolus by absorption. A lack of permeability of the alveolar epithelium for the substance, however, would virtually exclude its absorption.

6. It is well known that inhaled particles may be found in lymph nodes that are in series with lymph vessels that drain from the lungs. For material to enter these vessels, it must first be absorbed or transported from the alveolar epithelium to the interstitial space. It is known that terminal lymphatics are present in the interstitial space distal to the level of alveolar ducts. Inasmuch as lymphatic capillaries are highly permeable, it is no problem for particles to enter their interior. Once the particles have entered the lymph capillaries, they are directed to the lymph nodes, where they are either blocked by size or phagocytized by the mononuclear phagocyte system of the lymph nodes.

It has been noted above that phagocytosis facilitates the removal of particles by the alveolar clearance mechanism. It should also be recognized that phagocytosis by macrophages renders particles incapable of irritating or otherwise injuring the alveolar surface epithelium and also prevents penetration of dust particles into the lung interstitial space.

The fate of particles that settle upon the alveolar surface may be summarized according to four possibilities, as follows:

1. Particles may be transported to the mucous blanket of the tracheobronchial mucosa and thence to the pharynx, where they may be swallowed. This possibility includes free particles on the surface and those that have been phagocytized by macrophages or internalized by endocytosis into alveolar epithelial cells that subsequently desquamate.

2. Particles may be transported to the satellite lymph nodes that are in series with lymph vessels that serve the lungs (from which some may escape into the blood).

3. Particles may be dissolved and transferred in solution, either into the lymph or into the blood.

4. Some particles may fail to be phagocytized or may not be soluble. Instead, they may stimulate a local connective tissue reaction and be sequestered (isolated) within the lung. In this event, a pneumoconiosis may develop from continued exposure. This is a fibrous induration of the lung resulting from inhalation of certain dusts. Examples are asbestosis and silicosis. Also, dogs and cats that live in highly industrialized cities may show signs of anthracosis caused by inhalation of coal dust.

OTHER FUNCTIONS OF THE RESPIRATORY SYSTEM

The respiratory system has functions other than providing for alveolar ventilation. Of particular interest among animals are panting and purring. Panting is prevalent among many animal species; panting in the dog is described below. Perhaps it is similar in the other animals when it occurs. Purring is noted in some members of the feline family and is both audible and palpable in most domestic cats. The nasal cycle is also described below.

Panting

The respiratory center of the dog responds not only to the usual stimuli but also to body core temperature. The integration of these inputs permits the respiratory center to respond to metabolic needs by regulating alveolar ventilation and to dissipation of heat by regulating dead-space ventilation. Dead-space ventilation is increased by panting, which provides for cooling of the body by evaporation of water from the mucous membranes of the tissues involved.

Passage of air through the nasal cavity allows for more intimate association of air and mucosa than movement of air in the open mouth. Accordingly, it is reasoned that if, during panting, air moved in and out through the mouth only, the tongue and oral surfaces would not humidify the air sufficiently. Correspondingly larger volumes of air would need to be moved to provide cooling equivalent to that of fully saturated air. This would increase the expenditure of energy, and the heat load would increase. If air moved in and out only through the nose, the heat and water vapor added to the air during inhalation would be partially recovered by the body during exhalation. This would happen because of a countercurrent exchange system that would operate between the airstream and the nasal surfaces. Body cooling in this instance would be lessened.

Studies have shown that there are three patterns of panting: (1) inhalation and exhalation through the nose; (2) inhalation through the nose, exhalation through the nose and mouth; and (3) inhalation through the nose and mouth and exhalation through the nose and mouth.

It can be seen that the least cooling would be accomplished by nasal inhalation and exhalation (pattern 1). This pattern has been observed in resting dogs when the ambient temperature was below 26°C and also when they ran at slow speeds in the cold. Patterns 2 and 3 are observed when dogs rest quietly at ambient temperatures above 30°C and during exercise, except when exercise occurs at very low temperatures. Air direction through the nose and out the mouth would accomplish the greatest cooling, but where greater tidal volume is needed inhalation through the mouth and nose is necessary. There appears to be a continual oscillation between patterns 2 and 3. The proportion of time that pattern 3 is used instead of pattern 2 increases as temperature and speed are increased; pattern 3 is associated with greater alveolar ventilation requirements.

By changing the relative amounts of air exhaled through the nose or through the mouth, the dog can modulate the amount of heat dissipated without changing frequency or tidal volume. The advantage of a constant frequency is that added energy is not then needed to change from the intrinsic panting frequency (about 300 pants per minute) of the respiratory system. A change in the tidal volumes, especially an increase in tidal volume, could be undesirable because of its effect on hyperventilation and subsequent alkalosis. Apparently, this extreme may be prevented by the achievement of cooling with change in air direction (from pattern 1 to pattern 2). Tidal volume increase may be achieved when needed by a change from pattern 1 or 2 to pattern 3.

The airflow characteristics described for panting imply that the nasal mucosa, rather than the oral surfaces and the tongue, is the principal site of evaporation. Accordingly, an adequate supply of water must be provided to the nasal mucosa, and this may be derived from glandular secretions (nasal and orbital), vascular transudate, or both. The secretion from the lateral nasal glands has been studied to determine whether these glands serve to supply additional water during panting. There are two of these glands, one in each maxillary recess. Each gland empties through a single duct that opens about 2 cm inside the nostril. This rostral location is advantageous for caudal distribution of secretion when the airflow is directed into the nose and out through the mouth. The rate of secretion increases with increasing ambient temperature. An increase from 25 to 40°C increases the amount secreted 40 times. It has been suggested that this role of the lateral nasal glands is analogous to that of sweat glands in humans.

Purring

The following explanation of purring is derived from a reported study in the domestic cat. The study used electromyographic and tracheal pressure recording techniques and showed that the purr results from a highly regular, alternating activation of the diaphragm and intrinsic laryngeal muscles at a frequency of 25 times per second during both inspiration and expiration. The study showed that purring probably results from some oscillating mechanism within the central nervous system. Each repeated cycle has three phases: (1) glottal closing, (2) glottal opening and sound production, and (3) glottal opening (low glottal resistance and high airflow).

Glottal closing occurs when the adductor muscles of the larynx contract (i.e., the vocal cords become approximated). Each of the 25 successive sounds associated with 1 second of purring is produced when a pressure difference created on either side of the closed glottis is dissipated at the time of glottal opening (i.e., there is a sudden separation of the vocal cords). Glottal opening may be passive, but there is speculation that contraction of the laryngeal abductor muscles during inspiration occurs simultaneously with contraction of the diaphragm.

During the inspiratory phase of the respiratory cycle, there is also intermittent contraction of the diaphragm. In other words, diaphragmatic contraction alternates with laryngeal adductor contraction (glottal closure). The alternating contraction of the laryngeal adductors and of the diaphragm prevent extreme negativity in tracheal pressure at the time of glottal closure and also promote inspiratory flow during the time the glottis is open. Airflow during inspiration is provided by the intermittent contraction of the diaphragm and the lung expansion that follows. Repeated cycling and sound production continue until inspiration is complete.

During the expiratory phase of the respiratory cycle, the recoil tendency of the lungs creates tracheal pressure that is greater than pharyngeal pressure when the glottis is closed. When the laryngeal adductors relax, the glottis opens, the higher tracheal pressure forces air through the vocal cords, a sound is produced, the glottis closes (the vocal cords become approximated), tracheal pressure increases, and the cycle repeats until expiration is completed.

The reason for purring in cats is not known. It is known to occur at times when they are contented, when they are sick, and when they are sleeping. It seems possible that the intermittent nature of the inspiratory and expiratory phases of the respiratory cycle when a cat is purring may provide improved ventilation and prevent atelectasis during times of shallow breathing. In other words, purring may provide a function similar to complementary breaths.

Nasal cycling

The nasal cycle involves alternating congestion and decongestion of the nasal airways that reciprocate from one side to the other. Congestion, when it occurs, produces a change in resistance to airflow. As one nasal chamber becomes more open and its mucosal glands increase their secretion, the opposite nasal chamber becomes engorged as the erectile tissue of that side of the nose fills with blood and the mucosal gland secretion diminishes. The phenomenon was first observed in humans and more recently has been demonstrated in rats, rabbits, and pigs. Because of morphological similarities of the nasal cavity and nasal mucosa between humans and pigs, the latter may be valuable for experimentally determining the function of this cycle in humans. The period from the beginning of congestion to its end was about $2\frac{1}{2}$ hours. When one nasal cavity was most congested, the other was least congested. Human subjects usually are not conscious of the unilateral congestion because the total airway resistance remains steady.

In addition to the nasal cycle just described, another type of air resistance has been observed in humans and pigs. This type is associated with spontaneous increases or decreases in nasal resistance that accompany changes in respiration. In humans, the changes in respiration are in response to exercise and changes in arterial P_{CO_2}. Whereas the reciprocating cycle had a duration of $2\frac{1}{2}$ hours, the spontaneously induced increase or decrease in nasal air resistance persisted for 5 to 10 minutes. It was superimposed on the reciprocating cycle and involved both nasal cavities at the same time.

The changes in nasal cavity resistance are believed to be regulated by changes in the activity of autonomic innervation to the nasal erectile tissue. It is further believed that the sympathetic division of the autonomic nervous system has the major role in this regulation.

Recognition of the nasal cavities as highly organized physiological organs is relatively recent. Further studies of their activities will provide insight about their physiological significance and functions and also their relationship to other organs.

DESCRIPTIVE TERMS

States of breathing

The following terms are useful for describing the breathing pattern:

Eupnea is the state of ordinary quiet breathing.

Dyspnea is difficult or labored breathing.

Hyperpnea is a condition of breathing in which the frequency, the depth, or both are increased.

Tachypnea is excessive rapidity of breathing.

Bradypnea is abnormal slowness of breathing.

Hypopnea is breathing in which the frequency, depth, or both are decreased.

Polypnea is a rapid, shallow, panting type of respiration.

Hypoxia

Hypoxia is a decrease below normal P_{O_2} in air, blood, or tissue, short of anoxia. *Anoxia* literally means "without oxygen" and should not be used when the condition may be one of decreased P_{O_2} for which *hypoxia* is more appropriate. *Hypoxemia* is a decrease in the O_2 concentration of the arterial blood. Four types of hypoxia are recognized:

1. *Ambient hypoxia*, in which the arterial blood is insufficiently saturated with oxygen because of a low P_{O_2} in the atmosphere being breathed. This occurs naturally at high altitudes.
2. *Anemic hypoxia*, in which there is a decrease in the oxygen capacity of the blood because of a shortage of functioning hemoglobin. The partial pressure of oxygen in arterial blood and the percentage saturation of the hemoglobin are normal. Oxygen delivery to the tissues may be inadequate. Anemic hypoxia occurs after hemorrhage, in various anemias, and when some of the hemoglobin is changed to methemoglobin or is combined with carbon monoxide.
3. *Stagnant hypoxia*, also known as *ischemic hypoxia*, in which the blood flow through the whole body or a tissue is diminished. The oxygen content of arterial blood is normal, but the tissues fail to receive enough oxygen because of diminished blood flow.
4. *Histotoxic hypoxia*, in which the cells are unable to use the oxygen that is supplied. The amount of oxygen in arterial blood is normal, but because the cells are unable to use it, the amount is above normal in venous blood.

Other terms

Hypercapnia and *hypocapnia* are increased and decreased Pa_{CO_2}, respectively, in the blood.

Cyanosis is a bluish or purplish coloration of the skin and mucous membranes. The color reflects the degree of deoxygenation of hemoglobin. When observed throughout the body, it relates to improper oxygenation of blood. When seen locally, it is probably caused by blood flow obstruction.

Asphyxia is a condition of hypoxia combined with hypercapnia. It is apparent that hypoxia and hypercapnia may occur as single entities, but only their combination results in asphyxia. Breathing into a closed space provides a good example, and this results in what is commonly called suffocation.

Hyperbaric oxygenation is the provision of oxygen to the body at relatively high partial pressure of oxygen. The P_{O_2} may be extreme to the point that oxygen toxicity occurs. When this happens, there is a marked elevation of the P_{O_2} in the cells (hyperoxia) and the activity of many enzymes involved in tissue metabolism is affected.

Atelectasis is failure of the alveoli to open or remain open and usually involves one or more relatively small areas of lung. The usual cause of atelectasis is occlusion of the bronchus or bronchiole that supplies the area. This results most often from plugs of mucus or purulent exudate. When the bronchus closes, the air contained in the alveoli at the time is absorbed and the airless alveoli collapse because of the surrounding pressures.

Pneumonia is an acute inflammation of the lung that occurs in all species from a variety of causes. In the first stage the capillaries are distended with blood and the alveoli become filled with serous fluid. The serous fluid becomes mixed with erythrocytes, various leukocytes, and fibrin. Final resolution involves liquefaction of the alveolar debris, its removal, and regeneration of the alveolar epithelium.

REFERENCES

Adams, D.R., DeYoung, D.W., and Griffith, R. 1981. The lateral nasal gland of dog: its structure and secretory content. *J. Anat.* 132:29–37.

Albers, C., Usinger, W., and Scholand, C. 1975. Intracellular pH in unanesthetized dogs during panting. *Respir. Physiol.* 23:59–70.

Biscoe, T.J., Purves, M.J., and Sampson, S.R. 1970. The frequency of nerve impulses in single carotid body chemoreceptor afferent fibres recorded in vivo with intact circulation. *J. Physiol.* 208:121–31.

Bisgard, G.E., and Vogel, J.H.K. 1971. Hypoventilation and pulmonary hypertension in calves after carotid body excision. *J. Appl. Physiol.* 31:431–37.

Blatt, C.M., Taylor, C.R., and Habal, M.B. 1972. Thermal panting in dogs: The lateral nasal gland, a source of water for evaporative cooling. *Science* 177:804–805.

Clark, J.M., and Lambertsen, C.J. 1971. Pulmonary oxygen toxicity: A review. *Pharmacol. Rev.* 23:37–133.

Clements, J.A. 1962. Surface phenomena in relation to pulmonary function. *Physiologist* 5:11–28.

Comroe, J.H., Jr. 1974. *Physiology of Respiration*, 2d ed. Year Book, Chicago.

Crosfil, M.L., and Widdicombe, J.G. 1961. Physical characteristics of the chest and lungs and the work of breathing in different mammalian species. *J. Physiol.* 158:1–4.

Davenport, H.W. 1974. *The ABC of Acid-Base Chemistry*. 6th ed. University of Chicago Press, Chicago.

Eccles, R. 1978. The domestic pig as an experimental animal for studies on the nasal cycle. *Acta Otolaryngol.* 85:431–36.

Eccles, R. 1978. The central rhythm of the nasal cycle. *Acta Otolaryngol.* 86:464–68.

Federation Proceedings. 1950. Standardization of definitions and symbols in respiratory physiology. *Fed. Proc.* 9:602–605.

Felts, J.M. 1964. Biochemistry of the lung. *Health Phys.* 10:973–79.

Fidone, S.J., and Gonzalez, C. 1986. Initiation and control of chemoreceptor activity in the carotid body. In N.S. Cherniak and J.G. Widdicombe, eds., *Handbook of Physiology*. Sec. 3, vol. 2., *The Respiratory System*. Am. Physiol. Soc., Bethesda, Md.

Fitzgerald, R.S., and Tahiri, S. 1986. Reflex responses to chemoreceptor stimulation. In N.S. Cherniak and J.G. Widdecombe, eds., *Handbook of Physiology*. Sec. 3, vol. 2, *The Respiratory System*. Am. Physiol. Soc., Bethesda, Md.

Flandrois, R., Lacour, J.R., and Osman, J. 1971. Control of breathing in the exercising dog. *Respir. Physiol.* 13:361–71.

Gillespie, J.R., Tyler, W.S., and Eberly, V.E. 1966. Pulmonary ventilation and resistance in emphysematous and control horses. *J. Appl. Physiol* 21:416–22.

Godleski, J.J., and Brain, J.D. 1972. The origin of alveolar macrophages in mouse radiation chimeras. *J. Exp. Med.* 136:630–43.

Goldberg, M.B., Langman, V.A., and Taylor, C.R. 1981. Panting in dogs: paths of air flow in response to heat and exercise. *Respir. Physiol.* 43:327–38.

Guyton, A.C. 1991. *Textbook of Medical Physiology*. 8th ed., W.B. Saunders, Philadelphia.

Guyton, A.C., Crowell, J.W., and Moore, J.W. 1956. Basic oscillating mechanism of Cheyne-Stokes breathing. *Am. J. Physiol.* 187:395–98.

Hales, J.R.S., and Findlay, J.D. 1968. Respiration of the ox: Normal values and the effects of exposure to hot environments. *Respir. Physiol.* 4:333–52.

Hall, W.C., and Brody, S. 1933. XXVI. The energy increment of standing over lying and the energy cost of getting up and lying down in growing ruminants (cattle and sheep); comparison of pulse rate, respiration rate, tidal air, and minute volume of pulmonary ventilation during lying and standing. *Mo. Agr. Exp. Stat. Res. Bull.* 180:8–31.

Ham, A.W., and Cormack, D.H. 1979. *Histology*. 8th ed. J.B. Lippincott, Philadelphia.

Hamlin, R.L., and Smith, C.R. 1967. Characteristics of respiration in healthy dogs anesthetized with sodium pentobarbital. *Am. J. Vet. Res.* 28:175–78.

Hasegawa, M., and Kern, E.B. 1977. The human nasal cycle. *Mayo Clin. Proc.* 52:28–34.

Hatch, T.F., and Gross, P. 1964. *Pulmonary Deposition and Retention of Inhaled Aerosols*. Academic Press, New York.

Hernandez, A. 1987. Hypoxic ascites in broilers: A review of several studies done in Colombia. *Avian Dis.* 31:658–61.

Koterba, A.M., Kosch, P.E., Beech, J., and Whitlock, T. 1988. Breathing strategy of the adult horse (*Equus caballus*) at rest. *J. Appl. Physiol.* 64:337–46.

Leusen, S. 1972. Regulation of cerebrospinal fluid composition with reference to breathing. *Physiol. Rev.* 52:1–56.

Loeschcke, H.H. 1973. Respiratory chemosensitivity in the medulla oblongata. *Acta Neurobiol. Exp.* 33:97–112.

Loeschcke, H.H. 1974. Central nervous chemoreceptors. In J.G. Widdicombe, ed., *MTB International Review of Science*. Vol. 2, *Respiratory Physiology*. University Park Press. Baltimore, Md.

McCutcheon, F.H. 1951. The mammalian breathing mechanism. *J. Cell. Comp. Physiol.* 37:447–85.

Michel, C.C. 1974. The transport of oxygen and carbon dioxide by the blood. In J.G. Widdicombe, ed., *MTB International Review of Science*. Vol. 2. *Respiratory Physiology*. University Park Press, Baltimore, Md.

Mitchell, R.A., and Berger, A.J. 1981. Neural regulation of respiration. In C. Lenfant, ed., *Lung Biology in Health and Disease*. Vol. 17, *Regulation of Breathing*, Part 1. Marcel Dekker, New York.

Morrow, P.E. 1960. Some physical and physiological factors controlling the fate of inhaled substances. I. Deposition. *Health Phys.* 2:366–78.

Morrow, P.E. 1973. Alveolar clearance of aerosols. *Arch. Intern. Med.* 131:101–8.

Park, J.F., Clarke, W.J., and Bair, W.J. 1970. Respiratory system. In A.C. Anderson, ed., *The Beagle as an Experimental Dog*. Iowa State University Press, Ames.

Perkins, J.F., Jr. 1958. Historical development of respiratory physiology. In W.O. Fenn and H. Rahn, eds., *Handbook of Physiology*. Sec. 3, Vol. 1, *Respiration*. Am. Physiol. Soc., Washington.

Radford, E.P., Jr. 1957. Recent studies of mechanical properties of mammalian lungs. In J.W. Remington, ed., *Tissue Elasticity*. Am. Physiol. Soc., Washington.

Radford, E.P., Jr. 1964. The physics of gases. In W.O. Fenn and H. Rahn, eds., *Handbook of Physiology*. Sec. 3, vol. 1. *Respiration*. Am Physiol. Soc., Washington.

Rahn, H., and Farhi, L.E. 1964. Ventilation, perfusion, and gas exchange—the V_A/Q concept. In W.O. Fenn and H. Rahn, eds., *Handbook of Physiology*. Sec. 3, vol. 1, *Respiration*. Am. Physiol. Soc., Washington.

Randall, G.C.B. 1978. Perinatal mortality: Some problems of adaption at birth. In C.A. Brandley and C.E. Cornelius, eds., *Advances in Veterinary Science and Comparative Medicine*, vol. 22. Academic Press, New York.

Remmers, J.E., and Gautier, H. 1972. Neural and mechanical mechanisms of feline purring. *Respir. Physiol.* 16:351–61.

Ruiz, A.V. 1973. Ventilatory response of the panting dog to hypoxia. *Pflügers Arch.* 340:89–99.

Schmidt-Nielsen, K., Bretz, W.L., and Taylor, C.R. 1970. Panting in dogs: Unidirectional air flow over evaporative surfaces. *Science* 169:1102–4.

Slonim, N.B., and Hamilton, L.H. 1976. *Respiratory Physiology*, 3d ed. C.V. Mosby, St. Louis.

Stearns, R.C., Barnas, G.M., Walski, M., and Brain, J.D. 1987. Deposition and phagocytosis of inhaled particles in the gas exchange region of the duck, *Anas platyrhynchos*. *Respir. Physiol.* 67:23–36.

Tenney, S.M., and Remmers, J.E. 1963. Comparative quantitative morphology of the mammalian lung: Diffusing area. *Nature* 197:54–56.

Torrance, R.W. 1974. Arterial chemoreceptors. In J.G. Widdicombe, ed., *MTB International Review of Science*. Vol. 2. *Respiratory Physiology*. University Park Press, Baltimore, Md.

West, J.B. 1979. *Respiratory Physiology—The essentials*. 2d ed. Williams & Wilkins, Baltimore, Md.

West, J.B. 1991. *Respiration*. In J.B. West, ed., *Best and Taylor's Physiologic Basis of Medical Practice*. 12th ed. Williams & Wilkins, Baltimore, Md.

Youmans, W.B. 1958. Role of respiratory responses to changes in arterial blood pressure (editorial). *Anesthesiology* 19:552–54.

CHAPTER 14

Respiration in Birds | by M. Roger Fedde

ANATOMY OF THE RESPIRATORY SYSTEM

The lungs

In contrast to the mammalian respiratory system, the avian respiratory system has lungs that do not expand or contract during the respiratory cycle and compliant air sacs that act as bellows to ventilate the lungs. The avian respiratory system is shown diagrammatically in Fig. 14.1. The lungs serve as the gas-exchange portion of the respiratory system. They are located in the dorsal thoracic region, and each contains only three bronchial subdivisions: (1) a single intrapulmonary primary bronchus, (2) secondary bronchi, and (3) tertiary bronchi, or parabronchi. There are three sets of secondary bronchi: medioventral, mediodorsal, and lateroventral. Four medioventral secondary bronchi first leave

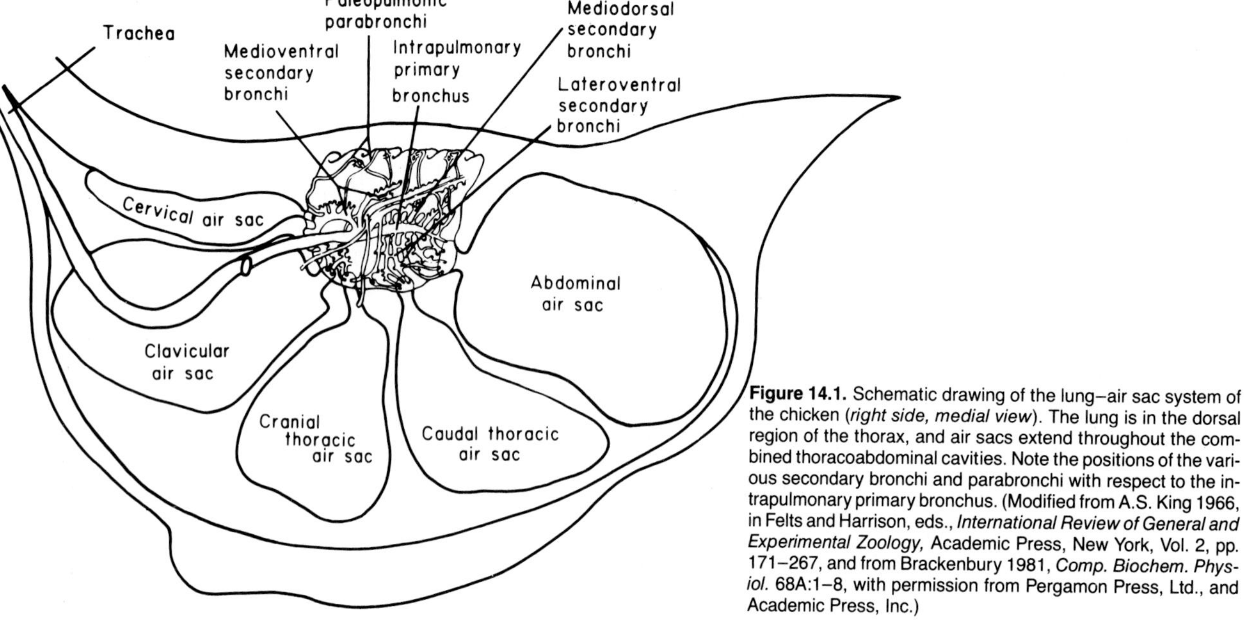

Figure 14.1. Schematic drawing of the lung–air sac system of the chicken (*right side, medial view*). The lung is in the dorsal region of the thorax, and air sacs extend throughout the combined thoracoabdominal cavities. Note the positions of the various secondary bronchi and parabronchi with respect to the intrapulmonary primary bronchus. (Modified from A.S. King 1966, in Felts and Harrison, eds., *International Review of General and Experimental Zoology,* Academic Press, New York, Vol. 2, pp. 171–267, and from Brackenbury 1981, *Comp. Biochem. Physiol.* 68A:1–8, with permission from Pergamon Press, Ltd., and Academic Press, Inc.)

the primary bronchus and spread over the medioventral surface of the lung. The eight to twelve mediodorsal secondary bronchi leave after the primary bronchus has coursed through the substance of the lung; these secondary bronchi spread over the dorsolateral surface of the lung. The several lateroventral secondary bronchi leave the primary bronchus opposite the mediodorsal bronchi and travel to the lateroventral regions of the lung. The tertiary bronchi, or parabronchi, connect mediodorsal and medioventral secondary bronchi and also course from some of the secondary bronchi to the air sacs. A detailed diagram of the tubular system of the chicken lung is shown in Fig. 14.2.

A model of the avian lung–air sac system is shown in Fig. 14.3. Those parabronchi (structures that contain the gas-exchange tissue in their walls) that course between mediodorsal and medioventral secondary bronchi are nearly parallel and are collectively called the paleopulmonic parabronchi; those that course from the mediodorsal and lateroventral secondary bronchi and intrapulmonary primary bronchus to the caudal air sacs are collectively called the neopulmonic parabronchi. These latter parabronchi are interconnected into a meshwork that covers the entire lateral surface of the lung in the chicken and strong-flying songbirds and may constitute 20 to 25 percent of the total lung volume. Penguins and emus, however, do not have neopulmonic parabronchi.

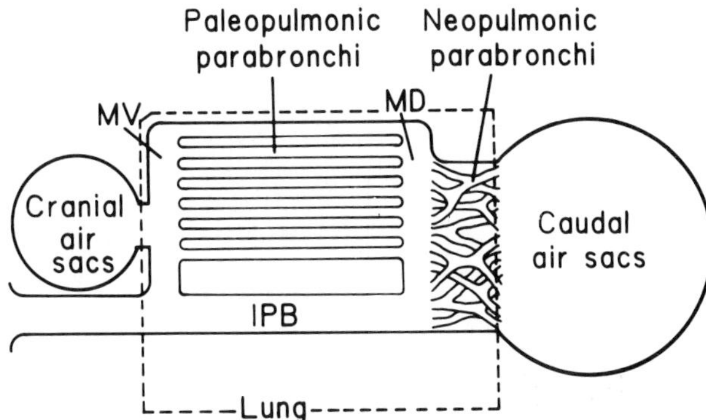

Figure 14.3. A simplified model of the avian respiratory system that aids in visualizing the bronchial organization and air sac connections (not drawn to scale). MV, medioventral secondary bronchi; MD, mediodorsal secondary bronchi; IPB, intrapulmonary primary bronchus. (Modified from Scheid et al. 1974, *Respir. Physiol.* 22:123–36.)

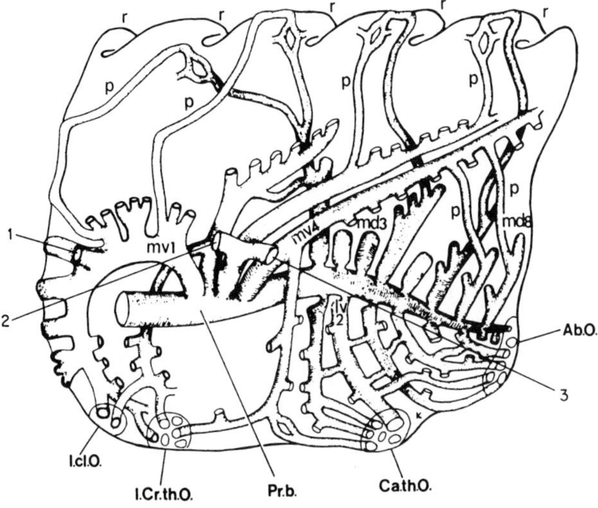

Figure 14.2. Schematic drawing of the tubular arrangement in the lung of the chicken. The structures shown represent the lumina of the various bronchi. Medial view of the right lung. mv, medioventral secondary bronchi (labeled 1 and 4); md, mediodorsal secondary bronchi (labeled 3 and 8); lv, lateroventral secondary bronchi (labeled No. 2); p, parabronchi; Ab.0., ostium of the abdominal air sac; Ca.th.O., ostium of caudal thoracic air sac; l.cl.O., lateral ostium of the clavicular air sac; l.Cr.th.O., lateral ostium of the cranial thoracic air sac; Pr.b., primary bronchus; r, impressions of ribs 2 to 6; 1, direct connection to the cervical air sac; 2, medial direct connection to clavicular air sac; 3, direct connection to the cranial thoracic air sac. From J. McLelland, 1989, in King and McLelland, eds., *Form and Function in Birds,* Academic Press, New York, Vol. 4, pp. 221–79 as modified from A.S. King 1966, in Felts and Harrison, eds., *International Review of General and Experimental Zoology,* Academic Press, New York, Vol. 2, pp. 171–267.

Exchange of oxygen and carbon dioxide between gas and blood in the lung occurs in the mantle of the parabronchi (Fig. 14.4). Gas molecules move through the lumen of a parabronchus by convection, but they move from the parabronchial lumen into the atria, infundibula, and air capillaries via diffusion. The air capillaries, which emanate from the infundibula, are small, cylindrical tubes (from 3 to 10 μm in diameter in various species of birds) that branch extensively and make close contact with the pulmonary blood capillaries. The surface area for gas exchange varies widely among species, from a low value of about 10 cm²/g of body weight in the domestic chicken to a high value of 87 cm²/g in the hummingbird. Comparable values for bats, shrews, and humans are 63, 33, and 18 cm²/g, respectively. The harmonic mean thickness of the tissue barrier between air and blood is also less for birds than for mammals. The harmonic mean thickness is defined as the mean of the reciprocal of the barrier thickness at each point in the barrier and is a value most relevant to the passive transport of gases across the barrier. It ranges from 0.314 μm for the domestic chicken to 0.099 μm for the hummingbird, compared with values of 0.206, 0.338, and 0.62 μm, for bats, shrews, and humans, respectively. These features, along with others to be discussed later, help make avian lungs very efficient gas exchanges.

Mixed venous blood from the pulmonary arteries enters the parabronchial mantle from interparabronchial arteries and flows in blood capillaries toward the lumen of the parabronchus (Fig. 14.4). Oxygen is added and carbon dioxide is removed from the blood as it passes through the blood capillaries. The oxygenated blood is collected into pulmonary venules beneath the epithelium of the parabronchial lumen.

Air sacs

Large, thin-walled air sacs emanate from some secondary bronchi (Figs. 14.1 and 14.2). These are illustrated in

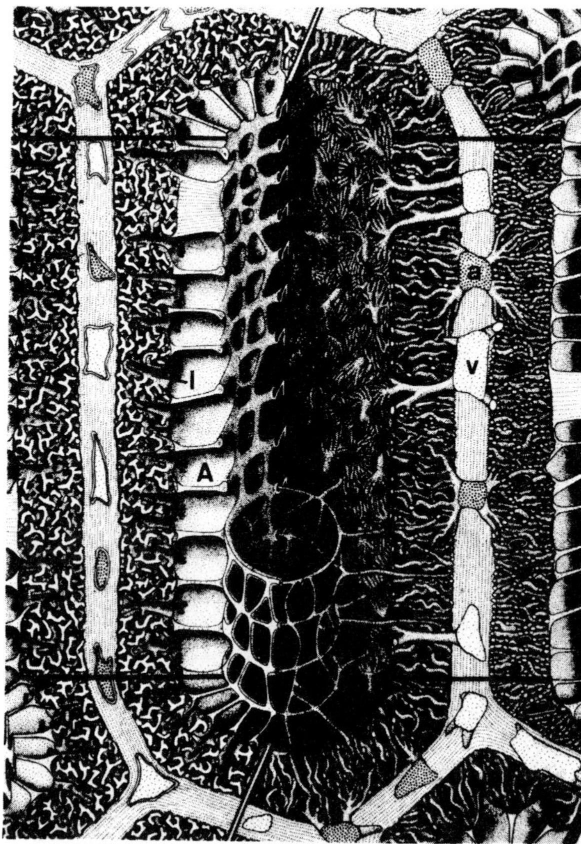

Figure 14.4. A schematic drawing of an avian parabronchus showing the open, round lumen in the center surrounded by a mantle of tissue providing close association between gas and blood. The left part of the drawing illustrates only the spaces containing gas: A, the atria; I, the infundibuli; and the tiny air capillaries emanating from the infundibuli. The right part of the drawing illustrates only the blood vessels: a, interparabronchial arteries that branch into intraparabronchial arterioles, for carrying mixed venous blood to the gas exchange surface, and the tiny blood capillaries; v, septal veins that collect the oxygenated blood after gas exchange from the venules at the base of the atria. By superimposing the air spaces and the blood spaces in the drawing, one can appreciate the extensive surface for close contact of gas and blood in the lung. (From Duncker 1974, *Respir. Physiol.* 22:1–19).

relation to other body organs in the duck in Fig. 14.5. A cranial group (the cervical, clavicular, and cranial thoracic air sacs) connects to the medioventral secondary bronchi; a caudal group (caudal thoracic and abdominal air sacs) connects to lateroventral and mediodorsal secondary bronchi and to the intrapulmonary primary bronchus. All except the clavicular air sacs are paired; in the chicken, duck, pigeon, and turkey there are nine air sacs.

Diverticula arise from some air sacs and penetrate into many of the bones. Although most of the bones in some birds are pneumatic (even the bones of the skull and distal phalanges in the frigate bird), the most prominent pneumatic bone in domestic species is the humerus. The suprahumeral diverticulum of the clavicular air sac extends into this bone, and it is possible for a bird to ventilate its

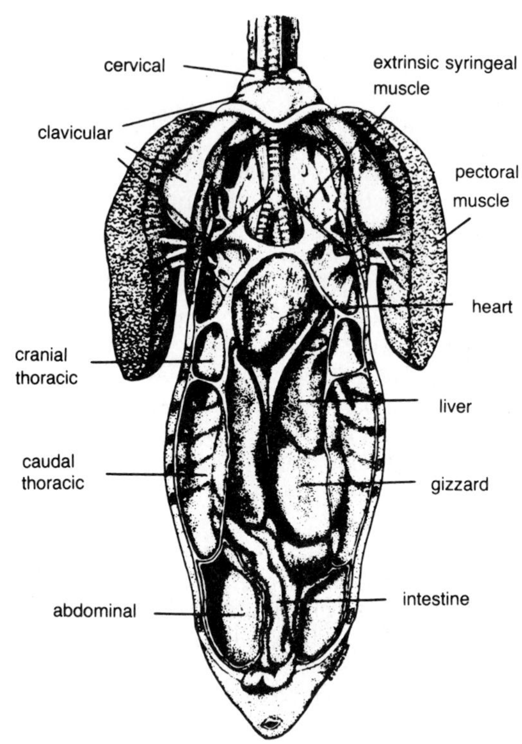

Figure 14.5. Location of air sacs in relation to other organs of the duck. (Modified from Sappey, *Recherches sur l'appareil respiratoire des oiseaux,* Bailliere, Paris, 1847.)

lung through a broken humerus. The precise function of the air sac extensions into the bones is not known.

The gas volume of the air sacs is approximately 10 times larger than that of the lungs, with the total respiratory system volume reaching as much as 500 ml in large male chickens. Essentially no gas exchange occurs in the walls of the air sacs.

DEFENSE MECHANISMS

In the mammalian lung, defense against disease relies heavily on the moving mucous blanket (mucociliary escalator) for the rapid elimination of inhaled foreign materials that are deposited on bronchial walls containing cilia (these end at the beginning of the respiratory bronchioles). Those foreign substances that reach parts of the lung beyond the respiratory bronchioles are engulfed by highly mobile alveolar macrophages, which in turn are ultimately eliminated by the mucociliary escalator. The mucociliary escalator in the avian lung is also effective in rapidly removing foreign materials from those parts of the lung that contain ciliated epithelium and from the extrapulmonary primary bronchi and trachea. However, many parts of the lung (parabronchi, atria, infundibula, and air capillaries) do not contain ciliated epithelia. Furthermore, in the nondiseased lung, phagocytic macrophages generally are not found in the gas spaces.

Recent studies have provided insights into the defense mechanisms of the nonciliated regions of the lung. Aerosolized iron oxide particles that are carried into the lung by convective gas movement deposit on the walls of the parabronchi, the atria, and the proximal regions of the infundibula. These particles are trapped by the trilaminar substance (a multilayer surfactant-like lining derived from atrial epithelial cells) that coats the atria and the infundibula. Both the foreign particles and the trilaminar substance are engulfed by the epithelial cells in the region of the atria and the infundibula forming phagosomes. The resulting phagosomes inside these cells appear to be transported to the basal side of the epithelial cells, and at least some of their contents are passed on to interstitial macrophages. The fate of the macrophages is not known.

Thus the entire epithelial surface in the parabronchi, the atria, and at least part of the infundibula can act in a phagocytic capacity. This potentiates the clearance of foreign materials and greatly decreases the chances of bacterial colonization. Much more needs to be learned about the process, especially about the mechanisms that control the rate of phagocytosis and the destruction of the contents of the phagosomes.

MECHANICS OF BREATHING

Body volume changes

Changes in the body volume are caused by contraction of the inspiratory and expiratory muscles, both sets of which are active and equally important (even in resting ventilation). Birds, unlike mammals, have no diaphragm, and skeletal muscles in the body wall provide the energy to change the body volume. The body volume increases during inspiration because of the ventral-cranial movement of the sternum and the lateral movement of the ribs (Fig. 14.6). The sternum-coracoid complex pivots at the shoulder, and the sternal tip moves in an arc as the bird breathes.

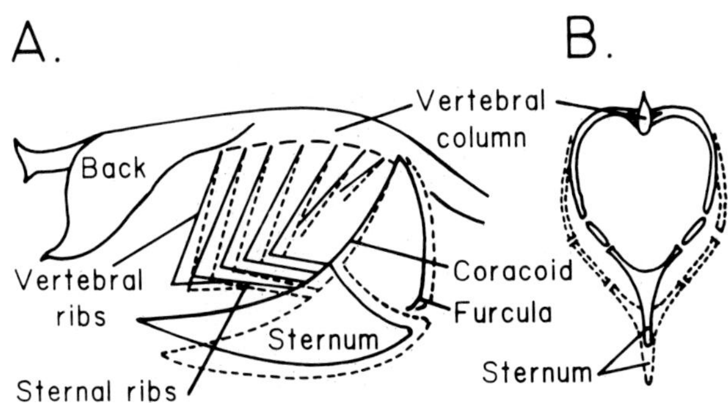

Figure 14.6. Changes in the position of the thoracic skeleton during inspiration (*dotted lines*) and expiration (*solid lines*) in a standing bird. (*A*) Lateral view; (*B*) cross-sectional view of the thorax. (Modified from Zimmer 1935, *Zoologica* 33 (Heft 88), 1–69.)

Gas pathway through the lungs

During inspiration, the body volume (both thoracic and abdominal) increases. This produces decreased pressure in the air sacs, relative to that of the atmosphere, and gas moves through the lungs into the air sacs. Conversely, during expiration, the body volume decreases, air sac pressure increases relative to that of the atmosphere, and gas is forced out of the air sacs and back through the lungs to the environment. Thus gas flows *through* the avian lungs during both phases of the respiratory cycle.

During inspiration, gas is partitioned in the lung. Some gas moves into the mediodorsal secondary bronchi, through the paleopulmonic parabronchi, and into the cranial air sacs; the remainder of the gas moves through neopulmonic parabronchi, lateroventral secondary bronchi, or intrapulmonary primary bronchus into the caudal air sacs (Fig. 14.7A). During expiration, gas from the caudal air sacs passes again through neopulmonic parabronchi and either the lateroventral secondary bronchi or the intrapulmonary primary bronchus (in the opposite direction as during inspiration) and then moves into the mediodorsal secondary bronchi and passes through the paleopulmonic parabronchi

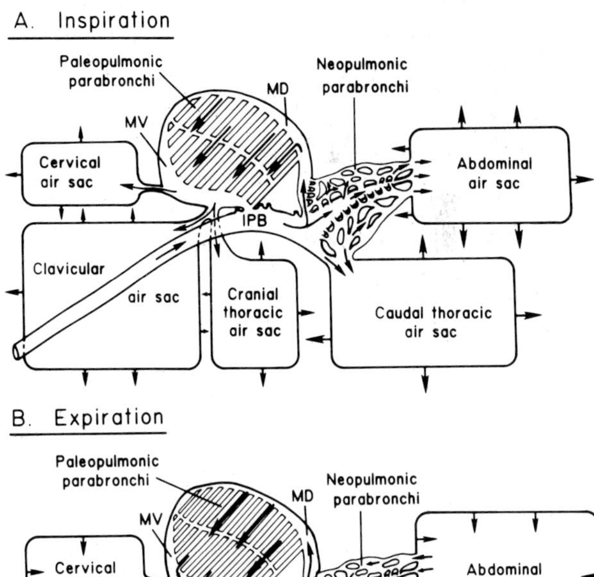

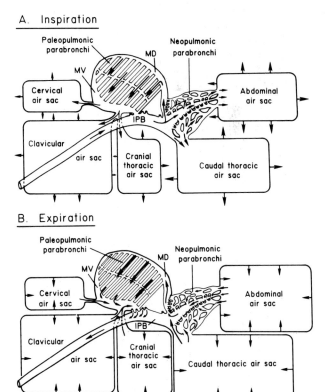

Figure 14.7. Diagram representing the pathway of gas flow through the avian lung during inspiration (*A*) and expiration (*B*). MV, medioventral secondary bronchus; MD, mediodorsal secondary bronchus; IPB, intrapulmonary primary bronchus. (Modified from Duncker 1971, *Ergebn. Anat. Entwickl.-Ges.* 45(6): 1–171.)

(in the same direction as during inspiration) (Fig. 14.7B). Gas from the cranial air sacs moves into the medioventral secondary bronchi and out the lung during expiration without again passing over gas-exchange surfaces. The unidirectional movement of gas through the paleopulmonic parabronchi, the major gas-exchange portion of the lung, reduces respiratory air shunts and thereby increases the efficiency of ventilation. This is advantageous to pulmonary gas exchange.

The unique pattern of gas flow through the avian lung results from forces applied to the gas molecules by the gas stream motion (aerodynamic inspiratory and expiratory valving). This valving occurs at the origin of the medioventral secondary bronchi, the mediodorsal secondary bronchi, and the laterobronchi. Recent investigation into the mechanisms of this valving indicates that gas flow rate through the primary bronchus, gas density, and geometry of the primary bronchus upstream from the site of valving are of principal significance.

GAS EXCHANGE

Cross-current exchange system

Because the mixed venous blood passes through the parabronchial mantle at right angles to the convective flow of gas through the lumen of the parabronchus (Fig. 14.4), a cross-current exchange system is formed (Fig. 14.8). The efficiency of gas exchange by this arrangement is greater than that by the alveolus of the mammalian lung.

The excellent gas-exchanging properties of the avian lung are observed when ventilation of the lung is high, as occurs in response to hypoxemia. When ventilation is high, the partial pressure of oxygen in the arterial blood may be only 2 to 3 torr (1 torr = 1 mm Hg pressure) less than that in the humidified gas entering the parabronchi. This small difference between the partial pressure of oxygen in the inspired gas and that in the blood implies that, under these conditions, there is essentially no diffusion limitation at the gas-blood barrier, no limitation of the chemical reaction rate of hemoglobin with oxygen, and almost a perfect balance of ventilation to perfusion in the lung.

The cross-current gas exchange system may constitute one of the factors that allow some birds to fly successfully at high altitudes, where the oxygen partial pressure is very low.

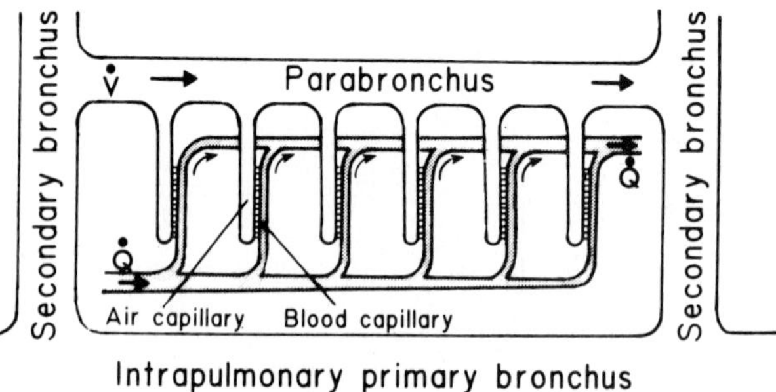

Figure 14.8. Schematic model of the cross-current gas exchange system in the avian lung. $\dot{V}$ represents the convective flow of gas through the parabronchus and $\dot{Q}$ is the blood perfusion of the parabronchus. (Modified from Scheid and Piiper 1970. *Respir. Physiol.* 9:246–62.)

Results of gas exchange

The end result of gas exchange in the lung is reflected by the oxygen and carbon dioxide blood gas tensions and pH of the arterial blood (Pa_{O_2}, Pa_{CO_2}, pHa). Arterial blood gases and pH from various species of unanesthetized birds are presented in Table 14.1. Arterial pH is generally higher, and Pa_{CO_2} generally lower, in resting birds than in most mammals despite the potential for higher gas exchange efficiency of the bird lung. A complete explanation for this observation is lacking.

CONTROL OF BREATHING

Ventilatory stability during rest

The ventilatory control system acts to adjust the amount and pattern of ventilation to achieve relatively constant arterial blood gases during resting conditions (Table 14.2). That action apparently is accomplished by the influence of many afferent inputs from both peripheral and central receptors on the central respiratory oscillator in the brain, which in turn controls the motoneurons that innervate the respiratory muscles.

Ventilatory adjustments during heat stress, exercise, and hypoxia

During heat stress in birds, respiratory frequency markedly increases, while tidal volume decreases and panting ultimately occurs. Total ventilation under these conditions may increase six- to sevenfold. Surprisingly, in some

Table 14.1. Arterial blood gases and pH in unanesthetized birds

Bird	P_{O_2} (torr)	P_{CO_2} (torr)	pH
Mute swan*	91.3	27.1	7.50
White pelican†	—	28.5	7.50
Domestic goose‡	96.8	31.5	7.52
Bar-headed goose§	91.0	35	7.44
Duck¶	82	38	7.49
Turkey vulture†	—	27.5	7.51
Black bantam hen†	—	29.9	7.48
White rock rooster†	—	29.2	7.53
White leghorn hen¶	82	33	7.52
Herring gull†	—	27.2	7.56
Pigeon†	—	28.5	7.52
Pigeon#	—	25.0	7.45
Roadrunner†	—	24.5	7.58

*Bech and Johansen 1980.
†Calder and Schmidt-Nielsen 1968.
‡Scheid, Fedde and Piiper 1989.
§Fedde, Orr, Shams and Scheid 1989.
¶Kawashiro and Scheid 1975.
#Bernstein and Samaniego 1981.

Table 14.2. Typical values of respiratory variables in resting, unanesthetized birds

Birds	Body weight (kg)	Respiratory frequency (breaths/min)	Tidal volume (ml)	Minute ventilation (ml/min)
Mute swan*	9.8	3.1	539	1595
Goose†	5.0	14.0	157	1700
Chicken‡				
Male	4.2	17	46	777
Female	3.4	27	31	766
Chicken§				
Female	1.6	23	33	760
Pekin duck¶	2.0	11.9	55	650
Pigeon#	0.34	28	3.9	108
Robin**	0.070	37	—	—
House sparrow††	0.025	59	—	—

*Bech and Johansen 1980.
†Scheid et al. 1989.
‡King and Payne 1964.
§Piiper et al. 1970.
¶Bouverot et al. 1974.
#Bernstein and Samaniego 1981.
**Lewis 1967.
††Calder 1968.

birds (ostrich, Bedouin fowl, Abdim's stork, rock partridge, Pekin duck, pigeon), this marked change in total ventilation does not result in a change in arterial blood gases and pH. The respiratory control system functions to maximize the ventilation of the upper airway dead space (which enhances evaporative water loss and, therefore, cooling of the body), while minimizing or preventing overventilation of the parabronchi. In some birds (chickens), parabronchial ventilation markedly increases during panting, resulting in severe hypocapnia and alkalosis. The reasons for the differences among species are not known.

During the activities of running or flying, birds hyperventilate and arterial P_{CO_2} decreases. In addition, when birds are exposed to the hypoxia of high altitude, they markedly overventilate, and arterial P_{CO_2} may drop below 8 torr. Thus during flight at high altitude, birds are probably severely alkalotic, but they appear to be able to tolerate this condition, along with severe hypoxia, much better than mammals.

Central respiratory oscillator

The respiratory neuronal pool responsible for the rhythmic action of the respiratory muscles is in the brain stem, probably in the region of the pons and the rostral part of the medulla oblongata. Very few studies have been conducted to locate these neuronal pools or to elucidate their interconnections. Neurophysiological studies of these neurons have only recently begun, and results are as yet incomplete.

Input to the central respiratory oscillator

The magnitudes of the output and/or cycle frequency of the respiratory oscillator may be influenced by neural input from several possible sources.

1. A humoral influence from changes in the blood affects chemoreceptors and may alter breathing. Chemoreceptors in the carotid bodies of birds respond to low oxygen partial pressures, and an increase in their neural discharge acts primarily to increase respiratory frequency, with some increase in tidal volume. Other chemoreceptors located in the lungs increase their discharge frequency when the carbon dioxide partial pressure in their microenvironment is lowered; apparently they are capable of influencing ventilation on a breath-to-breath basis and will inhibit ventilation when activated. Still other chemoreceptors located in the brain are excited by increases in carbon dioxide partial pressure or H^+ concentration. All of these chemoreceptors monitor gas partial pressure or pH and apparently function to maintain relatively constant values in the arterial blood.

2. A neurogenic influence on breathing originates apparently from mechanoreceptors or chemoreceptors in muscles or joints of the body. These receptors are activated by movement or by the buildup of metabolites in the muscles and appear to produce a strong drive to increase ventilation during exercise. Furthermore, descending neural input to the respiratory oscillator from higher brain areas also increases ventilation during exercise. In addition, mechanoreceptors in the air sacs or viscera, which are stimulated by changes in body volume, have recently been shown to have the capability of altering respiratory frequency and tidal volume. These receptors may be involved in a volume-sensitive reflex that is important in the control of breathing.

3. A cardiogenic influence from mechanoreceptors in the ventricular wall of the heart may act to modulate respiration. These receptors respond to changes in blood pressure. They have also been shown to increase their discharge when the carbon dioxide partial pressure decreases.

4. A thermal influence from thermoreceptors in the skin, muscle, spinal cord, and hypothalamus has an important effect on the respiratory oscillator. Receptors sensitive to heat in these locations lead to the rapid, shallow breathing pattern of panting.

Despite an understanding of some of the receptors that provide input into the central nervous system and despite some insight into the resulting respiratory pattern when these receptors are activated, it is still not well understood how these inputs interact under practical conditions. In some manner, these receptors induce modification of the respiratory pattern to meet the moment-by-moment needs of the bird for gas exchange and temperature regulation.

PRACTICAL CONCERNS

1. Because of the necessity of ventral-cranial movement of the sternum for the bird to change its body volume in the process of moving gas through its lungs, one must be extremely careful not to restrain a bird in such a way that sternal movement is impeded, or it will not be able to ventilate its lungs adequately.

2. Control of breathing and the consequent regulation of arterial P_{CO_2} and HCO_3^- concentration appear to be directly involved in the degree of calcification of the eggshell. Under conditions of hyperventilation, as often occurs in heat stress, thin eggshells are formed. Management techniques that lead to elevation of plasma HCO_3^- concentration in the chicken could have a beneficial effect in reducing egg breakage.

3. During surgical procedures in which either the thoracic or the abdominal cavity is opened (i.e., caponization), air sacs are ruptured, and the bird's ability to ventilate its lungs may be severely compromised. Further, with opened air sacs, gas anesthetics are not very effective if the bird is breathing spontaneously. This problem can be solved by use of the unidirectional ventilation technique to ensure adequate gas exchange and anesthetic delivery to the lung during these surgical procedures. With this technique, a continuous airstream can be delivered into an endotracheal tube. The air passes over gas-exchange surfaces of the lungs and exits from the bird through the opened air sacs. Low concentrations of anesthetic gas can be incorporated into the airstream to provide the required level of anesthesia.

4. Birds have a very low safety factor to most anesthetics, and it is easy to induce respiratory arrest. If this happens, the lungs can be artificially ventilated by gentle pumping action on the sternum, thereby compressing and expanding the thoracoabdominal cavity. Gas will then move through the lungs, and gas exchange can occur until the concentration of the anesthetic agent decreases and spontaneous breathing resumes.

5. Many diseases of birds involve the air sacs. Knowledge of the location and extent of the air sacs is important in the diagnosis of a number of avian diseases. Because inspired foreign materials are more likely to be deposited in the caudal air sacs (abdominal and caudal thoracic), these sacs are most likely to be involved in cases of respiratory disease.

6. Inspired foreign materials are deposited in greatest concentrations on the bronchial walls in the lung at locations where the gas velocity decreases, at points of abrupt angle changes in the bronchi, or where the gas first meets an increased surface area. Therefore sites of highest contamination should be near the origin of the mediodorsal secondary bronchi and their associated paleopulmonic parabronchi and in the neopulmonic parabronchi. The pulmonary defense system might be expected to be more developed or active in these regions of the lung.

7. If the trachea is occluded by endoscopic examination, by misdirection of a pill given orally, or during the surgical removal of an *Aspergillus* growth, spontaneous ventilation with effective gas exchange can be quickly established by means of a small incision in the thoracic inlet, opening of the clavicular air sac, and insertion of a short tube into that sac. When the trachea is clear, the tube can be removed and the skin sutured.

8. Fiberoptic endoscopes can be inserted easily into several of the air sacs (the caudal thoracic air sac can be entered by insertion of the scope between the last two ribs) for direct visualization of disease or for lavage with sterile saline solution. This may greatly aid in the diagnosis of a disease.

9. Intraperitoneal injections of drugs or other substances must be given very carefully. The injected material can be easily placed in an air sac, where it can do great damage.

10. Placing a bird on its back during examination or surgery often has serious consequences with respect to respiration. The inspiratory muscles may not have the strength (especially if the respiratory control centers are depressed by a general anesthetic) to lift the pectoral muscle mass and the viscera against the pull of gravity, and an unacceptably low tidal volume may result. If this body position is necessary, especially during surgery, unidirectional ventilation techniques may be used to provide adequate gas exchange.

11. Respiratory distress often occurs in turkeys with occlusion of the air ostia by exudate, fibrin, or lesions produced by aspergillosis. The foreign material acts as a valve so that air cannot exit from the air sacs.

REFERENCES

Abdalla, M.A. 1989. The blood supply to the lung. In A.S. King and J. McLelland, eds., *Form and Function in Birds,* vol. 4. Academic Press, New York. Pp. 281–306.

Ballam, G.O., Kunz, A.L., Clanton, T.L., and Michal, E.K. 1981. A stretch reflex in chickens at constant F_LCO_2. *Fed. Proc.* 40:453.

Banzett, R.B., Butler, J.P., Nations, C.S., Barnas, G.M., Lehr, J.L., and Jones, J.J. 1987. Inspiratory aerodynamic valving in goose lungs depends on gas density and velocity. *Respir. Physiol.* 70:287–300.

Barnas, G.M., Estavillo, J.A., Mather, F.B., and Burger, R.E. 1981. The effect of CO_2 and temperature on respiratory movements in the chicken. *Respir. Physiol.* 43:315–25.

Bech, C., and Johansen, K. 1980. Ventilation and gas exchange in the mute swan *Cygnus olor. Respir. Physiol.* 39:285–95.

Bech, C., Johansen, K., and Maloiy, G.M.O. 1979. Ventilation and expired gas composition in the flamingo, *Phoenicopterus ruber,* during normal respiration and panting. *Physiol. Zool.* 52:313–28.

Bernstein, M.H., and Samaniego, F.C. 1981. Ventilation and acid-base status during thermal panting in pigeons (*Columba livia*). *Physiol. Zool.* 54:308–15.

Black, C.P., and Tenney, S.M. 1980. Oxygen transport during progressive hypoxia in high-altitude and sea-level waterfowl. *Respir. Physiol.* 39:217–39.

Bouverot, P. 1978. Control of breathing in birds compared with mammals. *Physiol. Rev.* 58:604–55.

Bouverot, P., Hill, N., and Jammes, Y. 1974. Ventilatory responses to CO_2 in intact and chronically chemodenervated Peking ducks. *Respir. Physiol.* 22:137–56.

Brackenbury, J.H. 1987. Ventilation of the lung-air sac system. In T.J. Seller, ed., *Bird Respiration,* vol. I. CRC Press, Boca Raton, Fla. Pp. 39–69.

Brackenbury, J.H., Avery, P., and Gleeson, M. 1981. Respiration in exercising fowl. I. Oxygen consumption, respiratory rate and respired gases. *J. Exp. Biol.* 93:317–25.

Burger, R.E. 1980. Respiratory gas exchange and control in the chicken. *Poultry Sci.* 59:2654–65.

Butler, J.P., Banzett, R.B., and Fredberg, J.J. 1988. Inspiratory valving in avian bronchi: Aerodynamic considerations. *Respir. Physiol.* 72: 241–56.

Butler, P.J., West, N.H., and Jones, D.R. 1977. Respiratory and car-

diovascular responses of the pigeon to sustained, level flight in a wind-tunnel. *J. Exp. Biol.* 71:7–26.
Calder, W.A. 1968. Respiratory and heart rates of birds at rest. *Condor* 70:358–65.
Calder, W.A., and Schmidt-Nielsen, K. 1968. Panting and blood carbon dioxide in birds. *Am. J. Physiol.* 215:477–82.
Cohn, J.E., and Shannon, R. 1968. Respiration in unanesthetized geese. *Respir. Physiol.* 5:259–68.
Davey, N.J., and Seller, T.J. 1987. Brain mechanisms for respiratory control. In T.J. Seller, ed., *Bird Respiration*, vol. II. CRC Press, Boca Raton, Fla. Pp. 169–88.
Duncker, H.-R. 1972. Structure of avian lungs. *Respir. Physiol.* 14: 44–63.
Estavillo, J.A., and Youther, M.L. 1978. The effect of middle cardiac nerve stimulation upon the respiratory response to $PaCO_2$ in the chicken. In J. Piiper, ed., *Respiratory Function in Birds, Adult and Embryonic.* Springer-Verlag, New York. Pp. 175–81.
Fedde, M.R. 1978. Drugs used for avian anesthesia: A review. *Poultry Sci.* 57:1376–99.
Fedde, M.R. 1980. Structure and gas-flow pattern in the avian respiratory system. *Poultry Sci.* 59:2642–53.
Fedde, M.R. 1986. Respiration. In P.D. Sturkie, ed., *Avian Physiology*, 4th ed. Springer-Verlag, New York. Pp. 191–220.
Fedde, M.R. 1987. Respiratory muscles. In T.J. Seller, ed., *Bird Respiration*, vol. I. CRC Press, Boca Raton, Fla. Pp. 3–37.
Fedde, M.R., Burger, R.E., Geiser, J., Gratz, R.K., Estavillo, J.A., and Scheid, P. 1986. Effects of altering dead space volume on respiration and air sac gases in geese. *Respir. Physiol.* 66:109–22.
Fedde, M.R., Faraci, F.M., Kilgore, D.L., Jr., Cardinet, G.H. III, and Chatterjee, A. 1985. Cardiopulmonary adaptations in birds for exercise at high altitude. In R. Gilles, ed., *Circulation, Respiration and Metabolism.* Springer-Verlag, Berlin. Pp. 149–63.
Fedde, M.R., Kiley, J.P., Powell, F.L., and Scheid, P. 1982. Involvement of avian intrapulmonary CO_2 receptors in the control of breathing: Experiments with delayed blood flow to carotid body and brain in ducks. *Respir. Physiol.* 47:121–40.
Fedde, M.R., and Kuhlmann, W.D. 1978. Intrapulmonary carbon dioxide sensitive receptors: Amphibians to mammals. In J. Piiper, ed., *Respiratory Function in Birds, Adult and Embryonic.* Springer-Verlag, New York. Pp. 33–50.
Fedde, M.R., Orr, J.A., Shams, H., and Scheid, P. 1989. Cardiopulmonary function in exercising bar-headed geese during normoxia and hypoxia. *Respir. Physiol.* 77:239–62.
Fedde, M.R., and Peterson, D.F. 1970. Intrapulmonary receptor response to changes in airway-gas composition in *Gallus domesticus. J. Physiol. (London)* 209:609–25.
Fletcher, O.J. 1980. Pathology of the avian respiratory system. *Poultry Sci.* 59:2666–79.
Gleeson, M., and Molony, V. 1989. Control of breathing. In A.S. King and J. McLelland, eds., *Form and Function in Birds*, vol. 4. Academic Press, New York. Pp. 439–84.
Grubb, B., Colacino, J.M., and Schmidt-Nielsen, K. 1978. Cerebral blood flow in birds: Effect of hypoxia. *Am. J. Physiol.* 234:H230–H234.
Grubb, B., Mills, C.D., Colacino, J.M., and Schmidt-Nielsen, K. 1977. Effect of arterial carbon dioxide on cerebral blood flow in ducks. *Am. J. Physiol.* 232:H596–H601.
Kawashiro, T., and Scheid, P. 1975. Arterial blood gases in undisturbed resting birds: Measurements in chicken and duck. *Respir. Physiol.* 23:337–42.
Kiley, J.P., Kuhlmann, W.D., and Fedde, M.R. 1979. Respiratory and cardiovascular responses to exercise in the duck. *J. Appl. Physiol.: Respirat. Environ. Exercise Physiol.* 47:827–33.
Kiley, J.P., Faraci, F.M., and Fedde, M.R. 1985. Gas exchange during exercise in hypoxic ducks. *Respir. Physiol.* 59:105–115.
King, A.S., and Molony, V. 1971. The anatomy of respiration. In D.J. Bell and B.M. Freeman, eds., *Physiology and Biochemistry of the Domestic Fowl*, vol. 1. Academic Press, New York. Pp. 93–169.
King, A.S., and Payne, D.C. 1964. Normal breathing and the effects of posture in *Gallus domesticus. J. Physiol. (London)* 174:340–47.
King, A.S., and White, S.S. 1975. Aves respiratory system. In R. Getty, ed., *Sisson and Grossman's The Anatomy of the Domestic Animals*, vol. 2. W.B. Saunders, Philadelphia. Pp. 1883–1918.
Kunz, A.L. 1987. Peripheral mechanisms in the control of breathing. In T.J. Seller, ed., *Bird Respiration*, vol. II. CRC Press, Boca Raton, Fla. Pp. 129–67.
Lasiewski, R.C. 1972. Respiratory function in birds. In D.S. Farner and J.R. King, eds., *Avian Biology*, vol. 2. Academic Press, New York. Pp. 287–342.
Lewis, R.A. 1967. "Resting" heart and respiratory rates of small birds. *Auk* 84:131–32.
Linsley, J.G., and Burger, R.E. 1964. Respiratory and cardiovascular responses in the hyperthermic domestic cock. *Poultry Sci.* 43:291–305.
Maina, J.N. 1982. A scanning electron microscopic study of the air and blood capillaries of the lung of the domestic fowl *(Gallus domesticus). Experientia* 38:614–16.
Maina, J.N. 1988. Scanning electron microscope study of the spatial organization of the air and blood conducting components of the avian lung (*Gallus gallus* variant *domesticus*). *Anat. Rec.* 222:145–53.
Maina, J.N. 1989. The morphometry of the avian lung. In A.S. King and J. McLelland, eds., *Form and Function in Birds*, vol. 4. Academic Press, New York. Pp. 307–368.
Mather, F.B., Barnas, G.M., and Burger, R.E. 1980. The influence of alkalosis on panting. *Comp. Biochem. Physiol.* 67A:265–68.
Mensah, G.A., and Brain, J.D. 1982. Deposition and clearance of inhaled aerosol in the respiratory tract of chickens. *J. Appl. Physiol.: Respirat. Environ. Exercise Physiol.* 53:1423–28.
Michal, E.K., Ballam, G.O., and Kunz, A.L. 1981. Effects of CO_2 and air sac volume on the activity of medullary respiratory neurons of the chicken. *Physiologist* 24:131.
Milsom, W.K., Jones, D.R., and Gabbott, G.R.J. 1981. On chemoreceptor control of ventilatory responses to CO_2 in unanesthetized ducks. *J. Appl. Physiol.: Respirat. Environ. Exercise Physiol.* 50:1121–28.
Mongin, P. 1978. Acid-base balance during eggshell formation. In J. Piiper, eds., *Respiratory Function in Birds, Adult and Embryonic.* Springer-Verlag, New York. Pp. 247–59.
Pattle, R.E. 1978. Lung surfactant and lung lining in birds. In J. Piiper, ed., *Respiratory Function in Birds, Adult and Embryonic*, Springer-Verlag, Berlin. Pp. 23–32.
Piiper, J., Drees, F., and Scheid, P. 1970. Gas exchange in the domestic fowl during spontaneous breathing and artificial ventilation. *Respir. Physiol.* 9:234–45.
Powell, F.L., and Scheid, P. 1989. Physiology of gas exchange in the avian respiratory system. In A.S. King and J. McLelland, eds., *Form and Function in Birds*, vol. 4. Academic Press, New York. Pp. 393–437.
Powell, F.L., Geiser, J., Gratz, R.K., and Scheid, P. 1981. Airflow in the avian respiratory tract: Variations of O_2 and CO_2 concentrations in the bronchi of the duck. *Respir. Physiol.* 44:195–213.
Ramirez, J.M., and Bernstein, M.H. 1976. Compound ventilation during thermal panting in pigeons: A possible mechanism for minimizing hypocapnic alkalosis. *Fed. Proc.* 35:2562–65.
Rautenberg, W., May, B., Necker, R., and Rosner, G. 1978. Control of panting by thermosensitive spinal neurons in birds. In J. Piiper, ed., *Respiratory Function in Birds, Adult and Embryonic.* Springer-Verlag, New York. Pp. 204–10.
Richards, S.A., and Avery, P. 1978. Central nervous mechanisms regulating thermal panting. In J. Piiper, ed., *Respiratory Function in Birds, Adult and Embryonic.* Springer-Verlag, New York. Pp. 196–203.
Scheid, P. 1979. Mechanisms of gas exchange in bird lungs. *Rev. Physiol. Biochem. Pharmacol.* 86:137–85.
Scheid, P. 1981. Significance of unidirectional ventilation for avian pulmonary gas exchange. *Physiologist* 24:131.
Scheid, P., and Piiper, J. 1987. Gas exchange and transport. In T.J. Seller, ed., *Bird Respiration*, vol. I. CRC Press, Boca Raton, Fla. Pp. 97–129.

Scheid, P., and Piiper, J. 1989. Respiratory mechanics and air flow in birds. In A.S. King and J. McLelland, eds., *Form and Function in Birds,* vol. 4. Academic Press, New York. Pp. 369–91.

Scheid, P., Fedde, M.R., and Piiper, J. 1989. Gas exchange and air-sac composition in the unanesthetized, spontaneously breathing goose. *J. Exp. Biol.* 142:373–85.

Sébert, P., 1979. Mise en évidence de l'action centrale du stimulus CO_2−[H+] de la ventilation chez le Canard Pékin. *J. Physiol. (Paris)* 75:901–909.

Shams, H., and Scheid, P. 1989. Efficiency of parabronchial gas exchange in deep hypoxia: Measurements in the resting duck. *Respir. Physiol.* 77:135–46.

Stearns, R.C., Barnas, G.M., Walski, W., and Brain, J.D. 1987. Deposition and phagocytosis of inhaled particles in the gas exchange region of the duck, *Anas platyrhynchos*. *Respir. Physiol.* 67:23–36.

Wang, N., Banzett, R.B., Butler, J.P., and Fredberg, J.J. 1988. Bird lung models show that convective inertia effects inspiratory aerodynamic valving. *Respir. Physiol.* 73:111–24.

CHAPTER 15

Exercise Physiology | by Howard H. Erickson

Dogs and horses have developed into elite athletes through domestication and genetic selection for specific tasks; first, hunting, farming, and warfare and more recently, leisure activities. The greyhound originated in Babylon and Egypt more than 5000 years ago. It is the fastest breed within the canine species and is capable of attaining speeds of nearly 1000 meters per minute over 400 meters. In contrast, sled dogs (huskies), with their tremendous endurance capacity, are at the other end of the performance spectrum. They are capable of racing more than 1700 kilometers in 12 to 14 days.

Tribes in Mesopotamia and China domesticated horses more than 4500 years ago. Domestic horses were recorded in ancient Greece in 1700 BC and in Egypt in 1600 BC. The Romans standardized horses as a means of sport and recreation. In comparison with the dog, development of the horse for true speed is more recent. The British organized horse racing and developed the Thoroughbred, which has been selectively bred only within the last 300 years, from Arabian horses. The American Quarter Horse was developed in America during the early 1700s, largely from the Thoroughbred, and can attain speeds of 1200 meters per minute over 400 meters with peak speeds over 1400 meters/minute.

Both the racing greyhound and the equine athlete have maximal oxygen consumptions in excess of 160 ml/kg min, indicative of a high aerobic capacity. It is not known which physiological characteristics make the greyhound, the Quarter Horse, and the Thoroughbred faster than other breeds within their respective species. However, there is probably no single factor that limits exercise and performance. Peak performance capacity depends on maximizing the capacity of each body system to produce an overall maximal result. Physiological adaptation associated with exercise physical conditioning is a mechanism by which exercise capacity can be optimized. Progressive stress produces remarkable adaptations, enabling the animal to cope with increased physical demand and to attain maximum performance. In addition, considerable evidence suggests that genetic predetermination may be involved in setting the upper limit for performance potential.

The purpose of this chapter is to provide a basic understanding of the integrated physiological response to exercise and physical conditioning. The horse and the dog will be used as examples; parallels will be made between the physiology of the horse and the dog, and the human, where appropriate.

THE BLOOD

Red blood cell mobilization

Limits are imposed on muscle performance by the capacity to deliver oxygen and metabolic substrates to the working muscles and the efficiency of removal of waste products from the muscles. Blood is the pathway by which oxygen and substrates are supplied to the musculature and by which waste products, including heat, are removed. When an animal exercises, the changes observed in circulating blood are remarkably rapid. Most notable is a sharp increase in the unit volume of erythrocytes, leukocytes, and platelets.

Splenic contraction

The cardiovascular system has the ability to transport large quantities of oxygen to working muscle. In the horse and the dog, as well as several other species, the spleen acts as a reservoir for erythrocytes. Blood cells stored in the spleen can be mobilized into the circulation when there is an increased demand (Table 15.1). The release of stored erythrocytes from the spleen into the systemic circulation is under the influence of the sympathetic nervous system and circulating catecholamines. The smooth muscle capsule of the spleen is innervated by postganglionic sympathetic neurons. Any factor that increases sympathetic nervous activity or plasma catecholamines, such as asphyxia, hemorrhage, excitement, and exercise, will result in splenic contraction and increase the number of circulating erythrocytes. Consequently, exercise, as well as excitation, causes an increase in the circulating erythrocyte volume at an essentially unchanged or reduced plasma volume, resulting in an increase in the packed cell volume (PCV), hemoglobin concentration, and red blood cell count.

Other sites

Contraction of the spleen does not fully explain the increase in PCV after exercise. In the horse the PCV may increase from 40 to 50 percent to about 60 to 70 percent after exercise. A concomitant rise in blood viscosity may also occur at this time. A marked alteration in the cell/plasma ratio of the peripheral venous blood takes place during exertion, with an associated shift of intravascular to extravascular fluid. Erythrocytes can also be sequestered in other organs, such as the liver, gut, and lungs. In general, Thoroughbreds have resting erythrocyte indices (mean corpuscular volume, mean corpuscular hemoglobin, and mean corpuscular hemoglobin concentration) that are higher than those of Standardbred trotters and pacers or endurance horses. Hematologic values of greyhounds are also higher than those of other breeds. This adaptation makes possible increased oxygen carriage to the tissues during exercise.

Table 15.1. Splenic response to exercise in the horse and greyhound

	Thoroughbred		Greyhound	
Variable	Rest	Exercise	Rest	Exercise
Hb (g/dl)	12–14	21–24	19–20	23–24
PCV (%)	40–50	60–70	50–55	60–65

Data from Evans and Rose 1988, *Pflügers Arch.* 411:316–21; Snow, Harris, and Stuttard 1988, *Vet. Rec.* 123:487–89.

Blood volume

The potential of the spleen to increase the circulating red cell volume is impressive in both the dog and the horse. At rest, a large proportion of the erythrocytes are stored in the spleen. The increase in PCV is a function of exercise intensity; a linear relationship between PCV and speed exists up to a PCV of approximately 60 to 65 percent. This "autotransfusion" of erythrocytes during exercise boosts the oxygen-carrying capacity of the blood and is thought to be a significant factor contributing to the very high, maximal oxygen consumption of the horse and the dog compared with other species. Red cell volume, therefore, increases dramatically during exercise, as a result of the contribution of the splenic reservoir. However, exercise causes little change or a small reduction in plasma volume, which is attributed to fluid shift from the intravascular to extravascular compartment as a result of fluid loss through sweating and/or panting.

Physical training and oxygen-transport capacity

Physical training induces adaptations to increased metabolic demands in several respects. One limiting factor for fitness and endurance is the oxygen-transport capacity of the blood. This capacity is enhanced during training by an increase in the total volume of red cells. A relationship between state of training, cell volume, and other erythrocyte indices is well established, both in humans and in the horse. Plasma viscosity and fibrinogen levels are normally unaffected by training. Plasma viscosity values in the Thoroughbred are lower than in other breeds of horses and possibly all other animals.

When training is prolonged, however, the increase in red cell mass may become excessive. This increase in PCV results in reduced racing performance and has been attributed to overtraining. The increased blood viscosity may be associated with a reduction in capillary perfusion and inadequate delivery of oxygen to the tissues.

CARDIOVASCULAR SYSTEM

During strenuous exercise, the metabolic needs of working muscle increase dramatically. The ability of the heart to pump sufficient blood to meet the needs of the exercising horse and to provide effective redistribution of the blood to working skeletal muscle is essential for maintaining performance (Fig. 15.1). The extent to which delivery of oxygen to active muscles can be increased is thought by many to be a limiting factor in whole body exercise.

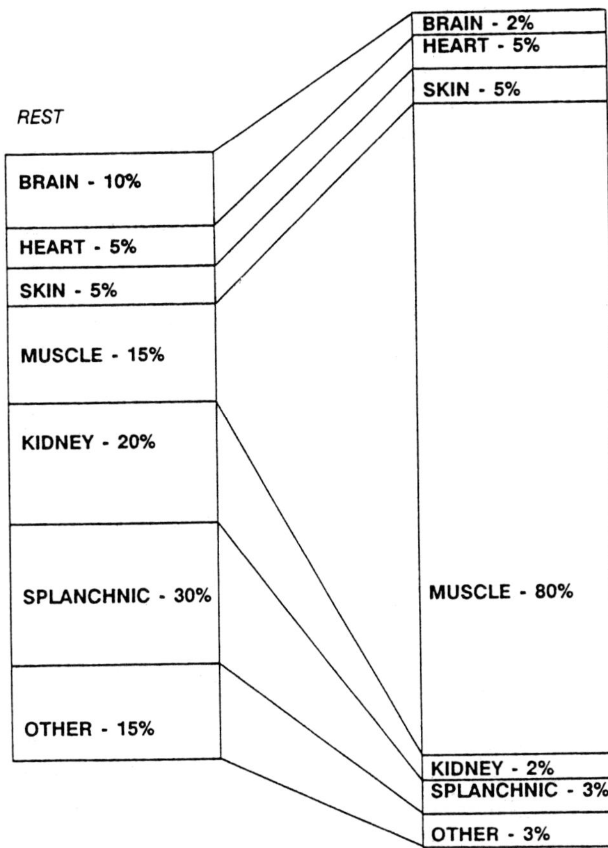

Figure 15.1. Representative changes in magnitude of blood flow (i.e., distribution of cardiac output) in the dog and horse to muscle and other organs from the resting state.

Cardiac output

Exercise results in increased cardiac output to meet the increased demands of working muscles for oxygen. The increase in cardiac output (Fig. 15.2) during exercise is a primary factor in the large increase in oxygen delivery in the canine and equine species. Cardiac output is the product of heart rate and stroke volume as follows:

$$\text{Cardiac output} = \text{Heart rate} \times \text{Stroke volume}$$

Because maximal heart rate is attained during severe exercise, stroke volume may limit the increase in cardiac output during exercise. During submaximal exercise, cardiac output increases linearly with work load and is principally due to increased heart rate. The three- to fourfold increase in cardiac output during maximal exercise in ponies is similar to that in dogs and humans. During submaximal work in horses, however, cardiac output can increase five- to eightfold.

The Thoroughbred and the racing Quarter Horse can augment their oxygen consumption 40-fold between rest and maximal exercise; this represents the highest aerobic scope in mammals. Cardiac output can increase about eightfold (Fig 15.2), whereas approximately a fivefold increase occurs in oxygen uptake (the arteriovenous oxygen content difference [a-v O_2 difference]) by the tissues. The a-v O_2 difference in Thoroughbred horses can exceed 23 volumes percent, whereas top human athletes can reach only 17 volumes percent when running at maximal intensity. Arterial oxygen content is a function of hemoglobin concentration of the blood and the efficiency of alveolar ventilation and gas exchange. An exercising horse can increase its oxygen-carrying capacity 60 percent through splenic contraction and still not increase viscous resistance enough to impede cardiac output. A high cardiac output is also aided in the elite athlete by a high ratio of heart weight to body

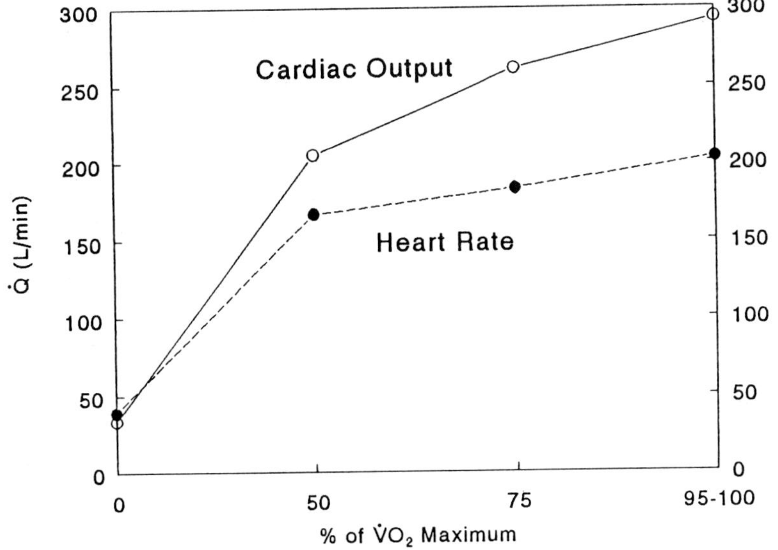

Figure 15.2. The response in cardiac output and heart rate in the horse during exercise on a high-speed treadmill. Q̇, cardiac output; $\dot{V}O_2$, oxygen consumption. (Data from M.K. Hopper 1989. Ph.D. dissertation, Kansas State University Library.)

weight (grams per kilogram). Average heart weight/body weight ratios are 8.6 and 12.0 g/kg, respectively, for the Thoroughbred and the greyhound, but only on the order of 4 g/kg for humans. Among elite athletes, the best-performing animals tend to have values considerably greater than these means.

Heart rate

The large increase in cardiac output is primarily due to the very high heart rates that can be attained in the horse and the dog. In the trained thoroughbred, resting heart rates in the mid 20s occur; however, the average is around 35 beats per minute. During maximal exercise, heart rate can increase to 240 to 250 beats per minute (Table 15.2) in the racing thoroughbred. In the dog, particularly in the racing greyhound, resting heart rates can be less than 100 and rise to 300 beats per minute or more during maximal exercise (Table 15.3). Heart rate rises rapidly at the onset of exercise, reaching a maximum in 30 to 45 seconds, and then often drops before reaching a plateau during steady-state work.

The anticipatory response to exercise is evidenced by an increased resting heart rate in the canine and equine athlete, as in humans. In addition, heart rate during submaximal exercise is affected by apprehension and anxiety. The psychogenic component of the heart rate response to exercise is proportionately larger at lower relative work loads. At a heart rate of less than 120 beats per minute in the horse there may be psychogenic factors such as fear; heart rates above 210 beats per minute begin to plateau with incremental work load as maximal heart rate is approached. Therefore, the heart rate response to graded exercise in the equine athlete is linear only between 120 and 210 beats per minute. After exercise, the heart rate decreases rapidly within the first minute or two after completion of the work effort.

Stroke volume

The literature contains contradictory statements concerning changes in stroke volume during exercise. Stroke volume has been reported to be increased or unchanged during exercise in the dog and increased during submaximal exercise in the horse (Fig. 15.3). Maintenance of stroke volume during exercise occurs by several physiological mechanisms. Increased sympathetic nervous activity during exercise results in both tachycardia and reduced end-systolic ventricular volumes by increasing myocardial contractility, so that ventricular emptying is more effective. Venous return during exercise is supplemented by mobilization of the splenic reserve of blood volume, muscle movement, and increased negativity of intrathoracic pressure. Increased stretch of myocardial fibers within physiologic limits leads to an increase in developed pressure and stroke volume through the Frank-Starling mechanism. The observed increases in left ventricular end-diastolic pressure and contractility during exercise, along with the increased venous return, assist in the maintenance of stroke volume, despite the decreased filling time associated with shortened diastole at increased heart rates. During severe exercise in free-running dogs, increases in end-diastolic left ventricular diameter and pressure have been observed, with a reduction in end-systolic diameter. Therefore stroke volume generally increases during exercise to aid in the augmentation of cardiac output and oxygen delivery to the body.

Table 15.2. Cardiovascular responses to exercise in 500 kg horse

Variable	Rest	Exercise	Exercise/rest ratio
Heart rate (beats per minute)	30	210–250	7–8
Cardiac output (L/min)	30	150–240	5–8
Systolic/diastolic arterial blood pressure (mm Hg)	130/80	230/110	1.6
Pulse pressure (mm Hg)	50	150–200	3–4
Pulmonary artery pressure (mm Hg)	20–30	80–90	3–4
Hemoglobin concentration (g/dl)	13	17–24	1.3–1.6
O_2 consumption (ml/min/kg)	3–4	120–160	30–40

Data from von Engelhardt 1977, 1979; Meixner et al. 1981; Rose 1985.

Table 15.3. Cardiovascular characteristics of greyhounds and of mongrels*

Variable	Conditioned greyhound*	Unconditioned mongrel*
Heart weight/body weight ratio (g/100 g)		
Adult	1.26	0.94
Neonatal	1.20	0.76 (coonhounds)
6 months	1.14	
Myocardial cell diameter (μm)	18.3	12.5
Mean arterial blood pressure (mm Hg)	118	98
Cardiac output (L/min) (resting)	4.4	2.7
Cardiac index (L/min/m²) (resting)	4.3	3.1
Stroke volume (ml) (resting)	55	27
Peripheral resistance (10 dynes/s/cm^{-5})	2.3	3.4
Carotid sinus OP† (mm Hg)	137	123
Plasma volume (ml/kg)	54	54
Blood volume (ml/kg)	114	79
Heart rate (beats per minute)		
Rest	29–48	61–117
Maximum exercise	290–420	220–325
Oxygen uptake (ml/kg/min)		
Rest	—	8
Maximum exercise	180	85

*Mean body weight for greyhounds, 26 kg; for mongrels, 20 kg.
†OP, operating point (the level at which carotid sinus perfusion pressure and systemic arterial pressure remain equal).
Data from Courtice 1943, Donald and Ferguson 1966, Detweiler et al. 1974, Cox et al. 1976, Alonso 1972, Carew and Covell 1978, Staaden 1980.

Myocardial contractility

During strenuous exercise in the dog and the pony, marked augmentation of myocardial contractility is observed, along with pronounced increases in both ventricular preload (increased end-diastolic volume) and afterload

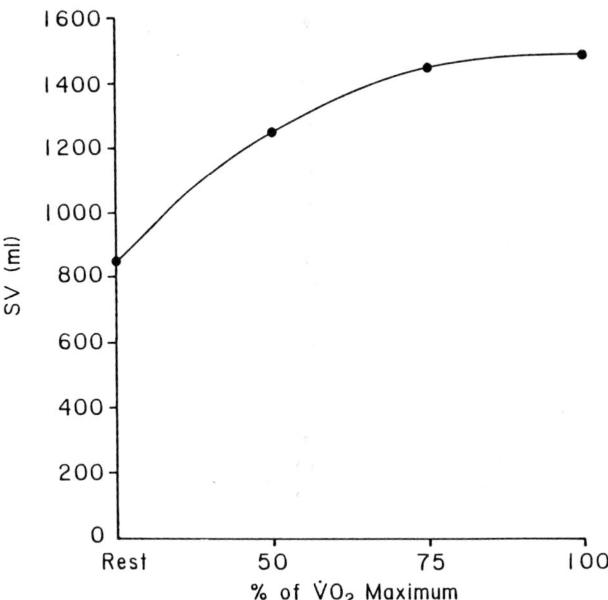

Figure 15.3. The response in stroke volume in the horse during exercise on a high-speed treadmill. SV, stroke volume; $\dot{V}O_2$, oxygen consumption. (Data from M.K. Hopper 1989. Ph.D. dissertation, Kansas State University Library.)

(mean arterial pressure). The net result is an increase in myocardial oxygen consumption, which is met by increases in both coronary blood flow and increased oxygen extraction. Exercise-induced tachycardia also contributes to the augmented myocardial oxygen requirement.

Blood flow

The main changes in distribution of blood flow during exercise are (1) increased pulmonary blood flow from opening of previously closed pulmonary capillaries, (2) coronary vasodilation resulting in increased coronary flow to provide oxygen for myocardial contraction, (3) vasodilation in working skeletal muscles, (4) vasoconstriction in the nonworking muscles and the splanchnic vasculature, and (5) increased blood flow to the skin (Fig. 15.1). These cardiovascular adaptations maintain the oxygen supply to tissues with increased oxygen requirements during exercise and body thermoregulation. Blood flow to the skin is dependent on environmental temperature and humidity.

Blood pressure

Ultrasound systems are often used to measure systemic arterial pressure at rest; during exercise, however, solid-state catheter transducer systems that use an exteriorized carotid artery provide more accurate measurements. During submaximal exercise, systemic arterial blood pressure is kept relatively constant by arterial baroreceptors in the wall of the aortic arch and in the carotid sinus. Light treadmill exercise has no significant effect on mean arterial pressure. During more strenuous treadmill exercise, however, significant increases in systemic arterial pressure occur (Table 15.2; Fig. 15.4). Chronic hypertension in ponies has been reported to result in enlargement of the heart, particularly the left ventricle.

During strenuous exercise, cardiac output (equal to total pulmonary blood flow) increases up to eightfold in the horse. This increase in pulmonary blood flow raises pulmonary arterial pressure from 20 to 30 mm Hg at rest to as much as 80 to 90 mm Hg during exercise (Table 15.2; Fig. 15.4). Assuming that left atrial pressure remains constant or increases, calculated pulmonary vascular resistance decreases. Presumably, in the horse, as in other species, the decrease in resistance results from a combination of dilation of perfused vessels and recruitment of previously unperfused vessels. Significant increases in right atrial pressure also occur (Fig. 15.4).

There are a number of differences in systemic hemodynamics between the racing greyhound and its mongrel counterpart (Table 15.3). Mean arterial pressure is significantly higher in greyhounds. This is associated with a significantly higher cardiac index and a lower calculated peripheral resistance.

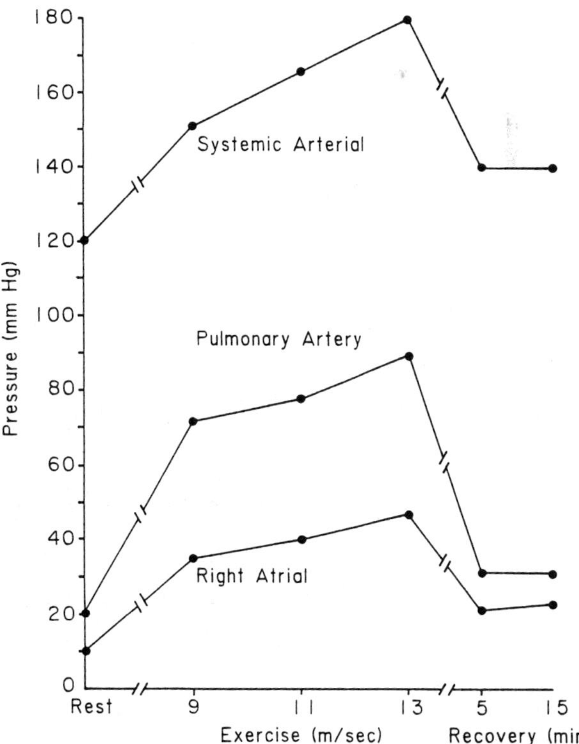

Figure 15.4. The response in mean systemic arterial pressure, mean pulmonary arterial pressure, and mean right atrial pressure in the horse at rest, during exercise, and during recovery on a high-speed treadmill. (From S.C. Olsen 1989, unpublished data.)

Cardiovascular adaptations to physical conditioning

Heart rate

In humans, physical conditioning or training results in sinus bradycardia at rest and a decreased heart rate during submaximal work. Most studies indicate that the resting heart rate of the horse does not change significantly after training (Table 15.4), although lower resting heart rates have been observed in endurance horses after training. It has been suggested that the lower resting heart rates observed are probably more attributable to decreased apprehension and nervousness than to a bradycardia. In horses and dogs, heart rates during submaximal exercise are lower after training. However, maximal heart rate in dogs is not usually altered.

Stroke volume

Cardiac enlargement is a well-recognized adaptation of highly conditioned human athletes and may be due to increased cardiac mass or to left ventricular volume that leads to increases in stroke volume. Cardiac output is maintained during submaximal exercise in the face of the reduction in heart rate after exercise training, indicating an increase in stroke volume.

Blood pressure

After training, there are consistent trends toward lower left ventricular pressure, arterial pressure, and left ventricular contractility at rest. In contrast to the decrease in pressures on the left side during exercise after training, mean right atrial pressure, which at rest is slightly lower than before training, increases steeply to significantly higher levels with increasing stages of exercise. This may be associated with an increased blood and plasma volume. After a period of exercise training, blood pressure is better regulated during exercise.

Blood volume

Long-term exercise training produces an expansion of blood and plasma volume. This adaptation to training provides an increased vascular volume to meet the increased cardiovascular and thermoregulatory needs during exercise. In the greyhound, after 14 days of training on a treadmill, plasma volume increases 27.5 percent, water intake 33 percent, and urine output 20.8 percent. The primary mechanism for the exercise training–induced hypervolemia is a net positive water balance from increased water consumption without significant contribution from an increase in renal water reabsorption. The same increase in plasma volume occurs in the horse after 14 days of training; however, daily water intake does not change during training. Packed cell volume and hemoglobin concentrations are lower in horses when they are in peak track condition, and the values increase when the horses are removed from the track.

Table 15.4. Cardiovascular effects after physical conditioning in the dog and horse

Variable	Effect: At rest	Effect: Maximum exercise
Heart rate	No change	Decreased
Stroke volume	Increased	Increased
O_2 uptake	Increased	Increased
Arteriovenous O_2 difference	No change	Increased
Heart volume	Increased	Increased
Blood volume	Increased	Increased
Blood pressure	Decreased	Decreased

Data from Gillespie and Robinson 1987, McKeever et al. 1987, Rose 1985, and Snow et al. 1983.

Electrocardiographic findings in racehorses

In the resting horse, heart rate is comparatively slow, and normal irregularities may occur in rhythm. The irregularities often disappear when heart rate increases, so that performance is not impaired. However, the persistence of arrhythmias at high heart rates during or immediately after exercise justifies a guarded prognosis, for circulatory efficiency is of major importance at these times.

Exercise has minimal effects on the QRS complex. However, the PR and QT intervals are shortened, and P waves are superimposed on the T waves that precede them. T waves can also change form during exercise, (e.g., increase in amplitude); this is associated with an increased potassium level. During recovery from exercise, premature ventricular beats or sinus arrythmia may occur. Measurement of the QRS interval has been used to determine heart size in racehorses and greyhounds.

Second-degee atrioventricular block

Second-degree partial atrioventricular (AV) block is the most common rhythm irregularity observed in horses at rest. It is clinically recognizable by the appearance of missed ventricular beats (Fig 15.5). In the majority of cases, the atrial or fourth heart sound can be heard. It is often accompanied by first-degree AV block and is generally Wenckebach type I with variations in PR interval, which often progressively lengthen to a missed beat. On auscultation, a corresponding increased separation can be noticed between the atrial contraction sound and the first heart sound.

One practice in assessment of the cardiac response to work is to gradually increase the amount of exercise, first at a trot, then at a canter, and later at a gallop. In most horses with partial AV block at rest, the missed beats disappear with exercise and do not recur until heart rate again approaches a resting value. Radiotelemetry or a treadmill may be used to detect missed beats, singles, and sometimes doubles for a short period immediately after exercise in a significant number of horses with partial AV block at rest. This transient period is usually followed by a regular

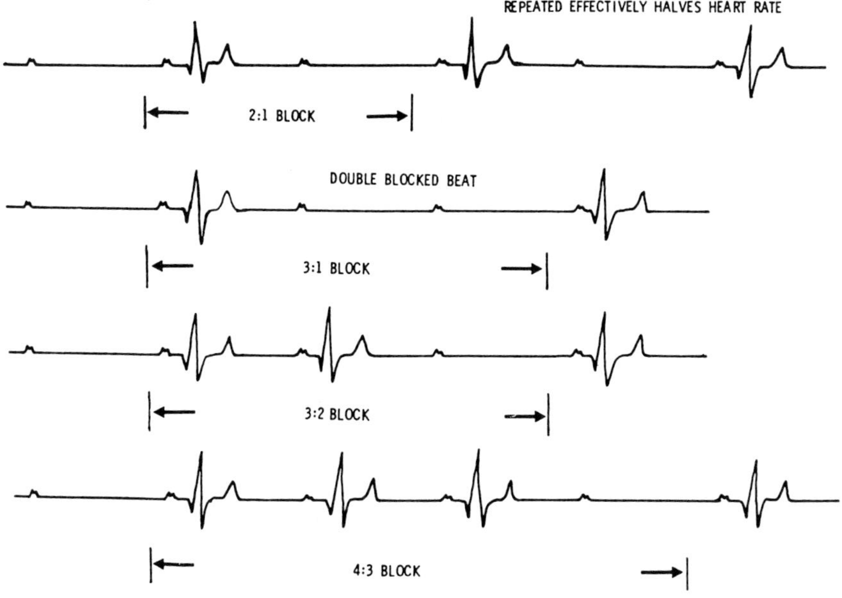

Figure 15.5. Conduction ratios in second-degree AV block in the horse at rest. A 2:1 block reduces the pulse rate by one-half the regular rhythm. A 3:1 block results in double blocked beats which are usually accompanied by single missed beats. An R-R interval plot would show normal/long/normal/long intervals with a 3:2 block, while a 4:3 block is characterized by two normal intervals and then a long interval. (From Holmes 1988, *Equine Cardiology,* University of Bristol, England.)

rhythm until heart rate approaches resting rate, when partial AV block reappears. The transient nature of this arrhythmia suggests that it may be a manifestation of excessive vagal action associated with the onset of heart rate slowing, just as vagal influence may explain the frequency of partial AV block in horses at low resting heart rates.

Whether second-degree AV block has a physiological or pathological basis is unresolved. It is the most common arrhythmia in the horse and is probably of little clinical significance. However, some regard second-degree AV block as a condition that may impair racing performance. Marked pathological changes have been noted in the myocardium of some horses with second-degree AV block. This condition can be minimized with atropine or exercise.

Atrial fibrillation

On auscultation, profound irregularity, absence of atrial contraction sounds, and variation in intensity of first and second heart sounds are indicative of atrial fibrillation. Figure 15.6 shows the variation of R-R intervals in a horse with atrial fibrillation.

During exercise at high heart rates, the arrhythmia persists but is less obvious. It quickly becomes more apparent again as heart rate begins to slow immediately after exercise. This cardiac abnormality is often associated with a history of poor performance and "fading" while racing and occurs more often in big horses.

Horses that show atrial fibrillation also have a significantly higher incidence of T wave abnormalities and second-degree AV block. Atrial fibrillation occurs more readily and probably with less serious underlying heart disease in the horse than in the dog. This arrhythmia may be complicated by murmurs, which are usually systolic and associated with the mitral valve. Mitral valve lesions may lead to atrial enlargement and atrial fibrillation.

RESPIRATORY SYSTEM

Respiratory function during exercise

The primary function of the respiratory system is the exchange of oxygen and carbon dioxide at a rate that is matched to metabolism. Horses have a very high aerobic scope, with the impressive ability to increase their oxygen consumption about 40-fold between rest and maximal exercise (Table 15.2). Gas exchange involves ventilation of the lungs, perfusion of the pulmonary capillaries with blood, matching of ventilation and blood flow, diffusion of gases between air and blood, and transport of gases to and from the muscles.

Ventilation

Ventilation is the bulk flow of gas into and out of the lungs. The resting horse is unusual in that it has a biphasic exhalation and occasionally a biphasic inhalation (see Chap. 13). Maximal expiratory flow has been measured in healthy horses to determine whether dynamic events in the pulmonary airways limit ventilation during maximal exercise. During maximal exercise, peak expiratory flow rates for a 540 kg horse range between 80 and 100 L/s. Catecholamine release, which accompanies exercise, dilates the bronchial tree and decreases resistance to airflow. Convective cooling associated with ventilation is also important in the regulation of body temperature in the horse. Environmental factors such as ambient temperature and humidity influence respiratory rate.

Horses change gait to minimize energy expenditure for any given running speed. At each gait there is an optimal

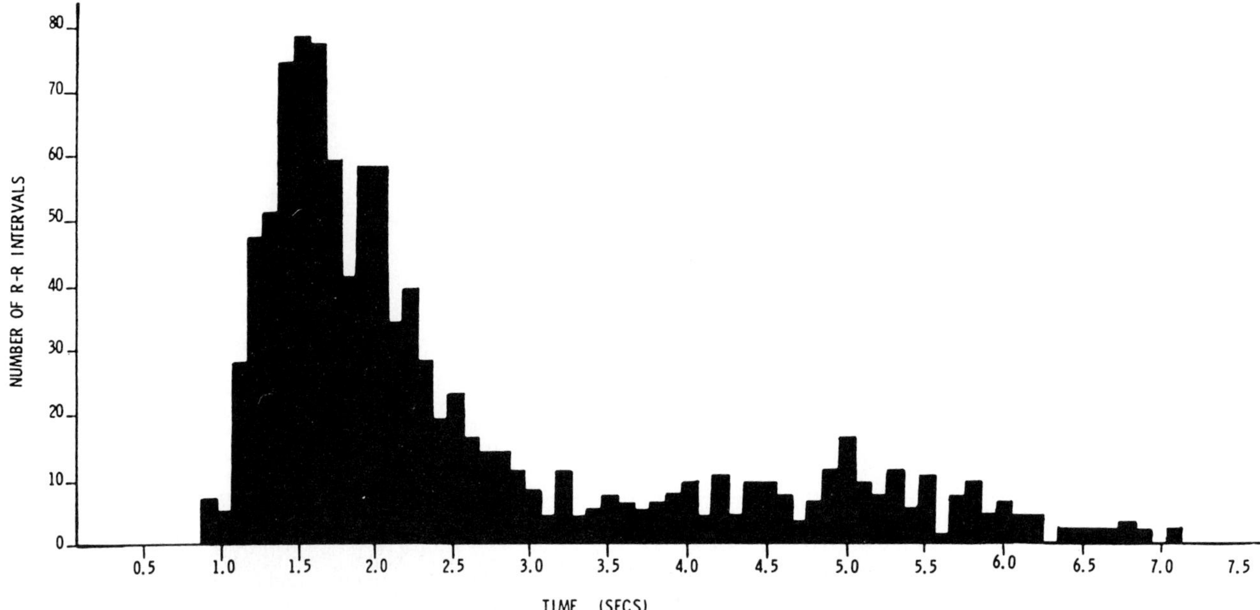

Figure 15.6. A histogram of 1024 R-R intervals measured at rest in a 20-year-old coach horse with atrial fibrillation. The histogram shows a wide distribution of R-R intervals. The resting heart rate averaged 26 beats per minute with some intervals of up to 7.94 seconds between beats. During these long periods of systolic standstill the jugular veins filled. During trotting and lunging, tachycardia occurred and the rhythm was regular. The arrhythmia was present almost immediately after work stopped. (From Holmes 1988, *Equine Cardiology,* University of Bristol, England.)

speed at which oxygen consumption is minimal. Both ponies and horses select a gait that maximizes their efficiency of movement. Despite this selection of gait to minimize energy expenditure, oxygen consumption increases almost linearly as speed increases. To accommodate this increase in oxygen consumption, there are increases in minute ventilation, cardiac output, and amount of hemoglobin in the blood. As exercise intensity increases, there is increased oxygen extraction, so that the approximately 40-fold increase in oxygen consumption that occurs during maximal exercise is satisfied by a 23-fold increase in minute ventilation and a five- to eightfold increase in cardiac output.

As running speed increases, minute ventilation increases linearly. This increase can be accomplished by an increase in either tidal volume, respiratory frequency, or both. At the walk and trot, respiratory frequency usually is not related to step frequency. At the canter and gallop, however, respiratory frequency and step frequency are synchronized, and this may be a mechanical advantage.

Oxygen consumption

The response of the oxygen transport system during locomotory exercise represents one of the most striking adaptations shown by horses for sustained aerobic performance. Thoroughbreds are able to augment their oxygen consumption more than 40-fold between rest and maximal exercise; this may be the highest aerobic scope in mammals (Fig. 15.7). Endurance-trained humans can increase oxygen consumption 18 to 24 times higher than resting values in response to strenuous exercise. Maximal $\dot{V}O_2$ of Thoroughbreds reaches approximately 160 ml/min/kg (or 70 L/min for a 440 kg animal) with an a-v O_2 difference of 23 volumes percent and a maximal cardiac output of 300 L/min. Maximum $\dot{V}O_2$ of trained humans does not exceed 80 ml/min/kg (or 5 to 6 L/min for a 70 kg individual). Therefore, Thoroughbred horses have an outstanding aerobic capacity with a mass specific $\dot{V}O_2$ maximum twice as high as in the best human athletes.

The kinetics of gas transport are more rapid in the dog and the horse than in humans. The rapidity of the increase in $\dot{V}O_2$ with the onset of exercise in these athletes appears to be associated with a rapid increase in minute ventilation and cardiac output, together with the release into the circulation of erythrocytes stored in the spleen. After a warm-up period before exercise, steady-state values for oxygen consumption are reached by 60 to 90 seconds of exercise at all intensities on a treadmill.

The oxygen-transfer chain is a functional chain for the transfer of oxygen from outside the body to metabolizing tissue (Fig. 15.8). This transfer chain includes O_2 uptake and diffusion (upper and lower respiratory tract function), O_2 binding to hemoglobin in red cells, O_2 transport (the cardiac pump function and circulation through the vascular system), O_2 delivery to the tissues (dissociation and diffusion), and O_2 utilization in mitochondria (oxidizable substrates and enzymes). The oxygen-transfer chain is only as strong as its weakest link.

Delivery of oxygen from the lungs to the tissues can be

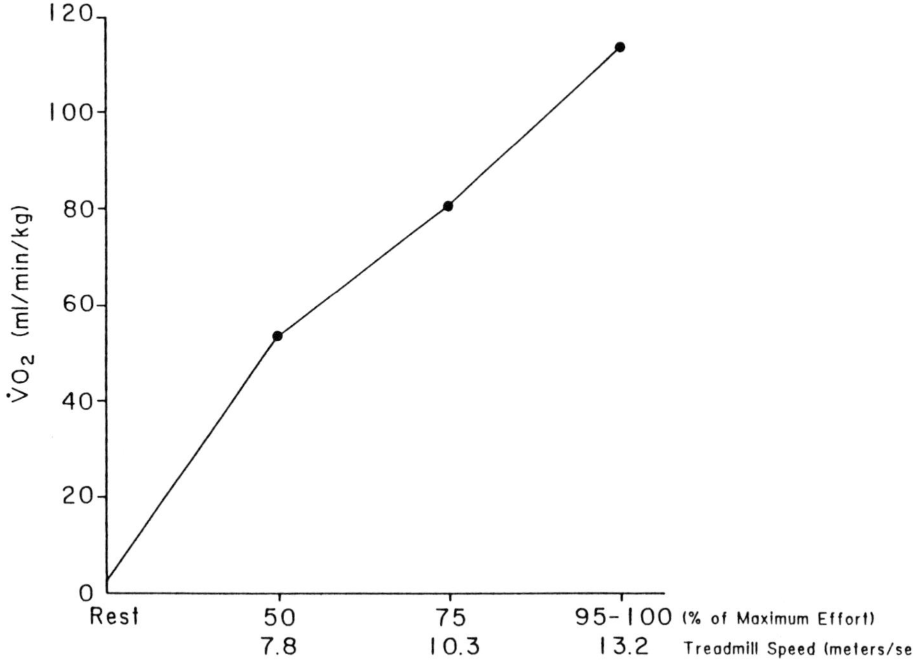

Figure 15.7. The response in oxygen consumption in the horse during exercise on a high-speed treadmill. $\dot{V}O_2$, oxygen consumption. (Data from M.K. Hopper 1989. Ph.D. dissertation, Kansas State University Library.)

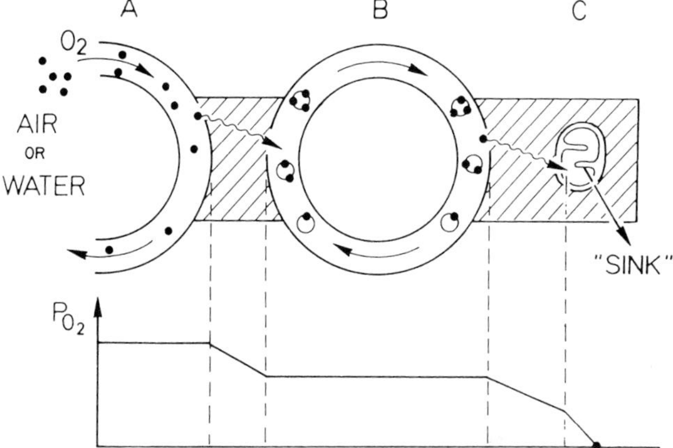

Figure 15.8. Cascade model describing oxygen flow from air (*A*) through the blood (*B*) to the mitochondria in cells (*C*), where it disappears into the "sink." The PO_2 falls step by step from environmental values to eventually zero in the sink. (Reprinted by permission of the publishers from *The Pathway for Oxygen* by Ewald R. Weibel, M.D., Cambridge, Mass.: Harvard University Press, Copyright 1984 by the President and Fellows of Harvard College.)

increased by three strategies during exercise: (1) increased cardiac output, (2) increased oxygen-carrying capacity of the blood (increased PCV), and (3) increased extraction of oxygen from the blood at the tissues (increased a-v O_2 difference). The approximately 40-fold increase in oxygen consumption during maximal exercise in the horse occurs with about an eightfold increase in cardiac output. However, each aliquot of blood has approximately a 50 percent increase in the amount of hemoglobin (oxygen capacity) because of splenic discharge of erythrocytes. The remainder of the increased oxygen demand is met by increasing oxygen extraction from the blood.

When a horse gallops from a standing start, the respiratory system responds immediately to the demands of greatly increased tissue respiration, whereas both heart function and hemoglobin mobilization respond more slowly to the metabolic demands of exercise. The apparent discrepancies between the respiratory responses on the one hand and the cardiovascular and hematologic responses on the other may be explained by the differences in the regulatory mechanisms involved. Ventilatory responses during exercise are under neural control by proprioreceptors in the locomotor apparatus, which overrides the inhibitory effect of decreased $Paco_2$ on central and peripheral chemoreceptors. Cardiac accelerator stimuli, on the other hand, originate both from the autonomic nervous system and from humoral catecholamines. Withdrawal of parasympathetic inhibition alone suffices to increase the heart rate to around 110. Increases in heart rate above this value are due to sympathetic stimulation and to circulating catecholamines. Erythrocyte mobilization is likewise under both neural and humoral control.

Respiration and locomotion

Respiratory frequency of mounted horses at rest varies between 15 and 45 breaths per minute, depending on the degree of preexercise restlessness of the animal. No relationship between respiratory frequency and step frequency is observed at the walk or the trot. It has been shown that, in normal horses, the respiratory and limb cycles are synchronized in phase (1:1) at the canter and gallop. Thus horses respire up to 130 to 140 times per minute during a fast gallop.

Tidal volume approximately doubles during the trot. When changing from the trot to the canter, most horses exhibit a slight decrease in tidal volume as a consequence of the higher respiratory frequency. Respiration in running horses differs from respiration in running humans. Bipedal locomotion has little repercussion on thoracic mechanics. Therefore humans can choose the most efficient combination of tidal volume and respiratory frequency. When running medium distances at near maximum speed, human athletes respire with a frequency of 50 to 60 breaths per min at a tidal volume of about 50 percent of vital capacity. In contrast, locomotion forces the galloping horse to respire at a very high rate with relatively shallow breaths. However, tidal volume rarely exceeds one-third of the vital capacity.

Blood gas tensions and acid-base balance

Horses develop metabolic acidosis during strenuous exercise. The decline in pH is not directly correlated with the rise in blood lactic acid. The respiratory response to exercise results in a fall in arterial Pco_2 in many species; however, Pco2 increases in the horse during strenuous exercise.

Arterial hypoxemia (low Po_2) occurs during strenuous exercise in the horse, in the racing greyhound, and in highly trained human athletes. The reasons for the development of hypoxemia are not clear, although there are several possible explanations, such as (1) increases in the blood-alveolar diffusion distance, which may be associated with the development of interstitial pulmonary edema and diffusion limited gas exchange; (2) hypoventilation; and (3) increased length of the airways, which may be an important factor in increasing airway resistance and inertia.

Hypoxemia has been observed during treadmill exercise tests in horses and presumably reflects changes in the perfusion and/or diffusion characteristics of the horses' lungs during exercise. Horses exercised at a lower speed (4 m/s) do not show significant changes in arterial Po_2 during exercise. In heavily exercising humans, arterial Po_2 is maintained at resting or at only slightly lower levels. The combined effect of a falling arterial Po_2 and pH and a rising temperature during exercise is a gradual fall in the oxygen saturation.

The development of exercise-induced arterial hypoxemia and hypercapnia appears to be closely related to exertion level. The increases in arterial Pco_2 and temperature and the fall in pH cause the oxyhemoglobin dissociation curve to shift to the right (Bohr shift). This shift results in a decreased affinity of hemoglobin for oxygen and facilitates the release of oxygen to the tissues.

The hypoxemia and hypercapnia observed in exercising horses are likely due to diffusion limitations and/or ventilatory inadequacies. In the event that alveolar Po_2 is reduced, the alveolar-pulmonary capillary diffusion gradient also would be decreased. This factor, when combined with the low oxygen saturation of the mixed venous blood being presented in the capillaries and the extremely high flow rate, may result in inadequate time for equilibration of red cells with alveolar Po_2 and incomplete oxygen saturation (Fig. 15.9). Prediction formulas have led to the conclusion that ventilatory factors are not likely to limit oxygen consumption in maximally exercising horses.

Hypercapnia may further influence the level of exertion of which a horse is capable by hindering the regulation of

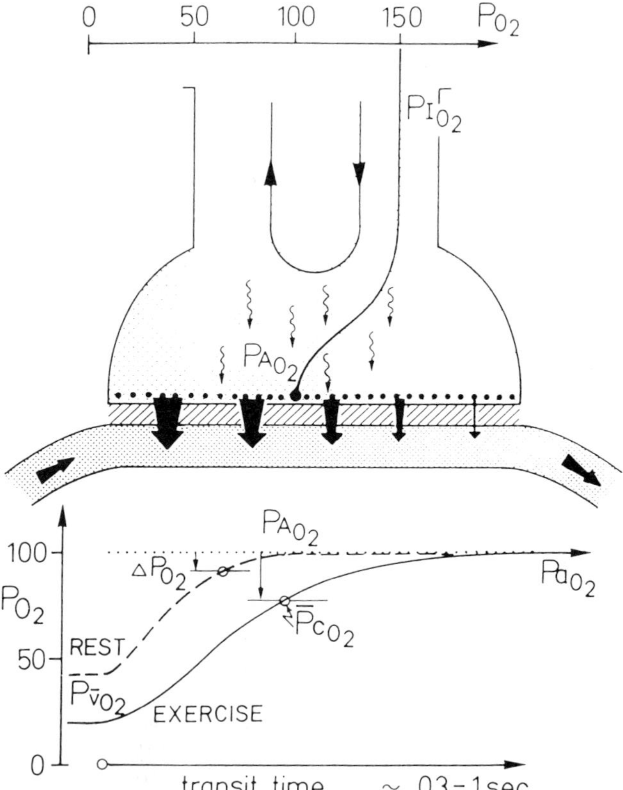

Figure 15.9 Change of Po_2 (mm Hg) in alveolar air and in capillary blood along the path from the pulmonary artery (venous blood) to the pulmonary vein (arterial blood). Heavy vertical arrows in lower part of upper illustration represent a decreasing flow rate of O_2 across the alveolar-capillary barrier as incoming venous blood equilibrates with alveolar air in becoming arterial blood. Arrows in the top part of the upper illustration show the movement of air in and out of the lung alveoli with each respiratory cycle. The lower illustration shows that pulmonary capillary blood for a person at rest (transit time about 1 second) is equilibrated with alveolar air after the first third of the capillary path, whereas during exercise (transit time about 0.3 second) the entire length of capillary path may be required for equilibration. As shown, the partial pressures at various locations are represented by $P_{I_{O_2}}$ (inspired oxygen = 150 mm Hg), $P_{A_{O_2}}$ (alveolar oxygen), $P_{\bar{v}_{O_2}}$ (mixed venous oxygen, $\bar{P}_{c_{O_2}}$ (mean capillary oxygen), and $P_{a_{O_2}}$ (arterial oxygen). $P_{a_{O_2}}$ is considered equivalent to the $P_{A_{O_2}}$ near 100 mm Hg. (Reprinted by permission of the publishers from *The Pathway for Oxygen* by Ewald R. Weibel, M.D., Cambridge, Mass.: Harvard University Press. Copyright 1984 by the President and Fellows of Harvard College.)

H^+, particularly that generated in the working muscles. The elevated arterial Pco_2 increases the diffusion gradient needed for rapid removal of acids. Impairment of this diffusion process may result in marked lowering of muscle cell pH and thereby alter the efficiency of muscle metabolism.

Exercise-induced pulmonary hemorrhage

Exercise-induced pulmonary hemorrhage (EIPH) is defined as bleeding from the lungs associated with exercise. Epistaxis or bleeding from the nose is a clinical sign observed in performance horses during or after exercise. There is a direct correlation between a horse's age and the incidence of EIPH. There is also a strong correlation between the distance raced and the frequency of EIPH. Thus older horses and those enduring prolonged bouts of intense exercise have a greater tendency to suffer EIPH.

Diagnosis of EIPH is usually confirmed by endoscopic observation of blood in the tracheobronchial airways within 30 to 90 minutes after the completion of exercise. During the course of the 1986 Hong Kong Thoroughbred racing season, 485 individual horses were examined with a flexible endoscope after racing to determine the incidence and severity of bleeding. Of these horses, 47 percent showed EIPH. For these horses examined more than three times, however, an incidence of 82 percent was recorded. Postmortem examinations performed on 117 of these horses showed that 82 percent had signs of previous hemorrhage in the posterior lobes of the lung. Histological examination revealed that 96 percent of these horses had evidence of previous alveolar hemorrhage and bronchiolitis.

The exact cause and anatomical identification of the vessels that rupture are unknown. Elevated pressure in pulmonary or bronchial vessels during exercise may distend these vessels and cause them to rupture and leak. Pulmonary vascular pressures are influenced by internal factors, such as high cardiac output and vascular resistance. Other factors associated with racing, such as large changes in intrapleural pressure and acceleration forces of the feet striking the ground, may also contribute to increased pulmonary vascular pressures and EIPH. The respiratory system of the competition horse is constantly exposed to dirt, allergy-causing particles, and infectious agents, which may contribute to bronchiolitis and EIPH.

MUSCULAR SYSTEM

Skeletal muscle adaptations

Adaptations in skeletal muscle occur at the gross, microscopic, and biochemical levels during exercise and after a period of exercise training. In the racing greyhound, skeletal muscle makes up 57 percent of the body mass (Table 15.5), considerably higher than the 44 percent found in other dogs and the 40 percent found in most mammals studied. Similarly, skeletal muscle makes up 52 percent of the total body weight in the thoroughbred compared with 42 percent in other horses.

Table 15.5. Percentage of live weight occupied by muscle, bone, and fat and the muscle/bone ratio in the horse and dog

	Muscle	Bone	Fat	Muscle/bone
Thoroughbreds	52	12	1.12	4.3
Other horses	42	12	2.11	3.5
Greyhounds	57	12	0.28	4.7
Other dogs	44	12	0.94	3.6

Modified from Gunn 1987.

Muscle fiber types

It was first observed that color and histological features of muscle correlate with their speed of contraction. On the basis of myosin ATPase activity at pH 9.4, two distinct types of fibers have been identified. Those with low activity at this pH have been classified as type I or slow-twitch (red) fibers, and those with high activity are classed as type II or fast-twitch (white) fibers. Type I fibers have slower contraction and relaxation times than type II fibers. In addition, type I fibers are highly oxidative and are more resistant to fatigue than type II fibers. Type II fibers can be further subdivided into subtypes IIA, IIB, and IIC. Type IIA represents more oxidative fibers, whereas type IIB is more glycolytic and type IIC appears to be intermediate in both oxidative and glycolytic capacity. In contrast to many species, including horses, all of the type II muscle fibers in dogs are highly oxidative.

Differences in the fiber composition of limb muscles can be seen among breeds of both species. These differences relate to performance characteristics for which the particular breed has been selected. In the horse, this difference is most prominent in the middle gluteal muscle, one of the largest and most important muscles for the generation of propulsive force (Table 15.6). Variations in fiber area and oxidative capacity also exist between and within breeds.

Although the proportions of slow-twitch and fast-twitch fibers are predominantly the result of genetic endowment, some evidence suggests that alterations in the properties of these fibers and their subtypes occur in response to training. The transition is usually toward increases in the proportions

Table 15.6. Fiber composition in the middle gluteal of untrained animals from different breeds of horses (percent fiber type, mean ± SEM)

	n	ST	FTH	FT
Quarter horse	28	8.7 ± 0.8	51.0 ± 1.6	40.3 ± 1.6
Thoroughbred	50*	11.0 ± 0.7	57.1 ± 1.3	32.0 ± 1.3
	149†	14.7 ± 0.4	65.1 ± 0.5	20.2 ± 0.5
Arabian	6	14.4 ± 2.5	47.8 ± 3.2	37.8 ± 2.8
Standardbred	8	18.1 ± 1.6	55.4 ± 2.2	26.6 ± 2.0
Shetland pony	4	21.0 ± 1.2	38.8 ± 1.9	40.2 ± 2.7
Heavy hunter	7	30.8 ± 3.1	37.1 ± 3.3	32.1 ± 3.4
Donkey	5	24.0 ± 3.0	38.2 ± 3.0	37.8 ± 2.8

*Elite broodmares.

†Moderate 2 year olds.

ST, slow twitch (type I fibers; FTH, fast twitch, high oxidative fibers (type IIA); FT, fast twitch (type II fibers).

From Snow 1985.

of the more oxidative type IIA fibers (i.e., increased type IIA/IIB ratio). Dramatic increases in the number and sizes of mitochondria and concomitant increases in the oxidative enzymes involved in the oxidative production of adenosine triphosphate (ATP) have been reported in horses undergoing various forms of training.

Elite endurance horses show higher percentages of type I and IIA fibers and lower percentages of type IIB fibers in their middle gluteal muscles than average competitors. In human endurance events, several reports have equated a high proportion of slow-twitch fibers in active muscles with superior performance. In contrast, sprint athletes usually display a greater percentage of type IIB muscle fibers in their locomotory muscles.

Muscle fiber recruitment

For the maintenance of posture and at low exercise intensities, only type I fibers and some type IIA fibers must be recruited; hence it is desirable for these fibers to be fatigue-resistant. As the work load increases, development of more tension is necessary and more type IIA fibers are recruited. The very forceful contractions required for rapid acceleration and power generation result in the recruitment of more type IIB fibers. Increased exercise intensity will lead to progressive recruitment of the faster-contracting, more powerful fibers. If prolonged low-intensity exercise is performed, however, a progressive recruitment from type I through type IIB fibers takes place to maintain the required work level as the working muscle fibers fatigue.

Studies of glycogen depletion during exercise in horses demonstrate that different motor units or combinations thereof are systematically recruited, depending on the type of exercise the animal is performing. In prolonged submaximal exercise (such as trail or endurance rides), only the type I and some type IIA fibers are initially recruited. As the duration and intensity of the exercise increase, however, more type IIA fibers, followed by type IIB fibers, are recruited; as the animal approaches exhaustion, all the motor units, regardless of type, may be used. This suggests that, during prolonged submaximal exercise, some motor units become exhausted and drop out of the contractile process as others are added. In contrast, under conditions of exercise in which production of maximal muscle tension is required (for example, Quarter Horse or Thoroughbred racing), all or nearly all muscle fiber types are recruited from the commencement of exercise.

Alterations in muscle fiber types

Skeletal muscle has the capacity to adapt to a wide variety of contractile patterns in the everyday life of an animal. One property of this tissue that allows these adaptations is the greater suitability of some motor units than others for certain types of activity. For example, the higher oxidative potential of type I and IIA motor units, relative to type IIB units, makes them more suitable to prolonged activity when fuel reserves can be used to greatest advantage. Conversely, type IIB fibers are best suited for short, intense contractile patterns in which the production and tolerance of lactate are required. Thus it is not surprising that elite endurance horses have been found to have high proportions of type I and IIA fibers, whereas animals performing high-speed exercise (for example, racing Quarter Horses and Thoroughbreds) tend to have higher proportions of type IIA and IIB muscle fibers.

Fiber area

In addition to the importance of the proportions of type I and type II fibers to muscle function and in assessment of athletic ability, the cross-sectional area of individual fibers also plays a significant role because it influences force output. Thus, when the cross-sectional area of a muscle fiber becomes greater, the potential for force output increases. Therefore, when explosive acceleration is needed, recruitment of larger type IIB fibers rather than smaller type IIA fibers is desirable. As they are usually of low oxidative capacity, however, they are rapidly fatigued and of little use for endurance exercise, for which highly oxidative fibers are required. The Quarter Horse has the largest cross-sectional area of type IIB fibers, constituting about 54 percent of the muscle mass, whereas the contributions of type IIB fibers in Thoroughbreds and Standardbreds are 46 percent and 37 percent, respectively.

Capillary density

Capillaries are the interface between skeletal muscle and the vascular supply that makes the exchange of metabolic substrates and waste materials possible. Increases in capillary density with endurance training have been well documented in humans. These studies have shown a close correlation between maximal oxygen uptake and capillary density. However, studies in the horse and the dog are less conclusive. A correlation of fiber type distribution with gross performance capacity has been established in equine muscle. The capillary density is influenced by the mean fiber area, the capillary/fiber ratio. To some extent, capillary density is also influenced by the relative distribution of fiber types, which differ in diffusional capacities. Of the individual fiber types, the highest diffusional capacity (small fibers surrounded by many capillaries) is displayed by type I fibers and the lowest by type IIB fibers, which is in accordance with their respective capacities for aerobic metabolism.

Myoglobin

The overall evidence seems to be that myoglobin levels are highest in those species that engage in high levels of muscular activity. The Thoroughbred has at least twice as much myoglobin in its muscle as other species. Myoglobin has an oxygen-dissociation curve (Fig. 3.5) that is shifted to the left relative to hemoglobin. This feature facilitates the movement of oxygen from the blood into the myocyte and may play a considerable role in delivery of oxygen to the tissues. In addition, research has shown that myoglobin concentrations increase with prolonged endurance training, thus demonstrating an enhanced potential to support aerobic metabolism by increasing oxygen uptake.

Biochemical Changes

A general increase in enzymes representative of improved oxidative capacity has been reported after an aerobic training program. These changes are in parallel with an increased mitochondrial volume. The enzyme activities in limb muscles in Thoroughbred horses have been examined after a 10 to 15-week training period involving predominantly submaximal, but some high-speed exercise. The activities of nearly all enzymes increase. Thus substantial increases in both aerobic and anaerobic potential occur with training. The major effects of endurance training are increased use of fat with concomitant sparing of muscle glycogen, reduced blood lactate accumulation, and increased work capacity during prolonged submaximal work.

In resting muscle samples, type I fibers have lower glycogen content than either the type IIA or type IIB fibers. After endurance exercise, type I fibers show the most glycogen depletion. As the distance or the intensity increases, progressive recruitment of type IIA and IIB fibers occurs. The mechanism for the progressive fiber-type recruitment appears to be related to fiber contractile properties. Glycogen repletion occurs in the reverse pattern to depletion, with a preferential repletion of type IIB relative to type I fibers.

Biochemistry

Training regimens that improve performance in humans and animals have been shown to induce changes in the cardiovascular system and also in the skeletal muscles involved in exercise. Growth itself and spontaneous activity, rather than any kind of controlled superimposed activity, seem to be the most important factors inducing the changes in muscle characteristics.

In humans, lactate has been suggested as the major contributor in promoting muscle fatigue during intense, short-term exercise. In the horse, the dog, and other species, exercise depletes the muscle of glycogen. The prime precursor of lactate formation in skeletal muscle during intense short exercise is intramuscular glycogen. The fuels used in exercise are dependent on the involvement of the different muscle types. Glycogen utilization and lactate production are increased with greater speeds because the energy demands exceed the aerobic capacity of the muscle fibers involved.

Maximum oxygen consumption is generally recognized to be the best global descriptor of aerobic performance and capacity. Estimation of plasma lactate concentration after a standard workload is a useful indirect method of assessing aerobic capacity in horses. Endurance exercise induces a considerable increase in the volume density of mitochondria and lipids in humans. Mitochondrial densities are higher in trained racehorses than in untrained ones. The amount of mitochondria is closely related to the potential for oxygen consumption of skeletal muscle tissue.

Energy considerations

Maintenance of muscular contraction during exercise requires the provision of large amounts of chemical energy. Although various sources of energy are available, ATP is the universal intracellular vehicle of chemical energy within skeletal muscle.

Energy for muscular contraction

During muscular work, ATP is hydrolyzed to adenosine diphosphate (ADP) in skeletal muscle, with the release of inorganic phosphate and energy by the myosin ATPase. During this process, a large amount of chemical potential energy is released as kinetic energy. Once this energy is liberated, it can be used by the muscle contractile proteins to generate force. Under normal conditions, however, only a limited amount of ATP is present in skeletal muscle, which is sufficient to maintain muscular contraction for only a few seconds. There are two distinct processes that provide the intracellular replenishment of ATP: (1) oxidative (aerobic) phosphorylation in which the major substrates for aerobic phosphorylation are circulating nonesterified fatty acids and glucose, together with intramuscular glycogen and triglycerides and (2) anaerobic phosphorylation, in which ATP is regenerated from creatine phosphate, circulating glucose, and local glycogen stores.

Depending on the type of exercise, a balance occurs between the contributions of oxidative and anaerobic phosphorylation. Therefore, during short-term intense exercise such as sprinting, energy liberation will involve predominantly anaerobic pathways, whereas endurance exercise involves a greater contribution from oxidative phosphorylation.

Regulation of substrate utilization

Regulation of substrate utilization involves complex metabolic regulation within muscle cells. During periods when blood flow to muscle is adequate to provide oxygen and nonesterified fatty acids, fatty acids appear to be the preferred metabolic substrate. As a result, glucose and glycogen metabolism is inhibited. However, when fatty acid oxidation is unable to meet the energy needs of the muscle cells, whether because of excessive energy expenditure in the muscle or because of inadequate blood flow, the inhibition of glucose metabolism is removed and glycolysis proceeds.

Substrate utilization in the exercising horse

During exercise, the metabolic requirements of muscle vary according to the duration and/or intensity of the work. As a result of the fine metabolic control that occurs in skeletal muscle, there is a highly regulated system in which the most effective contribution of the various energy-producing pathways occurs at any given time. These contributions are directly related to the force and speed of muscular contraction, the availability of substrates, and/or the presence of metabolites. As exercise commences, the immediate energy source is locally available ATP. However, because only very limited stores of ATP occur in skeletal muscle, this source is rapidly depleted, if not replenished by other processes. Creatine phosphate is able to donate its high-energy phosphate and, therefore, becomes the next source of energy for working muscle. Creatine phosphate levels also are limited in skeletal muscle; if exercise continues, other mechanisms for the provision of energy are required. Glycolysis, with the production of pyruvate and to some extent lactate, provides the ongoing energy supply. Within approximately 30 seconds from the onset of exercise, the glycolytic processes reach peak energy production. Because equine muscle has a large capacity for glycogen storage, this substrate is able to provide a considerable source of energy during exercise.

Thus, according to the intensity of exercise, a balance of anaerobic and aerobic pathways occurs. It is the availability of oxygen in the cell and concentrations of the mitochondrial enzymes that determine the extent to which the metabolic processes can proceed aerobically and/or anaerobically.

Morphology and speed

Visual observations suggest that animals noted for their high speed of running are characterized by long legs in relation to other parts of their body, whereas animals noted for their strength rather than fleetness have proportionately shorter legs. Comparisons of bulldogs with greyhounds, leopards with cheetahs, and draft horses with thoroughbreds demonstrate this phenomenon.

In the greyhound, the Quarter Horse, and the Thoroughbred, the proportion of muscle in the femoral region is greater than in other breeds of these species. Thoroughbreds and Quarter Horses have a greater mass of their hind limbs nearer the hip joint than other breeds. This feature favors a high natural frequency of hind limb movement and facilitates a higher stride frequency and, consequently, a faster speed of running in these breeds than in others. At top speed the Thoroughbred takes about 2.5 strides per second and the Quarter Horse three strides per second. This greater muscle mass may be explained by both greater cell number and greater fiber area. In the dog, however, fiber areas are relatively small. The relatively small size of canine muscle fibers may be related to the high oxidative capacity of all fibers, which permits a high surface area/volume ratio for rapid diffusion of oxygen.

THERMOREGULATION AND FLUID BALANCE

Muscular activity requires the transduction of chemical energy to mechanical energy. Traditionally, it has been assumed that the superior human athlete (and presumably also the canine and equine athlete) has a maximal metabolic efficiency of approximately 25 percent. That is, only about 25 percent of the available chemical energy is convertible to work. The remaining energy is converted to heat, which must be conducted to the environment if the body temperature is to remain unchanged. When exercise is performed in environments of high temperature and/or humidity, the competing demands for evaporative cooling and maximal energy output may limit performance and, in some instances, lead to serious heat-associated disturbances.

Energetics of exercise

Exercise is generally divided into two major categories—aerobic and anaerobic. Oxygen consumption is a reliable and measurable indicator of the rate of metabolism. Oxygen consumption and heat production continue to be elevated during the recovery period and may remain elevated for an hour or more. At very high work intensities (i.e., short-term anaerobic exercise), the rate of heat production may exceed basal levels by 40 to 60 times. The thermoregulatory responses to the heat load generated at this work rate may limit performance, particularly when environmental temperature and humidity are high.

Thermoregulation

During exercise, the burden of dissipating the increased production of metabolic heat is placed on the thermoregulatory mechanisms. There are four principal means by which the body dissipates heat: conduction, convection, radiation, and evaporation. The evaporative route is the most efficient means of heat loss during exercise and may be the only means of heat dissipation in hot environments.

One of the most essential, but often overlooked, functions of blood circulation is the transport of excess heat from the interior of the body to the surface. As the body's heat content increases in response to the increased metabolism asssociated with exercise, the cutaneous blood vessels dilate. Venous return from the extremities takes place through more superficial veins, thus increasing heat conductance of the tissues. The increased cutaneous circulation elevates skin temperature, facilitating heat loss by both convection and radiation, provided environmental temperature is lower than skin temperature. In addition, evaporative heat loss is facilitated by cutaneous vasodilation. The circulatory system must accommodate the competing demands for increased cutaneous blood flow and the increased metabolic requirements of working muscles.

If the heat load is sufficiently large, sweat glands are activated, particularly in the horse. Sweating induced by exercise occurs in response to both circulating epinephrine and the sympathetic nervous system, but only the latter is involved in thermal sweating. Epinephrine-induced sweating in the horse is mediated by $beta_2$ receptors. Sweat promotes heat loss only when the sweat evaporates. At extremely high environmental temperatures, evaporative heat loss may not be able to keep pace with the exercise-induced heat load and the animal will gain heat from the environment. High humidity prevents complete evaporation. With incomplete evaporation, sweat production results in little or no heat transfer but can contribute to dehydration. In controlled endurance rides of 60 km, the mean weight loss in a horse may be 5 to 6 percent of body weight. Conditions of high environmental temperature and humidity thus pose a serious risk to the equine athlete, particularly during protracted submaximal exercise. Although sweating is the principal means of evaporative cooling in exercising horses, the respiratory tract also contributes to heat and water loss.

In the dog sweating is insignificant in thermoregulation and panting is more important. Panting is discussed in Chapter 13, which concerns respiration in mammals, and in Chap. 17, which deals with temperature regulation. Panting is an important temperature-regulating mechanism in many species, particularly in dogs. The respiratory frequency increases to 200 to 400 breaths per minute, and the tidal volume decreases during panting so that alveolar ventilation remains constant.

The thermoregulatory responses to exercise-generated heat load are not always sufficient to prevent elevation of body temperature. Muscle, rectal, and blood temperatures increase dramatically in the horse with increasing work intensity and duration; rectal temperatures as high as 41 to 43°C have been recorded in the horse (Fig. 15.10). Racing greyhounds in hot climates often exhibit symptoms of heat stroke, azoturia, exertional rhabdomyolosis, and/or cardiac failure during the summer racing season. During a 500-meter race, ear canal or tympanic membrane temperatures can increase from 36.5 to 41.6°C and rectal temperature from 38.0 to 41.6°C.

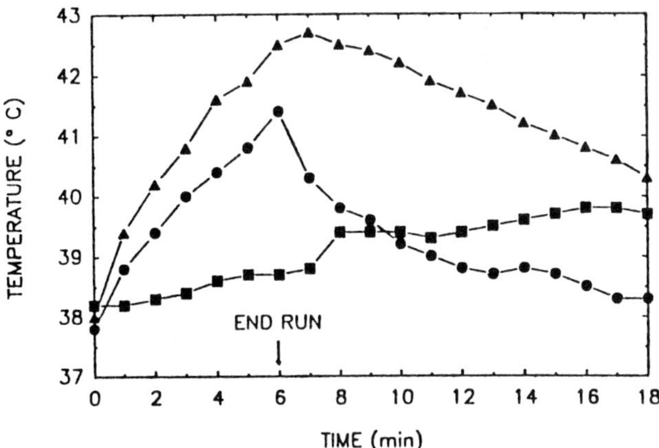

Figure 15.10 Temperatures recorded with thermocouples during and after 6-minute run in a standardbred horse exercising at 98 percent maximal rate of O_2 consumption. Triangles, temperatures 2.5 cm deep in the middle gluteal muscle; circles, temperatures in the pulmonary artery; squares, temperatures 25 cm deep in rectum. (From Jones et al. 1989, *J. Appl. Physiol.* 67:879–84.)

Sweat composition

Sodium ion (Na^+) is the principal cation in horse sweat and is present at concentrations similar to or higher than those in plasma. Potassium ion (K^+) concentrations in the sweat are typically 10 to 20 times greater than those in the plasma. There is also a very high concentration of chloride ion (Cl^-) in equine sweat. The relatively high ionic composition of equine sweat is in contrast to human sweat, which is almost invariably hypotonic relative to plasma. These differences in sweat composition are important in fluid and electrolyte alterations that result from heavy sweat losses during exercise in human and equine athletes. They are also important in the provision of fluid electrolyte supplements, particularly for endurance horses.

Fluid balance

During exercise, sweating is the principal route of both fluid and electrolyte loss in the horse. Sweat rates may approach 10 to 12 L/h during prolonged exercise in a hot environment. With massive fluid and electrolyte losses in sweat, excretion by other routes is probably altered. When sweat electrolyte losses are large, renal mechanisms for electrolyte conservation are brought into play in an attempt to maintain homeostasis.

Endurance-trained horses tend to maintain a lower resting PCV than horses trained for shorter, faster races. The lower PCV is not due to a decreased erythrocyte count or an increased storage of erythrocytes in the spleen but to an increased plasma volume. Both human and equine athletes develop an expanded plasma volume in response to endurance exercise training, which may serve to defend against excessive water losses during protracted work and heat stress.

HORMONAL RESPONSES

The supply, uptake, and utilization of substrates for the production of energy in working skeletal muscles are integral components of an organism's ability to carry out physical exercise. The adaptation by the organism to repeated bouts of exercise is reflected in the use it makes of the different substrates available. The onset of exercise is associated with changes in the plasma concentration of energy substrates and/or their delivery to working muscles in association with the changes that occur in cardiac output and blood flow distribution. The hormones produced by the various endocrine glands are important components of the control mechanism that regulates substrate supply and energy production. Excessive or inadequate levels of several hormones place constraints on exercise performance. In addition, the plasma levels of several hormones are increased with exercise as part of the integrated response to stress.

Signals from the working muscles or via reflexes originating from higher motor centers in the brain can modify the response of the endocrine glands directly via pituitary hormones or indirectly via the sympathoadrenal system. The initial response to the onset of exercise is enhancement of sympathoadrenal activity and secretion of ACTH and TSH, which result in a reduction in the plasma concentration of insulin and a rise in virtually all other hormones.

Thyroid gland

Thyroid hormones act at two major sites. In the mitochondria, thyroid hormone stimulates cellular respiration, leading to an increased rate of oxygen utilization and energy production. This is most evident in skeletal and cardiac muscle. At the nucleus, thyroid hormones increase the rate of RNA synthesis, which in turn leads to an increase in protein synthesis and in the concentration of many enzymes. There is probably a coordinated pituitary-thyroid response to repeated daily exercise that is largely influenced by the intensity of the exercise and is reflected in an increased production and turnover of thyroid hormones. Optimal levels of thyroid hormone are essential to achievement of maximal performance.

Adrenal gland

In common with other steroid hormones, glucocorticoids exert their effect at the nuclear level by increasing the production of RNA that supplies the code for protein synthesis. Among the enzymes produced are several that deaminate amino acids and stimulate glucose synthesis, hepatic glycogenolysis, and lipolysis. These actions facilitate metabolism to provide additional fuel for prolonged submaximal exercise, which might be compromised by inadequate levels of glucocorticoids. In the horse, the dominant glucocorticoid is cortisol. Cortisol levels are increased during and immediately after exercise in most species, including the horse (Fig. 15.11). In addition to the role of physical stress, psychologic stress may also influence the induction of cortisol secretion.

Circulating epinephrine initiates many of the metabolic events required for the maintenance of vigorous exercise. Epinephrine stimulates the conversion of muscle glycogen to glucose phosphate, activates tissue lipases, inhibits insulin release, stimulates the heart to increase rate and cardiac output, is involved in the redistribution of blood flow during exercise, facilitates neuromuscular transmission in skeletal muscle, stimulates contractile processes in fast-twitch fibers, relaxes bronchioles, and increases respiratory rate. Unlike thyroid and steroid hormones, catecholamines exert their effects within minutes.

The response of the sympathetic nervous system during exercise is reflected in the plasma concentrations of epinephrine and norepinephrine (Fig. 15.11). This response is generally proportional to the intensity of the work performed, with norepinephrine levels being increased significantly at lower work intensities than epinephrine levels. A ninefold increase in plasma norepinephrine has been noted

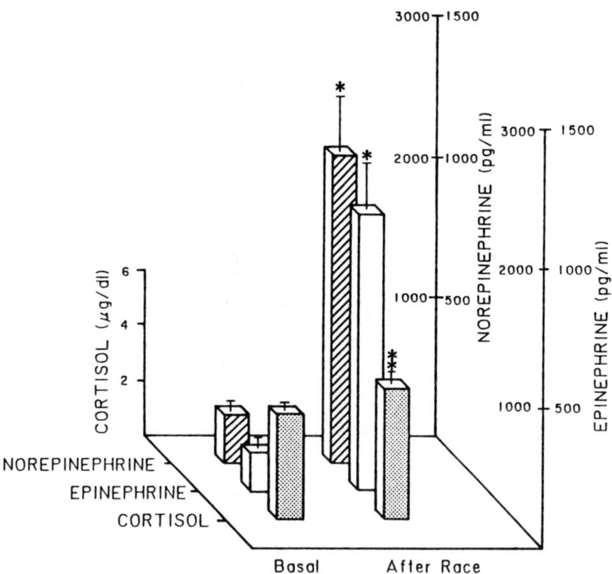

Figure 15.11 Plasma cortisol and catecholamine levels in the Thoroughbred horse before and after racing. Values are expressed as the mean of 10 determinations ± standard error of the mean. Significant differences from basal values are represented by $^{*}p < 0.0001$; $^{**}p < 0.05$. (Reprinted with permission from *Comp. Biochem. Physiol.* 91A:599–602 by Martinez, Godoy, Nareto and White, "Neuroendocrine changes produced by competition stress on the thoroughbred race horse." Copyright 1988, Pergamon Press plc.)

after brief maximal exercise in the horse and a 50 percent increase after an endurance ride. In contrast, there is little increase in plasma epinephrine during low-intensity work, whereas a marked increase occurs during heavy exercise, especially if it is accompanied by emotional stress. Although basal levels are unchanged, catecholamines increase less in trained subjects during exercise, unlike the adrenocortical hormones.

Other hormones

In the horse, as in humans and other species, both the intensity and the duration of exercise influence the changes in insulin and glucagon. It seems appropriate that each component contributes to an integrated response to stress. Other hormones involved in exercise stress are as follows: (1) ACTH stimulates the release of cortisol, which plays an important role in combatting stress and also increases the release of epinephrine; (2) lipotropic hormones mobilize lipids, which provide the fuel for prolonged muscular activity; and (3) endorphins may suppress the pain of fatigue and trauma (Fig. 15.12). A rapidly growing body of evidence suggests that the analgesia, euphoria, and motor stimulation of endogenous opioids play an important role in exercise performance in humans.

EVALUATION OF EXERCISE TOLERANCE AND FITNESS

Exercise tolerance is related to the functional capacity of both the cardiopulmonary and the musculoskeletal sys-

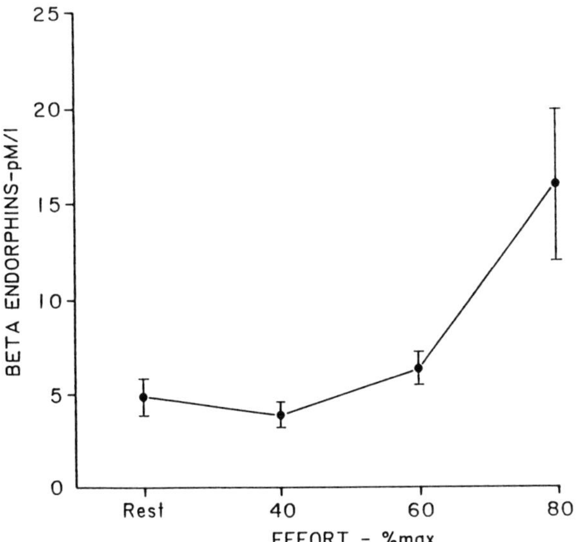

Figure 15.12 Changes in beta-endorphin levels (pM/L = pica moles per liter) in plasma at rest and at three levels of exercise expressed as percent of maximum capacity (percent maximum.) (From Bove 1989, *News Physiol. Sci.* 4:143–46.)

tems. Both dimensional and functional capacities of these organ systems can be limiting factors for maximal oxygen uptake and, consequently, for exercise performance. Aerobic energy production predominates during work that lasts more than about 1 minute. During heavy exercise, however, both aerobic and anaerobic energy production contributes to the work output. An increasing demand on energy production caused by continuous physical training induces a corresponding dimensional and functional adaptation of the cardiovascular system. It is possible to predict the degree of adaptation to physical work (i.e., exercise tolerance) from variables indicative of cardiovascular efficiency, such as the postexercise total hemoglobin level.

Blood volume is an expression of the dimensional capacity of the cardiovascular system; it is a limiting factor of the "oxygen-conduction system" that conveys oxygen from the air to the metabolically active tissues of the body. An unimpeded flow of oxygen to the tissues is also dependent on the functional capacities of the cardiovascular system. Thus blood volume can be correlated with values that describe those capacities.

In the horse, blood lactate generally does not increase significantly above the resting level until the heart rate exceeds 155 to 160 beats per minute. This indicates that work that causes a heart rate of 150 beats per minute is performed almost aerobically in most horses; thus V150 (the running speed or velocity at 150 beats per minute) is an expression of the aerobic capacity of the animal. A very steep increase in blood lactate occurs at an exercise heart rate of about 200 beats per minute, indicating that, above this level, anaerobic energy release starts to play a significant role in work output.

In summary, the cardiovascular system provides the link between pulmonary ventilation and oxygen usage at the cellular level. During exercise, efficient delivery of oxygen to working skeletal and cardiac muscles is vital for maintenance of ATP production by aerobic mechanisms. The equine cardiovascular response to increased demand for oxygen delivery during exercise contributes largely to the greater than 40-fold increase in oxygen consumption that occurs during maximal exercise. The large increases in cardiac output during exercise are primarily attributable to the relatively high heart rates that are achieved during exercise.

Higher work rates and oxygen uptake at submaximal heart rates after training imply an adaptation to training that enables more efficient oxygen delivery to and/or utilization by the working muscles. Such adaptations can be in either blood flow or a-v O_2 difference. Increases in blood hemoglobin concentrations during exercise after training are recognized, but at maximal exercise hypoxemia may reduce arterial oxygen content. More effective redistribution of cardiac output to muscles by increased capillarization and more efficient oxygen diffusion to cells may also be important means of increasing oxygen uptake after training.

NUTRITION

Energy

Energy is of particular importance for the exercising dog or horse because it is influenced by exercise. The amount of additional energy required during exercise depends on type of work, rate and length of work, condition of the animal, and environmental temperature. Exercise conditioning increases the resting metabolism; the anticipation of exercise also increases energy metabolism and raises dietary energy requirements.

The basic needs of the greyhound for racing are not vastly different from maintenance requirements. The average caloric intake is only 30 to 40 percent above estimated daily requirements. Food requirements for physical fitness involving short bursts of intensive exercise do not necessarily involve a high food intake.

Source of energy

The source of energy can influence performance. Energy requirements for horses are met with forage and forage-grain mixtures. A horse with high energy requirements cannot obtain all its energy from bulky hay. Endurance horses need more roughage; this dilates the intestinal volume and increases the intestinal water and electrolyte reserve. There is controversy concerning the effect of type of grain on performance in horses. Corn contains twice as much energy per volume as oats; however, digestive upsets and metabolic problems may occur if corn is substituted for oats. Fat has been suggested for athletic horses; the nonesterified fatty acids are a primary source of energy for horses during prolonged exercise. Fat also improves the performance of sled dogs racing over prolonged distances. Feeding high levels of fat during training may condition an animal to use fat more efficiently during endurance exercise because the enzymes are adapted to fat metabolism. During endurance events, fat is more likely to be a source of energy than glycogen. The addition of fat to equine diets protects against a decline in blood glucose during exercise.

Glycogen storage

Endurance capacity in the human athlete is directly related to the content of glycogen in the working muscles. Prolonged exercise may result in almost total depletion of glycogen in the muscle fiber bed. Glycogen storage is accomplished in human athletes by consumption of high-fat, high-protein diets during training to severely deplete glycogen stores. The athlete then eats a high-carbohydrate diet 3 days before the event to enhance storage. In the horse, studies of glycogen are very limited. Glycogen loading in horses appears to have limited value, particularly in short events, because glycogen stores are not depleted. Increased glycogen stores may be of value in endurance horses competing over long distances. Excessive glycogen loading may predispose a horse to exertional myopathy.

Protein

In the horse, there is little or no increase in dietary protein requirements during exercise. A small amount of nitrogenous compounds, including protein, are lost in sweat; however, the increased intake required to meet energy requirements provides sufficient protein. Plasma concentrations of urea and creatinine are consistently increased in endurance horses. The increase in urea is due primarily to a significant increase in the rate of protein catabolism. The greatest factor contributing to the rise in creatinine is the increased utilization of phosphocreatine by the working muscle. High-protein diets may actually be detrimental. Horses on a high-protein diet sweat more profusely, and their pulse and respiration rates are higher after long endurance events. If water is limited, a high-protein diet is not recommended because additional water is needed for the excretion of nitrogen.

Amino acid intake may affect the racing performance of greyhounds. Muscular work increases amino acid uptake and protein synthesis in muscle. Beef is the main source of protein in many kennels and is supplied as a broth. Fluid balance is critical in racing greyhounds because they do not drink very much water. Therefore, fluid needs to be supplied in the diet. Greyhounds dehydrate rapidly under hot summer conditions unless water is added to the diet.

Minerals

The exercising horse loses water, sodium, potassium, chloride, iron, and other elements in sweat. The heavily sweating horse may develop a negative electrolyte balance. During severe sweating, muscle may be the main source for replacement of potassium lost in sweat. Magnesium requirements are also increased in an exercising horse because magnesium is lost in sweat; magnesium is important in the muscle cell for ATPase activity. A growing horse that is being worked needs a higher level of calcium and phosphorus than is normally required for maintenance. A growing horse that is working is more susceptible to mineral deficiency than a growing horse that is not working, because exercise increases the rate of bone turnover. Selenium is required for the integrity of muscle and is used to treat exertional myopathy.

Vitamins

Vitamin supplements for athletes are popular, but their value is questionable. Good-quality hay contains an adequate level of vitamins to meet requirements in the horse, but poor-quality hay may require vitamin supplementation. Hay that is weathered or stored for a period of time (with loss of green color) may have a low level of vitamin A activity. Grains, such as oats, also contain little vitamin A. Racehorses are more susceptible to thiamine deficiency than other horses; thiamine is required for energy utilization. Vitamin E is important for exercise capacity; vitamin E deficiency significantly decreases endurance.

The nutritional requirements for dogs, including recommended minimal and maximal daily intakes of both minerals and vitamins, are well documented; however, the exact requirements for the racing greyhound have not been established. When one considers diet, physical stress of repeated racing, and parasites, greyhounds may benefit from supplementary vitamins and other additives.

REFERENCES

Aitken, M.M., Anderson, M.G., Mackenzie, G., and Sanford, J. 1974. Correlations between physiological and biochemical parameters used to assess fitness in the horse. *J. S. Afr. Vet. Assoc.* 454:361–70.

Allen, B.V., and Powell, D.G. 1983. Effects of training and time of day of blood sampling on the variation of some common haematological parameters in normal Thoroughbred racehorses. In D.H. Snow, S.G.B. Persson, and R.J. Rose, eds., *Equine Exercise Physiology*. Granta Editions, Cambridge, England. Pp. 328–35.

Alonso, F.R.A. 1972. Distribution of the cardiac output in the greyhound dog. Thesis, University of Pennsylvania.

Amend, J.F., Garner, H.E., and Rosborough, J.P. 1972. Physiological study of ventricular hypertrophy in a domestic pony. *J. Cardiovasc. Surg.* 13:131–37.

Amoroso, E.C., Scott, P., and Williams, K.G. 1963. The pattern of external respiration in the unanesthetized animal. *Proc. R. Soc. Lond. [Biol.]* 159:325–47.

Andersen, P., and Henriksson, J. 1978. Training induced changes in the subgroups of human skeletal muscle fibres. *Acta Physiol. Scand.* 99:123–25.

Archer, R.K. 1974. Haematology in relation to performance and potential: A general review. *J. S. Afr. Vet. Assoc.* 45:273–77.

Art, T., Lekeux, P., Gustin, P., Desmecht, D., Amory, H., and Paiva, M. 1989. Inertance of the respiratory system in ponies. *J. Appl. Physiol.* 67:534–40.

Astrand, P-O., and Rodahl, K. 1977. *Textbook of Work Physiology.* 2d ed. McGraw-Hill Book Co., New York.

Attenburrow, D.P. 1983. Respiration and locomotion. In D.H. Snow,

S.G.B. Persson, and R.J. Rose, eds., *Equine Exercise Physiology*. Granta Editions, Cambridge, England. Pp. 17–22.

Bayly, W.M., Gabel, A.A., and Barr, S.A. 1983a. Cardiovascular effects of submaximal aerobic training on a treadmill in Standardbred horses, using a standardized exercise test. *Am. J. Vet. Res.* 44:544–53.

Bayly, W.M., Grant, B.D., Breeze, R.G., and Kramer, J.W. 1983b. The effects of maximal exercise on acid-base balance and arterial blood gas tension in Thoroughbred horses. In D.H. Snow, S.G.B. Persson, and R.J. Rose, eds., *Equine Exercise Physiology*. Granta Editions, Cambridge, England. Pp. 400–407.

Bergsten, G. 1974. Blood pressure, cardiac output and blood-gas tension in the horse at rest and during exercise. *Acta. Vet. Scand. [Suppl.]* 48: 1–88.

Bjotvedt, G. 1985. Racing-induced cardiomyopathy in greyhounds. *Vet. Med.* 80:54–57.

Blomquist, C.G., and Saltin, B. 1983. Cardiovascular adaptations to physical training. *Ann. Rev. Physiol.* 45:169–89.

Bove, A.A. 1989. Hormonal responses to acute and chronic exercise. *News Physiol. Sci.* 4:143–46.

Brenon, H.C. 1956. Erythrocyte and hemoglobin studies in thoroughbred racing horses. *J. Am. Vet. Med. Assoc.* 128:343–45.

Cain, D.F., and Davies, R.E. 1962. Breakdown of adenosine triphosphate during a single contraction of working muscle. *Biochem. Biophys. Res. Commun.*, 8:361–66.

Carew, T.E., and Covell, J.W. 1978. Left ventricular function in exercise-induced hypertrophy in dogs. *Am. J. Cardiol.* 42:82–88.

Carlson, G.P. 1983. Thermoregulation and fluid balance in the exercising horse. In D.H. Snow, S.G.B. Persson, and R.J. Rose, eds., *Equine Exercise Physiology*.Granta Editions, Cambridge, England. Pp. 291–309.

Clausen, J.P. 1969. The effects of physical conditioning: A hypothesis concerning circulatory adjustments to exercise. *Scand. J. Clin. Lab. Invest.* 24:305–13.

Clark, L.L., Garner, H.E., and Hatfield, D. 1982. Plasma volume, electrolyte, and endocrine changes during onset of laminitis hypertension in horses. *Am. J. Vet. Res.* 43:1551–555.

Clausen, J.P. 1969. The effects of physical conditioning. A hypothesis concerning circulatory adjustments to exercise. *Scand. J. Clin. Lab. Invest.* 24:305–13.

Constantinopol, M., Jones, J.H., Weibel, E.R., Taylor, C.R., Lindholm, A. and Karas, R.H. 1989. Oxygen transport during exercise in large mammals. II. Oxygen uptake by the pulmonary gas exchanger. *J. Appl. Physiol.* 67:871–78.

Courtice, F.C. 1943. The blood volume of normal animals. *J. Physiol.* 102:290–305.

Cox, R.H., Bagshaw, R.J., and Detweiler, D.K. 1981. Arterial baroreceptor reflexes in young and old racing greyhounds. *Am. J. Physiol.* 240:H383–90.

Cox, R.H., Bagshaw, R.J., and Detweiler, D.K. 1985. Baroreceptor reflex cardiovascular control in mongrel dogs and racing greyhounds. *Am. J. Physiol.* 249:H655–62.

Cox, R.H., Peterson, L.H., and Detweiler, D.K. 1976. Hemodynamics in the mongrel dog and the racing greyhound. *Am. J. Physiol.* 230:211–18.

Davis, H.A. 1983. Nutrition and performance. In *Refresher Course for Veterinarians*. Proc. No. 64:29–33. Refresher Course on Greyhounds, University of Sydney, Sydney, Australia.

Davis, P.E. 1983. Greyhound management. In *Refresher Course for Veterinarians*. Proc. No. 64:237–252. Refresher Course on Greyhounds, University of Sydney, Sydney, Australia.

Detweiler, D.K., Cox, R.H., Alonso, F.R., Knight, D.H., Bagshaw, R., Jones, A., and Peterson, L.H. 1974. Hemodynamic characteristics of the young adult greyhound. *Fed. Proc.* 33:360.

Detweiler, D.K., Cox, R.H., Alonso, F.R., and Patterson, D.F. 1975. Characteristics of the greyhound cardiovascular system. *Fed. Proc.* 34:399.

Donald, D.W., and Ferguson, D.A. 1966. Response of heart rate, oxygen consumption, and arterial blood pressure to graded exercise in dogs. *Proc. Soc. Exp. Biol. Med.* 121:626–29.

Donald, D.E., Milburn, S.E., and Shepherd, J.T. 1964. Effect of cardiac denervation on maximal capacity for exercise in the racing greyhound. *J. Appl. Physiol.* 19:849–52.

Dukes, H.H. 1940. A case of heart-block in the horse. *Cornell Vet.* 30:248.

Duren, S.E., Jackson, S.G., Baker, J.P., and Aaron, D.K. 1987. Effect of dietary fat on blood parameters in exercised Thoroughbred horses. In J.R. Gillespie and N.E. Robinson, eds., *Equine Exercise Physiology 2*. ICEEP Publications, Davis, Calif. Pp. 674–85.

Erickson, H.H., Bishop, V.S., Horwitz, L.D., and Kardon, M.B. 1971. Left ventricular internal diameter and cardiac function during exercise. *J. Appl. Physiol.* 30:473–78.

Erickson, H.H., Sexton, W.L., Erickson, B.K., and Coffman, J.R. 1988. Oxygen transfer in the trained and untrained Quarter Horse. In N.C. Gonzalez and M.R. Fedde, eds, *Oxygen Transfer from Atmosphere to Tissues*, vol. 227. *Advances in Experimental Medicine and Biology*, Plenum Press, New York, Pp. 327–32.

Essén, B. 1978. Studies on the regulation of metabolism in human skeletal muscle using intermittent exercise as an experimental model. *Acta Physiol. Scand. [Suppl.]*, 454:1–64.

Essén-Gustavsson, B., Lindholm, A., McMiken, D., Persson, S.G.B., and Thornton, J. 1983. Skeletal muscle characteristics of young Standardbreds in relation to growth and early training. In D.H. Snow, S.G.B. Persson, and R.J. Rose, eds., *Equine Exercise Physiology.* Granta Editions, Cambridge, England. Pp. 200–10.

Essen-Gustavsson, B., McMiken, D., Karlstrom, K., Lindholm, A., Persson, S., and Thornton, J. 1989. Muscular adaptation of horses during intensive training and detraining. *Equine Vet. J.* 21:27–33.

Evans, D.L. 1985. Cardiovascular adaptations to exercise and training. *Vet. Clin. North Am. Equine Practice* 1:513–31.

Evans, D.L., and Rose, R.J. 1988. Cardiovascular and respiratory responses to submaximal exercise training in the thoroughbred horse. *Pflügers Arch.* 411:316–21.

Fregin, G.F., and Thomas, D.P. 1983. Cardiovascular response to exercise in the horse: a review. In D.H. Snow, S.G.B. Persson, and R.J. Rose, eds., *Equine Exercise Physiology*. Granta Editions, Cambridge, England. Pp. 76–90.

Garland, P.B., Randle, P.J., and Newsholme, E.A. 1963. Citrate as an intermediary in the inhibition of phosphofructokinase in rat heart muscle by fatty acids, ketone bodies, pyruvate, diabetes and starvation. *Nature* 200:169–70.

Gillespie, J.R. 1974. The role of the respiratory system during exertion. *J. S. Afr. Vet. Assoc.* 45:305–09.

Gillespie, J.R., and Pascoe, J.R. 1983. Respiratory function in the exercising horse. In D.H. Snow, S.G.B. Persson, and R.J. Rose, eds., *Equine Exercise Physiology*. Granta Editions, Cambridge, England. Pp. 1–6.

Gillespie, J.R., and Robinson, N.E., eds. 1987. *Equine Exercise Physiology 2*. ICEEP Publications, Davis, Calif.

Gillespie, J.R., Tyler, W.S., and Eberly, V.E. 1966. Pulmonary ventilation and resistance in emphysematous and control horses. *J. Appl. Physiol.* 21:416–22.

Gollnick, P.D. and Saltin, B. 1982. Significance of skeletal muscle oxidative enhancement with endurance training. *Clin. Physiol.* 2:1–12.

Griffiths, B.C.R. 1969. Nutrition of the Greyhound. *Vet. Rec.* 84:654–57.

Gunn, H.M. 1979. Total fibre numbers in a cross-section of m. semitendinosus of athletic animals and other members of their species. *J. Anat.* 128:821–28.

Gunn, H.M. 1981. Potential blood supply to muscles in horses and dogs and its relation to athletic ability. *Am. J. Vet. Res.* 42:679–84.

Gunn, H.M. 1983. Morphological attributes associated with speed of running in horses. In D.H. Snow, S.G.B. Persson, and R.J. Rose, eds., *Equine Exercise Physiology*. Granta Editions, Cambridge, England. Pp. 271–74.

Gunn, H.M. 1987. Muscle, bone and fat proportions and muscle distribution of Thoroughbreds and other horses. In J.R. Gillespie and N.E. Robinson, eds., *Equine Exercise Phsiology 2*. ICEEP Publications, Davis, Calif. Pp. 253–64.

Guy, P.S., and Snow, D.H. 1977. The effect of training and detraining on muscle composition in the horse. *J. Physiol.* 269:33–51.

Guy, P.S., and Snow, D.H. 1981. Skeletal muscle fiber composition in the dog and its relationship to athletic ability. *Research Vet. Sci.* 31:244–48.

Hales, J.R.S., and Dampney, R.A.L. 1975. The redistribution of cardiac output in the dog during heat stress. *J. Thermal. Biol.* 1:29–34.

Henckel, P. 1983. Training and growth induced changes in the middle gluteal muscle of young Standardbred trotters. *Equine Vet. J.* 15:134–40.

Henegan, T. 1977. Haematological and biochemical variables in the greyhound. *Vet. Sci. Commun.* 1:277–84.

Henckel, P. 1983. A histochemical assessment of the capillary blood supply of the middle gluteal muscle of Thoroughbred horses. In D.H. Snow, S.G.B. Persson, and R.J. Rose, eds., *Equine Exercise Physiology*. Granta Editions, Cambridge, England. Pp. 225–28.

Herrmann, G.R. 1926. The heart of the racing greyhound: Hypertrophy of the heart. *Proc. Soc. Exp. Biol. Med.* 23:856–57.

Hintz, H.F. 1983. Nutritional requirements of the exercising horse - a review. In D.H. Snow, S.G.B. Persson, and R.J. Rose, eds., *Equine Exercise Physiology*. Granta Editions, Cambridge, England. Pp. 275–90.

Hodgson, D.R. 1985. Energy considerations during exercise. *Vet. Clin. North Am. Equine Practice* 1(3):447–60.

Hodgson, D.R. 1985. Muscular adaptations to exercise and training. *Vet. Clin. North Am. Equine Practice* 1(3):533–48.

Hodgson, D.R., Rose, R.J., and Allen, J.R. 1983. Muscle glycogen depletion and repletion patterns in horses performing various distances of endurance exercise. In D.H. Snow, S.G.B. Persson, and R.J. Rose, eds., *Equine Exercise Physiology*. Granta Editions, Cambridge, England. Pp. 229–36.

Hodgson, D.R., Rose, R.J., Allen, J.R., and Dimauro, J. 1984. Glycogen depletion patterns in horses performing maximal exercise. *Res. Vet. Sci.* 36:169–73.

Hodgson, D.R., Rose, R.J., Allen, J.R., and Dimauro, J. 1985. Glycogen depletion patterns in horses competing in day 2 of a three day event. *Cornell Vet.* 75:366–74.

Holmes, J.R. 1974. An investigation of cardiac rhythm using an on-line radiotelemetry/computer link. *J.S. Afr. Vet. Assoc.* 45:251–61.

Holmes, J.R. 1982. A superb transport system: The circulation. *Equine Vet. J.*, 14:267–76.

Holmes, J.R. 1988. *Equine Cardiology*, Vol. IV, School of Veterinary Science, University of Bristol, England.

Hoppeler, H., Claassen, H., Howald, H., and Straub, R. 1983. Correlated histochemistry and morphometry in equine skeletal muscle. In D.H. Snow, S.G.B. Persson, and R.J. Rose, eds., *Equine Exercise Physiology*. Granta Editions, Cambridge, England. Pp. 184–92.

Hopper, M.K., Pieschl, R.L., Pelletier, N.G., and Erickson, H.H. 1991. Cardiopulmonary effects of acute blood volume alteration prior to exercise. In S.G.B. Persson, A. Lindholm, and L.B. Jeffcott, eds., *Equine Exercise Physiology 3*. ICEEP Publications, Davis, Calif. Pp. 9–16.

Hörnicke, H., Engelhardt, W. von, and Ehrlein, H.-J. 1977. Effect of exercise on systemic blood pressure and heart rate in horses. *Pflügers Arch.* 372:95–99.

Hörnicke, H., Meixner, R., and Pollman, U. 1983. Respiration in exercising horses. In D.H. Snow, S.G.B. Persson, and R.J. Rose, eds.,*Equine Exercise Physiology*. Granta Editions, Cambridge, England. Pp. 7–16.

Hoyt, D.F., and Taylor, C.R. 1981. Gait and the energetics of locomotion in horses. *Nature [Lond.]* 292:239–40.

Ilkiw, J.E., Davis, P.E., and Church, D.B. 1989. Hematologic, biochemical, blood-gas, and acid-base values in Greyhounds before and after exercise. *Am. J. Vet. Res.* 50:583–86.

Ingjer, F. 1979. Capillary supply and mitochondrial content of different skeletal muscle fiber types in untrained and endurance trained men. *Eur. J. Appl. Physiol.* 40:197–209.

Ingjer, F., and Brodal, F. 1978. Capillary supply of skeletal muscle fibers in untrained and endurance trained women. *Eur. J. Appl. Physiol.* 38:291–99.

Irvine, C.H.G. 1983. The role of hormones in exercise physiology. In D.H. Snow, S.G.B. Persson, and R.J. Rose, eds., *Equine Exercise Physiology*. Granta Editions, Cambridge, England. Pp. 377–88.

Jeffcott, L.B. 1974. Haematology in relation to performance and potential. 2. Some specific aspects. *J. S. Afr. Vet. Assoc.* 45:279–86.

Jenkins, W.L. 1974. Open discussion on respiration, biochemistry, electrolytes and performance. *J. S. Afr. Vet. Assoc.* 45:371–73.

Johnson, J.H., Garner, H.E., and Hutcheson, D.P. 1976. Ultrasonic measurement of arterial blood pressure in conditioned thoroughbreds. *Equine Vet. J.* 8:55–57.

Johnson, J.H., Garner, H.E., Hutcheson, D.P. and Merriam, J.G. 1973. Epistaxis. *Proc. Am. Assoc. Equine Pract.* 19:115–21.

Jones, W.E. 1989. *Equine Sports Medicine*. Lea & Febiger, Philadelphia.

Jones, J.H. 1989. Comparative exercise physiology: how do horses compare with other mammals? *Assoc. Equine Sports Med. Q.* 4:19–25.

Jones, J.H., Longworth, K.E., Lindholm, A., Conley, K.E., Karas, R.H., Kayar, S.R., and Taylor, C.R. 1989. Oxygen transport during exercise in large mammals I. Adaptive variation in oxygen demand. *J. Appl. Physiol.* 67:862–70.

Jones, J.H., Taylor, C.R., Lindholm, A., Straub, R., Longworth, K.E., and Karas, R.H. 1989. Blood gas measurements during exercise: errors due to temperature correction. *J. Appl. Physiol.* 67:879–84.

Kohnke, J.R. 1983. Nutrition of the racing greyhound. In *Refresher Course for Veterinarians*. Proc. No. 64:681–718. Refresher Course on Greyhounds, University of Sydney, Sydney, Australia.

Krzywanek, H., Wittke, G., Bayer, A., and Borman, P. 1970. The heart rates of Thoroughbred horses during a race. *Equine Vet. J.* 2:115–17.

Landgren, G.L., Gillespie, J.R., Fedde, M.R., Jones, B.W., Pieschl, R.L., and Wagner, P.D. 1988. O_2 transport in the horse during rest and exercise. In N.C. Gonzalez and M.R. Fedde, eds., *Oxygen Transfer from Atmosphere to Tissues*. Vol. 227 *Advances in Experimental Medicine and Biology*. Plenum Press, New York. pp. 333–36.

Lassen, E.D., Craig, A.M., and Blythe, L.L. 1986. Effects of racing on hematologic and serum biochemical values in greyhounds. *J. Am. Vet. Med. Assoc.* 188:1299–1303.

Lindholm, A. 1974. Glycogen depletion pattern and the biochemical response to varying exercise intensities in Standardbred trotters. *J. S. Afr. Vet. Assoc.* 45:341–43.

Lindholm, A. 1979. Substrate utilization and muscle fiber types in Standardbred trotters during exercise. In *Proceedings of the American Association of Equine Practitioners* 25:329–36.

Lindholm, A., Essén-Gustavsson, B., McMiken, D., Persson, S., and Thornton, J.R. 1983. Muscle histochemistry and biochemistry of Thoroughbred horses during growth and training. In D.H. Snow, S.G.B. Persson, and R.J. Rose, eds., *Equine Exercise Physiology*. Granta Editions, Cambridge, England. Pp. 211–17.

Lindholm, A., and Piehl, K. 1974. Fibre composition, enzyme activity and concentrations of metabolites and electrolytes in muscle of Standardbred horses. *Acta Vet. Scand.* 15:287–309.

Lindholm, A., and Saltin, B. 1974. The physiological and biochemical response of Standardbred horses to exercise of varying speed and duration. *Acta Vet. Scand.* 15:310–24.

Lindholm, A., Bjerneld, H., and Saltin, B. 1974. Glycogen depletion patterns in muscle fibres of trotting horses. *Acta Physiol. Scand.* 90:475–84.

Littlejohn, A., Bowles, F., and Aschenborn, G. 1983. Cardiorespiratory adaptations to exercise in riding horses with chronic lung disease. In D.H. Snow, S.G.B. Persson, and R.J. Rose, eds., *Equine Exercise Physiology*. Granta Editions, Cambridge, England. Pp. 33–45.

Lovell, David K. 1985. Exercise physiology: An overview. *Vet. Clin. North Am. Equine Practice* 1:439–45.

Maier-Bock, H., and Ehrlein, H.-J. 1978. Heart rate during a defined exercise test in horses with heart and lung diseases. *Equine Vet. J.* 10:235–42.

Manohar, M. 1988. Left ventraicular oxygen extraction during submaximal and maximal exertion in ponies. *J. Physiol.* 404:547–56.

Manohar, M., and Parks, C. 1983. Transmural coronary vasodilator reserve in ponies at rest and during maximal exercise. In D.H. Snow, S.G.B. Persson, and R.J. Rose, eds., *Equine Exercise Physiology.* Granta Editions, Cambridge, England. Pp. 91–104.

Marsland, W.P. 1968. Heart rate response to submaximal exercise in the Standardbred horse. *J. Appl. Physiol.* 24:98–101.

Martinez, R., Godoy, A., Naretto, E., and White, A. 1988. Neuroendocrine changes produced by competition stress on the thoroughbred race horse. *Comp. Biochem. Physiol.* 91A:599–602.

Mason, D.K., Collins, E.A., and Watkins, K.L. 1983. Exercise-induced pulmonary haemorrhage in horses. In D.H. Snow, S.G.B. Persson, and R.J. Rose, eds., *Equine Exercise Physiology.* Granta Editions. Cambridge, England Pp. 57–63.

McKeever, K.H., Schurg, W.A., and Convertino, V.A. 1985. Exercise training-induced hypervolemia in greyhounds: Role of water intake and renal mechanisms. *Am. J. Physiol.* 248:R422–25.

McKeever, K.H., Schurg, W.A., Jarrett, S.H., and Convertino, V.A. 1987. Exercise training-induced hypervolemia in the horse. *Med. Sci. Sports Exerc.* 19:21–27.

McMiken, D.F. 1983. An energetic basis for equine performance. *Equine Vet. J.*, 15:123–33.

Meixner, R., Hornicke, H. and Ehrlein, H. 1981. Oxygen consumption, pulmonary ventilation, and heart rate of riding horses during walk, trot, and gallop. In *W. Sanson, ed., Biotelemetry VI.* University of Arkansas Press, Fayetteville.

Meyer, H. 1987. Nutrition of the equine athlete. In J.R. Gillespie and N.E. Robinson, eds., *Equine Exercise Physiology 2.* ICEEP Publications, Davis, Calif. Pp. 644–73.

Milne, D.W. 1974. Blood gases, acid-base balance and electrolyte and enzyme changes in exercising horses. *J. S. Afr. Vet. Assoc.* 45:345–54.

Milne, D.W., Gabel, A.A., Muir, W.W., and Skanda, R.T. 1977. Effects of training on heart rate, cardiac output, and lactic acid in Standardbred horses, using a standardized exercise test. *J. Equine Med. Surg.* 1:131–35.

Needham, D.M. 1971. *Machina Carnis.* Cambridge University Press, Cambridge, England.

Newsholme, E.A. 1976. Carbohydrate metabolism in vivo: Regulation of the blood glucose level. *Clin. Endocrinol. Metab.* 5:543–78.

Nimmo, M.A., and Snow, D.H. 1983. Changes in muscle glycogen, lactate and pyruvate concentrations in the Thoroughbred horse following maximal exercise. In D.H. Snow, S.G.B. Persson, and R.J. Rose, eds., *Equine Exercise Physiology.* Granta Editions, Cambridge, England. Pp. 237–44.

Nimmo, M.A., Snow, D.H., and Munro, C.D. 1982. Effects of nandrolone phenpropionate in the horse. 3. Skeletal muscle composition in the exercising animal. *Equine Vet. J.* 14:229–33.

Olsen, S. C., Coyne, C.P., Lowe, B.S., Pelletier, N., Raub, E.M., and Erickson, H.H. 1992. Influence of furosemide on hemodynamic responses during exercise in horses. *Am. J. Vet. Res.* 53:742–47.

Parks, C.M., and Manohar, M. 1983. Transmural distribution of myocardial blood flow during graded treadmill exercise in ponies. In D.H. Snow, S.G.B. Persson, and R.J. Rose, eds., *Equine Exercise Physiology.* Granta Editions, Cambridge, England. Pp. 105–20.

Parks, C.M., and Manohar, M. 1983. Distribution of blood flow during moderate and strenuous exercise in ponies (*Equus caballus*). *Am. J. Vet. Res.* 44:1861–66.

Parmeggiani, A., and Bowman, R.H. 1963. Regulation of phosphofructokinase activity by citrate in normal and diabetic muscle. *Biochem. Biophys. Res. Commun.* 12:268–73.

Passoneau, J.V., and Lowry, O.H. 1963. P-Fructokinase and the control of the citric acid cycle. *Biochem. Biophys. Res. Commun.* 13:372–79.

Persson, S.G.B. 1967. On blood volume and working capacity in horses. *Acta Vet. Scand. [Suppl.]* 19:1–189.

Persson, S.G.B. 1968. Blood volume, state of training and working capacity of race horses. *Equine Vet. J.* 1:2–11.

Persson, S.G.B. 1983a. The significance of haematological data in the evaluation of soundness and fitness in the horse. In D.H. Snow, S.G.B. Persson, and R.J. Rose, eds., *Equine Exercise Physiology.* Granta Editions, Cambridge, England. Pp. 324–27.

Persson, S.G.B. 1983b. Evaluation of exercise tolerance and fitness in the performance horse. In D.H. Snow, S.G.B. Persson, and R.J. Rose, eds., *Equine Exercise Physiology.* Granta Editions, Cambridge, England Pp. 441–57.

Persson, S.G.B., and Bergsten, G. 1975. Circulatory effects of splenectomy in the horse. IV. Effect on blood flow and blood lactate at rest and during exercise. *Zentrabl, Vet. Med. [A]* 22:801–807.

Persson, S.G.B., Ekman, L., Lydin, G., and Tufvesson, G. 1973. Circulatory effects of splenectomy in the horse. I. Effect on red-cell distribution and variability of hematocrit in the peripheral blood. *Zentrabl. Vet. Med. [A]* 20:444–55.

Persson, S.G.B., Essen, B., and Lindholm, A. 1980. Oxygen uptake, red cell volume, and pulse/work relationship in different states of training in trotters. In *Proceedings of the 5th Meeting of the Academy Society of Large Animal Veterinary Medicine*, pp. 34–43.

Persson, S.G.B., Lindholm, A., and Jeffcott, L.B. 1991. *Equine Exercise Physiology 3.* ICEEP Publications, Davis, Calif.

Persson, S.G.B., and Lydin, G. 1973. Circulatory effects of splenectomy in the horse. III. Effect on pulse-work relationship. *Zentrabl. Vet. Med. [A]* 20:521–30.

Persson, S.G.B., and Ullberg, L.E. 1974. Blood volume in relation to exercise tolerance in trotters. *J. S. Afr. Vet. Assoc.* 45:293–99.

Purohit, R.C., Humburg, J.M., Teer, P.A., Norwood, G.L. and Nachreiner, R.F. 1975. Evaluation of hypertensive factors in the horse. *Proc. Am. Assoc. Equine Pract.* 21:43–51.

Purohit, R.C., Nachreiner, R.F., Humburg, J.M., Norwood, G.L., and Beckett, S.D. 1979. Effect of exercise, phenylbutazone, and furosemide on the plasma renin activity and angiotensin I in horses. *Am. J. Vet. Res.* 40:986–89.

Robinson, N. Edward. 1985. Respiratory adaptations to exercise. *Vet. Clin. North Am. Equine Practice* 1:497–512.

Rodiek, A.V., Russell, M.A., and Lawrence, L.M. 1982. The effect of training and intensity of exercise on heart rate and blood metabolites in the horse. *J. Anim. Sci. [Suppl. 1]* 55:384–85.

Rose, R.J. 1982. Haematological changes associated with endurance exercise. *Vet. Rec.* 110:175–77.

Rose, R.J. 1985. Exercise physiology. *Vet. Clin. North Am. Equine Practice* 1(3):437–617.

Rose, R. J., and Allen, J. R. 1985. Hematologic responses to exercise and training. *Vet. Clin. North Am. Equine Practice* 1:461–76.

Rose, R.J., Allen, J.R., and Brock, K.A. 1983. Effects of clenbuterol hydochloride on certain respiratory and cardiovascular parameters in horses performing treadmill exercise. *Res. Vet. Sci.* 35:301–05.

Rugh, K.S., Garner, H.E., Miramonti, J.R., and Hatfield, D.G. 1989. Left ventricular function and haemodynamics in ponies during exercise and recovery. *Equine Vet. J.* 21:39–44.

Rugh, K.S., Garner, H.E., Sprouse, R.F., and Hatfield, D.G. 1987. Left ventricular hypertrophy in chronically hypertensive ponies. *Lab. Anim. Sci.* 37:335–38.

Saltin, B., and Gollnick, P.D. 1983. Skeletal muscle adaptability: Significance for metabolism and performance. In L.D. Peachy, R.H. Adrian, and S.R. Grieger, eds., *Handbook of Physiology: Skeletal Muscle.* Baltimore, Williams & Wilkins. Pp. 555–631.

Saltin, B., Henricksson, J., Nygaard, E., Andersen, P., and Jansson, E. 1977. Fiber types and metabolic potentials of skeletal in sedentary man and endurance runners. *Ann. N.Y. Acad. Sci.* 301:3–29.

Schneider, H.P., Truex, R.C. and Knowles, J.O. 1964. Comparative observations of the hearts of mongrel and greyhound dogs. *Anat. Rec.* 149:173–80.

Senta, T., Smetzer, D.L., and Smith, C.R. 1970. Effects of exercise on certain electrocardiographic parameters and cardiac arrhythmias in the horse. A radiotelemetric study. *Cornell Vet.* 60:552–69.

Sexton, W.L., Erickson, H.H., and Coffman, J.R. 1987. Cardiopulmonary and metabolic responses to exercise in the Quarter Horse. In J.R. Gillespie and N.E. Robinson, eds., *Equine Exercise Physiology 2*. ICEEP Publications, Davis, Calif. Pp. 77–91.

Skarda, R.T., Muir, W.W., Milne, D.W., and Gabel, A.A. 1976. Effects of training on resting and postexercise ECG in Standardbred horses, using a standardized exercise test. *Am. J. Vet. Res.* 37:1485–88.

Smith, J.E., Erickson, H.H., and DeBowes, R.M. 1989. Changes in circulating equine erythrocytes induced by brief, high-speed exercise. *Equine Vet. J.* 21: 444–46.

Snow, D.H. 1983. Skeletal muscle adaptations: a review. In D.H. Snow, S.G.B. Persson, and R.J. Rose, eds., *Equine Exercise Physiology*. Granta Editions, Cambridge, England. Pp. 160–83.

Snow, D.H. 1983. Physiological factors affecting resting haematology. In D.H. Snow, S.G.B. Persson, and R.J. Rose, eds., *Equine Exercise Physiology*. Granta Editions, Cambridge, England. Pp. 318–23.

Snow, D.H. 1985. The horse and dog, elite athletes—Why and how? *Proc. Nutri. Soc.*, 44:267–72.

Snow, D.H., Baxter, P.B., and Rose, R.J. 1981. Muscle fibre composition and glycogen depletion in horses competing in an endurance ride. *Vet. Rec.* 108:374–78.

Snow, D.H., and Guy, P.S. 1976. Percutaneous needle muscle biopsy in the horse. *Equine Vet. J.* 8:150–55.

Snow, D.H., and Guy, P.S. 1979. The effect of training and detraining on several enzymes in horse skeletal muscle. *Arch. Int. Physiol. Biochem.* 87:87–93.

Snow, D.H., and Guy, P.S. 1980. Muscle fibre type composition of a number of limb muscles in different types of horse. *Res. Vet. Sci.* 28:137–44.

Snow, D.H., and Guy, P.S. 1981. Fibre type and enzyme activities of the gluteus medius in different breeds of horse. In J. Poortmans and G. Nisbet, eds., *Biochemistry of Exercise IV*. University Park Press, Baltimore. Pp. 275–82.

Snow, D.H., and Harris, R.C. 1984. *Proceedings of the First International Comparative Physiology and Biochemistry Congress, Vol. 1* (R. Gilles, editor). Berlin: Springer Verlag.

Snow, D.H., and Harris, R.C. 1985. Thoroughbreds and Greyhounds: Biochemical adaptations in creatures of nature and of man. In R. Gilles, ed., *Circulation, Respiration, and Metabolism*. Springer-Verlag, Berlin. Pp. 227–38.

Snow, D.H., Harris, R.C., Harman, J.C., and Marlin, D.J. 1987. Glycogen repletion following different diets. In J.R. Gillespie and N.E. Robinson, eds., *Equine Exercise Physiology 2*. ICEEP Publications, Davis, Calif. Pp. 701–10.

Snow, D.H., Harris, R.C., and Stuttard, E. 1988. Changes in haematology and plasma biochemistry during maximal exercise in greyhounds. *Vet. Rec.* 123:487–89.

Snow, D.H., Kerr, M.G., Nimmo, M.A., and Abbott, E.M. 1982. Alterations in blood, sweat, urine and muscle composition during prolonged exercise in the horse. *Vet. Rec.* 110:377–84.

Staaden, R.V. 1980. Cardiovascular system of the racing dog. In R.W. Kirk, ed., *Current Veterinary Therapy. VIII. Small Animal Pract.* Pp. 347–51.

Staaden, R.V. 1980. Exercise physiology. In *Electrocardiography and Cardiology, The J.D. Steel Memorial Refresher Course.* Proceedings No. 50:261–70. University of Sydney, Sydney, Australia.

Steel, J.D., Hall, M.C., and Stewart, G.A. 1976. Cardiac monitoring during exercise tests in the horse. 3. Changes in the electrocardiogram during and after exercise. *Aust. Vet. J.* 52:6–10.

Steel, J.D., and Stewart, G.A. 1974. Electrocardiography of the horse and potential performance ability. *J. S. Afr. Vet. Assoc.* 45:263–68.

Steel, J.D., Taylor, R.I., Davis, P.E., Stewart, G.A., and Salmon, P.W. 1976. Relationship between heart score, heart weight and body weight in greyhound dogs. *Austr. Vet. J.* 52:561–64.

Stewart, G.A., and Steel, J.D. 1974. Haematology of the fit racehorse. *J. S. Afr. Vet. Assoc.* 45:287–91.

Stewart, J.H., Rose, R.J., Davis, P.E., and Hoffman, K. 1983. A comparison of electrocardiographic findings in racehorses presented either for routine examination or poor racing performance. In D.H. Snow, S.G.B. Persson, and R.J. Rose, eds., *Equine Exercise Physiology*. Granta Editions, Cambridge, England. Pp. 135–43.

Stone, H.L. 1977. Cardiac function and exercise training in conscious dogs. *J. Appl. Physiol.* 42:824–32.

Straub, R., Detweiler, M., Hoppeler, H., and Claassen, H. 1983. The use of morphometry and enzyme activity measurements in skeletal muscles for the assessment of the working capacity of horses. In D.H. Snow, S.G.B. Persson, and R.J. Rose, eds., *Equine Exercise Physiology*. Granta Editions, Cambridge, England. Pp. 193–99.

Strauss, R.H. 1979. *Sports Medicine and Physiology.* WB Saunders, Philadelphia.

Sweeney, C.R., and Soma, L.R. 1983. Exercise-induced pulmonary haemorrhage in horses after different competitive exercises. In D.H. Snow, S.G.B. Persson, and R.J. Rose, eds., *Equine Exercise Physiology*. Granta Editions, Cambridge, England. Pp. 51–56.

Thomas, D.P., and Fregin, G.F. 1981. Cardiorespiratory and metabolic responses to treadmill exercise in the horse. *J. Appl. Physiol.* 50:864–68.

Thomas, D.P., Fregin, G.F., Gerber, N.H., and Ailes, N.B. 1980. Cardiorespiratory adjustments to tethered-swimming in the horse. *Pflügers Arch.* 385:65–70.

Thomas, D.P., Fregin, G.F., Gerber, N.H., and Ailes, N.B. 1983. Effects of training on cardiorespiratory function in the horse. *Am. J. Physiol.* 245:R160–65.

Thornton, John R. 1985. Hormonal responses to exercise and training. In *Vet. Clin. North Am. Equine Practice* 1:477–96.

Thornton, J., Essen-Gustavsson, B., Lindholm, A., McMiken, D., and Persson, S. 1983. Effects of training and detraining on oxygen uptake, cardiac output, blood gas tensions, pH and lactate concentrations during and after exercise in the horse. In D.H. Snow, S.G.B. Persson, and R.J. Rose, ed., *Equine Exercise Physiology*. Granta Editions, Cambridge, England. Pp. 470–86.

von Engelhardt, W. 1977. Cardiovascular effects of exercise and training in horses. *Adv. Vet. Sci. Comp. Med.* 21:173–205.

Wagner, P.D., Gillespie, J.R., Landgren, G.L., Fedde, M.R., Jones, B.W., DeBowes, R.M., Pieschl, R.L., and Erickson, H.H. 1989. Mechanism of exercise-induced hypoxemia in the horse. *J. Appl. Physiol.* 66:1227–33.

Waugh, S.L., Fregin, G.F., and Thomas, D.P., Gerber, N., Grant, B.D., and Campbell, K.B. 1980. Electromagnetic measurement of cardiac output during exercise in the horse. *Am. J. Vet. Res.* 41:812–15.

Webb, A.I., and Weaver, B.M.Q. 1979. Body composition of the horse. *Equine Vet. J.* 11:39–47.

Weber, J.M., Dobson, G.P., Parkhouse, W.S., Wheeldon, D., Harmon, J.C., Snow, D.H., and Hochachka, P.W. 1987. Cardiac output and oxygen consumption in exercising Thoroughbred horses. *Am. J. Physiol.: Regulatory, Integrative and Comparative Physiology* 253:R890–95.

Weber, J.M., Parkhouse, W.S., Dobson, G.P., Harman, J.C., Snow, D.H., and Hochachka, P.W. 1987. Onset of submaximal exercise in thoroughbred horses. *Can. J. Zool.* 65:2513–18.

Weems, C.W. 1984. Effects of acute strenuous exercise on body temperature and blood of racing greyhounds. *J. Anim. Sci.* 59:193.

Weibel, E.R. 1984. *The Pathway for Oxygen*. Harvard Univ. Press, Cambridge, Mass.

Wilmore, J.H., and Norton, A.C. 1974. *The Heart and Lungs at Work: A Primer of Exercise Physiology.* Beckman Instruments, Schiller Park, Ill.

PART III DIGESTION, ABSORPTION, AND METABOLISM

CHAPTER 16

General Functions of the Gastrointestinal Tract and Their Control and Integration | by Robert A. Argenzio

GENERAL FUNCTIONS OF THE GASTROINTESTINAL TRACT

The primary functions of the gastrointestinal tract and its accessory organs are digestion and absorption of nutrients essential to the animal's metabolic processes. In addition, the mucosa must discriminate against absorption of substances that would be toxic if they gained access to the body. The lumen of the gastrointestinal tract can therefore be considered as being "outside" the body. The epithelial cells lining the lumen are the only barrier between this outside environment and the blood. These cells, therefore, perform a variety of functions, including digestion, secretion, and absorption. They have enzymes capable of digesting sugars and peptides, and within them transport processes that promote uptake of specific luminal contents. The cell membranes and the junctional complexes between them provide such an efficient barrier that a specific transport process is required for many water-soluble substances.

Before many of the dietary constituents can be absorbed by the epithelium into the blood, they must be degraded (digested) in the intestinal lumen into substances that can then interact with the gastrointestinal cell enzymes or the transport carriers. This process, called *luminal digestion* (as opposed to digestion by the epithelial cell), requires a specific luminal environment. This environment is brought about by the secretions of accessory organs and the gastrointestinal mucosa. The salivary glands, pancreas, and liver provide secretions of electrolytes, water, digestive enzymes, and bile salts, all of which are necessary for luminal digestion. The gastrointestinal mucosa is also capable of secreting acid or base into the lumen and thereby establishing an optimal pH for the digestive enzymes. This *secretory* function, which provides the chemical environment for luminal digestion, is an active, energy-requiring process and is under control of the neuroendocrine system.

Another important function associated with digestion and absorption is transit. The transit of luminal contents must be regulated for specific digestive processes, and the digestive products must be maximally exposed to the epithelial cell surface for absorption. These requirements are brought about by the *motor* function of the gastrointestinal tract, which is also an energy-requiring process under neuroendocrine control.

Finally, the digested nutrients must be absorbed by the epithelium and transferred into the circulation. Of equal or greater importance is the reabsorption of all the isotonic digestive secretions provided by the accessory glands and the gastrointestinal mucosa. Because of the large volumes of electrolytes and water secreted into the lumen (especially in herbivores), failure to reabsorb them would result in dehydration and circulatory collapse leading to death. Therefore, the *absorptive* function, which includes both *absorption* of nutrients and *reabsorption* of endogenous secretions, is by far the most critical process of the gastrointestinal tract.

In summary, the primary functions of the gastrointestinal tract are digestion and absorption of nutrients. The motor and secretory events provide the necessary environment for these two functions. The digestive secretions are recovered by the reabsorptive process and returned to the extracellular fluid. These functions will be discussed separately in the next four chapters, but it is necessary to keep their interactions in mind.

COMPARATIVE ASPECTS OF DIGESTION

Proteins, fats, and carbohydrates do not occur in nature except in association with living matter; therefore, the higher animals are dependent on plants and other animals for these nutrients. Animals are conventionally classified on the basis of their eating habits in the natural state, although under domestication their diets may be considerably different from those eaten under natural conditions. Our discussion will be limited primarily to the common domesticated mammals.

In the carnivores, which obtain most of their food by eating other animals, digestion is mainly enzymatic in nature and microbial digestion is minimal. In contrast, the domesticated herbivores fall into two groups: (1) the ruminants, such as cattle, sheep, and goats, in which extensive microbial fermentation of the vegetable diet occurs in a specialized region of the digestive tract before digestion by alimentary enzymes and (2) those with simple stomachs, such as the horse, in which microbial fermentation takes place in the distal part of the digestive tract.

Although omnivorous animals feed on both plants and animals, their digestion is mainly alimentary enzymatic in nature, like that of the carnivores. The pig is usually considered to be omnivorous but under domestication is essentially herbivorous, and there is considerable microbial breakdown of plant material in the large intestine. The structure of the digestive tract varies greatly in different species because of the adaptations that have taken place in relation to diet. Because there is no need for extensive microbial fermentation, the tract of the carnivore is much shorter and of smaller relative capacity than that of the herbivore.

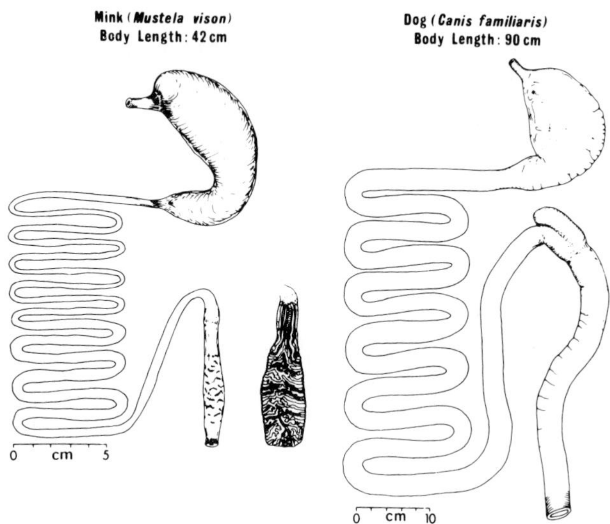

Figure 16.1. Gastrointestinal tracts of the mink and the dog (to different scales). Note simple, nonvoluminous large intestine. Terminal segment of mink also shown opened longitudinally. (Drawings by Erica Melack.)

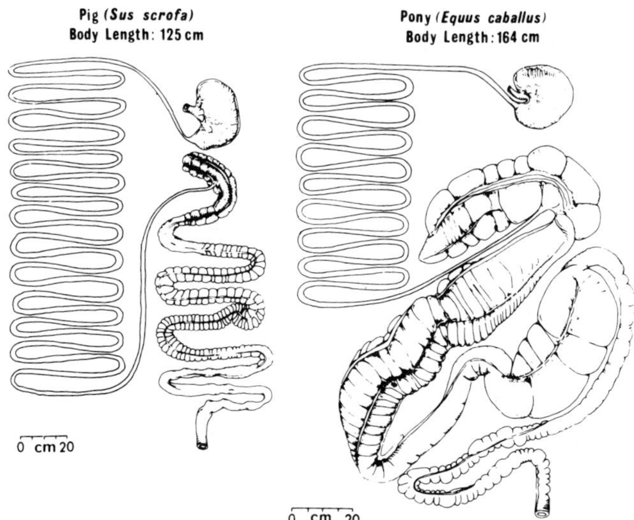

Figure 16.2. Gastrointestinal tracts of the pig and the pony. A major portion of the colon of pigs and other Artiodactyla is arranged in two spirals. The centripetal (ascending) spiral reverses itself to form the centrifugal (descending) spiral, as indicated by the slight downward bend near the center of the colon. The cecum and colon of the pony are also sacculated. The cecum of the pony is relatively voluminous, but its ventral and dorsal large colon are developed into even more voluminous compartments. The general structure of the pony large intestine is characteristic of Perissodactyla. (Drawings by Erica Melack.)

Gross structural differences in the gastrointestinal tract

Figures 16.1 to 16.4 illustrate the broad range of variations in the gastrointestinal tracts of mammals and demonstrate the profound influence of the dietary habits on structure. These digestive tracts were arranged in a similar manner and were drawn to scale to allow a direct comparison among species.

The digestive tract of the mink (Fig. 16.1) has a simple (noncompartmentalized) stomach and a relatively short intestine. The terminal segment of the intestine is larger than the upper intestine, but it is nonsacculated and does not contain a cecum or evidence of a sphincter or valve at its junction with the upper intestine. This general pattern is characteristic of arctoid (bearlike) carnivores. Some species in other mammalian orders (Insectivora, Edentata, Cetacea, Chiroptera, and Marsupialia) also have a simple stomach, no cecum, and little or no distinction between a small and a large intestine.

The digestive tract of the dog (Fig. 16.1), like that of the mink, is relatively short and simple, although the dog has an ileocecal valve and a small cecum. The pig (Fig. 16.2) has a simple stomach; however, the relative length of both its small and large intestines is considerably greater than that of either the mink or the dog. Furthermore, the pig cecum and a considerable part of the pig colon are sacculated as a result of longitudinal bands of muscle. As discussed below, these sacculations, or *haustra,* may serve as one means of prolonging the retention of digesta. The pony

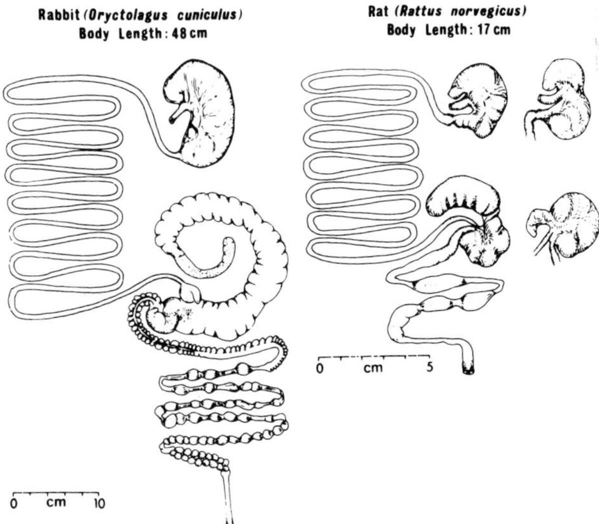

Figure 16.3. Gastrointestinal tracts of the rabbit and the rat. The appearance of the rat gastrointestinal tract 4 hours after a meal suggests a noncompartmentalized stomach and relatively voluminous cecum. However, an animal sacrificed immediately after a meal (*right*) demonstrates a constriction near the midpoint of the stomach, which results in partial compartmentalization. It also shows that while the stomach is more voluminous at this time, the terminal segment of cecum is much reduced in size. (Drawings by Erica Melack.)

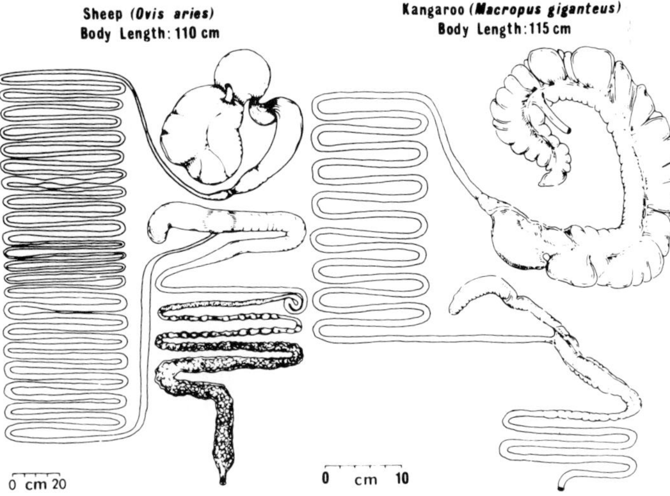

Figure 16.4. Gastrointestinal tracts of the sheep and the kangaroo. The kangaroo drawing was prepared from a photograph supplied by Dr. I.D. Hume (University of New England, Armidale, Australia), and the time between feeding and sacrifice is unknown. Note the similarity between the kangaroo stomach and the sacculated portions of the pig, pony, and rabbit colons. The point at which the spiral colon of the sheep reverses its direction is indicated in the same manner as that of the pig. (Drawings by Erica Melack.)

stomach (Fig. 16.2) is similar to that of the pig, but it is much shorter in relative length and the cecum and colon are much more voluminous. The equine species demonstrate an extreme in colonic capacity.

The rabbit stomach is simple in structure (Fig. 16.3); however, the cecum is extremely voluminous, and both the cecum and the proximal colon are sacculated. The rat cecum (Fig. 16.3) is also relatively voluminous, but the colon is neither sacculated nor particularly long. Furthermore, the rat stomach is partially compartmentalized. This characteristic, which is barely apparent in the rat, is evident in the sheep and the kangaroo (Fig. 16.4). The sheep small intestine appears to have the greatest relative length in comparison with the common domestic and laboratory mammals. However, neither the cecum nor the colon is sacculated or particularly voluminous. The sacculated appearance of the lower colon and rectum in the rabbit, rat, and sheep appears to be due to the presence of pelletized feces rather than the result of the haustral-type structures associated with longitudinal bands of muscle, as noted in the pig and the horse. The kangaroo stomach is voluminous and especially noteworthy because of its similarity, both in sacculation and in longitudinal bands of muscle, to the proximal large intestine of the pig, pony, and rabbit. The large intestine of the kangaroo is relatively short and nonvoluminous.

These species were chosen only to indicate the variation in the gastrointestinal tracts of mammals. Parallel changes apparently developed among marsupials and within a number of different orders of placental mammals. For example, the marsupial stomach can range from simple (opossum) to complex (kangaroo); this range is similar to that seen in the pig and sheep, two species of the order Artiodactyla. Both simple and complex stomachs are also evident among other orders, such as those that include the bats, edentates, rodents, and primates. The large intestines of these orders show similar variations in structure.

Capacity of gastrointestinal organs

Tables 16.1 and 16.2 list some species variations in the dimensions and capacity of various segments of the gastrointestinal tract. Since these are postmortem data, the values for capacity are questionable; a considerable exchange of water can occur between body fluid spaces and gut contents after death. As noted below, digesta volume can also vary by several orders of magnitude with time after feeding. However, these tables demonstrate marked species differences, especially between carnivores and herbivores and among various species of herbivores.

The marked effects of time after feeding on the volume of gastrointestinal contents in various segments of the pony digestive tract are shown in Fig. 16.5. The animals were fed at 12-hour intervals, and without exception the minimum volume of a segment was obtained 12 hours after feeding. The maximum volumes were related to digesta flow and secretions and varied with time after feeding. These were highest in gastric and proximal small bowel contents at 2 hours, in the middle small intestine at 4 hours, and in the remainder of the tract at 8 hours after the meal. At all times the large intestine represents 75 percent of the total volume capacity. These large volume changes are not evident in

Table 16.1. Lengths of parts of the intestine at necropsy

Animal	Part of intestine	Relative length (%)	Average absolute length (m)	Ratio of body length to intestine length
Horse	Small intestine	75	22.44	1:12
	Cecum	4	1.00	
	Large colon	11	3.39	
	Small colon	10	3.08	
	Total	100	29.91	
Ox	Small intestine	81	46.00	1:20
	Cecum	2	0.88	
	Colon	17	10.18	
	Total	100	57.06	
Sheep and goat	Small intestine	80	26.20	1:27
	Cecum	1	0.36	
	Colon	19	6.17	
	Total	100	32.73	
Pig	Small intestine	78	18.29	1:14
	Cecum	1	0.23	
	Colon	21	4.99	
	Total	100	23.51	
Dog	Small intestine	85	4.14	1:6
	Cecum	2	0.08	
	Colon	13	0.60	
	Total	100	4.82	
Cat	Small intestine	83	1.72	1:4
	Large intestine	17	0.35	
	Total	100	2.07	
Rabbit	Small intestine	61	3.56	1:10
	Cecum	11	0.61	
	Colon	28	1.65	
	Total	100	5.82	

Adapted from G. Colin, 1871. *Traité de physiologie comparée des animaux*, Baillière, Paris.

Table 16.2. Capacities of parts of the digestive tract at necropsy

Animal	Part of canal	Relative capacity (%)	Average absolute capacity (L)
Horse	Stomach	8.5	17.96
	Small intestine	30.2	63.82
	Cecum	15.9	33.54
	Large colon	38.4	81.25
	Small colon and rectum	7.0	14.77
	Total	100.0	211.34
Ox	Stomach	70.8	252.5
	Small intestine	18.5	66.0
	Cecum	2.8	9.9
	Colon and rectum	7.9	28.0
	Total	100.0	356.4
Sheep and goat	Rumen	52.9	23.4
	Reticulum	4.5	2.0
	Omasum	2.0	0.9
	Abomasum	7.5	3.3
	Small intestine	20.4	9.0
	Cecum	2.3	1.0
	Colon and rectum	10.4	4.6
	Total	100.0	44.2
Pig	Stomach	29.2	8.00
	Small intestine	33.5	9.20
	Cecum	5.6	1.55
	Colon and rectum	31.7	8.70
	Total	100.0	27.45
Dog	Stomach	62.3	4.33
	Small intestine	23.3	1.62
	Cecum	1.3	0.09
	Colon and rectum	13.1	0.91
	Total	100.0	6.95
Cat	Stomach	69.5	0.341
	Small intestine	14.6	0.114
	Large intestine	15.9	0.124
	Total	100.0	0.579

Adapted from G. Colin, 1871. *Traité de physiologie comparée des animaux*, Baillière, Paris.

animals that feed continuously, because of the relatively continuous secretory and motor activity of their gastrointestinal tracts.

Although the volumes are relatively large in comparison with digestive tract volumes in omnivores and carnivores, they represent only a small proportion of the total fluid load handled daily by the intestine. For example, the small and large intestines of the pony must reabsorb the equivalent of 40 percent of the body weight each day. These large volumes are due primarily to endogenous digestive secretions. Only a small percentage of this volume load is provided by the dietary and fluid intake.

Structural and functional characteristics

Simple-stomached carnivores may consume occasional meals of high energy content that are followed by a period of relative quiescence. Plant material, on the other hand, is low in energy content, and the herbivore must consume a large quantity to satisfy its energy requirements. The actual time spent eating is much greater in herbivores than in carnivores and, in grazing ruminants, may amount to 8 or more hours per 24-hour period. Rumination may occupy an equally long period. This type of feeding behavior is associated with essentially continuous activity of the secretory glands and the musculature of the tract. For example, the ruminant abomasum (often called the "true" stomach) nor-

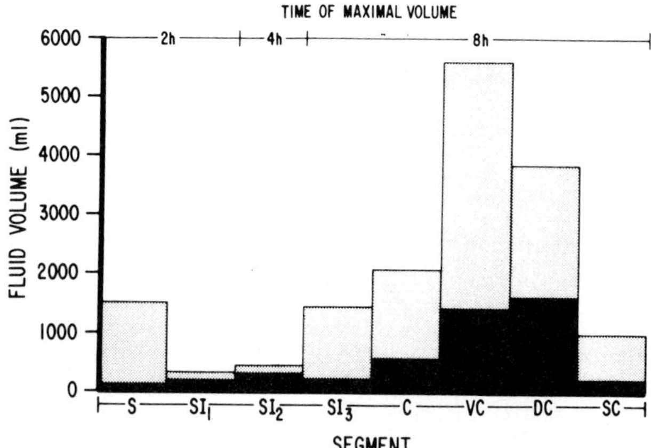

Figure 16.5. Maximal (*combined light and dark bars*) and minimal (*dark bars*) fluid volumes in various gastrointestinal segments of 160 kg pony. The sections examined were: stomach (S); proximal (SI_1), middle (SI_2), and distal (SI_3) thirds of small intestine; cecum (C); ventral colon (VC); dorsal colon (DC); and small colon (SC).

mally secretes acid gastric juice continuously because the flow of ingesta from the reticulorumen into the abomasum never ceases. Conversely, animals fed a concentrated feed once or twice daily, as in the preceding example of the pony, display cyclic gastrointestinal secretory and motor activity. Under pasture conditions, however, the horse will graze for a considerable proportion of each 24 hours.

The physiology of digestion in the ruminant, the horse, and, to a lesser extent, the pig must therefore be considered in relation to certain factors. These animals have an overriding necessity to maintain continuous fermentation and absorption in parts of the gastrointestinal tract where cellulose-containing materials can be broken down. Also, the physiology of digestion varies in relation to the feeding patterns used.

The major species differences in structural-functional relationships are most easily related to the rates of digesta passage through the various organs of the gastrointestinal tract. The efficiency of digestion and absorption is highly dependent on the rate at which digesta move through the tract, and this dependency is especially true for fermentative digestion.

Figure 16.6 shows the passage of a fluid marker through the tract of a carnivore (dog), an omnivore (pig), and a simple-stomached herbivore (pony). The liquid marker left the stomach and traversed the small intestine of each of the three species quite rapidly. Passage of fluid marker through the large intestine was much slower in the pig and the pony than in the dog. The spiral colon of the pig is analogous to the large colon in the pony; these appeared to be major sites of fluid marker retention. In the rabbit, fluid is retained only

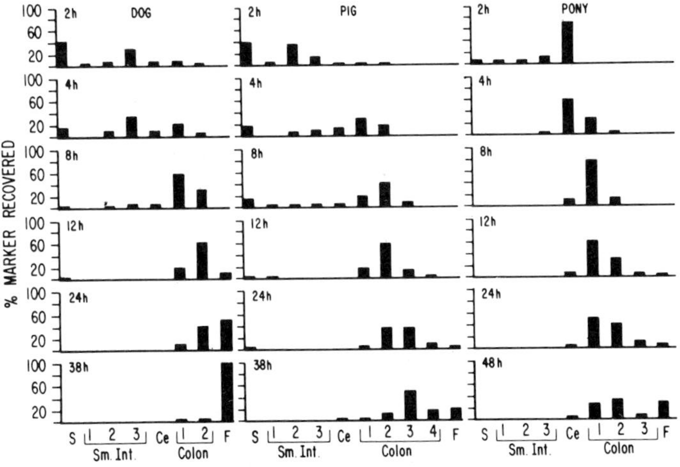

Figure 16.6. Passage of fluid marker through the digestive tract of the dog, the pig, and the pony. All animals were fed at 12-hour intervals, and markers were given by stomach tube at the time of the morning meal at time zero. Note that the last time scale for the pony is not the same as for the dog and the pig. S, stomach; Sm. int., small intestine; Ce, cecum; F, feces. Numbers represent approximately equal lengths of intestine and colon, proximal to distal. (Modified from Banta, Clemens, Krinsky, and Sheffy 1979, *J. Nutr.* 109:1592–1600; Clemens, Stevens, and Southworth 1975, *J Nutr.* 105:759–68; Argenzio, Lowe, Pickard, and Stevens 1974a, *Am. J. Physiol.* 226:1035–42.)

in the cecum, and passage through the colon is rapid (data not shown).

These comparisons indicate some substantial species differences in the rates of digesta passage through the gastrointestinal tract. The rate at which digesta pass through given segments of the tract should show some correlation with both anatomical structure and the degree of microbial digestion. Reinspection of large intestine structure in the dog, pig, pony, and rabbit (Figs. 16.1 to 16.4) shows that digesta tend to be retained in the sacculated segments. Passage of digesta may also be slowed by areas of constriction. For example, this occurs at the junction between the cecum and the colon of the rabbit, the junctions of the centripetal and centrifugal spiral colon of the pig, and the ventral and dorsal colon (pelvic flexure) of the pony. Regardless of the reason, prolonged passage of digesta allows greater time for both absorption and microbial digestion.

CONTROL AND INTEGRATION OF GASTROINTESTINAL FUNCTION

The integration of motor, secretory, and absorptive events in the gastrointestinal tract is brought about by complex actions and interactions of the neural and endocrine systems. This section presents an overview of these two control systems. Specific control of the various functions will be considered in detail in the next four chapters.

Neural mechanisms

Neural control of gastrointestinal function is brought about by the *sympathetic* and *parasympathetic* divisions of the *autonomic nervous system* (ANS) and by neurons of the submucosal and myenteric plexus. The latter is now considered separate from the ANS and is termed the *enteric nervous system* (ENS).

Central control pathways

The general scheme of extrinsic and intrinsic innervation of the gastrointestinal tract is depicted in Fig. 16.7. Autonomic outflow from the central nervous system (CNS) serves to modulate activity in the ENS. The vagal and sacral nerves contain afferent and efferent fibers of the parasympathetic division of the ANS. Sensory fibers of the vagus nerve have their cell bodies in the nodose ganglion, and some of these synapse in the dorsal nucleus of the vagus in the medulla. Axons from the dorsal nucleus project to the gastrointestinal tract, where they make *nicotinic, cholinergic* synapses with ganglion cells in the myenteric and submucosal plexus. *Acetylcholine* (ACh) is the major transmitter at these synapses.

Information transmitted from afferent receptors in the gastrointestinal tract to the dorsal vagal nucleus and back to ENS neurons act as a simple reflex arc. More complex functions are possible, however. For example, many vagal afferent fibers terminate in the nucleus of the solitary tract, whereas vagal efferents originate in the dorsal vagal nu-

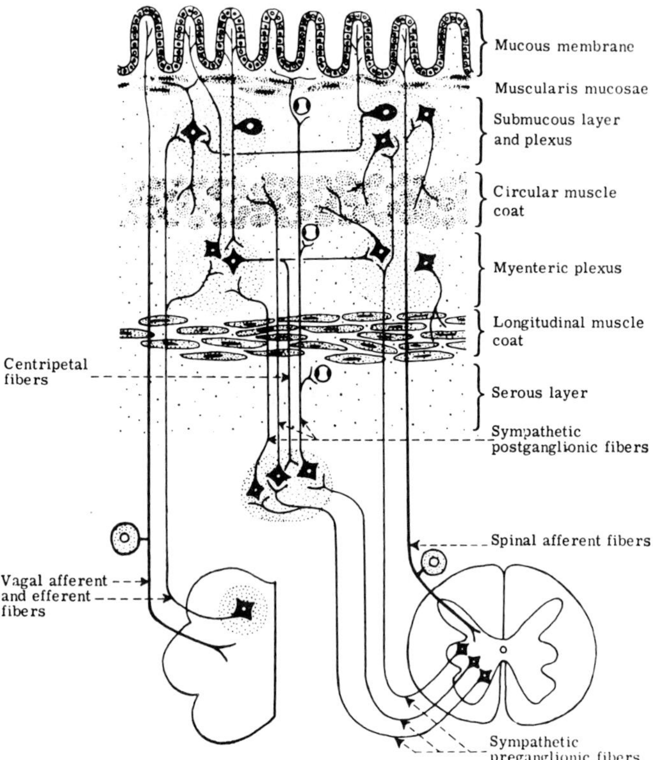

Figure 16.7. Scheme of the extrinsic and intrinsic innervation of the intestine. (From Schofield 1968, in *Handbook of Physiology,* Sec. 6, Code and Heidel, eds., *Alimentary Canal,* Vol. 4, *Mobility,* Am. Physiol. Soc., Washington.)

cleus. In many cases, one or more interneurons are interposed between these nuclei, allowing information to be processed and altered in the medulla before passing back to the stomach and intestine.

Many interneurons of the ENS are interposed between the vagal preganglionic fiber and the enteric neuron, which directly innervates the smooth muscle or epithelial cells. For example, it has been estimated that there are 10^8 neurons in the ENS and only 2×10^3 vagal efferent fibers. Thus, local integrative circuits of the ENS are organized for functional operations independent of preganglionic parasympathetic input. Cholinergic motor neurons innervating the muscle or epithelium act through *muscarinic,* cholinergic receptors by releasing ACh.

In the sympathetic nervous system, the sensory afferent neuron has its cell body in the dorsal root ganglia and synapses in the spinal cord. The efferent preganglionic neuron synapses in sympathetic ganglia outside the gastrointestinal tract (the paravertebral or prevertebral ganglia). Transmission at this synapse is mediated by ACh acting at nicotinic, cholinergic receptors. Postganglionic adrenergic neurons innervating the gastrointestinal tract are divided into three subsets depending on their chemical transmitters. Fibers containing *norepinephrine* and *somatostatin* (NE/SOM) supply primarily submucosal ganglia and mucosa and are involved with mucosal function. Fibers containing *NE and neuropeptide Y* (NPY) innervate blood vessels, while fibers containing *NE alone* project to the myenteric plexus and probably coordinate motility patterns. NE also is released onto cholinergic nerves to inhibit the release of ACh (Fig. 16.8). Conversely, ACh acting through muscarinic receptors on postganglionic sympathetic fibers inhibits the release of NE.

In general, parasympathetic fibers increase contractile activity and secretion. However, as discussed below ("Enteric Nervous System"), these fibers can also terminate on neurons that release inhibitory substances. Adrenergic innervation has the converse effects of inhibiting motility and blood flow, a blanketlike response to stress. Adrenergic nerves also indirectly inhibit secretion by inhibiting ACh release at presynaptic terminals. As discussed in Chapter 20, however, neurons releasing NE/SOM may increase intestinal absorption through direct innervation of the mucosa.

Enteric nervous system

The cell bodies of the ENS are located in the submucosal and myenteric plexus in the wall of the gastrointestinal tract. These neurons are of three types. *Motor neurons* innervate the muscle or epithelium and cause excitation or inhibition. *Interneurons* send information from one ganglion to another and even project to prevertebral ganglia outside the gastrointestinal tract. *Sensory* neurons receive signals from sensory receptors in the muscle or mucosa and convey this information to interneurons or motor neurons.

Motor neurons have been classified into two groups, depending on their chemical transmitters. *Cholinergic* motor neurons are excitatory and release ACh at nerve termi-

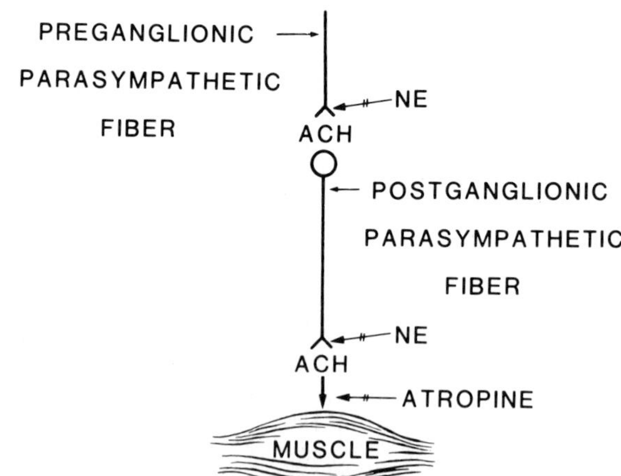

Figure 16.8. Inhibition of acetylcholine (ACh) release by norepinephrine (NE) at both preganglionic and postganglionic sites and inhibition of ACh access to postganglionic cholinergic receptors by atropine. ACH, acetylcholine. (Modified from Makhlouf 1974, *Gastroenterology* 67:159–84.)

nals. In smooth muscle, the longitudinal muscle is primarily under excitatory control, which results in contraction (shortening) of its fibers. Excitation of the epithelium by ACh results in secretion. *Vipergic* motor neurons release vasoactive intestinal peptide (VIP) at their terminals and are primarily inhibitory. For example, VIP causes relaxation of smooth muscle and is also a potent vasodilator. However, VIP results in secretion by the epithelium. Although the motor neurons discussed above have been classified into two groups with only two transmitters, it should be understood that many other chemical transmitters have been identified with these neurons. These may be released from the same neuron as the primary substance (e.g., ACh/substance P). At present, the physiological role of many of these substances is not well understood.

Enteric interneurons contain two groups of neurons. *Serotonergic* neurons contain *serotonin* or 5-hydroxytryptamine (5-HT). This substance activates both excitatory and inhibitory motor neurons. *Peptidergic* neurons contain peptides rather than amines. These include *enkephalins,* which have opioidlike activity. They suppress electrical activity of the neuronal cell body and thus decrease its excitability. For example, circular smooth muscle of the gastrointestinal tract is primarily under inhibitory control, in contrast to longitudinal muscle as discussed above. As shown in Fig. 16.9, discharge of an enkephalin containing neuron suppresses discharge of the inhibitory neuron, thereby removing the tonic inhibition of the muscle. Other peptidergic

INNERVATION OF CIRCULAR MUSCLE:
ENKEPHALINS ↑ CONTRACTION

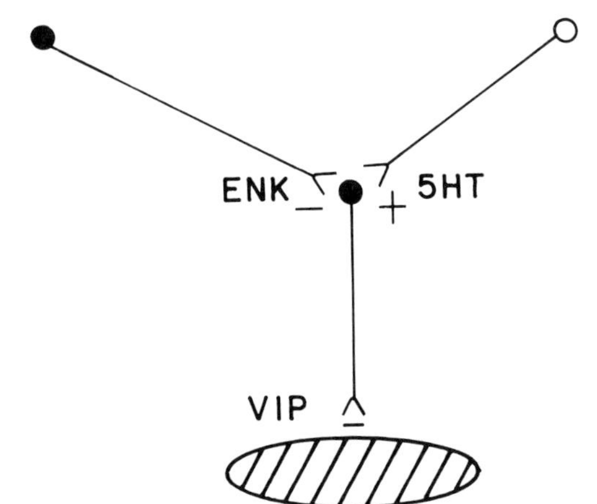

Figure 16.9. Enkephalins cause an increase in contractility of circular muscle by removing the dominant inhibitory tone.

neurons contain *somatostatin* (growth hormone–releasing inhibitory factor). This neurotransmitter suppresses spike discharge of cholinergic ganglion cells, thereby decreasing the release of ACh. It also activates inhibitory motor neurons. Diffuse discharge of such neurons could result in total paralysis of the smooth muscle of the gastrointestinal tract.

Cell bodies of *sensory neurons* of the gastrointestinal tract are located in three groups of ganglia: the *nodose* ganglia of the vagal nerves, the *dorsal root ganglia* of the spinal cord, and the *ganglia of the ENS.* Afferent fibers of the nodose and spinal ganglia transmit sensory information to the CNS. Intramural neurons of the ENS can transmit sensory information over local reflex arcs or project centrally to both prevertebral sympathetic ganglia and the CNS.

The modalities of the sensory system include force (pressure) and thermal and chemical receptors. Chemoreceptors respond to pH, amino acids, lipids, sugars, and osmolality. Sensory information in the form of action potentials is then processed in networks of the CNS, ENS, and prevertebral ganglia.

Prevertebral ganglia are sites of rapid exchange of information between different segments of the gastrointestinal tract. For example, signal transmission within the ENS rarely travels more than a few centimeters before encountering a synapse. The bypass routes through prevertebral ganglia overcome this problem for transmission over long distances. This pathway consists of projections from enteric neurons that synapse in prevertebral ganglia with postganglionic sympathetic neurons that project to the intestine. One function of these routes is the transmission of inhibitory reflexes from a distal region of intestine to a proximal site, thereby inhibiting motility and transit of intestinal contents into the distal segment.

Endocrine mechanisms

The gastrointestinal tract is the largest endocrine organ in the body. Enteroendocrine cells arising from the neural crest of the embryo are diffusively distributed throughout gastric, intestinal, and pancreatic tissue. These cells are known as amine precursor uptake and decarboxylation cells, and they synthesize peptide hormones and amines that are released from the cells on the appropriate stimulation.

There are two ways in which these peptide hormones can act. First, as shown in Fig. 16.10, they may be released from the endocrine cell and delivered into the blood, from where they exert their action on a distant organ. This is a true *endocrine function.* Second, they may be released from the cell and act in the immediate vicinity. This mode of action is termed *paracrine.* Peptides released from the nerve endings may have a neurotransmitter, neuromodulator, or neuroendocrine function. These peptides also may act in the local vicinity of the nerve or, less likely, enter the circulation.

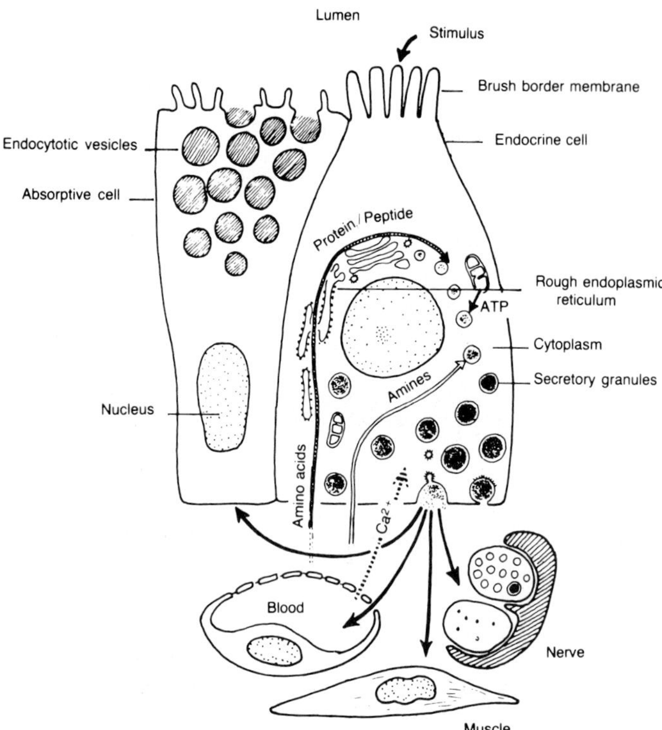

Figure 16.10. Diagram showing metabolism and function of intestinal endocrine cell. Stimulus from lumen acts on receptors of brush border membrane and results in release of hormones by exocytosis at basolateral membrane. These hormones can act locally, such as on the nerve, muscle, or adjacent cell, or can enter the general circulation. Secretory granules are formed in Golgi vesicles, grow in size, and move to storage sites in the cytoplasm. Endocrine cells have the ability for double production of peptides and amines. Synthesis of peptide hormones occurs through the rough endoplasmic reticulum-Golgi route. Adenosine triphosphate (ATP) enters granules and then serves for the incorporation of amines from the cytosol. (Modified from Fujita and Kobayashi 1978, in Bloom, ed., *Gut Hormones,* Churchill Livingston, New York.)

Although the primary target of many enteric hormones is most likely in the local vicinity of each, seven substances are thought to act as circulating hormones. These are the three classic gastrointestinal hormones: gastrin, secretin, and cholecystokinin (CCK). In addition to these, four other hormonal substances have been postulated: pancreatic polypeptide, gastric inhibitory polypeptide, motilin, and enteroglucagon.

Many of the endocrine cells show a characteristic distribution in the gastrointestinal tract, suggesting that they respond to different types of luminal stimuli. In fact, the precise stimulus that causes the release of several of the postulated hormones is not yet known, and their mechanism of action has been determined by infusion of the substances into the circulation.

Table 16.3 lists hormonal substances found in endocrine cells of the gastrointestinal tract, their distribution, their primary mechanism of action, and luminal factors that cause their release. The greatest distribution of endocrine cells occurs in the proximal intestine and decreases aborally. Enterochromaffin cells containing 5-HT make up the largest number of endocrine cells.

The primary functions are listed for each hormone. However, many secondary functions also characterize these agents. For example, gastrin and CCK, two structurally homologous hormones, have several functions in common. These include stimulation of gastric acid secretion, motility, enzyme secretion, and growth of pancreatic tissue and gastrointestinal mucosa. A second structurally homologous group includes secretin, gastric inhibitory polypeptide, and enteroglucagon. The general functions of this group are to inhibit gastric acid secretion, stimulate pancreatic fluid and bicarbonate secretion, stimulate intestinal secretion, stimulate biliary fluid secretion, and alter insulin release.

The major functions of the remaining agents listed in Table 16.3 have not been as well characterized. Motilin has been implicated in the initiation of the migrating myoelectric complex, a motility pattern associated with the interdigestive period in some species (Chap. 17). Serotonin and substance P (also released from nerves) are neuromodulators, stimulating activity of enteric neurons. Somatostatin acts as a paracrine substance to inhibit release of peptides from endocrine cells or enteric nerves.

As can be seen from Table 16.3, the major components of a meal stimulate the release of the major two classes of circulating hormones, although carbohydrates and glucose are ineffective in the case of gastrin, CCK, and secretin. The major stimulus for secretin release is acid perfusion of the duodenum.

Other endocrine/paracrine messengers such as neurotensin, motilin, and 5-HT can also be released by a meal or other stimuli. A number of these stimuli such as distention, hyperosmolality, and acid have been shown to act in a defined neuroendocrine reflex pathway. For example, Fig. 16.11 depicts such a reflex causing intestinal secretion. An epithelial sensory cell (A) liberates 5-HT in response to intraluminal stimuli and stimulates afferent neuron B. Synapse BC or CD is nicotinic. Neuron D secretes a neurotransmitter on enterocyte E. The best candidates for these neurotransmitters from efferent nerves are ACh and VIP. ACh involvement is shown by atropine blockade. Increased concentrations of VIP are seen in venous effluent on stimulation, and these are reduced with hexamethonium (a ganglionic blocker).

Neuroendocrine receptors

The action of neural or endocrine transmitters is mediated through receptors located on the target cell membrane or on the axons or cell bodies of intramural excitatory or inhibitory neurons. These receptors are postulated configurations of organic molecules that bind the neural or endocrine transmitters according to their degree of attraction, or

Table 16.3. Location of gastrointestinal hormonal substances and their primary mode of action

Product	Pancreas	Stomach O	Stomach A	Intestine U	Intestine L	Colon	Action	Stimulus for release
Gastrin	–	–	+	+	–	–	(S) Gastric secretion (S) Mucosal growth	Peptides, AA
CCK	–	–	–	+	±	–	(S) Pancreatic enzyme secretion (S) Gallbladder contraction	FA, AA
Secretin	–	–	–	+	±	–	(S) Pancreatic HCO_3 secretion	Acid
GIP	–	–	–	+	±	–	(I) Gastric secretion (S) Intestinal secretion (S) Insulin release	Gluc, AA, FA
Enteroglucagon	–	–	–	±	+	–	(S) Blood flow (S) Mitotic activity (S) Insulin release	Gluc, FA
Motilin	–	–	–	+	±	–	(S) MMC in antroduodenum	Variable
Neurotensin	–	–	–	±	+	+	(S) Vasodilation (I) Smooth muscle	Fat
5-HT	±	+	+	+	+	+	(S) Neuronal activity	Osmol, acid
Substance P	–	–	–	–	+	–	(S) Neuronal activity	Osmol, acid
Pancreatic polypeptide	+	–	–	–	–	–	(I) Pancreatic secretion	Protein
Somatostatin	+	+	+	+	±	±	(I) Peptide release	Fat, Protein

+ present; – absent; ± few; O, oxyntic; A, antrum; U, upper; L, lower; S, stimulate; I, inhibit; MMC, migrating myoelectric complex; AA, aminoacids; FA, fatty acids; Gluc, glucose; osmol, hyperosmolality.

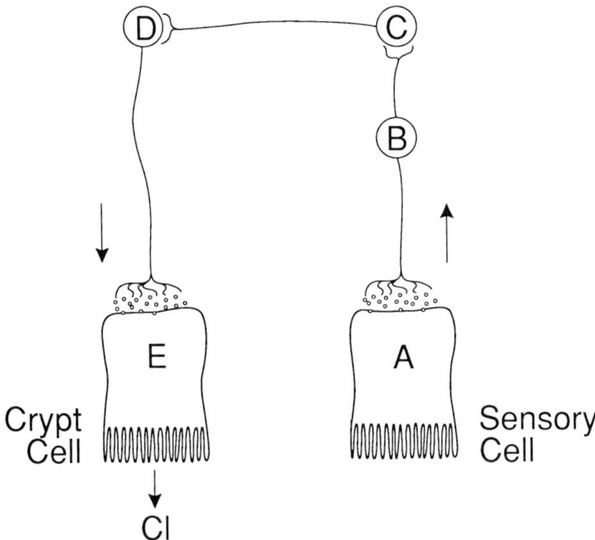

Figure 16.11. Reflex pathway involving endocrine cell and neural pathway. Luminal stimulus causes release of serotonin from endocrine cell (A), which stimulates afferent nerve (B). Interneuron (C) transmits signal to motor neuron (D), which then directly stimulates enterocyte (E) to secrete electrolytes into lumen. (Modified from Brunsson 1987. Acute inflammatory diarrhea in the small intestine. Thesis. Department of Physiology, University of Goteborg.)

affinity. The *efficacy* of these agents is determined by their ability to activate the intracellular machinery that brings about the physiological response. (Agents combining with receptors and having both affinity and efficacy are called *agonists;* agents that react with receptors but lack efficacy are called *competitive antagonists.*)

A number of the chemical transmitters have similar structures and can compete for the same receptor site. Thus the receptor binding depends on the relative concentration of the competing substances. Since the efficacy of these agents may be quite different, potentiation or inhibition of a response can be expected. The effect depends on the relative efficacy and concentration of the agents in the vicinity of the receptor.

For example, VIP has only approximately 17 percent of the efficacy of secretin on pancreatic HCO_3^- secretion in the dog. Both agents can interact with the same receptor site and are, therefore, competitive inhibitors or antagonists (Fig. 16.12). Thus at high concentrations VIP is a potent inhibitor of pancreatic HCO_3^- secretion. At very low secretin concentrations, however, VIP is a weak stimulus to

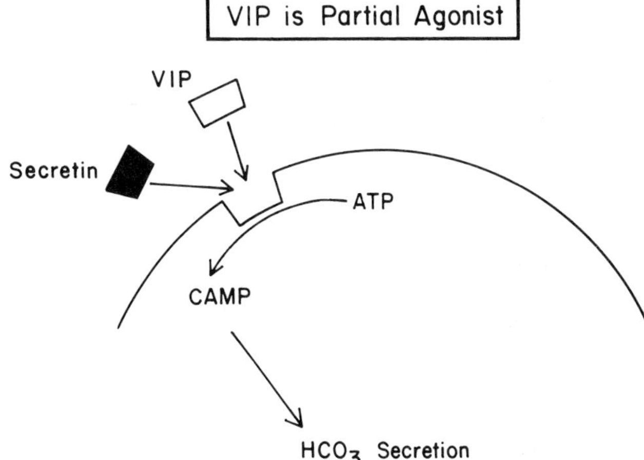

Figure 16.12. Interaction of secretin and VIP at receptor on pancreatic ductular cell. Both agents have equal affinity at receptor, but VIP is a weak stimulus of intracellular second messenger, cyclic AMP (CAMP). Thus VIP is a partial agonist for pancreatic bicarbonate secretion.

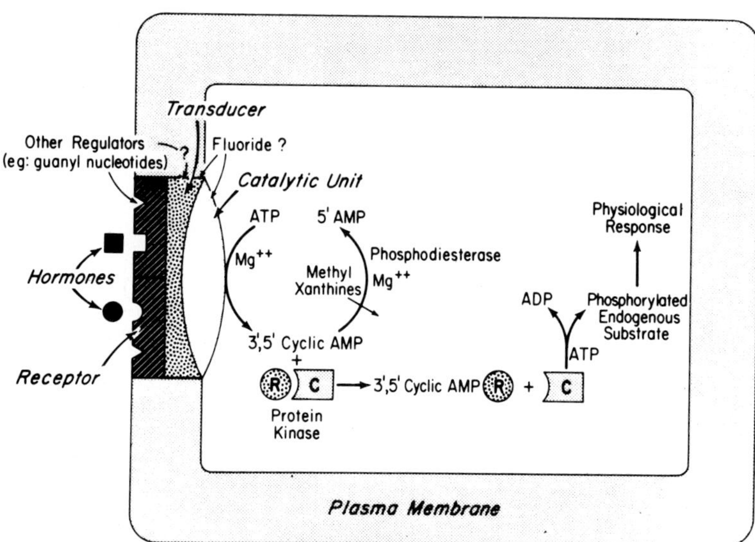

Figure 16.13. Schematic model of the adenylate cyclase–cyclic AMP system. Receptor on plasma membrane, when occupied by hormones, activates the catalytic unit, adenylcyclase, which then catalyzes the formation of cyclic AMP from ATP. Cyclic AMP then combines with the regulating (R) unit of a protein kinase and activates the catalytic (C) unit of the enzyme. The catalytic unit is then capable of phosphorylating an endogenous substrate. (From Kimberg 1974, *Gastroenterology* 67:1023–64.)

pancreatic HCO_3^- secretion and amplifies the secretin response. This type of control seems to be the rule in the gastrointestinal tract. Gastrointestinal hormones do not appear to be capable of exerting feedback control on their own release.

Stimulus response coupling

The coupling of neural or endocrine agents to the cellular response is brought about by intracellular messengers. These are the cyclic nucleotides—cyclic adenosine monophosphate (cAMP), cyclic guanosine monophosphate (cGMP), or intracellular calcium ions.

Cyclic nucleotide system

An example of the cAMP system is depicted in Fig. 16.13. The transmitters activate the enzyme adenyl cyclase which forms cAMP from adenosine triphosphate. Cyclic AMP activates a protein kinase (A kinase) which phosphorylates a membrane protein. Two examples of physiological responses involving cAMP are relaxation of smooth muscle and intestinal secretion. In the former, an adrenergic receptor is linked to the adenyl cyclase enzyme. The A kinase phosphorylates and hence activates a calcium pump protein. Calcium is then actively pumped from the cytosol into intracellular stores. With the falling concentration of cytosolic calcium, muscle relaxation occurs (Fig. 16.14). Intestinal secretion involving the cAMP system can be activated by the neurotransmitter, VIP, whose receptor is linked to adenyl cyclase. Similarly, prostaglandins, ubiquitous products that arise from arachidonic acid metabolism, activate adenyl cyclase and cause intestinal secretion (see Chap. 20).

Calcium and the phosphatidylinositol system

Calcium provides a link between electrical and chemical signals at the cell membrane and biochemical events within the cell that produce the response—cell shortening in the case of smooth muscle and secretion in the case of intestinal epithelium. Increased concentrations of cytosolic calcium can result either by release from intracellular stores or by entry from the extracellular fluid. Calcium then binds to a calcium-binding protein, calmodulin, which initiates the response (Fig. 16.15).

Release of calcium from intracellular stores is triggered by a muscarinic receptor, which is linked to a membrane phosphodiesterase. The activated phosphodiesterase hydrolyzes a membrane phospholipid, phosphatidylinositol

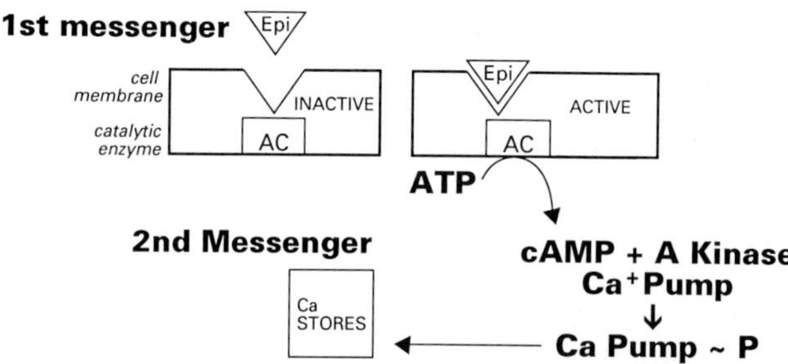

Figure 16.14. Chemico-mechanical coupling: Relaxation. Activation of cyclic AMP system by epinephrine (Epi) or norepinephrine causes relaxation of smooth muscle. Catalytic enzyme, adenyl cyclase (AC), generates cyclic AMP from ATP. The activated A kinase phosphorylates a calcium pump which then transports calcium from cytosol to intracellular stores. (Modified from Hendrix et al., 1987, in *Undergraduate Teaching Project in Gastroenterology and Liver Disease,* American Gastroenterological Association, Milner-Fenwick, Inc., Timonium, Md.)

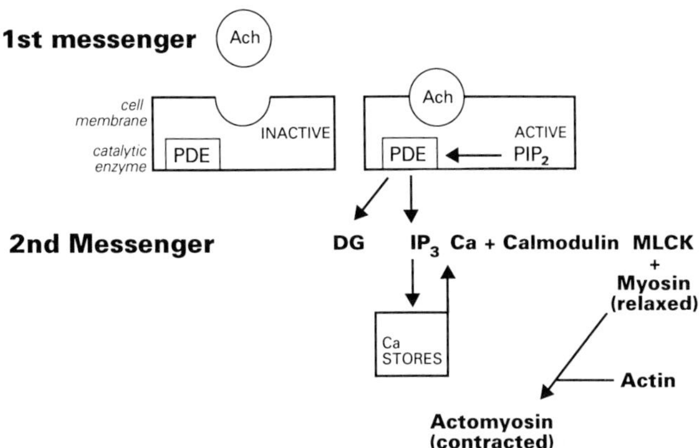

Figure 16.15. Chemico-mechanical coupling: Contraction. Phosphatidylinositol system increases intracellular calcium by releasing it from calcium stores. Activation of membrane phosphodiesterase (PDE) by ACh forms diacylglycerol (DG) and inositol triphosphate (IP_3) from a membrane phospholipid, phosphatidylinositol biphosphate (PIP_2). The increased calcium binds to calmodulin, which then activates myosin light chain kinase (MLCK). This enzyme phosphorylates myosin light chains (relaxed state). The phosphorylated myosin light chains form cross-bridges that bind actin to form actomysin (contracted state). Ach, acetylcholine. (Modified from Hendrix et al., 1987, in *Undergraduate Teaching Project in Gastroenterology and Liver Disease,* American Gastroenterological Association, Milner-Fenwick, Inc., Timonium, Md.)

biphosphate, into two second messengers—inositol triphosphate and diacylglycerol. The inositol triphosphate acts to release calcium into the cytosol.

Cytosolic calcium may also be elevated by the opening of voltage-dependent calcium channels. For example, depolarization of smooth muscle membranes opens a calcium channel, and calcium moves into the cell down a steep electrochemical gradient from the extracellular fluid. Cytosolic calcium then rises to a level that activates the contractile proteins (see Chap. 17).

REFERENCES

Argenzio, R.A., Lowe, J.E., Pickard, D.W., and Stevens, C.E. 1974. Digesta passage and water exchange in the equine large intestine. *Am. J. Physiol.* 226:1035–42.

Argenzio, R.A., and Southworth, M. 1975. Sites of organic acid production and absorption in gastrointestinal tract of the pig. *Am. J. Physiol.* 228:454–60.

Argenzio, R.A., Southworth, M., and Stevens, C.E. 1974. Sites of organic acid production and absorption in the equine gastrointestinal tract. *Am. J. Physiol.* 226:1043–50.

Banta, C.A., Clemens, E.T., Krinsky, M.M., and Sheffy, B.E. 1979. Sites of organic acid production and patterns of digesta movement in the gastrointestinal tract of dogs. *J. Nutr.* 109:1592–1600.

Bloom, S.E., and Polak, J.M. 1978. Gut hormone overview. In S.R. Bloom, ed., *Gut Hormones,* Churchill Livingston. Edinburgh. Pp. 3–18.

Cooke, H.J. 1987. Neural and humoral regulation of small intestinal electrolyte transport. 1987. In L.R. Johnson, ed., *Physiology of the Gastrointestinal Tract.* 2d ed. Raven Press, New York. Pp. 1307–50.

Davison, J.S. 1983. Innervation of the gastrointestinal tract. In J. Christensen, D.L. Wingate, P.S.G. Wright, eds., *A Guide to Gastrointestinal Motility.* J. Wright & Sons, Bristol. Pp. 1–47.

Grube, D., and Forssmann, W.G. 1979. Morphology and function of the entero-endocrine cells. *Horm. Metab. Res.* 11:589–606.

Hendrix, T.R., Castell, D.O., and Wood, J.D. 1987. Alimentary tract motility: Stomach, small intestine, colon, and biliary tract. In *Undergraduate Teaching Project in Gastroenterology and Liver Disease.* Produced by the American Gastroenterological Association, Milner-Fenwick Inc., Timonium, Md.

Johnson, L.R. 1977. Gastrointestinal hormones and their function. *Ann. Rev. Physiol.* 39:135–58.

Kalia, M., and Sullivan, J.M. 1982. Brainstem projections of sensory and motor components of the vagus nerve in the rat. *J. Comp. Neurol.* 211:248–64.

Konturek, S.J., Thor, P., Dembinski, A., and Krol, R. 1975. Comparison of secretin and vasoactive intestinal peptide on pancreatic secretion in dogs. *Gastroenterology* 68:1527–35.

Larsson, L-I. 1980. Peptide secretory pathways in GI tract: Cytochemical contributions to regulatory physiology of the gut. *Am. J. Physiol.* 239:G237–46.

Makhlouf, G.M. 1974. The neuroendocrine design of the gut. *Gastroenterology* 67:159–84.

Mer, N. 1985. Intestinal chemosensitivity. *Physiol. Rev.* 65:211–37.

Schofield, G.C. 1968. Anatomy of muscular and neural tissues in the alimentary canal. In *Handbook of Physiology.* Sec. 6, C.F. Code and W. Heidel, eds., *Alimentary Canal.* Vol. 4, *Motility.* Am. Physiol. Soc., Washington. Pp. 1579–1627.

Solcia, E., Capella, C., Buffa, R., Usellini, L., Fiocca, R., and Sessa, F. 1987. Endocrine cells of the digestive system. In L.R. Johnson, ed., *Physiology of the Gastrointestinal Tract.* 2d ed. Raven Press, New York. Pp. 111–30.

Szurszewski, J.H., and Krier, J. 1983. Thoracic and lumbar sympathetic neural pathways to the gastrointestinal tract. In P.J. Dyck, P.K. Thomas, E.H. Lambert, and R. Bunge, eds., *Peripheral Neuropathy.* W.B. Saunders, Philadelphia. Pp. 265–84.

Walsh, J.H. 1987. Gastrointestinal hormones. In L.R. Johnson, ed., *Physiology of the Gastrointestinal Tract.* 2d ed. Raven Press, New York. Pp. 181–253.

Wood, J.D. 1987. Physiology of the enteric nervous system. In L.R. Johnson, ed., *Physiology of the Gastrointestinal Tract.* 2d ed. Raven Press, New York. Pp. 67–109.

Wood, J.D. 1987. Neurophysiological theory of gastrointestinal motility. *Jpn. J. Smooth Muscle Res.* 23:143–86.

Wood, J.D., and Wingate, D.L. 1988. Gastrointestinal Neurophysiology. In *Undergraduate Teaching Project in Gastroenterology and Liver Disease.* Produced by American Gastroenterology Association, Milner-Fenwick Inc., Timonium, Md.

CHAPTER 17

Gastrointestinal Motility

by Robert A. Argenzio

From the time of its entrance into the mouth until the undigested residues leave the body, food is continuously subjected to movements that break it up and ensure its effective mixture with the digestive juices. The prehension, mastication, and subsequent swallowing of food form the first part of this process and constitute an ordered sequence of events that result in a bolus of food mixed with saliva entering the stomach.

PREHENSION

The seizing and conveying of food to the mouth is called *prehension.* Methods vary in different animals, but in all domestic animals the lips, teeth, and tongue are the principal organs of this function. The dog and cat often use their forelimbs to hold food, but it is passed into the mouth largely by the head and jaws.

The sensitive, mobile lips of the horse form its main prehensile structures and are used during feeding from a manger. During grazing, the lips are drawn back to allow the incisor teeth to sever the grass at its base. The lips of the other two common grazing animals—cows and sheep—have only limited movement; in these animals, the tongue is the main prehensile organ. It is long, rough, and mobile and can be readily curved around herbage, which is then drawn between the incisor teeth and dental pad and severed by movement of the head. Sheep have a cleft upper lip, which permits very close grazing; the incisor teeth and the tongue are its principal prehensile structures.

Under natural conditions, the pig digs up the ground with its snout (rooting), and food is carried to the mouth largely by the action of the pointed lower lip.

Cats and dogs convey fluids to the mouth by means of the tongue, the free mobile end of which forms a ladle. The other domestic animals draw liquid into the mouth by suction that is created by inspiration and tongue contractions.

MASTICATION

Mastication, or chewing, is the mechanical breakdown of food in the mouth. In the domesticated animals the incisor teeth are used to procure food by a tearing or scraping action, and the molar teeth are used for grinding food into small particles. The extent to which food is ground between the molars varies in different animals and is related to the nature of the diet. In carnivores molar grinding of food is imperfectly performed; in herbivores, however, a great deal of time is spent masticating. Although the main purpose of mastication is to break down food to provide a greater surface area for digestive juices, an important function of chewing is to mix food material thoroughly with saliva. Such mixing ensures adequate lubrication of the food bolus for its uninterrupted passage down the esophagus.

In carnivores and omnivores the jaw movements are mainly in a vertical plane and produce a shearing action. Tough, coarse plant food, however, requires far more mechanical grinding; therefore there is considerable lateral movement of the jaws in herbivores. The upper jaw is wider than the lower jaw, and mastication occurs on only one side at a time. Because of this lateral movement, the teeth wear with chisel-shaped grinding surfaces. The sharp edge of the lower teeth is innermost, and that of the upper teeth is outermost. The oblique tables of the teeth of herbivores are composed of substances of different degrees of hardness, and the grinding efficiency of the tables is increased by their uneven wear.

DEGLUTITION

Deglutition, or swallowing, is the passage of food from the mouth, through the pharynx and esophagus, to the stomach, and it involves a coordinated series of events in all these different regions. It commences as a voluntary act but becomes reflex during its execution, and it is a relatively rapid event that involves many structures.

Movements of the mouth and tongue are important in swallowing; after mastication and insalivation, the mouth and tongue bring the food bolus into a position that is on a midline between the tongue and the hard palate and suitable for swallowing. At this stage the food is in contact with receptors in the mucous membrane of the posterior part of the mouth and the posterior wall of the pharynx. Impulses from the receptors pass along the glossopharyngeal nerve, the superior laryngeal branch of the vagus nerve, and the maxillary division of the trigeminal nerve to the swallowing center in the medulla. Afferent impulses to the swallowing center also arise from the lower part of the pharynx and the upper surface of the epiglottis. Stratified squamous epithelium lines the mouth, tongue, and pharynx and the esophagus and is able to withstand the mechanical trauma associated with the ingestion of hard food materials.

The swallowing or deglutition center is formed by a collection of nerve cells located in the floor of the fourth ventricle of the brain, and it is stimulated by afferent impulses originating from the receptors described above. Different afferent patterns may stimulate the center, but once it is stimulated, the complete sequence of events associated with swallowing is evoked by a discharge of impulses through the motor nuclei of cranial nerves V, IX, X, XI, and XII (see Table 39.1). These nerves supply the tongue, the floor of the mouth, the fauces, and the laryngeal muscles.

The pattern of movements brought about by the rapid sequential discharge of impulses along the motor nerves in response to stimulation of afferent receptors by the food bolus lasts about 0.5 second. It begins with a series of events that have as their objective the closing off of the nasopharynx and the trachea from the mouth cavity to prevent entrance of food material into these areas. This closure is accomplished by elevation of the soft palate so that it lies close to the posterior pharyngeal wall and by repositioning of the larynx so that its opening into the pharynx is partially shielded. At the same time, the arytenoid cartilages, to which are attached the posterior ends of the vocal cords, are brought closer together by contraction of the laryngeal muscles, and the larynx is further occluded by contraction of the adductor muscles of the vocal cords. Respiration is inhibited at this stage. The end result of all these events is that the mouth and the pharynx form a completely closed chamber.

The sequence that occurs next is concerned with the transfer of the bolus from the back of the mouth to the upper end of the esophagus. The main driving force for this movement is derived from the contraction of the mylohyoid and hyoglossus muscles; the former presses the tongue against the hard palate, and the latter draws the root of the tongue backward. A sharp increase in intrapharyngeal pressure develops because of a reduction in volume of the closed pharyngeal cavity. This increase in pressure is followed by and is probably responsible for the sudden relaxation of the pharyngoesophageal junctional area. This area is guarded by a sphincteric mechanism that has a high resting tonicity and is normally closed. Relaxation appears to be due to inhibition of its normal tonic contraction. In humans, the sphincter opens 0.2 to 0.3 second after the beginning of a swallow, remains open 0.5 to 1.2 seconds, and then closes (Fig. 17.1).

The food bolus is squirted through the sphincter area by the backward movement of the base of the tongue and by contraction of the upper pharyngeal musculature, after which the sphincter immediately closes again. There is an initial receptive relaxation of the cranial end of the esophagus for reception of the bolus. Closure of the sphincter is accompanied by an increase in intrasphincter pressure to a level much greater than in the closed, resting sphincter, and at the same time a peristaltic wave begins at the anterior end of the esophagus. After the bolus has passed along the esophagus, the danger of reflux passage of food material into the pharynx and air passages recedes and the upper esophageal sphincter pressure falls to its normal resting level.

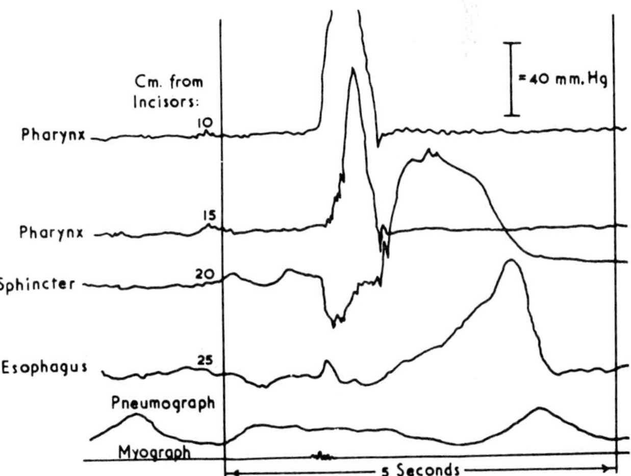

Figure 17.1. Pressures in the human pharynx and upper esophagus during a swallow. The beginning of a swallow is signaled by the myograph, which records action potentials in the jaw muscles. Respiration is interrupted. Pressure in the pharynx rises to a high level, and this increased pressure travels quickly down the pharynx. The pharyngoesophageal sphincter relaxes when pharyngeal pressure is high. As soon as the pressure in the pharynx has fallen to baseline level, pressure in the sphincter rises, and it remains high for more than 1 second. While the sphincter is tightly closed, the peristaltic wave begins to move slowly down the esophagus. (From *Physiology of the Digestive Tract,* by Horace W. Davenport. Copyright © 1961, Year Book Medical Publishers, Inc. Used by permission of Year Book Medical Publishers.)

ESOPHAGUS

In extending from the pharynx to the stomach, the *esophagus* crosses the thorax and perforates the diaphragm. Its wall is made up of four layers: an outer connective tissue coat, a muscular coat, submucosa, and mucosa. In many animals striated muscle fibers constitute the circular and longitudinal muscles throughout the length of the esophagus, but in others a varying proportion of the caudal esophagus is composed of smooth muscle. The distribution of striated and smooth muscle in the various species is shown in Fig. 17.2.

Between the muscle coats and the stratified squamous epithelial lining is the relatively thick submucosal layer, which throws the surface epithelium into folds. In the empty esophagus these folds are in close apposition, and they obliterate the lumen. During the passage of a bolus of food, the folds are flattened out and the esophageal lining becomes smooth.

The esophagus is normally closed at the pharyngoesophageal junction by the upper esophageal sphincter, and, although there is no anatomically defined sphincter at the gastroesophageal junction in some species, intramural pressure studies have demonstrated an intrinsic or functional sphincter at this region in all.

Innervation

The main motor nerve supply to the esophagus is from the vagus nerves. Although there is considerable variation among different species, the basic arrangement is for the cervical region to receive fibers from the recurrent laryngeal nerves; the remainder of the esophagus receives fibers from the thoracic vagal trunks. In the dog and cat, nerve fibers leaving the vagus cranial to the recurrent laryngeal nerve exert considerable control over the cervical esophagus.

Where the walls of the esophagus are made up of smooth muscle, a myenteric nerve plexus is present, and its ganglion cells serves as relay stations between the vagal preganglionic fibers passing to the muscle cells. A myenteric plexus does not exist in species in which the esophagus is made up entirely of striated muscle, although in dogs, rabbits, and small rodents ganglion cells are present between the muscle layers. Motor end plates connected to efferent fibers constitute the main innervation of the striated muscle. Sympathetic fibers supplying the esophagus arise mainly from the stellate ganglion and enter the plexal mazes, but whether they ultimately innervate the muscle is not known.

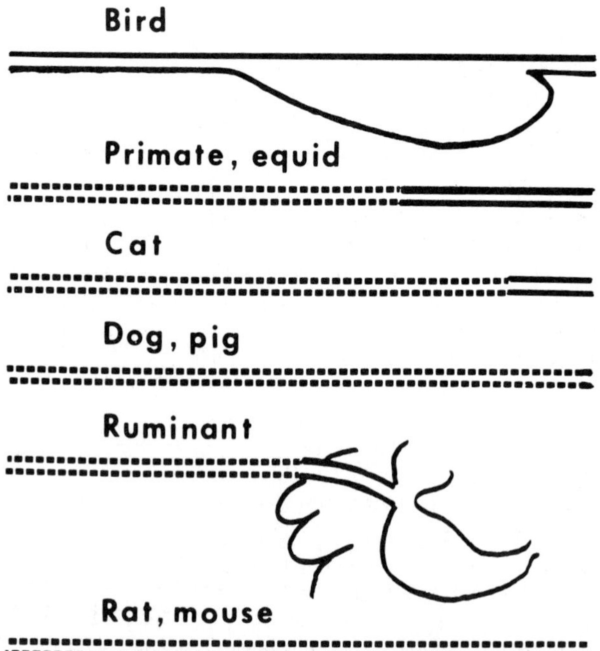

Figure 17.2. Distribution of esophageal striated muscle (*dotted line*) and smooth muscle (*solid line*) in some common species.

Movements of the esophagus

The movement of the esophagus associated with swallowing is a *peristaltic wave* that travels from the upper esophageal sphincter to the lower esophageal sphincter. Peristaltic contraction of the esophagus elicited only by a swallowing movement is termed *primary peristalsis*. Local esophageal stimulation by the introduction of a bolus or foreign body into the esophageal lumen will, however, elicit a peristaltic movement known as *secondary peristalsis*. Apart from the site of elicitation, there is no intrinsic difference between the two types of peristalsis. The significance of secondary peristalsis appears to be that if the primary wave initiated by a swallow succeeds only in passing the bolus into the upper portion of the esophagus, then the bolus itself will cause a series of reflex contractions that will drive the bolus onward.

The power of the peristaltic wave in carnivores is shown by the ease with which large pieces of meat and large bones that are occasionally swallowed are transported along the esophagus. Measurements of the force exerted by the contractile wave in the dog have shown that it is sufficient to overcome an opposing force equal to a weight of 400 g.

The rate at which the peristaltic wave, provoked by swallowing of a food bolus, passes along the esophagus appears to vary in different animals and is probably related to differences in innervation and the proportions of smooth and striated muscle in the esophagus. A bolus travels faster with striated muscle. The movement of a bolus along the dog's esophagus occurs at 5.0 cm per second, and the total transit time is 4 to 5 seconds.

GASTROINTESTINAL SMOOTH MUSCLE

The smooth muscles of the gastrointestinal tract generally show spontaneous (myogenic) activity, conduction of

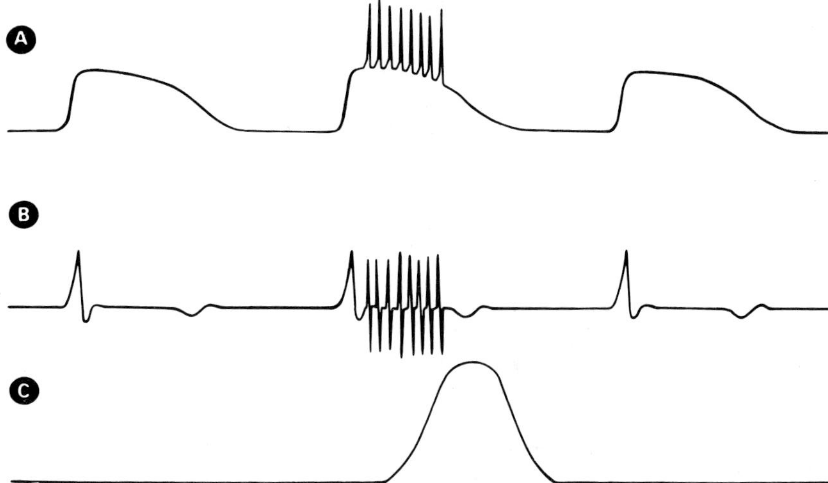

Figure 17.3. Diagram of relation between slow waves, spikes, and contractions. (*A*) Intracellular electrode. A burst of spike potentials appears on the second slow wave. (*B*) Extracellular electrode. The configuration of recorded waves approximates a derivative of the membrane potential change. (*C*) Tension record. Contractions coincide with bursts of spike potentials, which in turn are paced by slow waves. (From Christensen, reprinted, by permission, from the *N. Engl. J. Med.* 285:85–98, 1971.)

electrical impulses from fiber to fiber, and sensitivity to stretch. Their activity is modulated, but not initiated, by autonomic nerves. Exceptions are the smooth muscles of the ruminant forestomach and avian gizzard, which are primarily nerve activated. Within the cells are parallel myofilaments; individual filaments terminate at the cell wall at the tapering tips of the cell. Their contractions cause lateral indentations on the cell border, so that the cell seems to fold on itself like an accordion. The filaments may slide past one another, which accounts for (1) the great range of length over which tension can be exerted and (2) the decrease in wall tension subsequent to stretch (as in the stomach during eating). The latter is called *stretch relaxation* and can also be caused by inhibition of active contraction. That is, if tension is being maintained by active and regular spike discharge, stretch may inhibit spiking for a time during which the muscle relaxes to accommodate to the new length.

In smooth muscle, as in other excitable tissues, there is normally an electrical potential of about −50 mV (inside negative to outside) across the membranes of single cells. This fluctuates in two major ways. *Slow waves* are spontaneous, slow, transient depolarizations of the membrane potential, apparently conducted for varying distances along the tract (basal electrical rhythm). *Spikes* are faster transient depolarizations that can occur in bursts at the periods of maximal depolarization of a slow wave. These rapid transients precede and appear to initiate contraction (Fig. 17.3).

In the cat and the rabbit, longitudinal smooth muscle fibers at the peak of slow waves may show one or more prepotentials (or generator potentials) ahead of the spike. These have been likened to the prepotentials of cardiac pacemaker tissue and probably represent ion (Na^+, Ca^{2+}) conductance changes. Parasympathetic stimulation increases the rate at which these potentials depolarize the membrane, thus increasing the rate of spike discharge. Sympathetic stimulation prolongs the rate at which the generator potential depolarizes the membrane and thus slows the rate of spike discharge.

Slow waves set the maximal possible frequency of contractions. They are generated at a constant frequency at a given locus; however, the frequency of such pacemakers varies in different regions of the gastrointestinal tract. A sodium-potassium pump contributes to the resting potential; one hypothesis for slow waves is that they represent a rhythmic sodium pump. The nature of the primary pacemaker reaction is not known.

Spikes are normally required to activate contractions, and these depolarizations involve inward calcium currents. Cytosolic calcium may be raised to levels that initiate contraction by opening voltage-dependent calcium channels in the smooth muscle cell membrane (Fig. 17.4). Calcium moves into the cell down a steep electrochemical gradient. Vagal stimulation results in bigger bursts of spikes, probably by raising cytosolic calcium from intracellular stores, as discussed in Chapter 16. This results in more vigorous contractions. Sympathetic stimulation reduces spiking activity by moving cytosolic calcium into intracellular stores, as also discussed in Chapter 16.

Hyperpolarization of the muscle cell membrane (inside more negative) lowers cytosolic calcium by decreasing the number of open voltage-sensitive channels. Such hyperpolarization can be induced by the action of the neurotransmitter, VIP. When VIP binds to a receptor on the cell membrane, a potassium channel is opened. Potassium moves out of the cell, leaving an excess of negative charges behind and hence hyperpolarizing the membrane. Thus the resting membrane potential is moved farther from the threshold for a spike discharge.

Figure 17.5 shows electrical events in the duodenum of an unanesthetized cat with chronically implanted needle electrodes.

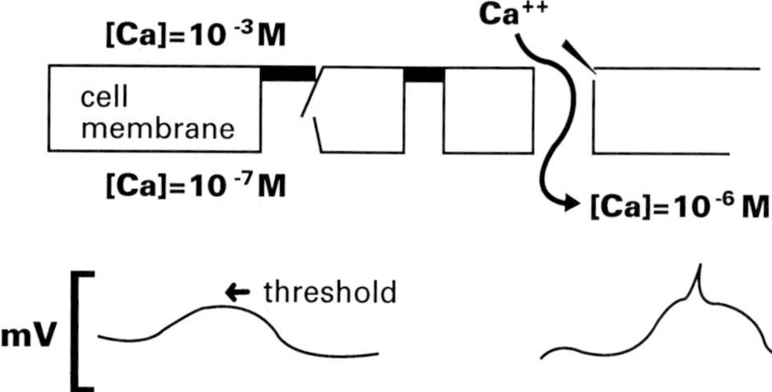

Figure 17.4. Electromechanical coupling: Contraction. Opening of voltage-dependent calcium channel. Cytosolic calcium may be raised to levels that initiate contraction by the opening of voltage-dependent calcium channels. On the left, maximal depolarization by the slow wave is subthreshold for calcium channel opening. On the right, threshold is reached and an action potential appears with rapid depolarization of the cell membrane. The voltage-sensitive calcium channel opens and calcium enters down a steep electrochemical gradient. Immediately afterward, an efflux of potassium occurs and repolarizes the membrane with resultant closure of the calcium channel. (Modified from Hendrix et al., 1987, in *Undergraduate Teaching Program in Gastroenterology and Liver Disease,* American Gastroenterological Association, Thorofare, N.J.)

PRESSURES IN HOLLOW ABDOMINAL VISCERA

The abdominal viscera are relatively mobile, and their specific gravity is approximately the same as that of water. The physical result is that the viscera apply hydrostatic pressure to the serosal surface of a given hollow viscus (e.g., the stomach) proportional to their vertical height.

If the stomach contents, for example, have nearly the same specific gravity as the abdominal viscera, then the stomach will behave as a water-filled bag suspended in water; that is, the transmural pressure approaches zero. As the animal eats or drinks, stomach filling results in a rise in hydrostatic pressure within it. The intra-abdominal hydrostatic pressure rises at the same time. Thus the difference in pressure across the stomach wall (transmural pressure) is small. The volume of the organ is increasing, however, so that wall tension is rising. In a hollow organ at constant transmural pressure (P), tension (T) in the wall is directly proportional to the radius (r) according to Laplace's law. For a sphere (which the stomach approximates), $P = 2T/r$; for a cylinder (which the intestine approximates), $P = T/r$.

This tension increase, proportional to the radius, is sensed by mechanoreceptors in the wall. For example, the afferent discharge of these receptors during active contraction of the organ is proportional to the developed tension and conveys the sensation of fullness (Fig. 17.6).

It is further apparent from Laplace's law that pressure in hollow organs is directly proportional to the tension in their walls. The tension in the wall of the digestive tract is maintained by active contraction of its muscle. Adjustments in active tension are the means by which pressure and volume are regulated. Stretch relaxation occurs as the organ fills. This involves both sliding of myofibrils past one another and inhibition of spiking. These allow accommodation to the new volume, and transmural pressure falls toward the value present before the volume increase. As the animal swallows, the gastric fundus also relaxes reflexly along with the lower esophageal sphincter; some additional volume for swallowed food (receptive relaxation) is thus provided.

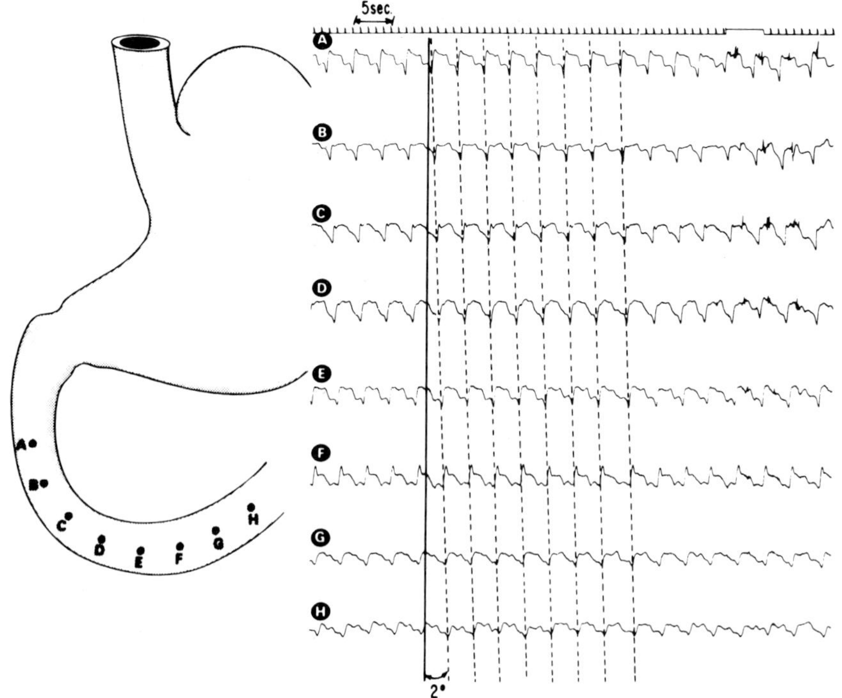

Figure 17.5. Electrical events in duodenum of unanesthetized cat. Note aboral progression of slow waves from A to H (*left*) and superimposed spikes (*right*). Angle between solid perpendicular line and dotted lines indicates time delay of progressive contraction. (From Christensen, reprinted, by permission, from the *N. Engl. J. Med.* 285:85–96, 1971.)

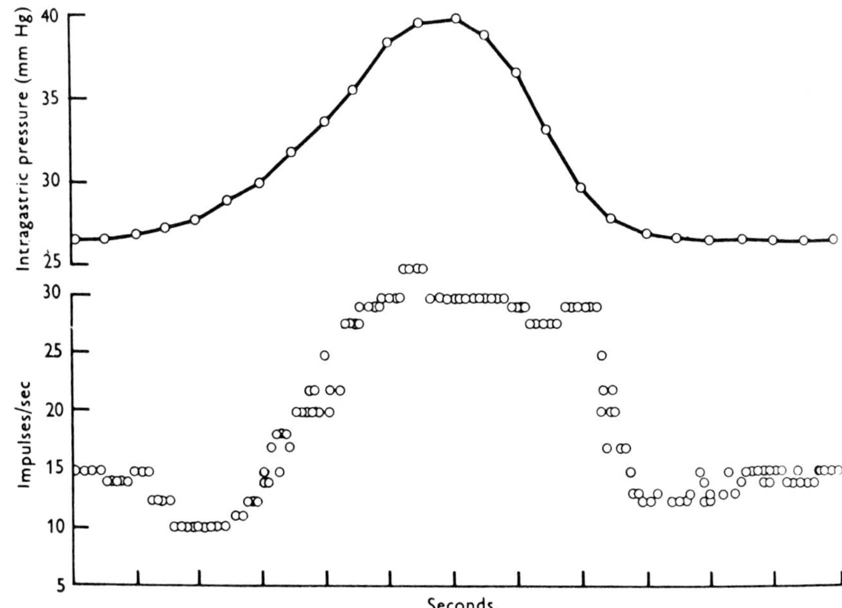

Figure 17.6. Intrareticular (intragastric) pressure, or reflex isometric contraction of reticulum (*top*), and frequency of discharge in single afferent vagal fiber (*bottom*) in the goat. (From Iggo 1955, *J. Physiol.* 128:593–607.)

MOTOR FUNCTIONS OF THE STOMACH

The functions of the stomach are (1) mixing and storage of the ingested food and (2) initiation of protein and fat digestion. Its most important function is storage of the food and the controlled release of its contents into the duodenum. For the purposes of mechanical function, the stomach may be divided into three zones, as shown in Fig. 17.7. The dorsal portion, or the *fundus,* is involved with reception and storage of contents and with adaptation to volume so that excessive pressure does not develop. The body, or *corpus,* serves as a mixing vat for the mixture of saliva and gastric juice with the food. The *antrum* is the gastric pump and regulates the propulsion of food past the pyloric sphincter and into the duodenum. However, the antral contractions also serve to retropel the contents and thereby to mix the ingesta and delay the passage of solid particles. This latter function is also shared by the pyloric sphincter.

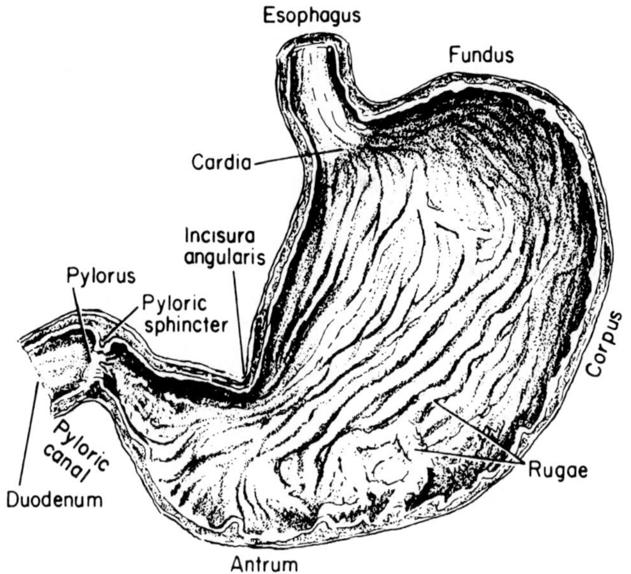

Figure 17.7. Physiologic anatomy of the stomach. The three main zones of mechanical function are the fundus, the corpus, and the antrum. (From Guyton, ed., 1981, *Textbook of Medical Physiology,* 6th ed, W.B. Saunders Co., Philadelphia.)

Rate of gastric emptying

There are considerable differences in the rate of gastric emptying among species, as discussed in Chapter 16. Liquid leaves the stomach at a faster rate than does particulate matter; thus the stomach is given time for necessary solubilization and partial digestion of its particulate contents. Table 17.1 shows the time required for one-half of the markers of fluid contents and of various sizes of particulate contents to leave the stomach of the dog and the pig. In all instances, fluid is emptied quite rapidly and particles are retained in proportion to their size. However, the rate at which fluid contents are delivered to the duodenum is regulated by duodenal receptors responding to the chemical composition of the meal.

The rate of gastric emptying is a function of the square root of the volume, and this is shown for the 160 kg pony in Fig. 17.8. When the square root of the residual volume is plotted against time, a straight line is obtained. These relationships suggest that the rate of emptying is dependent on the volume, and distention of the stomach is the primary stimulus to increase gastric motility. Most of the reflexes

Table 17.1. Gastric emptying half-time of dog and pig (in hours)

Species	Diet	Fluid marker	Particle markers (diameter × length in mm)		
			2 × 2	2 × 10	2 × 20
Dog	Cereal	1.7	3.1	9.4	10.0
Dog	Meat	1.8	10.1	10.7	11.1
Pig	Pelletized	2.0	8.8	12.6	14.2

Modified from Banta, Clemens, Krinsky, and Sheffy 1979, *J. Nutr.* 109:1592–1600, and from Clemens, Stevens, and Southworth 1975, *J. Nutr.* 105:759–68.

that control gastric motility are inhibitory, as discussed below.

Control of gastric motility

The maximum frequency of antral contractions is set by the slow wave, which in the dog and the horse occurs at the rate of four to five cycles per minute. Slow waves are initiated somewhere on the greater curvature of the stomach and spread distally with increasing velocity and voltage. In the terminal antrum, the velocity is highest so that vigorous contractions, if present, may occur. As discussed previously, the slow waves are present, whether or not the muscle contracts. They are the clock that sets the time when the muscle is allowed to respond. The mechanical response to the slow wave is governed by neural and hormonal influences. When the stomach is distended with food, mechanical receptors in the wall of the stomach are activated, and vagal tone to the stomach increases. Each slow wave may now bear spikes so that the maximal frequency of peristaltic contractions may be as great as four to five contractions per minute.

The inhibitory control of gastric emptying is brought about by an enterogastric reflex (neural mechanism) and an

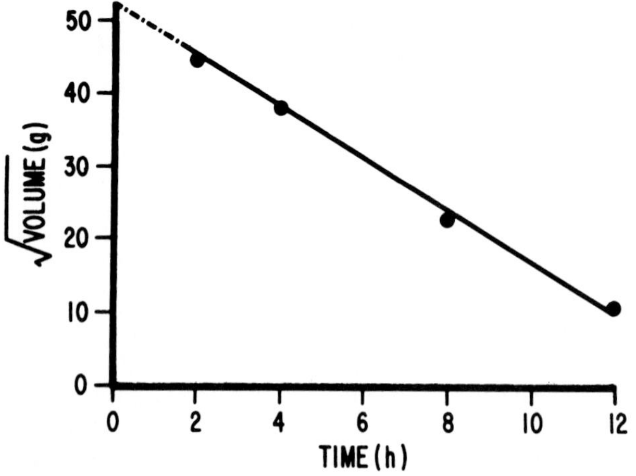

Figure 17.8. Rate of gastric emptying in 160 kg pony fed at 12-hour intervals. Extrapolation to zero time would indicate total volume of stomach contents due to ingestion of meal.

enterogastrone (endocrine mechanism). The receptors for these reflexes are present in the duodenum, and they monitor the chemical composition of the digesta leaving the stomach. The most important of these receptors are osmoreceptors in the duodenal mucosa. These are mucosal cells that respond with unusual sensitivity to the luminal osmolality. Hypertonic solutions of large solutes (glucose) cause the interstitial space to shrink, and this shrinking inhibits emptying of the stomach contents. Solutes of smaller molecular size are less effective, but nevertheless are inhibitory at hypertonic concentrations. Conversely, distilled water causes the interstitial space to swell and increases the rate of emptying. In an isotonic solution of NaCl there is no osmotic effect; however, an isotonic solution causes the interstitial space to swell to a maximum because there is net movement of salt followed by water into the interstitial space. Therefore gastric contents leave at a maximal rate when the osmoreceptor senses an isotonic solution in the duodenum.

This is a very fortunate control mechanism, because the osmolality of gastric contents can reach values as high as 1000 mOsm/kg water. Although such osmotic pressures can be sustained in gastric contents without provoking bulk water flow, this is not true of the highly permeable jejunum and duodenum, which osmotically equilibrate their contents rapidly with the blood (see Chap. 20). Therefore, if these hypertonic solutions were not delivered slowly into the duodenum, the animal would quickly become hypotensive through shifts of fluid from the extracellular space into the lumen. On the other hand, rapid emptying of isotonic or hypotonic solutions presents no immediate problem because these fluids are absorbed as the contents are moved along the small intestine, and the extracellular volume and osmolality are rapidly adjusted by the kidney.

A second set of receptors responds to acid in the duodenum. If the pH of duodenal contents becomes less than 3.5 to 4.0, an enterogastric reflex is immediately initiated and blocks further emptying of the acid contents until the duodenal fluid is neutralized by pancreatic and biliary secretions. Strength of the acid is not particularly important because acetic acid is next most effective to hydrochloric acid. The effectiveness of the acid is due to the molecular weight, presumably because the small anions can diffuse to the receptor more rapidly. Hydrogen ion is necessary, however, as the sodium salts of the acids are ineffective.

It is probable that the above inhibitory reflexes, as well as inhibition due to pain or distention of the duodenum, are mediated by sympathetic sensory and motor nerves. It also is possible that the peptidergic nervous system acting through inhibitory neurons, also participates in the control of gastric emptying.

The most powerful inhibitors of gastric emptying are lipids of 12 to 18 carbon atoms. Therefore, gastric emptying of fats is greatly prolonged; this allows sufficient time for the rather complex processes of fat digestion in the jejunum to take place. This response appears to be hormonally mediated. Release of cholecystokinin (CCK) in response to fat has been demonstrated, and CCK at physiological levels is inhibitory to gastric emptying.

Products of protein and carbohydrate digestion also inhibit gastric emptying. The response is primarily due to the osmoreceptor, as discussed above. However, at least one amino acid, L-tryptophan, inhibits gastric motility through its release of CCK.

In summary, there are feedback mechanisms mediated by neural and hormonal reflexes that inhibit gastric emptying. These two mechanisms inhibit emptying when there are hypertonic, acidic, or irritating contents perfusing the duodenum or when the contents contain too much lipid, carbohydrate, or protein. Thus the diverse spectrum of material present in the stomach is gradually released to the small intestine for digestion and absorption.

Interdigestive motility patterns

During digestion, large food particles are retained in the stomach because of the retropulsion achieved by the antropyloric region. There are special mechanisms, however, to empty fasting content and larger particles from the stomach and "sweep" them to the distal small intestine. This motility pattern, termed the *migrating myoelectric complex (MMC),* occurs in some species (dogs, humans) only during the fasting period. The MMC is divided into three phases (Fig. 17.9). During phase I, there is a quiescent period during which slow waves are present but no action potentials are generated. In phase II, there are intermittent action potentials. During phase III, there are intense bursts of spikes accompanying each slow wave. These result in strong antral contractions. Each phase usually migrates distally to the terminal small intestine. The pylorus does not close as these waves approach, as it does during the digestive period. Hence both solids and liquids are emptied from the stomach and carried rapidly to the large intestine.

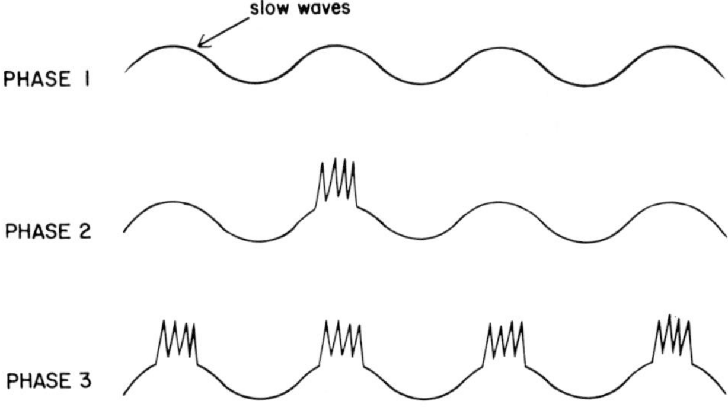

Figure 17.9. Migrating myoelectric complex of the stomach and small intestine. The three phases of the complex appear in carnivores and humans during the interdigestive (fasting) period. In herbivores and some omnivores, however, they are also present during the digestive period and are not interrupted by the meal. In some instances all three phases migrate all the way from the lower esophageal sphincter to the distal small intestine without interruption. Phase III is associated with powerful propulsive motility that sweeps the stomach and small intestine clean of particles and fasting content.

In carnivores, but not in herbivores, the MMC is interrupted on feeding, and a fed pattern, resembling phase II of the MMC, takes its place. In herbivores, the cyclic pattern is not interrupted by feeding, primarily because of the relatively continuous intake and low nutrient density of the feed. Conversely, carnivores consume meals of high nutrient density, which are low in bulk. In omniverous species, such as the pig, the pattern of motility can be varied by feeding either a herbiverous type of diet, or two to three discrete high-calorie meals a day.

The control of the MMC as well as the fed pattern differs in the proximal and distal gastrointestinal tract. In the stomach and proximal intestine, which includes the lower esophageal sphincter, stomach, and proximal duodenum, the hormone motilin appears to be involved in initiation of the MMC. However, the propagation of the MMC distally or, in some cases, initiation of MMC activity in the distal duodenum or jejunum is dependent on intrinsic nerves. For example, if motilin is not released, MMC activity will then be initiated in the distal duodenum and propagated distally.

In the stomach and proximal intestine, hormonal control may also be responsible for initiation of the fed pattern. Both gastrin and CCK have been implicated in this context. In contrast, extrinsic nerves are required for the fed pattern of motility in the distal intestine. For example, during vagal blockade, the MMCs are still generated but are not disrupted by a meal.

Emesis or vomiting

Carnivores and omnivores (except rodents) vomit easily. Swine, for example, frequently vomit with irritation of the pharynx or stomach, such as occurs with some indigestion or diarrheal states. In ruminants vomiting does not occur in the usual sense of the term but, rather, occurs as ejection of abomasal contents into the forestomach. This has been noted in intestinal obstruction. Vomiting in the horse is extremely rare, apparently because of the marked tonus of the lower esophageal sphincter. It is the only domestic species in which acute gastric dilatation can occur to the point of rupture of the stomach wall with or without vomiting.

A more detailed description of vomiting can be given for the cat. Electrical slow-wave amplitude in the duodenum decreases and is superseded by a long burst of intense spike activity spreading orad at about 3 cm/s, driving a mass of ingesta toward the mouth. This empties the proximal small intestine into the relaxed stomach. Repetitive inspiratory movements, with the glottis closed, result in filling of the relaxed thoracic esophagus with gastric content. This is followed by the repetitive and rhythmic reflux (*retching*) of contents from the thoracic esophagus into the stomach.

Retching drives the gastric contents forward and backward by inspiratory muscle contraction, with the glottis closed concurrent with rectus abdominis muscle contraction, followed by relaxation. The lowered intrapleural pressure, concurrent with raised intra-abdominal pressure, aspirates gastric content into the thoracic esophagus. Each such contraction lasts about 0.1 to 0.3 second. Relaxation of the inspiratory and abdominal muscles then occurs, allowing reflux into the stomach. Several such retching cycles precede the actual expulsive effort. Expulsion is brought about by a stronger and longer rectus abdominis muscle contraction occurring coincidentally with contraction of inspiratory muscles (including the diaphragm) against a closed glottis, as before, but this time ending with sudden relaxation of the diaphragm. This rapidly allows the intrapleural pressure to become positive by transmission of the pressure that has already been built up in the abdomen. Vomitus is expelled mostly through the mouth since the soft palate is elevated reflexly and closes off the posterior nares.

The neural centers of the emetic mechanism are located in the medulla. There are two anatomically and functionally distinct units. These are the vomiting center, which is located in the reticular formation, and the chemoreceptor trigger zone (CTZ) in the floor of the fourth ventricle. The vomiting center is activated directly by visceral afferent impulses arising anywhere in the gastrointestinal tract. These are conducted to the vomiting center from both vagal and sympathetic afferents. The efferent motor nerves are cranial nerves V, VII, X, and XII (see Table 39.1) to the upper gastrointestinal tract and the spinal nerves to the diaphragm and abdominal muscles.

The CTZ, on the other hand, receives central stimulation from chemical substances such as morphine, apomorphine, cardiac glycosides, and copper sulfate. The CTZ is not able to cause vomiting without connections to the vomiting center. Thus it acts as a relay station to initiate the vomiting act. Therefore, all emetic responses are mediated through the vomiting center, whether they originate at peripheral or central sites.

MOTILITY OF THE SMALL INTESTINE

Since the small intestine performs both digestive and absorptive functions, the flow of contents must be regulated to provide (1) mixing of luminal contents with pancreatic enzymes and bile; (2) luminal digestion of carbohydrates, fats, and proteins; and (3) maximal exposure of the digested nutrients to the mucosa of the small intestine. Although some of these processes require a certain amount of time, liquid contents are swept along the small intestine quite rapidly, as was shown in Chapter 15. The rate of gastric emptying, therefore, is of primary importance in preventing the small intestine from becoming overwhelmed.

Transit in the ileum is slowed as a result of a greater percentage of segmental contractions than occur in the jejunum. The ileocecal junction also provides some delay in transit, and contents are retained longer in the ileum than in the jejunum. By causing junctional tonus to rise, distention of the cecum also delays flow from the ileum.

The basic control system for small intestine motility is the electric slow wave. The primary pacemaker is located in the longitudinal muscle of the duodenum near the entrance of the bile duct. Slow waves are generated by the pacemaker at the rate of 17 to 18 per minute in the dog and the cat and 14 to 15 per minute in the horse. These waves are conducted aborally, but local pacemakers in the more distal areas will initiate slow-wave generation at a reduced frequency. Thus slow waves decrease in frequency and propagation velocity in the aboral direction. For example, only 10 to 11 per minute are observed in the horse ileum. Therefore transit is slowed in the lower small intestine.

Small intestine motility is mediated by both intrinsic and extrinsic innervation, which may increase or decrease the probability of spike discharge. The most important intrinsic reflex is the *peristaltic reflex*. Peristalsis induces mass propulsion and is due to sequentially timed contractions of both the longitudinal and circular muscles (Fig. 17.10). Contraction of the longitudinal muscle and inhibition of the circular muscle distal to the bolus induce shortening of the muscle and expand the lumen. At the same time, there is relaxation of the longitudinal muscle and contraction of the circular muscle proximal to the bolus. This reduces the lumen size and prevents backward flow.

Segmentation is a second reflex that can be initiated solely by intrinsic nerves (Fig. 17.11). This is primarily a result of intermittent circular muscle contractions occurring at different sites along the segment. Opiates induce this motility pattern, which is necessary for mixing and slowing the transit of contents during digestion.

Extrinsic reflexes also exist. Inhibitory reflexes caused by pain or distention can inhibit motility of the entire small

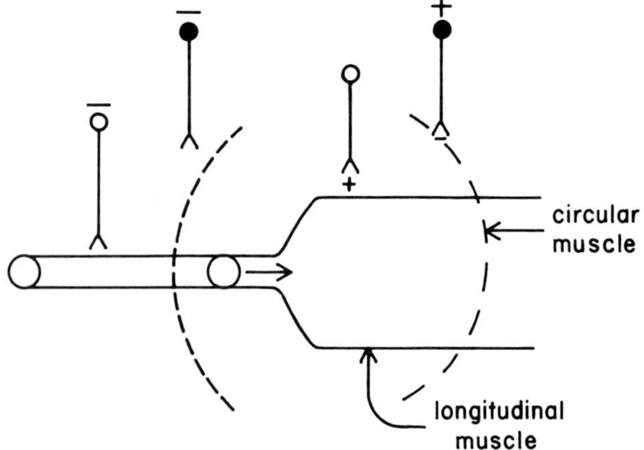

Figure 17.10. Peristaltic reflex. Inhibitory neurons (dark cell bodies) dominate control of circular smooth muscle. Their activation (+) distal to the bolus maintains the circular muscle in a relaxed state, whereas proximal to bolus they are inhibited (−). Longitudinal muscle distal to the bolus contracts under the influence of excitatory neurons (light cell bodies), while proximal to the bolus it relaxes because of inhibition of the excitatory neuron. This sequence can be propagated for variable distances and is controlled by programmed networks within the enteric nervous system.

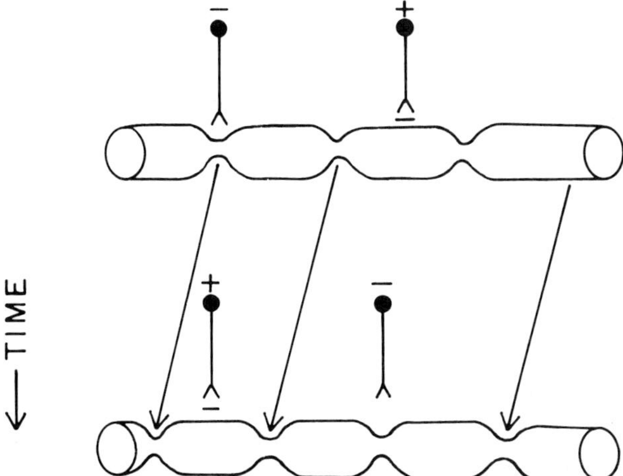

Figure 17.11. Segmentation reflex. This pattern of motility is controlled by inhibitory neuron influence on circular smooth muscle. When these neurons are stimulated (+) they inhibit contraction of circular muscle, and when they are inhibited (−) the muscle is allowed to contract. This sequence is not usually propagated in one direction; instead, these circular constrictions may appear anywhere on a given segment and result in mixing of the contents.

intestine. These reflexes are carried in the splanchnic nerves. Vagal afferents conduct stimuli from mechanoreceptors, and the vagal efferent stimulation is primarily excitatory.

Although endocrine control of motility is not well understood, it is known that gastrin and CCK stimulate and that

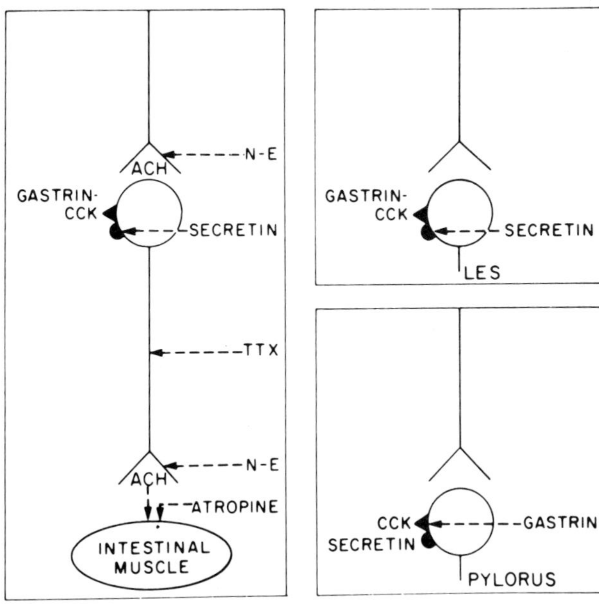

Figure 17.12. Scheme to demonstrate the mode of action of hormones on intestinal and sphincteric muscle. Agonists are placed on the left side and antagonists on the right side of each of the three sections illustrated. TTX, tetrodotoxin; N-E, norepinephrine; ACH, acetylcholine; LES, lower esophageal sphincter; PS, pyloric sphincter; CCK, cholecystokinin. (From Makhlouf 1974, *Gastroenterology* 67:159–84.)

secretin inhibits contractions of jejunal smooth muscle. This reciprocal response suggests that these hormones may be physiologically involved in the control of small intestine motility. There is good evidence that the action of gastrin and CCK is mediated by release of ACh from nerve terminals because it is abolished by nerve-blocking agents such as tetrodotoxin as shown in Fig. 17.12. Figure 17.12 also shows that norepinephrine released from postganglionic sympathetic nerve terminals is capable of inhibiting ACh release at the cholinergic synapse or nerve ending.

MOTOR FUNCTIONS OF THE LARGE INTESTINE

The functions of the large intestine are (1) microbial digestion and (2) reabsorption of electrolytes and water. Both of these functions require that transit of digestive contents be delayed, because both are relatively slow processes in contrast to the digestive and absorptive functions in the small intestine discussed above. Fermentative digestion requires a fluid environment with a high neutralizing capacity because the end products of microbial digestion are released to the luminal fluid in their acid form. Therefore, in species such as the horse in which microbial digestion is well developed, the large intestine carries out a complex and rather difficult function. Not only must it be capable of supplying a buffered fluid environment for digestion but it also must be capable of reabsorption of at least 90 percent of this fluid as well as some of the microbial end products before they are excreted. The motor activity of the large intestine provides one mechanism to accomplish these functions by ensuring that the contents are delayed long enough for all of these processes to occur.

Movements of the cecum and colon

Ingesta first enter the cecum of the horse and are then delivered into the colon. In others such as the sheep, a large proportion of ingesta first enters the colon, but some of this is retropelled into the cecum. In ruminants, rodents, and lagomorphs the cecum is the primary site of microbial digestion in the large intestine, and retrograde movement of contents from the proximal colon to the cecum is one means of delaying transit. In the horse no retrograde movement from the proximal colon to the cecum occurs, and contents leave the cecum rapidly (Fig. 16.6). The large colon of the horse, as well as the cecum, is the primary site of microbial digestion.

Figure 17.13 shows the anatomical arrangement in the horse of the ileocecal junction and the cecocolic ostium. The dorsal and ventral lips of the cecocolic ostium are usually closed and guard the entrance to the colon. The most common type of cecal contraction results in mass movement of ingesta from the cecal body to the base and then to the cupola. The cupola then isolates itself from the remainder of the base and its subsequent contraction forces some of the digesta into the colon.

Pressure recordings and myoelectrical measurements

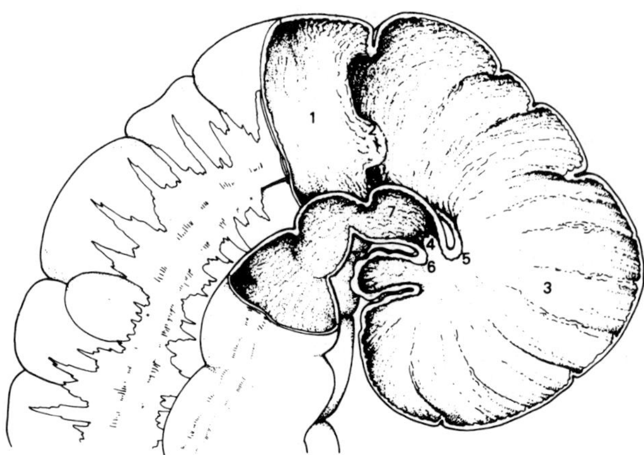

Figure 17.13. Physiological anatomy of horse cecum. (1) Caudal part of base of cecum; (2) ileal papilla with opening of ileum in center; (3) cupola; (4) cecocolic osteum with its (5) dorsal lips and (6) ventral lips; and (7) vestibule of right ventral colon. (From Dyce and Hartman 1976, *Res. Vet. Sci.* 20:40–46.)

have shown coordination of this progressive motility pattern from the ileum, through the cecum, and into the right ventral colon. Other patterns associated with mixing of ingesta are initiated locally and include spike bursts beginning at the apex and conducted to the cranial base, spike bursts beginning at the caudal base and conducted to the apex, and spike bursts beginning at the cranial base and conducted to the apex.

In general, two types of *contractile movement* are observed in the colon. First, there are stationary haustral contractions that perform a mixing function. Second, there are oral and aboral peristaltic movements. The stationary haustral contractions actually increase the resistance to flow; therefore, zones of high pressure and increased motor activity cannot be equated with aboral flow. There must be a withdrawal of this peripheral resistance for propulsion through the colon to take place.

Antiperistaltic movements also impede digesta flow. As discussed above, these seem to occur most commonly in the most proximal colon of ruminants and rodents and serve to fill the cecum. In the cat they occur at about the midpoint of the colon, but apparently no retrograde movement occurs in the colon of the dog. In the horse retrograde movement occurs at the pelvic flexure and thus delays movement of ingesta from the ventral colon to the dorsal colon. The pelvic flexure zone is also a site of narrowing of the large colon (Fig. 16.2). Thus there is probably also anatomical resistance at this point. The analogous zone in the pig colon (spiral colon flexure) is also a major point of resistance to digesta flow and thereby keeps the centripetal spiral colon filled. A second point of major resistance to flow is the junction between the dorsal colon and the small colon in the horse and at the termination of the spiral colon in the pig. Again, these zones are anatomically analogous in these species.

A third type of movement occasionally observed in the dog, cat, and human is an *aboral mass movement*. In the dog, mass movements start within 3 cm of the ileocolic junction and can evacuate the entire length of the colon, once peripheral resistance is withdrawn. In this case, very little force (e.g., gravity) is required to move ingesta over long distances. In the cat these movements are generated much lower in the colon.

Control of large intestine motility

Slow-wave activity in the colon and thus the direction and force of contraction differ from that in the small intestine. The frequency gradient of the slow wave is the reverse of that in the small intestine. A pacemaker in midcolon sends electrical slow waves in both directions, and a large percentage of these are conducted orally. In contrast, pacemakers in the proximal colon send slow waves aborally, but their lower frequency allows net propulsion of contents to occur in the oral direction in some instances. Thus aboral transit is delayed and a reservoir function has been assigned to the proximal colon. From mid to distal colon there is little or no frequency gradient. As in the small intestine, contractions of the muscle are associated with spike bursts. Spike bursts migrating variable distances in either direction are seen attending slow waves, and these are associated with both peristaltic and antiperistaltic activity.

The colon pacemaker generates a second type of signal that apparently is independent of slow wave activity. This is characterized by a prolonged burst of spikes migrating in the aboral direction and is attended by prolonged and powerful contractions of the circular muscle layer. This electrical activity is known as the *migrating spike burst* and is responsible for the mass movement of ingesta. The predominant electrical activity for the cat colon is shown in Fig. 17.14 and indicates a pacemaker position in approximately the midcolon. A similar pacemaker area is found in the pelvic flexure area in the horse.

The neural and endocrine control of colonic motility is not well understood. Cholinergic drugs prolong slow wave duration and increase the incidence of spike bursts of contractions. These effects are antagonized by atropine. Adrenergic drugs are inhibitory to spike activity in high doses. As in the small intestine, gastrin and CCK stimulate contractions of colonic smooth muscle, and secretin inhibits these contractions.

In summary, the colon displays stationary haustral, peristaltic, and antiperistaltic activity. The stationary haustral contractions perform a mixing function and delay the transit of contents. The resistance produced by haustral contractions must be withdrawn before peristaltic activity can drive the contents in the aboral direction. Antiperistaltic activity is responsible for the reservoir function of the proximal colon. The above factors explain the paradox that increased colonic motor activity is usually associated with constipation, whereas decreased activity is associated with diarrhea.

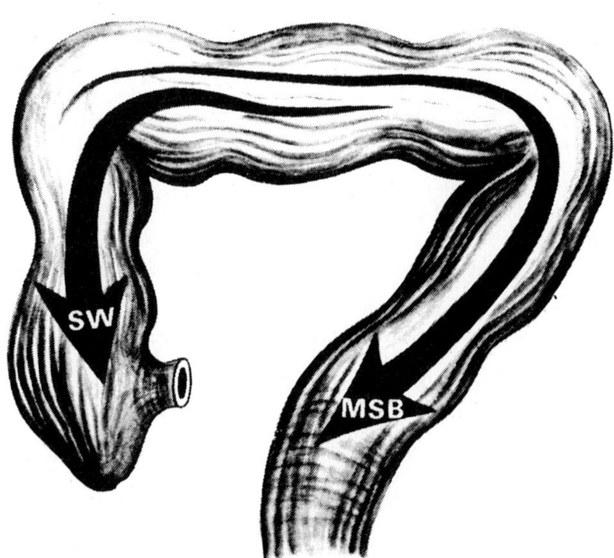

Figure 17.14. Proposed scheme for flow in the cat colon related to electrical events. Electrical slow waves (SW) are oriented in such a way that they appear to spread toward the cecum, away from a pacemaker whose position is highly variable but about midway along the colon. Since slow waves appear to pace rhythmic contractions, such contractions should produce flow with a polarity in the same direction (*arrow,* SW), although this polarity is probably not fixed. The migrating spike bursts (MSB) begin at a variable position in the middle or proximal colon and migrate toward the rectum. Since contractions accompany them, the contractions should produce flow with a polarity in the same direction (*arrow,* MSB). The migrating spike burst also has the capacity to reverse direction. (From Christensen, Anuras, and Hauser, *Gastroenterology* 66:240–47, © 1974, the Williams & Wilkins Co., Baltimore.)

Defecation

Defecation is a reflex act in which the feces are discharged from the terminal colon and rectum. It, like emesis, may be aided by abdominal press produced by muscle contraction with the glottis closed. It is subject to voluntary inhibition in trained animals and humans.

The efferent pathways of the defecation reflex are cholinergic. Thus, parasympathomimetic drugs make the reflex more vigorous. Distention of the terminal colon and rectum is the normal stimulus for the reflex, which includes strong peristaltic movements of the terminal colon, contraction of the longitudinal muscle of the rectum, and relaxation of the internal and external anal sphincters.

Frightened animals frequently defecate, presumably by facilitation of the reflex by centers in the brain. In humans, cord damage above the lumbosacral region results in transient incontinence. The reflex soon returns, and autonomous evacuation follows mass movement in the proximal colon. The latter is strongly influenced by ileal outflow, and this in turn is affected by eating.

REFERENCES

Argenzio, R.A., Lowe, J.E., Pickard, D.W., and Stevens, C.E. 1974. Digesta passage and water exchange in the equine large intestine. *Am. J. Physiol.* 226:1035–42.

Banta, C.A., Clemens, E.T., Krinsky, M.M., and Sheffy, B.E. 1979. Sites of organic acid production and patterns of digesta movement in the gastrointestinal tract of dogs. *J. Nutr.* 109:1592–1600.

Bortoff, A. 1976. Myogenic control of intestinal motility. *Physiol. Rev.* 56:418–34.

Burrows, C.F. 1980. Diseases of the colon, rectum, and anus in the dog and cat. In N.V. Anderson, ed., *Veterinary Gastroenterology,* Lea & Febiger, Philadelphia. Pp. 553–92.

Christensen, J. 1971. The controls of gastrointestinal movements: Some old and new views. *New Engl. J. Med.* 285:85–98.

Christensen, J. 1975. Myoelectric control of the colon. *Gastroenterology* 68:601–9.

Christensen, J. 1987. Motility of the colon. In L.R. Johnson, ed., *Physiology of the Gastrointestinal Tract.* 2d ed. Raven Press, New York. Pp. 665–93.

Christensen, J., Anuras, S., and Hauser, R.L. 1974. Migrating spike bursts and electrical slow waves in the cat colon: Effect of sectioning. *Gastroenterology* 66:240–47.

Christensen, J., Weisbrodt, N.W., and Hauser, R.L. 1972. Electrical slow waves of the proximal colon of the cat in diarrhea. *Gastroenterology* 62:1167–73.

Clemens, E.T., Stevens, C.E., and Southworth, M. 1975. Sites of organic acid production and pattern of digesta movement in the gastrointestinal tract of swine. *J. Nutr.* 105:759–68.

Code, C.F., and Carlson, H.C. 1968. Motor activity of the stomach. In *Handbook of Physiology.* Sec. 6, C.F. Code and W. Heidel. eds., *Alimentary Canal.* Vol. 4, *Motility.* Am. Physiol. Soc., Washington. Pp. 1903–16.

Connell, A.M. 1968. Motor action of the large bowel. In *Handbook of Physiology.* Sec. 6, C.F. Code and W. Heidel, eds., *Alimentary Canal.* Vol. 4, *Motility.* Am. Physiol. Soc., Washington, Pp. 2075–94.

Cooke, A.R. 1975. Control of gastric emptying and motility. *Gastroenterology* 68:804–16.

Cooke, A.R., and Christensen, J. 1973. Motor functions of the stomach. In M.H. Sleisenger and J.S. Fordtran, eds., *Gastrointestinal Disease.* W.B. Saunders, Philadelphia. Pp. 115–26.

Cooke, A.R., and Clark, E.D. 1976. Effect of first part of duodenum on gastric emptying in dogs: Response to acid, fat, glucose, and neural blockade. *Gastroenterology* 70:550–55.

Daniel, E.E., ed. 1974. *Proceedings, Fourth International Symposium on Gastrointestinal Motility.* Mitchell, Vancouver.

Davenport, H.W., ed. 1971. *Physiology of the Digestive Tract.* 3d ed. Year Book, Chicago.

Debas, H.T., Farooq, O., and Grossman, M.I. 1975. Inhibition of gastric emptying as a physiological action of cholecystokinin. *Gastroenterology* 68:1211–17.

Dinoso, V.P., Jr., Meshkin Pour, H., Lorber, S.H., Gutierrez, J.G., and Chey, W.Y. 1973. Motor responses of the sigmoid colon and rectum to exogenous cholecystokinin and secretin. *Gastroenterology* 65:438–44.

Dyce, K.M., and Hartman, W. 1976. A cinefluoroscopic study of the caecal base of the horse. *Res. Vet. Sci.* 20:40–46.

Farrar, T., and Ramirez, M. 1971. The effect of gastrointestinal hormones on small intestinal motility. In L. Demling and R. Ottenjunn, eds., *Gastrointestinal Motility.* Georg Thieme Verlag. Stuttgart. Pp. 192–93.

Fordtran, J.S. 1973. Vomiting. In M.H. Sleisenger and J.S. Fordtran, eds., *Gastrointestinal Disease.* W.B. Saunders, Philadelphia. Pp. 127–43.

Hancock, J. 1953. Grazing behavior of cattle. *Anim. Breed. Abstr.* 21:1–13.

Hendrix, T.R., Castell, D.O., and Wood, J.D. 1987. Alimentary tract motility: Stomach, small intestine, colon and biliary tree. In *Undergraduate Teaching Project in Gastroenterology and Liver Disease.* American Gastroenterological Association, Thorofare, N.J.

Hukuhara, T., and Neya, T. 1968. The movements of the colon of rats and guinea pigs. *Jpn. J. Physiol.* 18:551–62.

Hunt, J.N., and Knox, M.T. 1968. Regulation of gastric emptying. In *Handbook of Physiology.* Sec. 6, C.F. Code and W. Heidel, eds., *Ali-*

mentary Canal. Vol. 4, *Motility*. Am. Physiol. Soc., Washington. Pp. 1917–35.

Hwang. K. 1954. Mechanism of transportation of the content of the esophagus. *J. Appl. Physiol.* 6:781–96.

Hwang, K., Grossman, M.I., and Ivy, A.C. 1948. Nervous control of the cervical portion of the esophagus. *Am. J. Physiol.* 154:343–57.

Iggo, A. 1955. Tension receptors in the stomach and urinary bladder. *J. Physiol.* 128:593–607.

Ingelfinger, F.L. 1958. Esophageal motility. *Physiol. Rev.* 38:533–84.

Kelley, M.L., Wilbur, D.L., Schlegal, J.F., and Code, C.F. 1960. Deglutitive responses in the gastro-esophageal sphincter in healthy human beings. *J. Appl. Physiol.* 15:483–88.

Kosterlitz, H.W. 1968. Intrinsic and extrinsic nervous control of motility of the stomach and the intestines. In *Handbook of Physiology*. Sec. 6. C.F. Code and W. Heidel, eds., *Alimentary Canal*. Vol. 4, *Motility*. Am. Physiol. Soc., Washington. Pp. 2147–72.

Leek, B.F. 1972. Abdominal visceral receptors. In H. Autrum, ed., *Handbook of Sensory Physiology*. Vol. 3, pt. 1. E. Neil, ed., *Enteroreceptors*. Springer-Verlag, New York. Pp. 113–60.

Makhlouf, G.M. 1974. The neuroendocrine design of the gut. *Gastroenterology* 67:159–84.

McCarthy, L.E., and Borison, H.L. 1974. Respiratory mechanics of vomiting in decerebrate cats. *Am. J. Physiol.* 226:738–43.

Meyer, J.H. 1987. Motility of the stomach and gastroduodenal junction. In L.R. Johnson, ed., *Physiology of the Gastrointestinal Tract*. 2d ed. Raven Press, New York. Pp. 613–29.

Pickard, D.W., and Stevens, C.E. 1972. Digesta flow through the rabbit large intestine. *Am. J. Physiol.* 222:1161–66.

Rayner, V., and Wenham, G. 1986. Small intestinal motility and transit by electromyography and radiology in the fasted and fed pig. *J. Physiol.* 379:245–56.

Ross, M.W., Cullen, K.K., and Rutkowski, J.A. 1990. Myoelectric activity of the ileum, cecum, and right ventral colon in ponies during the interdigestive, nonfeeding and digestive periods. *Am. J. Vet. Res.* 51:561–66.

Ross, M.W., Donawick, W.J., Sellers, A.F., and Lowe, J.E. 1986. Normal motility of the cecum and right ventral colon in ponies. *Am. J. Vet. Res.* 47:1756–62.

Sellers, A.F., Lowe, J.E., and Brondum, J. 1979. Motor events in equine large colon. *Am. J. Physiol.* 237:E457–64.

Sellers, A.F., Lowe, J.E., Drost, C.J., Rendano, V.T., Georgi, J.R., and Roberts, M.C. 1982. Retropulsion-propulsion in equine large colon. *Am. J. Vet. Res.* 43:390–96.

Shedd, D.P., Scatliff, J.H., and Kirchner, J.H. 1960. The buccopharyngeal propulsive mechanism in human deglutition. *Surgery* 48:846–53.

Smith, C.C., and Brizzee, K.R. 1961. Cineradiographic analysis of vomiting in the cat. I. Lower esophagus, stomach and small intestine. *Gastroenterology* 40:654–64.

Smith, J., Kelly, K.A., and Weinshilboum, R.M. 1977. Pathophysiology of postoperative ileus. *Arch. Surg.* 112:203–9.

Szurszewski, J.H. 1987. Electrical basis for gastrointestinal motility. In L.R. Johnson, ed., *Physiology of the Gastrointestinal Tract*. 2d ed. Raven Press, New York. Pp. 383–422.

Tribe, D.E. 1955. The behavior of grazing animals. In J. Hammond, ed., *Recent Progress in the Physiology of Farm Animals*, vol. 2. Butterworth, London.

Weisbrodt, N.W. 1987. Motility of the small intestine. In L.R. Johnson, ed., *Physiology of the Gastrointestinal Tract*. 3d ed. Raven Press, New York. Pp. 631–63.

Weisbrodt, N.W., and Christensen, J. 1972. Electrical activity of the cat duodenum in fasting and vomiting. *Gastroenterology* 63:1004–10.

CHAPTER 18

Secretory Functions of the Gastrointestinal Tract | by Robert A. Argenzio

Secretion of electrolytes, water, and digestive enzymes is an active, energy-requiring process controlled by the neuroendocrine system. The salivary glands, stomach, pancreas, liver, and intestine are all capable of secreting large volumes of their respective fluids. Because the sequence of events that make up intestinal absorption and secretion are not easily separable, these processes will be considered together in Chapter 20. In addition, the energetics and mechanisms of cellular ion transport processes will be considered in detail in Chap. 20. Although these will be specifically related to the intestine, the same general principles apply to ion transport of other secretory tissues and, therefore, will not be considered in detail in this chapter.

The extracellular agents that initiate active secretory processes are the neurotransmitters of the autonomic nervous system and the gastrointestinal hormones. Central or reflex stimuli cause the increased release of these agents; the agents then activate the system by occupying specific receptors on the cell membranes, as was discussed in Chapter 16. Intracellular mechanisms are then activated, and these bring about a coordinated response that leads to the secretion of ions or enzymes by the target cells. These intracellular, biochemical events were also discussed in Chapter 16.

SALIVARY SECRETION

The salivary glands provide the digestive fluids for the first part of the digestive tract: the mouth and the forestomach (where present). The term *salivary glands* refers to the three main salivary glands, all of which are paired, and the numerous small glands found in the mucous membranes of the mouth. Saliva is the mixed secretion of all these glands. The three main glands are the parotid, the submaxillary (mandibular), and the sublingual.

Functional anatomy

A functional salivary unit called the *salivon* is shown in Fig. 18.1. The salivon is a converging system beginning most proximally with several acini that converge on an intercalated duct. Numerous intercalated ducts are drained by a striated duct or, in some cases (Fig. 18.1), directly into a granular tubule, and these empty into fewer excretory ducts. Finally, the excretory ducts converge to form a single main excretory duct, which leads from each gland and ends at the oral cavity.

Blood vessels and nerves enter the gland at the hilus. The flow of blood is in a direction opposite to flow of saliva; the arterial supply to the entire salivon may be countercurrent. The salivary glands receive efferent innervation from the sympathetic and parasympathetic divisions of the autonomic nervous system.

Function of saliva

In all mammalian species, facilitation of mastication and deglutition is a primary function of saliva. This is partic-

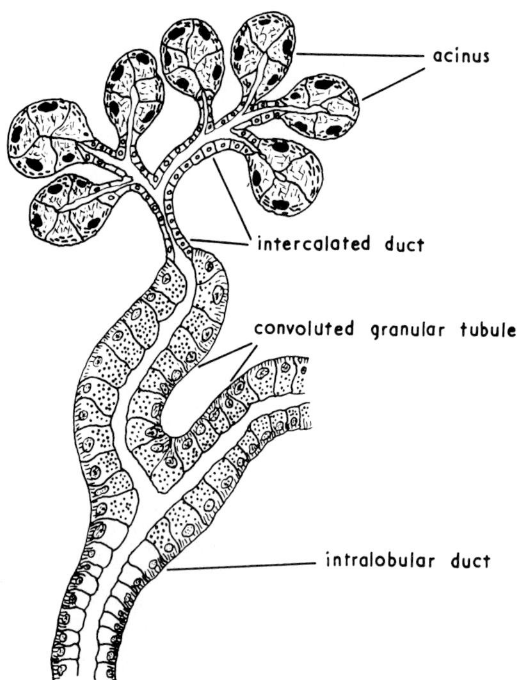

Figure 18.1. The acinar, granular tubule, and intralobular duct system (salivon) of the rat submaxillary salivary gland. (From Leeson 1961, in Burgen and Emmelin, eds., *Physiology of the Salivary Glands,* Edward Arnold Publishers, Ltd.)

ularly important in herbivores. For example, secretory flows as high as 50 ml/min have been recorded in a 150 kg pony during mastication, and the salivary glands of the cow secrete from 100 to 200 L/day. In the cat and the dog, salivary secretion has the special function of evaporative cooling, and the parotid gland of the dog under intense parasympathetic stimulation is capable of secreting at 10 times the rate (per gram of gland) of the parotid gland in humans. Thus regulation of body heat by this means is as effective as evaporation of sweat in humans.

In the ruminant, salivary secretion has an additional important function. It is essential to microbial digestion in the forestomach for two reasons. First, a fluid environment must be maintained for this process (Chap. 19). Because the forestomach has no secretory glands, this fluid is derived solely from salivary secretion. Second, large quantities of acid are produced in the rumen from microbial digestion; this acid must be rapidly neutralized to preserve normal rumen pH. Ruminant saliva is particularly rich in HCO_3 and PO_4 buffers and, therefore, has a powerful neutralizing capacity.

In ruminants, the parotid gland spontaneously secretes a large volume of fluid that is not under control of the secretory nerves. This is particularly fortunate because forestomach digestion is a continuous process and requires a continuous input of buffered fluid. During eating or ruminating, there is a fourfold increase in volume of secretion due to stimulation by the nerves. Thus, over the course of a day, the forestomach will receive net salivary secretion equivalent to two times the total extracellular fluid (ECF) volume. These figures emphasize the importance of large volumes of buffered fluid for the microbial process and also illustrate the importance of reabsorption of this fluid to preserve the ECF volume from which it was derived.

Composition of saliva

The ionic composition of saliva varies greatly among glands and species; however, two general types of parotid salivary secretion have been described in mammals. Fig. 18.2 shows the concentration of the main ions in the saliva of the dog and sheep as the salivary flow rate is increased. The basal (unstimulated) secretion from the submaxillary and parotid glands of nonruminants is markedly hypotonic. As the secretory flow increases, the concentration of sodium, chloride, and HCO_3 increases; at maximal flow rates the secretory fluid is approximately isotonic. In contrast, the composition of ruminant saliva is isotonic at any flow rate; however, there is a reciprocal change in PO_4 and HCO_3 concentrations as the flow rate increases. Therefore the ruminant saliva is highly buffered at all times, but the HCO_3 buffer system predominates during eating and ruminating.

Saliva also contains proteins; the chief digestive enzyme produced by the salivary glands is amylase, but this enzyme is absent in carnivores and ruminants.

Secretory process

Figure 18.3 shows the transepithelial transport of ions between the acinar and ductal fluid and the blood in ruminants. The primary secretion derived from the acinar cells is approximately the same as the blood except for the high

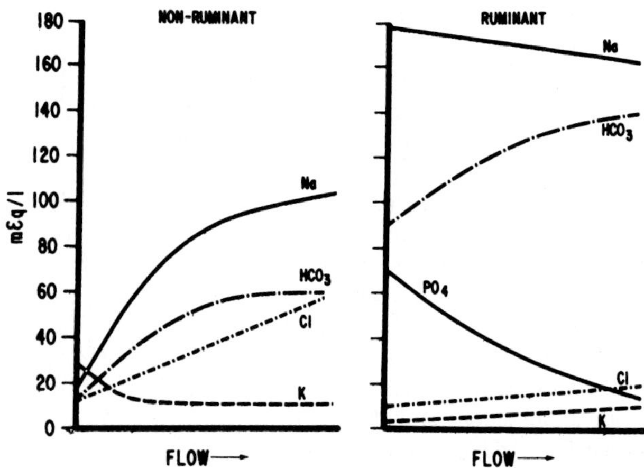

Figure 18.2. Concentration of major electrolytes in saliva of dog (nonruminant) or sheep (ruminant) as the salivary flow rate is increased. (Modified from Thaysen, Thorn, and Schwartz 1954, *Am. J. Physiol.* 178:155; and from Blair-West, Coghlan, Denton, and Wright 1968, in *Handbook of Physiology,* sec. 6, Code and Heidel, eds., *Alimentary Canal,* vol. 2, *Secretion,* Am. Physiol. Soc., Washington.)

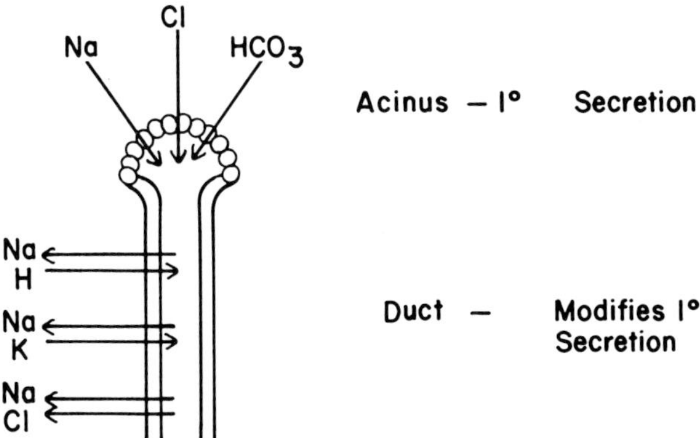

Figure 18.3. Primary electrolyte secretion by acinus (1° = primary) and exchanges of electrolytes along ducts of a salivary unit in nonruminants. At low rates of flow, duct modification would predominate and a relative increase in K concentration and a decrease in Na and Cl concentration would occur. The H ion entering duct fluid would react with the luminal bicarbonate, lowering its concentration.

PO_4 and HCO_3 concentrations that would be present in ruminant saliva. This secreted fluid is dependent primarily on active Na transport across the acinar cell from blood to lumen. Therefore, the changes observed in salivary composition are due to modification of the fluid along the ducts. More distally, Na and Cl are partially reabsorbed and K and H ions are secreted. The H ions neutralize the luminal HCO_3 and decrease its concentration. Thus, at high flow rates, the composition of saliva will approach the primary secretion; this is because there is less time for ductular exchange or reabsorption of ions. In the parotid salivary gland secretions of the dog, cat, rat, and human, the hypotonicity of the secretion at low flow rates is due to the ductular net reabsorption of ions with very little net fluid absorption occurring simultaneously.

Control of salivary secretion

The control of salivary secretion other than the spontaneous secretion of saliva is exerted solely by the nervous system. Parasympathetic fibers contribute a dense secretory innervation to the glands mediated by acetylcholine (ACh). In general, cholinergic stimulation results in a marked increase in salivary flow that is low in protein content. Adrenergic fibers from the sympathetic system are also present. These have less of an effect on flow rate, but they affect the salivary composition. Sympathetic nerves also carry vasoconstrictive fibers to the blood vessels of the salivary glands. Sympathetic saliva is especially rich in protein and mucin. The increase in secretory rate is brought about by both central stimulation from salivary centers in the medulla and reflex stimulation from mechanoreceptors in the mouth and stomach.

The coupling of cholinergic stimulation to salivary secretion is mediated by the Ca system as discussed in Chapter 16. In contrast, adrenergic stimulation is mediated by cyclic AMP. Calcium is not required to mediate the elevation in cAMP; however, Ca is required to produce the enzyme secretion in response to increased cAMP levels.

Although autonomic nerves govern the secretory flow and some of the salivary composition, mineralocorticoid hormones from the adrenal glands have a profound influence on the Na:K ratio of ruminant saliva. If Na is withheld from a sheep with a parotid fistula for 48 hours, urinary Na excretion falls to zero; in addition, salivary Na falls from 180 to 60 mEq/L and is reciprocated by an increase in K concentration. Therefore the normally large urinary excretion of K is shifted to the saliva in order to conserve Na. As illustrated previously, a large reservoir of Na is sequestered in the forestomach because of the tremendous amounts of Na and fluid secreted by the salivary glands. In addition to Na conservation by the salivary glands, the rate of salivary secretion also falls about 50 percent in a Na-depleted sheep, probably because of decreased blood flow through the gland. Because of these two effects, therefore, approximately 80 percent of the Na that otherwise would be delivered to the forestomachs, is conserved by the salivary glands and returned to the ECF.

The marked change in the Na:K ratio is due to increased levels of circulating aldosterone. In addition to stimulating the salivary glands, this hormone has pronounced stimulatory effects on active Na absorption in several tissues, including tissues of the kidney and colon. Aldosterone may act in the salivary glands by increasing the ductular reabsorption of Na in exchange for K.

GASTRIC SECRETION

The stomach secretes HCl and pepsinogen into the lumen and the hormone gastrin into the blood. The complex control of these secretions is regulated centrally as well as reflexly from mechanical and chemical receptors in the stomach and duodenum.

Functional anatomy

There are variations among species in the distribution and composition of the epithelium lining the stomach (Fig. 18.4). The simple stomach of both the human and the dog is lined with three major types of tissue: pyloric mucosa, proper gastric (oxyntic) mucosa, and cardiac mucosa. Pyloric mucosa lines the aboral portion of the simple stomach. Orad to this is a relatively large segment of proper gastric mucosa, which secretes both pepsinogen and HCl. Near the gastroesophageal junction, the proper gastric mucosa merges with the cardiac mucosa. The pig stomach is also a noncompartmentalized organ with the same orad progression of mucosal types, except that cardiac mucosa occupies a much larger percent of the pig stomach, and an additional small area of stratified squamous epithelium surrounds the gastroesophageal junction. The stomach of the horse is simple, but stratified squamous epithelium occupies a major part of its oral extremity. The distribution of gastric epithelium in the rat is similar to that of the horse. Because of a

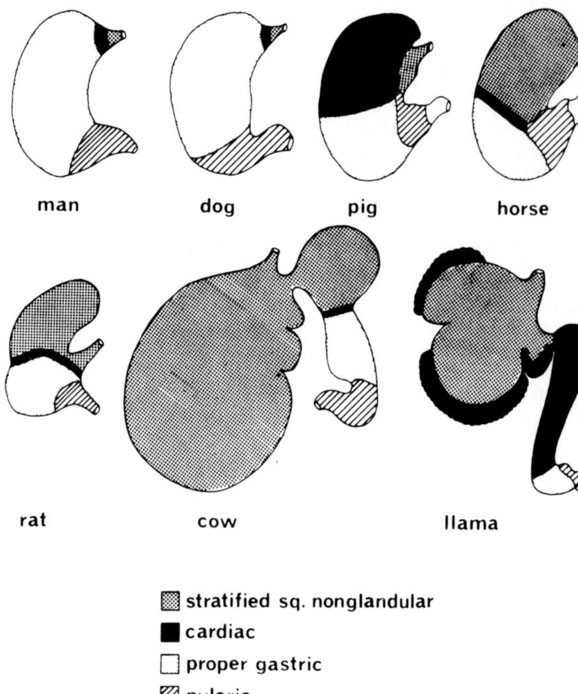

Figure 18.4. Variations in the type and distribution of gastric mucosa. Stomachs are not drawn to scale; for example, the capacity of the adult bovine stomach is approximately 70 times that of the human stomach, or 14 times the capacity per kilogram of body weight. (Modified from Stevens 1973, in Ussing and Thorn, eds., *Transport Mechanisms in Epithelia,* Munksgaard, Copenhagen.)

stricture at the junction of the cardiac glandular and stratified squamous epithelia, the rat stomach is partially divided into two compartments. The stomachs of the cow and the llama are extremely enlarged and compartmentalized. In the bovine stomach, typical of pecora, most of the additional surface area is lined with stratified squamous epithelium. The llama stomach, typically camelid, contains a large segment of cardiac mucosa in its third compartment as well as islands of this glandular epithelium within the areas of stratified epithelium that line its first two compartments.

The proper gastric mucosa contains the compound tubular glands that secrete HCl (parietal or oxyntic cells) and pepsinogen from the peptic or chief cells. This area of mucosa is of critical importance to the gastric digestive process, and it has received extensive study in a wide range of species. The glands of the pyloric region secrete mucus and some pepsinogen. The pyloric region also contains the gastrin cell, which, on appropriate stimulation, releases gastrin into the blood.

It is generally thought that cardiac glands secrete only mucus. In the pig, however, this relatively large area secretes HCO_3 in exchange for Cl. There is evidence of a similar exchange of anions by the cardiac mucosa lining the glandular pouches in the forestomach compartments of the llama.

Information on the function of stratified squamous tissue is largely limited to studies of the forestomach of ruminants. In these animals the stratified squamous tissue serves as a major site for absorption of volatile fatty acids (VFA), Na, and Cl. In addition, it may aid in neutralization of VFAs in rumen contents by secretion of HCO_3. Its stratified squamous structure is presumably protective in the same sense as the mucous secretion of the epithelium lining the remainder of the gastrointestinal tract.

Secretion of HCl

The parietal cells of the oxyntic zone actively secrete H and Cl ions in concentrations approximating 150 mM. Since the H ion concentration in gastric juice is some 3 to 4 million times greater than in the plasma, the large amount of energy (ca. 1500 calories per liter of gastric juice) derived principally from aerobic metabolism is required to transport H into the lumen. The mechanism by which the cell secretes HCl is shown in Fig. 18.5. Hydration of CO_2 in the parietal cell is responsible for the continuous production of H and HCO_3 ions. This reaction is catalyzed by the carbonic anhydrase enzyme present in high concentrations in these cells. The H ions are transported into the lumen by an active pump mechanism coupled to cellular metabolism.

Chloride is secreted into the lumen by a mechanism that may be coupled by some means to the H pump, inasmuch as the stoichiometry of secreted H and Cl is 1:1. The Cl ions available for transport appear to be derived from the operation of a Cl-HCO_3 exchange mechanism on the contraluminal membrane. Thus for every H ion secreted into the lumen, one HCO_3 ion diffuses into the blood in exchange for Cl (Fig. 18.6). This metabolic alkalosis that occurs during active acid secretion following a meal is known as the *alkaline tide.*

Gastric mucosal barrier

Because the H ion concentration in the gastric lumen is many times greater than that in the cell or lamina propria,

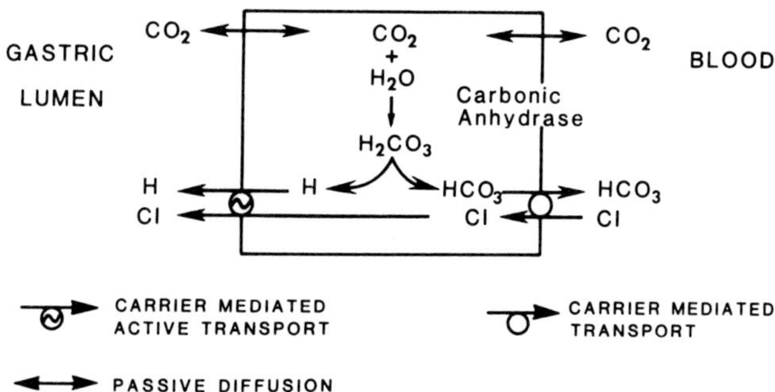

Figure 18.5. One possible mechanism for secretion of HCl by gastric parietal cell. The H and HCO_3 ions formed by the breakdown of carbonic acid are transported across opposing membranes by an active, energy-requiring process (H) and by a counter transport mechanism (HCO_3). (See Chap. 20 for description of carrier energetics.)

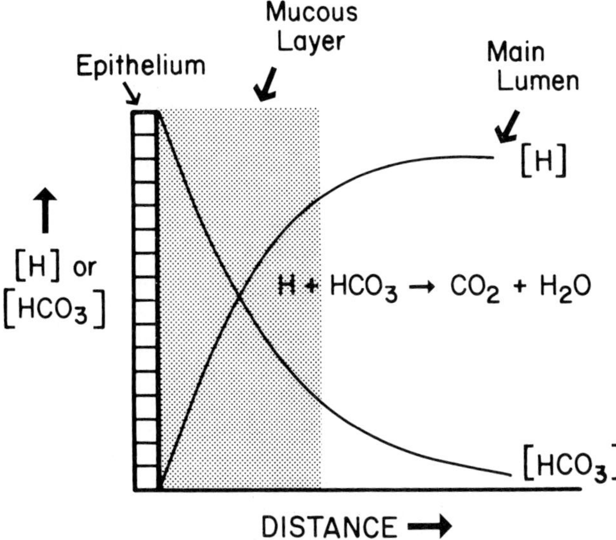

Figure 18.6. Mucus and bicarbonate produce a pH profile adjacent to epithelium. The mucus forms an unstirred layer adjacent to the surface epithelium in which bicarbonate is trapped. As bicarbonate diffuses into the mucus, it meets and neutralizes the H ion, which is diffusing down its concentration gradient from the bulk lumen contents.

there must be a means of preventing back-diffusion of the ion into the surrounding tissues. This barrier is due to several mechanisms. First, the electrical resistance of the apical cell membrane and junctional complexes of the oxyntic gland area are extremely high. This resistance, plus the lumen-negative electrical potential, restricts passive H ion movement. Second, mucus is secreted by the surface and neck cells in response to ACh and mechanical stimulation to form an unstirred layer adjacent to the mucosa. Third, bicarbonate ions are secreted by the surface epithelium and become trapped in the mucous gel. As shown in Fig. 18.6, H ions diffusing from the lumen toward the epithelium become neutralized in this zone and their concentration approaches zero next to the epithelium. Fourth, endogenous prostaglandins seem to be important in gastric mucosal defense. Although the precise mechanism by which prostaglandins protect the epithelium is not known, certain effects, such as increasing the mucosal blood flow and stimulating bicarbonate secretion by the surface cells, are probably of importance. In addition, these compounds may confer some degree of direct "cytoprotection" to the mucosa.

Although these mechanisms normally provide an effective barrier against both H ion and pepsin, there are certain agents capable of breaking the barrier, such as weak acids (aspirin, acetic acid), nonsteroidal anti-inflammatory drugs, and bile salts. The action of anti-inflammatory drugs may be due to their inhibition of endogenous prostaglandin synthesis. Once the barrier is broken, significant numbers of H ions diffuse back into the tissue. These cause mast cells to release histamine and increase capillary permeability. The result is formation of edema and movement of extracellular fluid into the lumen. Damage of cells causes leakage of K into the lumen and if the damage is severe, capillary bleeding occurs and blood appears in the lumen.

Recent studies have provided evidence of one additional mechanism in protection of gastric mucosa. This event, termed *restitution,* is a process by which the superficial epithelium is restored within minutes after complete denudation by various injurious agents. The process involves active migratory mechanisms of the epithelium; viable cells adjacent to damaged areas migrate onto the surface and spread out over the denuded area by extending *pseudopodia.* Thus a completely barren surface is rapidly covered with such cells, providing an effective barrier to large molecules in the lumen. This process is regarded by some as a *first line of defense* against mucosal injury.

Control of gastric acid secretion

Three main substances in the body stimulate the parietal cell to secrete acid. Each of these reaches the parietal cell by a different route. Acetylcholine is released from cholinergic neurons. The endocrine substance, gastrin, is released from the G cells in the pyloric gland area to the circulation, where it comes back to reach the parietal cell. The paracrine substance, histamine, is released from mast cells located in the vicinity of the parietal cell.

The interaction of ACh, gastrin, and histamine on the parietal cell is shown in Fig. 18.7, ACh and gastrin operate

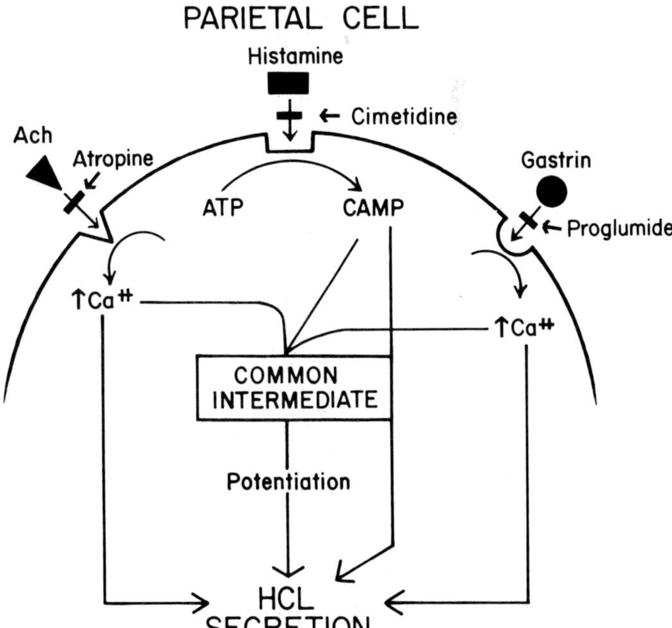

Figure 18.7. Acetylcholine, histamine, and gastrin all stimulate HCl secretion. The action of ACh or gastrin is potentiated by histamine, which is always present to some degree near the parietal cell. In the presence of histamine receptor blockade, ACh or gastrin elicits only weak responses. Accordingly, blockade of cholinergic receptors with atropine or gastrin receptors with proglumide would be less effective than those with cimetidine in inhibiting HCl secretion. Ach, acetylcholine.

through intracellular increases in calcium, which stimulate acid secretion. Histamine operates through the cAMP system. These two intracellular messengers interact in such a way with a common intermediate as to cause potentiation of acid secretion. Therefore, the combination of ACh and histamine or of gastrin and histamine causes a much greater secretion of acid than each agent alone. The highly effective action of histamine (H-2) receptor antagonists, such as cimetidine, in blocking acid secretion can be explained as a direct inhibition of the potentiating action of histamine on acid secretion stimulated by gastrin or ACh. It is assumed that a background of histamine is continuously acting on the parietal cell as a result of mast cell secretion. One protective effect of certain prostaglandins against acid injury of the mucosa is that they are capable of inhibiting the formation of cAMP in the parietal cell. Accordingly, they block both the basal and potentiating actions of histamine on acid secretion.

Phases of gastric secretion

The *cephalic phase* of gastric secretion is a result of central stimulation such as sight, smell, or taste of food and chewing or swallowing. Therefore this response is mediated entirely by the vagus nerve as depicted in Fig. 18.8. Postganglionic release of ACh stimulates the parietal cell to secrete acid as discussed above. In addition, the vagus nerve causes the release of gastrin from the G cell. The mediator of this effect appears to be the peptide *bombesin* that is released from enteric nerves. Gastrin then stimulates the parietal cell to secrete acid. As also shown in Fig. 18.8, vagal stimulation has yet another effect in stimulating acid secretion, and this is explained. Normally, the release of *somatostatin* has the paracrine effect of inhibiting release of gastrin from the G cell. Vagal stimulation inhibits the release of somatostatin, however, thereby removing the suppressor effect of somatostatin on gastrin release.

The *gastric phase* of secretion occurs as a result of the presence of food in the stomach. As shown in Fig. 18.9, this phase includes both vagal and local neural reflexes responding to gastric distention. In addition chemoreceptors on the G cell respond to peptides or amino acids in the gastric lumen. The end result is that both gastrin and ACh stimulate the parietal cell to secrete H.

The *intestinal phase* of secretion begins when food enters the duodenum. One or more hormones released from the duodenal mucosa stimulate gastric secretion. One of these is probably intestinal gastrin, which is present in duodenal as well as antral mucosa in some species (Table 16.3). In the cat, cholecystokinin (CCK) released from duodenal and jejunal mucosa is probably also involved; CCK is a full agonist of gastrin on H ion secretion in this species. In the dog, however, CCK is a partial agonist and competitive inhibitor (see "Neuroendocrine Receptors" in Chap. 16) of gastrin on H ion secretion. The intestinal phase also contains a cholinergic component to stimulate gastric secretion. Most intestinal responses, however, are inhibitory to gastric secretion, as discussed below.

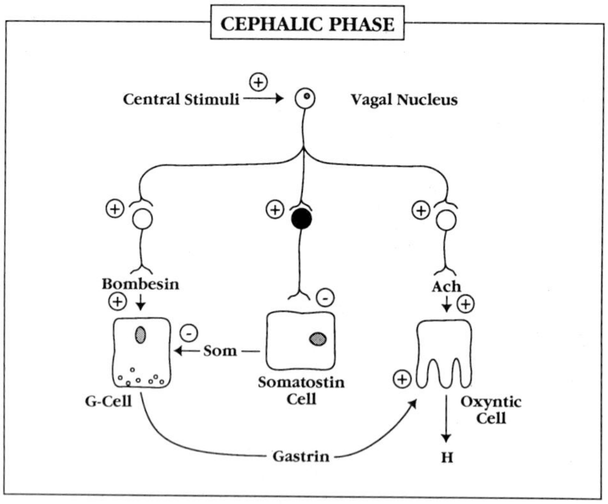

Figure 18.8. The cephalic phase is mediated by the vagus nerve. Vagal stimulation involves three mechanisms that directly or indirectly stimulate gastric acid secretion. Vagal efferent fibers innervate postganglionic cholinergic neurons that innervate the oxyntic (parietal) cell directly and cause HCl secretion. Vagal efferent fibers synapse with enteric neurons containing bombesin, which appears to be the mediator for gastrin release from the G cell. Gastrin then arrives at the oxyntic cell via the circulation. Vagal efferent fibers also synapse with inhibitory neurons innervating the somatostatin cell. Thus somatostatin release is inhibited.

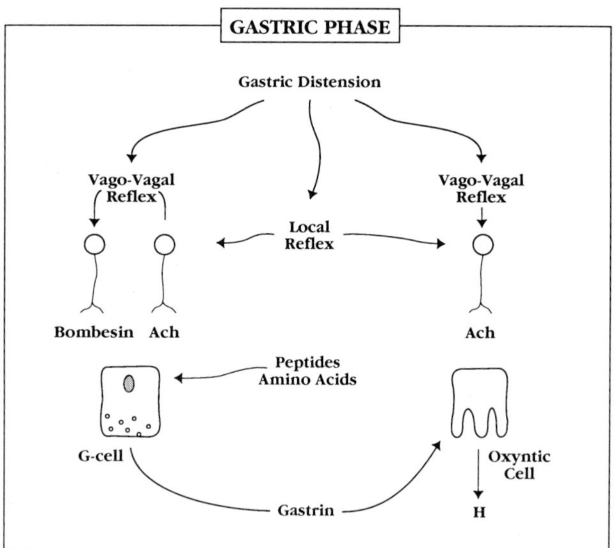

Figure 18.9. Gastric phase involves gastrin and ACh released by distention or protein digestion. The vagovagal reflex is conducted by afferent fibers in the vagi from the stomach to the vagal nuclei in the medulla. The efferent pathways are via postganglionic cholinergic neurons on both the oxyntic and G cells or on bombesin-containing neurons on the G cell. Local cholinergic reflexes that innervate both the oxyntic and the G cells are also activated. In addition, chemoreceptors on the G cell respond to protein digestion products in the lumen. Ach, acetylcholine.

Inhibition of gastric secretion

The most important mechanism to inhibit gastrin release is acidification of the stomach itself. When the stomach is stimulated to secrete acid at mealtime by antral release of gastrin, the luminal pH will decrease with time. When the pH of gastric contents approaches 2.0, gastrin release is almost totally suppressed. These events prevent continuous acid secretion by the stomach. The mechanism that inhibits gastrin release is release of somatostatin by antral acidification acting on the endocrine cells in the pyloric gland mucosa.

Inhibition from the intestine occurs in response to acid, fat, and hypertonic solutions. Therefore the same stimuli that inhibit gastric emptying also inhibit gastric secretion (Chap. 16). There is evidence of both neural and hormonal inhibition. The vagus appears to synapse with fibers inhibitory to gastrin release. Depending on the species, both secretin and CCK may be involved in the inhibitory response, and these two hormones are capable of potentiating each other's inhibitory action. Hormonal inhibition becomes manifest through competitive occupation of gastrin receptors on the parietal cell. For example, CCK is a weak stimulus to acid secretion in the dog when gastrin levels are low; when the gastrin mechanism is fully operative, however, CCK then becomes a potent inhibitor of the secretory response.

Secretion of pepsinogen and intrinsic factor

Pepsinogen, the inactive form of pepsin, is stored in granular form in the chief cells of the gastric mucosa. Pepsinogen is converted to pepsin in the presence of acid in the gastric lumen, beginning at about pH 5. Optimal activity occurs at pH 1.8 to 3.5 and initiates gastric protein digestion. Secretion of pepsinogen is stimulated by the same general stimuli as for HCl, except that secretin enhances pepsinogen secretion. The strongest stimulus for pepsin secretion is cholinergic stimulation.

Intrinsic factor is a mucoprotein secreted by the gastric mucosa. Its secretion is closely correlated with H secretion and is secreted by the same cell. Intrinsic factor interacts with vitamin B_{12}, the extrinsic factor, and forms a complex that binds to receptors in the ileum and facilitates vitamin B_{12} absorption.

PANCREATIC EXOCRINE SECRETION

The functions of the exocrine pancreas are (1) secretion of HCO_3 in an attempt to rectify the acid pH of gastric contents flowing into the duodenum and (2) secretion of enzymes for the luminal digestion of carbohydrate, fat, and protein.

Functional anatomy

The exocrine cells of the pancreas are arranged in acini. The acinar cells, characterized by the presence of zymogen granules, are responsible for the secretion of enzymes. Centroacinar cells appear to separate some of the granular cells from the lumen. These form the initial components of the glandular duct system. Duct lumina that lack acinar cells are designated intercalated ducts. These are collected into large intralobular ducts lined with columnar epithelial cells. The duct system is responsible for the secretion of water and electrolytes, particularly the smaller ducts that contain high levels of carbonic anhydrase. Figure 18.10 shows the functional unit, a pancreon, the origin of the primary secretion, and the passive equilibration of ions along the larger duct systems.

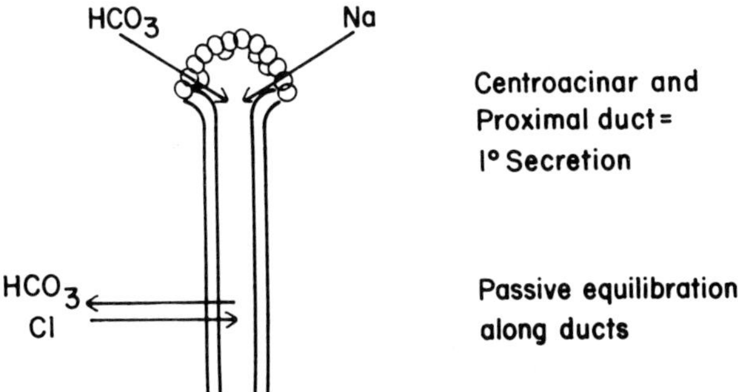

Figure 18.10. Functional unit of pancreas: the pancreon. The individual acinus is a sphere composed of pyramidal cells whose apices are pointed toward a central lumen. Each acinus is drained by a ductule, the most proximal cells of which are called centroacinar cells. The acinar cells are the source of pancreatic enzymes, and the centroacinar and proximal duct cells are the source of bicarbonate-rich fluid. Chloride and bicarbonate exchange passively between plasma and duct fluid.

Electrolyte composition and volume of secretion

The osmolality of pancreatic juice is isotonic at all rates of flow. The Na and K cations are similar in concentration to the plasma cations, and these remain constant at all flow rates. The remarkable distinguishing feature of pancreatic fluid is the HCO_3 concentration, which can reach values as high as 150 mM at maximum flow rates (Fig. 18.11). This HCO_3 anion forms an exact reciprocation with Cl so that at high flow rates the Cl concentration may be less than 20 mM. In the horse, which is an exception to the above situation, a change in the concentration of anions is not seen. The anion content is shared equally by Cl and HCO_3 at all flow rates. In addition, pancreatic secretion of the horse has a number of other unusual features. Even under maximal stimulation, for example, the rate of enzyme secretion is extremely small in comparison with other species. The resting flow of electrolytes and water, however, is already quite profuse and continuous and is further markedly increased when under stimulation. Thus the pancreas of the 100 kg pony secretes 10 to 12 L of fluid per day under normal feeding conditions.

Such high pancreatic flow rates are not seen in the cow (3 to 5 L/100 kg/day) or the sheep (0.5 to 1.0 L/100 kg/day). In the cat and the dog, very little basal pancreatic flow

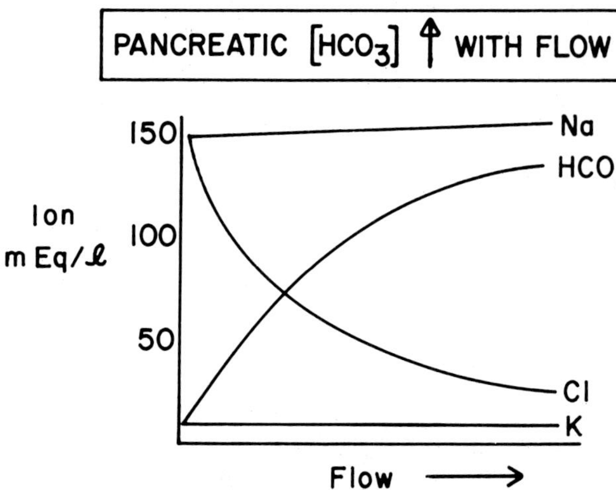

Figure 18.11. Bicarbonate concentration of pancreatic fluid increases with increased flow. At high rates of flow along the ducts there will be little time for passive exchange of Cl and HCO_3 ions, and the fluid will resemble the primary secretion, which is an isotonic solution of $NaHCO_3$.

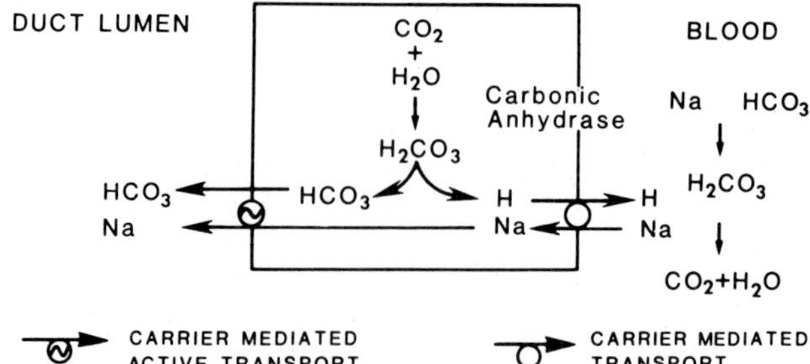

Figure 18.12. One possible mechanism for secretion of HCO_3 by pancreatic centroacinar and ductular cells. The H and HCO_3 ions formed by the breakdown of carbonic acid are transported across opposing membranes of the cell. The H enters the blood in exchange for a Na ion via a counter transport mechanism, and reacts with a HCO_3 ion in the blood to form CO_2. The intracellular HCO_3 ion and the Na ion are probably both actively transported into the lumen but the precise molecular mechanism is unknown.

occurs. When stimulated, however, the pancreas can produce high rates of flow (2 to 3 ml/min in the dog). Because of the feeding habits of these animals, a continuous flow of pancreatic juice is not necessary for HCl neutralization. Therefore it is fortunate that the pancreas can respond rapidly with large rates of flow of buffered fluid and enzymes during a meal, when an excess of HCl and undigested food is rapidly delivered to the duodenum.

Mechanism of electrolyte and water secretion

The pancreatic centroacinar cells and the proximal ductular cells appear to be responsible for active secretion of an isotonic $NaHCO_3$ solution. As this solution passes down the collecting ducts, it is modified by passive exchange of HCO_3 for Cl. At low rates of flow, the opportunity for this exchange would be greatest so that the Cl concentration of pancreatic juice would be highest at the lowest flow rate. This mechanism prevents the pancreas from secreting excess HCO_3 into the lumen during interdigestive periods when it is no longer needed to neutralize HCl.

One mechanism by which the primary secretion could be obtained is shown in Fig. 18.12. As in the gastric parietal cell, a continuous production of H and HCO_3 ions is maintained by the action of carbonic anhydrase, which facilitates the hydration of CO_2. Unlike the parietal cell, however, the H ion is extruded into the plasma in exchange for an Na ion, whereas the HCO_3 ion is transported into the lumen. Thus the secretory cell of the pancreas operates in reverse of the gastric parietal cell and almost exactly neutralizes the HCl in the proximal duodenum. Under normal conditions, therefore, all of the H secreted by the stomach is returned to the ECF, even though it is not the same H ion that was secreted by the stomach. In other words, all of the HCO_3 that entered the ECF during gastric secretion is now returned to the duodenum via the pancreas. Normally, these two mechanisms are so precisely regulated that net addition of acid or base to the ECF or lumen is eventually compensated; in some instances, however, an excess of HCO_3 is delivered into the duodenum. In the horse and the pig, this HCO_3 is needed in the large intestine as a source of buffer (see Chap. 19). In the dog and various other species, however, this excess HCO_3 is recovered by a mechanism in the jejunum (Chap. 20). Therefore in these animals the jejunum provides a reserve function to ensure that all of the pancreatic HCO_3 is returned to the ECF.

Fortunately, the neutralization of acid in the duodenum ($HCl + NaHCO_3 \rightarrow NaCl + CO_2 + H_2O$) is capable of removing all of the excess acidity from the lumen as CO_2 rapidly diffuses into the blood. By this means, the pancreas prevents extreme acidification of the duodenal and jejunal lumen, which would otherwise result in ulceration of these permeable epithelia. Furthermore, pancreatic enzymes cannot operate at the low pH of gastric contents, as was the case with pepsin, and neutralization of HCl in the duodenum establishes an optimal pH of about 6.8 for pancreatic enzyme action.

Mechanism of enzyme secretion

The pancreas secretes all of the enzymes necessary for protein, fat, and carbohydrate digestion. In the case of the protease trypsin, this is secreted in its inactive form, trypsinogen, which becomes activated in the intestinal lumen. Although trypsinogen can spontaneously change to trypsin in solution, this conversion is suppressed in the pancreatic gland by the presence of *trypsin inhibitor*. Otherwise, the active form of the enzyme would be capable of digesting the pancreatic tissue itself. The conversion of trypsinogen to trypsin is accelerated by contact with the enzyme enterokinase, which is present only in intestinal mucosa.

Pancreatic lipase is capable of hydrolyzing dietary triglycerides into constituents that can then be solubilized and absorbed by mechanisms discussed in Chapter 18. This enzyme appears to require bile acids, at least in part, for its activation. Pancreatic amylase hydrolyzes starch and is secreted in its active form.

The enzymes are stored in the apical cytoplasm of the acinar cells in storage granules (zymogen granules), each of which contains a full complement of digestive enzymes. These granules are moved to the apical cell membrane, and the contents are emptied into the lumen by the process of exocytosis, the mechanism of which is discussed in detail in Chapter 19. When the cell is stimulated to secrete enzymes, the rate of exocytosis is accelerated.

Neuroendocrine control of pancreatic secretion

Secretion of enzymes, electrolytes, and water is under control of the autonomic nervous system as well as the gastrointestinal hormones, CCK and secretin. All secretory nerves to the pancreas are cholinergic. Cholinergic stimulation also enhances the effect of secretin on the pancreas.

The cephalic and gastric phases of pancreatic secretion are controlled primarily by the nerves. In most species, cholinergic stimulation induces an increase in enzyme output by increasing the rate of zymogen discharge at the apical cell membrane. The vagus has a direct action on the pancreas; in addition, there are reflex arcs between the stomach and the pancreas that lead to pancreatic secretion after fundic distention. Therefore the cholinergic response is mediated reflexly as well as from central stimulation.

As indicated previously, cholinergic stimulation primarily increases enzyme output with little increase in secretion of electrolytes and water. Vagal stimulation in the horse and pig, however, results in a profuse flow of electrolytes and water. In these species, the pancreas receives a secretory innervation comparable to that received by the salivary glands. Vagal stimulation also increases enzyme secretion in these species, but the enzyme output (per gram of pancreatic tissue) in the horse is only 1/20 that in the pig.

Two hormones released from the intestine have major effects on pancreatic secretion. These are secretin and CCK. Secretin is released in response to acid perfusing the duodenum, and its effect on the pancreas is to increase the secretin of HCO_3 and water. Therefore the primary function of secretion is to neutralize the acid gastric contents.

Cholecystokinin is released in response to protein and fat in the duodenum, and its effect on the pancreas is to increase enzyme secretion. In addition to its strong stimulation of enzyme secretion, CCK is a weak stimulus of HCO_3 and water secretion when acting alone but markedly augments secretin-stimulated HCO_3 secretion. Similarly, secretin is a weak stimulus to enzyme secretion when acting alone but markedly augments CCK-stimulated enzyme secretion. These interactions, shown in Fig. 18.13, are important physiologically for the reason that *only small amounts of secretin are normally released because only the first few centimeters of duodenum are exposed to acid strong enough to release secretin.* Much larger amounts of CCK, however, are released because of the much larger area of intestine exposed to fat and protein. Therefore, the augmentation of pancreatic secretion can occur even with the small amount of secretin released during digestion.

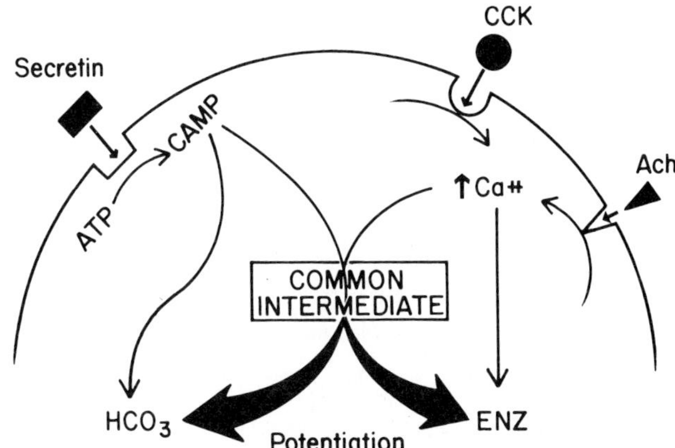

Figure 18.13. Secretin and CCK together result in potentiation of bicarbonate and enzyme output by the pancreas. Cholecystokinin and ACh primarily cause enzyme secretion by the acinar cell via the increases in intracellular Ca. Secretin acts primarily to increase bicarbonate output by the duct cells via the cyclic AMP system. When these agents are present together, however, bicarbonate and enzyme ouput is markedly increased because of interactions of the Ca and cAMP systems with a common intermediate. Ach, acetylcholine.

BILIARY SECRETION

Biliary secretions have the functions of (1) providing a source of bile acids that are necessary for fat digestion and absorption, (2) providing an excretory route for certain metabolites and drugs, and (3) providing an additional buffer for neutralization of H ion in the duodenum.

Structure of the liver lobule

A schematic representation of the liver lobule is shown in Fig. 18.14. Cords of hepatocytes are arranged more or less radially around a central vein. Between the hepatic cords course the sinusoids, which are endothelium-lined spaces analogous to capillaries in other organs. At the periphery of the lobule are the portal triads, consisting of a portal vein, a hepatic artery, and a bile duct. Blood from the hepatic artery and the portal vein flows centrally in the sinusoids, whereas bile drains peripherally into ductules and finally to the bile ducts in the portal triad. The sinusoids are lined with endothelial cells that have phagocytic capacity and are commonly known as Küpffer cells. Between the sinusoidal endothelium and the hepatocytes is the space of Disse. The sinusoidal endothelium has large pores that permit unrestricted passage of albumin from the sinusoidal plasma into the extravascular fluid that bathes the hepatocyte surface in the space of Disse. This facilitates the passage of albumin-bound molecules into the liver cell.

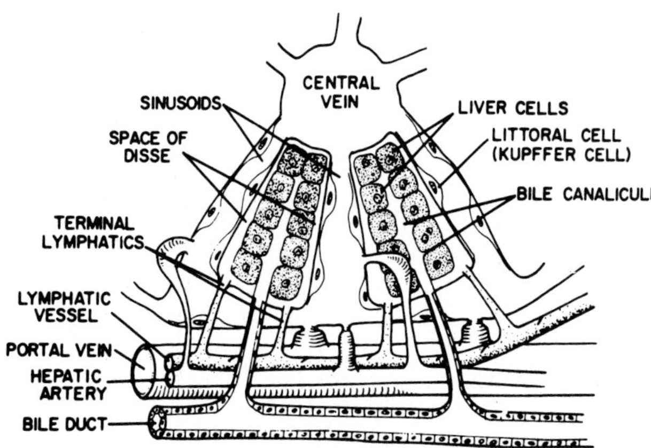

Figure 18.14. Basic structure of a liver lobule showing the hepatic cellular plates, the blood vessels, the bile-collecting system, and the lymph flow system. The latter comprises the spaces of Disse and the interlobular lymphatics. (From Guyton, Taylor, and Granger 1975, *Circulatory Physiology II. Dynamics and Control of the Body Fluids,* W.B. Saunders, Philadelphia.)

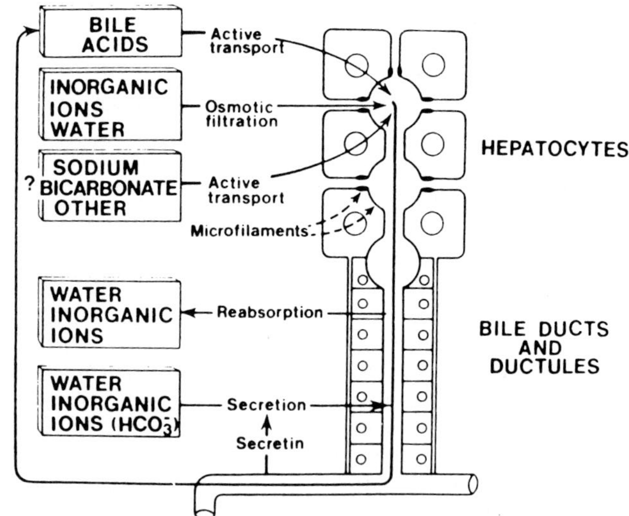

Figure 18.15. Bile formation. Major processes identified in bile formation: active transport of bile acids and osmotic filtration of water and inorganic ions (canalicular bile acid–dependent flow); active transport of inorganic ions (canalicular bile acid–independent flow); reabsorption in the bile ducts; secretion of a bicarbonate-rich fluid by the bile ducts, mainly in response to secretin. Microfilaments are also important for normal canalicular bile flow. (From Erlinger 1987, in Johnson, ed., *Physiology of the Gastrointestinal Tract,* Raven Press, New York.)

Bile acid synthesis and transport

Bile acids are synthesized in the liver from cholesterol under the action of the enzyme, 7α-hydroxylase. The activity of the enzyme is inversely proportional to the bile salts that are present. Therefore, as the concentration of bile salts perfusing the liver decreases, there is a corresponding increase in enzyme activity.

The bile acids formed in the liver are called primary bile acids and are usually cholic and chenodeoxycholic acids. These are conjugated with taurine or glycine to form taurocholic and glycocholic acids. The primary acids have a pK of about 6.0 The glycine conjugates have a pK of about 4.0, and the taurine conjugates have a pK of 2.0. Therefore, conjugation lowers the pK and forms charged complexes in the intestinal lumen, which has a pH of about 6.0. This ensures that the bile salts would not be passively absorbed to any extent in the upper intestine but would be retained in the lumen for the process of fat digestion and absorption. In the lower intestine, however, these bile salts are actively reabsorbed (see below).

Secondary bile salts result from bacterial deconjugation and dehydroxylation of unabsorbed bile salts in the colon. These are deoxycholic and lithocholic acids. At the pH of normal colonic contents, these secondary bile salts are relatively insoluble. They are precipitated from solution and excreted in the feces.

The bile salts are actively transported from the hepatocyte into the bile caniliculi by an energy-dependent process (Fig. 18.15). Cations and water follow passively, so that the bile is rendered iso-osmotic. This is known as the bile salt–dependent flow of bile and depends on recirculation of bile salts from the intestine (see below). Thus this bile salt–dependent flow will be greatest when bile salts are reabsorbed from the intestine and transported back to the liver for re-secretion. The second canalicular component is a bile salt–independent fraction of bile flow that is believed to be mediated by active Na transport. In the bile ducts and ductules there are both reabsorptive and secretory components of ions and water that further modify the composition of the canalicular bile. The secretory component is under the control of secretin, and its primary function is to deliver fluid rich in bicarbonate to the intestine.

Enterohepatic circulation of bile salts

The enterohepatic circulation of bile salts is shown in Fig. 18.16. There is active transport of bile salts in the ileum, and at least 90% of them are absorbed in this segment. Under normal conditions, hepatic synthesis equals fecal loss, but this is not nearly enough for fat digestion and the bile salts must therefore be recirculated. The normal pool of bile salts in the 70 kg human is about 4 g, and this pool turns over twice per meal or six to eight times in 24 hours. This constitutes a total usage of 32 g of bile salts, which is many times more than the hepatic synthetic rate. Therefore, if the enterohepatic circulation is interrupted, fat and fat-soluble vitamin malabsorption will be present.

Hepatic excretory function

Water-soluble organic compounds are carried in the plasma partially bound to the plasma proteins. Only the unbound fraction can be filtered at the renal glomerulus and excreted into the urine. In contrast, substances fully bound to the protein, including most lipid-soluble substances, cannot pass the glomerular filter. Such substances, nev-

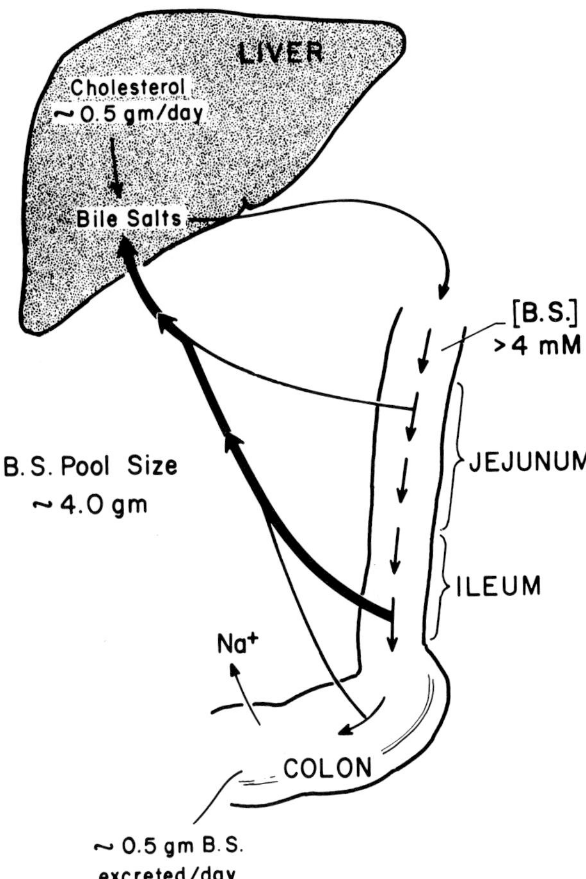

Figure 18.16. Enterohepatic circulation of bile salts (B.S.). Active transport of bile salts occurs in ileum, and about 90 percent of them are reabsorbed there. Some passive diffusion occurs in jejunum. Resecretion of bile salts by the liver is able to maintain sufficient concentrations in the intestine for fat digestion and absorption. Bile salt pool includes bile salts in the circulation, intestine, liver, and gallbladder and is about 4 g in the 70 kg human. (From Binder 1982, in Field, Fordtran, and Schultz, eds., *Secretory Diarrhea,* Am. Physiol. Soc., Bethesda, Md.)

ertheless, are readily removed from the protein at the sinusoidal membrane of the liver cell and thus can be excreted into the bile.

One such endogenous compound that the liver excretes is *bilirubin.* This pigment is one of the major end products of hemoglobin decomposition that are gradually released from the mononuclear phagocytic system into the plasma. This *free* bilirubin is bound to the plasma albumin and delivered to the hepatic cell. The steps in excretion of bilirubin into the bile are shown in Fig. 18.17 and, in general, represent mechanisms involved in hepatic clearance of all albumin-bound molecules. Uptake of bilirubin by the hepatocyte is due to the presence of a facilitated diffusion mechanism in the sinusoidal membrane of the hepatocyte. This mechanism is shared by many other organic compounds. In the hepatocyte, bilirubin is stored by binding to Y protein in the cytosol and then is conjugated, principally with glucuronic acid. The result *conjugated bilirubin* is actively secreted

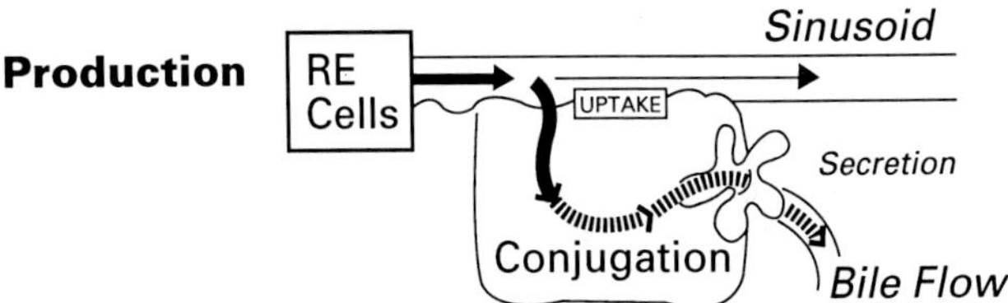

Figure 18.17. Bilirubin uptake and transport by hepatic cell. Bilirubin originates from hemoglobin breakdown by reticuloendothelial (RE) cells. It is bound to plasma albumin and taken up by the hepatocyte by a facilitated diffusion mechanism. The next step is conjugation with glucuronic acid, and the conjugated form is then secreted into the bile by an active transport mechanism. Secretion is normally the rate-limiting step that determines the maximum rate of transfer from blood to bile. (Modified from Ostrow et al. 1975.)

into the bile canaliculus by a transport process shared by some other organic acids but separate from the bile acid transport system.

After entering the intestine with the bile, bilirubin is converted by microbial action to *urobilinogen,* and some of this is reabsorbed into the blood by the intestine. About 95 percent of this urobilinogen is resecreted into the bile by the liver, and the remaining 5 percent is excreted into the urine. The remaining urobilinogen that is not reabsorbed by the intestine becomes oxidized in the feces to form *stercobilin,* which imparts the characteristic color to the feces.

Extrahepatic biliary tract

The functional anatomy of the extrahepatic biliary system is shown in Fig. 18.18. In the ruminant and the pig,

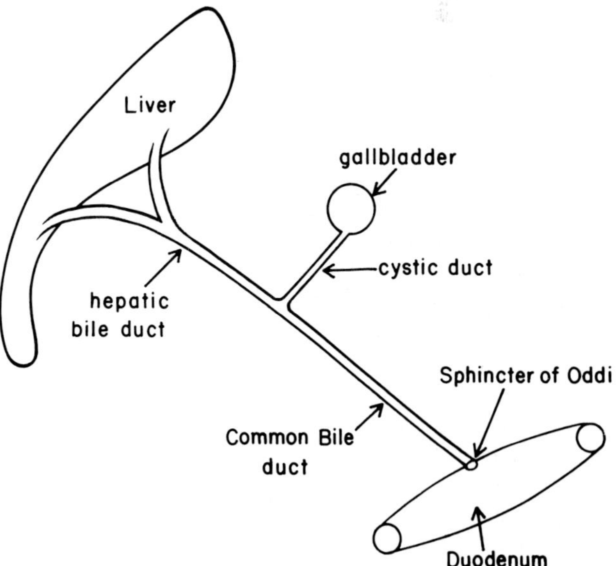

Figure 18.18. Extrahepatic biliary tract. In species that have a gallbladder, filling occurs during the interdigestive period when the sphincter of Oddi is closed and the gallbladder musculature is relaxed. During digestion, CCK is released from the intestine, and this hormone causes contraction of the gallbladder and relaxation of the sphincter, thus allowing gallbladder bile to enter the intestine. In species without a gallbladder (e.g., horse), a continuous flow of hepatic bile enters the duodenum.

there is a relatively continuous secretion of hepatic bile into the intestine. The sphincter of Oddi in these species is less well defined. In the horse, which does not have a gallbladder, there is a continuous secretion into the intestine. Other animals that do not have gall-bladders are the deer, elk, moose, giraffe, camel, elephant, pigeon, dove, and rat. In the dog and cat, a continuous secretion into the intestine is unnecessary because these species eat only once or twice a day. Therefore bile is stored in the gallbladder. During interdigestive periods, the sphincter is closed and the gallbladder muscle is relaxed. Therefore bile is backed up in the gallbladder. During digestive periods, the gallbladder contracts and the sphincter relaxes under the control of CCK. Accordingly, large amounts of gallbladder bile are delivered into the duodenum.

Different absorptive processes modify the concentration and relative composition of hepatic bile in the gallbladder during its storage. Hepatic bile consists of electrolytes and water and several organic compounds, such as cholesterol, lecithin, urobilinogen, and bile salts. Electrolytes and water are reabsorbed by gallbladder epithelium, and there is some passive absorption of lipid-soluble organic compounds such as cholesterol and lecithin from the gallbladder lumen. At the pH of gallbladder bile, however, the bile salts exist mainly in the charged form and are not soluble in the lipid membranes. Thus the bile salts may become concentrated some 10- to 20-fold in gallbladder bile.

REFERENCES

Admirand, W., and Way, L.W. 1973. Bile formation and biliary tract function. In M.H. Sleisenger and J.S. Fordtran, eds., *Gastrointestinal Disease*. W.B. Saunders, Philadelphia. Pp. 352–58.

Alexander, F., and Hickson, J.C.D. 1970. The salivary and pancreatic secretions of the horse. In A.T. Phillipson, ed., *Physiology of Digestion and Metabolism in the Ruminant*. Oriel, Newcastle upon Tyne. Pp. 375–89.

Banfield, W.J. 1975. Physiology of the gallbladder. *Gastroenterology* 69:770–77.

Binder, N.J. 1980. Pathophysiology of bile acid and fatty acid-induced diarrhea. In M. Field, J.S. Fordtran, and S.G. Schultz, eds. *Secretory Diarrhea*, Am. Physiol. Soc., Bethesda, Md. Pp. 159–78.

Blair-West, J.R., Coghlan, J.P., Denton, D.A., and Wright, R.D. 1968. Effect of endocrines on salivary glands. In *Handbook of Physiology*. Sec. 6, C.F. Code and W. Heidel, eds., *Alimentary Canal*, Vol. 2, *Secretion*. Am. Physiol. Soc., Washington. Pp. 633–64.

Brandborg, L.L. 1973. Pancreatic physiology. In M.H. Sleisenger and J.S. Fordtran, eds., *Gastrointestinal Disease*. W.B. Saunders, Philadelphia. Pp. 359–64.

Caple, I.W., and Heath, T.J. 1975. Biliary and pancreatic secretions in sheep: Their regulation and roles. In I.W. McDonald and A.C.I. Warner, eds., *Digestion and Metabolism in the Ruminant*, Univ. New Engl. Publ. Unit, Armidale, New South Wales, Australia. Pp. 91–100.

Debas, H.T. 1977. Regulation of gastric acid secretion. *Fed. Proc.* 36:1933–37.

Debas, H.T. 1987. Peripheral regulation of gastric acid secretion. In L.R. Johnson, ed. *Physiology of the Gastrointestinal Tract*. Raven Press, New York. Pp. 931–45.

Eckerlin, R.H., and Stevens, C.E. 1973. Bicarbonate secretion by the glandular saccules of the llama stomach. *Cornell Vet.* 63:436–45.

Erlinger, S. 1987. Physiology of bile secretion and the enterohepatic circulation. In L.R. Johnson, ed. *Physiology of the Gastrointestinal Tract*. Raven Press, New York. Pp. 1557–80.

Erlinger, S., and Dhumeaux, D. 1974. Mechanisms and control of secretion of bile water and electrolytes. *Gastroenterology* 66:281–304.

Gardner, J.D., Jackson, M.J., Batzri, S., and Jensen, R.T. 1978. Potential mechanisms of interactions among secretagogues. *Gastroenterology* 74:348–54.

Grossman, M.I. 1968. Neural and hormonal stimulation of gastric secretion of acid. In *Handbook of Physiology*. Sec. 6, C.F. Code and W. Heidel, eds., *Alimentary Canal*. Vol. 2, *Secretion*. Am. Physiol. Soc., Washington. Pp. 835–63.

Grossman, M.I. 1974. Candidate hormones of the gut. *Gastroenterology* 67:730–55.

Harper, A.A. 1968. Hormonal control of pancreatic secretion. In *Handbook of Physiology*. Sec. 6. C.F. Code and W. Heidel, eds., *Alimentary Canal*. Vol. 2, *Secretion*. Am. Physiol. Soc., Washington. Pp. 969–95.

Holler, H. 1970. Untersuchunger über Sekret und Sekretion der Cardiadrüsenzone in Magen des Schweines. *Zentralbl Veterinär-med*, ser. A, 17:685–711, 857–73.

Jacobson, E.D., L.R. Johnson, E.W. Moore. 1985. Gastric secretion. In *The Undergraduate Teaching Project in Gastroenterology and Liver Disease*. Produced by The American Gastroenterological Asso., Thorofare, N.J.

Jamieson, J.D. 1976. Anatomy of the pancreas. In J.M. Dietschy, ed., *Disorders of the Gastrointestinal Tract, Disorders of the Liver, Nutritional Disorders*. Grune & Stratton, New York. Pp. 190–93.

Janowitz, H.D. 1968. Pancreatic secretion of fluid and electrolytes. In *Handbook of Physiology*. Sec. 6, C.F. Code and W. Heidel, eds., *Alimentary Canal*. Vol. 2, *Secretion*. Am. Physiol. Soc., Washington. Pp. 925–33.

Johnson, L.R. 1966. Histamine liberation by gastric mucosa of pylorisligated rats damaged by acetic or salicyclic acids. *Proc. Soc. Exp. Biol. Med.* 121:384–89.

Kimberg, D.V. 1974. Cyclic nucleotides and their role in gastrointestinal secretion. *Gastroenterology* 67:1023–64.

Konturek, S.J. 1974. Gastric secretion. In E.D. Jacobson and L.L. Shanbour, eds., *MTP International Review of Science, Gastrointestinal Physiology*, Series 1, Vol. 4. University Park Press, Baltimore. Pp. 227–64.

Konturek, S.J., Thor, P., Dembinski, A., and Krol, R. 1975. Comparison of secretin and vasoactive intestinal peptide on pancreatic secretion in dogs. *Gastroenterology* 68:1527–35.

Ostrow, J.D. 1981. Hepatic excretory function. In *The Undergraduate Teaching Project in Gastroenterology and Liver Disease* produced by American Gastroenterological Asso. Thorofare, N.J.

Preshaw, R.M. 1974. Pancreatic exocrine secretion. In E.D. Jacobson and L.L. Shanbour, eds., *MTP International Review of Science, Gastrointestinal Physiology*, series 1, vol. 4. University Park Press, Baltimore. Pp. 265–91.

Rask-Madsen J., Lauritsen K. 1987. Enhancement of mucosal defence by prostaglandins: Rationale and clinical experience in ulcer disease. *Scand. J. Gastroenterol.* 22 (Suppl 128):34–42.

Schneyer, L.H., and Emmelin, N. 1974. Salivary secretion. In E.D. Jacobson and L.L. Shanbour, eds., *MTP International Review of Science, Gastrointestinal Physiology*, series 1, vol. 4. University Park Press, Baltimore, Pp. 183–226.

Schneyer, L.H., and Schneyer, C.A. 1968. Inorganic composition of saliva. In *Handbook of Physiology*. Sec. 6, C.F. Code and W. Heidel, eds., *Alimentary Canal*. Vol. 2, *Secretion*. Am. Physiol. Soc., Washington. Pp. 497–530.

Silen, W., Ito, S. 1985. Mechanisms for rapid reepithelialization of the gastric mucosal surface. *Annu. Rev. Physiol.* 47:217–29.

Singh, M., and Webster, P.D. 1978. Neurohormonal control of pancreatic secretion. *Gastroenterology* 74:294–309.

Soll, A.H., Rodrigo, R., and Ferrari, J.C. 1981. Effects of chemical transmitters on function of isolated canine parietal cells. *Fed. Proc.* 40:2519–23.

Stevens, C.E. 1973. Transport across rumen epithelium. In H.H. Ussing and N.A. Thorn, eds., *Transport Mechanisms in Epithelia*. Proc. Alfred Benzon Symposium V. Munksgaard, Copenhagen. Pp. 404–26.

Swanson, C.H., and Soloman, A.K. 1972. Evidence for Na-H exchange in the rabbit pancreas. *Nature New Biol.* 236:183–86.

Thomas, J.E. 1968. Neural regulation of pancreatic secretion. In *Handbook of Physiology.* Sec. 6, C.F. Code and W. Heidel, eds., *Alimentary Canal*. Vol. 2, *Secretion*. Am. Physiol. Soc., Washington. Pp. 955–68.

Thompson, W.J., Rosenfeld, G.C., and Jacobson, E.D. 1977. Adenyl cyclase and gastric acid secretion. *Fed. Proc.* 36:1938–41.

Walsh, J.H. 1973. Control of gastric secretion. In M.H. Sleisenger and J.S. Fordtran, eds., *Gastrointestinal Disease*. W.B. Saunders. Philadelphia. Pp. 144–62.

Young, J.A., and Schneyer, C.A. 1981. Composition of saliva in mammalia. *Aust. J. Exp. Biol. Med. Sci.* 59:1–53.

CHAPTER 19

Digestion and Absorption of Carbohydrate, Fat, and Protein | by Robert A. Argenzio

Although fat digestion and absorption occur exclusively in the small intestine, digestion and absorption of carbohydrate and protein occur in both the small and large intestines. The digestive processes and end products available for absorption, however, are quite different in these two environments. In the small intestine, dietary carbohydrates and proteins are enzymatically broken down by pancreatic and brush border enzymes. The resulting hexoses and peptides or amino acids are then absorbed by the small intestinal mucosa by specific active transport mechanisms. In contrast, carbohydrate and protein entering the large intestine are, by microbial action, converted chiefly to volatile fatty acids and ammonia, both of which are absorbed by passive diffusion mechanisms. The large intestine of most species does not have active transport mechanisms for hexoses or amino acids. (The dog and the newborn pig may be exceptions to this generalization.)

DIGESTIVE-ABSORPTIVE SURFACE

Figure 19.1 shows a segment of the human small intestine and the various levels of structural organization that amplify the available cross-sectional area for digestion and absorption. If viewed as a cylinder 280 cm long and 4 cm in diameter, the surface area would be about 3300 cm^2. The folds of Kerckring (valvulae conniventes) increase this surface by a factor of 3, which yields a surface area of 10,000 cm^2. The villi further increase the surface area tenfold. The microvilli projecting from the epithelial cell surface increase the surface area relative to the cylinder by a factor of 600. Therefore the total surface area available for digestion and absorption with the dimensions of a small intestine given above would be in the neighborhood of 200 m^2.

The microvilli (brush border) are responsible for the greatest amplification of the surface area, and it is on the brush border that the saccharidase and peptidase enzymes are located. Thus the mucosal phase of digestion occurs principally on the brush border surface, although a major proportion of dipeptidases are also located in the cytoplasm of the cell. In addition to these digestive enzymes, the brush border also contains specialized mechanisms for transporting the end products of digestion into the cytoplasm of the cell. Therefore the overall assimilation of food material includes a luminal and mucosal phase of digestion and a transport phase for delivery of the end products to the lymphatic or portal circulation.

CELLULAR TURNOVER AND RENEWAL

A cross-section of mucosa from the small intestine and the associated cell types is shown in Fig. 19.2. Five major cell types are present on the epithelium: (1) columnar absorptive cells, (2) mucous (goblet) cells, (3) enteroendocrine (enterochromaffin) cells, (4) Paneth cells, and (5) undifferentiated columnar cells. The first four types arise from undifferentiated columnar cells at the base of the crypts. The columnar absorptive cells outnumber the other major cell types. Thus cell division in the enteric epithelium is limited to the youngest cells at the base of the crypts of Lieberkühn. After at least two divisions within the crypt, the columnar cells migrate onto the villus and assume the role of the mature absorptive cell. With the exception of the

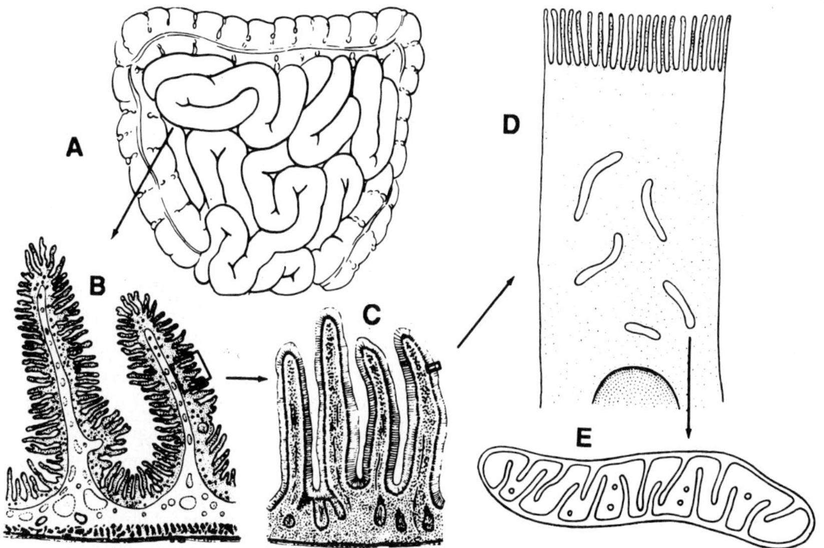

Figure 19.1. A diagram illustrating the devices at various levels of morphological organization in the alimentary tract which tend to increase efficiency by amplifying the area of the physiologically significant interfaces. First, the hollow viscus is greatly elongated (*A*). Its internal surface is further increased by the circumferential folds, or plications, of the mucosa visible with the naked eye (*B*). These, in turn, are covered with microscopic villi (*C*). The individual cells on the villi are covered with myriad microvilli (*D*). Also within the cell (*E*) the same principle of amplification can be seen in the plication of internal mitochondrial membrane. (From Fawcett 1962, Physiologically significant specialization of the cell surface, *Circulation* 26:1105–25, by permission of the American Heart Association, Inc.)

Paneth cell, the other cell types also migrate onto the villus, where they are finally extruded from the villous tip. The Paneth cells remain at the crypt base and finally degenerate and are phagocytized. Paneth cells contain secretory granules, which contain a lysozyme (a bacteriolytic enzyme) that partially degrades bacterial cell walls.

The enteric epithelium has the highest turnover rate of any normal tissue in the body and, therefore, a high capacity to regenerate. The turnover rate differs with age. For example, newborn pigs replace the small intestine villous epithelium in 7 to 10 days, whereas in 3-week-old pigs it is replaced in 2 to 4 days. Cell division and migration are slightly slower in the colon.

Cell division rates in the precursor compartment (crypt) are locally regulated by a feedback mechanism in the functional compartment (villus). Substances called *chalones* provide a feedback inhibition of cell division in the crypts. Thus cell proliferation becomes increased when the villous release of chalones decreases. This feedback mechanism is, in turn, governed by a number of extrinsic agents such as food and enteric secretions. Probably the most important extrinsic stimulus to cell division, however, is the action of tropic hormones. Current evidence indicates that gastrin stimulates DNA synthesis in the mucosa of the oxyntic gland area of the stomach and of the duodenum, ileum, and colon, and in fact this may be the most important effect of the hormone.

Of equal importance is the finding that many of the de-

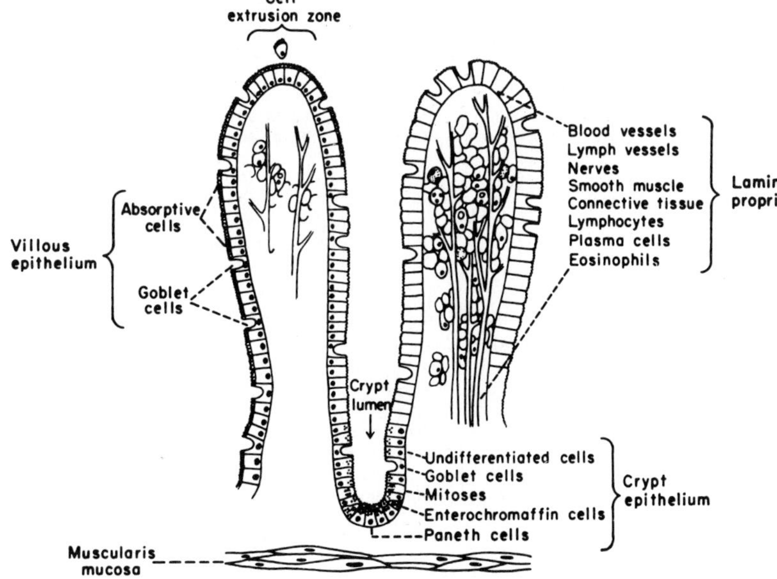

Figure 19.2. Schematic diagram of two sectioned villi and a crypt of Lieberkühn to illustrate the histological organization of the small intestinal mucosa. (From Trier 1968, in *Handbook of Physiology,* Sec. 6, Code and Heidel, eds., *Alimentary Canal,* Vol. 3, *Intestinal Absorption,* Am. Physiol. Soc., Washington.)

velopmental enzyme changes in the mucosa of the small intestine may be mediated by gastrin, and gastrin levels increase at the time of weaning. The oral ingestion of food and its presence in the gastrointestinal tract, however, are necessary to maintain endogenous gastrin secretion and thus the tropic effect of gastrin on the gut mucosa.

DIGESTION IN SMALL INTESTINE

With the exception of ruminants and other species in which the stomach is the major site of microbial fermentation, the principal digestive and absorptive mechanisms of soluble carbohydrate, fat, and protein are located in the proximal small intestine. Salivary amylase initiates starch digestion in the pig stomach, and some of the protein is hydrolyzed by the action of pepsin and HCl. Pepsin, however, is not essential for protein digestion. There are two general phases (*luminal* and *mucosal*) of small intestinal digestion, and these are considered separately below. Table 19.1 lists the enzymes operating at both the luminal and mucosal levels.

Carbohydrate digestion

Dietary carbohydrates are principally starches, sucrose, lactose, and fibrous carbohydrate. Starch is a glucose-containing polysaccharide consisting of a chain of α-1,4-glucosyl units. Most starches are of the branched (amylopectin) type and also contain α-1,6 branching linkages. Sucrose and lactose are disaccharides consisting of glucose and fructose (sucrose) and glucose and galactose (lactose), respectively. Fibrous carbohydrate includes hemicelluloses (pentose or hexose polymers) and cellulose, which contains the unbranched β-1,4-linked glucose polymers.

The *lumen phase* of starch digestion consists of enzymatic hydrolysis by pancreatic α-amylase of the α-1,4 interior linkages of the starch molecule to yield final oligosaccharide products in the duodenal lumen (Fig. 19.3). Because α-amylase has low specificity for the outermost linkages of the molecule and does not cleave the 1,6 branching links, the final products of amylase digestion are 1,4-linked trisaccharides and disaccharides (maltotriose and maltose) and a group of branched oligosaccharides containing both α-1,6 and α-1,4 linkages and known as α-dextrins (Fig. 19.4). *No free glucose is formed by pancreatic amylase hydrolysis.* In addition, pancreatic amylase is incapable of hydrolyzing β-linked glucose polymers, and therefore fibrous carbohydrates containing this linkage are not digested in the small intestine.

The products of luminal carbohydrate digestion cannot

Table 19.1. Major digestive enzmes

Source	Enzyme	Activator	Substrate	Action or products*
Salivary glands	Salivary α-amylase		Starch	Hydrolyzes α-1,4, linkages, producing α-limit dextrins, maltotriose, and maltose
Gastric mucosa	Pepsin (pepsinogen)	HCl, pepsin	Protein	Cleaves peptide bonds formed by carboxyl groups of aromatic amino acids, aspartate, and glutamate
Exocrine pancreas	Trypsin (trypsinogen)	Enterokinase	Protein	Cleaves peptide bonds formed by carboxyl groups of arginine and lysine
	Chymotrypsin (chymotrypsinogen)	Trypsin	Protein	Cleaves peptide bonds formed by carboxyl group of aromatic amino acids
	Elastase (proelastase)	Trypsin	Protein	Cleaves peptide bonds formed by carboxyl group of aliphatic amino acids
	Carboxypeptidase A (procarboxypeptidase A)	Trypsin	Protein	Cleaves carboxy terminal amino acids with aromatic or branched aliphatic side chains
	Carboxypeptidase B (procarboxypeptidase B)	Trypsin	Protein	Cleaves carboxy terminal amino acids with basic side chains
	Pancreatic lipase		Triglycerides	Monoglycerides and fatty acids
	Pancreatic esterase		Cholesterol esters	Cholesterol and fatty acids
	Phospholipase A_2 (prophospholipase A_2)	Trypsin	Lecithin	Lysolecithin
	Pancreatic α-amylase	Cl^-	Starch	Hydrolyzes α1,4 linkages, producing α-limit dextrins, maltotriose, and maltose
	Ribonuclease		RNA	Nucleotides and oligonucleotides
	Deoxyribonuclease		DNA	Nucleotides and oligonucleotides
Intestinal mucosa	Enteropeptidase (enterokinase)		Trypsinogen	Trypsin
	Aminopeptidase		Peptides	Cleaves N terminal amino acid from peptide
	Dipeptidases		Dipeptides	Two amino acids
	Maltase		Maltose, maltotriose	Glucose
	Lactase		Lactose	Galactose and glucose
	Sucrase		Sucrose	Fructose and glucose
	1,6-Glucosidase		1,6-Glucosides	Glucose
	α-Limit dextrinase		α-Limit dextrins	Glucose
	Phospholipase		Phospholipids	Glycerol, fatty acids, phosphate, and choline or other bases
	Nuclease, nucleotidases, and nucleosidases		Nucleic acids, nucleotides, nucleosides	Pentoses, purines, and pyrimidines

*Major end products of hydrolytic reactions are indicated.

Modified from Ganong 1979, *Review of Medical Physiology,* 9th ed., Lange Medical Publications, Los Altos, and Harper, Rodwell and Mayes 1979, in *Review of Physiological Chemistry,* 17th ed., Lange Medical Publications, Los Altos.

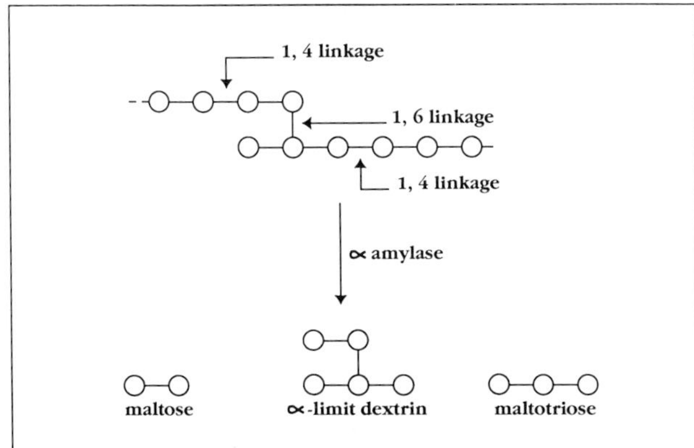

19.3. Intraluminal starch digestion. Pancreatic amylase hydrolyzes α-1,4 linkages at random and is an endo-glycosidase. It does not attack the α-1,6 linkages of amylopectins; nor can it attack the β linkages of fibrous carbohydrates.

be absorbed by the mucosa but must be further degraded into monosaccharides before they can be transported into the epithelial cell. As shown in Fig. 19.4, the *mucosal phase* of this degradation is accomplished by specific saccharidases in the brush border of the epithelial cell. These enzymes are incorporated into the luminal membrane of the cell and migrate to the tip of the microvilli. Therefore hydrolysis takes place in the juxtaluminal position. Except for lactose, these saccharides are hydrolyzed so efficiently that the rate-limiting step is usually absorption of the monosaccharides by the transport mechanism. Lactose is broken down more slowly; therefore its hydrolysis is rate limiting in its overall assimilation.

When an isotonic solution of 500 ml containing glucose and NaCl is rapidly administered into the proximal jejunum, an immediate increase in the plasma glucose concentration is obtained, as shown for the pig and calf in Fig. 19.5. This indicates how rapidly glucose is absorbed by the jejunum, even though its transport is the rate-limiting step in the overall assimilation process. In the calf, however, a major rate-limiting step, which is probably more important than glucose transport, appears to be in amylase hydrolysis of starch. In the normal suckling calf, these factors would be of little concern because the calf can readily hydrolyze the lactose of its mother's milk and can absorb glucose as rapidly as the pig (Fig. 19.5). These factors need to be considered in the formulation of diets to supplant the mother's milk.

In carnivores, and less so in omnivores normally fed a relatively low-fiber diet, most of the soluble carbohydrate is hydrolyzed and absorbed before the ingesta reach the terminal jejunum. In herbivores the amount of soluble carbohydrate digested in the small intestine depends on a number of factors including the relative percentage of dietary fiber. For example, if a horse is fed a corn diet, which is low in fiber, about 75 percent of the soluble carbohydrate will be digested and absorbed in the small intestine. Conversely, with a high-fiber diet such as an alfalfa–beet pulp mixture, only about 40 percent of the soluble carbohydrate will be digested in the small intestine. Thus the fiber content may protect the soluble material to some extent from release and enzymatic hydrolysis. In addition, fibrous material is moved through the intestine at a greater rate because of the stimulation of motility from its increased bulk. Furthermore, amylase output is relatively low in the horse; therefore luminal digestion of starch becomes the rate-limiting step.

The final stage in carbohydrate assimilation is transport of the monosaccharides into the epithelial cell. In the cases of glucose and galactose, this is accomplished by a specific transport mechanism on the luminal membrane requiring the presence of sodium. These hexoses can be transported into the cell against a concentration gradient by a process called *active transport*. Fructose cannot enter the cell against its concentration gradient, but a carrier mechanism facilitates its entry into the cell when the fructose concentration in the lumen is greater than that in the cell. Metabolism of fructose by the cell maintains its lower intracellular concentration. Once these monosaccharides gain entrance

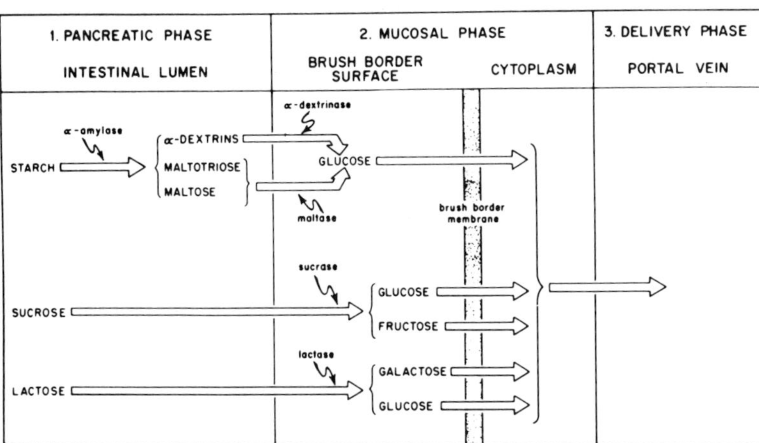

19.4. Summary of carbohydrate digestion and absorption. Initially, starch is hydrolyzed in the duodenal lumen by pancreatic α-amylase. Further hydrolysis of initial products and the dietary disaccharides takes place at the brush border membrane through the action of several oligosaccharidases. The final products of the enzymatic processes are transported into the cell through the brush border membrane. Glucose and galactose use an active transport system, and fructose is transported by facilitated diffusion. Then the monosaccharides diffuse down their concentration gradient into the portal vein system. (From Nervi 1976, by permission, in J.M. Dietschy, ed., *Disorders of the Gastrointestinal Tract, Disorders of the Liver, Nutritional Disorders,* Grune & Stratton, New York, pp. 35–37.)

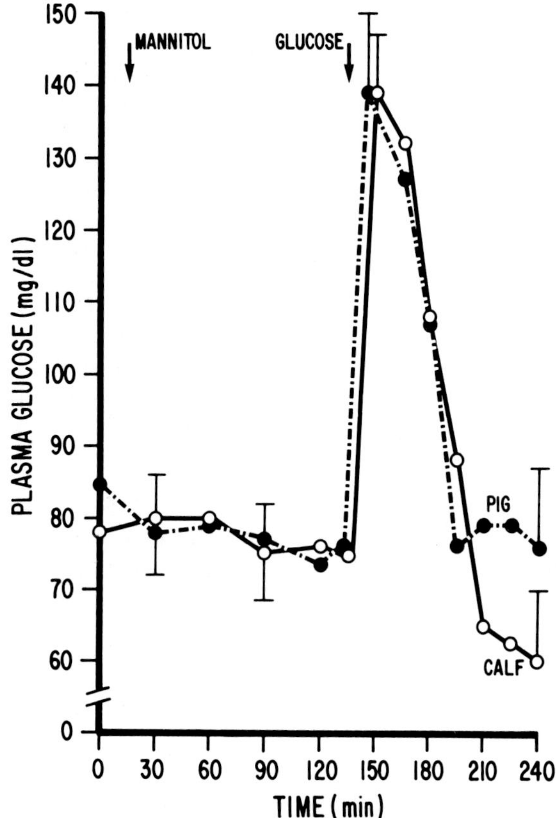

Figure 19.5. Plasma glucose concentration (±SE) after administration of an isotonic electrolyte solution containing either mannitol or glucose (time of injection indicated by arrows) into the proximal jejunum of the pig and calf. (Modified from Argenzio 1980, *Am. J. Vet. Res.* 41:2000–6, and unpublished data.)

into the epithelial cell, they can then diffuse down their concentration gradient into the portal blood for delivery to the general body tissues.

In ruminants the active transport mechanism for glucose becomes rudimentary after rumen function develops. Under normal conditions, very little glucose is delivered to the small intestine of the adult ruminant because most of the starch has already been digested and absorbed in the forestomach.

Protein digestion

Digestion of protein occurs principally in the proximal small intestine, although pepsin hydrolysis of protein begins in the stomach and lasts 1 to 2 hours because of the acid pH. Figure 19.6 shows the phases of protein digestion occurring in the lumen and on the mucosal surface. There are two groups of inactive proteases secreted by the pancreas into the duodenum: (1) *endopeptidases,* which are trypsinogen, chymotrypsinogen, and elastase, and (2) *exopeptidases,* which are carboxypeptidases A and B. Activation of trypsinogen by the enzyme enterokinase takes place at the brush border. Enterokinase attacks the proenzyme trypsinogen to form active trypsin. Trypsin then activates the remaining trypsinogen as well as the other proenzymes.

The main products of pancreatic protease hydrolysis are neutral and basic amino acids and *oligopeptides,* which are small peptides that contain various amino acid mixtures. Oligopeptides containing six or fewer amino acids are resistant to further hydrolysis by pancreatic enzymes and, therefore, accumulate in the lumen of the intestine after a meal. Further hydrolysis of the oligopeptides must occur because peptides of more than three amino acids cannot be absorbed by the epithelium. This further hydrolysis takes place at the brush border. The end products of the brush border oligopeptidases are amino acids, dipeptides, and tripeptides.

Absorption of amino acids into the epithelial cell occurs by specialized transport mechanisms much the same as for hexose transport. There are at least two separate active transport systems, one for neutral and one for basic amino acids. In addition to these, it has been established that systems are present to transport dipeptides and tripeptides into the cell, and it is likely that most of the dietary protein is

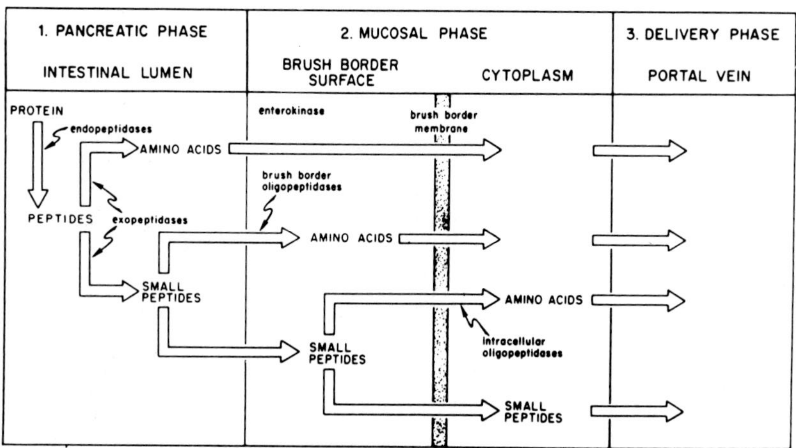

Figure 19.6. Schematic figure representing the different phases of protein digestion and absorption. (1) Endogenous and dietary proteins are hydrolyzed by pancreatic peptidases in the duodenal and jejunal lumen. Note that enterokinase, the activating duodenal enzyme, is located at the brush border surface. Trypsin is liberated through the action of enterokinase on trypsinogen; the liberated trypsin then activates the bulk of the pancreatic propeptidases. (2) Brush border oligopeptidases are able to attack only small neutral peptides. Other small peptides cross the brush border membrane and are hydrolyzed by soluble cytoplasmic oligopeptidases. There are several amino acid transport systems in the brush border membrane. (3) The final products of the mucosal phase, amino acids and a small fraction of oligopeptides, diffuse outside the mucosal cells down the concentration gradient to be delivered through the portal vein system. (From Nervi 1976, by permission, in J.M. Dietschy, ed., *Disorders of the Gastrointestinal Tract, Disorders of the Liver, Nutritional Disorders,* Grune & Stratton, New York, pp. 35–37.)

absorbed in this form rather than in the form of free amino acids. Fortunately, greater than 85 percent of the hydrolase activity against dipeptides resides in the cytoplasm of the cell so that about 90 percent of the peptides entering the cell are further hydrolyzed to free amino acids. As also shown in Fig. 19.6, the remaining 10 percent of the unhydrolyzed peptides can diffuse across the basolateral membrane into the blood.

As with hexose transport, most of the peptide and amino acid transport systems require the presence of sodium in the jejunal lumen. These sodium-dependent systems are also responsible for the absorption of a number of water-soluble vitamins and bile acids; because of the general importance of this process, it will be discussed in detail in Chap. 10.

Fat digestion

Most of the dietary fat is in the form of water-insoluble triglycerides, and these are emulsified by the action of bile salts. Large fat globules are released slowly into the duodenum because of feedback inhibition of gastric emptying by lipids in the duodenum (Chap. 17). Thus the complex process of fat digestion is allowed a greater time for completion than carbohydrate or protein digestion.

Lipid digestion in the intestinal lumen requires the participation of both pancreatic and biliary secretions (Fig. 19.7). Pancreatic lipase acts at the oil-water interface of the emulsion particles releasing a β-monoglyceride and two free fatty acids from the 1- and 3- positions of the triglyceride. These products are also water insoluble but are amphipaths, that is, part polar and water soluble and part nonpolar and lipid soluble.

The solubilization of the end products of lipase digestion is dependent on the action of bile acids. These acids act as a detergent and bring the water-insoluble material into solution by forming a negatively charge aggregate called a *micelle*. The water-insoluble material is dissolved in the interior of the micelle. Normally, for formation of a micelle, there must be present in the jejunum a concentration of bile acids of at least 2 mM; this is called the *critical micellar concentration*. The postprandial concentration of bile acids in the proximal jejunum is usually at least 4 mM and therefore is more than sufficient to promote solubilization of lipids. In the conversion of fats from an emulsion to a micelle, the diameter of the particles is reduced 100 times and the surface area increased more than 10,000 times. The micelles is diffuse from the emulsion particle to the brush border of the epithelium, where the fat is released to diffuse across the lipid membrane into the cell.

The fatty acids and monoglycerides are reesterified to triglycerides inside the epithelium. The triglycerides are then associated with cholesterol, cholesterol esters, phospholipids, and small amounts of protein to form *chylomicrons*. Formation of the chylomicron, which is analogous to the water-soluble micelle, facilitates the transport of water-insoluble triglyceride. Without the protein coat, fat is unable to leave the cell.

DEVELOPMENTAL ASPECTS OF DIGESTION

This section will discuss some of the peculiar aspects of digestion in the neonatal animal and how these functions change as the animal is weaned. The immediate postnatal period and the time of weaning are particularly critical periods in digestive function in certain species. Furthermore, the early weaning practices in modern-day feeding programs may introduce additional stresses on digestive function.

Antibody absorption and transmission of immunity

Absorption of intact protein by the neonatal intestine represents one means of antibody transfer, that is, the transfer of passive immunity. *Antibodies* are large protein molecules, found in the γ-globulin fraction of the blood serum. They react specifically with antigenic substances that stimulated their production so that the animal gradually develops immunity to the antigenic substance. The production of antibodies in response to an antigenic stimulus is low at birth. The newborn animal would be quickly overcome by invasive organisms before it had time to produce antibodies to combat them were it not for the γ-globulin that the fetus

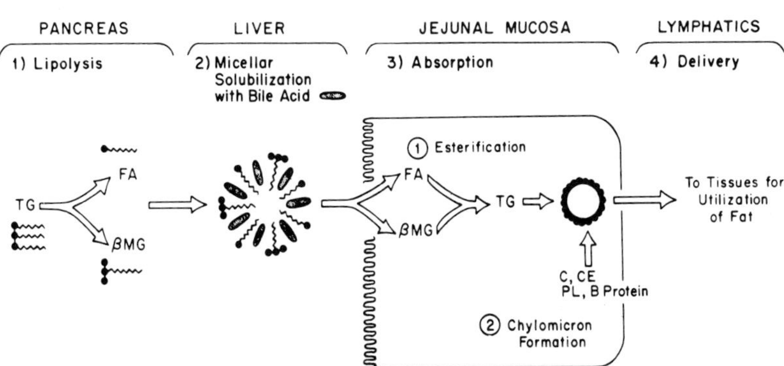

Figure 19.7. Diagrammatic representation of the four major steps in the digestion and absorption of dietary fat. These are (1) the lipolysis of dietary triglyceride (TG) by pancreatic enzymes; (2) micellar solubilization of the resulting long-chain fatty acids (FA) and β-monoglycerides (βMG) by bile acids secreted into the intestinal lumen by the liver; (3) absorption of the fatty acids and β-monoglyceride into the mucosal cell with subsequent reesterification and formation of chylomicrons; and (4) delivery of the chylomicrons from the mucosal cell into the intestinal lymphatic system. During the process of chylomicron formation, small amounts of cholesterol (C), cholesterol ester (CE), certain apoproteins (B protein) and phospholipid (PL), as well as TG, are incorporated into this specific lipoprotein fraction. (From Westergaard 1976, by permission, in J.M. Dietschy, ed., *Disorders of the Gastrointestinal Tract, Disorders of the Liver, Nutritional Disorders*, Grune & Stratton, New York, pp. 38–39.)

or neonatal animal receives from the mother. In some species, these are partially or wholly obtained after birth through the colostrum. In others, they are obtained before birth by way of placental transfer. The serum γ-globulins comprise five classes of immunoglobulins: IgG, IgM, IgA, IgD, and IgE.

Only the neonatal intestine has the ability for uptake of large amounts of intact protein. In the adult mammal, relatively small and nutritionally insignificant amounts of protein can be absorbed intact: in certain disease states, however, the adult intestine may become more permeable to macromolecules.

The neonatal small intestine ingests macromolecules by an endocytotic mechanism, the general scheme of which is shown in Fig. 19.8. The first stage is adsorption of macromolecules to the microvillous membrane of the small intestinal adsorptive cell. When these molecules reach a certain critical concentration at the microvillous border, invagination of the membrane occurs and small vesicles are formed (second stage). This uptake process is energy dependent; the energy is required for replacement of the cell membrane. The third stage is migration of the membrane-bound vesicles (phagosomes) to the supranuclear region of the cell. Here the vesicles coalesce with lysosomes to form large vacuoles termed *phagolysosomes*. In these, intracellular digestion occur. Some of the macromolecules escape breakdown, however and migrate to the basolateral surface of the cell membrane. Here, a reverse endocytosis (exocytosis) occurs, and the macromolecules gain access to the intercellular space and the lymphatic system.

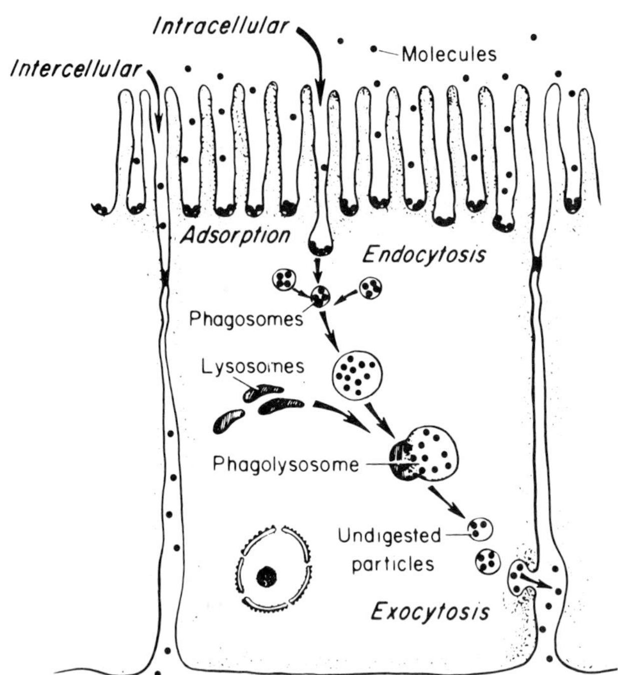

Figure 19.8. General mechanisms for macromolecule uptake and transport by the intestine. *Intracellular uptake:* After adsorption and endocytosis by the microvillous membrane, macromolecules are transported in small vesicles and larger phagosomes. Intracellular digestion occurs when lysosomes combine to form phagolysosomes. Intact molecules that remain after digestion are deposited in the intercellular space by a reverse endocytosis (exocytosis). *Intercellular uptake:* Alternatively, macromolecules may cross the "tight junction" barrier between cells and diffuse into the intercellular space. (From Walker and Isselbacher 1974, *Gastroenterology* 67:531–50.)

In the postpartum period all of the maternal immunoglobulins in ruminants, pigs, and horses are received from the colostrum by the intestinal transfer process described above. These animals are therefore hypogammaglobulinemic at birth. During the immediate postnatal period there is a short period in which the intestinal mucosa is highly permeable to *all* macromolecules in contact with the mucosa. The increased uptake of immunoglobulins by the intestine lasts only a short time, and then the intestine "closes" to prevent further bulk passage of proteins.

Rodents, on the other hand, derive passive immunity from intrauterine transport as well as from postpartum intestinal absorption. These species have a prolonged period of *selective transport* of γ-globulins; this is in contrast to the nonselective transport of all macromolecules, such as occurs in ruminants. Early closure can be demonstrated by giving corticosteroids to these animals and is probably related to premature cell maturation induced by steroids.

Passive immunity in humans is acquired almost entirely from intrauterine transport, and there is very little absorption of γ-globulins across the intestine. The primary mechanisms of transmission of passive immunity in various species and the times of intestinal closure are shown in Table 19.2.

Enzymatic development

The development and changes of digestive enzyme secretion are of practical significance because of the formulation of milk-replacer diets. It is important to realize that the activity level of the spectrum of enzymes used to attack the food material is not static; the activity of many of them

Table 19.2. Transmission of passive immunity*

Species	Prenatal	Postnatal
Horse	0	+++ (24 h)
Pig	0	+++ (24–36 h)
Ox, goat, sheep	0	+++ (24 h)
Wallaby (*Setonix*)	0	+++ (180 d)
Dog, cat	+	++ (1–2 d)
Fowl	++	++ (<5 d)
Hedgehog	+	++ (40 d)
Mouse	+	++ (16 d)
Rat	+	++ (20 d)
Guinea pig	+++	0
Rabbit	+++	0
Human, monkey	+++	0

*0, no absorption or transfer; + to +++, degrees of absorption or transfer.
From Brambell 1970, *The Transmission of Passive Immunity from Mother to Young*, American Elsevier, New York.

increases or decreases in response to a change in the concentration of the substrate available.

Many of the studies on enzyme development have been conducted on the pig because of the practical importance to early-weaning diets. Therefore this species will primarily be considered except for some of the important species differences discussed below.

Salivary amylase is low in very young pigs, increases slightly by the time the pigs are 2 to 3 weeks old, and then falls to a low level. This enzyme is therefore relatively unimportant in starch digestion in the pig and is not present in carnivores and ruminants.

The gastric glands of the newborn pig contain both peptic and parietal cells, but the proteolytic activity of gastric mucosa is low at birth and for the first 2 weeks of life. This situation is fortunate, because otherwise the colostral antibodies would be exposed to digestion before they could be absorbed by the intestine. In addition, colostral secretions have been shown to contain a trypsin-inhibitory factor that also helps to preserve the protein antibodies from pancreatic enzyme hydrolysis. The levels of pepsin in stomach tissue are shown in Fig. 19.9 and indicate that after 2 weeks the pepsin activity increases rapidly. Coinciding with this increase in pepsin output is an increase in HCl production by the parietal cells. Acidic conditions in the stomach are necessary for gastric proteolytic digestion. However, the major hydrolytic activity of carbohydrate, protein, and fat is supplied by the pancreas.

The enzyme content of the pancreas also shows considerable change as the pig develops. The changes in trypsin, chymotrypsin, amylase, and lipase from birth to the age of 8 weeks are shown in Figs. 19.10 and 19.11. Also shown is the total consumption of milk protein, carbohydrate, and fat

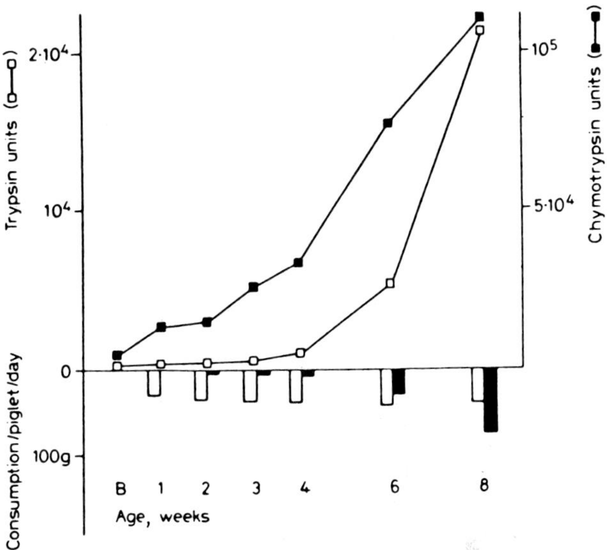

19.10. Total enzymatic activities of chymotrypsin and trypsin in the piglet from birth (B) until the eighth week of age. The bar graph shows average consumption of milk protein (open bars) and creep feed proteins (closed bars). (From Corring, Aumaitre, and Durand 1978, *Nutr. Metab.* 22:231–43.)

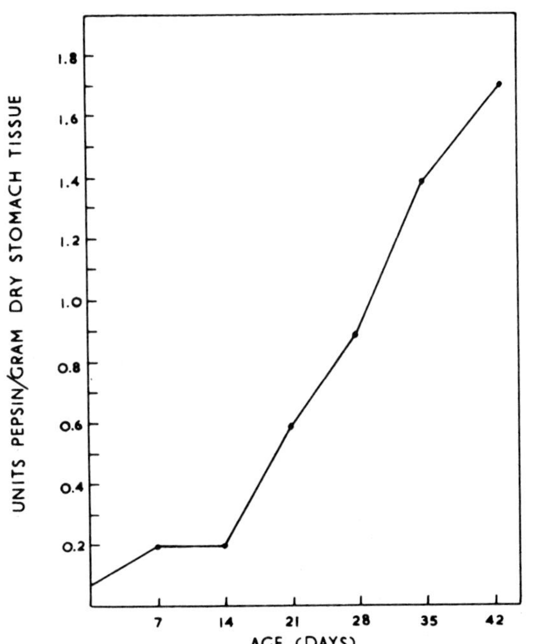

19.9. Pepsin level in dry stomach tissue from baby pigs of various ages. (From Lewis, Hartman, Liu, Baker, and Catron 1957, *J. Agric. Food Chem.* 5:687–90.)

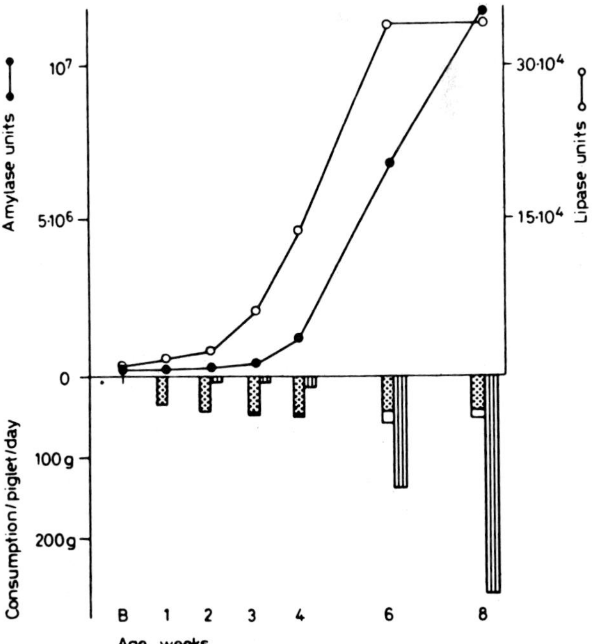

19.11. Total enzymatic activities of lipase and amylase in the piglet from birth (B) until the eighth week of age. The bar graph shows average consumption of milk fat (dotted bars), creep feed fat (open bars), and creep feed carbohydrates (lined bars). (From Corring, Aumaitre, and Durand 1978, *Nutr. Metab.* 22:231–43.)

as well as the amount of these substances, which were creep fed up to the time of weaning. The stimulation of enzyme activity coincides with the change in composition of the diet due to the intake of creep feed.

In adult nonruminants, with the exception of the horse, tremendous amounts of pancreatic amylase are delivered into the duodenum, and starch digestion is usually complete by the time the ingesta have reached the distal duodenum. However, owing in part to low levels of pancreatic amylase, the calf is unable to use starch. This low activity persists in the adult bovine and is important because in feeding practices where intake of grain is high, as much as 35 to 40 percent of the starch may reach the abomasum and small intestine.

Six different carbohydrases have been found in the brush border of the small intestine of the pig. These are lactase, trehalase, isomaltase, sucrase, and two maltases that are distinguishable by their different heat sensitivities.

Lactase activity is high at birth and throughout the first 2 to 3 weeks of life, after which time it declines rapidly. In contrast, sucrase and maltase activities are low at birth and then rise with age. These estimations have provided a rational explanation for the inability of the young pig to digest certain carbohydrates in artificial diets and have shown the importance of relating the composition of the diet (for example, its lactose content) to the animal's enzymatic capabilities. The activity of the six carbohydrate enzymes in the pig small intestine from 20 to 4000 days of age is shown in Fig. 19.12. Although the enzyme changes in pigs weaned early were significantly faster than in sow-reared pigs, age appears to be more important than diet in the development of these enzymes.

Thus, although the young pig has the ability to break down starch far in excess of what is normally fed, the amount of maltose that is hydrolyzed is very small compared with the amounts of starch broken down to maltose. Similarly, sucrase is low at birth but increases with age in the pig, whereas in the calf *sucrase is entirely absent from the intestinal mucosa*. Thus, while the young calf can readily use lactose, it has limited ability to use sucrose or starch.

DIGESTION IN LARGE INTESTINE

Digestion of carbohydrate and protein in the large intestine is brought about by the action of the microbial enzymes. No enzymatic digestion occurs in the large intestine of mammals.

Development of large intestine and microbial digestion

The gastrointestinal tract of the newborn animal is relatively devoid of microorganisms, but these are rapidly acquired after birth and a characteristic population soon de-

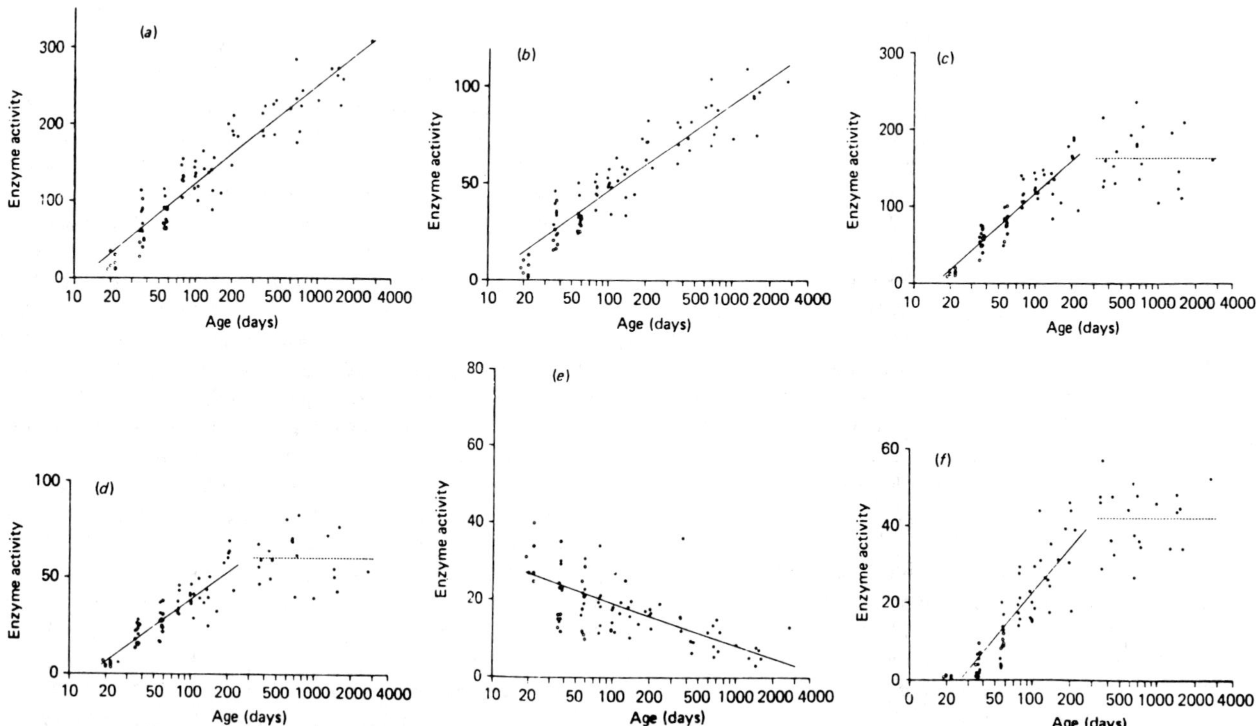

19.12. The mean brush border enzyme activities (units per gram of protein) for 21 samples from each of 84 pigs. Age is on a logarithmic scale. (*a*) Sucrase; (*b*) isomaltase; (*c*) maltase 2; (*d*) maltase 3; (*e*) lactase; (*f*) trehalase. (From Kidder and Manners 1980, *Br. J. Nutr.* 43:141–53.)

velops. In herbivores, foodstuffs are broken down in the digestive tract by the growth and development of microorganisms. This mechanism is characteristic of herbivore digestion, and the absorbed fermentation products constitute an important source of the animal's energy.

In ruminants the large forestomach constitutes a fermentation vat; in nonruminant herbivores the cecum and colon are large, well-developed organs where microbial digestion takes place. In ruminants enzymatic digestion occurs *after* the food material has been attacked by microorganisms, and the microbial bodies themselves are eventually digested by the animal. Fermentation digestion follows enzymatic digestion in the simple herbivore, so that only the fermentation products and not the bacterial bodies are available for digestion and absorption by the host.

Because of the overriding importance of the fermentation process in the ruminant stomach, a great deal is known about the organisms (see Chap. 22), fermentation reactions, and the absorptive mechanisms concerned. The short-chain volatile fatty acids (VFAs) (acetic, propionic, and butyric acids) are the most important fermentation products that are readily absorbed and used by the ruminant. The same VFA *concentrations* and relative proportions of the three VFAs are found in the cecum and colon of all species, but much greater *quantities* are found in herbivorous and omnivorous species. The widespread occurrence of the three VFAs suggests that this mixture is a characteristic result of fermentation in the alimentary tract; although the significance of VFAs as an energy source is fully established in ruminants, their importance in other species has not been fully assessed.

Microbial digestion is of little importance in carnivores because the digestive processes are practically complete in the small intestine. The colon is short and nonsacculated and the cecum is relatively undeveloped. A microbial population is present in the large intestine, however, and the VFA end products are the same as in the herbivore. Figure 19.13 shows the concentration of these VFAs throughout the gastrointestinal tract of the dog, pig, and pony. The large intestine is the primary site of production of VFAs in these species, and these organic acids constitute the major anions in colonic contents.

The functional and structural development of the large intestine coincides with the development of microbial digestion. The capacity of the stomach represents a much greater proportion of the capacity of the total gastrointestinal tract in the young, suckling foal than in the adult. The stomach of the suckling foal also empties more slowly after a meal. In the weaned foal, however, the stomach empties rapidly, and most of the delay in digesta transit occurs in the large intestine. This delay is necessary for the relatively slow process of microbial digestion and also for the reabsorption of the large volumes of digestive secretions. Thus in the adult pony the mean transit time of liquid from the stomach to the cecum is approximately 2 hours, whereas

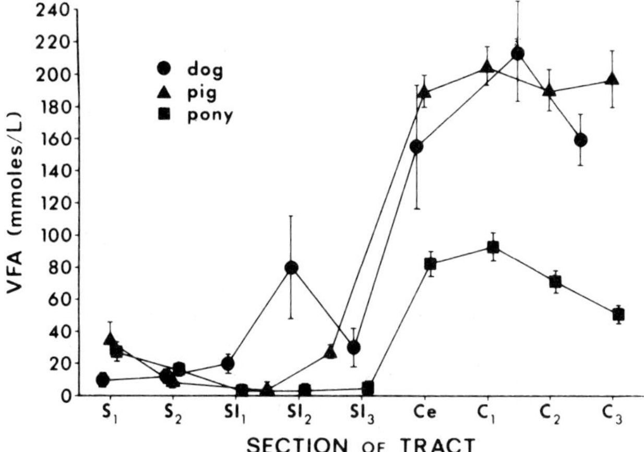

19.13. Mean volatile fatty acid (VFA) concentrations in segments of the dog, pig, and pony gastrointestinal tracts. Standard error (SE) is indicated with tick marks above and below each value. Each value represents the average from 12 animals that were killed in groups of 3 animals each at 2, 4, 8, and 12 hours after feeding. The sections examined were the oral (S_1) and aboral (S_2) halves of the stomach, two or three equal segments of the small intestine (SI_1, SI_2, and SI_3); the cecum (Ce); and two or three segments of the colon (C_1, C_2, and C_3). The pig colon was divided into proximal (C_1), centripetal (C_2), and centrifugal-plus-terminal (C_3) segments. In the pony, C_1 represents the ventral large colon, C_2 the dorsal large colon, and C_3 the small colon. Dogs were fed a meat diet, pigs were fed a high-concentrate diet and ponies were fed a conventional, pelletized horse diet. (Modified from Argenzio, Southworth, and Stevens 1974b, *Am. J. Physiol.* 226:1043–50; Argenzio and Southworth 1975, *Am. J. Physiol.* 228:454–60; Banta, Clemens, Krinsky, and Sheffy *J. Nutr.* 109:1592–1600.)

the transit time through the large colon is approximately 50 hours. This remarkable delay in digesta transit through the large colon is due to the motor function of the colon and to the great distensibility of the organs. The mechanisms responsible for these features were discussed in detail in Chapter 17.

Microbial digestion differs from enzymatic digestion in three ways. First, fibrous carbohydrate sources that have the beta-linked glucose polymers and are not broken down by mammalian enzymes are readily attacked by microbial enzymes. Furthermore, the end products of microbial carbohydrate digestion are not hexoses, but VFAs. This is fortunate because the adult colon is incapable of absorbing hexoses but can readily absorb the VFAs, which can then be used for a source of energy by the epithelium or general body tissues. Second, the microbes are capable of synthesizing microbial protein from nonprotein nitrogen sources such as urea. This protein may, in turn, be hydrolyzed to yield essential amino acids. Third, the microbes can synthesize the B vitamins. All of these processes have been studied at length in the ruminant stomach and will be discussed in detail in Chapter 21. Some principal physiological factors necessary for a contribution of the large intestine to energy and nitrogen conservation will be considered. The energy contribution from microbial digestion is of considerable importance in most herbivores and some omnivores.

Functional requirements for microbial digestion

Four major conditions are required for an environment capable of supporting an important degree of microbial digestion: (1) neutralization of the acidic end products released by the microbes into the luminal fluid; (2) a relatively long digesta-retention time to allow such slow processes as cellulose hydrolysis to occur; (3) a fluid environment capable of diluting the released end products to prevent feedback inhibition of their own production; and (4) continuous removal of the end products by absorption. In this chapter the first and fourth conditions will be considered. The motor function establishing the long retention time has been discussed in Chapter 17, and production of a fluid environment by intestinal secretion will be discussed in Chapter 20.

Carbohydrate digestion

Both soluble and insoluble carbohydrates are degraded by microbial enzymes, chiefly to hexoses (Fig. 19.14). The major difference in the digestion of these two sources, however, is the much longer time required to degrade cellulose. Soluble carbohydrate (starch) is fermented rapidly. Therefore, regardless of the carbohydrate source in the food, the hexoses that are produced are metabolized by the bacteria to VFA and gases, which are the end products of carbohydrate fermentation. A typical fermentation balance of hexose can be approximated by the following equation:

$$57.5\ (C_6H_{12}O_6) \rightarrow 65\ CH_3COOH + 20\ CH_3CH_2COOH + 15\ CH_3CH_2CH_2COOH + 60\ CO_2 + 35\ CH_4 + 25\ H_2O$$

(The first three constituents on the right-hand side of this equation are acetic acid, propionic acid, and butyric acid, respectively.) Only small amounts of lactate and succinate are produced under normal conditions. The ratios of the three major acids produced will vary according to the type of carbohydrate in the food. For example, a high-starch diet will result in a greater proportion of propionic acid than a high-fiber diet, which yields more acetate.

Under certain feeding conditions, such as when horses are fed a highly soluble carbohydrate diet once or twice a day, the production of acid may exceed the absorptive capacity of the large intestinal mucosa. For example, as much as 1.5 moles of acid accumulates in the large colon per day in ponies fed such a diet. Since this acid is produced faster than it is absorbed, it must be neutralized by the large intestinal buffer systems. Regulation of the luminal pH is one of the most important mechanisms in preserving normal function of the large intestine.

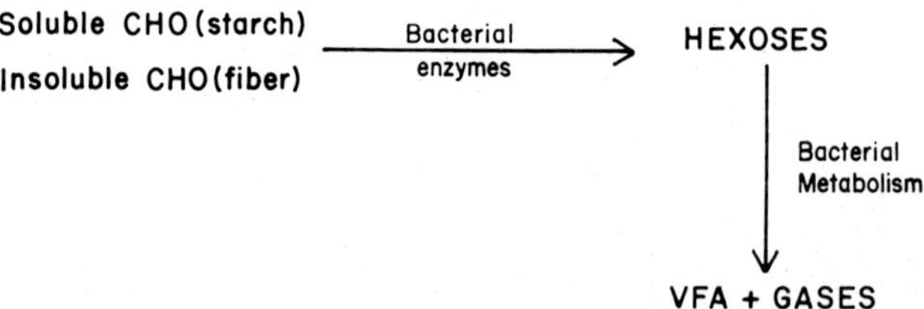

Figure 19.14. Carbohydrate digestion in large intestine. Both soluble and fibrous carbohydrates are broken down by microbial enzymes in the contents of the large intestine. The bacteria then ferment the hexoses to the end products shown.

Buffer systems of the large intestine

There are two major buffer systems operating in the large intestine: the HCO_3 and PO_4 buffers. The concentration of these buffers in the gastrointestinal tract for the horse, pig, dog, and cat is shown in Fig. 19.15. As discussed in Chapter 17, a substantial quantity of pancreatic HCO_3 is delivered into the duodenum; in the horse and pig, some of this contributes to the neutralizing capacity of the contents of the large intestine. In addition, the ileum is capable of secreting HCO_3 so that the fluid delivered to the cecum may have an HCO_3 concentration as high as 100 mM. In the dog and cat, the HCO_3 concentration entering the large intestine is not nearly as great; rather, PO_4 appears to be the major buffer.

When the HCO_3-buffered fluid enters the cecum and colon, it immediately reacts with the acids produced according to the following equation:

$$NaHCO_3 + HA \rightarrow NaA + CO_2 + H_2O$$

The net result is the disappearance of HCO_3 and replacement with the sodium salt of the organic acid. In addition to the neutralization by ileal fluid, the large intestine is also capable of secreting HCO_3. Therefore, the HCO_3 buffer system can precisely control the luminal pH.

In addition to the HCO_3 buffers, PO_4 also may contribute to the neutralization of the contents. In the ruminant, large

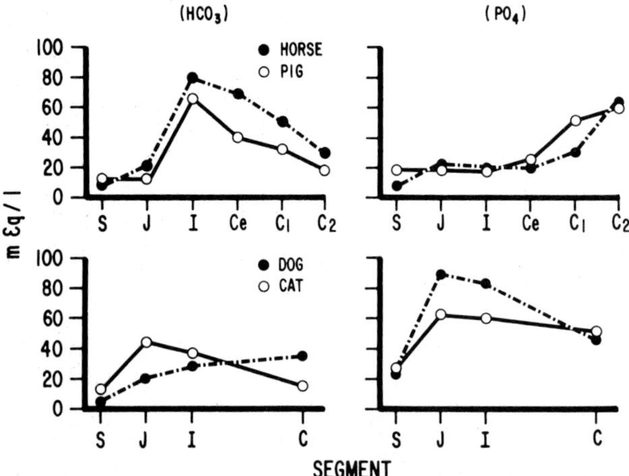

Figure 19.15. Concentrations of HCO_3 and PO_4 in gastrointestinal tracts of horse, pig, dog, and cat. S, stomach; J, jejunum; I, ileum; Ce, cecum; C_1, proximal colon; C_2, distal colon; C, colon plus rectum. Upper illustrations show values for the horse and pig. Lower illustrations show values for the dog and cat. (Modified from Alexander 1962, *Res. Vet. Sci.* 3:78–83, and 1965, *Res. Vet. Sci.* 6:238–44.)

amounts of PO_4 are secreted in the saliva, but in nonruminants the origin of intestinal PO_4 is primarily the diet. Phosphate is poorly absorbed by the intestine; therefore, as fluid is progressively absorbed, the concentration of PO_4 increases in the luminal contents. Phosphate reacts with the organic acids according to the following equation:

$$Na_2HPO_4 + HA \rightarrow NaH_2PO_4 + NaA$$

Thus the hydrogen ion will be excreted in the feces (as in the case of PO_4) rather than liberated as CO_2 (as in the case of the HCO_3 buffers).

Absorption of weak electrolytes

Absorption of a weak acid or a weak base is dependent on the un-ionized form of the compound as shown in Fig. 19.16. Most biological membranes are impermeable to the charged form of the weak electrolyte. In the case of the weak acid, the unprotonated form is ionized, whereas the protonated form of the weak base is ionized.

Lactic acidosis

Two situations that may arise and that can lower the luminal pH are depicted in Fig. 19.17. In the first case, there may be an *increase* in grain feeding in animals already adapted to a grain diet. In this situation, the rate of VFA production may be so intense that it overwhelms the buffer systems and lowers the luminal pH. When this occurs, the normal VFA-producing bacteria are killed and there is an increase in lactic acid–producing bacteria that thrive at a low pH. Lactic acid is poorly absorbed from colonic contents, however, and its increased rate of production leads to an increase in the effective osmotic pressure. The latter causes mucosal damage and results in osmotic flow of water from blood to lumen.

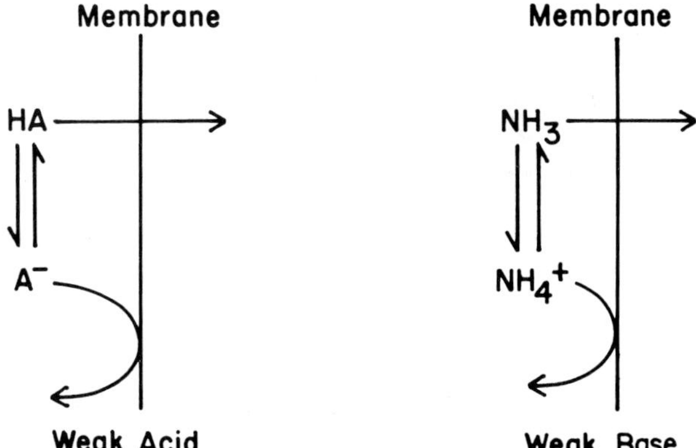

Figure 19.16. Absorption of weak electrolytes occurs in the un-ionized form. This form is lipid soluble in contrast to the charged form, which is water soluble. Thus the lipid-soluble component can diffuse across the lipid membranes of intestinal epithelial cells and gain access to the circulation. Large water-soluble molecules that are charged are excluded by membranes unless a specialized transport system is present. Horizontal arrows represent absorption. Curved arrows represent membrane exclusion.

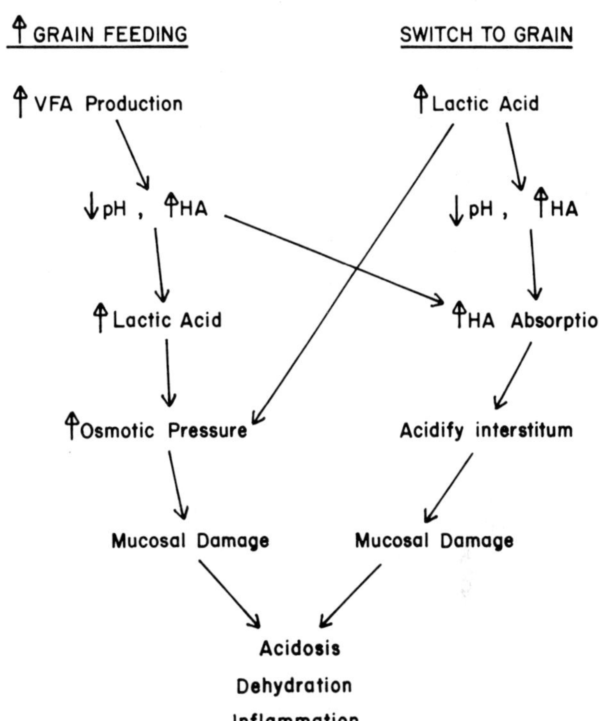

Figure 19.17. Generation of lactic acid and lowering of luminal pH in large intestinal contents. Overfeeding of starch or abrupt changeover in diet can result in lowering of the luminal pH and increased lactic acid production. These conditions can cause damage to the mucosa from acidification or hyperosmolality.

In the second case there is an abrupt switch to grain in animals that are not adapted. In this case lactic acid production increases immediately because the bacteria that metabolize lactic acid to VFAs are not yet present. Because lactic acid is a stronger acid than VFAs, it donates its hydrogen ion to the VFAs, causing a greater rate of VFA absorption because of the increase in undissociated acid as discussed above. The increased VFA absorption acidifies the interstitum and causes mucosal damage, as discussed under "Gastric Mucosal Barrier" (Chap. 18). Experimentally, it has been found that a pH of 5.0 or less begins to cause damage to the colonic mucosa.

Protein digestion

The processes of protein digestion in the large intestine are poorly understood but presumably are similar to forestomach digestion of protein (Chap. 21). In the rumen, microbial protein can be synthesized from nonprotein nitrogen sources such as urea. In addition, much of the dietary protein is broken down to peptides and amino acids and then resynthesized into microbial protein. In the ruminant, however, microbial protein can be digested and absorbed in the small intestine by the mammalian enzyme systems, whereas in the large intestine it is doubtful that an active

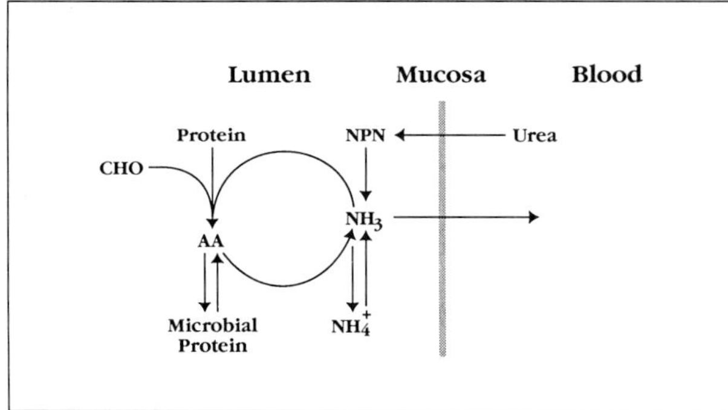

Figure 19.18. Generation and disposal of ammonia in large intestinal contents. Ammonia may be used for microbial protein synthesis, or it may be absorbed across the epithelium. When soluble carbohydrate is limiting, relatively more of the ammonia will be absorbed since carbohydrate components are needed for amino acid synthesis. Similarly, more ammonia will be absorbed if the lumen contents are alkaline. Although amino acids may arise from hydrolysis of protein, the absence of active transport systems for amino acids in colonic epithelium precludes their use for nutritional support of the host. Nevertheless, protein synthesis is important for the maintenance of microbial populations and the production of energy for the host in the form of volatile fatty acids.

amino acid or a peptide transport system is present. Except in species practicing coprophagy, it is unlikely that any major nutritional benefit is derived from protein synthesized by microbes in the large intestine.

Nitrogen use by the large intestine is important from the standpoint of NH_3 production and absorption (Fig. 18.18). Large amounts of NH_3 are produced in the cecum and colon. The source of this NH_3 is urea and also bacterial breakdown of dietary protein and amino acids. Urea in the blood can diffuse into the intestine down a concentration gradient. Urease enzymes, elaborated by the bacteria in the large intestine, immediately convert the urea to NH_3 so that urea concentrations in the large intestine are kept low. Some of the NH_3 produced may be used for microbial protein synthesis, and some may be absorbed.

As discussed previously, the rate of ammonia absorption is dependent on pH. Thus, in contrast to the VFAs, an increase in luminal pH gives rise to a greater rate of absorption. As can be seen from Fig. 19.18, the amount of NH_3 available for absorption is also dependent on the relative rate of NH_3 incorporation into microbial protein. Thus, when microbial protein synthesis is impaired, such as when a poorly fermentable source of carbohydrate is present, free ammonia levels may increase.

REFERENCES

Adibi, S.A. 1978. Intestinal absorption of amino acids and peptides. *Viewpoints on Digestive Diseases* 10(4):1–4.

Alexander, F. 1962. The concentration of certain electrolytes in the digestive tract of the horse and pig. *Res. Vet. Sci.* 3:78–83.

Alexander, F. 1965. The concentration of electrolytes in the alimentary tract of the rabbit, guinea pig, dog, and cat. *Res. Vet. Sci.* 6:238–44.

Argenzio, R.A. 1975. Functions of the equine large intestine and their interrelationship in disease. *Cornell Vet.* 65:303–30.

Argenzio, R.A. 1980. Glucose-stimulated fluid absorption in the pig small intestine during the early stage of swine dysentery. *Am. J. Vet. Res.* 41:2000–6.

Argenzio, R.A., and Hintz, H.F. 1972. Effect of diet on glucose entry and oxidation rates in ponies. *J. Nutr.* 102:879–92.

Argenzio, R.A., and Southworth, M. 1975. Sites of organic acid production and absorption in gastrointestinal tract of the pig. *Am. J. Physiol.* 228:454–60.

Argenzio, R.A., Southworth, M., Lowe, J.E., and Stevens, C.E. 1977. Interrelationship of Na, HCO_3, and volatile fatty acid transport by equine large intestine. *Am. J. Physiol.* 233:E469–E478.

Argenzio, R.A., Southworth, M., and Stevens, C.E. 1974. Sites of organic acid production and absorption in the equine gastrointestinal tract. *Am. J. Physiol.* 226:1043–50.

Banta, C.A. Clemens, E.T., Krinsky, M.M., and Sheffy, B.E. 1979. Sites of organic acid production and patterns of digesta movement in the gastrointestinal tract of dogs. *J. Nutr.* 109:1592–1600.

Brambell, F.W.R. 1970. *The Transmission of Passive Immunity from Mother to Young*. Elsevier, New York.

Bryant, M.P. 1970. Normal flora-rumen bacteria. *J. Clin. Nutr.* 23:1440–47.

Combe, N.B., and Smith, R.H. 1973. Absorption of glucose and galactose and digestion and absorption of lactose by the preruminant calf. *Br. J. Nutr.* 30:331–44.

Corring, T., Aumaitre, A., and Durand, G. 1978. Development of digestive enzymes in the piglet from birth to 8 weeks. I. Pancreas and pancreatic enzymes. *Nutr. Metab.* 22:231–43.

Crane, R.K. 1968. Absorption of sugars. In *Handbook of Physiology.* Sec. 6, C.F. Code and W. Heidel, eds., *Alimentary Canal.* Vol. 3, *Intestinal Absorption.* Am. Physiol. Soc., Washington. Pp. 1323–51.

Gillette, D.D., and Filkins, M. 1966. Factors affecting antibody transfer in the newborn puppy. *Am. J. Physiol.* 210:419–22.

Gray, G.M. 1973. Mechanisms of digestion and absorption of food. In M.H. Sleisenger and J.S. Fordtran, eds., *Gastrointestinal Disease.* W.B. Saunders, Philadelphia. Pp. 250–57.

Gray, G.M. 1980. Assimilation of dietary carbohydrate. *Viewpoints on Digestive Diseases* 12(3):1–4.

Herschel, D.A., Argenzio, R.A., Southworth, M., and Stevens, C.E. 1981. Absorption of volatile fatty acid, Na, and H_2O by the colon of the dog. *Am. J. Vet. Res.* 42:1181–24.

Huber, J.T. 1968. Development of the digestive and metabolic apparatus of the calf. *J. Dairy Sci.* 52:1–13.

Jackson, M.J., Shiau, Y.F., Bane, S., and Fox, M. 1974. Intestinal transport of weak electrolytes: Evidence in favor of a three-compartment system. *J. Gen. Physiol.* 63:187–213.

Johnston, J.M. 1968. Mechanism of fat absorption. In *Handbook of Physiology.* Sec. 6, C.F. Code and W. Heidel, eds., *Alimentary Canal.* Vol. 3, *Intestinal Absorption.* Am. Physiol. Soc., Washington. Pp. 1353–75.

Kidder, D.E. and Manners, M.J. 1980. The level and distribution of carbohydrases in the small intestine mucosa of pigs from 3 weeks of age to maturity. *Br. J. Nutr.* 43:141–53.

Lewis, C.J., Hartman, P.A., Liu, C.H., Baker, R.O., and Catron, D.V. 1957. Digestive enzymes of the baby pig: Pepsin and trypsin. *J. Agric. Food Chem.* 5:687–90.

Moir, R.J. 1968. Ruminant digestion and evolution. In *Handbook of Physiology.* Sec. 6, C.F. Code and W. Heidel, eds., *Alimentary Canal.* Vol. 5, *Bile, Digestion, Ruminal Physiology.* Am. Physiol. Soc., Washington. Pp. 2673–94.

Moon, H.W. 1971. Epithelial cell migration in the alimentary mucosa of the suckling pig. *Proc. Soc. Exp. Biol. Med.* 137:151–54.

Morris, I.G. 1968. Gamma globulin absorption in the newborn. In *Handbook of Physiology.* Sec. 6, C.F. Code and W. Heidel, eds., *Alimentary Canal.* Vol. 3, *Intestinal Absorption.* Am. Physiol. Soc., Washington. Pp. 1491–1512.

Nervi, F.O. 1976. Normal mechanisms of carbohydrate and protein absorption. In J.M. Dietschy, ed., *Disorders of the Gastrointestinal Tract,*

Disorders of the Liver, Nutritional Disorders. Grune & Stratton, New York. Pp. 35–37.

Powell, D.W. 1979. Transport in large intestine. In G. Giebish, D.C. Tosteson, and H.H. Ussing, eds., *Membrane Transport in Biology*. Springer-Verlag, New York. Pp. 781–809.

Rose, R.C. 1980. Water soluble vitamin absorption in intestine. *Ann. Rev. Physiol.* 42:157–71.

Scharrer, E. 1975. Developmental changes of sugar and amino acid transport in different tissues of ruminants. In I.W. McDonald and A.C.I. Warner, eds., *Digestion and Metabolism in the Ruminant*. Univ. of New Eng. Publ. Unit, Armidale, New South Wales, Australia. Pp. 49–59.

Siddons, R.C., Smith, R.H., Henschel, M.J., Hill, W.B., and Porter, J.W.G. 1969. Carbohydrate utilization in the pre-ruminant calf. *Br. J. Nutr.* 22:333–41.

Stevens, C.E., Argenzio, R.A., and Clemens, E.T. 1980. Microbial digestion: Rumen versus large intestine. In Y. Ruckebusch and P. Thivend, eds., *Digestive Physiology and Metabolism in Ruminants*. A.V.I. Publishing Co., Inc., Westport, Conn. Pp. 685–706.

Trier, J.S. 1968. Morphology of the epithelium of the small intestine. In *Handbook of Physiology*. Sec. 6, C.F. Code and W. Heidel, eds., *Alimentary Canal*. Vol. 3, *Intestinal Absorption*. Am. Physiol. Soc., Washington. Pp. 1125–75.

Toofanian, F. 1976. Small intestinal infusion studies in the calf. *Br. Vet. J.* 132:215–20.

Walker, D.M. 1959. The development of the digestive system of the young pig. *J. Agric. Sci.* 52:357–63.

Walker, W.A., and Isselbacher, K.J. 1974. Uptake and transport of macromolecules by the intestine: Possible role in clinical disorder. *Gastroenterology* 67:531–50.

Westergaad, H. 1976. Normal mechanisms of lipid absorption. In J.M. Dietschy, ed., *Disorders of the Gastrointestinal Tract, Disorders of the Liver, Nutritional Disorders*. Grune & Stratton, New York. Pp. 38–39.

Williamson, R.C.N., and Chir, M. 1978a. Intestinal adaptation: Structural, functional and cytokinetic changes. *New Engl. J. Med.* 298:1393–1402.

Williamson, R.C.N., and Chir, M. 1978b. Intestinal adaptation: Mechanisms of control. *New Engl. J. Med.* 298:1444–50.

Wooton, J.F., and Argenzio, R.A. 1975. Nitrogen utilization within equine large intestine. *Am. J. Physiol.* 229:1062–67.

CHAPTER 20

Intestinal Transport of Electrolytes and Water | by Robert A. Argenzio

The most critical function of the intestine, quite apart from its digestive and absorptive functions, is the reabsorption of the digestive secretions delivered into the proximal part of the intestine. In addition to the secretory fluids provided by the accessory organs and the stomach (Chap. 18), the intestine itself is capable of net secretion under certain conditions. Collectively, the sum of these secretory fluids forms a substantial fraction of the extracellular fluid (ECF) volume from which they are derived, and the ions present in the secretions also originate from the ECF. These secretions must be almost entirely recovered to preserve the ECF volume and arterial pressure.

ENTEROSYSTEMIC CYCLE

The net movement of fluid into and out of the intestine lumen every 24 hours is known as the *enterosystemic cycle* of fluid; this is shown for the pony in Fig. 20.1. It is important to realize that these figures represent net movements of fluid and not total diffusion fluxes into and out of the lumen. For example, the lumen of the intestine will daily exchange several times the total volume of body water, but most of this is simply bidirectional exchange of water or solute molecules across the intestine wall with little net loss or gain. Nevertheless, as shown in Fig. 20.1, a substantial fraction of the total body water is presented to the lumen every 24 hours as *net* fluid secretion and represents a potential loss of fluid from the body. In fact, the sum of these secretions approximates the entire ECF volume of the pony in Fig. 20.1.

Although such large volumes are not secreted in carnivores and omnivores, these fluids still comprise a substantial volume and are greatly influenced by the type of diet. A high-fiber diet in the pig, for example, will increase these secretory fluid volumes to values comparable (per unit of body weight) to those of the horse. It is also important to note that the major reabsorptive sites are the distal small intestine and large intestine. It can be readily seen from the values shown in Fig. 20.1 that complete failure of even the large intestine to reabsorb these secretions (as would occur in upper intestinal obstruction or certain types of diarrhea) would result in death in less than 24 hours from circulatory collapse. For example, a 30 percent loss of the ECF volume is sufficient to cause death. This would amount to 10 to 11 L in the 175 kg pony described above. This value approximates the amount of fluid reabsorbed by the large intestine in 24 hours.

FUNCTIONAL ANATOMY

Figure 20.2 shows two intestinal absorptive cells that are absorbing solute and fluid under normal conditions. Solute and water traverse the intestinal epithelium through two parallel pathways. The first of these (the *intracellular pathway*) is through the cell, and the apical cell membrane and basolateral membrane must be traversed. This pathway is also called the active transport path, because most water-soluble substances traversing the cell membranes are subjected to some type of specialized transport process. The second pathway (the *extracellular pathway*) is between the cells and through the tight junctions; this is the pathway through which many water-soluble substances are passively transported. The major barriers to transepithelial solute and water transport for actively transported substances are the

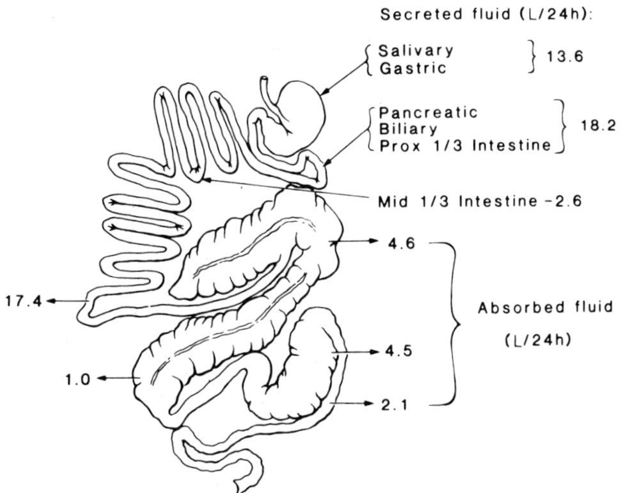

Figure 20.1. Enterosystemic circulation of fluid in 175 kg ponies; values shown are liters of fluid. Animals were in steady state with regard to intake of feed and marker, which were fed at 2-hour intervals for at least 2 weeks prior to study. Data from six animals. (From Schmall and Argenzio, unpublished data.)

cell membranes and, for passively transported substances, the tight junction. The basement membrane and lamina propria provide very little resistance to flow under normal conditions.

Also shown in Fig. 20.2 are active solute "pumps" located along the lateral and basal membranes of the transporting cells. These mechanisms pump Na into the lateral intercellular spaces by an active, energy-requiring process. This Na pumping initiates four sequential events that are responsible for most of the salt and water absorption by the intestine. First, the net Na delivery raises the effective osmotic pressure in the intercellular space. Second, it delivers a net positive charge into the space, and this charge attracts negatively charged ions that further increase the effective

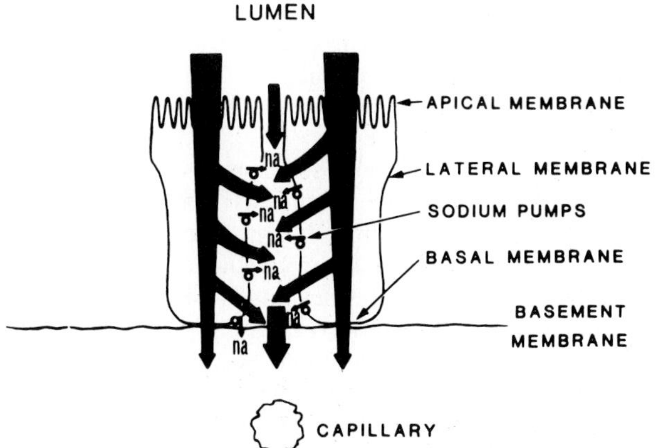

Figure 20.2. Pathways for transepithelial transport of solute and water. The active sodium pump mechanism at lateral and basal membranes establishes the electrochemical and osmotic gradient for passive ion and water flows. (Modified from Argenzio 1978, *J. Am. Vet. Med. Asso.* 173:667–72.)

osmotic pressure. Third, the increased effective osmotic pressure in the intercellular space results in water flow into the space through the cell membranes and tight junctions, and this in turn raises the hydrostatic pressure in the intercellular space. Fourth, the increased hydrostatic pressure drives solute and water across the basement membrane into the capillary.

As can be appreciated, the resistance to flow across the junction between the cells must be greater than the resistance across the basement membrane for the intercellular pressures to drive solute and fluid toward the capillary. Otherwise, so much cycling of solute and water back into the lumen would occur that the pump mechanism would be rendered ineffective. This important permeability characteristic of the junction is discussed below.

Permeability characteristics of the intestine

The permeability characteristics of the gastrointestinal tract vary greatly from the stomach to the rectum. The cell membranes of the epithelial cells are relatively impermeable to diffusion of charged ions and offer a high resistance barrier. Conversely, the so-called tight junctions actually are low-resistance pathways for movement of some ions. The relative passive permeability of the epithelium is, therefore, determined by the permeability of the tight junction. The permeability of the apical cell membrane is determined by specialized transport processes located on the membrane or by ion-selective pores in the membrane.

The stomach has such a tight epithelium that it is almost impermeable even to water. This characteristic prevents the large bulk flow of water into the stomach that otherwise would occur in response to the high effective osmotic pressures generated in gastric contents during digestion. In marked contrast to the stomach, the duodenum and the jejunum display the most permeable epithelia in the tract. Fortunately, as was discussed in Chap. 17, the hypertonic gastric contents are delivered slowly into the duodenum, thereby preventing rapid shifts of fluid from the extracellular space into the lumen. Because of this high-permeability characteristic, the osmolality of duodenal and jejunal contents equilibrates rapidly with that of the blood.

From the jejunum to the colon, the epithelium becomes progressively less permeable, so that in the distal colon relatively large osmotic and concentration gradients can be sustained between lumen and blood, as shown in Fig. 20.3. For this reason, fecal contents can have K concentrations as high as 80 to 90 mEq/L, while the Na concentration can be as low as 40 to 50 mEq/L. In the herbivore, whose intake of K is relatively high, this differential permeability is one means of getting rid of excess K while conserving Na.

One other characteristic of the junctional complex is important, and this is its ion selectivity. In the small intestine, the junction is cation-selective. A considerable amount of the Na that is transported into the intercellular space may leak back across this cation-selective junction into the lu-

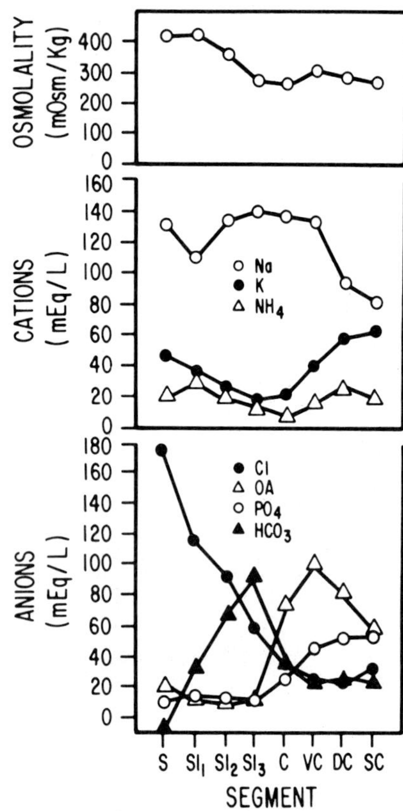

Figure 20.3. Digesta osmolality and ion concentrations along gastrointestinal tract of the pony. Data represent mean values over a 12-hour period between meals. S, stomach; SI_1, SI_2, SI_3, three equal segments of small intestine; C, cecum; VC, ventral colon; DC, dorsal colon; SC, small colon; OA, organic acids, including acetate, propionate, butyrate, and lactate. Data from 24 ponies. (From Argenzio 1975, *Cornell Vet.* 65:303–30.)

men. Consequently, the concentration of Na in the lumen of the small intestine never gets much below the plasma concentration, whereas the luminal Cl concentration may decrease along the small intestine (Fig. 20.3). A relatively high Na concentration is necessary in the small intestine, however, for reasons discussed below. The colonic tight junction, besides being relatively impermeable, is not Na-selective (but does appear to be K-selective), and very little Na leaks back into the lumen. Sodium is conserved by the colon, whereas Cl is conserved primarily by the small intestine.

PASSIVE FORCES GOVERNING ABSORPTION

A driving force of some kind is necessary to move salt and water from the intestinal lumen back into the blood. Most of the salt and water transport is a consequence of an active force requiring metabolic energy. Passive driving forces also develop across the intestine; in most cases these passive forces are secondary to active forces, but in other cases they result from the luminal fluid composition or certain pathological conditions. The passive forces that do not require a direct source of energy to affect net transport of salt and water will be considered first.

Osmotic pressure

The osmotic pressure difference that develops across a semipermeable membrane (membrane permeable only to water, not salt) will be equal to the product RTΔC, where R is the gas constant, T the absolute temperature, and ΔC the molar concentration difference across the membrane. The intestinal epithelium is not strictly semipermeable but is permeable to some solutes, and this permeability is in turn dependent on the epithelial zóne. In such instances, the *effective* osmotic pressure will be less than the theoretical osmotic pressure, depending on the relative permeability of the membrane to the solute. As noted previously, the tight junction or cell membrane is much less permeable to ion movement than is the basement membrane. Consequently, the effective osmotic pressure that develops across the tight junction or cell membrane, in response to solute concentration differences between the lumen and the intercellular space or cell, will be much greater than the effective osmotic pressure that develops across the basement membrane. For this reason, water flows into the hypertonic intercellular space from the cell or lumen rather than from the subepithelial tissue fluid.

For the same reason, some solutes present in the lumen (glucose, for example) are so rapidly absorbed across the apical cell membrane by a specialized process that their contribution to the effective osmotic pressure will be far less than would be predicted from their molar concentration. On the other hand, solutes (e.g., mannitol or sulfate) that are very poorly absorbed will exert almost their full theoretical osmotic pressure. Accordingly, if the epithelium is less permeable to solutes present in the lumen than to those in the blood, these will be a net movement of water into the lumen, even though the measured osmolality on both sides of the epithelium is identical. These factors also indicate that even though hypertonic or hypotonic solutions are present in the lumen, a driving force for net water movement is not necessarily present.

Hydrostatic pressure

As discussed above, hydrostatic pressures develop in the intercellular space from osmotically induced bulk water flow. Normally the hydrostatic pressure of subepithelial tissue is very low, so that the intercellular pressure is sufficient to drive solute and water into the capillary. In some edematous conditions, however, such as partial venous obstruction, the tissue pressure may become high enough to reverse the pressure gradient between the capillary and the intercellular space. In conditions in which the tissue fluid hydrostatic pressure becomes 5 cm of water or greater, pressure-induced secretion into the intestine may occur. In contrast, even very high luminal pressures cannot result in the converse situation. This is presumably due to the geometry of the epithelial cells, tight junctions, and intercellular spaces.

Solvent drag

In some circumstances an osmotic or hydrostatic pressure gradient across the epithelium is sufficient to induce net water movement. In such cases solute will become entrapped in the fluid stream and can even be transported against concentration or electrical gradients. This is a very important mechanism for net solute transport in the jejunum because the junctional complexes are so leaky that very little "sieving" of the fluid will occur.

Electrochemical gradient

Most transporting epithelia display electrical potential differences and ion concentration differences across their membranes as a result of active ion transport processes or diffusion of charged ions. In the intestine, the blood is normally positively charged in respect to the lumen contents. This is the net result of the algebraic sum of the potential differences across the apical and basolateral cell membranes arranged in series. The potential difference (PD) will cause a distribution of diffusible ions as depicted in Fig. 20.4. If movement of the ion is attributable solely to passive diffusion, its distribution at equilibrium may be calculated from the Nernst equation:

$$\text{EMF (mV)} = 61.5 \log [\text{concentration ratio}].$$

Accordingly, as shown in Fig. 20.4, a cation that distributes by passive diffusion will move from blood to lumen until its higher concentration in the lumen exactly offsets the electrical PD. Conversely, there will be a net movement of an anion in the opposite direction. The distribution of many ions across the intestinal epithelium does not satisfy the Nernst equation, however, and thus the ion must be subjected to some kind of active transport.

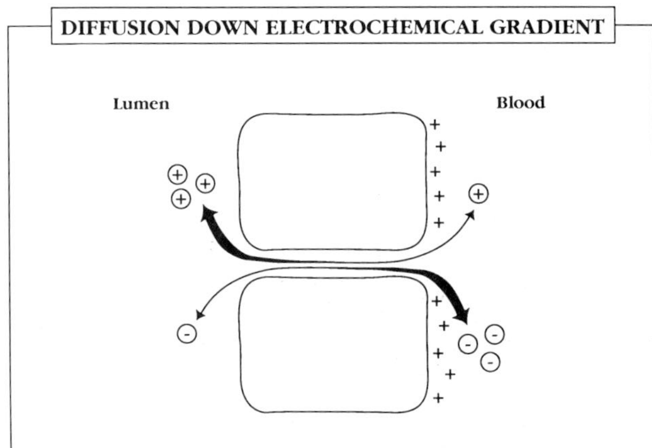

Figure 20.4. Diffusible ions move passively down an electrochemical gradient. A positive charge on the blood side of the tissue will cause diffusible cations to move into the lumen and anions to move toward the blood. Concentration differences of ions also cause a passive movement of the ion to a lower concentration. At equilibrium, there is no net movement of ions, and the combined electrochemical potential is therefore 0. If an ion distributes strictly by passive diffusion, its concentration ratio across the epithelium at equilibrium can be predicted from the Nernst equation if the electrical potential is known and, conversely, the electrical potential can be predicted if the concentration ratio is known.

ACTIVE TRANSPORT

By far the most important function of the intestinal epithelial cell is its active transport of Na from lumen to blood. This single mechanism not only is responsible for transepithelial Na transport but also is the principal mechanism for creating conditions for absorption of most electrolytes and a number of nonelectrolytes as well. Figure 20.5 shows a single small intestinal epithelial cell transporting Na from lumen to blood, as well as the Na and Cl concentrations and electrical PDs across the cell membranes.

The internal Na concentration of this cell (Fig. 20.5) is maintained at an extremely low level, and this is due to the Na pump at the basolateral membrane, which actively pumps Na from the cell to the blood. This pump mechanism requires a direct source of energy furnished by adenosine triphosphate because it must pump Na against both a tenfold concentration gradient and an electrical potential of 50 mV.

In contrast, entry of Na into the cell from the lumen is down an electrochemical gradient of nearly equal magnitude. Entry of Na into the cell is a passive process and does not require a direct source of energy. In fact, the diffusion process may *serve* as a source of energy for transport of other substances, as discussed below.

SMALL INTESTINE ABSORPTION

Large quantities of salt and water of both dietary and endogenous origin are absorbed by the small intestine. In addition, the majority of dietary substrates, fat- and water-soluble vitamins, and minerals are absorbed here. The absorption of most water-soluble compounds is by passive

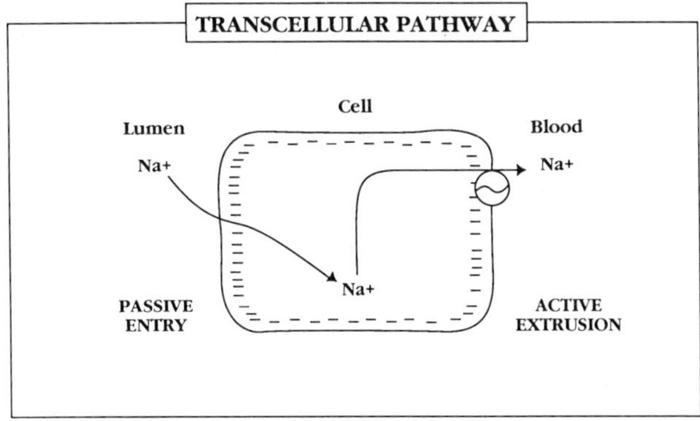

Figure 20.5. The active transport pathway is through the cell. Sodium moves into the cell down a combined electrochemical gradient, and therefore the uptake does not require a source of energy. In contrast, exit of Na from cell to blood is against an electrochemical gradient and requires a source of energy. This energy is supplied from adenosine triphosphate, which energizes the Na pump, shown as the circle on the basolateral membrane.

diffusion via the intercellular route or by active transcellular transport. Compounds absorbed against an electrochemical gradient require a source of energy; in most cases this is supplied by the Na pump.

Coupling of Na gradient to electrolyte and nonelectrolyte absorption

The Na gradient across the cell may serve as a source of free energy for other transport processes. Figure 20.6 shows three examples of how this is brought about. In the upper portion of the figure is shown a mechanism that is transporting the electrically neutral salt complex, NaCl, into the cell. As discussed above, entry of Na into the cell is a passive process that does not require a direct source of energy. In contrast, the entry of Cl requires a source of energy because it is entering the cell *against* a combined electrochemical gradient. Such movement, however, may be energized by the Na gradient through a carrier mechanism located on the apical cell membrane. This transport process is specific and requires an obligatory one-to-one interaction of both ions with the transport mechanism. The energy from the Na gradient is more than sufficient to drive Cl against its gradient into the cell. Such a process is not

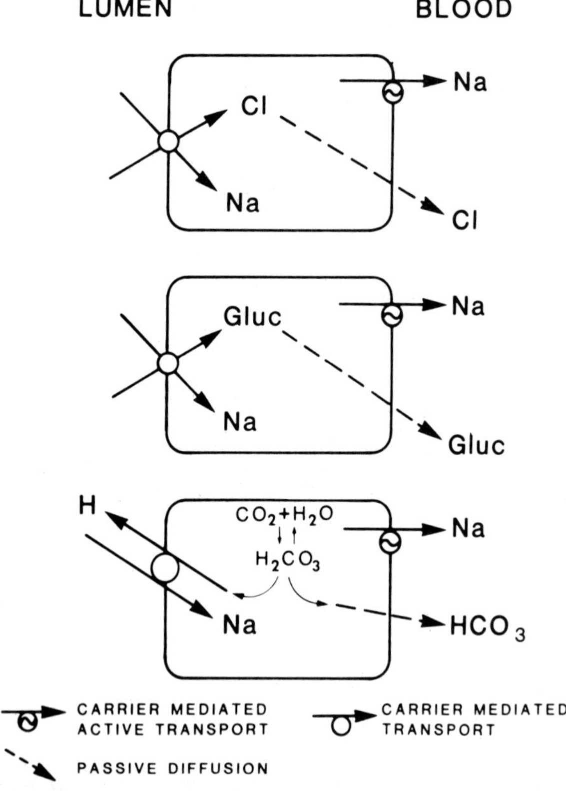

Figure 20.6. Coupled transport mechanisms using sodium gradient as a source of energy for transport across the luminal border of the epithelial cell. Secondary active transport (*top*), nonelectrolyte transport (*middle*), and countertransport (*bottom*) are depicted. Gluc, glucose.

active in the strict sense of the term because a direct source of metabolic energy is not consumed. It is, however, secondarily dependent on the active Na pump mechanism that establishes the Na gradient, therefore the process is termed *secondary active transport*.

There are present similar but substrate-specific mechanisms that couple the Na gradient to *nonelectrolyte transport,* as also shown in Fig. 20.6. In this case, glucose is transported into the cell against its chemical gradient by coupling itself to the Na gradient. Such Na-dependent mechanisms are capable of transporting a variety of sugars, amino acids, bile salts, and even more water-soluble vitamins against their respective electrochemical gradients into the cell. Once these substances gain entry into the cell, they may diffuse down their electrochemical gradients from cell to blood. All of these substrate-coupled mechanisms are present only in the small intestine. None are seen in the adult colon. It is fortunate that the Na concentration remains high in the small intestine, as discussed previously, for this provides the driving force for absorption of most end products of carbohydrate and protein digestion.

A third type of mechanism that uses the Na gradient, termed *countertransport,* is shown in the lower portion of Fig. 20.6. Such a mechanism may be capable of transporting an intracellular H ion against its electrochemical gradient into the lumen in exchange for Na. The operation of such a mechanism is dependent on the pH difference as well as the Na gradient across the membrane. As can be seen, this is one means by which the epithelium can acidify the lumen and alkalize the ECF, that is, by asymmetrical transport of the hydration products of CO_2. In some species, such as the dog, the operation of this mechanism in the jejunum is one means of recovering excess pancreatic HCO_3, even though it is not the same HCO_3 ion that was secreted by the pancreas. In the horse and the pig, pancreatic HCO_3 is not reabsorbed but contributes to the neutralization of organic acids in the cecum and colon.

In addition to the countertransport of Na and H, a similar but Na-independent mechanism can exchange Cl for intracellular HCO_3 across the luminal membrane. Such a process is driven by the electrochemical gradient of HCO_3 across the lumen membrane, which may be sufficient in some cases to energize Cl uptake into the cell. This mechanism has the virtue of alkalizing the luminal contents and is a very important mechanism in the ileum and large intestine of herbivores and omnivores. In Fig. 20.3 it can be seen that the concentration of HCO_3 is increasing in the distal small intestine, while that of Cl is decreasing. In all probability, this is the result of a Cl-HCO_3 exchange mechanism in this region. As discussed in Chapter 19, the organic acids produced in the cecum and colon of these animals must be rapidly neutralized or absorbed to prevent the consequences of luminal acidification. Secretion of HCO_3 by the distal intestine ensures a proper degree of neutralization of these acids under normal conditions.

COLONIC ABSORPTION

The colon absorbs Na, Cl, and volatile fatty acids (VFAs) (Fig. 20.7). Sodium is absorbed by two mechanisms, depending on the region of intestine examined. In the proximal colon Na is absorbed by a Na-H exchange process, which is an electrically neutral process inasmuch as its operation does not contribute to the transmural PD. In contrast, Na absorption in the distal colon is electrogenic because its movement is not coupled to an anion in the same direction or to a cation in the opposite direction; consequently, it is a source of electric charge across the epithelium.

Chloride is absorbed in exchange for HCO_3 on the luminal membrane. Such a process helps to buffer the luminal acidity; Cl concentrations in the colonic lumen are normally low, however, and quantitatively the process is relatively unimportant.

The absorption of a VFA (acetate) is depicted in Fig. 20.8. As discussed in Chapter 19, absorption of a weak acid occurs in the un-ionized form. At the normal luminal pH, more than 99 percent of the VFAs would be in the charged form, and their rapid absorption requires a source of H ions. This source of H is supplied by two mechanisms, as shown in the figure. First, hydration of CO_2 generates a H and a HCO_3 ion; absorption of HA maintains a gradient for this reaction to occur. Second, the Na-H exchange process in proximal colon generates a source of H. Thus the Na gradient is indirectly linked to colonic VFA absorption.

The colon both absorbs and secretes K in mammals that have been studied. Under normal conditions, the proximal colon secretes K, whereas the distal colon absorbs K. Aldosterone increases K secretion in the proximal colon and induces K secretion in the distal colon. Thus the distal colon is capable of both absorption and secretion of K, and it participates in the overall regulation of K balance.

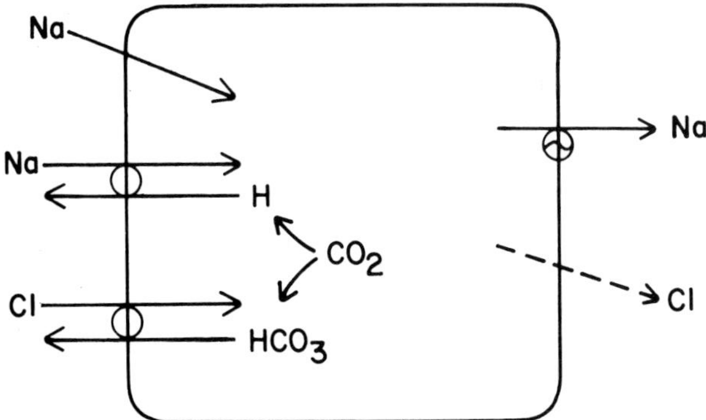

Figure 20.7. The colon absorbs Na, Cl, and VFAs. Sodium is absorbed from the lumen into the cell by an electrogenic mechanism in the distal colon and by a Na-H exchange process in the proximal colon, depicted on the left-hand side of the cell. Chloride is absorbed by Cl-HCO_3 exchange in both proximal and distal colon. The H and HCO_3 ions are produced in the cell from hydration of CO_2, and this reaction is facilitated by carbonic anhydrase. Sodium is pumped out of the cell into the blood by the Na pump; however, Cl is able to diffuse from cell to blood down its electrochemical gradient.

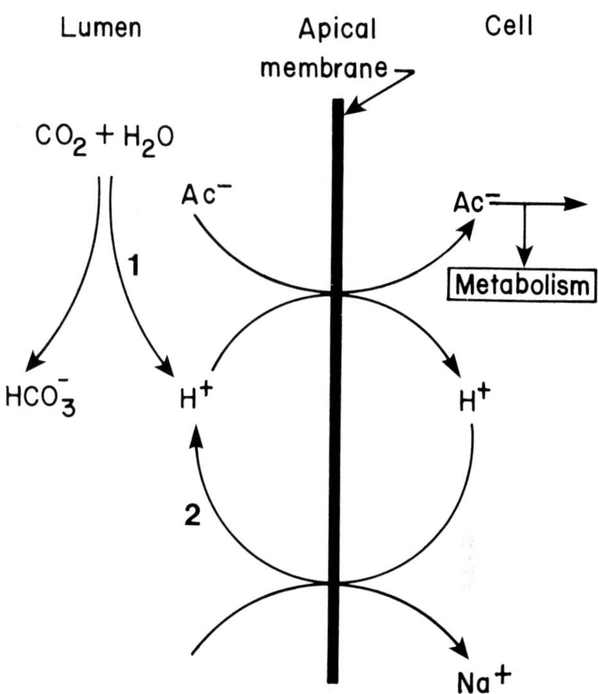

Figure 20.8. Absorption of volatile fatty acid by colonic mucosa. Un-ionized acetate is generated at the apical membrane by H derived from luminal CO_2 and from Na-H exchange. The acid dissociates inside the cell, and the H ion is recycled back into the lumen to form more undissociated VFA. Hydration of CO_2 provides an alternative source of H ions, however, so that, even if Na absorption is inhibited, VFA can still be absorbed. The VFA is partially metabolized by the cell, and the remainder is delivered into the blood. Thus, a concentration gradient for absorption of undissociated acid across the luminal membrane is maintained.

INTESTINAL SECRETION

Secretion by the intestine is a physiological event. In the case of herbivores and omnivores, an alkaline fluid furnished by the distal small intestine and the proximal large intestine is necessary for the microbial digestive process. Unfortunately, this mechanism, which is usually controlled precisely through physiological systems, can also be activated by certain bacterial toxins elaborated in the intestinal lumen. In such conditions uncontrolled secretory diarrhea develops; this pathological process is a leading cause of death in neonatal calves and pigs and an important cause of diarrhea in other species, including humans.

Mechanism of intestinal secretion

Secretory processes are a function of the crypt epithelium, whereas absorptive processes are confined to the villous epithelium of the small intestine and to the surface epithelium of the colon (Fig. 20.9). Normally there is an

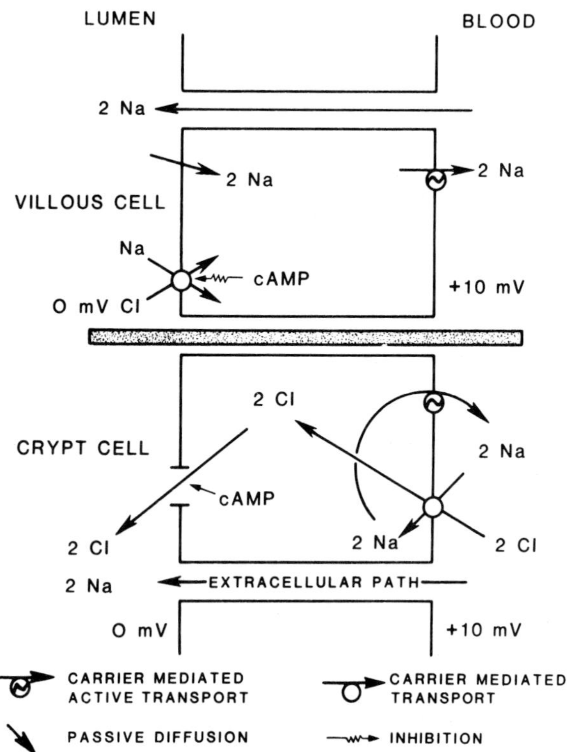

Figure 20.9. Antiabsorptive and secretory effects of cAMP. Many secretory stimuli affect both the absorptive processes on the villus as well as inducing secretion in the crypts. Therefore the neutral NaCl absorptive mechanism on the villus is interrupted. An increase in anion conductance in the crypts leads to net Cl secretion, which in turn pulls Na into the lumen as a result of the increased electrical potential across the epithelium.

underlying secretion by these crypt cells, which clears the crypt and washes mucous secretions to the surface. This crypt secretion is usually masked by a greater rate of absorption by the villous and surface epithelium, so that the overall effect is net absorption. When a secretory stimulus is present, however, hypersecretion by the crypt can result in net secretion.

As shown in Fig. 20.9, there are two components to most secretory stimuli. Such stimuli also affect absorptive processes on the villi and result in the abolition of the neutral NaCl absorptive process. The action is specific for the electrically neutral process, and the substrate-coupled Na absorptive processes are unaffected. Simultaneously, there is an activation of a Cl (or HCO_3) secretory process in the crypt that is electrogenic and results in an increase in the transmural PD. This increased PD forces Na movement into the lumen, and the net result is secretion of NaCl and water into the intestinal lumen.

CONTROL OF INTESTINAL ION TRANSPORT

Absorptive and secretory events of the intestine are partially controlled by and partially independent of the neural and endocrine systems. For example, the substrate-linked Na absorptive mechanisms discussed above appear to operate completely independently of neuroendocrine control and depend only on the concentrations of Na and substrate in the lumen.

Neural control

It is now reasonably well established that, in general, adrenergic stimulation enhances absorption, whereas cholinergic stimulation induces secretion by the intestine. Referring to Fig. 20.10, it is apparent that postganglionic cholinergic nerve fibers are in close proximity to the epithelium and, therefore, probably innervate the epithelial cells directly. In contrast, it is unclear whether adrenergic fibers innervate the cells directly or simply modulate cholinergic activity in the submucosal ganglia.

The intestine appears to be under a degree of cholinergic tone because atropine, which prevents access of acetylcholine to postganglionic cholinergic receptors, enhances net absorption. A low amount of basal secretion may be normal. Cholinergic agents increase secretion by the electrolyte transport mechanisms outlined above. Adrenergic agents, on the other hand, increase the activity of the coupled NaCl absorptive process but, as stated previously, this could as well be the result of an interruption of cholinergic tone on this mechanism.

Other enteric neurons provide regulatory input to the cholinergic or motor neurons. For example, serotoninergic interneurons originating in the myenteric ganglia provide excitatory input to the motor neurons stimulating Cl secretion. In contrast, enkephalinergic interneurons provide in-

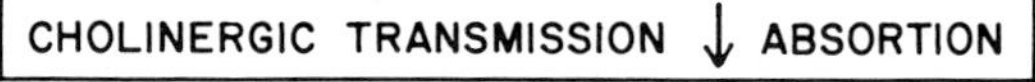

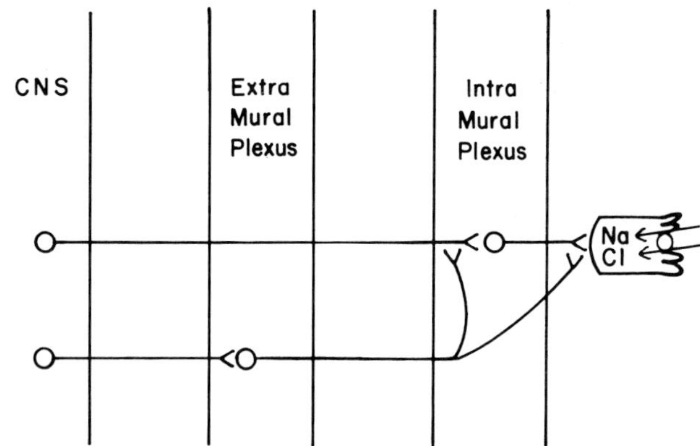

Figure 20.10. Cholinergic agonists decrease absorption or elicit secretion. The epithelium is innervated by cholinergic nerves that decrease the action of the NaCl absorptive process on the villi and elicit Cl secretion in the crypts. Depending on the strength of the stimulus, either decreased net absorption or net secretion may be observed. Adrenergic agonists modify cholinergic transmission from both preganglionic and postganglionic nerve endings. Recent evidence suggests that postganglionic adrenergic nerves also innervate the epithelial cell directly (not shown).

hibitory input by reducing excitability of motor neurons and reducing secretion (see Chap. 16).

Hormonal control

A number of hormonal mechanisms are capable of increasing absorption or inducing intestinal secretion, and many of these may be physiologically involved in the regulation of ion transport. Consideration will be given to those in which evidence of a physiological role is fairly certain.

Several gastrointestinal endocrine/paracrine substances cause the intestine to secrete when given in pharmacological concentration. It is not clear whether these substances are physiologically involved; the best case can be made for enterochromaffin cells elaborating serotonin, as degranulation of these cells has been observed during digestion. As discussed in Chapter 16, these substances may act in a reflex pathway involving enteric neurons.

In contrast to gastrointestinal hormones that all seem to favor secretion, systemic hormones (i.e., glucocorticoids, angiotensin, aldosterone, and catecholamines) promote absorption. Catecholamines stimulate neutral NaCl absorption in the jejunum, ileum, and proximal colon. The release of adrenergic agonists in the intestine appears to be mediated in two ways. First, it is mediated by a neurogenic reflex that originates in the carotid baroreceptors and cardiac mechanoreceptors and ends in splanchnic or mesenteric nerves. Second, the release comes through the production of renin and the subsequent angiotensin II–mediated release of norepinephrine (NE) from peripheral sympathetic nerves.

Fig. 20.11 shows how the renin-angiotensin-aldosterone system regulates absorption in all areas of the intestine. Stimulation of jejunal absorption is secondary to release of NE from enteric sympathetic nerves. Angiotensin II may act either within the brain or at sympathetic nerve terminals to liberate NE. In the ileum, angiotensin appears to have a direct effect in enhancing the operation of the neutral NaCl absorptive process. The hormone also controls colonic absorption through the release of aldosterone. Aldosterone increases electrogenic Na absorption in the distal colon, and recent evidence suggests that it also may acutely stimulate the action of the neutral NaCl absorptive process in the proximal colon.

Activation of the renin-angiotensin-aldosterone system may play a particularly important role in herbivorous animals that lose a considerable volume of fluid into the intestine during digestion. For example, Fig. 20.12 shows the plasma renin and aldosterone concentrations in the pony after a meal. Loss of approximately 15 percent of the ECF within 30 minutes after the meal caused the release of renin and subsequent release of aldosterone. Although this system was shown to have potent effects on the kidney at the observed concentrations, it is likely that intestinal absorption also was stimulated by angiotensin and colonic absorption by aldosterone. For example, aldosterone at the concentrations shown in Fig. 20.12 caused a twofold increase in Na absorption in in vitro experiments on the ventral, dorsal, and small colon in the pony.

The lower portion of Fig. 20.12 shows net fluid movement across the mucosa of the ventral colon during a period between meals. Net secretion is observed during the first 8 hours after feeding, and it is during this time that large quantities of VFAs are produced in the colon during microbial digestion. Net absorption is observed during the final 4 hours of the cycle, and it is at this time that the *action* of aldosterone becomes maximal. Thus it is possible that aldosterone exerts a major influence on colonic absorption after volume depletion caused by the meal. It is important to realize that fluctuations in plasma volume, renin and aldosterone concentrations, and net water movement across the colonic wall are not observed in ponies that were fed small portions of the meal for 2- or 4-hour intervals. Thus, when the grazing condition is simulated, acute losses of ECF into the intestine do not occur and there is a steady, low rate of absorption from the colonic contents.

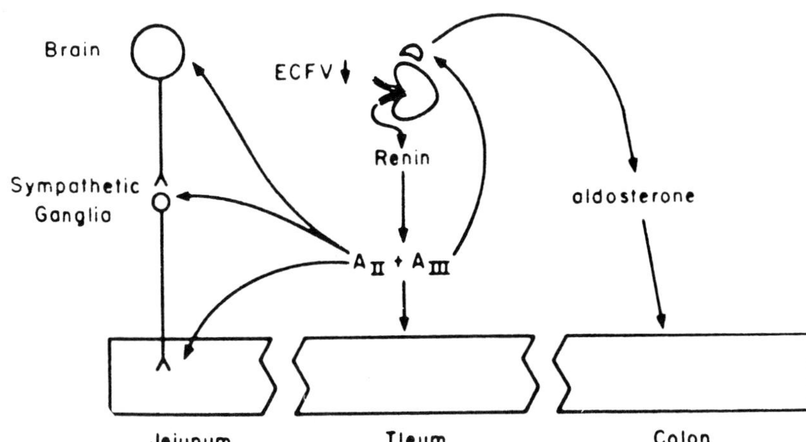

Figure 20.11. Renin-angiotensin-aldosterone stimulation of Na absorption in intestine and colon. Decreases in the extracellular fluid volume (ECFV) increase renin release from the kidney, with the subsequent formation of angiotensin II and III. Angiotensin releases norepinephrine, which stimulates Na absorption from the jejunum. Angiotensin may directly stimulate absorption in the ileum. Angiotensin stimulation of aldosterone production by the adrenal glands mediates a delayed Na absorptive mechanism in the colon. (From Levins 1985, *Am. J. Physiol.* 249:G3–G15.)

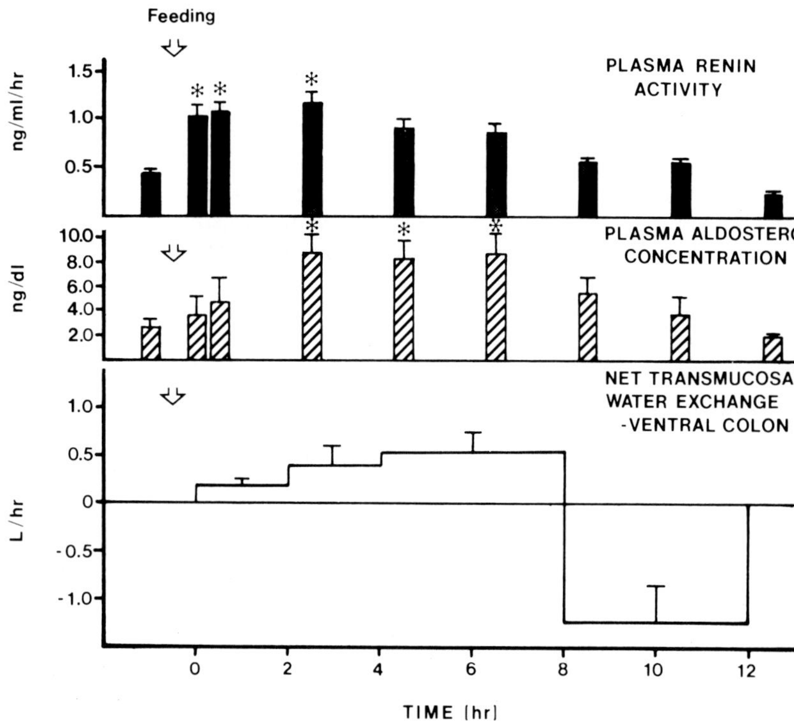

Figure 20.12. Activation of renin-angiotensin-aldosterone system in pony by ingestion of meal. Concentrations of renin and aldosterone are superimposed on ventral colonic fluid movement during the 12 hours between meals. Aldosterone action would coincide with net water absorption during the last 4 hours of the cycle and thus may be an important regulator of these cyclic changes in water movement observed in ponies fed twice daily. In animals fed every 2 hours, such cyclic changes in water movement are not seen. (From Argenzio and Clarke 1989, *Acta Vet. Scand. Suppl.* 86:1–234.)

Immune control

It is now becoming clear that cells of the lamina propria are the major sites of eicosanoid synthesis and that electrolyte transport is under a degree of eicosanoid tone. Eicosanoids are metabolites of arachidonic acid metabolism and include products of the cyclooxygenase pathway, such as prostaglandins, and products of the lipoxygenase pathway, such as leukotrienes. Components of this system are as follows.

1. *Mast cells,* whose degranulation causes secretion of several mediators. These are eicosanoids, histamine and serotonin, all substances that induce intestinal secretion.

2. *Macrophages* secrete eicosanoids and, in addition, can activate intracellular machinery, which may be mediated by reactive oxygen metabolites.

3. *Polymorphonuclear cells,* including neutrophils and eosinophils. These cells secrete mainly lipoxygenase products, some of which can cause intestinal and colonic secretion.

4. *Fibroblasts, endothelium, and muscle.* Bradykinin is a potent stimulus of eicosanoid production by intestinal lamina proprial elements. It is known that fibroblasts and endothelium have bradykinin receptors and respond with increased prostaglandin production.

Figure 20.13 shows that some of these agents released by inflammatory cells may interact with the enteric nervous system as well as stimulating the enterocyte directly. For example, the secretory response stimulated by these immune cells can be partially abolished with the nerve-blocking agents atropine, hexamethonium, and tetrodotoxin. Thus components of the nervous, endocrine, and immune systems all interact in the regulation of intestinal ion transport; however, many of the local stimuli that initiate mediator release and the relative physiological importance of each of these mediators are still uncertain.

Stimulus-secretion coupling

Figure 20.14 shows a simplified scheme of the intracellular mechanisms that control secretion. There are two major intracellular control systems: the cyclic guanosine monophosphate (cGMP) and the cyclic adenosine monophosphate (cAMP) systems. The cGMP system is located on the luminal membrane, whereas the cAMP system is located on the basolateral membrane.

Agents that activate either guanyl cyclase or adenyl cyclase enzymes bring about an increase in cGMP and cAMP, respectively, through a series of biochemical reactions. These agents in turn phosphorylate specific A or G protein kinases, and these protein kinases may in part be responsible for the transport events on the luminal membrane (Fig. 20.14).

Alternatively, secretion can result from an increase in intracellular free Ca (Fig. 20.14). This Ca may arise either from cyclic nucleotide-dependent release of stored Ca within the cell or from increased Ca entry across the basolateral membrane. Ca may act in part by activating a calcium-

Inflammatory Cell Products Elicit Secretion

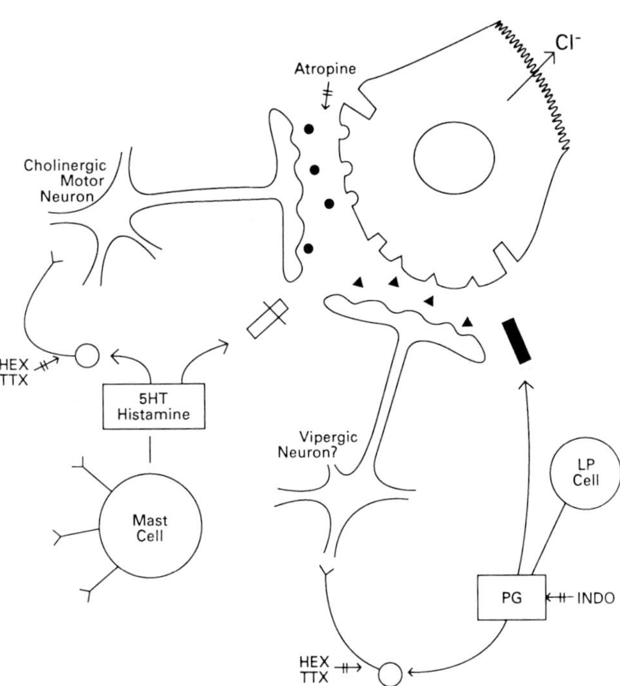

Figure 20.13. Inflammatory cell products elicit secretion. Mast cells and other cells in the lamina propria (LP cell) release mediators that act directly on receptors on enterocytes or indirectly via nerves that then stimulate the enterocyte. For example, the secretory response to serotonin, histamine, and prostaglandins (PG) is partially blocked with nerve-blocking agents such as atropine, hexamethonium (HEX), and tetrodotoxin (TTX). Similarly, indomethacin, an inhibitor of prostaglandin synthesis, inhibits the secretory response, as do histamine and serotonin antagonists.

dependent regulator protein, known as calmodulin, which is capable of activating membrane-phosphorylating protein kinases.

The mechanism that activates the coupled NaCl uptake process on the basolateral membrane of the secretory cell is not known. It is possible that this mechanism is in operation normally but is not "unmasked" until the luminal membrane conductance to Cl increases. Under normal conditions, the Cl may simply diffuse back across the basolateral membrane, which is more permeable to Cl than is the apical membrane, until the secretory stimulus is applied. Therefore, it is possible that the single effect required in the secretory cell to bring about net secretion is an increase in anion conductance of the luminal membrane.

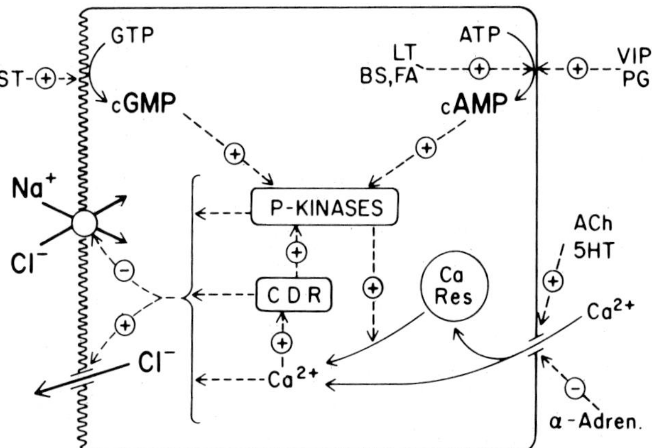

Figure 20.14. Postulated intracellular control mechanisms regulating small intestinal ion transport (NaCl uptake process and Cl conductance on lumen membrane). Stimulation is indicated by a plus sign and inhibition by a minus sign. ST, heat-stable *Escherichia coli* enterotoxin; P-kinases, protein kinases; CDR, calcium-dependent regulator protein, or calmodulin; Ca Res, calcium reservoir; LT, heat-labile *E. coli enterotoxin;* BS, bile salts; FA, fatty acids; VIP, vasoactive intestinal polypeptide; PG, prostaglandins; ACh, acetylcholine; 5HT, serotonin; α-Adren., alpha-adrenergic agonist, ATP, adenosine triphosphate; GTP, guanosine triphosphate; cAMP, cyclic adenosine monophosphate; cGMP, cyclic guanosine monophosphate. (From Powell and Field 1980, in Field, Fordtran, and Schultz, eds., *Secretory Diarrhea,* Am. Physiol. Soc., Bethesda, Md.)

REFERENCES

Argenzio, R.A. 1981. Effect of heat stable enterotoxin of *Escherichia coli,* cholera toxin, and theophylline on ion transport in porcine colon. *J. Physiol.* 320:469–87.

Argenzio, R.A. 1988. Fluid and ion transport in the large intestine. In A. Dobson and M.J. Dobson, eds., *Aspects of Digestive Physiology in Ruminants.* Cornell University Press, Ithaca. Pp. 140–55.

Argenzio, R.A., and Lebo, D.F. 1982. Ion transport by the pig colon: Effect of theophylline and dietary sodium restriction. *Can. J. Physiol. Pharmacol.* 60:929–35.

Argenzio, R.A., Lowe, J.E., Pickard, D.W., and Stevens, C.E. 1974. Digesta passage and water exchange in the equine large intestine. *Am. J. Physiol.* 226:1035–42.

Argenzio, R.A., and Whipp, S.C. 1979. Inter-relationship of sodium, chloride, bicarbonate, and acetate transport by the colon of the pig. *J. Physiol.* 295:365–81.

Binder, H.J., and Sandle, G.I. 1987. Electrolyte absorption and secretion in the mammalian colon. In L.R. Johnson, ed., *Physiology of the Gastrointestinal Tract.* Raven Press, New York. Pp. 1389–1418.

Castro, G.A. 1982. Immunological regulation of epithelial function. *Am. J. Physiol.* 243:G321–G329.

Charney, A.N., and Donowitz, M. 1976. Prevention and reversal of cholera enterotoxin-induced secretion by methylprednisolone induction of Na-K-ATPase. *J. Clin. Invest.* 57:1590–99.

Clarke, L.L., Argenzio, R.A., and Roberts, M.C. 1990. Effect of meal feeding on plasma volume and urinary electrolyte clearance in the pony. *Am. J. Vet. Res.* 51:571–76.

Clarke, L.L., Ganjam, V.K., Fichtenbaum, B., Hatfield, D., and Garner, H.E. 1988. Effect of feeding on renin-angiotensin-aldosterone system of the horse. *Am. J. Physiol.* 254:R524–R530.

Cooke, H.J. 1987. Neural and humoral regulation of small intestinal electrolyte transport. In L.R. Johnson, ed., *Physiology of the Gastrointestinal Tract.* Raven Press, New York. Pp. 1307–50.

Curran, P.F. 1965. Ion transport in intestine and its coupling to other transport processes. *Fed. Proc.* 24:993–99.

Curran, P.F., and McIntosh, J.R. 1962. A model system for biological water transport. *Nature* 193:347–48.

Field, M. 1979. Intracellular mediators of secretion in the small intestine. In H.J. Binder, ed., *Mechanisms of Intestinal Secretion.* Liss, New York, pp. 83–91.

Field, M. 1980. Regulation of small intestinal ion transport by cyclic nucleotides and calcium. In M. Field, J.S. Fordtran, and S.G. Schultz, eds., *Secretory Diarrhea*. Am. Physiol. Soc., Bethesda, Md. Pp. 21–30.

Fordtran, J.S. 1973. Diarrhea. In M.H. Sleisenger and J.S. Fordtran, eds., *Gastrointestinal Disease*. W.B. Saunders, Philadelphia. Pp. 291–319.

Hubel, K.A. 1976. Intestinal ion transport: Effect of norepinephrine, pilocarpine and atropine. *Am. J. Physiol.* 231:252–57.

Levans, N. 1985. Control of intestinal absorption by the renin-angiotensin system. *Am. J. Physiol.* 249:G3–G15.

Morris, A.I., and Turnberg, L.A. 1980. The influence of a parasympathetic agonist and antagonist on human intestinal transport in vivo. *Gastroenterology* 79:861–66.

Nellans, H.N., Frizzell, R.A., and Schultz, S.G. 1974. Brush border processes and transepithelial Na and Cl transport in rabbit ileum. *Am. J. Physiol.* 226:1131–41.

Partridge, I.G. 1978. Studies on digestion and absorption in the intestines of growing pigs. 4. Effects of dietary cellulose and sodium levels on mineral absorption. *Br. J. Nutr.* 39:539–45.

Phillips, S.F., and Devroede, G.J. 1979. Functions of the large intestine. In R.K. Crane, ed., *MTP International Review of Physiology, Gastrointestinal Physiology 3*, vol. 19. University Park Press, Baltimore, Md. Pp. 263–90.

Powell, D.W. 1979. Transport in large intestine. In G. Giebish, D.C. Tosteson, and H.H. Ussing, eds., *Membrane Transport in Biology*. Springer-Verlag, New York. Pp. 781–809.

Powell, D.W. 1987. Bacteria, nerves, endocrine, immune and epithelial cells: Who waltzes with whom in the intestine. *Z. Gastroenterol.* 25:614–16.

Powell, D.W. 1987. Intestinal water and electrolyte transport. In L.R. Johnson, ed., *Physiology of the Gastrointestinal Tract*. Raven Press, New York. Pp. 1267–1305.

Powell, D.W., and Field, M. 1980. Pharmacological approaches to treatment of secretory diarrhea. In M. Field, J.S. Fordtran, and S.G. Schultz, eds., *Secretory Diarrhea*. Am. Physiol. Soc., Bethesda, Md. Pp. 187–209.

Powell, D.W., and Tapper, E.J. 1979. Autonomic control of intestinal electrolyte transport. In H.D. Janowitz and D.B. Sacher, eds., *Frontiers of Knowledge in Diarrheal Diseases*. Projects in Health, Inc., Upper Montclair, N.J. Pp. 37–52.

Schultz, S.G. 1979. Transport across small intestine. In G. Giebisch, D.C. Tosteson, and H.H. Ussing, eds., *Membrane Transport in Biology*. vol. 4. Springer-Verlag, New York. Pp. 749–80.

Schultz, S.G. 1980. Cellular models of sodium and chloride absorption by mammalian small and large intestine. In M. Field, J.S. Fordtran, and S.G. Schultz, eds., *Secretory Diarrhea*. Am. Physiol. Soc., Bethesda, Md. Pp. 1–9.

Turnberg, L.A., Bieberdorf, F.A., Morawski, S.G., and Fordtran, J.S. 1970. Interrelationships of chloride, bicarbonate, sodium and hydrogen transport in the human ileum. *J. Clin. Invest.* 49:557–67.

Turnberg, L.A., Fordtran, J.S., Carter, N.W., and Rector, F.C., Jr. 1970. Mechanism of bicarbonate absorption and its relationship to sodium transport in the human jejunum. *J. Clin. Invest.* 49:548–56.

Yablonski, M.E., and Lifson, N. 1976. Mechanism of production of intestinal secretion by elevated venous pressure. *J. Clin. Invest.* 57:904–15.

CHAPTER 21

Digestion in the Ruminant Stomach | by Barry F. Leek

INTRODUCTION

The functional anatomy of the ruminant stomach

Ruminants, so named because they ruminate (chew the cud), have a stomach that consists of a nonsecretory forestomach and a secretory stomach compartment (the abomasum). The forestomach consists of three compartments (the reticulum, the rumen, and the omasum) and serves as a fermentation vat for the microbial fermentation of the ingesta, mainly by hydrolysis and anaerobic oxidation. The fermentation end products (volatile fatty acids, etc.) that the ruminant absorbs and uses as its prime metabolic substrates are quite different from the end products of digestion (glucose, etc.) in nonruminants. The abomasum, like the stomach of nonruminant animals, is largely concerned with the hydrolysis of protein by pepsin in an acid medium.

The main anatomical feaures are shown in Fig. 21.1. The *reticulum* is approximately spherical, and the esophagus enters dorsomedially at the cardia. The reticular groove runs ventrally from the cardia to the reticuloomasal orifice. In young ruminants the lips of this groove can be brought into apposition by contraction of the underlying musculature, so that a tube is formed whereby ingested milk bypasses the ruminoreticulum. The reticulum is partially separated from the cranial sac of the rumen by the ruminoreticular fold, which, even when contracted, leaves a large orifice between the reticulum and the rumen. For this and other reasons, the ruminoreticulum operates as a combined functional unit despite the clear anatomical differences between these two compartments. The *rumen* is divided into dorsal and ventral sacs by an incomplete partition formed by the cranial and caudal pillars and the right and left longitudinal pillars. The dorsal part is divided into (1) the cranial sac lying between the ruminoreticular fold and the cranial pillar, (2) the dorsal sac, and (3) the caudodorsal blind sac. In sheep the ruminoreticular fold is placed high in the forestomach and acts as the main barrier between the reticulum and the raft of fibrous contents in the

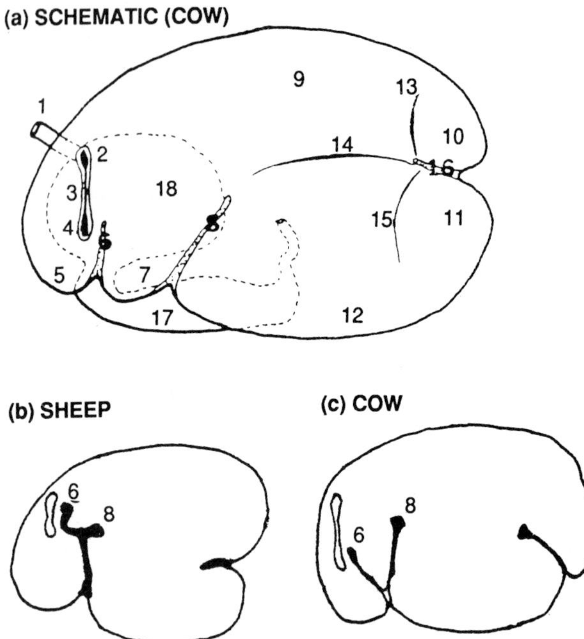

Figure 21.1. *(a)* A schematic diagram of a sagittal section through a bovine ruminoreticulum, viewed from the left side, to show the main anatomical features: 1, esophagus; 2, cardiac opening; 3, reticular groove; 4, reticuloomasal opening; 5, reticulum; 6, ruminoreticular fold; 7, cranial sac of the rumen; 8, cranial pillar; 9, dorsal sac of the rumen; 10, caudodorsal blind sac; 11, caudoventral blind sac; 12, ventral sac of the rumen; 13, dorsal coronary pillar; 14, right longitudinal pillar; 15, ventral coronary pillar; 16, caudal pillar; 17, abomasum; 18, omasum. Dotted lines show the outline of the omasum and abomasum, which lie on the right side of the reticulum and rumen. The outlines of a sagittal section through the ruminoreticulum of a sheep *(b)* and a cow *(c)* in specimens fixed in situ. The main barrier to flow between the reticulum and the main mass of ruminal contents is the ruminoreticular fold (6) in sheep and the cranial pillar (8) in cattle.

dorsal ruminal sac. In cattle the fold has a much lower position and the main barrier is provided by the cranial pillar, which has a more vertical inclination. The ventral part of the rumen consists of the ventral sac and the caudoventral blind sac, which lies ventral to the caudal pillar. The ruminoreticulum occupies the entire left side of the abdomen and, depending on the degree of stomach filling, also extends ventrally on the right side.

The *omasum* is a kidney-shaped structure and is relatively larger in cattle than in sheep and goats. On the luminal side of its lesser curvature is the short omasal canal that connects the reticuloomasal orifice with the omasoabomasal orifice. The body of the omasum consists of many leaves (laminae) attached at the greater curvature with their free edges parallel to and in contact with the omasal canal. The leaves bear small papillae, which further enhance the internal surface area/volume ratio of the omasum.

The *abomasum* consists of fundic, body, and pyloric regions. The mucosa is thrown up in about 12 high folds (rugae), which run spirally over the fundic and body parts and are absent from the pyloric region. A constriction, the pylorus, separates the pyloric region from the duodenum.

Microscopically, the ruminant stomach consists of the serosal, muscular, and luminal layers. In contrast to the ruminant esophagus, which has striated muscle throughout its entire length, the stomach has only smooth muscle, distributed in layers oriented in different directions. In the forestomach compartments the luminal surface is a stratified squamous epithelium with slight keratinzation. In the abomasum it is a mucosal epithelium pitted with peptic glands. The surface area/volume ratio of all the compartments is increased by characteristic folding of the luminal surfaces (e.g., the spiral folds of the abomasum and the papillated laminae of the omasum). The luminal surface of the rumen is densely studded with club-shaped papillae, and the reticulum is so named because its luminal surface is thrown up in a "honeycomb" network of low hexagonal ridges. These ridges are papillated in sheep but smooth in cattle.

The ruminant stomach is highly vascularized, and the blood flow to the luminal epithelium is greatly increased when fermentation end products are being absorbed. The arterial supply to the forestomach and most of the abomasum is via the left gastric branch of the celiac artery. A branch of the hepatic artery supplies the abomasoduodenal junction. The venous blood drains into the hepatic portal vein and passes to the liver before being returned to the caudal vena cava by the hepatic veins.

The ruminant stomach is innervated by vagal and splanchnic nerves, both of which provide sensory (afferent) and motor (efferent) pathways. The vagal motor (parasympathetic) nerve fibers to the forestomach originate in the right and left gastric centers within the dorsal vagal nuclei of the medulla oblongata in the hindbrain. The right and left vagi in the thoracic region divide into dorsal and ventral branches. The dorsal branches of each side unite to form the dorsal vagal trunk, which innervates all regions of the ruminant stomach. Likewise, the two ventral branches unite to form the ventral vagal trunk, which supplies all regions of the ruminant stomach except the dorsal ruminal sac. Discharges in the vagal motor nerves are essential for the major contraction cycles of the forestomach (the primary and secondary cycles). The splanchnic motor (sympathetic) nerve fibers supply all regions of the ruminant stomach. When stimulated they inhibit motility, but when they are removed or blocked with drugs no effect is observed and thus they appear not to be tonically active.

The ratio of afferent/efferent fibers, if similar to that in cats and rabbits, is 10:1 in the vagi and 3:1 in the splanchnic nerves. Therefore, although most emphasis is placed on the motor roles of these nerves, on numerical grounds they are predominantly *sensory* nerves! The vagal nerves transmit sensory information from two known kinds of sensory receptor: (1) tension receptors and (2) epithelial/mucosal receptors. In all stomach compartments the tension receptors are slowly adapting mechanoreceptors located in the muscle layer "in series" with the contractile elements (smooth muscle cells). They are excited by passive distention of the viscus and especially by active contraction of the smooth muscle. The epithelial receptors of the forestomach lie close to the basement membrane of the luminal epithelium and behave both as rapidly adapting mechanoreceptors and as chemoreceptors. They are concentrated particularly in the conical papillae surmounting the hexagonal ridges of the reticulum (in sheep) and between the club-shaped papillae of the cranial ruminal sac. Their greatest excitation is produced by repetitive light moving, tactile stimuli (rapid light brushing) and by a range of chemicals: acids, alkali, hypotonic salt solutions, and hypertonic salt solutions. The mucosal receptors of the abomasum have similar properties and are most concentrated in the body and pyloric regions. The epithelial/mucosal receptors are innervated by unmyelinated fibers, many of which acquire fine myelination by the time they reach the cervical region. The tension receptors are innervated by finely myelinated (B) fibers. These fibers, together with B fibers of the motor nerves, probably account for the much greater number of myelinated fibers in the vagi of ruminants than in those of nonruminants. Both tension-receptor and epithelial/mucosal-receptor sensory nerve fibers project to the left and right dorsal vagal motor nuclei and to the reticular formation lying lateral and dorsal to these nuclei.

The splanchnic nerves transmit sensory information from serosal receptors and possibly from tension receptors. The serosal receptors are particularly dense at the attachment of the mesenteries. They are slowly adapting mechanoreceptors, and their responses to many forms of stimuli resemble, and could be confused with, those of tension receptors.

The development of the ruminant stomach

Ungulates, the hooved mammals, are the most numerous and important group of large, grass-eating herbivores (Fig. 21.2). In grasses the physical support of the stems and leaves is provided by thick walls that encase each cell and are composed of carbohydrates, cellulose, and related compounds, some of which are replaced with age by lignin. Only microbes (bacteria, fungi, and protozoa) and a few invertebrates can digest cellulose and, with very great difficulty, lignin. Ungulates have established a symbiotic relationship with suitable microbes through the development of anatomical structures that serve as fermentation chambers. By this means, the major carbohydrates of grasses become nutritionally available.

The ungulates show a range of anatomical developments. In the odd-toed ungulates (Perissodactyla), typified by the horse family (Equidae), the fermentation vat is the greatly enlarged hindgut (cecum and colon), which receives digesta after gastrointestinal digestion has occurred. This device seems to be rather inefficient; of the 158 known genera, only 6 remain. Among the even-toed ungulates (Ariodactyla), the swine family (Suidae) represents a small transitional group, in which there is not only an enlarged large intestine but also an enlarged stomach. Part of the stomach is nonsecretory, so that microbes can start the fermentation process before peptic digestion begins. The nonsecretory area is not partitioned off from the secretory area in pigs, but it is in some other transitional animals, such as the hippopotamus. The development of a more complex forestomach occurs in the pseudoruminants (Tylopoda), represented by camels and llamas, in which the forestomach has two interconnecting compartments corresponding to a reticulum and a rumen but lacks a typical omasum. Although these animals chew the cud, the dentition includes upper and lower canine teeth. Finally, there are the true ruminants (Ruminantia), which have a three-compartment forestomach (reticulum, rumen, and omasum) in addition to a secretory stomach compartment (the abomasum) and a unique dentition, in which the upper incisor and canine teeth are absent and the lower canine teeth have joined with and taken the form of incisor teeth. These are in apposition to a dental pad in lieu of incisor teeth in the upper jaw. The true ruminants continue to be the most successful large grass-eating mammals. Of about 250 known genera, 68 still exist, notably the 4 containing the main domestic, agricultural species.

The benefits and costs of ruminant digestion

The ecological success of ruminants is due to the benefits of a pregastric fermentation vat, the forestomach. This (1) allows the use of diets that may be too fibrous for nonruminant animals; (2) confers the ability to break down cellulose, thus releasing the enclosed cell contents but, more important, allowing cellulose, itself the most abundant carbohydrate form present in the plant, to become a major nutrient; (3) allows the synthesis of high-biological-value microbial protein from low-biological-value plant protein, from dietary nonprotein nitrogen, and from recycled nitrogenous metabolic end products (e.g., urea); and (4) provides all components of the vitamin B complex, provided that adequate cobalt is available for vitamin B_{12}. In the wild, therefore, ruminants can compete successfully with nonruminant grass eaters and can, in addition, occupy niches where the quality of the grass would be too low to support the nonruminants—for example, above the Artic Circle (musk oxen), in high mountains (llamas, yaks), and in the hot deserts (camels, goats).

Each ruminant species can be placed on an ecological spectrum. At one end are the selective feeders, typified by antelopes and giraffes, which ingest the most nutritious parts of the plants. At the other end of the spectrum are the relatively nonselective, coarse grazers, such as cattle. Between these extremes would be an intermediate group, such as goats. Sheep are on the borderline between the intermediate types and the coarse grazers. The selective feeders

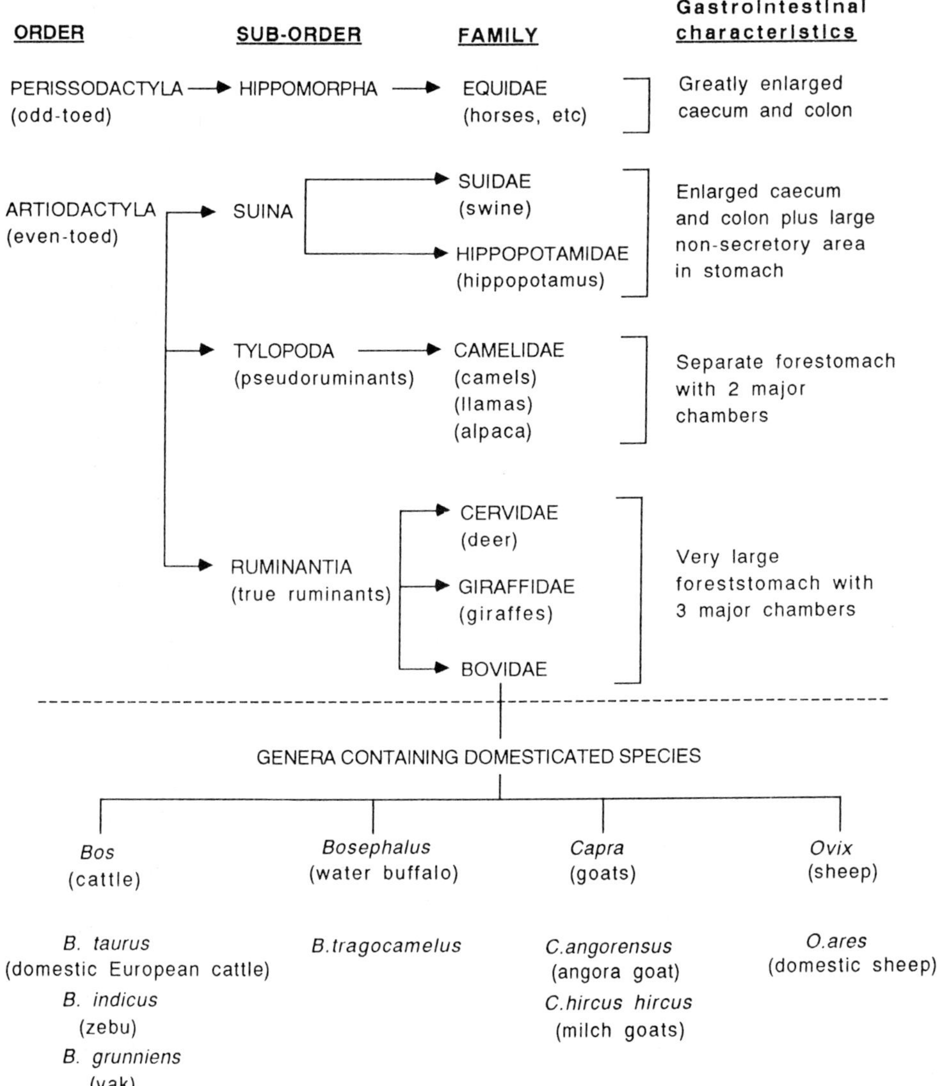

Figure 21.2. The classification of the large, mainly grass-eating, hooved mammals (ungulates). Microbial fermentation occurs in a greatly enlarged hindgut in the Equidae, in both an enlarged hindgut and a nonsecretory gastric region in a transitional group containing swine, and mainly in a separate, large forestomach with two major compartments in pseudoruminants (Tylopoda) and with three major compartments (reticulum, rumen, omasum) in true ruminants (Ruminantia). Within the true ruminants, the family Bovidae contains not only the majority of wild ruminants but also the four genera to which the main agriculturally important species belong. (Adapted from Hume and Warner 1980, in Ruckebusch and Thivend, eds., *Digestive Physiology and Metabolism in Ruminants,* AVI Publishing Co., Westport, Conn.)

tend to eat more frequently, ruminate more often for short periods, and have a relatively smaller forestomach, particularly a small omasum. Fermentation occurs faster, so that the transit time for digesta in the forestomach is short. Conversely, the coarse grazers tend to eat most intensively on a few occasions each day, ruminate infrequently in long bouts, and have a voluminous forestomach, with a particularly large omasum. Fermentation is slow, and the transit time is long.

The costs or disadvantages of ruminant digestion are that (1) the ruminant needs to spend a large part of its day chewing, i.e., chewing food (4–7 hours a day) or chewing the cud (about 8 hours a day), and adequate food needs to be supplied at regular intervals; (2) the ruminant needs complicated mechanisms to keep the fermentation vat working efficiently, e.g., (a) the regular addition of large quantities of alkaline saliva, (b) powerful mixing movements in the forestomach, (c) mechanisms for the elimination of the gases of fermentation (eructation), for the regurgitation of the cud (rumination), for absorption of end products, and for the onward passage of portions of the ferment to the omasum; and (3) pathways of intermediary metabolism must be geared to use of the peculiar end products of fermentation. In the case of all carbohydrates (cellulose, starch, etc.) and some proteins, these are the volatile fatty acids (mainly acetic, propionic, and butyric acids). Of these, only propionic acid is capable of being converted to glucose, for which the ruminant has a high requirement during milk production and during the later stages of fetal growth. In the wild state the costs are of little concern.

Under intensive systems of farming where starch-based feedstuffs ("concentrates") replace a significant fraction of the cellulose-based feedstuffs ("roughage"), the digestive mechanisms may be unable to cope with demands made by the ensuing greatly increased fermentation, leading to a variety of digestive and metabolic disorders.

MICROBIAL FERMENTATION

The dietary substrates

The major components of the most common types of ruminant feedstuffs are shown in Table 21.1. The atmospheric nitrogen-fixing legumes have a high protein content, but in nonleguminous plants carbohydrates make up about 66 percent of the dry matter (DM), both in roughages (straw and grasses) and in grains, the main components of concentrate feeds. In grains most of the carbohydrate is nonstructural and is intracellular as stored energy (starches and fructosans) or synthetic intermediaries (simple sugars). The starches are polysaccharide chains of glucose units arranged linearly with α-1,4 glucose linkages without side chains (in amylose) or with side chains (in amylopectin), the branch points being provided by α-1,6 linkages (Fig. 21.3). The fructosans are polysaccharides composed of fructose units, but the typical linkage is a β-1,2, as in inulin. The α-1 linkages, in contrast to the β-1 linkages, are readily hydrolyzed by enzymes (amylases) that are present in the alimentary tract secretions of most animals as well as in microbes and plants. In roughages most of the carbohydrate is structural and is found in the plant cell wall, except for the pectin, which has an intracellular structural function. The plant cell wall is made up of cellulose fibers embedded in a hemicellulose matrix. Cellulose is a β-1,4 glucose-linked polysaccharide. Hemicelluloses are polysaccarides composed principally of β-1,4 linked xylose units, xylose being a pentose (5-carbon ring). Pectin is mainly a β-1,4-galacturonan (i.e., a polysaccharide based on units composed of galactose with uronic acid). The β-1 linkages are difficult to hydrolyze, and the necessary enzymes (cellulase, hemicellulase, pectin lyase, and fructanase) are found only in microbes and plants. It is for this reason that herbivores benefit from a symbiotic fermentative relationship with suitable microbes. When plant walls age, the hemicellulose is replaced by lignin, which, even in the ruminant, is scarcely degraded.

Table 21.1. The principal components of ruminant foodstuffs showing typical average values of the percent composition in the dry matter

	C-1 linkage	Straw	Grasses	Grains	Legumes
Carbohydrates					
Nonstructural					
Starch	α	-	1	64	7
Other	α and β	7	13	2	8
Subtotal		7	14	66	15
Structural					
Cellulose	β	32	24	8	14
Hemicellulose	β	31	20	4	7
Pectin	β	3	2	-	6
Subtotal		66	46	12	27
Other components					
Crude protein		4	14	12	24
Lipids		2	4	4	6
Lignin		10	7	2	5
Other		8	14	5	21
Subtotal		24	39	23	56

Adapted from Czerkawski 1986. *An Introduction to Rumen Studies*, Pergammon Press, Oxford.

The fermenting mass

The microbes consist mainly of a mixed, interdependent population of bacteria but also yeastlike fungi and protozoa. Because of the impervious covering of most plant surfaces, the microbes can ferment only after they have gained access to the interior of the plant through the leaf pores and cut ends, hence the importance of chewing food and cud. A little trapped oxygen is taken in with food and water, and some oxygen diffuses across the forestomach wall, but it is quickly used up by facultative anaerobic species of bacteria. The majority of the microbes, particularly the protozoa, are strictly anaerobic, and therefore the main fermentation pathways are hydrolysis and anaerobic oxidation, involving the removal of hydrogen rather than the addition of oxygen. Thus the ruminal environment has a great need for a variety of hydrogen-accepting reactions in order to reoxidize reduced coenzymes, such as $NADPH + H^+ \rightarrow NADP^+ + 2\,[H]$. Only in exceptional circumstances is the potential hydrogen liberated as gaseous hydrogen.

Primary bacteria are those that degrade the actual constituents of the diet and, depending on their preference for celluloses or for starch, are termed cellulolytic or amylolytic, respectively (Fig. 21.4). *Secondary bacteria* use as their substrate the end products of the primary bacterial degradations, and this group includes the lactate-utilizing propionate bacteria, which produce some of the propionate, and the hydrogen-utilizing methanogenic bacteria, which produce methane gas. Little is known about the importance of ruminal *fungi* in fermentation. The *protozoa* feed on ruminal bacteria, plant starch granules, and other readily digestible materials, including perhaps the dietary polyunsaturated fatty acids (PUFAs), linoleic and linolenic acids. Protozoa are very sensitive to abnormal intraruminal conditions, and their presence in a ruminal fluid sample is a good indicator of its normality. Most of the protozoa are sequestered in the raft (collection) of fibrous digesta in the dorsal ruminal sac. Here they (1) form a reservoir of microbial protein useful at times of intermittent food supply; (2) help to prevent an overproliferation of bacteria at times of starch loading by engulfing starch particles, thereby curbing the undesirably high rates of starch degradation by amylolytic bacteria; and (3) when they pass out of the forestomach and undergo digestion in the lower gastrointestinal tract, they provide the ruminant host animal (a) with a better quality of microbial protein than would be the case with bacteria, (b) with small amounts of unfermented starch, and

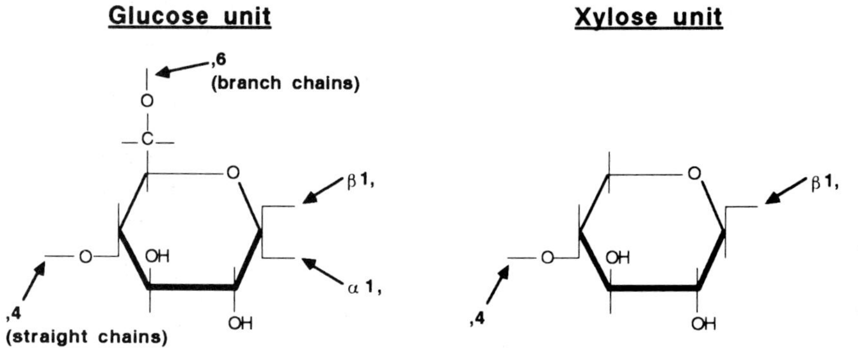

Figure 21.3. The structure of glucose and xylose, showing the potential linkage points. Sugars and starch use the α-1 linkage, whereas cellulose, hemicellulose, fructosans, and pectins use the β-1 linkage. These link to C-4 in straight chains and C-6 at each point of branching. Glucose units form the basis of sugars, starch, and cellulose. Xylose units make up hemicellulose and pectin. Fructosans are based on fructose.

(c) possibly with some PUFAs that would otherwise have been hydrogenated by the ruminal bacteria and therefore made unavailable to the ruminant itself. Different microbes have different pH optima. The protozoa, primary cellulolytic bacteria, and most secondary bacteria require a pH of 6.2 or greater, whereas the amylolytic bacteria are active in more acidic conditions, around pH 5.8. At even lower pH values, the usually insignificant lactic acid–producing lactobacilli become the dominant type, and this makes ruminal conditions even more acidic and unfavorable to the normal mixed population of ruminal microbes. In general, the numbers of microbes increase with the quantity and quality of the diet, protozoa being particularly plentiful when starch-rich diets are fed. When there are sudden major changes in diet, it takes about 2 weeks for the new population of microbial species and numbers to become established. For this reason, changes in diet need to be made gradually.

The digesta in the ruminoreticulum do not form a homogeneous mass. The most recently ingested food is added to a raft of fibrous material that occupies most of the dorsal ruminal sac and floats on the underlying soupy fluid, in which there are suspended only very fine particles, each no longer than 2 mm. Above the raft is a layer of ruminal gas, composed mainly of CH_4 and CO_2. During the clinical examination of a normal ruminant, palpation of the sublumbar fossa should detect the gas layer lying above the doughy textured fibrous raft. Excessive gas accumulation is called bloat (see below); excessive hardness of the raft is a sign of ruminal impaction, and softness or absence of the raft indicates that the animal has not recently consumed roughage. The ruminal digesta may be considered as being distributed in four fractions, each having a very different composition: (1) the fibrous raft particles with high densities of microbes inside, the microbes moving into fresh particles as the old ones disintegrate; (2) the liquid fraction of the raft, which

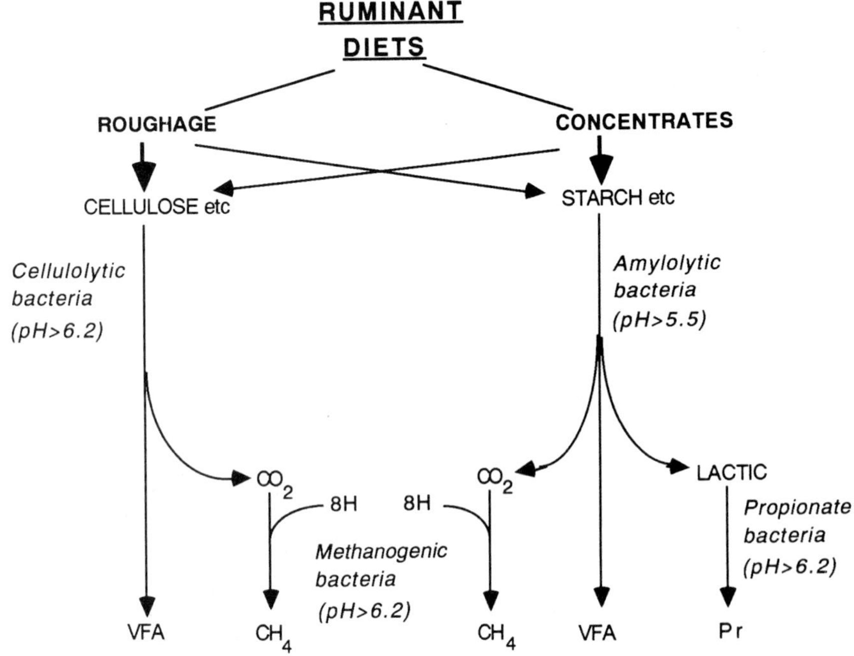

Figure 21.4. The primary microbes required for the fermentation of roughage and concentrates to VFAs are cellulolytic and amylolytic bacteria, respectively. Secondary bacteria use some of the other end products. For example, methanogenic bacteria reoxidize reduced coenzymes by using the hydrogen to convert carbon dioxide (and formate) to methane and proprionate bacteria prevent the accumulation of lactic acid, but only at relatively high pH values.

shuttles mainly soluble materials in (e.g., salivary constituents) and out (e.g., fermentative end products); (3) the soupy material that occupies the reticulum and the cranial and ventral sacs of the rumen; and (4) the boundary layer lying against the luminal surface of the ruminoreticulum, across which certain blood:rumen fluid exchanges occur in both directions. The soupy material receives all ingested food and water, saliva, reswallowed cuds and the end products from the raft. It floats light, particulate ingesta across from the cardia to join the raft. It provides the material for the cud "bolus" and the material that flows out of the reticulum into the omasum through the reticuloomasal opening. Clinically, it is the soupy material that is sampled, but this may not give an accurate indication of the microbial composition and fermentative activity of the raft.

Fermentation pathways

Figure 21.5 presents a simplified scheme of the main fermentation pathways, showing only the key intermediates. The volatile fatty acids (VFAs) are partly dissociated and partly undissociated, depending on pH. The terms *acetic acid* and *acetate* are therefore freely interchangeable. For convenience, fermentation may be considered as the first three stages of a four-stage microbial process. The *first* stage involves the hydrolysis of the plant polysaccharides to their constituent monosaccharides and then the conversion of these to fructose-1,6-bisphosphate. This is reached via glucose for starch and cellulose, via fructose for fructosans, and via xylose for hemicelluloses and pectin. The *second* stage involves the Embden-Meyerhof pathway for the anaerobic oxidation of fructose 1,6-bisphosphate to pyruvate via phosphoenolpyruvate. The *third* stage covers the reactions that produce the final metabolites of fermentation. Phosphoenolpyruvate is the origin of the pathway leading to the acetate, some butyrate, and a transient intermediate—formate—which is converted to methane. Pyruvate is the origin of the pathways that (1) via β-OH-butyrate, produce butyrate; (2) via oxaloacetate and succi-

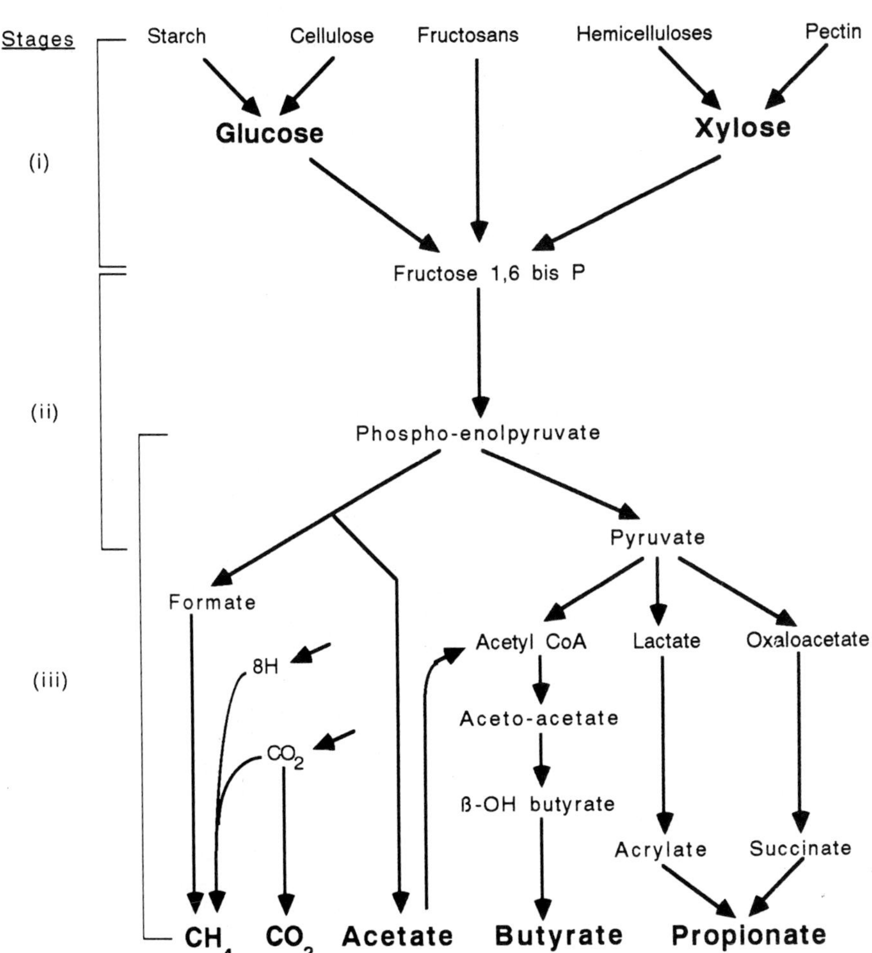

Figure 21.5. In the fermentation of dietary carbohydrates, stage i is the hydrolysis of the polysaccharides to fructose 1,6 bisphosphate, stage ii is anaerobic oxidation by the Embden-Meyerhof pathway to phosphoenolpyruvate and pyruvate, stage iii is the formation of the VFAs. Stage iv of the microbial process, which is not shown, is the synthesis of new bacterial products, such as protein. Hydrogen is used in the formation of methane (as shown) and also in the formation of butyrate and propionate (not shown).

nate ("the randomizing pathway"), produce propionate; and (3) via lactate and acrylate ("the direct reductive pathway"), also produce about 10% but sometimes up to 30% of the total propionate. The formation of methane and of propionate is an important means of reoxidizing reduced coenzymes, so that they may become available again for oxidative (dehydrogenation) reactions. The *fourth* stage of microbial activity is the synthesis of microbial compounds, particularly amino acid formation, using the above stage 1 to 3 intermediates coupled with transamination.

The fermentation of cellulose

The degradation of the β-1 linked compounds (cellulose, hemicelluloses, fructosans, pectin) is performed by several species of primary cellulolytic bacteria, which are capable of all four stages of fermentation described above except methane formation. This is carried out by secondary methanogenic bactera. The cellulolytic bacteria have a low metabolic rate, so the fermentation of cellulose is slow and, as they take about 18 hours to double their numbers (the "doubling time"), population changes are also slow. For protein synthesis, cellulolytic bacteria do not require a supply of amino acids but need NH_3, the stage 2 and 3 intermediates, and small amounts of iso-acids, which arise from the deamination of the branched amino acids in dietary plant proteins. The optimum pH is 6.2 to 6.8, which matches the typical ruminal pH of a roughage-fed animal. The methanogenic bacteria have a similar optimum pH, and they require a supply of formate, CO_2, and reducing units (2H) to produce methane and a supply of amino acids to meet their protein requirements. The mixed population of cellulolytic and methanogenic microbes leads to the production of CO_2, CH_4, and the VFAs. The VFAs derived from the fermentation of cellulose are generally in the ratio 70:15:10 for acetate, propionate, and butyrate, respectively.

The fermentation of starch

The degradation of the α-1 linked starches (amylose and amylopectin) and the simple sugars (e.g., sucrose, maltose) is performed by several species of primary amylolytic bacteria, some of which are capable of all four stages of fermentation, except for methane formation, and others of which carry out stages 1 and 2 but cease with the production of one of the metabolic acids, most commonly lactic acid. Unlike the cellulolytic bacteria, the amylolytic bacteria have faster fermentation rates, have much shorter doubling times (0.25–4 hours), and have a lower pH optimum of 5.5 to 6.6. This matches the lower ruminal pH values of ruminants on high-concentrate (starch-rich) diets and is due to higher VFA concentrations with an increase in the relative proportions of propionate, giving a typical acetate/propionate/butyrate ratio of 55: 25: 15. Amylolytic bacteria require not only a supply of NH_3 but also some amino acids for protein synthesis. Secondary bacteria are required for methane formation (methanogenic bacteria) and for the conversion of the lactic and other metabolic acids to propionate (propionate bacteria). Both of these groups of secondary bacteria require amino acids for their protein synthesis, have a long doubling time (16 hours) and an optimum pH of 6.2 to 6.8, which is higher than that required by the amylolytic bacteria. Therefore when sudden changes are made from roughage to concentrate feeds, the amylolytic bacteria quickly increase both their numbers and the overall rate of fermentation, causing a rapid accumulation of VFAs and lactic acid. This leads to a lowering of ruminal pH, which is within the pH optimum of the amylolytic bacteria but is too low for both kinds of secondary bacteria. Therefore lactic acid, a stronger organic acid than the VFAs, increases still further while the potential for hydrogen disposal declines and may provide some degree of negative feedback on further amylolytic activity. The numbers of protozoa increase when concentrates are fed, probably because of the greater availability of starch granules and of bacteria that feed on them. The protozoa thereby curb bacterial amylolysis until the pH falls below 5.5, at which point protozoa are quickly inactivated and later die.

The fermentation of dietary protein

Proteolytic bacteria represent only 12 to 38 percent of the total ruminal bacteria, and normally only about a half of the dietary protein is degraded in the rumen. The original idea that soluble but not insoluble proteins could be fermented is not tenable. Instead, dietary proteins are now classified as "rumen-degradable proteins" (RDPs) or as "rumen-undegradable protein" (RUPs). Certain natural proteins (e.g., those in maize) and other processed (protected) proteins (e.g., those denatured by heat treatment or tanned by the application of formaldehyde) escape ruminal degradation but can be readily hydrolyzed by the gastrointestinal proteolytic enzymes. Bacterial proteolysis commences with extracellular protease activity to produce peptides, which are phagocytized and subjected to further hydrolysis within the bacterial cell. The end products are amino acids, some of which are taken up by other microbes and the remainder of which are deaminated to produce ammonia and various metabolic acids. These are fermented to VFAs and include small amounts of branched-chain VFAs (the isoacids: isobutyrate and isovalerate), which arise from leucine, isoleucine, and valine and are required as minor nutrients by the cellulolytic bacteria.

Ammonia arises not only from the deamination of amino acids but also from the conversion of dietary and endogenous nonprotein nitrogen (NPN) compounds. These include plant amides, nitrites, nitrates, and endogenous urea which enters with saliva and diffuses across the rumen wall into the ruminal fluid. The urease activity, which is high at the ruminal wall: fluid boundary and in the fibrous raft in the dorsal ruminal sac, rapidly degrades urea to ammonia. This is an important substrate for microbial protein synthesis, subject to adequate amounts of α-ketoglutarate (for amination to glutamate) and of suitable VFAs (including the isoacids) being available to provide the carbon skeletons onto which the amino groups can be added (by transamination from glutamate). In practice, feeding regimens must, on the one hand, provide sufficient crude protein (true protein plus NPN) and readily fermentable carbohydrates to ensure that the ruminal microbes have adequate amino acids, ammonia, and carbon skeletons to meet the requirements of microbial protein synthesis for the maintenance of population numbers and, on the other hand, ensure that excessive protein breakdown to VFAs and ammonia does not occur. Overfeeding of protein is a wasteful use of an expensive commodity, and it leads to the overproduction of ammonia. In addition, it takes energy to convert NH_3 to urea (in the liver) and also creates a risk of ammonia toxicity.

In addition to the fermentation of dietary protein, there is a continuous recycling of the protein of dead microbes, especially in the fibrous raft. Essentially none of the amino acids produced in the forestomach becomes immediately available to the ruminant. Instead, from the material that flows out of the forestomach into the abomasum and small intestine, the ruminant acquires unfermented dietary proteins and microbes, the protein of which has a higher biological value (i.e., contains more essential amino acids) than the plant proteins of the diet.

The fermentation of dietary lipids

Dietary lipids occur as structural lipids in the leaves of forage plants and as storage lipids in oilseeds. The forage plant lipids are found in cell membranes and comprise 3 to 10 percent of the DM. Fewer than 50% of the total lipids are free fatty acids, and the majority are phospholipids, with palmitic, linoleic, and linolenic acids being the predominant fatty acids. In oilseeds, 65 to 80 percent of the lipids are free fatty acids with palmitic, oleic, and linoleic acids being predominant. Ruminal microbes rapidly hydrolyze dietary lipids and, using the unsaturated fatty acids (oleic, linoleic, and linolenic) as hydrogen acceptors, quickly convert most of them to stearic acid. Most plant unsaturated fatty acids are in the *cis* form. Ruminal microbes also synthesize microbial lipids from VFAs, and many of these are in the *trans* form. Diets generally do not contain more than 5% DM as lipid. Higher values adversely affect (1) food palatability, (2) the consistency of concentrate pellets at high and low temperatures, and (3) cellulolytic activity.

Other important ruminal reactions

A byproduct of ruminal fermentation is the vitamin B complex, provided that adequate cobalt (Co) is available for vitamin B_{12} production. This vitamin is required not only by the ruminant but also by some of its microbes. Feeding Co is therefore more effective than injecting the ruminant with vitamin B_{12}.

To synthesize the sulfur-containing amino acids (methionine, cystine/cysteine), a suitable dietary supply of sulfur (S) is required. Cystine/cysteine may be a factor limiting the growth of wool because of its high content in keratin (the wool fiber). In areas of molybdenum (Mo) excess, the ruminal bacteria form copper (Cu) thiomolybdenates, which reduce the availability of both Cu and S. Excess S forms insoluble cupric sulfide and also renders Cu unavailable. A deficiency of Cu, a cofactor of tyrosinase, leads to reduced melanin formation (a reddening of the coat of black animals) and loss of crimp in wool ("steely" wool).

Because of microbial actions, some dietary constituents that would be toxic for nonruminants are rendered harmless in ruminants (e.g., oxalates are converted to formate and CO_2). Conversely, dietary nitrate is reduced to the more toxic nitrite ion. When absorbed, the nitrite ion oxidizes the

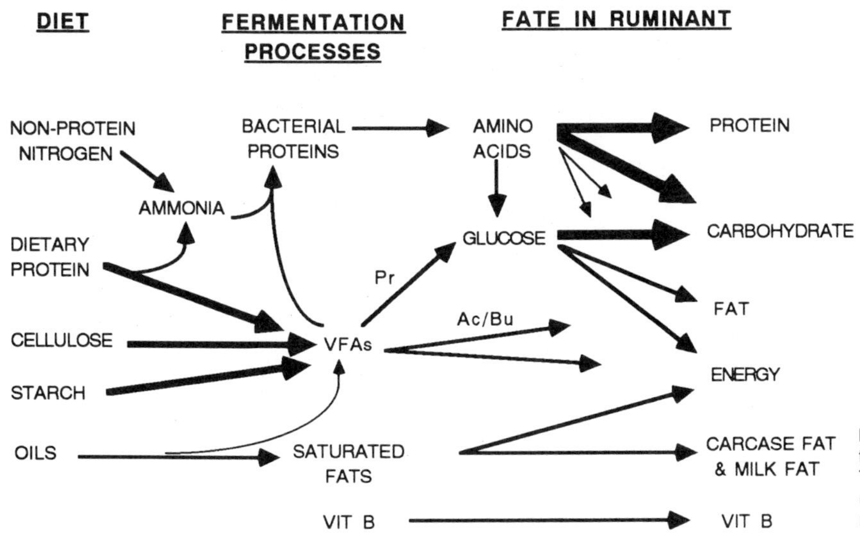

Figure 21.6. An overview of the fermentation and fate in the ruminant of the main dietary components. The principal volatile fatty acids (VFAs) are acetic (Ac), propionic (Pr), and butyric (Bu) acids. They are mainly present in the dissociated form.

ferrous ion of hemoglobin to the ferric ion, producing methemoglobin, which has no oxygen-carrying capacity.

Summary (Fig. 21.6)

Most of the plant material eaten by a ruminant is carbohydrate. In the case of roughage, these are structural carbohydrates, composed of β-1 linked glucose units (cellulose) or β-1 linked xylose units (hemicellulose), which are degraded slowly by cellulolytic bacteria to VFAs. In the case of concentrates based on grain, the main carbohydrate (starch) is composed of α-1 linked glucose units, which are rapidly degraded by amylolytic bacteria to VFAs and metabolic acids, particularly lactic acid. Plant proteins are also fermented largely to VFAs and ammonia. The cellolytic and amylolytic bacteria are *primary* bacteria. Important *secondary* bacteria include those that prevent the accumulation of lactic acid by converting it to propionate and those that convert hydrogen (using CO_2) to methane, thereby allowing reduced coenzymes to be re-oxidized and hence made available again as hydrogen acceptors. The most active level of fermentation occurs in the fibrous raft of digesta located in the dorsal ruminal sac. The microbes are located mainly inside the fibrous particles of the raft, and this reduces the rate at which microbes would be lost from the ruminoreticulum in the fluid that passes into the omasum and the abomasum. Some of the fermentation intermediaries are combined with the amino groups in the synthesis of microbial protein. The amino groups come from ammonia that arises from the deamination of plant proteins or from the urease hydrolysis of salivary and transruminal diffused urea. The unsaturated fatty acids of plant lipids are almost fully hydrogenated (saturated). All constituents of the vitamin B complex are synthesized. The strong reducing capacity of the rumen may result in dietary constituents and orally administered drugs becoming less toxic (oxalates), more toxic (nitrites), or less available (Cu and S when Mo is present).

THE FATES OF THE END PRODUCTS OF FERMENTATION

Volatile fatty acids

The fermentative end products of all carbohydrates are mainly acetic, propionic, and butyric acids, with a significant increase in the proportion of propionic acid when starch-rich concentrates are fed. The fermentation of proteins yields these acids together with valeric acid (having a 5-carbon chain) and the branched VFAs (isoacids)—isobutyric and isovaleric acid. These additional VFAs account for less than 5% of the total. They are probably more valuable to the microbes for protein synthesis using NPN than to the ruminant directly.

Even though all three forestomach compartments have a stratified squamous epithelial lining, most of the VFAs produced are absorbed across the forestomach wall. The VFAs are weak acids (pK = 4.6), so that the Henderson-Hasselbalch equation would give an anion/undissociated acid ratio of 100:1 at a typical rumen pH of 6.6. For this reason, individual VFAs are often referred to by the name of their anion. Absorption rates are higher (1) when ruminal pH is reduced, so that more of the compound is present as the undissociated acid, and (2) as the chain length increases, so that the rate of absorption is Bu>Pr>Ac. About one-half of the VFAs absorbed by passive diffusion are in the undissociated state, and the remainder are effectively absorbed as anions by facilitated diffusion in exchange for bicarbonate (hydrogen carbonate) ions (Fig. 21.7). The granulosum cells of the forestomach epithelium contain carbonic anhydrase, which promotes the formation of carbonic acid. This compound dissociates into bicarbonate ions and hydrogen ions. The latter associate with VFA anions to form undissociated VFAs, which can diffuse more easily across the epithelium, leaving bicarbonate ions in the ruminal fluid. This mechanism not only facilitates VFA absorption but also reduces the ruminal pH by exchanging the anions of stronger acids (VFAs) for those of a weaker acid (carbonic acid). About one-half of the VFAs produced are neutralized in this way, and the remainder by the salivary alkali.

During absorption through the forestomach walls, most of the butyric acid in sheep and rather less in cattle is metabolized (oxidized) to the ketone body, β-hydroxybutyrate (β-OH Bu). The remaining butyric acid is carried to the liver and is metabolized similarly. Thus the absorbed butyric acid appears in the general circulation almost entirely as β-OH Bu. This ketone body is readily metabolized by most tissues of the body and is used to provide the first four carbon units in the mammary synthesis of about half of the short- and medium-chain fatty acids (C4-C14) characteristic of ruminant milk. About 30 percent of the propionate is also metabolized by the forestomach wall to form lactic acid. Therefore some of the lactic acid in portal venous blood originates as propionate in the rumen. The portal venous lactate and the remainder of the propionate are almost completely removed by the liver. Here propionate is converted to oxaloacetate and used in the Krebs' cycle or, together with the lactic acid, is converted to glucose, either for release into the circulation or for storage in the liver as glycogen. Propionate is the only VFA capable of being used for gluconeogenesis. A small amount of acetate is metabolized to CO_2 by the forestomach wall, but the remainder is not changed during absorption or passage through the liver. Acetate, the most abundant VFA in the general circulation and the prime metabolic substrate, is taken up by most body tissues to form acetyl Co-A for use in the citric acid cycle. In the mammary gland it is used in the synthesis of the short- and medium-length fatty acids. It is used for about half of the first four carbon units in each fatty acid chain (i.e., those not derived from β-OH butyrate) and for all of the remaining carbon units in the chain.

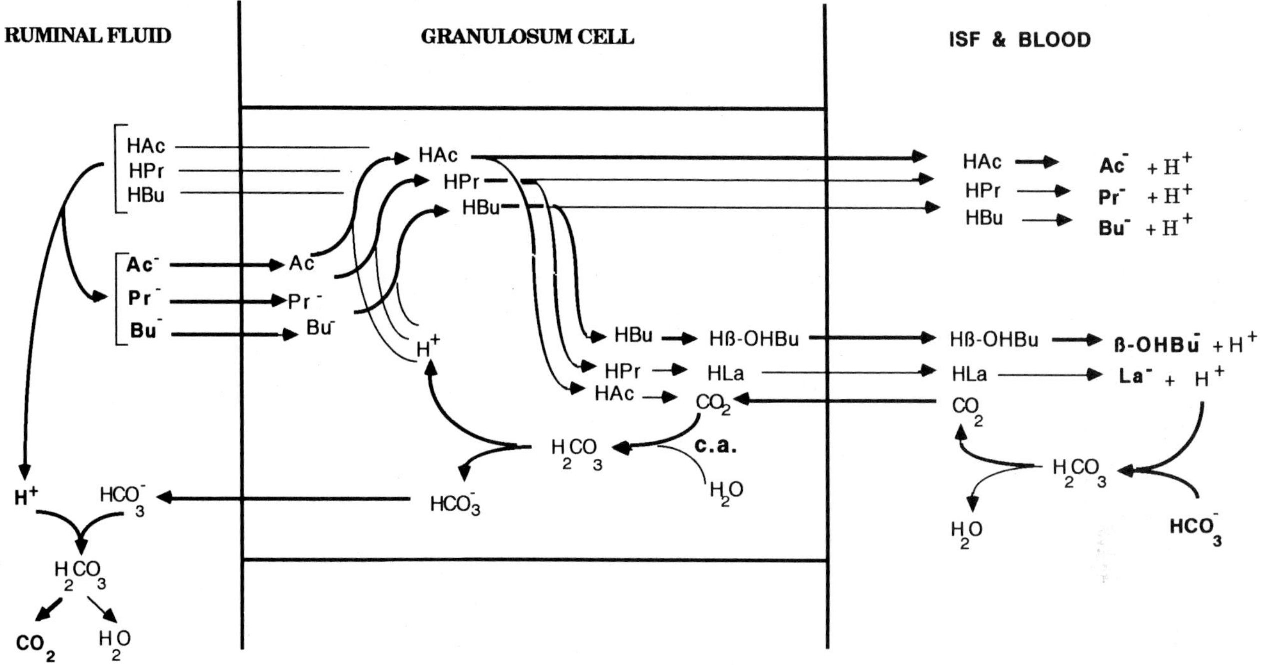

Figure 21.7. In the ruminal fluid (at pH 6.8) the ratio of dissociated to undissociated VFAs is 100:1. The main barrier to the absorption of VFAs is the granulosum cell layer of the ruminoreticulum. Whereas the luminal boundary of the cells is permeable to both dissociated and undissociated VFAs, the interstitial fluid (ISF) boundary is essentially permeable only to undissociated VFAs. In the cells the acetate (Ac^-), propionate (Pr^-) and butyrate (Bu^-) anions associate with H^+ ions produced from carbonic acid to form undissociated acetic acid (HAc), propionic acid (HPr), and butyric acid (HBu). A little of the HAc is catabolized to CO_2, half of the HPr is catabolized to lactic acid (HLa), and (in sheep) most of the HBu is catabolized to undissociated β-OH butyric acid (Hβ-OH Bu). These products diffuse across the ISF boundary and are buffered by bicarbonate, so that the material carried in the portal blood to the liver is mainly Ac^- with smaller amounts of Pr^-, La^-, β-OH Bu^-, and Bu^-. Carbon dioxide produced by catabolism and absorbed from the blood forms carbonic acid in the granulosum cells with the enzymic assistance of carbonic anhydrase (c.a.). The bicarbonate anions diffuse into the ruminal fluid and help to buffer the H^+ ions produced by the dissociating VFAs. In the process, additional CO_2 is added to the rumen.

Lactic acid

Along with VFAs, lactic acid is produced by certain of the amylolytic bacteria during the degradation of starch. Normally the lactic acid is present transiently, and, therefore, only in low concentrations, as it is used by secondary bacteria to produce propionate. At low ruminal pH values, the proprionate bacteria, but not the amylolytic bacteria, are inactivated, so lactic acid in both D(−) and L(+) isomeric forms accumulates. Lactic acid is a stronger acid (pK = 3.8) than the VFAs (pK = 4.6), so that ruminal pH tends to fall very quickly. Lactic acid is absorbed at only 10 percent of the VFA rate, and the more common L(+) isomer is metabolized to pyruvate (en route to glucose and glycogen) by the liver faster than the D(−) isomer. Unmetabolized acid will cause a metabolic acidosis.

Gases

The production of gases reaches a peak of up to 40 L/h in cattle 2 to 4 hours after a meal, when the fermentation rate is at its maximum. The principal gases are CO_2 (60%), CH_4 (30 to 40%) and variable amounts of N_2, with traces of H_2S, H_2, and O_2. They are eliminated almost entirely by eructation. Carbon dioxide arises (1) from the decarboxylations of fermentation and (2) from the neutralization of H^+ by the HCO_3-ions entering the rumen in the saliva and across the ruminal wall during VFA absorption. Methane arises from the reduction of CO_2 and formate by the methanogenic bacteria. These reactions are beneficial because they provide a hydrogen sink so that the oxidative (dehydrogenation) coenzymes can be recycled and wasteful because methane is a high-energy compound and its elimination from the body as a waste product represents the loss of about 8 percent of the total digestible energy of the diet. Hydrogen sulfide arises from the reduction of sulfates and from sulfur-containing amino acids. It is a potentially toxic gas, even in small amounts. Normally H_2 gas is present in traces and in significant amounts only where there is abnormal fermentation after a sudden large increase in concentrate feeding. Oxygen gas enters the rumen trapped in ingested food and water and by diffusion from the blood. It is quickly used by the facultative anaerobic bacteria, so that ruminal concentrations are always low. This is essential for the majority of ruminal microbes, which are strict anaerobes.

Ammonia

Ammonia arises from the deamination of dietary proteins, NPN, and urea derived from the saliva and, across the forestomach wall, from the blood. Feeding up to 30 percent total nitrogen as a urea supplement is usually well tolerated. If adequate and suitable VFAs are present, NH_3 is incorporated into microbial protein; otherwise, it is absorbed, particularly if the ruminal pH is alkaline. The NH_3 (now actually NH_4^+) must be removed from the portal blood and converted to urea; otherwise, ammonia toxicity develops (see below).

Other end products

Amino acids arising from fermentation are used by other microbes and are not immediately available to the ruminant. Microbes that pass out of the forestomach are digested in the gastrointestinal tract. Lysis of bacteria is started in the abomasum by the action of a lysozyme in the abomasal secretions. Microbes yield protein of high biological value, lipids (including some PUFAs), polysaccharides (as starches), and vitamins. The protein content of the microbes is about 27 percent and 45 percent of the total DM in the case of bacteria and protozoa, respectively. The long-chain fatty acids, having been hydrogenated by the ruminal bacteria, are absorbed and taken up by adipose tissue and by the lactating mammary gland. The intraruminal hydrogenation of unsaturated fatty acids causes ruminant carcass and milk fat to have a greater ratio of saturated to unsaturated fatty acids than nonruminant carcass and milk fat.

Summary

The main end products of carbohydrate and protein fermentation are the VFAs. They are absorbed directly across the forestomach wall, where butyrate and, to a lesser extent, proprionate undergo some metabolic changes before further metabolism in the liver. Some acetate is fully oxidized. VFAs and their metabolites enter the general circulation as acetate (from acetate), glucose (from propionate), and β-OH Bu (from butyrate) to become the principal metabolic substrates in ruminants. Lactic acid, in both isomeric forms, usually occurs as a transient intermediate. With high-starch diets, however, it may accumulate in the forestomach from which it is only slowly absorbed and then largely converted to glucose in the liver. The principal gases are methane, produced by methanogenic bacteria, and carbon dioxide, produced during fermentative oxidative decarboxylations and from the neutralization of VFA hydrogen ions by bicarbonate entering the rumen in the saliva and through transruminal exchange for VFA anions. The gases are eliminated by eructation. Dietary protein and NPN are synthesized into microbial protein of high biological value. After microbes flow out of the forestomach, their proteins, lipids, vitamins, and small amounts of stored starch are digested and become available in the lower gastrointestinal tract. Feeding of excess protein or urea supplements may produce high levels of intraruminal ammonia, leading potentially to ammonia toxicity.

THE RUMINANT'S CAPACITY TO INFLUENCE THE DIRECTION AND RATE OF GASTRIC DIGESTION

The ancillary requirements of fermentation

Fermentation is a continuous-flow (not batch) process. It requires (1) the regular addition of new macerated substrate (chewed food), (2) the steady removal of the end products of fermentation (VFAs, bacterial products, gases), (3) the onward propulsion of the unfermented material to the abomasum and intestines, (4) mixing devices to facilitate the addition of new substrate and buffers, to aid in the absorption of VFAs, and to prevent local accumulations of inhibitory end products, and (5) stable intraruminal conditions of temperature, osmotic pressure, and pH. It is only through its ability to regulate some of these ancillary requirements that the ruminant can exert limited influence over the direction and rate of fermentation. In some cases this regulation is not a direct response to a particular requirement but is incidental to the response to a parallel requirement. For example, the increased provision of saliva and, hence, of salivary buffers is not a direct response to reductions in intraruminal pH but is a reflex response to increased chewing and rumination evoked by the more fibrous diets.

Food intake

The quantity and quality of food ingested are the consequence of the mechanisms that control appetite and food selection with the modifications imposed by on-farm feeding practices. Appetite, which determines the amount of substrate available for fermentation, generally reflects the metabolic demands of the animal for food energy subject to a limited intake of DM imposed by the ruminoreticular capacity. The daily dry matter intake (DMI) for cattle on a mixed-feed diet in mid and late lactation can be estimated from the live weight (W) in kilograms and the milk yield (Y) in kilograms per day according to the formula: $DMI = 0.025\ W + 0.1\ Y$.

Food selection, which determines the quality of the substrate available for fermentation, will be the consequence of innate and acquired food preferences coupled with the animal's ability to differentiate between different foods by means of sight and smell before ingestion and taste mechanisms after ingestion of food samples. The extent of food selection practiced will be greatest in the selective feeders and least in the roughage/coarse grazers. Thus goats, sheep, and cattle are listed in order of decreasing food selectivity. Taste mechanisms depend on sensory receptors in the tongue and elsewhere, which, in the case of sheep, are able to discern (1) food temperatures (cold and warm thermoreceptors), (2) food shape and texture (slowly and rapidly adapting mechanoreceptors situated particularly on the small fungiform papillae), and (3) food composition (acid, salt, bitter, and sweet chemoreceptors). Receptors excited by sweet stimuli are restricted to the trough surrounding the circumvallate papillae. In addition to separate acid-sensitive and salt-sensitive receptors, there are receptors that are excited equally well by salt and by acidic solutions, including normal ruminal fluid, as would be present in a cud. The "salt" and "salt/acid" receptors are presumably of additional importance in relation to certain specific appetites, such as the appetite for salt in salt-deprived animals.

On the farm, food selection by the ruminant may be less significant than feeding practices in affecting the balance between cellulose and starch types of fermentation. The composition of the rations will determine the roughage (cellulose)/concentrate (starch) ratio, and this may be relatively constant on ad libitum feeding regimes. When large amounts of concentrates are fed infrequently (e.g., twice daily), there may be undesirable major fluctuations in amylolytic fermentation with a risk of developing conditions of low pH and temporary depression of cellulolytic and secondary fermentations for a significant part of each day (see below).

Prehension, mastication, and deglutition

Prehension (grasping of food) is an important element of selective feeding in the concentrate/selective feeding ruminants, for which the general characteristics are a long, pointed tongue and jaw, mobile thin and/or cleft lips, and a wide mouth. The roughage/coarse grazing ruminant has a shorter, rounded tongue and jaw, a thick muzzle, and a narrower mouth. The food is jammed between the labial surface of the incisor teeth of the lower jaw and the dental pad of the upper jaw. Then a forward movement of the muzzle bends the food over the sharp edges of the incisor teeth, which cut through it.

Mastication involves the premolar and molar teeth. The lower jaw is much narrower than the upper jaw, and the flat condyles of the temporomandibular joints allow considerable lateral movement. The teeth of the lower jaw are beveled, so that they are lower on the outer side and higher on the inner side, with the converse occurring in the upper jaw. Thus each chew begins with the lower jaw below and lateral to the upper jaw on one side. As the chew develops, the lower teeth move upward and inward against the upper teeth, so that food is subjected to a mixture of shearing and grinding actions. During its formation the wall of each tooth is invaginated so that the occlusal (grinding) surfaces are a mixture of dentine, enamel, and cement, each of which wears at a different rate. This ensures that the surfaces remain irregular, but it necessitates persistent pulp activity to maintain tooth growing during most of the animal's life.

In a laboratory recording of jaw movements, chewing of food is easily recognized by fast, irregular chews of variable amplitude, whereas during rumination the cud is chewed much more slowly and evenly, usually on one side, although occasionally a cud is changed to the opposite side. The direct importance of mastication is to break the stem and leaf fragments of food and to cut solids into small particles to increase the number of portals of entry for the ruminoreticular microbes. The indirect importance of mastication is that movements of the teeth excite sensory buccal mechanoreceptors, which provide the most potent natural excitatory inputs to both the salivary and gastric centers. Thus chewing movements, above all other stimuli, lead to increased salivation, particularly on the side on which the chewing is occurring, and to increases in the rate and the amplitude of primary and secondary cycle contractions of the ruminoreticulum. Foodstuffs that require little chewing on ingestion and that evoke little rumination subsequently fail to boost salivation and forestomach motility. They may have adverse digestive consequences.

Deglutition (swallowing) in ruminants is similar to that in nonruminants (see below) except that the ruminant esophagus consists mainly of striated muscle throughout its entire length and, therefore, peristaltic movements based on intrinsic nervous networks do not occur. Esophageal motility is required for the swallowing of ingesta, cuds, and liquids, for the regurgitation of cuds and (rarely) of vomitus, and for eructation of ruminal gases. The different sequences for these movements appear to be coordinated in centers in the hindbrain. When food is swallowed, the various segments of esophagus contract in sequence to produce a contraction wave that propels the ingesta aborally. The walls of the esophagus contain mechanoreceptors (tension receptors) that are excited sequentially as the food bolus distends successive parts of the esophagus. This sensory feedback mechanism appears to ensure that the force and rate of the propulsive wave match the requirements of a particular bolus. If the wave of contraction overtakes the bolus, the latter becomes stationary and the ensuing localized distention reflexly triggers a secondary wave of motility, which is usually confined to the distal third of the esophagus.

Salivation

Ruminants produce a high daily output of saliva (6 to 16 L/d in sheep; 60 to 160 L/d in cattle). The secretions from the major glands are isotonic with blood plasma, have no significant amylase content, change their composition in response to salt depletion, contain urea and alkali, and maintain a continuous basal secretion even after total denervation. The characteristics of the various salivary glands of sheep are summarized in Table 21.2. The major glands are the parotid glands, which produce about one-half of the total daily salivary output, the inferior molar glands, and the palatine, buccal, and pharyngeal glands. Their secretion responds strongly to mechanical stimulation of the mouth, esophagus, and ruminoreticulum. In contrast, the submaxillary, sublingual, and labial glands produce small

Table 21.2. Salivary glands and their properties (sheep)

Salivary glands	Total salivary volumes (L/d)	Characteristics	Sites of reflexogenic stimuli
Parotids	3–8	Serous, isotonic, strongly buffered	Mouth, esophagus, ruminoreticulum
Inferior molars	0.7–2	Serous, isotonic, strongly buffered	Mouth, esophagus, ruminoreticulum
Palatine, buccal, pharyngeal	2–6	Isotonic, strongly buffered	Mouth, esophagus, ruminoreticulum
Submaxillary	0.4–0.8	Mucous, hypotonic, weakly buffered	Mouth during feeding, not cudding
Sublingual, labial	~0.1	Very mucous, hypotonic, weakly buffered	Mouth
Total volume = 6–16 L/d			

Adapted from Kay 1958, *J. Physiol.* 144:463–75.

quantities of hypotonic, mucous, weakly buffered saliva. The submaxillary and labial glands are strongly stimulated only by feeding and give no response to esophageal or ruminoreticular stimulation.

Although parotid saliva is isotonic with blood plasma, there are much higher concentrations of K^+ (13 mM), HCO_3^- (112 mM), and $HPO_4^{=}$ (48 mM) and correspondingly lower concentrations of Na^+ (170 mM) and Cl^- (11 mM). At high rates of secretion the K^+ and $HPO_4^{=}$ concentrations fall slightly and the Na^+, HCO_3^- and Cl^- concentrations rise, suggesting a two-stage process in saliva formation: acinar secretion followed by ionic exchanges in the small ducts leading from the acini. In salt-depleted animals there is a replacement of Na^+ by K^+ because of the action of aldosterone.

The high salivary content of HCO_3^- and $HPO_4^{=}$ accounts for its high alkalinity (pH 8.1) and is an important mechanism for the neutralization of about one-half of the VFAs in the forestomach. The pK values for HCO_3^- and $HPO_4^{=}$ systems, being 6.1 and 6.8, respectively, help to buffer the ruminal contents in the normal pH range of 5.5 to 7.0. The high content of phosphate also represents a form of recycling, the microbes having a high demand for phosphate to synthesize nucleoproteins, phospholipids, nucleotide coenzymes, etc. Salivary nitrogen, 77% of which comes from urea, provides a useful additional source of NPN for microbial protein synthesis. The high urea content of ruminant saliva may be a critical factor for survival in situations of severe protein deficiency, when even the kidneys can increase renal tubular reabsorption of urea to facilitate its recycling.

A basal level of parotid secretion occurs even in the totally denervated or atropinized gland. Reflex-evoked increases in salivation are due to the excitation of the secretory (acinar) cells by acetylcholine liberated by the parasympathetic nerve endings, and this may be blocked by atropine. Electrical stimulation of the sympathetic nerve supply after atropinization produces a transient increase in salivary output followed by a compensatory reduction. This effect is due to the norepinephrine-induced contraction of the contractile myoepithelial (basket) cells that surround the acini and small ducts. It leads to an expulsion of stored saliva rather than to an increase in secretion. The increase in parotid blood flow does not exactly parallel the increase in parotid secretion and depends on a noncholinergic parasympathetic mechanism, which is not affected by atropine.

Salivary reflexes are integrated in salivary centers located in the hindbrain. The major reflex excitatory input arises from postulated buccal mechanoreceptors located in or near the tooth sockets, and the sensory pathways project mainly to the salivary center on the same side as the receptor stimulation. Thus chewing of ingesta or cud causes a large increase in salivary secretion, particularly from the ipsilateral parotid glands, one of which in cattle may increase its rate from 2 ml/min to 30 to 50 ml/min. Experimentally, the parotid and other major glands also increase their secretory rates in response to distention of the esophagus, reticulum, reticuloomasal orifice, and ruminoreticular fold as a result of excitation of tension receptors located in these sites. In contrast, little increase is evoked by lightly stroking the ruminoreticular epithelium. Such stimulation primarily excites epithelial receptors and has a lesser effect on tension receptors. Tension receptor–induced reflex effects account for the small increases in salivation that occur at the time of each reticular contraction and for the transient large increase in salivation that occurs when the cardia and esophagus are distended by the cud during the act of regurgitation. Reflex increases in salivation may be inhibited by concurrent stresses and excitement.

In ruminants the primary role of salivation appears to be the supply of copious and continuous amounts of alkaline saliva to buffer the ruminal VFAs and to provide a very aqueous suspension of those solids that are not compressed in the fibrous raft. In the selective feeders whose diet is more concentrated and the fermentation rate higher, the relative size of the salivary glands and their rates of secretion are correspondingly higher. Secondary roles of salivation include (1) the recycling of urea as a source of NPN for microbial protein synthesis and of phosphate for microbial nucleic acid/nucleoprotein and membrane phospholipid synthesis, (2) action as a wetting agent for ingesta, and (3) the provision of a possible antifoaming agent for the rumen.

Ruminoreticular motility

The patterns of motility

At approximately 1-minute intervals the various regions of the ruminoreticulum undergo powerful contractions in a more or less fixed sequence, known as the primary cycle, mixing cycle or A sequence (Figs. 21.8 and 21.9). A typical primary cycle lasts about 20 seconds and consists, in turn, of (1) a biphasic (double) contraction of the reticulum, (2) a caudally moving monophasic contraction of the dorsal ru-

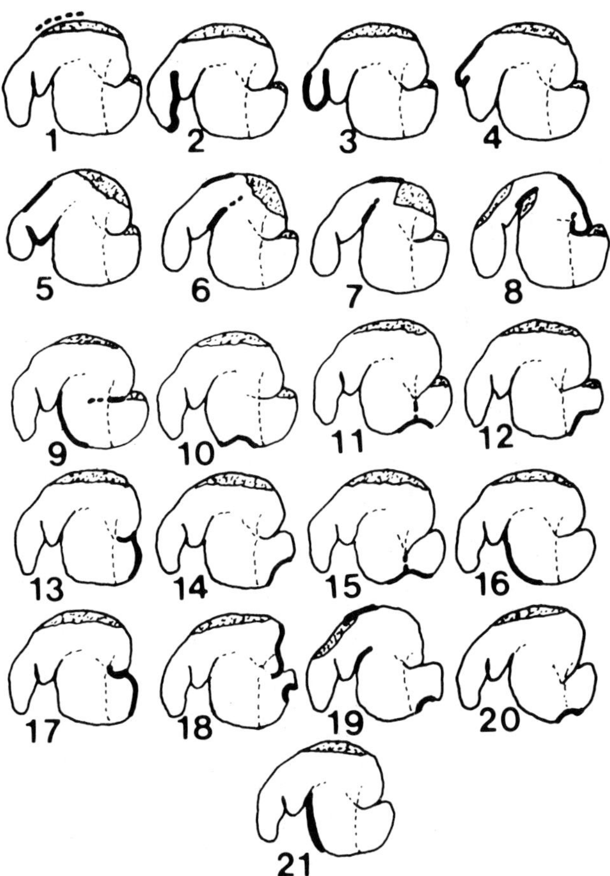

Figure 21.8. Contraction sequences in the ruminoreticulum of the resting sheep, based on drawings derived from tracings made directly from radiographs. Dashed lines represent ruminal pillars. Stippled regions represent the gas layer. The heavy dotted line represents the point of attachment of the rumen to the dorsal abdominal wall. The heavy solid line represents the region of wall actually contracting: 1, *Resting stage* between contraction cycles. 2–16, *Primary cycle,* commencing with the caudal wall of the reticulum and ruminoreticular fold (1) followed in turn by a double contraction of the reticulum (3–4), a contraction of the cranial sac, cranial pillar, and dorsal sac (5–7), a contraction of the caudodorsal blind sac and of the cranial and caudal pillars (8), a contraction of the longitudinal folds and cranial region of the ventral ruminal sac (9), spreading caudally (10–14) and then cranially (15–16). 17–21, *Secondary cycle,* typically occurring after alternate primary cycles, starting with a contraction of the caudal pillar and caudoventral blind sac (17) followed in turn by contractions of the caudodorsal blind sac (18), the (mid-) dorsal sac (19), the caudoventral blind sac (20), and the cranial region of the ventral sac (21). Eructation occurs occasionally during the primary cycle when the cardia is covered by a gas layer (8), but it occurs more commonly during the secondary cycle (19). (Modified from Wyburn 1980, in Ruckebusch and Thivend, eds., *Digestive Physiology and Metabolism in Ruminants,* AVI Publishing Co., Westport, Conn.)

minal sac, and (3) a contraction of the ventral ruminal sac. The reticulum relaxes completely in cattle and incompletely in sheep between the two phases of its biphasic contraction. Usually at the end of alternate primary cycles, a different cycle may occur. This is known as a secondary cycle, eructation cycle, or B sequence and consists of sequential contractions of (1) the caudoventral ruminal blind sac, (2) a cranially moving contraction of the caudodorsal ruminal blind sac followed by the middorsal ruminal sac, and (3) a contration of the ventral sac. During and shortly after feeding (Fig. 21.10) the rates of primary and secondary cycles almost double. During rumination, the rate of primary cycles has a value lying between the resting (not feeding, not ruminating) rate and the feeding rate, and the primary/secondary cycle ratios are as at rest. During rumination the reticular contraction is triphasic, the first phase often being referred to as the "extrareticular contraction." It precedes the usual biphasic contraction, and at its peak the cardia opens to allow the new cud to be drawn into the caudal part of the esophagus. Ventral sac contractions during rumination are more likely to be absent from both the primary and secondary cycles of cattle and from only those primary cycles that are immediately followed by a secondary cycle in sheep.

Ingesta enter the forestomach through the cardia lying in the dorsomedial wall of the reticulum. Heavy (metallic) foreign bodies fall to the bottom of the reticulum and tend to remain there. Most ingesta have a low density because of their fiber content and trapped air. Ingesta float high up in the reticulum and cranial sac of the rumen until the next biphasic reticular and cranial sac contractions carry them caudally to join the fibrous raft. There they become enmeshed in the raft as it is kneaded and slowly rotated anticlockwise (as seen from the left side) during the powerful dorsal ruminal sac contractions. Saliva, ingested water, and swallowed cud join the soupy material in the reticulum. This flows in turn into the cranial sac and then either back into the reticulum or on into the dorsal and ventral sacs. The contraction of the ventral sac forces its soupy fluid contents along the ventral and cranial surfaces of the fibrous raft to mix with the fluid in the cranial ruminal sac and reticulum. The material that leaves the reticulum via the reticuloomasal orifice is a random portion of the soupy material that is common to the reticulum, cranial sac, and ventral

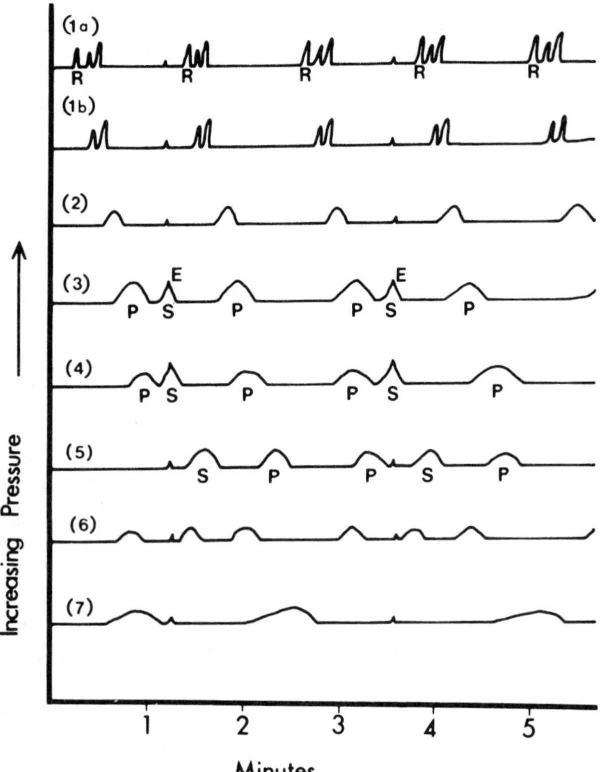

Figure 21.9. Diagram of typical pressure patterns recorded from different parts of the bovine forestomach. *(1a)* Triphasic contraction of the reticulum occurring only during rumination. Regurgitation (R) occurs at the peak of the first phase or "extra reticular contraction." *(1b)* Biphasic contraction of the reticulum, which occurs at all times other than during rumination. Relaxation between the first and second phases is complete in cattle but is incomplete in sheep. *(2)* Cranial ruminal sac, which commences during the second reticular phase but persists beyond it. It is not involved in the secondary cycle sequence. *3)* Dorsal sac contractions of the primary (P) and secondary (S) cycles. Eructation (E) most frequently occurs in secondary cycles at this point. *(4)* Caudodorsal blind sac, which contracts after the (mid-)dorsal sac in the primary cycle and before it in the secondary cycle. *(5)* Ventral sac contractions, which typically follow the dorsal sac contractions in both primary and secondary cycles. In cattle, more frequently than in sheep, the ventral sac contraction of the primary cycle may be absent. *(6)* Omasal canal. In cattle, but not in sheep, the contractions are variable and do not have a fixed time relationship with ruminoreticular contractions. *(7)* Omasal body. This undergoes episodic slow contractions, which are independent of the ruminoreticular contractions. Pressure increments, shown as upward deflections on the trace, do not exceed 30 mm Hg.

sac and happens to be in the reticulum at the time the orifice is open and when there is a suitable pressure gradient from the reticulum to the omasum. The particles in the omasum are the same size as those in the reticulum, so the orifice does not have a sieving role.

Most fermentation occurs in the raft, and it is therefore the site of origin of most of the gases of fermentation. During the kneading of the raft by the dorsal ruminal sac contractions, its dorsal surface splits, and this facilitates the release of free gas into the gas layer above the raft. Not much of the gas is absorbed, and most must be eliminated by eructation (belching). During the secondary cycles, to a greater extent than during the primary cycles, the dorsal sac contraction causes the gas layer to be moved cranially into the reticulum while the raft and fluid material are forced ventrally and held back primarily by the cranial pillar in cattle or by the ruminoreticular fold in sheep. If the gas layer reaches the cardia and clears it of fluid, the eructation mechanism is evoked (see below).

The reflex basis of motility.

The contraction sequences that make up the primary and secondary cycles result from coordinated motor nervous discharges traveling in different efferent vagal nerve fibers to their respective regions of reticulum and rumen. Because of their dependence on activity in extrinsic (vagal) nerves, the primary and secondary cycles are often referred to as extrinsic contractions and, after the destruction of more than 50 percent of the vagal nerve supply to the ruminoreticulum, extrinsic contractions are proportionately abolished. Total vagotomy or cholinergic blockade results in total loss of contractions (ruminoreticular stasis). Feeble intrinsic contractions responsible for the smooth muscle tone in the forestomach wall arise from nervous activity in its intrinsic nerve networks. When extrinsic contractions are absent the intrinsic contractions become more forceful, but they do not produce a recognizable cyclical sequence and cannot compensate for the loss of extrinsic contractions. In such a case the animal dies, unless, experimentally, it is given special feeding directly into the ruminoreticulum and abomasum.

The efferent (motor) vagal activity responsible for the extrinsic contractions originates from the bilaterally paired gastric centers in the medulla oblongata of the hind-brain. Experimental evidence suggests the existence of two groups of neuronal circuits responsible for controlling, respectively, the rates and amplitudes of the primary and secondary cycles. The gastric centers do not have spontaneous activity and need to be driven by excitatory inputs in excess of inhibitory inputs from other parts of the nervous system. Inputs from unidentified higher brain-stem centers are excitatory, and those from lower brain-stem centers are inhibitory. Splanchnic nerve inputs do not appear to be tonically active but are potentially inhibitory. The principal inputs to the gastric centers are from the forestomach, abomasum, and duodenum by way of the vagus nerves, the excitatory inputs normally dominating the inhibitory inputs (Fig. 21.11). When the animal is feeding and ruminating, a particularly potent excitatory input to the gastric centers arises from buccal mechanoreceptors during the act of chewing, which accounts for the more frequent and more forceful cyclical movements that occur at these times.

The known sensory receptor mechanisms responsible for the vagal inputs are of two kinds: tension receptors and epithelial/mucosal receptors. The tension receptors are located in the muscle layer of all parts of the forestomach,

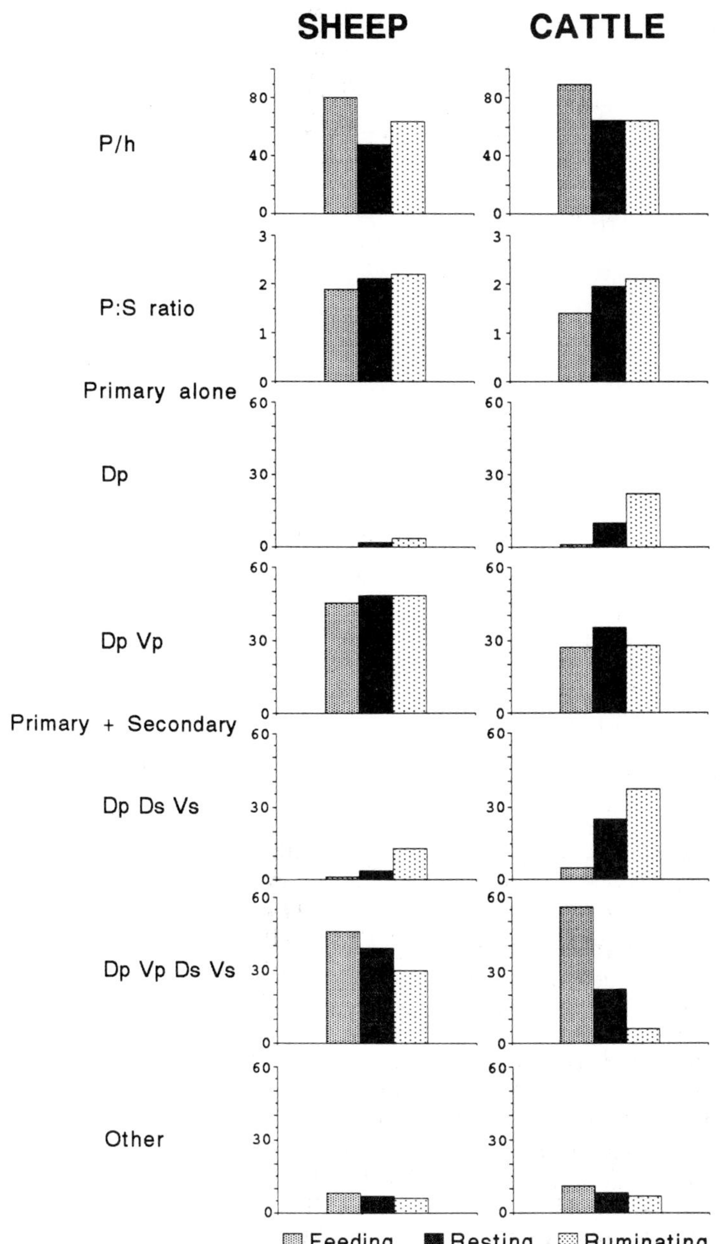

Figure 21.10. The characteristics of the primary and secondary cycle contraction of the rumen in sheep and cattle that are feeding, ruminating, and resting (not feeding, not ruminating). P/h, number of primary cycles occurring per hour; P:S ratio, primary/secondary cycle ratio; Dp, dorsal sac contraction only, during primary cycle; Dp Vp, dorsal and ventral sac contractions, during primary cycle; Dp Ds Vs, dorsal sac contraction only, during primary cycle, followed by dorsal and ventral sac contractions, during secondary cycle. Dp Vp Ds Vs, dorsal and ventral sac contractions. during primary cycle and during secondary cycle. The numerical values for contractions of the various sacs refer to the occurrence of a particular sequence, expressed as a percentage of the total number for each state (feeding, resting, ruminating). In sheep the primary cycle rate increases with rumination and especially with feeding. The primary/secondary cycle ratio hardly changes, although secondary cycles become slightly more frequent during feeding. In primary cycles, a ventral sac contraction usually occurs after each dorsal sac contraction, except in some of the primary cycles during rumination. In cattle the primary cycle rate and especially the secondary rate increase significantly only during feeding. The ventral sac contractions are frequently absent from the primary cycles, particularly when cattle are ruminating. (Based on data from Phillipson and Reid 1960, *Proc. Nutr. Soc.* 19:XXVII, and Ohga, Ota and Nakatato 1965, *Jap. J. Vet. Sci.* 27:151–60.)

abomasum, and intestine, produce slowly adapting responses, and behave as if they are "in series" with the contractile elements (smooth muscle cells). Tension receptors monitor the tension present in the muscular wall, through being excited by passive distention of the region in which they are located, by active contractions, and by drug-induced contractures of the surrounding smooth muscle. The epithelial receptors are located close to the basement membrane of the luminal epithelium of the forestomach, and the mucosal receptors are located close to the luminal mucosa of the abomasum and small intestine. They are unusual in that they are excited both by mechanical stimuli and by certain chemical stimuli. They have a low threshold to mechanical stimulation and are particularly sensitive to any moving light tactile stimulus. They give rapidly adapting responses to mechanical stimuli (e.g., brief "on-off" responses to low and moderate levels of sustained distention, repeated discharges of action potentials when the receptive field is lightly brushed, and an irregular discharge during contractions of the region). At high levels of sus-

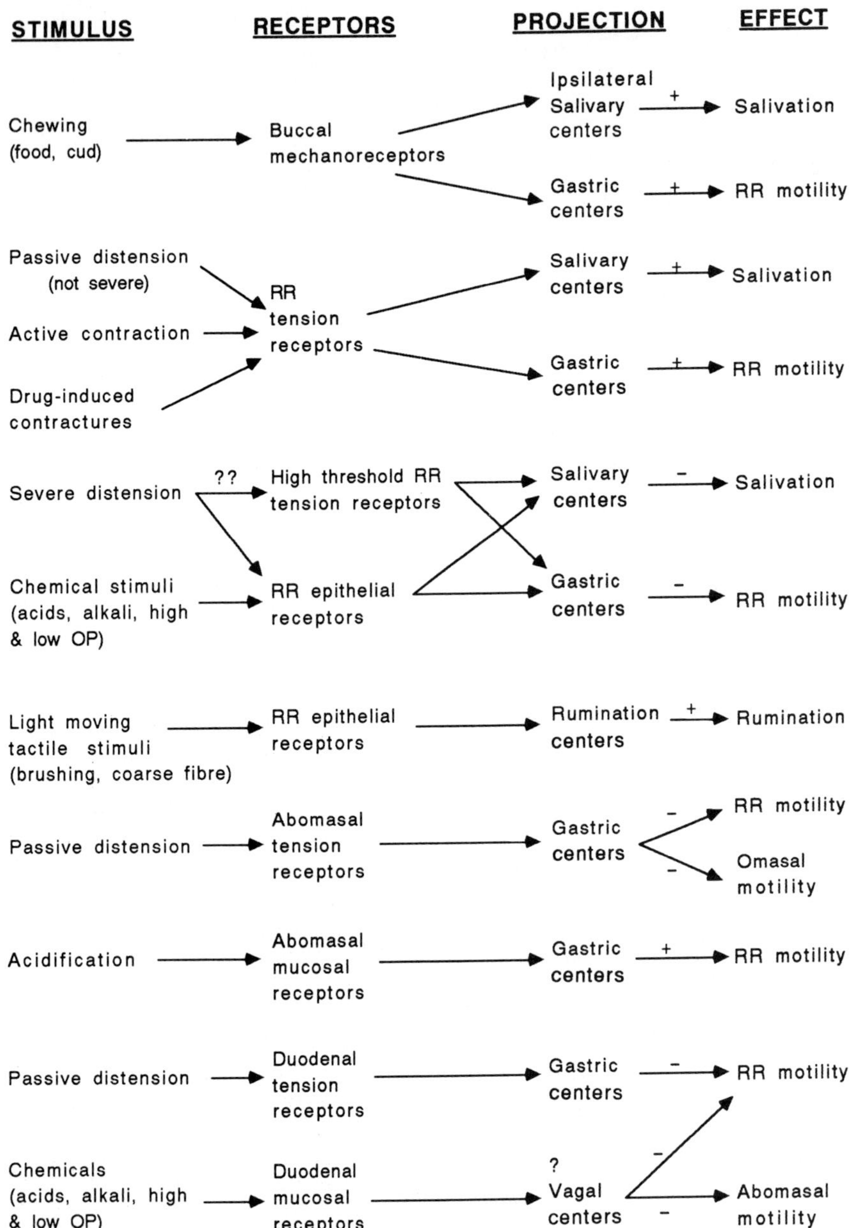

Figure 21.11. A summary of those alimentary tract sensory receptor mechanisms known to exert reflex effects on salivation and ruminoreticular motility. (Based on Leek 1986 in Milligan, Grovum, and Dobson, *Control of Digestion and Metabolism in Ruminants.* Prentice-Hall, Englewood Cliffs, N.J.)

tained distention, they produce a more persistent but somewhat irregular discharge. In the reticulum of sheep they are found particularly in the conical papillae surrounding the hexagonal ridges. They give sustained discharges when excited by certain chemicals (i.e., acids, alkalies, hypertonic and hypotonic salt solutions, and water). The acid sensitivity of these receptors is not due to the hydrogen ion concentration (pH) of an individual acid solution but is more closely related to its titratable acidity. In the case of weak acids, therefore, the presence of salts of that acid raise the pH but do not lessen the effectiveness of the acid itself. Strong acids are effective only at low pH values. The epithelial receptors in the forestomach and the mucosal receptors in the abomasum lie about 150 μm below the luminal surface, and this long diffusion distance favors low-molecular-weight weak acids, particularly those with high membrane permeabilities, such as butyric acid. Some high-molecular-weight acids (e.g., citric acid) and acids with low permeabilities (e.g., lactic acid) are relatively ineffective in the direct excitation of epithelial/mucosal receptors. When mixed with ruminal contents they may be more effective in exciting epithelial receptors than when they are used in isolation. This is due to an indirect action whereby the VFAs in the ruminal fluid are rendered more undissociated by a stronger acid (such as lactic acid), so that the titratable acidity of the VFAs increases above the threshold for receptor activation.

In the forestomach, tension receptors are most apparent (1) in the medial walls of the reticulum and of the cranial ruminal sac, (2) in the ruminoreticular fold, (3) in the cranial pillar, and especially (4) on the outer side of the lips of the reticular groove, around the cardia and around the reticuloomasal orifice. A few tension receptors have been detected elsewhere in the rumen and along the omasal canal. Low and moderate levels of passive reticular distention and of ruminoreticular fold stretching have been shown to excite tension receptors and gastric center neurons, leading to increases in the rate and amplitude of primary and secondary cycle contractions. These excitatory inputs also go to the salivary centers to produce the increased salivation that occurs under these circumstances. Tension receptor inputs are evoked actively during relatively isometric contractions, particularly when the ruminioreticular contents are insufficiently fluid. These give beneficial effects through reflexly compensatory increases in salivation and in the force and amplitude of the contractions themselves.

High levels of reticular distention, in contrast, lead reflexly to a reduction in ruminoreticular motility and salivation, even though tension receptor activity is at a peak. This paradox may be due to the excitation of separate high-threshold tension receptors with an inhibitory action, although no such receptors have been observed; to the gastric centers changing their response from excitation to inhibition in response to high inputs; or, more likely, to the persistent discharge of epithelial receptors evoked at high levels of distention dominating the concurrent excitatory effect of the tension receptor input. Sustained epithelial receptor discharges are also encountered in experimentally induced "ruminal acidosis" and reflexly lead to progressive reductions in ruminoreticular motility to the point of total stasis. It seems unlikely that the chemosensitive properties of these receptors have any role in regulating normal ruminal pH, but their activation may become important during the early stages of clinical ruminal acidosis. The reduction in ruminoreticular motility may, in turn, reduce fermentation and thereby reverse the developing acidosis and effect a spontaneous cure. The reflex inhibitory effects on ruminoreticular motility of situations (e.g., severe reticular distention and ruminal acidosis) that are associated with sustained discharges from epithelial receptors must be contrasted with other situations that excite epithelial receptors only intermittently and reflexly evoke rumination (see below).

The reflex roles of the abomasum

In the abomasum, vagally innervated mucosoal receptors are located in the fundic and pyloric regions and show combined mechanosensitive and chemosensitive properties similar to those of the ruminoreticular epithelial receptors. The normal levels of abomasal acidity are above the threshold for the epithelial receptors, and their activation would account for reflex excitation of primary cycle movements of the ruminoreticulum when the abomasal contents are acidified experimentally with VFAs and with HCl. Perhaps this reflex mechanism serves to promote abomasal filling from the forestomach when abomasal acid secretion exceeds substrate inflow. Distention of the abomasum reflexly inhibits primary cycle movements of the ruminoreticulum by two independent sensory pathways: (1) a vagal pathway to the gastric centers, which carries the input from tension receptors in the muscular wall of the abomasum, and (2) a splanchnic pathway, which carries the input perhaps from tension receptors but more likely from serosal receptors lying at the serosal mesenteric boundaries. Perhaps these reflexes serve to limit the onward propulsion of the forestomach material into the abomasum and thereby prevent overfilling.

Clinical disorders of motility

In many clinical situations, ruminoreticular motility is disturbed because of changes in the excitability of the gastric centers, in the normal sensory inputs to the centers, or in the efferent nervous activation of the forestomach smooth muscle. Fever, excitement, pain at any site in the body, and all anesthetics, sedatives, and tranquilizers depress the gastric centers, leading to subnormal motility or total lack of cyclical motility ("ruminal stasis"). Clinical conditions that exhibit anorexia ("animal off its feed") will produce subnormal motility because of the lack of normal excitatory sensory inputs arising from buccal mechanoreceptor activation during eating and ruminating and from ruminoreticular tension receptor activation during moderate ruminoreticular distention. High levels of ruminoreticular acidity (pH 5.8 or lower, as may occur in ruminal acidosis after grain engorgement) lead to subnormal motility to the point of complete stasis due to inhibitory sensory inputs from persistent activation of the acid-sensitive ruminoreticular epithelial receptors. High levels of ruminoreticular distention that arise during severe bloat or during ruminal impaction of indigestible fibrous material may have similar consequences, again probably because of the persistent activation of epithelial receptors at high mechanical thresholds or, alternatively and less likely, because of the activation of high-threshold tension receptors. Displacement of the abomasum leads to severe distention with gases and fluid resulting in ruminal stasis as a reflex consequence of abomasal tension receptor activation. Experimentally, the loss of more than 50 percent of the vagal nerve supply to the forestomach leads progressively to greater degrees of reduced motility, and this is the explanation generally but erroneously given as the basis for the ruminal stasis described as "vagus indigestion." In practice, such a degree of vagal damage has never been convincingly demonstrated in this condition. At autopsy, many cases of vagus indigestion show chronic inflammatory lesions of the ruminoreticular wall. The main effect of these is to interfere with the normal excitation of the sensory nervous receptors responsible for evoking the various gastric reflexes, particularly those related to motility. The motor pathway is susceptible to blockade by ganglionic blocking agents (hexamethonium, tetraethylammonium) and by postganglionic muscarinic blocking agents (atropine). Neuromuscular transmission is particularly sensitive to hypocalcaemia, and ruminal stasis may be seen at a very early stage of incipient "milk fever" and may, indeed, be the earliest sign of the disorder.

Eructation

The gases of fermentation accumulate in the gas layer above the fibrous raft in the dorsal ruminal sac. They are eliminated at frequent intervals, every 1 to 2 minutes, by eructation. Normally the cardia, the entrance to the esophagus from the reticulum, is covered by soupy reticular fluid. As a prelude to eructation, the gas layer is moved cranially by the secondary (occasionally the primary) cycle contraction of the dorsal ruminal sac. The ruminal contents are held back by the ruminoreticular fold in sheep or by the cranial ruminal pillar in cattle, and the reticular fluid is forced ventrally so that the cardia is no longer covered with fluid. The cardia and the lower esophageal sphincter open and the relaxed esophagus fills with gas. A rapid orally moving wave of esophageal contraction, together with opening of the cranial esophageal sphincter and elevation of the soft palate to close the nasopharyngeal orifice, allows much of the gas to be expelled through the mouth. This cycle may be repeated several times while the gas surrounds the cardia. Some gas from the pharynx enters the trachea and the pulmonary system and is absorbed into the blood. This provides the most common route by which aromatic chemicals in the rumen reach the mammary gland to produce undesirable milk taints.

Moderate distention of the ruminoreticulum with digesta, fluid, or gas excites tension receptors in the reticulum and cranial ruminal sac and provides a potent reflex stimulus for increases in the rates and amplitudes of both primary and secondary cycle contractions. These bring the gas layer to the region of the cardia. Here distention will trigger the remaining sequence of events necessary for eructation, but only if the cardia is fully cleared of fluid and froth. If present, fluid and froth, sensed perhaps by epithelial receptors, exert a dominant reflex inhibitory effect on the eructation mechanism. Thus the cardia and/or the caudal esophageal sphincter does not open and the gas remains trapped in the ruminoreticulum. Experimentally, by insufflating the rumen with gas through a cannula, it can be shown that the eructation mechanism is potentially capable of eliminating gas at rates far in excess of those volumes produced even at peaks of fermentation. Nevertheless, the clinical condition of "bloat," the distention of the rumen through the accumulation of gas, occurs quite frequently (see below).

Rumination

Rumination ("chewing the cud") is a unique characteristic of the true ruminants (deer, giraffes, and bovidae) and pseudoruminants (chevrotains, camels, and llamas). It is most pronounced in the relatively nonselective, coarse-grazing members of the bovidae (cattle) fed high-roughage diets, when it may occur in about 10 major bouts occupying up to 10 hours a day. With low-roughage diets or diets in which the roughage is finely ground, total rumination time may be as short as 3 hours a day or less. The incidence of rumination has a circadian rhythm and is most commonly associated with the state of drowsiness, the highest incidences occurring during the afternoon and in the middle of the night. Many lactating ruminants ruminate while they are suckling their young or are being milked.

Rumination involves a stereotyped sequence of events with complex coordination of its various components. Regurgitation ("bringing up the cud") starts with an inspiratory effort, with the tongue and soft palate raised to block the buccal cavity and nasopharyngeal orifice, respectively, so that an increased negative pressure develops in the thorax. Simultaneously, the reticulum produces an extra contraction in advance of the usual biphasic contraction. At the peak of the extra contraction, the cardia and the caudal esophageal sphincter open and a cud of the soupy reticular contents is drawn into the relaxed esophagus under the influence primarily of the heightened negative intrathoracic pressure. The extra reticular (regurgitation) contraction is not essential; it may be abolished by atropine without any effect on rumination. An orally directed wave of esophageal contraction carries the cud (a column of soupy fluid) toward the mouth, the glottis closing briefly as the cud traverses the pharynx into the mouth, where the tongue and the jaw are lowered to receive it. Often the head is pushed forward momentarily at this point. Earlier accounts of regurgitation describe an inspiratory effort with the *glottis* closed to achieve the increased negative pressure within the thorax, but it has been clearly demonstrated that the airways are closed during the inspiratory effort by elevation of the soft palate, the glottis closing only momentarily as the cud traverses the pharynx. The tongue is raised to squeeze out of the cud the liquid fraction, which is immediately swallowed. If no solid fraction remains in the mouth no chewing takes place, and this event is generally described as "pseudorumination." If a solid fraction does remain, as is usually the case, this is chewed with slow, regular chewing movements for about 40 seconds, during which time saliva is added and several swallows occur. Finally, chewing ceases and the remains of the cud and added saliva are swallowed. There are no jaw movements for about 5 seconds until the cycle is repeated, with the next cud being regurgitated into the mouth. Usually, during any particular bout of rumination, chewing occurs on only one side of the jaw. In some animals, such as camels, it is common for the cud to be chewed alternatively on the left and on the right with successive chews. As with eating, chewing the cud excites buccal mechanoreceptors and leads to reflex excitation of salivation, particularly from the parotid glands, and of primary and secondary cycle movements of the ruminoreticulum.

The solid fraction of the cud normally consists of the relatively small particulate matter in the soupy contents of the reticulum at the time of regurgitation. These particles are likely to be in a more advanced stage of fermentation than the material in the fibrous raft in the dorsal ruminal sac. Nevertheless, the rechewing causes further reduction in particle size, which provides new portals of entry for the fermentation microbes, and an increase in particle density through the expulsion of entrapped atmospheric and fermentation gases. Both size reduction and increase in density promote the chances of a particle being in a position favorable for passage into the omasum. When the cud is swallowed, it reenters the reticulum and becomes dispersed once again in the soupy material. Cud chewing leads to a three- to fivefold increase in salivation and its associated benefits. The increase in ruminoreticular motility may have both benefits and disadvantages. The benefits include greater mixing and eructation. Conversely, with certain kinds of feed, a disadvantage may be increased motility, which leads to greater onward propulsion of contents through the reticuloomasal orifice. Thus the mean intraruminal retention time, and hence the extent of fermentation of the ingesta, is reduced, leading to increased food intake and reduced digestibility. In construction of diets containing a mixture of roughage (which will promote rumination) and concentrates, it is worthwhile to engineer the particle density and size (determined by the degree of grinding of the concentrate components) so that each kind of concentrate particle receives the benefit of its optimum intraruminal retention time, depending for instance, on whether its protein component is primarily RDP or RUP.

Rumination represents one of the behavioral states of a ruminant and occupies about one-third of its lifetime. The coordinated series of stereotyped events occurs only during certain central nervous states and requires a peripheral sensory trigger (Fig. 21.12). The coordinated events of rumination include (1) modification of gastric center activity, in the case of cud regurgitation, to produce the extra contraction of the reticulum (the regurgitation contraction that forms the first part of the triphasic contraction), (2) modification of respiratory center activity to produce the inspiratory effort with closure of the upper airway, and (3) the esophageal activity needed to produce the cardiac opening at the peak of the extra contraction of the reticulum and the orally directed wave of propulsion to bring the cud to the mouth. The presence of the cud evokes the typical slow, regular chewing movements (50 to 55 chews per minute) and the increases in salivation and ruminoreticular motility. However, cud chewing ceases and swallowing always occurs not less than 2 seconds before the start of the next extra reticular contraction, during which there is regurgitation of the next cud. Thus, a second cud is never in the mouth at the same time as the first cud. It is convenient to ascribe the coordination of the events to rumination centers in the brain, the hypothalamus being a likely site because (1) decorticate but not decerebrate sheep can ruminate, (2) rumination can be excited experimentally by electrical stimulation of the anterior region of the hypothalamus, and (3) rumination often occurs during suckling and milking, possibly by radiation of nervous excitability to the rumination centers from the hypothalamic component of the milk ejection ("let-down") pathway. In a ruminant eating a typical feed there is a potent central nervous behavioral drive to ruminate. Animals that are prevented from ruminating by the application of masks or ties around the jaw will undertake a compensatory long bout of rumination even to the detriment of eating food when the impediments are removed. Similarly, although an animal that is alerted experi-

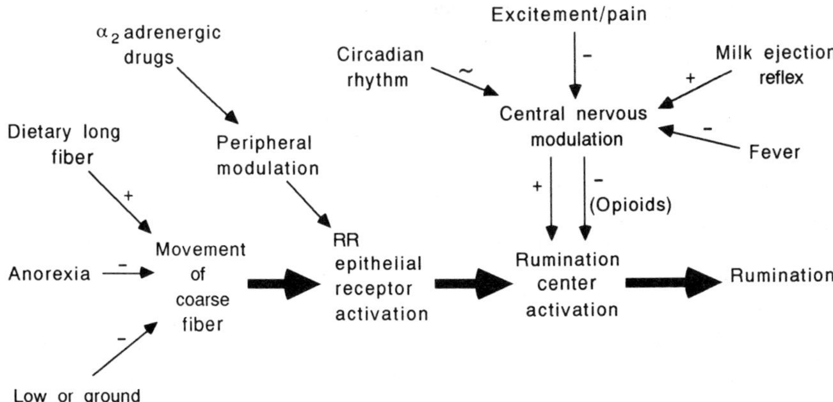

Figure 21.12. Rumination is the reflex consequence of ruminoreticular epithelial receptor activation by the "brushing" movement of coarse fiber against the luminal epithelium. Situations that reduce the presence in the ruminoreticulum of coarse fiber of suitable length reduce the incidence of rumination. The reflex may be facilitated or suppressed by central nervous modulation arising from a variety of factors. (Based on Leek and Stafford unpublished and 1989, *J. Vet. Med.*, A36:230–35.)

mentally will stop ruminating on the first few occasions, later it will persist with rumination even when subjected to high levels of disturbance. Rumination can be evoked in response to suitable conditioning stimuli.

Despite the potential central nervous drive, rumination normally will occur only if the rumination centers themselves receive an adequate peripheral excitatory drive from epithelial receptors in the ruminoreticulum. If a typical diet is fed in a finely ground form, little or no rumination will occur. To achieve normal rumination patterns, the average length of forage particles must be greater than 5 mm. At the other extreme, particles greater than 300 mm, as might occur after ingestion of long-cut silage, cannot be regurgitated. In this situation unsuccessful attempts at rumination ("pseudorumination") may occur over an abnormally lengthened period of 12 hours or more per day. In this case the long particles are producing an exaggerated peripheral excitatory drive to the rumination centers, but the cuds themselves are mainly liquid and are swallowed immediately after being regurgitated.

Experimentally, rumination can be restored in an animal fed a finely ground diet by insertion of low-density, long fibrous material such as chopped straw or pieces of polypropylene string through a ruminal cannula. Alternatively, working with a hand or probe through such a ruminal fistula, one can readily evoke rumination by light, moving, tactile stimulation in the region of the cardia, the cranial ruminal pillar, and the medial parts particularly of the ruminoreticular fold and reticular wall. These sites are richly supplied with epithelial receptors, and the above maneuvers provide the most effective form of epithelial receptor excitation. The sensitivity of these receptors can be enhanced transiently by bolus administration of certain drugs that have an alpha$_2$-adrenergic action. These include epinephrine, norepinephrine, and dopamine, all of which may be given intravenously, and xylazine, which must be given locally into the celiac or left gastric arteries to avoid its rumination-inhibiting central nervous system sedative effect. Although the drug action and the ensuing enhanced epithelial receptor activity last only a few seconds, this is often sufficient to trigger a bout of rumination that lasts several minutes. Thus the occurrence of rumination appears to be the consequence of the rumination centers receiving a peripheral excitatory trigger arising from stimulation of ruminoreticular epithelial receptors by coarse fibrous digesta. The trigger will not always cause rumination, because the central excitatory state of the rumination centers varies at different times of the day and night, at different levels of wakefulness, and with different behavioral states, (e.g., during suckling). Opioid mechanisms appear to affect this central excitatory state, and the opioid antagonist, naloxone, often facilitates the evocation of rumination.

Rumination is one of the cardinal and most obvious signs of health. Except when diets deficient in suitably long fiber are fed to normal animals, the absence of rumination is indicative of abnormality. It is absent in stressful situations, and in those diseases in which (1) the animal has not eaten for a day or more, (2) ruminoreticular motility is subnormal, or (3) there is a fever.

Omasal function

The typical, spheroidal omasum is absent in the pseudoruminants and is largest in the coarse-grazing true ruminants (e.g., cattle). Reticular material enters the omasum via the reticuloomasal orifice, particularly when the orifice is wide open during the second phase of the primary cycle contraction of the reticulum. After the reticular contraction, the orifice becomes tightly closed for several seconds and subsequently undergoes cycles of closure and partial opening, during which additional small amounts of reticular contents flow into the omasum. In sheep and goats, after a reticular contraction there is a sequence of omasal contractions, starting with the omasal canal, which tends to force omasal contents between the leaves of the omasum. This is followed by a prolonged contraction that spreads over most of the body of the omasum, being finally terminated at the onset of reticular contraction of the next primary cycle (Fig. 21.9). The contractions of the omasal body tend to empty the material trapped between the omasal leaves. In cattle, the omasal body contractions are variable and do not have the same cyclical rhythmicity as the reticular contractions. They are powerful and prolonged and are not always terminated before or because of the onset of the next primary cycle contraction.

Most of the particles of digesta found in the omasum are less than 1 mm in length, as are those in the reticular contents adjacent to the reticuloomasal orifice. Therefore, contrary to an earlier theory, the reticuloomasal orifice does not have a sieving action and the size of the orifice does not determine the dimensions of the material entering the omasum. The physicochemical conditions inside the omasum are similar to those in the cranial and ventral regions of the ruminoreticulum, so that fermentation and absorption are also similar. Relative to the volume of contents, the large surface area presented by the omasal leaves makes this an important site of absorption of VFAs, electrolytes, and water, although it does not seem to have special advantages over the ruminoreticulum when absorption is calculated per unit of luminal surface area. Unlike what happens in the ruminoreticulum, however, chloride makes a more important contribution than bicarbonate in the anion exchange for the absorption of VFAs. Therefore concentrations in the omasum, when compared with those in the ruminoreticulum, are 3 times higher for chloride and 0.5 times lower for bicarbonate.

The functional significance of the omasum is (1) that it is a site of fermentation with an importance related to its cubic capacity, (2) that it is a site of absorption with an importance related to its luminal surface area, and (3) that it helps to regulate the onward propulsion of digesta between the reticulum and the abomasum. In general, diets that lead to the most chewing, both during ingestion and during rumination, will lead to the highest rates and amplitudes of reticular contractions, to the highest aggregated duration of reticuloomasal orifice opening, and to the highest rates of transomasal flow of digesta. Increasing the liquid content of the ruminoreticulum also increases transomasal flow rates.

Abomasal function

The abomasum is a pepsinogen- and hydrochloric acid–secreting organ, which is embryologically and functionally homologous with the stomach of nonruminants. Unlike the nonruminant stomach, the abomasum receives a continuous, though variable, inflow of forestomach material. This consists of a continuous trickle of fluid, supplemented occasionally with gushes of fluid containing fine particles and with the slow extrusion of lumps of more solid matter. The total inflow in sheep amounts to 4 to 8 L/d. Despite this variability of inflow (rate and composition), the outflow from the abomasum to the duodenum is remarkably constant in both rate (11 L/d in sheep) and composition. Thus the abomasum functions not only as the site of acidic enzymic digestion but also as an inflow stabilizer for the duodenum. Pyloric distention, rises in abomasal pH, and (most particularly) VFA solutions are potent stimuli for gastrin release and secretion of hydrochloric acid. Secretion is strongly inhibited by an increase in the acidity of the pyloric region or of the duodenum. Gastric juice from the fundic region, amounting to 4 to 6 L/d may have an acidity close to pH 1.0, particularly at low rates of secretion. Conversely, pepsinogen concentrations are relatively constant, which means that pepsinogen output varies in step with gastric juice volume. Pyloric secretions are slightly alkaline, have little peptic activity, and are of small volume (0.5 L/d). Abomasal contents are maintained at around pH 3 as a result of the various interactions.

The fundus and body of the abomasum show tonal variations with little obvious movement, whereas the pyloric part undergoes typical peristaltic movement at about 6 contractions per minute. These movements persist after total vagotomy and splanchnotomy. They are therefore based on an intrinsic mechanism, which is significantly affected by extrinsic mechanisms: (1) excitation by vagal stimulation and parasympathomimetic drugs, blocked by atropine, (2) inhibition by splanchnic nerve stimulation and epinephrine, and (3) inhibition by gastrointestinal hormones. These mechanisms in the fundic and body regions provide the abomasum with the capacity for receptive relaxation to accommodate the variable inflows from the omasum and, in the pyloric part, provide motility for mixing and for onward propulsion of material into the duodenum at a relatively steady rate. Abomasal motility is increased by feeding and even by the sight of food, but for the most part the abomasum represents a link in a chain of negative-feedback mechanisms that curb gastric motility and hence the rate of propulsion of gastric contents. Duodenal distention and the presence of abomasal contents strongly inhibit pyloric motility reflexly through a duodenal tension receptor mechanism. Stimuli such as acids and hypoosmotic and hyperosmotic solutions in the duodenum excite mucosal receptors and retard abomasal emptying. This effect is reduced by vagotomy, implicating a vagal reflex pathway. Long-chain fatty acids also inhibit abomasal emptying, but, by analogy with nonruminants, an intestinal hormonal mechanism may be involved in this case. Pyloric motility appears to reduce the tone of the fundic and body regions. Distention of the abomasum, by stimulating tension receptors with sensory pathways in both vagal and splanchnic nerves, has a powerful inhibitory effect on ruminoreticular and omasal canal motility. This mechanism allows abomasal filling to become self-limiting when the capacity for receptive relaxation is reached. Acidification of the abomasum, by stimulating acid-sensitive mucosal receptors, has a potent reflex excitatory effect on ruminoreticular motility via vagovagal pathways. Presumably this is a "feed-foward" mechanism that corrects for underfilling of the abomasum.

Clinically, abomasal dysfunction is the cause of, or is involved in, many gastrointestinal disorders. Duodenal infections probably sensitize the sensory receptors responsible for the feedback inhibition of abomasal motility. Gastrin production caused by certain abomasal worms (*Ostertagia* sp.) and abomasal ulceration also reduce motility. Impaired motility by whichever cause leads to abomasal distention, resulting in (1) a predisposition to right-sided abomasal displacement and (2) subnormal forestomach motility, usually evident as a persistent tympany, which is often mild but occasionally severe and fatal.

Summary

The ruminant's capacity to influence the direction and rate of gastric digestion depends primarily on the type, texture, and volume of the diet selected or fed. Diets, such as those consisting of long roughage, provide a positive drive to the system as a result of the reflex consequences of chewing the ingesta initially and the cud later. The consequences include increases in salivation, ruminoreticular motility, eructation, rumination, omasal, abomasal, and, to a lesser extent, duodenal filling. The positive drives resulting from mastication are partly countered by the negative-feedback mechanisms, which retard motility and the rate of flow of digesta through the forestomach into the abomasum and on into the duodenum. Distention of the duodenum is a potent stimulus for the inhibition of abomasal and forestomach motility. In turn, abomasal distention and extreme ruminoreticular distention strongly inhibit forestomach motility. In addition to the regulatory effect of one location on more proximal or distal locations, each location itself has a degree of control over the level of its own activity.

Sensory mechanisms in the ruminoreticulum can influence the levels of motility, of salivary inflow, of further maceration of food particles (through rumination), and of eructation. Abomasal mechanisms can maintain the acidity of its contents near to pH 3 and can adjust its reservoir capacity to buffer the variable rates of inflow in order to give less variable rates of outflow.

INTENTIONAL AND UNINTENTIONAL CHANGES IN RUMINAL FUNCTION

Protected nutrients

Certain RUP plants, maize in particular, are poorly fermented in the forestomach but are readily digested in the abomasum and intestine. Similarly, many denatured proteins escape fermentation. Commercially, this has been exploited by subjecting RDP proteins to denaturation by formaldehyde (formalin). This process prevents the microbial degradation of high-quality proteins, so that their content of essential amino acids becomes directly available to the ruminant in the small intestine. An extension of the manufacture of protected proteins is the protection of other dietary supplements that would normally be fermented (e.g., lipids). These can be encapsulated in a coating of protected protein. This device would (1) prevent the saturation of polyunsaturated fatty acids and (2) allow higher levels of lipids to be fed, with the benefits of their high-energy content but without their fermentation-depressing effects.

Selective antibiotics in feed

About 8 percent of the energy content of the total digestible nutrients ends up as the waste product, methane. An antibiotic in the feed that would selectively suppress the methane-producing bacteria would reduce the amount of wasted energy. The ionophore, monensin, achieves this objective, presumably by affecting electrolyte transport across the cell walls of methanogenic and other bacteria while not disturbing monensin-resistant propionate-producing bacteria. In this way, less energy is lost as methane and more energy is conserved as propionate by the succinate pathway. In addition, monensin inhibits some of the bacteria responsible for proteolysis and deamination, so that improved efficiency of dietary protein utilization may also accrue.

Probiotics

A probiotic feed supplement involves the addition, in a dried form, of selected active microbes whose fermentation pathways are particularly desirable in a particular dietary situation. Being foreign to the natural microbial population, the probiotic microbes used in the forestomach undergo only limited proliferation, cannot become established permanently, and need to be added repeatedly. Certain species of yeast have been shown to have commercially advantageous effects on the fermentation of concentrate-enriched roughage diets. Preliminary studies suggest that the yeasts absorb partially hydrolyzed starch molecules, perhaps at the 3-9 glucose unit chain length. The immediate consequence of this is to reduce the availability of preferred substrate for the lactate-producing bacteria. As a result, less lactic acid is produced, ruminal pH does not fall below the limit for cellulolytic bacterial activity, and cellulolysis is not impaired. Reduced lactate production also reduces the rate of hydrogen production and hence methane formation. The growth, limited multiplication, and death of the added yeasts increase the total protein biomass in the rumen, and some of this ultimately becomes available to the ruminant. Overall, the yeast supplement increases the yield of VFAs and microbial protein and decreases the yield of lactate and methane. This represents an increased efficiency of feed utilization.

Concentrate-enriched diets

When the energy and protein requirements of domestic ruminants are increased to satisfy productive situations (lactation, pregnancy, growth), part of the roughage component of the diet is replaced by the feeding of grain or grain-based concentrates. This allows the ingestion of a greater amount of potential energy and protein without exceeding the DMI limit to appetite. Although, paradoxically, the potential energy from a unit amount of concentrates (5 mol VFAs per kilogram of DM digested) is less than that from roughage (7.5 mol VFAs per kilogram of DM digested), concentrates more than compensate for this by virtue of their greater digestibility (75 to 90 percent) as compared with roughage (45 to 70 percent) and of producing much higher fermentation rates via the amylolytic pathways than would roughage via the cellulolytic pathways. If adequate plant protein or NPN is available, the plentiful supply of VFAs coupled with the short doubling time of the amylolytic bacteria allows high rates of microbial protein synthesis through microbial proliferation. This is subsequently reflected in a greater availability of microbial protein products of high biological value to the ruminant host. The amylolytic pathways yield substantial amounts of lactic acid. If the intraruminal conditions remain above pH 6.2, the lactic acid will be converted by propionate bacteria to propionic acid, which will therefore form a higher proportion of the VFA mixture. This is an important advantage in situations, such as lactation, when increased rates of gluconeogenesis are required. Intraruminal conditions below pH 6.2 inactivate the propionate bacteria, resulting in an accumulation of lactic acid, a stronger acid than the VFAs, which renders the forestomach contents progressively more acidic. This misfortune is exacerbated by the concurrent decrease in the physiological mechanisms, which normally stabilize forestomach activity (Fig. 21.13).

Grain and other concentrates undergo less chewing on ingestion than roughage diets, and their particle size is too small to evoke much rumination. As a consequence, there is a reduced reflex excitatory drive from the buccal mechan-

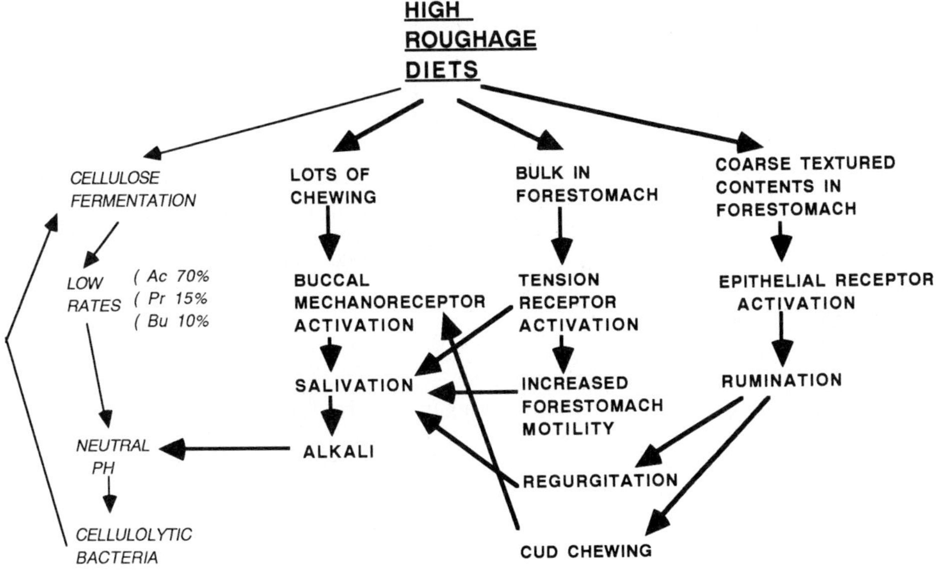

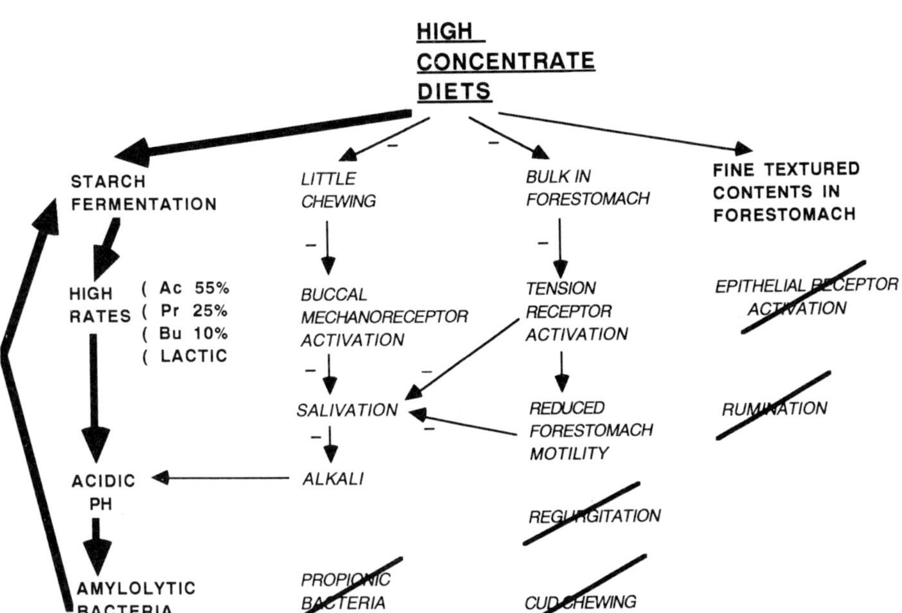

Figure 21.13. With high-roughage diets, high rates of salivation are evoked by several reflex mechanisms. This gives adequate alkali to buffer the VFAs produced at low rates by the slow cellulolytic fermentation. With high-concentrate diets, much smaller amounts of saliva and hence of alkali are produced because the reflex stimuli for salivation are less than with the high-roughage diet. Paradoxically, the low availability of alkali occurs under conditions of high VFA production rates with the added risk of lactic acid accumulation.

oreceptors to the salivary and gastric centers. Reduced salivation is thus occurring at a time of higher than normal ruminal acidity when the need for salivary alkali is heightened. Under these conditions the gastric centers receive not only a reduced excitatory drive from the mouth but also an increased inhibitory drive from the acid-sensitive epithelial receptors of the ruminoreticulum. The ensuing reduced forestomach motility results in less mixing and less absorption, so that the potential for VFA:bicarbonate exchanges across the forestomach epithelium is lessened at a time when increased amounts of bicarbonate into the ruminoreticulum would be advantageous to combat the rising acidity. Ultimately, ruminoreticular motility ceases (ruminal stasis). In some cases this is sufficient to retard fermentation, and the animal returns to normal as the intraruminal pH rises. In other cases the high intraruminal osmolality arising from the fermentation of large nutrient molecules into many small end-product molecules causes large movements of water into the forestomach, leading to tissue dehydration and diarrhea. The high acidity gives rise to a systemic metabolic acidosis and also breaks down the integrity of the forestomach lining, leading to multiple ulceration of the epithelium (rumenitis) and the entry of largely anaerobic bacteria into the portal venous system. At best these bacteria cause multiple liver abscesses, and at worst they swamp the animal's immune system and cause a fatal toxemia. Clinically, this condition is known as "ruminal acidosis."

Ruminal acidosis

Classically, pronounced ruminal acidosis is seen when cattle (more so than sheep) are suddenly changed from a roughage diet to a high-concentrate diet or when cattle gain accidental access to a grain store, accounting for the alternative name for ruminal acidosis, the "grain engorgement syndrome." Less pronounced but perhaps cumulatively more important is the subclinical ruminal acidosis that occurs 1 to 3 hours after a meal of concentrates. This is the most common way of providing the milk yield–related ration of concentrates to dairy cows. During this period, amounting perhaps to one-fourth of each day, concurrent cellulolytic fermentation is suppressed. This phenomenon is known as the negative associative effect on cellulolysis of feeding concentrates. This is due in part to the reduction of intraruminal pH to values below the limit for cellulolysis and in part to the preferential acquisition of metabolic substrates by the more competitive amylolytic microbes.

Given a suitable period for adaptation (up to 4 weeks), cattle can manage a diet that is composed largely or even wholly of concentrates. In this situation the increase in lactate-producing bacteria must be matched by an increase in lactate-utilizing bacteria, so that lactate accumulation does not become a problem. Protozoa increase in line with the concentrate content of the diet. This is advantageous inasmuch as the protozoa feed on the rapidly proliferating lactate-producing bacteria and also, by absorbing starch granules, reduce the amount of substrate available for these microbes. If lactate production is too rapid, however, so that the pH falls below 5.5, protozoa are inactivated and die out, so that this advantage is lost. In practice, the absence of protozoa from a sample of ruminal contents is usually indicative of a recent period of low intraruminal pH.

Good-quality silage has a pH of about 4 and has a high lactic acid content. Silage-based rations, particularly when supplemented with concentrates, make high-yielding dairy cows prone to ruminal acidosis, especially if the fibrous texture of the ingesta leads to little mastication and rumination and, hence, reflexly excites insufficient additional saliva (and alkali).

Acute pulmonary edema in cattle

Acute pulmonary edema, also called "foggage" or "fog fever," occurs naturally 2–10 days after mature cattle are switched suddenly from poor to lush pastures, such as to the aftermath growth (foggage) in hay and silage fields. The animals suffer obvious respiratory distress and, with no effective treatment known, about a third of the affected ones die. The avidly consumed lush pastures lead to abnormal ruminal fermentation, the significant feature being the conversion of tryptophan to 3-methylindole, which is absorbed into the portal blood. When it reaches the lung, this compound is oxidized to an active compound, which binds to and kills alveolar and certain bronchial cells in the lung. The cells slough off, allowing the airways to fill with frothy edematous fluid, so that the lungs at necropsy are enlarged, heavy, and rubbery.

Ketosis

Ketosis is a generic term for any condition in which ketone bodies, particularly acetone and acetoacetate, are readily detectable in the body fluids (blood, milk, and urine) and in the expired breath. The formation of ketone bodies in liver mitochondria occurs when acetyl-coenzyme A is being formed at a greater rate than it can be metabolized in Krebs' tricarboxylic or citric acid cycle (Chaps. 24 and 27). This is due to the inadequate provision of oxaloacetate to prime the cycle and occurs either when oxaloacetate precursors, predominantly propionate, are deficient or when the available oxaloacetate is preferentially channeled by a hormonally controlled rate-limiting enzyme reaction toward phosphoenol pyruvate for the purpose of gluconeogenesis, thus reducing its availability for the citric acid cycle.

The primary ketotic diseases are pregnancy toxemia or twin-lamb disease, which occurs just before parturition in ewes that are carrying more than one fetus, and acetonemia, which occurs at peak lactation in high-yielding dairy cows. Pregnancy toxemia typically occurs close to parturition, particularly if there is an added nutritional or metabolic stress, such as food restriction or the onset of colder weather. The high metabolic demands of the twin-lamb pregnancy, exacerbated by the cold and/or by a reduced availability of glucogenic fermentation products (propionic acid), trigger the onset of disease, which is often fatal. In acetonemia, the demands of the mammary glands for glucose as the precursor of lactose at peak lactation cause the available oxaloacetate to be used for gluconeogenesis at the expense of the needs of the citric acid cycle. The early stages in the development of this disease are exacerbated when the cow loses its appetite for concentrates, which would provide a relatively greater proportion of propionate, before it loses its appetite for roughage. As the disease progresses, the milk yield falls rapidly, so that the ketosis and its cause therefore decline. The disease is usually not fatal, but the slowness of the self-cure and the consequential loss of peak milk production make therapy worthwhile. This includes dosing with propionate, intravenous administration of glucose, and the injection of the gluconeogenic corticosteroid hormones.

Low-milk-fat syndrome

Low-milk-fat syndrome has no detrimental effect on the ruminant itself, but only on the butterfat content of its milk. When concentrate-rich diets are fed to high-yielding dairy cows around the peak of lactation, the predominantly amylolytic intraruminal fermentation pathways will increase the proportion of propionate in the VFA mixture. The accelerated glucogenic pathways result in reduced adipose tissue lipolysis and low blood levels of the free fatty acids needed as precursors for the synthesis of some of the milk lipids. The solution lies in increasing cellulolysis by increasing the proportion of dietary roughage.

Ammonia toxicity

Ammonia toxicity arises most commonly when excessive amounts of urea are fed, particularly at a time of low amylolytic fermentation. Occasionally toxicity may arise as a result of grazing young, high-protein pastures. Ruminal urease rapidly deaminates urea to ammonia. In the presence of adequate amounts of intraruminal VFAs, as would be present after the feeding of starch-rich diets, the ammonia is used in the synthesis of microbial protein. With cellulolytic fermentations, (1) the VFA production rate is much lower, so that there is less substrate for protein synthesis, (2) the rate of microbial growth and division is much slower, so that the rate of microbial protein synthesis is less, and (3) the higher intraruminal pH values favor ruminal absorption of ammonia. The toxicity of ammonia arises after its absorption and is due in small part to a systemic metabolic alkalosis and in large part to central nervous system intoxication by ammonia. Toxicity is countered by oral administration of VFAs and by feeding of grain. The reduced ruminal acidity slows ammonia absorption, and the VFAs provide carbon skeletons for microbial protein synthesis.

Bloat

Normal animals, even when the rumen is experimentally insufflated with gas, can eliminate ruminal gases by eructation at rates that far exceed those reached by maximal fermentation. Bloat, the distention of the ruminoreticulum by accumulated gas, is therefore due to a failure of the eructation mechanism. In "simple bloat" or "free gas bloat" the gas is present as a gas layer, and in "frothy bloat" the gas exists as bubbles in a liquid foam.

The most common simple bloats arise from esophageal dysfunction. Eructation is defective when there is obstruction of the esophagus, which may be internal (choking), e.g., due to a foreign object stuck in the thoracic part of the esophagus, or external as a result of enlargement of the mediastinal lymph nodes, e.g., with tuberculosis, actinobacillosis, or carcinomas. Esophageal spasm as a cause of bloat is an early sign of tetanus (lockjaw) in cattle.

Bloats also arise from ruminoreticular dysfunction, through failure of the cardia to be cleared of ruminoreticular contents. The reflex inhibition of cardiac opening caused by these contents dominates the reflex cardiac opening because of cardiac distention. In simple bloats, the failure of cardiac clearing is the consequence of partial or complete ruminoreticular stasis, caused by reflex inhibition of ruminoreticular motility. This may arise from overdistention of the ruminoreticulum with indigestible material (ruminal impaction), chronic mild ruminal acidosis, gross distention of the abomasum (abomasal displacement), or distention of the duodenum (as a sequel to duodenal infection). In frothy bloat, there is ruminoreticular hypermotility except in the last stage. At this point distention is extreme, but the animal's inability to clear the foam from around the cardia results, as above, in the dominant reflex inhibition of cardiac opening.

There are three contributory factors underlying the formation of a stable foam in the pathogenesis of frothy bloat: (1) dietary, (2) microbial, and (3) animal factors. Frothy bloat is most common in animals consuming fresh, young legumes (clover, alfalfa) or being fed in corn feedlots. The foaming agent in the legumes is related to the leaf more than to the stem, to fresh more than to wilted material, to young rather than old material, and to high chloroplast content. The actual chemical responsible for the foaming is debatable. Frothy leguminous bloat rarely develops until the animal has been grazing legumes for 3 to 7 days, during which time there is a change in the microbial population, including the development of a large protozoal complement. In feedlot bloat certain protozoa develop a capsule, and this causes a microbial slime that has foaming properties. However, defaunation (selective destruction of protozoa) may reduce but does not totally prevent frothy bloat. Animal factors exist because, in a group of animals given the same feed, certain individuals show a higher risk than others in the development of frothy bloat. Why sheep and low-risk cattle are less prone to bloat than high-risk cattle is not known. Among the possible reasons advanced are differences in selection of the plant material ingested, the extent of chewing and salivation, and the animal's influence on the intraruminal environment and hence on the microbial population that becomes established. The animal factors are inheritable, as indicated by the fact that identical twins show similar high- or low-risk tendencies.

Summary

Most of the intentional and unintentional changes in fermentation are brought about primarily by changes in the microbial population and in the ensuing direction and rate of fermentation. Physiological changes, such as the time spent chewing and ruminating, salivary flow, and ruminoreticular motility, are secondary. Intentional changes, usually in the interest of greater productivity, include (1) increase in the proportion of concentrate feed (in order to increase the amount of VFAs and particularly the proportion of the only glucogenic VFA, propionate), (2) feeding of urea supplements along with concentrates (to promote microbial protein synthesis), (3) administration of selective antibiotics, such as monensin (to reduce methane energy losses and to promote increased propionate production), (4) use of probiotics, such as yeast cultures (to reduce the negative associative effect of concentrates on cellulolysis), and (5) feeding of nutrients in a form that will largely protect them from fermentation without affecting enzymic degradation lower down the gastrointestinal tract.

Unintentional changes in fermentation and ruminoreticular activity occur (1) when the concentrate feed level is too high (leading to ruminal acidosis, rumenitis, multiple liver absesses, and sometimes death), (2) when high tryptophan levels in grass lead to bovine pulmonary emphysema (fog fever), (3) when the available glucogenic substrates are deficient (ketosis) or are excessive (low-milk-fat syndrome), and (4) when eructation mechanisms are defective because of either esophageal dysfunction (esophageal obstruction, spasm) or failure to clear the cardia of ruminal fluid (ruminal hypomotility and stasis) or foam (frothy bloat).

GASTRIC DIGESTION IN THE YOUNG RUMINANT

In the young ruminant, the development of gastric digestion may be considered as having four phases: (1) the newborn phase (0 to 24 hours), (2) the preruminant phase (1 day to 3 weeks), (3) the transitional phase (3 to 8 weeks) and (4) the preweaning and postweaning phase (8 weeks to adulthood).

The newborn phase (0 to 24 hours)

At birth the forestomach is small and nonfunctional. It represents only 39 percent of the total stomach on a wet-weight basis, it contains no microbes, and the ruminoreticular papillae and omasal leaves are very rudimentary. The diet consists solely of colostrum (first milk), which is particularly rich in immune globulins. The abomasum secretes no acid or pepsinogen during the first day, so gastric digestion does not occur. This allows the immune globulins (IgM antibodies, γ-globulins) of the colostrum to pass through the stomach without being digested. An antitrypsin factor in the colostrum also prevents their degradation in the intestine. Subsequently, the colostral antibodies are absorbed intact through the intestinal mucosa by a phagocytic mechanism. In this way a newborn ruminant acquires a passive immunity to those diseases against which its dam (or the donor of the colostrum) has a resistance. Normally the serum γ-globulin concentration is 50 percent of maximum about 5 hours after birth. The facility to transport the immune globulins without digestion and to absorb them intact is limited to the first 24 to 48 hours after birth and is terminated if milk rather than colostrum is given.

Colostrum is also a rich source of vitamins A, D, and E and of calcium and magnesium. Lactose is readily digested in the intestine to provide potential energy substrates, glucose and galactose. Colostrum contains the usual mammary gland microbes (mainly lactobacilli), and these increasingly gain access to the intestine with each sucking period. Fecal contamination of the environment provides a source of *Escherichia coli,* streptococci, and *Clostridium welchii,* which are detectable in the intestine within 8 to 16 hours of birth. Their access is also facilitated by the lack of abomasal acid. The early microbes are mainly anaerobic.

Failure to acquire colostral antibodies renders the newborn animal susceptible immediately to acute infections ("joint-ill" and "navel-ill") and later to diarrhea (scours). Failure to acquire energy substrate from lactose before the limited liver glycogen reserves are exhausted is a common cause of death due to hypothermia, particularly in lambs born in a cold environment, when brown adipose tissue metabolism has a high demand for glucose.

The preruminant phase (1 day to 3 weeks)

During the preruminant period the principal food is milk. During the latter half of this period the young ruminant may taste solid foods, but these make little contribution to its nutrient intake. The act of sucking promotes salivary secretion and sucking from a teat, when compared with drinking from a bucket, leads to a great flow of saliva. The saliva contains an esterase (pregastric esterase), which starts the hydrolysis of the milk lipids.

As the milk passes through the pharynx, it stimulates chemoreceptors with afferent pathways in the glossopharyngeal nerve (ninth cranial nerve). These receptors can be stimulated experimentally with solutions containing Na^+ ions in calves or Cu^{2+} ions in lambs. The sensory input is integrated in the medulla oblongata, and the efferent vagal nerve output leads to closure of the reticular groove and to relaxation of the reticuloomasal orifice and omasal canal. Contraction of the spiral lips of the reticular groove causes their shortening and apposition to produce a temporary tube connecting the cardiac and reticuloomasal orifices. Thus the milk, which has evoked the reflex closure of the reticular groove, bypasses the ruminoreticulum, flows quickly through the relaxed rudimentary omasum, and ends up in the abomasum. The integrative mechanism in the medulla is subject to modulation by inputs from other parts of the brain, such as the appetite centers and memory for conditioned reflexes. Normally, the unconditioned reflex is facilitated by the behavioral mechanisms responsible for the hunger drive but not by those for the thirst drive. When an adequately hydrated young ruminant drinks milk in response to a hunger drive, this is accompanied by head butting (of the udder), vigorous tail wagging, and reflex closure of the reticular groove. When a dehydrated animal drinks milk in response to a thirst drive, there is no head butting, no tail wagging, and no reflex closure of the groove. The hunger drive appears to be the main determinant of reflex groove closure, and closure is not consistently affected by other factors such as head position and whether feeding involves sucking from a teat or drinking from a bucket.

The act of sucking and the presence of milk in the abomasum evoke abomasal secretions. Thus, like salivation, the secretion is proportional to the number of sucks; therefore teat feeding is more effective than bucket feeding. The abomasal secretions consist of the proteolytic enzyme, rennin or chymosin (not pepsinogen at this stage), and hydrochloric acid. Rennin acting on milk at pH 6.5 for 3 to 4 minutes can produce a hard clot or curd consisting of the butterfat and the curd proteins (caseinogens) precipitated as calcium caseinate. The remaining fraction of the milk—whey—consists of the whey proteins (albumins and globulins) and the milk sugar (lactose). The whey enters the duodenum in bursts after each suck and spends little time in the abomasum. If the milk entering the abomasum encounters acidic conditions of pH 5 or less, it forms a soft curd because of the acid, not the rennin. The hard curds undergo very slow degradation over the next 12 to 18 hours. The butterfat is hydrolyzed to fatty acids and glycerol by (1) a lipase of mammary gland origin present in the milk and (2) the pregastric esterase of the saliva. The precipitated caseinate undergoes further proteolysis by the rennin at an optimum pH of 3.5. As the clot is digested by the enzymes, the end products flow steadily into the duodenum. New clots form aggregates with the remains of earlier clots.

In the intestine the curd and whey proteins undergo complete proteolysis. The lactose is hydrolyzed by lactase to glucose and galactose. The intestine does not have significant maltase activity, so starch products cannot be digested. Intermediary metabolism is based on glucose, and blood glucose levels are insulin-sensitive.

At this stage, physiological aberrations predispose the animal to two commercially important diseases—scour and "milk drinking in veal calves." If calves are bucket-fed too infrequently, the rapid ingestion of a large volume of milk increases the risk of forming a defective curd in the abomasum. This results in overloading of the intestine with protein and leads to bacterial overproliferation, culminating in diarrhea (scours). Similarly, feeding of poorly formulated milk substitutes may cause an inadequate curd, leading to excessively fast abomasal emptying, protein overload, etc. In addition, starch products, because they cannot be digested unless there has been a suitable adaption period for development of maltase also give rise to bacterial overproliferation with similar consequences.

In some veal calves, there may be inadequate closure of the reticular groove, so that clotted milk mixed with hair and straw is found in the ruminoreticulum. The animals have no appetite, are bloated, try to vomit and, because of lipase action in the clot, produce large quantities of fatty acids that are not absorbed but appear in the feces and give them the appearance of kaolin (steatorrhea).

The transitional phase (3 to 8 weeks)

During the transitional period, peak volumes of milk are ingested, and these are handled as described above. Simultaneously the animal starts to ingest progressively larger amounts of roughage, which is responsible for the initiation of salivary gland and ruminoreticular developments.

The salivary glands, particularly the parotid glands, increase their size and volume of secretion, which becomes alkaline in composition. The ruminoreticulum accelerates its acquisition of microbes. The early microbes, at 1 week after birth, are largely milk contaminants (lactobacilli), which produce mainly lactic acid and give very low ruminoreticular pH values. The transitional ruminant acquires its complement of more normal microbes from the ingestion of food and water contaminated with ruminal microbes voided in the eructate, cud, and feces by older ruminants sharing the same environment. Microbial fermentation of roughage produces VFAs, which are essential for the development of the ruminoreticular papillae and of the omasal leaves. Gases are produced and necessitate operation of the eructation mechanism. The bulk factor of the roughage is responsible for the size and muscular development of the ruminoreticulum, for the onset of cyclic motility, and for effective rumination. Abortive attempts at rumination occur in animals at about 10 days of age, but little is actually regurgitated or chewed.

This period is critical for establishing the potential degree of development of the ruminoreticulum. By the end of the period the ruminoreticulum will have the basic features and proportions of its adult form (Fig. 21.14). Correspondingly, intermediary metabolism will be moving away from being glucose-based toward being VFA-based, with blood glucose levels becoming less insulin-sensitive.

The preweaning and postweaning phases (8 weeks to adulthood)

The start of the preweaning phase concides approximately with the start of the natural decline in lactation, so that progressively less milk is available up to the point of weaning. Unless the animal continues to receive milk regularly, reflex closure of the reticular groove becomes erratic and is usually absent in older animals. The empty stomach mass assumes a progressively greater proportion of the total empty gastrointestinal mass as the animal approaches adulthood. The rates and forms of forestomach motility cycles attain the characteristics of adult animals. Pepsinogen replaces rennin in the abomasal secretions.

Summary

For the newborn ruminant (0–24h), colostrum provides immunoglobulins for protection against disease, lactose as a ready source of energy, vitamins, and bivalent cations. The lack of proteolytic activity and hydrochloric acid secretion avoids the degradation of the immunoglobulins, and a

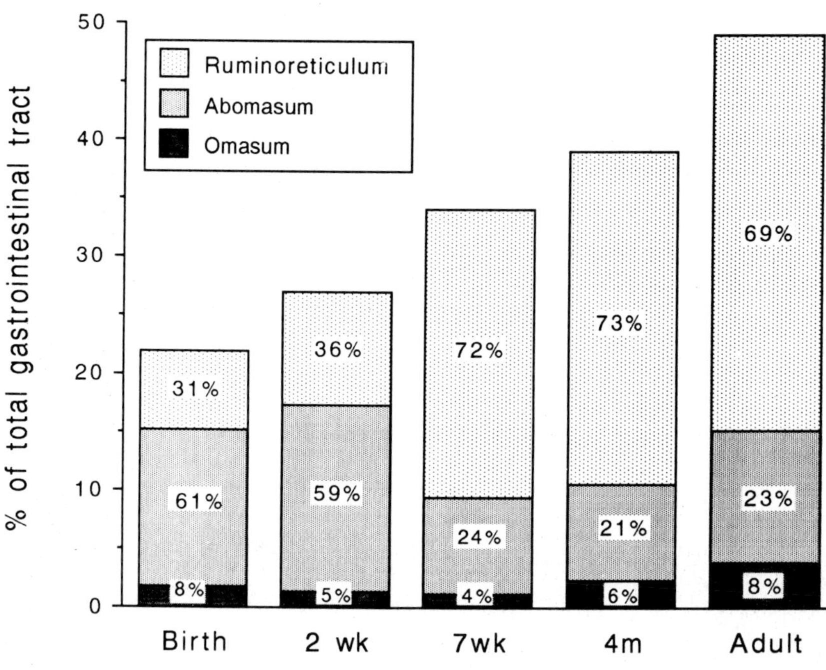

Figure 21.14. The ruminant stomach represents a proportion of the total gastrointestinal tract, measured as weight tissue mass, which increases steadily from 22 percent at birth to 49 percent in adult sheep. Within the stomach itself, the biggest change is during the transitional period (2–7 weeks of age in this study) during which the forestomach more than doubles its relative size and the abomasum decreases by more than one-half. (Based on data from Wardrop and Coombe 1960, *J. Agric. Sci.* 54:140–43.)

short-lived phagocytic mechanism in the intestine allows them to be absorbed intact. In the preruminant phase (1d–3wk), reflex closure of the reticular groove and adequate curd formation in the abomasum are essential. The whey proteins and lactose pass rapidly to the intestine. The curd fat and protein are degraded gradually, and the products pass slowly into the intestine to complete their digestion and absorption. Milk replacers that do not form a satisfactory curd or contain starch products are likely to exceed the intestine's capacity for digestion, allow bacterial overproliferation, and lead to diarrhea. In the transitional phase (3–8wk), ingestion of milk with reticular groove bypass of the ruminoreticulum and curd formation in the abomasum occur in parallel with accelerated developments in the forestomach. These include the acquisition of microbes through contact with older ruminants, the development of papillae and omasal leaves through epithelial metabolism of VFAs, and development of forestomach muscles largely through the bulk effect of roughage. Ruminoreticular motility, eructation, rumination, and copious alkaline salivation become established. Intermediary metabolism switches from being glucose-based and insulin-sensitive to being VFA-based and insulin-insensitive. The remainder of the preweaning period sees a reduced reliance on milk as the source of nutrients and a greater dependence on roughage. The various gastric compartments are nearing adult proportions, and the ruminant stomach grows disproportionately greater than the intestine as the animal approaches its adult size.

REFERENCES

Church, D.C., ed. 1988. *The Ruminant Animal: Digestive Physiology and Nutrition.* 2d ed. Prentice-Hall, Englewood Cliffs, N.J.

Czerkawski, J.W. 1986. *Introduction to Rumen Studies.* Pergammon Press, Oxford.

Dougherty, R.W., ed. 1965. *Physiology of Digestion in the Ruminant.* Butterworth, Washington, D.C.

Kay, R.N.B. 1963. Reviews of the progress of dairy science. Part 1A. The physiology of the rumen. *J. Dairy Res.* 30:261–88.

Leek, B.F. 1983. Clinical diseases of the rumen: a physiologist's view. *Vet. Rec.* 113:10–14.

McDonald, I.W., and Warner, A.C.I., eds. 1975. *Digestion and Metabolism in the Ruminant.* Univ. of New Eng. Publ. Unit., Armidale, Australia.

Milligan, L.P., Grovum, W.L., and Dobson, A., eds. 1986. *Control of Digestion and Metabolism in Ruminants.* Prentice-Hall, Englewood Cliffs, N.J.

Ooms, L.A., Degryse, A.D., and van Miert, A.S.J.P.A.M., eds. 1987. *Physiological and Pharmacological Aspects of the Reticulo-rumen.* Martinus Nijhoff Publishers, Dordrecht.

Phillipson, A.T., ed. 1970. *Physiology of Digestion and Metabolism in the Ruminant.* Oriel, Newcastle-upon-Tyne.

Ruckebusch, Y., and Thivend, P., eds. 1980. *Digestive Physiology and Metabolism in Ruminants.* AVI Publishing Co., Westport, Conn.

CHAPTER 22

Microbiology of the Rumen and Small and Large Intestines | by Milton J. Allison

Gastrointestinal tracts of higher animals are colonized by a great diversity of microorganisms. The use of fibrous vegetation by herbivores depends on the metabolic activities of populations of anaerobic microbes that colonize fermentation sites, such as the rumen and the large intestine. These are enlarged compartments, where particle-transit time is retarded enough to allow the relatively slow microbial digestion of fiber to occur. Highly concentrated populations of bacteria occupy these regions, and some of these sites are also colonized by protozoa and anaerobic fungi. The large intestines of humans and other omnivores are also populated by concentrated populations of microbes. The gastrointestinal tract can be considered the most intimate environment that animals are exposed to and thus an environment that has a profound impact on the physiology and health of the host animal. Since intestinal microbes play a major role in regulation of the intestinal environment, these organisms and their metabolic activities must be considered in any comprehensive study of digestive physiology. This chapter will be concerned primarily with these complex anaerobic microbial populations, and emphasis will be on the best-studied system—the rumen.

FORESTOMACH FERMENTATIONS

When microbial fermentation occurs in the simple stomach, it is generally limited to an ethanolic or lactic acid type of fermentation that has a relatively minor impact on the digesta or the nutrition of the animal. Some animals, however, use microbial populations to ferment and significantly modify the digesta before it reaches the acidic stomach. These fermentations occur at a nearly neutral pH and depend upon development of a sac or chamber that provides for physical separation of the digesta from the acid-secreting region. Ruminants are the most diverse (about 155 species) and best known of the herbivores with extensive forestomach fermentation systems. A ruminantlike fermentation also occurs in animals with complex three-chambered stomachs—the Tragulidae (chevrotains) and Camelidae (camel, llama, alpaca, guanaco, and vicuna)—and in hippopotamuses, tree sloths (Cholopus and Bradypus), leaf-eating monkeys of the subfamily Colobinae, the macropod marsupials, and one neotropical leaf-eating bird, the hoatzin (*Opisthocomus hoazin*).

The reticulorumen is a fermentation chamber in which complex and dense populations of bacteria and protozoa convert plant materials to volatile fatty acids (VFAs), methane, carbon dioxide, ammonia, and microbial cells. Some of the advantages of the ruminant model of fermentation are as follows:

1. The site of the fermentation (before the acidic abomasum) allows for digestion and then absorption of fermentation products that are of value to the host (e.g., microbial cells, VFAs, and B vitamins).

2. Both quality and quantity of dietary protein can be upgraded since poor quality protein and other dietary nitrogenous compounds are used by the microbes for synthesis of good-quality microbial protein.

3. Selective retention of coarse particles extends fermentation time and allows for further mechanical breakdown during rumination (cud chewing).

4. The considerable amounts of fermentation gas (mostly carbon dioxide and methane) can be readily released from the system by eructation.

5. Microbial attack on feedstuffs is optimized by the large input of saliva to provide a highly buffered medium (usual pH is between 6 and 7) with a consistency that permits effective mixing by ruminal contractions.

6. Toxic substances in the diet may be attacked by the microbes before they are presented for absorption in the small intestine.

NUMBERS AND KINDS OF RUMINAL MICROBES

Most of the available information about ruminal microbes has been obtained from studies of cattle and sheep. Ruminal populations of both cattle and sheep are strongly regulated by diet, and similar (but not necessarily identical) distributions of predominant microbial species are found in the rumens of cattle and sheep that are fed similar diets. For example, all of 24 species of protozoa from a steer fed an alfalfa ration were able to colonize in protozoa-free sheep that were fed the same alfalfa diet, while fewer than one-half of these species colonized sheep fed a concentrate diet.

Knowledge about microbial populations in wild ruminants is largely limited to that obtained by microscopic observations, which permit distinctions at a species level for protozoa but which are less definitive for bacteria. A few cultural studies indicate that the predominant bacteria in rumen contents from deer, reindeer, elk, and moose are species that are also found in cattle and sheep. Marked differences have been observed between ciliate protozoal populations in wild ruminants. Geographic limits to the distribution of protozoal species in domestic ruminants probably reflect importation origins and the relative isolation of areas, such as New Zealand and Brazil, where these differences were noted.

Some of the most important bacterial species in cattle and sheep and their fermentative properties are listed in Table 22.1. All of these bacteria are anaerobes, and most are carbohydrate fermenters. Included are gram-negative and gram-positive cells; sporeformers and non-sporeformers; and motile and nonmotile cells, which may be shaped as rods, cocci, or spirochetes. Most are species that were discovered in ruminal contents; however, a number of these species have since been found in samples from other environments. Obligately anaerobic mycoplasmas (cells enclosed by membranes rather than by rigid walls) are also present in ruminal contents. Although these are minor components of the population, they are of interest because they are unique organisms that have not been detected in environments other than the rumen. They ferment starch and other carbohydrates, but their contribution to the overall fermentation is probably minor.

A comparison of numbers and relative volumes of bacteria and protozoa (Table 22.2) indicates that while protozoa are far less numerous than bacteria, they are so much larger than the bacteria that they may occupy a volume nearly equal to that occupied by the bacteria. The most important ruminal protozoa are anaerobic ciliates that are differentiated on the basis of morphology. Most belong to two groups: the holotrichous protozoa, with the entire body surface covered by cilia, and the entodiniomorphid protozoa, with cilia congregated in tufts or syncilia that do not cover much of the body surface. Numbers and kinds of protozoa are markedly affected by diet, and variability among protozoal populations with time and among animals

Table 22.1. Fermentative properties of ruminal bacteria

Species	Function*	Products†
Fibrobacter (Bacteroides) succinogenes	C,A	F,A,S
Ruminococcus albus	C,X	F,A,E,H,C
Ruminococcus flavefaciens	C,X	F,A,S,H
Butyrivibrio fibrisolvens	C,X,PR	F,A,L,B,E,H,C
Clostridium lochheadii	C,PR	F,A,B,E,H,C
Streptococcus bovis	A,S,SS,PR	L,A,F
Ruminobacter (Bacteroides) amylophilus	A,P,PR	F,A,S
Prevotella (Bacteroides) ruminocola	A,X,P,PR	F,A,P,S
Succinimonas amylolytica	A,D	A,S
Selenomonas ruminantium	A,SS,GU, LU,PR	A,L,P,H,C
Lachnospira multiparus	P,PR,A	F,A,E,L,H,C
Succinivibrio dextrinosolvens	P,D	F,A,L,S
Methanobrevibacter ruminantium	M,HU	M
Methanosarcina barkeri	M,HU	MC
Treponema bryantii	P,SS	F,A,L,S,E
Megasphaera elsdenii	SS,LU	A,P,B,V,CP,H,C
Lactobacillus sp.	SS	L
Anaerovibrio lipolytica	L,GU	A,P,S
Eubacterium ruminantium	SS	F,A,B,C
Oxalobacter formigenes	O	F,C
Wolinella succinogenes	HU	S,C

*C, cellulolytic; X, xylanolytic; A, amylolytic; D, dextrinolytic; P, pectinolytic; PR, proteolytic; L, lipolytic; M, methanogenic; GU, glycerol-utilizing; LU, lactate-utilizing; SS, major soluble sugar fermenter, HU, hydrogen utilizer; O, oxalate-degrading.

†F, formate; A, acetate; E, ethanol; P, propionate; L, lactate; B, butyrate; S, succinate; V, valerate; CP, caproate; H, hydrogen; C, carbon dioxide; M, methane.

Modified from Hespell 1981, in Underkolfer and Wulf, eds., *Developments in Industrial Microbiology,* Society for Industrial Microbiology, Arlington, Va.

Table 22.2. Approximate average volumes and numbers of microbial groups in the rumen of sheep fed alfalfa and wheaten chaff

Organism	Average individual cell volume (μm^3)	Number per milliliter	Percentage of total microbial volume*
Ciliate protozoa			
Isotricha, Epidinium, Diplodinium sp.	1,000,000	1.1×10^4	33.55
Dasytricha, Diplodinium sp.	100,000	2.9×10^4	8.78
Entodinium sp.	10,000	2.9×10^5	8.79
Polyflagellated fungal zoospores	500	9.4×10^3	0.01
Oscillospiras and fungal zoospores	250	3.8×10^5	0.26
Selenomonads	30	1.0×10^8	0.09
Small bacteria	1	1.6×10^{10}	48.52

*Total microbial volume was about 0.036 ml per milliliter of rumen fluid.
Modified from data of Warner 1962, *J. Gen. Microbiol.* 28:129–46.

tends to be greater than for bacterial populations. In general, the diversity of ciliate species is lower in deer or other browsing ruminants than in grazing ruminants that feed less selectively on more fibrous foods. Ciliates in the forestomach of the hippopotamus are different from those found in ruminants.

It has been demonstrated that organisms once thought to be flagellate protozoa are actually fungal zoospores. The zoospores attach to plant fragments and form rhizoids that penetrate the plant tissue. Rhizoids are the precursors of sporangia which, when mature, release new zoospores. Increased numbers of free zoospores can be detected 15 minutes to 1 hour after feeding. The zoospores are motile, and their chemotactic response to soluble carbohydrate probably facilitates rapid attachment to plant particles. The significance of the fungi is not yet known, but there is general agreement they are less important than the bacteria. In animals on low-fiber diets the fungal biomass appears to be very low, but fungi may account for as much as 8 percent of the total biomass in the rumen in animals on high-fiber diets. Anaerobic fungi have been found in large intestine fermenters (horses and elephants), in both domestic and wild ruminants, and in other forestomach fermenters (kangaroo). They are the only known fungi that are strictly anaerobic.

ECOLOGY

The rumen is essentially an open ecosystem, and there are probably few, if any, microbial species that have not had an opportunity to grow there. This is probably true for the small and large intestine as well, even though the acid stomach presents an appreciable but frequently hurdled barrier. In the course of time, the microbes best able to survive and compete have been selected and transmitted to succeeding generations. Gastrointestinal habitats for microbes are dynamic, since conditions are continually modified by the diet and by the metabolic activities of both the host and the microbes themselves. Many characteristics collectively determine the capacity of organisms to survive, compete, grow, and thus colonize at specific sites in the tract. The definition of these microbial properties as well as the animal factors that regulate gastrointestinal populations continues to be a major challenge for scientists studying gastrointestinal function and disease.

Newborn animals provide intestinal habitats that are open for colonization. Grooming behavior among cud chewers no doubt facilitates microbial transfer, and strictly anaerobic bacteria (including cellulose digesters) have been found in animals less than 1 week old. Differences in diet (and thus in habitats), however, dictate that microbial populations in very young ruminants differ markedly from those in adults. Transmission of protozoa between ruminants depends on close or direct contact, and thus early isolation of calves and lambs from adults prevents colonization of the young by protozoa. Normal rumen bacteria, however, may be isolated from aerosols in stables, and they are more readily transmitted between animals than are the protozoa.

Two axioms of the ecology of open natural ecosystems are that (1) one cannot change bacterial numbers or composition by inoculating with exotic species and (2) the numbers and composition of microbial populations can be changed by changing the environment. It is fortunate that established gastrointestinal populations create conditions that tend to exclude all but the most competent of invaders. Animals protected from exposure to microbes (germ-free or gnotobiotic animals reared in isolators) are more susceptible to some disease agents than are conventional animals with a normal intestinal flora. For example, about ten *Salmonella* cells can kill a germ-free mouse, but it would take 1 million such cells to kill a conventional mouse. A main reason for this difference appears to be the suppression of growth of the pathogen by the normal flora, but higher phagocytic activity and immunoglobulin levels in normal animals than in germ-free animals may also be involved. The increased susceptibility to agents that produce intestinal disease when the normal gastrointestinal flora has been changed by per os antibiotic treatment is further evidence of the protective role of the normal flora. Attempts to supplement the natural colonization of the intestine have led to proposals that live microbial preparations be used as feed supplements. These are intended to benefit the host animal by improving its intestinal microbial balance. A diversity of such "probiotics" have been marketed, and most contain lactobacilli or streptococci. There does not appear to be a consensus on which microbes are effective, and the efficacy of probiotics as growth promoters in farm animals has generally not been well documented in field trials.

Considering the openness of the system and the complexity of factors regulating colonization, the discovery of exotic natural microbes that have particularly desirable physiological capabilities including the ability to colonize the rumen, seems improbable. The experience with Leucaena (discussed later) indicates, however, that the concept of geographic limits to the distribution of functional ruminal microbes needs further consideration. It would also be premature to predict either success or failure of experiments designed to use genetic engineering technology to introduce added desirable capabilities into existing ruminal species.

The practice of transferring a bolus (the cud of a ruminating animal) or fresh rumen contents from a healthy animal has long been recommended for reestablishment of normal ruminal microbial populations after acute digestive disturbance (e.g., lactic acidosis). When such conditions have led to loss of appetite, massive transfers of ruminal contents may provide both a fermentable feed and a more suitable microbial environment. The fermentation that occurs then contributes to restoration of both ruminal motility and the appetite that is needed for resumption of normal fermentation. Commercial preparations that contain rumen microbes have been widely sold, but their efficacy has not been well documented. Such preparations are probably of less value than inoculations with fresh rumen contents, since ruminal population growth is more likely to be limited by lack of a suitable environment in the rumen than by lack of a suitable inoculum.

Anaerobiosis (life in the absence of oxygen) is a fundamental property that limits both the kinds of microbe able to colonize fermentative gastrointestinal ecosystems and the kinds of reaction that can occur. While small quantities of free oxygen can sometimes be detected in the rumen, especially after feeding, oxygen is metabolically removed by both bacteria and by protozoa so that dissolved oxygen is generally too low to be detected (10^{-6} or less). Carbohydrates or products from carbohydrate metabolism supply energy for growth of most ruminal microbes. Some bacteria, however, are specialists that obtain energy through fermentation of amino acids and other compounds that are supplied in the diet or that are produced by their microbial associates. Short-chain VFAs are the major end products of the fermentation since, in the absence of oxygen, carbon skeletons cannot be completely oxidized to CO_2. Similarly, since oxygen-linked electron transport systems do not function, the yield of energy in the form of adenosine triphosphate (ATP) per mole of substrate catabolized is generally low. Ruminal microbes are able to tolerate large amounts of VFAs that would be inhibitory to many bacteria from non-intestinal habitats. Although a large part of the carbon in feeds is converted to organic acids, the ruminal environment usually is only slightly acidic (pH 5.5 to 7.0). The large amount of saliva (more than 100 L per day in an adult bovine) that flows to the rumen provides phosphate and bicarbonate ions that, with the VFAs, buffer against pH change.

Maintaining the colonization of the rumen depends on the ability of microbes to grow rapidly enough to avoid being washed out by the flow of material through the system. That is, a steady state requires an average microbial doubling time that is not longer than the material turnover time (quantity entering per unit time divided by quantity present in the system). Estimates of turnover time for the fluid fraction are as high as twice a day, while particle turnover is generally slower, with particle size serving as a main regulating factor. Most rumen bacteria have the genetic capacity to grow at rates that are much greater than would be needed to maintain them while ciliate protozoa generally grow more slowly than the bacteria. It is difficult to measure actual growth rates in vivo, but since the availability of substrate (nutrients) is an important limit to growth, average growth rates vary greatly with time after feeding. Since the passage rate of the solids fraction is less than that of the fluid fraction, the ability to attach to plant particles has survival value for microbes that might not always have generation times that are shorter than the fluid turnover time. Selective retention on particles seems to be particularly important for the protozoa.

As indicated in Table 22.1, most of the predominant ruminal bacteria use any of a number of substrates as energy sources (generalists), but some species use only one or a few substrates (specialists). Different substrate preferences and sequential substrate utilization patterns are important in the competitive ruminal environment and help to explain why a species that is a generalist with great versatility in the substrates that it can attack, does not completely displace its competitors.

A predator-prey relationship exists between certain protozoal species and between many protozoa and bacteria. Antagonisms between protozoa have also been shown in a certain (type A) population of ciliates that tends to be dominant in domestic ruminants. When animals with type B populations of ciliates were inoculated with rumen fluid from a type A animal, type B populations were replaced by type A. Reasons for such population changes are still poorly understood.

Although competition for nutrients is a usual state in the system, cross-feeding between species is also well documented. Examples of the latter include the production of monosaccharides, oligosaccharides, amino acids, ammonia, branched-chain fatty acids, heme, and B vitamins by certain species. These compounds are used by other species, some of which have absolute nutritional requirements for the compounds. A mutualistic relationship may well exist between certain protozoa and the bacteria (methanogens and others) that have been observed attached to and apparently growing on the surface of the protozoa (Fig. 22.1). While some of the interactions between ruminal microbes have been described, it seems clear that further study will reveal many other examples of interesting ecological relationships between ruminal species.

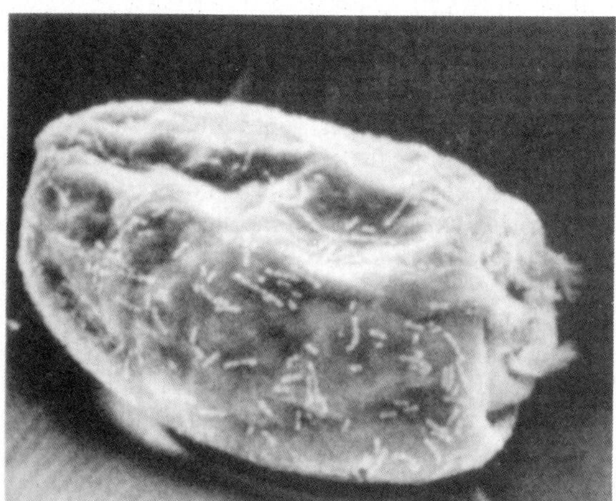

Figure 22.1. Scanning electron micrograph of *Diplodinium anisacanthum* with attached bacteria. ×1400. (Ogimoto and Imai 1981, *Atlas of Rumen Microbiology,* Japan Scientific Societies Press, Tokyo.)

CULTIVATION OF GASTROINTESTINAL ANAEROBES

Most of the bacteria in the rumen and large intestine are strict anaerobes, and initial isolation and culture of most of them have depended heavily on the use of culture methods that rigorously exclude oxygen and are designed to simulate conditions in the natural habitat. The Hungate roll tube method, as modified by various workers, is still the basic procedure in most laboratories studying pure cultures of rumen bacteria. Anaerobic glove box techniques may also be employed, but anaerobic jar methods that are adequate for culture of clostridia are generally not suitable for many of the more fastidiously anaerobic gastrointestinal bacteria. Culture of the methane producers depends on especially rigorous methods to exclude oxygen and the inclusion of hydrogen gas or formate as oxidizable substrate. Rumen fluid is commonly used to supply vitamins and other nutrients in media designed for nonselective enumeration and isolation of the predominant rumen flora. In addition to rumen fluid, media usually contain mineral salts, cysteine, and/or sodium sulfide as reducing agents, resazurin as an oxidation-reduction indicator, and a mixture of carbohydrates (glucose, cellobiose, starch, and xylan) to provide energy needed for growth. The gas phase is usually carbon dioxide. Media that will allow for selective culture of a given genus or species of predominant rumen bacteria are generally not available.

Batch cultures of mixed rumen microbes have been used extensively to estimate the digestibility of feed constituents or to study other metabolic activities. A wide variety of continuous culture systems have been developed to study metabolism of the mixed population under controlled conditions. Useful information may be obtained with such cultures, even though complete duplications of in vivo conditions and reaction rates are not obtained.

FUNCTIONS OF RUMINAL BACTERIA

The overlap of functions among organisms (e.g., the first five species are cellulose digesters) and the metabolic versatility of some species as well as the specialization of others, with regard to substrates that are attacked are illustrated in Table 22.1. Some of the end products of singly grown pure cultures (e.g., formate, succinate, ethanol, hydrogen, and lactate) are further metabolized by other species and are thus intermediates rather than end products of the mixed population.

The Embden Meyerhof glycolytic pathway is the major pathway for hexose catabolism by rumen microbes. Most ruminal pentose appears to be metabolized by the pentose phosphate cycle coupled to glycolysis, with some metabolized by the phosphoketolase pathway. Pyruvate, a key intermediate, is metabolized by a variety of mechanisms to yield acetate, butyrate, hydrogen, carbon dioxide, and propionate (Fig. 22.2). Propionate is formed by two distinct pathways. Most of the propionate is produced by the pathway involving succinate (a product of many species). Succinate does not accumulate significantly in the mixed population but is decarboxylated to yield propionate by such organisms as *Selenomonas ruminantium*. The direct reduction pathway via acrylyl coenzyme A is found in *Megasphaera elsdenii*, and the relative amount of propionate formed by this pathway increases when high-concentrate diets are fed.

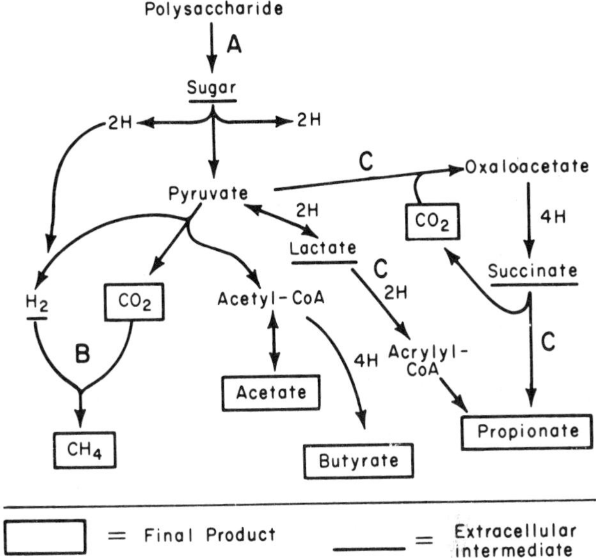

Figure 22.2. Complex foodweb of diverse bacterial species involved in carbohydrate fermentation. H, an electron plus a proton or electrons from reduced-pyridine nucleotides; A, carbohydrate-fermenting species; B, methanogenic species; C, lactate-fermenting species which often also ferment carbohydrates.

Concentrations of hydrogen in the rumen are low because of its consumption by the methanogens. Low H_2 concentrations prevent feedback inhibition of further H_2 production so that more of the electrons generated in glycolysis can be excreted by individual cells as H_2. When methanogenesis is inhibited, however, the use of H_2 as a hydrogen sink is less favored and less carbon can flow to acetate and CO_2 because reduced pyridine nucleotides in cells must be reoxidized and propionate and succinate serve as hydrogen sinks. These interspecies hydrogen transfer reactions explain how propionate production is increased when methanogensis is inhibited.

Proteins are hydrolyzed by bacteria, protozoa, and anaerobic fungi. Of these, the bacteria are most important. A main function of the protozoa appears to be metabolism of bacterial protein rather than hydrolysis of exogenous soluble protein. The types of protease found in rumen contents are many and varied, but most of these enzymes are closely associated with bacterial cells. There is considerable interest in inhibition of microbial proteases so that more dietary protein will "bypass" the rumen and be available for the host animal.

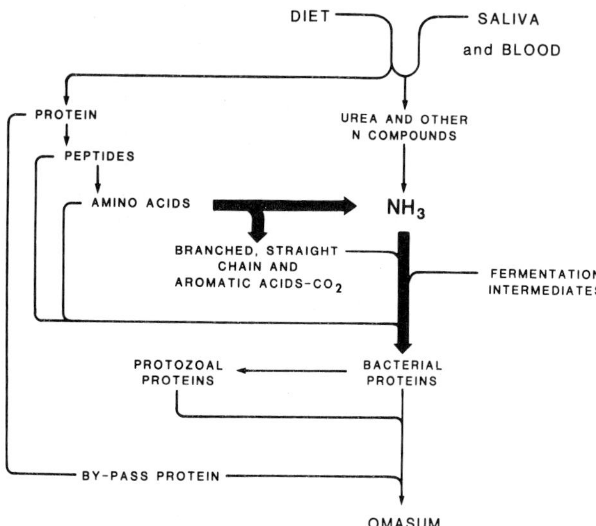

Figure 22.3. Transformations of nitrogenous substances in the rumen. Ammonia is produced during microbial metabolism of diverse substrates and is a major source of the nitrogen used for biosynthesis of microbial cells.

Urea enters the rumen in feeds, in saliva, and by direct translocation from the blood across the rumen wall. Urease is produced in small amounts by a number of species of obligate anaerobes and by facultatively anaerobic bacteria that are less numerous but produce higher amounts of urease. It is not yet clear which of these are most important. Experiments showing that ruminant growth and milk production are possible with urea as the sole source of dietary nitrogen agree with the concept that ammonia has a central role in ruminal nitrogen metabolism (Fig. 22.3). Many ruminal bacteria are able to grow with ammonia as the main source of nitrogen, and thus must have enzymes that enable them to synthesize a complete mixture of amino acids as well as other nitrogen compounds. Some ruminal bacteria, however, require amino acids, and others require branched-chain or other fatty acids that are produced by other microbes in the population. The protozoa are less metabolically independent; bacterial cells supply a major part of their nitrogen needs.

Glutamate dehydrogenase and glutamine synthetase are the bacterial enzymes that are most important for ammonia fixation. Of the two enzymes, glutamine synthetase has the higher affinity for ammonia and thus is probably more important when ammonia levels are low. Efficient use of ammonia depends on a balanced supply of the fermentable carbohydrate that is needed to furnish both the carbon skeletons for amino acid biosynthesis and the energy for this process. To help achieve this balance, animal nutritionists have developed model systems and computer programs for diet formulation that consider the nitrogen content and the energy available from fermentation of various feedstuffs as well as the protein requirements of the animal.

On most, if not all, rations a major portion of the total amino acids absorbed from the ruminant digestive tract is supplied as microbial cell protein. The extent of the contribution by microbes to the protein needs of the host has been determined from estimates of the amount of microbial protein entering the proximal duodenum. Various compounds, such as diaminopimelic acid or D-alanine, that are present in microbial cells but are not usually found in feeds have been used as markers to estimate the microbial contribution to such samples. The quantity of microbial protein available for digestion is particularly critical when protein demand is high (e.g., during rapid growth or in late pregnancy and early lactation). Considerable attention has thus been given to factors that influence the efficiency of microbial cell synthesis. Yields of cells (expressed as Y_{ATP} and equivalent to grams of cells per mole of adenosine triphosphate (ATP) available from the fermentation) have been estimated to range from about 10 to 21. These calculations involve assumptions concerning amounts of ATP produced per mole of end products (VFAs and CH_4) by substrate linked phosphorylations and by anaerobic electron transfer reactions.

FUNCTIONS OF RUMINAL PROTOZOA

Ruminal ciliate protozoa are metabolically versatile and capable of using all major plant constituents. The entodiniomorphid protozoa engulf particulate matter and have enzymes that attack cellulose, hemicellulose, etc., whereas the holotrichs generally depend on nonstructural polysaccharides (especially starches and soluble sugars). End products of fermentation by protozoa include various organic acids, CO_2, and hydrogen. A number of species of protozoa have been cultivated in vitro, but extended axenic culture (without bacteria) has not been accomplished. Although bacterial predation is an important feature of protozoal life in the rumen, and amino acids from ingested bacteria are used extensively for synthesis of protozoal proteins, at least some protozoa are able to synthesize amino acids de novo.

Elimination of protozoa from the rumen (defaunation) may be accomplished by treatment with chemicals (e.g., $CuSO_4$ or surface-active agents). Protozoa-free ruminants may also be maintained by keeping young animals isolated from faunated animals from birth. Delineation of the role of protozoa in the mixed population is complicated, however, by the fact that bacteria are present in significantly greater concentrations in defaunated animals. This may be due to bacteria filling vacated ecologic niches as well as to the absence of predators.

While there is conclusive evidence that protozoa are not essential for ruminant digestion, it is also clear that they do have a major influence on the overall microbial process. Protozoa account for as much as one-third of ruminal cellulolysis, and there is evidence that their presence enhances the cellulolytic activity of the bacteria. Furthermore, in defaunated animals, where there is less organic matter digestion, levels of ruminal ammonia are lower because degradation of dietary protein is reduced. This means that more dietary protein may be available for intestinal digestion in protozoa-free ruminants. This concept, plus a reduction in the amount of bacterial protein by protozoal predation, explains the considerable interest in the possibility of regulating ruminal protozoal populations. When starch or soluble sugars are present in excess, a number of species of protozoa rapidly assimilate these substrates and incorporate them into intracellular reserve polysaccharides. A favorable function is thus served because the protozoa compete with lactic acid-producing bacteria for these readily fermented substrates, and this competition is thought to reduce the probability of overgrowth of the lactic acid producers and the risk of lactic acidosis.

MANIPULATIONS OF RUMINAL MICROBES

As the basic understanding of functions of ruminal microbes improves, so does the potential for purposeful modification of these functions for more efficient animal production. Attempts have thus been made to discover ways to manipulate the microbial population to enhance fiber degradation and microbial protein synthesis, to minimize the degradation of feed protein and the production of methane. A comprehensive discussion of this rapidly changing area is not possible here, but a few examples will illustrate the practical value and potential of such manipulations.

Ruminal microbes may provide the animal with adequate protein for maintenance and during periods of slow growth or early pregnancy. At other times, when protein demand is high, animal productivity can sometimes be enhanced by increasing the amount of dietary protein that escapes degradation in the rumen. Considerable effort has thus been directed toward searches for chemicals that would inhibit the activity of microbial proteases or deaminases as well as toward studies of treatment of feedstuffs that would inhibit ruminal proteolysis. Feed treatments for this purpose include use of various drying procedures, heat, or treatment with chemicals. An example of this effort is evidence of increased efficiency of growth with formaldehyde-treated feeds. Formalized protein has also been used to coat and protect fats from microbial attack so as to enhance yields of milk and to increase amounts of unsaturated fatty acids in milk or animal fat.

Various chemicals have been tested for their capacity to inhibit methanogenesis in the hope that diversion of hydrogen to other end products could save some of the 10 percent of dietary energy that is lost as methane. Other compounds have been screened in tests for a capacity to increase the ratio of ruminally produced propionate to acetate. As discussed above, the *interspecies hydrogen transfer* concept explains the close link between enhanced propionate production and the inhibition of methanogenesis.

The best example of successful manipulation of the rumen through addition of microcomponents to the diet is the experience with monensin. Monensin is an ionophore that promotes transport of monovalent cations (particularly sodium) across lipid barriers (membranes), and gram-positive bacteria are more sensitive to it than are gram-negative organisms. The biochemical basis for increased feed efficiency with monensin is not completely understood, but it is clear that monensin inhibits microbial methane production, proteolysis, and amino acid degradation and that it causes an increase in the ruminal propionate/acetate ratio. Changes in animal tissue metabolism may also be involved with its activity. Success with monensin as an enhancer of feedlot productivity has led to a multitude of trials with other ionophores and related antibiotics.

BLOAT

When proprioreceptors in mucosa around the cardia are in contact with fluid or foam, an eructation-inhibition reflex is initiated. With eructation blocked, gas produced by rumen microbes cannot escape and the buildup of pressure ("acute tympany") can be sufficient to interfere with movement of the diaphragm and also cause circulatory impairment, both contributing to the cause of death. In *legume bloat,* soluble plant proteins and saponins are major contributing factors to the formation of a stable froth that is composed of a mixture of gas bubbles and small particles. Alfalfa, red clover, and white clover are the principal bloat-causing legumes. Rapid release of proteins from the degradation of the forage and rapid production of gas by the microbes are directly correlated with bloat-producing potential, and the inhibition of microbial activity by tannins may explain their antibloat activity. In *feedlot bloat,* the formation of an extracellular dextran slime by amylolytic bacteria in the rumen is thought to be important in the development of the stable foam. Animals differ in susceptibility to bloat, and thus animal, plant and microbial factors are all involved. Research on control of bloat involves selection of plants that do not cause bloat, selection of bloat-resistant animals, and application of various antifoaming agents.

PRODUCTION AND MODIFICATION OF TOXIC SUBSTANCES IN THE RUMEN

Some poisonous plants are more toxic to nonruminants than they are to ruminants, because in ruminants a microbial attack on toxic compounds occurs before exposure to gastric digestion and absorption (Table 22.3). In this regard, ruminal microbes could be considered as a "first line of defense" against toxic compounds in feedstuffs and the degradation of toxic materials by ruminal microbes probably has had an important role in the competitive success of ruminant species. In some cases, dietary changes may lead to selection of microbial populations that degrade specific toxic substances more rapidly. Such adaptations are in reality manipulations of microbial population, and better knowledge of the factors that are involved could improve management decisions about dietary change.

In contrast to these beneficial actions, ruminal microbes

Table 22.3. Substances detoxified in the rumen

Substance	Source	Reactions	Organisms
Nitrite	Nitrate	Reduced to ammonia	Various bacteria and protozoa
Oxalate	*Oxalis* and *halogeton*	Decarboxylated to formate	*Oxalobacter formigenes*
Ochratoxin A	Moldy feeds	Hydrolysis	Unidentified microbes
3-Nitropropanol and 3-nitropropionic acid	Miserotoxin in many *Astragalus* sp.	Nitro-group reduction to amine	*Coprococcus, Megasphaera, Selenomonas*
Phytoestrogens	Subterranean clover and red clover	Degraded to p-ethylphenol	Unknown
Gossypol	Cottonseed meal	Bound to soluble protein	Unknown
Pyrrolizidine alkaloids heliotrine	*Heliotropium*	Reductive fission	*Peptococcus heliotrinreducans*
3-Hydroxy-4(1H)-pyridone	Mimosine from leucaena	Unknown	*Synergistes jonesii, Clostridium* sp.

can also produce toxic compounds (Table 22.4). In some cases, these products may be subsequently detoxified by the microbes, but the latter reactions may not occur rapidly enough to prevent accumulation of harmful concentrations of the toxic intermediate. Toxic substances that are released by hydrolysis of glycosidic bonds include cyanide, 3-nitropropanol and 3-nitropropionic acid, and goitrin. Other toxic compounds produced by rumen microbes include intermediates in the metabolism of various constituents in feeds—e.g., 3-methylindole from tryptophan, 3-hydroxy-4(1H)-pyridone(3,4DHP) from mimosine, nitrite from nitrate—or an end product that is overproduced (D-lactic acid). It is not possible to describe all of the interactions here, but some that are more pertinent to practical problems are discussed.

Table 22.4. Toxic substances produced in the rumen

Substance	Source	Organisms involved
3-Methylindole (skatole)	Tryptophan in feeds	*Lactobacillus* sp.
Nitrite	Reduction of nitrates in feed	*Selenomonas ruminantium; Veillonella alcalescens*
Lactic acid	Rapidly degraded carbohydrates (in high-concentrate diets)	*Streptococcus* spp.; *Lactobacillus* spp.
3-Hydroxy-4(1H)-pyridone	Degradation product of mimosine	Unidentified gram-negative rod
Cyanide	Hydrolysis of cyanogenic glycosides	Gram-negative rods and gram-positive diplococci
Dimethyl disulfide	Degradation product of S-methylcysteine sulfoxide (*Brassica* anaemia factor)	*Lactobacillus* spp.; *Veillonella alcalescens; Anaerovibrio lipolytica; Megasphaera elsdenii*
Equol	Demethylation and reduction of formononetin (a phytoestrogen)	Unknown
Thiaminase	Microbial enzymes	*Clostridium sporogenes; Bacillus* spp. and various anaerobes
3-Nitropropanoic acid and 3-nitropropanol	Hydrolysis of miserotoxins	Unknown
Goitrin	Hydrolysis of glucosinolates found in rapeseed meal and other crucifers	Unknown

Lactic acidosis

High levels of lactic acid accumulate in the rumen and subsequently in the blood if animals are overfed with, or are abruptly switched to, grain or other readily fermented carbohydrate. This lactic acidosis is a potentially lethal condition that is also known as grain overload or acute indigestion. A drastic shift in microbial populations from a predominance of gram-negative bacteria to a population dominated by gram-positive lactic acid producers (*Streptococcus bovis* and *Lactobacillus* sp.) occurs in the rumen and in the cecum and colon of overfed animals. The rapid growth of *S. bovis* may be explained, at least in part, by the markedly increased concentrations of glucose and the high growth rate of *S. bovis* when appropriate substrate levels are high. Ruminal pH characteristically drops from more than 6 to 5 or less. Normal rumen microbes are generally unable to compete when the pH is less than about 5.5, and the resulting population is dominated by the more acid-tolerant lactobacilli.

Ruminal lactic acid concentrations may exceed 100 mM, and such accumulations markedly increase the osmolality of the rumen so that water is drawn into the gastrointestinal tract from the systemic circulation. The severe dehydration and circulatory collapse that may follow can occur within a period of 1 or 2 days. The proportion of lactate present as the D(−) isomer may increase from about 20 percent at pH 6 to 50 percent when ruminal pH is less than 5. The less rapid metabolism and clearance by the animal of the D(−) isomer, as compared with the L(+) isomer of lactate, are no doubt important in the disease. Other toxic factors such as histamine or endotoxin, which is produced by lysis of the gram-negative anaerobes at low ruminal pH, may also be involved. Ethanol accumulates in the rumens of overfed animals but probably does not contribute significantly to pathological changes.

Gradual adaptation to high concentrate rations may occur without the above population shift. This can be explained by the selection of higher proportions of VFA-producing organisms that are able to rapidly use the carbohydrate as well as by the selection of increased numbers of lactic acid users. The capacity of certain bacteria and of protozoa to assimilate excess, readily available carbohydrate and to store it as intracellular polysaccharide for future use may also be important, as this reduces the availability of sugar for *S. bovis*. Transfer of rumen contents from animals adapted to high-grain diets to unadapted animals protects against lactic acidosis, but even adapted populations may be overwhelmed. Several studies suggest that certain antibiotics, particularly those selective against *S. bovis,* may provide protection against lactic acidosis.

Nitrate-nitrite toxicity

Drought stress and overfertilization of cereals and row crops can lead to production of feedstuffs with toxic levels of nitrate. A number of species of rumen bacteria and at least some of the protozoa reduce nitrate to nitrite and then reduce nitrite to ammonia. Reduction of both nitrate and nitrite depends on a supply of hydrogen-donating substrates such as can be supplied by readily fermented carbohydrate. With moderate levels of dietary nitrate, there is usually no accumulation of the toxic intermediate, nitrite, in the rumen. High levels of dietary nitrate, however, frequently result in the accumulation of nitrite in the rumen which, when absorbed, unites with hemoglobin to form methemoglobin (see Chap. 3). The impairment of oxygen transport leads to clinical signs of toxicity with methemoglobin levels of 40 to 60 percent and to death at levels 75 percent or higher. Gradual increases in dietary nitrate lead to selection of populations of ruminal microbes that reduce both nitrate and nitrite at a greatly increased rate. Animals with such adapted populations are able to tolerate amounts of dietary nitrate that would be lethal to unadapted ruminants. The change in proportions of specific ruminal microbes that is the basis for this adaptation is not yet understood.

Organic nitro-compounds

Organic nitro compounds, 3-nitropropionic acid (NPA) and 3-nitropropanol (NPOH) occur as glycosides in various species of *Astragalus,* (e.g., crown vetch and timber milk vetch). The glycoside of NPOH is also known as miserotoxin. The glycosides are rapidly hydrolyzed by ruminal microbes; the toxic nitro-compounds can be absorbed directly from the rumen, or they can be metabolized by ruminal microbes. NPOH is absorbed more rapidly than NPA, and its conversion to NPA (the toxic metabolite) occurs in the liver. Microbial metabolism of NPOH and NPA in the rumen involves reduction of the aliphatic nitro group to the corresponding amines, 3-aminopropanol, and β-alanine, respectively. This activity explains the higher tolerance of ruminants than non-ruminants to these compounds. Efforts are under way to define conditions that will maximize rates of nitro-compound reductions in the rumen.

Oxalic acid toxicosis

Salts of oxalic acid are present at low levels in most plants, but the oxalate content of some plants (e.g., *Oxalis* and *Halogeton*) may exceed 10 percent of the plants' dry weight. Acute toxicity and major losses of animals can occur after entry to pastures where these plants are prevalent. When oxalate is present in soluble form (sodium or potassium salts or free acid) rather than as the insoluble calcium salt, it is readily absorbed; acute intoxications involve marked reductions in circulating ionized calcium as well as severe damage to rumen epithelium and renal tissue from the calcium oxalate crystals that form. Animals gradually switched to high-oxalate diets, however, acquire a tolerance to such high levels of oxalate. This adaptation is due to increased rates of oxalate degradation in the rumen. The organism responsible for this is a recently discovered species, *Oxalobacter formigenes*. The obligate requirement of this organism for oxalate as an energy source explains the selection of increased numbers when the oxalate content of the diet is increased. *O. formigenes* is a specialist organism, but since many plants contain small amounts of oxalate low populations of oxalate degraders are maintained in rumens of animals fed normal diets. Although *O. formigenes* concentrations in sheep fed a high oxalate diet may not exceed more than 1 percent of the concentration of total bacteria, the rate of oxalate degradation can still be high enough to protect the animal from toxicity. Organisms similar to ruminal strains of *O. formigenes* have also been isolated from the cecum of swine and from human feces.

Acute bovine pulmonary emphysema

Acute bovine pulmonary edema and emphysema may develop after cattle are moved from dry range to lush green pasture. A similar disease is induced by intraruminal dosage with tryptophan or with either indoleacetic acid or 3-methylindole, which are the products of tryptophan metabolism by rumen microbes. Ruminal production of 3-methylindole is critical since intravenous dosage with 3-methylindole also produced the disease but intravenous dosage with tryptophan or indoleacetic acid did not. A lactobacillus capable of converting indoleacetic acid (but not tryptophan) to 3-methylindole has been isolated from the rumen. Monensin, which inhibits these conversions in animals loaded with tryptophan, also prevents development of the disease under field conditions.

Mimosine toxicity

Leucaena leucocephala is a leguminous tropical shrub/tree that grows rapidly and provides leaves and seeds that are a nutritious forage for ruminants in certain parts of the world. High levels of productivity with leucaena as a major dietary component have been noted, but in some geographic areas severe toxicity is observed if leucaena makes up more than 30 percent of the diet. The explanation for this is that mimosine, a toxic amino acid in leucaena, is degraded to nontoxic products by microbes that are in the rumens of animals where high-leucaena diets are tolerated. In areas where toxicity is seen, however, ruminal degradation of mimosine does not proceed beyond the toxic (goitrogenic) intermediate, 3,4 DHP. It has been found that when rumen bacteria able to degrade 3,4 DHP from a goat in Hawaii were inoculated intraruminally into cattle in Florida or Australia, these organisms became established and provided protection so that 100 percent leucaena diets could be well tolerated. Furthermore, the 3,4 DHP degraders readily disseminated to other animals in the herd. The 3,4 DHP-degrading bacteria are the first known example of geographic limits to the distribution of truly functional rumen bacteria.

SMALL-INTESTINE MICROBES

Concentrations of viable bacteria in contents of small intestine (10^4 to 10^6 per gram) are much lower than are found in the rumen or large intestine. Segmented filamentous microbes colonize the small intestinal epithelium in normal rodents, but it is generally accepted that most of the bacteria in the small intestine are transients and that the impact of microbes on digestion in the small intestine is minimal. In a variety of pathological conditions, the small intestine becomes colonized by specific enteric pathogens or by populations similar to those in the colon (small-intestine overgrowth).

LARGE-INTESTINE MICROBES

The large intestines of most terrestrial mammals are colonized by populations of obligately anaerobic bacteria. The density of these organisms is about the same as found in the rumen—10^{10} to 10^{11} per gram. Generalizations about microbial populations in the large intestine are more difficult than generalizations concerning ruminal populations because of the diversity of animal species and diets and the relative lack of information concerning large intestinal populations. In the large intestine (as in the rumen), bacteria are found in intimate association with epithelial tissue. The specificity and significance of this association are not yet understood. There is, however, evidence that populations associated with epithelial tissue are somewhat different from luminal populations. Microbial fermentation is a major component of digestion in the large intestine, and the main products include carbon dioxide, acetate, propionate, and butyrate. Methane, hydrogen, or both, may also be formed.

It is probable that microbial interactions and other factors that regulate selection of ruminal bacteria are also important in the large intestine. Mixing is less complete in the less fluid environment of the large intestine and the continuous culture model used for consideration of selective phenomena in the rumen is less appropriate for the large intestine.

Although many workers have studied bacterial populations in feces from various animals, it is unlikely that fecal populations are representative of populations of the entire large intestine. In the pig, it is clear that gram-negative anaerobes constitute a greater proportion of the culturable population in the cecum than in the feces where gram-positive bacteria are predominant.

Much of the published information on fecal or large-intestine bacteria involves broad groupings of organisms at the genus or family level. In some studies the predominant anaerobic organisms have simply been grouped and enumerated as "total anaerobes," and in others inadequate anaerobic techniques have been employed. In spite of these deficiencies, it is clear that the indigenous populations of the large intestines of pigs and ruminants include several species that are among the predominant species of the rumen. Genera of bacteria that are frequently found among the predominant organisms in large-intestine populations include *Bacteroides, Fusobacterium, Streptococcus, Eubacterium, Ruminococcus,* and *Lactobacillus.* Spirochetes of the genus *Treponema* are frequently observed, and coliforms, particularly *Escherichia coli,* may be present at higher concentrations than are found in the rumen. In normal animals, however, coliforms are not usually among the most prevalent species.

Anaerobic protozoa that are similar, but not identical, to rumen ciliates inhabit the large intestines of horses, rhinoceroses, tapirs, and elephants. Anaerobic protozoa have also been found in the gorilla, chimpanzee, and rodents. Concentrations of ciliates in the large intestine of the horse (10^3 to 10^6 per gram) are of the same order of magnitude as concentrations in the rumen. Little is known about the role of protozoa in the large intestine.

The nutritional significance of microbial fermentations in the large intestine is less readily appreciated than that in pregastric fermentation sites, where synthesized microbial protein and vitamins pass to the absorptive small intestine. A number of animals that are large-intestine fermenters are, however, able to salvage these products through coprophagy and there is abundant evidence that organic acids produced by microbes in the large intestine make important contributions to the energy metabolism of both ruminant and nonruminant herbivores.

REFERENCES

Allison, M.J. 1989. Characterization of the flora of the large bowel of pigs: A status report. *Anim. Feed Sci. Tech.* 23:79–90.

Allison, M.J., and Rasmussen, M.A. 1992. The potential for plant detoxification through manipulation of the rumen fermentation. In L.F. James, R.F. Keeler, E.M. Bailey Jr., P.R. Cheeke, M.P. Hegarty, eds. *Poisonous Plants,* Proc. Third Int. Symp. Iowa State University Press, Ames. Pp. 367–76.

Bauchop, T. 1977. Foregut fermentation. In R.T.J. Clarke and T. Bauchop, eds., *Microbial Ecology of the Gut.* Academic, London. Pp. 223–50.

Broderick, G.A., Wallace, R.J., and Orskov, E.R. 1991. Control of rate and extent of protein degradation. In T. Tsuda, Y. Sasaki, R. Kawashima, eds., *Physiological Aspects of Digestion and Metabolism in Ruminants.* Harcourt Brace Jovanovich, New York. Pp. 541–92.

Dawson, K.A., and Allison, M.J. 1988. Digestive disorders and nutritional toxicity. In P.N. Hobson, ed., *The Rumen Microbial Ecosystem.* Elsevier Science Publishers, New York. Pp. 445–60.

Dehority, B.A. 1986. Microbes in the foregut of arctic ruminants. In L.P. Milligan, W.L. Grovum, and A. Dobson, eds., *Control of Digestion and Metabolism in Ruminants.* Prentice-Hall, Englewood Cliffs, N.J. Pp. 307–25.

Dehority, B.A., and Orpin, C.G. 1988. Development of, and natural fluctuations in, rumen microbial populations. In P.N. Hobson, ed., *The Rumen Microbial Ecosystem.* Elsevier Science Publishers, New York. Pp. 151–184.

Fonty, G., and Joblin, K.N. 1991. Rumen anaerobic fungi: their role and interactions with other rumen microorganisms in relation to fiber digestion. In T. Tsuda, Y. Sasaki, R. Kawashima, eds., *Physiological Aspects of Digestion and Metabolism in Ruminants.* Harcourt Brace Jovanovich, New York. Pp. 655–80.

Hobson, P.N., and Wallace, R.J. 1982. Microbial ecology and activities in the rumen. *Critical Rev. in Microbiol.* 9:165–225.

Howarth, R.E., Cheng, K.J., Majak, W., and Costerton, J.W. 1986. Ruminant bloat. In L.P. Milligan, W.L. Grovum, and A. Dobson, eds., *Control of Digestion and Metabolism in Ruminants.* Prentice-Hall, Englewood Cliffs, N.J. Pp. 516–27.

Hungate, R. E. 1966. *The Rumen and Its Microbes.* Academic Press, New York.

Mackie, R.I. 1987. Microbial digestion of forages in herbivores. In J.B. Hacker and J.H. Ternouth, eds., *The Nutrition of Herbivores.* Academic Press, Orlando, Fla.. Pp. 233–65.

Macy, J. M., and Probst, I. 1979. The biology of gastrointestinal bacterioides. *Ann. Rev. Microbiol.* 33:561–94.

McBee, R.H. 1977. Fermentation in the hindgut. In R.T.J. Clarke and T. Bauchop, eds., *Microbial Ecology of the Gut.* Academic, London. Pp. 185–222.

Ogimoto, K., and Imai, S. 1981. *Atlas of Rumen Microbiology.* Japan Scientific Societies Press, Tokyo.

Orpin, C.G., and Joblin, K.N. 1988. The rumen anaerobic fungi. In P.N. Hobson, ed., *The Rumen Microbial Ecosystem.* Elsevier Science Publishers, New York. Pp. 129–50.

Prins, R.A. 1977. Biochemical activities of gut micro-organisms. In R.T.J. Clarke and T. Bauchop, eds., *Microbial Ecology of the Gut.* Academic, London. Pp. 73–183.

Prins, R.A., Lankhorst, A., and van Hoven, W. 1984. Gastro-intestinal fermentation in hervibores and the extent of plant cell-wall digestion. In F.M.C. Gilchrist and R.I. Mackie, eds., *Herbivore Nutrition in the Subtropics and Tropics.* The Science Press, Craghall, South Africa. Pp. 408–34.

Russell J.B. 1984. Factors influencing competition and composition of the rumen bacterial flora. In F.M.C. Gilchrist and R.I. Mackie, eds., *Herbivore Nutrition in the Subtropics and Tropics.* The Science Press, Craighall, South Africa. Pp. 313–45.

Russell, J.B., and Wallace, R.J. 1988. Energy yielding and consuming reactions. In P.N. Hobson, ed., *The Rumen Microbial Ecosystem.* Elsevier Science Publishers, New York. Pp. 185–216.

Stewart, C.S., and Bryant, M.P. 1988. The rumen bacteria. In P.N. Hobson, ed., T*he Rumen Microbial Ecosystem.* Elsevier Science Publishers, New York. Pp. 21–76.

Williams, A.G., and Coleman, G.S. 1988. The rumen protozoa. In P.N. Hobson, ed., *The Rumen Microbial Ecosystem.* Elsevier Science Publishers, New York. Pp. 77–128.

Wolin, M.J., and Miller, T.L. 1988. Microbe-microbe interactions. In P.N. Hobson, ed., *The Rumen Microbial Ecosystem.* Elsevier Science Publishers, New York. Pp. 343–60.

Van Nevel, C.J., and Demeyer, D.I. 1988. Manipulation of rumen fermentation. In P.N. Hobson, ed., *The Rumen Microbial Ecosystem.* Elsevier Science Publishers, New York. Pp. 387–444.

CHAPTER 23

Avian Digestion | by Gary E. Duke

ANATOMY OF THE ALIMENTARY CANAL

The anatomy of the avian alimentary canal differs most notably from that of mammals in the mouth area, in the presence of a crop in the esophagus, and in the presence of a muscular stomach (ventriculus or gizzard). The mouth and pharynx are not sharply delimited in birds, and in most species there is no soft palate. The hard palate is cleft and thus communicates with the nasal cavities. There are no teeth, their functions being performed by the horny beak and the gizzard, and there is a great variety of tongue and beak adaptations. Salivary glands and taste buds are present, and their number and locations vary.

The size and length of the digestive tract vary considerably among species, depending upon dietary habits. For example, the small intestine is much longer in herbivorous birds than in carnivorous birds. The size of the tract of an individual bird may also change. Size decreases in hen waterfowl during breeding, and size increases in many herbivorous species during the winter when wild foods are of poor quality and greater quantities must be eaten. Parasitic infections (e.g., *Eimeria acervulina*) increase tract weight and length in chickens, and antibiotics decrease intestinal weight. In adult chickens the length of the entire digestive tract may be 210 cm or more (Table 23.1).

The avian esophagus is generally comparatively long and rather large in diameter, being larger in species that swallow larger food items. There is a dilatation of the esophagus, the crop (Fig. 23.1), in most species, although it is absent in some (e.g., insectivorous birds and owls). The form of the crop may vary from a simple enlargement of the esophagus to one pouch (e.g., fowl) or two (e.g., pigeons) pouches off the esophagus.

The glandular stomach or proventriculus (Fig. 23.1) of birds functions primarily in secretion, although it may also have a storage function in those birds that lack crops and in some fish-eating species (e.g., herons). The muscular stomach is highly specialized for grinding in those species that eat hard foods or for mixing digestive secretions with food in carnivorous species. In most species the muscular stomach is composed of two pairs of muscles called the *musculi intermedii* and the *musculi laterales*, or more recently termed the *thin* and *thick muscle pairs*, respectively (Fig. 23.1). These pairs of muscles are not present in most carnivorous birds (e.g., hawks, owls, herons), whose stomachs are somewhat similar to that of a mammalian carnivore.

The small intestine of birds has a duodenum like that in mammals, but beyond the duodenum there is no sharp histological distinction into a jejunum and ileum. The vestige of the yolk sac (Meckel's diverticulum) may be found about midway in the small intestine. The mucosa of the small intestine is like that of mammals except that in general the villi are taller, more slender, and more numerous in birds.

Table 23.1. Length of the digestive tract of chickens (five birds)

	At 20 days (cm)	At 1.5 years (cm)
Entire digestive tract	85	210
Angle of beak to crop	7.5	20
Angle of beak to proventriculus	11.5	35
Duodenum (complete loop)	12	20
Ileum and jejunum	49	120
Cecum	5	17.5
Rectum and cloaca	4	11.25

Modified from Calhoun 1954, *Microscopic Anatomy of the Digestive System of the Chicken*, Iowa State Univ. Press, Ames.

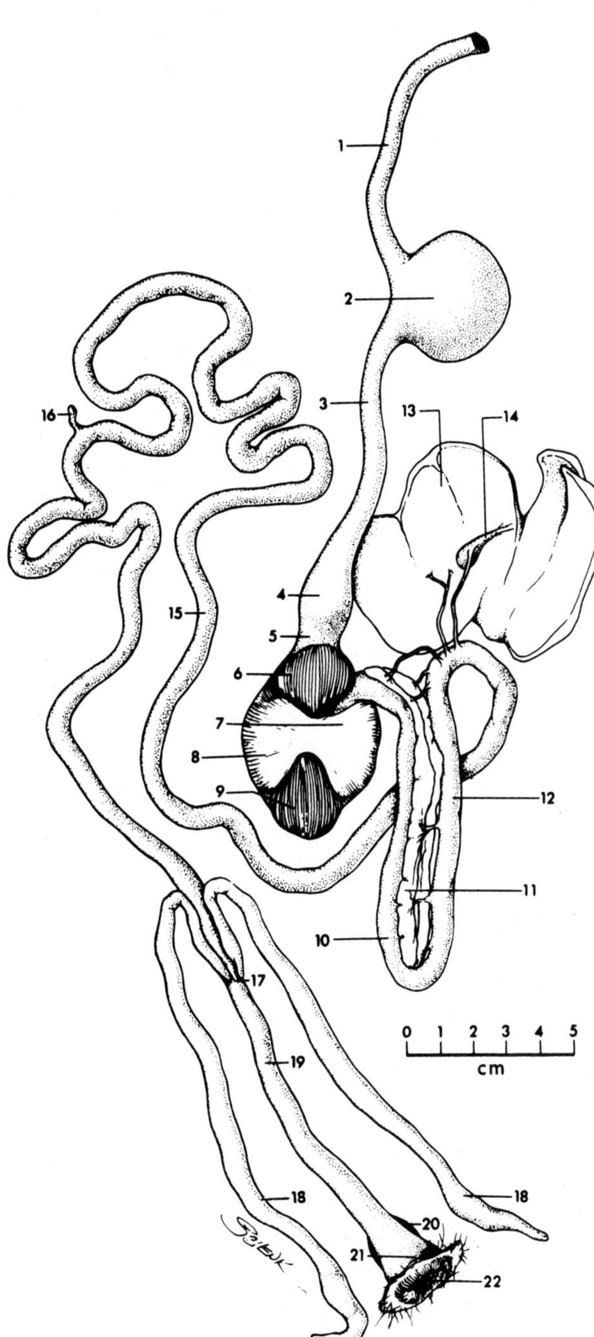

Figure 23.1. Digestive tract of a 12-week-old turkey weighing 2.24 kg. 1, precrop esophagus; 2, crop; 3, postcrop esophagus; 4, glandular stomach; 5, isthmus; 6, thin craniodorsal muscle; 7, thick cranioventral muscle; 8, thick caudodorsal muscle; 9, thin caudoventral muscle (6–9, muscular stomach); 10, proximal duodenum; 11, pancreas; 12, distal duodenum; 13, liver; 14, gallbladder; 15, ileum; 16, Meckel's diverticulum; 17, ileocecocolic junction; 18, ceca; 19, colon; 20, bursa of Fabricius; 21, cloaca; 22, vent.

There are no intestinal submucosal glands in the chicken, although in some species there are tubular glands that are homologous to these glands in mammals. Electron microscopic examination of chicken villi reveals a well-defined network of blood capillaries but no lacteals.

Located at the junction of the small and large intestines are the ceca, which in birds, unlike in most mammals, are usually paired. Their size is influenced by dietary habits, and ceca are not present in all species (e.g., hawks and songbirds). In birds the large intestine is relatively short and is not demarcated into a rectum and a colon, as it is in mammals.

Another organ concerned with digestion is the liver, which is bilobed. The left hepatic duct communicates directly with the duodenum, whereas the right duct sends a branch to the gallbladder, or it may be enlarged locally as a gallbladder. Gallbladders are present in chickens, ducks, and geese, but not in some other species, including the pigeon. The gallbladder gives rise to a bile duct, which empties into the duodenum near the terminus of the distal loop. The pancreas lies within the duodenal loop. It consists of at least three lobes, and its secretions reach the duodenum via three ducts.

Innervation of the avian intestinal tract and accessory organs is not well understood. The vagus nerves serve the esophagus, stomach, small intestine, pancreas, and gallbladder, much as in mammals. The lower tract is served by the intestinal nerve, also called the nerve of Remak. This nerve trunk runs nearly the entire length of the small and large intestines and is an autonomic nerve unique to birds. Electrical stimulation of the nerve evokes discharges both orally and aborally from the stimulation site. The orally projecting nerves are cholinergic whereas those that project aborally are believed to be noncholinergic and nonadrenergic. The caudal mesenteric nerve joins the intestinal nerve to serve the colon.

Neurotransmitters associated with enteric plexuses also have not been well studied, but axons containing the catecholamines, the peptidergic compounds (metenkephalin, somatostatin, substance P, vasoactive intestinal peptide, cholecystokinin, bombesin), and γ-aminobutyric acid have all been identified as neurotransmitters.

REGULATION OF FOOD INTAKE

In birds as in mammals, hypothalamic centers are involved in the control of appetite. Ventromedial hypothalamic lesions produce hyperphagia, and lateral hypothalamic lesions result in aphagia. A number of other factors affect feeding; for example, high environmental temperatures, high dietary energy levels, and high dietary protein levels all result in decreased food consumption, whereas low ambient temperatures, molting, and egg production increase food intake. If a diet is high in protein but low in energy value, food consumption will increase over normal levels. Apparently, energy content of a diet is a more important regulator of food intake than protein content. Protein content of the diet is important, however, and chickens are able to select between isocaloric diets with differing protein contents. They have been shown to choose a 16 percent protein diet over diets containing 8, 12, or 23 percent protein. Chicks are even able to select diets adequate in methionine over those with a methionine deficiency or excess.

Several processes have been shown to be involved in the regulation of feeding in fowl. Crop distention decreases food intake, but this is probably not a primary regulator. Also, glucoreceptors in the crop and intestine, duodenal osmoreceptors, and intestinal amino acid receptors, when stimulated by glucose, hypertonic saline, or amino acids, respectively, will depress feeding, but these are not considered primary regulators of food intake.

Glucostatic regulation of feeding appears to play a dominant role in mammals. In this process, increased levels of circulating glucose are "sensed" by hypothalamic cells and feeding is suppressed. Decreased levels of blood glucose will increase the consumption of feed. Chickens apparently employ a similar but less sensitive process, and glucostatic regulation by the liver may be more important in fowl. Intraperitoneal injections of glucose or glucose infusion into the hepatic portal circulation depress feeding. The latter effect has been shown in an egg-laying strain of hens but not in a heavier broiler breed. Lipostatic and aminostatic actions in the regulation of feeding have not been well studied in birds, but these mechanisms probably function to some extent.

The influence of central administration of neurochemicals on feeding is much less well understood in birds than in mammals. Intracerebroventricular (ICV) injections of epinephrine stimulates feeding in broilers but has no effect in layers. In broilers, 5-hydroxytryptamine decreases feeding in fully fed birds but not in birds fasted for 24 hours, whereas in layers it decreases feeding in both fed and fasted subjects. Broilers are fast-growing, meat-producing birds, whereas layers are slow-growing egg producers. Thus differences in their regulation of feeding might be expected. Turkeys are also fast-growing meat producers, but they respond differently than either broilers or layers. ICV injections of both epinephrine and 5-hydroxytryptamine decrease food intake in turkeys.

Several hormones or peptides have been shown to influence feeding in fowl. Cholecystokinin injected intracerebroventricularly decreases feeding in broilers. Melatonin also decreases feeding. Since melatonin is released at night and appears to be involved in inducing sleep, a depression of feeding as well seems appropriate. ICV injection of angiotensin II in turkeys increases drinking but has no effect on feeding. ICV injection of prolactin decreases feeding in turkey hens during periods of egg production but not during periods when hens are out of production. The opioid peptide β-endorphin given by ICV injection increases feeding in both meat-type and egg-type chickens. Avian pancreatic polypeptide given by ICV injection increases feeding in layers, and the related peptides—neuropeptide Y and peptide YY—increase feeding in broilers. Finally, and very interestingly, food intake is significantly decreased by an ICV injection of plasma from a fully fed bird. Apparently there is a satiety factor (or factors) in the plasma of free-feeding fowl (layers); this factor can be detected by the central nervous system and it influences feeding.

MOTILITY

Deglutition and esophageal and crop motility

During swallowing the tongue, hyoid apparatus, and larynx actively move food or fluid into the esophagus. Stimulation of the pharyngeal roof or tongue by food results in reflex closure of the glottis and choanal slit. Food is moved through the esophagus by peristalsis. Swallowing is coordinated with gastric motility, so that the swallowed bolus passes into the esophagus at the beginning of contraction of the thick muscles of the muscular stomach. It is not known what determines whether swallowed boluses enter the crop or go on to the stomach. The contractions of the crop (peristaltic waves) vary considerably in rhythm and amplitude and are influenced by the nervous state of the bird, hunger, and other factors.

Gastroduodenal motility

A complex gastroduodenal contraction sequence is seen in chickens and turkeys. In this sequence the pair of thin muscles of the muscular stomach (Fig. 23.1) contract first. Second, two to three peristaltic waves pass through the duodenum. Next, the pair of thick muscles contract. Finally, a peristaltic wave passes through the glandular stomach (Fig. 23.2). In the contractions of the thin and thick muscles, a wave of contraction proceeds in a counterclockwise direction (as viewed in Fig. 23.1) across each muscle. This inherent rhythmicity is apparently neurogenic. Contractions of the glandular stomach and duodenum are dependent on intrinsic neural connections with the muscular stomach, and contractions of these organs cease if myenteric neurons at the pylorus and isthmus are destroyed by application of benzalkonium chloride (which affects neural tissue but not muscles). Total extrinsic denervation causes the glandular stomach and duodenum to contract only slightly out of sequence; therefore extrinsic innervation does not appear to be involved in initiation of contractions or significant in regulation of the sequence.

During each gastroduodenal contraction sequence ingesta flow from the muscular stomach into the duodenum at the end of the contraction of the thin muscles and orally into the glandular stomach during contraction of the thick muscles. The latter flow produces pressure changes in the glandular stomach preceding its contraction (Fig. 23.2). During contraction of the glandular stomach, ingesta are returned to the muscular stomach.

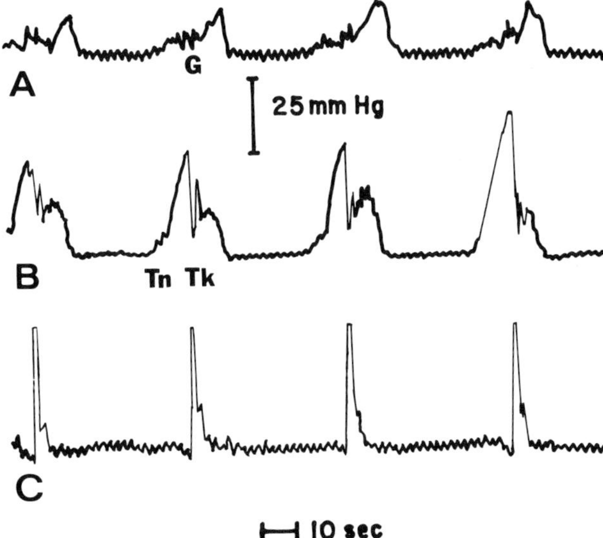

Figure 23.2. Tracings of a typical record of intraluminal pressure changes recorded from the glandular stomach *(A)*, muscular stomach *(B)*, and distal duodenum *(C)*. Tn, start of thin muscle contraction; Tk, start of thick muscle contraction; G, start of glandular stomach contraction. (From Duke, Kostuch, and Evanson 1975a, *Am. J. Dig. Dis.* 20:1047–58.)

Two other orad movements of luminal contents are associated with the normal function of the avian gastroduodenal apparatus. A reflux of duodenal and upper ileal contents into the muscular stomach occurs about four times per hour in turkeys. This apparently permits remixing of intestinal ingesta with gastric secretions. Predaceous birds (e.g., owls, hawks, herons) regularly egest a pellet of bones and hair or feathers of their prey from the stomach. Several species of birds (e.g., vultures) egest gastric contents, apparently by vomiting. The emesis of vultures appears to be a reaction to disturbance or fright rather than a part of the normal digestive process.

In the glandular and muscular stomachs of fowl two to three contractions occur per minute. Frequency of duodenal contraction in turkeys is six to nine contractions per minute, but two to three contractions occur in rapid succession in conjunction with each gastroduodenal contraction cycle. The mean amplitude of intraluminal pressure changes in the glandular stomach of turkeys eating commercial mash diets was found to be approximately 35 mm Hg. Mean amplitudes measured in the muscular stomach of fowl on these diets range from 40 to 150 mm Hg, with the higher average pressures being recorded during contraction of the thick muscle pair. In the domestic goose, the common buzzard, and the great horned owl, amplitudes of 265 to 280, 8 to 26, and 60 to 170 mm Hg, respectively, have been reported. In the latter two species, mean amplitudes varied with the quantity eaten and with the time at which measurements were made after eating (i.e., amplitudes decreased with time).

Hunger or starvation decreases the frequency of gastric contractions in fowl, and the duration of contractions tends to increase; the latter is decreased when fibrous or coarse food is ingested. The presence of grit in the gizzard increases the amplitude of contractions.

Inherent myogenic electric slow waves (basic electric rhythm), which are recorded from the mammalian gastrointestinal tract, have not been recorded from the stomach of turkeys. Slow waves have been recorded throughout the intestines and ceca of turkeys, but they are not believed to have a regulatory (pacesetter) function in the duodenum because the intrinsic neural system coordinates motility in the stomach and duodenum. Also, as many as three duodenal contractions may occur during a single duodenal slow wave, indicating that slow waves are not setting the pace of contractions.

The esophagus, crop, proventriculus, and gizzard are innervated by the vagi, parasympathetic nerves that are principal motor nerves to these organs, and by sympathetic fibers. Stimulation of the peripheral ends of the vagus nerves increases motility, and ligation of these nerves (particularly the left vagus) decreases motility for 2 to 3 days but has little effect thereafter (see above).

Grit (i.e., small stones) is present in the muscular stomach of most graminivorous and herbivorous birds. It is used for grinding hard foods between the thick muscles of the muscular stomach. Grit apparently is not essential for normal digestion, but digestion of hard foods is slower and the total digestibility of a diet may be decreased without it. Normally grit is ingested regularly, but if it is not available, food is retained longer in the muscular stomach.

Ileal, colonic, and cecal motility

Little is known about ileal motility in birds. Peristalsis and segmenting contractions have been observed radiographically. In the ileum of the turkey, contractions normally occur at a mean frequency of about four per minute, with an average amplitude of about 16 mm Hg; however, periods of more intense activity, with contractions of higher amplitude and with a frequency of about six per minute, have also been observed. Electrical slow wave frequency is also six per minute, and slow waves are believed to be regulatory in the ileum of the turkey. Regularly occurring (every 1.3 hours) migrating motor complexes (MMCs) have been recorded from the ileum of turkeys. Interestingly, while they could not be recorded from other parts of the digestive tract of turkeys, they could be in chickens. In turkeys, MMCs were recorded during both the fed and fasted states in poults but only rarely in the fed state in adults. In many species of mammals MMCs occur only in the fasted state. The duration of the complexes is longer in adult turkeys than in poults.

The most striking feature of colonic motility is antiperistalsis, which is believed to occur almost continuously. This activity appears to have two functions: (1) movement of urine from the cloaca into the colon and ceca for water absorption and (2) filling of the ceca. The antiperistaltic contractions arise from the cloaca and occur at a rate of 10 to 14 contractions per minute in chickens and turkeys. Antiperistalsis ceases immediately before defecation, during which the entire colon appears to contract simultaneously. Peristalsis, with a frequency of three contractions per minute, has also been recorded from the colon in turkeys. Electric slow waves associated with and believed to regulate each type of activity have been recorded. The occurrence of slow waves and contractile activity simultaneously moving orad and aborad in the same segment of intestine are unique.

Two types of contraction have been recorded from the ceca of turkeys: those with low amplitude and a frequency of 2.6 contractions per minute (minor) and those with much higher amplitude occurring at the rate of 1.2 contractions per minute (major). Radiographic studies have shown that minor contractions were performing a mixing function, and the major contractions were associated with peristaltic or antiperistaltic activity. Minor contractions of the ceca were often coordinated with ileal contractions and with peristaltic contractions in the colon; these three types of contraction (cecal, ileal, colonic) occurred at the same frequency but slightly out of phase. The function of this coordination is not known. A series of major contractions, primarily antiperistaltic, was associated with cecal evacuation, and a single major contraction occurred at the time of colonic evacuation (defecation). Cecal peristalsis and antiperistalsis have also been observed in chickens and owls. These peristaltic and antiperistaltic contractions appear to be myogenic in origin.

Cecal droppings of most avian species can easily be distinguished from the greenish, granular-textured intestinal droppings by their chocolate brown color and homogenous texture. One or two cecal droppings occur per day in gallinaceous species, while 25 to 50 intestinal droppings are formed.

There is a diurnal rhythm in cecal motility, with the highest daily frequency of contraction occurring in late afternoon and the lowest frequency occuring with the onset of darkness.

The time required for food to pass through the entire alimentary canal is generally longest in herbivores and shortest in carnivores and frugivores. Within 2.5 hours after feeding, a nonabsorbable chromic oxide marker given to fowl can be detected in the excreta, and most of it can be recovered from the excreta within about 24 hours. Marked cecal excreta can, however, be detected for 2 to 3 days after feeding of the marker. The rate of passage can be influenced by the fat content, consistency, hardness, and water content of the food and by the amount consumed. Apparently age also influences passage rate, because food passes through young chicks faster than through adults. The rate of passage through the adult turkey is, however, similar to that of the adult chicken.

SECRETION AND DIGESTION

Buccal, crop, and esophageal

The number and arrangement of salivary glands vary among species. In general, species that eat wet foods have fewer glands than those that eat dry food with little natural lubrication. The salivary glands of most birds have only mucus-secreting cells; serous cells have been reported in a few species, however, and amylase has been found in the saliva of poultry. In most avian species little maceration of food occurs, and food spends little time in the mouth. Hence, even if amylase is present in saliva, little digestion can occur in the mouth. Likewise, food passes quickly through the esophagus, and its major secretion is mucus for lubrication of this passage.

Mucus is also secreted by the crop in fowl (gallinaceous birds), but amylase probably is not. Amylase found in the crop may originate from the salivary glands, ingested food, bacteria in the crop or regurgitated duodenal contents. It is believed that a significant amount of starch digestion occurs in the crop of the chicken as a result of bacterial action. However, when collected crop contents of chickens are incubated after the bacteria are killed with chloroform, sucrose is still digested, indicating that nonbacterial digestion of carbohydrates also occurs in the crop.

Both serous and mucous salivary glands occur in pigeons, and mucus, amylase, and invertase have been found in the crop mucosa of that species. Perhaps the crop of the pigeon is more active in chemical digestion than that of fowl. In any case, after leaving the crop, ingesta receive much more thorough mechanical and chemical digestion in the stomach and intestines.

Gastric

Two types of gland predominate in the glandular stomach–(1) simple mucosal glands that secrete mucus and (2) compound submucosal glands that secrete mucus, hydrochloric acid and pepsinogen. Apparently, the compound glands are functionally homologous to both the chief and parietal cells of the mammalian stomach. Although gastric juice is secreted by the glandular stomach, preliminary acid proteolysis occurs mostly in the muscular stomach. In most species mechanical digestion also occurs predominantly in this organ. The pH of gastric juice ranges from about 0.5 to 2.5, being slightly higher in omnivores and herbivores than in carnivores, and is appropriate for good peptic activity. Values for gastric pH may also vary considerably, depending on method of collection and analysis of the juice and on the hunger of the bird.

The chicken secretes about 8.8 ml of gastric juice per kilogram of body weight per hour which is considerably higher than the amount secreted by humans, dogs, rats, and monkeys. Likewise, the acid concentration is higher, but the pepsin content per volume is lower than in most mammals. The total pepsin output, however, in pepsin units per kilogram of body weight per hour (2430) is higher than in mammals.

Intestinal, pancreatic, and biliary

The small intestine is the primary site of chemical digestion, and a number of digestive enzymes are secreted by its cells. The intestinal mucosa has been shown to have proteolytic activity in chickens and pigeons, and aminopeptidases and carboxypeptidases have been found in the duodenal mucosa of chickens. Intestinal amylase has been found in chickens, and maltase and sucrase of intestinal origin have been found in a number of species. Intestinal esterase activity has also been reported. Lactase activity is not present.

Intestinal pH ranges from about 5.6 to 7.2 in those species in which pH has been measured. The pH of the avian intestinal tract increases from the oral to the aboral end, and the pH of each portion of the tract is regulated by secretory activity within that portion. A pH of approximately 6 to 8 is optimal. Bacterial production of acid metabolites lowers pH in the crop, ceca, and colon.

Digestion of nutrients in the intestine occurs as a result of pancreatic enzymes and microbial activity as well as by intestinal secretions. The pancreas secretes both digestive enzymes and an aqueous solution containing buffering compounds. The latter secretion acts to neutralize the acid gastric chyme, thus providing a pH of 6 to 8. The pancreas is the major source of amylase and lipase. Pancreatic proteolytic activity is also important. Trypsin and chymotrypsin are the main enzymes, but dipeptidase, aminopeptidase, and carboxypeptidase activities have also been found in pancreatic extracts of chickens. The pancreatic secretory rate is relatively greater in fowl than in dogs, rats, and sheep, and it is less affected by fasting in fowl than it is in these mammals.

The secretion of bile into the duodenum aids in the neutralization of chyme. Bile salts are required for the emulsification of fats, a process that aids in their digestion. In fowl, as in mammals, bile salts are reabsorbed in the lower ileum and recirculated to the liver to be used again. Amylase is present in the bile of a number of species.

Cecal function

Only about 10 percent of most diets eaten by Galliformes (an order that includes domestic fowl, pheasants, grouse, partridges, etc.) receives cecal action, and fowl survive well after cecectomy. Nevertheless, several important functions are believed to occur in the ceca, most notable of which is the microbial digestion of cellulose. Wild Galliformes apparently derive a significant proportion of their daily energy needs from bacterial fermentation of fiber, especially during the winter when only poor-quality foods are available. Although domestic fowl are generally considered to be less capable in this regard, this view may have arisen mainly because usually high-fiber diets have not been fed before experimental studies of cecal function in poultry. Such a procedure has been shown to stimulate development of a cecal flora more capable of fiber breakdown. Captive grouse maintained on commercial diets are much less able to digest natural diets than are their wild counterparts.

Urine is moved from the cloaca into the colon, from which it may pass into the ceca via colonic antiperistalsis. Absorption of water from the cecal contents appears to be another major function of the ceca, and immediately after cecectomy water balance may be seriously affected. Within 4 to 12 weeks, however, the water-resorption capacity returns to normal, presumably via accommodation(s) of the lower intestine.

This refluxing of urine also exposes the cecal microflora to urea and uric acid which are degraded. The nitrogen is not recycled for use by the host, however, and apparently is used only by the microflora. Microbial synthesis of vitamins also occurs in the ceca, but the vitamins apparently are not absorbed by the host. When chicks are raised in both conventional and germ-free environments on diets lacking in various B-complex vitamins, normal amounts of the omitted vitamins are subsequently found in the cecal contents of conventionally raised birds, but only negligible amounts are found in the ceca of germ-free birds. Signs of dietary deficiency due to omission of the vitamins, however, are no less severe in conventionally raised birds, indicating that they derive little benefit from the vitamins synthesized by their cecal microbes. However, feces of chickens are a source of vitamin B_{12} and other B vitamins.

REGULATION OF MOTILITY AND SECRETION

Salivary secretion increases in response to eating. Similarly, the presence of food in the esophagus stimulates secretion of mucus, and the presence of food in the mouth and in the esophagus initiates motility in these areas. Regulation of the movement of food into or out of the crop is not understood, but it is probably controlled reflexly by the fullness of the rest of the tract below the crop.

Regulation of gastric activities is also very complex. There appear to be both a "cephalic" and a "gastric" phase of regulation of gastric motility and secretion in birds as in mammals. In fasted turkeys, the sight of food results in significant increases in frequency of gastroduodenal contractious (cephalic); subsequent ingestion results in further significant increases in both frequency and amplitude of gastric contractions (gastric). The sight of food also causes an increase in the volume of gastric secretion in ducks and an increase in acid secretion in barn owls. Sham-feeding of chickens results in increased gastric secretion. Increased

Table 23.2. Distribution of endocrine cells showing immunoreactivities (+) for peptides and hormones and their known functions in the digestive system of chickens

Peptide or hormones	Provent.	Gastrointestinal tract regions					
		Gizzard	Pylorus	Duodenum	Ileum	Cecum	Rectum
aPP*	+	–	–	+	+	–	–
	↓ S(vol)	↓ M					
Peptide YY	–	–	–	+	+	–	–
Glucagon	++	–	±§	±	±	–	–
	↓ S						
Glicentin	–	–	–	+	+++	+	+
Secretin	–	–	–	+	+	–	–
	↑ ↓ S‡			↑ S			
VIP†	–	–	–	++	++	+	+
Cholecystokinin	–	±	–	+	+	–	–
	↑ S(H^+)						
Bombesin	+++	+	–	–	–	–	–
Neurotensin	–	–	+++	+	+	±	++
Gastrin	–	–	+++	++++	+	–	–
	↑ S(H^+)						
Motilin	–	±	±	++	±	–	–
Somatostatin	++	–	++++++	+	±	–	–
Substance P	–	–	–	+++	++	+	±

+, Relative presence of substance.
–, Substance not present.
↓, Depress.
↑, Stimulate.
S, Secretion.
M, Motility.
*Avian pancreatic polypeptide.
†Vasoactive intestinal peptide.
‡Secretin stimulates pepsin and depresses H^+ secretion.
§References differ on its presence.
From Burhol 1974, 1982; Yamada et al. 1983; Rawdon 1984.

gastric secretion also occurs in chickens as a result of feeding, and in turkeys there is a direct relationship between the protein content of a diet and the proteolytic activity and rate of production of gastric juice. The latter (effects of feeding and protein content) findings indicate the presence of a gastric phase in the control of gastric secretion.

Secretion of gastric acid is enhanced by hypoglycemia in mammals. The cephalic phase of gastric secretion in fowl may also be mediated by such a mechanism.

Control of a gastric phase may be neural or hormonal. Stimulation of the vagus is a well-known initiator of or enhancement to both gastric secretion and motility. With the use of immunocytochemistry, radioimmunoassay, and/or ultrastructural studies, endocrine cells secreting many peptides and hormones have been located in the avian stomach and intestine (Table 23.2).

There is also a duodenal phase of gastric regulation in which the nature and volume of duodenal contents inhibit gastric activity. In mammals this happens through the action of neural and humoral mechanisms (enterogastric reflex and enterogastrone, respectively). In birds the mechanisms are unknown, but both neural and humoral elements appear to be involved. Distention of the duodenum causes a decrease in gastric secretion in chickens and a decrease in gastric motility in turkeys. Intraduodenal injections of small volumes of corn oil, 1600 mOsm NaCl (pH 7), 0.1 N HCl, and 10 percent amino acid solutions all inhibit gastric motility in turkeys. The inhibition requires 2 to 3 minutes with oil but occurs immediately after injection of the other solutions, implying the existence of a humoral mechanism for the oil and a neural mechanism for the others. After bilateral section of the vagal innervation of the glandular stomach of fowl, duodenal distention produces much less inhibition of gastric secretion than in normal birds, indicating a neural mechanism. Serotonin may act as a humoral mediator in avian gastric regulation. When the actions of endogenous serotonin are blocked (by injection of UML 491, a serotonin blocker), there is less inhibition of gastric secretion after duodenal distention.

The inherent motility of the entire small intestine is increased by vagal stimulation, as is intestinal secretion. The latter is increased more by duodenal distention or by injection of hormones.

Although several hormones have been shown to be released postprandially (Table 23.2), their full significance in normal regulation of secretion and motility in birds is still very unclear.

When a fasted chicken eats, pancreatic secretion begins immediately (i.e., a cephalic phase). If the bird's vagus nerve is severed at the pancreatic level, no immediate secretion occurs, although pancreatic secretion eventually increases. The delayed secretion is probably humorally induced. Secretin, which is responsible for stimulation of the initial secretion of the aqueous component of pancreatic juice in mammals, has been isolated from the intestinal mucosa of turkeys. Cholecystokinin (CCK), which causes prolonged secretion of both aqueous and enzyme components of mammalian pancreatic juice, has also been found in birds (Table 23.2).

Avian secretin has been shown to stimulate increased pancreatic secretion (aqueous component) but not increased enzyme secretion. Avian vasoactive intestinal peptide (VIP) is, however, a more potent stimulator in this regard. The active COOH-terminal octapeptide of mammalian CCK (CCK 8) stimulates both aqueous and enzyme secretion from the avian pancreas. Simultaneous injection of avian secretin and CCK 8 produced no more response than CCK 8 alone. It is believed that secretin plays an insignificant role in normal regulation of the avian pancreas and that VIP is involved in secretory regulation in a role analogous to secretin in mammals.

The rate of bile secretion in chickens increases on eating and, while the mechanism is not known, CCK is probably responsible.

ABSORPTION

The absorption of nutrients from the intestines of chickens has been relatively well studied. The upper ileum is the most important site of absorption of the end products of digested fats, carbohydrates, and proteins. Bile salts are absorbed largely in the lower ileum; amino acids coming from exogenous proteins are mostly absorbed in the upper half of the ileum; and the breakdown products from endogenous proteins are absorbed primarily in the lower half of the ileum.

The absorption of D-glucose, D-galactose, D-xylose, 3-methyl glucose, α-methyl glucoside, and possibly D-fructose is active. Seven other monosaccharides are apparently passively transported. Chickens have a sodium-dependent mobile carrier system for active transport of sugars similar to that of mammals, and the system becomes functional before hatching. Maximum glucose absorption capacity is apparently reached within the first week of life, and capacity decreases thereafter.

Amino acids are also transported by carrier-mediated processes in birds, but the transport does not appear to decrease with age. In birds, as in mammals, most proteinaceous products are absorbed as peptides but appear in the mesenteric blood as amino acids. Neutral amino acids are transported more rapidly than basic or acidic amino acids. There may be more than one transport system for each type of amino acid (neutral, basic, or acidic), and a single amino acid may be handled by more than one transport system. For example, glutamic acid may be transported either by diffusion or by a carrier-mediated route, while intestinal transport of cystine occurs only by the latter process. Amino acids handled by the same transport system, however, usually inhibit each others' transport. In chickens, transport of L-leucine is inhibited by the presence of L-valine, L-isoleucine, or L-methionine in the same solution. Likewise, L-lysine transport is inhibited by the presence of L-arginine, L-phenylalanine, or L-histidine. D-amino acids usually inhibit the transport of corresponding L-amino acids.

The in vivo absorption rate of L-amino acids is not dependent on molecular weight but amino acids with large nonpolar side chains (e.g., methionine, valine, leucine) are absorbed more readily than those with polar side chains.

Determination of the concentration of glucose and amino nitrogen in portal vein blood and wing vein blood, may show that within 15 minutes after eating there is a significantly higher concentration of these substances in the portal blood, indicating a high rate of digestion and absorption.

Apparently the amounts of fat digested and absorbed in birds and mammals are similar. The processes of absorption, however, are somewhat different between the two vertebrate classes. In mammals fat is absorbed into the lymph lacteals of the villi, whereas in birds fats are absorbed into the blood of the villi. Approximately 80 to 95 percent of the fatty acids present in the intestine of adult chickens are absorbed, but newly hatched chicks absorb less.

Environmental conditions may affect absorption. Turkeys held at 35°C without prior acclimatization absorb less potassium and phosphate than at 24°C, and at 8°C (cold stress) they absorb less calcium and more nitrogen than at 24°C. The depressed absorption during heat stress may be due to altered mesenteric blood flow. At 37°C, mesenteric blood flow is decreased by about 50 percent in chickens.

REFERENCES

Allen, P.C. 1984. Physiological responses of chicken gut tissue to infection with *Eimenia acervulina*. *Avian Dis* 28:868–76.

Bensadoun, A., and Rothfeld, A. 1972. The form of absorption of lipids in the chicken *Gallus domesticus*. *Proc. Soc. Exp. Biol. Med.* 141:814–19.

Bolton, W. 1965. Digestion in crop. *Br. Poult. Sci.* 6:97–102.

Bottje, W.G., and Harrison, P.C. 1986. The effect of high ambient temperature and hypercapnia on post prandial intestinal hyperemia in domestic cockerels. *Poultry Sci.* 65:1606–14.

Burhol, P.G. 1974. Effect of glucagon on gastric secretion in fistula chickens. *Scand. J. Gastroenterol.* 9:411–14.

Burhol, P.G. 1982. Regulation of gastric secretion in the chicken. *Scand. J. Gastroenterol.* 17:321–23.

Chaplin, S.B., and Duke, G.E. 1988. Effect of denervation on initiation and coordination of gastroduodenal motility in turkeys. *Am. J. Physiol.* 255:G1-G6.

Coates, M.E., Ford, J.E. and Harrison, G.F. 1968. Intestinal synthesis of vitamins of the B-complex in chicks. *Br. J. Nutr.* 22:493–500.

Denbow, D.M. 1985. Food intake control in birds. *Neurosc. Biobehav. Rev.* 9:223–32.

Dimaline, R., and Dockray, G.J. 1979. Potent stimulation of the avian exocrine pancreas by porcine and chicken vasoactive intestinal peptide. *J. Physiol.* 294:153–63.

Duffy, D.C., Furness, B.L., Laugksch, R.C., and Smith, J.A. 1985. Two methods of measuring food transit rates of seabirds. *Comp. Biochem. Physiol.* 82A:781–85.

Duke, G.E., Dziuk, H.E. and Evanson, O.A. 1972. Gastric pressure and smooth muscle electrical potential changes in turkeys. *Am. J. Physiol.* 222:167–73.

Duke, G.E., and Evanson, O.A. 1972. Inhibition of gastric motility by duodenal contents in turkeys. *Poult. Sci.* 51:1625–36.

Duke, G.E., Evanson, O.A., and Huberty, B.J. 1980. Electrical potential changes and contractile activity of the distal cecum of turkeys. *Poult. Sci.* 59:1925–34.

Duke, G.E., Kostuch, T.E., and Evanson, O.A. 1975. Gastroduodenal electrical activity in turkeys. *Am. J. Dig. Dis.* 20:1047–58.

Duke, G.E., Kostuch, T.E., and Evanson, O.A. 1975. Electrical activity and intraluminal presure in the lower small intestine of turkeys. *Am. J. Dig. Dis.* 20:1040–46.

Dziuk, H.E., and Duke, G.E. 1972. Cineradiographic studies of gastric motility in the turkey. *Am. J. Physiol.* 222:159–66.

Grubb, B.R., Driscoll, S.M., and Bently, P.J. 1987. Electrical PD, short-circuit current and fluxes of Na and Cl across avian intestine. *J. Comp. Physiol. B* 157:181–86.

Herpol, C. 1967. Zuurtegraad en vertering in de maag van vogels. *Natuurwet. Tijdschr.* 49:201–15.

Hodgkiss, J.P. 1984. Evidence that enteric cholinergic neurones project orally in the intestinal nerve of the chicken. *Q. J. Exp. Physiol.* 69:797–807.

Hodgkiss, J.P. 1984. Peristalsis and antiperistalsis in the chicken caecum are myogenic. *Q. J. Exp. Physiol.* 69:161–70.

Holthuizen, A.M.A. and Adkisson, C.S. 1984. Passage rate, energetics and utilization efficiency of the cedar waxwing. *Wilson Bull.* 96:680–84.

Hurwitz, S., and Bar, A. 1968. Regulation of pH in the intestine of the laying fowl. *Poult. Sci.* 47:1029–30.

Joyner, W.L., and Kokas, E. 1971. Action of serotonin on gastric (proventriculus) secretion in chickens. *Comp. Gen. Pharmacol.* 2:145–50.

Kan, C.A. 1975. The intestinal absorption of amino acids and peptides with special reference to domestic fowl. *World's Poult. Sci. J.* 31:46–56.

Kokue, E., and Hayama, T. 1972. Effects of starvation and feeding on the exocrine pancreas of the chicken. *Poult. Sci.* 51:1366–70.

Lai, H.C., and Duke, G.E. 1978. Colonic motility in domestic turkeys. *Am. J. Dig. Dis.* 23:673–81.

Lerner, J., Burrill, P.H., Sattelmeyer, P.A., and Janicki, C.F. 1976. Developmental patterns of intestinal transport mechanisms in the chick. *Comp. Biochem. Physiol.* 54A:109–12.

Lerner, J., and Messier, D.L. 1978. Specificity relationships in cystine transport in the chicken intestine. *Comp. Biochem. Physiol.* 60A:497–501.

Long, J.F. 1967. Gastric secretion in unanesthetized chickens. *Am. J. Physiol.* 212:1303–7.

MacNab, J.M. 1973. The avian caeca: A review. *World's Poult. Sci. J.* 29:251–63.

Meglasson, M.D. and Hazelwood, R.L. 1983. Adrenergic regulation of Avian pancreatic polypeptide secretion in vitro. *Am. J. Physiol.* 244:E408-E413.

Mueller, L.R. 1989. Investigations of the avian migrating motor complex. M.S. thesis. University of Minnesota.

Nagasaki, M., Takewaki, T., and Ohashi, H. 1983. Nerve pathways in the rectal region of the nerve of Remak of the chicken. *Jpn. J. Vet. Sci.* 54:443–52.

Nakagawa, H., Nishimura, M., and Urakawa, N. 1983. 2-Deoxy-D-glucose stimulated acid secretion from chicken proventriculus. *Jpn. J. Vet. Sci.* 45:721–26.

Noyan, A., Lossow, W.J., Brot, N., and Chaikoff, I.L. 1964. Pathway and form of absorption of palmitic acid in the chicken. *J. Lipid Res.* 5:538–41.

Pritchard, P.J. 1972. Digestion of sugars in the crop. *Comp. Biochem. Physiol.* 43A:195–205.

Rawdon, B.B. 1984. Gastrointestinal hormones in birds—morphological, chemical and developmental aspects. *J. Exp. Zool.* 232:659–70.

Wolfenson, D., Sklan, D., Graber, Y., Kedar, O., Bengal, I., and Hurwitz, S. 1987. Absorption of protein, fatty acids and minerals in young turkeys under heat and cold stress. *Br. Poult. Sci.* 28:739–742.

Yamada, J., Kitamura, N., and Yamashita, T. 1983. Avian gastrointestinal endocrine cells. In S. Mikamu, K. Homma, and M. Wada, eds, *Avian endocrinology: Environmental and Ecological Perspectives*. Japan Sci. Soc. Press, Tokyo/Springer-Verlag, Berlin, pp. 67–79.

CHAPTER 24

Carbohydrate Metabolism | by Donald C. Beitz

Dietary carbohydrates provide well over one-half of the energy needed for performance of metabolic work, growth, repair, secretion, absorption, excretion, and mechanical work in most warm-blooded animals. The mechanism through which energy is developed, trapped, and delivered to the active functional machinery in individual cells is called *intermediary metabolism. Metabolism,* therefore, is the sum of all anabolic and catabolic reactions in a living organism that pertain to use of all nutrients, such as glucose, amino acids, fatty acids, purines, pyrimidines, H_2O, and O_2. Metabolic expression of the whole organism results from integration of the multitude of individual reactions into a dynamic metabolic circuitry of intricate design that is finely tuned. Disruption of the maintenance of this fine tuning results in abnormal metabolism and often in diseased states.

Carbohydrate metabolism includes all reactions that carbohydrates undergo, whether provided in the diet or formed in the body from noncarbohydrate sources. Most dietary carbohydrates are in the form of polysaccharides (starch, occasionally small amounts of glycogen, and, in some species, cellulose, hemicellulose, and the pentosans). Other dietary carbohydrates include disaccharides (maltose, sucrose, and lactose) and monosaccharides (glucose, fructose, galactose, mannose, and certain pentoses). Except for small amounts of glucose and fructose, monosaccharides are not important dietary sources of energy.

An overview of carbohydrate metabolism is presented in Fig. 24.1. Details of this overview are presented in the rest of the chapter and in biochemistry texts. On entry into the cell, glucose has several metabolic fates, depending on cell type and energy status of the cell. Glucose may be catabolized to pyruvate (aerobic) or lactate (anaerobic) by a series of reactions known as glycolysis. Oxygen-using cells oxidize pyruvate to form acetyl CoA and CO_2; the acetyl CoA can enter the citric acid cycle for complete oxidation to CO_2. Acetyl CoA is a precursor for several compounds, such as fatty acids and cholesterol. Particularly in liver and muscles, glucose may be polymerized and stored as glycogen. Furthermore, glucose may be oxidized via the pentose phosphate pathway to form ribose phosphate or triose phosphates. Triose phosphates give rise to the glycerol moiety of acylglycerols. Also, intermediates of carbohydrate metabolism provide carbon skeletons for synthesis of nonessential amino acids. Metabolism of other carbohydrates not illustrated in Fig. 24.1 will be described later as well.

In nonruminants, dietary starch and glycogen are hydrolyzed enzymatically in the gastrointestinal tract as described in Chap. 19, and the resulting glucose is transported to the liver. In herbivorous animals, cellulose, hemicellulose, and pentosans are converted, to the extent that they are digested, to short-chain or volatile fatty acids (VFAs) by microbial fermentation in the alimentary canal. Acetate, propionate, and butyrate predominate. The first two are most abundant, with relative amounts of these varying with time after eating, composition of the diet, and the pH and microbial composition of the ruminal, cecal, or intestinal contents. In adult ruminants and nonruminant herbivores, relatively small amounts of dietary carbohydrates escape fermentation. Because ruminants derive the major portion of their energy from VFAs, glucose and other

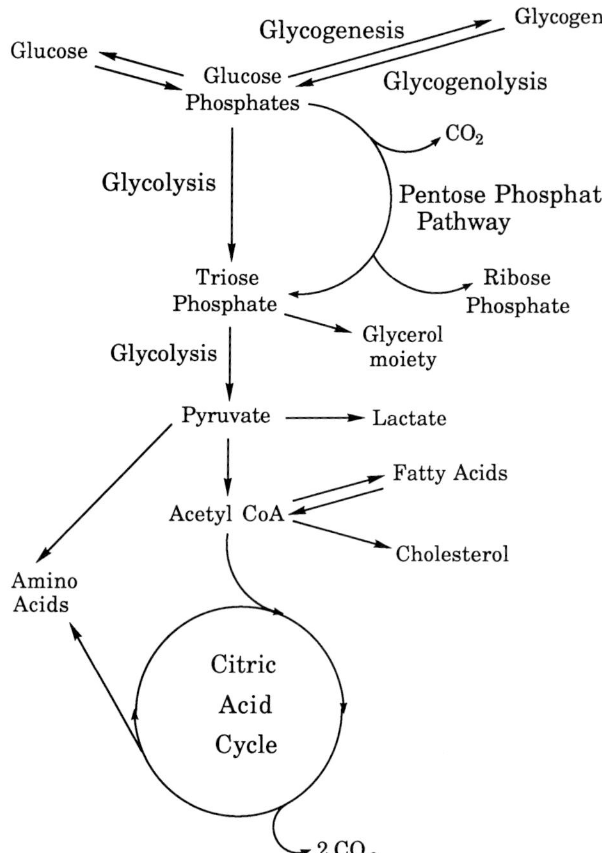

Figure 24.1. Overview of carbohydrate metabolism in animal cells. Most arrows represent sequences of reactions.

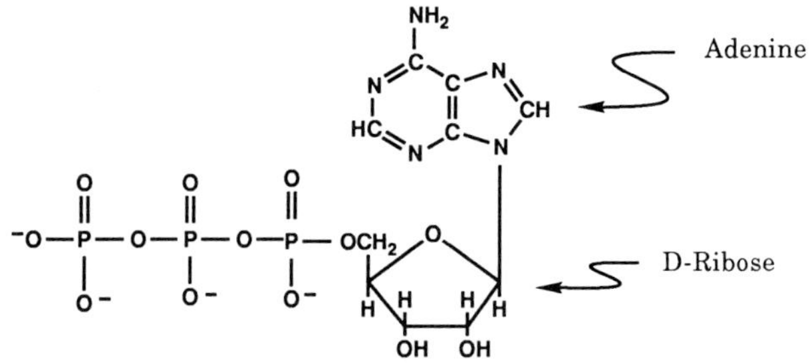

Figure 24.2. Structure of adenosine triphosphate.

monosaccharides, as such, play only a secondary role in the energy metabolism of these animals.

BLOOD GLUCOSE

The characteristic carbohydrate of blood and of other tissue fluids is glucose. Occasionally small amounts of galactose and fructose are present after absorption from the intestine and before their conversion to glucose in intestinal mucosa and liver.

Glucose in blood and in certain tissue fluids is drawn upon by all cells of the body to produce useful energy or adenosine triphosphate (ATP) (Fig. 24.2). The dependence of different tissues on circulating blood glucose, however, varies greatly. Erythrocytes and the mature brain are critically dependent. Under certain circumstances (e.g., as in starved animals), however, the brain is able to oxidize significant quantities of blood ketone bodies for ATP generation. Other tissues, such as skeletal muscle but not liver, are capable of deriving considerable amounts of the chemical energy they need from oxidation of ketone bodies and fatty acids and thus are less dependent on blood glucose.

The concentration of glucose in blood is an important factor in determining the glucose concentration in the interstitial fluid, which in turn has an influence on the rate of transport of this hexose into individual cells. Under postabsorptive conditions, blood glucose concentrations vary considerably among species (see Chap. 3). Variability among animals within a given species is observed often and is related to nutritive state and to carbohydrate stores within the animal.

Blood glucose concentrations in mature ruminants are substantially lower than those in nonruminants. Although the newborn ruminant has blood glucose values similar to those of nonruminant mammals, these values decrease sharply during the first few weeks of life and then decrease more slowly until adult values are reached.

Maintenance of stable glucose concentrations in blood is a finely regulated mechanism in which the liver, extrahepatic tissues, and several hormones, including insulin, glucagon, epinephrine, glucocorticoids, and thyroid hormone, play a major role.

Sources

Absorption of monosaccharides resulting from digestion of dietary carbohydrates constitutes a major, though variable, source of blood glucose in nonruminants. Digestive and absorptive rates may be highly variable, even among animals of the same species on similar dietary regimens. After a high-carbohydrate meal, the blood glucose concentrations may be considerably above that in the fasting state, but in a relatively short time concentrations return to a prefeeding level. A second continuing and variable source of blood glucose results from endogenous synthesis in the liver from glucogenic amino acids and glycerol and, in addition, propionate in ruminants.

Uses

Subsequent to active transport of blood glucose into cells, a hexokinase-catalyzed reaction produces glucose-6-phosphate (G-6-P) according to the need for G-6-P by the cells. The phosphorylation of glucose "traps" the glucose in the cell for subsequent metabolism because only nonphosphorylated glucose can exit a cell. This G-6-P, in turn, can be converted into cellular glycogen, catabolized by way of pyruvate and the citric acid cycle to provide useful energy, metabolized by way of the pentose phosphate pathway, used in biosynthesis of other carbohydrate derivatives (e.g., glycolipids, nucleic acids, lactose, and complex polysaccharides), or converted into triacylglycerols for energy storage in nonruminants. As discussed in Chapter 25, ruminants do not store glucose carbon as fatty acids in triacylglycerols.

Normally, only trace amounts of glucose are excreted into urine, even when a high-carbohydrate diet is fed. Several diseases, however, result in significant urinary excretion of glucose (glucosuria) because of a hyperglycemic condition. Disease conditions that cause glucosuria often result from hormone imbalances (see Chaps. 27, 34, and 37), as in diabetes mellitus in humans, dogs, and other animals where insufficient insulin is available for promotion of glucose entry especially into skeletal muscle and adipose tissue. Prolonged insufficiency of insulin is accompanied by greater rates of fatty acid release from adipose tissue and subsequent conversion of the fatty acids to ketone bodies by the liver. Excessive accumulation of ketone bodies in blood results in their excretion into urine and thus stress on the acid-base balance of the body. This ketoacidosis may be treated with insulin. Excessive administration of insulin, on the other hand, will result in hypoglycemia and associated neurological symptoms.

PATHWAYS OF CARBOHYDRATE METABOLISM

Oxidative phosphorylation

The oxidative degradation of carbohydrates, as well as of lipids and amino acids, terminates in a series of oxidation-reduction reactions in which electrons flow from organic substrates to O_2, yielding free energy for ATP generation from adenosine diphosphate (ADP) and inorganic orthophosphate (Pi) by a process known as *oxidative phosphorylation* (Fig. 24.3). Reduced coenzymes also are used in reduction reactions of synthetic pathways. The ATP generated by oxidative phosphorylation is then available for support of critical processes of life, such as synthesis of nucleic acids and proteins, muscle contraction, ion transport, and thermogenesis. The respiration assembly, located on the inner membrane of mitochondria, contains numerous electron carriers responsible for transfer of electrons from reduced nicotinamide adenine dinucleotide (NADH) or reduced flavin adenine dinucleotide ($FADH_2$) to O_2 (Fig. 24.4). The free energy of the oxidation of NADH with O_2, which yields oxidized nicotinamide adenine dinucleotide (NAD^+) and H_2O, is -52.6 kcal/mole. Oxidation within the respiration assembly leads to the pumping of protons from the mitochondrial matrix and to the generation of a membrane potential (proton-motive force). The ATP is synthesized when protons return to the matrix via an enzyme complex known as ATP synthase or ATPase. The proposed mechanism for coupling of oxidative reactions to ATP synthesis is the basis of the much-supported chemiosmotic theory of oxidative phosphorylation. Thus oxidation of reduced coenzymes and phosphorylation of ADP are coupled by the proton gradient across the inner mitochondrial membrane.

Electrons are transferred from NADH and $FADH_2$ to O_2 through flavins, iron-sulfur complexes, quinones, and hemes that are prosthetic groups of proteins (Fig. 24.4). Oxidation of several substrates generates NADH or $FADH_2$. Electrons of NADH are transferred to NADH-Q reductase complex (*Q* for ubiquinone), which is also called NADH dehydrogenase complex. Prosthetic groups of this enzyme complex include flavin mononucleotide and several nonheme iron atoms that function in sequence in the electron transfer. Ubiquinone or coenzyme Q accepts electrons from NADH-Q reductase and also from other flavin-linked dehydrogenases, such as succinate dehydrogenase ands fatty acyl CoA dehydrogenase. Except for one nonheme iron protein, the electrons carried between coenzyme Q and O_2 are all *cytochromes,* which are proteins containing a heme prosthetic group. Like the nonheme iron, heme iron is a one-electron carrier. Cytochromes b and c, in addition to a nonheme iron, are components of the QH_2-

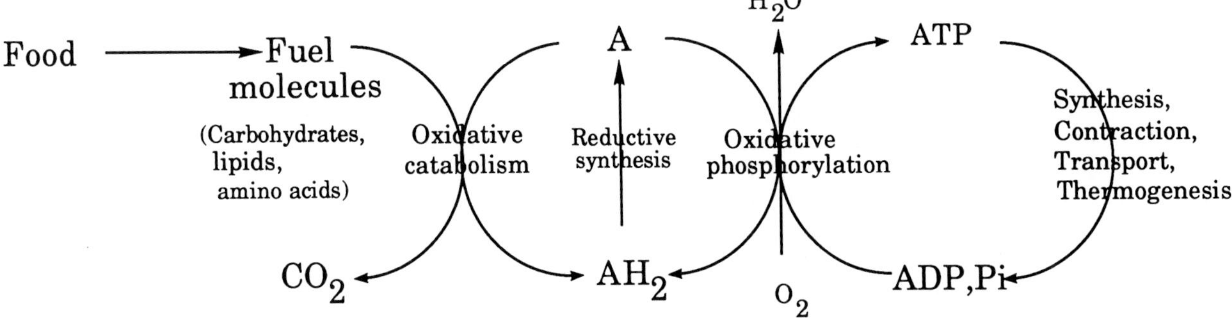

Figure 24.3. Overall view of aerobic metabolism in animals. Oxidative catabolic reactions release free energy that is captured in the form of high-energy phosphate bonds in ATP for driving reactions of synthesis (e.g., growth, muscle contraction, ion transport, and thermogenesis).

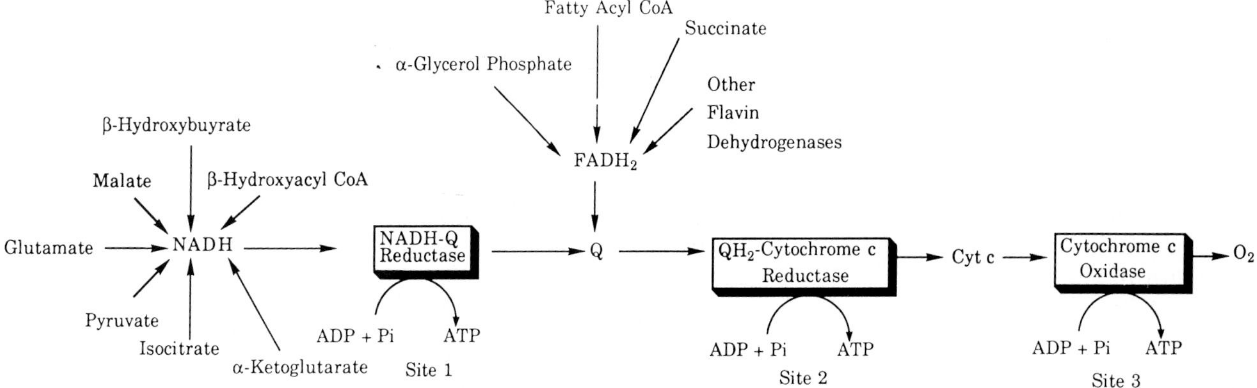

Figure 24.4. Electron transfer and oxidative phosphorylation in the respiratory assembly. Electron transfer from NADH and $FADH_2$ to O_2 occurs by enzyme-catalyzed, oxidation-reduction reactions. The NADH-Q reductase complex catalyzes transfer of electrons, in order, from NADH to FMN, several nonheme iron atoms, and Q (coenzyme Q or ubiquinone). The QH_2-cytochrome c reductase catalyzes electron transfer, in order, from Q to cytochrome b, nonheme iron, cytochrome c_1, and cytochrome c. Cytochrome c oxidase catalyzes electron transfer, in order, from cytochrome c to cytochrome a, cytochrome a_3, and O_2. Proton gradients are generated by the three complexes that are enclosed by the rectangles and represent sites of ATP generations.

cytochrome c reductase complex. Cytochrome c transfers electrons to the cytochrome c oxidase complex, which contains cytochromes a and a_3. Electrons finally are transferred from cytochrome a_3 to O_2 with the formation of water as follows: $O_2 + 4\ H^+ + 4\ e^- \rightarrow 2\ H_2O$. More specifically, aerobic oxidation of 1 g of glucose to CO_2 yields 0.55 g of H_2O. Oxidation of 1 g of protein yields 0.41 g of H_2O, and 1 g of lipid yields 1.07 g of H_2O.

Protons are "pumped" at the three sites indicated in Fig. 24.4. The proton gradient generated by a pair of electrons drives the synthesis of one molecule of ATP at each site. Thus, three molecules of ATP are generated per electron pair transferred from $NADH_2$ to O_2; consequently, a phosphate/oxygen (P/O) ratio of 3 is observed.

Rotenone and amytal inhibit generation of the proton gradient at site 1, antimycin A inhibits gradient generation at site 2, and cyanide, azide, and carbon monoxide block gradient generation at site 3. 2,4-Dinitrophenol disrupts the tight coupling of electron transport and phosphorylation. In the presence of this uncoupler, electron transport from NADH to O_2 proceeds normally, but ATP is not synthesized and the generated free energy is released as heat.

Under most physiological conditions, electron transport does not occur unless ADP is simultaneously phosphorylated to ATP. Besides a source of electrons, oxidative phosphorylation requires O_2, Pi, and ADP; concentration of the latter seems to be an important physiological regulator of oxidative phosphorylation. The formation of three ATPs when an electron pair of NADH is transferred to O_2 conserves 21.9 kcal/mole (7.3 × 3) of the total free energy of 52.6 kcal/mole. Thus the mechanism of biological oxidation of foodstuffs allows the free energy of oxidation to be captured as ATP in an efficient and controlled fashion. The noncaptured free energy is released as heat and thus contributes to the maintenance of body temperatures.

Glycogenesis

Glycogen, a highly branched polymer of glucose, is present as granules in cytosol of practically all tissues in all species of animals. Most glucose residues in glycogen are linked by α-1,4-glycosidic bonds. Branches are generated by α-1,6-glycosidic bonds that represent about 10 percent of the glycosidic bonds. Although highly variable in size, the average molecular weight of glycogen is around 5 million. Polymerization of glucose as glycogen allows an animal cell to store large quantities of glucose with lesser influence on osmotic pressure of intracellular fluids. Glycogen may occupy between 2 and 8 percent of the wet weight of the liver, depending on nutritional status. If an animal has fasted for 24 hours or longer, the liver may be almost depleted of glycogen. A dietary intake of glycogenic materials such as glucose results in a rapid glycogenesis or biosynthesis of liver glycogen. In the normal animal, even when excess carbohydrate is available in the diet, the concentration of liver glycogen is relatively constant, despite being continuously formed and degraded. Thus liver glycogen serves as an important reservoir for maintenance of blood glucose concentration.

Muscle glycogen content varies from about 0.5 to 1 percent of wet weight; because of the large muscle mass, most body glycogen, however, is found in this tissue. Muscle glycogen concentrations in muscle usually are more constant than those in liver. Muscle glycogen and the glycogen of other extrahepatic tissues are used extensively in metabolic processes and are restored primarily by synthesis from blood glucose. The principal function of muscle glycogen is to act as a readily available source of glucose for oxidation and ATP synthesis within the muscle itself.

Both the quantity and the composition of food consumed influence the quantity of liver glycogen. Animals fed high-carbohydrate diets tend to have greater liver glycogen con-

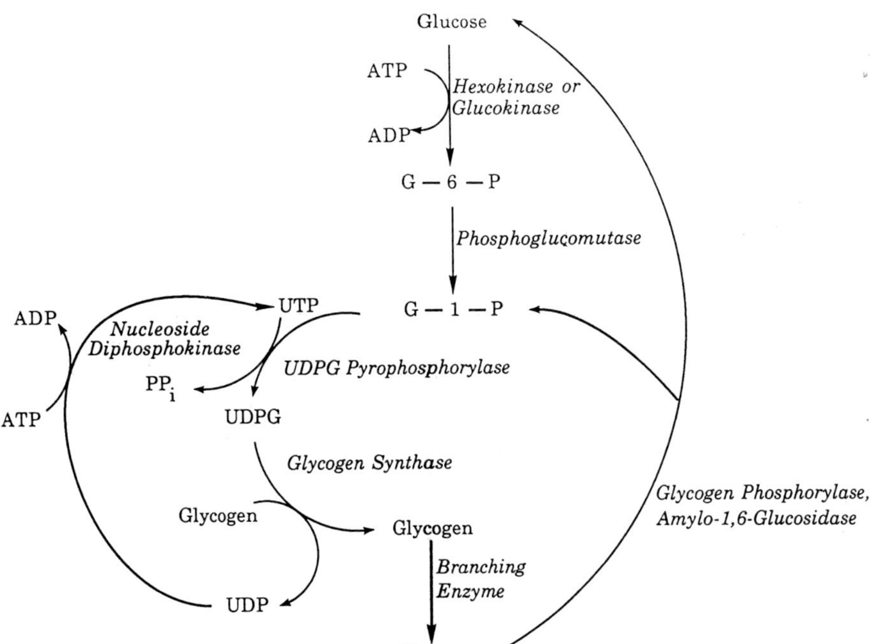

Figure 24.5. Metabolism of glycogen in animal cells.

centrations than those fed diets that are lower in carbohydrate. Exercise and abnormal conditions such as hypoxia and acidosis decrease the quantity of glycogen in liver. In addition, liver glycogen content is under endocrine regulation. Under normal circumstances, epinephrine and glucagon have glycogenolytic activity. Insulin and the glucocorticoids favor accumulation of liver glycogen. Uptake of glucose from blood by skeletal muscle is dependent on insulin, whereas uptake by the liver is not; therefore muscle glycogen increases more significantly after insulin injection than does liver glycogen.

For glycogenesis to occur (Fig. 24.5), G-6-P is converted reversibly to glucose-1-phosphate (G-1-P). In the presence of uridine diphosphoglucose pyrophosphorylase, G-1-P reacts reversibly with uridine triphosphate to form uridine diphosphoglucose (UDPG) and pyrophosphate (PPi). Rapid enzymatically catalyzed hydrolysis of PPi to 2 Pi makes UDPG synthesis essentially irreversible. Synthesis of the amylose chain of glycogen is catalyzed by glycogen synthase and involves a transfer of UDPG to the hydroxyl group at the C-4 of the nonreducing ends of preexisting glycogen chains, of at least four glucose residues (primers), to form the α-1,4-glucosidic linkage. As described below, uridine diphosphate derivatives of hexoses function in other pathways of hexose metabolism.

The highly branched structure of glycogen is a result of activity of a branching enzyme, amylo-(1,4→1,6)-transglucosidase. The branching enzyme cleaves fragments (minimal length of six glucose residues) of the glycogen chain at α-1,4 linkages and transfers them to the same or another glycogen molecule to form α-1,6 linkages at least four glucose residues away from a preexisting branch. Thus a branch with a nonreducing C-4 group is established, increasing the number of residues available for formation of α-1,4-glucosidic bonds. Each branch is extended by the action of glycogen synthase, and further branching and extension continue so that the highly branched glycogen molecule is produced. With regard to the energy cost of glycogenesis, one high-energy phosphate bond is used for incorporation of a G-6-P into glycogen.

Glycogen synthase exists in phosphorylated and dephosphorylated forms. Its active form, glycogen synthase *a,* is produced by action of a phosphoprotein phosphatase on glycogen synthase *b*. Conversion of the active form to the less active form requires ATP and protein kinase, which is stimulated by cyclic AMP (cAMP). The cAMP arises from the stimulatory effect of epinephrine (effect greatest in skeletal muscle) and of glucagon (response greatest in the liver) on adenylate cyclase, the plasma membrane enzyme responsible for cAMP formation from ATP. The effect of these two hormones is to decrease glycogen synthesis. Glycogen synthase *b* is activated allosterically by G-6-P, whereas glycogen synthase *a* is not. In addition, high concentrations of glycogen inhibit the action of phosphatase on glycogen synthase *b*. Insulin increases capacity of muscle to synthesize glycogen by activation of glycogen synthase *b*.

Glycogenolysis

In contrast to hydrolytic fragmentation of polysaccharides in the gastrointestinal tract, the α-1,4 glucosidic bonds of glycogen are degraded phosphorolytically within cells to G-1-P by the action of glycogen phosphorylase in the presence of Pi (Fig. 24.5). Phosphorylase degradation of glycogen begins at nonreducing ends of each chain, releasing G-1-P successively until four glucose residues of a branch remain. The phosphorolytic cleavage of glycogen is energetically advantageous because the glucose residues are released as G-1-P rather than as glucose. For glycogen degradation to continue, another enzyme (oligotransferase) redistributes the chain to leave a single glucose residue at the α-1,6 linkage. The resulting compound, called a limit dextrin, then is attacked hydrolytically at the α-1,6 linkage by amylo-1,6-glucosidase (debranching enzyme), and free glucose is removed. Subsequently, phosphorylase action continues with release of additional G-1-P until another branch point is approached. The transfer, hydrolytic, and phosphorolytic reactions result in glycogenolysis to produce mostly G-1-P and a lesser amount of glucose. The G-1-P may be converted to G-6-P and then, as described later, the G-6-P may enter the glycolytic or pentose phosphate pathways or, through the action of glucose-6-phosphatase in liver, contribute directly to blood glucose.

Glycogenolysis is under metabolite, nucleotide, hormone, enzyme, and cation control. Skeletal muscle has two forms of glycogen phosphorylase; *a* is active, *b* is inactive. The *b* form becomes active when adenosine monophosphate (AMP) concentrations are high, whereas both ATP and G-6-P inhibit phosphorylase *b*. In contrast, phosphorylase *a* is active, regardless of the concentrations of AMP, ATP, and G-6-P. Phosphorylase *b* is converted by phosphorylase kinase to phosphorylase *a* by phosphorylation of a serine residue of each subunit. Phosphorylase kinase, like phosphorylase, is converted from a low-activity form to a high-activity form by phosphorylation that is catalyzed by cAMP-dependent protein kinase. Conversion of *b* to *a* also is triggered by increased concentrations of Ca^{2+} in the cytosol that stimulates both muscle contraction and the partial activation of kinase. The Ca^{2+} binds to calmodulin, which is a subunit of the phosphorylase kinase. Thus glycogen breakdown and muscle contraction are linked by transient increases in free Ca^{2+} concentrations. Therefore the epinephrine-cAMP system stimulates the formation of fully active phosphorylated kinase, which converts phosphorylase *b* to *a*. Deactivation of glycogenolysis results from the conversion of the phosphorylase *a* to *b*.

Regulation of liver glycogenolysis is similar to that in muscle except that the principal hormone that stimulates cAMP formation is glucagon. Liver phosphorylase *b*, however, is not activated by AMP. Low blood glucose concentrations result in greater glucagon release from alpha cells of the pancreas, so that liver glycogen is used to normalize blood glucose concentrations.

Eight different glycogen-storage disease (types I to VIII) have been characterized in humans. For each, an enzyme involved in glycogen metabolism is defective, resulting in abnormal storage of glycogen in the liver, muscle, and kidney and often abnormal control of blood glucose concentration.

Glycolysis

Glycolysis is the sequence of reactions by which glucose is converted to pyruvate by enzymes in the cytosol of all cells of an animal. The generated pyruvate can follow different routes for continued metabolism, depending on availability of O_2. When both O_2 and mitochondria are available, the complete aerobic degradation of pyruvate to CO_2 and H_2O occurs as described below. If the supply of O_2 is insufficient, as in contracting skeletal muscle, or if mitochondria are absent, as in erythrocytes, pyruvate is reduced to lactate (anaerobic glycolysis). The ATP generated by anaerobic glycolysis is used for muscle contraction and other functions during sudden strenuous exercise. During glycolysis, some free energy of the glucose molecule is conserved in the form of ATP. This is illustrated by the following balanced equations for anaerobic glycolysis in active skeletal muscle:

$$
\begin{array}{rl}
a: & \text{Glucose} \rightarrow 2\ \text{lactate} + 2\ \text{H}^+ \\
b: & 2\ \text{Pi} + 2\ \text{ADP} \rightarrow 2\ \text{ATP} + 2\ \text{H}_2\text{O} \\
\hline
\textit{Sum}: & \text{Glucose} + 2\ \text{Pi} + 2\ \text{ADP} \rightarrow 2\ \text{lactate} \\
 & \quad + 2\ \text{H}^+ + 2\ \text{ATP} + 2\ \text{H}_2\text{O}
\end{array}
$$

The reactions of glucose conversion to pyruvate (glycolysis) are depicted in Fig. 24.6. In the first stage of glycolysis, glucose is converted to fructose-1,6-biphosphate by phosphorylation, isomerization, and a second phosphorylation. Each phosphorylation step uses the terminal high-energy phosphate bond of ATP. In the second phase, fructose-1,6-bisphosphate is cleaved with aldolase to dihydroxyacetone phosphate and 3-phosphoglyceraldehyde. Dihydroxyacetone phosphate can be isomerized readily into 3-phosphoglyceraldehyde. The latter then is oxidized and phosphorylated to form 1,3-biphosphoglycerate, which is a high-energy phosphate compound and has high-energy transfer potential. After transfer of the acyl phosphate to form ATP (substrate-level phosphorylation), the 3-phosphoglycerate undergoes phosphoryl shift and dehydration to produce phosphoenolpyruvate, which is a second compound of glycolysis with a high-energy transfer potential. A transfer reaction then results in the generation of ATP (substrate-level phosphorylation) and pyruvate.

Under anaerobic conditions, the NADH generated during glycolysis must be oxidized to NAD^+ by pyruvate, a reaction catalyzed by lactate dehydrogenase and resulting in L-lactate formation. Because of the limited supply of cellular NADH, formation and exit of lactate from the cell allow for continuation of glycolysis. In animal tissues under aerobic conditions (except erythrocytes and some tumors), the NADH formed by the dehydrogenation of 3-phosphoglyceraldehyde ultimately is reoxidized to NAD^+ by O_2 within the mitochondria by way of the electron-transport system.

Because inner membranes of mitochondria are impermeable to NADH, special shuttle systems carry the reducing equivalents of cytosolic NADH into the mitochondria for eventual transfer to O_2. The most active NADH shuttle, which functions in liver, kidney, and heart, is called the malate-aspartate shuttle. Cytosolic oxaloacetate accepts the cytosolic reducing equivalents and forms malate, which then is carried through the inner membrane on a decarboxylate carrier system. Once in mitochondria, malate is oxidized to oxaloacetate, forming mitochondrial NADH, which then can transfer a pair of electrons to the respiratory chain. Transamination reactions involving glutamate and asparatate result in regeneration of cytosolic oxaloacetate.

In skeletal muscle and brain, the α-glycerol phosphate shuttle prevails. In this shuttle, cytosolic NADH reduces dihydroxyacetone phosphate to form α-glycerol phosphate. After transfer into mitochondria, α-glycerol phosphate is oxidized by a flavin adenine dinucleotide (FAD)-linked dehydrogenase, resulting in $FADH_2$ and dihydroxyacetone phosphate. Return of the dihydroxyacetone phosphate to cytosol allows for shuttle continuation.

Flux of glucose carbon through glycolysis is controlled by the supply of glucose and several enzymes, primarily phosphofructokinase, of the glycolytic scheme. Hexokinase is inhibited by G-6-P. Phosphofructokinase is inhibited allosterically by citrate and ATP and activated by AMP and fructose-2,6-biphosphate. Synthesis of fructose-2,6-bisphosphate is inhibited by a cAMP-dependent protein kinase. Activity of phosphofructokinase is the primary determinant of the rate of glycolysis because this enzyme catalyzes the first irreversible reaction unique to glycolysis (the "committed" step). Pyruvate kinase, a secondary control point, is inhibited by high concentrations of ATP.

Oxidation of pyruvate to acetyl CoA and CO_2

The pyruvate produced by glycolysis is cotransported into mitochondria of all respiring cells with a proton by a pyruvate transporter and is decarboxylated oxidatively to form acetyl CoA and CO_2 by the pyruvate dehydrogenase complex (Fig. 24.7). This enzyme system is an integrated complex of three enzymes with cofactor requirements of NAD^+, thiamine pyrophosphate (TPP), FAD, CoA, and lipoic acid. In the first reaction catalyzed by the pyruvate dehydrogenase complex, pyruvate is decarboxylated and the α-hydroxyethyl derivative becomes linked to TPP of pyruvate dehydrogenase. As the second reaction, the same enzyme catalyzes transfer of hydrogen atoms and the acetyl group from TPP to the oxidized form of lipoic acid on dihydrolipoyl transacetylase, forming an acetyl thioester with the reduced lipoic acid. Transfer of the acetyl group to CoA constitutes the third reaction. The fourth reaction in-

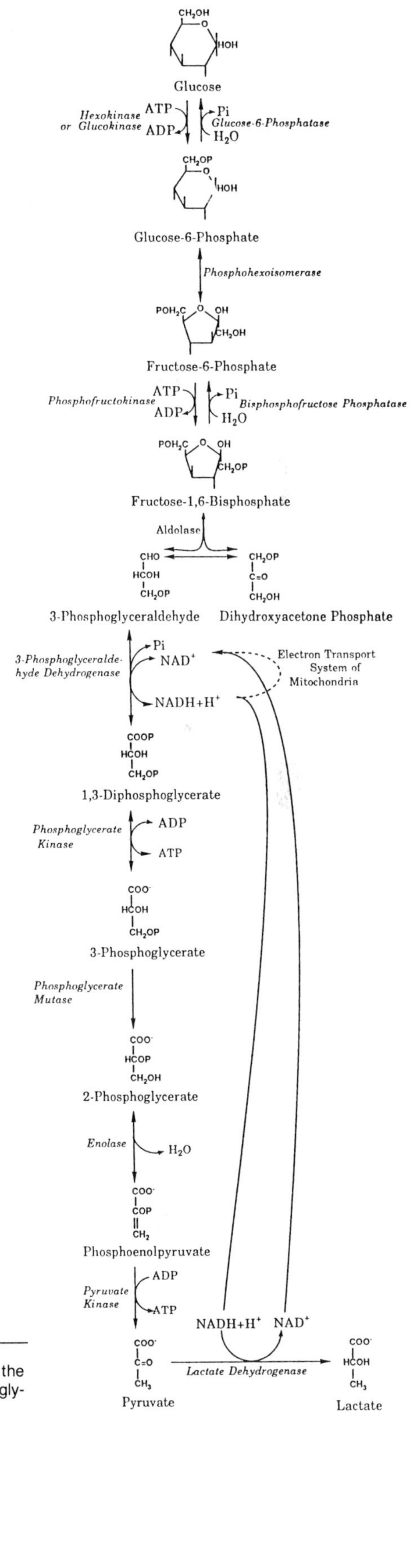

Glucose
Hexokinase or Glucokinase: ATP → ADP
Glucose-6-Phosphatase: H_2O → Pi
Glucose-6-Phosphate
Phosphohexoisomerase
Fructose-6-Phosphate
Phosphofructokinase: ATP → ADP
Bisphosphofructose Phosphatase: H_2O → Pi
Fructose-1,6-Bisphosphate
Aldolase
3-Phosphoglyceraldehyde ⇌ Dihydroxyacetone Phosphate
3-Phosphoglyceraldehyde Dehydrogenase: Pi, NAD^+ → $NADH+H^+$
Electron Transport System of Mitochondria
1,3-Diphosphoglycerate
Phosphoglycerate Kinase: ADP → ATP
3-Phosphoglycerate
Phosphoglycerate Mutase
2-Phosphoglycerate
Enolase: → H_2O
Phosphoenolpyruvate
Pyruvate Kinase: ADP → ATP
Pyruvate → Lactate (Lactate Dehydrogenase; $NADH+H^+$ → NAD^+)

Figure 24.6. Reaction of glycolysis. The NADH generated in the pathway is oxidized largely by the electron transport system of mitochondria (-----) or by lactate dehydrogenase during anaerobic glycolysis (———).

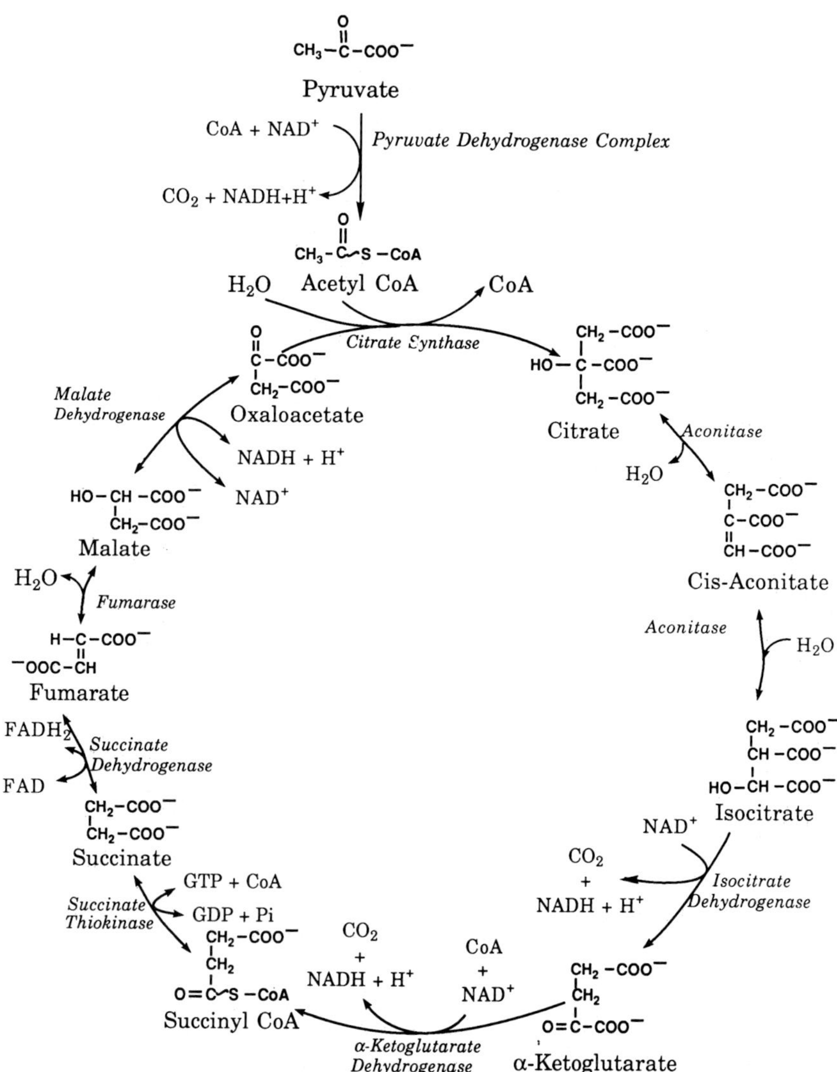

Figure 24.7. Oxidative decarboxylation of pyruvate and the citric acid cycle.

volves a third enzyme, dihydrolipoyl dehydrogenase, which catalyzes transfer of hydrogen atoms from the reduced lipoic acid to FAD attached to the enzyme. The fifth reaction involves the transfer of hydrogen atoms from $FADH_2$ to NAD^+, forming NADH and H^+. The NADH then may be oxidized by the electron-transport system.

Acetyl CoA is a versatile intermediary metabolite. In addition to being oxidized to CO_2 by the citric acid cycle (discussed in the next section), acetyl CoA may be used for formation of long-chain fatty acids, cholesterol, bile acids, steroid hormones, ketone bodies, and a variety of acetylated compounds.

Pyruvate dehydrogenase is regulated by phosphorylation-dephosphorylation. High ATP concentration decreases activity of pyruvate dehydrogenase by serving as a stimulatory modulator of pyruvate dehydrogenase kinase, which catalyzes phosphorylation of the dehydrogenase. An increase in free Ca^{2+} results in increased dephosphorylation by a phosphatase. Acetyl CoA, ATP, and NADH allosterically inhibit pyruvate dehydrogenase.

Citric acid cycle

The citric acid cycle (also known as the Krebs or tricarboxylic acid cycle) is confined to the matrix of mitochondria in respiring tissues of all animals. This cycle consists of a series of reactions that result in the oxidation of acetyl units to CO_2 with associated reduction of coenzymes. Transfer of reducing equivalents from these coenzymes to O_2 results in substantial amounts of ATP synthesis. The cycle (Fig. 24.7) is initiated by condensation of the acetyl unit of acetyl CoA with oxaloacetate to form citrate. Aconitate is an intermediate of citrate conversion to isocitrate. Isocitrate, an isomer of citrate, then is decarboxylated oxidatively to produce α-ketoglutarate, which subsequently is decarboxylated oxidatively by a mutlienzyme complex resembling that of the pyruvate dehydrogenase complex. The resulting succinyl CoA is converted to succinate, a process that generates guanosine triphosphate (GTP) from the energy-rich thioester linkage in succinyl CoA. Succinate is oxidized to fumarate, which then is hydrated to produce malate. Finally, malate is oxidized to oxaloacetate by malate dehydrogenase to complete the cycle. Significant quantities of this enzyme also exist in the cytosol.

In one "turn" of the citric acid cycle, two carbon atoms enter as the acetyl unit and two carbon atoms leave as CO_2, four pairs of hydrogen atoms (or electrons) are produced (three NAD^+ are reduced, one FAD is reduced), one high-energy phosphate bond (GTP) is generated by substrate-level phosphorylation, and two H_2O molecules are consumed. The GTP reacts with ADP to form ATP plus guanosine diphosphate.

Considerable energy in the form of ATP becomes available to the organism by oxidation of the NADH and $FADH_2$ produced by the oxidative reactions of the citric acid cycle. Unlike the glycolytic pathway, which can proceed aerobically or anaerobically, the continual flux of acetyl units through the citric acid cycle is dependent on electron transport to O_2 for reoxidation of the reduced coenzymes generated by reactions of the cycle. Oxidative phosphorylation coupled to transport of electron pairs of NADH and $FADH_2$ to O_2 results in formation of 11 moles of ATP per mole of acetyl CoA oxidized to 2 moles of CO_2. The net result is the formation of 12 moles of ATP (11 moles via oxidative phosphorylation, 1 mole from substrate-level phosphorylation) for each complete turn of the citric acid cycle, starting with acetyl CoA. Obviously, the citric acid cycle is of major importance in the production of ATP for cellular processes.

The oxidation of glucose to 6 CO_2 and 6 H_2O yields 36 or 38 ATP molecules as illustrated in Table 24.1. Assuming 36 ATP molecules per glucose, the P/O ratio of glucose oxidation by way of glycolysis through citric acid cycle is 3.0. The P/O ratio refers to moles (molecules) of phosphate used in ATP synthesis per one-half mole (one-half molecule) of oxygen (O_2) used. The corresponding free energy change for complete glucose oxidation is 686 kcal/mole. Therefore the overall efficiency of trapping useful chemical energy from glucose as ATP is 38 percent—(36 × 7.3/686) × 100. The *respiratory quotient (RQ)*, an index of metabolism defined as moles of CO_2 produced per mole of O_2 consumed, is 1.0 for oxidation of glucose to 6 CO_2. The RQ for fats and proteins is about 0.71 and 0.80, respectively. Thus the RQ of the whole body of an animal reflects relative use of carbohydrates, fats, and proteins for oxidative purposes.

The citric acid cycle is a central pathway that integrates total cellular metabolism. Both catabolism and anabolism of carbohydrates, lipids, and amino acids involve this vital aerobic reaction sequence. Acetyl CoA is derived from carbohydrate degradation, from oxidative breakdown of long-chain fatty acids, and from catabolism of ketone bodies and several amino acids. Oxaloacetate, fumarate, succinyl CoA, and α-ketoglutarate also are produced in the degradation of amino acids.

Table 24.1. ATP yield from oxidation of glucose to CO_2

Reaction sequence	ATP yield per glucose*
Glucose → glucose-6-phosphate	−1
Fructose-6-phosphate → fructose-1,6-bisphosphate	−1
1,3-Bisphosphoglycerate → 3-phosphoglycerate	+2
2 Phosphoenolpyruvate → 2 pyruvate	+2
Oxidation by electron transport system of:	
2 NADH formed by glycolysis assuming	
Glycerol phosphate shuttle or	+4
Malate-asparate shuttle	(+6)
2 NADH from 2 pyruvate → 2 acetyl CoA	+6
2 NADH from 2 isocitrate → 2 α-ketoglutarate	+6
2 NADH from 2 α-ketoglutarate → 2 succinyl CoA	+6
2 FADH from 2 succinate → 2 fumarate	+4
2 NADH from 2 malate → 2 oxaloacetate	+6
Succinyl CoA → 2 succinate (GTP)	+2
Net yield per glucose	36(38)

*Per molecule or per mole of glucose.

Several components of the citric acid cycle play vital anabolic roles, many of which are discussed also in Chapters 25 and 26. Oxaloacetate serves as a precursor of phosphoenolpyruvate in gluconeogenesis and is the carbon skeleton for aspartate and asparagine syntheses. Pyruvate, although not an intermediate of the citric acid cycle per se, serves as a carbon source for several amino acids. Citrate, when produced in greater than normal amounts, is transported from mitochondria and is cleaved to oxaloacetate (returns to mitochondria after reduction to malate) and acetyl CoA in the cytosol (used in synthesis of long-chain fatty acids and sterols). Succinyl CoA is involved in some acylation reactions and in biosynthesis of the porphyrin ring system of heme. α-Ketoglutarate is converted readily to glutamate, a precursor of several other amino acids. Biosynthesis of purine and pyrimidine nucleotides also involves compounds derived from the citric acid cycle.

Intermediates of the citric acid cycle that are "drawn off" for anabolic reactions must be replenished for continual cycle activity. This is accomplished by the pyruvate carboxylase-catalyzed reaction: pyruvate + CO_2 + ATP + H_2O → oxaloacetate + ADP + Pi + 2 H^+. Acetyl CoA present in excess allosterically activates pyruvate carboxylase to promote cycle activity. In addition to pyruvate carboxylation as a method of oxaloacetate replenishment (anaplerosis), the phosphoenolpyruvate carboxykinase-catalyzed reaction is important in skeletal and cardiac muscles: phosphoenolpyruvate + CO_2 + GDP → oxaloacetate + GTP. For gluconeogenesis, this reaction proceeds in reverse.

A variety of controls governs the citric acid cycle. The citric acid cycle is controlled at three sites: (1) concentration of acetyl CoA, as controlled by pyruvate dehydrogenase, regulates citrate formation, and ATP allosterically inhibits citrate synthase, (2) isocitrate dehydrogenase is stimulated allosterically by ADP but is inhibited by ATP and NADH, and (3) α-ketoglutarate dehydrogenase is inhibited by succinyl CoA, NADH, and ATP. The cyclic process is adjusted carefully to meet the need for ATP in the cell. For example, when the concentration of mitochondrial ATP is high, acceptance of acetyl CoA into the cycle is decreased.

Pentose phosphate pathway

The combined glycolysis and citric acid cycle reactions in association with reactions of the oxidative phosphorylation system are largely responsible for ATP production from carbohydrates. Another type of metabolic energy, namely, reducing potential as NADPH, is required for reductive biosyntheses. The major metabolic system used for generation of NADPH, and also of ribose-5-phosphate, is called the pentose phosphate pathway. The pathway also is called hexose monphosphate shunt, pentose shunt, or phosphogluconate pathway. Enzymes for the pathway are in cytosol of those cells in which this process is important, including liver, adipose tissue, mammary gland (particularly during lactation), adrenal gland, erythrocytes, and the cornea and lens of the eye. As much as 30 percent of glucose oxidation to CO_2 in the liver occurs by way of the pentose phosphate pathway during highly lipogenic situations; the percentage can be even greater in adipocytes. Enzymes of the pathway are virtually absent in skeletal muscle.

In the pentose phosphate pathway (Fig. 24.8), NADPH is generated by the oxidative conversion of G-6-P to gluconolactone-6-phosphate and of gluconate-6-phosphate to ribulose-5-phosphate. The pentose phosphate pathway also involves nonoxidative interconversion of four-, five-, six-, and seven-carbon sugars. Recycling of ribulose-5-phosphate to G-6-P, as indicated in Fig. 24.8, allows for complete oxidation of G-6-P to CO_2 with the concomitant generation of NADPH. The stoichiometric description of the pathway, written as a cycle as in Fig. 24.8, is as follows: G-6-P + 12 $NADP^+$ + 7 $H_2O \rightarrow$ 6 CO_2 + 12 NADPH + 12 H^+ + Pi. The NADPH serves primarily in biosynthesis of long-chain fatty acids and cholesterol, in hydroxylation of fatty acids and steroids, and in maintaining a cellular pool of reduced glutathione, as in erythrocytes. Glutathione

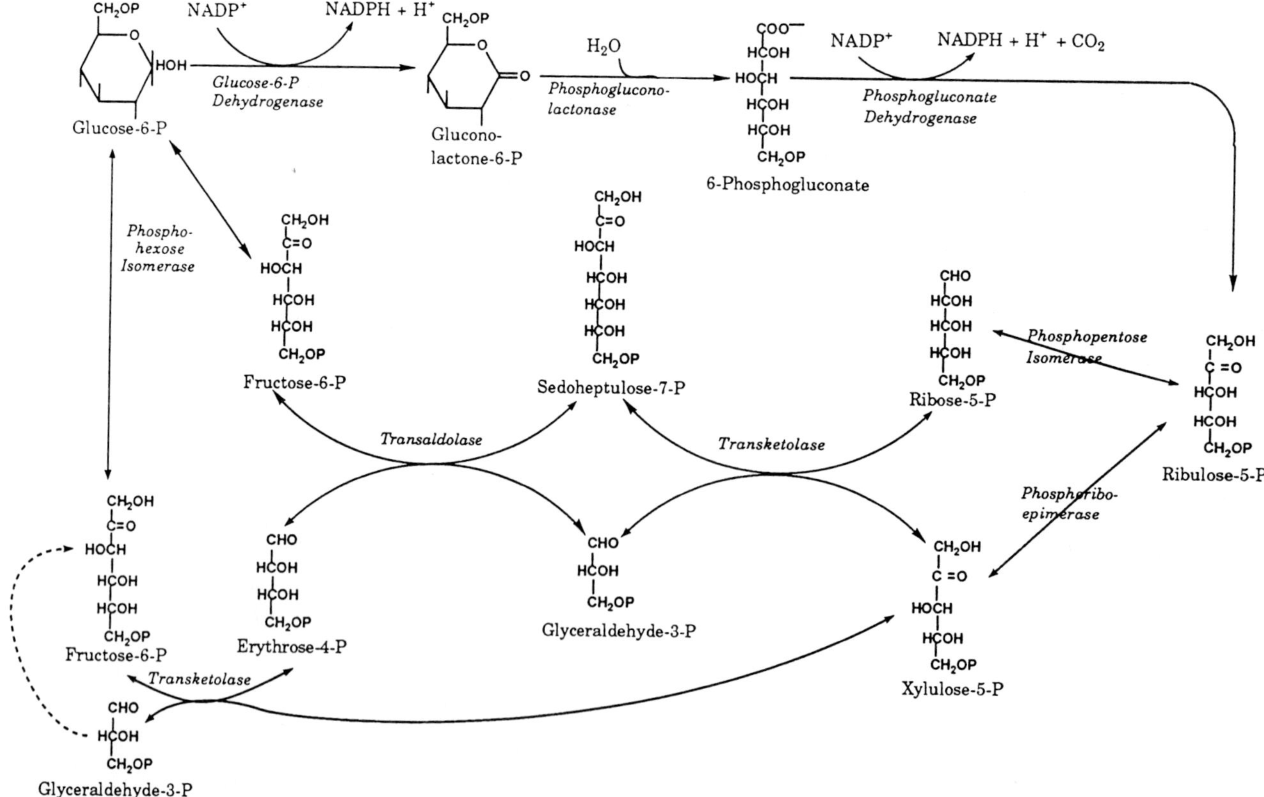

Figure 24.8. Pentose phosphate pathway. Broken line indicates that a second glyceraldehyde-3-P isomerizes to form dihydroxyacetone-P and the glyceraldehyde-3-P and dihydroxyacetone-P combine to form fructose-1,6-bisphosphate, which is converted to fructose-6-phosphate (see Fig. 24.6).

peroxidase catalyzes the oxidation of reduced glutathione by H_2O_2, and glutathione reductase catalyzes reduction of oxidized glutathione by NADPH. Because accumulation of H_2O_2 may decrease the life span of erythrocytes, pentose phosphate cycle activity and fragility of erythrocytes are related inversely.

When more ribose-5-phosphate than NADPH is needed, G-6-P is converted by way of the glycolytic pathway to fructose-6-phosphate and 3-phosphoglyceraldehyde; transketolase and transaldolase then convert these products to ribose-5-phosphate by reversal of the nonoxidative phase of the pathway according to the following stoichiometric formula: 5 G-6-P + ATP $\rightarrow$ 6 ribose-5-phosphate + ADP + H^+. Ribose-5-phosphate is a key intermediate in the formation of several important biomolecules such as NAD^+, CoA, ATP, FAD, RNA, and DNA.

Regulation of the pentose phosphate pathway involves primarily the irreversible and rate-limiting dehydrogenation of G-6-P. The supply of $NADP^+$ is the most important regulator. Also, NADPH acts as a competitive inhibitor for G-6-P dehydrogenase.

Gluconeogenesis

Gluconeogenesis, glucose synthesis from noncarbohydrate compounds, provides for the glucose needs of the body when dietary carbohydrate is insufficient. Clearly, gluconeogenesis assumes increasing importance during fasting when liver glycogen becomes depleted. A continual supply of glucose ($\sim$160 g/day for the human) is necessary as a source of energy, especially for the nervous system ($\sim$120 g of glucose per day for the human) and erythrocytes, as a source of acylglycerol-glycerol, and for anaplerosis. Also, skeletal muscle functioning under anaerobic conditions requires glucose as a fuel source. Glucose is needed for lactose synthesis during lactation and is actively taken up by the fetus. The animal body has the enzymatic machinery in the liver to ensure a continual supply of glucose by glucose synthesis. Gluconeogenic pathways also provide a mechanism for clearance from blood of lactate produced by muscles and erythrocytes and of glycerol produced by adipose tissue. The liver is the principal organ responsible for gluconeogenesis. Some occurs in the cortex of the kidney, and the importance of the cortex as a site of gluconeogenesis increases during fasting situations.

Gluconeogenesis is not a simple reversal of glycolysis because of the essential irreversibility of three glycolytic reactions: (1) glucose to G-6-P, (2) fructose-6-phosphate to fructose-1,6-bisphosphate, and (3) phosphoenolpyruvate to pyruvate. Moreover, glycolysis is a highly exergonic process.

Circumvention of these virtually irreversible reactions is accomplished by (1) conversion of pyruvate to phosphoenolpyruvate by way of oxaloacetate, (2) hydrolysis of fructose-1,6-bisphosphate to form fructose-6-phosphate, and (3) hydrolysis of G-6-P to produce glucose (Fig. 24.9). Because of the presence of pyruvate carboxylase in the mitochondria, pyruvate is transported into the mitochondria for carboxylation and returns to cytosol as malate in the course of the gluconeogenic process in most species. In those species, such as the rabbit and chicken, in which the phosphoenolpyruvate carboxykinase is in the mitochondria rather than in the cytosol, the phosphoenolpyruvate synthesized from oxaloacetate is returned to the cytosol. The balance of the reactions of gluconeogenesis occurs in the cytosol, and they are reversible reactions common to glycolysis. Glucose-6-phosphatase, bound to endoplasmic reticulum, is present only in those tissues (liver, kidney, and intestinal epithelium) that provide glucose to blood.

The corresponding glycolytic reactions paired with each of the three sets of unique reactions of gluconeogenesis illustrated in Fig. 24.9 represent substrate or futile cycling. For example, the sum of the hexokinase- and glucose-6-phosphatase-catalyzed reactions is ATP + $H_2O \rightarrow$ ADP + Pi. Thus this and other substrate cycles are potentially important heat generators. During most physiological situations, however, futile cycling is minimized by regulatory metabolites.

A total of six high-energy phosphate bonds and two NADHs is expended in the gluconeogenic conversion of two pyruvates to glucose. The ATPs are required to shift the energetically unfavorable process (direct reversal of glycolysis) to a favorable one (gluconeogenesis). During periods of gluconeogenesis, the ATP for gluconeogenesis most frequently is derived from the oxidation of fatty acids.

Gluconeogenesis is controlled at the enzyme level primarily at two reaction steps. First, pyruvate carboxylase is virtually inactive in the absence of acetyl CoA, its positive allosteric activator. Thus accumulation of mitochondrial acetyl CoA, such as from fatty acid oxidation, promotes gluconeogenesis. Furthermore, acetyl CoA will inhibit pyruvate dehydrogenase to diminish futile cycling. Second, fructose-1,6-bisphosphatase is strongly inhibited by AMP and fructose-2,6-bisphosphate. Again, futile cycling at this stage is minimized because AMP and fructose-2,6-bisphosphate stimulate phosphofructokinase.

The chief gluconeogenic substances in monogastric animals are the amino acids. Most amino acids may be converted to α-keto acids by deamination and transamination reactions (see Chap. 26). Pyruvate, oxaloacetate, and α-ketoglutarate are converted to glucose by the gluconeogenic reactions illustrated in Fig. 24.9. In addition, several nitrogen-free compounds derived from amino acids by deamination may be converted to one of these three α-keto acids and thus serve as carbohydrate precursors.

Lactate produced in active skeletal muscle and erythrocytes also is an important gluconeogenic compound. After transport to the liver by blood, lactate is oxidized to pyruvate and subsequently converted to glucose. The overall process of lactate production in muscle, conversion to glu-

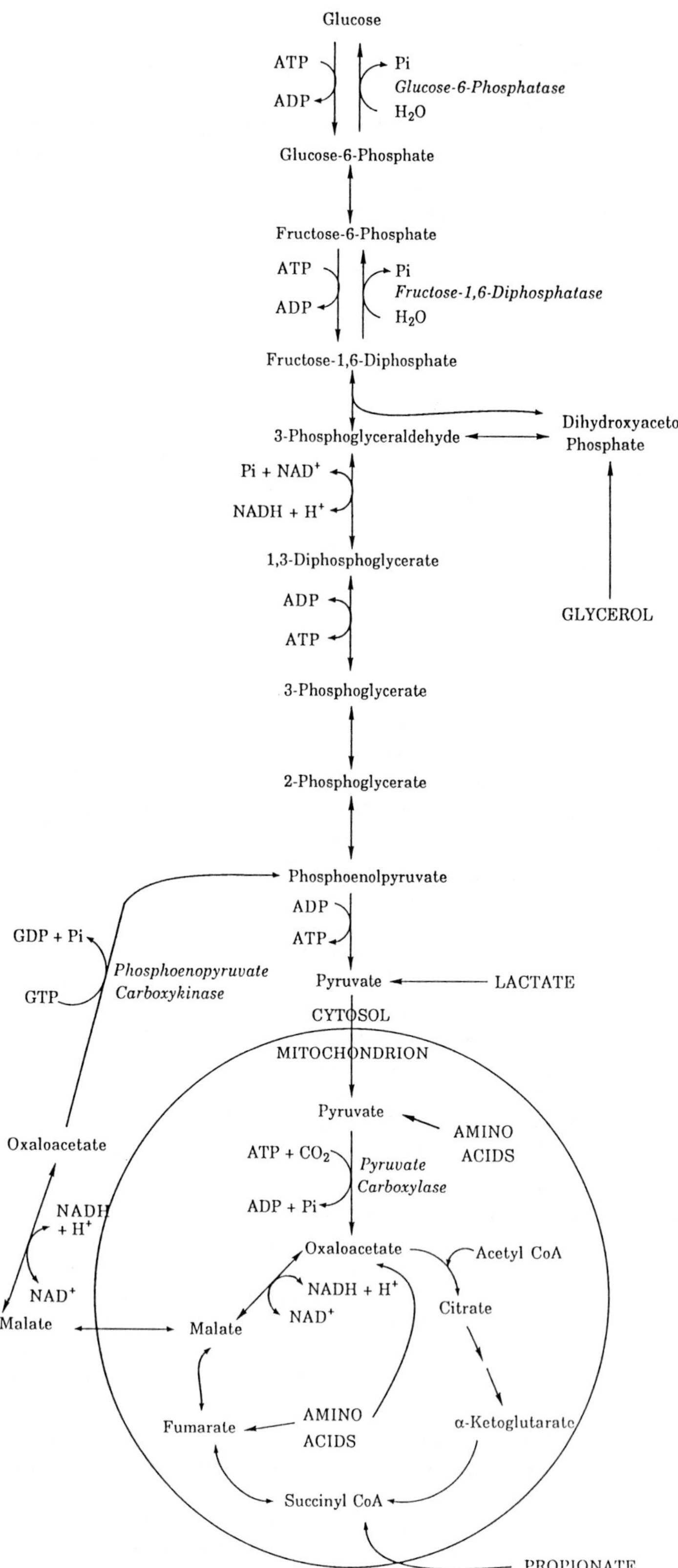

Figure 24.9. Pathway for gluconeogenesis. Names of enzymes of gluconeogenesis that are unique from reversal of glycolysis are indicated. All reactants of every reaction are not indicated.

$$\text{Propionate + ATP + CoA} \xrightarrow[\textit{Acyl CoA synthase}]{} \text{propionyl CoA}$$

$$\text{Propionyl CoA + ATP + } CO_2 + H_2O \xrightarrow[\textit{Propionyl CoA carboxylase}]{} \text{D-methylmalonyl CoA + ADP + Pi}$$

$$\text{D-Methylmalonyl CoA} \underset{\textit{Methylmalonyl CoA racemase}}{\rightleftharpoons} \text{L-methylmalonyl CoA}$$

$$\text{L-Methylmalonyl CoA} \underset{\textit{Methylmalonyl CoA mutase}}{\rightleftharpoons} \text{succinyl CoA}$$

$$\text{Succinyl CoA} \rightarrow \rightarrow \text{oxaloacetate} \rightarrow \rightarrow \text{glucose}$$

Figure 24.10. Conversion of propionate to glucose. See Fig. 24.9 for elaboration of the reactions within the last sequence.

cose in the liver, and return of glucose to muscle is called the Cori cycle.

Glycerol derived from acylglycerol hydrolysis may be converted to glucose; glycerol, however, is of minor significance as a precursor of carbohydrate. Glycerol is phosphorylated by glycerol kinase, which is located primarily in the liver, to form 3-glycerol phosphate. A specific dehydrogenase then catalyzes the dehydrogenation of the glycerol phosphate to form NAD^+ and dihydroxyacetone phosphate, which is a glycolytic intermediate.

Propionate and other odd-carbon fatty acids are glucogenic. Carbon atoms are removed, two at a time, from the longer odd-carbon fatty acids by beta oxidation, finally resulting in formation of propionyl CoA. Propionyl CoA is converted to succinate by the CO_2 fixation and molecular rearrangement reactions depicted in Fig. 24.10. In ruminant animals, gluconeogenesis is of continual importance because most dietary carbohydrates are fermented primarmily to VFAs in the alimentary tract, and the propionate and the lesser amounts of valerate contribute to glucose synthesis in the liver. Propionate, including that produced by oxidation of valerate, is converted to glucose in the ruminant liver according to reactions summarized in Fig. 24.9. Acetyl CoA is not glucogenic because it cannot be converted to pyruvate.

Glucuronic acid pathway

The glucuronic acid pathway consists of a number of reactions whereby glucose is converted to glucuronic acid, ascorbic acid, and pentose intermediates. This pathway, which is located primarily in the liver, also is an alternative oxidative pathway for glucose. Without stating all intermediates, G-6-P is converted to UDPG. After two oxidation steps involving NAD^+, UDP-glucuronate is formed to function in the synthesis of chondroitin sulfate or of conjugates (glucuronides) of steroid hormones, certain drugs, or bilirubin. Alternatively, the UDP-glucuronate may form glucuronate and then L-gulonate. Except in humans, guinea pigs, and many fishes, gulonate is converted to ascorbate. Gulonate also may be decarboxylated oxidatively to generate L-xylulose, which ultimately enters the pentose phosphate pathway as D-xylulose-5-phosphate. To complete a cycle, G-6-P would be regenerated. Important physiological functions of reactions of this pathway include synthesis of ascorbic acid or vitamin C, drug detoxification and excretion, secretion of bilirubin into the small intestine via the bile, synthesis of uronic acids for glycoprotein and proteoglycan synthesis, and synthesis of pentoses and pentose derivatives.

Catabolism of nonglucose hexoses

Fructose, galactose, and mannose are other significant hexoses of animal metabolism. Relationship of their metabolism to that of glucose is shown in Fig. 24.11. After transport of dietary fructose to the liver, fructose-1-phosphate is formed by action of fructokinase. An aldolase then forms dihydroxyacetone phosphate and D-glyceraldehyde. The major pathway for glyceraldehyde is formation of 3-phosphoglyceraldehyde by triose kinase. In humans, much dietary fructose is converted to glucose in intestinal mucosal cells. Free fructose is present in seminal plasma and fetal blood of ungulates and whales. The source of this fructose is glucose by way of sorbitol as an intermediate.

Galactose, which may be derived from dietary lactose or milk sugar after hydrolysis by lactase (β-galactosidase), is converted readily into glucose in the liver. First, galactose is phosphorylated to galactose-1-phosphate by galactokinase. After reaction with UDPG, UDP-galactose and G-1-P are formed by galactose-1-phosphate uridyl transferase, an enzyme that is deficient in galactosemic patients. Next, epimerization at C-4 results in production of UDPG, which then can be converted to G-6-P, a glycolytic inter-

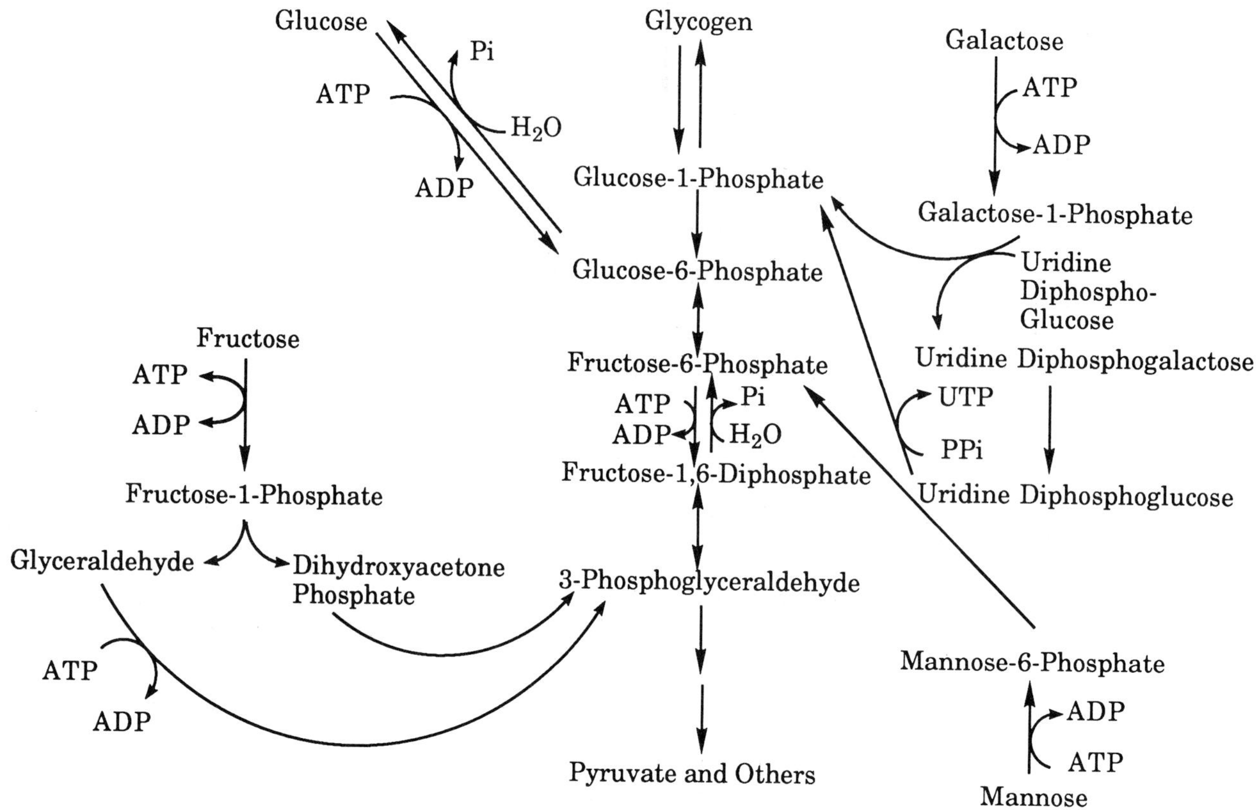

Figure 24.11. Interrelations of fructose, galactose, glucose, and mannose metabolism.

mediate. Reversal of this epimerization reaction results in formation of UDP-galactose from UDP-glucose, a necessary reaction for lactose synthesis in the lactating mammary gland. Insufficient lactase in the small intestine results in greater fermentation of lactose by intestinal organisms and thus greater gas and VFA production and diarrhea, as in lactose intolerance in humans.

Lactose synthesis in mammary glands occurs by way of formation of an α-1,4 bond between the galactose of UDP-galactose and free glucose by lactose synthetase. Lactose synthesis by a lactating animal is quantitatively highly significant. For example, production of 50 kg of milk daily by a dairy cow requires synthesis of 2.4 kg of lactose daily.

Mannose, absorbed after digestion of different polysaccharides and glycoproteins of foods, is phosphorylated largely in liver by hexokinase to form mannose-6-phosphate. Fructose-6-phosphate is formed by isomerization of the mannose-6-phosphate.

Synthesis of complex carbohydrates

Hexoses undergo a variety of reactions, including amination, acetylation, and epimerization, for synthesis of the monomer units that are used for synthesis of a variety of complex polysaccharides as illustrated in Fig. 24.12. Amino sugars are distributed widely throughout the animal body as part of the structural elements of tissue. Glycoproteins and proteoglycans are molecules of protein to which oligosaccharides or polysaccharides are attached covalently. The polysaccharide or glycosaminoglycan of proteoglycans consists of repeating disaccharide units in which D-glucosamine or D-galactosamine is present. Furthermore, most disaccharide units contain a uronic acid and sulfate groups. One example of a glycosaminoglycan is hyaluronic acid, which occurs in synovial fluid, vitreous humor, umbilical cord, skin, and bone. This polymer consists of alternating units of glucuronate and *N*-acetylglucosamine. Other glycosaminoglycans containing glucuronate and *N*-acetylgalactosamine are the sulfates of chondroitin, dermatan, heparin, and keratin and are found in association with protein in cartilage, large blood vessels, tendons, heart valves, mucus, and skin. Amino sugars are also constituents of glycoproteins, which include several enzymes, hormones, blood group substances (agglutinins), collagen, interferons, and immunoglobulins.

Metabolism of volatile fatty acids

Ruminants (e.g., cattle, sheep, and goats) and pseudorumimants (e.g., horses and rabbits) rely extensively on

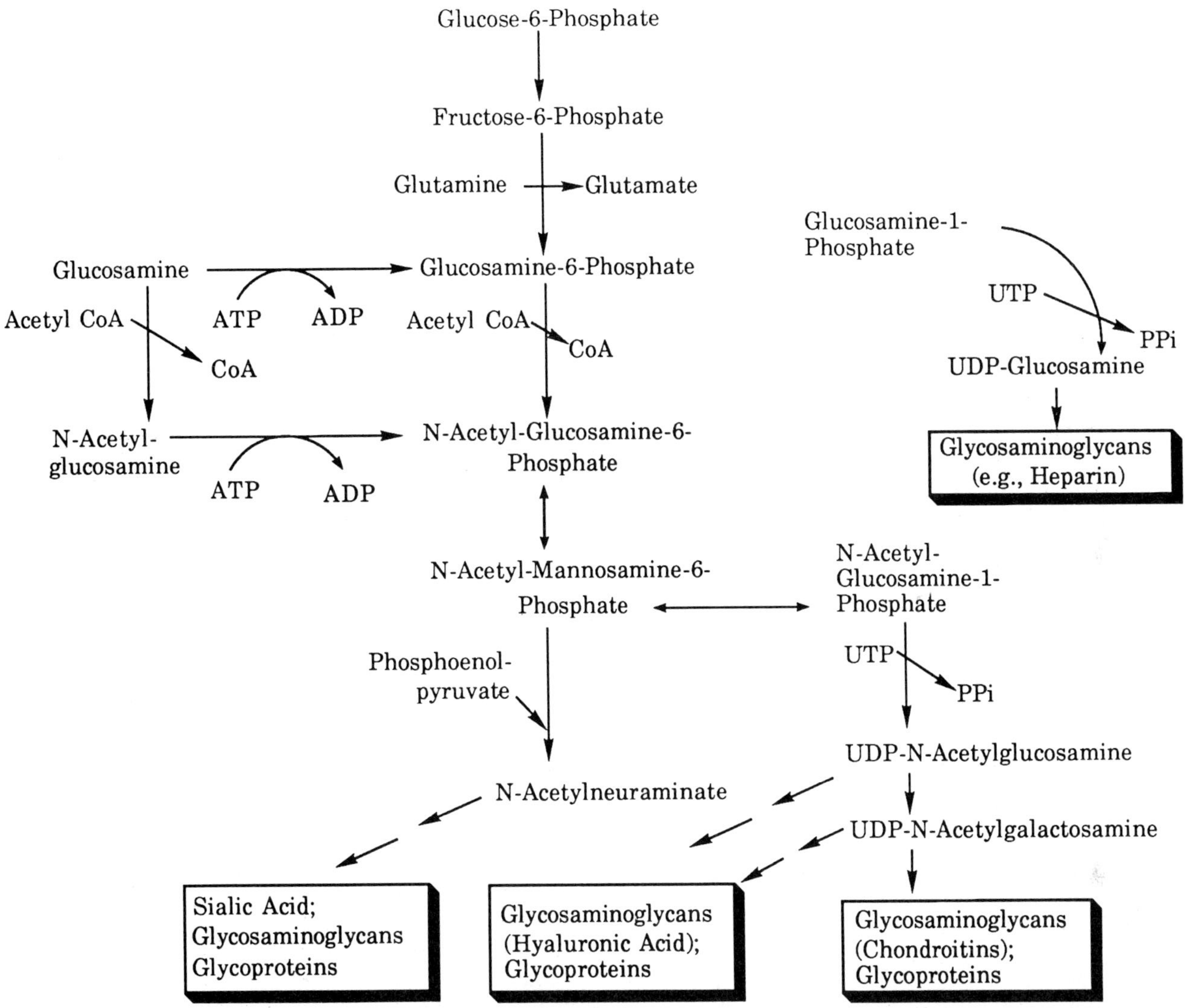

Figure 24.12. Synthesis of several complex carbohydrates from common intermediates.

the production of acetate, propionate, butyrate, and valerate by anaerobic fermentation of dietary carbohydrates and other feed constituents within the rumen and the cecum. Lesser production of the same end products occurs via fermentation in the large intestine of all animals. Depending on diet composition, VFAs may contribute up to 80 percent of the total energy needed by a ruminant. Because fermentation is usually extensive, a dairy cow, for example, usually has available for absorption from the small intestine less than 10 percent of her daily glucose requirement and thus must rely extensively on gluconeogenesis to meet this glucose need. The production of VFAs from dietary carbohydrates and their subsequent utilization is depicted in Fig. 24.13.

Other dietary constituents also contribute carbon for VFA synthesis. For example, when cellulose rather than starch is the major dietary carbohydrate for cattle, acetate is the major VFA produced. Increasing the proportion of starch will increase ruminal production of propionate and valerate and decrease production of acetate and butyrate. In addition to production of the VFAs, the fermentation of dietary constituents by numerous species of bacteria and protozoa in the digestive tracts of animals results in production of CO_2 and methane. These two gases are lost to the environment, whereas the VFAs are efficiently absorbed and transported via the portal circulatory system to the liver.

Before the VFAs are metabolized by tissues, they must be activated by specific synthases according to the following reaction: VFA + CoASH + ATP → VFA CoA + AMP

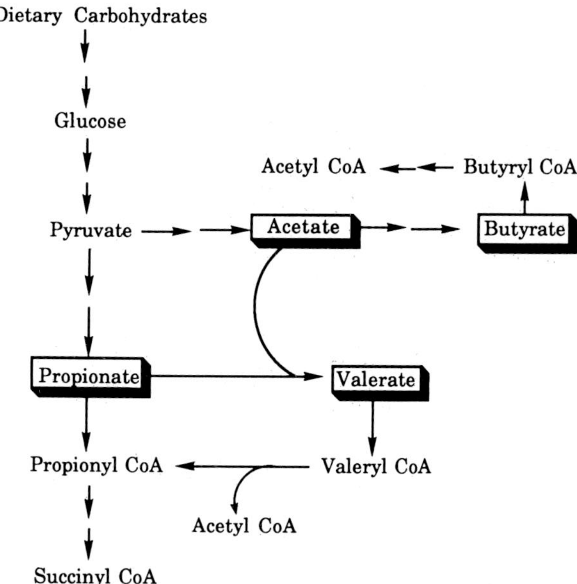

Figure 24.13. Summary of volatile fatty acid metabolism. Acetate, propionate, butyrate, and valerate (in boxes) are the primary end products of microbial fermentation and are absorbed from the digestive tract and converted to acetyl CoA and succinyl CoA by animal tissues for subsequent metabolism.

+ PPi. The liver efficiently removes the propionate, butyrate, and valerate from portal blood, but much acetate passes through the liver to peripheral tissues for subsequent metabolism. Propionate is a major precursor for glucose synthesis in the liver. Approximately half of the butyrate absorbed through the rumen wall is converted to β-hydroxybutyrate, which is metabolized by peripheral tissues rather than by liver.

REFERENCES

Beitner, R. 1985. *Regulation of Carbohydrate Metabolism.* Vol. I and II. CRC Press, Inc. Boca Raton, Fla.

Blaxter, K. 1989. *Energy Metabolism in Animals and Man.* Cambridge University Press, Cambridge.

Fahey, G.C., Jr., and Berger, L.L. 1988. Carbohydrate nutrition in the ruminant. In D.C. Church, ed., *The Ruminant Animal: Digestive Physiology and Nutrition.* Prentice Hall, New Jersey. Pp. 269–97.

Hatefic, Y. 1985. The mitochondrial electron transport and oxidative phosphorylation system. *Annu. Rev. Biochem.* 54:1015–70.

Hems, D.A., and Whitton, P.D. 1981. Control of hepatic glycogenolysis. *Physiol. Rev.* 60:2–38.

Jequier, E., Acheson, K., and Schutz, Y. 1987. Assessment of energy expenditure and fuel utilization in man. *Annu. Rev. Nutr.* 7:187–208.

Larner, J. 1990. Insulin and the synthesis of glycogen synthesis: The road from glycogen structure to glycogen synthase to cyclic AMP-dependent protein kinase to insulin mediators. *Adv. Enzymol.* 63:173–231.

Lindahl, V., and Höök, M. 1978. Glycosaminoglycans and their binding to biological macromolecules. *Annu. Rev. Biochem.* 47:385–417.

Martin, B.R. 1987. *Metabolic Regulation: A Molecular Approach.* Blackwell Scientific Publications, Boston.

Martin, C.R. 1985. *Endocrine Physiology.* Oxford University Press, New York.

Marshall, R.D. 1972. Glycoproteins. *Annu. Rev. Biochem.* 41:673–702.

McGarry, J.D., Kuwajima, M., Newgard, C.B., and Foster, D.W. 1987. From dietary glucose to liver glycogen: The full circle. *Annu. Rev. Nutr.* 7:51–73.

Mela-Riker, L.M., and Bukoski, R.D. 1985. Regulation of mitochondrial activity in cardiac cells. *Annu. Rev. Physiol.* 47:645–63.

Newsholme, E.A., Chaliss, R.A.J., and Crabtree, B. 1984. Substrate cycles: Their role in improving metabolic control. *Trends Biochem. Sci.* 9:277–80.

Pilkis, S.J., El-Maghrabi, M.R., and Claus, T.H. 1988. Hormonal regulation of hepatic glyconeogenesis and glycolysis. *Annu. Rev. Biochem.* 57:755–84.

Randle, P.J., Steiner, D.F., and Whelan, W.F. 1981. *Carbohydrate Metabolism and Its Disorders,* Vol. 3. Academic Press, Inc., New York.

Roehrig, K.L. 1985. *Carbohydrate Biochemistry and Metabolism.* AVI Publishing Co., Inc. Westport, Conn.

VanSchaftingen, E.V. 1986. Fructose 2,6-biphosphate. *Adv. Enzymol.* 59:315–95.

Wheeler, T.J., and Hinkle, P.C. 1985. The glucose transporter of mammalian cells. *Annu. Rev. Physiol.* 47:503–17.

Williamson, J.R., and Cooper, R.H. 1980. Regulation of the citric acid cycle in mammalian systems. *FEBS Lett.* 117:K73–K85.

Wood, T. 1985. *The Pentose Phosphate Pathway.* Academic Press, Inc. New York.

Young, J.W. 1977. Gluconeogenesis in cattle: Significance and methodology. *J. Dairy Sci.* 60:1–15.

CHAPTER 25

Lipid Metabolism | by Donald C. Beitz

Lipids in animals are those compounds that are relatively insoluble in water and are soluble in nonpolar solvents, such as diethyl ether and chloroform. Lipids to be discussed are those related to fatty acids and include triacylglycerols (formerly triglycerides), cholesterol, steroids, phospholipids, sphingolipids, and eicosanoids. Ketone bodies that are incomplete oxidation products of fatty acids will be discussed also. Lipids function in at least five ways in an animal body. Two readily evident roles of lipids are (1) in the oxidation of fatty acids to CO_2 as a major means of metabolic energy production and (2) as necessary constituents (most notably the phospholipids and sphingolipids) of cell membranes. In addition, other quantitatively less important but functionally significant roles include the use of surface-active properties of some complex lipids for maintenance of lung alveolar integrity and for solubilization of nonpolar compounds in body fluids. Also, like eicosanoids and steroid hormones, lipids play physiologically important regulatory roles in metabolism.

An overview of lipid metabolism in animals is presented in Fig. 25.1. The diet contains fuel molecules that can provide fatty acids from acylglycerols or acetyl CoA from carbohydrates, amino acids, or ethanol. Fatty acids may be oxidized to acetyl CoA and to CO_2, or they may be used in the synthesis of eicosanoids, triacylglycerols, phospholipids, or sphingolipids. Acetyl CoA may be used for synthesis of cholesterol and other steroids, ketone bodies, or fatty acids. Ketone bodies and fatty acids may be oxidized to acetyl CoA and to CO_2.

LIPID TRANSPORT AND DEPOSITION

During absorption of dietary or endogenous lipids from the gastrointestinal tract (see Chap. 19), most lipids enter the lacteals as chylomicrons along with some very-low-density lipoproteins (VLDLs). These complexes are formed in the intestinal mucosal cells and consist largely of a central core of triacylglycerols. The core also contains all of the cholesteryl esters and some free cholesterol, whereas the lipoprotein envelope consists largely of phospholipids along with some protein (apolipoprotein) and free cholesterol. This envelope undergoes compositional change by exchange with lipids and proteins in the extracellular fluids. The lymph carrying intestinally derived lipoproteins enters the systemic blood by way of the thoracic lymph duct. The short- and medium-chain fatty acids and the free glycerol resulting from complete hydrolysis of triacylglycerols within the intestinal lumen are absorbed into portal blood and thereby are transported directly to the liver.

Blood plasma lipids

Lipids in blood plasma may arise from intestinal absorption of ingested lipids, mobilization of lipids from storage in adipose tissue, or synthetic processes. Most plasma lipids are present as chylomicrons and other higher-density lipoproteins. In addition, nonesterified or free fatty acids are transported as a complex of fatty acid and albumin. Properties of the major plasma lipoproteins are summarized in Table 25.1. The relative proportions of the different

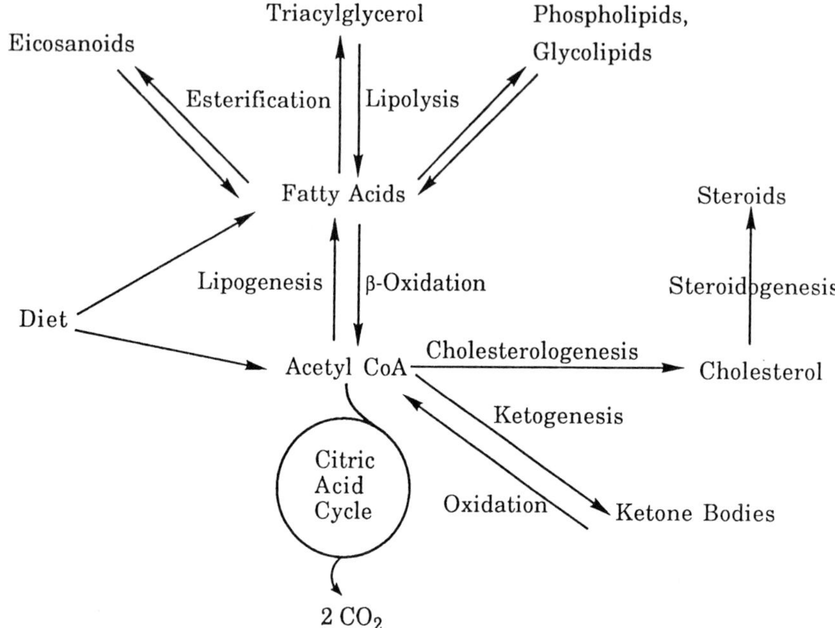

Figure 25.1. Overview of lipid metabolism.

classes of lipoproteins and, to a lesser extent, the composition of different classes of lipoproteins vary among different animal species. For example, most plasma cholesterol in cattle is contained in high-density lipoproteins (HDLs) whereas most of the cholesterol in humans is contained in the low-density lipoproteins (LDLs).

Large differences in plasma lipid components exist among species and among individuals within species. Factors that influence plasma lipid concentrations include quantity and type of dietary lipid, time after consumption of food, health and age of the animal, and hormone balance. The cholesterol/cholesteryl ester and the cholesterol/phospholipid ratios tend to be relatively constant within a given animal species. These ratios seem to be under hepatic control, whereas triacylglycerol concentrations can vary greatly, depending in large part on dietary intake, storage in or mobilization from adipose tissues, and synthesis in the liver.

Under normal conditions, concentrations of nonesterified fatty acids are considerably below those of other plasma lipids. Fatty acids are released to plasma from adipose triacylglycerol through the action of hormone-

Table 25.1. Composition of lipoproteins of human plasma

				Composition						
						Percentage of total lipid†				
Fraction*	Source	Diameter (nm)	Density (g/ml)	Protein (%)†	Total lipid (%)†	Triacylglycerol	Phospholipid	Cholesteryl ester	Cholesterol	Nonesterified fatty acids
Chylomicrons	Intestine	100–1000	<0.960	1–2	98–99	88	8	3	1	—
VLDL	Liver and intestine	30–90	0.960–1.006	7–10	90–93	56	20	15	8	1
IDL	VLDL and chylomicrons	25–30	1.006–1.019	11	89	29	26	34	9	1
LDL	VLDL and chylomicrons	20–25	1.019–1.063	21	79	13	28	48	10	1
HDL_2	Liver and intestines, VLDL? chylomicrons?	10–20	1.063–1.125	33	67	16	43	31	10	—
HDL_3	Liver and intestines, VLDL? chylomicrons?	7.5–10	1.125–1.210	57	43	13	46	29	6	6
Albumin-free fatty acid	Adipose tissue		>1.281	99	1	0	0	0	0	100

*VLDL, very-low-density lipoproteins; IDL, intermediate-density lipoproteins; LDL, low-density lipoproteins; and HDL, high-density lipoproteins.
†Expressed on a weight basis.
Modified from Murray, Granner, Mayes, and Rodwell, 1988, *Harper's Biochemistry,* 21st ed., Appleton & Lange, Norwalk, Conn.

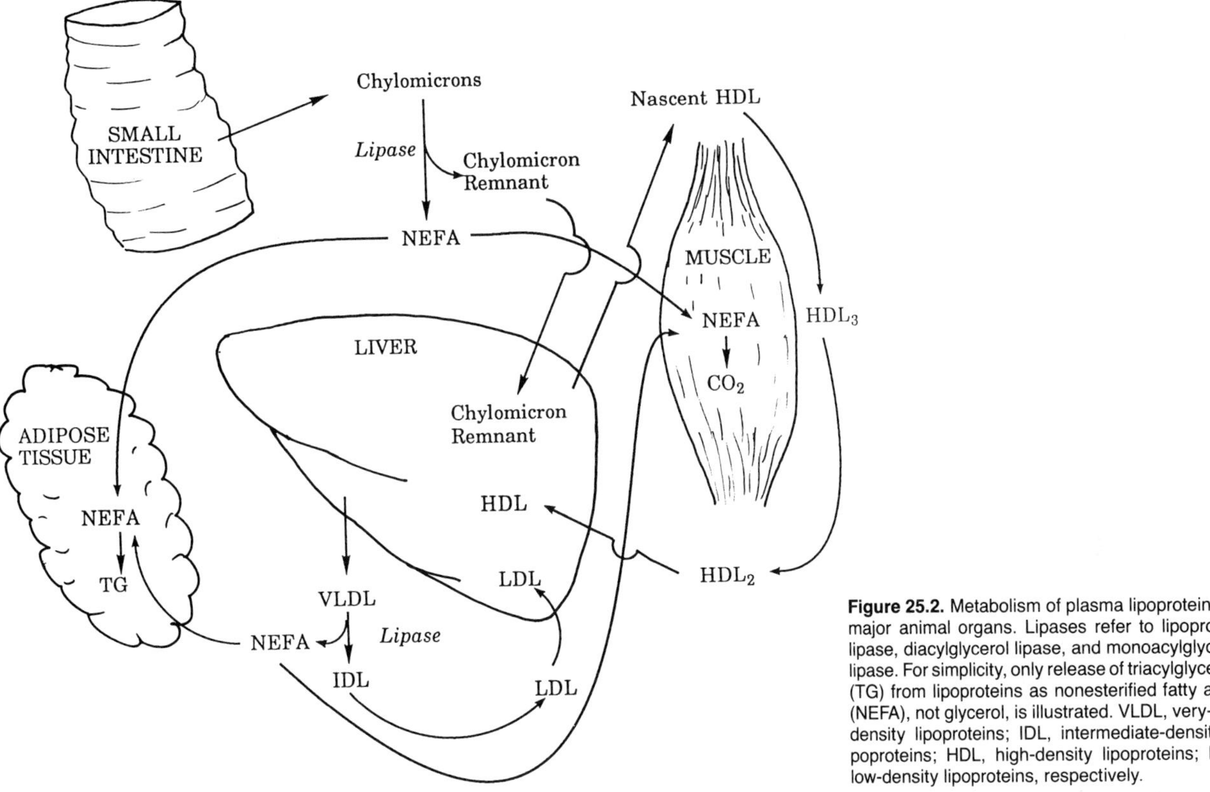

Figure 25.2. Metabolism of plasma lipoproteins by major animal organs. Lipases refer to lipoprotein lipase, diacylglycerol lipase, and monoacylglycerol lipase. For simplicity, only release of triacylglycerols (TG) from lipoproteins as nonesterified fatty acids (NEFA), not glycerol, is illustrated. VLDL, very-low-density lipoproteins; IDL, intermediate-density lipoproteins; HDL, high-density lipoproteins; LDL, low-density lipoproteins, respectively.

sensitive lipase. The fatty acids then physically bind to plasma albumin and are transported to the heart, skeletal muscles, liver, and other tissues for oxidation or conversion to other lipids. Although the concentrations of plasma nonesterified fatty lipids are low, their turnover rates are extremely rapid (1 to 3 minutes in most species). Whereas the heart uses these acids as a significant source of energy, the brain seems unable to use the nonesterified fatty acids for generation of adenosine triphosphate (ATP) but does incorporate unesterified fatty acids into its polar lipids.

Transport and storage

A simplified scheme for the transport and storage of lipids is presented in Fig. 25.2. Individual reactions within tissue cells are discussed below. Chylomicron triacylglycerols are removed rapidly from plasma by extrahepatic tissues and, to only a limited extent, by the liver. The mechanism in extrahepatic tissues involves a hydrolytic enzyme, lipoprotein lipase, which is anchored to the luminal side of the capillary wall with proteoglycan chains called heparan sulfate and functions extracellularly. This enzyme is found in adipose tissue, heart and skeletal muscles, the diaphragm, the lactating mammary gland, the spleen, the lung, and the kidney medulla but not in the brain. Intravenous injection of heparin releases lipoprotein lipase into the circulation, which results in a more rapid clearing of lipemia. Both phospholipids and apolipoprotein C-II are cofactors for lipoprotein lipase. Both cofactors plus the substrate are constituents of chylomicrons and of the VLDLs. Triacylglycerols within lipoproteins are hydrolyzed progressively to diacylglycerol and monoacylglycerol; the latter is hydrolyzed by a separate monoacylglycerol hydrolase, which circulates primarily in plasma. Some released fatty acids and glycerol return to plasma, but most fatty acids enter intercellular spaces and are absorbed by tissue cells.

Actions of lipoprotein lipase on chylomicrons result in loss of about 90 percent of triacylglycerols and loss of apolipoprotein C, which associates with HDLs. The chylomicron remnant then is taken up by the liver through apolipoprotein E-specific, receptor-mediated endocytosis.

The VLDLs, synthesized primarily within the liver and to a lesser extent in the small intestine, transport triacylglycerol to extrahepatic tissues, where hydrolysis of triacylglycerol occurs through the action of lipoprotein lipase. The liberated fatty acids are absorbed rapidly and are esterified or oxidized by the tissues. Liberation of triacylglycerols from the VLDLs forms VLDL remnants or intermediate-density lipoproteins, which then become converted, while still in blood plasma, to LDLs. Most LDLs seem to arise from VLDLs; some, however, are synthesized and secreted directly by the liver. The liver seems responsible for at least 50 percent of LDL removal from plasma. There is a great deal of interest in the control of LDL concentration because the concentration of LDLs in plasma is correlated positively with the development of coronary atherosclerosis.

The HDLs are synthesized and secreted by both liver and intestine. Lecithin-cholesterol acyl transferase, which catalyzes formation of cholesteryl esters and lysolecithin from cholesterol and lecithin (phosphatidylcholine) extracellularly, assists with the maturation in plasma of the newly secreted nascent HDL to form HDL_3 and then HDL_2. This transferase and its activator (apolipoprotein A_2) are constituents of HDLs. The major source of the cholesterol in HDLs is extrahepatic tissues. The mature HDLs then become endocytosed by the liver, thus illustrating the scavenger role of HDLs in effecting a flow of extrahepatic cholesterol to the liver. Unlike those of LDLs, HDL concentrations are related inversely to the incidence of coronary atherosclerosis.

Storage of lipids as triacylglycerols occurs in virtually all tissues. Under normal circumstances, however, adipose tissue is most important quantitatively as a lipid-storage depot. Stored triacylglycerols result from reaction of fatty acids (from action of lipoprotein lipase on triacylglycerols or from de novo synthesis) with α-glycerol phosphate (mostly derived from glucose). The relative contributions of diet-derived triacylglycerol and endogenously synthesized triacylglycerol to storage lipid depend on diet composition and amount of intake.

Liver and adipose tissue are two major tissues that are very important in the homeostasis of lipid metabolism of the nonlactating animal. Specific roles of both and the role of the mammary gland in lactating animals will be discussed before specific pathways of lipid metabolism are described.

Liver

Because of the dual afferent blood supply of the liver (the portal vein carrying blood from the alimentary tract, spleen, and pancreas and the hepatic artery), the water-soluble end products of lipid digestion, such as short- and medium-chain fatty acids and the peripherally circulated lipids, are subjected to liver functions. In addition, the liver facilitates absorption of lipids from the intestine by production of bile acids from cholesterol; bile acids are transferred to the alimentary tract through the bile duct. The liver has active enzyme systems for (1) synthesis of fatty acids (low in some species, as indicated later), cholesterol, phospholipids, triacylglycerols, bile acids, and less toxic or more water-soluble forms of compounds eventually excreted by way of urine or feces and (2) oxidation of fatty acids to CO_2 or to ketone bodies. Furthermore, the main source of plasma lipoproteins other than chylomicrons is the liver. Triacylglycerols normally do not accumulate in the liver but are packaged with phospholipids, cholesterol, cholesteryl esters, and apolipoproteins to form primarily VLDLs and nascent HDLs for secretion into the blood by reverse pinocytosis. When mobilization of nonesterified fatty acids from adipose tissue exceeds VLDL secretion by the liver, as in lactation ketosis in dairy cattle, pregnancy toxemia in ewes, diabetes mellitus, and starvation, triacylglycerols accumulate in the liver and cause a fatty liver. Metabolic blocks that cause the fatty liver may occur at the stage of (1) apolipoprotein synthesis, (2) assembly of lipid and apolipoproteins into lipoproteins, (3) synthesis of phospholipids (e.g., choline deficiency), or (4) the secretory mechanism. When excess lipid accumulation becomes chronic, fibrosis develops and leads to cirrhosis and impaired liver function.

Adipose tissue

Adipose tissue is a specialized type of connective tissue that has a central role in energy metabolism of the entire animal. Fuel molecules, when absorbed in excess of daily maintenance requirements, are stored in adipose tissue as triacylglycerol. When the animal has an energy deficit, the triacylglycerols are hydrolyzed to glycerol and fatty acids that are then used as metabolic fuel by many tissues. These two major functions of adipose tissue are under the control of the nervous and endocrine systems.

Within any animal species, the fatty acid composition of triacylglycerols in adipose tissue tends to be constant. Drastic changes in the type of lipid fed to nonruminant animals, however, will alter the fatty acid composition of stored triacylglycerols. For example, pigs fed peanuts or soybeans deposit a more unsaturated fat than do those fed a typical and lower-fat diet. On the other hand, pigs fed a diet containing highly saturated fats tend to deposit triacylglycerols that contain more unsaturated fatty acids than did the diet because of desaturation of some saturated long-chain fatty acids. Accordingly, an animal will desaturate fatty acids in an effort to deposit a fat typical of that animal species. The fatty acid composition of triacylglycerols in adipose tissue of ruminant animals is remarkably nonresponsive to dietary changes, because most dietary unsaturated fatty acids become saturated by ruminal microbes before absorption.

As mentioned earlier, adipose tissue, through action of lipoprotein lipase, is capable of transferring fatty acids of plasma triacylglycerols into its constituent fat cells or adipocytes for triacylglycerol resynthesis and storage. Nonesterified fatty acids in plasma also may be absorbed and stored. In addition, fatty acids synthesized in situ from glucose, acetate, and (or) other metabolites may be converted to triacylglycerols for storage. Adipose tissue is the major anatomical site of de novo fatty acid synthesis in cattle, sheep, goats, swine, rabbits, cats, and dogs, whereas the liver is the major anatomical site in humans and birds. Adipose tissue and liver are highly active sites of de novo fatty acid synthesis in rodents. The major anatomical site of fatty acid synthesis in the horse is not known. Because of this site specificity for de novo fatty acid synthesis, lipoprotein lipase activity plays a major role in the eventual storage in adipose tissue of triacylglycerols from both diet and the liver.

Several hormones are involved in controlling the process of de novo fatty acid and triacylglycerol syntheses and of hydrolysis of triacylglycerol (lipolysis) in fat cells of adipose tissue. For example, insulin stimulates fatty acid and triacylglycerol synthesis primarily by increasing glucose permeation through the cell membrane and secondarily by increasing activity (probably at the gene level) of several lipogenic enzymes. This hormone also increases the influx of nonesterified fatty acids into adipose tissue, presumably by activation of lipoprotein lipase. In summary, insulin promotes lesser nonesterified fatty acid concentrations in blood plasma and greater rates of triacylglycerol or fat deposition in adipose tissue.

Lipolysis of triacylglycerols and the subsequent release of nonesterified fatty acids from adipose tissue to plasma are stimulated by norepinephrine, epinephrine, glucagon, and adrenocorticotropic hormone. These lipolytic hormones result in activation of hormone-sensitive lipase, which catalyzes hydrolysis of triacylglycerol to produce diacylglycerols and fatty acids. On the other hand, insulin decreases activity of hormone-sensitive lipase. The diacylglycerols that are generated by action of this enzyme are hydrolyzed to fatty acids and glycerol through the catalytic action of cellular diacylglycerol and monoacylglycerol lipases, both of which are considerably more active than is hormone-sensitive lipase. Adipose tissue of most animal species has low glycerol kinase activities so that most glycerol that is formed by lipolysis diffuses to plasma.

Lipolytic hormones combine with receptor sites on the cell membrane and activate adenylate cyclase, which converts adenosine triphosphate (ATP) to cyclic AMP (cAMP). The latter activates a protein kinase that catalyzes phosphorylation of inactive hormone-sensitive lipase to form the active enzyme. Glucocorticoids and thyroid hormones have no direct lipolytic effect, but they facilitate or permit action of other lipolytic hormones. Prostaglandin E_1, nicotinic acid, and insulin inhibit lipolysis, probably by decreasing the amount of available cAMP. Insulin also decreases mobilization of fatty acids to plasma by increasing reesterification of cellular fatty acids to re-form triacylglycerols through increased glucose uptake, as mentioned before. There is considerable variation in degree of effect on lipolysis by different hormones among different animal species. For example, lipolysis in human adipose tissue is unresponsive to most hormones except catecholamines, whereas lipolysis in the rabbit, guinea pig, pig, and chicken is nearly unresponsive to catecholamines. Glucagon is an important lipolytic regulator in birds.

In starvation and in diabetes mellitus, where carbohydrate insufficiency exists at the tissue level, fatty acid and triacylglycerol syntheses are decreased sharply; hormone-sensitive lipase activity continues, resulting in increased amounts of nonesterified fatty acids being transported to the liver and other tissues. Under the same conditions, activity of lipoprotein lipase in adipose tissue decreases. The overall result of carbohydrate deprivation is a hyperlipemia that results primarily from increased concentrations of lipoproteins formed in liver from fatty acids derived originally from adipose triacylglycerols.

Brown adipose tissue in newborn and hibernating animals and in cold-exposed animals (nonshivering thermogenesis) is involved in heat production after norepinephrine stimulation of intracellular lipolysis. Released fatty acids are oxidized to CO_2 and thereby generate reducing equivalents for reduction of O_2 by the electron-transport system. The proton gradient generated by electron transport to O_2 is dissipated by a thermogenic protein called *thermogenin*. Thus oxidation of fatty acids to CO_2 in brown adipose tissue results in greater amounts of heat than in other tissues. Futile cycling of triacylglycerol synthesis and hydrolysis is a minor heat-generating mechanism in both white and brown adipose tissues.

Mammary gland

The mammary gland of the lactating animal is highly active in triacylglycerol synthesis and secretion into milk. Total lipid concentration of different milks ranges from about 1.5 percent in horses to around 50 percent in seals. Nearly all milk lipid is triacylglycerol. Fatty acids in secreted triacylglycerols are derived from (1) circulating triacylglycerols through action of lipoprotein lipase, (2) circulating nonesterified fatty acids originating from adipose tissue, and (3) de novo fatty acid synthesis in the mammary gland. Approximately 50 percent of fatty acids in bovine milk fat are synthesized de novo in the mammary gland. The rest is derived from the diet or from adipose tissue as preformed fatty acids. Glucose is the principal precursor of fatty acid in nonruminant animals. Acetate and lesser amounts of β-hydroxybutyrate are the two principal precursors of fatty acid in the ruminant mammary gland.

TRIACYLGLYCEROL METABOLISM

Triacylglycerols are the most significant group of lipids from the standpoint of energy metabolism of animals. Triacylglycerols may be provided by diet or may be synthesized from nonlipid sources largely in the liver, adipose tissue, and the lactating mammary gland.

De novo synthesis of fatty acids

In avian and mammalian species, fatty acids are synthesized in the lipogenic cell cytosol from acetyl CoA, a substrate that may be derived from carbohydrates and amino acids as well as from fatty acids. Acetyl CoA that is generated in the mitochondrion cannot cross the inner mito-

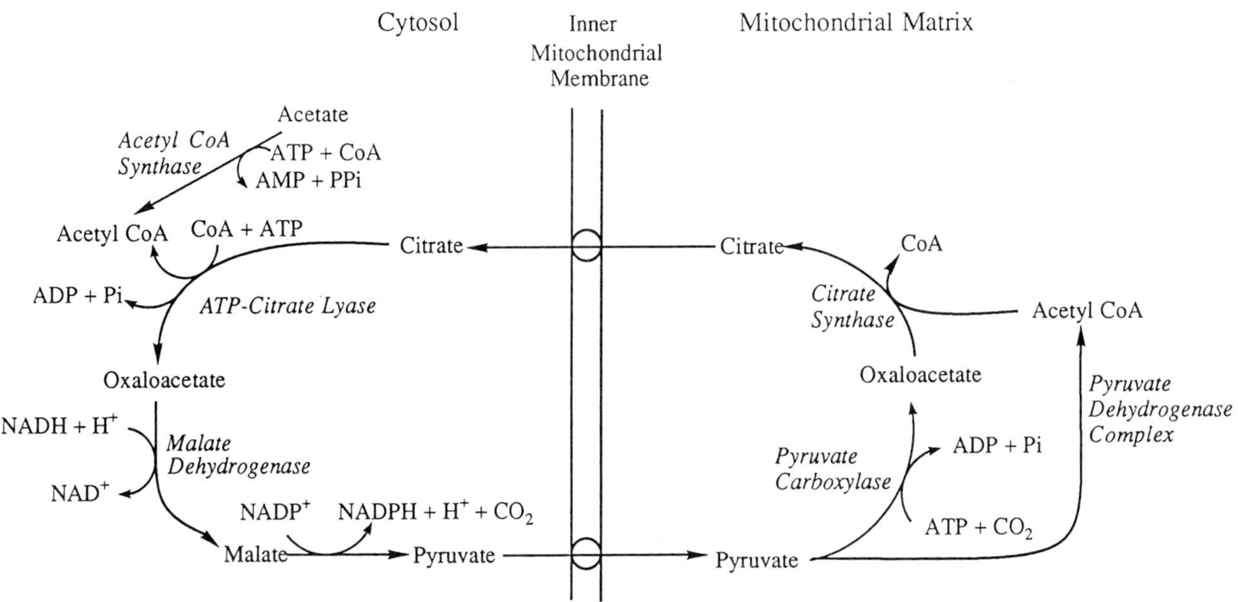

Figure 25.3. Citrate cleavage pathway. The circles within the membrane represent the tri- and dicarboxylate carrier systems.

chondrial membrane. Therefore citrate "carries" acetyl groups from mitochondria to cytosol where ATP-citrate lyase catalyzes the formation of cytosolic acetyl CoA and oxaloacetate. Return of the oxaloacetate to the mitochondrion completes the citrate cleavage pathway illustrated in Fig. 25.3. In ruminants acetate is the major precursor of fatty acid synthesis. For some yet-to-be explained mechanism, glucose is not a significant precursor of cytosolic acetyl CoA in ruminant lipogenic tissues, which serves as a precursor of long-chain fatty acids and steroids. Acetate is activated in the cytosol, obviating the need for citrate cleavage pathway enzymes. Furthermore, the citrate cleavage pathway decreases in importance for fatty acid synthesis as a milk-fed animal is weaned and develops a functional rumen. Lactate can be a significant precursor in ruminants as well and probably is converted to pyruvate and thus citrate before conversion to long-chain fatty acids.

The sequence of reactions involved in the synthesis of palmitate, the major fatty acid produced from acetyl CoA, is shown in Fig. 25.4. Other fatty acids are made by modifications of the palmitate. Carboxylation of acetyl CoA to form malonyl CoA is the initial and rate-limiting reaction in fatty acid synthesis and is catalyzed by acetyl CoA carboxylase. The enzyme system that catalyzes the synthesis of long-chain fatty acids from acetyl CoA, malonyl CoA, and nicotinamide adenine dinucleotide phosphate (NADPH) is a tightly associated multienzyme complex called fatty acid synthase, which exists as a dimer. The growing fatty acyl chain is attached as a thioester to a 4′-phosphopantetheine that is covalently linked to a unique protein called acyl carrier protein (ACP), which is a constituent of the fatty acid synthase. The thiol of a cysteine residue forms a thioester link with the primer, acetyl CoA. This acetyl CoA reacts with the β carbon of the malonyl CoA attached to the 4′-phosphopantetheinyl thiol of ACP to form an acetoacetyl moiety. Reduction, dehydration, and reduction, in order, generate a butyryl group that becomes transferred to the cysteinyl thiol of fatty acid synthase. Each subsequent elongation sequence includes binding of another malonyl CoA to the 4′-phosphopantetheinyl thiol of ACP, condensation with the growing fatty acyl group, reduction, dehydration, and reduction again and again until palmityl-fatty acid synthase is formed. Palmitate finally is released by hydrolysis.

The reduction reactions of de novo fatty acid synthesis require NADPH, which is derived from the pentose phosphate pathway and from the cytosolic oxidation of malate to pyruvate CO_2 in the citrate cleavage pathway. In summary, NADPH produced in the citrate cleavage pathway arises by transhydrogenation of cytosolic reduced nicotinamide adenine dinucleotide (NADH). Because of low malic enzyme activity, cytosolic oxidation of malate to pyruvate is a minimal NADPH producer in adipose tissue and lactating mammary tissue of ruminants. Although probably not a major source, another NADPH source is the cytosolic NADPH-isocitrate dehydrogenase.

The equation for synthesis of palmitate from acetyl CoA as primer and malonyl CoA is as follows: Acetyl CoA + 7 malonyl CoA + 14 NADPH + 14 $H^+ \rightarrow$ palmitate + 7 CO_2 + 6 H_2O + 8 CoA + 14 $NADP^+$. When available, propionyl CoA and butyryl CoA may serve as primers. Long-chain fatty acids that have an odd number of carbon atoms

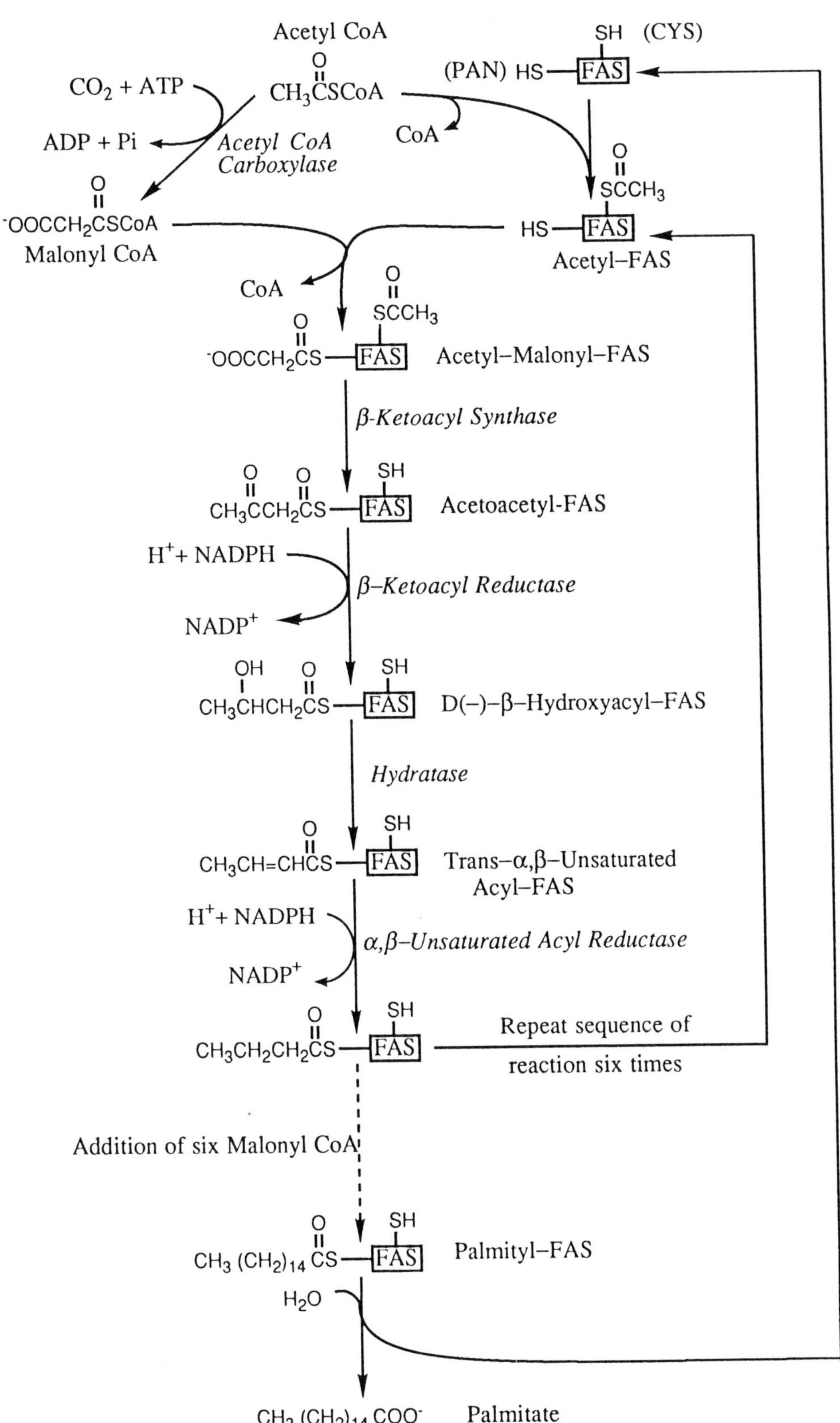

Figure 25.4. De novo synthesis of long-chain fatty acids. The cysteinyl (CYS) thiol groups (SH) of fatty acid synthase (FAS) are indicated. Broken line represents addition of six malonyl CoA sequentially by repetition of above reactions that show condensation of malonyl CoA with growing fatty acyl-FAS. Two fatty acyl chains are synthesized simultaneously on the dimeric FAS.

result when propionyl CoA is used as primer; propionate and butyrate are used more frequently in ruminants and pseudoruminants in which great amounts of these two acids are absorbed from the gastrointestinal tract.

Biosynthesis of long-chain fatty acids is under nutritional, hormonal, and metabolite influences. During fasting or ingestion of high-fat diets, fatty acid synthesis is decreased to very low rates. Greater synthetic rates occur after ingestion of high-carbohydrate diets or during intermittent eating (fasting followed by feeding). Insulin stimulates biosynthesis, whereas a diabetic state sharply decreases fatty acid synthesis. Several metabolites affect the specific enzymes involved. For example, ATP stimulates ATP-citrate lyase, citrate and isocitrate allosterically stimulate acetyl CoA carboxylase, and palmityl CoA allosterically inhibits both acetyl CoA carboxylase and fatty acid synthase. Acetyl CoA carboxylase is controlled by a cAMP-mediated phosphorylation-dephosphorylation mechanism. Glucagon promotes phosphorylation (deactivation), and insulin promotes dephosphorylation (activation). Phosphorylation-dephosphorylation mechanisms are independent of the allosteric regulation. Long-term regulation of fatty acid synthesis by diet involves control over concentration of acetyl CoA carboxylase and fatty acid synthase.

Fatty acid elongation and unsaturation

Animals can synthesize all commonly occurring fatty acids except linoleate ($C_{18}\Delta^{9,12}$) and linolenate ($C_{18}\Delta^{9,12,15}$). The nomenclature indicates that linoleate contains a carbon-carbon double bond between the No. 9 and 10 and the No. 12 and 13 carbon atoms. Thus linoleate may be called an unsaturated fatty acid; alternatively, saturated fatty acids contain only carbon-carbon single bonds in their chemical structure. Palmitate synthesized de novo or those fatty acids that originate from the diet may be modified by elongation, desaturation, and hydroxylation. A system for elongation of fatty acids by acetyl CoA addition occurs in mitochondria; the elongation reactions catalyzed by enzymes associated with the endoplasmic reticulum (microsomal system), however, seem to be the principal system for fatty acid elongation. This microsomal system consists of the addition of acetyl units as malonyl CoA to saturated (C_{10} to C_{16}) or unsaturated (C_{18}) fatty acids and uses NADPH as a reductant. The sequence of reactions is similar to that catalyzed by fatty acid synthase, except that intermediates are CoA thioesters rather than 4-phosphopanthetheinyl thioesters.

Although animals have enzyme systems to desaturate fatty acids, they cannot introduce a double bond beyond C-9 of a long-chain fatty acid. As examples of desaturation, palmitoleate may be produced from palmitate, and oleate may be synthesized from stearate. Each of these monoenoic fatty acids is a 9,10-unsaturated compound. The desaturase (mixed-function oxidase) system is associated with endoplsmic reticulum and is exemplified by the following reaction: Stearoyl CoA + NADPH(NADH) + H^+ + O_2 → oleoyl CoA + $NADP^+(NAD^+)$ + 2 H_2O. Double bonds can be introduced at the Δ^4, Δ^5, Δ^6, and Δ^9 positions in fatty acids by desaturases in several animal tissues.

A variety of unsaturated fatty acids can be formed from oleate by additional elongation and (or) desaturation reactions. Oleate gives rise to the omega-9 (ω-9) series of unsaturated fatty acids. The designation *omega-9* means that the ninth carbon from the methyl end of the fatty acid is a part of a double bond. Elongation and desaturation of the two essential fatty acids, linoleate and linolenate, result in a variety of other polyunsaturated fatty acids. The ω-6 polyunsaturated fatty acids, such as archidonate ($C_{20}\Delta^{5,8,11,14}$) are synthesized from linolenate. The ω-3 polyunsaturated fatty acids such as $C_{20}\Delta^{5,8,11,14,17}$ and $C_{22}\Delta^{4,7,10,13,16,19}$ that are present in marine fish oils are synthesized from linolenate. An important function of polyunsaturated fatty acids is to serve as a precursor of eicosanoids, which will be discussed later. In addition, polyunsaturated fatty acids are necessary constituents of a variety of structural lipids.

Triacylglycerol synthesis

Triacylglycerols are the major form of lipid in the animal body. They are transported between tissues in lipoproteins and are stored as an energy reserve in adipose tissue. Most triacylglycerol synthesis occurs in adipocytes, liver, intestinal mucosa, and lactating mammary glands. Three pathways have been proposed for synthesis of triacylglycerols. The first two (Fig. 25.5) involve phosphatidate as an intermediate, whereas the third does not include phosphorylated intermediates. In each case, activated fatty acids (fatty acyl CoA) are essential to the formation of glyceryl ester linkages. Fatty acyl CoA is synthesized by the following reaction: Fatty acid + ATP + CoA → fatty acyl CoA + AMP + PPi. In all pathways, a diacylglycerol is produced and subsequently esterified to form a triacylglycerol. α-Glycerol phosphate of the phosphatidate pathway is generated by reduction of dihydroxyacetone phosphate of the glycolytic pathway or by phosphorylation of glycerol with ATP by glycerol kinase. Alternatively, in the liver dihydroxyacetone phosphate may be esterified with an activated fatty acid before reduction of the carbon moiety (dihydroxyacetone phosphate pathway). The fatty acid on the No. 2 position of glycerol is usually unsaturated. The phosphatidate pathway predominates in the synthesis of triacylglycerol in most tissues, whereas monoacylglycerol (monoacylglycerol pathway) serves as a major substrate for triacylglycerol synthesis in mucosal epithelial cells during formation of chylomicrons and VLDL.

Triacylglycerol catabolism

Triacylglycerol catabolism to CO_2 is an important generator of useful energy in animals. Depot triacylglycerols are hydrolyzed readily by tissue lipases, as described before, and the released fatty acids are oxidized in situ or are trans-

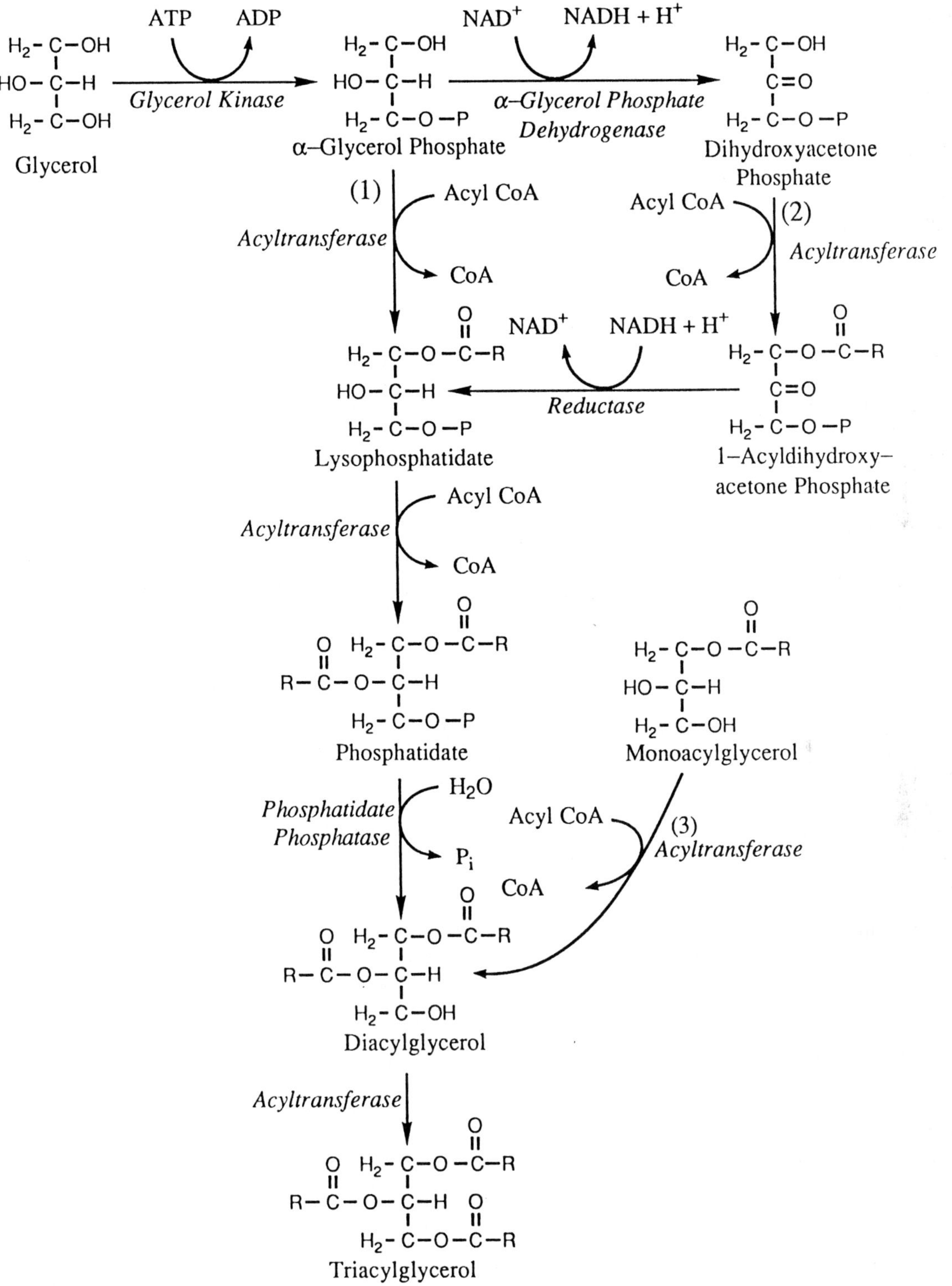

Figure 25.5 Biosynthesis of triacylglycerols by way of the phosphatidate (1), dihydroxyacetone phosphate (2), and monoacylglycerol (3) pathways.

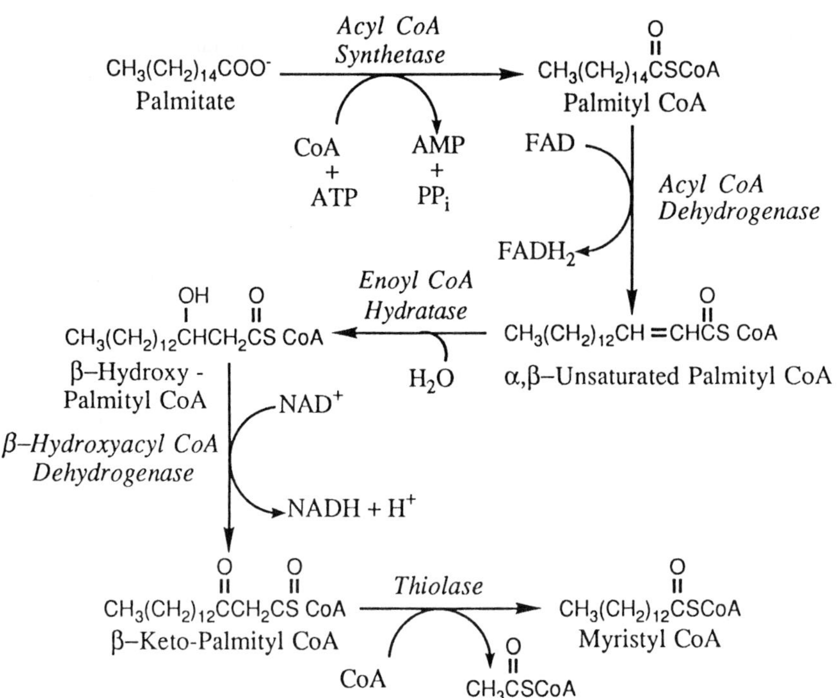

Figure 25.6. The beta oxidation of palmitate to myristyl CoA. Complete oxidation to acetyl CoA units requires repetition of reactions beginning with the acyl CoA dehydrogenase and terminating with thiolase.

ported to other tissues as albumin–fatty acid complexes. Within cells, long-chain fatty acids are attached to a fatty acid–binding protein before they are metabolized. Liver, heart, and resting skeletal muscle rely extensively on oxidation of fatty acids to CO_2. Released glycerol is transported primarily to the liver for formation of α-glycerol phosphate. This metabolite can be used for acylglycerol synthesis or can be oxidized to dihydroxyacetone phosphate for use in oxidative metabolism or conversion to glucose.

Degradation of fatty acids proceeds primarily by a process of beta oxidation that results in a stepwise removal of two carbons as acetyl CoA from the carboxyl end of the acid (Fig. 25.6). Before oxidation can begin, the fatty acid must first be activated by conversion to acyl CoA. At least three acyl CoA synthetases or thiokinases are known, each specific for a set of fatty acids. One requires short-chain (C_2 or C_3) fatty acids, a second is specific for intermediate-chain (C_4 to C_{12}) fatty acids, and a third acts on long-chain (C_{10} to C_{22}) fatty acids. Short-chain fatty acids also diffuse across the outer and inner mitochondrial membranes into the mitochondrial matrix for activation by an intramitochondrial thiokinase.

Activation of intermediate- and long-chain fatty acids occurs on the outer mitochondrial membrane, whereas beta oxidation involves mitochondrial matrix enzymes. Because the fatty acyl CoA molecules cannot traverse the inner mitochondrial membrane, carnitine (γ-trimethyl-β-hydroxybutyrobetaine) carries the acyl group across the membrane. The acyl group of fatty acyl CoA is transferred to the hydroxyl group of carnitine by carnitine acyltransferase I to form fatty acyl carnitine, which diffuses across the inner mitochondrial membrane. Activity of this enzyme regulates the rate of fatty acyl entry into mitochondria and thus the rate of oxidation of fatty acids to CO_2. On the matrix side, the fatty acyl group is transferred to CoA by carnitine acyltransferase II.

The saturated fatty acyl CoA is degraded by way of a sequence of reactions involving, in order, oxidation (linked to flavin adenine dinucleotide or FAD), hydration, oxidation (linked to nicotinamide adenine dinucleotide or NAD^+), and thiolysis by CoA to produce acetyl CoA and a fatty acyl CoA with two carbons less than the starting compound (Fig. 25.6). The beta oxidation process may be repeated to completely degrade the original even-carbon fatty acids to acetyl CoA. The beta oxidation of odd-number carbon fatty acids yields a propionyl CoA from the methyl end. Oxidation of palmityl CoA to acetyl CoA has the following stoichiometric formula: Palmityl CoA + 7 CoA + 7 FAD + 7 NAD^+ + 7 $H_2O \rightarrow$ 8 acetyl CoA + 7 $FADH_2$ + 7 NADH + 7 H^+. Reduced coenzymes may transfer electrons to O_2 in mitochondria and generate 35 moles of ATP per mole of palmityl CoA oxidized to 8 moles of acetyl CoA. Oxidation of 8 moles of acetyl CoA to CO_2 and H_2O by the citric acid cycle results in an additional 96 moles of ATP. Accounting for the equivalent of two high-energy phosphate bonds for palmitate activation, oxidation of 1 mole of palmitate to CO_2 and H_2O results in generation of 129 moles of high-energy phosphate bonds. Recovery of useful chemical energy by biological oxidation of palmitate, therefore, is about 43 percent—(129 × 7.3/2340) × 100.

Unsaturated fatty acids are oxidized also. The process involves all of the same enzymes used in beta oxidation of saturated fatty acids plus two additional ones, an isomerase to isomerize, if necessary, a beta, gamma double bond to an alpha, beta one, and an epimerase to epimerize the D(−)-β-hydroxyacyl CoA intermediate to the normal L(+)-β-hydroxyacyl CoA intermediate of the beta oxidation pathway. This combination of mitochondrial enzymes catalyzes the degradation of unsaturated fatty acids to acetyl CoA at rates similar to those for saturated fatty acids.

Acetyl CoA from oxidation may be used in a variety of ways, including entry into the citric acid cycle, acetylation reactions, steroid synthesis, and ketone body formation.

An enzyme system associated with endoplasmic reticulum, especially of the brain, degrades long-chain fatty acids one carbon at a time by oxidation of the α-carbon (alpha oxidation). This pathway is also one route for synthesis of α-hydroxy fatty acids (e.g., cerebronic acid) that are important constituents of sphingolipids. This pathway usually is relatively unimportant in total energy metabolism.

As indicated in the previous chapter, oxidation of 1 g of an average lipid mole results in the production of 1.07 g of water (metabolic water). Because glucose is a more highly oxidized compound, more metabolic water is produced per unit of weight by oxidation of lipids to CO_2 than is glucose.

Although the physiological significance is not known, another method of degrading long-chain fatty acids in the liver is by omega oxidation in which the methyl carbon is oxidized to a carboxyl group. Cytochrome P_{450}, NADPH, and O_2 are required to convert the terminal methyl group to a hydroxymethyl group by monooxygenase. Additional oxidation produces the dicarboxylic acid that then can be beta-oxidized from either end. A curious observation is that potentially one succinate can be derived from each fatty acid if beta oxidation occurs, giving gluconeogenic potential to even-carbon fatty acids.

SYNTHESIS OF KETONE BODIES

Fatty acyl CoAs generated in liver cytosol have two major fates. One is oxidation in mitochondria, and the other is conversion to triacylglycerols and phospholipids in the extramitochondrial compartment. Relative fluxes through the two pathways are largely dependent on entry of fatty acyl CoAs into mitochondria by way of a carnitine-mediated, rate-controlling step of fatty acid oxidation. Entry into mitochondria commits cellular fatty acids to oxidation. Carnitine acyltransferase I, the enzyme responsible for entry of fatty acyl groups into mitochondria, is inhibited allosterically by malonyl CoA. Concentration of cytosolic malonyl CoA is high during conditions of energy excess, and thus fatty acid entry into mitochondria and subsequent oxidation and ketogenesis are low. Conversely, during conditions of glucose shortage and thus lower cytosolic malonyl CoA concentrations, fatty acid oxidation and ketogenesis are promoted.

Oxidation of fatty acids in liver mitochondria occurs by two routes. First, as already described, fatty acids are oxidized to CO_2 by a combination of beta oxidation and citric acid cycle reactions. Second, fatty acids are oxidized incompletely to acetyl CoA, and then acetyl CoA is diverted from oxidation to CO_2 in the liver by formation of ketone bodies (acetoacetate, β-hydroxybutyrate, and acetone), which are oxidized to CO_2 in nonhepatic tissues. Acetate also seems to be released from the liver in ruminant animals during conditions of increased ketogenesis. Concentration of ketone bodies in blood plasma normally is very low (<1 mg/dl) but may become elevated markedly, even to a level as great as that of glucose, when rates of ketogenesis exceed rates of ketone body oxidation by peripheral tissues. The resulting ketosis, which sometimes occurs during fasting, pregnancy, lactation, and diabetes mellitus, may become pathological largely because of the associated acidosis (see Chaps. 27 and 37).

Key factors in abnormally great rates of ketogenesis are the high rates of fatty acid uptake by the liver and the shortage of glucose within the liver. The glucose shortage decreases generation of citric acid cycle intermediates (anaplerosis). Also, maximal stimulation of gluconeogenesis during a glucose shortage and a greater ratio of NADH to NAD^+ in mitochondria contribute to a decreased supply of mitochondrial oxaloacetate. Thus, the concentration of mitochondrial oxaloacetate seems to be a major determinant of whether the acetyl CoA generated from beta oxidation of fatty acids enters the citric acid cycle or is used for ketogenesis. During great fatty acid supply, the beta oxidation increases the ratio of NADH to NAD^+ in mitochondria, which in turn increases the reduction of oxaloacetate to malate for gluconeogenesis. As mentioned earlier, the concentration of malonyl CoA in cytosol is another factor that, by regulation of fatty acid entry into mitochondria, seems to control the rate of ketogenesis in the liver.

The first reaction in ketogenesis from acetyl CoA is catalyzed by thiolase and produces acetoacetyl CoA (Fig. 25.7). Most acetoacetyl CoA condenses with acetyl CoA to yield β-hydroxy-β-methylglutaryl CoA (HMG CoA); a much lesser amount undergoes hydrolysis to form acetoacetate. Cleavage of acetyl CoA from HMG CoA yields acetoacetate, which may be reduced by NADH to form D-β-hydroxybutyrate. The L isomer, as a CoA thioester, is an intermediate of beta oxidation of fatty acids. The availability of NADH governs the production of β-hydroxybutyrate from acetoacetate. Some acetoacetate spontaneously decarboxylates to generate acetone. β-Hydroxybutyrate also is produced by rumen epithelium from

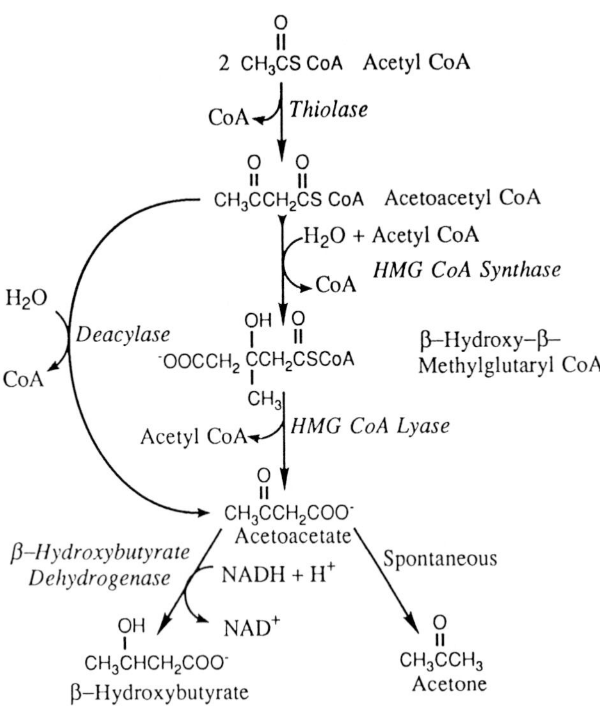

Figure 25.7. Synthesis of the common ketone bodies. HMG CoA, β-hydroxy-β-methylglutaryl CoA.

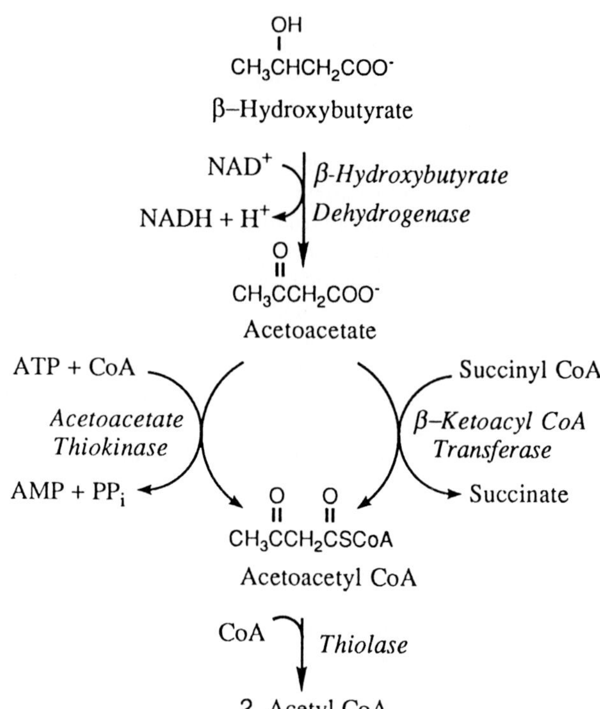

Figure 25.8. Conversion of β-hydroxybutyrate and acetoacetate to acetyl CoA.

about half the butyrate that is absorbed from the rumen field.

OXIDATION OF KETONE BODIES

Peripheral tissues, especially skeletal muscle, may derive a significant fraction of their energy needs from the oxidation of ketone bodies to CO_2 within their mitochondria. Moreover, heart muscle and renal cortex use acetoacetate in preference to glucose. Although glucose is the major fuel in a well-nourished animal, the brain increases acetoacetate oxidation, but not to the exclusion of glucose, during starvation and diabetes mellitus.

For oxidation of ketone bodies to acetyl CoA (Fig. 25.8), β-hydroxybutyrate is oxidized by NAD^+ to form acetoacetate, which is converted to acetoacetyl CoA by reacting with primarily succinyl CoA or, to a lesser extent, with ATP and CoA. Subsequent thiolysis with CoA yields 2 acetyl-CoA. Acetone is used poorly in tissues by several proposed pathways: Acetoacetate may be generated by reversal of decarboxylation of acetone, or propanediol (propylene glycol) may be formed from acetone, which then is converted to pyruvate or is cleaved to form formate and acetate. Because it lacks the ability to acylate acetoacetate with CoA, the liver does not oxidize ketone bodies to CO_2.

STEROID METABOLISM

The most abundant sterol in animal tissue is cholesterol, which originates from the diet if it contains animal-derived foods and from biosynthesis from acetyl CoA. Animals that consume only plants and plant-derived foods must synthesize all the cholesterol in their bodies. Most other steroids are derived from cholesterol, or one of its precursors, including vitamin D that is formed in the skin during exposure to ultraviolet light. Cholesterol is a necessary component of all cell surfaces and intracellular membranes, is a constituent of myelin of nerve tissues, and is a precursor of bile acids and numerous steroid hormones.

Absorption of dietary cholesterol is solely via the lacteals and is dependent on bile salts in the intestinal lumen. After absorption into mucosal cells, some free cholesterol is converted to cholesteryl esters. Both free and esterified forms of cholesterol subsequently appear in lymphatic chylomicrons; the latter form of cholesterol generally predominates.

Biosynthesis

Acetyl CoA serves as the sole source of all carbons of biosynthetic cholesterol. Although the liver (accounting for ~50 percent of the total) and intestines (~15 percent of the total) usually are the major anatomical sites, virtually all nucleated cells of the body are capable of cholesterol synthesis. The skin, adrenal cortex, ovaries, testes, and placenta also synthesize this sterol largely for conversion to other steroids. The responsible enzymes are associated primarily with endoplasmic reticulum or are in the cytosol.

The sequence of reactions for the synthesis of cholesterol

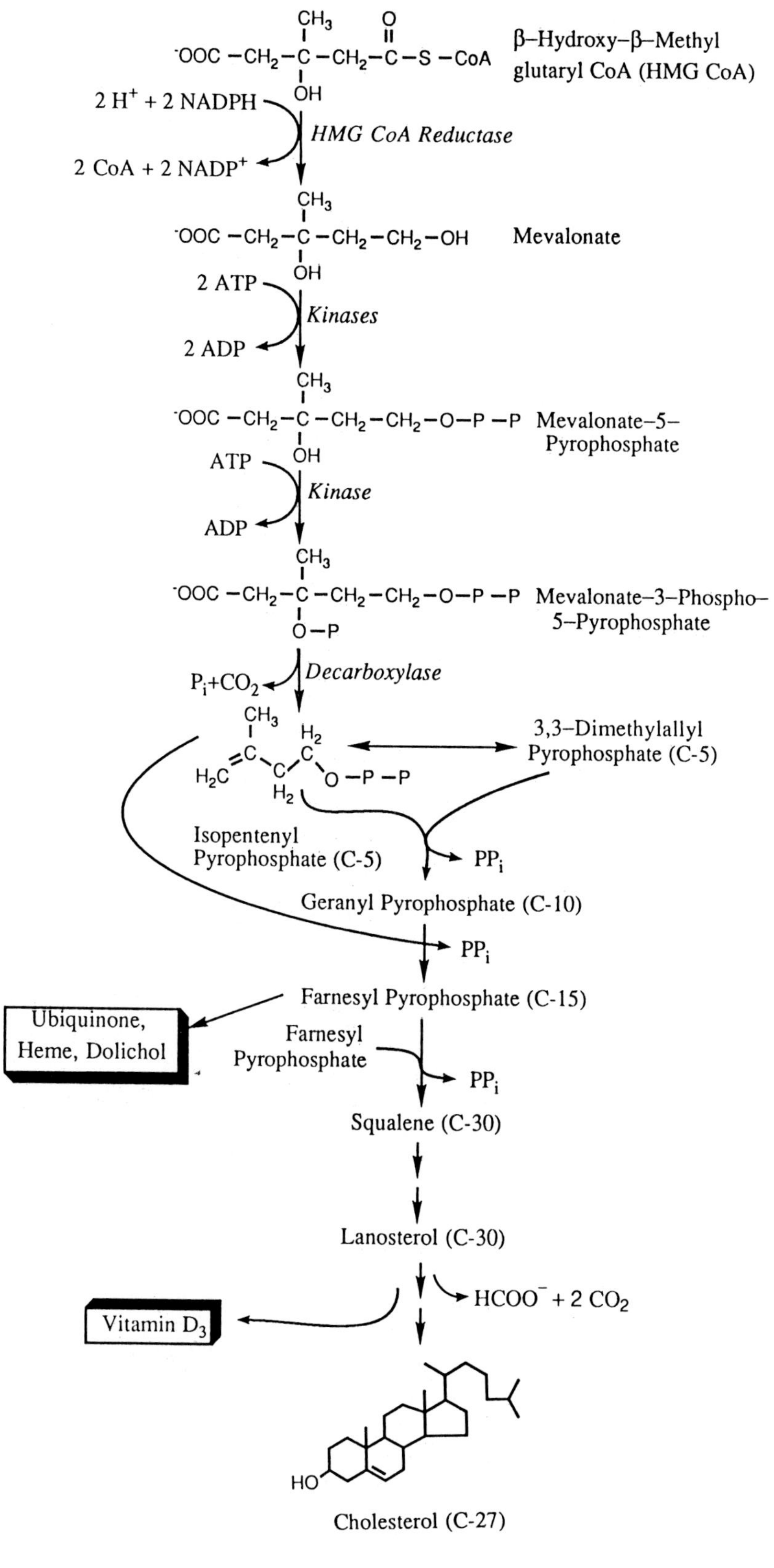

$^{-}OOC-CH_2-C(CH_3)(OH)-CH_2-C(=O)-S-CoA$ β-Hydroxy-β-Methyl glutaryl CoA (HMG CoA)

$2H^+ + 2NADPH$ → *HMG CoA Reductase* → $2CoA + 2NADP^+$

$^{-}OOC-CH_2-C(CH_3)(OH)-CH_2-CH_2-OH$ Mevalonate

2 ATP → *Kinases* → 2 ADP

$^{-}OOC-CH_2-C(CH_3)(OH)-CH_2-CH_2-O-P-P$ Mevalonate–5–Pyrophosphate

ATP → *Kinase* → ADP

$^{-}OOC-CH_2-C(CH_3)(O-P)-CH_2-CH_2-O-P-P$ Mevalonate–3–Phospho–5–Pyrophosphate

Decarboxylase → $P_i + CO_2$

$H_2C=C(CH_3)-CH_2-CH_2-O-P-P$ Isopentenyl Pyrophosphate (C-5) ↔ 3,3–Dimethylallyl Pyrophosphate (C-5)

→ PP_i

Geranyl Pyrophosphate (C-10)

→ PP_i

Farnesyl Pyrophosphate (C-15) → Ubiquinone, Heme, Dolichol

Farnesyl Pyrophosphate → PP_i

Squalene (C-30)

Lanosterol (C-30)

→ $HCOO^- + 2CO_2$

→ Vitamin D_3

HO

Cholesterol (C-27)

Figure 25.9. Biosynthesis of cholesterol. Synthesis of β-hydroxy-β-methylglutaryl CoA from 3 acetyl CoA is illustrated in Fig. 25.7. Conversion of the C-5 intermediate to cholesterol is illustrated in abbreviated form.

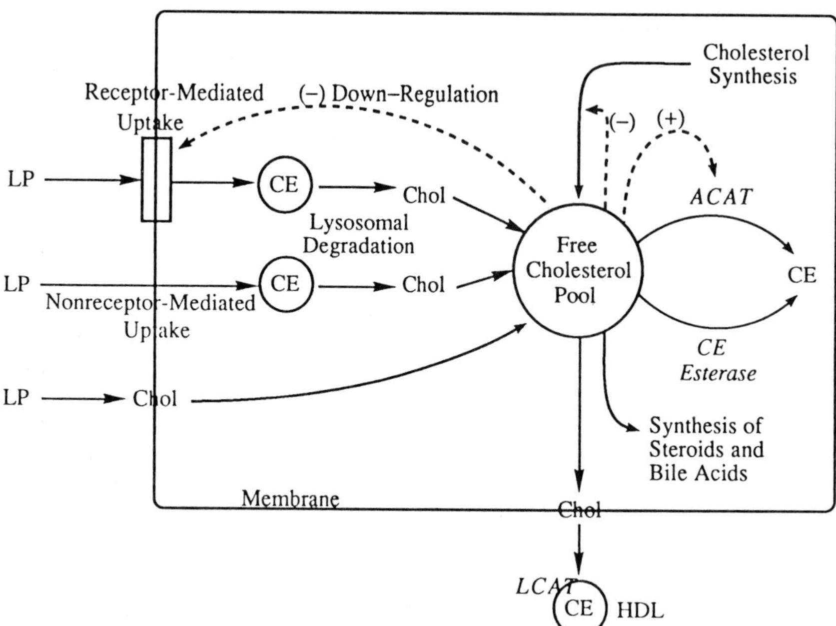

Figure 25.10. Metabolic processes that regulate the intracellular pool of free cholesterol. LP, plasma lipoproteins; Chol, cholesterol; CE, cholesteryl ester; ACAT, acyl CoA: cholesterol acyltransferase; LCAT, lecithin: cholesterol acyltransferase. Broken lines indicate positive or negative impacts on specific process.

from acetyl CoA is illustrated in Fig. 25.9. The HMG CoA synthesized in the mitochondria becomes converted to ketone bodies, whereas the HMG CoA synthesized in cytosol is converted to cholesterol. On reduction with NADPH by the rate-controlling HMG CoA reductase, mevalonate is formed. Phosphorylation with ATP and subsequent loss of phosphate and CO_2 yield isopentenyl pyrophosphate. A rearrangement catalyzed by an isomerase gives 3,3-dimethylallyl pyrophosphate. Condensation of the latter two compounds yields geranyl pyrophosphate. Condensation of an additional isopentenyl pyrophosphate with the geranyl pyrophosphate yields farnesyl pyrophosphate, a C_{15} compound. Two farnesyl pyrophosphates then interact, under reducing (NADPH) conditions, to form squalene, a C_{30} hydrocarbon. Conversion of squalene to lanosterol involves cyclization and methyl group transfers and requires O_2 and NADPH. The formation of cholesterol from lanosterol is rather complicated and may involve more than one pathway. This synthetic process involves removal of three methyl groups, reduction of one double bond by NADPH, and migration of the other double bond to the 5,6-position. Intermediates from squalene to cholesterol probably are attached to a carrier protein. As illustrated in Fig. 25.9, ubiquinone, heme, dolichol, and vitamin D_3 are synthesized from intermediates of the cholesterol synthetic pathway.

As for most metabolic pathways, regulation of cholesterol biosynthesis occurs at an early step in the synthetic sequence. Increased intracellular cholesterol derived from diet via cholesterol-rich chylomicron remnants or from uptake of LDL or HDL results in decreased activity of HMG CoA reductase, the rate-controlling enzyme of cholesterol synthesis. The following five metabolic processes can increase the concentration of intracellular free cholesterol: (1) uptake of cholesterol-containing lipoproteins such as LDL, HDL, and chylomicron remnants (mostly dietary cholesterol) by cell membrane receptors, (2) uptake of the same lipoproteins by a nonreceptor-mediated pathway, (3) direct transfer of cholesterol from lipoproteins to cell membranes, (4) de novo cholesterol synthesis, and (5) hydrolysis of intracellular stores of cholesterol esters. Lysosomes participate in the degradation of the lipoproteins after internalization. The following three processes can decrease the intracellular concentration of free cholesterol: (1) efflux of cholesterol from membrane to lipoproteins such as nascent HDL or HDL_3 as promoted by lecithin: cholesterol acyltransferase activity, (2) esterification of cholesterol by acyl CoA: cholesterol acyltransferase (cholesterol + fatty acyl CoA → cholesteryl ester + CoA), and (3) use of cholesterol for synthesis of other steroids and bile acids, as in the liver. These eight mechanisms for control of the intracellular pool of free cholesterol are illustrated in Fig. 25.10.

The mechanism of change of activity of HMG CoA reductase, however, remains to be elucidated. Phosphorylation/dephosphorylation via a cAMP-dependent mechanism of the reductase seems to be one significant control mechanism because insulin and thyroid hormone increase reductase activity and glucagon and glucocorticoids decrease it. Regulation of the concentration of the HMG CoA reductase is controlled at the gene level and by control of enzyme turnover.

Catabolism

The fates of cholesterol include (1) excretion as cholesterol in bile, (2) conversion to bile acids, (3) production of 18-, 19-, and 21-carbon steroid hormones, and (4) pathological deposit, as in cholesterol calculi in the gallbladder and cholesterol-containing plaques in arteries. From a quantitative standpoint, the conversion of cholesterol to bile acids is most significant. Bile acid synthesis from cholesterol, which occurs exclusively in the liver, includes shortening of the side chain from eight to five carbons, oxidation of the terminal side-chain carbon to a carboxyl, saturation of the Δ^5 double bond, inversion of the β-hydroxyl at C-3 to the α orientation, and hydroxylation of C-7 and (or) C-12. The principal rate-limiting step of bile acid synthesis is the first reaction of cholesterol conversion to bile acids. This reaction is catalyzed by 7-α-hydroxylase and is inhibited by bile acid accumulation. The bile acids (as CoA derivatives) become conjugated with taurine or glycine. The conjugated bile acids are excreted in bile, and most are reabsorbed actively in the lower intestinal tract after having participated significantly in lipid digestion and absorption. While in the intestinal lumen, most primary bile acids become deconjugated and partly dehydroxylated to secondary bile salts by intestinal microbes. Bile salts that escape reabsorption (~500 mg per day for adult humans) and cholesterol from diet, bile, or digestive tract sloughing that is not absorbed (~600 mg per day for adult humans) represent the only two significant means of excretion of body cholesterol. Much lesser amounts of cholesterol are lost as skin sloughing (~85 mg per day in adult humans) and steroid hormones in the urine (~50 mg per day in adult humans).

Cholesterol is the precursor of five major classes of steroid hormones. These classes and their major sites of synthesis are as follows: progestagens, corpus luteum; estrogens, ovary; androgens, testis; and glucocorticoids and mineralocorticoids, adrenal cortex. The biosynthesis of these hormones is presented in Fig. 36.1.

Cholesterol, atherosclerosis, and heart disease

Epidemiological studies have documented that in humans there is a positive correlation between risk of heart disease and (1) total cholesterol concentration, (2) total cholesterol in LDL, and (3) ratio of cholesterol in LDL and HDL. These correlations seem logical on the basis of previous discussions of LDL as carriers of cholesterol to extrahepatic tissues, such as coronary tissue and cerebral arteries, and of HDL as reverse transporters of cholesterol from extrahepatic tissues to the liver. Several dietary modifications have been recommended to decrease risk; these include decreased total fat intake, decreased saturated fat intake, increased ratio of polyunsaturated to saturated fatty acids in dietary fat, and decreased cholesterol intake. These changes may result in decreased concentrations of total cholesterol or LDL cholesterol in plasma. Aerobic exercise is thought to increase the HDL value of plasma, which results in a decreased risk of heart disease. Dietary additives include lovastatin, which is a competitive inhibitor of HMG CoA reductase, nicotinic acid, which inhibits lipolysis in adipose tissue and thus VLDL secretion by the liver, and anion exchange resins such as colestipol and cholestyramine, which decrease reabsorption of bile salts from the intestine. Hereditary factors play the greatest role in control of one's plasma cholesterol concentration. Several inherited genetic defects in lipoprotein metabolism are known and result in abnormal lipoprotein patterns in blood and often greater susceptibility to atherosclerosis, which is characterized by deposition of cholesterol and cholesteryl esters in arterial walls.

METABOLISM OF PHOSPHOLIPIDS

The phospholipids (also called phosphoglycerols, phosphoglycerides, and phosphatides) that are most abundant in animal tissues are phosphatidylcholine (also called lecithin), phosphatidylethanolamine, and phosphatidylserine. By definition, sphingomyelin is a phospholipid, but its metabolism will be discussed in a subsequent section along with other sphingolipids. Phospholipids tend to be soluble in both water and nonpolar solvents and thus serve as structural bridges between proteins and nonpolar lipids. Phospholipids are essential components of all cellular membrane systems. Normal lung function depends on an unusual phospholipid, dipalmitoylphosphatidylcholine, to act as a surfactant and prevent atelectasis at the end of expiration. The lack of this component of lung surfactant is responsible for respiratory distress in premature newborns. Phosphatidylinositol is a precursor of inositol phosphates that act as second messengers in hormone action. Also, an alkylphospholipid functions as the platelet-activating factor. Membrane phospholipids provide precursor fatty acids for eicosanoids, which include prostaglandins, prostacylins, thromboxanes, and leukotrienes. Detergent properties of phospholipids in bile are important in lipid absorption from the intestines. Phospholipids are integral components of lipoproteins; without their availability, as in a choline deficiency, VLDLs are not secreted normally and fatty livers result.

Biosynthesis

All cells possess the capability to synthesize phospholipids. Only the liver and the intestine synthesize significant quantities of phospholipid for release into the blood. Phosphatidylcholine may be synthesized by two major pathways (Fig. 25.11); the first makes use of choline directly, and the second is by methylation of phosphatidylethanolamine. The first pathway to be discussed involves phosphorylation of choline with ATP to yield phosphocholine, which reacts with cytidine triphosphate to produce pyrophosphate and cytidine diphosphocholine (CDP-choline). The latter interacts with 1,2-diacylglycerol to generate phosphatidylcholine and cytidine monophosphate. The second pathway, which is confined to the liver, involves methylation of phosphatidylethanolamine with *S*-adenosylmethionine, wherein the methyl groups are successively added to form phosphatidylmonomethylethanolamine, phosphatidyldimethylethanolamine, and finally phosphatidylcholine.

The biosynthesis of phosphatidylserine involves either

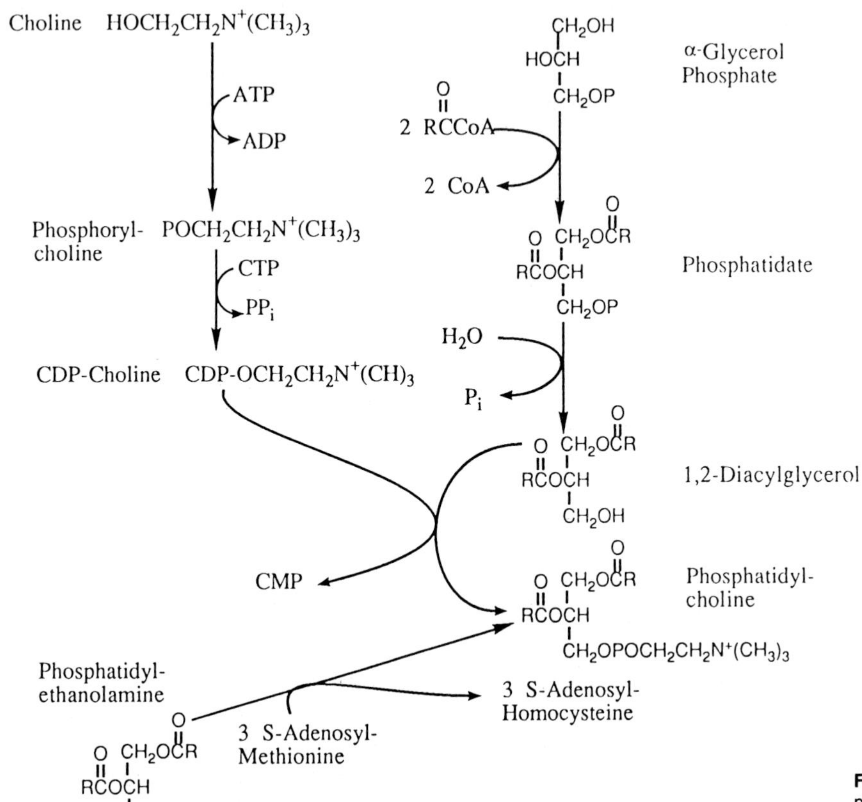

Figure 25.11. Pathways for biosynthesis of phosphatidylcholine. Synthesis of phosphatidate is illustrated in Fig. 25.5. Names of enzymes were omitted.

an exchange reaction between the ethanolamine of phosphatidylethanolamine and free serine (a common amino acid of proteins) or a reaction of CDP-diacylglycerol with serine (Fig. 25.12).

Phosphatidylethanolamine may be synthesized by two pathways (Fig. 25.12). The first involves phosphorylation of ethanolamine with ATP and subsequent reactions analogous to those for synthesis of phosphatidylcholine. The second and less important pathway is simply a decarboxylation of phosphatidylserine.

CDP-diacylglycerol serves as an essential precursor for several other phosphatides, including phosphatidylinositol, phosphatidylglycerol, and diphosphatidylglycerol (cardiolipin). The synthetic pathways for these three phospholipids plus those for others (glycerol ether phospholipids, plasmalogens, and platelet activating factor) can be found in most biochemistry texts.

Catabolism

Hydrolytic reactions are prominent in phospholipid remodeling and degradation. Phospholipases that catalyze hydrolysis of both ester and phosphoester linkages are located primarily in endoplasmic reticula, mitochondria, and lysosomes of cells.

Degradation may be illustrated with phosphatidylcholine. Fatty acid moieties are removed through the combined actions of phospholipases A_1 and A_2. The A_1 enzyme promotes removal of the fatty acid from the α or 1 position, whereas A_2 catalyzes removal of the fatty acid from the β or 2 position. Remodeling of phosphatidylcholine and other phospholipids occurs when phospholipase A_1 or A_2 catalyze removal of a fatty acid, which forms lysophospholipid that then accepts another fatty acyl CoA by the action of fatty acyl transferase. The product from the sum of the actions of phospholipases A_1 and A_2 is two fatty acids and glycerylphosphorylcholine, which is hydrolyzed further to α-glycerol phosphate and choline in a reaction promoted by phospholipase D. Phospholipase C catalyzes hydrolysis of phosphatidylcholine to yield diacylglycerol and phosphorylcholine. Similar hydrolytic reactions are thought also to occur with the other phospholipids.

Liberated fatty acids are catabolized oxidatively for energy or reused for synthesis of different lipids, such as the eicosanoids. Choline, ethanolamine, serine, and inositol may be reused for phospholipid synthesis or used in other pathways as discussed in Chapter 26. Glycerol phosphate is converted readily to dihydroxyacetone phosphate, an intermediate in the glycolysis sequence, or used in triacylglycerol or phospholipid synthesis.

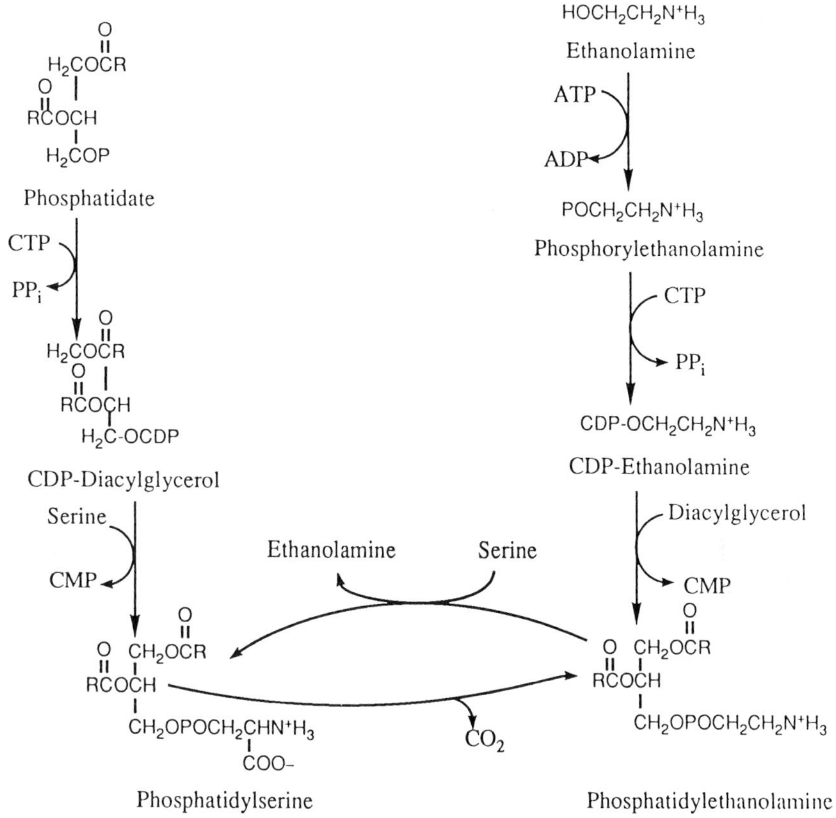

Figure 25.12. Pathways for biosynthesis of phosphatidylserine and phosphatidylethanolamine.

METABOLISM OF EICOSANOIDS

Arachidonate, which is the most prevalent, and other C_{20} fatty acids are precursors of the physiologically and pharmacologically active eicosanoids that include the prostaglandins, prostacyclins, thromboxanes, and leukotrienes. The precursor fatty acid usually is derived from the 2 position of membrane phospholipids by phospholipase A_2 (Fig. 25.13). The fatty acid precursor, which may contain three, four, or five double bonds, may be converted to the several known leukotrienes by cyclooxygenase activity and subsequent reactions involving glutathione. Alternatively, the fatty acid precursor may be converted to a prostaglandin endoperoxide and subsequently to prostacyclins, prostaglandins, or thromboxanes. Details of synthesis and catabolism of individual eicosanoids are illustrated in most biochemistry texts.

Thromboxanes are synthesized in platelets and cause vasoconstriction and platelet aggregation. Prostacyclins are produced by blood vessel epithelial cells and are potent inhibitors of platelet aggregation. Thus these two classes of eicosanoids are antagonistic and may play a role in myocardial infarction through control over blood clot formation. Prostaglandins are synthesized in a variety of tissues, including smooth muscles, and cause contraction of smooth muscle in animals. Thus prostaglandins have therapeutic uses in the prevention of contraception, induction of parturition, termination of pregnancy, prevention or alleviation of gastric ulcers, control of inflammation and of blood pressure, and relief of asthma and nasal congestion. Leukotrienes are synthesized in leukocytes, platelets, and macrophages; they cause vascular permeability and attraction and activation of leukocytes, and they regulate inflammatory and hypersensitivity reactions.

METABOLISM OF SPHINGOLIPIDS

The sphingolipids, including the phosphosphingolipids and the glycosphingolipids, are membrane constituents of cells, are present in plasma lipoproteins, are receptors for bacterial toxins (e.g., cholerotoxin), and are constituents of blood group substances. They are particularly significant in nerves. Their structure contains sphingosine [$CH_3(CH_2)_{12}CH{=}CHCHOHCHNH_2CH_2OH$] rather than glycerol. This amino alcohol is synthesized by enzymes associated with endoplasmic reticulum through condensation of palmityl CoA with serine and with the loss of CO_2, followed by reduction with NADPH and dehydrogenation by FAD to form the *trans* double bond. Acylation of the amino group of sphingosine by reaction with fatty acyl CoA

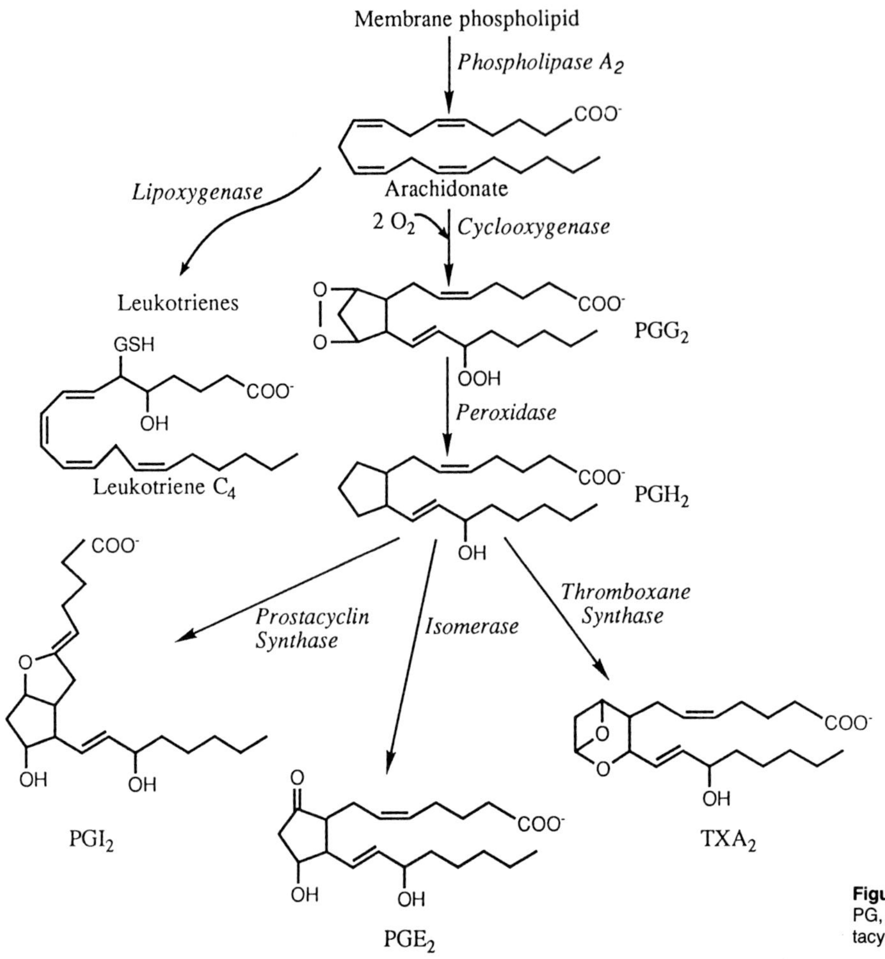

Figure 25.13. Synthesis of eicosanoids in animals. PG, prostaglandin; TX, thromboxane; PGI_2, prostacyclin I_2; GSH, reduced glutathione.

produces ceramides. The terminal hydroxyl group of ceramides is substituted to form the different sphingolipids.

Ceramides react with CDP-choline or phosphatidylcholine to yield the phosphosphingolipid called sphingomyelin. Furthermore, ceramides react with uridine diphosphate (UDP)-glucose or UDP-galactose to form cerebrosides, which are important glycosphingolipids. Cerebrosides may react with phosphoadenosine-phosphosulfate (active sulfate) to form sulfatides or sulfocerebrosides. An oligosaccharide unit that contains at least one sialic acid or N-acetylneuraminic acid linked to ceramide by a glucose residue forms gangliosides, another type of glycosphingolipid.

Degradation of sphingolipids is initiated by specific hydrolases. Sphingomyelin yields phosphorylcholine and ceramide. Cerebrosides are cleaved to monosaccharides and ceramide. Gangliosides, through the sequential action of glycosyl hydrolases found in lysosomes, yield ceramide and monosaccharide (free and amino-derivative) units. The enzyme ceramidase promotes hydrolysis of ceramides to form free fatty acids and sphingosine. The latter may be reused for sphingolipid synthesis or catabolized to palmitate. Several serious diseases of humans are caused by abnormal degradation as well as synthesis of sphingolipids, especially in the nervous system. For example, in multiple sclerosis, certain phospholipids (especially ethanolamine plasmalogen) and sphingolipids are present in decreased amounts in the white matter of the brain. Patients with Tay-Sachs disease, which is one of at least 11 identified inherited sphingolipidoses, lack the ability to degrade ganglioside GM_2 properly.

RELATION OF LIPIDS TO OTHER NUTRIENTS

Fig. 25.14 presents some of the relationships of the major types of lipids to other nutrients. Acetyl CoA is the key component relating carbohydrate and lipid metabolism. The major sources of acetyl CoA are glucose, fatty acids derived primarily from triacylglycerols, and amino acids. The major pathways of use of acetyl CoA are (1) oxidation by way of the citric acid cycle, (2) conversion to β-hydroxy-

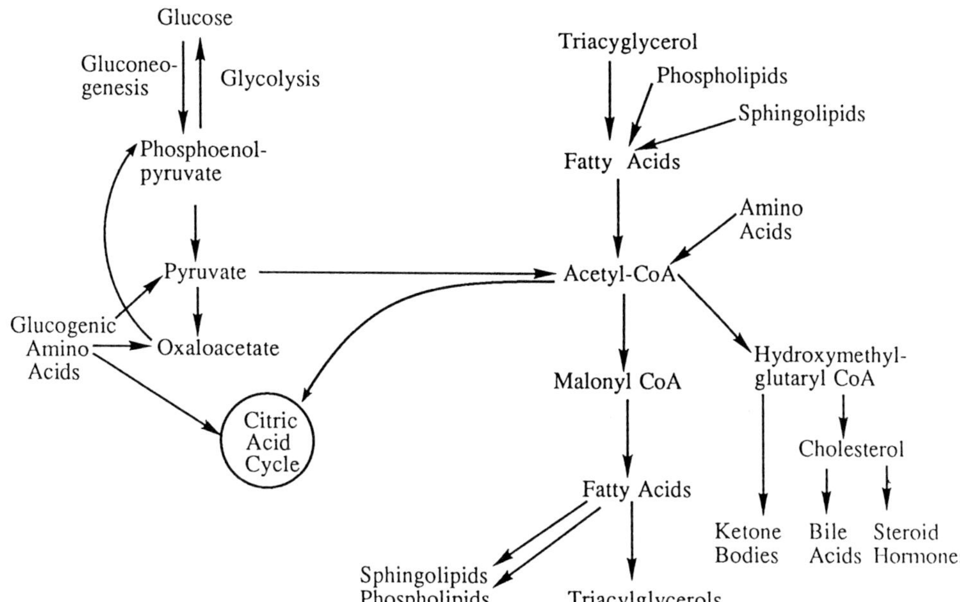

Figure 25.14. Metabolic relations of the major lipids to other nutrients.

β-methylglutaryl CoA and subsequent formation of ketone bodies and (or) cholesterol, which is a precursor of bile acids and steroid hormones, and (3) synthesis of long-chain fatty acids that are used in the formation of triacylglycerols, phospholipids, and sphingolipids.

When glucose catabolism is depressed (as in insulin deficiency and fasting), acetyl CoA oxidation by the citric acid cycle is decreased and there is a marked tendency to convert available resources, particularly glucogenic amino acids (see Table 26.1), into blood glucose through gluconeogenesis. Other processes are affected as well. These include a decrease in fatty acid synthesis, an increase in lipolysis in adipose tissue to provide fatty acids that are beta oxidized for ATP generation, and an increase in ketone body formation from acetyl CoA in the liver. Although both ketone bodies and cholesterol arise from HMG CoA, cholesterol synthesis is under metabolic control; thus, the great bulk of the excess acetyl CoA in the liver is converted to ketone bodies.

Under normal conditions, an increase in blood glucose stimulates the release of insulin that increases glucose uptake by adipose tissue and fatty acid reesterification and also suppresses activity of hormone-sensitive lipase in adipose tissue. The consequences in adipose tissue are decreased release of free fatty acids to the blood and increased triacylglycerol formation. Glucose catabolism in adipose tissue provides α-glycerol phosphate and acetyl CoA (used in the formation of long-chain fatty acids) for triacylglycerol synthesis. Ketone body formation is depressed when the rate of glucose catabolism is high.

REFERENCES

Bishop, W.R., and Bell, R.M. 1988. Assembly of phospholipids into cellular membranes: Biosynthesis. *Annu. Cell Biol.* 4:519–610.

Brown, M.S., and Goldstein, J.L. 1985. The LDL receptor and HMG-CoA reductase—Two membrane molecules that regulate cholesterol homeostasis. *Curr. Top. Cell. Regul.* 26:3–16.

Byers, F.M., and Shelling, G.T. 1988. Lipids in ruminant nutrition. In D.C. Church, ed., *The Ruminant Animal: Digestive Physiology and Nutrition.* Prentice Hall, Englewood Cliffs, N.J. Pp. 298–312.

Chapman, M.J. 1980. Animal lipoproteins: Chemistry, structure, and comparative aspects. *J. Lipid Res.* 21:789–853.

Clegg, R.A. 1988. Regulation of fatty acid uptake and synthesis in mammary and adipose tissues: Contrasting roles for cyclic AMP. *Curr. Top. Cell. Regul.* 29:77–128.

Davidowicz, E.A. 1987. Dynamics of membrane lipid metabolism and turnover. *Annu. Rev. Biochem.* 5:42–62.

Goldberg, A.C., and Schoenfeld, G. 1985. Effects of diet on lipoprotein metabolism. *Annu. Rev. Nutr.* 5:192–212.

Green, P.H.R., and Glickman, R.M. 1981. Intestinal lipoprotein metabolism. *J. Lipid Res.* 22:1153–73.

Havel, R.J. 1980. Lipoprotein biosynthesis and metabolism. *Ann. N.Y. Acad. Sci.* 348:16–29.

Havel, R.J. 1986. Functional activities of hepatic lipoprotein receptors. *Annu. Rev. Physiol.* 48:119–34.

Himms-Hagen, J. 1990. Brown adipose tissue metabolism and thermogenesis: Interdisciplinary studies. *FASEB J.* 4:2890–98.

Jeffcoat, R. 1979. The biosynthesis of unsaturated fatty acids and its control in mammalian liver. *Essays Biochem.* 15:1–36.

Littledike, E.T., Young, J.W., and Beitz, D.C. 1981. Common metabolic diseases of cattle: Ketosis, milk fever, grass tetany, and downer cow complex. *J. Dairy Sci.* 64:1465–82.

McGarry, J.D., and Foster, D.W. 1980. Regulation of hepatic fatty acid oxidation and ketone body production. *Annu. Rev. Biochem.* 49:395–420.

Nilsson-Ehle, N., Garfinkel, A.S., and Schotz, M.C. 1980. Lipolytic enzymes and plasma lipoprotein metabolism. *Annu. Rev. Biochem.* 49:667–94.

Nimmo, H.G. 1981. The hormonal control or triacylglycerol synthesis. *Mol. Aspects Cell Reg.* 1:135–52.

Quig, D.W., and Zilversmit, D.B. 1990. Plasma lipid transfer activities. *Annu. Rev. Nutr.* 10:169–94.

Rudney, H., and Sexton, R.C. 1986. Regulation of cholesterol bicsynthesis. *Annu. Rev. Nutr.* 6:245–72.

Srere, P.A. 1975. The enzymology of the formation and breakdown of citrate. *Adv. Enzymol.* 43:57–101.

Stoffel, W. 1971. Sphinogolipids. *Annu. Rev. Biochem.* 40:57–82.

Sweetser, D.A., Heuckeroth, R.O., and Gordon, J.I. 1987. The metabolic significance of mammalian fatty acid-binding protein. *Annu. Rev. Nutr.* 7:331–59.

Vahoney, C.V., Chanderbhan, R., Kharroubi, A., Noland, B.J., Pasbeszyn, A., and Scallen, T.J. 1987. Sterol carrier and lipid transfer proteins. *Adv. Lipid Res.* 22:83–115.

van den Bosch, H. 1974. Phosphoglyceride metabolism. *Annu. Rev. Biochem.* 43:243–77.

Vernon, R.G. 1980. Lipid metabolism in the adipose tissue of ruminant animals. *Prog. Lipid Res.* 19:23–106.

Whitehurst, G.B., Beitz, D.C., Cianzio, D., and Topel, D.G. 1981. Fatty acid synthesis from lactate in growing cattle. *J. Nutr.* 111:1454–61.

Williamson, D.H. 1979. Recent developments in ketone body metabolism. *Biochem. Soc. Proc.* 7:1313–21.

Willis, A.L. 1981. Nutritional and pharmacological factors in eicosanoic biology. *Nutr. Rev.* 39:239–301.

CHAPTER 26

Protein and Amino Acid Metabolism | by Donald C. Beitz

Proteins are essential organic constituents of all cells and constitute approximately 18 percent of the body weight of animals. An overview of the metabolism of proteins and their constituent amino acids is given in Fig. 26.1. The purpose of this chapter is to describe each of the indicated metabolic pathways in the overview. Proteins are complex polymers that range in molecular weight from about 5000 to 1 million. Some peptides consist of only two (e.g., carnosine) or three (e.g., glutathione) amino acids. The monomer units of proteins are L-amino acids linked together by peptide bonds in which nitrogen of the amino group of one amino acid is linked to the carbonyl group of a neighboring amino acid through the loss of water. The sequence of amino acids, as genetically controlled through the DNA, determines the physical, chemical, and biological properties of proteins. In addition to the primary structure controlling biological function, secondary (helical and pleated-sheet regions), tertiary (three-dimensional conformation), and quaternary (multichain) structures of proteins determine biological activity. Proteins function as (1) regulators of metabolism, such as enzymes and hormones, (2) structure components, as for membranes, muscles, and connective tissue, (3) transport materials, such as O_2 by hemoglobin and electrons by cytochrome c, (4) osmoregulators, such as albumin, (5) nucleic acid constituents, as in nucleoproteins, and (6) body defenders, such as the immunoglobulins and interferons.

Dietary proteins are hydrolyzed in the intestinal lumen and in the mucosal cells of the gastrointestinal tract by the action of numerous proteases and peptidases, resulting in production of free amino acids that, for the most part, are transported to the liver by way of the portal blood (see Chap. 19). The liver then plays a major role in the type and amount of amino acids available to nonhepatic tissues. In addition to this dietary supply, amino acids derived from catabolism of tissue proteins, which must be replenished continually, represent a significant input to the pool of amino acids in the body. Typically, protein catabolism contributes two to three times more amino acids than does the diet.

Although intracellular amino acids are not necessarily in equilibrium with circulating amino acids, the blood pool serves as a major source of specific amino acids for synthesis of protein. In many animal species, the total amino acid concentration in blood plasma ranges between 35 and 65 mg/dl. Glutamine, alanine, and glycine (in decreasing order) are usually the three most prevalent ones. In addition, many other nitrogenous compounds essential for proper tissue function (purines, pyrimidines, neurotransmitters, and heme) are formed from amino acids absorbed from the blood pool. Decarboxylation of amino acids results in pro-

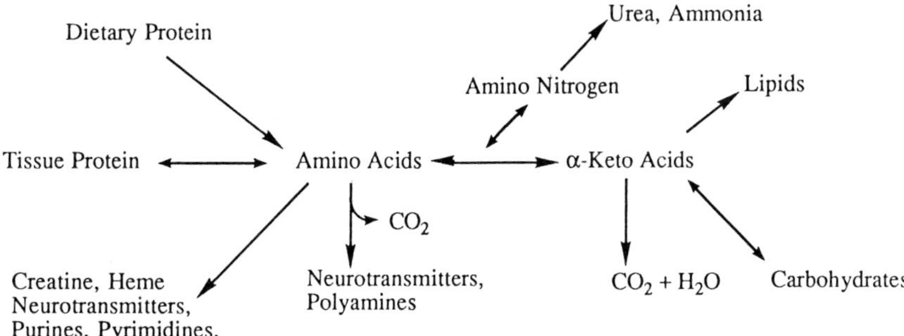

Figure 26.1. An overview of protein and amino acid metabolism.

duction of necessary amines such as neurotransmitters and polyamines.

Free amino acids undergo catabolism in most tissues but especially in the intestinal mucosa, liver, skeletal muscle, kidney, and brain. The catabolic process commonly involves removal of the amino group and use of the resulting α-keto acids for oxidation to CO_2 and adenosine triphosphate (ATP) generation (physiological fuel value of 4 kcal/g) and for synthesis of glucose and lipids. In most terrestrial vertebrates, a large part of the released ammonia is converted into urea and excreted. In terrestrial reptiles and birds, the amino groups are converted to uric acid for excretion. Many aquatic animals excrete excess nitrogen as ammonium ions.

Many amino acids can be synthesized from corresponding α-keto acids, from closely similar compounds, or from essential amino acids by animal tissues. Several, however, must be provided by the diet to maintain normal growth and function. Essential and nonessential amino acids that commonly occur in proteins are listed in Table 26.1. Microorganisms in the rumen of a ruminant animal normally are able to synthesize both essential and nonessential amino acids for production of microbial protein. Digestion of microbial protein and absorption of amino acids in the small intestine of a ruminant animal then make both essential and nonessential amino acids available for body functions and growth. Microbes in the ceca of pseudoruminants, such as the rabbit and the horse, and in the large intestine also synthesize amino acids; only small amounts of these amino acids, however, become available to animal tissues. Essentiality of some amino acids varies with species and physiological states. For example, birds also require glycine in the diet, and arginine and histidine are not required by adults of several animal species.

Brain, skeletal muscles, intestines, and liver are the major tissues involved in removal of excess amino acids. Much of the nitrogen of amino acids is transported between tissues by a few major compounds indicated in Fig. 26.2. Skeletal muscles export excess nitrogen largely as glutamine and alanine, whereas the intestines transfer excess nitrogen to the liver to a great extent as alanine, citrulline, and ammonia. In mammals the liver actively removes alanine, citrulline, ammonium ions, and other amino acids from the blood for urea synthesis. Glutamine is a neutral, relatively nontoxic amino acid that crosses plasma membranes readily and is an important "carrier" of ammonium ions from several tissues, such as those of the brain and skeletal muscles. Much of the plasma glutamine is absorbed by the small intestine, and nitrogen is transported to the liver as citrulline and alanine for eventual urea synthesis. Also, alanine is an important nitrogen transporter, especially from skeletal muscle and intestines.

Table 26.1. Essential and nonessential amino acids for humans

Essential	Nonessential
Arginine*	Alanine
Histidine*	Asparagine
Isoleucine	Aspartate
Leucine	Cysteine
Lysine	Glutamate
Methionine	Glutamine
Phenylalanine	Glycine
Threonine	Hydroxylysine†
Tryptophan	Hydroxyproline†
Valine	Proline
	Serine
	Tyrosine

*Not essential for adults.
†Not used during protein synthesis.

REMOVAL OF AMINO GROUPS FROM AMINO ACIDS

Amino groups are removed from amino acids by several different reactions. The removed amino groups ultimately can be used to synthesize a variety of other compounds. The emphasis in this section is on the generation of ammonium ions, which directly provide one of the two nitrogens for urea synthesis.

Transamination

The most common method of removing the amino group from an amino acid is by transfer of the amino group to an

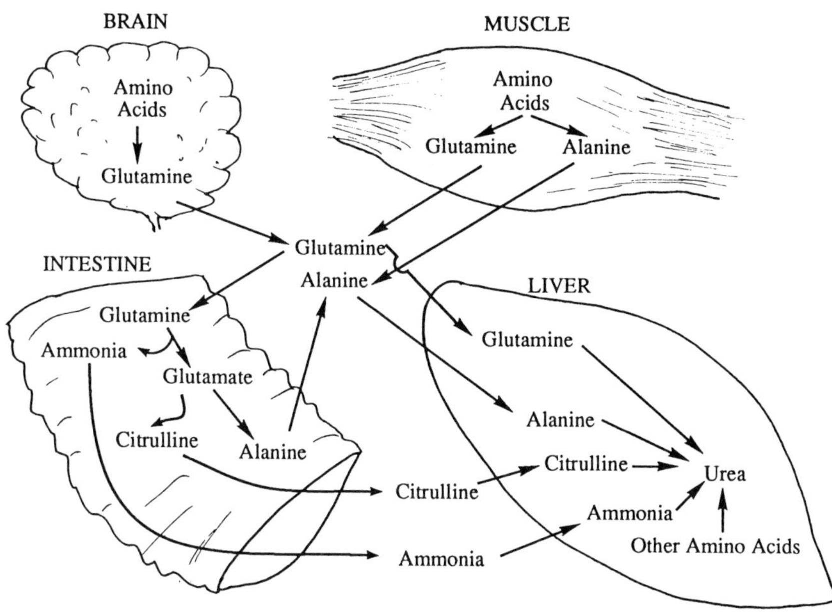

Figure 26.2. Major transfer routes of excess nitrogen among brain, skeletal muscle, small intestine, and liver during postabsorptive state.

α-keto acid (acceptor) by a transaminase (also called aminotransferase). The reaction is reversible, and transaminases are distributed widely in animal tissues, especially tissues of the brain, heart, kidney, and liver. Some transaminases are mitochondrial, some are cytosolic, and others are found in both cell compartments. The coenzyme for the transaminases is pyridoxal phosphate. Only lysine, threonine, and the imino acids, proline and hydroxyproline, do not undergo transamination.

Transamination is illustrated by the reaction catalyzed by aspartate transaminase: Aspartate + α-ketoglutarate → oxaloacetate + glutamate. For most transaminations, α-ketoglutarate is the amino acceptor and forms glutamate. Alternatively, transminase action, coupled with glutamate dehydrogenase activity (described later), results in formation of ammonium ions from the "transaminated" amino group.

Transamidation

The amide nitrogen of glutamine serves as a source of amino groups in synthesis of amino sugars as illustrated with the following reaction: Fructose-6-phosphate + glutamine → glucosamine-6-phosphate + glutamate.

Use of the glucosamine-6-phosphate for synthesis of other complex carbohydrates is discussed in Chapter 24.

Oxidative deamination

Several specialized enzyme systems are capable of oxidative deamination of amino acids. One of these is D-amino acid oxidase. This enzyme is widespread in animal tissues and is quite active, but it is of little known significance in view of the shortage or almost complete absence of D-amino acids in mammalian tissues. Activity of its counterpart, L-amino acid oxidase, on the other hand, is low, and the enzyme is restricted to the liver and kidney. The D-amino acid oxidases are flavoproteins that contain flavin adenine dinucleotide (FAD), whereas the L-amino acid oxidases contain flavin mononucleotide (FMN) as the coenzyme (Fig. 26.3). The two hydrogen atoms removed from the amino acid are passed to oxygen to form hydrogen peroxide, which subsequently is decomposed rapidly by cellular catalase. The overall reaction is as follows: Amino acid + $\frac{1}{2}$ $O_2 \rightarrow$ α-keto acid + NH_4^+.

A third enzyme involved in oxidative deaminations is L-glutamate dehydrogenase, which is distributed widely in animal tissues. Glutamate dehydrogenase catalyzes a reversible reaction illustrated in Fig. 26.4. Thus the enzyme catalyzes amination of ammonium ions as well as deamination. Glutamate dehydrogenase is present in the mitochondrial matrix and is controlled allosterically; ATP and guanosine triphosphate (GTP) are inhibitors, whereas adenosine diphosphate (ADP) and guanosine diphosphate (GDP) are activators. Thus, these metabolites, by affecting

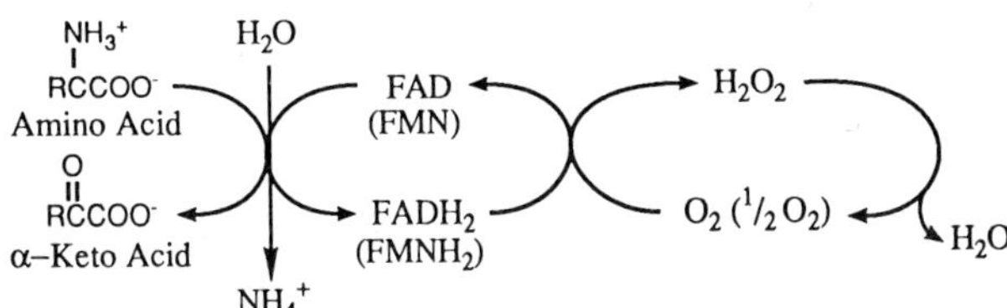

Figure 26.3. Oxidative deamination by D- or L-amino acid oxidases. The reaction on the far right is catalyzed by catalase. The generalized structure for an amino acid is shown on the left.

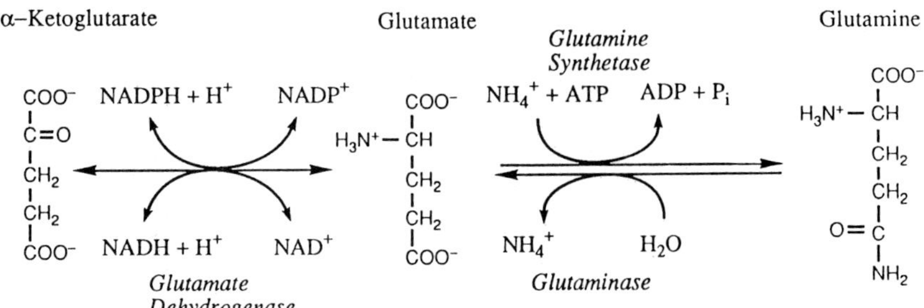

Figure 26.4. Oxidative deamination by glutamate dehydrogenase and interconversion of glutamate and glutamine. NADH will serve as reductant in dehydrogenase reaction as well.

glutamate dehydrogenase, also regulate citric acid cycle activity by control of α-ketoglutarate concentration.

Most of the ammonia pool is derived from a combination of transamination of amino acids with α-ketoglutarate forming glutamate, which is deaminated oxidatively by glutamate dehydrogenase. Ammonium ions may be released to the blood or used to aminate glutamate by glutamine synthetase (Fig. 26.4), which then is released to the blood. Ammonium ions and glutamine absorbed by the liver and ammonia generated in the liver are converted to urea in mammals or to uric acid in birds.

Direct deamination

Only histidine is directly deaminated by a mechanism similar to dehydration of an alcoholic intermediate, as in de novo fatty acid synthesis. Direct deamination of histidine, catalyzed by histidase, results in formation of urocanate and ammonium ions, as illustrated later.

Deamination by dehydration

A significant contribution to the total ammonia production results from the action of amino acid dehydratase, which requires the coenzyme pyridoxal phosphate. Substrates for this enzyme include serine and threonine.

Hydrolytic deamination

Ammonium groups are released from asparagine and glutamine by hydrolysis catalyzed by asparaginase (asparagine + $H_2O \rightarrow$ aspartate + NH_4^+) and glutaminase (Fig. 26.4).

Many ammonium ions generated in skeletal muscle are formed by hydrolysis of adenosine monophosphate (AMP) in the purine nucleotide cycle, as shown in Fig. 26.5. Ammonium ion generation by this mechanism increases markedly when AMP is high, as in contracting or exhausted muscle. The AMP concentration increases during contraction because of the myokinase reaction, which converts 2 ADP (produced from ATP) to an ATP and an AMP. The purine nucleotide cycle, when associated with fumarase, malate dehydrogenase, and glutamate-oxaloacetate transaminase, provides a method by which (1) the nitrogen of aspartate and therefore of other amino acids can appear as an ammonium ion, (2) citric acid cycle intermediates can be replenished, and (3) reduced nicotinamide adenine dinucleotide (NADH) is generated. The following reactions demonstrate those three activities:

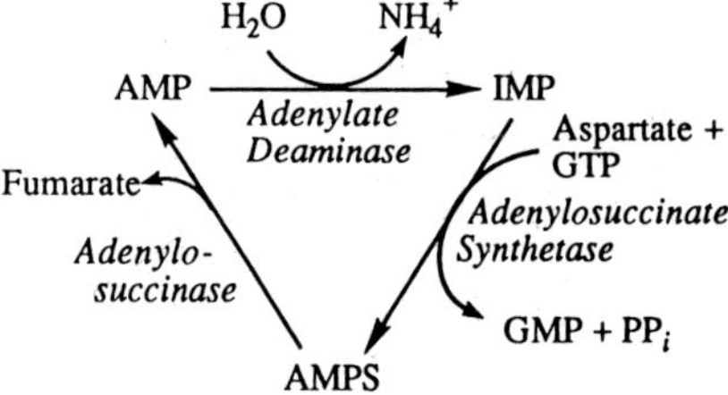

Figure 26.5. The purine nucleotide cycle. AMP, adenosine monophosphate; IMP, inosine monophosphate; AMPS, adenylsuccinate.

$$\text{Aspartate} + \text{GTP} + H_2O \xrightarrow[\text{Purine nucleotide cycle}]{} \text{fumarate} + NH_4^+ + \text{GDP} + \text{PPi}$$

$$\text{Fumarate} + H_2O \xrightarrow[\text{Fumarase}]{} \text{malate}$$

$$\text{Malate} + \text{NAD}^+ \xrightarrow[\text{Malate dehydrogenase}]{} \text{oxaloacetate} + \text{NADH} + H^+$$

$$\text{Glutamate} + \text{oxaloacetate} \xrightarrow[\text{Transaminase}]{} \text{aspartate} + \alpha\text{-ketoglutarate}$$

$$\text{Sum: Glutamate} + \text{GTP} + 2\,H_2O + \text{NAD}^+ \rightarrow \alpha\text{-ketoglutarate} + NH_4^+ + \text{GMP} + \text{NADH} + H^+$$

Glutamate may have derived its amino group from other amino acids by transamination. Thus the purine nucleotide cycle and amino acid degradation provide a mechanism for continued energy generation in contracting muscle.

FATE OF AMMONIA

The fate of ammonia (98.5 percent of ammonia in body fluids exists as an ion at physiological pH) produced by the different deamination reactions varies with the type of animal and its habitat. Because ammonia is highly toxic (70 μM is the upper limit of normal range in humans), probably as a result of depletion of α-ketoglutarate through gluta-

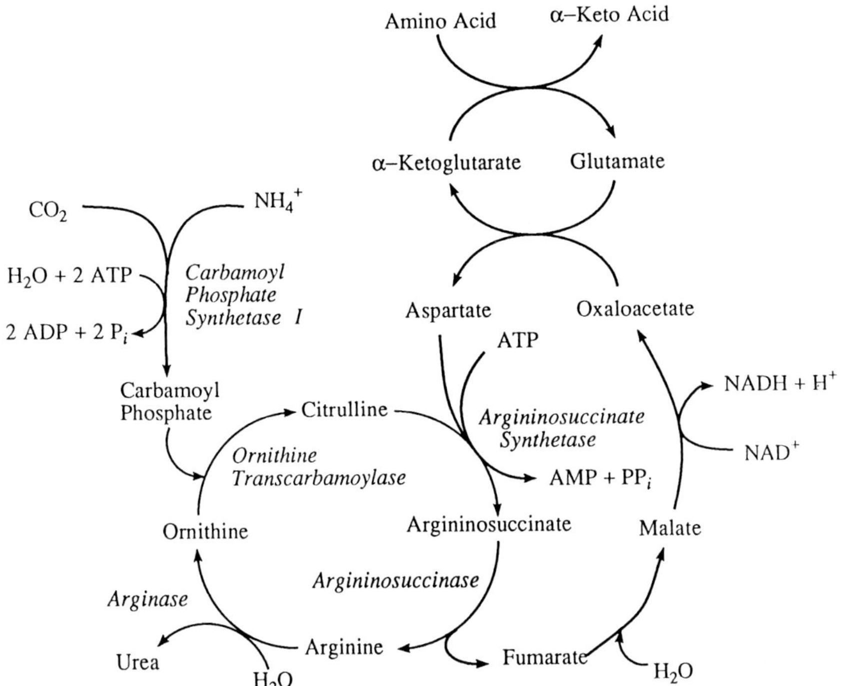

Figure 26.6. Urea cycle plus reactions showing transfer of nitrogen from amino acids to form aspartate.

mate dehydrogenase, animal tissues are equipped with different mechanisms to convert ammonia into nontoxic materials, either for further use in anabolism by the animal or for excretion. The most significant means of excreting excess nitrogen are (1) urea formation and excretion in terrestrial vertebrates (ureotelic), (2) uric acid synthesis in birds and land-dwelling reptiles (uricotelic), and (3) direct elimination in the urine of aquatic animals (ammonotelic).

Biosynthetic reactions

Some ammonia resulting from deamination of amino acids is used for the formation of biologically useful nitrogenous compounds. The processes initially involved in fixation of ammonia throughout the body are (1) reductive amination of α-ketoglutarate to form glutamate (Fig. 26.4) and (2) amination of glutamate to produce glutamine (Fig. 26.4). Glutamine synthesis from glutamate is especially important in the brain because that tissue is extremely sensitive to ammonia. Glutamate and glutamine then participate in a variety of reactions, such as protein biosynthesis and biosynthesis of other low-molecular-weight, nitrogen-containing compounds.

Urea formation

Deamination of amino acids occurs primarily in the liver, and the resulting ammonium ions may be converted to urea in the liver in most terrestrial vertebrates (Fig. 26.6) and then excreted by the kidneys into the urine. Eighty to 90 percent of nitrogen excretion by an adult human occurs via urea. An adult who consumes a typical 100 g of protein daily must then convert approximately 16 g of nitrogen to urea daily to maintain protein homeostasis. It has been estimated that approximately one-fourth of the urea produced daily in humans enters the intestinal lumen, where bacterial urease produces ammonia by hydrolysis of urea. The resulting ammonium ions, then, are absorbed and transported to the liver, chiefly for resynthesis of urea, completing the recycling of urea between the liver and the intestines. Less than 5 percent of the urea nitrogen is excreted in the feces. Ammonium ions and carbon dioxide (derived primarily from the citric acid cycle) interact with ATP to form carbamoyl phosphate in the mitochondria. Primary generators of mitochondrial ammonium ions are glutamate dehydrogenase and glutaminase. Carbamoyl phosphate synthetase I requires *N*-acetylglutamate for activity. *N*-Acetylglutamate is synthesized in greater amounts when greater amounts of amino acids are present, thus providing a signal to increase urea synthesis during amino acid excess.

The carbamoyl group is transferred from carbamoyl phosphate to ornithine to form citrulline, a reaction catalyzed by ornithine transcarbamoylase of mitochondria. After transport of citrulline to cytosol, argininosuccinate synthetase then catalyzes the condensation of aspartate with citrulline to produce argininosuccinate. This synthesis is driven by cleavage of ATP into AMP and inorganic pyrophosphate (PPi) and the subsequent hydrolysis of PPi to 2 Pi. Argininosuccinase then cleaves argininosuccinate into fumarate and arginine. The latter is cleaved hydrolytically by arginase to form urea and ornithine, thus completing the cycle. Arginase is found in large amounts only in the liver in animals that excrete urea. Fumarate formed in the argininosuccinase reaction is hydrated readily to malate and reoxidized to oxaloacetate for acceptance of an amino group, usually from glutamate, to regenerate aspartate.

Thus urea is formed from ammonium ions, CO_2, and the α-amino nitrogen of aspartate. Glutamate that transaminates with oxaloacetate to regenerate aspartate is formed easily by transamination of α-ketoglutarate with most amino acids. Aspartate, therefore, serves to channel α-amino nitrogen from amino acids to urea. The synthesis of urea is an energy-consuming process that requires the cleavage of four high-energy phosphate bonds as follows: $NH_4^+ + CO_2 + 3\ ATP + \text{aspartate} \rightarrow \text{urea} + \text{fumarate} + 2\ ADP + AMP + PPi + 2\ Pi$. Although rare, metabolic disorders of urea synthesis are caused when any one of the five enzymes named in Fig. 26.6 is deficient. The clinical symptoms of vomiting, irritability, lethargy, intermittent ataxia, and mental retardation are caused by ammonia intoxication. Low-protein diets and frequent small meals result in lower blood ammonia concentrations and thus fewer symptoms.

Uric acid synthesis

Birds, lizards, and snakes (uricotelic animals) excrete excess amino nitrogen as uric acid. The pathway for synthesis of uric acid involves generation of aspartate, glutamine, and glycine for the de novo synthesis of purine nucleotides. The purine moiety then is converted to uric acid for excretion by the kidneys. Synthesis of purines and their degradation to uric acid are summarized later.

Direct excretion

Urinary ammonium is derived in the distal tubules of the kidneys of mammals, largely from the hydrolysis of glutamine by glutaminase and secondarily from the deamination of other amino acids. The resultant keto acids are used chiefly for gluconeogenesis. Ammonia formed in renal tubular cells reacts with hydrogen ions to form ammonium ions during metabolic acidosis. Ammonium ion excretion is negligible during alkalosis. Excretion of ammonium ions helps conserve sodium ions, which are the chief cations in the regulation of electrolyte concentration and acid-base balance in the blood. Such replacement of sodium ions with ammonium ions occurs to a greater extent during ketosis when ketone bodies are being eliminated through the urine. Aquatic animals that excrete excess nitrogen as ammonium ions (ammonotelic) produce most excretory ammonia by the action of glutaminase on glutamine.

BIOSYNTHESIS OF AMINO ACIDS

Both nonessential and essential dietary amino acids are necessary for animal life. The essential amino acids must be provided in the diet because of the inability of the animal to synthesize them in adequate quantities. The principal reason for the inability of animals to synthesize these acids is the lack of synthesis of the proper α-keto acids for transamination. The following section emphasizes the metabolic pathways for synthesis of the nutritionally nonessential amino acids. Glutamate dehydrogenase, glutamine synthetase, and transaminases play central roles in amino acid synthesis. For pathways of synthesis of the nutritionally essential amino acids, the reader is referred to a standard biochemistry text. The biosynthesis of the nonessential

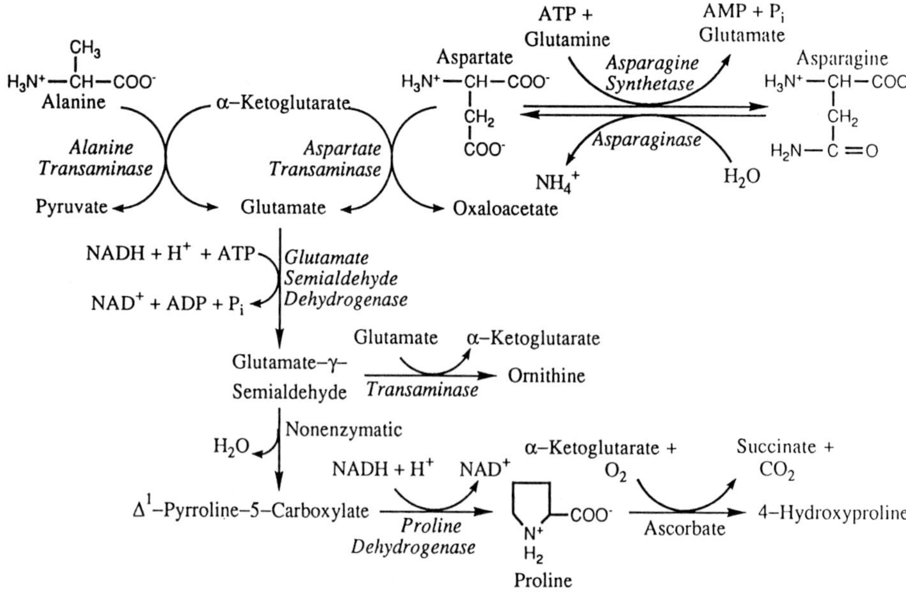

Figure 26.7. Formation of alanine, glutamate, asparagine, aspartate, hydroxyproline, ornithine, and proline. Synthesis of glutamate from glutamine by glutaminase and from α-ketoglutarate by glutamate dehydrogenase is shown in Fig. 26.4.

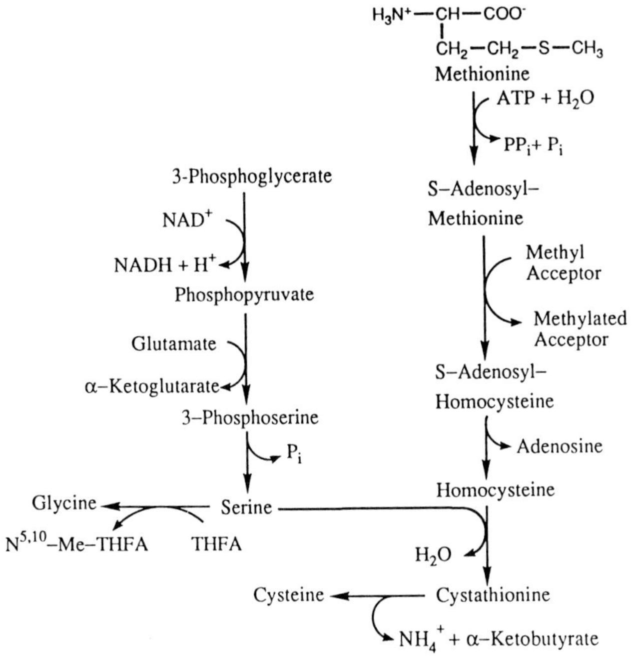

Figure 26.8. Synthesis of serine, glycine, and cysteine. Names of enzymes have been omitted. THFA, tetrahydrofolate; $N^{5,10}$-Me-THFA, 5,10-methylenetetrahydrofolate.

amino acids in animal tissues requires precursors derived primarily from carbohydrate metabolism.

Alanine, asparagine, aspartate, glutamate, glutamine, hydroxyproline, and proline

Alanine, aspartate, and glutamate may be synthesized by transamination reactions as illustrated in Fig. 26.7. Glutamate also may be synthesized by the glutamate dehydrogenase- and glutaminase-catalyzed reactions (Fig. 26.4). Glutamine may be synthesized by amination of glutamate (Fig. 26.4), which is a principal mechanism of ammonia removal in the brain and liver. Glutamate also is a precursor of proline after reduction of the γ-carboxyl group, nonenzymatic cyclization to Δ^1-pyrroline-5-carboxylate, and reduction to proline. Asparagine is generated from aspartate by transfer of the amino group from glutamine.

4-Hydroxyproline is a constituent amino acid of collagen only, the most abundant protein of animals. Hydroxyproline accounts for almost one-half of the amino acids of collagen (one-third is glycine). During maturation of the collagen, proline residues in peptide linkages to the amino group of an adjacent glycine may become hydroxylated by proline hydroxylase, which requires O_2, α-ketoglutarate, and ascorbate (Fig. 26.7). Additional prolines situated next to the amino side of the hydroxyprolines then may become hydroxylated.

Transamination of glutamate-γ-semialdehyde with glutamate results in ornithine synthesis and represents a method of replenishment of urea cycle intermediates (Fig. 26.7).

Cysteine, glycine, and serine

Carbon atoms of serine are derived primarily from 3-phosphoglycerate, an intermediate of glycolysis (Fig. 26.8). Cysteine derives its carbon and nitrogen atoms from serine and the sulfur moiety from methionine, an essential amino acid. Methionine is converted to homocysteine by way of *S*-adenosyl intermediates. In summary, the sulfur of methionine replaces the oxygen of the serine hydroxyl in a transsulfuration process for synthesis of cysteine. This relationship of cysteine and methionine explains why dietary cysteine decreases the requirement for methionine.

The principal reaction for glycine synthesis is from serine. The responsible enzyme, serine hydroxymethylase, is a pyridoxal phosphate enzyme. Two other synthetic means are (1) the transamination of glutamate with glyoxylate to form glycine and α-ketoglutarate and (2) formation from choline, which includes demethylation reactions. Insufficient transamination of glyoxylate seems to be the cause of excess oxidation of glyoxylate to oxalate, which can accumulate as calcium oxalate in the urinary systems. This disorder is called primary hyperoxaluria.

Tyrosine and hydroxylysine

In addition to cysteine, tyrosine and hydroxylysine are synthesized from nutritionally essential amino acids. If their precursor amino acids are deficient, then these three amino acids can approach dietary essentiality. Tyrosine is synthesized from phenylalanine by phenylalanine hydroxylase. This enzyme is a mixed-function oxygenase that is present in the liver. One atom of O_2 is added in the *para* position, and the other oxygen is reduced by tetrahydrobiopterin to form H_2O and dihydrobiopterin. A reductase catalyzes regeneration of the tetrahydrobiopterin by reduction of the dihydrobiopterin with reduced nicotinamide adenine dinucleotide phosphate (NADPH). Thus tyrosine synthesis is represented as follows: Phenylalanine + O_2 + NADPH + H^+ → tyrosine + $NADP^+$ + H_2O.

Synthesis of hydroxylysine occurs by way of a reaction similar to that for hydroxyproline in which the lysine in peptide linkage of procollagen is hydroxylated at C-5. The hydroxyl group of hydroxylysine in collagen becomes a point of covalent attachment of glucose and galactose units during maturation of collagen.

METABOLIC FATE OF AMINO ACIDS

As illustrated in Fig. 26.1, amino acids undergo a great variety of reactions. Metabolic fates of amino acids in animals include the synthesis of proteins and use as fuels in energy metabolism and as precursors of numerous nitrogen-containing compounds such as neurotransmitters, creatine, glutathione, purines, and pyrimidines. When an animal consumes more nitrogen than is excreted, it is described as being in positive nitrogen balance, as during growth and pregnancy. An excess of nitrogen excretion over intake causes negative nitrogen balance.

During nitrogen equilibrium, the human adult must resynthesize about 300 g of the 8000 to 10,000 g of body protein per day to replace the same amount of body protein that undergoes protein catabolism or turnover. Energy for this protein synthesis represents a significant fraction of the daily energy requirements for body maintenance.

Protein synthesis

The animal body may store both glycogen and fat but has little capacity for storage of reserve proteins. Generally speaking, intake of protein beyond daily needs results in formation of increased urea, uric acid, or ammonium ion accompanied by conversion of the carbon skeleton of most amino acids to carbohydrates and lipids or to CO_2 for ATP generation. On the other hand, if dietary intake is less than normal daily needs, catabolism of body proteins proceeds with a loss of body nitrogen until nitrogen balance at a lower level has been achieved. Return to adequate amounts of protein intake results in resynthesis of "mobilized" tissue proteins.

The mechanisms of protein synthesis are complex. Protein synthesis may be considered to occur in four phases: activation, initiation, elongation, and termination.

During the activation phase, individual L-amino acids become attached by ester linkage to the ribose portion of the adenosine residue at the 3′ terminus of specific transfer RNAs (tRNAs) by the action of specific aminoacyl-tRNA synthetases. This action is driven by ATP. At least one specific tRNA and one specific aminoacyl-tRNA synthetase are available for each amino acid. Activation proceeds as a two-step reaction sequence:

Amino acid + ATP + enzyme
$\rightleftharpoons$ aminoacyl-AMP-enzyme + PPi

Aminoacyl-AMP-enzyme + tRNA
$\rightleftharpoons$ aminoacyl-tRNA + AMP + enzyme

Sum: Amino acid + ATP + tRNA $\rightleftharpoons$ aminoacyl-tRNA + AMP + PPi.

Ubiquitous pyrophosphatases shift equilibrium far to the right.

The initiation phase includes dissociation of the ribosome into its large and small subunits, binding of the initiator, methionine-$tRNA_i^{Met}$ ("Met" refers to methionine and "i" refers to initiator) to the small subunit–messenger RNA (mRNA) complex in response to the initiator codon (a nucleotide triplet, usually AUG) on the mRNA, and finally association of the large ribosomal subunit with the small subunit–initiation complex. The methionine-$tRNA_i^{Met}$ occupies the peptidyl (P) site on the ribosome. Initiation (protein) factors participate in generation of the initiation complex. Hydrolysis of GTP to GDP and Pi is involved in the binding of the methionine-$tRNA_i^{Met}$ at the P site. The second aminoacyl-tRNA binding site on the ribosome (A site) is available for the elongation phase to proceed.

The elongation phase starts with the binding of aminoacyl-tRNA at the A site on the ribosome of the initiation complex by a process that requires GTP hydrolysis and an elongation factor. Peptidyl transferase, associated with the large ribosomal subunit, then catalyzes formation of the peptide bond between the amino group of the incoming aminoacyl-tRNA and the carbonyl of methionine of the methionine-$tRNA_i^{Met}$ bound at the P site. The dipeptidyl-tRNA now occupies the A site on the ribosome, whereas the P site carries the deacylated $tRNA_i^{Met}$. The dipeptidyl-tRNA is then translocated to the P site with concomitant release of the deacylated tRNA. This translocation step requires GTP hydrolysis to GDP and Pi and another elongation factor. Another round of elongation occurs with the binding of another aminoacyl-tRNA as dictated by the next codon on the mRNA. The elongation cycle continues until a termination codon is "in" the A site. Thus proteins are synthesized from the amino terminal end to the carboxyl terminal end.

Termination of protein synthesis occurs when a termination codon on mRNA is positioned appropriately on the ribosome for recognition by the protein release factor rather than by a tRNA. The termination codon activates a large ribosomal subunit enzyme to catalyze hydrolysis of the bond between the polypeptide chain and the tRNA at the P site. The polypeptide then leaves the ribosome, and the ribosome dissociates into two subunits for subsequent involvement in initiation of another sequence of protein synthesis. The termination process requires hydrolysis of a GTP to GDP and Pi.

The net reaction of protein synthesis can be written as follows:

$$\underset{\text{Growing peptide}}{RHN{-}\overset{R_1}{\overset{|}{C}}H{-}COO^-} + \underset{\text{Amino acid}}{{}^+H_3N{-}\overset{R_2}{\overset{|}{C}}H{-}COO^-} \xrightarrow[\text{Ribosomes}]{\text{tRNA, mRNA,ATP,GTP,}}$$

$$\underset{\text{Peptide bond}}{RHN{-}\overset{R_1}{\overset{|}{C}}H{-}\overset{O}{\overset{\|}{C}}{-}NH{-}\overset{R_2}{\overset{|}{C}}H{-}COO^-}$$

Several protein factors and enzymes also are needed. Protein synthesis is highly energy intensive and requires at least four high-energy phosphate bonds per peptide bond formed.

Some proteins are destined for export to extracellular space. Specificity of proteins for export derives from synthesis of a "signal" peptide attached to the amino terminal of the growing peptide. Signal peptides facilitate binding of the functioning ribosome to endoplasmic reticulum and "secretion" of protein into endoplasmic reticulum for packaging and eventual export from the cell.

After protein synthesis is completed, certain modifications can occur: Methionine or additional amino acids are removed from the amino terminal; disulfide linkages are formed; lysine and proline residues are hydroxylated in collagen; mono- or polysaccharides may be attached to aspartate, serine, and threonine residues to form glycoproteins; phosphorylation of some protein occurs; and certain polypeptide chains may be cleaved to provide biologically active proteins.

Catabolism of carbon skeletons of amino acids

After removal of nitrogen atoms of amino acids by transamination or deamination, the resulting α-keto acids are converted to intermediates common to carbohydrate and lipid metabolism. As illustrated in Fig. 26.9 and Table 26.2, only leucine and lysine generate nonglucogenic intermediates (acetyl CoA and acetoacetyl CoA) that are not capable of being converted to glucose. Others generate at least one intermediate that is capable of gluconeogenesis. Therefore, in common terminology, leucine and lysine are considered to be ketogenic amino acids whereas others are considered to be glycogenic or ketogenic and glycogenic. *Nonglycogenic* may be a more descriptive term for ketogenic amino acids because even the glycogenic amino acids can contribute carbon to intermediates that ultimately could develop into ketone bodies. As seen in Fig. 26.9, a common property of catabolism of amino acids is the formation of intermediates that can be (1) converted to glucose, (2) oxidized to CO_2 by the citric acid cycle, or (3) converted to ketone bodies and lipids. In fact, all amino acids except hydroxylysine are degraded to just seven different inter-

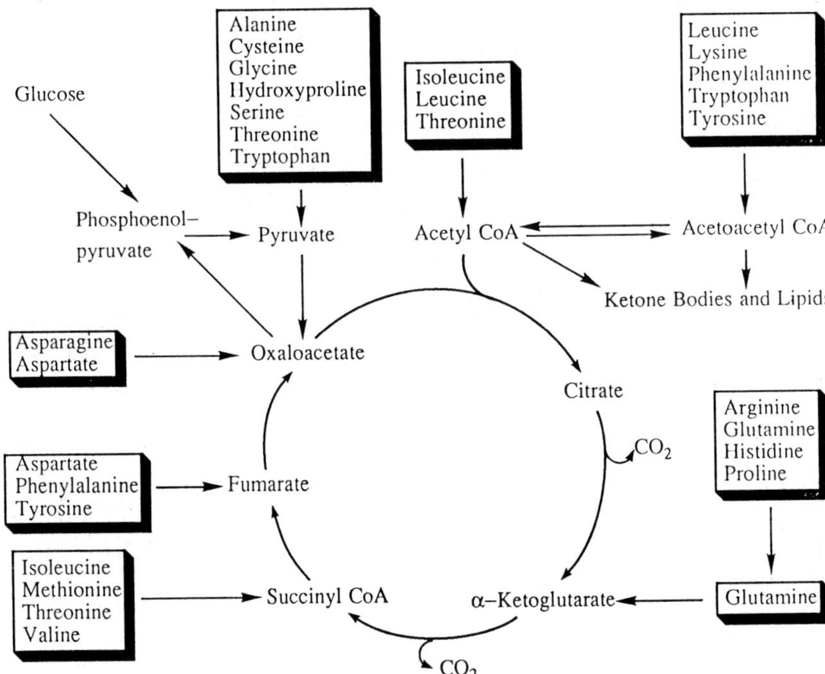

Figure 26.9. Integration of amino acid catabolism with intermediates common to citric acid cycle.

Table 26.2. Classification of amino acids according to catabolic fates

Glucogenic	Glucogenic and ketogenic	Ketogenic
Alanine	Isoleucine	Leucine
Arginine	Phenylalanine	Lysine
Asparagine	Threonine	
Aspartate	Tryptophan	
Cysteine	Tyrosine	
Glutamate		
Glutamine		
Glycine		
Histidine		
Hydroxyproline		
Methionine		
Proline		
Serine		
Valine		

mediates of carbohydrate and lipid metabolism. Amino acids, therefore, provide carbon for synthesis of a variety of compounds, including triacylglycerols, glycogen, ketone bodies, and steroids. Hydroxylysine is not degraded by animal tissues but is excreted in the urine intact or as an *O*-glycosylated compound.

The catabolism of endogenous proteins and amino acids is minimized when dietary carbohydrates and lipids are readily available to meet energy needs. Carbohydrates seem more effective amino acid sparers, probably because the need for gluconeogenesis is less, a greater supply of α-keto acids for synthesis of nonessential amino acids becomes available, and carbohydrates provide a greater stimulus for insulin secretion, which promotes protein anabolism. In energy-deficit situations, body proteins and thus amino acids are needed to maintain normal blood glucose concentrations by way of gluconeogenesis.

Amino acids catabolized to pyruvate

Pyruvate is the entry point for alanine, cysteine, hydroxyproline, serine, threonine, and tryptophan (Fig. 26.9). By transamination with α-ketoglutarate, alanine generates pyruvate (Fig. 26.7). With subsequent action of glutamate dehydrogenase on the generated glutamate, alanine (as well as other transaminated amino acids) then results in ammonium ion generation as alanine + $NAD^+ \rightarrow$ pyruvate + NH_4^+ + NADH + H^+.

More alanine than any other amino acid is absorbed from blood by the liver. Much of the alanine is derived from skeletal muscle, where alanine constitutes from 7 to 10 percent of amino acids in muscle proteins but accounts for more than 30 percent of the amino acids delivered from skeletal muscle to the liver. Much of the alanine is synthesized by transamination after catabolism of muscle protein. Thus a glucose-alanine cycle between skeletal muscle and liver is evident and may be represented as

$$\text{Glucose (muscle)} \xrightarrow[\text{Glycolysis}]{} \text{pyruvate} \xrightarrow[\text{Transamination}]{} \text{alanine (to liver)}$$

$$NH_4^+ \xrightarrow[\text{Urea cycle}]{} \text{urea}$$

$$\text{Alanine (liver)} \xrightarrow[\substack{\text{Transamination}\\ \text{and glutamate}\\ \text{dehydrogenation}}]{} \text{pyruvate} \xrightarrow[\text{Gluconeogenesis}]{} \text{glucose (to muscle)}$$

Cysteine is converted to pyruvate by a variety of pathways, with its constituent sulfur atom emerging as SSO_3^{2-}, SCN^-, H_2S, or SO_3^{2-} (Fig. 26.10). The major pathway seems to be by way of cysteinsulfinate formation, which, after transamination, produces pyruvate and sulfite. Sulfite oxidase catalyzes the oxidation of sulfite to sulfate with reduction of cytochrome c. Thus one high-energy phosphate bond is generated per sulfite oxidized to sulfate. Cystinuria, cystinosis, and homocystinuria are caused by defects in cysteine catabolism.

Catabolism of glycine, serine, and threonine can be considered together (Fig. 26.11). Threonine is catabolized to glycine and acetaldehyde (oxidized to acetyl CoA) by threonine aldolase or is deaminated by threonine dehydratase to form α-ketobutyrate, which is decarboxylated oxidatively to form propionyl CoA. Propionyl CoA is converted to succinyl CoA by reactions illustrated in Fig. 24.10. Glycine, including that derived from threonine, is converted to serine by hydroxymethyl transferase. Serine is deaminated by serine dehydratase to form pyruvate. The major pathway for glycine catabolism is conversion to CO_2, NH_4^+, and methylenetetrahydrofolate.

4-Hydroxyproline catabolism results in generation of pyruvate and glyoxylate by the reactions shown in Fig. 26.12. Glyoxylate may be used by transamination to form glycine.

Tryptophan is catabolized to a variety of end products as indicated in Fig. 26.13. Catabolism is initiated with tryptophan pyrrolase to form *N*-formylkynurenine. Formate is removed by hydrolysis to produce kynurenine that is deaminated by transamination. Kynurenine may be used for synthesis of nicotinic acid as well as acetoacetyl CoA and alanine. Thus tryptophan catabolism decreases the dietary requirement of nonruminant animals for niacin and removes the requirement in the rat, rabbit, dog, and pig.

Amino acids catabolized to oxaloacetate

Asparagine undergoes hydrolytic deamination by asparaginase to form aspartate (Fig. 26.7). Aspartate may transfer its amino group to α-ketoglutarate to form oxaloacetate and glutamate.

Amino acids catabolized to fumarate

Aspartate, phenylalanine, and tyrosine, when catabolized, result in the production of fumarate. Aspartate conversion to fumarate occurs by way of the urea cycle reactions wherein aspartate combines with citrulline to ultimately form arginine and fumarate (Fig. 26.6).

Phenylalanine catabolism is initiated by formation of tyrosine by action of phenylalanine hydroxylase (Fig. 26.14). Subsequent oxidative decarboxylation, oxidation, isomerization, and hydrolysis reactions result in formation of

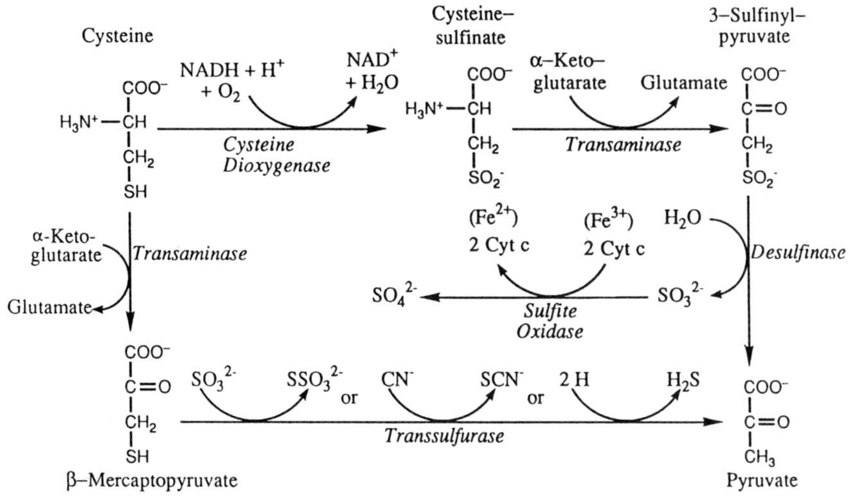

Cysteine; Cysteine–sulfinate; 3–Sulfinyl–pyruvate; Cysteine Dioxygenase; Transaminase; Desulfinase; Sulfite Oxidase; Transsulfurase; β–Mercaptopyruvate; Pyruvate

Figure 26.10. Catabolism of cysteine. Three possible forms of sulfur are produced by the transsulfurase reaction.

fumarate and acetoacetate, which is activated to form acetoacetyl CoA. Classic phenylketonuria is caused by a deficiency of phenylanine hydroxylase. Patients with the disorder must be fed a diet low in phenylalanine to minimize (1) production of phenylpyruvate, phenyllactate, and phenylacetate and (2) mental retardation in the young developing brain.

Amino acids catabolized to succinyl CoA

This group of amino acids that are catabolized to succinyl CoA includes isoleucine, methionine, threonine, and valine. Methionine degradation begins by formation of *S*-adenosylmethionine, which results in formation of cysteine, ammonium ion, and α-ketobutyrate after transmethylation, deadenosylation, and cystathionase activity (Fig. 26.8). The α-ketobutyrate is converted to succinyl CoA by way of propionyl CoA (Fig. 26.11). Threonine is converted to succinyl CoA via α-ketobutyrate by reactions illustrated in Fig. 26.11.

Catabolism of valine and isoleucine proceeds by a similar sequence of reactions (Fig. 26.15). Both undergo transamination, oxidative decarboxylation, and dehydro-

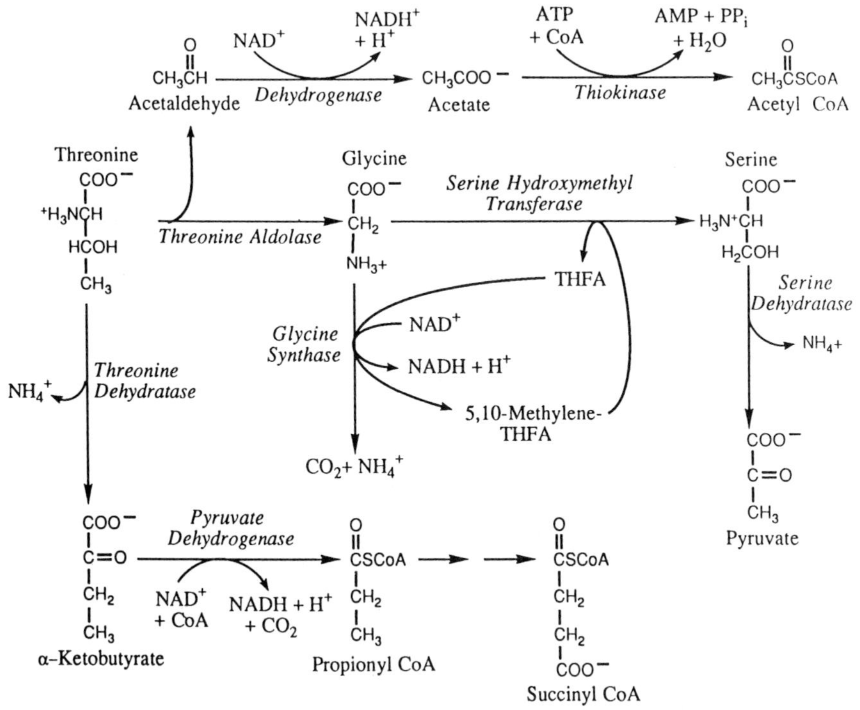

Acetaldehyde; Dehydrogenase; Acetate; Thiokinase; Acetyl CoA; Threonine; Glycine; Serine; Serine Hydroxymethyl Transferase; Threonine Aldolase; Glycine Synthase; Serine Dehydratase; Threonine Dehydratase; 5,10-Methylene-THFA; Pyruvate Dehydrogenase; α-Ketobutyrate; Propionyl CoA; Succinyl CoA; Pyruvate

Figure 26.11. Catabolism of glycine, serine, and threonine. For elaboration of the conversion of propionyl CoA to succinyl CoA, see Fig. 24.10.

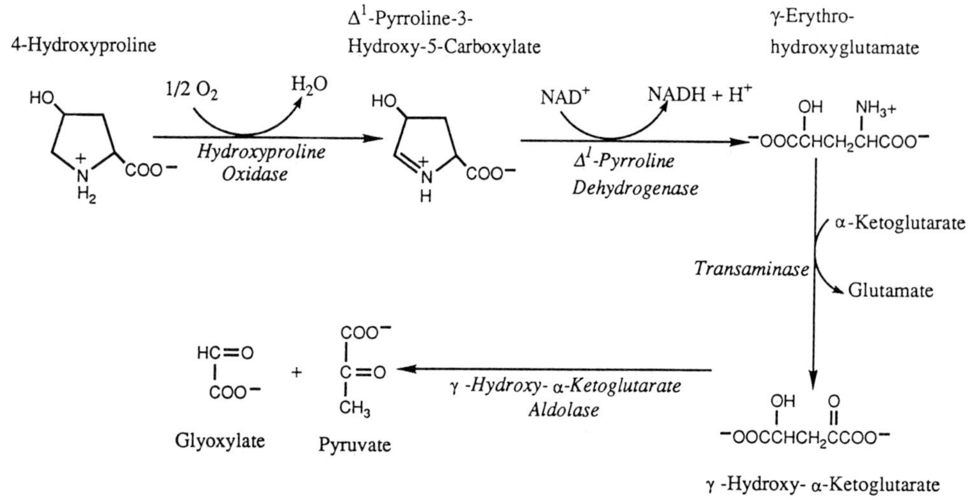

Figure 26.12. Catabolism of hydroxyproline.

genation to form methylacrylyl CoA and tiglyl CoA, respectively. Both of these intermediates then are converted to succinyl CoA by way of propionyl CoA. Catabolism of these two branched-chain amino acids plus catabolism of leucine occurs primarily in skeletal muscle, brain, heart, lung, and spleen; little catabolism of these amino acids occurs in the liver.

Amino acids catabolized to α-ketoglutarate

Catabolism of arginine, histidine, glutamine, and proline yields glutamate; after oxidative deamination or transamination, α-ketoglutarate is generated from the glutamate. Glutamine is converted directly to glutamate by hydrolytic deamination catalyzed by glutaminase (Fig. 26.4). This reaction is especially important in the kidney to generate ammonia for excretion during ketoacidosis.

Arginine catabolism begins with action of arginase to catalyze formation of urea and ornithine. Ornithine undergoes transamination to form glutamate-γ-semialdehyde, which may be dehydrogenated to form glutamate (Fig. 26.7).

The pathway for histidine catabolism is initiated by a direct deamination of histidine, catalyzed by histidase (Fig. 26.16), to form urocanate and ammonium ions. Urocanate undergoes hydration, ring cleavage, and removal of a formimino group to form glutamate, which is then converted to α-ketoglutarate.

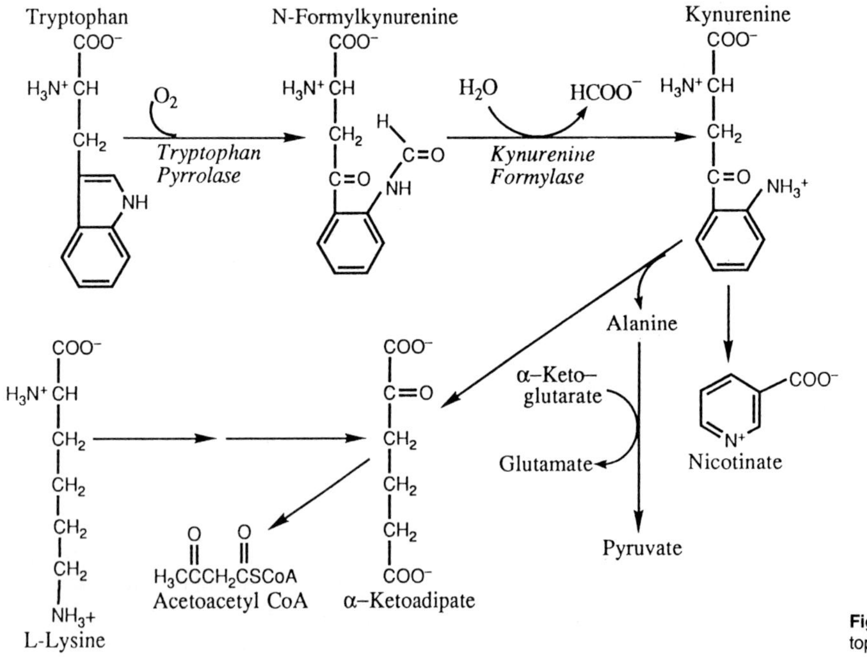

Figure 26.13. Summary of catabolism of tryptophan and lysine.

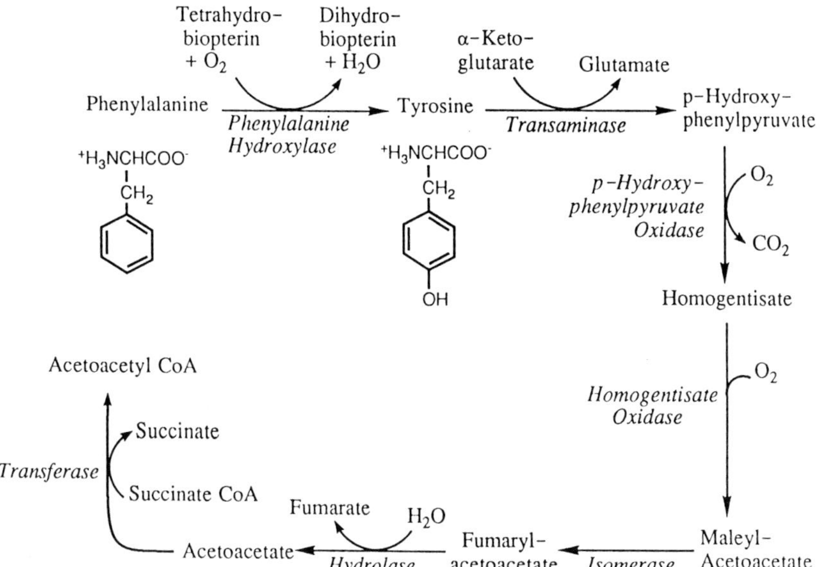

Figure 26.14. Catabolism of phenylalanine and tyrosine.

Proline catabolism to glutamate occurs by way of reversal of its biosynthetic pathway (Fig. 26.7).

Amino acids catabolized to acetyl CoA

Isoleucine is catabolized to acetyl CoA and succinyl CoA as indicated in Fig. 26.15. Leucine is degraded to an acetyl CoA and an acetoacetate. The first three steps of leucine catabolism resemble the first three catabolic reactions of valine and isoleucine. Ultimately, HMG CoA is formed in the mitochondrial matrix. Lyase activity results in the production of the two nonglucogenic end products. Threonine yields, in addition to succinyl CoA, acetyl CoA when catabolized (Fig. 26.11). Maple syrup urine disease in humans is the most highly characterized disorder of branched-chain amino acid catabolism. The characteristic odor of urine is caused by the α-keto acids of the catabolic pathway that accumulate because of insufficient α-keto acid decarboxylase.

Amino acids catabolized to acetoacetyl CoA

Leucine (Fig. 26.15), lysine (Fig. 26.13), phenylalanine (Fig. 26.14), tryptophan (Fig. 26.13), and tyrosine (Fig. 26.14) yield acetoacetyl CoA when catabolized. Unique in this group are lysine and leucine, which yield only nonglucogenic end products and thus commonly are classified as ketogenic amino acids.

Use of amino acids to synthesize several essential nitrogenous compounds

Synthesis of a group of selected nitrogen-containing compounds from individual amino acids, as summarized in Fig. 26.17, is discussed below. Not included in this diagram are a group of small peptides with highly specialized functions. Principal anatomical sites of synthesis will be indicated.

Aspartate, glycine, and glutamine

Aspartate, glycine, and glutamine provide carbon and nitrogen for synthesis of purines and pyrimidines, which is discussed below. In addition, glycine participates in synthesis of porphyrins by condensing with succinyl CoA to form α-amino-β-ketoadipate, which then is decarboxylated to form δ-aminolevulinate. Condensation of two δ-aminolevulinates forms porphobilinogen. Condensation of four porphobilinogens forms a tetrapyrrole that undergoes ring modifications and chelation with ferrous iron to form heme. Heme then combines with specific proteins to form the different cytochromes and hemoglobin. Defects in different reactions of heme synthesis cause a variety of prophyrias that are characterized by increased excretion of porphyrins or their precursors.

Glycine also participates in detoxification processes by forming conjugates, such as with benzoyl CoA (formed from benzoate) to generate hippurate. Liver is the major site of hippurate synthesis. Excretion of hippurate into urine after a test dose of benzoate serves as the basis for a liver function test. Glycine also conjugates with cholyl CoA to form glycocholate, a common secretory form of bile acid. Glycine is also a constituent of glutathione, which is a tripeptide containing glutamate, cysteine, and glycine.

Glycine, arginine, and methionine participate in synthesis of creatine according to a sequence of reactions shown in Fig. 26.18. Creatine phosphate functions as a reserve store of high-energy phosphate by a reversal of the creatine phos-

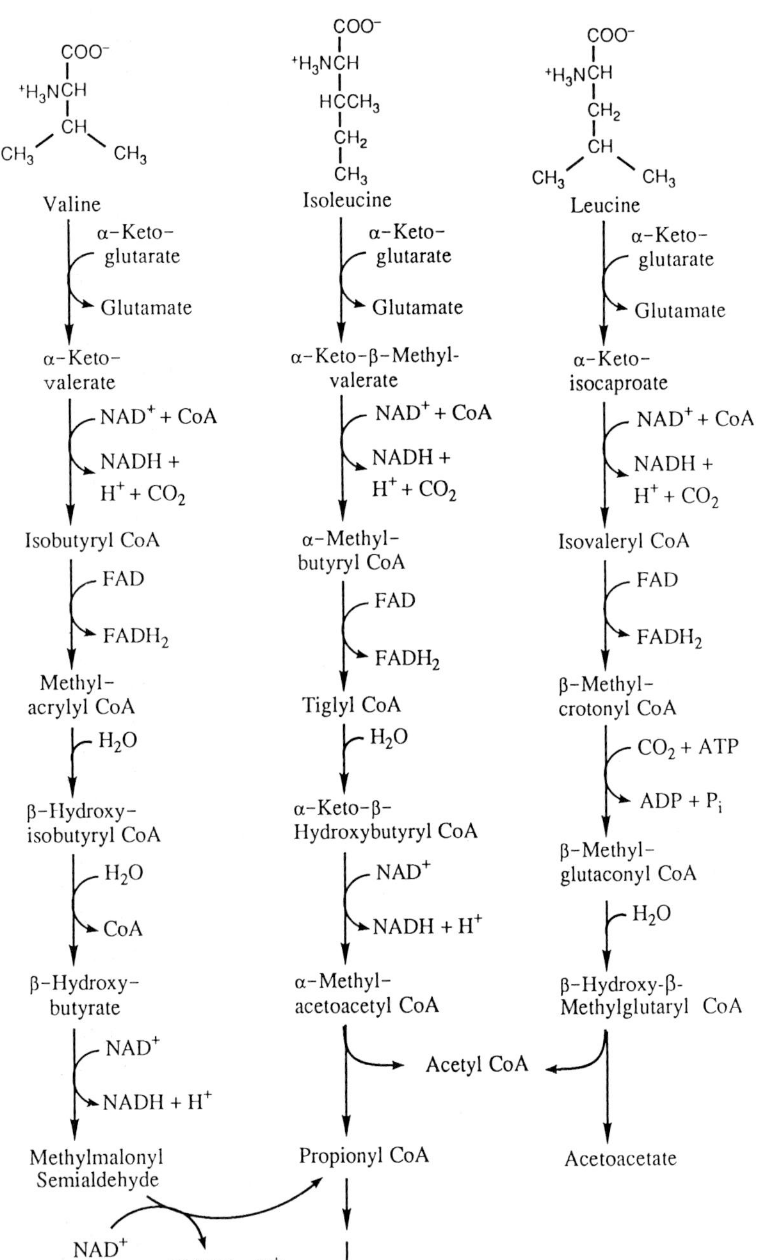

Figure 26.15. Catabolism of branch-chain amino acids. The first three reactions are common for the three amino acids; the same enzyme catalyzes the similar reaction for each of the three amino acids. Names of specific enzymes were omitted. See Fig. 24.10 for elaboration of conversion of propionyl CoA to succinyl CoA and Fig. 25.8 for elaboration of conversion of acetoacetate to acetoacetyl CoA.

phokinase reaction. Creatinine is formed nonenzymatically from creatine phosphate at a remarkably constant daily rate in proportion to muscle mass and is excreted in the urine.

Histidine

Histidine is converted to histamine by a decarboxylation catalyzed by aromatic α-amino acid decarboxylase or a specific histidine decarboxylase. Histamine is a powerful vasodilator that is secreted by mast cells in allergic reactions and in response to trauma. Carnosine, β-alanyl-histidine, is found in muscle and brain and can replace dietary histidine. Methylation of carnosine forms anserine. The function of these two dipeptides is poorly understood. It is suggested that they serve as intracellular buffers in muscle and activators of myosin ATPase. Brain carnosine may be a neurotransmitter; 1- and 3-methylhistidines are

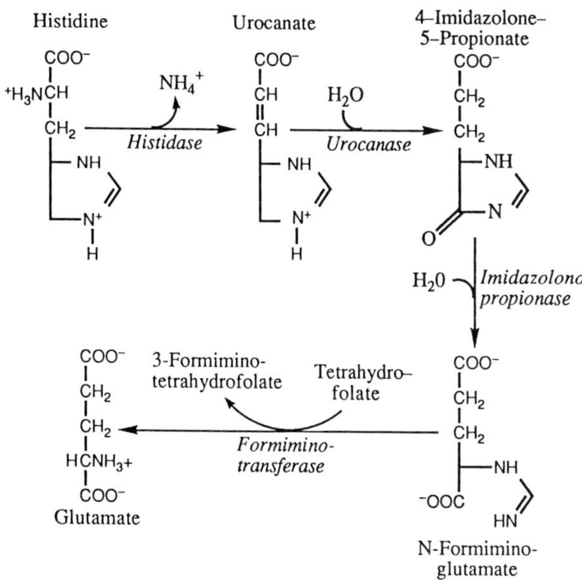

Figure 26.16. Catabolism of histidine.

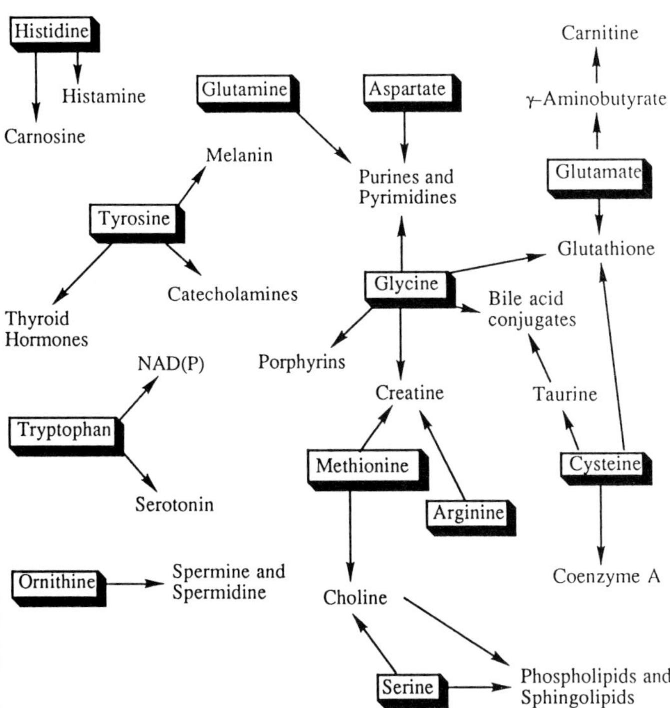

Figure 26.17. Summary of conversions of several amino acids to biologically active, nitrogen-containing compounds.

modified histidines found in skeletal muscle protein. Because these two compounds are used poorly by most animals, a change in their urinary excretion rates indicates altered rates of muscle protein catabolism in most animal species.

Tryptophan

As already indicated, tryptophan is a precursor of nicotinic acid (Fig. 26.13). In addition, tryptophan is a precursor of the neurotransmitter serotonin (5-hydroxytryptamine). Tryptophan is hydroxylated and decarboxylated to form serotonin by enzymes located in serotonergic tissues where serotonin is found rather than being synthesized in one tissue and transported to a second for action.

Melatonin (*N*-acetyl-5-methoxytryptamine) is a hormone that is synthesized in the pineal gland and peripheral nerves from tryptophan and is responsible for regulation of skin pigment (melanin) production. Albinism results when melanin synthesis in melanocytes of skin and eyes is abnormally low.

Tyrosine

The catecholamine neurotransmitters, dopamine, norephinephrine, and epinephrine, are synthesized in the medulla of the adrenal glands and sympathetic ganglia from tyrosine by the sequence of reactions shown in Fig. 26.19. Human patients with Parkinson's disease are administered L-dopa, which will cross the blood-brain barrier to replenish the abnormally low supply of dopamine in their brains. Melanin, the pigment of skin and hair, is synthesized in skin and in nervous tissues, such as substantia nigra of the brain stem, from dopa as an intermediate. Tyrosine is also a direct precursor of the thyroid hormones, which are iodinated tyrosine compounds. Follicle cells of the thyroid gland concentrate iodide and form the iodotyrosines that are linked covalently into a protein called thyroglobulin. Proteolysis results in release of tri- and tetraiodinated thyronines (T_3 and T_4) to plasma.

Ornithine

Ornithine is not a constituent of protein but participates directly in urea synthesis from amino acids and in synthesis of polyamines. Ornithine decarboxylation results in formation of putrescine, which, after additional modification, results in spermidine and spermine. Because of their polycationic form at cellular pH, these three polyamines serve as stabilizing agents for polyanionic structures such as DNA and cell membranes in animal cells.

Glutamate

Decarboxylation of glutamate in inhibitory synapses by glutamate decarboxylase results in production of γ-aminobutyrate, which functions as a neurotransmitter. γ-Aminobutyrate also is a precursor for synthesis of carnitine. Three successive methylations of γ-aminobutyrate with *S*-ade-

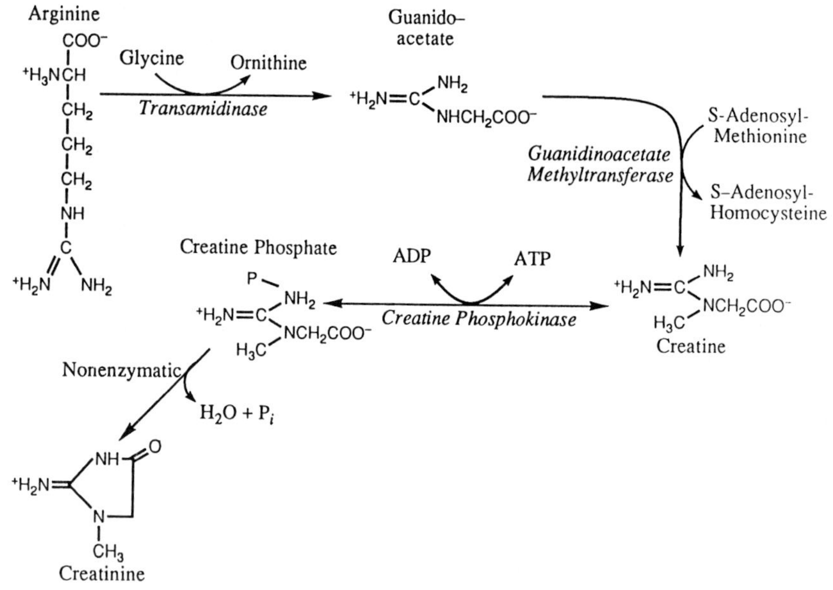

Figure 26.18. Synthesis of creatine, creatine phosphate, and creatinine.

nosylmethionine generates γ-butyrylbetaine, which is hydroxylated to form carnitine.

Serine

As mentioned in Chapter 25, serine is a constituent of phosphatidylserine and sphingomyelins. Further, serine may be decarboxylated to form ethanolamine. The latter compound may be methylated progressively to form choline, a constituent of phospholipids, sphingolipids, and the important neurotransmitter, acetylcholine.

Methionine

Methionine as *S*-adenosylmethionine provides methyl groups for synthesis of carnitine, choline, polyamines, and a variety of other metabolic intermediates.

Cysteine

Cysteine is involved in the synthesis of coenzyme A and of taurine, which conjugates with cholyl CoA in the liver to form taurocholate, an important primary bile acid.

NITROGEN METABOLISM IN RUMINANTS

Ruminants have a unique ability to utilize nonprotein nitrogen compounds such as urea and biuret as a source of nitrogen for amino acids. This unique ability occurs because rumen microbes are capable of synthesizing all essential and nonessential amino acids from nonprotein nitrogen and appropriate carbon and sulfur sources. Depending on the type of protein, most dietary proteins are hydrolyzed with high efficiency by the ruminal microbes to amino acids, which are used directly for protein synthesis by the microbes or are degraded to ammonia and their respective "carbon skeletons." The ammonia and carbon skeletons then may be used for resynthesis of amino acids for microbial use. Some ammonia is transferred to the liver for ureogenesis, and the carbon skeletons are converted to volatile fatty acids. Incompletely degraded proteins pass through the rumen to the abomasum and small intestine for additional hydrolysis. Depending on the time since the animal ate and the amount of dietary protein, the ammonia concentration in the rumen usually ranges between 5 and 8

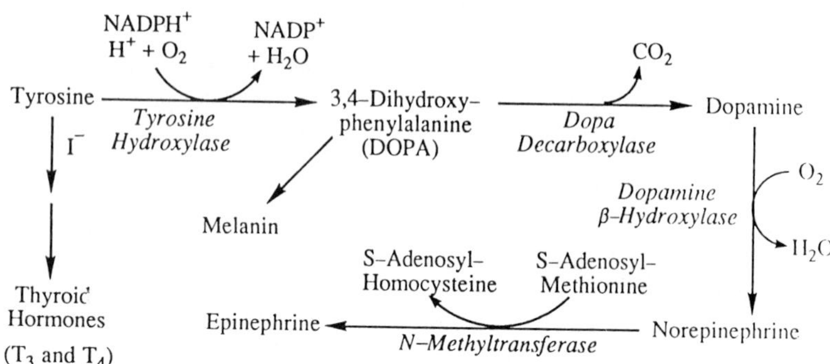

Figure 26.19. Conversion of tyrosine to catecholamines, melanin, and thyroid hormones.

mg/100 ml. Ammonia fixation into amino acids by rumen microbes is initiated primarily by the reactions catalyzed by glutamate dehydrogenase and glutamine synthetase. Some urea is recycled to the rumen for ammoniogenesis. Cattle can grow, reproduce, and lactate, although not at optimal rates, when the diet contains only nonprotein nitrogen as a source of nitrogen.

The sources of amino acids for use by the ruminant, therefore, are (1) those proteins that escape hydrolysis by the rumen microbes and (2) those proteins that are constituents of microbes that reach the abomasum or true stomach and small intestine for digestion (Chap. 19). Microbes in the cecum, as in pseudoruminants, and in the large intestine synthesize microbial proteins from dietary proteins that escape hydrolysis and subsequent absorption in the small intestine. These microbes, however, contribute only a minor amount of amino acids to the animal because little hydrolysis of microbial proteins and subsequent amino acid absorption occurs in the lower tract.

PURINE AND PYRIMIDINE NUCLEOTIDE METABOLISM

All animal cells contain purine and pyrimidine nucleotides. They are involved in a variety of metabolic processes that are summarized as follows:

1. *Energy metabolism*. ATP is the main form of chemical energy available for such metabolic work as to (1) drive metabolic reactions, (2) phosphorylate compounds such as protein, and (3) provide energy for muscle contraction, active transport, and maintenance of cell membrane integrity.

2. *Nucleic acid synthesis*. RNA and DNA are composed of mononucleotides in which primarily ATP, cytidine triphosphate (CTP), GTP, and uridine triphosphate (UTP) are polymerized, after pyrophosphate removal, to form RNA and deoxy forms of ATP, CTP, CTP, and thymidine triphosphate (dATP, dCTP, dGTP, and dTTP), to form DNA.

3. *Physiological mediation*. Examples of nucleotides as mediators of physiological processes include cyclic AMP as "second messenger" in hormone action, ADP in blood platelet aggregation, and adenosine in coronary blood vessel dilation.

4. *Coenzyme component*. NAD, NADP, FAD, FMN, and CoA are necessary coenzymes for numerous metabolic reactions.

5. *Activated intermediates*. Activated intermediates often are carried by nucleotides. Examples are uridine diphosphoglucose (UDPG), UDP-glucuronate, CDP-choline, CDP-ethanolamine, CDP-diacylglycerol, and *S*-adenosylmethionine.

6. *Allosteric effectors*. Intracellular concentrations of AMP, ADP, ATP, NAD^+, and NADH are responsible for regulation of many pathway-controlling enzymes. In normal cells, total concentrations of nucleotides (e.g., ATP + ADP + AMP) are fixed within narrow limits, although the concentration of individual ones may vary considerably. Usually, nucleoside triphosphate concentration exceeds that of the monophosphate form.

Metabolism of purine nucleotides

Purine nucleotides (e.g., ATP and GTP) and pyrimidine nucleotides (e.g., UTP, CTP, and TTP) may be synthesized de novo from amino acids, formate, CO_2, and ribose with a relatively high input of energy, or they may be synthesized by efficient "salvage" pathways in which dietary or endogenous purines (e.g., adenine and guanine) and pyrimidines (e.g., uracil, cytosine, and thymine) are reused. Treatment of cancer is possible with the use of such drugs as methotrexate, 5-fluorouracil, and 6-mercaptopurine that inhibit the synthesis of purine and pyrimidine nucleotides, which are needed in relatively high amounts in rapidly dividing, cancerous tissues.

De novo synthesis

The direct precursors of the purine nucleotides are summarized in Fig. 26.20. Glycine, aspartate, and glutamine provide all nitrogens and some carbons. The ribose phosphate is derived from the pentose phosphate pathway.

The original ribosyl unit on which the purine molecule is constructed is 5-phosphoribosyl-1-pyrophosphate (PRPP), which is synthesized from ribose-5-phosphate and ATP. A series of 10 reactions in which intermediates are attached to a phosphoribosyl group (derived from PRPP) leads to synthesis of the purine nucleotide called inosine-5-monophosphate (IMP). The IMP is converted to either GMP or to AMP, which then can gain two high-energy phosphates apiece to form GTP and ATP, respectively.

Salvage of purines

Purines from the diet or from turnover of cellular nucleic acids can be reused or salvaged, resulting in an energy conservation for the cell. The reactions are as follows:

$$\text{Guanine} + \text{PRPP} \rightarrow \text{GMP} + \text{PPi}$$

$$\text{Hypoxanthine} + \text{PRPP} \rightarrow \text{IMP} + \text{PPi}$$

$$\text{Adenine} + \text{PRPP} \rightarrow \text{AMP} + \text{PPi}.$$

Hypoxanthine is produced from adenine and can be reconverted to AMP or to GMP by way of IMP synthesis. Salvage activity is necessary for normal life functions; this is demonstrated by the interruption of normal functions in the Lesch-Nyhan syndrome in humans, which results from a lack of salvage activity because of deletion of a single gene. Patients with this syndrome have symptoms of cerebral palsy, self-mutilation (biting of fingers and lips), and severe overproduction of uric acid that results in hyperuricemia.

Conversion of ribonucleotides to deoxyribonucleotides

Deoxyribonucleotides, the building blocks of DNA, are synthesized from purine- and pyrimidine-containing

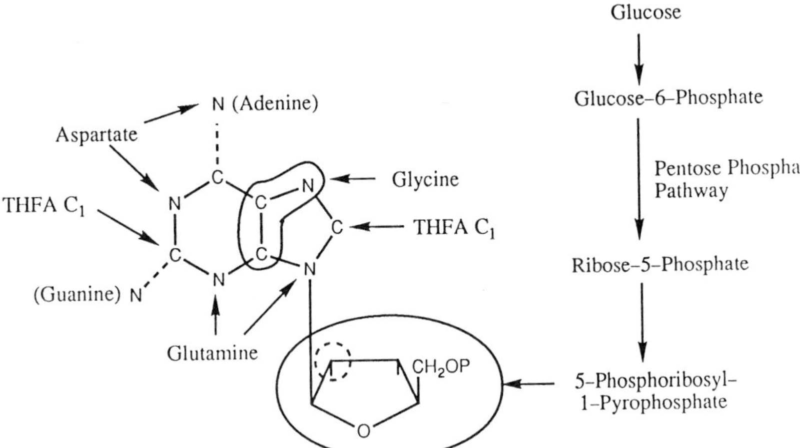

Figure 26.20. Biosynthesis of purine nucleotides. The THFA C_1 refers to a formyl group for transfer from tetrahydrofolate. The encircled carbon atom of the pentose may be hydroxylated (ribose) or hydrogenated (deoxyribose).

ribonucleotides in which C-2 of ribose is reduced by thioredoxin reductase. Electrons for reduction are transferred from NADPH to the disulfide group of thioredoxin and then to the ribose moiety to form the deoxyribose.

Degradation of purines

Uric acid is the end product of purine degradation in primates (including humans) and some reptiles (Fig. 26.21) and of amino acid degradation in birds. Uric acid formation is initiated when nucleotides are dephosphorylated to form nucleosides. Pentose units are removed, and the purine is modified appropriately to form the uric acid. Nonprimate mammals and some reptiles further degrade uric acid to allantoin. Allantoin is generated by uric acid oxidation with removal of a CO_2 from the purine ring. The Dalmatian dog excretes only a small part of its purines in the form of allantoin, even though its liver is fairly rich in urico-oxidase. It seems that the renal threshold for uric acid in this breed of dogs is abnormally low, and uric acid escapes rapidly into the urine before the liver enzyme has had time to oxidize it to allantoin.

Abnormally high rates of uric acid synthesis or low rates of renal excretion result in the development of gout, a disease that afflicts about 0.3% of the human population. Most cases of primary gout are caused by excessive purine synthesis rather than by increased purine nucleotide catabolism. Allopurinol, a competitive inhibitor of xanthine oxidase, is commonly used in treatment of gout because it inhibits urate formation. Hypoxanthine and xanthine, which are more soluble than uric acid, also are excreted during allopurinol therapy.

Metabolism of pyrimidine nucleotides

De novo synthesis

Pyrimidines are synthesized de novo from amino acids and carbamoyl phosphate (Fig. 26.22). Carbamoyl phosphate is synthesized from CO_2 and glutamine in the cytosol of cells by carbamoyl phosphate synthetase II. The carbamoyl synthetase I of the mitochondria of the liver is responsible for carbamoyl phosphate for urea synthesis. Uridine monophosphate (UMP) is formed by condensation of carbamoyl phosphate with aspartate, ring closure of the product, addition of PRPP, and decarboxylation. After transfer of the amide group from glutamine to UMP, CMP is generated. The deoxythymidine monophosphate (dTMP) is

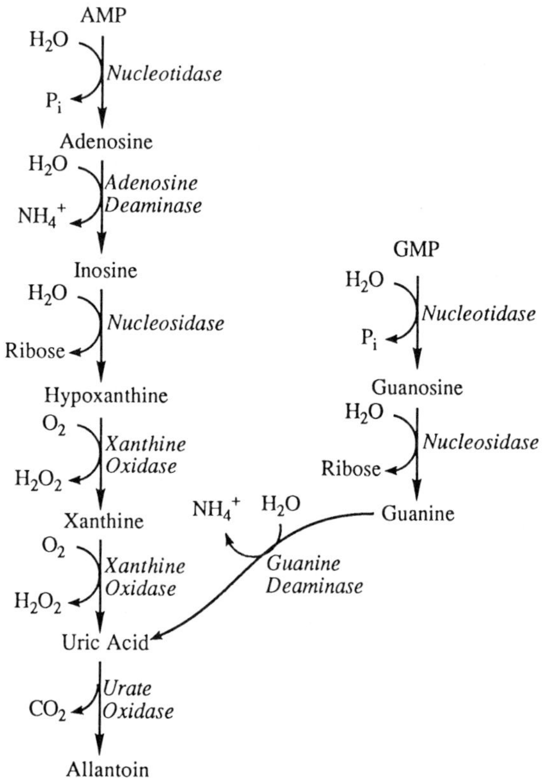

Figure 26.21. Degradation of common purine nucleotides. AMP, adenosine monophosphate; GMP, guanosine monophosphate.

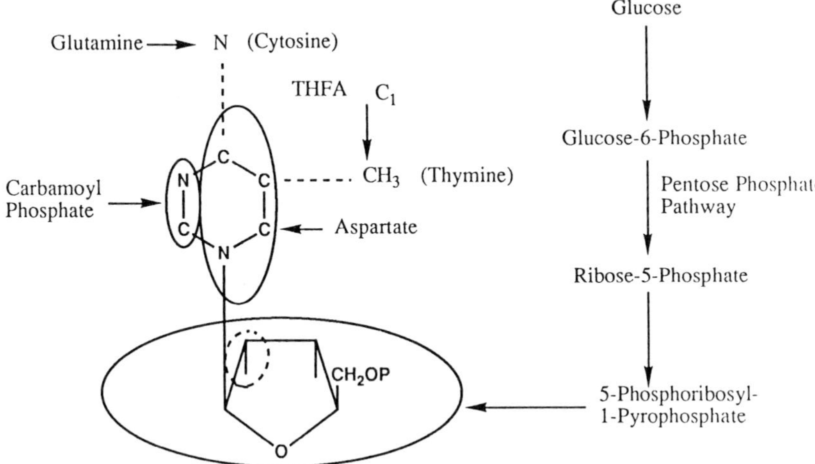

Figure 26.22. Biosynthesis of pyrimidine nucleotides. The THFA C_1 refers to a methyl group for transfer from tetrahydrofolate. The carbon atom of the pentose encircled with a broken line may be hydroxylated (ribose) or hydrogenated (deoxyribose).

synthesized when deoxyuridine monophosphate (dUMP) is methylated.

Salvage of pyrimidines

Like purines, pyrimidines derived from the diet or from turnover of endogenous nucleic acids may react with PRPP to form pyrimidine nucleotides.

Degradation of pyrimidines

Cytosine of nucleotides or nucleosides is converted by deamination to uracil. Then the uracil is cleaved from UMP or dUMP. Cleavage of deoxyribose-3-phosphate from deoxythymidine monophosphate (dTMP) produces thymine. Uracil and thymine are degraded by similar reactions to form β-alanine and β-aminoisobutyrate, respectively, for excretion by way of the urine. Both CO_2 and ammonium ions are produced from pyrimidine catabolism.

NUCLEIC ACIDS AND NUCLEOPROTEINS

Amino acids provide carbon and nitrogen for nucleoside and deoxynucleoside triphosphate synthesis and thus contribute to synthesis of DNA and RNA. Most nucleic acid in animal cells is complexed with primarily basic proteins to form nucleoproteins. Synthesis of DNA (replication) occurs by a mechanism in which a new DNA strand that matches each original strand is synthesized. The DNA provides the template to direct the synthesis of messenger, transfer, and ribosomal RNA (transcription). These three types of RNA, then, function in protein biosynthesis (translation), which is the major fate of the amino acid pool of animals.

REFERENCES

Bender, D.A. 1985. *Amino Acid Metabolism*. 2d Ed. John Wiley & Sons, New York.

Christensen, H.N. 1982. Interorgan amino acid nutrition. *Physiol. Rev.* 62:1193–1233.

Cooper, A.J.L., and Plum, F. 1987. Biochemistry and physiology of brain ammonia. *Physiol. Rev.* 67:470–519.

Henderson, J.F., and Paterson, A.R.P. 1973. *Nucleotide Metabolism: An Introduction*. Academic Press, New York.

Jones, M.E. 1980. Pyrimidine nucleotide biosynthesis in animals. *Annu. Rev. Biochem.* 49:253–79.

Kaldor, G. 1969. *Physiological Chemistry of Proteins and Nucleic Acids in Mammals*. W.B. Saunders, Philadelphia.

Krebs, H.A. 1964. The metabolic fate of amino acids. In H.N. Munro and J.B. Allison, eds., *Mammalian Protein Metabolism*. Vol. 1. Academic Press, New York. Pp. 125–76.

Larner, J. 1971. *Intermediary Metabolism and Its Regulation*. Prentice-Hall, Englewood Cliffs, N.J. Pp. 219–47.

Lowenthal, A., Mori, A., and Marescau, B. 1982. *Urea Cycle Diseases*. Plenum Press, New York.

Meijer, A.J., Lamers, W.H., and Chamuleau, A.F.M. 1990. Nitrogen metabolism and ornithine cycle function. *Physiol. Rev.* 70:701–48.

Moldave, K. 1985. Eukaryotic protein synthesis. *Annu. Rev. Biochem.* 54:1109–50.

Mortimore, G.E., and Poso, A.R. 1987. Intracellular protein catabolism and its control during nutrient deprivation and supply. *Annu. Rev. Nutr.* 7:539–64.

Nyhan, W.L. 1984. *Abnormalities in Amino Acid Metabolism in Clinical Medicine*. Appleton-Century-Crofts, Norwalk, Conn.

Owens, F.N., and Zinn, R. 1988. Protein metabolism in ruminant metabolism. In D.C. Church, ed., *The Ruminant Animal: Digestive Physiology and Nutrition*. Prentice Hall, Englewood Cliffs, NJ. Pp. 227–49.

Saheki, T., Kobayashi, K., and Inoue, I. 1987. Hereditary disorders of the urea cycle in man: Biochemical and molecular approaches. *Rev. Physiol. Biochem. Pharmacol.* 108:22–68.

Scriver, C.R., Stanbury, J.B., Wyngaarden, J.B., and Frederickson, D.S. 1989. *The Metabolic Basis of Inherited Diseases*. McGraw-Hill Book Co., New York.

Snell, K. 1980. Muscle alanine synthesis and hepatic gluconeogenesis. *Biochem. Soc. Trans.* 8:205–31.

Stipanuk, M.J. 1986. Metabolism of sulfur-containing amino acids. *Annu. Rev. Nutr.* 6:179–209.

Wellner, D., and Meister, A. 1981. A survey of inborn errors of amino acid metabolism and transport in man. *Annu. Rev. Biochem.* 50:911–68.

CHAPTER 27

Disorders of Carbohydrate and Fat Metabolism | by Emmett N. Bergman

In domestic animals the principal metabolic disorders associated with carbohydrate, fat, and protein metabolism are bovine ketosis, ovine pregnancy toxemia, spontaneous hypoglycemias such as hypoglycemia in newborn pigs, diabetes mellitus in dogs, and numerous fatty liver syndromes that affect both mammals and birds.

RUMINANT KETOSIS

In ruminants ketosis and an associated hypoglycemia occur most frequently in high-producing dairy cows (acetonemia) and in pregnant ewes (pregnancy toxemia, twin-lamb disease). Ketosis of varying intensity may occur in all animal species, however, and can be induced by starvation, high-fat and low-carbohydrate diets, impaired liver function, anesthesia, and endocrine disorders such as diabetes mellitus. Females of any species are more susceptible to ketosis than males, and this predisposition is exaggerated during lactation or pregnancy. The minimum number of fetuses required for the development of intense ketosis is two in the sheep, three in the guinea pig, and eight in the rat. The ketosis syndrome of the guinea pig and rat is very similar to that of the sheep.

In all pregnant and lactating animals, in fact, there is a continuous withdrawal of metabolites, especially glucose and amino acids, by the fetuses and by the mammary gland. Under normal circumstances, maternal adjustments are adequate, but the animal becomes susceptible to a state of accelerated starvation. Inadequate feed intake or unusually large withdrawals of metabolites can overwhelm the body's ability to mobilize its metabolic fuels. A major difference between pregnancy and lactation is that the total energy demands for lactation are larger, but they are highly variable and dependent on the lactating animal's supply of metabolites and nutrients. Thus, when there is an energy shortage or hypoglycemia, milk production decreases. Fetal metabolism, however, is more independently controlled and less susceptible than the mammary gland to changes in the maternal hormonal and metabolic environment. For example, fetal insulin plays a major role in the metabolism of the fetus itself and is already present at early stages of gestation.

Ketosis usually affects cows within 6 weeks after calving. The mortality rate is low, but since ketosis causes a marked loss in milk production and body weight, it results in a great economic loss to the dairy farmer. Bovine ketosis has been classified into primary and secondary (or complicated) ketosis. Secondary ketosis may be induced or aggravated by a poor appetite resulting from any one of a variety of pathological conditions, such as metritis, gastrointestinal disturbances, mastitis, and nephritis. Ketosis of sheep usually occurs during the last month of pregnancy, when fetal growth is the most rapid. It is most common in ewes carrying twins or triplets, and practically all of the ewes die unless parturition occurs or the lambs are removed by a cesarean operation. Ketosis can often be produced experimentally in sheep by undernutrition during pregnancy, but ketosis in cows is more difficult to induce. Administration of thyroid hormones along with a low-energy or high-protein diet is the only method found to produce severe ketosis in cattle.

Ketoses of cattle and sheep thus are not identical diseases, but they have at least three features in common: (1) a negative energy balance due to high production or inadequate food consumption, (2) a reduction of carbohydrate in the blood (hypoglycemia) and liver (glycogen depletion), and (3) an increased fat metabolism. The first two features undoubtedly influence the third, and the body compensates in the direction of excessive fat metabolism and ketosis.

Glucose metabolism

Tissue requirements for glucose

In ruminants, a blood glucose concentration of 30 to 60 mg/dl is required for normal physiological processes. Below this amount, ketosis and clinical signs become evident, although the severity of illness depends on the duration as well as the degree of hypoglycemia. Glucose is needed by the body for at least the following five components: (1) nervous system, (2) fat, (3) muscle, (4) fetuses, and (5) mammary gland.

The nervous system, in particular, is completely dependent on a regular supply of glucose for its oxidative requirements. This is made quite clear by the coma that results from severe hypoglycemia and the rapidity of recovery if glucose is injected. During prolonged glucose shortage or starvation, the brain in most animal species will begin to use ketone bodies and free fatty acids for at least part of its energy requirements. This is not true in ruminants, however, and no reduction occurs in the brain's need for glucose. Recent estimates show that in ruminants the nervous system uses 10 to 15 percent of the glucose produced in the whole body.

Glucose also is indispensable, although in small amounts, for the turnover and synthesis of body fat in that it serves as a glycerol precursor and as an essential reducing agent (formation of reduced nicotinamide adenine dinucleotide phosphate, or NADPH). Even further, glucose is needed for the production of muscle glycogen, which serves as a source of anaerobic energy during exercise.

The greatest demand for glucose is during late pregnancy and lactation. Glucose is the predominant metabolite used by the fetus for energy. In addition, the placentas of all ungulates convert some of the glucose to fructose, and the glycogen content of the fetal liver, lung, and muscle increases to very high levels just before term. Further, the glycogen amounts are not greatly reduced by starvation of the mother. Lactation also poses a great demand for glucose since milk contains about 90 times as much sugar as does blood, and glycerol has to be synthesized for production of milk fat. A high-producing milk cow requires more than 1800 g of glucose per day, and 70 to 90 percent is used for milk production. Normal sheep synthesize about 100 g of glucose per day, but during late pregnancy this basal rate goes up to about 180 g per day. When the rate of synthesis is too low, hypoglycemia develops, and the animal becomes ketotic.

Sources of glucose

In animals with simple stomachs dietary carbohydrates such as starch and sucrose are sources of glucose. In roughage-fed ruminants, however, dietary carbohydrates, including cellulose, are fermented in the rumen to form volatile fatty acids (VFAs). Thus only small amounts of glucose are absorbed, and gluconeogenesis (synthesis of glucose from nonhexose sources) is of prime importance for ruminant metabolism. The supply of glucose precursors and the organs that synthesize glucose can be limiting factors for the animal's overall productivity and even for its survival. The liver is the major gluconeogenic organ and produces about 85 percent of the glucose in ruminants. The cortices of the kidneys produce about 15 percent of the glucose under normal conditions. Evidence indicates, however, that the kidneys may produce even more glucose during starvation and thus seem to be emergency-type organs for glucose production.

Only four groups of metabolites are important for gluconeogenesis in ruminants: propionate, protein, glycerol, and lactate. Other glucose precursors are present only in small amounts, and their contribution is limited (Fig. 27.1).

Acetic, propionic, and butyric acids are the most important of the VFAs, but propionic acid is the only VFA that can be used for gluconeogenesis (Fig. 27.2). It is the major source of glucose and glycogen in the ruminant. The percentage of the total glucose formed from propionate varies with the diet, from a maximum of about 70 percent under heavy grain feeding to none at all during starvation. Acetic

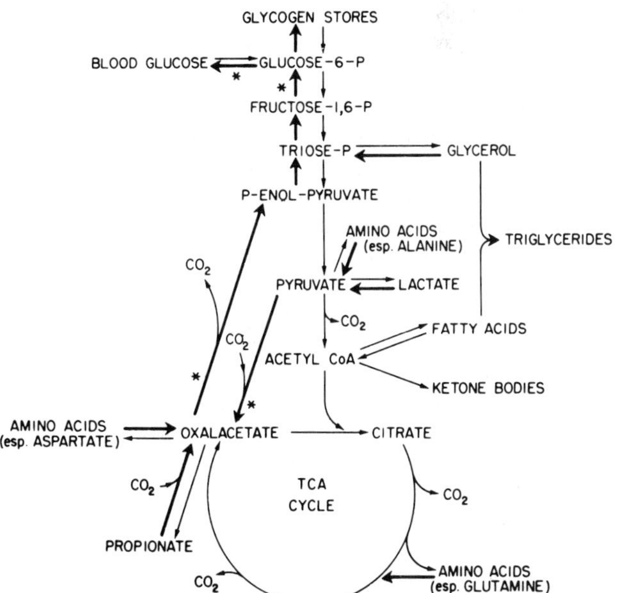

Figure 27.1. Major metabolic pathways in ruminant liver. Since insufficient glucose is absorbed, one of the main functions of the liver is gluconeogenesis. These reactions are shown by heavy arrows; four major pacemaker reactions are indicated by asterisks. TCA, tricarboxylic acid.

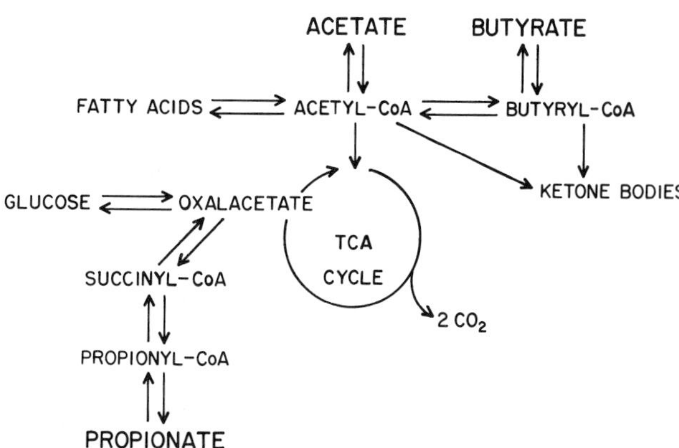

Figure 27.2. Major metabolic pathways for metabolism of volatile fatty acids. Propionate is glucogenic, whereas acetate and butyrate are ketogenic. TCA, tricarboxylic acid.

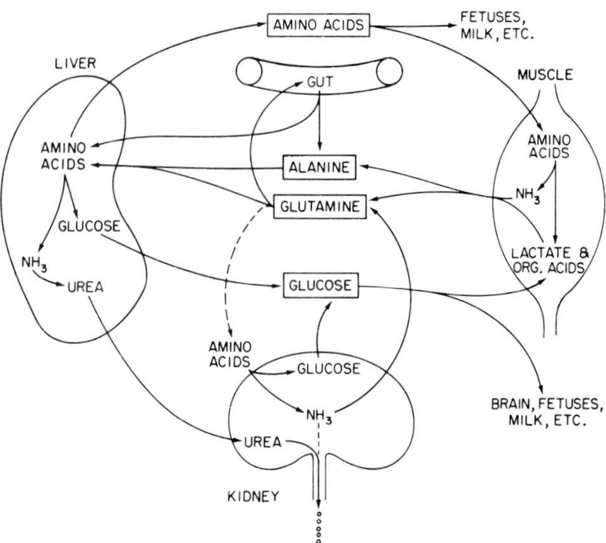

Figure 27.3. Alanine and glutamine as major forms of amino acid transport or gluconeogenesis in ruminants. Both are continuously released by muscle and removed by the liver. In addition, glutamine is an important energy source for the intestine. The kidneys normally release glutamine into the blood, but broken lines indicate that glutamine is removed during fasting or acidosis. In this case, ammonia is produced for neutralization of acids in the urine. (From Bergman 1973, *Cornell Vet.* 63:341–82.)

and butyric acids, as well as longer-chain fatty acids, cannot contribute to a net synthesis of carbohydrate. Unlike propionate, they either form ketone bodies or enter the tricarboxylic acid (TCA) cycle as acetyl CoA. In this case, both carbon atoms are lost as CO_2 and a net gain of oxaloacetate is not possible.

Other than propionate, the most important source of glucose is protein. Recent estimates show that protein accounts for a range of about 20 percent of the glucose synthesis in feeding ruminants to about 50 percent during complete starvation. Alanine and glutamine are the principal amino acids involved (Fig. 27.1) and account for more than one-half of the glucogenicity of all the amino acids. Aspartic acid also is highly glucogenic, but its blood concentration is too low to be significant.

Figure 27.3 shows that, although nearly all amino acids are absorbed into the blood, variable amounts are removed by the liver or are transported to peripheral tissues. Alanine is absorbed in unusually large amounts; more important, both alanine and glutamine are continuously formed from other amino acids in the muscles. Both are then released to the blood and removed by the liver for glucose synthesis. In normal ruminants the kidneys also release glutamine, but during fasting and acidosis this renal release function switches to that of removal. In these conditions ammonia is needed to neutralize acids in the urine, and the amino groups of glutamine serve as the major source of ammonia. Additional glucose is then produced in the kidneys from the carbon chain of glutamine to augment that formed by the liver. Release of alanine and glutamine by muscle is greatly increased during fasting to continue this use of glutamine by the kidneys and conversion of alanine to glucose by the liver.

Lactic acid and glycerol are sources of glucose, but little is produced during normal digestion. During starvation, however, glycerol from mobilized body fat largely replaces propionate as an important glucogenic compound. The synthesis of glucose from the above compounds is controlled by several pacemaker reactions (see Fig. 27.1), which in turn are influenced by specific enzymes and hormones.

Fat metabolism

Rumen volatile fatty acids

Acetic, propionic, and butyric acids are the major VFAs produced by rumen fermentation. Acetate is not used by the liver but is readily oxidized in the TCA cycle by the muscles and is also used for synthesis of fat (lipogenesis) by the adipose tissue and mammary gland (Fig. 27.2). Its concentration in the blood during ruminant ketosis can be either higher or lower than normal. No specific defect in acetate utilization has been found in ketosis, and the probable reason for any decreased metabolism is that less acetate is being absorbed because of the decreased feed consumption. Long-chain fatty acids are mobilized from adipose tissue in ketosis and, because of their high concentration in the blood, would be metabolized in place of acetate. Under conditions of excessive fat metabolism and acetyl CoA formation, however, acetate sometimes can be released from the tissues (endogenously) in increased amounts, resulting in high blood concentrations.

Practically all of the absorbed propionate and butyrate are removed by the rumen epithelium and liver before they reach the general blood circulation. Propionate is glucogenic, whereas butyric acid is ketogenic. Most of the butyric acid is converted to ketone bodies by the rumen epithelium during absorption.

Adipose tissue and fat transport

The body's reserve of glucose and glycogen is limited, and, in terms of calories, it can sustain the animal for only a few hours. Adipose tissue, on the other hand, serves as a vast storage depot for calories. The major functions of adipose tissue can be summarized as follows: (1) synthesis of triglycerides (triacylglycerides), (2) storage of triglycerides, and (3) release of free fatty acids (FFAs) and glycerol into the blood. The plasma FFA concentration, therefore, can be regarded as an index of fat mobilization and metabolism. The quantity of FFAs in plasma is small, but its turnover is extremely rapid, on the order of 2 to 3 minutes.

Acetate is the major precursor of adipose tissue triglycerides in ruminants. Glucose, however, still plays an essential role: First, it forms α-glycerophosphate, which is the precursor of glycerol with which fatty acids are esterified for triglyceride storage. Adipose tissue has no glycerokinase, and therefore free glycerol cannot be used. Second, glucose furnishes NADPH via the pentose pathway; NADPH is specifically required as a reducing agent at recurring steps in the synthesis of fatty acids.

The processes of fat synthesis and degradation are under nervous and endocrine control. During periods of exercise, stress, or excitement, the body's energy requirements are temporarily increased. Therefore the sympathetic nerve supply and the release of epinephrine by the adrenal medulla increase the rate of lipolysis and release FFAs to the bloodstream. Thus the body tissues are flooded with an easily oxidizable substrate for their energy needs.

During starvation, and especially during hypoglycemia, there is a decreased rate of glucose utilization, which results in a decreased synthesis of triglycerides. In addition, the pituitary gland increases its output of growth hormone (somatotropic hormone, STH) and adrenocorticotropic hormone (ACTH), which increase the rate of formation of FFAs and glycerol from the stored triglycerides. Thus the effect of decreased glucose utilization, which is especially marked during hypoglycemia, is an increase in the rate of FFA release from adipose tissue cells. The liver is then flooded with FFA, much of which is oxidized to acetyl CoA. These two-carbon fragments condense into ketone bodies, which appear in the bloodstream in increased concentrations. An increased plasma FFA concentration has been demonstrated quite clearly in both bovine and ovine ketosis and is the primary factor in the development of ketosis.

Ketone body metabolism

In normal ruminants, the concentration of blood ketone bodies is only 2 to 4 mg/dl. During hypoglycemia and increased fat mobilization, however, the ketone concentration will rise, usually above 10 mg/dl.

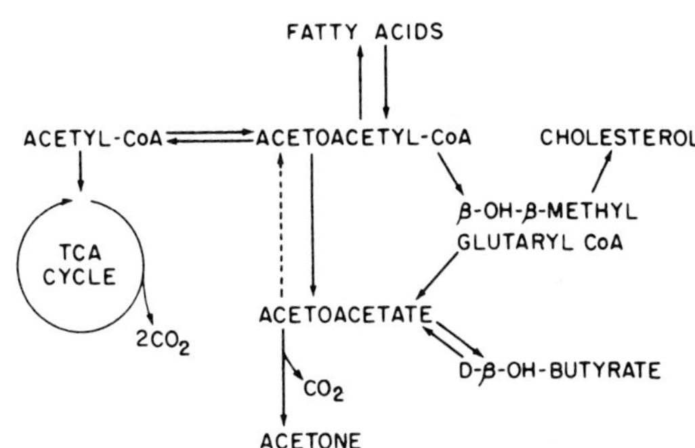

Figure 27.4. Major metabolic pathways in the formation, utilization, and interconvertibility of ketone bodies. The reaction indicated by the broken line does not occur in liver. TCA, tricarboxylic acid.

Production of ketone bodies

The ketone bodies are acetoacetic acid (CH_3COCH_2-COOH), β-hydroxybutyric acid ($CH_3CHOHCH_2COOH$), and acetone (CH_3COCH_3). All of these compounds arise from acetoacetyl CoA, which is a normal intermediate in fatty acid oxidation but which also is readily formed from acetyl CoA (Fig. 27.4). The liver is the primary site of ketone body production during ketosis; once acetoacetate is formed, however, the liver cannot reconvert it efficiently to acetoacetyl CoA. This is because the liver is deficient in the necessary activating enzyme system. In the normal ruminant, smaller amounts of ketone bodies also are produced from butyrate and acetate by the rumen epithelium during the process of absorption. Furthermore, certain feeds, such as silage, may at times have a high butyric acid content and therefore augment ketone body production.

Acetoacetate is the parent ketone body (see Fig. 27.4), but most of it is reduced to β-hydroxybutyrate by the coenzyme, reduced nicotinamide adenine dinucleotide. The reaction is reversible and the compounds are interconvertible, but wide variations in the ratio of the two acids may be encountered. The conversion of acetoacetate to β-hydroxybutyrate may play a special role in the transport of ketone bodies by the blood, since acetoacetate is unstable. It undergoes irreversible decarboxylation to form acetone at a rate of about 5 percent per hour. Acetone metabolism is of little importance to the animal unless the ketosis is severe and of long duration.

Utilization of ketone bodies

Since ketone bodies are produced by the liver but are used by other tissues, ketosis could conceivably be the result of underutilization by the extrahepatic tissues or overproduction by the liver. The underutilization theory was widely accepted at one time, but many studies have now demonstrated extensive extrahepatic use of ketone bodies, even in severely ketotic states. Except for the liver, they readily enter the TCA cycle for oxidation to CO_2 (Fig. 27.4).

By the infusion of isotopically labeled ketone bodies, it has been possible to estimate the production and utilization of ketone bodies by the whole animal. Studies on sheep show that the rates of production and utilization of ketone bodies in ketotic sheep are proportional to their concentration in the blood, but only up to a total ketone concentration of about 20 mg/dl. Therefore ketone body concentrations up to this amount reflect the rate of ketone production. Utilization, in turn, is regulated by the blood ketone concentration. Maximal ketone body utilization occurs at about 20 mg/dl, and after reaching this maximum, small increments in production result in similar increases in blood concentration. The maximal utilization rate of ketone bodies in sheep is about the same in naturally occurring ketosis as it is in artificial ketosis. Sheep can derive at least 30 percent of their energy from ketone bodies.

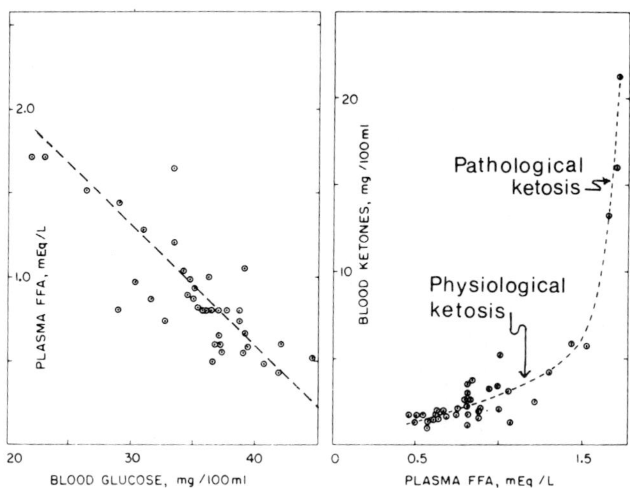

Figure 27.5. Relationship between plasma free fatty acids (FFA), blood glucose, and blood ketone bodies in pregnant sheep. (Calculated from Reid and Hinks 1962, *Aust. J. Agric. Res.* 13:1124–36.)

Excretion and toxicity of ketone bodies

Ketone bodies are excreted mainly in urine (ketonuria) and milk. A third avenue is that of acetone via the breath. All are easily detectable by simple qualitative chemical tests or by the odor. The amount excreted varies with the severity of ketosis, and excretion in urine far exceeds that in milk or breath. The total amount excreted, however, probably never exceeds 10 percent of that produced.

Since ketone bodies are acids, an excessive accumulation in the body can produce a metabolic acidosis. The acidosis in ruminant ketosis, however, is much less severe than that in diabetes mellitus. β-Hydroxybutyrate is nontoxic, but high concentrations of acetoacetate and acetone can result in depression of the central nervous system and contribute to the development of clinical signs. The concomitant hypoglycemia, however, is the major factor involved in the onset and development of the disease.

Metabolic interrelationships

Physiological versus pathological ketosis

The metabolism of glucose, fat, and ketone bodies is intimately related. When the concentration of blood glucose decreases to hypoglycemic levels, the ketone bodies increase, frequently to high but erratic concentrations.

Figure 27.5 shows that the plasma concentrations of FFAs, which represent the mobilization of body depot fat, and glucose are inversely proportional to each other. In other words, when the blood glucose concentration is normal, the FFA concentration is low and of only minor importance, but as blood glucose falls to hypoglycemic proportions the FFA concentration increases in a linear relationship.

Figure 27.5 also shows the relationship of FFAs to ketone bodies. Blood ketones increase as the FFA concentration increases, but the increase is not linear. When the FFA concentration becomes more than about 1.5 mEq/L, the ketone body concentration increases rapidly and can reach almost any magnitude. It is at this point that the body shifts from what is called a physiological ketosis to a pathological ketosis. Before this, ketogenesis is controlled merely by FFA mobilization from the adipose tissue in response to a low blood glucose level, with only part of the FFAs forming ketone bodies. The more severe or pathological ketosis is most likely due to a hepatic factor, a shift in the pattern of FFA utilization in the liver.

Free fatty acid use and oxalacetate deficiency

The liver is a major user of FFAs. It removes about 25 percent, regardless of the actual quantities released. In the liver, however, there are only three major pathways for FFA catabolism (see Fig. 27.1): (1) oxidation to CO_2 in the TCA cycle, (2) partial oxidation to ketone bodies, and (3) esterification to triglycerides. If the first pathway is decreased, ketogenesis and liver fat formation increase out of proportion to the FFAs being presented. If the condition also is of sufficient duration, a grossly fatty liver occurs. Reduced hepatic function associated with fatty livers occurs frequently in ruminant ketosis.

An important theory as to how the first FFA pathway (oxidation to CO_2) is decreased involves oxalacetate deficiency. Oxalacetate plays a dual role in gluconeogenesis and the production of CO_2 (see Fig. 27.1). It is needed to combine with acetyl CoA for CO_2 production and is involved in the metabolism of all glucose precursors except glycerol. Thus, if oxalacetate becomes deficient, a shift in liver FFA metabolism to that of ketogenesis and fat formation occurs. There are several hypotheses for hepatic oxalacetate deficiency, but the most likely is a shortage of glucose precursor (propionate, amino acids, or lactate).

Adequately fed ruminants are not short of glucose precursors. If they are not eating, however, or if large amounts of feed are needed for high productivity, an excessive drain of precursors will occur, resulting in hypoglycemia and ketosis. Feed intake may also be reduced even further in ruminants with clinical signs of hypoglycemia and ketosis, because vital areas of the nervous system become depressed by the hypoglycemia, ketosis, or other metabolic disturbances.

Hormonal control

The hormonal control of metabolism is complex, but it occurs in two general areas: (1) extrahepatic tissues to alter the supply of precursors and (2) the liver to control precursor uptake and metabolic pathways.

Control of precursor supply

If hypoglycemia occurs (Fig. 27.6), the first response is a decreased secretion of insulin, increased secretion of glucagon, and stimulation of the hypothalamus to increase the secretion of epinephrine from the adrenal medulla. These will increase glycogenolysis in the liver but will also cause mobilization of glycerol and FFAs from adipose tissue. Glycerol will increase glucose synthesis, and more FFAs will provide an alternate fuel for oxidation by the body. Amino acid release from muscle is also stimulated, and additional glucose precursors, especially alanine and glutamine, become available for gluconeogenesis.

These hormonal reflexes are rapid; if a glucose shortage

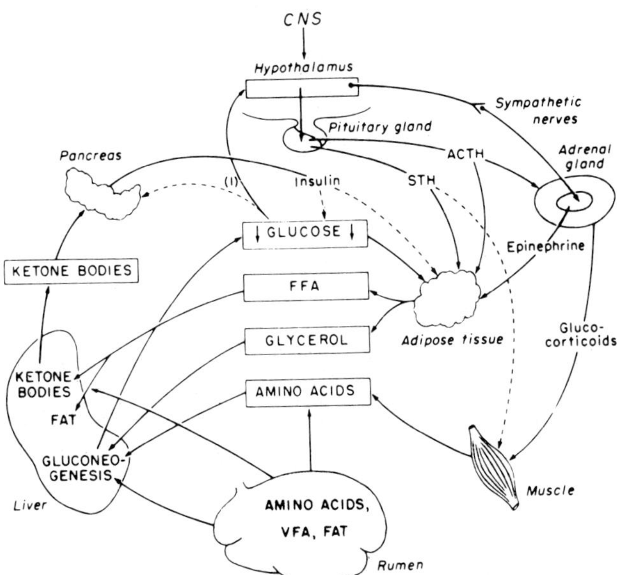

Figure 27.6. Metabolic interrelationships and hormonal control. Broken lines indicate inhibition. Hypoglycemia initiates a complex of hormonal adjustments (1) that are mediated by the pancreas, hypothalamus, and pituitary gland. Direct effects of hormones on the liver are not shown. Epinephrine and glucagon accelerate glycogenolysis, and glucagon and glucocorticoids increase gluconeogenesis. Insulin also inhibits and glucagon increases amino acid release from muscle. CNS, central nervous system; ACTH, adrenocorticotropic hormone; STH, somatotropic (growth) hormone; FFA, free fatty acid; VFA, volatile fatty acid.

persists, more long-range actions are necessary. The anterior pituitary secretes STH and also ACTH, which increases glucocorticoid secretion by the adrenal cortex. These hormones all act in a "permissive role," but their overall effect is a maintained and high release of glycerol, FFAs, and amino acids from the peripheral tissues. The action of glucocorticoids probably is one of the most beneficial effects of the various hormones, since more amino acids are mobilized as precursors for gluconeogenesis. Plasma glucocorticoid concentrations are elevated in bovine and ovine ketosis, and they reduce milk secretion in lactating animals. They also have an anti-insulin effect and thus decrease glucose utilization so that the general body tissues rely more on FFA oxidation for their caloric needs.

Control of liver metabolism

The hormonal regulation of metabolism within the liver is important, and four major rate-limiting or pacemaker enzymes are involved (see Fig. 27.1): (1) glucose-6-phosphatase for release of free glucose into the blood; (2) fructose-1,6-diphosphatase; (3) pyruvate carboxylase for formation of oxalacetate from pyruvate; and (4) phosphoenolpyruvate (PEP) carboxykinase for conversion of oxalacetate to phosphoenolpyruvate. All of these reactions are influenced by hormones as well as by diet. Glucocorticoids and glucagon accelerate their rates, and insulin depresses them.

The third reaction (pyruvate carboxylase) is of particular importance, since the enzyme is specifically catalyzed by most acyl CoA compounds. Propionate and butyrate are converted to propionyl CoA and butyryl CoA by the liver, and increases in these compounds, as after feeding, will increase oxalacetate and gluconeogenesis. The reaction also is particularly sensitive to glucagon. Phosphoenolpyruvate carboxykinase activity probably is a major factor only in long-term adaptations of gluconeogenesis, such as occurs during fasting, diabetes, or prolonged glucocorticoid administration. It is not changed during ruminant ketosis.

Thus, in ketosis, there seems to be an insufficient production of oxalacetate within the liver to maintain the needed high rate of glucogenesis. The animal's ability to mobilize precursors seems inadequate. Further research is needed on the control of feed intake and on the control of the peripheral supply of precursors.

Therapy for ketosis

There are several forms of therapy for ketosis, but none is consistently successful. Cows often recover without treatment, but the recovery time is longer and there is a greater loss in milk production than when they are treated. Sheep, as a rule, respond poorly to treatment unless it is given in the early stages of the disease. This poor outcome is probably due to irreversible damage to the central nervous system or other organs from the prolonged hypoglycemia. Termination of the pregnancy is the surest way to remedy the disease.

Any treatment that will raise or maintain a normal blood glucose concentration is a logical measure for ketosis. The oral administration of sugar is of little or no value, however, since microorganisms in the rumen ferment the compound into VFAs. Glycerol and propylene glycol are commonly used since they resist fermentation and, after absorption, will form glucose and glycogen. Intravenous injections of 500 ml of 50 percent glucose solutions are successful in a high percentage of cases of bovine ketosis, but more persistent cases require repeated injections at short intervals. The resultant hyperglycemia from a single injection is short lived and raises the blood sugar concentration for only about 2 hours. About 10 percent of the injected glucose is eliminated in the urine. The administration of glucose by continuous intravenous infusion for several days has practical limitations, but ketosis can be controlled successfully by this technique. Fructose or invert sugar has been suggested as a possible replacement for glucose because it is converted more rapidly into glycogen and slightly less is excreted in the urine.

Adrenal glucocorticoid hormones are efficacious in the treatment of ketosis since they stimulate the animal to produce its own glucose at the expense of body protein. The action of these hormones in elevating the blood glucose concentration is more prolonged than in the case of an intravenous injection of glucose. This is desirable since considerable time may be required for metabolic adaptations.

In many instances ketosis may be prevented by increasing the feed intake, especially the grain ration, before inappetence has had a chance to occur. In the high-producing animal a deficiency of total digestible nutrients can be a considerable factor in the onset of the disease. The energy requirements at the peak of lactation are large. It is difficult, and in some cases impossible, for the cow to ingest enough total digestible nutrients to meet these energy needs. Molasses, when added to the ration, may increase feed intake since it increases palatability. Sodium propionate has proved of some value in the prevention of ketosis. Propionate is glucogenic, but only small amounts can be added to the feed since it is relatively unpalatable.

SPONTANEOUS HYPOGLYCEMIAS

Spontaneous hypoglycemias occur in a variety of metabolic disorders (Table 27.1). The severity of clinical signs depends on both the degree and the duration of the hypoglycemia. If the decrease in blood sugar is rapid, early signs are largely attributed to epinephrine release. There can be trembling, chills, paresthesia, tachycardia, increased blood pressure, and dilated pupils. If the hypoglycemia is severe, the central nervous system is affected, and such nervous symptoms as muscle twitching, impaired locomotion, visual disturbances, fainting, convulsions, and coma can occur.

Table 27.1. Principal types of hypoglycemia

Basic condition	General mechanism
Pregnancy and lactation, especially in ruminants	Insufficient gluconeogenesis for high production
Neonatal, especially pigs or if premature	Insufficient gluconeogenesis and precursor storage
Hyperinsulinism	
Insulin administration	Insulin overdose
Islet cell tumors	Organic hyperinsulinism
Rapid glucose absorption	Functional hyperinsulinism
Deficient adrenal cortex or anterior pituitary	Insufficient gluconeogenesis
Mesenchymal tumors	Inhibition of glucagon
Liver disease	Impaired gluconeogenesis or glycogenesis
Excessive alcohol	Impaired gluconeogenesis and depleted glycogen
Glycogen storage diseases (e.g., von Gierke's disease)	Impaired glycogenolysis

Prolonged and severe hypoglycemia will result in permanent cerebral damage.

Hypoglycemia of newborn pigs

Neonatal hypoglycemia can occur in all animal species, especially if the newborn is premature or of low weight. The liver and muscles of the fetus have high levels of glycogen near term, which help to tide the newborn over the transitional period until efficient suckling is established. Thereafter, its principal fuel is fat; otherwise, stored fat and protein must become available to maintain metabolism.

Newborn pigs are more susceptible to hypoglycemia than are animals of other species. The first week of life constitutes the critical period of susceptibility, especially if the pigs are kept in a cool environment or if milk is not easily obtainable. The pig is unique in that it has only small amounts of adipose tissue at birth (about 1 percent of body weight), and therefore can mobilize only limited amounts of FFA. There is no deficiency in hepatic glucogenic enzymes but, since the animal is forced to rely on glucose metabolism, gluconeogenesis cannot keep pace with the glucose demands. In early stages of the disease glucose therapy will alleviate the clinical signs, but in the terminal stages it is ineffective. The same disorder can be produced experimentally by fasting for 36 to 48 hours (Fig. 27.7). Weanling pigs, however, show only a moderate fall in blood sugar level, even when fasted for 3 to 4 weeks.

Hyperinsulinism

An overdose of insulin in the treatment of diabetes is a frequent cause of hypoglycemia (Table 27.1). It can produce a coma similar to that seen in diabetic coma caused by too little insulin. A correct differential diagnosis of the two conditions therefore is critical.

Hyperinsulinism also can be due to an organic structural change (e.g., insular carcinoma) or to a functional derangement. It has been diagnosed on many occasions in dogs and humans but only rarely in other species. It seems probable

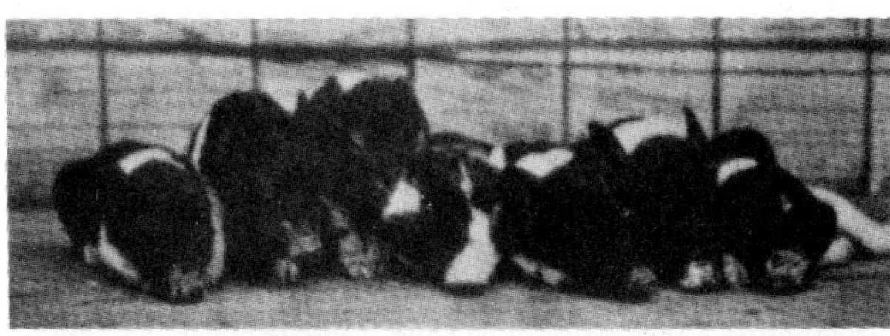

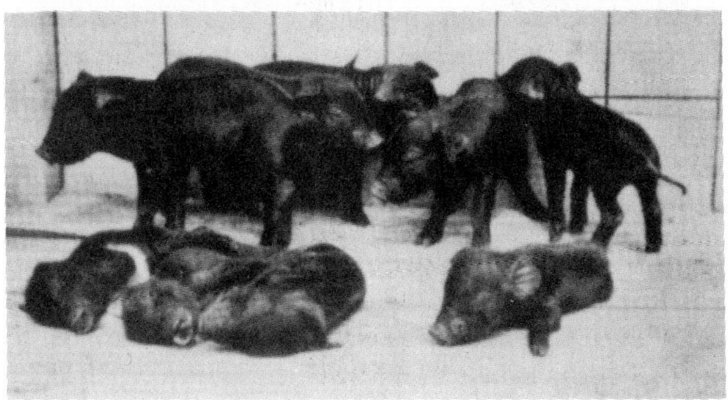

Figure 27.7. Hypoglycemia in newborn pigs. (*Top*) Severe spontaneous hypoglycemia; (*bottom*) hypoglycemic coma produced by fasting. Increasing stupor and finally coma are manifested as the blood glucose continues to fall below 40 mg/dl. Convulsions may or may not be observed. The normal range of blood glucose level in newborn pigs is 60 to 140 mg/dl. (Courtesy of Drs. Sampson, Hanawalt, Hester, and Graham, College of Veterinary Medicine and Agricultural Experiment Station, University of Illinois.)

that, because of difficulties in diagnosis, the disorder occurs more frequently than is generally supposed.

Organic hyperinsulinism has been studied more completely in the human. The tumors arise from the islets of Langerhans of the pancreas and contain large numbers of beta cells. Tumors in the dog usually have been malignant, and considerable metastases occur to the liver. If the tumor is benign, surgical extirpation will remedy the condition. Since most tumors in the dog have been malignant, however, the disorder usually will reappear after several months. The administration of alloxan, which leads to selective necrosis of the beta cells in the normal pancreas, has been unsuccessful as a therapeutic measure. The condition in dogs is characterized by a persistent hypoglycemia, but at certain times, such as during fasting or exercise, the usual control mechanisms are overwhelmed and the hypoglycemia becomes more intense. Acute clinical attacks caused by the hypoglycemia can occur at any time, but they occur more often if the animal is fed only once a day or if exercise is particularly vigorous. The attacks are characterized by weakness, unresponsiveness, staggering, and convulsions. Injections of glucose temporarily relieve the attacks.

Functional hyperinsulinism occurs more frequently than the organic type. In this condition insulin is secreted at a normal rate during fasting but in excessive amounts after such usual stimuli as ingestion of carbohydrate or changes in activity of the autonomic nervous system. The hypoglycemic syndrome has been observed in dogs, especially the hunting breeds; affected animals usually have a highly nervous temperament and an insatiable desire to hunt. Starvation is well tolerated but the blood glucose concentration falls to hypoglycemic levels 2 to 4 hours after ingestion of carbohydrate. Frequent feedings with a low-carbohydrate diet will minimize the alimentary hyperglycemia and also minimize insulin secretion.

Miscellaneous hypoglycemias

Hypoglycemia can be caused by deficiencies of the anterior pituitary gland or adrenal cortex. From Fig. 27.6 it is apparent that ACTH, somatotropic hormone (STH), and the glucocorticoids exert a physiological action on the mobilization of FFAs, glycerol, and amino acids from adipose tissue and muscle protein, thereby promoting the formation of ketone bodies and glucose. Furthermore, these factors are related to an endocrine balance involving a close relationship with insulin and glucagon. In deficiencies of the adrenal cortex, anterior pituitary gland, or of glucagon, gluconeogenesis is impaired. Animals with these deficiencies, when fasted, undergo a rapid decline in liver glycogen and hypoglycemia develops; in fact, a deficiency of the adrenal cortex (Addison's disease) may be easily mistaken for hyperinsulinism. Similar but more drastic disturbances occur in animals with an anterior pituitary deficiency.

Spontaneous hypoglycemia also occurs in a wide variety of liver diseases and is due to an interference with the glycogenic, gluconeogenic, or glycogenolytic enzyme systems. Some diseases that can cause extensive liver damage are viral hepatitis, diffuse carcinomas, fatty degeneration, cirrhosis, and hepatic poisons, such as carbon tetrachloride.

Glycogen storage diseases (types I to VIII) are characterized by excessive deposition of glycogen in the liver, kidneys, muscle, and other tissues. They are primarily hereditary diseases of children, and symptoms include hypoglycemia, enlargement of the liver, and ketosis. Deficiencies of at least four liver enzymes have been found, although the most common type is von Gierke's (type I), which is due to a deficiency of glucose-6-phosphatase. Thus glycogen can be formed, but only little glucose can be regenerated. A condition similar to von Gierke's disease has been reported to occur in puppies.

DIABETES MELLITUS

Diabetes mellitus is due to an absolute or relative lack of insulin. The disease can be brought about by one or more predisposing factors, including hereditary tendency, pancreatitis, obesity, hyperfunction of the anterior pituitary gland or adrenal cortex, and any factor that causes degeneration of the islets of Langerhans. Diabetes mellitus has been reported in cattle, horses, pigs, and sheep but is most frequently found in dogs and cats. Herbivorous animals are more resistant and can live for longer periods without insulin. Diabetes is divided mainly into two different types: the more severe type I or juvenile-onset diabetes that usually begins early in life and the milder type II or maturity-onset diabetes. Type II diabetes results mainly from the insulin resistance that occurs during obesity. Reduction of body weight along with exercise is the best method of controlling type II diabetes and, in fact, insulin administration may not even be necessary.

Experimental diabetes mellitus

Diabetes mellitus can be produced by a number of experimental procedures. Total pancreatectomy has been performed in many animal species, but it has been studied most thoroughly in the dog and the rat. If as much as one-eighth of the pancreas is left intact, however, the animal does not become diabetic. Feeding a high-carbohydrate diet or repeated administrations of glucose produces a permanent diabetes, especially if part of the pancreas has been removed or previously damaged. The increased glucose metabolism and hyperglycemia will overwork the remaining beta cells and produce an exhaustion atrophy. The injection of excessive amounts of insulin over several weeks' time can also produce diabetes by disuse atrophy.

The intravenous injection of alloxan or streptozotocin leads to a selective necrosis of the beta cells of the pancreatic islets, and the secretion of glucagon and pancreatic juice remains undisturbed. These chemicals, therefore, provide a quick and easy method of producing experimental diabetes mellitus.

A temporary and in some cases permanent diabetes can be produced by the prolonged administration of STH, ACTH, or adrenal glucocorticoids. All of these hormones tend to produce hyperglycemia, which will stimulate insulin secretions and produce an exhaustion and degeneration of the beta cells. In addition, anterior pituitary and adrenal hormones exert an anti-insulin effect and reduce the ability of the animal to use glucose. The prolonged actions of STH are commonly called "pituitary diabetes," and the actions of ACTH or glucocorticoids are called "steroid diabetes."

A temporary diabetes that lasts for only a few hours also can be produced by injection of anti-insulin serum or by compounds that inhibit insulin release, such as mannoheptulose and 2-deoxyglucose.

Metabolic alterations

The mechanism of insulin action is complex (see Chap. 34). There are many metabolic alterations in diabetes mellitus, but the central feature is hyperglycemia. It is due to reduced entry of glucose into cells of adipose tissue and muscle and to increased glucose production by the liver. Thus there is an extracellular glucose excess but an intracellular glucose deficiency, or "starvation in the midst of plenty." In hyperglycemia (more than 180 mg/dl) the renal tubules are unable to reabsorb all the filtered glucose, and glucose is excreted into the urine (glucosuria). This produces an osmotic diuresis, and the loss of water (polyuria) causes dehydration in spite of an increased thirst and water intake (polydipsia).

In severe insulin deficiency, mobilization of FFAs occurs, and the concentration of blood ketone bodies greatly increases. These compensatory changes are similar to those responsible for ruminant ketosis (see Fig. 27.6) but are more marked. In addition, the blood glucagon value usually is elevated in diabetes as a result of the loss of the restraining influence of insulin on the secretion of glucagon by the alpha cells in the islets of Langerhans of the pancreas. The increased glucagon level not only increases gluconeogenesis but also accelerates the carnitine transport mechanism that is needed for transporting fatty acids into liver mitochondria. More FFAs thus can be catabolized, and large amounts of acetyl CoA are released, resulting in accelerated ketogenesis. Severe ketoacidosis occurs and this, together with the large urine volume, results in a depletion of electrolytes. The acidosis, dehydration, hyperosmolarity, and hypotension will eventually cause renal failure, hyperventilation, and deterioration of cerebral function.

The plasma sodium concentration usually remains normal because of the reduction in extracellular fluid volume. The plasma potassium level may be increased because of the intracellular loss of amino acids for use in gluconeogenesis. In other cases the plasma potassium level is decreased (hypokalemia) as a result of the large losses of potassium that can occur during polyuria. With insulin administration, potassium reenters the cells along with glucose, and it is not unusual for severe hypokalemia to occur. This is an inherent danger, and potassium may have to be administered along with insulin in the treatment of ketoacidosis.

Glucose tolerance tests are frequently used to test the ability of the animal to use glucose and are of great value in the diagnosis of diabetes mellitus or hyperinsulinism. In this procedure the animal is fasted for 24 hours and then given an intravenous injection of 0.5 g of glucose per kilogram of body weight. The height to which the blood sugar value rises and the rate of its return to normal are then measured. In the normal animal the preinjection glucose concentration is reached in about 2 hours, but if a decreased tolerance is present, which is indicative of diabetes, 3 or more hours may be required. An increased tolerance (i.e., is a faster rate of return to normal) is observed in hyperinsulinism, and the tolerance curve is followed by a hypoglycemic phase at least $\frac{1}{2}$ hour in duration. The glucose tolerance curve tests primarily the ability of the pancreas to respond and provide additional insulin when needed.

The basic goal in treating diabetes is to supply the correct amount of exogenous insulin. If this is not done, severe muscle wasting can occur, or a chronically fatty liver can result in liver disease. Cataracts are another common sequela and are frequently seen in small-animal practice. The lens of the eye is freely permeable to glucose, even without insulin, and its cells convert glucose to fructose and sorbitol. In chronic diabetic hyperglycemia these sugars remain in the cell and cause an osmotic accumulation of water, resulting in lenticular swelling, aggregation of proteins, opacity, and eventual blindness.

FATTY LIVERS

Liver fat metabolism

The liver plays a major role in fat metabolism. It removes much of the FFA released by adipose tissue and, in addition to oxidation in the TCA cycle or formation of ketone bodies, the liver converts large amounts of FFA into triglycerides. The triglycerides are either secreted into the circulation as lipoproteins or accumulate in the liver as stored fat. Lipoproteins are the major circulating form of fatty substances and are used extensively by adipose tissue as well as by muscle and mammary gland. They also are important for transporting cholesterol throughout the body. The synthesis of the protein moiety of the lipoproteins occurs only in the liver and is a rate-limiting step for the hepatic release of lipoproteins. Thus there is an active shuttle of fatty substances between the liver and extrahepatic tissues. Except in ruminants, the liver also actively participates in liponeogenesis from amino acids and glucose.

Causes of fatty liver

Fat normally constitutes about 5 percent of the weight of the liver, but in many instances it can rise to 30 percent or more. Excessive fat in the liver is sometimes called a fatty infiltration or fatty degeneration; this accumulation is not a disease per se but, rather, a symptom of deranged fat metabolism." It may be due to an overproduction or an underutilization, that is, an increased transport of fat to the liver or a defective transport of fat away from the liver.

Fatty livers may be caused by any one of the following: (1) high-fat or high-cholesterol diet; (2) increased liponeogenesis by the liver from excessive carbohydrate intake or excessive administration of certain vitamins, such as biotin and thiamine; (3) increased mobilization of fat from adipose tissue as a result of high milk production, starvation, insulin deficiency, hypoglycemia, hyperactivity of the sympathoadrenal system, or increased output of glucagon, STH, ACTH, and adrenal steroids; (4) liver damage due to hepatitis, cirrhosis, necrosis from vitamin E deficiency, or liver poisons such as carbon tetrachloride and chloroform; and (5) deficient transport of fat from the liver because of excessive glucagon or specific nutritional deficiencies, such as lack of choline, inositol, protein, essential fatty acids, pyridoxine, and pantothenic acid.

The rate of transport of fat away from the liver depends on the ability of the liver to synthesize the protein moiety of the lipoproteins. Without this ability, fat cannot be released into the circulation. Substances that improve lipoprotein synthesis and thus prevent many nutritionally induced fatty livers are said to have a lipotropic action. Among these lipotropic factors are choline, inositol, and lipocaic, of which choline is generally the most effective. Deficiencies of B vitamins are related primarily to the use of essential fatty acids for lipoprotein synthesis.

Exposure to toxic chemicals or infections, or even deficiencies that cause fatty livers, eventually lead to excessive production of fibrous tissue in the liver. This is called cirrhosis, and the liver is shrunken, distorted, and orange-brown in color. Cirrhosis also is commonly seen in cases of prolonged protein deficiency and begins after the central lobular cells have been ruptured by excessive fat. The ruptured cells atrophy, and scars are formed. The scars may spread and even include areas around the large portal veins. A reduction in portal blood flow and portal hypertension can occur.

Fatty livers in birds

Fatty livers are commonly found in laying hens and are associated with a 30 percent decrease in egg production and a mortality rate as high as 2 percent per month. The fat content of the liver can exceed 50 percent, and the liver becomes so enlarged that hepatic hemorrhages and rupture frequently occur. The syndrome can be produced experimentally in high-producing flocks by the feeding of diets high in carbohydrate and energy. It also can be partially reversed by the feeding of more fiber, such as wheat bran, to reduce the intake of digestible carbohydrate and energy. In some societies, fatty goose livers are considered a delicacy and are deliberately produced by the force-feeding of large quantities of cereal grains.

Apparently, fatty livers develop in birds when a high carbohydrate intake stimulates hepatic lipogenesis and triglyceride formation beyond the liver's maximal ability to synthesize lipoproteins for secretion into the plasma. Furthermore, the hormone glucagon probably is involved. Glucagon is secreted by the avian pancreas to a much greater extent than in mammals, and it has been shown to limit or even decrease the synthesis of the protein portion of the lipoproteins. The major effect of glucagon on the liver, in addition to glycogenolysis, is enhancement of protein catabolism for use in gluconeogenesis. This is an adverse effect as far as fat metabolism is concerned and could increase the incidence of fatty liver. In any case, both nutritional and hormonal factors are involved.

REFERENCES

Aafjes, J.H. 1964. Volatile fatty acids in blood of cows with ketosis. *Life Sci.* 3:1327–34.

Baird, G.D. 1981. Metabolic modes indicative of carbohydrate status in the dairy cow. *Fed. Proc.* 40:2530–35.

Bardens, J.W., Bardens, G.W., and Bardens, B. 1961. A von Gierke–like syndrome in puppies. *Allied Vet.* 32:4–7.

Barton, T.L. 1967. Fatty liver studies in laying hens. Dissertation, Michigan State University.

Bauman, D.E. 1984. Regulation of nutrient partitioning. In F.M.C. Gilchrist and R.J. Mackie, eds., *Herbivore Nutrition in the Subtropics and Tropics*. Science Press, Craighall, South Africa.

Beck, A.M., and Krook, L. 1965. Canine insuloma. *Cornell Vet.* 55:330–39.

Bergman, E.N. 1971. Hyperketonemia-ketogenesis and ketone body metabolism. *J. Dairy Sci.* 54:936–48.

Bergman, E.N. 1982. Hypoglycemia associated with pregnancy and lactation. In J.C. Woodard and M. Bruss, eds., *Comparative Aspects of Nutritional and Metabolic Diseases*. CRC Press, Boca Raton, Fla.

Bergman, E.N. 1990. Energy contributions of volatile fatty acids from the gastrointestinal tract in various mammalian species. *Physiol. Rev.* 70:567–90.

Bergman, E.N., and Heitmann, R.N. 1980. Integration of whole-body amino acid metabolism. In P.J. Buttery and D.B. Lindsay, eds., *Protein Deposition in Animals*. Butterworth, London.

Bergman, E.N., Reulein, S.S., and Corlett, R.E. 1989. Effects of obesity on insulin sensitivity and responsiveness in sheep. *Am. J. Physiol.* 257(5 Pt 1):E772–81.

Bergman, E.N., and Sellers, A.F. 1960. Comparison of fasting ketosis in pregnant and nonpregnant guinea pigs. *Am. J. Physiol.* 198:1083–86.

Bergman, E.N., and Wolff, J.E. 1971. Metabolism of volatile fatty acids by liver and portal-drained viscera in sheep. *Am. J. Physiol.* 221:586–92.

Bloom, A., and Ireland, J. 1980. *Color Atlas of Diabetes*. Year Book, Chicago.

Brockman, R.P. 1986. Pancreatic and adrenal hormonal regulation of metabolism. In L.P. Milligan, W.L. Grovum, and A. Dobson, eds., *Control of Digestion and Metabolism in Ruminants*. Prentice Hall, Englewood Cliffs, N.J.

Couch, J.R. 1968. Fatty liver syndrome. *Feedstuffs* 7:48–51.

DeOya, M., Prigge, W.F., Swenson, D.E., and Grande, F. 1971. Role of glucagon on fatty liver production in birds. *Am.J.Physiol.* 221:25–30.

Elliot, J.M. 1980. Propionate metabolism and vitamin B_{12}. In Y. Ruckebusch and P. Thivend, eds., *Digestive Physiology and Metabolism in Ruminants*. Int. Med. Publishers, Lancaster, Pa.

Hibbitt, K.G., and Baird, G.D. 1967. An induced ketosis. *Vet. Rec.* 81:511–17.

Kaneko, J.J., and Rhode, E.A. 1964. Diabetes mellitus in a cow. *J. Am. Vet. Med. Assoc.* 144:367–73.

Katz, M.L., and Bergman, E.N. 1966. Acid-base and electrolyte equilibrium in ovine pregnancy ketosis. *Am. J. Vet. Res.* 27:285–92.

Kolterman, D.G., Insel, J., Saekow, M., and Olefsky, J.M. 1980. Mechanisms of insulin resistance in human obesity: Evidence for receptor and postreceptor defects. *J. Clin. Invest.* 65:1272–84.

Lindsay, D.B., and Pethick, D.W. 1983. Adaptation of metabolism to various conditions: metabolic disorders. In P.M. Riis, ed., *Dynamic Biochemistry of Animal Production. World Animal Science A3*. Elsevier, Amsterdam.

McCann, J.P., and Bergman, E.N. 1988. Endocrine and metabolic factors in obesity. In A. Dobson and M.J. Dobson, eds., *Aspects of Digestive Physiology in Ruminants*. Cornell Univ. Press, Ithaca, N.Y.

Morrow, D.A. 1976. Fat cow syndrome. *J. Dairy Sci.* 59:1625–29.

Pell, J.M., and Bergman, E.N. 1983. Cerebral metabolism of amino acids and glucose in fed and fasted sheep. *Am. J. Physiol.* 244:E282–89.

Reid, I.M. 1981. Fatty liver in dairy cows: Incidence, severity, pathology and functional consequences. In D. Giesecke, G. Dirksen, and M. Stangassinger, eds., *Metabolic Disorders in Farm Animals*. Institute for Physiology, Veterinary Faculty of the University of Munich, W. Germany.

Reid, R.L. 1968. The physiopathology of undernourishment in pregnant sheep with particular reference to pregnancy toxemia. *Adv. Vet. Sci.* 12:163–238.

Reid, R.L., and Hinks, N.T. 1962. Studies on the carbohydrate metabolism of sheep. *Aust. J. Agric. Res.* 13:1124–36.

Scow, R.O., Chernick, S.S., and Brinley, M.S. 1964. Hyperlipemia and ketosis in the pregnant rat. *Am. J. Physiol.* 206:796–804.

Stogdale, L. 1986. Definition of diabetes mellitus. *Cornell Vet.* 76:156–74.

Swiatek, K.R., Kipnis, D.M., Mason, G., Chao, K., and Cornblath, M. 1968. Starvation hypoglycemia in newborn pigs. *Am. J. Physiol.* 214:400–405.

Tokarnia, C.H. 1961. Islet cell tumor of the bovine pancreas. *J. Am. Vet. Med. Assoc.* 138:541–47.

Unger, R.H., and Orci, L. 1979. Glucagon: Secretion, transport, metabolism, physiologic regulation of secretion, and derangements in diabetes. In L.J. DeGroot, ed., *Endocrinology*, vol. 2. Grune & Stratton, New York.

Wilkinson, J.A. 1957. Spontaneous diabetes in domestic animals. *Vet. Rev. Annot.* 3:69–96.

CHAPTER 28

Vitamins | by Richard C. Ewan

Vitamin A
Vitamin D
Vitamin E
Vitamin K

Thiamine
Riboflavin
Niacin
Pantothenic acid
Biotin

Choline
Folic acid
Vitamin B_6
Vitamin B_{12}
Ascorbic acid

Vitamins are organic compounds that are required in small quantities and, in general, they function as metabolic catalysts or regulators. Vitamins are not used to provide energy or amino acids for protein deposition. They can be classified on the basis of solubility as fat-soluble (vitamins A, D, E, and K) or water-soluble (the B vitamins and vitamin C). Research to detail the role of vitamins in intermediary metabolism and in the physiological regulation of cellular functions is an active field.

Although the physiological effects of vitamin deficiencies are described in historical writings, Hopkins first suggested in 1906 that there were "accessory food factors" that were essential and could not be classified as carbohydrate, fat, or protein. Funk, in 1912, used the term *vitamine* (an amine essential to life) to describe an accessory food factor. In 1913 McCollum and Davis described a fat-soluble factor A that was required for growth, and in 1915 they further suggested the presence of a water-soluble factor B that was essential for growth. Emmett and Luros, in 1920, suggested after heat treatment of the water-soluble B that there was more than one factor present in the complex. In the same year, Drummond suggested that most vitamines were not amines and that the "e" at the end of the name should be dropped. McCollum and others demonstrated, in 1922, that the fat-soluble A contained a second factor, which was designated vitamin D. In the ensuing years, water-soluble B was differentiated into numerous factors (the B complex), as was fat-soluble A.

In considering the vitamin requirement of an animal, it is necessary to distinguish between a physiological and a dietary requirement. All vitamins are physiologically required by higher animals and play an essential role in metabolism. In some instances, the vitamin is synthesized within the body tissues, as vitamin C is in many animals. Of special significance is the synthesis of the B vitamins and vitamin K by rumen microorganisms. For this reason, ruminants, after the rumen microflora is established, are not dependent on dietary sources of the B vitamins or vitamin K. In nonruminants, intestinal microbial synthesis of many vitamins occurs in the large intestine, but these, for the most part, are not readily available to the host because of lack of absorption unless coprophagy is practiced. When synthesis of vitamins is inadequate, the animal is dependent on the diet to meet physiological requirements.

For the vitamin content of various feeds and foods, see National Research Council (1971) and Ensminger and Olentine (1978). For requirements of vitamins by animals, see National Research Council (1977–1989).

The vitamins discussed are listed in Table 28.1 with the generic term that is the general designation for activity associated with the vitamin, the chemically active compounds, and other (older) terms that have been used for the particular activity. Other organic compounds—inositol, *p*-amino benzoic acid, and carnitine—have been suggested as vitamins in special situations but are not included because they have not been demonstrated to be essential for domestic animals.

VITAMIN A

Vitamin A was initially described as a fat-soluble factor required for growth of animals fed diets prepared from purified carbohydrates, protein, and minerals. Although pure vitamin A is a pale yellow compound, vitamin A activity was associated with bright yellow compounds found in plants. This was resolved by Steenbock, who demonstrated that carotene fed to rats had vitamin A activity. Carotenoids are of plant origin and are the source of many of the bright red and yellow colors of plant products. While many com-

Table 28.1. Vitamin nomenclature

Generic term	Active compounds	Other terms
Vitamin A	All-trans retinol All-trans retinal All-trans retinoic acid	Axerophthol
Vitamin C	*l*-Ascorbic acid *l*-Dehydroascorbic acid	Cevitamic acid, hexuronic acid, antiascorbutic factor
Vitamin D	Cholecalciferol Ergocalciferol	Vitamin D_3 Vitamin D_2
Vitamin E	Alpha-tocopherol	Antisterility factor
Vitamin K	Menaquinone Phylloquinone Menadione	Vitamin K_2 Vitamin K_1 Vitamin K_3
Thiamine	Thiamine	Vitamine B_1, vitamin F, aneurin(e), antineuric factor
Riboflavin	Riboflavin	Vitamin B_2, vitamin G, riboflavine, lactoflavin(e)
Niacin	Nicotinic acid Nicotinamide	Vitamin PP, anti-black tongue factor
Pantothenic acid	*d*-pantothenic acid	Pantothen, filtrate factor
Folate	Folic acid Tetrahydrofolic acid	Folacin, vitamin M, vitamin B_c norite eluate factor, factor R
Vitamin B_6	Pyridoxine Pyridoxal Pyridoxamine	Adermin, vitamin Y
Vitamin B_{12}	Cyanocobalamin	Cobalamin
Biotin	*l*-(+)-biotin	Vitamin H, coenzyme R, factor S, factor W, factor X
Choline	Choline	Bilineurine

pounds (more than 600) are classified as carotenoids, only carotenoids that contain an intact beta-ione ring have biological activity. Beta-carotene contains two beta-ione rings and has the greatest biological activity. Carotenoids with one beta-ione ring have approximately one-half the biological activity of beta-carotene, and carotenoids lacking a beta-ione ring have no biological activity.

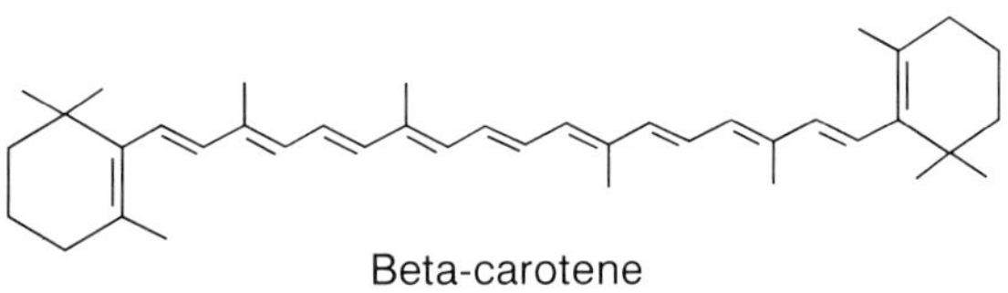

Beta-carotene

CH_2 OH

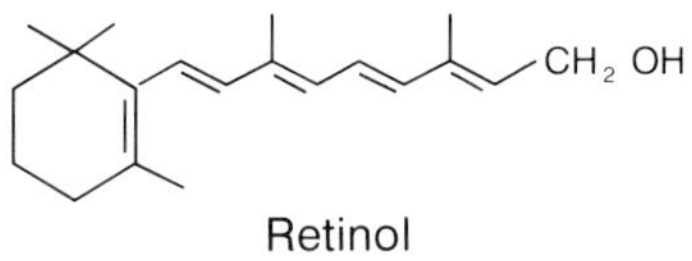

Retinol

Carotenoids are converted in the intestinal mucosa to vitamin A by carotene dioxygenase by cleavage at the 15–15′ double bond. If the reaction were 100% efficient, one molecule of beta-carotene would yield two molecules of vitamin A. The rat and the chicken are the most efficient in converting carotene to vitamin A; cattle, sheep, and pigs are intermediate; and carnivores (foxes, minks)) are least efficient. The cat does not convert carotene to vitamin A and is dependent on a source of vitamin A. Carotenoids are absorbed intact by cattle, sheep, and chickens, and they can be deposited in tissues. In the chicken, carotenoids provide the yellow coloration to the shanks, beak, and egg yolk. Oxygenated carotenoids, common in yellow corn, do not contribute to vitamin A activity but can contribute to the coloration of tissues.

The functional group of vitamin A can be an alcohol (retinol), aldehyde (retinal), or acid (retinoic acid). Retinol and retinal have full biological activity, but retinoic acid has partial activity. The double bonds in the side chain are all in the *trans* configuration, and stereoisomers of vitamin A or carotene containing *cis* double bonds have reduced biological activity.

Vitamin A is added to diets as retinyl esters (generally palmitate), and retinyl esters are hydrolyzed in the intestinal lumen to retinol. Retinol, from the diet or from conversion of carotenoids, is esterified in the intestinal cell (primarily as palmitate), incorporated into the chylomicrons, and transported to the systemic circulation via the lymphatic system. Retinol esters remain with the chylomicron remnant and are hydrolyzed to retinol in the liver and absorbed by the hepatocytes. In the hepatocytes, retinol can be stored as retinol esters in lipid droplets. The liver stores vitamin A during periods of excess intake and releases vitamin A when it is needed by the tissues. The liver also synthesizes retinol-binding protein that functions to solubilize retinol for transport to the tissues. If needed, the retinyl esters are hydrolyzed to retinol, which is bound by retinol-binding protein in the hepatocytes, and this complex is released into the bloodstream. Retinol-binding protein is combined with four subunits of another protein, prealbumin, in the blood, and this complex transports retinol to the tissues. The complex also has binding sites for thyroxine and transports the hormone to peripheral tissues.

In the tissues, cells have receptor sites for the retinol-binding protein-retinol complex, and retinol is transferred into the cells. The cells contain binding proteins for retinol and retinoic acid that differ from the plasma retinol-binding protein. In the tissues, retinol can be reversibly oxidized to retinal. Retinal can be further oxidized to retinoic acid in the cells. Retinoic acid, however, cannot be reduced to retinal. Retinoic acid can function to maintain body growth and epithelial tissues but cannot sustain other functions of vitamin A. Retinoic acid is further metabolized by shortening of the side chain by oxidation or by the introduction of oxygen into the ring. Glucuronides can be formed from the oxidation products and are excreted in bile or urine.

Vitamin A functions in the visual process, maintenance of epithelial tissue, bone development, and maintenance of reproduction. The role of vitamin A in the visual process has been well defined biochemically. Night blindness is a result of vitamin A deficiency. Adaptation to darkness requires the pigment, rhodopsin, in the rods of the retina.

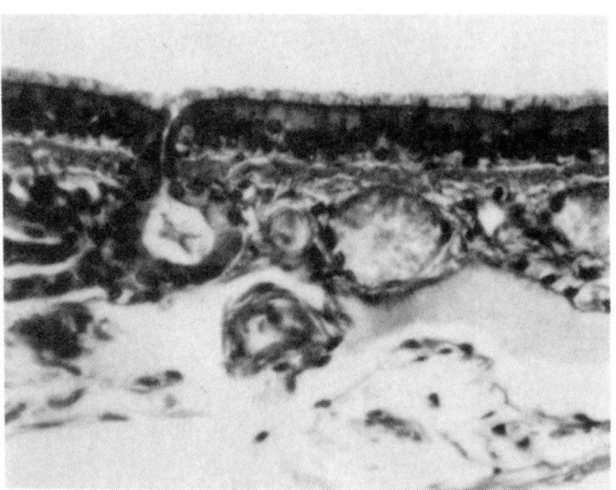
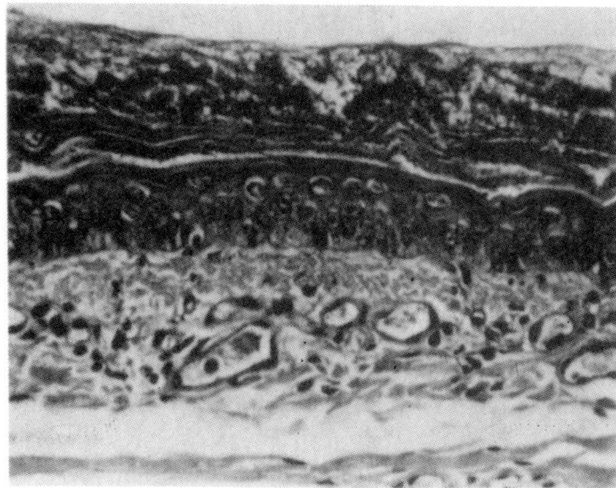

Figure 28.1. (*Left*) Tissue from the trachea of a normal mink and (*right*) from a vitamin A–deficient mink shows a squamous metaplasia of the normal ciliated, cylindric epithelium. Hematoxylin and eosin. × 300. (Courtesy Prof. L. Krook, Cornell University.)

Rhodopsin is composed of the protein, opsin, and an isomer of vitamin A, 11-*cis* retinal. On exposure to light, the 11-*cis* retinal isomerizes to all-*trans* retinal, is dissociated from the protein opsin, and initiates a neural signal recognized as sight. All-*trans* retinal in the absence of light is isomerized to the 11-*cis* isomer by an isomerase and rebound by opsin to complete the visual cycle. Color vision is associated with three pigments that contain 11-*cis* retinal as a component with different proteins that result in sensitivities to red, green, or blue wavelengths of light.

In the absence of vitamin A, normal cuboidal epithelial cells do not develop but become flattened, keratinized squamous cells (Fig. 28.1). Because cells of epithelial origin line the intestinal, urinary, and reproductive tracts, the function of these organs is impaired by a deficiency of vitamin A. Changes in the epithelial tissue of the eye result in xerophthalmia and can cause blindness independent of the function of vitamin A in the visual process. The altered epithelial cells are more susceptible to invasion by microorganisms, and the incidence and severity of disease increase. The biochemical link between vitamin A and differentiation of epithelial cells has not been determined. Evidence has been reported to suggest that retinol phosphate may be required for the incorporation of carbohydrate into glycoproteins synthesized by many epithelial cells. The interpretation of recent evidence has indicated a possible nuclear binding site for vitamin A, which implies that vitamin A may play a role in the regulation of protein synthesis. The specific proteins that may be regulated by vitamin A, however, have not been identified.

During growth, vitamin A deficiency causes defects in the remodeling of bone. Passages for nerves in bone fail to enlarge as the nerves grow. Mechanical pressure on nerves results in distortion, herniation, and degeneration of the nerves or central nervous system. This effect causes nervous lesions and can produce blindness by mechanical pressure on the optic nerve. Increased cerebrospinal fluid pressure has been reported in cattle, sheep, and pigs and has been attributed to defects in bone remodeling. Vitamin A stimulates the activity of osteoclasts in tissue culture studies, and this may explain the lack of remodeling observed in bone development.

Reproductive failure occurs during vitamin A deficiency and may, in part, be the result of abnormal differentiation of epithelial cells in the reproductive tract. Change in the vaginal cells of vitamin A–deficient rats from squamous cells to cuboidal cells with resupplementation of vitamin A has been used as a biological assay for vitamin A activity. Some evidence has been reported to suggest that, in cattle, carotene may be required in addition to vitamin A for normal reproduction. Ruminants can absorb intact carotene that may be deposited in tissues. It is difficult, however, to establish that there is a specific function for carotene other than as a source of vitamin A.

Consumption of excess amounts of vitamin A can result in toxicity in humans and animals. The livers of some arctic animals (seals and polar bears) accumulate high levels of vitamin A, and consumption of 300 to 500 g can produce acute toxicity. Acute toxicity in humans results in headache, vomiting, diarrhea, and giddiness. Chronic toxicity is dependent on the level and duration of intake and causes production of excess mucus by epithelial cells and increased osteoclastic activity.

Vitamin A activity is expressed in terms of international units (IU), which have been defined as 0.3 μg of *trans*-retinol, 0.344 μg of *trans*-retinyl acetate, 0.366 μg of *trans*-retinyl palmitate, or 0.6 μg of carotene. Recommended levels of intake by most species range from 1000 to 2000 IU daily. Foods of animal origin (milk fat, egg yolks, and liver) are sources of vitamin A, whereas plant products are sources of carotene but not vitamin A.

VITAMIN D

The fat-soluble, antirachitic factor was named vitamin D by McCollum in 1925. McCollum and coworkers had demonstrated earlier that "fat-soluble A" in cod liver oil con-

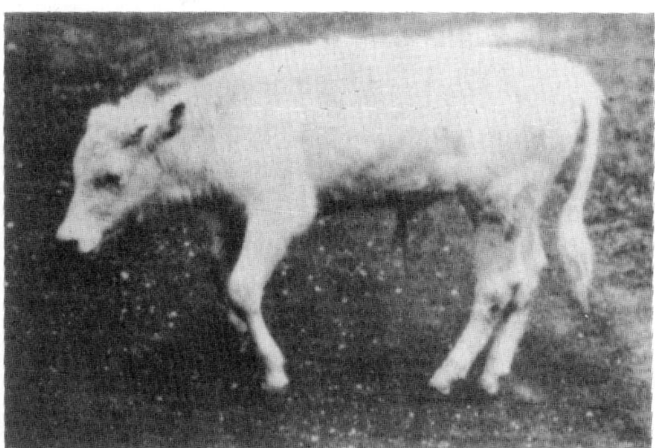

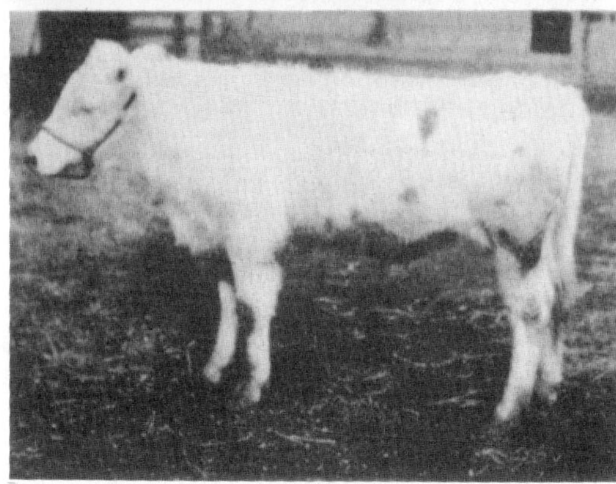

Figure 28.2. (*Top*) Calf suffering from clinical rickets. (*Bottom*) The same calf after having been on a rachitogenic diet and a vitamin D supplement for 6 months. (From Rupal, Bohstedt, and Hart 1933. *Wis. Ag. Exp. Sta. Res. Bull.* 115.)

tained two active compounds; the vitamin A activity that was destroyed by heating of the oil and the antirachitic activity that was stable to heating. Two compounds—one from plants and one from animal tissue—can be converted to metabolically active forms of vitamin D. Plants produce ergosterol, whereas animals synthesize 7-dehydrocholesterol. With exposure to ultraviolet light (230 to 330 nm), these compounds are converted to vitamin D_2 (ergocalciferol) or vitamin

R
R =
ERGOCALCIFEROL
R
CH_2
R =
CHOLECALCIFEROL
OH
OH
PRECURSOR
VITAMIN D

D_3 (cholecalciferol), respectively, through cleavage in the B ring of the sterol precursor and isomerization of the compound. Thus irradiation of plant products will result in formation of ergocalciferol, and exposure of humans and animals to sunlight will result in the production of cholecalciferol.

In humans and animals, dietary vitamin D_2 or vitamin D_3 is absorbed from the intestinal tract with other lipid-soluble components of the diet and transported to the blood by the lymphatic system. Endogenous vitamin D_3 is transported from the skin to the liver by a specific transport protein. Vitamin D is transformed by a hydroxylase in the liver to form 25-OH-vitamin D. Both vitamin D_2 and D_3 can be hydroxylated. Further metabolism of 25-OH-vitamin D requires transport of the compound to the kidney by a specific transport protein. In the kidney, 25-OH-vitamin D is further hydroxylated to form the active compound, 1,25-$(OH)_2$-vitamin D, or the inactive form, 24,25-$(OH)_2$-vitamin D. The hydroxylation at the 1 or 24 position of vitamin D is regulated by the parathyroid hormone and plasma concentration of phosphorus. Under conditions that require additional calcium and phosphorus, the major compound that is formed is 1,25-$(OH)_2$-vitamin D.

The major function of the active form of vitamin D, 1,25-$(OH)_2$-vitamin D, is to increase the extracellular levels of calcium and phosphorus. Thus 1,25-$(OH)_2$-vitamin D acts to increase intestinal absorption of calcium and phosphorus and, with the influence of parathyroid hormone, to increase resorption of calcium and phosphorus from bone. The action of 1,25-$(OH)_2$-vitamin D on intestinal absorption is best understood. The intestinal cell contains receptor proteins that facilitate the uptake and transport of 1,25-$(OH)_2$-vitamin D to the nucleus. The active vitamin initiates the synthesis of several proteins (calcium-binding protein and others) that are required for the absorption of calcium from the ingesta in the small intestine and transfer to the blood. Phosphorus absorption is also increased by 1,25-$(OH)_2$-vitamin D, but this process differs from the calcium absorptive process and is not as well defined.

A lack of vitamin D in growing animals results in rickets (Fig. 28.2), which is characterized by a decrease in extracellular levels of calcium and phosphorus. Under these conditions there is a lack of calcification in the skeletal system, and bone deformities occur. In adults, a lack of vitamin D results in osteomalacia through the mobilization of calcium and phosphorus from the skeletal system to maintain the extracellular levels of calcium and phosphorus.

Milk fever in dairy cattle occurs with the onset of lactation because large amounts of calcium are secreted in milk and the affected animals are not able to maintain extracellular levels of calcium. Affected animals are treated by infusion of calcium salts. The incidence of the condition can be reduced with massive doses of vitamin D before parturition or with lesser amounts of vitamin D metabolites. The condition can be prevented by feeding a calcium-deficient diet for the last 2 weeks of gestation, which seems to enhance the intestinal absorption of calcium and resorption processes for the mobilization of calcium from skeletal tissue.

With the recognition of the metabolic processes that result in the formation of 1,25$(OH)_2$-vitamin D, treatment of several types of bone disorder in humans became possible. In patients without functional kidneys, renal rickets, and renal osteodystrophy occur because the kidneys do not produce 1,25$(OH)_2$-vitamin D. Administration of 1,25$(OH)_2$-vitamin D_3 during dialysis is effective in normalizing calcium metabolism in these patients. Genetically determined vitamin D-resistant rickets in humans has also been successfully treated with physiological amounts of 1,25$(OH)_2$-vitamin D. Compounds with fluorine introduced into the side chain of 1,25$(OH)_2$-vitamin D are more resistant to degradative oxidation and are active for a longer time than 1,25$(OH)_2$-vitamin D.

Dietary requirements for vitamin D are expressed in international units and range from 125 to 1000 IU/kg of diet. One IU is defined as 0.025 μg of vitamin D_2 or D_3. Vitamin D_2 and D_3 have similar activities for humans and animals, but for poultry vitamin D_3 is about 10 times more active than vitamin D_2. Therefore an international chick unit is defined as 0.025 μg of vitamin D_3.

The difference in activity of vitamin D_2 and D_3 in the chick is the utilization of the 25 hydroxylated form of the vitamin. Vitamin D_2 can be hydroxylated by the hydroxylase in chick liver, but 25-OH-vitamin D_2 is not readily transported from the liver and is excreted in the bile. It has been suggested that the protein that transports the 25 hydroxylated form has a low affinity for 25-OH-vitamin D_2, resulting in excretion of the compound.

Consumption of excess amounts of vitamin D can result in vitamin D toxicity. Vitamin D toxicity causes a dramatic increase in the concentration of 25-OH-vitamin D and a decrease in the concentration of 1,25-$(OH)_2$-vitamin D in blood.

VITAMIN E

The failure of reproduction in rats fed purified diets was recognized as a vitamin deficiency by Evans and Bishop in 1922. The active compound was recognized as fat soluble and was designated as vitamin E. Evans also suggested the term *tocopherol* from the Greek terms *toco* "childbirth" and *pherol* ("to carry, bear") and isolated the compound from wheat-germ oil in 1936.

Vitamin E and *tocopherol* are terms used to refer to a group of structurally related compounds. There are eight structural isomers that vary by the number of methyl groups in the 6-hydroxy-chroman nucleus and the degree of unsaturation of the isoprene side chain. The variation in the number of methyl groups is distinguished by α-, β-, γ-, and δ-tocopherol. *Tocopherol* is used to refer to a saturated side chain, and *tocotrienol* is used to designate the presence of the unsaturated side chain. There are also three asymmetrical carbons in the molecule that can be in the *d* or *l* configuration. Of all the asymmetrical possibilities, the natural form isolated from vegetable oil is in the *d* form at all the asymmetrical carbon atoms. Natural or free tocopherol is easily oxidized, and the oxidation can be accelerated by the presence of copper or iron. In contrast, the esters of tocopherol are relatively stable under various oxidizing conditions. α-tocopheryl acetate is generally used to supplement diets.

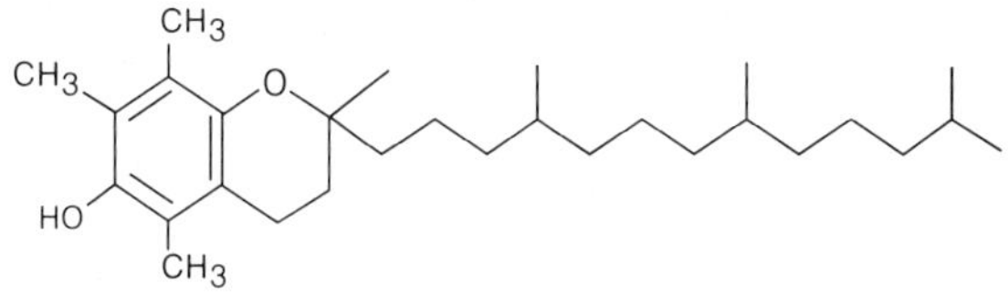

CH_3 CH_3 O HO CH_3

α-tocopherol

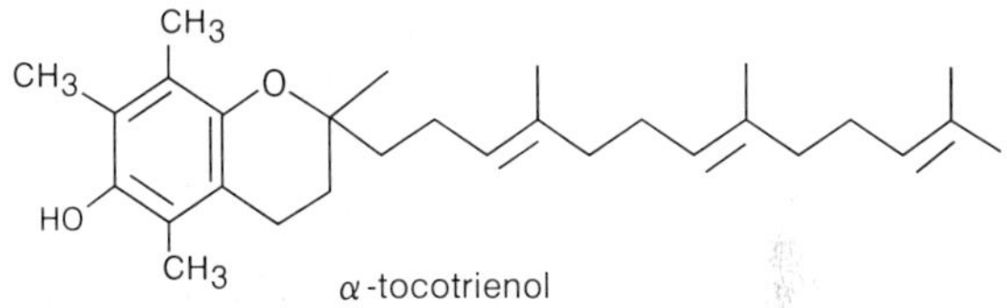

CH_3 CH_3 O HO CH_3

α-tocotrienol

Vitamin E is fat soluble, and its absorption is dependent on normal fat absorption. Tocopheryl esters are hydrolyzed in the intestinal lumen and the free tocopherols are incorporated into the chylomicrons for absorption via the lymphatic system. The absorption of tocopherols requires the presence of bile salts, as illustrated by the lack of tocopherol absorption in humans with fat malabsorption syndromes. Tocopherol is present in all tissues, but it is not clear whether it is taken up from chylomicrons directly by tissues or whether it remains with the chylomicron remnant that returns to the liver. Tocopherol in blood can be associated with the lipoproteins, but no specific transport protein has been identified. In liver a specific binding protein has been described, but the function of the protein has not been established. A major route of excretion for tocopherol is via bile from the liver. Some tocopherol is reabsorbed from the intestine. The side chain can be shortened by oxidation and the resultant compounds excreted in the urine.

In tissues it has been suggested that tocopherol is present in the lipid bilayer of cell membranes. It is suggested that the side chain of tocopherol interweaves with the long-chain fatty acids with the chroman nucleus at the surface of the cell membrane. In this location, tocopherol functions as an antioxidant to protect the cell membrane from the damaging effects of free radicals. Polyunsaturated fatty acids contain the configuration of $-CH=CH-CH_2-CH=CH-$ in which the hydrogen in the central carbon atom is easily abstracted, resulting in the formation of a free radical. The electrons in the radical rearrange, and oxygen is added to form a peroxide. Peroxides can break down to form two free radicals, resulting in a self-propagating chain reaction. Antioxidants function by contributing hydrogen to the free radical and stabilizing it. The antioxidant becomes a free radical but has the property of being able to rearrange to a stable compound and thus break the propagation reaction.

Tocopherol is the major biological, fat-soluble antioxidant in animal tissues.

The action of tocopherol as an antioxidant is supplemented by the presence of glutathione peroxidase in the soluble component of the cell. Glutathione peroxidase catalyzes the conversion of organic peroxides and hydrogen peroxide to alcohols or water thus preventing the peroxides from damaging cellular components. Glutathione peroxidase contains selenium as a component of its active site and provides an explanation of the observations that selenium is effective in preventing some of the deficiency conditions that are also prevented by tocopherol.

A dietary deficiency of vitamin E results in clinical disorders that vary according to species. In many species, muscular degeneration is associated with vitamin E deficiency. The degeneration is a Zenker's degeneration of both skeletal and cardiac muscle fibers. In poultry encephalomalacia (an ataxia resulting from hemorrhage and edema in the cerebellum) is associated with vitamin E deficiency. In rodents reproductive failure is typical, with resorption of the fetus in midgestation in the female and degeneration of the germinal epithelium in the male.

One IU of vitamin E is defined as 1 mg of *dl*-alpha-tocopheryl acetate. Biological assays with rats have provided conversions of other forms of vitamin E to international units, in units per milligram, as follows: *d*-alpha tocopherol, 1.49; *d*-alpha tocopheryl acetate, 1.36; *d*- alpha-tocopheryl succinate acid, 1.21.

VITAMIN K

Chicks fed a purified, ether-extracted diet were reported by Dam in 1934 to develop subcutaneous hemorrhages. Dam further established that the condition was related to a lack of a fat-soluble factor and proposed the name vitamin K (for the Danish word, *koagulation*). In 1939 vitamin K was isolated from alfalfa and putrefied fish meal. The vitamin synthesized by plants is termed phylloquinone or vitamin K_1, whereas bacteria synthesize menaquinone or vitamin K_2. Both compounds are derivatives of naphthoquinone and vary in the isoprene side chain, with phylloquinone containing saturated isoprene units whereas menaquinone contains a double bond in each isoprene unit. Both side chains can vary in the number of isoprene units in the side chain. The ring system itself (or menadione) has biological activity and has been used to supplement animal diets. This also emphasizes that animals require vitamin K because they do not synthesize the ring system.

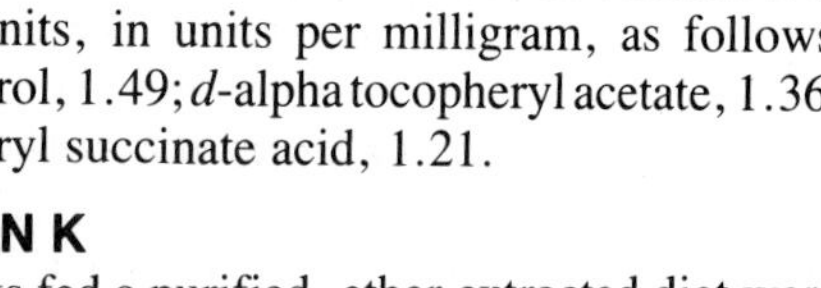

Phylloquinone

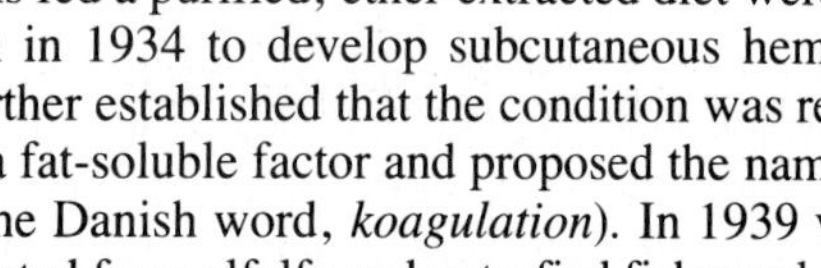

Menaquinone

Vitamin K is fat soluble, and therefore absorption of the vitamin is dependent on normal fat absorption. Vitamin K is absorbed into the lymphatic system with the chylomicrons and transported to tissues. Some absorption of vitamin K_2 from the large intestine has been reported. Vitamin K isomers with isoprene side chains of varying lengths have been isolated from the liver in a number of species. Thus it is suggested that the liver can modify the side chain of the compound. The vitamin is metabolized by oxidation of the side chain and the oxidized products are excreted.

Vitamin K functions in the synthesis of calcium-binding proteins. Those that have been studied most are the proteins that are involved in the coagulation of blood. They include prothrombin, factor VII, factor IX, and factor X. These proteins are synthesized by the liver as precursor proteins, and they do not have biological activity. The proteins are activated by the incorporation of CO_2 into glutamic acid residues in the precursor protein to form γ-carboxyglutamic acid. The quinone form of vitamin K is reduced to the hydroquinone and the hydroquinone catalyzes the incorporation of CO_2 through a hydroperoxide intermediate. The hydroquinone is converted to a 2,3 epioxide during the carboxylation, and the epioxide is converted to the quinone to complete the cycle. In vitro studies of the hydroxylation reaction indicate that menadione does not catalyze the reaction and that vitamin K compounds with four or five isoprene units in the side chain have the greatest activity.

All of the vitamin K–dependent coagulation factors have a region in the protein that is rich in γ-carboxyglutamic acid. The presence of γ-carboxyglutamic acid gives the proteins the property of binding calcium and is necessary for the proper configuration for activation of the protein. When vitamin K is lacking, inactive proteins that can be converted to active proteins with vitamin K supplementation accumulate.

Dietary requirements for vitamin K range from 0.05 to 2 mg/kg of diet. Intestinal microorganisms synthesize vitamin K, and ruminants do not have a dietary requirement because of ruminal biosynthesis of the vitamin. In nonruminants, the site of synthesis is in the cecum and large intestine, where absorption is limited, but if the animal practices coprophagy the synthesized vitamin is readily available. In poultry the rapid rate of passage of ingesta through the large intestine limits the synthesis of vitamin K and a dietary source of the vitamin is necessary. Prolonged administration of sulfa drugs or antibiotics will reduce the intestinal synthesis of vitamin K and result in an increase in the dietary requirement. Dietary supplements are generally supplied as menadione or one of the more water-soluble derivatives of menadione (menadione bisulfite, menadione dimethylpyrimidinol bisulfite).

A natural antagonist (dicoumarin) to vitamin K was isolated from moldy sweet clover hay. This and related compounds are structurally similar to the ring system in vitamin K and prevent conversion of the epioxide to the quinone form of vitamin K. These compounds have been used as rodenticides (warfarin) and as anticoagulants in medicine.

THIAMINE

Beriberi, now recognized as a thiamine deficiency in humans, was described in the Chinese literature several centuries ago. Eijkman, in 1897, recognized that the consumption of polished rice was the cause of polyneuritis in birds and of beriberi in humans. In 1915 McCollum and Davis suggested the term *water-soluble B*. Emmett and Luros suggested that there were two factors in the water-soluble B from the observation that heating the fraction destroyed biological activity with some diets but not others. Jansen and Donath obtained a crystalline substance with great antineuritic activity in 1926. Williams, in the mid-1930s, established the structural formula.

Thiamine is composed of a pyrimidine and a thiazole ring system. It is highly soluble in water and is readily destroyed by heat, especially in the presence of alkali. Thiamine in diets may be the free or phosphorylated form, but any phosphorylated thiamine is hydrolyzed to free thiamine before absorption. Free thiamine at low concentrations is absorbed by an active transport mechanism that differs from the active transport systems for sugars or amino acids. In plasma, thiamine is transported in the free form and no specific transport protein has been identified as being associated with the transport of thiamine in plasma. A binding protein has been observed in birds and rats; this protein is associated with reproduction and is thought to facilitate the transport of thiamine to the egg or the fetus.

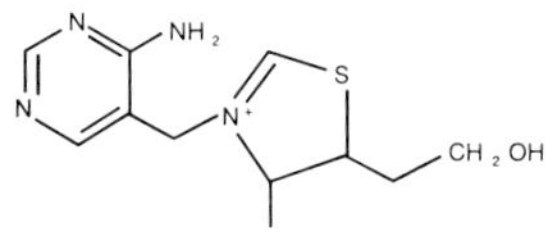

Thiamine

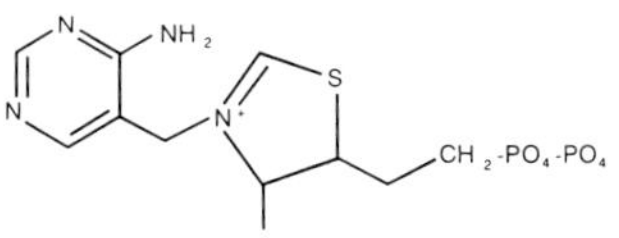

Thiamine Pyrophosphate

In tissues, thiamine is phosphorylated by adenosine triphosphate (ATP) to form thiamine pyrophosphate and, in this form, serves as a cofactor for the enzymes that require it. Thiamine pyrophosphate serves as a cofactor in the conversion of pyruvate to acetyl CoA and in the conversion of α-ketoglutarate to succinyl CoA. These reactions proceed by a similar mechanism that releases CO_2 and requires lipoic acid to transfer the carbon skeleton to CoA. Similar reactions that require thiamine pyrophosphate are involved in the metabolism of the keto acids formed in the metabolism of leucine, isoleucine, and valine. The other type of reaction that requires thiamine pyrophosphate is in the pentose shunt, where the cofactor is required for the transfer of two carbon fragments by transketolase enzymes. When there is a deficiency of thiamine, pyruvic and lactic acid are elevated in body fluids, the activity of thiamine-dependent enzymes declines, and urinary excretion of thiamine is minimal.

Thiamine pyrophosphate is metabolized by dephosphorylation and cleavage of the ring systems, resulting in the urinary excretion of 2-methyl-4-amino-5-pyrimidine carboxylic acid and 4-methyl-thiazole-5-acetic acid. As intake increases above the dietary requirement, free thiamine can also be excreted.

Alteration of the chemical structure of thiamine results in compounds that can inhibit its activity. Substitution of other nitrogenous bases for the thiazole ring result in antivitamins such as pyrithiamine and neopyrithiamine. Substitution of a hydroxyl for the amino group in the pyrimidine ring results in an antivitamin, oxythiamine. Pyrithiamine interferes with the phosphorylation of thiamine whereas oxythiamine is phosphorylated and competes with thiamine pyrophosphate for the binding sites of enzymes. Some plants, microorganisms, and fish contain enzymes called thiaminases. There are two types of thiaminase, one type that destroys thiamine by cleaving the thiazole ring and a second type that substitutes a nitrogenous base such as nicotinic acid or picolinic acid for the thiazole ring, resulting in the production of antivitamins. Thiaminase activity in certain species of fish fed raw to foxes results in thiamine deficiency that is termed Chastek paralysis. Bracken ferns also contain thiaminase activity that causes thiamine deficiency when fed to horses. Ruminants normally have an abundant supply of thiamine provided by the microorganisms in the rumen, but in some situations thiaminase activity increases in the rumen and intestine and results in a thiamine deficiency called polioencephalomalacia. Parenteral administration of thiamine is used to treat animals with polioencephalomalacia caused by its deficiency.

Dietary requirements of thiamine for animals and birds range from 0.8 to 2 mg/kg of diet. Thiamine requirements of humans are expressed in milligrams per day and are a function of caloric intake. This reflects the requirement of thiamine for normal energy metabolism. Most diets fed to nonruminants contain adequate amounts of thiamine, and vitamin supplements generally do not contain thiamine.

RIBOFLAVIN

The discovery of riboflavin developed from three areas of research. Riboflavin was the heat-stable component of the water-soluble B complex, and the investigation of the nature of this complex was one area. A second area was the study of a respiratory enzyme ("old yellow enzyme") that required riboflavin as a cofactor, by Warburg and Christian. The third area was the study of fluorescence of natural products; Wagner-Jauregg, in 1933, isolated fluorescent riboflavin from egg white. The chemical structure was identified and synthesis of riboflavin was accomplished in 1934 and 1935 by two laboratories (Kuhn et al. and Karrer et al.). Riboflavin is composed of ribose and an isoalloxine ring system. It is relatively stable to heat in neutral solutions but is highly sensitive to light with the formation of lumiflavin that does not have biological activity.

Riboflavin (oxidized) Riboflavin (reduced)

Riboflavin is absorbed from the intestine by an active transport process at low concentrations and by diffusion at high concentrations. Phosphorylated forms of riboflavin in the diet are hydrolyzed before absorption. As with thiamine, the transport of absorbed riboflavin to tissues does not require a specific transport protein. An estrogen-induced transport protein that facilitates the transport of riboflavin to the egg and the fetus, respectively, has been described in the chicken and the rat. In the chicken genetic lines lacking this transport protein have been identified.

In the tissues riboflavin is required for the synthesis of two cofactors—flavin mononucleotide (FMN) and flavin adenine dinucleotide (FAD). The formation of FMN requires phosphorylation of the ribose with ATP as the source of the phosphate. Further reaction with ATP adds the ribose-adenine structure to form FAD. In most tissues, the major form of riboflavin is FAD, with lesser amounts of FMN.

The coenzymes of riboflavin function in the oxidation of substrates to generate ATP through the electron transport system. Thus the coenzymes of riboflavin are essential for the utilization of substrates. In the reactions, the nitrogens in positions 1 and 5 of the isoalloxine ring are oxidized and reduced. Most reactions end with the oxidation of oxygen to form water, but the oxidation of amino acids and purines forms hydrogen peroxide. The methyl group in position 8 of the isoalloxine ring has been identified as the binding site of riboflavin to a histidine or cystine residue in the enzymatic protein.

The coenzyme forms of riboflavin are metabolized by hydrolysis of the adenine-ribose and phosphate to give free riboflavin. The free vitamin is excreted in the urine or secreted into the intestine via the bile. No metabolic destruction of the compound has been described.

Inadequate intake of riboflavin in nonruminants causes dermatitis, loss of hair, loss of appetite, and the development of cataracts or lens opacities. In chickens marginal deficiency causes damage to the sciatic and brachial nerves, and the birds walk on their hocks with their toes curled inward ("curled toe paralysis"). A direct explanation of the deficiency conditions based on the biochemical functions of riboflavin is not available.

The requirements for riboflavin range from 1.8 to 4 mg/kg of diet. Cereal grains and plant proteins are low in riboflavin, and therefore riboflavin is included in vitamin premixes for nonruminants. Ruminants obtain adequate supplies of riboflavin from microbial synthesis in the rumen.

Modification of the structure of riboflavin results in compounds that have no activity or that are antagonistic to riboflavin. The substitution of other pentoses for ribose reduces activity while substitution of hexoses for ribose results in antivitamins. Changes in the positions of the methyl groups in the isoalloxine ring also result in antivitamin formation.

NIACIN

Nicotinic acid or niacin was prepared chemically by oxidation of nicotine with nitric acid by Hubner in 1867. The condition in humans that was eventually recognized as a deficiency of niacin was called "pellagra." In 1916 Goldberger suggested that the lack of a component in the diet caused pellagra and implicated the three "M's" as meat, molasses, and maize as major constituents in the diet. Wheeler et al., in 1922, produced "black tongue" in dogs by feeding diets that caused pellagra in humans. Recognition of niacin as a vitamin was the result of the work of Elvehjem et al. who demonstrated in 1937 that niacin would cure black tongue in dogs. Niacin was later shown to be effective in the prevention of pellagra in humans.

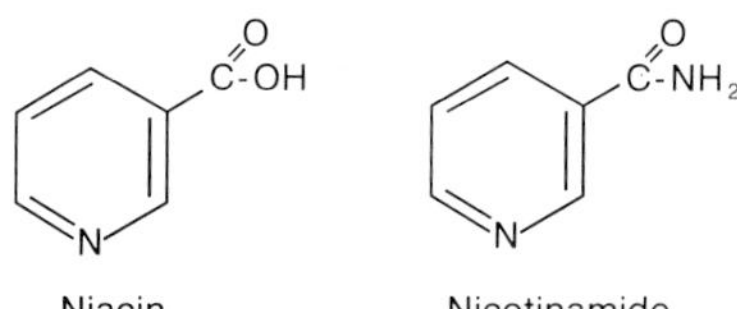

Niacin Nicotinamide

Niacin is a derivative of pyridine, and the acid and amide have biological activity. Niacin is soluble in water and stable in the dry state. The absorption mechanism for niacin has been described as an active transport process at low concentrations and by diffusion. No transport proteins have been reported. In tissues niacin is used to synthesize nicotine adenine dinucleotide (NAD) and nicotine adenine dinucleotide phosphate (NADP). Niacin in the cofactors NAD and NADP is in the form of nicotinamide, with the nitrogen for the amide function being supplied by glutamine.

Niacin as NAD or NADP functions in oxidation-reduction systems and transfers electrons into the electron-transport system with the generation of ATP. The site of oxidation-reduction is the 4 position in nicotinamide in NAD or NADP. A wide variety of reactions require NAD or NADP as cofactors, and many of the reactions are reversible. The reactions can be classified as follows: (1) primary alcohols to aldehydes, (2) secondary alcohols to ketones, (3) aldehydes to acids, (4) oxidation-reduction of sulfhydryls, and (5) conversion of amines to imines. The wide variety of reactions that require NAD or NADP as cofactors emphasizes the importance of these compounds in the utilization of energy for maintenance and growth of the organism.

The cofactors of niacin are metabolized by liberation of nicotinamide. The nitrogen in the pyrimidine ring is methylated to form N^1-methyl-nicotinamide as a major metabolite in nonruminants and is excreted in urine. In ruminants nicotinamide is conjugated with glycine to form nicotinuric acid as a urinary excretory product. In birds nicotinamide is conjugated with the nitrogen in the 2 and/or 5 position of ornithine for excretion.

Niacin requirements in animals and birds range from 11 to 70 mg/kg of diet. In contrast, requirements in humans are expressed in milligrams per day. There are no units associated with requirements for niacin. While cereal grains contain substantial amounts of niacin, biological assays indicate that only about one-third of the total niacin is available to nonruminants. Therefore niacin is included in vitamin premixes for nonruminants. Ruminants benefit from the synthesis of niacin by microorganisms and do not require dietary supplements.

Dietary requirements for niacin can be influenced by the level of tryptophan in the diet. Tryptophan can be converted to niacin metabolically. Theoretically, the conversion could yield 1 mg of niacin from 1.7 mg of tryptophan, but, physiologically, conversions are much lower. In humans 60 mg of tryptophan are required to generate 1 mg of niacin, and in the chicken 45 mg of tryptophan yields 1 mg of niacin.

PANTOTHENIC ACID

The isolation of pantothenic acid was achieved through the efforts of three research groups. Williams et al. were evaluating essential nutrients for yeast, Snell et al. were studying the essential nutrients for lactic acid bacteria, and Woolley et al. were investigating the antidermatitis factor for chicks present in the heat-stable component of the B complex. Cleavage products of the purified compound were identified as beta-alanine and lactone. The structure was confirmed by Williams and Major in 1940. The vitamin in pure form is a pale yellow oil, but the sodium, potassium, and calcium salts are crystalline and soluble in water.

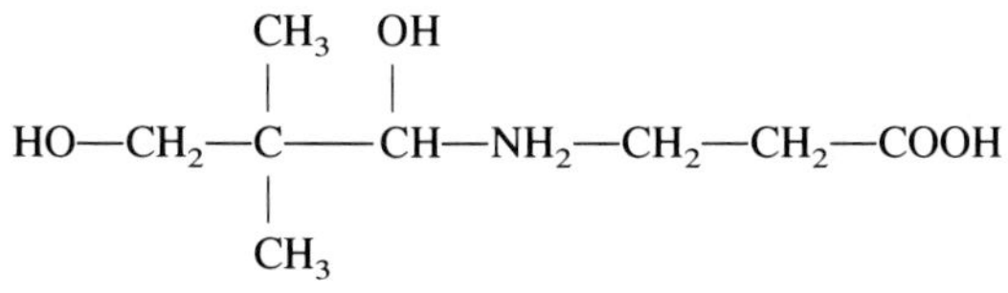

$$HO{-}CH_2{-}\overset{\displaystyle CH_3}{\underset{\displaystyle CH_3}{\overset{|}{\underset{|}{C}}}}{-}\overset{\displaystyle OH}{\overset{|}{C}H}{-}NH_2{-}CH_2{-}CH_2{-}COOH$$

d-Pantothenic acid

Pantothenic acid contains an asymmetrical carbon atom at the position of the hydroxyl group in the center of the molecule. Only the *d* form of the compound has biological activity. The mechanism of absorption of pantothenic acid has been described as involving both an active transport process and passive diffusion. No transport compounds have been described for pantothenic acid.

Pantothenic acid is required for the synthesis of coenzyme A (CoA) and the acyl carrier protein. In the synthesis of CoA, pantothenic acid is phosphorylated, followed by the addition of cysteine. The cysteine residue is decarboxylated to form pantotheine-4′-phosphate. Adenine and ribose are added from ATP, and in the final step a phosphate is added in the ribose to complete the synthesis. The active site of CoA is the sulfhydryl group contributed by cysteine. Substrates bind to the sulfhydryl functional group, and generally the beta carbon is involved in the reaction. CoA is required for fatty acid oxidation, entry of acetate and pyruvate into the citric acid cycle, steroid synthesis, and ketone body metabolism. Fatty acid synthesis also requires pantothenic acid as pantotheine-4′phosphate bound to protein to form the acyl carrier protein in the fatty acid synthetase complex. CoA clearly has a major role in the utilization of a wide variety of substrates in the production of energy.

The requirements of birds and animals for pantothenic acid range from 8 to 16 mg/kg of diet. Calcium pantothenate is generally used as the supplemental form in vitamin premixes (1.087 g of *d*-calcium pantothenate is equivalent to 1 g of *d*-pantothenic acid). Omega-methyl-pantothenic acid and pantoyl taurine are antivitamins for pantothenic acid. These compounds, however, are not found in natural products.

BIOTIN

The discovery of the vitamin, biotin, resulted from three lines of research involving a yeast growth factor (coenzyme R), the toxicity associated with feeding raw egg white (vitamin H), and a second growth factor for yeast isolated from dried egg yolk (biotin). In 1940 the three factors were recognized as the same compound, and in 1942 duVigneaud characterized biotin and published its structure. Harris et al. verified the structure by synthesis in 1943.

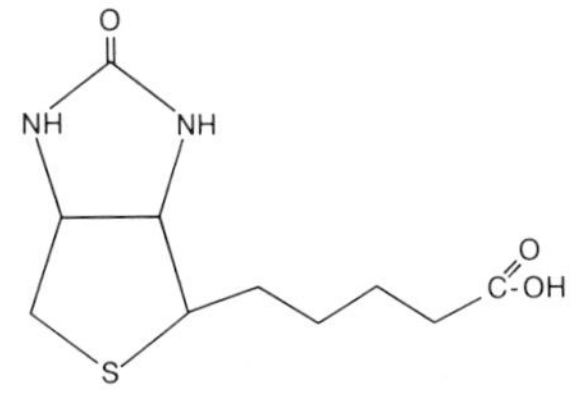

O
NH NH
C-OH
S

d-(+)-Biotin

The structure of biotin includes two five-membered rings and results in three asymmetrical carbon atoms. Only *d*-biotin has biological activity, and other isomers do not have biological activity. Absorption of biotin has been described as an active transport process that requires the presence of sodium ions. This has led to the speculation that a sodium carrier complex is involved, but such a complex has not been characterized. No specific transport protein has been described.

In tissues, biotin is required as a cofactor for enzymes that incorporate carbon dioxide into substrates. Biotin is bound to the enzyme through a peptide linkage to the terminal amino group of lysine residue in the enzymatic protein. In the enzymatic reaction, bicarbonate forms an intermediate with the nitrogen in the ring of biotin and is subsequently transferred to the substrate. Some of the reactions catalyzed by biotin enzymes include the conversion of acetate to malonate for fatty acid synthesis, of pyruvate to oxaloacetate, and of propionate to methyl malonate.

Biotin is metabolized by oxidation of the sulfur in the ring to the sulfoxide or sulfone or by oxidation of the side chain to form bisnorbiotin (removal of two carbon atoms). These compounds and free biotin are excreted in urine.

Requirements for biotin range from 100 to 300 μg/kg of diet for domestic animals. Biotin is synthesized by microorganisms in the lower intestine, and if coprophagy is not prevented it is difficult to produce a dietary deficiency. Sulfa drugs have also been used to suppress intestinal synthesis in the development of deficiencies. In chickens the rate of passage of intestinal contents is more rapid than in other species, reducing synthesis of biotin in the intestine. A deficiency can be produced by omission of biotin from the diet.

Cereal grains are reasonable sources of biotin, and the biotin in corn and soybean meal are available to the chicken. Chicken bioassays suggest that in other cereal grains (wheat, barley, oats, and milo) little biotin is available (30 percent or less). Some studies with pigs have suggested that, with a diet based on ingredients other than corn and soybean meal, supplementation with biotin may be beneficial.

Biotin deficiency can be produced by feeding raw egg white. Egg white contains a protein (avidin) that binds biotin, forming a complex that is not broken down during digestion. Avidin is not normally saturated with biotin, so that feeding egg white results in binding of any dietary biotin, thereby inducing a deficiency.

CHOLINE

Choline was first isolated from hog bile by Strecker in 1849. The nutritional significance of choline was discovered in 1932 by Best et al., who reported that fatty livers in dogs after pancreatectomy could be prevented with dietary lecithin. The effective component in lecithin was choline. In 1941 duVigneaud provided the link between sulfur amino acids and choline by demonstrating that homocysteine could be converted to methionine with methyl groups from choline.

$$\begin{array}{c} CH_3 \\ | \\ CH_3-N^{+}-CH_2-CH_2-OH \\ | \\ CH_3 \end{array}$$

Choline

The classification of choline as a vitamin is questionable because it is required in greater quantities than other vitamins, is a component of phospholipids (lecithin), and is a neurotransmitter (acetylcholine). In addition, choline is synthesized by the body in the presence of adequate amounts of the precursors, such as phosphatidyl serine and labile methyl groups from methionine. Excess methionine can spare the dietary requirement for choline by serving as a methyl donor.

Choline is absorbed by a carrier-mediated process at low concentrations and by diffusion at high concentrations. No specific transport mechanism has been described for translocation of absorbed choline to other tissues.

Choline has functions in tissues as a component of lecithin and can be incorporated directly into a 1,2-diglyceride after phosphorylation by ATP and formation of cytidine diphosphocholine. A deficiency of choline results in the accumulation of lipid in the liver because of a lack of phospholipid to transport fat from the liver to tissues. It functions in nerve impulse transmission as acetylcholine. The final function is as a source of methyl groups for methylation reactions. In this process, choline is oxidized to betaine and can be used to convert homocysteine to methionine. The other methyl groups can be transferred to other substrates through reactions that require reduced folic acid. The resulting carbon skeleton is glycine, which can then be used for protein synthesis.

Requirements for choline range from 400 to 1900 mg/kg of diet, depending on species and stage of the life cycle. Vitamin premixes for nonruminants will normally contain choline.

FOLIC ACID

A number of factors that were growth stimulants for microorganisms and chickens and prevented anemia in monkeys and chickens were eventually demonstrated to be a form of folic acid. In 1944 Mitchell prepared highly purified crystalline preparations, and in 1946 Angier et al. proposed the chemical structure and confirmed it by synthesis. Folic acid is composed of a pteridine nucleus, *p*-aminobenzoic acid, and glutamic acid.

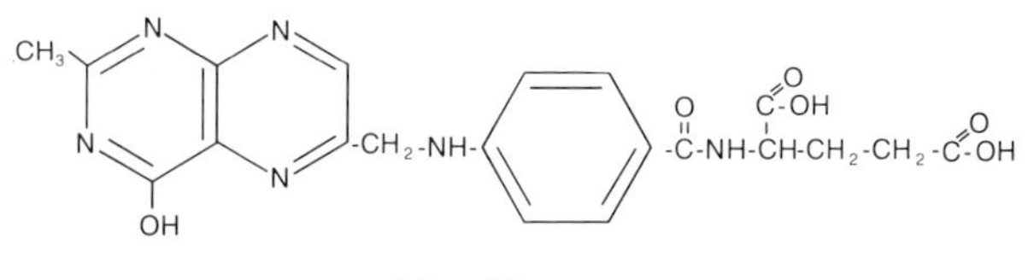

Folic acid

Folic acid is present in dietary ingredients with multiple residues of glutamic acid. The multiple residues are hydrolyzed by γ-glutamylcarboxypeptidase during digestion to release folic acid. Folic acid is taken up by the intestinal cell by active transport and diffusion. It may be reduced to tetrahydrofolic acid in the intestinal cell. Folic acid or its reduced form is released into the bloodstream. Specific binding proteins for folic acid that increase during a deficiency and in pregnancy have been described in blood. Folic acid is taken up by the liver and can be combined with additional residues of glutamic acid to form polyglutamates. The polyglutamates in the liver are storage forms of the vitamin and are mobilized by hydrolysis of the glutamic acid. Folic acid is reduced to tetrahydrofolic acid and a methyl group added to form N^5methyl-tetrahydrofolic acid. This form of folic acid can be released by the liver and transported to the tissues.

In tissues, tetrahydrofolic acid is involved in transfer of one-carbon units and in hydroxylation. Reactions involving methyl group transfer include the synthesis of methionine, serine, thymidine, and purine bases. Hydroxylation of phenylalanine, tyrosine, and tryptophan requires tetrahydrofolic acid and results in synthesis of norepinephrine and serotonin. Tetrahydrofolic acid also serves as an acceptor of a one-carbon unit during degradation of histidine.

Urine is the major route of excretion of folic acid metabolites. The identification of *p*-acetamidobenzoyl glutamate and a number of compounds with the pteridine nucleus as urinary metabolites suggests extensive degradation.

Requirements for folic acid range from 0.25 to 1 mg/kg of the diets of animals and poultry. Because of ruminal synthesis, folic acid is not required in the diets of ruminants. Omission of folic acid in the diet of chickens will result in development of folic acid deficiency. Rats and pigs, however, require the presence of sulfa drugs or other compounds to induce folic acid deficiency. Deficiency of folic acid results in a macrocytic type of anemia that is similar to the pernicious anemia in humans that results from vitamin B_{12} deficiency.

VITAMIN B_6

In 1934 György defined vitamin B_6 activity as that part of the B complex responsible for the cure of a specific dermatitis observed in rats. The vitamin was described as a nitrogenous base in 1936. Within 2 years, the compound was isolated by a number of laboratories. The chemical structure was proposed and verified by synthesis in 1939. Work with microorganisms indicated that there was more than one form of pyridoxine. Three biologically active forms are recognized: pyridoxol, a primary alcohol; pyridoxal, the aldehyde form; and pyridoxamine, the amine form.

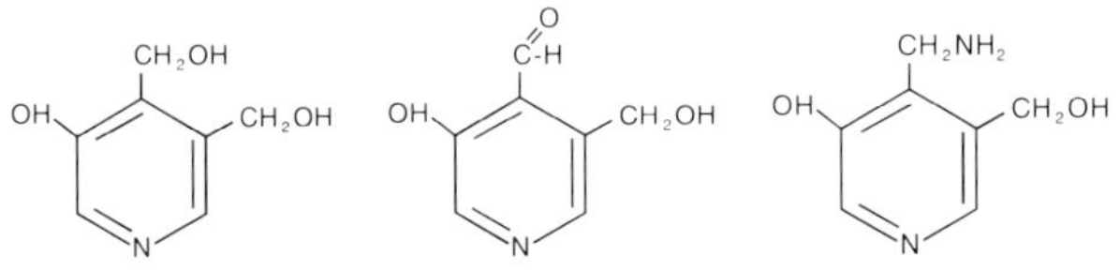

CH_2OH, OH, CH_2OH, N — Pyridoxol

O, C-H, OH, CH_2OH, N — Pyridoxal

CH_2NH_2, OH, CH_2OH, N — Pyridoxamine

During digestion phosphorylated forms of vitamin B_6 are hydrolyzed, and the free vitamin enters the intestinal cell by passive diffusion. In the intestinal cell vitamin B_6 may be phosphorylated, but this reaction is not necessary for absorption to occur. Vitamin B_6 is present in the blood as free pyridoxol or pyridoxal and pyridoxal phosphate bound to albumin. There is no specific transport protein for vitamin B_6.

In the tissues the three forms of vitamin B_6 can be phosphorylated and converted to the coenzyme form of the vitamin, pyridoxal phosphate. Pyridoxal phosphate serves as a cofactor for a large number of enzymes that are involved in the metabolism of amino acids. In all of the reactions involving amino acids, pyridoxal phosphate forms a Schiff's base intermediate that serves to activate the amino acid for further reaction. The enzyme systems that require pyridoxal phosphate can be classified by the type of reaction catalyzed: (1) transaminases that catalyze the exchange of the amino group from an amino acid to a keto acid; (2) decarboxylation to form amines from amino acids; (3) racemization to transform *d* amino acids to *l* amino acids; (4) oxidation of amines; and (5) deamination and beta elimination (serine and cysteine). Metabolism of tryptophan to niacin requires a number of pyridoxal phosphate–dependent enzymes, and in a deficiency intermediates in this pathway are excreted in the urine. The metabolism of phenylalanine and tyrosine is also dependent on several vitamin B_6 enzymes.

While pyridoxol and pyridoxal can be interconverted, oxidation of the aldehyde to the acid, 4-pyridoxic acid, is not reversible and the acid is excreted in the urine. Free vitamin B_6 can also be excreted in the urine.

Requirements for vitamin B_6 range from 1 to 6 mg/kg of diet for animals and poultry. Generally, adequate amounts of the vitamin are present in diets of nonruminants. Vitamin B_6 in feed ingredients is biologically available, so vitamin premixes do not contain the vitamin. The requirements of ruminants are satisfied by microbial synthesis in the rumen.

VITAMIN B_{12}

The study of pernicious anemia in humans, which is characterized as a megaloblastic anemia, was the major area of research that led to the discovery of vitamin B_{12}. In 1926 Minot and Murphy recognized that the consumption of liver by humans was effective in treating pernicious anemia. Castle et al., in 1930, hypothesized that the effectiveness of liver in treating pernicious anemia was due to a combination of an intrinsic factor produced by the stomach and a dietary extrinsic factor. Progress in concentrating and identifying the dietary factor was slow because patients with pernicious anemia were required to test the activity of any fractions for activity. In 1948 Schorb reported that the vitamin was required for the growth of a microorganism providing a microbiological assay. The complicated nature of the structure of vitamin B_{12} was established in 1956, and the structure of the coenzyme form was reported in 1961.

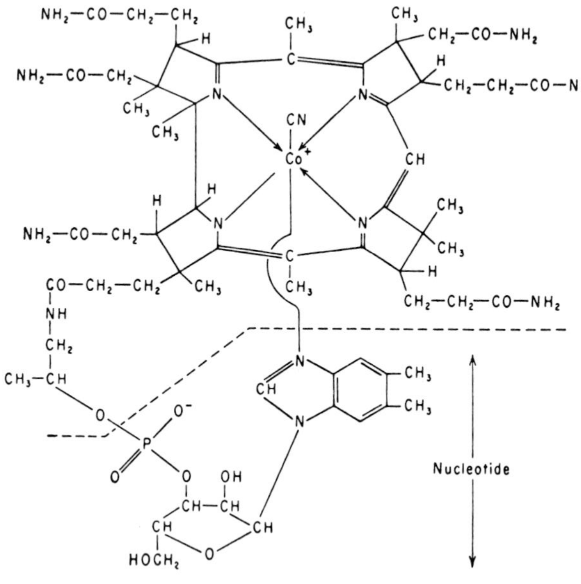

Cyanocobalamin

While the structure of vitamin B_{12} is complex, there are three major components of the structure. A corrin ring system that is similar to the porphyrin ring system in hemoglobin is a major component. Cobalt is coordinated to the N in the center of the corrin ring system. Below the plane of the corrin ring system is a 5,6-dimethylbenzimidazole ring that is coordinated to the cobalt and, through ribose, to one of the rings in the corrin ring. A number of forms of vitamin B_{12} are known and vary by the functional group that is coordinated to the cobalt above the corrin ring system. The functional group can be cyanide (cyanocobalamin), hydroxyl (hydroxylcobalamin), nitrate (nitrocobalamin), or other groups. This position is also the site of formation of the coenzyme forms of vitamin B_{12}.

The absorption of vitamin B_{12} requires the presence of a protein synthesized by the parietal cells of the stomach, called intrinsic factor. Intrinsic factor binds vitamin B_{12}, and the complex is bound by receptors in the ileum. Calcium may also be required for binding at the receptor site. Vitamin B_{12} is absorbed by the intestinal cell, and the intrinsic factor is either released into the intestine or also taken up by the intestinal cell. The absorbed vitamin B_{12} enters the bloodstream and is bound by a transport protein, transcobalamin II, that transports the vitamin to the tissues. The liver synthesizes transcobalamin II and another protein, transcobalamin I. Transcobalamin I binds methylcobalamin and, because of its slow turnover, it has been suggested that it functions as a storage form of the vitamin. Other binding proteins have been described, but no specific functions for the other binding proteins have been determined.

In tissues, vitamin B_{12} forms two coenzyme forms. One is 5′deoxyadenosylcobalamin and is a coenzyme for methylmalonyl CoA mutase enzyme. This enzyme catalyzes the conversion of propionate via *l*-methylmalonyl CoA to succinyl CoA. This reaction is necessary for ruminants to use propionate arising from volatile fatty acid production in the rumen, and vitamin B_{12} deficiency reduces the utilization of propionate. The second coenzyme is methylcobalamin, and it functions in the methylation of homocysteine to form methionine.

Vitamin B_{12} is excreted by the liver in bile. If vitamin B_{12} intake is reduced, the absorption mechanisms are very effective in the reabsorption of the vitamin that is excreted in bile.

Requirements for vitamin B_{12} range from 3 to 50 μg/kg of diet for nonruminants. Microorganisms in the rumen normally synthesize vitamin B_{12} but require a source of cobalt. In ruminants cobalt deficiency will result in a vitamin B_{12} deficiency, characterized by anorexia, depressed growth, and anemia (Fig 28.3).

Vitamin B_{12} is not synthesized by plants, so diets that are formulated only from plant materials require supplementation with vitamin B_{12}. Feeds and feed ingredients from animal origin are reasonably good sources. Vitamin B_{12} deficiency was not observed in nonruminants until attempts were made to use all-plant diets. Pigs and chicks fed all-plant diets grew slowly, and the growth rate could be restored by the inclusion of feed ingredients of animal origin. Supplementation of plant diets with vitamin B_{12} eliminated the need for feeds of animal origin.

ASCORBIC ACID

Scurvy, the condition caused by inadequate intake of ascorbic acid (vitamin C), has been known for centuries. It occurred epidemically during wars, famines, and long voyages when there was a shortage of fruits and vegetables.

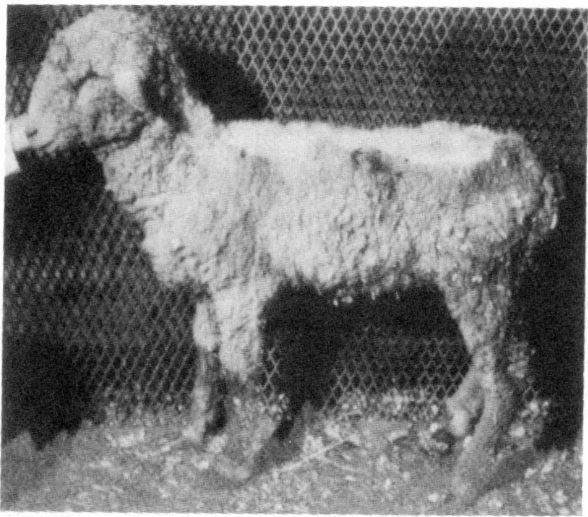

Figure 28.3. Vitamin B_{12} deficiency in the lamb induced by limiting the intake of cobalt. This lamb was approximately 50 percent of normal weight and severely anemic.

Pure ascorbic acid was isolated by Waugh and King in 1932 and was shown to prevent scurvy. Ascorbic acid is a hexuronic acid and has the property of being reversibly oxidized to dehydroascorbic acid.

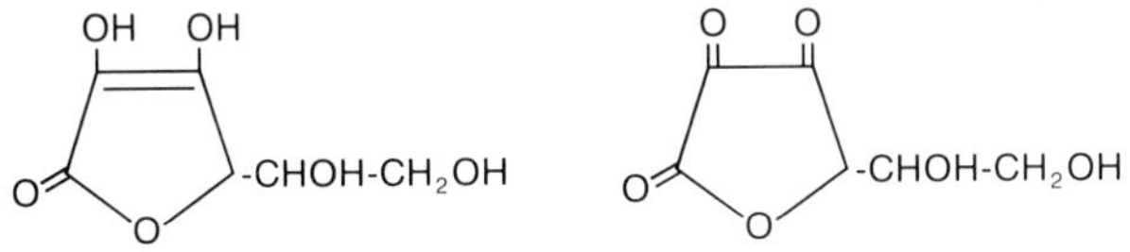

L-Ascorbic Acid — L-Dehydroascorbic acid

In species that require a dietary source, ascorbic acid is absorbed by an active transport mechanism that is similar to the active transport of glucose. The active transport process can be saturated so that the efficiency of absorption decreases if dietary intake is high. In species that do not require ascorbic acid, absorption is by diffusion. No specific transport proteins have been described for ascorbic acid.

Ascorbic acid is present in all tissues and is found in high concentrations in the adrenal cortex and the pituitary gland. The predominant form in tissues is ascorbic acid, and dehydroascorbic acid is present at low levels. A major function of ascorbic acid is the hydroxylation of proline and lysine in collagen to allow formation of the normal helical structure of the compound. The reaction also requires α-ketoglutarate and ferrous iron. This function explains the defects of capillary fragility, weak bones, and slow healing of wounds observed in scurvy. In the metabolism of tyrosine, ascorbic acid functions as a reducing agent but is not the only reducing agent that is effective. Intermediates of tyrosine metabolism are excreted in urine during a deficiency. The property of reversible oxidation-reduction allows ascorbic acid to function as an antioxidant. It has also been suggested that this property facilitates iron absorption and utilization by reducing ferric to ferrous iron.

The metabolism of ascorbic acid is initially oxidation to dehydroascorbic acid and further oxidation to *l*-diketogulonic acid. Diketogulonic acid in humans is converted to threonic acid and oxalic acid. In the guinea pig diketogulonic acid is decarboxylated to produce carbon dioxide and lyxonic or xylonic acid. Urinary metabolites include ascorbic acid, dehydroascorbic acid, ascorbate-2-sulfate, and oxalic acid.

Ascorbic acid is a dietary requirement for humans, monkeys, guinea pigs, and some species of fish. A few species of birds, the fruit bat, flying fox, and some insects have a dietary requirement for ascorbic acid. The domestic animals and poultry do not have a dietary requirement. Ascorbic acid is synthesized in the liver of most species and in the kidneys of amphibians and reptiles. Those species that require a dietary source of ascorbic acid lack the enzyme, L-gulono-gamma-lactone oxidase, that converts the gulonolactone to ascorbic acid.

REFERENCES

Angier, R.B., Boothe, J.H., Hutchins, B.L., Mowat, J.H., Semb, J., Stokstad, E.L.R., Subbarow, Y., Waller, C.W., Cosulich, D.B., Fahrenbach, M.J., Hultiquist, M.E., Kuh, E., Northey, E.H., Seeger, D.R., Sickels, J.P., and Smith, J.M., Jr. 1946. The structure and synthesis of the liver *L. casei factor. Science* 103:667–9.

Benkovic, S.J. 1980. On the mechanisms of action of folate- and biopterin-requiring enzymes. *Ann. Rev. Biochem.* 49:227–51.

Bowman, B.B., McCormick, D.B., and Rosenberg, I.H. 1989. Epithelial transport of water-soluble vitamins. *Ann. Rev. Nutr.* 9:187–99.

Castle, W.B., Townsend, W.C., and Heath, W.C. 1930. Observations on the etiologic relationship of achylia gastrica to pernicious anemia, III. The nature of the reaction between normal human gastric juice and beef muscle leading to animal improvement and increased blood formation similar to the effect of liver feeding. *Am. J. Med. Sci.* 180:305–35.

Dakshinamurti, K., and Chauhan, J. 1988. Regulation of biotin enzymes. *Ann. Rev. Nutr.* 8:211–33.

Dam, H. 1934. Haemorrhages in chicks reared on artificial diets: New deficiency disease. *Nature* 133:909–10.

Dam, H. 1935a. The antihaemorrhagic vitamin of the chick. *Biochem. J.* 29:1273–85.

Dam, H. 1935b. The antihaemorrhagic vitamin of the chick: Occurrence and chemical nature. *Nature* 135:652–3.

Dam, H., Geiger, A., Glavind, J., Karrer, P., Karrer, W., Rothschild, E., and Salomon, H. 1939. Isolierung des Vitamins K in hochgereinigter Form. *Helv. Chim. Acta* 22:310–3.

Dam, H., and Schonheyder, F. 1934. A deficiency disease in chicks resembling scurvy. *Biochem. J.* 28:1355–9.

DeLuca, H. 1988. The vitamin D story: A collaborative effort of basic science and clinical medicine. *FASEB J.* 2:224–36.

Diplock, A.T. 1985. *The Fat Soluble Vitamins: Their Biochemistry and Applications.* Heineman, London.

Diplock, A.T. 1989. Vitamin E: Biochemistry and health implications. *Ann. New York Acad. Sci.* 570:555.

duVigneaud, V., Melville, D.B., György, P., and Rose, G.S. 1940. On the identity of vitamin H with biotin. *Science* 92:62–3.

duVigneaud, V., Ressler, C., and Rachele, J.R. 1950. The biological synthesis of "labile methyl groups." *Science* 112:267–71.

Elvehjem, C.A., and Koehn, C.J., Jr. 1935. Studies on vitamin B_2; the non-identity of vitamin B_2 and flavins. *J. Biol. Chem.* 108:709–28.

Elvehjem, C.A., Madden, R.J., Strong, F.M., and Woolley, D.W. 1937. Relation of nicotinic acid and nicotinic acid amide to canine black tongue. *J. Am. Chem. Soc.* 59:1767–68.

Englard, S., and Seifer, S. 1986. The biochemical functions of ascorbic acid. *Ann. Rev. Nutr.* 6:365–406.

Ensminger, M.E., and Olentine, C.G., Jr. 1978. *Feeds and Nutrition.* Ensminger, Clovis, Calif.

Evans, H.M. 1962. The pioneer history of vitamin E. *Vitam. Horm.* 20:379–87.

Fernholz, E. 1938. On the constitution of α-tocopherol. *J. Am. Chem. Soc.* 60:700–705.

Funk, C. 1912. The etiology of the deficiency diseases. *J. State Med.* (Roy. Inst. Pub. Health, London) 20:341–68.

Goldblith, S.A., and Joslyn, M.A. 1964. *Milestones in Nutrition.* Avi. Westport, Conn.

Goodwin, T.W. 1986. Metabolism, nutrition, and function of carotenoids. *Ann. Rev. Nutr.* 6:273–97.

György, P., and Pearson, W.N. 1967. *The Vitamins,* vol. VI and VII. Academic Press, New York.

Harris, S.A., Wolf, D.E., Mozingo, R., and Folkers, K. 1943. Synthetic biotin. *Science* 97:447–8.

Jansen, B.C.P., and Donath, W.F. 1926. On the isolation of the anti-beriberi vitamin. *Proc. R. Acad. Sci. Amsterdam* 29:1390–1400.

Jukes, T.H. 1939. The pantothenic acid requirements of the chick. *J. Biol. Chem.* 129:225–31.

Karrer, P., Morf, R., and Schöpp, K. 1931. Zur Kenntnis des Vitamins-A aus Fischtranen. *Helv. Chim. Acta* 14:1431–6.

Karrer, P., Schöpp, K., and Benz, F. 1935. Synthesen von Flavinen. *Helv. Chim. Acta* 18:426–9.

Kuhn, R., Reinėmund, K., Weygand, F., and Strobele, R. 1935. Uber die Synthese des Lactoflavins (Vitamin B_2). *Beriche Deutsch. Chem. Gesellsch.* 68:1765–71.

Link, K.P. 1943–44. The anticoagulant from spoiled sweet clover hay. *Harvey Lect.* Vol. 39 ser. 39:162–216.

Link, K.P. 1959. The discovery of dicumarol and its sequels. *Circulation* 19:97–107.

Lipmann, F. 1945. Acetylation of sulfanilamide by liver homogenates and extracts. *J. Biol. Chem.* 160:173–90.

Lipmann, F. 1954. Pantothenic acid. III. Biochemical systems. In W.H. Sebrell and R.S. Harris, *The Vitamins: Chemistry, Physiology, Pathology, Methods,* Vol. 2. Academic, New York. Pp. 598–625.

Machlin, L.J. 1980. *Vitamin E: A comprehensive treatise*. Marcel Dekker, Inc., New York.

McCollum, E.V. 1957. *A History of Nutrition*. Houghton Mifflin, Boston.

McCollum, E.V., and Davis, M. 1913. The necessity of certain lipids in the diet during growth. *J. Biol. Chem.* 15: 167–75.

McCollum, E.V., Simmonds, N., Becker, J.E., and Shipley, P.G. 1925. Studies on experimental rickets. XXVI. A diet composed principally of purified foodstuffs for use with the "Line Test" for vitamin D studies. *J. Biol. Chem.* 65:97–100.

McDowell, L.R. 1989. *Vitamins in Animal Nutrition*. Academic Press, New York.

Mitchell, H.K., Snell, E.E., and Williams, R.J. 1941. The concentration of folic acid. *J. Am. Chem. Soc.* 63:2284.

National Research Council. 1971. *Atlas of Nutritional Data on United States and Canadian Feeds*. Nat. Acad. Sci., Washington, D.C.

National Research Council. 1977–1989. *Nutrient Requirements of Domestic Animals*. 1–XIV. Nat. Acad. Press, Washington, D.C.

Price, P.A. 1988. Role of vitamin K-dependent proteins in bone metabolism. *Ann. Rev. Nutr.* 8:565–83.

Olson, R.E. 1984. The function and metabolism of vitamin K. *Ann. Rev. Nutr.* 4:281–37.

Sable, H.Z., and Gubler, C.J. 1982. Thiamine: Twenty years of progress. *Ann. New York Acad. Sci.* 378:470.

Sebrell, W.H., and Harris, R.S. *The Vitamins: Chemistry, Physiology, Pathology, Methods*. Academic, New York. Vol. 1 (1967), vol. 2 (1968), vol. 3 (1971), vol. 5 (1972).

Smith, E.L. 1960. *Vitamin B_{12}*. Methuen, London.

Smith, S.E., and Loosli, J.K. 1957. Cobalt and vitamin B_{12} in ruminant nutrition. *J. Dairy Sci.* 40:1215–27.

Steenbock, H. 1919. White corn vs. yellow plant pigments. *Science* 50:352–3.

Suttie, J.W. 1985. Vitamin K-dependent carboxylase. *Ann. Rev. Biochem.* 54:459–77.

Wald, G. 1960. The visual function of vitamin A. *Vitam. Horm.* 18:117–30.

Warburg, O., and Christian, W. 1932. A new oxidation enzyme and its absorption spectrum. *Biochem. Z.* 254:438–58.

Warburg, O., and Christian, W. 1934. The problem of the coenzyme. *Biochem. Z.* 274:112–6.

Wasserman, R.H., and Taylor, A.N. 1968. Vitamin D-dependent calcium-binding protein. *J. Biol. Chem.* 243:3987–93.

Waugh, W.A., and King, C.G. 1932. Isolation and identification of vitamin C. *J. Biol. Chem.* 97:325–31.

Web, R.A., and Holick, M.F.. 1988. The role of sunlight in the cutaneous production of vitamin D_3. *Ann. Rev. Nutr.* 8:375–99.

White, H.B., and Merrill, A.H., Jr. 1988. Riboflavin-binding proteins. *Ann. Rev. Nutr.* 8:279–99.

Williams, R.J., Lyman, C.M., Goodyear, G.H., Truesdail, J.H., and Holaday, D. 1933. "Pantothenic acid," a growth determinant of universal biological occurrence. *J. Am. Chem. Soc.* 55:2912–27.

Williams, R.R., and Cline, J.K. 1936. Synthesis of vitamin B_1. *J. Am. Chem. Soc.* 58:1504–1505.

Woolley, D.W., Waisman, H.A., and Elvehjem, C.A. 1939. Nature and partial synthesis of the chick antidermatitis factor. *J. Am. Chem. Soc.* 61:977–78.

PART **IV** | **MINERALS AND BONES**

CHAPTER **29**

Minerals | by Virgil W. Hays and Melvin J. Swenson

All forms of living matter require inorganic elements, or minerals, for their normal life processes. Minerals that have demonstrable bodily functions either in elemental form or incorporated into specific compounds are calcium, phosphorus, magnesium, sodium, potassium, sulfur, chlorine, iron, copper, cobalt, iodine, manganese, selenium, zinc, chromium, fluoride, molybdenum, nickel, silicon, and vanadium. Virtually all elements have been found in animal tissues, and several additional ones may have physiological significance. There is some evidence that arsenic, lithium, and tin play a functional role in animal physiology; however, their essentiality has not been established. Although aluminum, barium, boron, bromine, cadmium, and strontium occur in animal tissue, their biological significance is unknown.

The functions of minerals in animal physiology are interrelated; seldom can they be considered as single elements with independent and self-sufficient roles. The definite relationship of calcium and phosphorus in the formation of bones and teeth and the interrelationships of iron, copper, and cobalt (in vitamin B_{12}) in hemoglobin synthesis and red blood cell formation are examples. Sodium, potassium, calcium, phosphorus, and chlorine serve individually and collectively in the body fluids. However, some elements serve very specific roles, such as iodine in thyroxine and cobalt as an integral part of vitamin B_{12}. Thyroxine and vitamin B_{12}, however, are intimately involved in processes related to many other organic and inorganic nutrients.

Cobalt, copper, iodine, and selenium deficiencies in the soil and flora in certain areas of the world have led to deficiencies of these minerals in domestic animals. Also, excesses of selenium in the soil may result in levels in certain seleniferous plants that can contribute to toxicity in animals. Nutritional disorders involving the mineral elements may arise as simple deficiencies or excesses of particular elements, but they occur more often as deficiencies or toxicities conditioned by the extent to which other organic or inorganic nutrients are present in the diet. These conditioning factors may themselves be a reflection of the soils on which the plants are grown, or they may be related to the presence of specific plants that are seleniferous or goitrogenic.

CALCIUM AND PHOSPHORUS

Calcium and phosphorus serve as the major structural elements of skeletal tissue, with more than 99 percent of the total body calcium and more than 75 percent of the total phosphorus being found in the bones and teeth. They are present in the bone principally as apatite salt and as calcium phosphate and calcium carbonate. In addition to being the structural framework, bone also is the calcium and phosphorus reservoir of the body. The calcium and phosphorus found in the trabecular portion (substantia spongiosa) of bones are in dynamic equilibrium with that of body fluids and other tissues of the body. During periods of dietary deficiency or when the requirement is increased, as during pregnancy and lactation, calcium and phosphorus are readily mobilized from the bones to maintain normal and nearly constant levels (especially of calcium) in blood and other soft tissue (see Chap. 34).

Normally, blood plasma or serum contains 5 mEq of calcium per liter (9 to 11 mg/dl for most species). The laying hen, however, has calcium levels between 15 and 20 mEq/L of plasma (estrogens increase plasma calcium). The values of calcium in erythrocytes have been reported to vary from approximately 0.05 to 1.35 mEq/L of cellular water.

From 45 to 50 percent of the plasma calcium is in the soluble ionized form, whereas 40 to 45 percent is bound with protein, primarily albumin and other plasma proteins. The remaining 5 percent is complexed with nonionized inorganic elements depending on blood pH. Plasma calcium is essential for the coagulation of blood (see Chap. 4). In cerebrospinal fluid, calcium is present in the diffusible (ionic) form and is equal in concentration to the ionic form in blood plasma. It is also required for membrane permeability, neuromuscular excitability, transmission of nerve impulses, and activation of certain enzyme systems. A reduced extracellular blood calcium level increases the irritability of nerve tissue, and very low levels may cause spontaneous discharges of nerve impulses leading to tetany and convulsions. Hypocalcemia may cause weakness of the heart similar to that caused by hyperkalemia. Excess calcium depresses cardiac activity and leads to respiratory and cardiac failure; it may cause the heart to stop in systole. Normally, though, calcium ions increase the strength and duration of cardiac muscle contraction.

Phosphorus has more known functions than any other mineral element in the animal body. In addition to uniting with calcium and carbonate to form compounds that lend rigidity to bones and teeth, it is located in every cell of the body and is vitally concerned in many metabolic processes, including those involving the buffers in body fluids. Practically every form of energy exchange inside living cells involves the forming or breaking of high-energy bonds that link oxides of phosphorus to carbon or to carbon-nitrogen compounds. Since every biological event involves gain or loss of energy, one can readily grasp the great physiological role of phosphorus.

ABSORPTION AND UTILIZATION

Dietary calcium and phosphorus are absorbed chiefly in the upper small intestine, particularly the duodenum; the amount absorbed is dependent on source, calcium-phosphorus ratio, intestinal pH, lactose intake, and dietary levels of calcium, phosphorus, vitamin D, iron, aluminum, manganese, and fat. As is the case with most nutrients, the greater the need, the more efficient the absorption. Absorption increases somewhat, though not proportionally, with increased intake. Absorption of calcium and phosphorus is facilitated by a low intestinal pH, which is necessary for their solubility. Thus normal gastric secretion of hydrochloric acid or H^+ is necessary for efficient absorption. Achlorhydria decreases absorption of these minerals. The low pH of the duodenum accounts for the greater absorption in that area. Lactose has also been reported to enhance the absorption of calcium.

A major and possibly the sole function of vitamin D is its role in the intestinal and cellular absorption of calcium (see Chap. 28). Growing, pregnant, and especially lactating animals require liberal amounts of calcium and phosphorus, and in some species the ratio may be critical. A ratio of calcium to phosphorus of 1 : 1 to 2 : 1 is usually recommended. The ratio is far more critical if the level of phosphorus is marginal or inadequate or if vitamin D is limited.

Insoluble calcium salts such as calcium oxalate formed from oxalic acid pass through the intestine without being absorbed. The amounts consumed by domestic animals fed natural feedstuffs are usually not great enough to cause serious problems. Plants known to concentrate oxalic acid are rhubarb (leaves), sheep sorrel, sour dock, curly dock, and greasewood. When these plants are eaten in sufficient quantities, poisoning may occur, with an increase in coagulation time of blood.

A large part (60 to 80 percent) of the total phosphorus of cereal grains and oil seeds exists organically bound as phytic acid. Phytic acid, the hexaphosphoric acid ester of inositol, is present in cereal and legume seeds primarily as the Ca-Mg salt called phytin. Phytic acid may form insoluble salts with free calcium. Zinc may also be complexed with the calcium-phytate and lead to inefficient utilization of dietary zinc. Liberal calcium intake will compensate for the reduced availability of calcium, but it aggravates the zinc deficiency. Such a relationship has frequently led to parakeratosis in pigs.

The organically bound phosphorus, phytin phosphorus, is largely unavailable to monogastric animals, whereas ruminants are capable of using it relatively well. The species difference is explained by the presence of the enzyme phytase from rumen microorganisms, which hydrolyzes the organically bound phosphorus and renders it available for absorption. This, coupled with the slower growth rate of ruminants, accounts in part for the rather large difference in phosphorus requirements of ruminant and nonruminant animals (Table 29.1). The availability of phytate phosphorus to nonruminants varies with plant source, as a result of naturally occurring phytase enzymes in certain seeds (e.g., wheat) but little or no phytase in other seed (e.g., cottonseed).

An excess of dietary fat or poor digestion of fat also may reduce calcium absorption through the formation of insoluble calcium soaps; however, small amounts of fat may improve calcium absorption.

An excess of iron, aluminum, or magnesium interferes with phosphorus absorption through the formation of insoluble phosphates.

Calcium and phosphorus absorbed from the intestine by the portal route are circulated through the body and readily withdrawn from the blood for use by the bones and teeth during periods of growth. Some incorporation into bone occurs at all ages. The plasma calcium level is regulated by the parathyroid hormone and thyrocalcitonin (see Chap. 34). The plasma phosphorus level is inversely related to the blood calcium level. Thyrocalcitonin decreases plasma calcium and phosphate levels while parathyroid hormone in-

Table 29.1. Some dietary mineral requirements

Species	Body weight (kg)	Ca (%)	P (%)	Na (%)	Cl (%)
Chickens					
Starting chicks		1.0	0.45	0.15	0.15
Laying hens		3.4	0.32	0.15	0.15
Pigs	30	0.60	0.5	0.1	0.08
Lactating sows	200	0.75	0.6	0.2	0.16
Beef steers	300	0.41	0.32	0.08	0.08
Pregnant beef cows	500	0.19	0.19	0.08	0.08
Lactating beef cows	500	0.28	0.22	0.08	0.08
Veal calves	100	0.70	0.60	0.1	0.20
Dairy herd replacements	400	0.41	0.30	0.1	0.20
Lactating dairy cows*	550	0.64	0.41	0.18	0.25
Horses					
Weanlings		0.55	0.30	0.10	—
Lactating mares		0.47	0.30	0.10	—

*Requirement varies depending on level of milk production. Data from National Research Council 1984–1989, *Nutrient Requirements of Domestic Animals,* Nat. Acad. Sci., Washington, D.C.

Table 29.2. Calcium and phosphorus supplements fed to livestock*

Supplement	Ca (%)	P (%)
Bone meal, steamed	24–28	12–14
Calcite	34	0
Calcium carbonate (limestone)	38	0
Curacao Island phosphate	34	14
Diammonium phosphate	0	20–23
Dicalcium phosphate	20–24	18.5
Disodium phosphate†	0	20.5
Defluorinated rock phosphate	32	18
Monocalcium phosphate	15–21	21
Monosodium phosphate‡	0	22.4
Oyster shell	38	0
Phosphoric acid	0	24
Sodium tripolyphosphate§	0	25.3
Soft rock phosphate	18	9

*Analysis of feed grade products varies.
†Contains 32.4% sodium.
‡Contains 19.2% sodium.
§Contains 32.1% sodium.

creases them. Excess calcium and phosphorus are excreted by the kidney. Calcium and phosphorus excreted in feces are largely the unabsorbed dietary minerals; some comes from the digestive juices, including bile.

Insufficient intake of calcium, phosphorus, or vitamin D will result in rickets in young animals. In adults, calcium deficiency may cause osteomalacia, a generalized demineralization of bones, not to be confused with osteoporosis, a metabolic disorder resulting in decalcification of bone with a high incidence of fractures (see Chap. 30).

Parturient paresis, or milk fever, in cows is also associated with calcium metabolism. The malady usually occurs with the onset of profuse lactation, and the most consistent abnormality is acute hypocalcemia with the blood calcium declining from the normal of 5 mEq/L to levels of 2 to 3 mEq/L. Serum magnesium levels may be elevated or depressed, low levels are accompanied by tetany and high levels by a flaccid paralysis.

The feedstuffs used markedly affect the adequacy of both calcium and phosphorus in animal diets. Grains are low in calcium for all livestock regardless of the soil. Forage crops are relatively high in calcium, with legumes containing 1 to 2 percent. The calcium-phosphorus ratio in legumes ranges from 6 : 1 to 10 : 1, which often upsets the balance of these two elements and increases the requirement for phosphorus. The calcium-phosphorus ratio in bone is about 2 : 1, and in milk it is about 1.3 : 1. With adequate phosphorus, animals, particularly ruminants, are quite tolerant of rather wide ratios. For herbivores and omnivores, it is advisable to not have less calcium than phosphorus in the diet. There is evidence, however, that phosphorus levels that exceed calcium levels may be beneficial to carnivores by reducing urine pH and reducing incidence or preventing urolithiasis.

Phosphorus-deficient areas are prevalent in the Great Lakes region and the Pacific Northwest and extend into the Dakotas and Nebraska. The application of fertilizers to the soil and the movement of feedstuffs from one area to another alter the picture of localized mineral deficiencies to some extent. Fertilization of soil, however, may not always be accompanied by an improvement in quality or even by the maintenance of existing levels of minerals. Thus phosphorus supplements in livestock nutrition are of particular importance. Table 29.2 provides data on calcium and phosphorus supplements fed to livestock.

MAGNESIUM

Approximately 70 percent of the magnesium in the animal body is in bone. In addition, cardiac muscle, skeletal muscle, and nerve tissue depend on a proper balance between calcium and magnesium ions. Magnesium is an active component of several enzyme systems in which thiamine pyrophosphate is a cofactor. Oxidative phosphorylation is greatly reduced in the absence of magnesium. Magnesium is also an essential activator for the phosphate-transferring enzymes myokinase, diphosphoyridinenucleotide kinase, and creatine kinase. It also activates pyruvic acid carboxylase, pyruvic acid oxidase, and the condensing enzyme for the reactions in the citric acid cycle (see Chap. 24).

Deficiency of magnesium was first studied intensively in the rat but has since been produced in other species. Acute magnesium deficiency results in vasodilation, with erythema and hyperemia appearing after a few days on the deficient diet. Neuromuscular hyperirritability increases with the continuation of the deficiency and may be followed eventually by cardiac arrhythmia and generalized tremors. The symptoms of magnesium deficiency resemble those of a low-calcium tetany.

Tissue analysis of animals fed a deficient diet reveals a drop in plasma magnesium levels to 30 to 50 percent of normal within 7 to 9 days. Blood plasma concentrations of magnesium are normally 2 to 3 mEq/L. The concentration in other soft tissue is not altered appreciably, however. Bone apparently acts as a reservoir for magnesium, but the mobilization from bone is relatively slow. Thus a dietary deficiency may result in a marked reduction in blood magnesium before the level in bone is affected. If the deficiency is sufficiently severe, tetany and other clinical signs may result. On continued deficiency, the magnesium content of bone decreases and the calcium content increases. The bone magnesium is rapidly replenished when the animals are fed a diet high in magnesium.

A common form of magnesium-deficiency tetany is called *grass tetany* or wheat-pasture poisoning. Although this condition closely resembles the magnesium-deficiency syndrome and can be corrected by the administration of magnesium salts, it is not a typical magnesium deficiency. The condition occurs in ruminants grazing on rapidly growing young grasses or cereal crops and develops very quickly. Unlike other magnesium deficiency conditions, the magnesium in the bone is not normally depleted in grass tetany. The magnesium content of soils where grass tetany occurs is usually within normal ranges. A high level of fertilization results in high levels of nitrogen and potassium in the plants and tends to reduce the uptake of magnesium by the plant. In turn, the high level of potassium interferes with the absorption of magnesium, and the high levels of dietary nitrogen provided by the plants increase the excretion of magnesium. These effects lead to a physiological deficiency of magnesium and can result in tetany and death. The physiological deficiency can be prevented by magnesium supplementation of a salt or grain mixture. Adequate consumption, of course, is critical.

The prolonged feeding of a whole milk diet, which is deficient in magnesium, to calves results in a type of magnesium deficiency that is different from grass tetany and resembles classic magnesium deficiencies observed in other species. On continued feeding of the deficient diet, a reduction in serum magnesium occurs, and magnesium content of the bone may decline.

The dietary requirement for magnesium has not been well established. The National Research Council (1984–1989) estimates a requirement of 400 ppm of the diet for the pig, 600 ppm for the chick, 700 ppm for the calf, and 2000 to 2500 ppm for lactating cows. With the exception of milk diets of calves and the pasture conditions mentioned above for lactating cows, most diets composed of natural ingredients contain sufficient quantities of magnesium.

SODIUM

In animals sodium is present largely as the sodium ion. The major functions of the sodium ion concern regulation of crystalloid osmotic pressure, acid-base balance, maintenance of membrane potentials, transmission of nerve impulses, and the absorptive processes of monosaccharides, amino acids, pyrimidines, and bile salts (see Chaps. 18, 19 & 20). The role of sodium in regulation of osmotic pressure may be typified by consideration of the electrolyte distribution of blood plasma in mEq/L, which is approximated for humans as follows:

$$Na^+(155) + K^+(5) + Ca^{2+}(5) + Mg^{2+}(3)$$
$$= Cl^-(105) + HCO_3^-(30) + \text{proteinate}(18) + \text{other}(15)$$

The sodium ion is the chief cation of extracellular fluids. Intracellularly, potassium and magnesium are the principal cations. Of the osmotically effective bases of extracellular fluids, sodium makes up more than 90 percent of the total. Thus changes in osmotic pressure are largely dependent on the sodium concentration. Under stress conditions, a loss of sodium may be compensated for by an increase in potassium, but the organism is limited in its capacity to substitute bases, and major losses of sodium lead to a significant lowering of osmotic pressure and, therefore, to a loss of water or dehydration. Restoration is incomplete until both the base and water are replaced.

The role of sodium in acid-base balance, though important, is secondary to its role in maintaining osmotic pressure. The portion of sodium equivalent to the bicarbonate present (about 30 mEq/L of plasma water as shown above) represents most of the available base that can be used for the neutralization of acids entering the bloodstream, and, in conjunction with carbonic acid, it affects the pH of blood. It is more accurate, however, to regard changes in acid-base balance in terms of the anions present than in terms of sodium. Thus an acidosis or alkalosis with variation in plasma bicarbonates and carbon dioxide tension can exist without significant changes in sodium content. (Acid-base balance and osmotic pressure regulation are more thoroughly covered in Chap. 32.)

Commonly used vegetable feedstuffs do not contain sufficient quantities of sodium to meet the animal's need of 0.10 to 0.20 percent of the diet (Table 29.1). This inadequacy is overcome by inclusion of sodium chloride (common salt) in the diet or by allowing the animal to consume salt ad libitum. Sodium is readily absorbed as the sodium ion and circulates throughout the body. Excretion takes place mainly through the kidney as sodium chloride or phosphate. There are appreciable losses in perspiration, and the quantities lost by this route vary rather markedly with the humidity of the environment and among animal species.

Excessive intake of sodium chloride may result in salt toxicity. The sodium ion is primarily responsible for the toxicity, since sodium acetate or sodium propionate affects the animals in a manner similar to that of sodium chloride. The amounts required for toxicity vary tremendously and are largely dependent on the availability of water to the animals. Mature cows will tolerate more than 450 g per day without ill effects, and sows and chicks will tolerate 8 to 10 percent of the diet as salt, provided ample water is available. Toxicity most often results when animals are deprived of salt and then have access to a brine solution or loose salt without access to sufficient water.

POTASSIUM

Potassium is the major cation of body cells and apparently serves the same general functions relating to osmotic pressure to regulation and acid-base balance in the cells as does sodium in the extracellular fluids. Blood plasma of humans contains about 5 to 6 mEq/L of potassium. Approximately 75 to 80 percent of the cation content of red cells is made up of potassium (about 125 to 170 mEq/L of cellular water) in many animals. However, lesser amounts are present in the erythrocytes of dogs, cats, cattle, sheep, goats, and other animals (see Chap. 3). Potassium deficiency leads to an increase in the basic amino acid concentration of the tissue fluids and some increase in cellular sodium levels as a means of maintaining cation-anion balance.

Potassium functions in the maintenance of acid-base balance, regulation of osmotic pressure, and development of cellular membrane potentials, as does sodium. When the extracellular potassium is low, transmission of nerve impulses becomes impaired, and muscular paralysis develops. Potassium influences the contractibility of smooth, skeletal, and cardiac muscle and has an effect on muscular irritability that, like that of sodium, tends to antagonize the effect of the calcium ion. Under conditions of salt restriction, however, calcium appears highly important in helping to maintain the potassium content of tissue. Potassium aids in the transfer of phosphate from adenosine triphosphate to pyruvic acid and probably has a role in numerous other basic cellular enzymatic reactions.

Since potassium is the major intracellular cation, its depletion is associated with many functional and structural abnormalities, including impaired neuromuscular functions of skeletal, smooth, and cardiac muscle. Cardiac arrhythmias and impaired carbohydrate tolerance are abnormalities seen in potassium deficiency. Altered electrocardiograms have been reported in potassium-deficient calves. There was a pronounced increase in the QRS duration, to twice the normal time. The increase in time for the QRS complex to form was attributed to degenerative lesions in the Purkinje fibers. Excess potassium causes dilatation of the heart. When extracellular potassium reaches three or more times the normal value, heart block develops. The heart stops in diastole. This is why inorganic potassium salts are usually not recommended for intravenous administration. When plasma potassium is low (2.5 to 3.0 mEq/L), however, a veterinarian should give potassium salts intravenously to increase the concentration to normal values (3.4 to 5.0 mEq/L). In hypokalemia the electrocardiogram shows a decrease in heart rate, an increase in PR interval, and an increase in QRS duration and eventually leads to atrioventricular block. When lactating dairy cows have hypokalemia, milk production is lowered markedly and may be restored with intravenous potassium therapy. Along with this treatment, proper dietary changes should be made to correct the potassium deficiency.

Potassium deficiency affects the collecting tubules of the kidney, resulting in an inability to concentrate urine, and also causes alterations of gastric secretions and intestinal motility.

Because of their related roles in regulating cation balance and osmotic pressure in intracellular and extracellular fluids, it has been suggested that the relative quantities of sodium and potassium in the diet are critical. However, plant products contain many times as much potassium as sodium, yet animals do well on such diets. The potassium requirement of chicks and pigs is approximately 0.20 to 0.4 percent of the diet; the requirement is affected to some extent by the growth rate of the animal and the protein level of the diet. Rapidly growing animals apparently have a higher requirement for potassium, and increasing the protein level increases the requirement. The turkey, for example, has a relatively high requirement for potassium (0.4 to 0.7 percent of the diet) . The requirement of ruminants has not been established accurately; however, it is recommended that their diets contain 0.8 percent. The requirement of lactating dairy cows is even higher, 0.9 to 1.0 percent (Table 29.5).

CHLORINE

The principal anion in extracellular fluid is chloride. It is the chief anion of the gastric juice and is accompanied by the hydrogen ion in nearly equal amounts. The chloride of the gastric secretions is derived from blood chloride and is normally reabsorbed during later stages of digestion in the lower intestine.

Excessive depletion of chloride ions through losses in the gastric secretions or by deficiencies in the diet may lead to alkalosis due to an excess of bicarbonate, since the inadequate level of chloride is partially replaced or compensated for by bicarbonate. On a chloride-deficient diet, the excretion of chloride in the urine or perspiration is markedly reduced.

A close relationship exists between chloride and sodium ions. Chloride is involved in the regulation of extracellular osmotic pressure and makes up more than 60 percent of the anions in this fluid compartment. Thus the chloride ion is important in acid-base balance. The concentration of the chloride ion is subject to more variation than that of sodium, since other anions, especially bicarbonates, can exchange for the chloride. The optimum dietary intakes of sodium and chloride approximate a 1 : 1 ratio. Excess chloride and a constant level of sodium can result in acidosis, whereas an excess of sodium and a constant level of chloride can result in alkalosis. The ratios in Table 29.1 appear satisfactory, provided there is an adequate level of both elements in the diet.

Chloride is excreted in the feces, sweat, and urine primarily as sodium or potassium chloride, although it may be accompanied by ammonium ions when base needs to be conserved (see Chap. 31).

IODINE

Iodine functions in animals as a basic component of the thyroid hormones, tri-iodothyronine and tetra-iodothyronine (see Chap. 34). Although the specific roles of thyroid hormones are not clear, it is accepted that they play a vital role in oxygen utilization, energy metabolism, and regulation of metabolic rate; thus they are involved in all body functions. In the absence of pathological conditions, the major factor affecting the secretion of thyroxine and related compounds by the thyroid gland is the dietary intake and biological availability of iodine. The ion is freely diffusible, is readily absorbed from the gastrointestinal tract, and is excreted mainly in the urine at a relatively constant rate, provided the dietary intake is sufficient. Plasma iodide is trapped by the thyroid gland and oxidized to a form available for incorporation into thyroxine by combination with thyroglobulin. Proteolysis results in release of thyroxine and its intermediates. Deiodination of the hormone intermediates supplies reactive iodine for reincorporation into the thyroglobulin protein. Much of the released iodine reenters the iodide pool, so that little is wasted, especially if the diet is limited in iodine.

Iodine deficiency has been stated to be the most widespread of all mineral deficiencies in grazing stock. It can be due to a deficiency of iodine in the diet or the presence of dietary constituents that interfere with the use of iodine by the thyroid gland. As a result, the production and general health of farm animals are markedly affected. Reproductive failures have long been attributed to iodine deficiency. The birth of dead, weak, or hairless young, early embryonic death and resorption of the fetus, later fetal death and abortion, abnormal estrous cycles, and poor conception rates have all been associated with low-iodine diets or interference with iodine absorption by goitrogenic substances.

Plants are highly variable in iodine content, depending on the species, soil type (including its iodine content), fertilization, and climate. Iodine-deficient areas are found in the interior of all countries, especially in areas where wind or rainfall are unable to carry traces from the sea and where the soil has been depleted by leaching by heavy iodine-poor rains or where there is little rainfall (Fig. 29.1). Feedstuffs or forages produced in these areas may be deficient in iodine and affect the growth and reproduction of livestock (see Chap. 34).

Animals fed a prepared feed or concentrate may be provided with supplemental iodine by incorporation of iodine into the salt, mineral mixture, or other concentrates. It is more difficult to assure adequate intake by grazing animals. The most effective way is to incorporate a stabilized form of iodine into the salt offered the animals. Calcium iodate, stabilized potassium iodide, or pentacalcium orthoperiodate are preferable because they are less subject to losses from leaching or volatilization.

Goitrogenic activity has been found in many plants, including virtually all cruciferous plants, soybeans, linseed, peas, and peanuts. The goitrogenic substances in the plant material include thioglycosides, thiocyanates, and perchlorates. Thiocyanate and perchlorate ions act by inhibiting the selective concentration of iodine by the thyroid. Their actions are reversible with iodine. Thioglycosides from brassica seeds and other goitrogens of the thiouracil type act by inhibiting hormonogenesis in the thyroid gland, and their effects are either not reversible or only partly so with iodine supplementation.

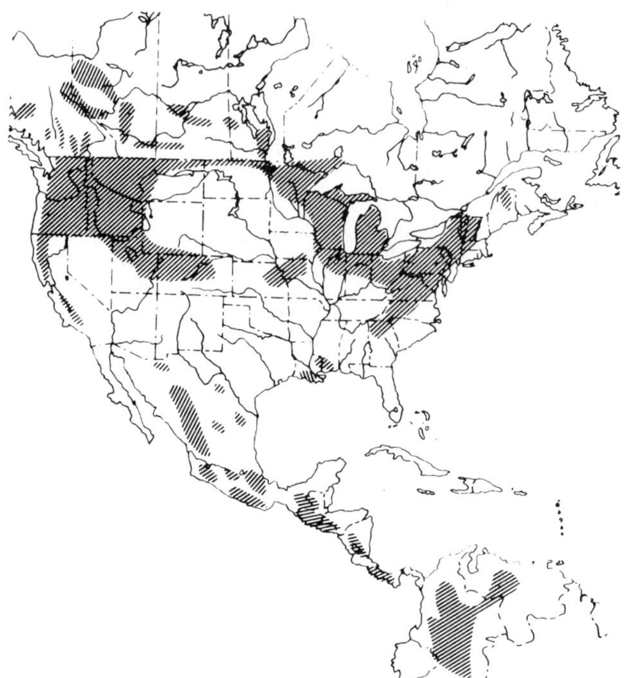

Figure 29.1. Areas of endemic goiter caused by deficiency of iodine in the United States and adjoining countries. (From Kelly and Sneeden 1960, *Endemic Goiter,* World Health Organization, Geneva.)

Goitrogens have been demonstrated in the milk of cows that have ingested cruciferous plants in grazing or as fodder. The goitrogenic factor in the milk of such animals is not corrected by supplemental iodine. This could contribute to the endemism of goiter in humans in areas in which the animals consume such feedstuffs and their milk is subsequently consumed.

The iodine requirement of animals has not been clearly established. The requirement for chicks is approximately 0.3 ppm of the diet or the equivalent of 75 to 95 μg/1000 kcal of metabolizable energy. An estimated requirement is 1 to 2 μg/per day for rats, which, on a caloric basis similar to the above, would be approximately 30 to 65 μg/1000 kcal. In the absence of a goitrogenic substance in the diet, 0.2 to 0.4 ppm of iodine appears sufficient for monogastric animals and nonlactating ruminants. Since lactating cows may excrete up to 10 percent of the intake in the milk, the recommended level for dairy cows is 0.6 ppm. The feeding of iodized salt containing 0.01 percent stabilized iodine or 0.0076 percent iodine at the rate of 0.25 to 0.50 percent of the diet or by allowing ad libitum consumption of iodized salt will prevent signs of iodine deficiency. The animals will tolerate 50 to 100 times the actual requirement without ill effects, and if feedstuffs include goitrogenic substances, dietary levels well above the minimum requirement may be not only desirable but also necessary.

SULFUR

Sulfur is usually not considered in discussions of inorganic metabolism, since only an insignificant part of the sulfur ingested is inorganic. By far the greatest portion of sulfur is in the amino acids, cystine and methionine (see Chap. 26). Proteins vary widely in sulfur content, depending on their amino acid composition, but average about 1 percent sulfur. The sulfur amino acid requirement for the monogastric animals is approximately 3 to 4 percent of the total protein requirement. Thus the sulfur requirement would approximate 0.6 to 0.8 percent of the total protein. For metabolic purposes, however, this is necessary as the preformed amino acid; hence sulfur deficiencies are reflected as sulfur-containing amino acid deficiencies.

Ruminants depending largely on nonprotein nitrogen sources, such as urea, biuret, or ammonium phosphate, may need supplemental inorganic sulfur. This sulfur is used by the microorganisms for synthesis of methionine and cystine. Inadequate sulfur intake reduces feed intake, digestibility, rate of weight gain, and milk production. In diets containing nonprotein nitrogen, it is recommended that the nitrogen-sulfur ratio be maintained at 10 : 1 to 12 : 1.

The end products of sulfur metabolism are taurine and sulfuric acid. The sulfuric acid is either neutralized and excreted as inorganic sulfates in the urine or conjugated with phenol, glucuronic acid, or indoxyl. The taurine is conjugated with choleic acid and excreted in the bile.

Other sulfur compounds of biological significance include cyanate in saliva and other fluids, ergothioneine of the red blood cells, glutathione, which is present in all cells, and chondroitin sulfate, which serves a structural function in cartilage, bone, tendons, blood vessel walls, and so forth. The primary function of sulfur is as the disulfide linkage, -S-S-, of such organic compounds.

FLUORINE

Fluorine is an important mineral in the formation of bones and teeth. A proper intake is essential to achieve maximum resistance to dental caries. Fluorine deficiency in terms of soft-tissue lesions or specific metabolic functions has not been reported under natural conditions; however, there is evidence that low fluoride intake retards growth rate, reduces fertility, and results in anemia. Fluorine deficiency is not likely to be of practical significance in animals.

A fluorine concentration of about 1 to 2 ppm added to the drinking water will result in a marked reduction in dental caries in humans. Apparently fluorine, which is deposited in the enamel of teeth during their formation, increases crystal size and perfection in the biological apatites, and reduces the solubility of enamel in the acids that are produced by the bacteria implicated in tooth decay. Fluorides may also inhibit bacterial action. In the growing animal, fluorine replaces the hydroxyl group in the formation of the apatite structure, but there is only limited metabolic exchange of fluorine in the previously formed bone. In the mature animal, the incorporation is apparently limited to the latter mechanism.

Intestinal absorption of fluorine is highly variable, depending in a large part on the solubility of that ingested. Mammalian species differ little in their susceptibility to fluorine, but poultry have a higher tolerance, probably because of a lower absorption and increased excretion of the element. In general, animals will tolerate a considerably higher level of fluorine in natural feedstuffs or in rock phosphate than in the highly soluble forms such as sodium fluoride (Table 29.3).

Fluorine is widely but unevenly distributed in nature. Water normally contains traces, but the fluorine content may vary markedly. Water that is high in fluoride content is usually from deep wells in which the fluorine comes from deep rock formations and not from surface contamination. Surface water rarely contains as much as 1 ppm and more often contains about 0.1 ppm. By contrast the deep well water from the Texas panhandle and Colorado, where chronic fluorine toxicity is endemic, may contain 2 to 5 ppm. If the water is allowed to stand in tanks, evaporation may result in a much higher concentration.

Fluorine content of the soil may affect the fluorine content of forages; however, plant materials seldom contain more than 1 to 2 ppm, even though the levels in the soil or the phosphate fertilizers used may be considerably higher. Contamination of the plant material from soil being splashed or blown onto the plant or from irrigation water that is high in fluorine content may leave fluorine deposits on the plants and may result in fluorosis even though the actual plant material contains safe amounts of bound fluorine. Excessive fluorine intakes may also result from grazing too close, when the animals actually consume sufficient amounts of soil or dust to result in fluorosis.

Table 29.3. Safe levels of fluorine in the total diet (ppm)*

Species	NaF or other soluble fluoride (ppm)	Phosphatic limestone or rock phosphate (ppm)
Dairy cow	40	60–100
Beef cow	50–100	65–100
Sheep	60–150	60–150
Chickens	200	300–400
Turkeys	15	
Swine	150	100–200

*From National Research Council 1960, *The Fluorosis Problems in Livestock Production,* Nat. Acad. Sci., Washington, D.C.; and National Research Council 1980, *Mineral Tolerance of Domestic Animals,* Nat. Acad. Sci., Washington, D.C.

Table 29.4. Levels of daily fluorine ingestion from raw rock phosphate compatible with growth

Species	F per kg body weight per day (mg)
Cattle	2–3
Swine	8
Poultry	35–70

Data from National Research Council 1960, *The Fluorosis Problems in Livestock Production,* Nat. Acad. Sci., Washington, D.C.

The more common fluorosis results when the animals consume foods that have been contaminated with or supplemented with fluoride-bearing minerals, or when they inhale or ingest fumes and dusts emitted from industrial plants. In the processing of rock phosphates, in smelting of aluminum and other ores, and in ceramic industries, dust or fumes containing fluorides may be given off. This fluorine in large amounts may result in increased concentrations in the forages and water in the surrounding area.

The principal fluorine-containing minerals in animal feeds are the phosphatic limestones or rock phosphate. Most of the rock phosphate used in animal feeds has been defluorinated to the extent that it will not result in toxic levels (Table 29.4). However, other ration components and water may contribute appreciable amounts.

The signs of fluorine toxicity are similar for all species. Quantities of fluorine that show no gross ill effects at first may eventually be harmful. The animal is protected by increased urinary excretion and by deposition in the skeletal tissue. When the upper limits of the protective mechanisms are reached, the soft tissues are flooded with fluorine, resulting in metabolic disturbances and finally death. Voluntary reduction in food intake occurs as the critical stage is reached. Thus typical signs of starvation are observed in acute fluorine toxicity.

Various clinical signs of fluorosis become apparent before the critical stage is reached. The teeth become modified in shape, size, and color; they become pitted; and the pulp cavities may be exposed due to fracture or wear (Fig. 29.2). These abnormalities occur only in animals exposed to excess fluorine before eruption of the permanent teeth. Fluorine is an enzyme inhibitor. When this happens in odontoblasts and osteoblasts, teeth and bone deformities occur. Exostoses of the jaw and long bones develop and the joints become thickened and ankylosed, resulting in lameness. As these conditions become more advanced, there is a reduction in food consumption, accompanied by reduced growth or weight loss. Reproductive performance is not affected by fluorosis unless food intake is severely depressed. Signs of fluorosis are rarely seen in the newborn or suckling animal, as placental and mammary transfer of fluorine is limited.

No single sign of fluorosis is proof of toxicity. The results of chemical analysis of the bone, teeth, and urine, in conjunction with evidence of chalkiness, mottling, erosion of enamel, enamel hypoplasia, and excessive wear of the teeth, as well as evidence of anorexia, inanition, and bone changes, are all important in recognizing fluorine toxicosis.

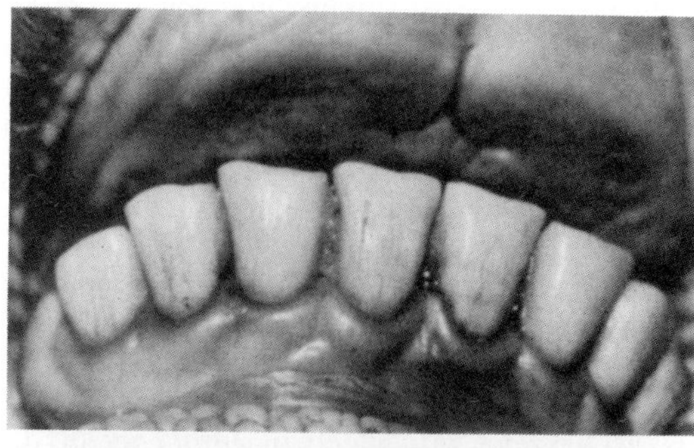

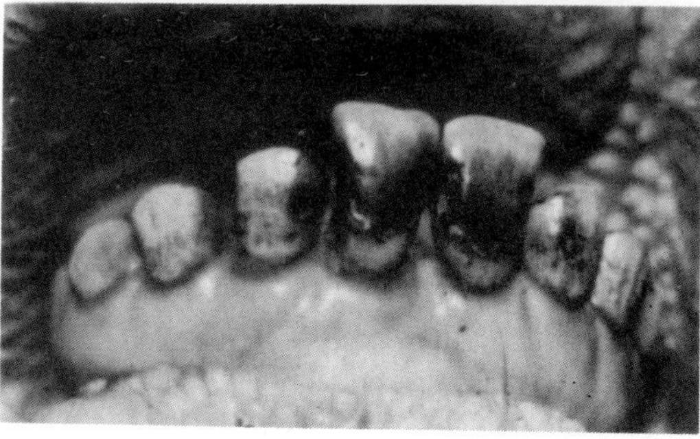

Figure 29.2. (*Top*) Teeth of cow fed ration containing 7 ppm fluorine. (*Bottom*) Teeth of cow fed ration containing 107 ppm fluorine; note excess chalkiness, staining, deep erosions, and hypoplasia of enamel and teeth. (From Hobbs et al. 1954, *U. Tenn. Agric. Exp. Sta. Bull.* 235.

SELENIUM

The nutritional significance of selenium is well established but still somewhat confounded by its potential toxic effects. The beneficial level for animals is approximately 0.1 to 0.3 ppm of the diet; levels of 5 to 8 ppm are toxic.

Certain plants grown on soils containing high levels of selenium (0.5 to 40 ppm) concentrate selenium and are potentially hazardous to animals. In areas where soil is high in selenium, white muscle disease and other signs of selenium deficiency are not serious problems (Fig. 29.3). Selenium is incorporated into the plant primarily by replacement of sulfur in the amino acids, methionine and cystine. Toxic levels in plants result in blind staggers in horses and the sloughing of hair and hoofs in horses and cattle. The animals become lame, and death in such cases is mainly due to starvation resulting from the locomotive impediment.

Selenium deficiency results in white muscle disease (a muscular dystrophy), a malady that has resulted in a high mortality rate among young calves and lambs. This disease is characterized by a myopathy that affects both heart and skeletal muscle, frequently accompanied by abnormal cal-

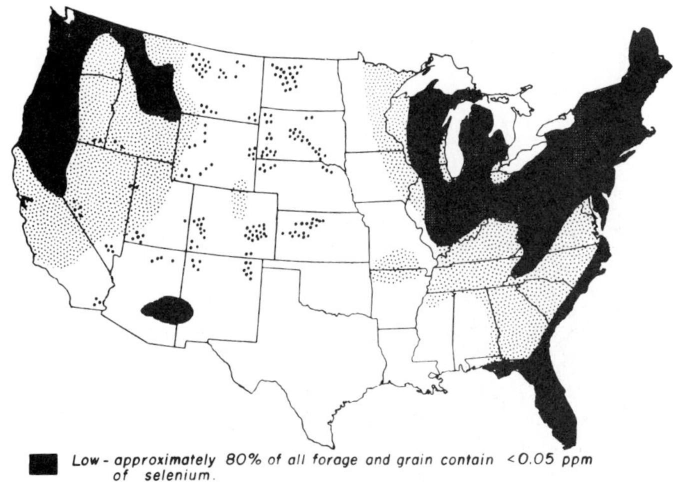

■ *Low - approximately 80% of all forage and grain contain <0.05 ppm of selenium.*

▒ *Variable - approximately 50% contains >0.1 ppm.*

□ *Adequate - 80% of all forages and grain contain >0.1 ppm of selenium.*

• *Local areas where selenium accumulator plants contain >50 ppm.*

Figure 29.3. Distribution of selenium in forages and grains in the United States. (Reproduced from Kubota and Allaway, Geographic distribution of trace element problems, in Mortvedt, Giordano, and Lindsay, eds., 1972, *Micronutrients in Agriculture,* Soil Science Society of America, Madison, Wis., pp. 525–54, by permission of the Soil Science Society of America.)

cification. In less acute form, selenium deficiency interferes in the normal growth process of sheep and cattle. Selenium deficiency also disrupts the normal reproductive process, apparently affecting ovulation and fertilization resulting in a higher incidence of embryonic death. Selenium deficiency has been associated with a higher incidence of retained placentas resulting in delayed onset of estrus and impaired conception. In pigs, selenium deficiency results in liver necrosis (hepatosis dietetica), which results in high mortality. Mulberry heart disease in swine has been attributed to selenium deficiency, but more recent evidence suggests that the selenium deficiency is complicated by other factors.

Organic and inorganic selenium compounds function in preventing certain disease conditions that in the past have been associated with vitamin E deficiency. Selenium will prevent liver necrosis in rats, white muscle disease in lambs, and exudative diathesis in chicks. It will not protect against certain other manifestations of vitamin E deficiency (e.g., muscular dystrophy in rabbits, encephalomalacia in chicks, or reproductive failure in rats, turkeys, and chickens).

A selenium deficiency in rats, chicks, and sheep causes a marked reduction in the activity of glutathione peroxidase in various tissues. Selenium apparently protects the organism from oxidative damage to cell membranes by functioning as a component of an enzyme system that reduces or destroys peroxides, whereas vitamin E protects against damage by preventing the formation of the lipid hydroperoxides.

The activity of selenium appears to be closely related to the antioxidative properties of α-tocopherol (vitamin E) and coenzyme Q (ubiquinone). It enhances the overall activity of the α-ketoglutarate oxidase system, probably by affecting the decarboxylation reaction.

MOLYBDENUM

Molybdenum is a component of several metalloenzyme systems, including xanthine oxidase, aldehyde oxidase, nitrate reductase, and hydrogenase. Its occurrence in these metalloflavoproteins demonstrates that it is an essential nutrient. However, a definite requirement for molybdenum has been difficult to establish because no characteristic syndrome of molybdenum deficiency has been recognized and animals have performed normally on extremely low dietary levels of molybdenum.

Evidence of a need for molybdenum has been found in studies involving the mineral element tungsten, which acts as an antagonist to molybdenum. A growth response to molybdenum in chicks fed diets containing 0.5 to 0.8 ppm occurs if tungsten is also added to the diet. Also, a response to supplemental molybdenum has been reported when chick diets contained 1 ppm of molybdenum. Naturally occurring molybdenum is largely unavailable. A growth response in lambs from supplemental molybdenum added to a diet containing 0.4 ppm has been reported; however, the molybdenum apparently renders its influence through a stimulatory effect on the microbial degradation of cellulose in the rumen.

There is evidence also that low molybdenum intake is a predisposing cause of renal xanthine calculi. A high incidence of such calculi occurred in sheep restricted to the Moutere Hills pastures of the south island of New Zealand. The pasture forages of the area contained 0.03 ppm molyb-

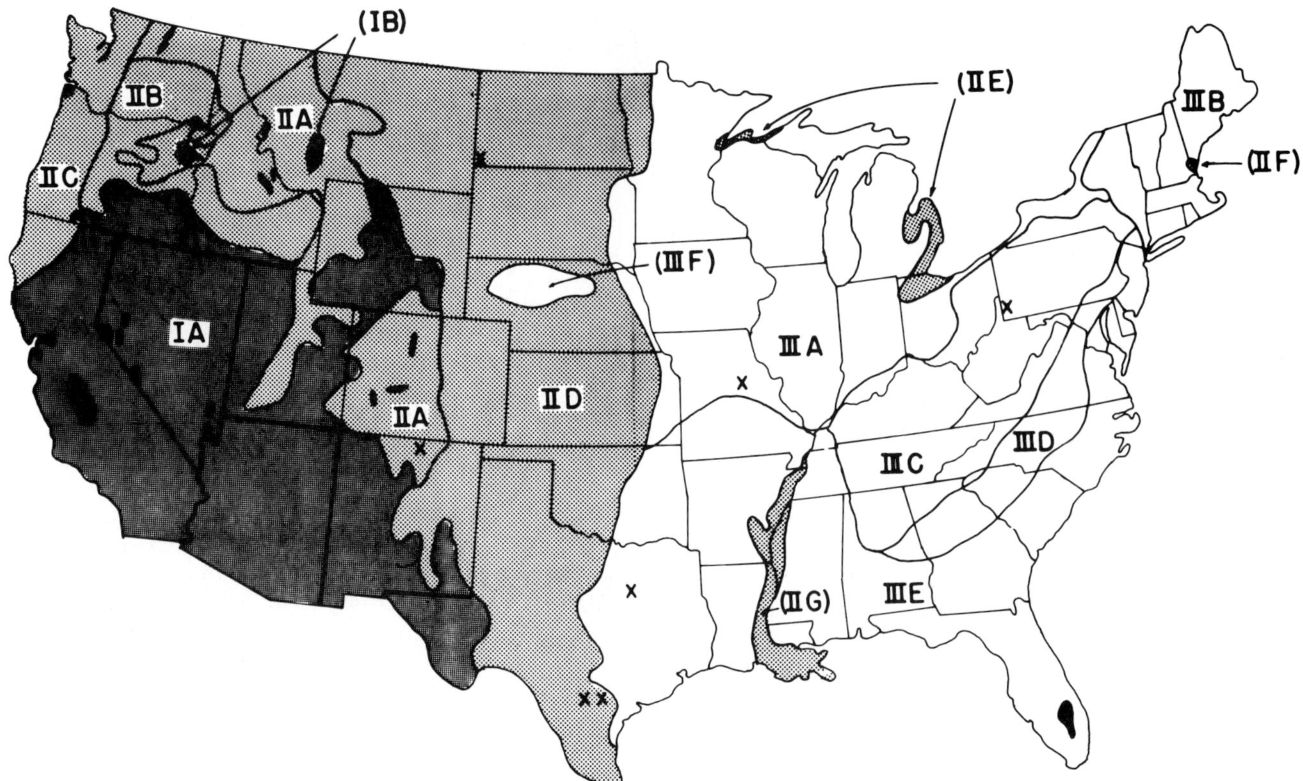

Generalized Regional Pattern of molybdenum concentration (median) in legumes.
I. Areas with background levels of 6 to 8 ppm.
II. Areas with background levels of 2 to 4 ppm.
III. Areas with background levels of 1 ppm or less.

Figure 29.4. Concentration of molybdenum in legumes grown in the United States and its relationship to reported incidences of molybdenosis. Areas marked with a solid black symbol or X represent general location of naturally occurring molybdenum-toxic areas or industrial molybdenoses, respectively. (Adapted from Kubota 1977, in Chappell and Peterson, eds., *Geochemistry, Cycling and Industrial Uses of Molybdenum,* Marcel Dekker, New York, by courtesy of Marcel Dekker, Inc.)

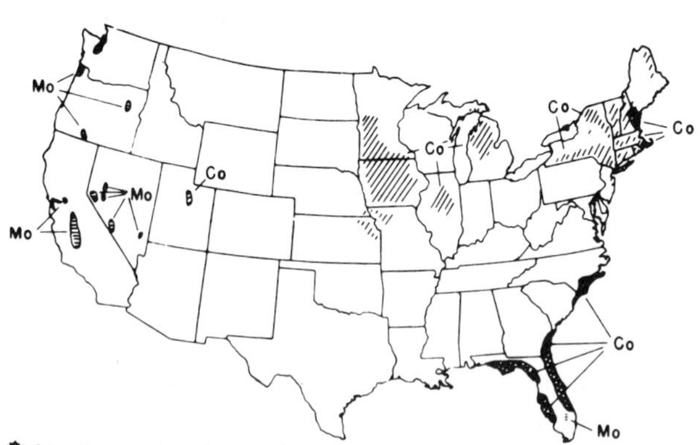

Co Areas where legumes* are low in cobalt (historic areas of cobalt deficiency)

/// Co Areas where legumes are moderately low in cobalt

Mo General areas of molybdenum toxicity

*Grasses generally have low amounts of cobalt.

Figure 29.5. Soil status of cobalt and molybdenum in the United States. (Courtesy of J. Kubota.)

denum or less. Sheep grazing these pastures also had subnormal molybdenum levels in the liver. The incidence of calculi was lower in areas nearby in which the forages contained 0.4 ppm or more of molybdenum. The incidence was also lower in the calculi areas after fertilization of the pastures; however, changes in molybdenum concentration of the forages were accompanied by other changes in composition, including an increase in protein content. Figures 29.4 and 29.5 give the geographical picture of molybdenum deficiencies and toxicities in the United States.

A reciprocal antagonism exists between molybdenum and copper. Molybdenum, in the presence of sulfates, limits copper retention in cattle and sheep; however, neither molybdenum nor sulfates alone affect copper retention. Chronic copper poisoning associated with high levels of copper in the liver of ruminants has been observed under conditions of moderate intake of copper but very low dietary levels of molybdenum and sulfate. Conversely, excessive levels of molybdenum and sulfate may lead to characteristic signs of copper deficiency, even with apparently adequate intake of copper.

Supplemental copper has been beneficial in counteracting a diarrhea of cattle, teart or peat scours, caused by excessive intake of molybdenum from forages grown on peat or muck soils high in molybdenum. The diarrhea has been established as a molybdenosis caused by the ingestion of excessive amounts of molybdenum and may be reproduced by administration of excessive quantities of sodium or ammonium molybdate. It may be counteracted by orally or intravenously administered copper.

Molybdenum is a component of the intracellular iron-containing enzymes, xanthine oxidase and aldehyde oxidase. These enzymes play a role in iron utilization as well as in electron transport in cellular metabolism. Xanthine oxidase is involved in the uptake and release of iron from ferritin in the intestinal mucosa and in the release of iron from ferritin in the liver, placenta, and erythropoietic tissues to the ferrous form.

IRON

Iron functions in the respiratory processes through its oxidation-reduction activity and its ability to transport electrons. Iron exists in the animal body mainly in complex forms bound to protein as heme compounds (hemoglobin or myoglobin), as heme enzymes (mitochondrial and microsomal cytochromes, catalase, and peroxidase), or as nonheme compounds (flavin-Fe enzymes, transferrin, and ferritin). Only negligible amounts of free inorganic iron are found in the animal body. Ionic iron tends to form complexes with six coordinate bonds, linking with oxygen or nitrogen disposed in appropriate groupings. The porphyrins, tetrapyrrole compounds, combine with iron in this way, their nitrogen atoms satisfying four of the coordinate valences (see Fig. 3.2). Heme, one such complex of protoporphyrin and iron, links with a number of different proteins to form compounds that are active in mammalian respiration: hemoglobin, myoglobin, the cytochromes, cytochrome oxidase, peroxidases, and catalases. Hemoglobin and the catalases contain four heme groups per molecule; whereas, myoglobin, the cytochromes, and peroxidases contain one heme group per molecule (see Chap. 3). The protein component of these compounds determines their specific function, but heme is the functional group and iron serves as the carrier of oxygen or transporter of electrons in each. In iron-deficient animals, the mitochondria of skeletal muscle cells exhibit impaired respiratory function. Thus, iron plays a major role at the cellular level.

Hemoglobin iron represents approximately 60 percent of the total body iron. Thus any factor influencing the hemoglobin level in the blood greatly affects the total iron status of the body. Myoglobin represents only about 3 percent of the total iron but is appreciably higher in some species (e.g., horse and dog). Approximately 7 percent of the total iron in the body of the dog is in the myoglobin fraction. Species differences in total body iron per unit of metabolic size are relatively small in adults but appreciable in the newborn. Individual variation in iron content within a species can be large in the iron-storage organs, such as liver, spleen, and kidney, but is relatively small in other organs of the body.

Iron exists in the blood mainly as hemoglobin in the erythrocytes and as transferrin in the plasma. Small quantities of ferritin and nonheme iron also exist in the erythrocytes. Figure 29.6 outlines iron metabolism.

The nonhemoglobin iron in blood, transferrin, is bound to β-globulin. Two atoms of ferric iron unite with the plasma protein, which serves as an iron carrier in the vascular system. There are at least three different transferrin proteins, and normally only about 40 percent of the transferrin protein is bound with iron, the remainder being known as the latent iron-binding capacity. The plasma iron concentration is normally 100 to 300 μg/dl. In iron deficiency of pigs and other animals it may be as low as 40 to 50 μg/dl. When plasma iron is low, ferritin in hepatic and other cells is released. Adrenocortical hormones (glucocorticoids) play a part in regulating the level of plasma iron. During stress, when the hypothalamus, adenohypophysis, and adrenal cortex are activated, regardless of the source, the plasma iron decreases. Simultaneously with the lowering of the plasma iron, the erythrocyte sedimentation rate may increase (see Chap. 3).

In monogastric species iron is absorbed principally as the ferrous state from the duodenum (Fig. 29.6). Iron in foods occurs predominantly in the ferric form and also in combination with organic compounds. Therefore it must be released from the organic molecule and reduced before absorption. The fact that ferric salts are relatively well utilized indicates that gastrointestinal conditions are favorable to such reduction.

Reducing substances in the food, such as ascorbic acid and cysteine, may aid in the reduction of iron from the ferric to the ferrous state and enhance iron absorption. Dietary factors may also interfere with iron absorption (e.g., higher levels of phosphates reduce absorption). Phytates also interfere with the absorption of this element by the formation of insoluble iron-phytate, but it is questionable whether the normal phytates of feeds are of much practical significance in this respect.

Iron absorption is quantitatively controlled by body requirements. With reduced iron stores or increased erythropoiesis, iron absorption is enhanced, whereas in the presence of adequate iron stores and normal erythropoiesis, iron absorption is diminished. Evidence suggests that an active transferrinlike carrier exists to facilitate the transfer of iron across the mucosal cell membrane. An increase in this carrier is present in animals with iron deficiency.

Disease resistance of pigs may be lowered in iron deficiency. In such cases pigs may succumb more quickly to respiratory and enteric diseases. On the other hand, there is evidence that excessive levels of oral iron increase susceptibility of pigs to certain bacterial diseases. Increased mortality has been observed in young pigs challenged with *Escherichia coli* and given large doses of oral iron (200 mg)

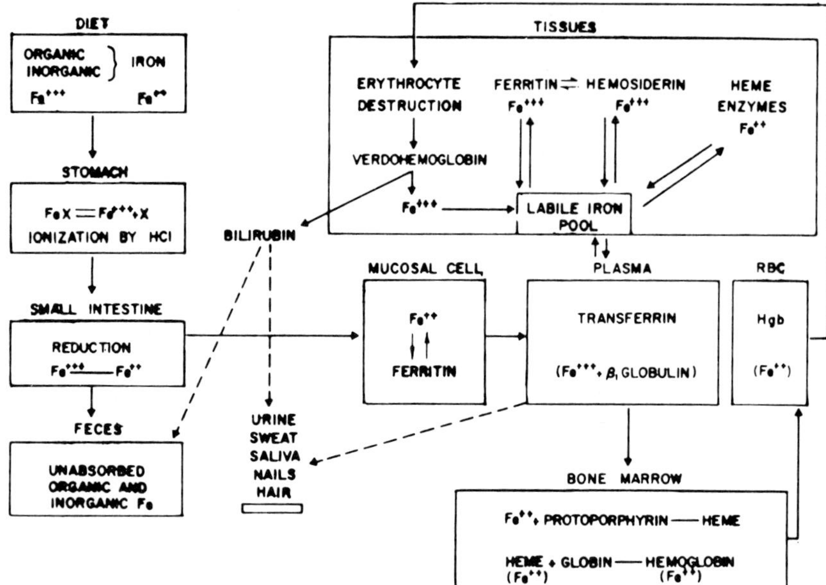

Figure 29.6. Outline of iron metabolism. (From Wintrobe 1961, *Clinical Hematology,* 5th ed., Lea & Febiger, Philadelphia.)

as compared with those not given the iron. Differences in mortality were not noted when similar amounts of iron were injected intramuscularly. Also, iron toxicity may occur with indiscriminate use of excess iron. In these cases, chelating agents may aid in the recovery of patients with iron poisoning.

Except for what is known about the suckling pig, much remains to be learned about the iron requirements of domestic animals. The abundance of iron in natural feedstuffs and macromineral supplements largely explains the limited interest shown in establishing iron requirements, especially for ruminants.

The pig is born with low iron stores and develops an iron-deficiency anemia if not provided with supplementary iron. The factors responsible for the onset of anemia in the baby pig are its relatively low stores of iron at birth (approximately 45 to 50 mg per pig), its high growth rate early in life, and the low level of iron in sow's milk. Pigs reach 4 to 5 times their birth weight by 3 weeks of age. Such a rapid increase in body size requires a retention of 7 to 16 mg of iron per day. Since sow's milk will provide only about 1 mg per day, a source of supplemental iron must be provided. The absorption rate of iron is relatively low; thus about 15 mg of oral iron must be provided daily to maintain adequate erythropoiesis and iron stores. When one injection of iron dextran is given intramuscularly shortly after birth, 100 to 150 mg of elemental iron is needed to maintain adequate hemoglobin in the pig.

Figure 29.7 depicts the decrease in hemoglobin concentration, packed red cell volume, or red blood cell numbers per unit of volume that develops in pigs (and all mammals) after birth. This decrease can be corrected in part by supplying a readily available source of iron, such as injectable iron compounds or dietary iron supplements. The decrease in these levels from birth as shown by both lines (solid and broken) in Fig. 29.7 occurs in all newborn mammals. The difference depicted by A between the broken and solid lines is considered pathological. The decrease in blood values shown by the broken line is sometimes referred to as "physiological anemia." Iron supplements will improve the blood values from the solid line to the broken line but not any farther.

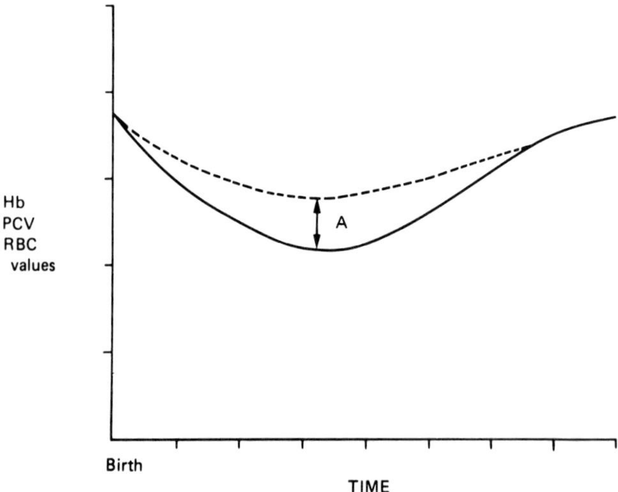

Figure 29.7. Hemoglobin (Hb), packed red cell volume (PCV), and red blood cell (RBC) values in the newborn animal and during the early part of its life. These changes take place in the first 6 to 8 weeks of life in pigs and lambs and approximately 3 months in calves. (See text for explanation of A.)

In rapidly growing pigs, the total blood volume (red cell mass plus plasma) per unit of body weight remains nearly constant. If pigs are provided adequate iron, the red cell mass increases nearly proportional to the increase in body weight. In anemic (iron-deficient) animals, the blood values decline because red cell synthesis declines. Since there is no significant change in total blood cell volume, the reduced rate of red cell synthesis and the diluting effect of increase in plasma volume accentuate the anemia, as shown by the solid line, and accounts for the pathological anemia shown as A in Fig. 29.7. The recovery to normal values is accounted for by adequate iron supplied as supplemental feeds.

COPPER

Copper is an integral part of the cytochrome system. The enzymes tyrosinase, laccase, ascorbic acid oxidase, cytochrome oxidase, plasma monoamine oxidase, erythrocuprin (ceruloplasmin), uricase, and superoxide dismutase contain copper, and their activity is dependent on this element.

Copper is present in blood plasma as a copper-carrying plasma protein called erythrocuprin. Essentially all of the copper in plasma is in combination with protein. Erythrocuprin provides a link between copper and iron metabolism. The oxidation of ferrous iron to the ferric form is increased 10 to 100 times by erythrocuprin, depending on the demands of the erythropoietic organs for iron. Plasma iron values are governed by the availability of iron from the reticuloendothelial cells and the rate at which iron is released from them. Erythrocuprin mediates the release of iron from ferritin and hemosiderin. Approximately half of the copper in blood is in the erythrocytes either loosely bound as amino acid complexes or as a functional component of superoxide dismutase.

The dietary requirement for copper is affected by the level of certain other minerals in the diet, being increased in ruminants by excessive molybdenum. Excess dietary copper results in an accumulation of copper in the liver with a decrease in blood hemoglobin concentration and packed cell volume. Liver function is impaired in copper poisoning. Jaundice results from hemolysis of erythrocytes; death occurs unless treatment is begun. Treatment is based on the rationale that excess molybdenum may cause copper deficiency. In fact, molybdenum in conjunction with the sulfate ion is effective in treating copper poisoning in ruminants. A high level of sulfide, but not sulfate ions, in the diet of pigs will protect against toxic effects of excess copper.

In the monogastric animal, copper is absorbed mainly in the upper part of the small intestine, where the pH of the contents is still acid. The availability of copper is influenced by the chemical form, the sulfides being less available than the carbonate, oxide, or sulfate. In general, copper is poorly absorbed, with only about 5 to 10 percent of the ingested copper being absorbed and retained. Under normal conditions 90 percent or more of the ingested copper appears in the feces. Most of the fecal copper is unabsorbed dietary copper, but some of it comes from bile, which is the major pathway of copper excretion. Biliary obstruction increases the excretion of the copper through the kidney and intestinal wall.

Clinical disorders associated with copper deficiencies include anemia, bone disorders, neonatal ataxia, depigmentation and abnormal growth of hair or wool, impaired growth and reproductive performance, heart failure, and gastrointestinal disturbances. The incidence of these disorders varies widely among species. For example, in sheep the depigmentation and abnormal growth of wool are frequently observed first. Neonatal ataxia occurs frequently in lambs from copper-deficient ewes, but it has never been noted in pigs or dogs.

Copper functions in the utilization of iron in an early stage of hematopoiesis. In iron deficiency, the number of cells is not affected, but the cells are smaller (microcytic) and usually hypochromic, whereas, copper deficiency reduces the number of cells but not their hemoglobin concentration. However, the nature of copper-deficiency anemias varies with species. In rabbits and pigs it is hypochromic and microcytic and indistinguishable from iron deficiency. In lambs it is hypochromic and microcytic; in cattle, ewes, and chicks it is hypochromic and macrocytic; and in dogs, it is normochromic and normocytic. Such varied differences suggest other complicating environmental or nutritional factors in addition to species variation. Copper deficiency results in an increase in iron in the liver, whereas an excess of copper results in a decrease in iron content of the liver, reflecting the role of copper in the utilization of iron.

Spontaneous bone fractures have been observed in sheep and cattle grazing copper-deficient pastures. The fractured bones exhibit a mild degree of osteoporosis along with other defects. In pigs, copper deficiency results in a failure of deposition of calcium salts in the normal cartilage matrix.

A long-recognized nervous disorder of lambs is associated with copper deficiency. Various names, including swayback, lamkruis, renguera, and Gingin rickets, have been given to this condition. All these disorders appear to be pathologically the same as the neonatal enzootic ataxia. The changes in ataxia may include symmetrical cerebral demyelination, degeneration of motor tracts in the spinal cord, and changes in the neurons of the brain stem. The lesions are irreversible and may commence as early as 6 weeks before birth and continue until delivery. The condition is frequently observed in lambs but has also been reported in cattle and goats. It has not been reported in pigs.

Lack of pigmentation and marked changes in the growth and physical appearance of hair, fur, or wool may result from copper deficiency. The mechanism is related to the biochemical conversion of tyrosine to melanin, since this conversion is catalyzed by copper-containing oxidases. The

Table 29.5. Dietary mineral requirements

Element	Pigs	Chicks	Turkeys	Calves	Dairy Cattle	Beef Cattle	Sheep
Potassium (%)	0.2–0.3	0.2–0.4	0.4–0.7	0.65	0.9–1.0	0.65	0.5–0.8
Iron (ppm)	40–100	50–80	50–80	50–100	50	50	30–50
Copper (ppm)	3–6	6–8	6–8	10	10	8	7–11
Manganese (ppm)	2–4	30–60	60	40	40	40	20–40
Magnesium (ppm)	400	400–600	600	700–1000	2000	1000	1200–1800
Zinc (ppm)	50–100	35–65	40–75	40	40	30	20–33
Iodine (ppm)	0.14	0.3–0.4	0.4	0.25	0.6	0.5	0.1–0.8
Selenium (ppm)	0.1–0.3	0.1–0.2	0.2	0.3	0.3	0.2	0.1–0.2
Cobalt (ppm)	—	—	—	0.1	0.1	0.1	0.1–0.2

Data from National Research Council 1984–1989, *Nutrient Requirements of Domestic Animals,* Nat. Acad. Sci. Washington, D.C. Requirements vary depending on stage of maturity and level of production.

deficiency leads to progressively less crimp in wool until the fibers emerge as straight hairlike growth that has been referred to as stringy or steely wool. The fact that straight wool has more sulfhydryl groups and fewer disulfide groups suggests that copper is required for the oxidation of -SH to -S-S- (disulfide) groups in keratin synthesis.

Copper deficiency has also been associated with cardiac hypertrophy and sudden cardiac failure. The copper requirement varies among species to some extent but is influenced to a greater degree by its relationship with and the intake of other mineral elements, such as iron, molybdenum, and sulfate. The minimum requirements are probably less than those presented in Table 29.5 if other elements are present in optimum amounts.

COBALT

An established function of cobalt is its role as a component of the vitamin B_{12} molecule. Approximately 4.5 percent of the molecular weight of B_{12} (cyanocobalamin) is contributed by elemental cobalt (see Chap. 28). It is firmly bound in the vitamin B_{12} molecule.

Cobalt is readily absorbed into the bloodstream and excreted primarily in the urine. Excessive intake results in polycythemia, which is apparently due to the inhibition by cobalt of certain respiratory enzyme systems (e.g., cytochrome oxidase and succinic dehydrogenase).

Although ruminants require a dietary source of cobalt, it appears that it is used solely as a part of the B_{12} molecule and that the animal is completely dependent on the microflora within the rumen for vitamin B_{12} biosynthesis. Deficiencies of cobalt in ruminants result in anorexia, wasting of the skeletal muscle, fatty livers, hemosiderosis of the spleen, and anemia.

A coenzyme form of B_{12} is required in the conversion of methylmalonate to succinate, an intermediate step in the metabolism of propionic acid. Thus cobalt, as a component of B_{12}, is required for a reaction that is more prevalent in the energy (propionate) metabolism of ruminants than in nonruminants. This probably accounts for the apparent high requirement for cobalt or B_{12} by the ruminant. Vitamin B_{12} also plays a role in methylating choline and thymine. The latter is required in the synthesis of DNA, which regulates cell division and growth.

Nonruminants require preformed vitamin B_{12} to meet their metabolic needs; in ruminants, however, practical control of B_{12} deficiency may be achieved by supplementation of the diet with cobalt or by treating the pastures with cobalt salts or ore. (See Fig. 29.5 for cobalt-deficient areas.) Also, cobalt deficiency in ruminants has been successfully alleviated by use of cobalt oxide pellets, which remain in the reticulum or rumen fluid. In the case of young animals, however, the pellets may become coated with calcium phosphate deposit, rendering the cobalt unavailable to the animal.

The estimated dietary requirement of vitamin B_{12} for pigs and chicks is 0.01 to 0.02 ppm (10 to 20 μg/kg diet), which would represent only 0.0005 to 0.0010 ppm of cobalt. There is little evidence that chicks and pigs require cobalt in addition to that needed as B_{12}. The estimated cobalt requirement for ruminants is 0.07 to 0.11 ppm of the diet or several times that included in the required B_{12} for nonruminants. This difference is related to the inefficiency of the biosynthesis of vitamin B_{12} in the rumen and the additional amount required for the energy metabolism of methylmalonate.

ZINC

Zinc is distributed widely in plant and animal tissues and is a functional component of several enzyme systems, including carbonic anhydrase, carboxypeptidase, alkaline phosphatase, lactic dehydrogenase, and glutamic dehydrogenase.

Carbonic anhydrase is present in erythrocytes, kidney tubules, gastrointestinal mucosa, and glandular epithelium. In erythrocytes it functions by combining carbon dioxide and water in peripheral capillary blood and then releasing carbon dioxide from pulmonary capillary blood into the alveoli. These changes are based on pressure differences of carbon dioxide.

Primary roles of zinc appear to be in the fundamental

process of cell replication and gene expression and in nucleic acid and amino acid metabolism.

Zinc is important in an enzymic system necessary for the synthesis of ribonucleic acid (RNA). RNA is present in cytoplasm and in the nucleoli and chromosomes of the nuclei and is essential for the growth of germinal and somatic cells. Zinc in relatively large quantities in the testes and the prostate gland is important in the maturation of spermatozoa.

Zinc occurs in all living cells. The zinc found in the pancreas exhibits an active metabolic turnover, a large proportion being secreted in pancreatic juice. The addition of zinc to insulin solutions results in a delay in the physiological action of insulin and prolongs the hypoglycemia produced when injected. Apparently zinc is bound to the insulin molecule but its function is uncertain.

Elemental zinc prevents and cures parakeratosis (thickening or hyperkeratinization of the epithelial cells of the skin and esophagus) in swine, and a similar malady in chicks and other species. Excess calcium in the diet, however, hastens the onset of parakeratosis. An animal's dietary requirement for zinc is higher with plant protein diets than with animal protein diets. This difference is associated with the phytic acid content of the plant protein source, since the addition of phytic acid to casein diets, which are known to be low in phytic acid, also increases the dietary zinc requirements.

Zinc deficiency in pigs results in a marked depression of appetite and growth rate. Continued deficiency leads to parakeratosis. Zinc deficiency in the chick is similarly characterized by poor growth, severe dermatitis, especially of the feet, and poor feathering. In addition, zinc-deficient chicks exhibit abnormal respiration and a shortening and thickening of long bones. The abnormal bone development appears to arise from a failure of cartilage cell development in the epiphyseal plate region of the long bones and decreased osteoblastic activity in the thin bony collar. The severity of the lesions and the growth depression in chicks and pigs are directly related to the extent to which zinc content of the diet falls below the optimum level. Zinc deficiency has been produced experimentally in calves. The signs are similar to those of other species: rough and scaly skin, breaks in the skin around the hoofs, and a dull, listless appearance.

The absorption of zinc is inefficient. Thus the dietary requirement is much greater than the metabolic requirement. According to studies involving infused zinc, the estimated metabolic requirement for pigs is equivalent to 3 to 4 ppm of the diet, whereas 30 to 40 ppm in the diet, or higher levels in the presence of phytic acid, is required to prevent parakeratosis and allow for normal growth. The oxide, carbonate, and sulfate forms of zinc are efficiently used, whereas the sulfide form is poorly used.

Zinc, whether ingested or injected, is excreted primarily in the feces. Zinc found in the feces consists largely of unabsorbed dietary zinc, and the balance is from pancreatic excretions. Urinary excretion of zinc and several other metals is increased if chelating agents such as ethylenediamine tetraacetic acid (EDTA) are given in combination with the mineral.

MANGANESE

Little is known of the chemical form or combinations in which manganese exists in the animal body. Manganese deficiency is associated with a number of defects, including ataxia, skeletal deformities, and impairments in growth, reproduction, eggshell formation, and blood clotting. Some of these defects are related to the role of the manganous ion as the most effective activator of glycosyltransferase enzymes in the synthesis of mucopolysaccharides and glycoproteins.

Numerous enzyme systems are activated by manganese in vitro, a property shared in most cases by other bivalent ions, particularly magnesium. The fact that manganese is concentrated in the mitochondria has led to the suggestion that, in vivo, manganese is involved in the partial regulation of oxidative phosphorylation.

Manganese is distributed throughout the body, but the total quantity is much lower than for other elements, amounting to only about one tenth the copper content. Manganese is not concentrated in any specific organ or tissue, but it is found in higher concentrations in bone, liver, kidney, and pancreas (1 to 3 ppm of fresh tissue) than in skeletal muscle (0.1 to 0.2 ppm). The concentrations in the bone, liver, and hair can be altered considerably by varying the manganese intake.

Manganese deficiency has been demonstrated in several species of animals, including laboratory animals, pigs, poultry, and possibly cattle. Its severity depends greatly on the degree and duration of the deficiency and on the maturity of the animal. Lameness, enlarged hock joints, and shortened legs in pigs, leg deformities with overknuckling in cattle, perosis or slipped tendon in chicks, poults, and ducklings, and nutritional chondrodystrophy in chick embryos have all been attributed to manganese deficiency. Perosis in chicks is the most commonly observed manganese deficiency. It is characterized by enlarged and malformed tibiometatarsal joints, twisting and bending of the tibia and the tarsometatarsus, thickening and shortening of the long bones, "parrot beak" resulting from shortening of the lower jaw, and high embryonic mortality. Other factors such as deficiencies of choline or biotin may result in some of the same signs, and an excess of calcium may aggravate the conditions. In other species similar congenital defects in embryonic bone development result from manganese deficiency.

The manganese requirements for growth, health, and reproduction are more precisely defined for poultry than they are for mammals. The dietary requirement is approximately 30 to 60 ppm for growth and 30 ppm for hatchability (embryo development and emerging from the shell). The requirements are less precisely established for turkeys but are estimated to be similar to those for chickens. The requirements for pigs are much lower than those for birds and are approximately 2 to 4 ppm of the diet for growth and possibly higher (10 ppm) for reproduction.

Manganese deficiency is not encountered in cattle and is seldom seen in pigs fed diets composed of natural ingredients. However, excess calcium added to nonlegume rations without added trace minerals inhibits the estrous cycle, including ovulation, in cattle. Excess calcium does not alter the normal estrous cycle if alfalfa hay or trace minerals, including manganese, are added to the ration.

Corn is extremely low in manganese (4 to 12 ppm); thus animals fed high-corn diets, especially if supplemented with animal by-products that are also low in manganese content, may receive inadequate amounts. The high requirement of poultry and the low levels of manganese in many of the ingredients of poultry diets make manganese supplementation of paramount importance.

Animals appear to be highly tolerant of excess dietary manganese. Growth of rats is unaffected by intakes as high as 1000 to 2000 ppm, but higher levels have been reported to interfere with phosphorus retention. Hens tolerate 1000 ppm without ill effects, but 4800 ppm is toxic to young chicks. Pigs tolerate 4000 ppm with only slight depressions in growth rate and no other signs of ill effects.

CHROMIUM

Chromium has been found in nucleoproteins isolated from beef liver and also in RNA preparations. It may play a role in the maintenance of the configuration of the RNA molecule, as chromium has been shown to be particularly effective as a cross-linking agent for collagen. Also, chromium has been identified as the active component of the glucose tolerance factor, a dietary factor required to maintain normal glucose tolerance in the rat. Chromium has been shown also to catalyze the phosphoglucomutase system, and to a limited extent it activates the succinic dehydrogenase-cytochrome system. Evidence is accumulating on the role and essentiality of chromium, and there are indications that deficiencies may exist, particularly in children suffering from protein-calorie malnutrition. The chromium content of foodstuffs varies widely and is present in combination with a small organic molecule, the glucose-tolerance factor. Humans and rats appear to have a limited capacity to synthesize this physiologically active form of chromium. There is growing evidence that chromium intakes are insufficient in some populations, resulting in severe impairment of glucose tolerance that can be dramatically corrected by chromium supplements. There is little evidence that chromium has practical significance in the nutrition of farm animals, but this may reflect only the lack of research on this element.

SILICON

Silicon is one of the most abundant elements in plant and animal tissue. The economic losses resulting from silicon urolithiasis in grazing steers and wethers have stimulated research on the metabolism of silicon in ruminants. Herbivorous animals consume relatively large quantities of silica (silicon dioxide) daily. Most of the insoluble silica passes unabsorbed through the alimentary tract, but appreciable amounts are absorbed and excreted in the urine. Normally, the silica is eliminated without ill effects, but in some animals a portion is deposited as granules in the kidney, bladder, or urethra to form uroliths or calculi. These can block urine passages, which may result in death. These calculi may be composed of various minerals, especially magnesium, phosphorus, and silicon.

Silicon has been shown to be essential for normal growth and skeletal development in rats and chicks. It is an essential component of certain mucopolysaccharides (hyaluronic acid and chondroitin-4-sulfate), which are important constituents of connective tissue. Silicon appears to function as a biological cross-linking agent contributing to the structure and resiliency of connective tissue. The level required is low, and one would not expect a deficiency in animals fed other than purified diets.

OTHER TRACE ELEMENTS

Tin has been shown to improve growth in rats fed riboflavin-deficient diets. No specific clinical or physiological changes in the animals were noted, and the improvement in growth rate could not be confirmed in rats fed the same diet adequately supplemented with riboflavin.

There is increasing evidence that nickel is an essential element. Clear evidence of growth impairment has not been demonstrated in animals fed diets resulting in normal growth. Chicks maintained in a controlled environment on a diet containing less than 0.05 ppm nickel developed increased skin pigmentation of the legs, swollen hocks, and thickening of the legs near the joints. None of these manifestations were apparent in chicks fed the same diet supplemented with 3 to 5 ppm nickel. There is limited evidence of depressed growth in cattle, goats, sheep, and pigs fed diets very low in nickel. Severe nickel deficiency results in altered iron metabolism and depressed hematopoiesis.

A precise biochemical or physiological role for vanadium has not been determined but has long been suspected because of its effects on phospholipid oxidation and inhibition of cholesterol biosynthesis. There is evidence that vanadium is necessary for normal feather development in chicks and normal growth in chicks and rats. The required level appears to be very low, 0.1 to 2 ppm or less.

The mineral elements that have been unequivocally proven as essential dietary nutrients represent only a portion of the total number that occur regularly in animal tissues. Arsenic, bromine, barium, and strontium should be included with those that have strong possibilities of being metabolically essential.

Bromine has been reported to increase the growth rate of chicks and mice. There is evidence also that the thyroid glands of rabbits concentrate bromine during periods of dietary iodine insufficiency. This suggests that the thyroid gland does not distinguish perfectly between iodine and bromine. The bromine does not prevent the development of goiter, however, and it is rapidly replaced by iodine when the latter is restored to the diet.

The omission of either barium or strontium from diets has been reported to result in growth depressions in rats and guinea pigs; however, these early reports have not been confirmed or invalidated. The omission of strontium also resulted in an impairment of calcification of the bones and teeth and in a higher incidence of carious teeth. These observations are yet to be confirmed. Strontium^{90} is one of the most abundant and potentially hazardous radioactive byproducts of nuclear fission. Although animals are less efficient than plants in the absorption of strontium, radioactive strontium is absorbed and deposited in tissues, especially in the bones. It is also readily transmitted to the fetus and secreted in the milk. Strontium and calcium have a similar and interrelated physiological behavior. Calcium however, is preferentially absorbed from the intestinal tract, and strontium is preferentially excreted, especially in the urine, thereby providing a substantial factor of protection against ^{90}Sr.

Arsenic has been reported to stimulate the growth of tissue cultures and to improve growth and reproduction in goats and minipigs. The dietary levels required to result in the apparent deficiencies were less than 10 ppb. On the other hand, the beneficial effects of various organic arsenicals on the performance and health of pigs and poultry have been shown. The action of these compounds closely resembles that of antibacterial agents and appears to be largely related to the control of harmful intestinal organisms.

There is limited evidence that other mineral elements may be of physiological significance. An aggregation of cadmium in specific association with protein macromolecules has been fractionated from horse kidney cortex, suggesting a biological role for cadmium. Rubidium and cesium are also found in animal tissue and resembles potassium in their distribution and excretory pattern. Relatively high levels of rubidium occur in soft tissue, whereas skeletal tissue contains very little. Addition of rubidium or cesium to potassium-deficient diets has been reported to prevent the lesions characteristic of potassium depletion in rats and for short periods of time support nearly normal growth.

Aluminum and titanium are found in animal tissue, but as yet satisfactory elucidation of a physiological role for them has not been demonstrated. Because of the abundance of aluminum in the environment, there is increasing concern about aluminum toxicity as evidenced by pulmonary damage if inhaled and neurophysiological abnormalities if ingested or infused. The toxic signs are associated with impaired kidney function.

Table 29.6. Suggested supplements to chemically defined (purified) diets

Element	Diet level (ppm)
Boron	2
Chromium	3
Molybdenum	1
Nickel	0.1
Silicon	250
Tin	3
Vanadium	0.2
Fluorine	20

From National Research Council 1984. *Nutrient Requirements of Poultry,* Nat. Acad. Sci. Washington, D.C.

There are many metabolic and absorptive interrelationships among the mineral elements, which contribute to variations in degree of physiological response to deficient or toxic levels. These relationships make it very difficult to determine the optimum dietary level for the individual elements as nutrients. Tables 29.1 and 29.5 present the estimated dietary requirements for those nutrients for which relatively reliable data are available. The recommended dietary level of any element should seldom be considered independent of the level of other essential nutrients. Dietary requirements have not been established for several of the mineral elements for which there is substantial evidence of a physiological function. The poultry subcommittee of the National Research Councils' Committee on Nutrient Requirements (1984), has proposed guideline levels (Table 29.6) for certain elements. These guideline levels are suggested for situations in which chicks are fed purified (chemically defined) diets. Feed ingredients used in animal diets normally would provide ample amounts of these elements, hence supplementation of practical diets is not advised.

REFERENCES

Allman, R.T., and Hamilton, T.S. 1948. Nutritional deficiencies in live stock. *FAO Agric. Stud.* No. 5.

Askew, H.O. 1958. Molybdenum in relation to the occurrence of xanthin calculi in sheep. *New Zealand J. Agric. Res.* 1:447–54.

Baumann, E.J., Sprinson, D.B., and Marine, D. 1941. Bromine and the thyroid. *Endocrinology* 28:793–96.

Bennetts, H.W., and Chapman, F.E. 1937. Copper deficiency in Western Australia: A preliminary account of the aetiology of enzootic ataxia of lambs and an anaemia of ewes. *Aust. Vet. J.* 13:138–49.

Bentley, O.G., and Phillips, P.H. 1951. The effect of low manganese rations upon dairy cattle. *J. Dairy Sci.* 34:396–403.

Bowland, J.P., Braude, R., Chamberlain, A.G., Glascock, R.F., and Mitchell, K.G. 1961. The absorption, distribution, and excretion of labeled copper in young pigs given different quantities, as sulphate or sulphide, orally or intravenously. *Br. J. Nutr.* 15:59–74.

Burley, R.W. 1954. Sulphydryl groups in wool. *Nature* 174:1019–20.

Carlisle, E.M. 1974. Essentiality and function of silicon. In W.G. Hoekstra, J.W. Suttie, H.E. Ganther, and W. Mertz, eds., *Trace Element Metabolism in Animals.* 2d ed.University Park Press. Baltimore.

Clements, F.W. 1957. A goitrogenic factor in milk. *Med. J. Aust.* 2:645–46.

Clements, F W., and Wishart, I.W. 1956. A thyroid blocking agent in the etioloyy of endemic goiter. *Metabolism* 5:623–39.

Cohen, I., Hurwitz, S., and Bar, A. 1972. Acid-base balance and sodium-to-chloride ratio in diets of laying hens. *J. Nutr.* 10:1–7.

Creek, R.D., Parker, H.E., Hauge, S.M., Andrews, F.N., and Carrick, C.W. 1954. The iodine requirement of young chickens. *Poult. Sci.* 33:1052.

Edfors, C.H., Ullrey, D.E., and Aulerich, R.J. 1989. Prevention of urolithiasis in the ferret (*Mustela putrius furo*) with phosphoric acid. *J. Zoo and Wildlife Med.* 20:12–19.

Ellis, W.C., and Pfander, W.H. 1960. Further studies on molybdenum as a possible component of the "alfalfa ash factor" for sheep. *J. Anim. Sci.* 19:1260.

Follis, R.H., Jr. 1943. Histological effects in rats resulting from adding rubidium or cesium to a diet deficient in potassium. *Am. J. Physiol.* 138:246–50.

Follis, R.H., Jr., Bush, J.A., Cartwright, G.E., and Wintrobe, M.M. 1955. Studies on copper metabolism. XVIII. Skeletal changes associated with copper deficiency in swine. *Bull. Johns Hopkins Hosp.* 97:405–14.

Gallup, W.D., and Noms, L.C. 1939. The effect of a deficiency of manganese in the diet of a hen. *Poult. Sci.* 18:83–88.

Gillis, M.B. 1948. Potassium requirement of the chick. *J. Nutr.* 36:351–57.

Grashuis, J., Lehr, J.J., Beuvery, L.L.E., and Beuvery-Asman, A. 1953. "De Schothorste" Inst. Moderne Veevoeding, Netherlands. Cited by E. J. Underwood in *Trace Elements in Human and Animal Nutrition*, 2d ed. Academic Press, New York, 1962. P. 197.

Green, J.D., McCall, J .T., Speer, V.C., and Hays, V.W. 1962. Effect of complexing agents on utilization of zinc by pigs. *J. Anim. Sci.* 21:997.

Gubler, C.J., Cartwright, G.E., and Wintrobe, M.M. 1957. Studies on copper metabolism. XX. Enzyme activities and iron metabolism in copper and iron deficiencies. *J. Biol. Chem.* 224:533–46.

Gustavson, K.H. 1958. A novel type of metal-protein compound. *Nature* 182:1125–28.

Hahn, P.F. 1937. The metabolism of iron. *Medicine* 16:249–66.

Heller, V.G., and Penquite, R. 1937. Factors producing perosis in chickens. *Poult. Sci.* 16:243–46.

Heppel, L.A., and Schmidt. C.L.A. 1938. Studies on the potassium me tabolism of the rat during pregnancy, lactation, and growth. *Univ. Calif. (Berkeley) Pub. Physiol.* 8:189–205.

Hobbs, C.S., Moorman, R.P.,Jr., Griffith, J.M., West, J.L., Merriman, G.M., Hansard, S.L., Chamberlain, C.C., MacIntire, W.H., Hardin, L.J., and Jones, L.S. 1954. Fluorosis in cattle and sheep. *Univ. Tenn. Ag. Exp. Sta. Bull.* 235.

Hoekstra, W G. 1975. Biochemical function of selenium and its relation to vitamin E. *Fed. Proc.* 34:2083–89.

Hoekstra, W.G., Suttie, J.W., Ganther, H.E., and Mertz, W., eds. 1974. *Trace Element Metabolism in Animals.* 2d ed. University Park Press, Baltimore.

Horecker, B.L., Stotz, E., and Hogness, T.R. 1939. The promoting effect of aluminum, chromium, and the rare earths in the succinic dehydrogenase- cytochrome system. *J. Biol. Chem.* 128:251–56.

Huff, J.W., Bosshardt, D.K., Miller, O.P., and Barnes, R.H. 1956. A nutritional requirement for bromine. *Proc. Soc. Exp. Biol. Med.* 92:216–19.

Hurwitz, S., Cohen, I., Bar, A., and Bornstein, S. 1973. Sodium and chloride requirements of the chick: Relationship to acid-base balance. *Poult. Sci.* 52:903–9.

Jensen, A.H., Terrill, S.W., and Becker, D.E. 1961. Response of the young pig to levels of dietary potassium. *J. Anim. Sci.* 20:464–67.

Kägi, J.H.R., and Vallee, B.L. 1960. Metallothionein: A cadmium- and zinc-containing protein from equine renal cortex. *J. Biol. Chem.* 235:3460–65.

Kadis, S., Udeze, F.A., Polanco, J. and Dreesen, D.W. 1984. Relationship of iron administration to susceptibility of newborn pigs to enterotoxic colibacillosis. *Am. J. Vet. Res.* 45:255–59.

Kelly, F.C., and Snedden, W.W. 1960. Prevalence and geographical distribution of endemic goitre. In *Endemic Goiter.* World Health Organization Monograph Series, No. 44. Geneva. Pp. 27–233.

Kirchgessner, M., Roth-Maier, D.A., and Sporl, R. 1981. Untersuchungen zun Trachtigkaitsanabolismus der Apurenelamente Kupfer, Zink, Nickel und Mangan bei Zuchtsaver. *Arch. Tierenahr.* 31:21.

Klein, G.L., Ott, S.M., Alfrey, A.C., Sherrard, D.J., Hazlet, T.K., Miller, N.L., Maloney, N.A., Berquist, W.E., Ament, M.E., and Coburn, J.N. 1982. Aluminum as a factor in the bone disease of long-term parenteral nutrition. *Trans. Assoc. Amer. Phys.* 95:155.

Kruse, H.D., Orent, E.R., and McCollum, E.V. 1932. Studies on magnesium deficiency in animals. I. Symptomatology resulting from magnesium deprivation. *J. Biol. Chem.* 96:519–39.

Kubota, J. 1977. Molybdenum status of U.S. soils and plants. In W. Chapell and K. Peterson, eds., *The Geochemistry, Cycling and Industrial Uses of Molybdenum.* vol. 2. Marcel Dekker, New York. Pp. 555–81.

Kubota, J., and Allaway, W.H. 1972. Geographic distribution of trace element problems. In J.J. Mortvedt, P.M. Giordano, and W.L. Lindsay, eds., *Micronutrients in Agriculture.* Soil Science Society of America. Madison, Wis. Pp. 525–54.

Leach, R.M., Jr. 1974. Biochemical role of manganese. In W.G. Hoekstra, J.W. Suttie, H.E. Ganther, and W. Mertz, eds., *Trace Element Metabolism in Animals* 2d ed. University Park Press, Baltimore.

Leach, R.M., and Norris, L.C. 1957. Studies on factors affecting the response of chicks to molybdenum. *Poult. Sci.* 36:1136.

Leach, R.M., Jr., Dam, R., Ziegler, T.R., and Norris, L.C. 1959. The effect of protein and energy on the potassium requirement of the chick. *J. Nutr.* 68:89–100.

Leibholz, J., Speer, V.C, and Hays, V.W. 1962. Effect of dietary manganese on baby pig performance and tissue manganese levels. *J. Anim. Sci.* 21:772-76.

Mahoney, J.R. Jr., Hallaway, P.E., Hedlund, B.E., and Eaton, J.W. 1989. Acute iron poisoning. Rescue with macromolecular chelators. *J. Clin. Invest.* 84:1362–66.

Marine, D., and Lenhart, C.H. 1909a. Further observations on the relation of iodine to the structure of the thyroid gland in the sheep, dog, hog, and ox. *Arch. Intern. Med.* 3:66–77.

Marine, D., and Lenhart, C.H. 1909b. Relation of iodine to the structure of human thyroids: Relation of iodine and histologic structure to diseases in general, to exophthalmic goiter, to cretinism and myxedema. *Arch. Intern. Med.* 4:440–93.

Mertz, W. 1974. Chromium as a dietary essential for man. In W.G. Hoekstra, J.W. Suttie, H.E. Ganther, and W. Merty, eds., *Trace Element Metabolism in Animals.* 2d ed. University Park Press, Baltimore.

Mertz, W., ed. 1987. *Trace Elements in Human and Animal Nutrition.* 5th ed. Academic Press, New York.

Messer, H.H., Armstrong, W.D., and Singer, L. 1974. Essentiality and function of fluoride. In W.G. Hoekstra, J.W. Suttie, H.E. Ganther, and W. Mertz, eds., *Trace Element Metabolism in Animals.* 2d ed. University Park Press, Baltimore.

Meyer, J.H., Grummer, R.H., Phillips, P.H., and Bohstedt, G. 1950. Sodium, chlorine, and potassium requirements of growing pigs. *J. Anim. Sci.* 9:300–306.

National Research Council. 1984–1989. Nutrient Requirements of Domestic Animals: I(1984), Poultry; II(1988), Swine; III(1988), Dairy Cattle; IV (1984), Beef Cattle; V(1989), Horses. Nat. Acad. Sci., Washington, D.C..

National Research Council. 1980. *Mineral Tolerance of Domestic Animals.* Nat. Acad. Sci., Washington, D.C.

National Research Council. 1974. *Effects of Fluorides in Animals.* Nat. Acad. Sci., Washington D.C..

National Research Council. 1960. *The Fluorosis Problems in Livestock Production.* Nat. Acad. Sci., Washington, D.C.

Neher, G.M., Doyle, L.P., Thrasher, D.M., and Plumlee, M.P. 1956.

Radiographic and histopathological findings in the bones of swine deficient in manganese. *Am. J. Vet. Res.* 17:121–28.

Nielsen, F.H. 1974. Essentiality and function of nickel. In W.G. Hoekstra J.W. Suttie, H.E. Ganther, and W. Mertz, eds. *Trace Element Metabolism in Animals* 2d ed. University Park Press, Baltimore.

O'Dell, B.L., Newberne, P.M., and Savage, J.E. 1958. Significance of dietary zinc for the growing chicken. *J. Nutr.* 65:503–18.

O'Dell, B.L., and Savage, J.E. 1957. Potassium, zinc, and distillers dried solubles as supplements to a purified diet. *Poult. Sci.* 36:459–60.

Pierson, R.E., and Aanes, W.A. 1958. Treatment of chronic copper poisoning in sheep. *J. Am. Vet. Med. Assoc.* 133:307–11.

Reid, B.L., Kurnick, A.A., Svacha, R.L., and Couch, J.R. 1956. The effect of molybdenum on chick and poultry growth. *Proc. Soc. Exp. Biol. Med.* 93:245–48.

Richards, C.E., Brady, R.O., and Riggs, D.S. 1949. Thyroid hormonelike properties of tetrabromthyronine and tetrachlorthyronine. *J. Clin. Endocrinol.* 9:1107–21.

Roy, J.H.B., Shillam, K.W.G., Hawkins, G.M., and Long, J.M. 1959. The effect of white scours on the sodium and potassium concentration in the serum of newborn calves. *Br. J. Nutr.* 13:219–26.

Rygh, O. 1949. Research on trace elements. I. Importance of strontium, barium, and zinc. *Bull. Soc. Chim. Biol.* 31:1052–61.

Schwarz, K. 1974. New essential trace elements (Sn, V, F, Si): Progress report and outlook. In W. G. Hoekstra, J.W. Suttie, H.E. Ganther, and W. Mertz et al., eds., *Trace Element Metabolism in Animals.* 2d ed. University Park Press, Baltimore.

Schwarz, K., and Mertz, W. 1959. Chromium (III) and the glucose tolerance factor. *Arch. Biochem. Biophys.* 85:292–95.

Spears, J.W., Jones, E.E., Samsell, L.J., and Armstrong, D.W. 1984. Effect of dietary nickel on growth, urease activity, blood parameters and tissue mineral concentrations in neonatal pigs. *J. Nutr.* 114:845–52.

Streef, G.M. 1939. Sodium and calcium content of erythrocytes. *J. Biol. Chem.* 129:661–72.

Streeten, D.H.P., and Williams, E.M.V. 1952. Loss of cellular potassium as a cause of intestinal paralysis in dogs. *J. Physiol.* 118:149–70.

Strickland, L.H. 1949. The activation of phosphoglucomutase by metal ions. *Biochem. J.* 44:190–97.

Swenson, M.J., Goetsch, D.D., and Underbjerg, G.K.L. 1962. Effects of dietary trace minerals, excess calcium, and various roughages on the hemogram, tissues, and estrous cycles of Hereford heifers. *Am. J. Vet. Res.* 23:803–808.

Sykes, J.F., and Alfredson, B.V. 1940. Studies on the bovine electrocar diogram. I. Electrocardiographic changes in calves on low potassium rations. *Proc. Soc. Exp. Biol. Med.* 43:575–79.

Talbot, R.B., and Swenson, M.J. 1970. Blood volume of pigs from birth through 6 weeks of age. *Am. J. Physiol.* 218:1141–44.

Tucker, H.F., and Salmon, W.D. 1955. Parakeratosis or zinc deficiency disease in the pig. *Proc. Soc. Exp. Biol. Med.* 88:613–16.

Valberg, L.S., Card, R.T., Paulson, E.J., and Szivek, J. 1965. The metal composition of erythrocytes in different species and its relationship to the lifespan on the cells in the circulation. *Comp. Biochem. Physiol.* 15:347–59.

Venn, J.A.J., McCann, R.A., and Widdowson, E.M. 1947. Iron metabolism in piglet anemia. *J. Comp. Path. Ther.* 57:315–25.

Wacker, W.E.C., and Vallee, B.L. 1959. Nucleic acids and metals. I. Chromium, manganese, nickel, iron, and other metals in ribonucleic acid from diverse biological sources. *J. Biol. Chem.* 243:3257–62.

Weinberg, E.D. 1978. Iron and infection. *Microbiol. Rev.* 42:45–66.

Wilgus, H.S., Jr., Norris, L.C., and Heuser, G.F. 1937. The role of certain inorganic elements in the cause and prevention of perosis. *Science* 84:252–53.

Willis, W.T., and Dallman, P.R. 1989. Impaired control of respiration in iron-deficient muscle mitochondria. *Am. J. Physiol.*257(6):C1080–5.

Wooley, J.G., and Mickelson, O. 1954. Effect of sodium, potassium, and calcium on the growth of young rabbits fed purified diets containing different levels of fat and protein. *J. Nutr.* 52:591–600.

CHAPTER 30

Bones, Joints, and Synovial Fluid | by R. H. Wasserman, F. A. Kallfelz, and George Lust

GENERAL ASPECTS OF BONE PHYSIOLOGY AND METABOLISM*

The skeleton is the primary supporting connective tissue of vertebrates and is comprised of bones of different sizes and shapes. Because of its relative permanence and resistance to decay, one is tempted to consider bone in the living animal to be a "dead" tissue that is relatively inert after it is formed. On the contrary, bone is dynamic throughout life, modifying its structure in response to internal and external stresses. It differs from other types of connective tissue in its higher mineral content, which is responsible for its hardness and rigidity, and is characterized by the presence of unique cells: the osteoblasts, osteoclasts, and osteocytes. These cells are responsible for the formation, resorption and remodeling of bone, and their behavior is influenced by various hormones, growth factors, vitamins, and dietary minerals. Through hormonal action, for example, the minerals of bone can be withdrawn when exogenous sources are limited and, in this way, aid in maintaining a relatively constant concentration of calcium ions in blood.

The three main functions served by bones and the bone cells of the skeleton are (1) helping to maintain, through *homeostatic regulation,* a constant ionic environment within the organism; (2) *supporting* and *protecting* soft tissues and organs, including bone marrow and the brain; and (3) with muscles and tendons, providing a means of bodily *locomotion,* and *movement* of parts of the body (e.g., the grasping facility of the hands).

The skeleton can also accumulate potentially toxic exogenous mineral ions, including lead, aluminum, radioactive strontium, and radium. The concentration of these minerals in bone can have direct deleterious effects on the skeleton, leading to improper bone formation, excessive bone resorption, and, for the radionuclides, the induction of cancer.

Anatomical considerations

The architecture and form of the various bones of the vertebrate skeleton are determined genetically and are due to the metabolic and synthesizing properties of bone cells. The specific functioning of these cells are described below. For now, however, suffice it to say that their coordinated activities result in the proper formation of bone during the growth period of the animal, the maintenance of bone in the mature animal, and the modification of bone in response to external and internal stresses.

Anatomical features of a growing long bone are diagrammed in Fig. 30.1. This bone can be arbitrarily divided into three regions: the shaft, termed the *diaphysis;* the ends

The authors gratefully acknowledge the contributions of Mrs. Norma Jayne in the preparation of the manuscript.

*The author of this section is R. H. Wasserman.

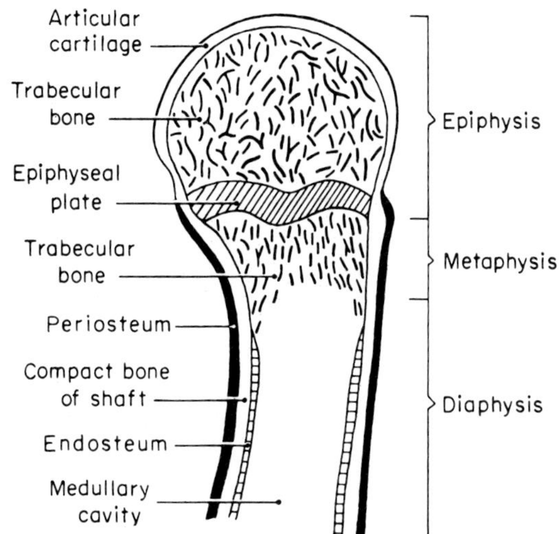

Figure 30.1. Anatomy of a growing long bone.

of the bone, the *epiphyses;* and an intermediate section, the *metaphyses.* In the growing animal, a highly cartilaginous region is located between the epiphyses and the diaphysis, the *epiphyseal plate* or *growth apparatus.*

The diaphysis is composed of the compact *cortical* bone in the form of a cylinder that surrounds the *medullary cavity,* which contains the bone marrow. The medullary cavity, particularly in the metaphyseal region, also contains *spongy* or *cancellous* bone that is made up of fine spicules of bone called *trabeculae* (Fig. 30.2). The epiphyses are composed of cancellous bone surrounded by a thin layer of compact bone. The strength and rigidity of long bones are due to the hardness and rigidity of the compact bone of the shaft and the epiphysis and to the underlying scaffolding arrangement of the cancellous bony spicules, the trabeculae. These trabeculae run parallel to the lines of maximum stress, in accordance with sound engineering principles.

The compact bone of the shaft and elsewhere has an internal structure that reflects its pattern of formation as well as changes that occur during remodeling of bone. The diagram of the section of the shaft of a long bone in Fig. 30.3 shows the internal features of compact bone. The channels that generally run parallel to the long axis of the bone are the *Haversian canals,* which contain blood vessels supported by connective tissue. The blood vessels within the Haversian canals communicate with the external surface and the medullary cavity by way of the *canals of Volkmann.*

The unit of structure of compact bone is the *Haversian system* or *osteon,* which consists of a central Haversian canal surrounded by concentric layers of bone, the *lamellae.* The bone cells within the bony substance, the *osteocytes,* are contained within melon-shaped cavities, the *lacunae,* and communicate with each other and with the Haversian canal through a branching network of *canaliculi.* The *canaliculi* and *lacunae* are extravascular, and tissue fluids for the maintenance of the osteocytes move from the blood vessels through the canaliculi. Mechanisms to facilitate fluid transport may be present, such as the periodic contraction of the entrapped bone cells.

The trabeculae of spongy bone also contain concentric lamellae with enclosed lacunae and osteocytes. As in com-

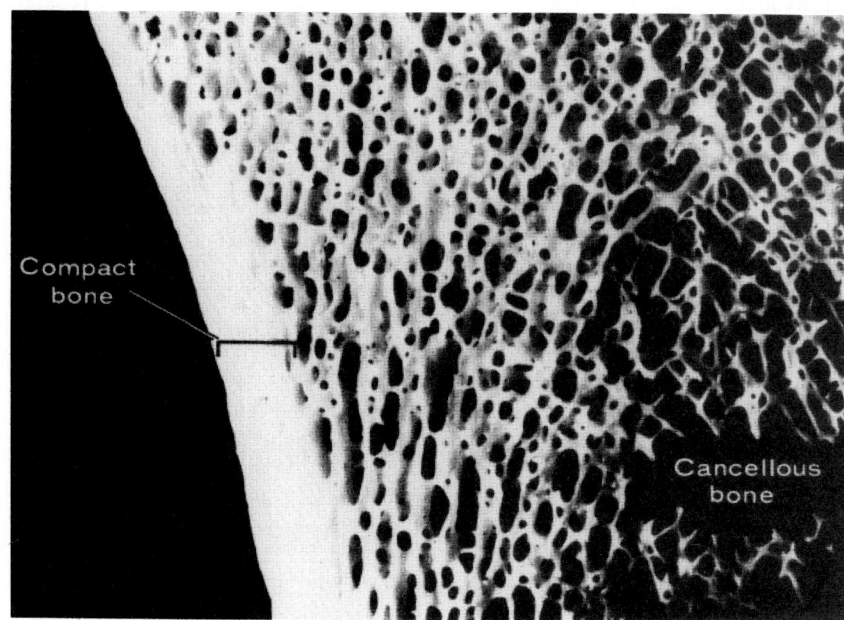

Figure 30.2. A thick ground section of the tibia illustrating the cortical compact bone and the lattice of trabeculae of the cancellous bone. (From Fawcett 1986, *Bloom and Fawcett's A Textbook of Histology,* W.B. Saunders, Philadelphia.)

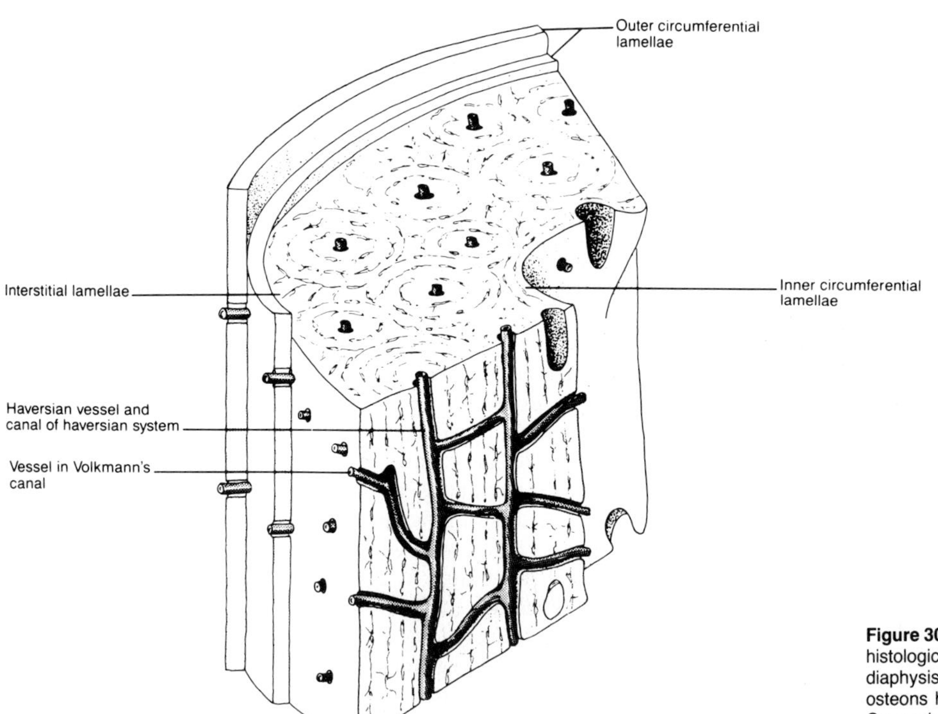

Figure 30.3. Diagrammatic representation of the histological organization of compact bone in the diaphysis of an adult long bone. The number of osteons has been reduced for simplicity. (From Cormack 1987, *Ham's Histology,* 9th ed., J.B. Lippincott, Philadelphia.)

pact bone, the lacunae intercommunicate via canaliculi, but the Haversian system is absent.

The flat bones of the skull are composed of compact bone on both surfaces with a layer of cancellous bone between them. The smaller and irregularly shaped bones, such as the digits of the hand, also consist primarily of spongy bone, circumferentially bounded by a cortex of compact bone.

Bone, except where covered with cartilage at articulating surfaces, is covered externally with a dense connective tissue layer, the *periosteum,* that is attached to bone by collagenous bundles known as *Sharpey's fibers* and by small blood vessels. The aspect of the periosteum lying closest to the bone surface contains cells that have bone-forming potential. The medullary cavity of bone is covered with a layer of thin connective tissue, the *endosteum.* Endosteum also lines the cavities of the Haversian canals of compact bone and covers the trabeculae of spongy bone.

Cells

The cells of bone

Four different types of cells are specifically associated with bone (Fig. 30.4). Bone surfaces are populated with *osteoblasts,* bone *lining cells, osteoclasts* and, entrapped within the mineralized matrix, the *osteocytes.*

The primary function of *osteoblasts* is the synthesis and secretion of components of the organic matrix of bone and, in addition, participation in the mineralization of the organic matrix. The cells are cuboidal in configuration and have an abundant rough endoplasmic reticulum, numerous mitochondria, and a prominent Golgi apparatus, all features of cells engaged in protein synthesis and protein export (Fig. 30.5A). Osteoblasts produce collagen, the major component of the organic matrix and other organic components of the matrix.

The *osteocytes* (Fig. 30.5B) are derived directly from osteoblasts that become surrounded by bone matrix. Osteocytes, within mineralized bones, reside in lacunae and communicate with other osteocytes and with bone surface cells through cytoplasmic processes and gap junctions. These processes occupy the canaliculi that permeate throughout the mineralized matrix of bone. Osteocytes have the potential of either forming bone tissue or resorbing the bony surface of their lacunae; the particular function is determined by extracellular stimuli. In the *formative phase* osteocytes have prominent rough endoplasmic reticula, and in the *resorptive phase* the endoplasmic reticulum is less apparent and many lysosomes, which contain hydrolytic enzymes, are present.

The *osteoclasts* are bone-resorbing cells; they are large motile cells and are often multinucleated (Fig. 30.5C). Where attached to the bone surface, they display fingerlike projections, the *ruffled border,* that extend into the bone surface. Encircling the ruffled border and adjacent to the bone surface is a clear zone, so named because this part of the cell is devoid of prominent organelles but does contain microfilaments. In active osteoclasts, numerous cyto-

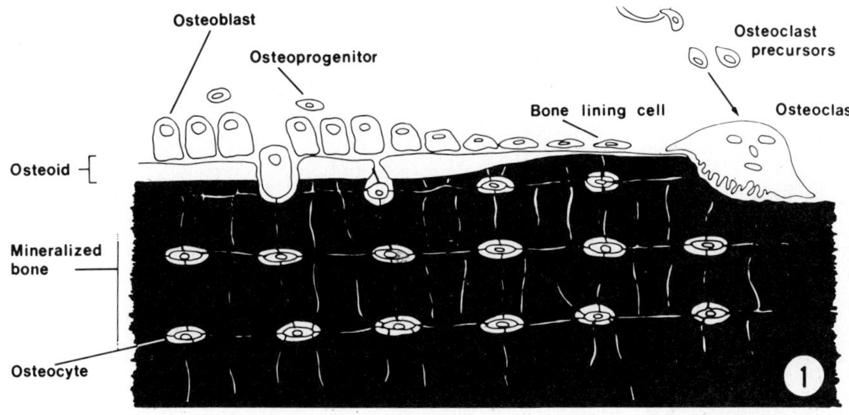

Figure 30.4. Topographic relationships among bone cells. (Modified from a drawing by T. Chambers. From Marks and Popoff 1988, *Am. J. Anat.* 183:1–44.)

plasmic vacuoles are located within the cytoplasm. These vacuoles are primary and secondary lysosomes, which are intimately involved in the bone-resorbing function of these cells.

Bone-lining cells (Fig. 30.5D) cover bone surfaces that are not undergoing formation or resorption. These cells are flatter than osteoblasts, appear to be relatively inactive, and are thought to constitute a "pseudomembrane," separating the bone surface from the extracellular fluids in regions not covered by other types of bone cells. It has been presumed that bone-lining cells might be precursors of osteoblasts and might have a regulatory function in the process of bone formation.

The cartilage cells of bone

The cartilage cells, or *chondrocytes,* are prominent in the epiphyseal plates of long bones during periods of growth and persist in the cartilage at articulating surfaces. As growth proceeds in this region, the chondrocytes transform into enlarged *hypertrophic chondrocytes* that participate in the mineralization of the cartilage matrix.

The origin of bone cells

The question of the source of the differentiated bone cells has had the attention of bone biologists for a number of years. The earlier theories, based on morphological examination, radioactive tracer studies, and other experimental approaches, proposed a common lineage of osteoblasts and osteoclasts. The osteoblasts, initially derived from committed primitive stem cells called *osteoprogenator* cells in connective tissue, were considered to be the direct precursors of osteoclasts. According to this theory, differentiation and coalescence of osteoblasts led to the formation of the large, multinucleated osteoclasts. It was also proposed that osteoclasts could revert back to the osteoblastic phenotype. A different view is now held.

Osteoblasts are clearly derived from local, nonmigrating stromal cells, which reside in the connective tissue that is associated with the periosteal and endosteal surfaces of bone and in the connective tissue that covers the surfaces of the Haversian canal. These osteogenic precursor cells, under the influence of physical and chemical stimuli in their microenvironment, differentiate into either the osteoblastic or chondrocytic cell lines (Fig. 30.6). It is proposed that a preosteoblastic stage immediately precedes the formation of the mature osteoblast. Both preosteoblasts and osteoblasts contain high concentrations of the hydrolytic enzyme, *alkaline phosphatase,* characteristic of the osteoblastic phenotype. The presence of this enzyme is also characteristic of chondrocytes in the region of the cartilage growth plate that is being calcified.

Osteoclasts originate from stem cells that are not locally associated with the bone tissue. Evidence of the extraskeletal origin of osteoclasts comes from a number of ingenious experiments. One of the latter is a study of the bone disease, *osteopetrosis,* a metabolic bone disease characterized by an excessive amount of mineral in bone, which is due to reduced bone resorption. The bone-resorbing osteoclasts in this disease are defective or absent. In a mutant strain of mice that gives rise to osteopetrotic progeny, it was demonstrated that a parabiotic union between an osteopetrotic mouse and a normal littermate reversed the disease. In the *parabiosis* procedure, a common blood supply is surgically developed between the two parabionts and allows the transfer of blood cells from one animal to the other. The result of this study provided substantial evidence that osteoclasts originate from sites other than bone tissue. It is now held that the precursors of osteoclasts are stem cells in the hematopoietic tissue of bone marrow and spleen. The committed preosteoclasts differentiate into bone-resorbing monocytes and then fuse to form the large multinucleated osteoclasts.

Macrophages, the mononuclear phagocytic cells from bone marrow, are considered by some to be another possible precursor of osteoclasts.

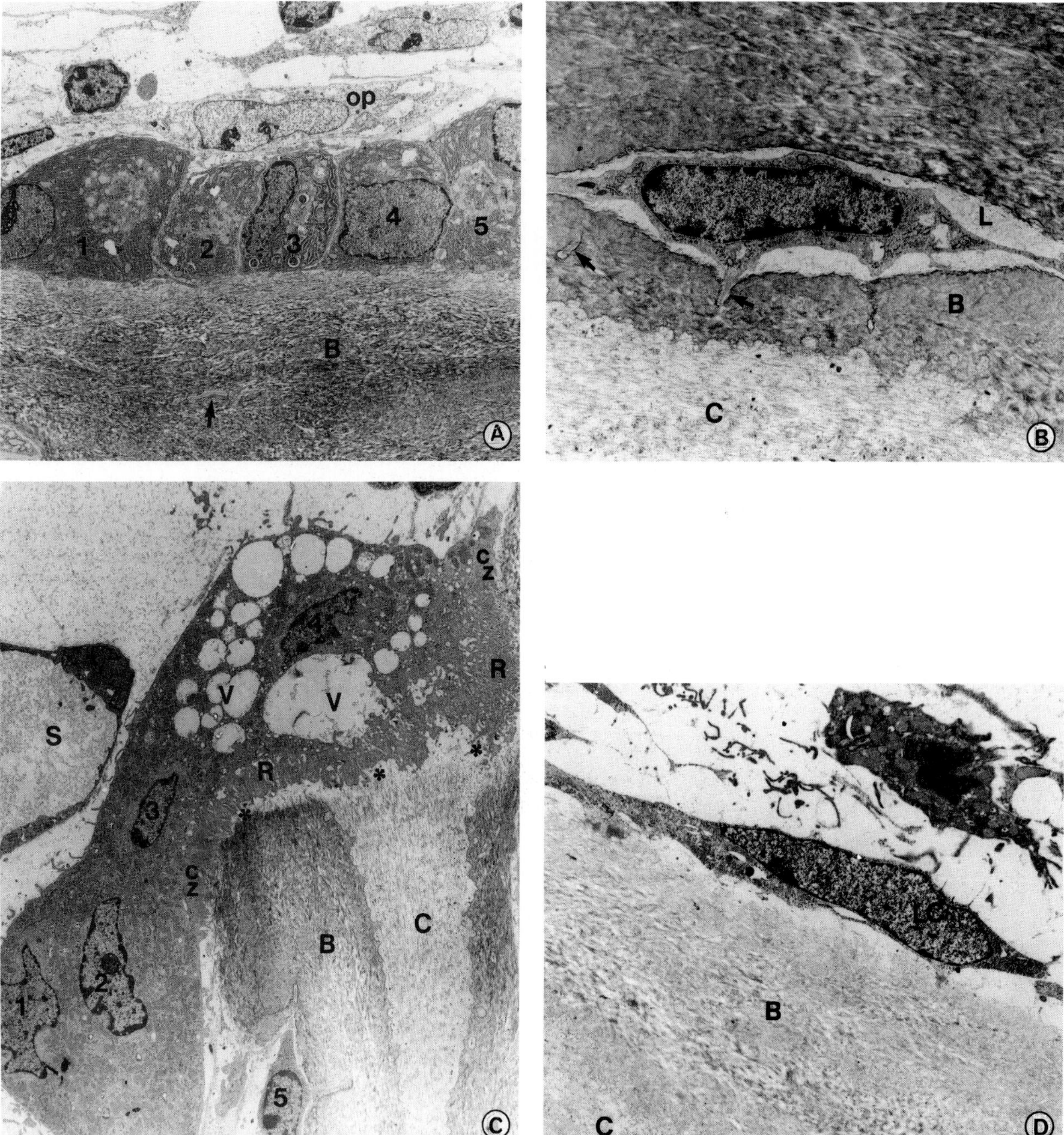

Figure 30.5. (*A*) Transmission electron micrograph of five osteoblasts (numbered). All have abundant rough endoplasmic reticulum, and cells 1, 2, and 5 show a prominent Golgi apparatus. These cells, cut in different planes of section, lie on a bone (B) surface, separating it from a thin osteoprogentor top cell. The arrow identifies an osteocyte process with a canaliculus, perhaps belonging to the cell seen in the lower left-hand corner of the figure. ×1825. (*B*) Electron micrgraph of an osteocyte. This cell, situated in a lacuna (L) within bone (B) extends several processes (*arrows*) through canaliculi that penetrate bone. Cartilage (C) previously calcified, is located at the bottom of the figure. Notice the different morphology of collagen fibrils in bone (banded, type I) and cartilage (no bands, type II). ×4680. (*C*) Electron micrograph of an osteoclast. Four nuclei (numbered 1 to 4) are seen in this section. This large cell is attached to both bone (B) and calcified cartilage (C) by clear zones (cz) and a ruffled border (R) The bone and cartilage surfaces below the ruffled border are frayed (*asterisks*) compared with smooth surfaces beneath clear zones. Active osteoclasts have a vacuolated cytoplasm next to the ruffled border.These vacuoles (V) are large and visible by light microscopy, and their presence is a reliable indicator of bone resorption. Large venous sinuses (S) are often seen next to osteoclasts. An osteocyte (5) is seen in the lower part of the figure. ×2.25. (*D*) Electron micrograph of a bone-lining cell. These cells (LC) cover bone (B) surfaces and are flat and elongated with little rough endoplasmic reticulum. (C) Cartilage. ×3400. (From Marks and Popoff 1988. *Am. J. Anat.* 183:1–44.)

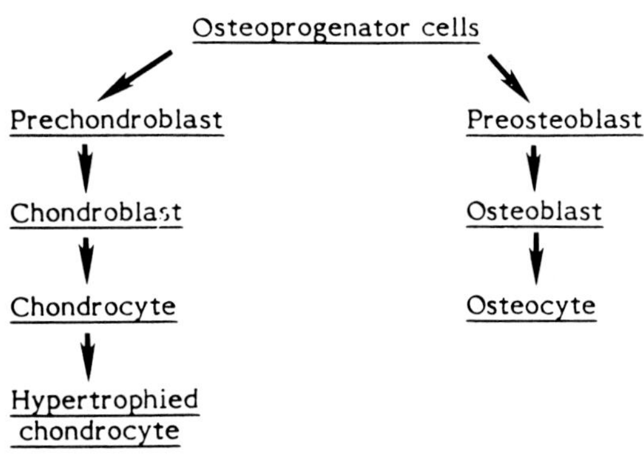

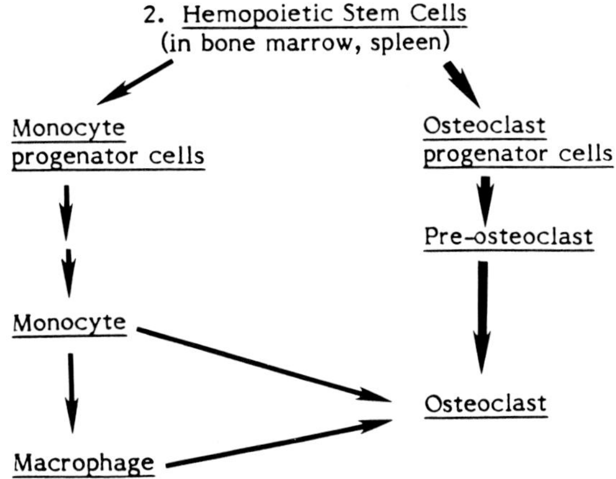

Figure 30.6. Diagram of views of the lineage of osteoblasts and osteoclasts. (Modified from Marks and Popoff 1988. *Am. J. Anat.* 183:1–44.)

Overall composition of bone

Adult bone is, on a wet-weight basis, approximately 25 percent water, 45 percent ash, and 30 percent organic matter. Calcium constitutes about 37 percent of the ash content and phosphorus, about 18.5 percent. On a dry-weight basis, the mineral content of bone is between 65 and 70 percent and the organic fraction is roughly 30 to 35 percent. Of the organic fraction, about 90 percent is collagen, which, on heating in aqueous solution, is converted to gelatin.

The chemical composition of bone changes during embryonic development and postfetal growth and maturation. The mineral content increases progressively as the water content decreases. The reciprocal relationship between the mineral and water fractions suggests that, as bone formation proceeds, there is a progressive displacement of water by mineral.

The mineral composition of bovine cortical bone is given in Table 30.1. Also included in this table are the concentrations of carbon dioxide (as carbonate) and citric acid. It can be seen that several different elements are incorporated in the mineral phase of bone, but by far the major constituents are calcium and phosphorus.

Table 30.1. Composition of dry, fat-free, bovine cortical bone

Constituents	Percentage	mEq/g
Cations		
Calcium	26.7	13.3
Magnesium	0.44	0.36
Sodium	0.73	0.32
Potassium	0.056	0.014
Anions		
Phosphorus	12.5	
as PO_4^{2-}		12.1
Carbon dioxide	3.5	
as CO_3^{2-}		1.6
Citric acid	0.36	
as Cit^-		0.14
Chloride	0.08	0.02
Fluoride	0.07	0.04
Molar ratio Ca/P		1.656

Adapted from Armstrong and Singer, as given by McLean and Budy, *Radiation, Isotopes, and Bone,* Academic Press, New York, 1964.

Intercellular matrix

The matrices of cartilage and bone, the two primary skeletal tissues, differ significantly in consistency and composition (Fig. 30.7). The fibrous protein, collagen, is the major organic constituent of bone and is less prominent in cartilage. Bone collagen is primarily of the type I variety, and the collagen of cartilage is of the type II variety. In contrast to bone, proteoglycans are the major components of cartilage. The proteoglycans in the two tissues differ both structurally and in their chemical composition (Fig. 30.8). In cartilage, the proteoglycans are large molecules with a complex structure and, because of their water-adsorbing characteristics, contribute to the permeable gel-like consistency of cartilage. Because of the permeable nature of cartilage, except where mineralized, the embedded chondrocytes receive nutrients and oxygen by diffusion from extracellular fluid.

The proteoglycan molecules are smaller in bone than in cartilage, thus contributing to the denser, closer packing of the bone matrix. The close packing of the matrix of bone and its high mineral content hinder diffusional processes; therefore bone cells are necessarily situated very near blood vessels, which give access to nutrients and oxygen either directly or by way of the conduits (canaliculi) that permeate the bone tissue.

The matrix of bone, in addition to mineral, collagen, and proteoglycans, also contains a number of different organic constituents, some of which are considered to have important roles in either promoting mineralization or controlling the degree of mineralization by their inhibitory actions.

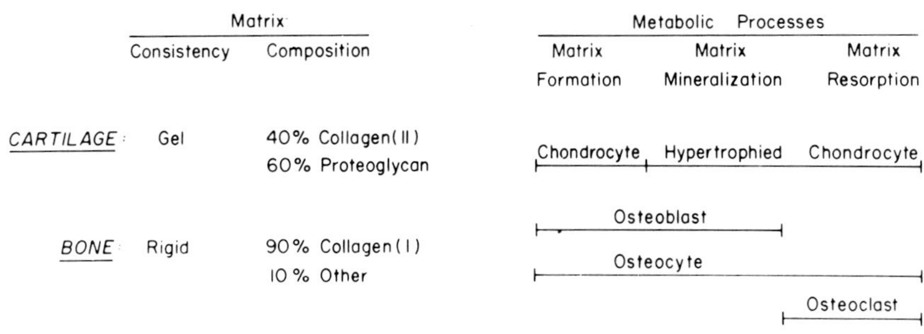

Figure 30.7. Distinguishing features of matrices and major cell functions in cartilage and bone. (From Marks and Popoff 1988. *Am. J. Anat.* 183:1–44.)

The mineral phase

The type of mineral found in bone, in calcified cartilage, and in the dentine and enamel of teeth is mainly hydroxyapatite. Hydroxyapatite is approximated by the formula $Ca_{10}(PO_4)_6(OH)_2$ and is a member of the apatite series of minerals that are characterized by a distinctive X-ray diffraction pattern. However, these biological minerals are not *pure* hydroxyapatite and contain some of the mineral ions listed in Table 30.1. Some of these elements, however, are not incorporated into the crystal structure of bone mineral but are adventitiously associated with mineralized matrix of bone. About 70 percent of the citrate, 60 percent of magnesium, and 50 percent of the sodium of the body are present in the skeleton.

Bone mineral is in the form of large numbers of small crystals, and this configuration yields enormous surface areas. It has been estimated that the surface area of the bone crystals in the skeleton of a 70 kg human exceeds 1200 acres and that the surface area of 1 g of bone mineral is more than 100 m^2. Because of these extremely large surface areas, reactions at the crystalline surface provide for a rapid interchange of ions between interstitial fluid and bone.

The organic phase

It is the bone mineral in the matrix of bone that gives bone its special properties of hardness and rigidity, but it is the organic matrix, primarily collagen, that provides the framework for mineralization and gives bone its architectural form. For bone and cartilage, it is the collagen in these connective tissues that determines its anatomical configuration.

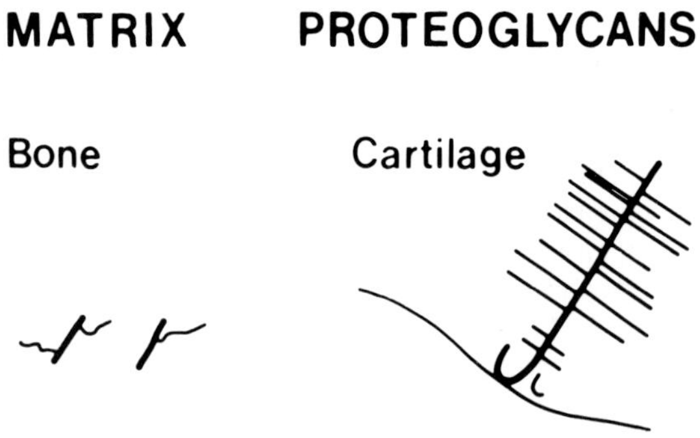

Collagen. The collagens are a *heterogeneous* class of fibrous proteins that share common physical and chemical properties. Collagen is usually the primary component of extracellular matrix and gives support and tensile strength to skin, bone, tendon, and cornea of vertebrates. In addition to this structural role, the collagens are also directly or indirectly involved in cell attachment and differentiation, and they have chemotactic properties.

Type I collagen, the primary collagen of bone, is synthesized within *osteoblasts* and *osteocytes* as precursor proteins, which are modified intracellularly before extrusion into the extracellular milieu. The collagen fibril is comprised of three collagen molecules that are "wrapped around each in ropelike fashion," yielding the tight triple-helical configuration. This arrangement yields an asymmetrical fibrous protein complex that gives the strength and rigidity usually associated with collagen fibers and bundles. Type I collagen has two different but similar protein chains.

The amino acid composition of collagen is unique. About 33 percent of the amino acid residue is glycine, and about 22 percent is proline and hydroxyproline. Because of its high content of hydroxyproline (about 10%), the content of this amino acid in urine has been used as a measure of bone resorption. Another amino acid in collagen of functional importance is hydroxylysine, which participates with norleucine in covalent cross-linkages between adjacent collagen fibrils during the course of its maturation, stabilizing the fibrils and contributing to the three-dimensional character and properties of the extracellular matrix.

The collagen of bone has a characteristic banding pattern caused by the staggered assembly of the fibrils of type I collagen. The staggered configuration results in "holes" in the multimolecular fibrillar complex into which the mineral is thought to be initially deposited and provides a framework for subsequent mineral deposition (Fig. 30.9).

The triple-helical molecule of Type II collagen of cartilage comprises three amino acid chains of identical com-

MATRIX PROTEOGLYCANS

Bone

Cartilage

Figure 30.8. Proteoglycans in cartilage and bone differ significantly in both size and components. The bone variety has a smaller core protein with one or two glycosaminoglycan (GAG) side chains. The cartilage variety is heterogeneous with respect to both number and length of GAG side chains. (From Marks and Popoff 1988. *Am. J. Anat.* 183:1–44.)

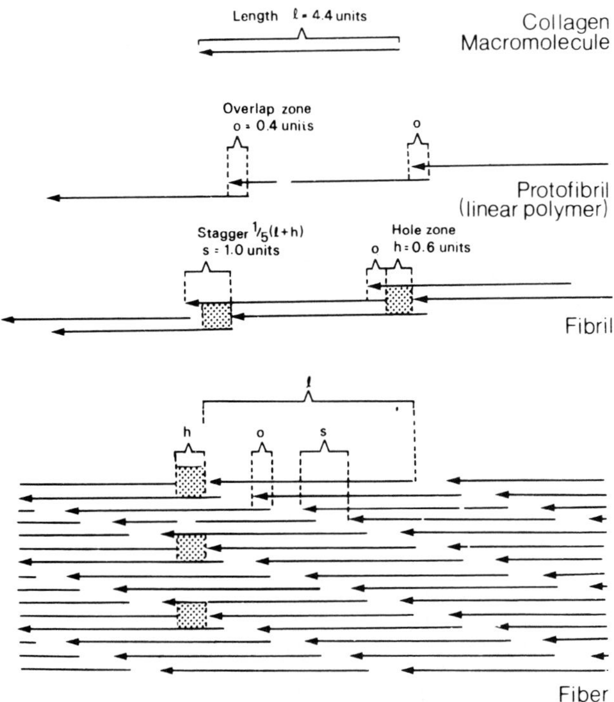

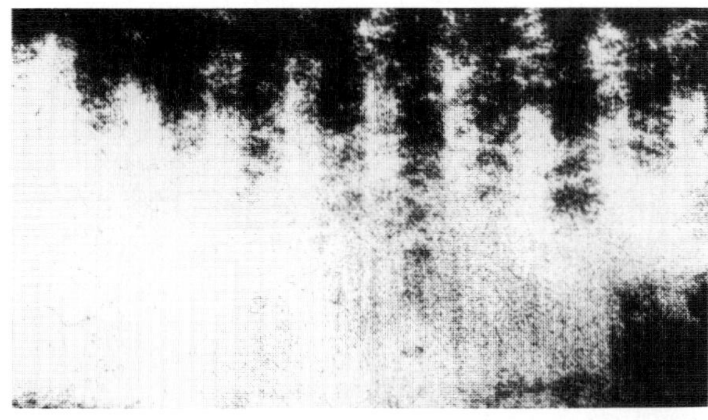

Figure 30.9. Diagram of the overlapping staggered arrangement of molecules in a collagen fiber, showing the small discontinuities or holes that are thought to be sites of nucleation of apatite crystals in the mineralization of bone. (Modified from Glimcher and Krane 1968, in Gould and Ramachandran, eds., *A Treatise on Collagen,* Vol. II. Academic Press, New York. From Fawcett 1986, *Bloom and Fawcett's A Textbook of Histology,* W.B. Saunders, Philadelphia.)

position, thus differing in this respect from Type I collagen.

Type X collagen, a smaller collagen, is also present in cartilage. It is synthesized primarily by hypertrophic chondrocytes (see below) and is localized in hypertrophic cartilage of the growth plate, which becomes calcified before true bone formation takes place. Because much of the synthetic potential of hypertrophic chrondrocytes is devoted to synthesizing type X collagen, and because of its restricted localization, it is suggested that this molecule has a significant developmental function. Two possible functions of type X collagen have been proposed. It might represent a "disposable" collagen that facilitates the turnover of hypertrophic cartilage and(or) it might have a role in the process of calcification of cartilage. (This is discussed further in the "Joint and Synovial Fluid" section.)

Proteoglycans. As the name implies, proteoglycans are composed of both protein (*proteo-*) and carbohydrate (*glycans*), and are ubiquitously found in connective tissues throughout the body. In cartilage, the proteoglycans are large molecules, of which 5 percent is a core protein and 95 percent is carbohydrate. The cartilage proteoglycans have the capacity to adsorb a considerable amount of water, which contributes to the gel-like consistency of cartilage.

In bone, the proteoglycans are smaller molecules than in cartilage with 25 to 40 percent as the core protein and 60 to 75 percent as carbohydrate. (A diagrammatic representation of bone and cartilage proteoglycans is given in Fig. 30.8.) Two types of these small proteoglycans are present in bone and, in in vitro studies, have been shown to bind to collagen fibrils and, functionally, possibly to control the formation and final configuration of the fibrillar network of collagen (further discussed in the "Joints and Synovial Fluid" section).

Osteocalcin. The bone-specific protein, osteocalcin, also known as bone Gla protein or BGP, contains three γ-carboxyglutamic acid residues. These residues bind calcium ions and form complexes with bone mineral. Carboxylation of three glutamate residues is a vitamin K–dependent posttranslational modification of the protein. The rate of its synthesis by osteoblasts is increased by 1,25-dihydroxycholecalciferol (1,25[OH]$_2$D$_3$), the most active metabolite of vitamin D. It has been proposed that osteocalcin acts as an inhibitor of hydroxyapatite precipitation from supersaturated solutions and blocks the transformation of the more soluble forms of calcium phosphate salts to hydroxyapatite.

Osteocalcin is also found in blood, and its concentration in blood is greater in diseases characterized by increased bone turnover (e.g., Paget's disease, primary hyperparathyroidism, and renal osteodystrophy).

In addition to a possible role in bone mineralization, osteocalcin has chemoattractive activity for mononuclear leukocytes and thereby might be involved in the regulation of bone resorption.

Matrix Gla protein. Matrix Gla protein (MGP) is larger than osteocalcin and also contains vitamin K–dependent γ-carboxyglutamic acid residues. MGP has been identified in long bones, calvaria, and dentin. In bone, this protein is found tightly bound to another noncollagenous protein, the bone morphogenetic protein of Urist (see below).

It is of interest that, in failure of vitamin K utilization brought about by treatment of animals with warfarin, the amount of osteocalcin and MGP in the skeleton is considerably diminished, but the skeleton does not show major changes. Although the warfarin experiments question the essentiality of the bone-associated vitamin K–dependent proteins in bone metabolism, subtler effects of these proteins in the skeleton might be present but not yet detectable by present techniques.

Bone sialoprotein. Sialoprotein contains about 12 percent of sialic acid (N-acetylneuraminic acid) and was one of the first noncollagenous proteins isolated from bone matrix. Sialic acid is a sugar derivative with one negatively charged carboxyl group. Actually, the sialoprotein initially identified in 1963 by Herring was later shown to consist of two similar molecules, sialoprotein I and sialoprotein II. Sequence analysis of sialoprotein I revealed a pentapeptide sequence identical to the cell-binding region of fibronectin. Since this bone protein binds strongly to hydroxyapatite, it might serve as a bridge between bone cells and bone mineral. Sialoprotein II, according to recent analysis, is a proteoglycan.

Phosphoproteins. Several phosphorylated proteins have been identified in bone matrix. One of these is the phosphorylated glycoprotein, *osteonectin,* the most abundant noncollagenous protein produced by osteoblasts. Osteonectin is also present in nonosseous tissues and, therefore, is not bone specific. Osteonectin binds both calcium ions and hydroxyapatite and also binds tightly to collagen. Because of these properties and other observations on its behavior, osteonectin might have some function in the control of mineralization, although its exact function is not known.

Bone morphogenetic proteins. Bone matrix also contains a number of mitogenic and growth factors that influence the activity of bone cells. Among these are the *bone morphogenetic proteins,* proteins derived from bone matrix, which have osteoinductive properties (i.e., they stimulate bone formation). The early studies by Urist and colleagues demonstrated that the implantation of demineralized bone matrix into muscle results in the formation of true bone in that tissue. New bone formation occurs by a series of steps. These steps include the chemotactic recruitment of mesenchymal cells to the site, the differentiation of these cells into chondrocytes, the formation of cartilage by the chondrocytes, invasion of the cartilage by blood vessels, and replacement of cartilage by bone. The complete process takes about 3 to 4 weeks after the demineralized bone matrix has been implanted. Bone-derived growth factors stimulate the proliferation and activity of the differentiated bone cells.

Osteogenin, another matrix-derived protein that is homologous with BMP, also induces cartilage and bone formation in vivo.

The implantation of demineralized bone matrix, mineralized bone matrix, or bone powder has been shown, with some success, to heal nonunion bone fractures and defects in the skull. The therapeutic potential of bone matrix implantation in animals and humans has attracted considerable interest, and investigations in this direction are well under way. In addition, the mitogenic activity of bone matrix proteins was recently demonstrated to be decreased in vitamin D deficiency and might constitute one of the several effects of vitamin D on bone and mineral metabolism.

Lipids. Bone matrix contains lipids, some of which are associated with *matrix vesicles,* to be discussed subsequently. Matrix vesicles, derived from bone and cartilage cells, are intimately involved in the calcification of cartilage and perhaps bone.

Intramembranous bone formation

The process of intramembranous bone formation is exemplified by bone formation under the periosteum of long bones and the formation of the flat bones (calvaria) of the skull. The latter is illustrated in Fig. 30.10. At the site where bone is to be formed, one observes mesenchymal cells that are connected by cell processes. Bundles of col-

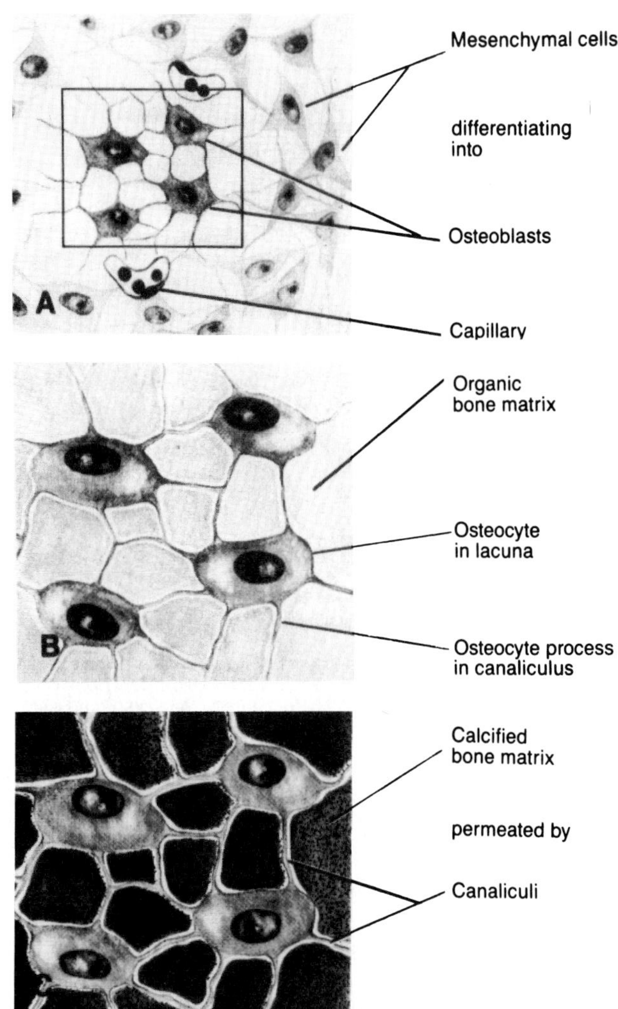

Figure 30.10. Schematic diagram showing three stages of intramembranous ossification. (From Cormack 1987, Bone, in *Ham's Histology,* 9th ed., J.B. Lippincott, Philadelphia, Chap. 12.)

lagenous fibrils run between the cells in all directions, and a semifluid matrix bathes both cells and fibrils. Just before mineralization, the mesenchymal cells are transformed to osteoblasts, the intercellular matrix increases in density and amount, and the matrix becomes more homogeneous. After these transformations, the mineral content of the matrix rapidly increases, forming bone. The osteoblasts on the exterior surface continue to form matrix, and thus the bone increases in thickness. Some osteoblasts become surrounded by calcified matrix and develop into osteocytes.

Endochondral (intracartilaginous) bone formation

Events occurring in the epiphyseal plate, the growth apparatus of long bones, illustrates endochondral bone formation. In general terms, the cartilage is first synthesized by chondrocytes and is later removed in a systematic manner to be replaced by bone. The growth apparatus, as diagrammed in Fig. 30.11, encompasses the region that includes the epiphyseal cartilage and the underlying spongy (cancellous) bone of the metaphysis. This region can be separated into arbitrary zones, each designating the progression of events in this type of bone formation. At the epiphyseal front, the chondrocytes form the cartilage matrix and subsequently begin to multiply and form into columns separated from each other by "horizontal" bands of cartilage. In the "vertical" direction, the cells are separated by a thin capsule of matrix. As growth proceeds, the older cartilage cells hypertrophy (i.e., become enlarged) and incorporate stores of glycogen. Through the action of these hypertrophic chondrocytes, the interstitial matrix in the zone of provisional calcification becomes mineralized, and this calcified cartilage provides structural continuity between the epiphyseal cartilage and the underlying cancellous bone in the metaphyseal region.

The next event is the penetration of blood vessels and

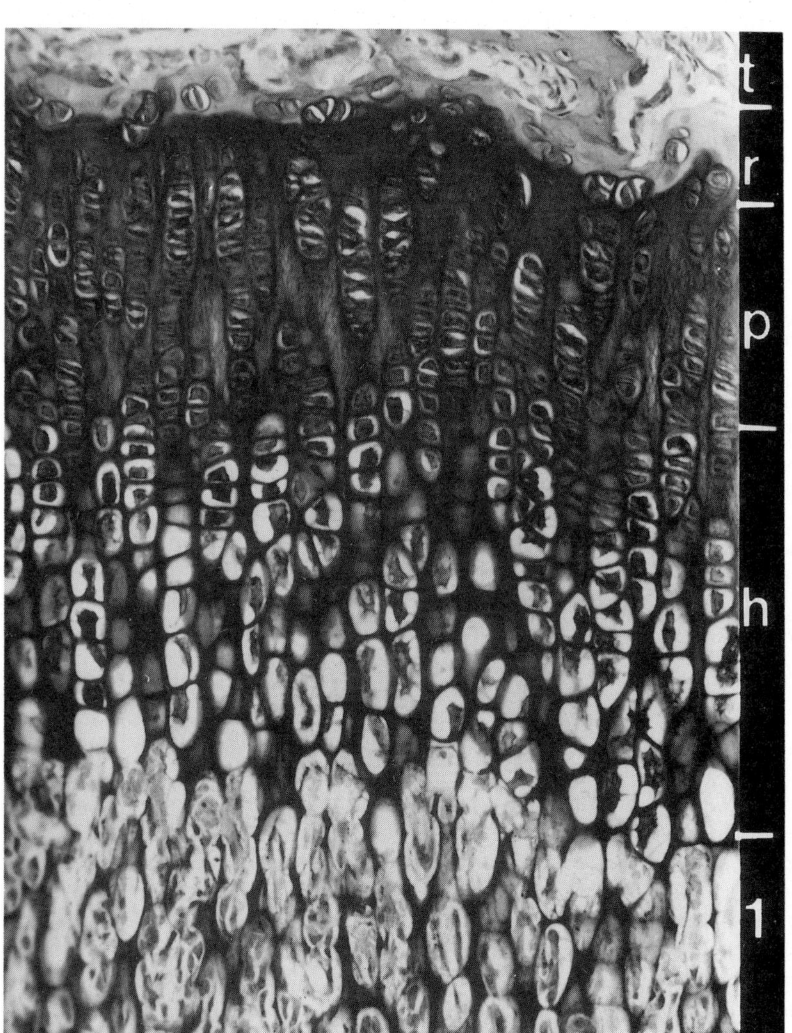

Figure 30.11. Detail of epiphyseal growth plate. t, proximal terminal plate. Epiphyseal plate is r + p + h. r, reserve zone; p, proliferation zone; h, hypertrophic zone. In the reserve zone, the cells are few and small with abundant matrix. In the proliferative zone, the cells enlarge and arrange in columns. In the hypertrophic zone, the cells become larger and vesiculate. The most distal cells die and are penetrated by vessels. The cores between the hypertrophic cells extend into the metaphysis. These cores serve as the framework on which bone is laid down to the primary spongiosa (1). Hematoxylin and eosin. Original magnification ×180; enlarged × 1.2. (Courtesy of L. Krook, Dept. of Pathology, New York State College of Veterinary Medicine, Ithaca, N.Y.)

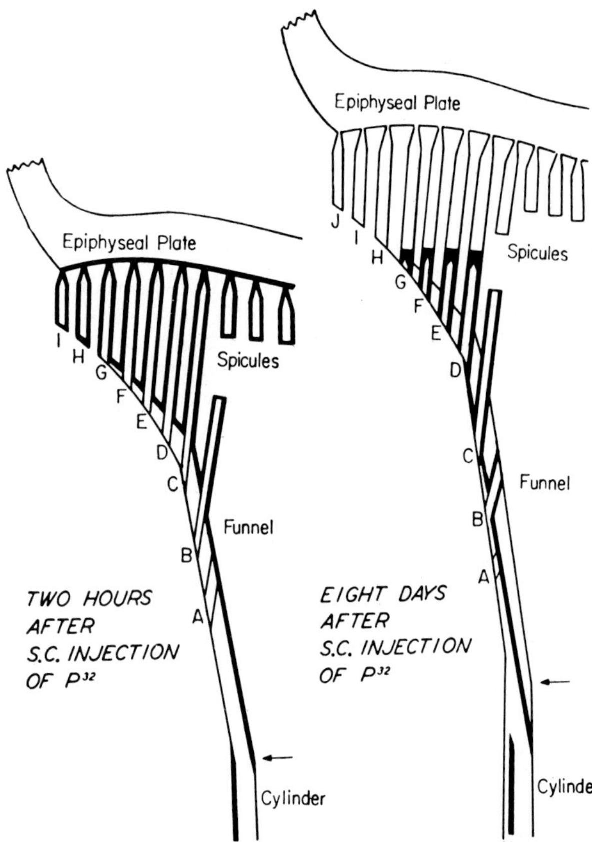

Figure 30.12. Visualization of features of the pattern of growth of rat tibia by autoradiographic method. On the left, a diagram represents part of the head of the tibia of a 50 g rat 2 hours after a subcutaneous injection of radiophosphorus. The heavy lines indicate the surfaces where deposition of radiophosphorus takes place. On the right, a diagram represents the corresponding region of the tibia 8 days later. The reactive areas have been drawn as heavy lines in a position corresponding to that in the left diagram. The solid reactive band bordering the epiphyseal plate soon after injection—which is due to ^{32}P accumulation in the zone of calcified cartilage (*left*)—persists as a broken line across some of the spicules (*right*); the rest of the line has been eroded. The reactive coating on the spicules soon after injection (*left*) persists on the lower parts of some of the spicules (*right*); when the individual spicules are traced from one diagram to the other, their role in making up the wider end of the funnel becomes apparent. The reactive line found on the endosteum of the funnel soon after injection (*left*) becomes deeply embedded in the bone along most of the length of the funnel and is even resorbed at the wider end (*right*). The reactive line found on the periosteal surface of the cylinder soon after injection (*left*) becomes embedded in the bone (*right*). (From Leblond, Wilkinson, Belanger, Robichon 1950, *Am. J. Anat.* 86:289–341.)

connective tissue into the zone of the calcified cartilage. The uncalcified interstitial material is removed, and the vertical columns of calcified cartilage remain. Accompanying the invading connective tissue are *osteoprogenitor* cells that differentiate into mature osteoblasts. These cells participate in the formation of bone on remnants of the calcified cartilage scaffolding in the *primary spongiosa* zone. As bone continues to grow, the primary spongiosa undergoes modification by removal of the calcified matrix and replacement by bone in the form of bony spicules, the trabeculae, of the metaphysis. The lower ends of the trabeculae in the midportion of the metaphysis are continuously being resorbed by osteoclasts that are relatively numerous in this region. However, the metaphyseal trabeculae that are located at the periphery and adjacent to the cortical shaft become incorporated in the shaft as growth continues. Fig. 30.12 illustrates some of these events during the process of bone formation at the epiphyseal plate.

Modeling and remodeling

The shape of the bones of the skeleton, predetermined genetically for the various functions to be served, represents an excellent example of biological engineering. The cavity of the cranium increases in size during maturation to accommodate the growing brain, and this comes about by the appositional laying down of new bone on the outer surface of the cranial bones and the coordinated removal of bone at the inner surface.

Similarly, the shape of long bones of young vertebrates remains about the same as that of the mature animal. As with the cranium, the growth of a long bone (e.g., the femur) is not simply a matter of adding more matrix to the outer surface. If this were the case, the femur in the adult would be excessively heavy and the medullary cavity housing the bone marrow would be unacceptably small. Again, there is a coordinated formation of new bone at its outer surfaces and resorption of bone at the inner surfaces. An early study that demonstrated the manner of growth of the developing femur of the rat used the technique of *autoradiography* to follow the events that occurred during bone growth. Radiocalcium is injected into young rats and is rapidly deposited into bone that is being formed at the time. The deposited radiocalcium remains associated with that newly formed bone until it is resorbed during the growth process. The localization of radiocalcium in bone at any period after its injection can be visualized by autoradiography. After removal from the animal, the bone is cut longitudinally and placed on photographic film. The beta particles emitted from radiocalcium expose the film, and when the film is developed the location of the radiocalcium can be readily visualized. As shown in Fig. 30.13, features of the process of growth of the rat femur were deduced from the autoradiographic images. Much of the 30-day femur was replaced by newly forming bone at 100 days and still more at 200 days. This approach illustrates two points: (1) the shape of the femur does not grossly change during growth and (2) the marrow cavity enlarges during the growth process to assure a sufficient amount of bone marrow to meet requirements for blood cell formation.

The curvatures at either end of the femur result from different rates of bone formation and resorption at the convex and concave surfaces. An increase in the width of cortical bone occurs since bone formation under the periosteum takes place at a somewhat more rapid rate than resorption under the endosteum.

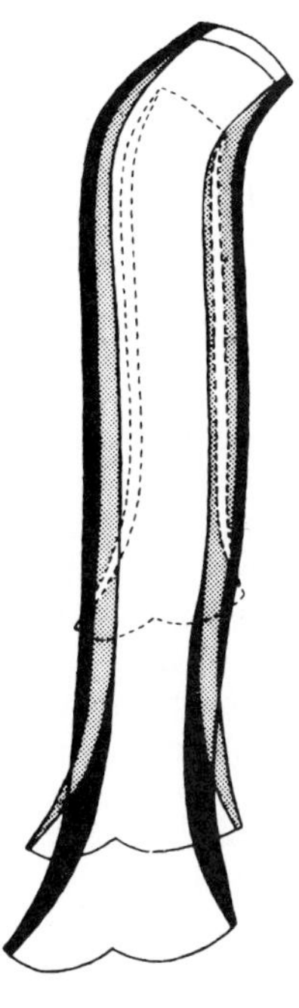

Figure 30.13. Three stages in the growth of the femur in the rat. (From Tomlin, Henry, and Kon 1953, *Br. J. Nutr.* 7:235–52. By courtesy of the British Journal of Nutrition.)

Even as bone is growing in size, internal reconstruction is taking place, principally through the formation, destruction, and remodeling of the Haversian systems (osteons). Osteoclasts associated with blood vessels erode through the endosteal surface, forming channels oriented with the long axis of the shaft (Fig. 30.14). A layer of osteoblasts forms on the surface of the eroded tunnel, and successive layers of lamellar bone are laid down, enclosing osteocytes within their lacunae. As the blood vessels grow and branch with accompanying osteoclasts and osteoblasts, new channels are made and new osteons form to surround them. These initial osteons are termed the Haversian system of the first generation. Subsequently, the first-generation osteons may be eroded by similar processes and replaced by Haversian systems of the second and later generations (Fig. 30.3). The newer osteons usually cut across more than one of the older osteons, giving rise to a complicated pattern of lamellae that are generally concentric. A cement line separates adjacent osteons at their boundaries.

Wolff's law of the skeleton

The morphology of bone, in addition to being genetically programmed for its general shape and length, is also affected by external and internal stresses and factors. The internal factors that affect the mass of bone include hormones, growth factors, and nutritional status. The response of the skeleton to external stresses is encompassed in *Wolff's law,* which simply states that the organization of bone is controlled in large measure by mechanical activity. The organization of bone can change to meet mechanical and other stresses placed on the skeleton, and it represents a balance between bone formation and bone resorption. Bone atrophy accompanies loss of muscle mass and decreased mobility; in contrast, an increase in muscle mass and exercise is accompanied by an increase in bone mass. Osteoporosis, for example, is less prevalent in women of greater

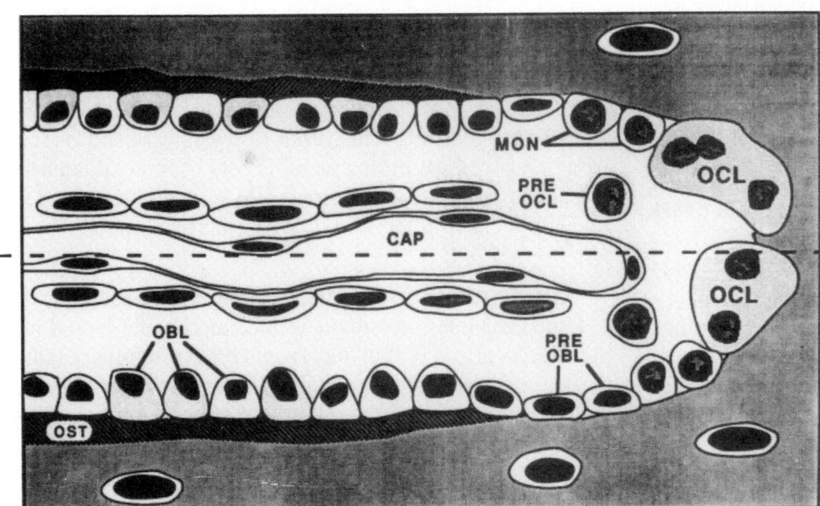

Figure 30.14. Diagram of the histology of bone remodeling. The figure is a camera lucida drawing of an osteon. An endosteal bone remodeling unit is basically an osteon bisected along its longitudinal axis (---) with marrow and/or a layer of bone lining cells forming the bisection surface. Two osteoclasts (OCL) form the apex of the resorptive or cutting cone. The reversal zone, where radial resorption occurs, is occupied by spindle-shaped preosteoblasts (PREOBL), large mononuclear preosteoclasts (PREOCL) and smaller reversal phase monocytes (MON). The bone-forming or closing cone contains osteoblasts (OBL) on an osteoid surface (OST). Loose vascular connective tissue with capillaries (CAP) is the source or transmitter of precursors of these cells. (From Huffer 1988, Morphology and biochemistry of bone remodeling: Possible control by vitamin D, parathyroid hormone and other substances, *Lab. Invest.* 59:418–41. © U.S.-Canadian Academy of Pathology, Inc.)

body weight and muscle mass than women of lower body weight and muscle mass. Obese persons usually have a large skeletal mass and are less frequently osteoporotic than thinner persons.

An interesting illustration of the operation of Wolff's law comes from a comparison of the bone mass of the humeri of professional tennis players. The humerus of the racquet-holding, serving arm had a 35 percent greater cortical thickness than the humerus of the arm that merely threw the ball into the air. In contrast, immobilization and bed rest, as shown by clinical studies, resulted in a 0.9 percent loss of vertebral bone mass per week of confinement.

The site in bone that detects the alteration in mechanical stress has not been conclusively identified. One possibility relates to the piezoelectrical property of bone mineral and collagen. Stresses placed on crystals with this property give rise to an electric potential that, in bone, might represent the signal that influences bone cell metabolism. Another possible sensor is the osteocyte network. Osteocytes embedded in bone within their lacunae are in an excellent strategic position to act as strain gauges and to secrete informational factors that influence osteoclastic or osteoblastic function or both.

Mineralization of cartilage and bone matrix

The organic matrix of cartilage and bone, as mentioned, provides the three-dimensional framework for the precise deposition of mineral. The deposition of mineral in the matrix of these specialized tissues is dependent on a number of factors. Collagen per se cannot alone account for the initiation of calcification, since type I collagen seen in bone is present in nonmineralizing tissues. A conclusion to be drawn from this fact is that the noncollagenous proteins in the matrix are important factors in determining the locality and extent of mineralization.

The concentrations of calcium and phosphorus in blood and in the extracellular fluid bathing the bone surfaces are important determinants of mineralization. If the concentrations of these ions in body fluids are low, mineralization does not occur or occurs at a slow rate. In vitamin D deficiency, for example, the intestinal absorption of these mineral ions is decreased. Mineralization of bone and cartilage is depressed, but the synthesis of the organic matrix continues, yielding the characteristic symptoms and signs of rickets and osteomalacia.

The process of mineralization can be arbitrarily divided into two parts: (1) the formation of the initial mineral and its the proper deposition in the organic matrix and (2) the subsequent and complete deposition of mineral. A number of theories to explain these processes have appeared over the years, and complete agreement on the validity of any one theory has not been attained. In fact, more than one explanation might be required to account for the complex process of mineralization at each and every site.

The prominent theories are based primarily on either physicochemical considerations (the nucleation theory) or the direct involvement of cellular and enzymatic events (the matrix vesicle theory). Briefly stated, the problem for bone researchers is to explain how calcium and phosphorus in the extracellular fluid make the transition from the soluble state to the solid crystalline state and deposit in precise localities within bone and cartilage.

The nucleation theory

The operation of the nucleation theory depends on evidence that the ion concentrations of calcium and phosphate in the extracellular fluid bathing the organic matrix are supersaturated with respect to formation of the primary bone salt, hydroxyapatite, although in a metastable state. The deposition of hydroxyapatite can be induced by the presence of either preformed crystals of hydroxyapatite (*homogeneous nucleation*) or an organic molecule with appropriate surface-oriented groupings complementary to hydroxyapatite (*heterogeneous nucleation*). The attraction and concentration of the soluble minerals on the surfaces of these nucleating substances provide energetically favorable circumstances for the formation and initial deposition of bone mineral.

The fibrous protein, collagen, as shown by X-ray diffraction and electron diffraction, has a crystalline structure and can act as a nucleating center for the deposition or precipitation of calcium phosphate salts. Reconstituted native collagen (64 nm repeating unit) from skin and tendon induces crystal nucleation when added to metastable calcium-phosphate solutions. When the molecular structure of the isolated collagen is altered, the ability to induce nucleation or crystallization is lost. The deposition of the mineral phase appears to occur in spaces or holes located within the collagen fibers of the organic matrix. These spaces might provide not only nucleation sites but also a suitable micro-environment for a phase transition to occur (i.e., from a solution phase to a solid state).

Sialoproteins, phosphoproteins, and osteocalcin have calcium-binding properties, and their potential as nucleation centers for hydroxyapatite formation has been proposed. It has also been suggested that members of this group of proteins might also control crystal size and crystal growth, as well as serving as inhibitors of mineral deposition at inappropriate sites. Lipids are another class of molecules implicated in the initiation of calcification.

Matrix vesicles in the mineralization process

Matrix vesicles are small, round, membrane-bound organelles localized within the organic matrix of mineralizing tissues and are truly extracellular. Matrix vesicles arise by budding of the plasma membrane of chondrocytes and osteoblasts to form noninverted vesicles.

Ultrastructural studies of growth plate cartilage reveal that matrix vesicles are restricted to the region of calcification and that the first crystals of mineral appearing in these

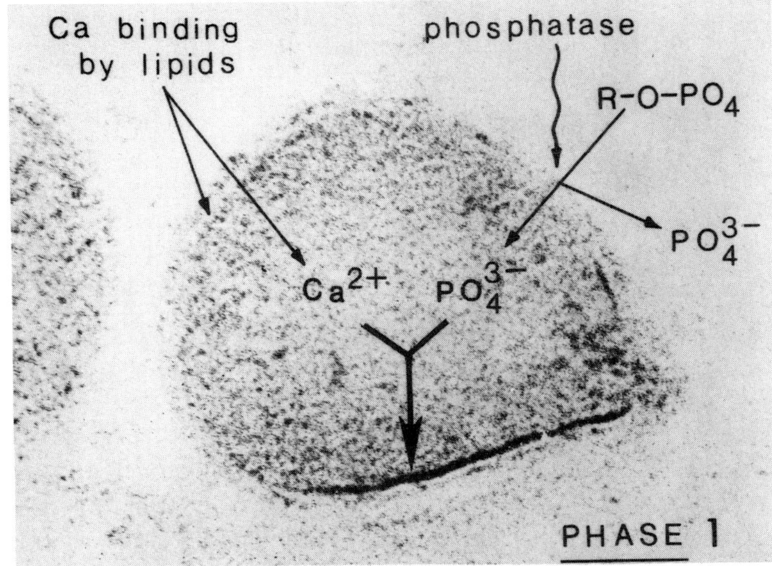

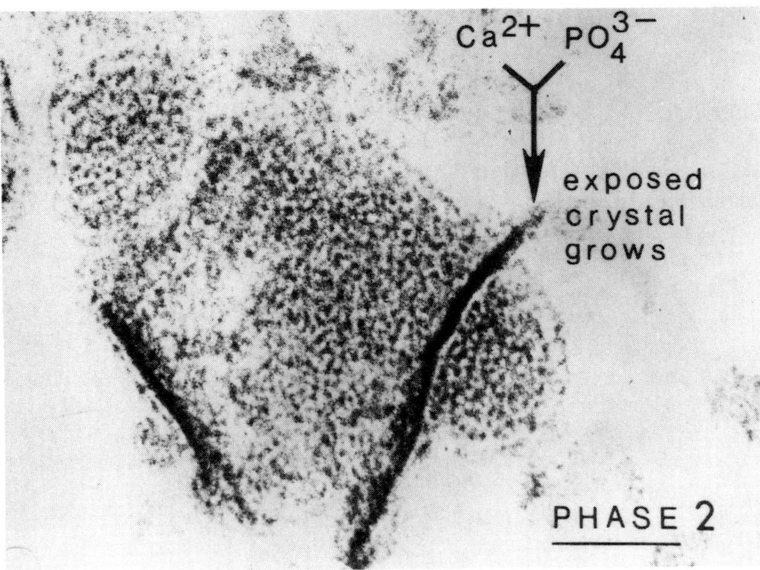

Figure 30.15. Scheme for mineralization in matrix vesicles. During phase 1, intravesicular calcium concentration is increased by its affinity for lipids of the vesicle membrane interior. Phosphatase (e.g., alkaline phosphatase, pyrophosphatase, or adenosine triphosphatase) at the vesicle membrane acts upon ester phosphate of matrix or vesicle fluid to produce a local increase in PO_4 in the vicinity of the vesicle membrane. The intravesicular ionic product ($Ca^{2+} \times PO_4$) is thereby raised, resulting in initial deposition of Ca and PO_4 near the membrane. With accumulation and growth, intravesicular crystals are exposed to the extravesicular fluid, which in normal animals is supersaturated with respect to apatite, enabling further crystal proliferation. Matrix vesicles pictured are in rat growth plate cartilage. (Reprinted from Anderson 1978, *Metab. Bone Dis. Relat. Res.* 1:83. Copyright 1978, with permission from Pergamon Press Ltd, Headington Hill Hall, Oxford 0X3 0BW, UK.)

calcifying regions are within the matrix vesicles. These initial crystals are in close association with the inner membrane of the vesicle; later, crystals of mineral are observed on the external surface of these vesicles (Fig. 30.15). Matrix vesicles have been identified in cartilage, bone, dentin, fracture callus, and calcifying tumors. The constituents and properties of matrix vesicles provide considerable support for an important role in the calcification mechanism. These vesicles contain a high concentration of *alkaline phosphatase,* an enzyme that catalyzes the hydrolysis of a number of phosphorylated organic compounds. This enzyme was shown many years ago to be present in calcifying regions of bone. Glycogen is known to accumulate in hypertrophic chondrocytes and to disappear before cell degeneration takes place. During glycogen breakdown, organic phosphate esters that might serve as substrates for alkaline phosphatase and as sources of inorganic phosphate are formed.

The presence of alkaline phosphatase in the membrane of matrix vesicles and the possible mediated transport of phosphate into the vesicle interior provide a mechanism for restricting phosphate ions to a small, confined space. The membrane also provides a barrier to prevent the dissolution of the more soluble initial mineral crystals before their conversion to hydroxyapatite. It has also been suggested that phosphatase enzymes are involved in the uphill transport of calcium into these vesicles.

The membrane of the matrix vesicle is enriched in acidic phospholipids, particularly phosphatidyl serine. These phos-

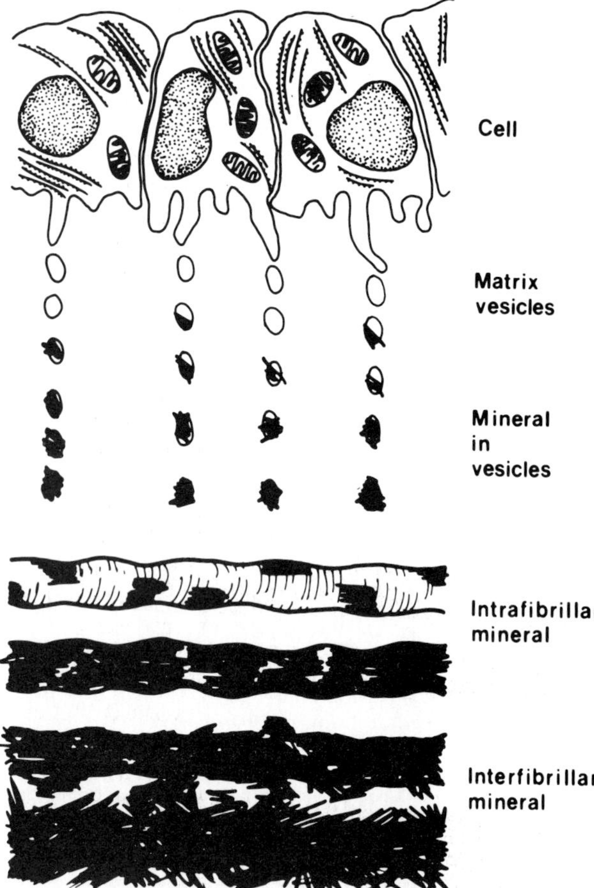

Figure 30.16. Hypothetical scheme of cell-mediated biological mineralization. The contribution of mitochondrial mineral deposits (seen as dark granules in some mitochondria) to mineralization, the mechanism of vesicle movement, and the intermediates between vesicular and intrafibrillar mineralization are unknown. (From Marks and Popoff 1988, *Am. J. Anat.* 183:1–44.)

pholipids have the ability to bind calcium and calcium-acidic phospholipid-phosphate complexes have the capacity to initiate hydroxyapatite precipitation. With alkaline phosphatase and its potential for providing increased concentrations of phosphate or calcium ions to the matrix vesicle, the conditions are suitable for new crystal formation. Figure 30.16 depicts a scheme of biological mineralization based on a significant role of matrix vesicles in the initiation of the calcification process. As shown, the initial mineral formed by matrix vesicles or other mechanisms first deposits in "hole" regions of the collagen fiber. Subsequent deposition of mineral occurs in close association with the three-dimensional framework of collagen.

Another function visualized for alkaline phosphatase and other phosphatases of the matrix compartment is the removal of *inhibitors* of calcification. These inhibitors of calcification are present in bone and include pyrophosphate and adenosine triphosphate. Hydrolysis of these inhibitors by phosphatases could promote and continue mineral deposition and crystal growth.

Mitochondria

The mitochondria of bone and cartilage cells also have the capacity to accumulate calcium, and this particular function of mitochondria also bears on the overall mechanism of calcification. Before calcification of the epiphyseal growth plate, the mitochondria of chondrocytes become loaded with calcium and phosphate. During calcification, the mitochondria lose their calcium and phosphate, presumably providing a source of mineral for the process of calcification. The calcium and phosphate released from mitochondria could also provide mineral for subsequent accumulation by matrix vesicles.

Bone resorption

Resorption is the dissolution of the matrix of bone through the action of bone cells. Both classes of matrix constituents—the insoluble and soluble organic constituents—need to be degraded and solubilized. The products therefrom (i.e., the peptides and amino acids from bone proteins and the mineral ions) are subsequently transferred to the systemic circulation. Osteoclasts are mainly responsible for bone resorption, but osteoblasts, traditionally assigned a role exclusively in bone formation, also participate directly and indirectly in the bone resorptive process.

Mature osteoclasts, as previously described, are large, mobile, multinucleated bone cells that are attached to bone surfaces that are undergoing resorption. Figure 30.17 shows an osteoclast on a bone surface and an underlying cavity resulting from its resorbing activity. Resorption occurs in the region of the ruffled border, the specialized fingerlike projections that extend from the plasma membrane of the osteoclast into the bone surface undergoing resorption. The tight binding of the osteoclast at the bone surface with the ruffled border encloses a sealed space where bone-resorbing activity takes place. It is into this confined region that acid is secreted to degrade and dissolve bone mineral and into which proteolytic enzymes are secreted to degrade and dissolve the organic matrix (Figs. 30.18 and 30.19). The secreted proteases have a pH optimum in the acid range and are derived from primary lysosomes that are prominent in osteoclasts during active resorption. The intracellular lysosomes fuse with the membrane of ruffled border and, by exocytosis, release their acid proteases and acid phosphatases into the acid environment at the bone surface. The completely solubilized components enter the osteoclast by diffusion or mediated transport processes and are then extruded into the extracellular fluid on the vascular side of the cell. Partially degraded mineral and organic constituents could also be transferred into the cell by endocytosis; the endocytotic vesicles coalesce with primary lysosomes, forming secondary lyso-

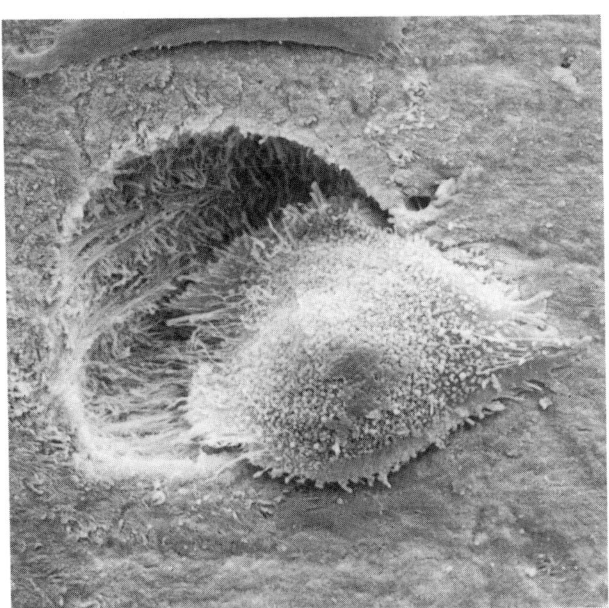

Figure 30.17. Higher-magnification scanning electron micrograph of a human osteoclast overlying a resorption cavity. The cavity base consists of partially demineralized organic fibrils. In the pit wall and base are seen blind-ending fibrils, the continuity of which has clearly been interrupted during resorption. Osteoclasts resorb both mineral and organic components of bone unaided by other cell types. Bar, 8 μm. (From Chambers 1989, The origin of the osteoclast. In *Bone and Mineral Research,* Elsevier Science Publishing Co., Amsterdam.)

somes, where further breakdown of the engulfed particles occurs.

Recent studies have provided biochemical details of some of the events in bone resorption. The secretion of acid appears to be analogous to the process of acid secretion in the stomach (Fig. 30.20). Carbonic anhydrase and a proton-pumping adenosine triphosphatase have been identified in bone-resorbing cells. Carbonic anhydrase catalyzes the formation of carbonic acid (H_2CO_3) from carbon dioxide, a by-product of cell metabolism, and water. Carbonic acid dissociates into bicarbonate (HCO_3^-) and hydrogen ions (protons). The latter are actively transported into the confined space at the bone surface by an adenosine triphosphate–dependent proton pump. The acid environment facilitates the solubilization of bone mineral and provides for the optimal activity of lysosomally derived acid proteases and phosphatases. The release of lactic and citric acids by osteoclasts might contribute to the acidity at the bone surface in accordance with the earlier "acid theory" of Neuman.

Collagenase, the enzyme that degrades collagen with high specificity, is known to be secreted by osteoblasts under the influence of parathyroid hormone (PTH). Osteoblastic collagenase is thought to partially remove osteoid from the bone surface. Although there is not complete agreement on the function of this process, it is proposed by some that it increases the chemoattractive potential of the bone surface for osteoclasts. The classic collagenase is a metalloprotease with an optimal pH in the neutral range and, for this reason, is thought not to have a significant role

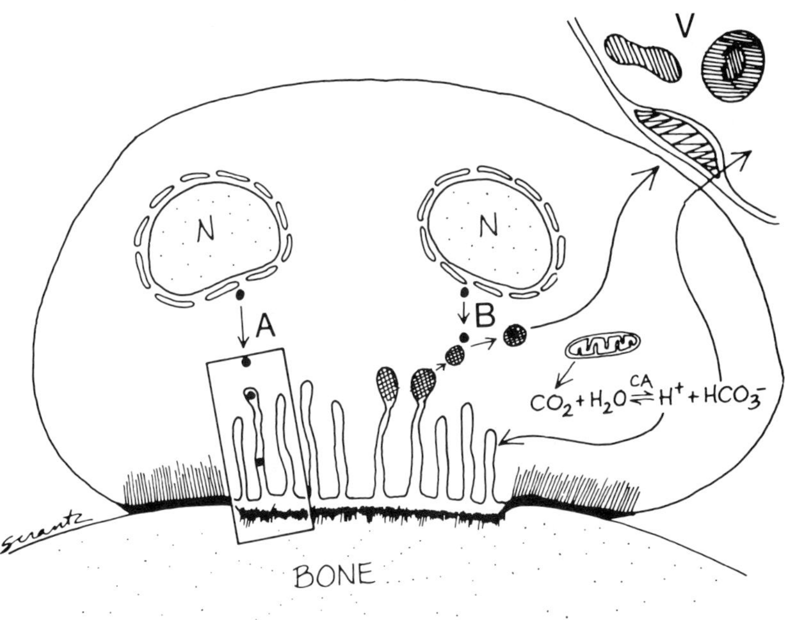

Figure 30.18. Diagram of the mechanism of bone resorption by osteoclasts. Enzymes packaged in the perinuclear Golgi region (A) move to the ruffled border region, where they are released into the confined space next to mineralized tissue. Products of resorption are taken back up into the cell (B) further digested in secondary lysosomes, and released in adjacent venous sinuses (V) Products of cell respiration are catalyzed by carbonic anhydrase (CA, located in ruffled border) to produce hydrogen ions, which acidify the confined extracellular compartment below the ruffled border, thus providing an optimal environment for the action of acid hydrolases. The outlined area is shown at higher magnification in Figure 30.19. (From Marks and Popoff 1988, *Am. J. Anat.* 183:1–44.)

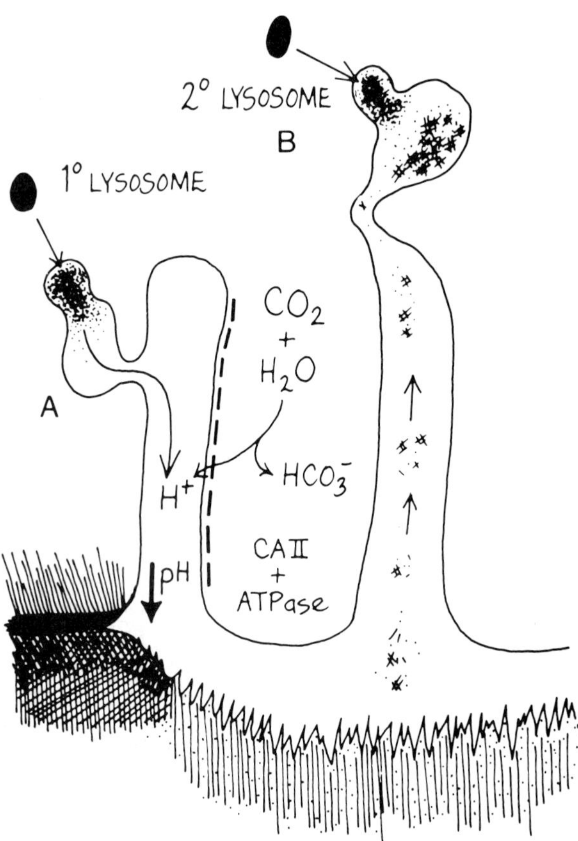

Figure 30.19. The exocytic and endocytic pathways of bone resorption. (From Marks and Popoff 1988, *Am. J. Anat.* 183:1–44.)

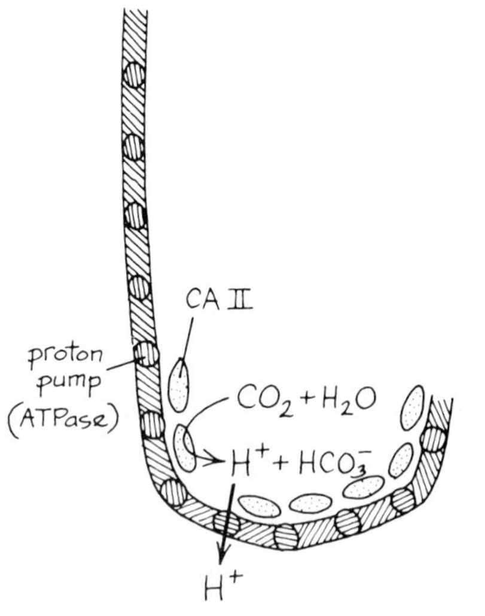

Figure 30.20. Higher magnification of the plasma membrane in the region of the ruffled border illustrating the intramembranous location of the ATPase and the location of carbonic anhydrase II (CA-II) on the cytoplasmic side of the membrane. (From Marks and Popoff 1988, *Am. J. Anat.* 183:1–44.)

in osteoclastic bone resorption, which occurs in an acid environment. The acid hydrolases secreted by osteoclasts are presumably sufficient to account for osteoid degradation and dissolution without a requirement for neutral collagenase.

The osteocytes are also capable of resorbing bone from the surfaces of the lacunae in which the osteocyte resides. The term applied here is *osteocytic osteolysis* in contrast to *osteoclastic osteolysis*. Replacement of the resorbed lacunar bone is also carried out by the osteocyte, and these two osteocytic processes (i.e., bone removal and bone replacement) participate in the remodeling of the bone. Both osteoclastic osteolysis and osteocytic osteolysis are stimulated by parathyroid hormone, providing the means for maintaining normal serum calcium levels.

Bone repair

The process of repairing a broken bone exemplifies the dependence of bone formation on an adequate blood supply, the signal that attracts the bone-forming cells to the break, and the phenomenon of bone remodeling that yields a mended bone that is almost indistinguishable from the intact bone. This discussion will deal only with a *simple fracture* (Fig. 30.21).

To facilitate the repair of a simple fracture, the two broken ends of the bone are mechanically realigned and stabilized by either external (a cast) or internal (pinning) fixation. At the break, the soft tissues, including the periosteum and the endosteum, are torn and some of the blood vessels are severed. Severe bleeding at the break is followed by clot formation. Some of the torn blood vessels are those that enter the Haversian canal at the fracture line and those that supply the periosteum and the endosteum. Because of the interruption of the circulation, there is a lack of oxygen and nutrients, and the osteocytes in the region of the break die. This is revealed histologically by the presence of empty lacunae. The periosteum and the bone marrow also become necrotic because of the interrupted blood supply.

Initially, there is an acute inflammatory reaction, and subsequently phagocytes begin to remove the components of the blood clot, the blood cells, and dead tissue. As blood vessels proliferate and begin to move into the region of the break, the process of osteogenesis (new bone formation) begins. This emphasizes the requirement of an adequate blood supply for bone formation.

Two general types of bone repair have been described: indirect and direct. Indirect bone repair involves *callus* formation, and the direct process of bone repair involves the direct appositional union of the broken ends of the fractured bone.

The *callus* is comprised of a *collar* of repair tissue that forms around the external surface of the fragment and, as it grows, forms a bridge across the break (the *external callus*). Similarly, callus forms in the medullary cavity and also forms a bridge termed the *internal callus*.

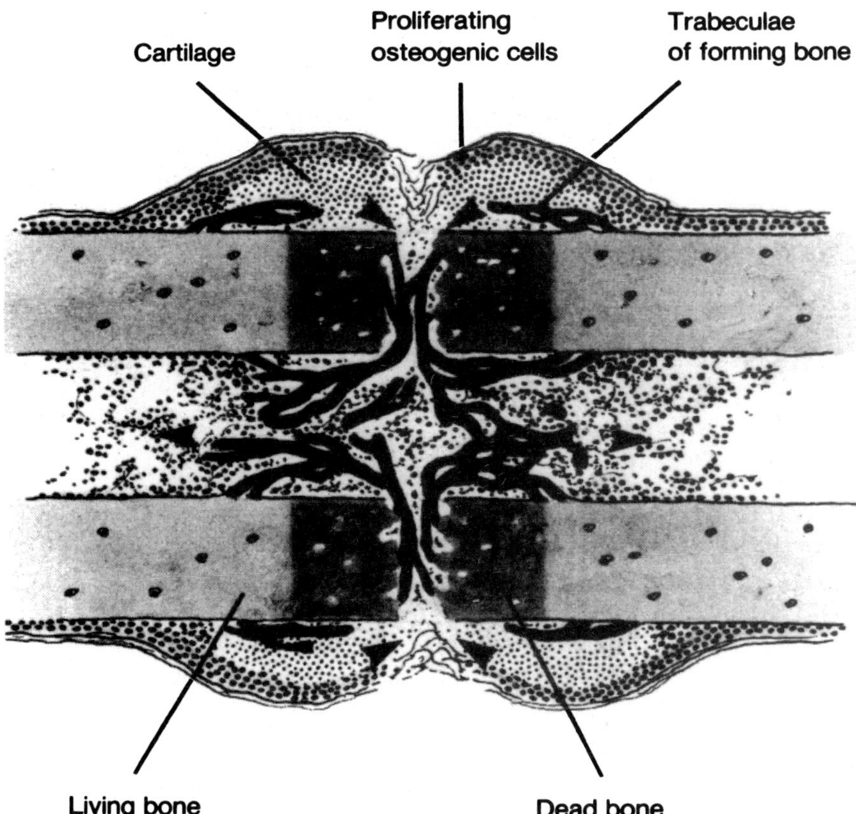

Figure 30.21. Summary diagram of healing rib fracture. New cancellous bone is shown in black; cartilage is indicated in light stipple. Arrowheads indicate the direction of growth of trabeculae of new bone in the external and internal callus. (From Cormack 1987, Bone, in *Ham's Histology,* 9th ed., J.B. Lippincott, Philadelphia.)

The healthy intact periosteum is the origin of the osteogenic cells for external callus formation. These cells begin to proliferate and extend in both directions toward the break. Where there is a rich supply of periosteal capillaries in the deeper regions of the periosteum, the osteogenic cells differentiate into osteoblasts that produce true bone of the cancellous type. These trabecular fragments, firmly attached to the preexisting bone, grow from each fragment of the break and eventually fuse. Where the blood supply is inadequate in the outer layers of growing callus, the osteogenic cells differentiate into chondrocytes to form cartilage within this avascular environment.

As depicted in Fig. 30.21, three regions of the external callus are identifiable: the bony trabeculae cemented to the bone tissue, an intermediate cartilaginous zone, and the outer zone comprising proliferating osteogenic cells. The peripheral, external calluses, by growth and eventual fusion, have sufficient strength to stabilize the fracture. The internal calluses also grow and fuse, but this fusion yields a weaker union than that of the external callus.

The cartilage that first forms in the avascular region of the callus is subsequently replaced by true bone. The transformation of this cartilage into bone is similar to that which occurs in the epiphyseal growth plate of long bones during growth. The chondrocytes hypertrophy, and the cartilage matrix becomes calcified. When blood vessels extend into this region, the calcified cartilage is removed and replaced with trabecular bone by the action of osteoblastic cells.

As part of the process of bone repair, the dead bone closest to the break is resorbed by osteoclasts and is replaced by new bone. After a firm union is established by the growth and fusion of both external and internal calluses, there is extensive remodeling and the newly formed trabecular bone is transformed into dense cortical bone.

The formation of the callus must certainly depend on the secretion of various growth and mitogenic factors. One of the most likely mitogenic factors is the bone morphogenetic proteins that have osteoinductive potential. This class of proteins, as previously described, has the property of attracting osteogenic precursor cells that transform into bone-forming cells. Also, angiogenic factors are certainly important in stimulating the growth of blood vessels into the repair tissue, providing a source of oxygen and nutrients to support bone cell activity.

In addition to bone repair through callus formation, a direct union can occur in compact bone at the site of the break. A prerequisite for this process of bone repair appears to be rigid stabilization of the two ends of the fracture in close apposition by mechanical devices (e.g., the use of pins, lag screws, and compression plates). With these constraints in place, blood vessels and accompanying osteogenic cells from the Haversian canals can extend into the dead bone. Osteoclasts form resorption tunnels in the dead bone, after which osteoblasts lay down new bone. Osteons are formed and extend across the break in a manner that is analogous to the joining of parts of wooden furniture with the use of wooden pegs. This union of the fractured ends of bone is a comparatively slow process, and the newly formed bone is often of the immature type. Thereafter, extensive remodeling occurs to complete the repair process and to form mature, strong bone.

Regulation of bone metabolism and mineral homeostasis

The growth and metabolism of the skeleton are controlled by a number of factors that include systemic hormones, systemic and local growth factors, and mitogenic factors. Affected by these substances are the development of the skeleton, the control of the growth of the skeleton, and the turnover and renewal of bone by the coordinated activity of osteoblasts, osteocytes, and osteoclasts.

Systemic hormones are more specifically involved in the homeostatic regulation of plasma calcium levels through their effects on bone as well as on other organs (intestine, kidney). Parathyroid hormone was the first of these *calciotropic* hormones to be discovered, and subsequently two other hormones that act directly on bone—$1,25(OH)_2D_3$ and calcitonin—became known.

Growth and mitogenic factors that control bone cell multiplication, differentiation, and metabolism have attracted considerable attention recently. These include the prostaglandins and various polypeptide growth factors, such as epidermal growth factor, insulinlike growth factor, the interleukins, and transforming growth factor.

Systemic hormones

Parathyroid hormone. Parathyroid hormone is secreted from parathyroid glands in response to a low blood calcium concentration. A major effect of PTH, and consonant with its calcium homeostatic function, is the stimulation of the resorption of bone by osteoclasts. This action supplies calcium ions to the circulatory system, contributing to the maintenance of normal plasma calcium levels. Both the activity and the number of osteoclasts are increased by PTH. Despite these effects, PTH receptors have not been found in *mature* osteoclasts. PTH, however, does directly affect the osteoblasts, and the stimulation of osteoclasts is thought to be due to factors elaborated by osteoblasts in response to PTH. Figure 30.22 shows some of the features of the proposed interactions between osteoblasts and bone-resorbing cells. The increase in the osteoclastic cell population, on the other hand, might be a direct effect of PTH on the differentiation and fusion of monocytes that are precursors of mature osteoclasts.

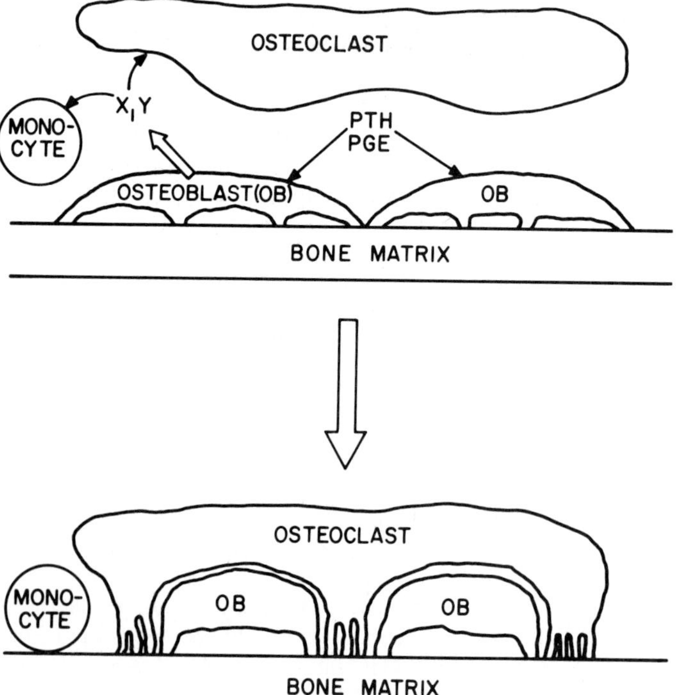

Figure 30.22. Schematic representation of osteoblast involvement in hormone-stimulated bone resorption. This proposed scheme visualizes a direct effect of parathyroid hormone (PTH) and other resorbing agents, such as prostaglandins (PGE), on the osteoblast. The osteoblast, through a change in shape, exposes bone matrix. Osteoclasts now have access to the bone matrix, and resorption is initiated. The products of this digestion attract osteoclast precursor cells, the monocytes. Hormone action on osteoblasts could also cause the release of a substance (x,y) from the osteoblast, which more directly influences the resorptive activity of the osteoclast and monocytes. (From Rodan and Martin 1981, *Calcif. Tissue Int.* 33:349–51.)

In osteoblasts, PTH stimulates the formation of the second messenger, cyclic adenosine monophosphate (cAMP), and this reaction has been useful in characterizing the cells of osteoblastic lineage. Cyclic AMP elaborated by osteoblasts has been considered to be one of the paracrine factors affecting osteoclastic activity. The injection of a derivative of cAMP (dibutyryl cAMP) into animals stimulates bone resorption, and the addition of dibutyryl cAMP increases the resorption of bone in tissue culture. Prostaglandins, particularly PGE_2, have also been suggested as local factors controlling bone resorption. At certain concentrations, PTH stimulates the synthesis of PGE_2 by osteoblasts.

Activation of osteoclasts causes the rapid development of the ruffled border at the bone surface and the appearance of a number of vacuoles within the cytoplasm. There are also increases in acid production and the synthesis and secretion of hydrolytic enzymes, events that are intimately associated with osteoclastic bone resorption.

Osteoblasts, in response to PTH stimulation, change shape and shrink, exposing bone matrix that seemingly contains chemotactic substances that attract osteoclasts to the bone surface. The synthesis of collagen and other matrix proteins by osteoblasts is inhibited, and the secretion of collagenase and other proteolytic enzymes is stimulated. Collagenase is elaborated as a latent enzyme that is activated by proteolytic cleavage. A protease implicated in the activation process is plasminogen-activating factor (PAF). PAF converts plasminogen to plasmin, another protease that converts latent collagenase to the active form. PAF production by bone cells is stimulated by PTH, $1,25(OH)_2D_3$, and other factors.

Some of the latent collagenase binds to matrix proteins, including collagen, and is later released and activated during osteoclastic bone resorption. The activity of neutral collagenase would depend on its being located at a site in the matrix remote from the acid environment.

Although the catabolic effect of PTH has been emphasized thus far, PTH also has anabolic activity in terms of new bone formation. The bone-resorbing catabolic effect of PTH occurs on the continuous exposure of bone tissue to relatively high concentrations of PTH. The anabolic activity of PTH, in contrast, is associated more with the intermittent exposure of bone cells to low concentrations of the hormone. Under these conditions, both the number and the activity of the bone-forming osteoblasts are increased. Bone cell–derived growth factors, such as insulinlike growth factor (IGF) and transforming growth factor-beta, have been implicated in the anabolic effect of PTH.

In the kidney PTH inhibits phosphate reabsorption, thereby increasing the urinary excretion of this anion (*the phosphaturic response*) and, in addition, increases the reabsorption of calcium by the kidney tubule.

PTH indirectly increases the intestinal absorption of calcium and phosphorus through its stimulatory effect on the synthesis of the vitamin D hormone as discussed in the section on vitamin D.

Calcitonin. Calcitonin is produced and secreted by the C cells of the thyroid gland in mammals and the ultimobranchial gland in birds and lower vertebrates. The primary stimulus for secretion is hypercalcemia. This antihypercalcemic polypeptide hormone inhibits bone resorption, and this action appears to be a direct effect of the hormone on osteoclasts that do contain calcitonin receptors. There is a retraction of the cell membrane, with the "ruffled" border becoming less prominent. The osteoclast also separates from the bone surface and becomes less mobile, and lysosomal enzyme formation is inhibited. The formation of multinucleated mature osteoclasts from monocytic precursor cells might also be prevented. Biochemically, calcitonin action is associated with the increased synthesis of cAMP.

Exposure of bone tissue to calcitonin only transiently inhibits bone resorption and, on continued exposure to the hormone, bone resorptive activity resumes. This "escape" phenomenon is not well understood but could be due to two events: (1) the downregulation of calcitonin receptors on the osteoclasts and(or) (2) the formation of a population of osteoclasts that are resistant to calcitonin. The "escape" reaction is prevented by the coincubation of bone cells with calcitonin and either glucocorticoids or elevated concentrations of the phosphate ion.

Because of its inhibitory effects on bone resorption, calcitonin has been examined as a potential therapeutic agent to offset the bone loss that occurs in postmenopausal osteoporosis.

Vitamin D. Vitamin D deficiency causes rickets in the growing animal and osteomalacia in the adult. Both diseases are characterized by a depressed mineralization of the skeleton while synthesis of uncalcified matrix, the osteoid, continues. The result is bone with a low ash (mineral) content. Although the primary cause of rickets and osteomalacia is vitamin D deficiency, other disorders produce similar pathological conditions, such as steatorrhea in which there is a malabsorption of vitamin D by the intestine, renal tubular defects, or chronic uremia. In rickets and osteomalacia, the blood calcium level is either normal or low, the blood phosphate level is low, and the blood alkaline phosphatase level is either high or normal.

A source of vitamin D is the diet, which could contain the plant form of the vitamin, vitamin D_2 (ergocalciferol), or the animal form, vitamin D_3 (cholecalciferol). Another source is the endogenous production of vitamin D_3 by the exposure of skin to sunlight or other sources of ultraviolet rays. The acquired vitamin D_3* is converted biochemically

*Both vitamin D_2 and vitamin D_3 are similarly transformed, respectively, to $25(OH)D_2$ and $25(OH)D_3$, $1,25(OH)_2D_2$ and $1,25(OH)_2D_3$, and $24,25(OH)_2D_2$ and $24,25(OH)_2D_3$. The vitamin D_2 forms have the same qualitative biological effects as the vitamin D_3 forms, but responses can be quantitatively different. For brevity in the following discussion, reference will be made primarily to the vitamin D_3 forms.

into a number of metabolites, three of which are of especial biological significance. These are 25-hydroxycholecalciferol (25 [OH]D_3). 1,25 $(OH)_2D_3$, and 24,25-dihydroxycholecalciferol (24,25$[OH]_2D_3$ The 25(OH)D_3 metabolite, produced in the liver, is the major circulating form of the vitamin and is primarily bound in blood to the vitamin D–binding protein. The serum level of this metabolite has been used as an indicator of vitamin D status. The 25(OH)D_3, metabolite is further hydroxylated in the kidney, forming the most biologically active metabolite, 1,25$(OH)_2D_3$ considered to be the hormonal form of the vitamin. The formation of 1,25$(OH)_2D_3$, is stimulated by a direct effect of PTH on kidney cells. Thus a hypocalcemic condition that promotes the release of PTH also results in the PTH-stimulated synthesis of the vitamin D hormone, 1,25$(OH)_2D_3$ (Fig. 30.23).

The other dihydroxylated metabolite, 24,25$(OH)_2D_3$, is also produced by renal cells. Its production is highest in normocalcemic states and decreases during periods of hypocalcemia when the synthesis of 1,25$(OH)_2D_3$ increases. The role of 24,25$(OH)_2D_3$ in mineral homeostasis and bone metabolism has been controversial, although some reports have suggested a direct effect of this metabolite on the skeleton.

A major site of action of 1,25$(OH)_2D_3$ is the intestine, which stimulates the absorption of calcium and phosphorus that contributes to the maintenance of serum calcium and phosphorus concentrations. The antirachitic and anti-osteomalacic effects of vitamin D are thought to be due primarily to this physiological effect, supplying calcium

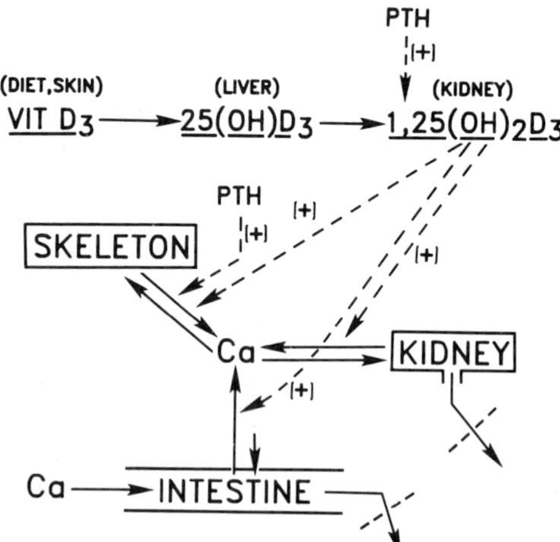

Figure 30.23. Major homoestatic effects of vitamin D_3. Diagrammed are the two hydroxylation steps that yield the vitamin D hormone, 1,25-dihydroxyvitamin D_3 (1,25$[OH]_2D_3$). Parathyroid hormone (PTH), as well as other factors (not shown), increases the rate of conversion of 25-hydroxyvitamin D_3 (25[OH]D_3) to 1,25$(OH)_2D_3$. 1,25$(OH)_2D_3$ stimulates bone resorption, as does PTH. 1,25$(OH)_2D_3$ also stimulates the intestinal absorption and the renal tubules reabsorption of calcium (Ca).

and phosphorus to the body for subsequent incorporation into bone during the mineralization process.

The resorption of bone is also stimulated by 1,25$(OH)_2D_3$ and, in many ways, acts similarly to PTH by increasing the activity and the number of bone-resorbing cells. The osteolytic function of 1,25$(OH)_2D_3$, like that of PTH, contributes calcium to the blood circulatory system, providing the calcium essential for soft tissue metabolism and for the mineralization of bone at sites remote from where the calcium was derived. Receptors for 1,25$(OH)_2D_3$ are present in osteoblasts and are not yet found in mature osteoclasts. However, 1,25$(OH)_2D_3$ receptors are located in preosteoclasts and, again like PTH, appear to affect the differentiation and coalescence of these precursor cells into mature multinucleated osteoclasts. The increase in the resorbing activity of the resident cell population is also thought to result from the elaboration of factors from osteoblasts that secondarily influence osteoclastic activity.

In the target cells, 1,25$(OH)_2D_3$ acts like other steroids by inducing the synthesis of proteins by gene transcription. The first proteins shown to be induced are the vitamin D-dependent intestinal calcium-binding proteins. Two types of induced calcium-binding proteins, named the calbindins, have been identified—one in mammalian intestine with a molecular weight of about 9000 and a larger protein of about 28,000 to 30,000. The larger protein calbindin-D_{28K}, is present in the avian intestine, kidney, shell gland, and other tissues, and a homologous calbindin-D_{28K} is present in mammalian kidney, brain, and other organs. In the intestine, the calbindins are considered to participate in intestinal absorption of calcium. In vitamin D deficiency, the intestinal absorption of calcium is depressed and the calbindins are virtually absent, providing part of the evidence that implicates a role of the protein in the calcium absorptive process.

Calbindin D_{9K} has recently been identified in matrix vesicles of cartilage in close association with the inner aspect of the matrix membrane. Because of its high affinity, calcium-binding properties, it has been suggested that calbindin has a role in the formation of mineral within these vesicles.

Growth hormone. Growth hormone or somatotropin is a peptide hormone secreted from the anterior pituitary gland. Growth hormone deficiency causes dwarfism and, in excess, results in gigantism in the growing animal or acromegaly in the adult. Removal of the pituitary gland (hypophysectomy) decreases the width of the epiphyseal growth plate in cats and dogs; this effect could be partially reversed with the injection of anterior pituitary extracts. It has been suggested that this increase in thickness of the epiphyseal cartilage by growth hormone is due to stimulation of the proliferation of the chondrocytes. Although other hormones, such as insulin and thyroid hormone, influence bone growth, growth hormone is considered to be the primary hormone that affects the longitudinal growth of bone.

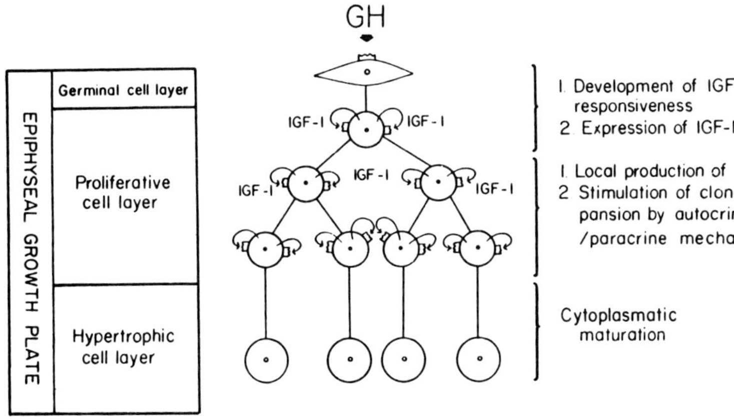

Figure 30.24. Hypothetical model for the stimulatory effect of GH on longitudinal bone growth. (From Isaksson, Lendahl, Nilsson, and Isgaard 1987, Mechanism of the stimulatory effect of growth hormone on longitudinal bone growth, *Endocr. Rev.* 8:426–438. © The Endocrine Society.)

A reliable assay of growth hormone depends on the dose-dependent increase in the width of the growth plate of hypophysectomized rats.

It is usually considered that the hormone does not act directly on responsive tissues but stimulates the synthesis and secretion of growth-stimulating factors from liver, the somatomedins. The somatomedins are also known as the insulin-like growth factors (IGFs). The latter designation is derived from the observation that somatomedins, like insulin, have antilipolytic effects on adipose tissue and increase the uptake of glucose and amino acids by skeletal muscle.

However, a current hypothesis suggests that both growth hormone and IGF have significant roles in controlling the growth of the epiphyseal growth plate (Fig. 30.24). Their effects are different but complementary. It is proposed that growth hormone causes the differentiation of prechondrocytes into chondrocytes, and and the chondrocytes become responsive to IGF. The differentiated chondrocyte synthesizes IGF itself and the secreted IGF binds to receptors, increasing the rate of proliferation of themselves (autocrine stimulation) or near neighbor cells (paracrine stimulation).

Estradiol. Much evidence of the effects of this steroid hormone on the skeleton comes from clinical experience with individuals afflicted with postmenopausal osteoporosis. In the postmenopausal state, there is an increase in bone turnover. The rate of bone resorption exceeds the rate of bone formation, yielding a net loss of bone mass. Replacement therapy with estrogens decreases bone resorption and, thus far, appears to be the most efficacious means of preserving the skeleton of the osteoporotic individual.

The biochemical and physiological mechanism of action of estrogens on bone metabolism is virtually unknown. Only recently, receptors for estrogen have been identified in isolated bone cells, cultured bone cells, and osteosarcoma cells of the osteoblastic phenotype. Continued studies of these estrogen-responsive cells might reveal how estrogen influences bone metabolism.

Glucocorticoids. Excess glucocorticoids are associated with net bone loss and contribute to the development of osteoporosis. It is proposed that the major effect of excess glucocorticoids is a depression of the absorption of calcium from the intestine. This results in secondary hyperparathyroidism, in which there is an increase in osteoclastic bone resorption and a decrease in bone formation. Glucocorticoids also decrease bone turnover in pathological states.

Thyroid hormones. Thyroid hormones are required for normal growth and development and act primarily through the stimulation and release of somatomedins by the liver. The somatomedins stimulate bone and cartilage growth and also exert direct effects on osteoclasts, increasing bone resorption.

Insulin. Insulin, secreted by the beta cells of the pancreas, is an important stimulator of bone matrix synthesis. In animals with experimental diabetes, there is a depressed growth of bone and cartilage and a decrease in skeletal mineralization. Part of the effect of insulin is mediated by somatomedins since insulin has a direct effect on the release of somatomedins from the liver. Insulin also stimulates the formation of $1{,}25(OH)_2D_3$ by renal tubules, and the insulin effect on mineralization might be mediated by way of the vitamin D hormone.

Other factors

The growth and mitogenic factors that influence bone cell metabolism have only recently come under intensive investigation. Some twenty factors, in addition to the more classic systemic hormones, have been identified, and their actions on the replication and metabolism of specific bone cell populations are being defined. Some of these are listed in Table 30.2. With few exceptions, information on the behavior of these factors has been derived from the study of cultured bone cells or cultured bone tissue. Although these in vitro approaches provide information about the potential significance of these factors in bone metabolism, additional studies are required to determine the extent and significance of their actions in the intact animal.

Table 30.2. Some growth factors isolated from bone matrix

1. Platelet-derived growth factor (PDGF)
2. Fibroblast growth factors (FGF)
   - Acidic FGF
   - Basic FGF
3. Insulin-like growth factors (IGF)
   - IGF-I
   - IGF-II
4. Transforming growth factors-β (TGF_β)
   - $TGF\beta_1$
   - $TGF\beta_2$
5. Osteoinductive factors or bone morphogenetic proteins (BMP)

From Canalis, McCarthy, and Centrella 1989, The role of growth factors in skeletal remodeling, *Endocrinol. Metab. Clin. North Am.* 18:903–18.

Locally derived factors, some synthesized in response to systemic factors, are produced by bone cells or bone-related cells and exert effects on the same type of cell or a different population of cells. In addition, some of factors derived from bone cells or the systemic circulation might become trapped within matrix of bone and activated on their release from bone matrix during the resorptive process. These latter include chemotactic and osteoinductive factors. All of these factors undoubtedly participate in the coordinated functioning of bone cells in growth and remodeling processes.

DISEASES AND DISORDERS OF BONE AND BONE METABOLISM*

One of the most common clinical abnormalities involving bone is a fracture or "broken bone." This has already been discussed under the heading of "Bone Repair." A large number of other diseases and metabolic disorders, however, can result in pathological changes in the skeleton. These include primary diseases of bone as well as abnormalities of other organ systems, which result in skeletal changes. Primary bone diseases such as osteitis, osteomyelitis, and bone tumors are beyond the scope of this discussion and will not be considered. The "secondary" diseases of bone, referred to as metabolic bone diseases, generally result from syndromes that cause alterations in the circulating concentrations of the previously discussed hormones, which are required for normal bone homeostasis.

Hyperparathyroidism

As already discussed, PTH is one of several systemic hormones that exert direct action on bone metabolism. Under normal circumstances the circulating level of PTH is controlled by modulation of secretion of this hormone from the parathyroid gland through feedback mechanisms based on the blood calcium concentration and perhaps other factors, including the vitamin D hormones. A number of abnormalities, however, can result in abnormal function of the parathyroid gland and, as a consequence, cause significant alterations of bone metabolism.

*The author of this section is F. A. Kallfelz.

Primary hyperparathyroidism

With primary hyperparathyroidism, which occurs almost exclusively in older animals, there is an excess and uncontrolled secretion of PTH and, therefore, increased circulating levels of this hormone caused by a lesion in the gland itself. Frequently primary hyperparathyroidism results from the presence of a parathyroid adenoma (a nonmalignant tumor). The clinical signs of this disease are related to the hypercalcemia that occurs and include muscle weakness, anorexia, and vomiting. Recently seizures have been described in a dog with primary hyperparathyroidism.

The increased circulating level of PTH that occurs in primary hyperparathyroidism promotes renal excretion of phosphorus and retention of calcium. In bone, excessive bone resorption occurs as a result of accelerated osteoclastic and osteocytic osteolysis, causing the occurrence of hypercalcemia in the presence of elevated blood PTH concentrations. The bone tissue that is lost is replaced by fibrous tissue, and the result is a condition known as fibrous osteodystrophy. Although this occurs throughout the skeleton, it is most prominent in bones that have a high content of cancellous bone tissue (see above), such as the mandible and the vertebrae.

Diagnosis of this disease is based on history and clinical signs as well as on the results of other diagnostic procedures (Table 30.3). Hypercalcemia is a primary finding but must be differentiated from other causes of this abnormality, such as vitamin D toxicity. An elevated blood phosphorus concentration is not found in this disease, since the input of phosphorus to the blood from bone resorption is offset by enhanced renal excretion induced by the elevated circulating concentrations of PTH. Radiographs will reveal skeletal demineralization, particularly in the mandible, skull, and vertebrae, and even fractures in chronic cases. If reliable immunoreactive parathyroid hormone (iPTH) assays are available, elevated circulating levels of this hormone will be found. Circulating concentrations of calcitonin (CT), if an assay is available, might be elevated because of the persistent hypercalcemia. Determination of the blood levels of vitamin D hormones would most likely reveal a normal concentration of $1,25(OH)_2D_3$ since the stimulatory effect of PTH on the 1-hydroxylase would be offset by the depressing effect of the hypercalcemia.

Treatment is based on elimination of the source of the excessive PTH, which requires surgical exploration and removal of the hyperfunctioning parathyroid gland. Generally only one of the four glands is involved, and the lesion is most often an adenoma of the affected gland that is manifested by a gross enlargement of that gland.

Secondary hyperparathyroidism

In addition to lesions in the parathyroid gland itself, other abnormalities can result in excessive secretion of PTH and thus cause many of the clinical signs seen in primary hyperparathyroidism. These conditions thus cause "secondary"

Table 30.3. Diagnostic criteria for selected plasma, biochemical parameters in metabolic bone disease

Disease condition*	Biochemical parameters					
	Ca	P	Alkaline phosphatase	iPTH	CT	$1,25(OH)_2D_3$
PHP	Elevated	Normal	Elevated	Elevated	Elevated	Normal
NSHP (Ca)	Normal-decreased	Normal	Elevated	Elevated	Decreased	Elevated
NSHP (D)	Decreased	Decreased	Elevated	Elevated	Decreased	Decreased
RSHP	Normal-decreased	Elevated	Elevated	Elevated	Decreased	Decreased
PSHP	Elevated	Normal	Elevated	Normal	Decreased	Decreased
HOP	Decreased	Normal-elevated	Decreased	Decreased	Decreased	Decreased
HCT	Normal-elevated	Normal	Decreased	Decreased	Elevated	Decreased
HVD	Elevated	Elevated	Normal	Decreased	Elevated	Normal-elevated†

*PHP, primary hyperparathyroidism; NSHP(Ca), nutritional secondary hyperparathyroidism due to calcium deficiency; NSHP(D), nutritional secondary hyperparathyroidism due to vitamin D deficiency; RSHP, renal secondary hyperparathyroidism; PSHP, pseudohyperparathyroidism; HOP, hypoparathyroidism; HCT, hypercalcitoninism; HVD, hypervitaminosis D; iPTH, immunoreactive parathyroid hormone; CT, calcitonin.

†Normal in most species, elevated in cattle.

hyperparathyroidism. The two such diseases seen most often are nutritional and renal secondary hyperparathyroidism.

Nutritional secondary hyperparathyroidism

A dietary deficiency of calcium or a lack of vitamin D can cause nutritional secondary hyperparathyroidism (NSHP). Although this is most often described in growing animals, it can also occur in adults, generally with somewhat different clinical signs. The pathophysiology of NSHP is related to the dietary deficiency. A lack of dietary calcium results in a relative hypocalcemia, which stimulates the parathyroid gland to secrete PTH. The increased concentration of this hormone, as well as the decreased concentration of calcium in the blood, stimulates increased production of $1,25(OH)_2D_3$ in the kidney.

Since there is a lack of dietary calcium, the elevated blood level of $1,25(OH_2)D_3$ is ineffective in increasing intestinal absorption of calcium; thus the blood level of calcium remains in the low range of normal. PTH and $1,25(OH)_2D_3$ do, however, stimulate bone resorption in an attempt to normalize the blood calcium level. Because of continuing loss of calcium by excretory mechanisms, the blood calcium does not return to a consistently normal level; thus the hormonal stimuli for continued bone resorption persist, causing eventual loss of bone to a level that results in pathological fractures and perhaps even death of the animal (Fig. 30.25). Because of the effect of PTH on the kidney, the blood concentration of phosphorus remains within the normal range (Table 30.3).

If the dietary deficiency involves vitamin D rather than calcium, and there is insufficient production of this hormone by the skin, then a deficiency of $1,25(OH)_2D_3$ occurs. The pathophysiology is similar to that seen in calcium deficiency, with the exception that the circulating concentration of $1,25(OH)_2D_3$ is reduced rather than elevated. In this case, of course, the lack of intestinal absorption of calcium is due to a deficiency of the active form of vitamin D rather than to a dietary deficiency of calcium. Since vitamin D is also needed for phosphorus absorption, the plasma P concentration may be in the low normal range (Table 30.3).

In either case, the continued removal of bone without replacement results in fibrous osteodystrophy of bone, as previously described for primary hyperparathyroidism. In growing animals, although the production of bone matrix continues, there is a lack of mineralization of this matrix, which is a classic sign of rickets. The chronic stimulation of

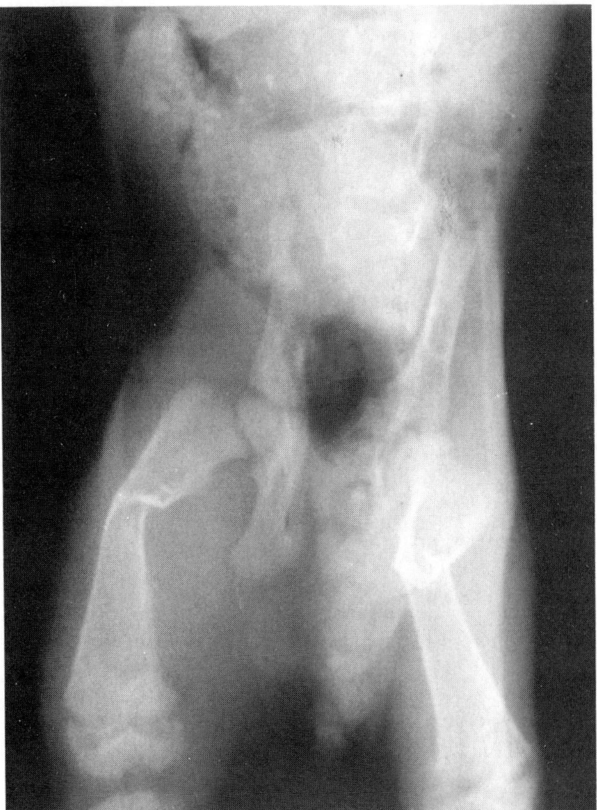

Figure 30.25. Pathological fractures of both femurs in a puppy suffering from nutritional secondary hyperparathyroidism. The puppy was being fed an all-meat diet, which is very low in calcium content.

the parathyroid glands occurring in NSHP results in their hypertrophy (enlargement). However, the enlarged parathyroid glands are rarely detectable on clinical examination.

The clinical signs of NSHP relate to the bone lesion. In young animals there is a cessation of growth. Because of a lack of available mineral for bone formation, the epiphyseal plates are soft, weak, and swollen. The cortices of long bones are seen to be very thin, and pathological fractures are common (Fig. 30.25). In adults, the epiphyseal plates have already closed. In this case, therefore, removal of bone occurs mainly from the sites already mentioned for hyperparathyroidism (i.e., the mandible, skull, and vertebrae with corresponding clinical signs of a swollen jaw).

Diagnosis of NSHP is based on the clinical signs, the clinical and dietary history and the results of other diagnostic procedures. Radiographs of patients with NSHP will demonstrate a lack of mineral density to the bone, thin cortices, and unmineralized epiphyses in young animals. Blood chemistry will probably reveal normal to low normal concentrations of calcium and phosphorus, since continued bone resorption tends to maintain these minerals even in the face of the phosphaturic effect of PTH. The blood level of alkaline phosphatase, an enzyme involved in bone metabolism, will be elevated (Table 30.3). The iPTH level in the blood will be elevated whereas that of $1{,}25(OH)_2D_3$ will depend on the dietary deficiency that is present. Plasma calcitonin (CT) concentration will be low since there is no stimulus for its release.

Treatment of NSHP requires correction of the dietary deficiency and repair of any bone abnormalities (e.g., fractures) that are present. In many cases, complete recovery is possible. However, if there has been irreversible damage, such as chronic spinal cord compression as a result of vertebral fractures, then the possibility of recovery to useful function may be negligible.

Renal secondary hyperparathyroidism

Renal secondary hyperparathyroidism (RSHP) presents a clinical picture somewhat similar to that seen in NSHP, but occurs in animals that are afflicted with chronic renal disease (CRD). CRD usually occurs in older dogs and cats and is associated with a progressive loss of functional nephrons. Eventually the number of functional nephrons is reduced below the number (about 25 percent of the total) necessary to sustain normal renal function. Once this occurs, the clinical signs of CRD appear.

Since the kidney is the major organ involved in phosphorus excretion, a significant loss of renal function as described above results in a retention of phosphorus and the occurrence of hyperphosphatemia (Table 30.3). The elevated blood phosphorus, by virtue of the dynamic equilibrium existing between calcium and phosphorus, causes hypocalcemia and a stimulation of PTH release.

The pathophysiology of RSHP differs to some extent from that of NSHP. The elevated PTH concentration that occurs as a result of the hypocalcemia associated with CRD induces the usual metabolic effects with one notable exception—a lack of increase in $1{,}25(OH)_2D_3$ concentration. This hormone fails to increase since much of the cell mass responsible for its production has been destroyed as a result of the renal disease. Osteocytic and osteoclastic bone resorption increases, releasing significant amounts of calcium and phosphorus into the blood, and this helps to normalize the blood calcium concentration. Since renal function is compromised, however, PTH does not have its usual phosphaturic effect and the increase in the blood phosphorus concentration is exacerbated, potentiating the hypocalcemia and stimulating further PTH release.

Thus a "vicious cycle" is induced, resulting in ever higher levels of PTH and increased bone resorption in fruitless continuing attempts to normalize the blood calcium concentration. The ability to normalize the blood calcium concentration is further compromised by the decreased availability of $1{,}25(OH)_2D_3$, which is needed for optimal intestinal absorption of calcium.

Since CRD usually occurs in older animals, the clinical signs of RSHP are similar to those seen in adult cases of NSHP. These include swelling of the mandible and skull and eventual thinning of the cortices of long bones (Fig. 30.26). Hypertrophy of the parathyroid glands, though usually not clinically detectable, is also present. Of course, the other clinical signs of renal disease will occur in association with those of RSHP. Diagnosis of this condition is based on history, clinical signs, and results of diagnostic procedures. While the blood calcium concentration in cases of RSHP is usually normal, for reasons already mentioned, the blood phosphorus level may be significantly elevated. Plasma concentrations of iPTH are elevated. The blood alkaline phosphatase concentration will also be abnormally high, but the plasma CT concentration will be decreased because

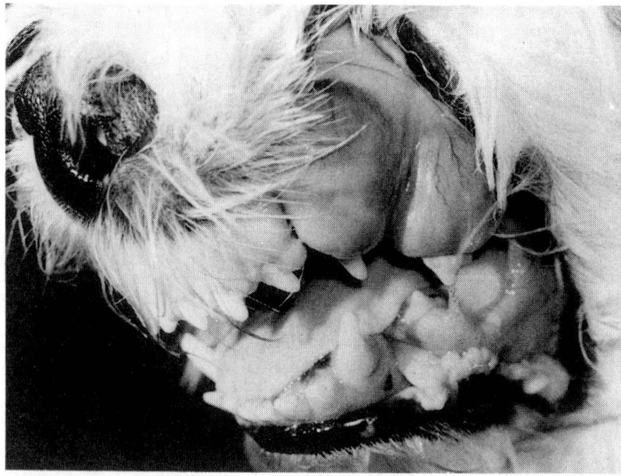

Figure 30.26. Swelling of the maxilla and mandible as a result of fibrous osteodystrophy of these bones in a dog suffering from chronic renal disease.

of the marginally low blood calcium concentration (Table 30.3).

Since the underlying cause of RSHP, reduced renal function, usually cannot be reversed, therapy for CRD and RSHP is based on attempts to offset the pathological changes that are occurring. With respect to RSHP, these are mainly due to hyperphosphatemia and a lack of $1,25(OH)_2D_3$. A low-phosphorus diet is helpful in restoring normophosphatemia. Feeding of phosphate binders, such as aluminum hydroxide, is not as effective. Treatment with $1,25(OH)_2D_3$ is used to restore the normal intestinal absorptive capacity for calcium. Additional management, which is outside the scope of this chapter, is necessary to deal with non-bone-related aspects of CRD.

Pseudohyperparathyroidism

There are a number of conditions described in dogs, cats, and other species in which hypercalcemia occurs in the absence of any evidence of hyperplasia or neoplasia of the parathyroid gland and in which there is no evidence of vitamin D toxicity. These conditions are caused by excessive production of PTH-like peptides or other bone-resorbing substances. This syndrome is referred to as pseudohyperparathyroidism. In clinical veterinary medicine this syndrome occurs most commonly in association with malignant tumors, specifically either tumors that involve the apocrine glands of the anal sac or lymphosarcoma. Recently hypercalcemia in association with squamous cell carcinoma in cats has been described.

The clinical signs of pseudohyperparathyroidism are related to the hypercalcemia and the same as those previously described for primary hyperparathyroidism. Diagnosis is based on clinical signs, including the presence of an appropriate tumor, and on the results of additional diagnostic procedures. In addition to hypercalcemia, blood chemical analysis may reveal an elevated concentration of alkaline phosphatase. Circulating levels of iPTH, however, have been shown to be very low (Table 30.3). Generalized bone demineralization is not as severe in this syndrome as it is in primary or secondary hyperparathyroidism. Also, in this disease the parathyroid glands are small, since chronic hypercalcemia suppresses both production and secretion of PTH.

Treatment of pseudohyperparathyroidism is directed at elimination of the tumor responsible for the hypercalcemia. This can be accomplished by surgical removal, radiation therapy, chemotherapy, or a combination of these modalities. A protein with some amino acid sequence similarities to human PTH has recently been identified in cases of humoral hypercalcemia of cancer in humans. The active principle has yet to be identified in dogs, however, although some of the characteristics of the principle have been identified.

Hypoparathyroidism

A number of situations can occur in which the normal secretion of PTH is reduced or prevented, resulting in hypoparathyroidism. Today the most common cause of this syndrome is inadvertent removal or compromise of the parathyroid glands during surgical removal of hyperplastic thyroid glands in cats. Other causes include autoimmune disease or invasion and destruction of the parathyroid glands by tumors. Recent evidence indicates that chronic elevation of the blood magnesium concentration may also result in hypoparathyroidism.

When the circulating level of PTH falls below normal, $1,25(OH)_2D_3$ production and bone resorption decrease dramatically, resulting in a reduction of the plasma calcium concentration to very low levels. Since the hyperphosphaturic effect of PTH is not present, blood phosphorus concentrations may rise, further compromising the blood calcium. The clinical signs are those of hypocalcemia and, in most species (cattle being an exception), include restless and nervous behavior followed by ataxia, recumbency, and intermittent tremors that progress to generalized tetany.

Diagnosis of hypoparathyroidism is based on history, clinical signs and other diagnostic procedures. With respect to blood chemistry, hypocalcemia and perhaps a tendency toward hyperphosphatemia will be noted. Since bone turnover is compromised, the alkaline phosphatase level in the blood will be below normal. Of course, circulating levels of iPTH and of $1,25(OH)_2D_3$ will be very low (Table 30.3). In chronic cases, because of the lack of stimulus for bone resorption, the mineral content of bone will increase, resulting in a condition known as osteopetrosis. This may be visible on radiographs as increased cortical thickness and an overall increase in density of the skeleton.

Acute hypoparathyroidism is a life-threatening disorder, and immediate intravenous therapy to restore the blood calcium concentration to normal is necessary. Long-term maintenance of patients with persistent lack of PTH is difficult and requires feeding of high-calcium, low-phosphorus rations. Since the primary stimulus for production of $1,25(OH)_2D_3$ is absent, treatment with vitamin D is of little value. The recent availability of the active form of vitamin D—calcitriol—as a therapeutic agent, holds promise for more effective management of this condition. It has recently been shown that, in cats, the blood calcium level will spontaneously return to normal several weeks after parathyroidectomy. The mechanism for this is not known, but it probably does not involve ectopic production of PTH, since the circulating concentration of iPTH remains at undetectable levels as the blood calcium concentration returns to normal.

Calcitonin

As previously mentioned, CT is an antihypercalcemic hormone that functions to decrease the blood calcium concentration during periods of hypercalcemia. The hormone is produced by the interstitial or C cells of the thyroid gland, and the primary stimulus for its secretion is an above-normal concentration of blood calcium. Other substances, however, have also been shown to stimulate secretion of CT; one of these is the hormone gastrin, which is produced by certain of the stomach-lining cells. The physiologic importance of CT is not as great as that of PTH and the vitamin D hormones since animals are able to maintain normal calcium homeostasis after thyroidectomy. However, a number of disease processes have been attributed to overproduction of this hormone.

Nutritional hypercalcitoninism

Animals that are fed rations containing much higher than required amounts of calcium have been shown to develop skeletal abnormalities, such as abnormal bone development and remodeling in growing animals and the presence of excessive amounts of bone, i.e., abnormally thick bone trabeculae and cortices in adults, a condition known as osteopetrosis. One of the first descriptions of this phenomenon in veterinary medicine involved bulls in an artificial insemination complex. For long periods of time, these animals had been fed a ration, containing relatively high amounts of calcium, that was designed for lactating dairy cows. In many of them abnormal bone mineral deposits (exostoses) developed, particularly on the vertebrae. In the affected bulls this led to actual fusion of the vertebrae and loss of mobility. In these animals the C cell regions of the thyroid glands were hypertrophied, and in some cases actual tumors (adenomas) of these cells were present. Hypercalcitoninism as a result of overfeeding of calcium was a likely cause of this problem.

In growing dogs, particularly in large breeds, a number of skeletal abnormalities, such as hip dysplasia and osteochondritis dissecans, are known to occur. It is also known that owners and breeders, for a number of reasons, frequently overfeed these animals. Several studies have now shown that overnutrition can predispose rapidly growing puppies to stunted growth and the development of skeletal abnormalities and that too much dietary calcium may be the primary factor. This syndrome is also classified as hypercalcitoninism, and similar abnormalities have been demonstrated in growing cattle, horses and sheep.

The pathophysiology of hypercalcitoninism is due to excessive production of CT, either as a direct result of hypercalcemia or secondary to excessive secretion of gastrin resulting from high gastric calcium content. Elevated blood gastrin concentrations are thought to induce persistently high CT secretion rates, even in the face of normal to low blood calcium concentrations. The CT acts as previously described to inhibit osteoclastic bone resorption but does not affect bone production. Thus osteopetrosis develops in the adult.

In addition to its effects on bone tissue, CT also has significant inhibitory effects on the development and maturation of both articular and epiphyseal cartilage. The combination of the effects of CT on cartilage development and bone resorption leads to significant abnormalities in bone formation and remodeling in the growing animal with hypercalcitoninism. This leads to stunted growth and an increased incidence of the skeletal diseases previously mentioned.

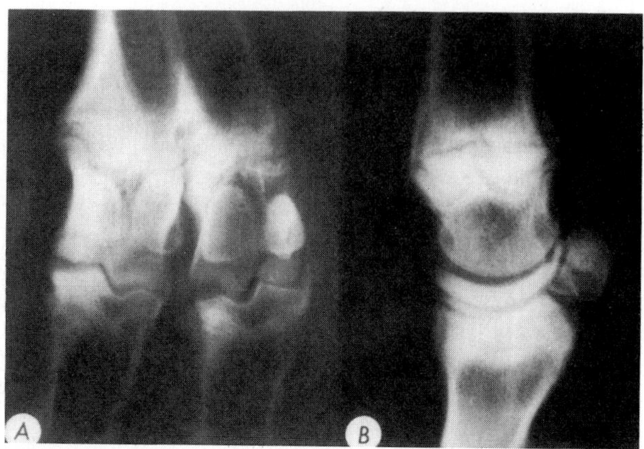

Figure 30.27. Dorsoplantar (*A*) and lateral (*B*) radiographs of the rear fetlock joints of a heifer suffering from nutritional hypercalcitoninism. Note the increased mineral density in the epiphyseal plate region in the distal metatarsus. (From Rostowski, Wilson, Allan, Deftos, Benson, Kallfelz, Minor, and Krook, 1981, *Cornell Vet.* 71:188–213.)

The diagnosis of hypercalcitoninism is based on history and clinical signs. Additional diagnostic testing may also be helpful. Radiographs may demonstrate abnormal bone development, thickened bone trabeculae and cortices, and epiphyseal plate abnormalities. (Fig. 30.27). Although the blood calcium level will probably be in the high normal range, the blood alkaline phosphatase concentration is frequently well below normal, as would be the concentrations of iPTH and of $1,25(OH)_2D_3$. On the other hand, circulating concentrations of CT would be elevated (Table 30.3). There is no specific treatment for this problem other than correction of the dietary abnormalities. If significant skeletal abnormalities have already occurred, they may very well be irreversible.

Hereditary osteopetrosis

As mentioned above, the primary bone abnormality in hypercalcitoninism is osteopetrosis resulting from the inhibition of bone resorption while bone formation continues. A hereditary disease has been described in cattle in which osteopetrosis occurs to a very significant degree. The syndrome begins in calves during intrauterine development. Affected calves are born prematurely and usually are stillborn. The primary abnormal finding is that all bones are much smaller than usual and are completely solid (i.e., there is no marrow cavity). Although this disease has not been further characterized, it is most likely due to either failure of osteoclasts to develop at all or a lack of the biochemical mechanisms needed to stimulate their activity. As a consequence, the resorptive phase of bone remodeling does not occur and severe osteopetrosis develops.

Of interest is the fact that this condition occurs normally in the manatee, an aquatic mammal. As a result of the absence of bone marrow cavities, this species must rely on extramedullary hematopoiesis for blood cell formation.

Vitamin D

As mentioned earlier, the vitamin D hormones, particularly $1,25(OH)_2D_3$, are extremely important in mineral and bone metabolism. Since vitamin D has important effects at several sites (intestine, kidney, bone), either a deficiency or an excess of this vitamin can cause very serious abnormalities.

Hypovitaminosis D

Vitamin D deficiency is generally considered to be a major cause of rickets and osteomalacia, defined previously in this chapter as a lack of mineralization of osteoid. In fact, however, the clinical signs and pathological changes seen in hypovitaminosis D are identical to those described above for NSHP; that is, a calcium deficiency also occurs as a result of the lack of intestinal absorption of this element in the absence of the active form of vitamin D. Thus, in addition to a failure of newly formed bone matrix to mineralize, there is also a PTH-stimulated enhanced resorption of preexisting bone, causing fibrous osteodystrophy to develop as well.

Primary vitamin D deficiency is rarely seen as a clinical entity in veterinary medicine. In large animals, even though poor-quality forages may contain inadequate amounts of vitamin D, production in the skin almost always is sufficient to meet the need. In small-animal practice, virtually all pet foods today contain more than adequate amounts of the vitamin, which is added as part of a vitamin and mineral supplement during production of the food.

As mentioned previously, conditioned deficiencies of vitamin D are possible in situations, such as fat-malabsorption syndromes, in which intestinal absorption of the vitamin is compromised. Genetic abnormalities in vitamin D metabolism (vitamin D–resistant rickets) can also occur and have been rather well characterized in humans. Although they probably do occur, these conditions have not as yet been documented in clinical veterinary medicine.

Hypervitaminosis D

An excess of vitamin D, vitamin D toxicity, does occur in animals and has been identified in several species. The cause of vitamin D toxicity is the inadvertent administration to, or consumption by, an animal of excessive amounts of vitamin D or its active metabolites. In cattle, toxicity has been reported to result from administration of inordinate amounts of vitamin D in an attempt to prevent parturient hypocalcemia (milk fever). Oversupplementation of grain mixtures with vitamin D has caused clinical toxicity in horses. In small animals, consumption of vitamin D–containing rodenticides or overzealous treatment of certain diseases (e.g. RSHP) with active metabolites of vitamin D can cause toxicity.

The pathophysiology of vitamin D toxicity is due partially to the severe hypercalcemia that results from exaggerated response to the vitamin. This produces the clinical signs and pathological changes described previously. In dogs, toxicity due to excessive administration of $1,25(OH)_2D_3$ has been shown to cause almost a complete cessation of food intake (anorexia). Additional pathological changes are also common in vitamin D toxicity. As a result of the severe hypercalcemia, precipitation of calcium phosphate salts occurs in soft tissues (dystrophic calcification). Renal tubules and the inner walls of large blood vessels are common sites for this to occur. As a result, kidney failure is a common finding in vitamin D toxicity.

In bone, death (necrosis) of bone cells has been described as a consequence of acute vitamin D toxicity. The dissolution of mineral from the dead bone thus contributes to the hypercalcemia that occurs in this syndrome. In horses with vitamin D toxicity, there may be precipitation of mineral in the tendons and ligaments of the extremities, causing contracted tendons as well as skeletal abnormalities.

Diagnosis of vitamin D toxicity, as of the other diseases discussed, is based on history, clinical signs, and other diagnostic work. In addition to observation of severe hypercalcemia and also hyperphosphatemia, assessment of vitamin D metabolite concentrations in the blood can be helpful. In most species, cattle being a possible exception, the circulating level of $25(OH)D_3$ is most indicative of vitamin D status, since conversion to the active metabolite is controlled and thus $1,25(OH)_2D_3$ concentration in the blood remains normal in vitamin D toxicity. The toxic effects, therefore, are really due to inordinately high concentrations of $25(OH)D_3$, even though this metabolite is much less potent than the active form of the vitamin. Circulating concentrations of iPTH would be low in vitamin D toxicity because of the persistent hypercalcemia, and alkaline phosphatase concentration would usually be normal.

Vitamin D toxicity is a serious disease that is difficult to treat because many of the pathological changes may be difficult, if not impossible, to reverse. Initially, it is most important to alleviate the hypercalcemia in order to relieve clinical signs and halt the progression of pathological changes. Treatment with exogenous calcitonin can be helpful in reducing the blood calcium concentration. Fluid therapy and diuretics are also used. Other steps include elimination of the source of the vitamin D, if necessary, and reduction of dietary calcium until the blood calcium concentration is stabilized.

Calcinosis in grazing animals

In several parts of the world, grazing animals are known to develop a syndrome called "calcinosis" from consumption of toxic plants. Calcinosis is the deposition of calcium salts in various soft tissues, such as the lining of large vessels, kidneys, tendons, and ligaments. Such changes are similar to those seen in vitamin D toxicity. Several plants, including *Solanum malacoxylon* in South America and *Cestrum diurnum* in the southern United States, have been shown to cause this syndrome. The active principle in both plants has been shown to be $1,25(OH)_2D_3$.

The hormonal form of vitamin D is present in these toxic plants in the form of a glycoside of the steroidal hormone, which is cleaved in the intestinal tract of the affected animal. The excess vitamin D hormone results in changes very similar to those already described for acute vitamin D toxicity. One exception is that, instead of osteonecrosis, osteopetrosis occurs in this syndrome. Apparently the vitamin D metabolite levels do not reach concentrations high enough to cause bone necrosis. Rather, the hypercalcemia results in chronic calcitonin secretion from the C cells, causing the skeletal picture of osteopetrosis as previously described.

Other systemic hormones

Although of much less significance, deficiencies or excesses of some of the other systemic hormones that affect bone metabolism can result in clinically observable abnormalities seen in veterinary practice. Genetic defects are well known to cause growth hormone deficiencies in dogs, resulting in "pituitary dwarfs." While the dogs generally survive, they remain small, have immature-type hair coats, and may exhibit secondary deficiencies of other hormones, such as those of the thyroid or adrenal glands. As would be expected, the bone abnormalities are related to a lack of normal development of the epiphyseal plate, resulting in short bones, particularly those of the appendicular skeleton, with lack of closure of the epiphyses at the appropriate age. There is no effective treatment for this problem, which is inherited as an autosomal recessive trait in German shepherd dogs.

As mentioned previously, a lack of estrogen is related to the net loss of bone mass that occurs in postmenopausal osteoporosis in women. This syndrome does not occur in veterinary medicine. It has been postulated, however, that a transient lack of estrogen may be involved in the pathogenesis of parturient hypocalcemia (milk fever) in cattle, but it is unlikely that estrogen deficiency is of great importance in this syndrome.

Deficiencies or excesses of other systemic hormones (e.g., thyroid, adrenal, pancreatic) definitely result in clinically recognized syndromes in veterinary medicine. However, the skeletal manifestations of these abnormalities are of minor clinical significance as compared with effects on other organ systems that are more essential for continuation of normal life functions.

JOINTS AND SYNOVIAL FLUID*

In anatomy a *joint* is the connection in the skeleton between any of its rigid component parts, whether bones or cartilages. *Articulation* is synonymous with joint. Terms such as *arthrology* (the study of joints) and *arthritis* (the inflammation of joints) are of Greek origin (*arthron*).

Vertebrate joints vary in structure and arrangement to serve specific functions but have certain features in common. On the basis of their most characteristic structural features, joints may be classified into three main types: fibrous, cartilaginous, and synovial. The present account deals mainly with synovial joints in mammals.

Since joints diseases are among the most frequent afflictions of animals, an understanding of the anatomy and physiology of joints is of particular importance. Such knowledge will help the clinician interpret the signs of joint diseases, interpret diagnostic tests, and appreciate the value and limitations of treatment.

Classification and description of joints

The present account deals mainly with synovial joints of mammals since these are the joints most commonly affected by disease processes.

Fibrous joints

The bones of a fibrous joint (sometimes called a synarthrosis) are united by fibrous tissue. There are two types of fibrous joint—sutures and syndesmoses. In the sutures of the skull, the bones are tightly connected by several fibrous layers. The mechanisms of growth at these joints are important in accommodating the growth of the brain. A syndesmosis is a fibrous joint in which the intervening connective tissue is much greater in amount than in a suture. Examples are the tibiofibular and tympanostapedial fibrous joints.

Cartilaginous joints

The bones of cartilaginous joints are united either by hyaline cartilage or by fibrocartilage.

Hyaline cartilage joints. In the hyaline cartilage joint, also called a synchondrosis, the bones are temporarily united by hyaline cartilage. This cartilage is a part of the embryonic cartilaginous skeleton that persists during postnatal maturation, and it serves as a growth zone for one or both of the bones that it joins. Most hyaline cartilage joints have been replaced by bone by the time growth ceases. Examples of hyaline cartilage joints are the epiphyseal plates of long bones and the sphenooccipital joint.

Fibrocartilaginous joints. The fibrocartilaginous type of joint, also known as amphiarthrosis, unites the skeletal elements by means of fibrocartilage during some phase of their existence. The fibrocartilage is usually separated from the bones by thin plates of hyaline cartilage. Fibrocartilaginous joints include the pubic symphysis and the disks between the bodies of the vertebrae.

An intervertebral disk forms a resilient body whose superior and inferior (or anterior and posterior) aspects are separated from the adjacent vertebral body by a thin hyaline cartilage plate, the latter a growth zone for the vertebral

*This section was authored by George Lust and is based on the chapter written by Ernest D. Gardner for the ninth edition of this textbook.

body. The anulus fibrosus consists of a series of lamellae of collagen bundles that are anchored to the margins of the hyaline plates and to the edges of the vertebral bodies. The innermost lamellae contain fibrocartilage. With advancing age, the entire disk tends to become cartilaginous. Degenerative changes of the disk are common in many domestic animals, especially large ones with relatively long lives. Where present, these degenerative changes predispose the disk to injury. In some animals (e.g., dachshunds), intervertebral disk disease appears to be brought about by abnormalities of the hyaline cartilage plates.

In many mammals, including humans, marked pelvic relaxation occurs late in pregnancy to facilitate passage of the fetus. This relaxation, which consists of a separation of the pubic symphysis and, in some, a loosening of the sacroiliac joints, is brought about by the hormone relaxin operating in conjunction with other hormones, especially estrogens. The pubic symphysis is a fibrocartilaginous joint in which the fibrocartilage may contain a cleft. Separation of this joint under the influence of relaxin is especially pronounced in guinea pigs and mice.

The sacroiliac joint is a synovial joint, and the relaxation of its capsule and ligaments is marked in sheep and cows under the influence of relaxin and estrogens.

Synovial joints

The movement of bones occurs at *synovial joints,* complex structures that allow gliding of one surface over another. This motion is facilitated by the efficient lubrication action of *synovial fluid* that has the consistency of egg white and the smooth surface of *articular cartilage* of each bone at the points of contact.

The synovial joint comprises the joint capsule within which are the different types of synovial membrane, the articulating surfaces of the bones of the joint, ligaments, other structures, and the synovial fluid, as depicted for the knee joint in Fig. 30.28. The synovial membranes are involved in the formation of synovial fluid. The articular cartilage of the hyaline type is synthesized by the embedded chondrocytes. The outer layer of the joint capsule consists of a fibrous layer (the fibrous capsule), and the inner surface is composed of the synovial membranes (synovial capsule). The fibrous capsule layer contains collagen fibers that extend from the fibrous layer of the periosteum of one bone to the periosteum of the other bone, contributing to the stability of the joint. Ligaments are extensions of the fibrous capsule and are either located within the interior of the capsule or separated therefrom by *bursa.* The *menisci* within the joint capsule, composed of fibrocartilage, have a

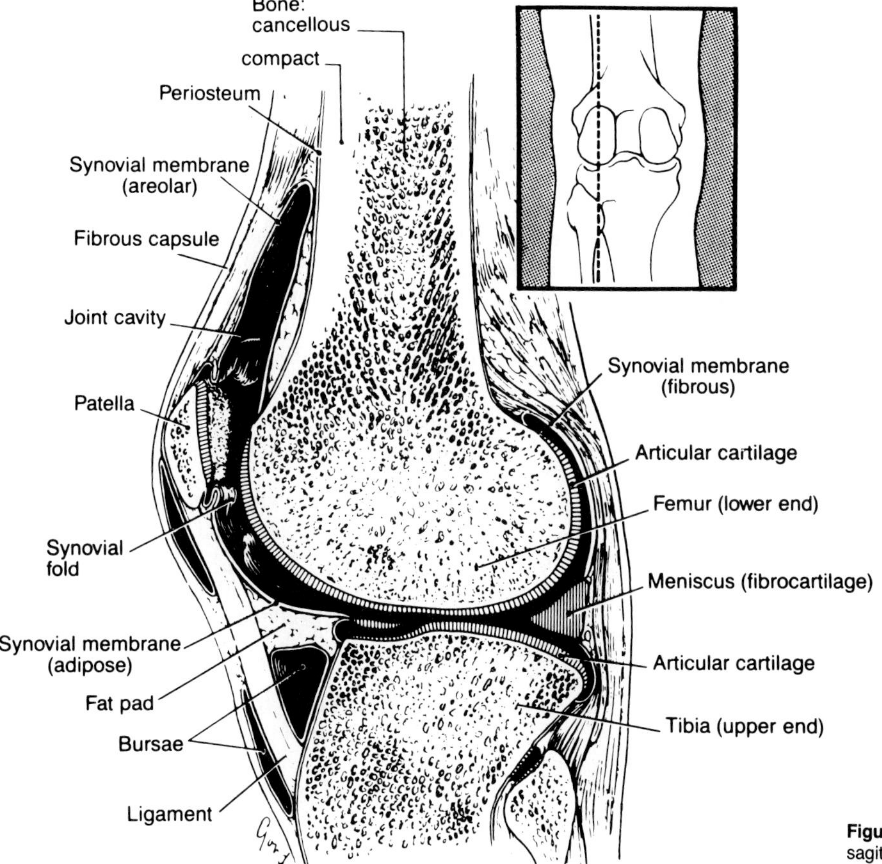

Figure 30.28. Diagram of a knee joint, cut in the sagittal plane indicated in the inset. (From Cormack 1987, Bone, in *Ham's Histology,* 9th ed., J.B. Lippincott, Philadelphia, Chap. 12.)

cushioning function. As shown for the knee joint (Fig. 30.28), the meniscus has a free inner border. In other joints, the meniscus lies between the articulating surfaces, dividing the synovial cavity into two separate cavities.

Synovial membrane and synovial fluid

Synovial membrane is a vascular connective tissue that lines the inner surface of the capsule but does not cover the bearing surfaces. It consists of formed elements such as cells and fibers, together with intercellular matrix.

The cells of the synovial membrane, the synoviocytes, are localized adjacent to the joint cavity and are grouped together in one to three layers to form a relatively smooth surface. A variable number of folds, villi, and fat pads project from the synovial membrane into the joint cavity. Immediately subjacent to these surface cells is a capillary network. The synovial membrane varies in thickness and contains fibroblasts, macrophages, mast cells, and fat cells, as well as blood and lymphatic vessels and a few nerve fibers. If a synovial membrane is removed, a new synovial membrane may form from this underlying tissue or from the joint capsule.

Synovial fluid is an ultrafiltrate of plasma to which hyaluronic acid is added as it is synthesized and secreted by synoviocytes. The lack of a basement membrane and the proximity of the capillaries to the inner surface of the synovial membrane surface facilitate the exchange of solutes.

Fluid exchange between plasma and synovial fluid seems to be governed by Starling forces, i.e., hydraulic or hydrostatic pressure differences and colloidal osmotic pressure differences between plasma and synovial fluid. Large molecules are prevented by the endothelium from leaving the capillary. The "permeability barrier" of the synovium to small molecules is maintained by the narrow space between the synoviocytes and the composition of the matrix of the synovial membrane. Molecules of less than 10,000 Da are usually in equilibrium between plasma and synovial fluid and generally cross the synovial membrane by simple diffusion. Glucose transport into the synovial fluid is an exception, however, as glucose enters normal joints faster than other small molecules, probably by a facilitated diffusion mechanism rather than by active transport. Molecules, like oxygen and carbon dioxide, diffuse freely into and out of the synovial fluid. These gases can diffuse through the synoviocytes as well as between them.

Synoviocytes consist of two main types. Type A cells are considered to be mainly phagocytic and pinocytic, and type B cells have mainly synthetic activity, although, to a certain degree, these various functions occur in both cell types. Synovial lining cells synthesize the extracellular matrix of the synovial lining, which contains collagen, proteoglycans, and fibronectin. *Lubricin* is also synthesized by synovial lining cells. Lubricin, a polydisperse glycoprotein with an apparent molecular weight of 160,000 Da also provides boundary lubrication to articular cartilage.

The viscosity of synovial fluid is due to its hyaluronic acid content. Hyaluronic acid is a single, long carbohydrate chain comprising repeating sequences of carbohydrate units. The acid nature of hyaluronic acid is derived from the carboxyl and sulfate groups associated with the constituent sugar residues and, at neutral pH, is negatively charged.

In solution, hyaluronic acid adopts the configuration of a stiffened, random-coiled sphere with a high affinity for water. The large molecular domains overlap and entangle, imparting a high viscosity to the synovial fluid. This viscous property enables the synovial fluid to resist strain, absorb some of the energy generated by movement, and function as a boundary lubricant of synovium.

The other constituents of synovial fluid are those that are normally present in blood plasma. In fact, synovial fluid, aside from its hyaluronic acid content, can be considered a dialysate of blood plasma. Synovial fluid also normally contains a few cells, mostly mononuclear, derived from the lining tissue. Many pathological processes (infections, rheumatic disorders, autoimmune disorders, neoplasms) affect the synovial membrane, and they generally alter the cellular content of the fluid. Withdrawal of synovial fluid and determination of its cellular and chemical content and physical characteristics can be a valuable diagnostic aid.

Articular cartilage

Adult articular cartilage is usually hyaline in nature, avascular and nerveless, with chondrocytes widely dispersed within the cartilage matrix. It is nevertheless a highly specialized connective tissue with biochemical and biophysical characteristics that enable it to play a dual role as a shock absorber and a bearing surface. Its matrix is hyperhydrated. The part of articular hyaline cartilage adjacent to bone is usually calcified. Articular cartilage, except for its calcified zone, is not visible in ordinary radiograms. Hence the so-called radiological joint space is wider than the true joint space.

During the growth period, articular cartilage provides the growth zone for endochondral ossification in the epiphysis and, like the epiphyseal cartilage, is under the influence of the somatotropic hormone of the adenohypophysis. During growth, articular cartilage is capable of regeneration and can repair defects. When growth in body length ceases, however, articular cartilage loses much of its capacity for repair, especially in the higher vertebrates. Some growth is still possible, though, and is brought into play in the slow remodeling of adult joints, which may result from mechanical or pathological stress.

Chondrocyte function and metabolism

Articular cartilage chondrocytes make up only a small proportion (about 1 to 5 percent) of the cartilage volume. Chondrocytes near the surface of cartilage have a flattened, fibroblastic appearance, and cells in the deeper layers are plump, with well-developed endoplastic reticula and Golgi apparatuses, secretory vacuoles, lysosomes, and mitochondria. These cells synthesize, regulate, and organize the cartilage matrix remote from blood vessels, nerves, and lymphatics in the mature animal. Chondrocytes synthesize and secrete (type II) collagen, proteoglycans, noncollagenous glycoproteins, chondronectin, small cationic polypeptides, and enzymes. After secretion into the extracellular matrix, the collagen becomes insoluble and a meshwork of fibrils is formed. Type IX collagen, also synthesized by the chondrocytes, forms aggregates with type II collagen during fibril formation.

Cartilage metabolism is predominantly anaerobic, and, although oxygen consumption is low (about 2 percent of vascular tissues), oxygen utilization makes a substantial contribution to the total energy requirements of the cell. Nutrients, including glucose, oxygen, and amino acids, used for synthesis of collagen and other matrix constituents must reach the cell by diffusion from the synovial fluid. Diffusion depends on the molecular size, shape, and charge of the molecule. Generally, molecules larger than hemoglobin (molecular weight about 68,000) are excluded. The intermittent "pumping action" of weight-bearing and joint motion results in movement of fluid into and out of the cartilage and facilitates diffusion. Chemical and hormonal stimuli from the synovium reach the chondrocyte through the synovial fluid.

The sequence of events in the synthesis of collagen was described briefly in a previous section. In articular cartilage, the collagen fibers nearest the articular surface are thin and tightly packed, and they are oriented parallel to the surface. In the deeper regions, the collagen fibers are thicker and exist in an oblique, criss-cross pattern. This configuration is well suited to respond to the stresses imposed by the movement of the joints, and the opposing articular cartilages can thus better withstand the shearing stress near their surfaces and compression forces deeper within the cartilage matrix.

Proteoglycans, prominent constituents of the cartilage matrix and products of chondrocyte synthesis, comprise a variable number of glycosaminoglycans bound to a core protein and can have molecular masses on the order of 10^6 Da. The glycosaminoglycans, previously termed mucopolysaccharides, are long unbranched chains of repeating disaccharide units. One of the two sugars of the disaccharide unit is an acetylated amino sugar, which accounts for its name. In articular cartilage, the glycosaminoglycans are primarily chondroitin-4-sulfate, chondroitin-6-sulfate, keratin sulfate, and dermatan sulfate. Chondroitin-4-sulfate and dermatan sulfate are characteristic of embryonic and immature cartilage. The content of chondroitin-6-sulfate and keratan sulfate in cartilage increases during maturation. Like hyaluronic acid, glycosaminoglycans are highly negatively charged because of the presence of carboxyl and sulfate groups, a property that has functional significance.

The core protein is the first part of the proteoglycan molecule synthesized. Subsequently, initiation of the glycosaminoglycan chain occurs at the attachement of the chain to the core protein by the synthesis of a sugar bridge. The sugar chain is elongated in the Golgi region of the chondrocyte. Sulfation is a late stage in the formation of proteoglycans and therefore provides a convenient means of monitoring proteoglycan synthesis by the use of radioactive labeling techniques with radioactive sulfate ($^{35}SO_4{}^{2-}$).

In the extracellular space, as many as 100 proteoglycan molecules assemble into extremely large aggregates by binding, through a binding region on the core protein, to a hyaluronic acid chain. This binding is noncovalent, stabilized by the so-called *link protein* at the point of attachment between the core protein and the hyaluronic acid backbone. The aggregates can have molecular weights of 10^8 or more, and the proteoglycan aggregates may better resist degradation and might inhibit the calcification of cartilage.

Proteoglycans form complexes with collagen predominantly by electrostatic interactions, which appear to give mechanical stability to the collagen fibers. The binding stability of these complexes varies with proteoglycan type. Chondroitin-4-sulfate and dermatan sulfate have a high affinity for collagen, but hyaluronic acid (chondroitin-6-sulfate) and keratin sulfate bind to a lesser degree. Chondroitin-4-sulfate, the major glycosaminoglycan of immature cartilage, with its high affinity for collagen, accelerates fiber formation of secreted collagen, favoring the production of fine collagen fibers. Conversely, keratin sulfate and chondroitin-6-sulfate, glycosaminoglycans more common in mature and aging cartilage, permit greater fiber growth, yielding the thicker fibers of the mature tissue. About 25 percent of the proteoglycans are associated with collagen, and the balance exists as proteoglycan aggregates.

The three-dimensional structure of proteoglycans bears on some of the functional properties of these molecules. The negative charges on adjacent glycosaminoglycan chains on the protein core tend to repel each other, thereby providing these aggregates with an extremely large molecular volume. The spaces provided by the extended glycosaminoglycan chains are occupied by water, providing considerable elastic resistance to compressive forces. These polyanionic complexes also contribute significantly to the osmotic pressure of the matrix, which bears on the resiliency of the matrix.

There is a slow turnover of the components of normal cartilage. The synthesis of collagen and proteoglycans is balanced by their rate of degradation in normal cartilage. Degradation of these macromolecules occurs by extracellular and intracellular processes. Cartilage contains several proteases responsible for the extracellular hydrolytic reactions. After the uptake of partially degraded fragments by endocytosis, further degradation occurs in the lysosomes of the chondrocytes. In the cartilage matrix there are low-molecular-weight proteins that inhibit the proteases. These protease inhibitors are thought to contribute to the normal balance between the formation and degradation of the components of cartilage. Degenerative diseases occur when the balance shifts and the degradation of cartilage matrix exceeds its formation.

Joint movements

The range of movements at joints is limited by the muscles, the ligaments and capsule, the shapes of the bones, and the opposition of soft parts.

The movements that occur at synovial joints may be classified as active, passive, and accessory. Active movements include (1) gliding or slipping movements, (2) angular movements about a horizontal or side-to-side axis (flexion and extension) or about an anteroposterior axis (abduction and adduction), and (3) rotary movements about a longitudinal axis (medial and lateral rotation). Whether one, several, or all types of movement occur at a particular joint depends on the shape and ligaments of that joint.

Passive movements are those produced by an external force, such as gravity or an examiner. Accessory movements (often classified with massive movements) are defined as movements for which the muscular arrangements are not suitable but which can be brought about with manipulation by an examiner. The production of passive and accessory movements is of value in testing and in diagnosing muscle and joint disorders.

If limbs of immature animals are immobilized, the tendinous and ligamentous support of the joint weakens, and the immobilized joint can overextend on weight bearing. In mature animals, contracture of the joint capsule and associated soft tissues occurs upon immobilization. Immobilization is associated with shrinkage of soft tissues as a result of decreased water content, accompanied by an increase in the synthesis of collagen and glycosaminoglycans. An increase in the amount of fibrous tissue occurs. These findings emphasize the importance of mechanical or physical interactions in maintaining tissue structure associated with the joint capsule.

Muscle contraction squeezes the joint together, sometimes producing forces equivalent to three or four times body weight. This force, as well as weight bearing, contributes to the maintenance of normal cartilage matrix; passive joint movement alone does not suffice. Limb amputation distal to the stifle in dogs, which permits movement but not weight bearing or muscle contraction across the joint, results in cartilage matrix changes in the stifle that are similar to those occurring in the cartilage of immobilized stifle joints. The changes in cartilage consist of decreased proteoglycan content of the matrix, cartilage thinning, and defects in proteoglycan aggregation due, in part, to abnormalities in the hyaluronate-binding region of the core protein.

Lubrication of joints

Lubrication mechanisms

It should be emphasized that synovial joints are mechanical structures that are specialized to permit more or less free movement. The lubricating mechanisms of these joints are such that the effects of friction on weight-bearing surfaces are minimized. The coefficient of friction during movement is less than that of ice sliding on ice. This is made possible by the nature of the lubricating fluid, by the nature and shapes of the bearing surfaces, and the response of the articular cartilage to compressive, tensile, and other forces during the movement of the joint.

The fluids that lubricate the joint are the synovial fluid and fluid elaborated from the articular cartilage during compression. Substances within synovial fluid that contribute to its lubricating properties are hyaluronic acid, which increases the fluid's viscosity, and the glycoprotein, lubricin. These factors are important for boundary lubrication at low loads. At higher loads, these are displaced from the articular surfaces, and another mechanism of lubrication becomes significant. Fluid is expressed from the cartilage during compression, and a layer of fluid forms between the two opposing surfaces. This mechanism is referred to as weeping lubrication. As a joint moves under load, fluid, expressed at the leading edge of contact between the juxtaposed articular cartilages, reenters the cartilage at the trailing edge. The fluid is imbibed in response to the increase in the osmotic force within the cartilage, and the fluid stops flowing when the osmotic pressure exerted by the trapped proteoglycans is resisted by the tension developed in the collagen network. The magnitude of the osmotic force depends on the density of the charged groups on the proteoglycans, the distribution of the charged groups along the branches of the proteoglycans, and molecular conformation of the proteoglycans. The magnitude of the resisting force depends on structural organization, tensile stiffness, and the strength of the collagen network. Knowledge of the contribution of these forces to this equilibrium and to weight bearing is pertinent to an understanding of how strain is less well tolerated in diseased cartilage.

Boundary lubrication of the synovial membrane is also important to decrease resistance to joint movement. Hyaluronic acid in the synovial fluid lubricates the synovial membrane.

Any mechanical system wears with time, and synovial joints are no exception. Even though the effects of friction are minimized, some wear and tear (also called use-destruction or attrition) is inevitable. The most common result is the wearing away of articular cartilage to varying degrees, occasionally to the extent of exposing, eroding, and polishing the underlying bone. Wear and tear may be exaggerated by such factors as body weight, abnormal movements or gait, trauma, and disease, and by pathological processes that change articular geometry, alter synovial

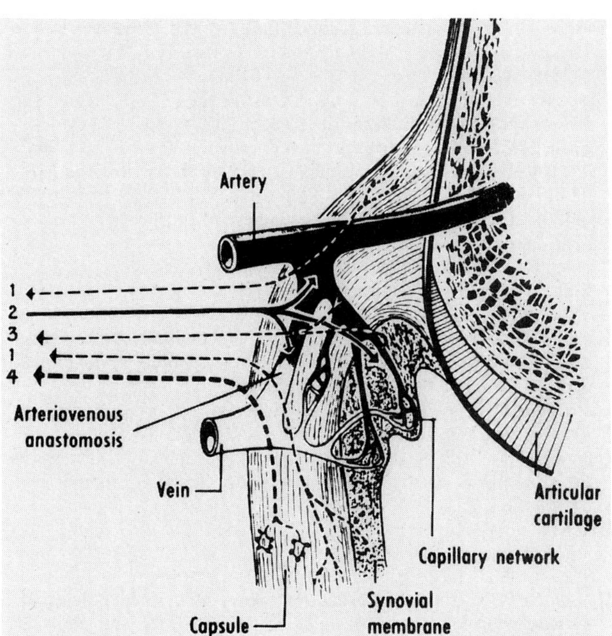

Figure 30.29. Blood and nerve supply of a synovial joint. An artery is shown supplying the epiphysis, joint capsule, and synovial membrane. Note the arteriovenous anastomosis. The articular nerve contains (1) sensory fibers (mostly pain) from the capsule and synovial membrane, (2) autonomic fibers (postganglionic, sympathetic to blood vessels), (3) sensory fibers (pain, and others with unknown functions) from the adventitia of blood vessels, and (4) proprioceptive fibers from Ruffini endings and from small lamellated corpuscles (not shown). Arrows indicate direction of conduction. (From Gardner, Gray, and O'Rahilly 1975, *Anatomy,* 4th ed. W.B. Saunders, Philadelphia.)

fluid, and interfere with cartilage metabolism. Osteoarthritic conditions aggravated by wear and tear occur in many domestic animals, including birds; when a thoroughbred is so afflicted, the animal may become useless for normal activity.

Blood and lymphatic supply

The arteries that supply a joint and adjacent bone arise more or less in common. Those that supply the bone usually enter the bone at or near the line of capsular attachment and form a prominent network around the joint. Articular vessels (Fig. 30.29) ultimately form a capillary network that is most prominent in the cellular and areolar areas of the synovial membrane. Both the joint capsule and the synovial membrane bleed profusely when injured. Arteriovenous anastomoses are also present in positions that would enable them to shunt blood past the capillary networks. However, their specific functions in joints are not known. Relatively little is known about the normal pattern of blood flow in joints and the control of such flow.

Lymphatic vessels accompany blood vessels and form plexuses in the synovial membrane and capsule. The lymphatic vessels that leave a joint drain into regional lymph nodes.

Diffusion takes place readily in either direction between the joint cavity on the one hand and the blood and lymphatic capillaries on the other. Most substances in the bloodstream, normal or pathological, easily enter the joint cavity. Conversely, when soluble substances are injected into the joint cavity, they diffuse rapidly through the synovial membrane and into capillaries. When colloidal solutions or fine suspensions are injected into the cavity, the rate of entrance into the synovial membrane and subsynovial tissue is inversely proportional to particle size.

The rate of diffusion and absorption of fluids is increased if the intra-articular pressure is increased, either by injection under high pressure or by movement. Moreover, in infected joints, bacteria may enter the circulation. Infection of a joint because of material introduced from the outside (as by trauma) may be followed by septicemia.

Nerve supply

The importance of a joint nerve supply lies in two main factors: the marked subjective effects (pain) and reflex changes that may accompany joint disease; and the role of joint nerves in posture, locomotion, and kinesthetic sense. Nerves to joints arise, either directly or indirectly, from the nerves that supply the overlying skin and the muscles that move the joint (Fig. 30.29). The major features of distribution, termination, and functions of articular nerves are as follows:

Proprioception in part is provided by a combination of slowly adapting mechanoreceptors (mostly located in the fibrous capsule) that signal changing pressure relationships around the joint and spindle receptors in related muscles and tendons. These receptors are most active near the limits of flexion and extension. Rapidly adapting receptors have been characterized as velocity- or acceleration-sensitive receptors. The importance of sensory innervation to the maintenance of normal joint function is shown by arthropathies that result from sensory loss in diseases.

REFERENCES

Allan, G.S., Huxtable, C.R.R., Howlett, C.R., Baxter, R.C., Duff, B., and Farrow, B.R.H. 1978. Pituitary dwarfism in German Shepherd Dogs. *J. Small Anim. Pract.* 19:711–27.

Anderson, H.C. 1989. Mechanism of mineral formation in bone. *Lab. Invest.* 60:320–30.

Akizuki, S., Mow, V.C., Muller, F., Pita, J.C., and Howell, D.S. 1987. Tensile properties of human knee joint cartilage. II. Correlations between weight bearing and tissue pathology and the kinetics of swelling. *J. Orthop. Res.* 5:173–86.

Balmain, N., Hotton, D., Cuisinier-Gleizes, P., and Mathieu, H. 1989. Immunoreactive calbindin-D_{9K} localization in matrix vesicle-initiated calcification in rat epiphyseal cartilage: An immunoelectron microscope study. *J. Bone Mineral Res.* 4:565–75.

Barland, P., Novikoff, A.B., and Hamerman, D. 1962. Electron microscopy of the human synovial membrane. *J. Cell Biol.* 14:207–20.

Barnes, D.M. 1987. Close encounters with an osteoclast. *Science* 236:914–16.

Barnett, C.H., Davies, D.V., and MacConaill, M.A. 1961. *Synovial Joints.* Clowes, London.

Baron, R. 1989b. Molecular mechanism of bone resorption by the osteoclast. *Anat. Rec.* 224:317–24.

Belanger, L.F., Robichon, J., Migicovsky, B.B., Copp, D.H., and Vincent, J. 1963. Resorption without osteoclasts (osteolysis). In R.F. Sognnaes, ed., *Mechanisms of Hard Tissue Destruction*. Am. Assoc. Adv. Sci., Washington, D.C. Pp. 531–56.

Blair, H.C., Teitelbaum, S.L., Ghiselli, R., and Gluck, S. 1989. Osteoclastic bone resorption by a polarized vacuolar proton pump. *Science* 245:855–57.

Boyan, B.D., Schwartz, Z., Swain, L.D., and Khare, A. 1989b. Role of lipids in calcification of cartilage. *Anat. Rec.* 224:211–219.

Broadus, A.E., Mangin, M., Ikeda, Insoogna, K.L., Weir, E.C., Burtis, W.S., and Stewart, A.F. 1988. Humoral hypercalcemia of cancer: Identification of a novel parathyroid hormone-like peptide. *N. Engl. J. Med.* 319:556–63.

Brandt, K.D., and Radin, E. 1987. The physiology of articular stress: Osteoarthrosis. *Hosp. Pract. [Off]* 22:103–107; 110–12; 117–19.

Canalis, E., McCarthy, T., and Centrella, M. 1989. The role of growth factors in skeletal remodeling. *Endocrinol. Metab. Clin. North Am.* 18:903–18.

Capen, C.C., and Martin, S.L. 1983. Calcium regulating hormones and diseases of the parathyroid glands. In S.J. Ettinger, ed., *Textbook of Veterinary Internal Medicine,* 2d ed. W.B. Saunders, Philadelphia. Vol. 2, pp. 1550–92.

Chambers, T.J. 1989. Origin of the osteoclast. In W.A. Peck, *Bone and Mineral Res./6,* Elsevier, Amsterdam. Pp. 1–25.

Clyne, M.J. 1987. Pathogenesis of degenerative joint disease. *Equine Vet. J.* 19:15–18.

Cooper, C.W., Schwesinger, W.H., Ontjes, D.A., Mahgoub, A.M., and Munson, P.L. 1972. Stimulation of secretion of pig thyrocalcitonin by gastrin and related hormonal peptides. *Endocrinology* 91:1079–89.

Copp, D.H., and Cheney, B. 1962. Calcitonin: A hormone from the parathyroid which lowers the calcium level of the blood. *Nature* 193:381–82.

Cormack, D.H. 1987. *Ham's Histology,* 9th ed. J.B. Lippincott, Philadelphia. Pp. 273–323.

Cutlip, R.C., and Cheville, N.F. 1973. Structure of synovial membrane of sheep. *Am. J. Vet. Res.* 34:45–50.

Davis, W.H., Jr., Lee, S.L., Sokoloff, L. 1978. Boundary lubricating ability of synovial fluid in degenerative joint disease. *Arthritis Rheum.* 21:754–56.

Dee, R. 1978. The innervation of joints. In L. Sokoloff, ed., *The Joints and Synovial Fluid,* Academic Press, New York. Pp. 177–204.

DeLuca, H.F. 1979. The vitamin D system in the regulation of calcium and phosphorus metabolism. *Nutr. Rev.* 37:161–78.

Dzanis, D.A., and Kallfelz, F.A. 1988. Recent knowledge of vitamin D toxicity in dogs. *Proc. ACVIM Forum,* 6:289–91.

Eronen, I., Videman, T. 1985. Effects of sodium diclofenac on glycosaminoglycan metabolism in experimental osteoarthritis in rabbits. *Scand. J. Rheumatol.* 14:37–42.

Eronen, I., Videman, T., Friman, C., Michelsson, J.E. 1978. Glycosaminoglycan metabolism in experimental osteoarthrosis caused by immobilization. *Acta Orthop. Scand.* 49:329–34.

Fawcett, D.W. 1986. *Bloom and Fawcett's A Textbook of Histology.* W.B. Saunders, Philadelphia. Pp. 199–238.

Flanders, J.A., Harvey, H.J., and Erb, H.N. 1987. Feline thyroidectomy: A comparison of postoperative hypocalcemia associated with three different surgical techniques. *Vet. Surg.* 16:362–66.

Freeman, M.A.R., ed. 1973. *Adult Articular Cartilage.* Pitman Medical, London.

Furey, J.G., Clark, W.S., and Brine, K.L. 1959. The practical importance of synovial fluid analyses. *J. Bone Joint Surg.,* ser. A, 41:167–74.

Gardner, E. 1972. The structure and function of joints. In J.L. Hollander and D.J. McCarty, Jr., eds., *Arthritis and Allied Conditions.* 8th ed. Lea & Febiger, Philadelphia.

Gardner, E. 1975. Joints. In E. Gardner, D.J. Gray, R. O'Rahilly, eds., *Anatomy,* 4th ed. W.B. Saunders, Philadelphia. Pp. 17–22.

Gardner, E. 1977. Joints and synovial fluid. In M.J. Swenson, *Dukes' Physiology of Domestic Animals,* 9th ed. Cornell Univ. Press, Ithaca, N.Y. Pp. 433–42.

Ghadially, F.N., and Roy, S. 1969. *Ultrastructure of Synovial Joints in Health and Disease.* Butterworth, London.

Glimcher, M.J. 1989. Mechanism of calcification: Role of collagen fibrils and collagen-phosphoprotein complexes *in vitro* and *in vivo. Anat. Rec.* 224:139–53.

Grant, M., and Prockop, D. 1972. Biosynthesis of collagen. *New Engl. J. Med.* 286:291–300.

Greene, H.J., Leipold, H.W., Hibbs, C.M., and Kirkbride, C.N. 1974. Congenital defects in cattle: Osteopetrosis. *J. Am. Vet. Med. Assoc.* 164:389–95.

Ham, A.W., and Harris, W.R. 1956. Repair and transplantation of bone. In G.H. Bourne, ed., *The Biochemistry and Physiology of Bone.* Academic Press, New York. Pp. 475–505.

Hamerman, D., Rosenberg, L.C., and Schubert, M. 1970. Diarthrodial joints revisited. *J. Bone Joint Surg.,* ser. A, 52:725–74.

Hammett, F.S. 1925. A biochemical study of bone growth. I. Changes in the ash, organic matter, and water during growth. *J. Biol. Chem.* 64:409–28.

Haschek, W.M., Krook, L., Kallfelz, F.A., and Pond, W.G. 1978. Vitamin D toxicity: Initial site and mode of action. *Cornell Vet.* 68:589–97.

Hauschka, P.V., Chen, T.L., and Mavrakos, A.E. 1988. Polypeptide growth factors in bone matrix. In D. Evered and S. Harnett, eds., *Cell and Molecular Biology of Vertebrate Hard Tissues,* Wiley, Chichester, N.Y. Pp. 207–25.

Haussler, M.R., Wasserman, R.H., McCain, T.A., Peterlik, M., Bursac, M., and Hughes, M.R. 1976. 1,25-dihydroxyvitamin D_3 glycoside: Identification of the calcinogenic principle of Solanum malacoxylon. *Life Sci.* 18:1049–56.

Hazewinkel, H.A.W., Goedegebuure, S.A., Poulos, P.W., and Wolvekamp, W. Th. C. 1985. Influences of chronic calcium excess on the skeletal development of growing great Danes. *J. Am. Anim. Hosp. Assoc.* 21:377–91.

Hedhammar, A., Wu, F.M., Krook, L.P., Schryuer, H.F., deLahunta, A., Whalen, J.P., Kallfelz, F.A., Nunez, E.A., Hintz, H.F., Sheffy, B., and Ryan, G.D. 1974. Overnutrition and skeletal disease: An experimental study in growing Great Dane dogs. *Cornell Vet.* 64 (Suppl. 5): 1–160.

Henderson, B., Pettipher, E.R. 1985. The synovial lining cell: Biology and pathology. *Semin. Arthritis Rheum.* 15:1–32.

Herman, H., and Dallemagne, M.J. 1961. The main mineral constituents in bone and teeth. *Arch. Oral Biol.* 5:137–44.

Herring, G.M. 1972. The organic matrix of bone. In G.H. Bowrne, ed., *The Biochemistry and Physiology of Bone,* Vol. 1. Academic Press, New York. Pp. 127–89.

Hirsch, P.F., Gauthier, G.F., and Munson, P.L. 1963. Thyroid hypocalcemic principle and recurrent laryngeal nerve injury as factors affecting the response to parathyroidectomy in rats. *Endocrinology* 73:244–52.

Huffer, W.E. 1988. Morphology and biochemistry of bone remodeling: Possible control by vitamin D, parathyroid hormone and other substances. *Lab. Invest.* 59:418–41.

Ihle, S.L., Nelson, R.W., and Cook, J.R. 1988. Seizures as a manifestation of primary hyperparathyroidism in a dog. *J. Am. Vet. Med. Assoc.* 192:71–72.

Irving, J.T. 1976. Interrelations of matrix lipids, vesicles, and calcification. *Fed. Proc.* 35:109–11.

Isaksson, O.G., Lindahl, A., Nilsson, A., and Isgaard. 1987. Mechanism of the stimulatory effect of growth hormone on longitudinal bone growth. *Endocr. Rev.* 8:426–38.

Jaffe, H.L. 1972. *Metabolic, Degenerative, and Inflammatory Diseases of Bones and Joints.* Lea & Febiger, Philadelphia.

Kerr, H.R., Warbuston, B. 1985. Surface rheological properties of hyaluronic acid solutions. In Fifth International Congress in Biorheology

Symposium: Some Biological Aspects of Joint Diseases. *Biorheology* 22:133–44.

Klausner, J.S., Bell, F.W., Hayden, D.W., et al. 1990. Hypercalcemia in two cats with squamous cell carcinomas. *J. Am. Vet. Med. Assoc.* 196:103–104.

Krane, S.M., Goldring, M.B., and Goldring, S.R. 1988. Cytokines. In D. Evered and S. Harnett, eds., *Cell and Molecular Biology of Vertebrate Hard Tissues.* Wiley, Chichester, N.Y. Pp. 239–56.

Krook, L.P., Barrett, R.B., Usui, K., and Wolke, R.E. 1963. Nutritional secondary hyperparathyroidism in the cat. *Cornell Vet.* 53:224–40.

Krook, L.P., Wasserman, R.H., Shively, J.N., Tashgian, A.H. Jr., Brokken, T.D., and Morton, J.F. 1975. Hypercalcemia and calcinosis in Florida horses: Implication of the shrub, Cestrum diurnum, as causative agent. *Cornell Vet.* 65:26–56.

LeBlond, C.P., Wilkinson, G.W., Belanger, L.F., and Robichon, J. 1950. Radio-autographic visualization of bone formation in the rat. *Am. J. Anat.* 86:289–341.

Levick, J.R. 1984. Blood flow and mass transport in synovial joints. In E.M. Renkin, and C.C. Michel, eds., The Microcirculation, *Handbook of Physiology: The Cardiovascular System.* Am. Physiol. Soc., Bethesda, Md:. Vol. IV, pp. 917–47.

Linsenmeyer, T.F. 1981. Collagen. In E.D. Hay, ed., *Cell Biology of Extracellular Matrix.* Plenum Press, New York. Pp. 5–37.

Mackay-Smith, M.P. 1962. Pathogenesis and pathology of equine osteoarthritis. *J. Am. Vet. Med. Assoc.* 141:1246–48.

Mankin, H.J. 1974. The reaction of articular cartilage to injury and osteoarthritis. *New Engl. J. Med.* 291:1285–92.

Marks, S.C., Jr., and Popoff, S.N. 1988. Bone cell biology: The regulation of development, structure and function of the skeleton. *Am. J. Anat.* 183:1–44.

Maroudas, A. 1970. Distribution and diffusion of solutes in articular cartilage. *Biophys. J.* 10:365–79.

Maroudas, A. 1976. Transport of solutes through cartilage: Permeability to large molecules. *J. Anat.* 122:335–47.

Maschio, G., Oldrizzi, L., Tessitore, N., D'Angelo, A., Volvo, E., Lupo, A., Loschiavo, C., Fabris, A., Ganmaro, L., Rugiw, C., and Panzetta, G. 1982. Effects of dietary protein and phosphorus restriction on the progression of early renal failure. *Kidney Int.* 22:371–76.

McCall, W.D., Jr., Farias, M.C., Williams, W.J., BeMent, S.L. 1974. Static and dynamic responses of slowly adapting joint receptors. *Brain Res.* 70:221–43.

McCutcheon, C.W. 1978. Lubrication of joints. In L. Sokoloff, ed., *The Joints and Synovial Fluid.* Academic Press, New York. Vol. 1, pp. 437–83.

McLean, F.C., and Urist, M.R. 1955. Bone: *An Introduction to the Physiology of Skeletal Tissue.* Univ. of Chicago Press, Chicago.

Meuten, D.J., Segre, G.V., Capen, C.C., Kociba, G.J., Voelkel, E.F., Levine, L., Tashjian, A.H. Jr., Chew, D.J., and Nagode, L.A. 1983. Hypercalcemia in dogs with adenocarcinoma derived from apocrine glands of the anal sac: Biochemical and histomorphometric investigations. *Lab. Invest.* 48:428–35.

Muller-Glauser, W., Humble, B., Glatt, M., Strauli, P., and Winterhalter, K.H. 1986. On the role of type IX collagen in the extracellular matrix of cartilage: Type IX collagen is localized to intersection of collagen fibrils. *J. Cell Biol.* 102:1931–39.

Neuman, W.F., and Neuman, M.W. 1958. *The Chemical Dynamics of Bone Mineral,* Univ. of Chicago Press, Chicago.

Peterlik, M., Bursac, K., Haussler, M.R., Hughes, M.R., and Wassermann, R.H. 1976. Further evidence for the 1,25-dihydroxyvitamin D-like activity of Solanum molycoxylon. *Biochem. Biophys. Res. Comm.* 70:797–804.

Posner, A.S. 1973. Bone mineral on the molecular level. *Fed. Proc.* 32:1933–37.

Price, P.A. 1989. GLA-containing proteins of bone. *Connect. Tissue Res.* 21:51–60.

Raisz, L.G. 1988. Hormonal regulation of bone growth and remodelling. In D. Evered and S. Harnett, eds., *Cell and Molecular Biology of Vertebrate Hard Tissues.* Wiley, Chichester, N.Y. Pp. 226–38.

Reddi, A.H., Muthukumaran, N., Ma, S., Carrington, J.L., Luyten, F.P., Paralkar, V.M., and Cunningham, N.S. 1989. Initiation of bone development by osteogenin and promotion by growth factors. *Connect. Tissue Res.* 20:303–12.

Robison, R. 1923. The possible significance of hexosephosphoric esters in ossification. *Biochem. J.* 17:286–93.

Rodan, G.A., and Martin, T.J. 1981. Role of osteoblasts in hormonal control of bone resorption: A hypothesis. *Calcif. Tissue Int.* 33:349–51.

Rostowski, C.M., Wilson, T.D., Allan, G.S., Deftos, L.J., Benson, K.W., Kallfelz, F.A., Minor, R.R., and Krook, L. 1981. Hypercalcitoninism without hypercalcitoninemia. *Cornell Vet.* 71:188–213.

Rubin, C.T., and Hausman, M.R. 1988. The cellular basis of Wolff's law: Transduction of physical stimuli to skeletal adaptation. *Rheum. Dis. Clin. North Am.* 14:503–17.

Schneider, L.E., Schedl, H.P., McCain, T., and Haussler, M.R. 1977. Experimental diabetes reduces circulating 1,25-dihydroxyvitamin D in the rat. *Science* 196:1452–54.

Schubert, M., and Hamerman, D. 1968. *A Primer on Connective Tissue Biochemistry.* Lea & Febiger, Philadelphia.

Schurz, J., and Ribitsch, V. 1987. Rheology of synovial fluid. *Biorheology* 24:385–99.

Scott, J.E., Conochie, L., Faulk, W.P., Bailey, A.J. 1975. Passive agglutination method using collagen coated tanned sheep erythrocytes to demonstrate collagen-glycosaminoglycan interactions. *Ann. Rheum. Dis.* 34 (suppl.): 38–39.

Seppälä, P.O., and Balazs, E.A. 1969. Hyaluronic acid in synovial fluid. *J. Gerontol.* 24:309–14.

Simpkin, P.A., and Pizzorno, J.E. 1974. Transsynovial exchange of small molecules in normal human subjects. *J. Appl. Physiol.* 36:581–87.

Simon, S.R. 1985. Biomechanics of joints. In E.D. Harris, W.N. Kelly, S. Ruddy, and C. Sledge, eds., *Textbook of Rheumatology.* W.B. Saunders, Philadelphia. Pp. 317–36.

Skoglund, S. 1973. Joint receptors and kinaesthesis. In A. Iggo, ed., *Somatosensory System.* Springer, Berlin.

Smith, E.L., and Gilligan, C. 1989. Mechanical forces and bone. In W.A. Peck, *Bone and Mineral/6,* Elsevier, Amsterdam. Pp. 139–73.

Stockwell, R.A. 1983. Metabolism of cartilage. In B.K. Hall, ed., *Cartilage.* Academic Press, New York. Vol. 1, pp. 253–80.

Swann, D.A. 1982. Structure and function of lubricin, the glycoprotein responsible for the boundary lubrication of articular cartilage. In P. Franchimont, ed., *Articular Synovium.* S. Karger, Basel. Pp. 45–58.

Swann, D.A., Silver, F.H., Slayter, H.S., Stafford, W., and Shore, E. 1985. The molecular structure and lubricating activity of lubricin isolated from bovine and human synovial fluids. *Biochem. J.* 225:195–201.

Teare, J.A., Krook, L., Kallfelz, F.A., and Hintz, H.F. 1979. Ascorbic acid deficiency and hypertrophic osteodystrophy in the dog: A rebuttal. *Cornell Vet.* 69:384–401.

Termine, J.D. 1988. Non-collagen protein in bone. In D. Evered and S. Harnett, eds., *Cell and Molecular Biology of Vertebrate Hard Tissues.* Wiley, Chichester, N.Y. Pp. 178–202.

Tomlin, D.H., Henry, K.M., and Kon, S.K. 1953. Autoradiographic study of growth and calcium metabolism in the long bones of the rat. *Br. J. Nutr.* 7:235–52.

Urist, M.R., DeLange, R.J., and Finerman, G.A.M. 1983. Bone cell differentiation and growth factors. *Science* 220:680–86.

Van Pelt, R.W. 1962. Anatomy and physiology of articular structures. *Vet. Med.* 57:135–43.

Van Pelt, R.W. 1962. Properties of equine synovial fluid. *J. Am. Vet. Med. Assoc.* 141:1051–61.

Van Pelt, R.W., and Connor, G.H. 1963. Synovial fluid from the normal bovine tarsus. *Am. J. Vet. Res.* 24:112–21, 537–44, 735-42.

Veis, A. 1988. Phosphoproteins from teeth and bone. In D. Evered and S.

Harnett, eds., *Cell and Molecular Biology of Vertebrate Hard Tissues*. Wiley, Chichester, N.Y. Pp. 161–77.

Videman, T. 1987. Connective tissue and immobilization. Key factors in musculoskeletal degeneration? *Clin. Orthop.* 221:26–32.

Wasserman, R.H., Corradino, R.A., and Krook, L.P. 1975. Cestrum diurnum: A domestic plant with 1,25-dihydroxycholecalciferol-like activity. *Biochem. Biophys. Res. Comm.* 62:85–91.

Wasserman, R.H., and Fullmer, C.S. 1989. On the molecular mechanism of intestinal calcium transport. In F.R. Dintzis and J.A. Laszlo, eds., *Mineral Absorption in the Monogastric GI Tract: Chemical, Nutritional and Physiological Aspects*. Advances in Experimental Medicine and Biology, Plenum Press, New York. Pp. 45–65.

Weir, E.C., Norrdin, R.W., Matus, R.E., Brooks, M.B., Broadus, A.E,. Mitnick, M., Johnston, S.D., and Insogna, K.L. 1988. Humoral hypercalcemia of malignancy in canine lymphosarcoma. *Endocrinology* 122:602–608.

Weller, R.E. 1984. Cancer associated hypercalcemia in companion animals. *Comp. Cont. Ed. Pract. Vet.* 6:639–44.

Widdowson, E.M., and Dickerson, J.W.T. 1964. Chemical composition of the body. In C.L. Comar and F. Bronner, eds., *Mineral Metabolism*. Academic Press, New York. Vol. 2, pt. 2A.

Wuthier, R.E. 1989. Mechanism of de novo formation by matrix vesicles. *Connect. Tissue Res.* 22:27–34.

PART **V** | **WATER BALANCE AND EXCRETION**

CHAPTER 31

The Kidneys | by William O. Reece

Two major functions of the kidneys are excretion of metabolic waste products and regulation of the volume and composition of the body's internal environment, the extracellular fluid. Other essential functions that have been recognized more recently are secretion of hormones and hydrolysis of small peptides. The hormones participate in the regulation of systemic and renal dynamics, red blood cell production, and calcium, phosphorous, and bone metabolism. Small peptide hydrolysis conserves amino acids, detoxifies toxic peptides, and regulates effective plasma levels of some peptide hormones. Because of these multiple functions, there are many clinical signs associated with renal disease.

HISTORICAL PERSPECTIVES

Claudius Galen (AD c130–c200), a Greek physician and writer on medicine, was the first to demonstrate that urine was formed in the kidneys and transmitted from them to the bladder by the ureters. Before this time there was much speculation about how fluid taken by mouth passed from the intestine to the bladder.

Theories about kidney function date from the thirteenth century, when William of Salicet (1210–1280) propounded his ideas of urine formation and gave his classic account of renal "dropsy," an early description of chronic nephritis. Sir William Bowman (1816–1892) published his theory of urinary secretion and his discovery of the capsule surrounding the Malpighian body (glomerulus), which he showed to be continuous with the urinary tubule, in 1842. He believed that water alone was secreted at the Malpighian body and that the dissolved constituents were secreted by the epithelium of the urinary tubules. According to his view, the quantity of water secreted at the capsule approximated the urine volume. Two years later, in 1844, Carl Ludwig (1816–1895) proposed that urine formation begins with the separation of a protein-free ultrafiltrate of plasma in the glomerulus. He believed that the hydrostatic pressure in the glomerulus was the force responsible for filtration and that the volume of filtrate formed was sufficient to account for the rate of excretion of all urinary solutes. He further believed that the filtrate was reduced in volume and the urinary constituents were concentrated by the tubular reabsorption of a large fraction of the filtered water. Ludwig rejected tubular secretion. In 1874, Rudolph Heidenhain (1834–1897) revived Bowman's theory that urine is formed by the combined secretory activities of the glomerular capillary tufts and of the renal tubules. Thereafter, the secretory theory was referred to as the Bowman-Heidenhain theory.

The so-called "modern theory" of urine formation was proposed by Arthur Cushny (1866–1926) in 1917. He reviewed all that had been written and concluded that ultrafiltration (not secretion) occurred at the glomerulus and that tubular reabsorption accounted not only for water but also for other plasma constituents. The fluid reabsorbed was considered to be of constant composition resembling protein-free plasma. Cushny also rejected tubular secretion.

Present-day views of urine formation recognize glomerular filtration, tubular reabsorption of a fluid of varying composition, and tubular secretion.

STRUCTURAL CONSIDERATIONS

The functional unit of the kidney is the nephron, and an understanding of its function is essential for understanding kidney function. Nephron numbers vary considerably among species, and approximate numbers for several species are given in Table 31.1. Within a species the nephron numbers are relatively constant. Considering the differences in size among various breeds of dog, it might be thought that the kidneys of large-breed dogs would contain more nephrons than the kidneys of small-breed dogs. This is not the case, however, and the larger kidney size in large dogs is compensated by their having larger nephrons rather than more nephrons.

Types of nephron

The mammalian kidney has two principal types of nephron, identified by (1) the location of their glomeruli and (2) the depth of penetration of the loops of Henle into the medulla. Those nephrons with glomeruli in the outer and middle cortices are called cortical nephrons. They are associated with a loop of Henle that extends to the junction of the cortex and medulla or into the outer zone of the medulla. Those nephrons with glomeruli in the cortex close to the medulla are known as juxtamedullary nephrons. Juxtamedullary nephrons are associated with loops of Henle that extend more deeply into the medulla; some extend as deep as the renal crest of unipyramidal kidneys (small ruminants, carnivores, and the horse) and to the papillae of multipyramidal kidneys (large ruminants and the pig). The relationship of each nephron type to the cortex and medulla is shown in Fig. 31.1. The juxtamedullary nephrons are more instrumental in developing and maintaining the osmotic gradient from low to high in the outer medulla to the inner medulla, respectively. It is important to note, however, that the tubular fluid of all nephrons (cortical and juxtamedullary) is emptied into shared collecting tubules and ducts that proceed through the medulla to the renal pelvis. Thus, regardless of the influence of different nephron types upon the tubular fluid, the final output of each nephron is subjected to the same factors affecting urine concentration (medullary influence). The percentage of nephrons that have long loops of Henle (juxtamedullary nephrons) varies among animal species (see Table 31.2) and ranges from 3 percent in the pig to 100 percent in the cat. In humans about 14% of the nephrons have long loops.

Table 31.1. Approximate number of nephrons in each kidney for several domestic animals and humans

Species	Nephrons/kidney
Cattle	4,000,000
Pig	1,250,000
Dog	415,000
Cat	190,000
Human	1,000,000

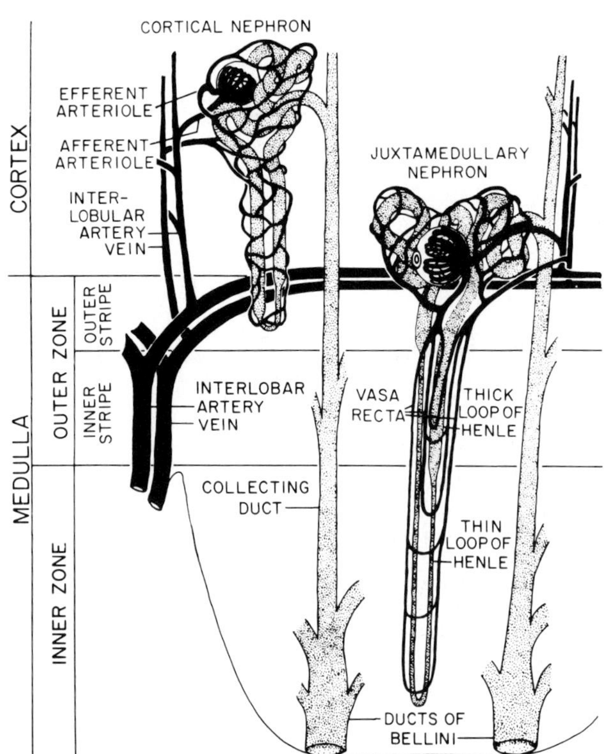

Figure 31.1. The relationship of cortical and juxtamedullary nephrons to the cortex and medulla. (From Pitts 1974, *Physiology of the Kidney and Body Fluids*, 3d ed. Yearbook Medical Publishers, Chicago.)

Table 31.2. Relationship of structure to concentrating capacity in mammalian kidneys

Animal	Kidney size* (mm)	Long-looped nephrons (%)	Relative medullary thickness†	Maximum freezing point depression in urine (°C)
Beaver	36	0	1.3	0.96
Pig	66	3	1.6	2
Human	64	14	3	2.6
Dog‡	40	100	4.3	4.85
Cat	24	100	4.8	5.8
Rat	14	28	5.8	4.85
Kangaroo rat	5.9	27	8.5	10.4
Jerboa	4.5	33	9.3	12
Psammomys	13	100	10.7	9.2

*Kidney size = cube root of the product of the dimensions of the kidney.
†Relative medullary thickness = medullary thickness in millimeters × 10/kidney size.
‡Beeuwkes and Bonventre have shown (1975) that the dog kidney does contain short-looped or corticomedullary nephrons; therefore, long-looped nephrons comprise fewer than 100% of the nephrons.
From Schmidt-Nielsen and O'Dell, 1961, *Am. J. Physiol.* 200:1119–24.

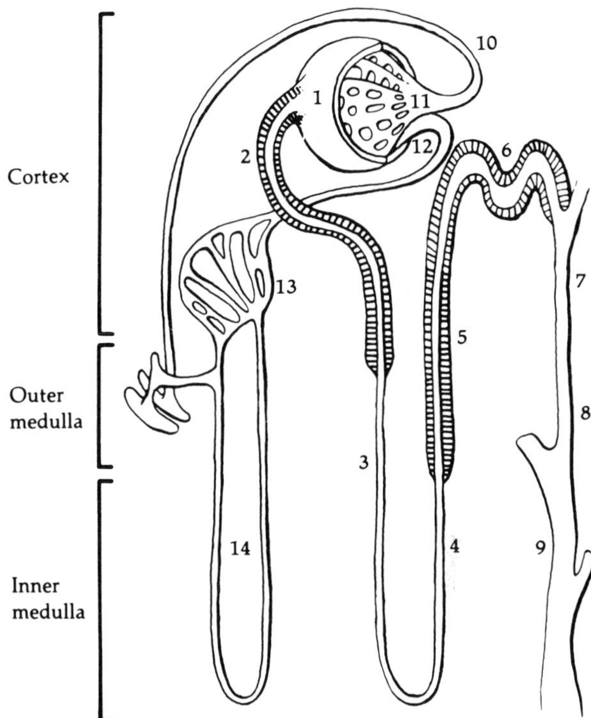

Figure 31.2. The nephron with blood supply. 1, glomerular capsule (Bowman's capsule); 2, proximal tubule; 3, thin descending limb of loop of Henle; 4, thin ascending limb of loop of henle; 5, thick ascending limb of loop of Henle; 6, distal tubule; 7, cortical collecting tubule; 8, outer medullary collecting duct; 9, inner medullary collecting duct; 10, afferent arteriole; 11, glomerulus; 12, efferent arteriole; 13, peritubular capillaries; 14, vas rectum. Connecting tubule (not shown) is the segment between the distal tubule (6) and its junction with the cortical collecting tubule (7). (From Reece 1991, *Physiology of Domestic Animals*, Lea & Febiger, Philadelphia.)

Nephron components

A typical nephron and its component parts is shown in Fig. 31.2. The glomerular capsule (Bowman's capsule) is the dilated blind end of the nephron. The renal corpuscle refers to the combined invagination of a capillary tuft, the glomerulus, into the glomerular capsule. Also, because of the intimate association of the capillary tuft with the glomerular capsule, the term *glomerulus* is often used to include both the capillary and nephron components. The nephron is continued from the glomerular capsule by the proximal tubule, composed of the proximal convoluted portion and the proximal straight portion. The convoluted portion is contained within the cortex, and the straight portion extends about halfway into the outer medulla. The loop of Henle consists of the descending thin limb that is continuous from the proximal straight tubule, the ascending thin limb that terminates at the junction of the inner and outer medullae (cortical nephrons lack a thin ascending limb), and the ascending thick limb that returns to its glomerulus of origin in the cortex and passes between the afferent and efferent arterioles. The distal nephron begins at this point and consists of the distal tubule, the connecting tubule, the cortical collecting tubule, the outer medullary collecting duct, and the inner medullary collecting duct. Embryologically, the distal tubule represents the last segment of the nephron. Physiologically, segments beyond the distal tubule are important structures associated with the processing of glomerular filtrate and, accordingly, are implied segments of the distal nephron. The cortical collecting tubule, the outer medullary collecting duct, and the inner medullary collecting duct, when considered as a unit, are referred to as the collecting tubule/duct. The outer and inner medullary collecting ducts represent the medullary extension of the straight portion of the cortical collecting tubule. The distal tubule, the connecting tubule, and the early cortical collecting tubule (before it becomes straight) are sometimes collectively referred to as the distal convoluted tubule.

Nephron blood supply

Blood to the nephrons is supplied by branches from the interlobular arteries (see Fig. 31.1). The afferent arteriole conducts blood to the glomerulus, and the efferent arteriole conducts blood away from the glomerulus. Blood leaving through the efferent arterioles is redistributed into another capillary bed known as the peritubular capillaries; these perfuse the nephron tubules. The vasa recta are capillary branches into the medulla from the peritubular capillaries and are associated with the long-looped nephrons. After perfusion of the kidneys, blood is returned to the caudal vena cava by the renal veins.

The juxtaglomerular apparatus

When the thick segment of the ascending limb of the loop of Henle returns to its glomerulus of origin in the cortex, it is noted that it passes in the angle between the afferent and

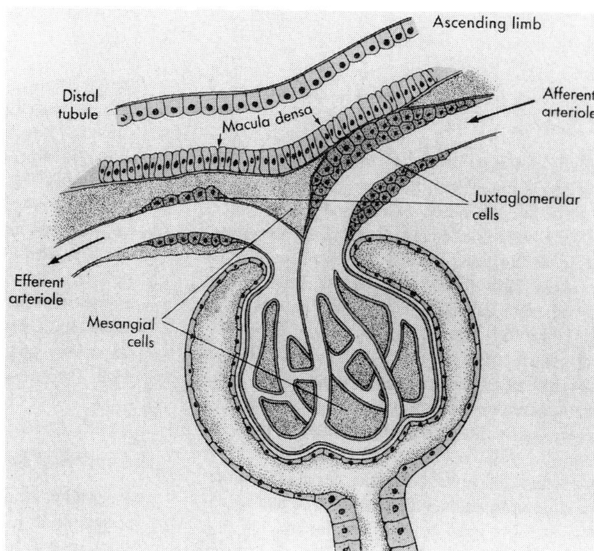

Figure 31.3. Juxtaglomerular apparatus, comprising the juxtaglomerular cells, macula densa, and extraglomerular mesangial cells. (From Duling 1988, in Berne and Levy, eds., *Physiology*, 2d ed., C.V. Mosby, St. Louis.)

efferent arterioles and continues as the distal tubule (Fig. 31.3). The side of the tubule that faces the glomerulus comes in contact with the arterioles; the contact epithelial cells of the tubules are more dense than the other epithelial cells and are collectively called the macula densa. The macula densa marks the beginning of the distal tubule. The smooth muscle cells of the afferent and efferent arterioles that make contact with the macula densa are specialized smooth muscle cells and are called juxtaglomerular (JG) cells or granular cells. The JG cells have secretory granules that contain renin, a proteolytic enzyme.

The space between the macula densa and the afferent and efferent arterioles as well as the space between the glomerular capillaries is known as the mesangial region and it consists of mesangial cells and mesangial matrix. Mesangial cells secrete the matrix, secrete the glomerular basement membrane, provide structural support, have phagocytic activity, and secrete prostaglandins. Mesangial cells also exhibit contractile activity and can influence blood flow through glomerular capillaries. Those cells located between the macula densa and the arterioles are known more specifically as extraglomerular mesangial cells, or lacis cells.

Because of their intimacy and functional relationship, the three components of the JG apparatus are (1) the macula densa, (2) the JG (granular) cells, and (3) the extraglomerular mesangial cells. The JG apparatus is involved in feedback mechanisms that assist regulation of renal blood flow and glomerular filtration rate.

Innervation

Innervation to the kidney is provided by fibers from the sympathetic division of the autonomic nervous system. Their activity assists regulation of renal blood flow, glomerular filtration rate, and salt and water reabsorption by the nephron. Nerve fiber endings lie adjacent to the smooth muscle cells of the major branches of the renal artery, as well as the afferent and efferent arterioles. Regulation of renal blood flow and glomerular filtration rate is accomplished by vasoconstriction initiated by reflexes through the vasomotor center in the medulla and pons. Innervation also includes the renin-producing granular cells of the afferent and efferent arterioles and the nephron proximal tubules and loops of Henle. Increased sympathetic tone elicits renin secretion from the granular cells and enhances sodium reabsorption from nephron segments.

OVERVIEW OF URINE FORMATION

From plasma to urine

The three processes involving the nephrons and their blood supply in urine formation are (1) glomerular filtration, (2) tubular reabsorption, and (3) tubular secretion (Fig. 31.4). As a result of glomerular filtration, an ultrafiltrate of plasma known as glomerular filtrate appears in Bowman's capsule. Because of tubular reabsorption and secretion, the composition of glomerular filtrate begins to change immediately on entering the proximal tubule and is thereafter known as tubular fluid. Tubular reabsorption and

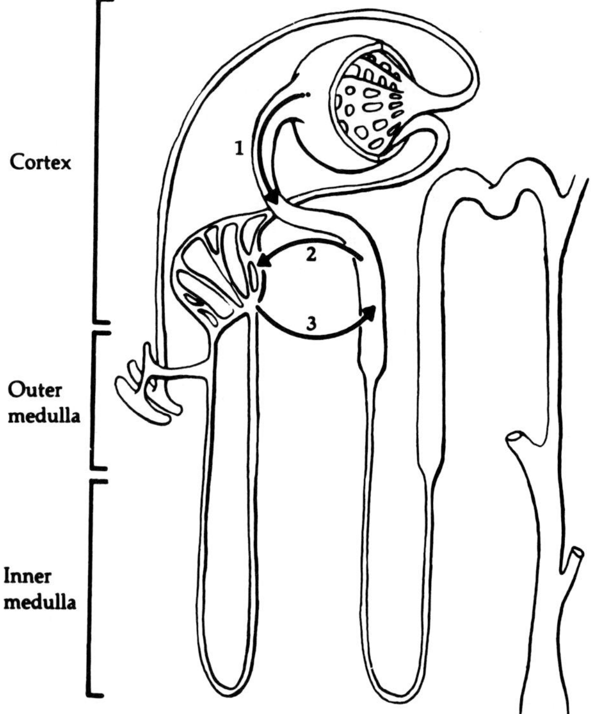

Figure 31.4. Nephron and processes involved in urine formation. Shown are the direction and location of glomerular filtration (1), tubular reabsorption (2), and tubular secretion (3) as they would occur in the glomerulus and proximal tubule. (From Reece 1991, *Physiology of Domestic Animals*, Lea & Febiger, Philadelphia.)

tubular secretion continue throughout the length of the nephron so that tubular fluid does not become urine until it enters the renal pelvis. With the possible exception of the addition of mucus in the horse, there are no compositional changes in urine beyond the collecting ducts.

Distribution of blood at the glomerulus

The renal blood flow (RBF) refers to the rate at which blood flows to the kidneys. Inasmuch as plasma is the fluid part of the blood, renal plasma flow (RPF) refers to that part of the RBF that is plasma. Glomerular filtrate is formed from plasma at the glomerulus, and the rate at which it is formed is known as the glomerular filtration rate (GFR) and is measured in milliliters per minute. Renal blood flow and RPF are also measured in milliliters per minute, and the GFR/RPF ratio is referred to as the filtration fraction (FF). The FF is the fraction (or percentage) of plasma flowing through the glomerulus that becomes glomerular filtrate. Correlation of the several factors of kidney function is illustrated for the canine in Table 31.3.

Kidney solute load

The amount of any substance contained in plasma that is presented to the kidneys each minute is known as the plasma load for that substance. Depending on its usual concentration unit, the load would be expressed as milligrams or milliequivalents per minute. If the plasma concentration for glucose is 80 mg/dl and the RPF is 200 ml/min (2 dl/min), the plasma load of glucose would be 160 mg/min (80 mg/dl $\times$ 2 dl/min).

The tubular load of a plasma substance is the part of the plasma load that filters into Bowman's capsule. It is the amount that will be presented to the tubules, regardless of whether or not it is reabsorbed. If the RPF and the plasma glucose concentration are 2 dl/min and 80 mg/dl, respectively, and the GFR is 0.4 dl/min (FF = 0.4/2 = 1/5), the tubular load could be calculated two ways, as follows:

(1) Tubular load = 0.4 dl/min $\times$ 80 mg/dl = 32 mg/min

(2) Tubular load = FF $\times$ Plasma load = 1/5 $\times$ 160 mg/min = 32 mg/min

Table 31.3. Approximate values for several kidney function variables in a 9.5 kg dog in normal state of hydration*

Variable	Value
Cardiac output (ml/min)	900
Blood flow to kidneys (% of cardiac output)	20
Renal blood flow (ml/min/kg)	18.9
Renal plasma flow† (ml/min/kg)	11.4
Glomerular filtration rate (ml/min/kg)	4
Filtration fraction (decimal equivalent)	0.35
Urine volume in 24 h‡ (ml)	500
Glomerular filtrate volume in 24 h (ml)	54,720
Volume of urine as percent of filtrate	0.92
Filtrate reabsorbed (%)	99.08

*Values used are close to those obtained in unanesthetized beagle bitches by Ewald (1967).

†Based upon plasma portion of hematocrit being approximately 60 percent.

‡Calculated from average rate of urine formation for dogs being 2.2 ml/kg/h.

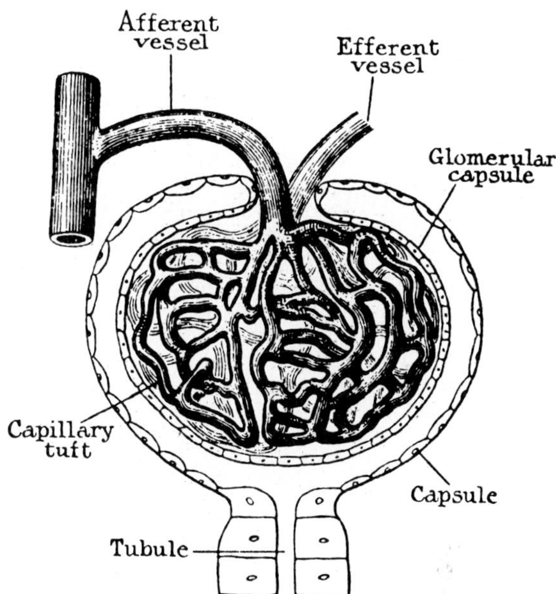

Figure 31.5. Early drawing of Malpighian corpuscle (renal corpuscle). (From Cushny 1917, *The Secretion of the Urine*, Longmans, Green & Co., London.)

GLOMERULAR FILTRATION

A drawing of the glomerulus as it appeared in Cushny's book in 1917 is shown in Fig. 31.5. Note the striking similarity to its current depiction nearly 70 years later (Fig. 31.6). Greater schematic detail, made possible by scanning electron microscopy (Fig. 31.7), permits visualization of the physical barriers to filtration.

Formation of the filtrate

The kidneys have the functional counterpart of two capillary beds, represented by the glomeruli and the peritubular capillaries. The glomeruli are considered to be a high-pressure system (high hydrostatic pressure favoring filtration), and the peritubular capillaries, which are perfused with blood coming from the glomerular capillary bed, are considered to be a low-pressure system (low hydrostatic pressure favoring reabsorption). As such, the glomeruli are similar to the arterial end of a typical muscle capillary, and the peritubular capillaries are similar to the venous end.

The formation of urine begins when an ultrafiltrate of plasma passes through the glomerular capillary endothelium, basement membrane, and Bowman's capsule epithelium into the urinary space of Bowman's capsule (Fig. 31.6). Energy for this filtration process is provided by the heart in the form of hydrostatic pressure (HP) within the glomerular capillaries and is opposed by the colloidal osmotic pressure (COP) of plasma proteins plus the HP of the filtrate.

The dynamics of filtration are illustrated in Fig. 31.8. According to the values shown, there is net filtration because the capillary HP of 60 mm Hg exceeds the combined values for capillary COP of 32 mm Hg and Bowman's

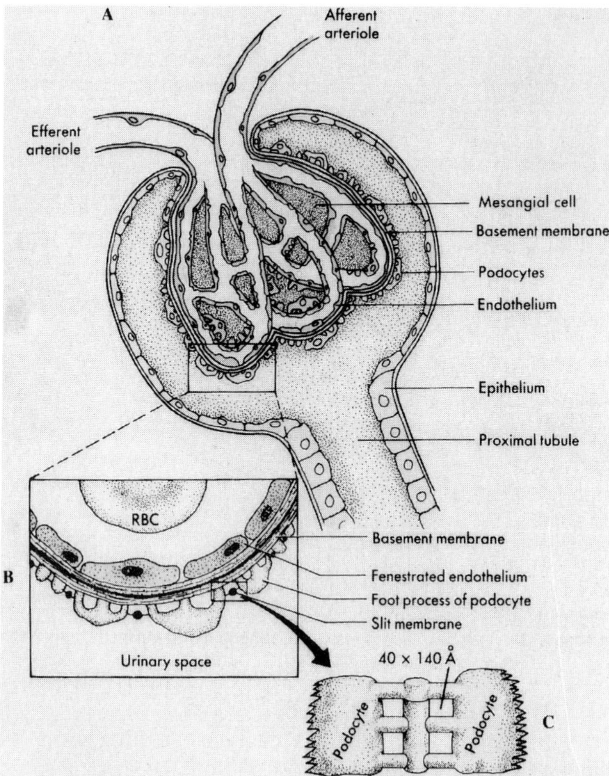

Figure 31.6. Current drawing of renal corpuscle (glomerulus and glomerular capsule). (*A*) Glomerular tuft invaginated into glomerular capsule (Bowman's capsule). (*B*) Filtration membrane. (*C*) Expanded view of slit membrane (rotated outward 90 degrees to show its inner face). (From Berne and Levy 1988, *Physiology*, 2d ed. C.V. Mosby, St. Louis.)

capsule urinary space HP of 18 mm Hg (60 − [32 + 18] = 10 mm Hg). Although some filtration of protein (a potential source of COP in Bowman's capsule) occurs (as in muscle capillaries), the filtrate does not accumulate as it does in muscle because the hydrostatic pressure in Bowman's capsule causes the filtrate to flow away from the capsule and through the nephron tubules. Therefore COP in Bowman's capsule urinary space is negligible.

Nature of the filtrate

The glomerular filtrate is called an ultrafiltrate of blood because the larger components (colloids and blood cells) are not filtered. Practically speaking, it is similar to plasma and interstitial fluid, except that it has a lower protein concentration than either of them.

Because of its fenestration (see Fig. 31.6), the capillary endothelium of the glomerulus is more porous than muscle capillary endothelium, and larger molecules are more readily filtered. Protein molecules are relatively restricted from filtration (similar to their restriction in muscle capillaries) because of their large molecular size, but they might not be excluded altogether. Proteins with a molecular weight of 70,000 and above are virtually excluded from the filtrate. Albumin, the smallest of the plasma proteins, has an average molecular weight of about 69,000, and 0.2 to 0.3 percent of its plasma concentration can appear in the filtrate. Hemoglobin has a molecular weight of about 68,000 and, when unbound, it appears in filtrate at a concentration equal to about 5 percent of its unbound concentration in plasma. The hemoglobin in plasma that arises from normal intravascular lysis of erythrocytes is bound by plasma haptoglobin (a plasma protein) so that the combined size prevents leakage at the glomerulus. If too much intravascular lysis occurs, plasma haptoglobin becomes saturated and hemoglobin begins to appear in the urine, a condition known as hemoglobinuria. If tubular hemoglobin concentration rises too high, coupled with continued water reabsorption from the tubules, hemoglobin can precipitate and block tubules. Blocked tubules can cause acute renal shutdown.

Factors that influence filtration

The GFR can be varied by changes in the diameter of the afferent or efferent arterioles. Dilation of the afferent arteriole increases the blood flow to the glomerulus, which in turn increases the hydrostatic pressure and the potential for filtration. Constriction of the efferent arteriole increases the glomerular hydrostatic pressure, just as blockage of a vein increases the hydrostatic pressure in capillaries behind it. At the same time, it reduces the RBF. Neural and humoral factors are recognized as being capable of affecting the above diameter changes. These will be discussed below at appropriate times.

For any given molecular size, positively charged molecules are more readily filtered than negatively charged molecules. This happens because of electrostatic repulsion by anionic sites in the glomerular basement membrane that are composed mostly of proteoglycans. These negatively charged proteoglycans repel similarly charged molecules. In the physiologic pH range, plasma albumin molecules are polyanionic; in addition to their large molecular size, this is an important aspect in restricting their filtration. Poor perfusion of the kidneys can result in a change in the electrostatic charge of the glomerular membrane, and molecules previously restricted from filtration can be filtered and gain entrance to the capsular space.

Autoregulation

RBF and GFR remain relatively constant regardless of large changes in mean systemic arterial pressure. Between the values of 80 and 180 mm Hg, the change is less than 10 percent (Fig. 31.9). This phenomenon is referred to as autoregulation of RBF and GFR. It is an intrinsic mechanism independent of outside nerve supply. Kidneys have been denervated and transplanted to other parts of the body, and they still retain autoregulation.

Two theories—the myogenic theory and the juxtaglo-

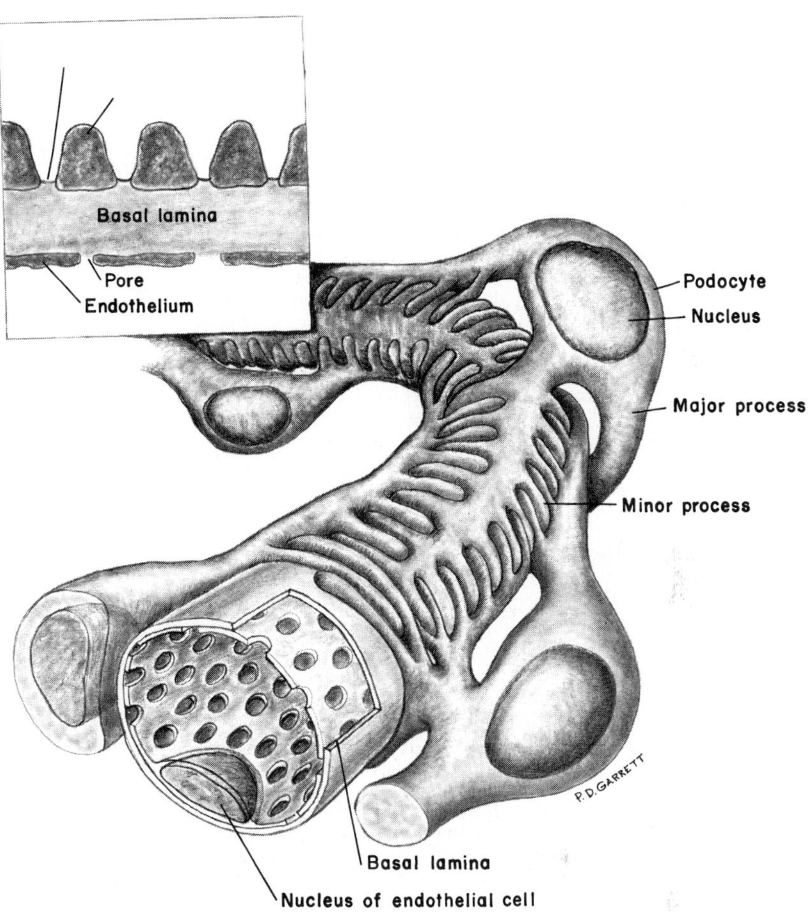

Figure 31.7. Schematic drawing from a scanning electron photomicrograph illustrating the ultrastructure of the glomerular filtration apparatus. (From Dellmann and Brown 1987, *Textbook of Veterinary Histology*, 3d ed., Lea & Febiger, Philadelphia. Courtesy E.J. King and D.A. Kinden.)

merular (JG) theory—have been proposed to explain autoregulation. According to the myogenic theory, increased blood pressure would expand an artery, and it would respond by contracting. In this way, RBF would be decreased and glomerular HP reduced. The reduced glomerular HP would reduce GFR. A reduction in blood pressure would cause less tension, and the blood vessel would dilate to increase RBF and glomerular HP with subsequent increased GFR.

In the JG theory it is believed that renal hypoperfusion, resulting from low blood pressure or blood volume depletion, causes the JG cells to secrete renin, a proteolytic enzyme. Renin acts on a plasma protein (angiotensinogen) to produce angiotensin I. Angiotensin I is rapidly converted to angiotensin II by converting enzyme, which has its highest concentration in the lung. In addition to its location in the lung, converting enzyme is also found in the luminal membrane of vascular endothelial cells and in the glomerulus itself, which provides for an intrarenal renin-angiotensin system. Systemically, angiotensin II influences hemodynamics by promoting renal Na^+ and water reabsorption, thereby expanding the plasma volume, and by producing arteriolar vasoconstriction, which elevates vascular resistance, thereby increasing systemic blood pressure. Locally, the intrarenal production of angiotensin II regulates GFR and RBF by constricting the efferent arterioles to a greater extent than the afferent arterioles. The net result is an elevation of the hydrostatic pressure in the glomerulus, which tends to maintain GFR in the event of hypoperfusion. The renal vasoconstriction also reduces RBF.

The mechanism of tubuloglomerular feedback (TGF) is also associated with the JG theory of autoregulation. TGF refers to alterations in GFR that can be induced by changes in tubular flow rate. It appears to be mediated by the macula densa cells of the JG apparatus. These cells sense changes in the delivery of Na^+ and Cl^- to their region. Therefore, if GFR is increased because of increased glomerular HP, the subsequent increase in macula densa flow and Na^+ and Cl^- delivery initiates a response that returns GFR and macula densa flow toward normal. The return toward normal is brought about by afferent arteriolar constriction (which lowers glomerular HP) and by contraction of the mesangium (which lessens filtration surface area).

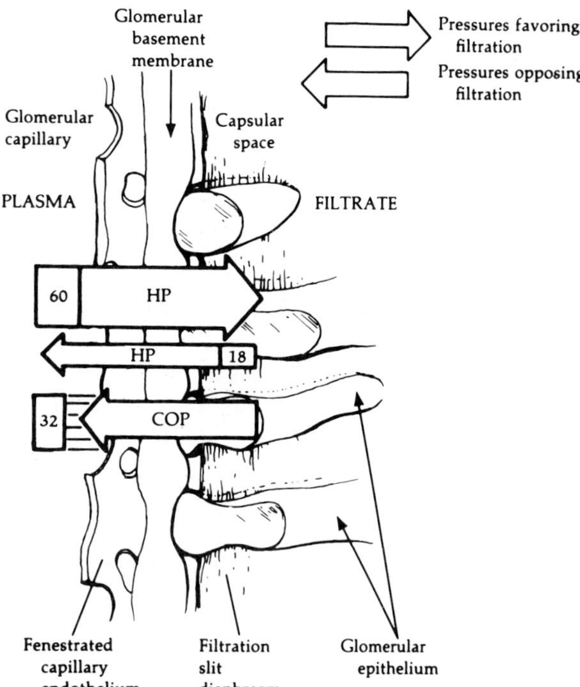

Figure 31.8. Dynamics of glomerular filtration. The capsular space is separated from plasma by a glomerular membrane through which filtration occurs. The extent of filtration is determined by the difference between the pressures favoring filtration and those opposing filtration. In this illustration, filtration occurs because 60 − (32 + 18) = 10 mm Hg. Values greater than or less than 10 mm Hg would correlate with more or less filtration, respectively. Pressure values (60, 32, 18) are in millimeters of mercury. HP, hydrostatic pressure; COP, colloidal osmotic pressure. Glomerular epithelium is represented by minor podocyte processes. (From Reece 1991, *Physiology of Domestic Animals*, Lea & Febiger, Philadelphia.)

TUBULAR TRANSPORT

Tubular transport refers to all phenomena associated with tubular fluid throughout the nephron and collecting tubule/duct length. Transport from Bowman's capsule to the renal pelvis is accomplished by a difference in HP. Tubular reabsorption involves transport of water and solute from tubular fluid to peritubular capillaries. Tubular secretion is associated with transport of solute from peritubular capillaries to the tubular fluid. The directions and structures traversed for both reabsorption and secretion are shown in Fig. 31.10.

Capillary dynamics in peritubular capillaries

Reabsorption of fluid into the peritubular capillaries is analogous to the reabsorption that occurs at the venous end of a muscle capillary. In other words, in contrast to filtration that occurs at the glomerulus, the capillary dynamics favor reabsorption. Assuming peritubular capillary HP and COP to be 17 and 30 mm Hg, respectively, and interstitial fluid HP and COP to be 6 and 10 mm Hg, respectively, reabsorption pressures (30 + 6 = 36 mm Hg) exceed filtration pressures (17 + 10 = 27 mm Hg) by 9 mm Hg (36 − 27 = 9 mm Hg). It is important to associate reductions in peritubular capillary HP and elevations in peritubular capillary COP with greater tubular reabsorption.

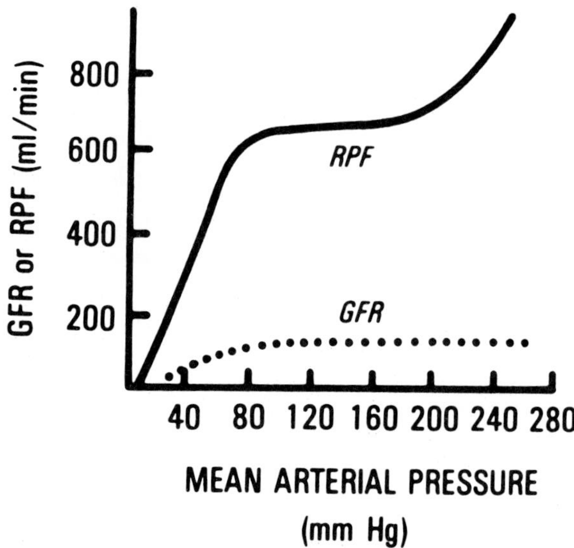

Figure 31.9. Schematic illustration of the autoregulation phenomenon. Note minimal change of renal plasma flow (RPF) and glomerular filtration rate (GFR) as mean arterial pressure increases between 80 and 180 mm Hg. (From Laiken and Fanestil 1985, in West, ed., *Best and Taylor's Physiological Basis of Medical Practice*, 11th ed., Williams & Wilkins, Baltimore. © 1985, the Williams & Wilkins Co.)

Tubular reabsorption

Substances important to body function, such as Na^+, glucose, and amino acids, enter tubular fluid by filtration at the glomerulus. Because of their relatively small molecular size, they pass easily through the glomerular membrane,

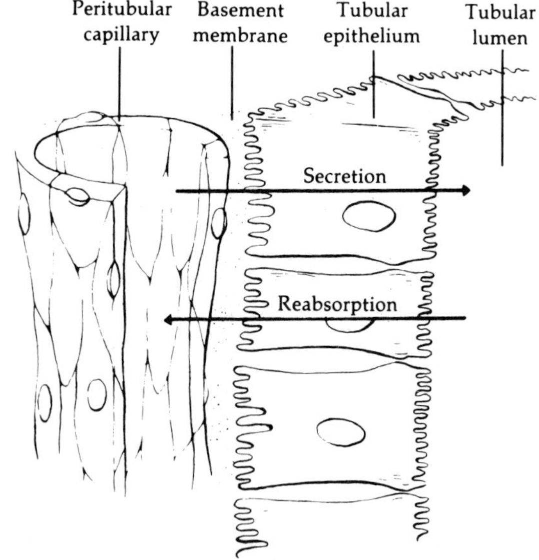

Figure 31.10. Tubular reabsorption and secretion. Longitudinal section of nephron tubule. Shown is the relationship among the tubular lumen, epithelial cell, and peritubular capillary. (From Reece 1991, *Physiology of Domestic Animals*, Lea & Febiger, Philadelphia.)

and their concentrations in the glomerular filtrate are about equal to their concentrations in plasma. Unless these substances are returned to the blood, they are excreted in the urine and lost from the body.

Active transport

In order that Na^+, glucose, and amino acids from the tubular fluid may be returned to the blood, energy is supplied by the Na^+-K^+ ATPase pump on the basolateral surfaces of the tubular epithelial cells. Two unidirectional mechanisms involving carrier proteins on the luminal surface are recognized. Transport by a carrier for a single compound (e.g., Na^+) is called *uniport.* Simultaneous transport of two compounds on the same carrier in the same direction (e.g., Na^+ plus glucose, or Na^+ plus amino acid) is known as *symport* or *cotransport. Antiport* or *countertransport* refers to the movement of a compound in one direction, driven by the movement of a second compound in the opposite direction (e.g., Na^+-H^+ antiport). These mechanisms whereby the concentration gradient for one compound creates a concentration gradient favoring transport of another compound are illustrated in Fig. 31.11.

Sodium reabsorption

Three major mechanisms are recognized for Na^+ reabsorption in the proximal tubule, this location accounting for about 65 percent of its return to the plasma (Fig. 31.12). The energy requirement underlying each of the mechanisms is derived from the Na^+-K^+ ATPase ("sodium pump") located in the basolateral membranes of proximal tubule epithelial cells.

Sodium ions are actively transported from the interior of the tubular epithelial cells to the peritubular space across the basolateral membranes. The intracellular Na^+ concentration is thereby lowered, creating a chemical gradient for Na^+ (lumen concentration higher) between the tubular lu-

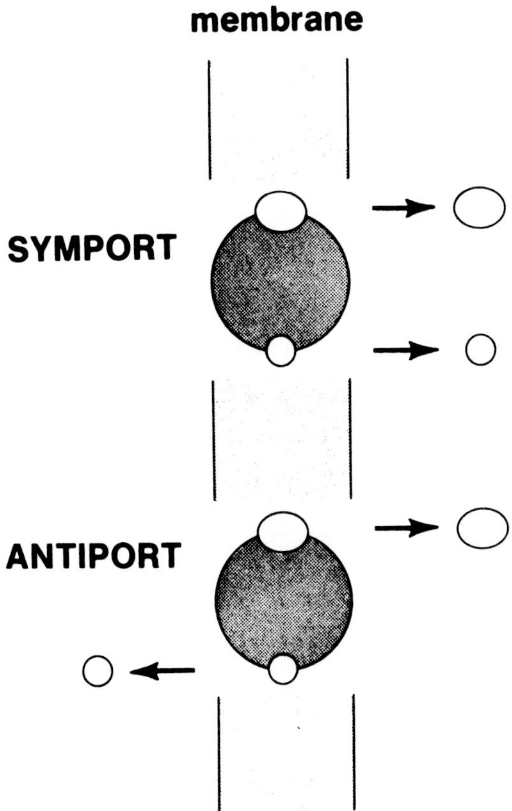

Figure 31.11. Membrane transport mechanisms. Symport (cotransport) is the transport of two compounds through a membrane in the same direction, with the flow of one down its preexisting gradient carrying the other against a gradient. Antiport (countertransport) also couples the transport of one compound to transport of the other, but in an opposite direction. (From McGilvery 1983, *Biochemistry: A Functional Approach*, 3d ed., W.B. Saunders, Philadelphia.)

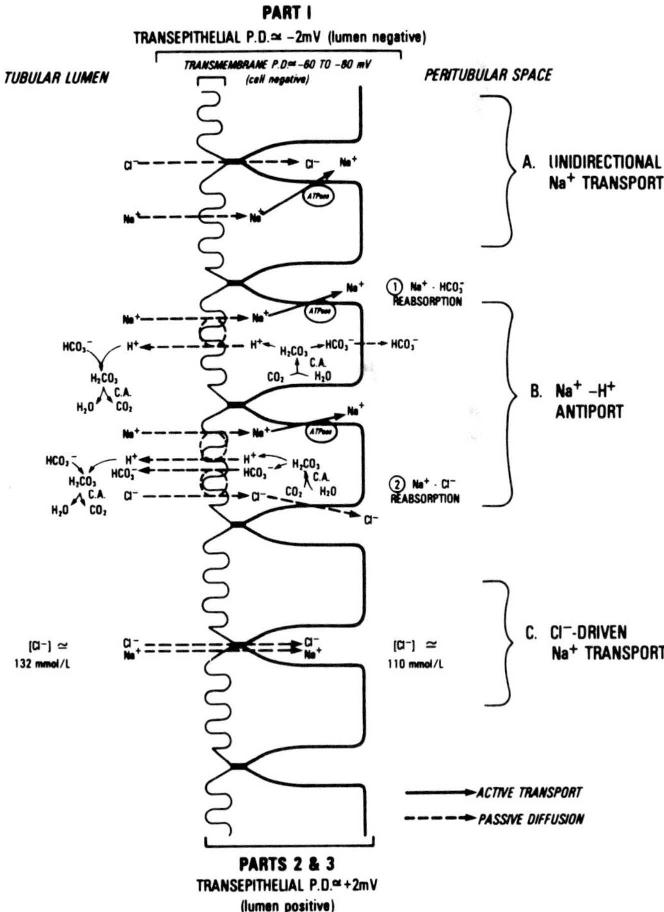

Figure 31.12. Mechanisms for Na^+ reabsorption in the proximal tubule. PD (potential difference) is shown as transepithelial (between peritubular space and tubular lumen) and transmembrane (between cell interior and tubular lumen). Parts 1 and 2 refer to the early and late proximal convoluted tubule, respectively, and part 3 refers to the proximal straight tubule (distal portion of proximal tubule). See text for details of these mechanisms. (From Laiken and Fanestil 1985, in West, ed., *Best and Taylor's Physiological Basis of Medical Practice*, 11th ed., Williams & Wilkins, Baltimore. © 1985, the Williams & Wilkins Co.)

men and the tubular epithelial cell. The active transport of Na^+ also creates a transmembrane electrical potential difference (cell negative) of about −70 mV. An electrochemical gradient is thus established, and, since the luminal membrane is not only permeable to Na^+ but also contains a carrier protein for Na^+, it readily diffuses (facilitated diffusion) from the lumen into the cell. This mechanism is uniport or unidirectional Na^+ transport (Fig. 31.12A). Chloride ion readily diffuses from the tubular lumen to the peritubular space through the tight junctions between tubular epithelial cells because of the transepithelial electrical potential difference (lumen negative) created by active transport of Na^+. Because of the relatively high permeability of the tubular epithelium to Cl^- (refer to parts 1 and 2 in Fig. 31.12), the transepithelial potential difference is only about −2 mV.

The second mechanism of Na^+ transport is antiport or countertransport. The diffusion of Na^+, because of its electrochemical gradient, is coupled through a carrier protein with H^+ diffusing in the opposite direction, from the cell interior to the tubular lumen (Fig. 31.12B). The HCO_3^- in the cell that resulted from H^+ formation can diffuse through the basolateral membranes into the peritubular space or move into the tubular lumen in countertransport to Cl^- diffusion into the cell. The former occurrence results in plasma recovery of $NaHCO_3$ (B① in Fig. 31.12), and the latter results in plasma recovery of NaCl (B② in Fig. 31.12).

A third mechanism of Na^+ reabsorption is known as chloride-driven Na^+ transport (Fig. 31.12C). In the more distal portions of the proximal tubule, the Cl^- concentration in the lumen increases as a result of more HCO_3^- (that formed in the cell) being reabsorbed into the peritubular space as anion rather than Cl^-. The Cl^- gradient now favors diffusion of Cl^- through the "leaky" tight junctions from the tubular lumen into the peritubular space, and this is accompanied by diffusion of Na^+ through the tight junctions in the same direction to maintain electrical neutrality. The transepithelial potential difference in these distal locations (refer to part 3 in Fig. 31.12) is about +2 mV (lumen positive).

About 25 percent of the tubular load of Na^+ is reabsorbed in the ascending thin and thick segment of the loop of Henle. Active transport of Na^+ in the ascending thick segment requires the presence of Cl^- in the lumen because entry of Na^+ into the tubular cell appears to be coupled to the entry of Cl^- (cotransport). Once in the cell, Na^+ is actively extruded across the basolateral surfaces by the Na^+-K^+ ATPase, and Cl^- diffuses passively to maintain electrical neutrality. Na^+-Cl^- cotransport in the loop of Henle is inhibited by the so-called loop diuretics, such as furosemide (diuretics increase output of urine).

The remaining 10 percent of filtered Na^+ is presented to the distal nephron. The mechanism of reabsorption is similar to the uniport mechanism found in the proximal tubule. In addition, Na^+ reabsorption in the collecting tubules and collecting ducts is stimulated by the hormone aldosterone.

Glucose and amino acid reabsorption

Glucose and amino acids are reabsorbed by symport or cotransport (Fig. 31.13). They are coupled with specific carriers that require Na^+ binding and diffuse to the cell interior because of the electrochemical gradient for Na^+. Inside the cell, the Na^+ and glucose or amino acid separate from the carrier. The Na^+ is then actively transported by the Na^+-K^+ ATPase to the peritubular space, and presumably specific carriers are present for facilitated diffusion of glucose and amino acids into the peritubular space. It is likely that several specific Na^+-amino acid carriers are present in the luminal membrane for amino acid transport.

Transport of water and nonactively reabsorbed solutes

After the diffusion of solute (Na^+, Cl^-, HCO_3^-, glucose, amino acids) into the peritubular space, an osmotic gradient is established whereby a greater effective osmotic pressure is present in the peritubular space. In response to the greater effective osmotic pressure in the peritubular space, water diffuses from the tubular lumen through the tight junctions (paracellular) and tubular cells (transcellular) into the peritubular space.

The reabsorption of about 65 percent of the Na^+ and its accompanying anions from the proximal tubules accounts for most of the effective osmotic pressure in the peritubular

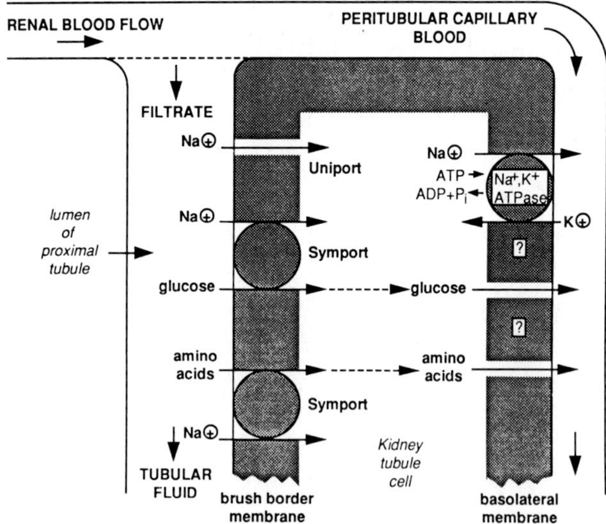

Figure 31.13. Symport (cotransport) mechanism for the reabsorption of glucose and amino acids in the proximal tubule. Also shown is a uniport (unidirectional) mechanism for Na^+ transport. The Na^+ gradient, created by the Na^+-K^+ ATPase, is used for the transport of glucose and amino acids into the cell. Transport of glucose and amino acids from the cell to the peritubular space (and thence to the blood) is by facilitated diffusion. (Question marks indicate that specific carriers are not known.) (Modified from McGilvery 1983, *Biochemistry: A Functional Approach*, 3d ed., W.B. Saunders, Philadelphia.)

space. Accordingly, 65 percent of the water is reabsorbed from the proximal tubule (an additional amount for the other osmotically active substances, i.e., glucose, amino acids). As the water is reabsorbed, urea and other nonactively reabsorbed solutes are concentrated in the tubular lumen. A chemical concentration gradient is established for urea and other nonactively reabsorbed solutes, and they are reabsorbed down their concentration gradient. The extent of their reabsorption is dependent on the permeability of the tubular epithelium for the solute. The urea permeability of the proximal tubular epithelium is much less than that for water, and thus more than half of the amount of urea in the glomerular filtrate continues beyond the proximal tubule.

Reabsorption of proteins and peptides

It was noted above that proteins with a molecular weight less than about 69,000 have a potential for becoming a part of the glomerular filtrate. Most of these proteins are reabsorbed in the proximal tubule and are not lost in the urine. However, a small quantity of protein is present in normal urine. The protein concentration in random samples from 157 dogs with no evidence of urinary tract disease averaged 23 mg/dl of urine. The protein in urine from normal dogs has been reported to contain 40 to 60 percent albumin. Other components include all fractions of globulins. In the illustration given in Table 31.3, in which a 9.5 kg beagle formed 500 ml of urine in 24 hours, the amount of protein lost would be about 115 mg/24 h.

Proteins (and polypeptides) are reabsorbed by endocytosis and subsequently degraded by cellular lysosomes to their constituent amino acids. The amino acids presumably move from inside the cell to the peritubular space by facilitated diffusion.

Small peptides are hydrolyzed at the luminal brush border of the proximal tubule and the resultant amino acids taken into the cell by the cotransport mechanism of the luminal membrane. Small peptide hydrolysis is a high-capacity mechanism capable of returning to the body large amounts of amino acids that might otherwise be lost in the urine as peptides or fail to be reabsorbed into the cell by endocytosis.

Other substances

No attempt will be made to define the mechanism of reabsorption for all substances. Those for which the most is known have been presented above. Kreb's cycle intermediates (i.e., lactate and citrate) are reabsorbed as well as the plasma cations and anions, Ca^{2+}, Mg^{2+}, K^+, and phosphate. Water-soluble vitamins present in plasma would otherwise be lost in the urine if mechanisms for reabsorption were not present.

Tubular secretion

Several substances are transported from the peritubular capillaries into the interstitial fluid and then to the tubular lumen via the tubular epithelial cells. The antiport of H^+ that accompanied Na^+ reabsorption in the proximal and distal tubule is one example. H^+ secretion continues to a lesser extent throughout the remainder of the nephron but does not appear to be coupled with Na^+ reabsorption.

Renal potassium transport is unique in that it is reabsorbed in some parts of the tubule and secreted in others. It is reabsorbed in the convoluted portion of the proximal tubule, secreted in the straight portion, and both reabsorbed and secreted in the distal nephron. When dietary potassium intake is extremely low there is greater reabsorption of K^+ in the distal nephron, and when dietary potassium intake is high there is greater K^+ secretion.

An exogenous substance, para-aminohippuric acid (PAH), is an organic acid that is used to measure renal plasma flow. It is used because, if plasma concentrations of PAH are maintained low enough, any PAH that is not freely filtered is virtually all secreted as it circulates through the peritubular capillaries. The system that secretes PAH is not specific but, rather, accounts for the secretion of a number of organic acids. Penicillin is lost from the body fluids because of tubular secretion. A longer-acting penicillin that has been developed persists in the body for longer periods of time because its rate of secretion has been slowed. A number of organic bases are also secreted by a nonspecific mechanism similar to that for organic acids.

Transport maximum

For substances, such as glucose, that are associated with a carrier for their transport from tubular lumen to peritubular fluid, there is a maximum rate at which they can be reabsorbed; this is known as the tubular transport maximum (T_m). When the T_m for the substance in a nephron is exceeded, the substance will appear in the urine. In the disease known as diabetes mellitus, the movement of glucose from plasma into body cells is impaired because of the lack of insulin. Glucose concentration in plasma therefore increases, causing the plasma and tubular loads of glucose to increase. When the increased tubular load exceeds the availability of carrier molecules for glucose reabsorption, the excess glucose continues its flow through the tubules into the urine. Because glucose is retained within the tubules, it contributes to the effective osmotic pressure of the tubular fluid, and water remains in the tubular fluid. Thus, in diabetes mellitus glucose can be detected in the urine and a greater volume of urine is formed. Because greater amounts of water are lost from the body in the urine, the afflicted animal drinks more water to compensate for the urine loss. Increased urine formation is known as *diuresis;* when it is caused by retention of water in the tubules because of increased effective osmotic pressure in the tubular lumen, it is known as *osmotic diuresis.*

Not all of the hundreds of thousands of nephrons have the same T_m. The first appearance of glucose in the urine does not represent the T_m for the kidney but, rather, the renal

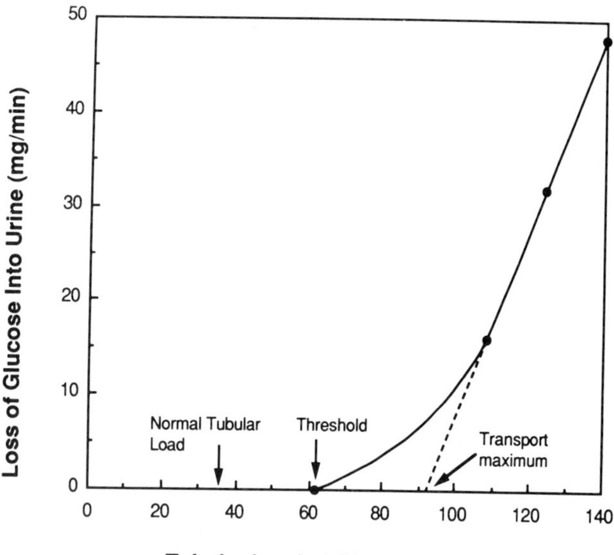

Figure 31.14. Example of renal threshold and transport maximum for glucose in the dog as related to its tubular load and loss into the urine. See text for details.

threshold. The T_m for the kidney is reached when all nephrons are reabsorbing to their maximum ability.

An example that illustrates renal threshold and T_m is given below and in Fig. 31.14 for a 10 kg dog that has an RPF and FF of 1.2 dl/min and 0.3, respectively. Assuming a plasma glucose concentration of 100 mg/dl, the plasma load for glucose is 120 mg/min (100 mg/dl × 1.2 dl/min) and the tubular load is 36 mg/min (120 mg/min × 0.3). It is expected that all of the glucose making up the tubular load will be reabsorbed and none will appear in the urine. If the plasma glucose concentration is increased to 175 mg/dl (plasma load = 175 mg/dl × 1.2 dl/min = 210 mg/min; tubular load = 210 mg/min × 0.3 = 63 mg/min), glucose begins to appear in the urine. The plasma glucose concentration at which glucose first begins to appear in the urine, 175 mg/dl, is known as the *renal threshold* for glucose.

The T_m for glucose will not be reached until all the symporters of all the nephrons in both kidneys are occupied. Experimentally, this occurs when increments of increase in tubular load result in like increments of increase in the urine. In the above example, if the plasma concentration is increased to 256 mg/dl (plasma load = 256 mg/dl × 1.2 dl/min = 307 mg/min; tubular load = 307 mg/min × 0.3 = 92 mg/min), the T_m for glucose is reached. After T_m definition, an increased plasma concentration of 44 mg/dl (plasma load increase = 44 mg/dl × 1.2 dl/min = 53 mg/min; tubular load increase = 53 mg/min × 0.3 = 16 mg/min) would increase urine glucose excretion 16 mg/min.

Glomerulotubular balance

A large part of the glomerular filtrate is reabsorbed in the proximal tubule and the transport processes are subjected to only a slight degree of control. In contrast, various hormones exert their influence on segments of the distal nephron to cause a fine adjustment of reabsorption that permits precise regulation of salt and water balance.

The amount of filtrate reabsorbed by the proximal tubule is consistently a certain percentage of the filtrate (about 65 percent for water and NaCl) rather than a constant amount for each unit of time. If the GFR is low, only a fractional amount of filtrate is reabsorbed in the proximal tubule (rather than most of it), and the remaining fraction (about one-third) continues to the distal nephron where the regulatory processes are given a chance to operate. If the GFR is high, the additional amount of filtrate does not continue to the distal nephron but, rather, only about one-third of it, and the limited capacity for regulation is not overloaded. This property of the proximal tubule to reabsorb a consistent fractional amount of the glomerular filtrate is known as *glomerulotubular balance*.

RENAL CLEARANCE

Renal clearance is a measurement of the kidney's ability to remove substances from the plasma. Clearance measurements are used not only to determine RBF, RPF, GFR, and FF (elements of kidney function) but also to understand how different substances are handled by the kidney tubules (reabsorbed or secreted), to determine the fraction of a substance that is reabsorbed, to estimate solute excretion and urine concentration, and to compare kidney function values for diagnostic purposes.

Renal clearance can be determined by the following general formula:

$$C_x = \frac{U_x\dot{V}}{P_x}$$

where C_x = clearance of substance x (milliliters per minute), U_x = concentration of x in urine (milligrams per minute), $\dot{V}$ = rate of urine formation (milliliters per minute), and P_x = concentration of x in plasma (milligrams per milliliter). Thus, if U_x = 130 mg/ml, $\dot{V}$ = 1 ml/min, and P_x = 2 mg/ml, then C_x = (130 × 1)/2 = 65 ml/min.

U_xV (130 mg/ml × 1 ml/min) is the rate at which substance x is excreted. Accordingly, dividing the excretion rate by the concentration of the substance in plasma (130 mg/min divided by 2 mg/ml = 65 ml/min) gives the amount of plasma that would be needed (completely cleared) each minute to provide the quantity that is excreted. Only a few substances are completely removed from the blood as they circulate through the kidney; thus the renal clearance measurement does not actually describe an event but only provides values for comparison. For example, a renal clearance value for urea of 50 ml/min does not mean that 50 ml of the RPF is completely cleared of urea and that the remainder continues through the kidney with none extracted. Rather, it means that every milliliter of the RPF contributes some urea to that which is excreted, but the amount excreted in the urine each minute would require all the urea in 50 ml of the RPF.

Measurement of glomerular filtration rate and renal plasma flow

A substance used to measure GFR must be freely filtered at the glomerulus and, further, it should not be reabsorbed or secreted by the tubular epithelium after it enters the nephron. Since the substance is freely filtered, its concentration in the filtrate will be the same as its concentration in the plasma. Furthermore, since it is not reabsorbed or secreted, the rate of its excretion into the urine will be the same as its tubular load. Inulin, a fructose polysaccharide, is the substance that is most commonly used, and it behaves as above for all vertebrates (Fig. 31.15). Creatinine is also commonly used but is not as versatile because in some species it is secreted by the tubules. It is generally successful in dogs, cats, sheep, and cattle. Analysis of both substances is quite easy. Creatinine is an endogenous substance that arises mostly from phosphocreatine in muscle under physiologic conditions. Free creatinine in the blood is not reused and is ultimately excreted in the urine at a constant rate. Therefore endogenous creatinine clearance is frequently used in the clinical evaluation of renal function. Normal plasma concentrations of creatinine in domestic animals average 1 to 2 mg/dl. Because of these relatively low values, critical evaluations require infusion of exogenous creatinine in order to increase measurement accuracy.

A substance used to measure RPF must be freely filtered at the glomerulus, must not be reabsorbed from the tubular lumen, and must be secreted by the tubular epithelium so that all of the substance in the blood perfusing the tubules is removed before the blood leaves the kidney. Thus, if all of the substance in the plasma that perfuses the kidneys is excreted in the urine, the rate of its excretion is the same as its plasma load. A substance widely used for this purpose is PAH (see discussion under "Tubular Secretion"). Inasmuch as there is a T_m for its secretion, the infusion must be adjusted so that the plasma concentration does not exceed the T_m.

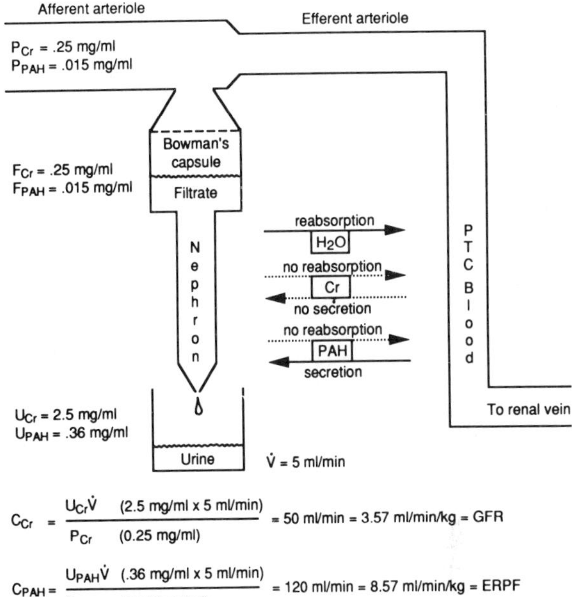

Figure 31.16. Schematic illustration of the determination of effective renal plasma flow (ERPF) by measurement of the renal clearance of para-aminohippuric acid (C_{PAH}) and of glomerular filtration rate (GFR) by measurement of the renal clearance of creatinine (C_{Cr}). See text for details. Cr, creatinine; P_{Cr}, creatinine concentration in plasma; U_{Cr}, creatinine concentration in urine; F_{Cr}, creatinine concentration in filtrate; PAH, para-aminohippuric acid; P_{PAH}, para-aminohippuric acid concentration in plasma; U_{PAH}, para-aminohippuric acid concentration in urine; F_{PAH}, para-aminohippuric acid concentration in filtrate; $\dot{V}$, rate of urine formation; PTC, peritubular capillary. Weight of dog for this illustration is 14 kg.

Simultaneous infusion of inulin (or creatinine) and PAH is usually accompanied by a timed urine collection and blood sampling at appropriate times (usually at the beginning, middle, and end of timed urine collection). Values for excretion rate and plasma concentration are the necessary components for calculating renal clearance and, because of the unique characteristics of the substances used, GFR and RPF can be determined. The excretion rate ($U \times \dot{V}$ of renal clearance formula) is calculated from values obtained from analysis for each substance in urine (U) in milligrams per milliliter) and from the timed urine collection ($\dot{V}$) in milliliters per minute. Plasma concentration (P) in milligrams per milliliter of each substance is obtained by analysis and the average of the collected samples is used for calculation. The determination of GFR and RPF by renal clearance methods is illustrated in Fig. 31.16. Effective RPF (ERPF)

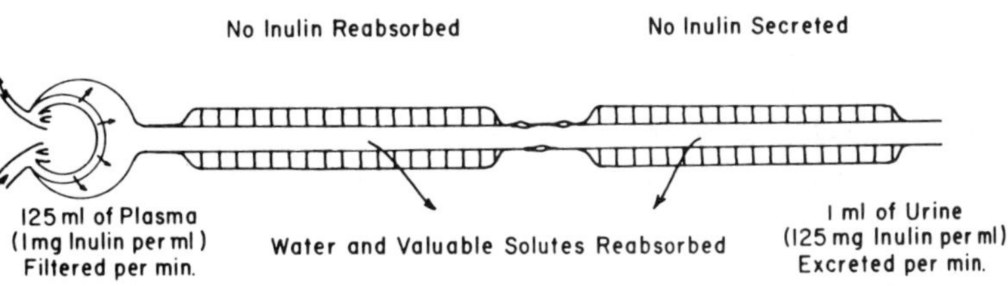

Figure 31.15. Schematic illustration of measuring glomerular filtration rate by the inulin clearance method. Note that the inulin filtration rate (1 mg $ml^{-1} \times 125$ ml min^{-1} = 125 mg/min) is equal to its excretion rate (125 mg $ml^{-1} \times 1$ ml min^{-1} = 125 mg/min). The GFR (inulin clearance) is equal to 125 ml/min [inulin excretion rate (125 mg ml^{-1})/plasma concentration of inulin (1 mg ml^{-1})]. (From Pitts 1974, *Physiology of the Kidneys and Body Fluids*, 3d ed., Yearbook Medical Publishers, Chicago.)

is shown because not all of the PAH is secreted from the blood that perfuses the kidney and RPF is underestimated (only 80 percent of canine RBF perfuses parts of kidney involved in secretion and filtration). The extraction of PAH in the dog (80 percent) is less than it is for humans (90 percent). RPF is estimated from ERPF by calculation. In Fig. 31.16, the estimated RPF would be 150 ml/min (ERPF/0.8 = 120/0.8 = 150).

Determining fraction of substance reabsorbed

In mammals urea is formed from NH_3 in the liver. Because urea is a small, nonionic substance, the glomerular membranes offer no barrier to it and it readily diffuses into the capsular space. The diffusion of water from the proximal tubule to the interstitial space is accompanied by diffusion of urea. Whereas 65 percent of the filtrate water may be reabsorbed from the proximal tubule, only 30 to 40 percent of the urea is reabsorbed at that location, indicating that proximal tubule epithelium is not as permeable for urea as it is for water.

The fate of urea in the more distal nephron segments depends on the rate of urine flow. Increased urine flow rates are accompanied by an increase in the amount of urea excreted into urine. Because of adequate hydration, less ADH is secreted, diffusion from the tubular fluid to the medullary interstitial fluid is reduced, and urea is excreted at a higher rate. Example: Simultaneous inulin and urea clearances are determined in an 18 kg dog that has been adequately hydrated:

$\dot{V} = 4$ ml/min; $U_{in} = 3.2$ mg/ml; $P_{in} = 0.2$ mg/ml; $U_{urea} = 3.2$ mg/ml; $P_{urea} = 0.3$ mg/ml

$$C_{in} = \frac{3.2 \text{ mg/ml} \times 4 \text{ ml/min}}{0.2 \text{ mg/ml}} = 64 \text{ ml/min}$$

$$C_{urea} = \frac{3.2 \text{ mg/ml} \times 4 \text{ ml/min}}{0.3 \text{ mg/ml}} = 43 \text{ ml/min}$$

The fraction of filtered urea that is excreted is determined by comparison of its renal clearance (C_{urea}) with inulin clearance (C_{in}).

$$\frac{C_{urea}}{C_{in}} = \frac{43}{64} = 0.67$$

In this example, 67 percent of the filtered urea was excreted into the urine.

During water deprivation, more ADH is secreted and the permeability of the inner medullary collecting duct increases, not only for water but also for urea. Although urea continues to be excreted, it is excreted at a slower rate.

Example: Simultaneous inulin and urea clearances are determined in an 18 kg dog deprived of water for 30 hours:

$\dot{V} = 0.3$ ml/min; $U_{in} = 42$ mg/ml; $P_{in} = 0.2$ mg/ml; $U_{urea} = 28$ mg/ml; $P_{urea} = 0.3$ mg/ml

$$C_{in} = \frac{42 \text{ mg/ml} \times 0.3 \text{ ml/min}}{0.2 \text{ mg/ml}} = 63 \text{ ml/min}$$

$$C_{urea} = \frac{28 \text{ mg/ml} \times 0.3 \text{ ml/min}}{0.3 \text{ mg/ml}} = 28 \text{ ml/min}$$

$$\frac{C_{urea}}{C_{in}} = \frac{28}{63} = 0.44$$

In this example, 44 percent of filtered urea was excreted into urine.

Determining reabsorption or secretion

A substance such as inulin in the plasma is freely filtered at the glomerulus. It is not reabsorbed from the tubular fluid; nor is it secreted into the tubular fluid from the peritubular capillaries. All that is filtered is excreted. Because it is freely filtered, any increase in plasma concentration results in a proportionately increased excretion rate. Plasma clearance does not change (Fig. 31.17). A substance such as glucose is freely filtered at the glomerulus, and as long as the renal threshold is not reached all that is filtered is reabsorbed and the renal clearance is zero. If the plasma concentration is increased to the point where the renal threshold is surpassed, however, part of the filtered glucose is excreted and renal clearance values begin to rise. These values can never equal the renal clearance values for inulin because some of the filtered glucose will always be absorbed (Fig. 31.17). A plasma substance such as PAH, which is freely filtered and is not reabsorbed from the tubules but is secreted into the tubules (increases the tubular load), will always have a renal clearance value greater than that of

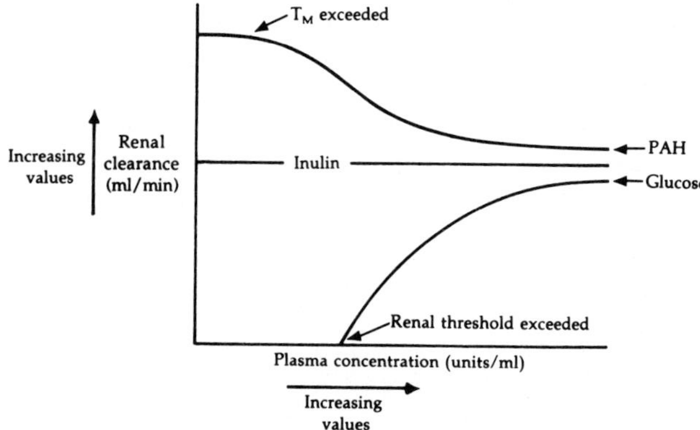

Figure 31.17. Relationship of renal clearance to increasing plasma concentrations of inulin (freely filtered, not reabsorbed, not secreted), glucose (freely filtered, reabsorbed, not secreted), and para-aminohippuric acid (PAH) (freely filtered, not reabsorbed, secreted). (From Reece 1991, *Physiology of Domestic Animals*, Lea & Febiger, Philadelphia.)

inulin because a greater proportion of the plasma load is excreted (Fig. 31.17).

The way in which the kidney handles a given substance known to be excreted into urine is summarized as follows:

$\frac{C_x}{C_{in}} = 1$; substance x was excreted solely by filtration

$\frac{C_x}{C_{in}} = <1$; substance x was both filtered and to some extent reabsorbed

$\frac{C_x}{C_{in}} = >1$; substance x was both filtered and secreted into urine

Estimates of solute excretion and urine concentration

Osmolal clearance

Osmolal clearance provides a quantitative estimate of solute excretion. These estimates are of value in evaluating the action of diuretics. Increased values indicate that water loss is associated with solute loss. During a renal clearance laboratory exercise with 17 normal dogs, the osmolality of the diluted timed urine collections was determined. The average urine osmolality (U_{osm}) was 240 mOsm/kg H_20. The rate of urine formation ($\dot{V}$) was arbitrarily set at 5 ml/min by dilution of urine formed in the timed period to a set volume. Plasma osmolality (P_{osm}) was determined from the plasma samples used for creatinine and PAH analysis and averaged 308 mOsm/kg H_2O. Accordingly,

$$C_{osm} = \frac{U_{osm}\,\dot{V}}{P_{osm}} = \frac{240 \text{ mOsm/kg } H_2O \times 5 \text{ ml/min}}{308 \text{ mOsm/kg } H_2O} = 3.9 \text{ ml/min}$$

The C_{osm} indicates that 3.9 ml of plasma was cleared of solute per minute.

Solute-free water clearance

Solute-free water clearance (C_{H_2O}) provides a quantitative estimate of urine concentration. Its determination requires knowledge of $\dot{V}$ and C_{osm}. In the laboratory exercise described above, values for C_{osm} and $\dot{V}$ from the 17 dogs were used to calculate an average C_{H_2O} as follows:

$C_{H_2O} = \dot{V} - C_{osm} = 5$ ml/min $-$ 3.9 ml/min $=$ 1.1 ml/min

The following interpretation can be placed on C_{H_2O} values:

$C_{H_2O} = 0$; urine and plasma have same solute concentration.

$C_{H_2O} =$ positive value; urine more dilute than plasma.

$C_{H_2O} =$ negative value; urine more concentrated than plasma.

Inasmuch as the dogs used for this experiment were hydrated so as to obtain best results for the renal clearance measurements, it is not surprising to see a positive value for C_{H_2O}.

CONCENTRATION OF URINE

The mechanism for concentration of the tubular fluid depends on the existence of a very high osmolality in the interstitial fluid of the renal medulla. The osmolality increases with the distance from the cortex, reaching a maximum in the innermost aspects of the medulla. The magnitude of this maximum value varies by species. In the dog, it is about 2400 mOsm/kg H_2O, compared with plasma osmolality of about 300 mOsm/kg H_2O. The maximum value in humans is about 1200 mOsm/kg H_2O. The high osmolality exists because of the countercurrent mechanism. It is established by the activities of the loops of Henle and is maintained by the special characteristics of the blood supply to the medulla (the vasa recta).

Countercurrent mechanism

A countercurrent system of tubules or vessels exists where the inflow of fluid runs parallel to, counter (opposite) to, and in close proximity to the outflow for some distance. These characteristics are common to the anatomical arrangements of the loops of Henle and the vasa recta. Accordingly, the countercurrent mechanism in the kidney comprises two countercurrent systems: the countercurrent multiplier (loops of Henle) and the countercurrent exchanger (vasa recta).

Countercurrent multiplier

In the countercurrent multiplier, the transport of tubular solute from the lumen of the ascending thick limb of the loop of Henle to the peritubular fluid, with retention of water in the tubule, dilutes the tubular fluid. It also creates an initial small, horizontal, osmotic gradient between the tubular and peritubular fluids. The osmotic gradient is amplified or "multiplied" vertically by countercurrent flow in the descending thin limb (permeable for water but not for solutes). Water diffuses from the lumen of the descending thin limb to the peritubular fluid in response to the horizontal gradient established by transport activities of the ascending thick limb. Therefore, the tubular fluid of the descending thin limb increases in osmotic concentration as it descends to the innermost region of the medulla (Fig. 31.18). When this tubular fluid enters the ascending thin limb (permeable for solute, impermeable for water), NaCl readily diffuses outward into the inner medullary interstitial fluid and urea diffuses inward into the tubular fluid. Continued active secretion by the ascending thick limb, concentration of tubular fluid in the descending thin limb, and diffusion from the lumen of the ascending thin limb into the inner medullary interstitial fluid establish the vertical os-

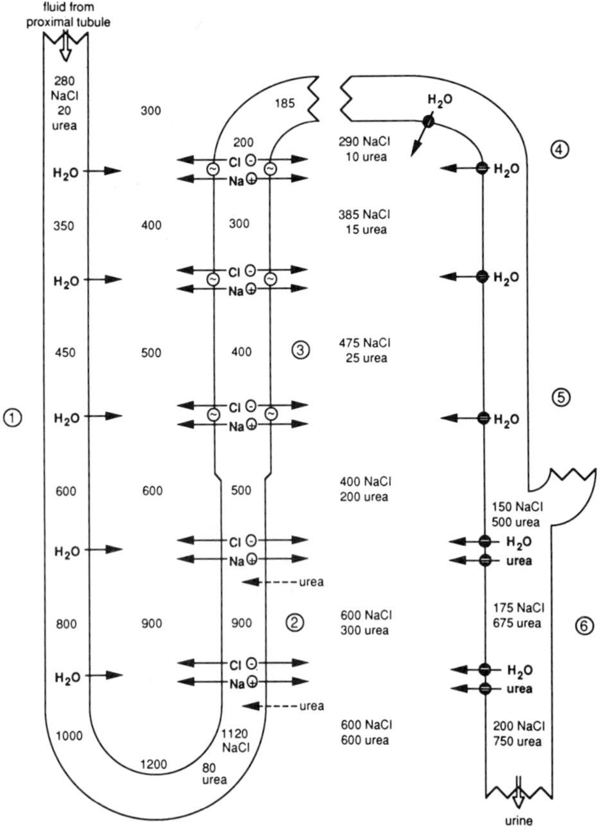

Figure 31.18. Countercurrent multiplication in the loop of Henle and recirculation of urea. Values shown (in milliosmoles per kilogram H_2O) are hypothetical but approximate those of humans under conditions of low water intake. Single numbers represent total osmolality. Identified numbers (NaCl, urea) represent specific contribution to total osmolality. Transport of NaCl and urea at the level of the thin segment of the ascending limb of the loop of Henle is by simple diffusion. Active transport of Na^+ in the ascending thick limb is coupled with the transport of Cl^- (symport). Water channels (also urea) on the right are open (influence of antidiuretic hormone). In this example, urine is being concentrated. Circled numbers identify locations as follows: 1, descending limb of the loop of Henle; 2, thin segment of ascending limb of loop of Henle; 3, thick segment of ascending limb of loop of Henle; 4, cortical collecting tubule; 5, outer medullary collecting duct; 6, inner medullary collecting duct. See text for details. (Modified from McGilvery 1983, *Biochemistry: A Functional Approach*, 3d ed., W.B. Saunders, Philadelphia.)

motic gradient. There are three reasons that passive reabsorption can occur from the lumen of the ascending thin limb:

1. The prior existence of the medullary gradient that caused reabsorption of water from the descending thin limb and the subsequent concentration of Na^+ and Cl^- delivered to the ascending thin limb.

2. About $\frac{2}{3}$ of the high osmolality of the peritubular fluid that favors diffusion of water from the descending thin limb is contributed by NaCl, and about $\frac{1}{3}$ is contributed by urea. Consequently, a diffusion gradient for NaCl develops (high concentration in tubule, low concentration in peritubular fluid).

3. The permeability of the thin segments of the loops of Henle changes at the hairpin turn, so that the ascending thin limb is permeable to solute (Na^+, Cl^-, urea) and impermeable to water. Reabsorption of Na^+ and Cl^- by passive diffusion from tubular fluid to peritubular fluid is now favored, and a progressive dilution of tubular fluid begins (loss of Na^+ and Cl^- coupled with water retention).

Diffusion of urea into the tubule from the peritubular fluid (a part of urea recirculation, see below) occurs in the ascending thin limb, but the tubule becomes impermeable to urea when it reaches the ascending thick limb.

Countercurrent exchanger

A countercurrent exchanger is a countercurrent system in which transport between the outflow and the inflow is entirely passive. The vasa recta act as countercurrent exchangers (Fig. 31.19). They are permeable to water and solutes throughout their length (similar to most tissue capillaries). In the descending limbs of the vasa recta, water is drawn by osmosis from the plasma of the vasa recta to the hyperosmotic peritubular fluid (created by countercurrent multiplier), and the solutes diffuse from the peritubular fluid into the vasa recta. In the ascending limbs, solutes diffuse back into the peritubular fluid and water is drawn by osmosis back into the vasa recta. The net result is that the solutes

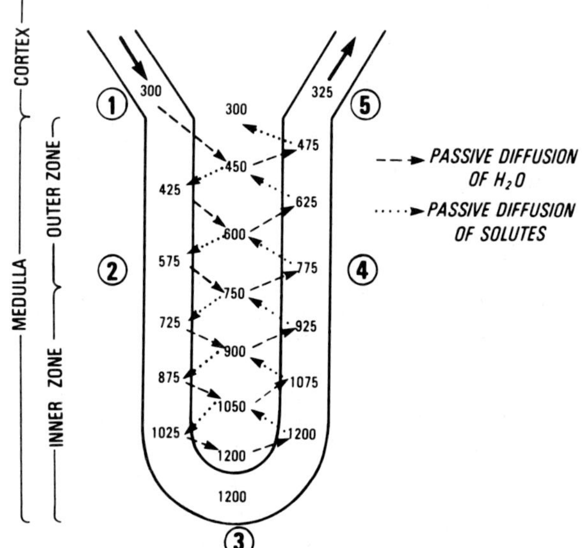

Figure 31.19. Countercurrent exchange in the vasa recta. Values shown (milliosmoles per kilogram H_2O) approximate those of humans. Blood enters from the cortex near circled number 1 with a milliosmolality of about 300 and descends through an increasingly hypertonic peritubular fluid (circled number 2). Water diffuses out and solute diffuses in until the hairpin turn is reached (circled number 3). Now the blood ascends through decreasing hypertonicity and water diffuses in and solute diffuses out (circled number 4). When blood returns to the cortex (circled number 5), the milliosmolality is only slightly higher than when it entered the vasa recta. (From Laiken and Fanestil 1985, in West, ed., *Best and Taylor's Physiological Basis of Medical Practice*, 11th ed., Williams & Wilkins, Baltimore. © 1985, the Williams & Wilkins Co.)

responsible for the vertical medullary gradient are mostly retained in the medulla. The vasa recta carry away slightly more solutes than are brought into them.

An increased rate of medullary blood flow would reduce the time required for diffusion of solute from the ascending limb back to the peritubular fluid. The result would be a gradual loss or "washout" of the medullary gradient. To prevent medullary loss of solute and to maintain the medullary gradient, the blood flow to the vasa recta is reduced (vasa recta comprise 10 to 20 percent of kidney blood flow), and it is often characterized as being rather sluggish. All of the excess salt removed from the peritubular fluid by the vasa recta must be replaced by the loops of Henle for the osmotic gradient to be maintained. There is also a good reason for countercurrent flow in the vasa recta. If blood from the descending limb of the vasa recta returned directly to the renal vein instead of counterflowing into the ascending limb, the solute of the renal medulla would be quickly removed instead of being retained.

Antidiuretic hormone

Tubular fluid entering the distal nephrons from the loops of Henle has an osmolality lower than that of plasma (osmolality of plasma is about 300 mOsm) because of the removal of NaCl that occurs in the ascending thin and thick limbs of the loops of Henle. Tubular fluid osmolality continues to be lowered (150 mOsm) in the distal tubule and the connecting tubule because of unidirectional active transport of Na^+ (accompanied by anion, mostly Cl^-) and continued tubular impermeability for water. Beyond the connecting tubules (in the collecting tubules/ducts), Na^+ reabsorption continues (stimulated by aldosterone), but permeability for water depends on the concentration of antidiuretic hormone (ADH). ADH increases the permeability for water.

The net effect of ADH activity is to return water from the tubular fluid to the extracellular fluid (ECF) and thus reduce the ECF effective osmotic pressure (rehydration), thereby minimizing the effects of water loss. ADH has a biologic half-life of 15 to 20 minutes and thus is effective only when secreted continuously. It is synthesized in the cell bodies of hypothalamic nuclei (supraoptic neurons) and transported to nerve fiber endings in the posterior lobe of the pituitary where it is stored in secretory granules. Its release into the blood is controlled by osmoreceptors in the hypothalamus that are close to the supraoptic nuclei. The osmoreceptors respond mostly to changes in ECF sodium concentration (very little to concentrations of potassium, urea, and glucose) and are sometimes called osmosodium receptors. Sodium and its accompanying anion constitute about 90 percent of the effective osmotic pressure of the ECF.

When ECF osmolality rises (Na^+ influence), the supraoptic neurons are more active and ADH release increases. When ECF osmolality falls, the neurons are less active and ADH release decreases. When ECF osmolality is normal, there is a constant, moderate rate of ADH release. Significant changes from the moderate rate occur when plasma osmolality is changed as little as 1 percent in either direction.

The rate of ADH secretion is influenced by other factors in addition to hydration of the ECF. Another aspect of water reabsorption is compensation for loss of blood volume and resultant low blood pressure. There are "volume receptors" in the walls of many large blood vessels that monitor the degree of filling of the cardiovascular system. When blood volume decreases, the receptors stimulate increased ADH secretion, and when blood volume increases, the receptors stimulate decreased ADH secretion. In both cases blood volume is adjusted toward normal by increases or decreases in water reabsorption, respectively.

It should be noted that significant changes in ADH release occur when plasma osmolality changes as little as 1% in either direction. Significant changes in ADH release caused by changes in blood volume do not occur until the changes in blood volume exceed 10%. When the blood volume change exceeds 10 percent, the volume responses may temporarily override the effect of the osmoreceptors.

Water reabsorption from distal nephrons

As noted, the distal tubules and the connecting tubules are not permeable to water, and the collecting tubules and collecting ducts are variably permeable to water, depending on the amount of ADH that is secreted.

Hypotonic tubular fluid entering the collecting tubules could be excreted as urine if water were not reabsorbed. This happens in diabetes insipidus, in which ADH is either absent or present in a severely decreased amount. Usually, when tubular fluid enters the collecting tubules, water is reabsorbed as it proceeds to the renal pelvis. As the tubular fluid proceeds through the collecting ducts (located in the renal medulla), it is exposed to effective osmotic pressures of increasing magnitudes (the vertical medullary gradient) in the peritubular fluid of the kidney medulla that were established by the countercurrent mechanism. It would be possible for the osmolality of the tubular fluid, and hence that of the urine, to approach the osmolality of the peritubular fluid in the innermost region of the medulla. In the dog this would approach 2400 mOsm and the urine/plasma osmolal ratio (2400:300) would be approximately 8:1. The urine would have a concentration eight times that of plasma. Some desert rodents attain a urine/plasma osmolal ratio of about 16:1. This ratio represents an extreme adaptation for body water conservation. Environmental water is usually not available for desert animals (water gain is mostly metabolic water), and water losses are minimized for survival.

Table 31.2 compares the percentage of juxtamedullary nephrons (long-looped nephrons) and the relative medullary thickness of different animals. The relative medullary thickness is derived from measurements of the depth of the medulla from the corticomedullary junction to its innermost depth, which protrudes into the renal pelvis. Relative medullary thickness is believed to be a better predictor of the ability to concentrate than percentage of long-looped nephrons. As judged by freezing point depressions (solute particles lower the freezing point of solutions), the jerboa, a mouselike rodent of North Africa and Asia, has the greatest concentrating capacity for urine. As compared with humans, it appears that its innermost medullary peritubular fluid osmolality would be about 4.6 times that of humans, or about 5500 mOsm.

Recirculation of urea

In addition to NaCl, urea also contributes to the high osmolality of the peritubular fluid in the kidney medulla. This is accomplished by a recirculation mechanism for urea between the collecting ducts and the loop of Henle. *Recirculation* means that urea diffuses from the inner medullary collecting ducts into the peritubular fluid and, from there, diffuses into the lumina of the thin segments of the ascending limbs of the loops of Henle (see Fig. 31.18). The ascending thick limb of the loop of Henle and the segments of the distal nephron to the inner medullary collecting duct are not permeable for urea, so that urea entering the ascending thin limbs of the loops of Henle is recycled through the tubules back to the inner medullary collecting duct. The permeability of the inner medullary collecting ducts for urea is dependent on ADH. With maximum ADH, water is removed from the tubule, concentrating the urea and creating a concentration gradient for its diffusion into the medulla because of the increased permeability. Even though vasa recta are permeable for urea, it is effectively trapped within the medulla because of the countercurrent flow. The high concentration of urea in the medulla caused by the recirculation mechanism not only assists the countercurrent multiplier (see above) but also ensures excretion of urea when urine output is low. For example, if urine is formed at the rate of 2 ml/min and it has a urea concentration of 2 mg/ml, then 4 mg of urea would be excreted each minute. If, however, urine formation is reduced to 1 ml/min (greater reabsorption of water), the concentration of urea is increased to 4 mg/ml and excretion is maintained at 4 mg/min. The concentration of urea remains high in the collecting ducts because the concentration is also high in the interstitial fluid (diffusion from the tubule limited by gradient). This example shows a constant excretion rate. As explained above, however, urea excretion depends on the rate of urine flow. However, even though the percentage of urea filtered to that which is excreted may be decreased (as in dehydration), a substantial rate of excretion is maintained.

Summary of countercurrent mechanism

The countercurrent mechanism exists to establish and maintain high osmolality in the interstitial fluid of the renal medulla. Because of the high osmolality, an osmotic gradient exists between the interstitial fluid of the renal medulla and the tubular fluid in the collecting ducts. In the presence of ADH, the membranes of the collecting tubules and collecting ducts are permeable to water and the osmotic gradient favors diffusion of water from the tubular fluid to the interstitial fluid of the renal medulla, resulting in recovery of water from the tubular fluid and the formation of urine with greater solute concentration.

A schematic representation of the countercurrent mecha-

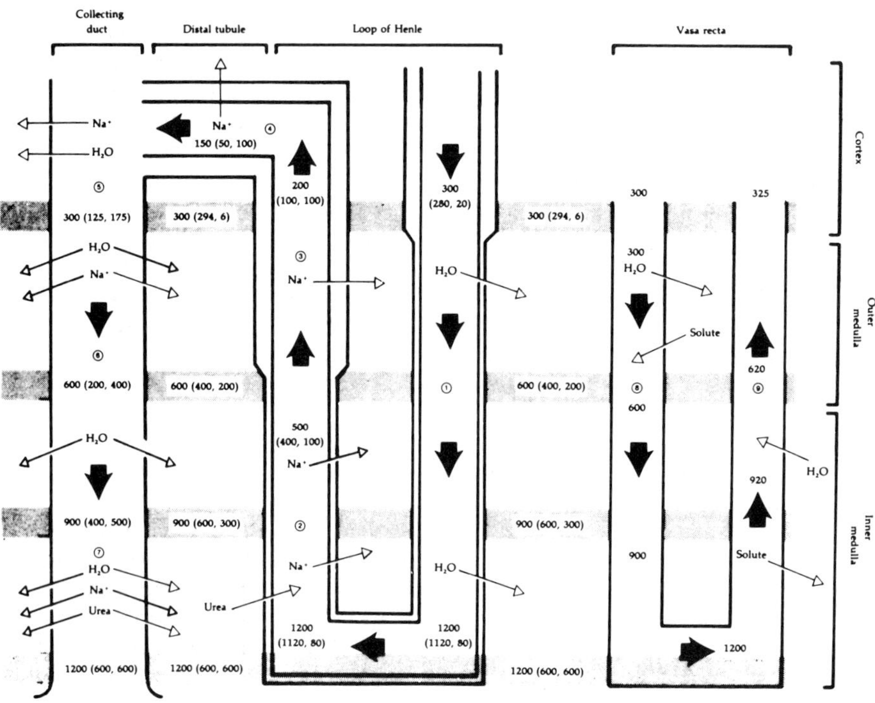

Figure 31.20. Functional aspects of the countercurrent mechanism. Values shown approximate those for humans. The movement of Na^+ from the tubule implies a similar movement of Cl^-. 1, Descending limb of the loop of Henle; 2, thin segment of ascending limb of loop of Henle; 3, thick segment of ascending limb of loop of Henle; 4, distal tubule; 5, cortical collecting tubule; 6, outer medullary collecting duct; 7, inner medullary collecting duct; 8, descending limb of vas rectum; 9, ascending limb of vas rectum. The values of the tubular fluid osmolality are shown for each part (in milliosmoles); the numbers in parentheses represent the contribution to the osmolality from NaCl and minor electrolytes and from urea, respectively. For example, at the end of the cortical collecting tubule (5), the osmolality is 300 mOsm (125, 175), with 125 mOsm contributed from NaCl and minor electrolytes and 175 mOsm contributed from urea. See text for further explanation. (From Reece 1991, *Physiology of Domestic Animals*, Lea & Febiger, Philadelphia.)

nism for the kidney is shown in Fig. 31.20; the nephron parts are identified by circled numbers. The osmolality values approximate those for humans.

The tubular fluid entering the descending limb of the loop of Henle (Fig. 31.20, *1*) from the proximal tubule has an osmolality of 300 mOsm, 280 contributed from NaCl and minor electrolytes and 20 from urea (280, 20). There is a high permeability for H_2O and no permeability for Na^+, Cl^-, and urea. Water diffuses outward (osmosis), and solutes remain within. The tubular fluid at the hairpin turn has an osmolality of 1200 (1120, 80).

The ascending thin limb of the loop of Henle (Fig. 31.20, *2*) is not permeable to H_2O, highly permeable to NaCl, and moderately permeable to urea. The tubule retains H_2O while NaCl diffuses outward and urea diffuses inward. The tubular fluid osmolality when it reaches the thick segment is 500 mOsm (400, 100).

The ascending thick limb of the loop of Henle (Fig. 31.20, *3*) is involved with active transport of NaCl from the lumen to the peritubular fluid, and it has a low permeability for the diffusion of H_2O and urea. The average osmolality of fluid in the lumen that is leaving the ascending thick limb and entering the distal tubule is about 200 mOsm (100, 100), which is hypotonic to plasma.

There is continued active transport of NaCl and low permeability for H_2O and urea in the distal tubule (Fig. 31.20, *4*). At the end of the distal tubule, and before the fluid enters the collecting tubule, the osmolality is about 150 mOsm (50, 100).

In the cortical collecting tubule, the outer medullary collecting duct, and the inner medullary collecting duct (Fig. 31.20, *5, 6,* and *7*), sodium reabsorption is stimulated by aldosterone, water reabsorption is influenced by ADH, and urea reabsorption (inner medulla only) is influenced by ADH.

With maximum ADH, as shown in Fig. 31.20, there is increased permeability for water and urea. At the end of the cortical collecting tubule the osmolality is 300 mOsm (125, 175), at the end of the outer medulla it is 600 mOsm (200, 400), and before it empties into the renal pelvis it is 1200 mOsm (600, 600).

With no ADH there would be no water and urea reabsorption, but there could be continued NaCl reabsorption under the influence of aldosterone. In this situation the osmolality of urine formed would be 130 mOsm (30, 100).

Both the descending and ascending limbs of vasa recta (Fig. 31.20, *8* and *9*) are permeable to water and solutes. Because there is an increasing osmolality in the interstitial fluid from the cortex through the inner medulla, there is osmosis of water outward from the descending limb and diffusion of solutes inward. After the hairpin turn, the plasma in the vasa recta is exposed to decreasing concentrations of solute in the peritubular fluid as it proceeds upward, the solute that was gained while going down is lost by diffusion as it ascends, and water diffuses by osmosis into the tubule. The osmolality of the plasma is only slightly higher (325 mOsm) than when it entered the vasa recta.

Medullary washout

It was mentioned above that to prevent a gradual loss or "washout" of the medullary gradient, not only is there countercurrent blood flow in the vasa recta, but also the blood flow has been characterized as sluggish (permits adequate time for diffusion). A loss of medullary gradient (solute concentration) reduces the ability to concentrate tubular fluid on its descent through the medullary collecting ducts.

Medullary washout can also be caused by diuretics that block active sodium chloride cotransport in the ascending limb of the loop of Henle. Examples of these diuretics are furosemide and ethacrynic acid, known also as loop diuretics. They produce diuresis because increased delivery of solute to the distal nephrons increases the effective osmotic pressure within the tubules and prevents reabsorption of a proportional amount of water. Also, failure to reabsorb NaCl from the loop of Henle into the medullary interstitium decreases the osmoconcentration of the medullary interstitial fluid (washout), reducing its potential for reabsorbing water from the tubular fluid in the medullary collecting ducts.

A contribution to medullary washout is also provided by urea during periods of diuresis. It was explained above that increased urine flow increases the renal clearance of urea whereby a greater amount of the urea filtered is excreted. A lesser amount is thus recirculated and the contribution of urea to medullary osmolality is decreased, which further diminishes the ability to concentrate tubular fluid in the collecting ducts.

REGULATION OF EXTRACELLULAR FLUID OSMOLALITY AND VOLUME

The ability to retain water in the ECF is due to its effective osmotic pressure. Since about 90 percent of the effective osmotic pressure of ECF is due to Na^+ and its associated anions, the central role played by Na^+ must be recognized when one is considering the regulation of ECF osmolality (osmoregulation) and ECF volume (volume regulation). In osmoregulation the ratio of Na^+ to water (osmoconcentration) is being regulated, and in volume regulation the absolute amounts of Na^+ and water that are present are being regulated. The differences between osmoregulation and volume regulation are shown in Table 31.4 relative to what is being sensed, the sensors, the effectors, and, finally, what is affected.

Osmoregulation

From day to day in any one animal the water content of the body is relatively constant. There is water balance because water intake is equal to water excretion. Water excretion without water intake would cause ECF hyperosmolality, and water intake without water excretion would cause hypo-osmolality. To prevent either, the plasma osmolality is maintained within narrow limits by appropriate adjustments of water excretion and intake. These adjustments are governed by centers in the hypothalamus that influence

Table 31.4. Differences between osmoregulation and volume regulation

	Osmoregulation	Volume regulation
What is being sensed	Plasma osmolality	Effective circulating volume
Sensors	Hypothalamic osmoreceptors	Carotid sinus Afferent arteriole Atria
Effectors*	Antidiuretic hormone Thirst	Renin-angiotensin-aldosterone system Sympathetic nervous system Atrial natriuretic peptide Pressure natriuresis Antidiuretic hormone
What is affected	Urine osmolality and, via thirst, water intake	Urine sodium excretion

*Thirst is also an effector in volume regulation (Laiken and Fanestil, 1985). From Rose 1989, *Clinical Physiology of Acid-Base and Electrolyte Disorders,* 3d ed., McGraw-Hill Publishing Company, New York. Reproduced with permission of McGraw-Hill, Inc.

both the secretion of ADH (water excretion) and thirst (water intake).

In the event of water load (intake exceeds excretion) the ECF is diluted, causing hypo-osmolality. The response of osmoreceptors in the hypothalamus is to inhibit the secretion of ADH and subsequently increase water excretion, returning the osmolality to normal.

When water loss exceeds water intake, the ECF is concentrated, resulting in hyperosmolality. A water deficit requires water intake for correction. The ECF hyperosmolality not only stimulates greater secretion of ADH so that water excretion is suppressed but also stimulates thirst so that the animal seeks water for ingestion (Fig. 31.21). The osmoreceptors respond to effective osmotic pressure; hence the osmolality increase must be due to substances restricted from diffusion into the osmoreceptor cells. For this reason, the osmoreceptor cells are often considered to be Na^+ receptors. Osmolality increase due to urea (freely diffusible) does not stimulate the osmoreceptors.

When defects occur in the ability to concentrate urine, as in diabetes insipidus (lack of ADH), water losses increase. This activates the thirst mechanism, promoting water intake, and prevents hyperosmolality that might otherwise occur from the excessive excretion of water.

Volume regulation

The maintenance of normal plasma volume, which varies directly with ECF volume, is essential for adequate tissue perfusion and is closely related to the regulation of sodium balance. Na^+ loading (excess) tends to produce ECF volume expansion (because of the increase in effective osmotic pressure), and Na^+ excretion by the kidneys rises in an attempt to lower the volume toward normal. Conversely, the kidneys retain Na^+ in the presence of ECF volume depletion. Change in volume is the signal that allows urinary Na^+ excretion to vary as needed with fluctuations in Na^+ intake.

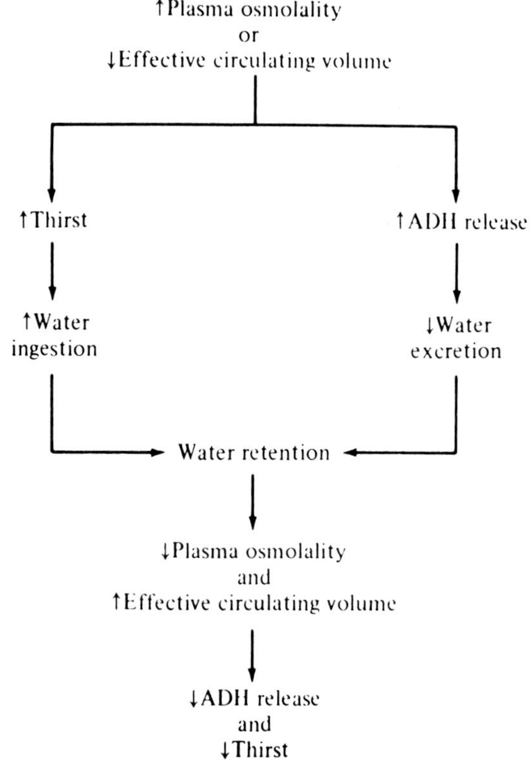

Figure 31.21. Cycle of events for the relief of hyperosmolality and hypovolemia. (From Rose 1989, *Clinical Physiology of Acid-Base and Electrolyte Disorders*, 3d ed., McGraw-Hill Publishing Company, New York. Reproduced with permission of McGraw-Hill, Inc.)

Receptors of volume change

The major receptors (sensors) of volume change are pressure receptors located in the afferent arterioles of the glomeruli, the atria of the heart, the carotid sinuses, and the aortic arch. Even though they are classified as pressure receptors, it is believed that they may be responding to stretch, a situation more appropriate to volume expansion or depletion.

The volume receptors in the kidney are located in the juxtaglomerular cells of the afferent arteriole and in macula densa cells of the distal tubule. In response to decreased volume (hypoperfusion), these receptors increase the activity of the renin-angiotensin-aldosterone system. The receptors located outside the kidney are concerned with the activity of the sympathetic nervous system, atrial natriuretic peptide (ANP), ADH, and thirst. Atrial natriuretic peptide is also referred to as atrial natriuretic hormone (ANH) and atrial natriuretic factor (ANF). Reduction in ECF volume results in an increase in sympathetic tone, a reduction in the release of ANP, an increase in secretion of ADH, and thirst, whereas volume expansion causes a decrease in sympathetic tone, increased ANP release, and a decrease in secretion of ADH. Note that decreased ECF volume can increase

ADH release and thirst independent of increase caused by hyperosmolality (see Fig. 31.21).

Renin-angiotensin-aldosterone system

The juxtaglomerular cells of the afferent arteriole of each glomerulus secrete the proteolytic enzyme renin. Renin converts plasma angiotensinogen (produced in the liver) to angiotensin I. Angiotensin I is converted to angiotensin II by converting enzyme, which is located in the lung, vascular endothelial cells (including the glomerulus), and other organs.

The major effects of angiotensin II reverse the ECF volume reduction and hypotension that are usually responsible for its production. Within the kidney, angiotensin II promotes Na^+ reabsorption and subsequent H_2O retention. Na^+ reabsorption is stimulated directly by angiotensin II in the proximal tubule and indirectly by enhanced secretion of aldosterone from the adrenal cortex. Aldosterone stimulates Na^+ reabsorption in the cortical collecting tubules and medullary collecting ducts. Systemically, angiotensin II causes arteriolar vasoconstriction, which increases vascular resistance and elevates systemic blood pressure. There is speculation that angiotensin II can stimulate thirst and release of ADH. A summary of the renin-angiotensin-aldosterone system response to hypovolemia and hypotension is shown in Fig. 31.22.

Sympathetic nervous system

Sympathetic tone and secretion of epinephrine and norepinephrine are enhanced during ECF volume depletion and are reduced during ECF volume expansion. The changes

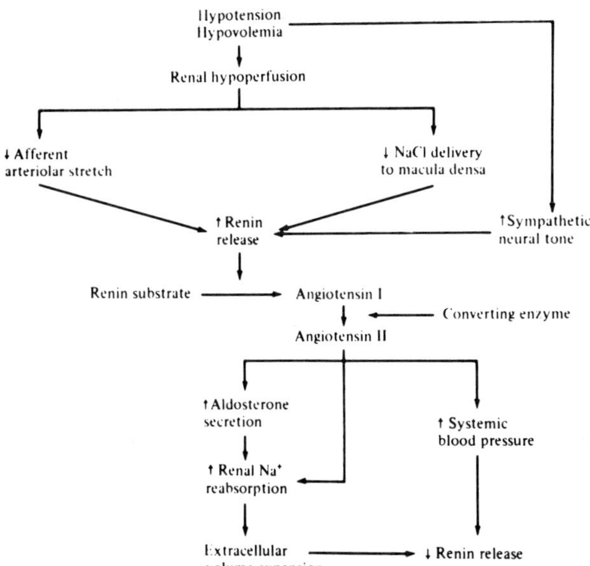

Figure 31.22. Renin-angiotensin-aldosterone system response to hypovolemia and hypotension. (From Rose 1989, *Clinical Physiology of Acid-Base and Electrolyte Disorders*, 3d ed., McGraw-Hill Publishing Company, New York. Reproduced with permission of McGraw-Hill, Inc.)

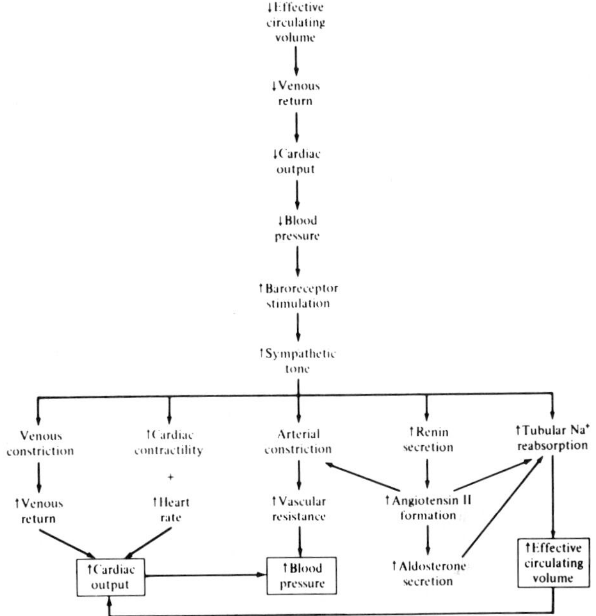

Figure 31.23. Renal and cardiovascular responses induced by the sympathetic division of the autonomic nervous system in response to reduced circulating volume. (From Rose 1989, *Clinical Physiology of Acid-Base and Electrolyte Disorders*, 3d ed., McGraw-Hill Publishing Company, New York. Reproduced with permission of McGraw-Hill, Inc.)

in pressure (or stretch) associated with volume depletion or expansion are sensed by the cardiac and arterial receptors. The receptors then change their rate of stimulation to the vasomotor centers in the brain stem.

The following series of events are related to increased sympathetic tone resulting from volume depletion:

1. Enhanced venous return due to venous constriction, coupled with increased activities of the heart, results in increased cardiac output.
2. Arteriolar constriction causes systemic blood pressure to increase.
3. Renin secretion increases (direct action of increased sympathetic tone on β_1-adrenergic receptors) causing angiotensin II generation that contributes to systemic vasoconstriction.
4. Renal tubular Na^+ reabsorption increases because of direct stimulation (α_1-adrenergic receptors) of proximal tubule and loop of Henle Na^+ reabsorption and as a result of aldosterone secretion caused by angiotensin II generation.

These changes are summarized in Fig. 31.23. Sympathetic tone is decreased during volume expansion, and the above changes are reversed and excess Na^+ is excreted.

Atrial natriuretic peptide

Following Na^+ load, the ECF volume expands and Na^+ excretion increases. It was formerly believed that the increase in Na^+ excretion resulted from increased GFR and reduced aldosterone secretion. However, when the GFR is prevented from increasing (constriction of the aorta to reduce blood pressure) and when aldosterone is administered in excess (to promote Na^+ reabsorption), excretion of the Na^+ load continues. The reason for the continued excretion was sometimes referred to as the "third factor" effect. Since the discovery of ANP, considerable work has been done to show its natriuretic and diuretic effects and specific sites of renal activity. There now appears to be good reason for ANP to be the so-called "third factor."

Myocardial cells of the atria release ANP when they are stretched during volume expansion (thus the need for natriuresis and diuresis). The following actions of ANP relate to its ability to excrete Na^+ and water:

1. ANP increases GFR by causing preglomerular vasodilatation and postglomerular vasoconstriction (filtration fraction increases).
2. ANP inhibits angiotensin II–stimulated proximal tubular sodium and water reabsorption.
3. ANP reduces Na^+ reabsorption in the collecting ducts and collecting tubules.
4. ANP inhibits aldosterone release induced by angiotensin II.
5. ANP diminishes response of collecting tubules and collecting ducts to ADH.

The exact role of ANP in a physiologic setting is yet unproven. It is not possible to remove its site of production, and until antagonists to ANP are developed, a complete definition of its physiologic role cannot be achieved.

Normal volume regulation

The unidirectional reabsorption of Na^+ in the collecting tubules and collecting ducts is influenced by aldosterone. Normally, about 10 percent of the tubular load of Na^+ (and associated anions) is delivered to the distal nephron, and the basal level of aldosterone provides for much of its reabsorption.

When Na^+ intake increases (initially expands ECF volume), aldosterone secretion decreases (via reduced renin secretion) and ANP secretion increases. Because both of these hormones affect the collecting tubules and collecting ducts, changes in reabsorption of Na^+ at these locations may be the principal means of volume regulation under conditions of normal Na^+ intake and Na^+ balance. Marked changes in volume necessitate other means for regulation, and the proximal tubules may play a greater role in Na^+ and water excretion under these conditions.

Pressure natriuresis

The pressure natriuresis phenomenon implies that increases in Na^+ and water excretion occur because of the blood pressure increase caused by volume expansion independent of neural and humoral involvement. It is a physical phenomenon thought to be mediated by increases in systemic blood pressure that are transmitted to the peritubular capillaries and vasa recta. Reabsorption of Na^+ and water into peritubular capillaries is passive and requires diffusion gradients. Consequently, since peritubular capillary pressure is increased, reabsorption is impaired and an increasing quantity of Na^+ and water escapes through the proximal tubular tight junctions from the intercellular spaces back into the tubular lumen.

The increased hydrostatic pressure in vasa recta suppresses reabsorption of water from the medullary interstitial space and, in turn, water does not diffuse as readily from the lumina of the water-permeable descending limbs of the loops of Henle into the medullary interstitial space. Accordingly, the concentration of Na^+ does not rise to the degree necessary for passive diffusion of Na^+ from the thin segments of the ascending limbs of the loops of Henle. Because of the decrease in Na^+ reabsorption in the proximal tubules and loops of Henle, an excess is presented to the distal nephron, and Na^+ and water excretion increases.

It is believed that pressure natriuresis is not a contributing factor in the normal day-to-day variations in ECF volume but may be important when there is impairment of neurohumoral mediators. It is believed that changes in aldosterone and ANP secretion ordinarily accomplish the modest ECF volume changes that are necessary.

Summary

The reduction in ECF volume that accompanies reduced Na^+ intake is followed by enhanced activity of the renin-angiotensin-aldosterone system and reduced secretion of ANP. Because of increased aldosterone secretion, more Na^+ is reabsorbed from the collecting tubules and ducts, and Na^+ excretion is diminished. In the event of greater Na^+ depletion and hypovolemia, reabsorption of Na^+ is enhanced in the proximal tubule by the action of angiotensin II and increased sympathetic tone (norepinephrine).

With volume expansion associated with increased Na^+ intake, ANP secretion is increased and aldosterone secretion is decreased. With a modest degree of expansion, enhanced Na^+ excretion occurs because of decreased Na^+ reabsorption in the distal nephron. When greater degrees of volume expansion occur, the effects of ANP and reduced sympathetic tone to inhibit Na^+ reabsorption in the proximal tubule are more apparent.

Finally, pressure natriuresis may be the determining factor for Na^+ excretion when one or more neurohumoral factors are abnormal. This situation can exist if there is excess aldosterone (as with an adrenal tumor). There is a limit to the amount of Na^+ retention that will occur because of excess aldosterone, inasmuch as the increased blood pressure resulting from volume expansion will enhance Na^+ excretion by pressure natriuresis. Intake and excretion of Na^+ will become equal, but blood pressure will be reestablished at a higher level.

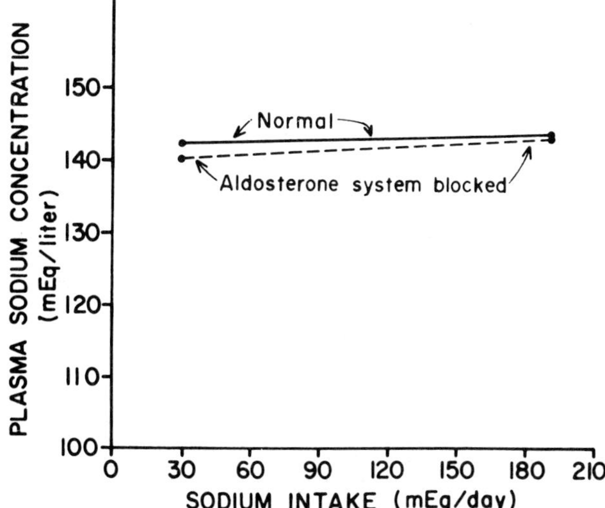

Figure 31.24. Response of canine plasma sodium concentration to increasing sodium intake in instances in which the aldosterone system is blocked and the ADH-thirst system is intact. (Courtesy of Dr. David B. Young, University of Mississippi School of Medicine, Jackson.)

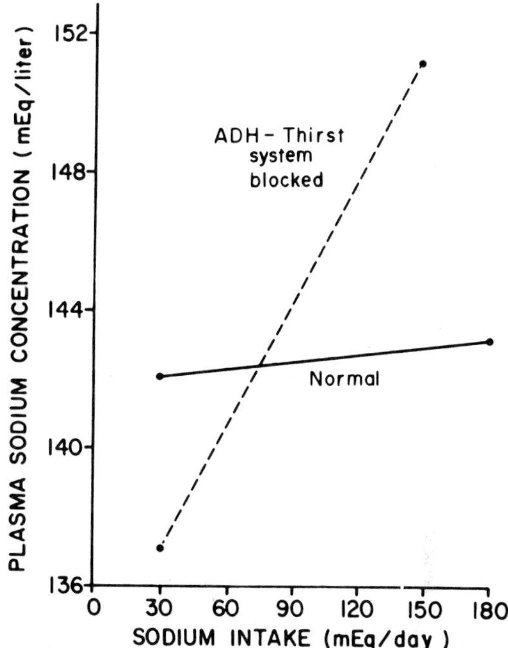

Figure 31.25. Response of canine plasma sodium concentration to increasing sodium intake in instances in which the ADH-thirst system is blocked and the aldosterone system is intact. (Courtesy of Dr. David B. Young, University of Mississippi School of Medicine, Jackson.)

REGULATION OF EXTRACELLULAR FLUID ELECTROLYTES

Sodium concentration

Reabsorption of Na^+ from the nephron (unidirectional, symport, antiport) was explained above. It was noted that the unidirectional reabsorption of Na^+ in the collecting tubules and collecting ducts was influenced by aldosterone concentrations. In the complete absence of aldosterone, seemingly 10 percent of the tubular load of Na^+ (and associated anions) could be lost in the urine. Conversely, with excess aldosterone, the last vestige of the tubular load of Na^+ can be reabsorbed.

Even though aldosterone is associated with Na^+ reabsorption, it is not a regulator of ECF Na^+ concentration. This lack of regulation by aldosterone in dogs is illustrated in Fig. 31.24. In this instance, the aldosterone system has been blocked, and it is noted that plasma Na^+ concentration remains stabilized near normal, even though sodium intake increases. In another experiment with dogs, the aldosterone system is left intact and the ADH-thirst system is blocked (Fig. 31.25). This latter experiment shows that plasma Na^+ concentration increases in proportion to increases in sodium intake and, coupled with the former experiment, demonstrates that ECF Na^+ concentration is regulated by the ADH-thirst system (as in osmoregulation) and not by aldosterone.

Potassium concentration

The regulation of ECF K^+ concentration is accomplished by either greater reabsorption or secretion in the distal nephron. Potassium is unique among substances in that it can be either reabsorbed or secreted. About 10 percent of the tubular load of K^+ is delivered to the distal nephron, and it is ordinarily reabsorbed at a rather constant rate. With low intake of K^+, there is net reabsorption with minimal secretion. With high K^+ intake, secretion exceeds reabsorption and K^+ is excreted in urine in order to maintain K^+ balance in the ECF.

Secretory mechanisms

An increase in plasma K^+ concentration is the major stimulus for aldosterone secretion. After its secretion, aldosterone causes the following in the distal nephron:

1. Increases in the activity of the Na^+-K^+ ATPase and associated transport of K^+ from the peritubular fluid across the basolateral borders and into the tubular cells, thereby increasing the magnitude of the concentration gradient for diffusion from the tubular cell into the lumen.
2. Stimulation of Na^+ reabsorption, which increases the transepithelial potential difference (lumen negative), thereby increasing the magnitude of the electrical gradient for diffusion of K^+ from the tubular cell into the lumen.

and

3. Increases in the permeability of the luminal membrane to K^+, thereby facilitating diffusion from the tubular cell into the lumen.

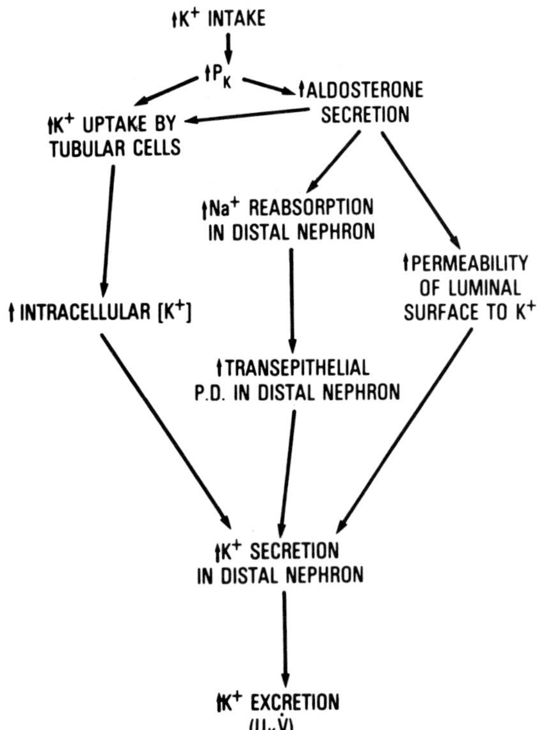

Figure 31.26. Pathways whereby plasma potassium concentration is restored after increases in potassium intake. P_K, plasma potassium concentration, U_K, potassium concentration in urine; $\dot{V}$, rate of urine formation; P.D., potential difference. (From Laiken and Fanestil 1985, in West, ed., *Best and Taylor's Physiological Basis of Medical Practice*, 11th ed., Williams & Wilkins, Baltimore. © 1985, the Williams & Wilkins Co.)

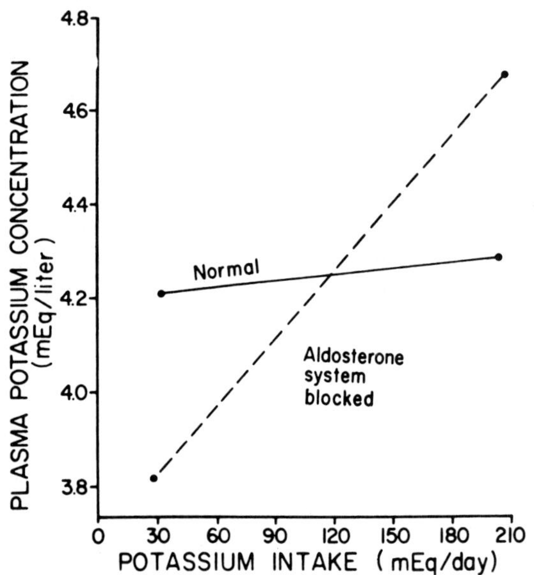

Figure 31.27. Response of canine plasma potassium concentration to increasing potassium intake in instances in which the aldosterone system is blocked and the aldosterone system is intact. (Courtesy of Dr. David B. Young, University of Mississippi School of Medicine, Jackson.)

The pathways linking increased plasma K^+ concentrations with increased K^+ excretion are shown in Fig. 31.26.

The importance of aldosterone in the regulation of ECF K^+ concentration is shown in Fig. 31.27. In the experiment depicted in this figure, dogs with intact adrenal glands were given increasing amounts of potassium, and plasma K^+ concentration increased very little. After adrenalectomy and infusion of a fixed amount of aldosterone, plasma K^+ concentration increased simultaneously with increases in K^+ intake.

Calcium concentration

About half of the plasma Ca^{2+} is bound to albumin and is not filtered at the glomerulus. Most of the remainder exists as ionic Ca^{2+}, and some is bound to citrate, bicarbonate, or phosphate. Most of the filtered Ca^{2+} (80 to 85 percent) is reabsorbed from the proximal tubule and medullary portions of the loop of Henle. The reabsorption in these parts is passive, following gradients established by NaCl and water.

Regulation of Ca^{2+} occurs primarily in the distal tubule and the connecting tubule. Parathyroid hormone and vitamin D stimulate Ca^{2+} reabsorption in these segments. A calcium-binding protein is produced by the action of vitamin D, and it is believed that this protein facilitates the entry of luminal Ca^{2+} into the cells. The intracellular Ca^{2+} is then returned to the peritubular fluid by the Ca^{2+}-ATPase pump in the basolateral membrane.

Magnesium concentration

A lesser percentage of Mg^{2+} (about 25 percent) is protein bound so that about 75 percent is filtered. The proximal tubule accounts for 25 to 30 percent of its reabsorption, and most of the remainder is reabsorbed from the loop of Henle. Alterations that occur in Mg^{2+} excretion are due to changes in the loop of Henle reabsorption. Specific factors that regulate plasma Mg^{2+} concentration have not been identified. It is believed that there may be a direct effect of plasma Mg^{2+} concentration on tubular function and its subsequent reabsorption.

Phosphate concentration

About 80 to 95 percent of the filtered phosphate is reabsorbed, and most reabsorption occurs in the proximal tubule. There is a specific Na^+-phosphate symporter in the luminal membrane for transport from the lumen into the cell. After cell entry, phosphate diffuses across the basolateral membrane into the peritubular fluid.

Two factors appear to regulate phosphate transport—the plasma phosphate concentration and the parathyroid hormone. Virtually no phosphate is excreted with a low phosphate load, and this is believed to be due to increased Na^+-phosphate symport activity. With a high phosphate load, urinary excretion increases because of a direct effect of phosphate concentration and also because of increased parathyroid hormone secretion that promotes excretion of excess phosphate.

MICTURITION

Associated structures and their function

During the formation of urine, the tubular fluid flows through the nephron tubules because of a hydrostatic pressure gradient that exists between Bowman's capsule and the renal pelvis. There is almost no hydrostatic pressure in the renal pelvis. The ureters are muscular (smooth muscle) tubes that convey urine by peristalsis from the renal pelvis of each kidney to the urinary bladder. The ureters enter the bladder at an oblique angle (ureterovesicular junction), thus forming a functional valve to prevent backflow when the bladder is filling (Fig. 31.28). The urinary bladder is a hollow, muscular (smooth muscle) organ that varies in size, depending on the amount of urine it contains at any one time. Emptying of the bladder is accomplished by contraction of the bladder musculature, which is arranged in three sheets. The muscle sheets converge on the neck of the bladder in such a way that their contraction also shortens and widens the neck, decreasing urethral resistance. Passive tension of elastic elements in the mucosa ordinarily keep the lumen of the neck closed.

The epithelial cell lining of the bladder, known as transitional epithelium, accommodates for the change in bladder size. When the bladder is empty the cells appear to be piled on one another, giving it a stratified appearance. A transition occurs on filling so that the piled-up appearance gives way to a thinner epithelial stratification.

The urethra is the caudal continuation of the neck of the bladder. It conveys the urine from the bladder to the exterior. The external sphincter lies beyond the bladder; it is composed of skeletal muscle that encircles the urethra at this point. The functional boundary between the bladder and the urethra is represented by this sphincter.

Escape of urine while the bladder is filling is prevented by contraction of the external sphincter and by tension passively exerted by elastic elements within the mucosa. When urine is expelled from the bladder, the external sphincter relaxes and the bladder muscles contract.

Micturition reflexes

Micturition is the physiologic term for emptying of the bladder. The bladder is allowed to fill before emptying because of reflex control in the sacral spinal cord and brain stem. Activation of the sacral spinal reflex occurs when receptors in the bladder wall are stretched during filling. This allows urine to be evacuated through the neck of the bladder and the external sphincter. Afferent impulses simultaneously received at the brain stem reflex center, however, prevent contraction of the bladder and relaxation of the external sphincter that would otherwise occur. In this manner, the bladder accommodates to the increasing volume and continues to fill. Successive spinal and brain-stem reflexes are aroused with subsequent accommodation. When a certain expanded volume is reached, the pressure rises sharply, creating the urge to void. In most animals the urge is usually obeyed, but it may be postponed in house-trained dogs. In the latter, voluntary control intervenes and micturition is permitted when appropriate. Once micturition proceeds, complete emptying is ensured because of another reflex (brain-stem) activated by flow receptors in the urethra. As long as urine is flowing, bladder contraction continues until there is no further flow (the bladder is empty).

The parasympathetic division of the autonomic nervous system is the sole motor supply to the muscle in the body and neck of the bladder. The sympathetic nerves have no effect on micturition but appear to constrict the neck of the bladder during ejaculation, thus directing the ejaculate through the penile urethra rather than allowing backflow into the bladder.

Descriptive terms

Urinary continence is the normal condition of storing urine in the bladder while it fills. Continence is maintained by continuous tone of the external sphincter muscle and by closure of the neck of the bladder, which is augmented by elastic tissue. An incontinent animal dribbles urine at frequent intervals instead of permitting the bladder to fill. Spinal injuries cranial to the sacrum are frequently the cause; in such injuries the brain-stem reflexes do not effectively prevent emptying, and thus emptying is initiated by the sacral reflexes as the bladder fills.

Polyuria refers to increased urine output, *oliguria* means decreased output, and *anuria* describes the condition of no urine output. *Dysuria* is a term used to describe difficult or painful micturition. *Stranguria* is slow, dropwise, painful discharge of the urine caused by spasm of the urethra and bladder. Stranguria is a clinical sign of feline urologic syndrome (FUS), caused by obstruction of the urethra by a plug

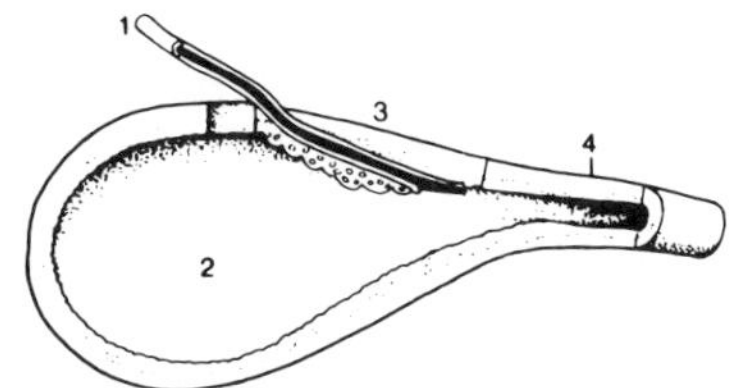

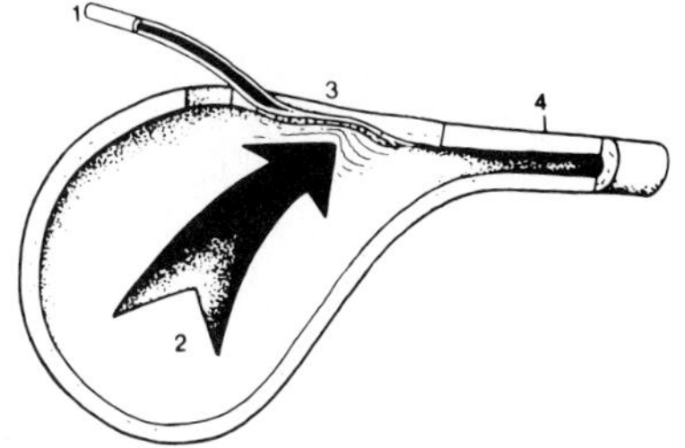

Figure 31.28. Ureterovesicular junction (entrance of ureter into urinary bladder). Because of the oblique passage of the ureter through the bladder wall, it is occluded when the pressure from accumulated urine rises (arrow). 1, Ureter; 2, bladder lumen; 3, bladder wall; 4, bladder neck. The external sphincter is just beyond the neck of the bladder. (From Dyce, Sack, and Wensing 1987, *Textbook of Veterinary Anatomy*, W.B. Saunders, Philadelphia.)

consisting of struvite (magnesium ammonium phosphate) crystals and mucoid material.

Behavioral and practical aspects

The following keen observations that describe micturition are quoted from a book written 70 years ago.[1] The word *horse,* as used herein, refers to the male.

"At the moment the bladder wall begins to contract, it is assisted by the abdominal muscles and a fixed diaphragm. The flow is never so powerful in the female as in the male, the final expulsion of the last drops from the urethra of the latter being effected by the rhythmical contraction of the perineal muscles and by the *accelerator urinae*. During the act both the horse and mare stand with the hind-legs extended and apart, resting on the toes of both hind feet, thereby sinking the posterior part of the body. The male animal also often advances the fore-legs in order to avoid their being splashed; in this position the penis is protruded, and the tail raised and quivering. The streams which flow from the two sexes are very different in size, depending on the relative diameters of the urethral canal. The mare after urinating spasmodically erects the clitoris, the cause of which is difficult to see; it may be due to the passage of a hot alkaline fluid over a remarkably sensitive surface. The horse can, under ordinary circumstances, pass urine only when standing still, though both sexes can defecate while trotting; but in a condition of oestrum the mare can empty her bladder while cantering. In the ox the urine simply dribbles away, owing to the curved character of the urethral canal, and is directed towards the ground by the tuft of hair found on the extremity of the sheath. The ox can pass his urine while walking. The cow arches her back to urinate, but instead of extending her hind-limbs, as does the mare, she brings them under her body, at the same time raising the tail.

The upright position is essential to micturition; no horse of either sex can evacuate the bladder while lying down—a point of extreme importance in practice. Further, it will be remembered that the fundus of an over-distended bladder hangs into the abdominal cavity, and is thus on a lower level than the urethra; this contributes to the difficulty of emptying an over-distended organ. As a horse cannot micturate at work, it is obvious that opportunity for this should be regularly afforded, or much suffering must result."

CHARACTERISTICS OF MAMMALIAN URINE

Composition

Urine is formed to keep the composition of the extracellular fluids constant, and generally most substances that are present in extracellular fluid are also present in urine. Also, the composition of urine varies, depending on whether substances are being conserved or excreted.

[1]Smith, F. 1921. *Manual of Veterinary Physiology,* 5th ed. Alex Eger, Chicago.

Color

Urine is usually yellow in color. The yellow color is derived from bilirubin that was excreted into the intestine and reabsorbed into the portal circulation as urobilinogen. Much of the urobilinogen is reexcreted by the liver into the intestine, but urobilinogen that bypasses the liver can be excreted by the kidneys into the urine. The various bilinogens are colorless but are spontaneously oxidized on exposure to oxygen. Thus urobilinogen, when partially oxidized, is known as urobilin, and it is largely responsible for the yellow color of urine.

Odor

The odor of urine is characteristic for a species and is probably influenced by diet. For example, the characteristic odor imparted to human urine after the ingestion of asparagus is caused by formation of the amide form of the amino acid, aspartic acid.

Consistency

Urine has a watery consistency in most species. Equine urine is somewhat thick and syrupy, however, because of the secretion of mucus from glands in the pelvis of the kidneys and the upper part of the ureters. The urine of the horse has high concentrations of carbonates and phosphates, which seem to precipitate on standing. The secretion of mucus probably provides a carrier for the carbonates and phosphates and prevents their collection in the renal pelvis.

Nitrogenous component

The principal nitrogenous constituent of mammalian urine is urea. Urea is formed by the liver from ammonia, which is produced during amino acid metabolism. The body expends considerable energy in producing urea so that the toxicity of ammonia can be avoided. Urea itself is relatively nontoxic.

Amount and specific gravity

The amount of urine excreted daily varies with diet, work, external temperature, water consumption, season, and other factors. Marked pathological variations may occur. The specific gravity of urine varies with the relative proportion of dissolved matter and water. In general, the greater the volume, the lower the specific gravity. Volumes and specific gravities for several domestic animals and humans are shown in Table 31.5.

AVIAN RENAL PHYSIOLOGY

In urine formation and elimination, birds have many similarities to mammals, but major differences are notable. Similarities include glomerular filtration followed by tubular reabsorption and tubular secretion whereby the filtrate is modified. Also, ureteral urine can have an osmolality that is above or below that of plasma. Differences from mammals

Table 31.5. Volumes and specific gravities of urine

Animal	Volume (ml/kg body wt/day)	Specific gravity mean and range
Cat	10–20	1.030 (1.020–1.040)
Cattle	17–45	1.032 (1.030–1.045)
Dog	20–100	1.025 (1.016–1.060)
Goat	10–40	1.030 (1.015–1.045)
Horse	3–18	1.040 (1.025–1.060)
Sheep	10–40	1.030 (1.015–1.045)
Swine	5–30	1.012 (1.010–1.050)
Human	8.6–28.6	1.020 (1.002–1.040)

Data from Altman and Dittmer 1961, *Blood and Other Body Fluids,* Fed. Am. Soc. Exp. Biol., Washington, D.C.

include the presence of two major nephron types, the presence of a renal portal system, formation of uric acid instead of urea as the major end product of nitrogen metabolism, and postrenal modification of ureteral urine.

To understand renal physiology of birds, it is important to review the anatomy of the avian urinary organs and relate form with function.

Gross anatomy

Avian kidneys are paired retroperitoneal structures that are closely fitted to the bony depressions of the fused pelvis. Each kidney is divided into cranial, middle, and caudal lobes. Ureters transport urine from the kidneys to the cloaca, which is the common collection site for the digestive, reproductive, and urinary organs (Fig. 31.29). Each lobe is comprised of lobules, as shown in Fig. 31.30. A lobule somewhat resembles a mushroom, with its cortex corresponding to the cap of the mushroom and its smaller medulla corresponding to the stem.

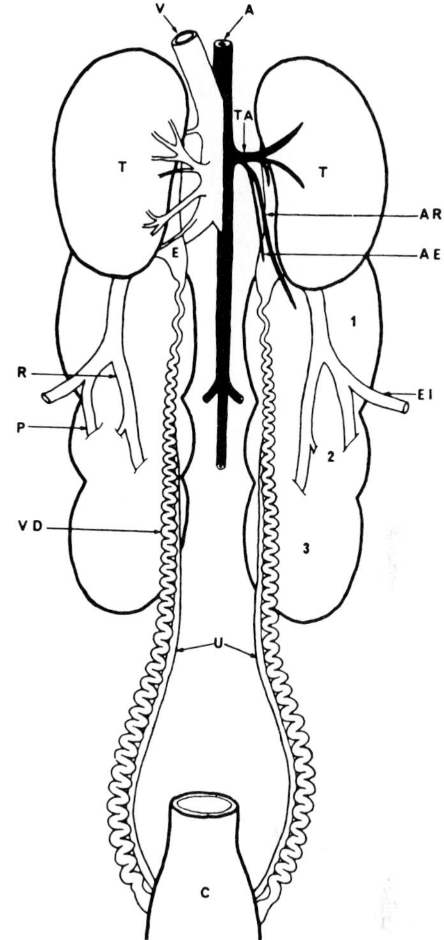

Figure 31.29. Ventral view of organs and associated structures of the dorsal abdominal cavity of a cockerel. A, abdominal aorta; AE, epididymal artery; AR, cranial renal artery; C, cloaca; E, epididymis; EI, external iliac vein; P, caudal renal portal vein; R, renal vein; T, testis; TA, testicular artery; U, ureters; V, posterior vena cava; VD, ductus deferens; 1, 2, and 3, cranial, middle, and caudal lobes of the left kidney, respectively. (From Hodges 1974, *The Histology of the Fowl,* Academic Press, New York.)

Nephron types

Avian kidneys are characterized by having two major nephron types, reptilian and mammalian (Fig. 31.31). The reptilian-type nephrons are located in the cortex and lack loops of Henle. An intermediate segment that connects the proximal and distal tubules and is believed to represent a primitive nephron loop has been described. Reptilian-type nephrons are not capable of concentrating urine.

The mammalian-type nephrons have well-defined loops of Henle that are grouped into a medullary cone (Fig. 31.30), the part of the lobule that corresponds to the stem of a mushroom. Other structures in the medullary cone are medullary collecting tubules and ducts and vasa recta, all of which enter at the wider cortical end of the cone. The extent of the vasa recta is shown in Fig. 31.32. A corticomedullary osmotic gradient exists in the peritubular fluid of the medullary cone that is established by the loops of Henle of the mammalian-type nephrons and maintained by the vasa recta. The osmotic gradient permits the excretion of urine that has an osmolality greater than plasma. All tubular fluid, whether from nephrons of the reptilian or the mammalian-type, is exposed to the osmotic gradient because of the exit of the collecting tubules and ducts through the cone to join the common ureteral branch.

There is some evidence that the avian kidney can alternate between the use of reptilian-type and mammalian-type nephrons, depending on the need for water conservation. For example, when birds are given a salt load (and thus the need to conserve water for diluting the added salt), a majority (about 80 percent) of the reptilian-type nephrons shut

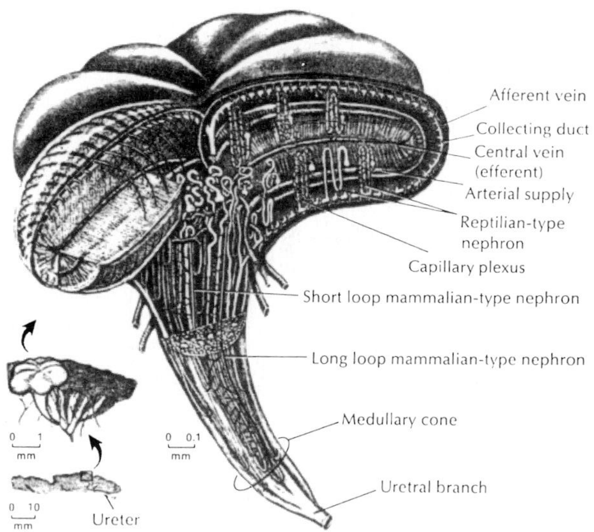

Figure 31.30. Avian kidney lobule (labeled illustration). The three lobes of each kidney comprise many lobules. The relative location of mammalian-type and reptilian-type nephrons are shown. (From Sturkie 1986, in Sturkie, ed., *Avian Physiology*, 4th ed., Springer-Verlag, New York.)

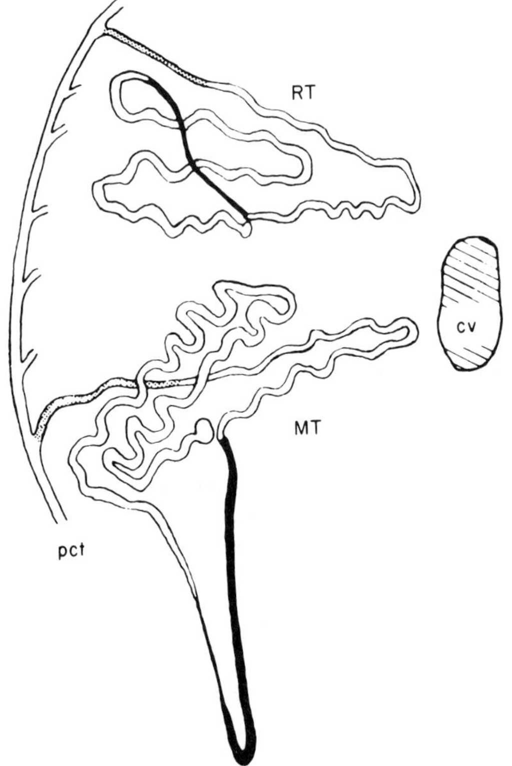

Figure 31.31. The location of avian reptilian-type (RT) and mammalian-type (MT) nephrons relative to an intralobular central vein (cv) and a perilobular collecting tubule (pct). The intermediate segment of the RT nephron and the nephron loop of the MT nephron are shown in black. The finely stippled areas are beginning collecting tubules. (From Johnson 1979, in King and McClelland, eds., *Form and Function in Birds*, Academic Press, San Diego.)

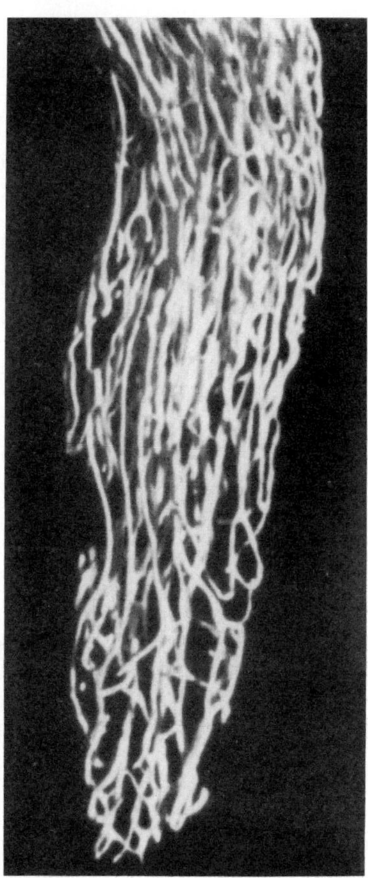

Figure 31.32. The vasa recta and associated capillary plexus from an avian kidney medullary cone. "Microfil" injection via ischiadic artery. (From Johnson 1979, in King and McClelland, eds., *Form and Function in Birds*, Academic Press, San Diego.)

down to zero filtration. Also, the whole-kidney GFR is reduced to about 40 percent of the control value; of that amount, an equal amount of filtrate comes from nephrons of the reptilian type and of the mammalian type. During control diuresis (both nephron types functional), 25 percent of the filtrate comes from mammalian-type nephrons and 75 percent from the reptilian-type nephrons.

Renal portal system

A unique feature of the avian kidney is its renal portal system for a portion of the blood supply that perfuses the tubules. Venous blood arriving by this means comes from the hind limbs via the external iliac and sciatic veins (Fig. 31.33). The renal portal blood enters the kidney from its periphery, supplying afferent blood to the peritubular capillaries. Within the peritubular capillaries, it is mixed with efferent arteriolar blood coming from the glomeruli (Fig. 31.34). The mixture perfuses the tubules and proceeds to the central vein of the lobule. It is estimated that the renal portal system supplies $\frac{1}{2}$ to $\frac{2}{3}$ of the blood to the kidney.

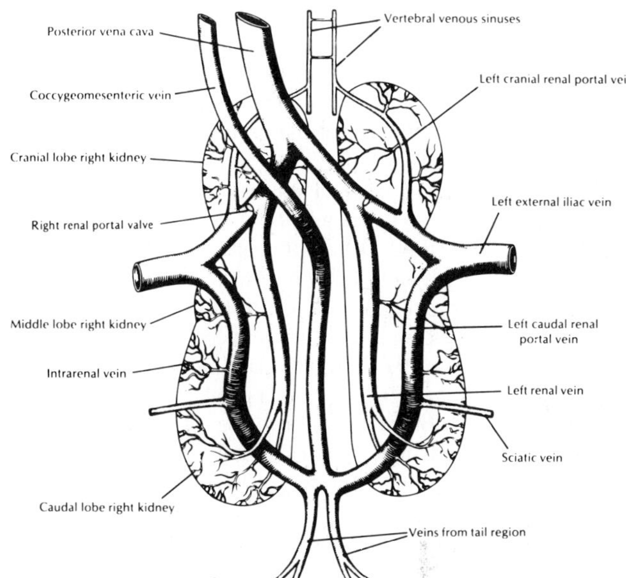

Figure 31.33. The veins associated with the renal portal system of birds. Blood arrives from the hind limbs via the external iliac and sciatic veins. Also shown is a renal portal valve. Its closure has potential for diverting more blood to the renal portal system. (From Sturkie 1986, in Sturkie, ed., *Avian Physiology*, 4th ed., Springer-Verlag, New York.)

A renal portal valve is located at the juncture of the right and left renal veins and their associated iliac veins (Fig. 31.33). Closure of the valve would have the potential of diverting more blood to the renal portal system. The physiologic significance of these valves has not been settled, but it seems likely that they may be controlled by factors that regulate blood flow to the kidneys.

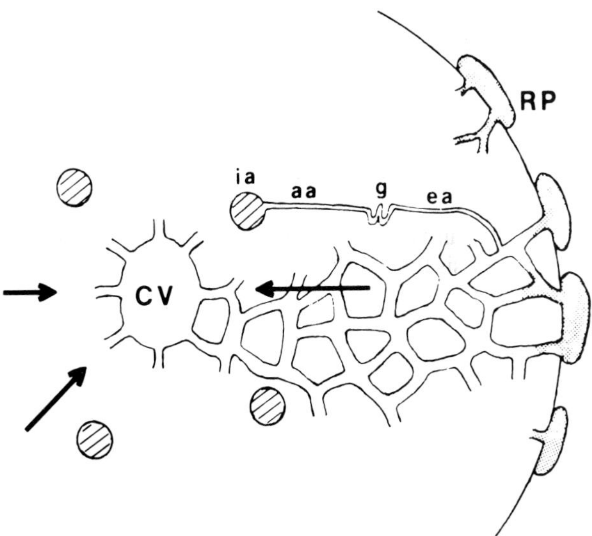

Figure 31.34. Intralobular blood flow. Intralobular artery (ia) blood supplies afferent arterioles (aa) going to glomeruli (g). Blood leaving the glomeruli via efferent arterioles (ea) enters the peritubular capillaries and mixes with blood from branches of the renal portal (RP) veins. Peritubular blood enters the central vein (CV) of each lobule. Arrows indicate direction of blood flow. (From Johnson 1979, in King and McClelland, eds., *Form and Function in Birds*, Academic Press, San Diego.)

Uric acid formation and excretion

The metabolism of proteins and amino acids results in the production of nitrogenous end products. Among the many different kinds of animals, ammonia, urea, or uric acid accounts for two-thirds or more of the total nitrogen excreted. Accordingly, animals are divided into three groups, depending on whether their main nitrogenous excretory product is ammonia, urea, or uric acid.

Ammonia is a very toxic substance and must be either rapidly excreted or converted to a less toxic substance, such as urea or uric acid. Among vertebrates, the ammonia-excreting group is confined to animals that are entirely aquatic. The ammonia, a relatively diffusible substance, is quickly discharged into the vast reservoir about them.

The urea-excreting group is found among mammals and amphibians that inhabit not only fresh water but also land. Ammonia is found in amphibian embryos, which develop in water, but at the time of metamorphosis they change and begin to produce urea as the end product of nitrogen metabolism. Mammalian fetuses give off excretory products to the mother, and the urea presents no excretory problems of water wasting (urea excretion obligates water excretion).

In dry-living reptiles and birds, uric acid is formed instead of urea because embryonic development takes place in eggs that have shells that are impervious to water. Since the embryo must develop on the limited supply of water present in the egg, it is better that the excretory products are deposited as insoluble materials (precipitated uric acid) that do not require water for their removal. It would be necessary to eliminate the liquid urine formed if urea were the end product.

Uric acid in birds is formed in the liver from ammonia.

Hepatectomy leads to the accumulation of ammonia and amino acids in the blood of birds, just as it does in mammals. It is also believed that the kidney, as well as the liver, may be a site for uric acid synthesis in birds.

Uric acid is freely filtered at the glomerulus and is also secreted by the tubules. Tubular secretion is the dominant process and accounts for about 90 percent of total excretion. The presence of the renal portal system provides a greater source of blood to the tubules for clearance than could be supplied by the efferent arterioles, and greater amounts can be secreted into the tubule. The greater amounts of uric acid in the tubules exceeds its solubility, and precipitation occurs. Uric acid continues through the tubules in the precipitated form and appears in the urine as a whitish coagulum. Because uric acid is no longer in solution, it does not contribute to the effective osmotic pressure of the tubular fluid, and obligatory water loss is avoided.

Modification of ureteral urine

Postrenal modification of ureteral urine is possible because of its exposure to membranes of the cloaca. It is also exposed to membranes of the colon and ceca because of retrograde flow caused by reverse peristalsis. Although the cloaca seems to be impermeable to water, water is reabsorbed from the colon. Water reabsorption from the colon follows the active reabsorption of Na^+. Even though there is some Na^+ reabsorption from the cloaca, it is not associated with water reabsorption. Water reabsorption does occur from the ceca and could involve urine water if retrograde flow progressed to that location.

Concentration of avian urine

The renal response to ADH in birds, like that in mammals, consists of an increased permeability of the collecting tubules and collecting ducts to water. The tubular fluid reaches osmotic equilibrium with the interstitial fluid surrounding the tubules, thus becoming hyperosmotic to plasma as collecting tubules and collecting ducts pass through the medullary cone. Urea plays virtually no role in the establishment of hypertonicity of the medullary cone interstitial fluid in birds. The hypertonicity is most likely created by NaCl transport from ascending limbs of loops of Henle. The maximum concentration that urine can attain is identical to the concentration of the interstitial fluids at the tip of the medullary cone, which is about 540 mOsm/kg H_2O. A maximum urine/plasma osmolal ratio would be about 1.58:1.

Urine characteristics and flow

Bird urine unmixed with feces is cream colored and contains thick mucus. Precipitated uric acid is mixed with the mucus. Mucus secretion probably facilitates transport of the precipitated solutes similar to the mucus in equine urine. Urine flows for several species under different conditions are shown in Table 31.6.

Table 31.6. Urine flows of selected avian species under certain specified conditions*

Species	Conditions	Urine flow (ml/kg/hr)†
Chicken	Dehydrated	1.08
	Hydrated	17.9
	Salt loaded	10.9
Chicken	Control	86.8 (ml/hr/bird)
	Diuresis	148.7 (ml/hr/bird)
Turkey	Control	3.3
	Hydrated	30.5
	Control	32. (μl/kg/min)
	Diuresis (epinephrine)	55. (ml/hr/bird)
Duck	Hydrated	7.8
	Hydrated	2.4
	Salt loaded	0.57
Gambel's quail	Mannitol diuresis	11.2
	Hydration	6.2
Budgerigar	Control	6.3
	Dehydration	1.68

*Most urine samples were not taken by ureter cannulation.
†Unless otherwise stated.
From Sturkie 1986, in Sturkie, ed., *Avian Physiology,* 4th ed., Springer-Verlag, New York.

REFERENCES

Altman, P.L., and Dittmer, D.S. 1961. *Blood and Other Body Fluids*, Federation of American Societies for Experimental Biology, Washington.

Andreoli, T.E., and Schafer, J.O. 1979. Effective luminal hypotonicity: The driving force for isotonic proximal tubular fluid absorption. *Am. J. Physiol.* 236:F89–96.

Barsanti, J.A., and Finco, D.R. 1979. Protein concentration in urine of normal dogs. *Am. J. Vet. Res.* 40:1583–8.

Beeuwkes, R., and Bonventre, J.V. 1975. Tubular organization and vascular tubular relations in the dog kidney. *Am. J. Physiol.* 229:695–713.

Blantz, R.C. 1987. The glomerular and tubular actions of angiotensin II. *Am. J. Kid. Dis.* 10 (suppl. I):2–6.

Boudreau, J.E., and Carone, F.A. 1974. Protein handling by the renal tubule. *Nephron* 13:22–34.

Boulpaep, E.L., and Sackin, H. 1977. Role of the paracellular pathway in isotonic fluid movement across the renal tubule. *Yale J. Biol. Med.* 50:115–31.

Cushny, A.R. 1917. *The Secretion of the Urine,* Longmans, Green & Co., New York.

De Bold, A.J., Borenstein, H.B., Veress, A.T., and Sonnenberg, H. 1981. A rapid and potent natriuretic response to intravenous injection of atrial myocardial extract in rats. *Life Sci.* 28:89–94.

Dellmann, H.-D., and Brown, E.M. 1987. *Textbook of Veterinary Histology*, 3d ed., Lea & Febiger, Philadelphia.

Dukes, H.H. 1955. *The Physiology of Domestic Animals.* 7th ed. Cornell University Press, Ithaca.

Duling, B.R. 1988. The kidneys. In R.M. Berne and M.N. Levy, eds., *Physiology*, 2d ed. C.V. Mosby, St. Louis.

Dyce, K.M., Sack, W.O., and Wensing, C.J.G. 1987. *Textbook of Veterinary Anatomy*, W.B. Saunders, Philadelphia.

Edwards, B.S., Zimmerman, R.S., Schwab, T.R., Heublein, D.M., and Burnett, J.C., Jr. 1988. Atrial stretch, not pressure, is the principal determinant controlling the acute release of atrial natriuretic peptide. *Circ. Res.* 62:191–5.

Ewald, B.H. 1967. Renal function tests in normal beagle dogs. *Am. J. Vet. Res.* 28:741–9.

Fulton, J.F., and Wilson, L.G. 1966. *Selected Readings in the History of Physiology*, 2d ed. Charles C Thomas, Springfield, Ill.

Gans, J.H., and Mercer, P.F. 1984. The kidneys. In M. J. Swenson, ed.,

Dukes' Physiology of Domestic Animals, 10th ed. Cornell University Press, Ithaca.

Guyton, A.C. 1991. *Textbook of Medical Physiology*, 8th ed. W.B. Saunders, Philadelphia.

Guyton, A.C., Coleman, T.G., Cowley, A.W., Jr., Scheel, K.W., Manning, R.D., and Norman, R.A. 1972. Arterial pressure regulation: Overriding dominance of the kidneys in long-term regulation and in hypertension. *Am. J. Med.* 52:584–94.

Hall, J.E. 1986. Regulation of glomerular filtration rate and sodium excretion by antiotensin II. *Fed. Proc.* 45:1431–7.

Hodges, R.D. 1974. *The Histology of the Fowl*. Academic Press, New York.

Jamison, R.L., and Maffly, R.H. 1976. The urinary concentrating mechanism. *N. Engl. J. Med.* 295:1059–67.

Johnson, O.W. 1979. Urinary organs. In A.S. King and J. McClelland, eds., *Form and Function in Birds*, Vol. 1. Academic Press, San Diego.

Katz, A.I. 1982. Renal Na-K-ATPase: Its role in tubular sodium and potassium transport. *Am. J. Physiol.* 242:F207–19.

Knepper, M.A., and Roch-Ramel, F. 1987. Pathways of urea transport in the mammalian kidney. *Kidney Int.* 31:629–33.

Laiken, N.D., Fanestil, D.D. 1985. Body fluids and renal function. In J.B. West, ed., *Best and Taylor's Physiological Basis of Medical Practice*, 11th ed. Williams & Wilkins, Baltimore.

McGilvery, R.W. 1983. *Biochemistry: A Functional Approach*, 3d ed. W.B. Saunders, Philadelphia.

Needleman, P., and Greenwald, J.E. 1986. Atriopeptin: A cardiac hormone intimately involved in fluid, electrolyte, and blood-pressure homeostasis. *N. Engl. J. Med.* 314:828–34.

Pitts, R.F. 1974. *Physiology of the Kidneys and Body Fluids*. 3d ed. Yearbook Medical Publishers, Chicago.

Reece, W.O. 1991. *Physiology of Domestic Animals*. Lea & Febiger, Philadelphia.

Rose, B.D. 1989. *Clinical Physiology of Acid-Base and Electrolyte Disorders*. 3d ed. McGraw-Hill, New York.

Sands, J.M., Nonoguchi, H., and Knepper, M.A. 1987. Vasopressin effects on urea and H_2O transport in inner medullary collecting duct subsegments. *Am. J. Physiol.* 253:F823–32.

Schmidt-Nielson, B., and O'Dell, R. 1961. Structure and concentrating mechanism in the mammalian kidney. *Am. J. Physiol.* 200:1119–24.

Smith, F. 1921. *A Manual of Veterinary Physiology*. 5th ed. Alexander Eger, Chicago.

Spring, K.R., and Kimura, G. 1979. Intracellular ion activities in *Necturus* proximal tubule. *Fed. Proc.* 38:2729–32.

Straffen, R.A. 1979. The urinary tract. In J. R. Brobeck, ed., *Best and Taylor's Physiological Basis of Medical Practice*. 10th ed. Williams & Wilkins, Baltimore.

Sturkie, P.D. 1986. Kidneys, extrarenal salt excretion, and urine. In P. D. Sturkie, ed., *Avian Physiology*. 4th ed. Springer-Verlag, New York.

Thames, M.D., Miller, B.D., and Abboud, F.M. 1982. Baroreflex regulation of renal nerve activity during volume expansion. *Am. J. Physiol.* 243:H810–14.

Tune, B.M., Burg, M.B., and Patlak, C.S. 1969. Characteristics of p-aminohippurate transport in proximal renal tubules. *Am. J. Physiol.* 217:1057–63.

Ullrich, K.J., Capasso, G., Rumrich, F., Papvassilious, F., and Kloss, S. 1977. Coupling between proximal tubular transport processes. *Pflugers Arch.* 368:245–52.

Warnock, D.G., and Rector, F.C., Jr. 1979. Proton secretion by the kidney. *Ann. Rev. Physiol.* 41:197–210.

Weidmann, P., Hasler, L., Gnadinger, M.P., Lang, R.E., Uehlinger, D.E., Shaw, S., Rascher, W., and Reubi, F.C. 1986. Blood levels and renal effects of atrial natriuretic peptide in normal man. *J. Clin. Invest.* 77:734–42.

Weiner, I.M., and Mudge, G.H. 1964. Renal tubular mechanisms for excretion of organic acids and base. *Am. J. Med.* 36:743–62.

CHAPTER 32

Acid-Base Balance | by T. Richard Houpt

The pH of the extracellular fluid is one of the most vigorously regulated variables of the body. The vital limits of pH variation for mammals are usually given as from pH 7.0 to 7.8. The normal pH range in arterial blood is 7.36 to 7.44, and the average pH is 7.4. The pH of a solution is defined as $pH = \log 1/[H^+]$. In terms of $[H^+]$, pH 7.8 represents 40 percent and pH 7.0 represents 250 percent of the $[H^+]$ at pH 7.4. It would appear from this that tissue cells are relatively tolerant to changes in $[H^+]$. The concentrations of hydrogen ion that determine pH are extremely low, however, and consequently the pH of the fluids is easily disturbed by addition of small amounts of strong acid or base.

ACID-BASE BALANCE

The relatively constant extracellular fluid (ECF) $[H^+]$ is the result of a balance between acids and bases. Acids are substances that donate hydrogen ions (i.e., protons) to a solution; bases are substances that accept and bind hydrogen ions from a solution. This balance is disturbed when acids or bases are added to or removed from the body fluids. A depression of blood pH to below the normal range is known as acidemia; a value above the normal pH range is called alkalemia. The disturbance caused by the addition of excess acid or the removal of base from ECF is known as acidosis. If it is due to the addition of excess base or the loss of acid, the disturbance is called alkalosis.

Under normal conditions, acids or bases are added continuously to the body fluids, either because of their ingestion or as the result of their production in cellular metabolism. In disease, such conditions as insufficient respiratory ventilation, vomiting, diarrhea, or renal insufficiency may cause an unusual loss or gain of acid or base. To combat these disturbances, the body uses three basic mechanisms: chemical buffering, respiratory adjustment of blood carbon dioxide concentration, and excretion of hydrogen or bicarbonate ions by the kidneys. The buffers and the respiratory mechanism act within minutes to prevent a large shift in $[H^+]$. If a nonvolatile acid or base is involved, renal excretion of hydrogen ions or bicarbonate ions begins immediately, but complete restoration of acid-base balance may take from a few hours to several days.

Metabolic problems

Carbonic acid

Within the body, the metabolism of most organic compounds containing carbon, hydrogen, oxygen, and nitrogen results in the formation of water, carbon dioxide, and urea. The carbon dioxide reacts with water to yield carbonic acid, which is quantitatively the most important acid formed in the catabolism of nutrients. In a large dog about 5000 mEq of hydrogen ions from carbonic acid are formed daily, as compared with about 100 mEq of hydrogen ions from all other acids. However, because of its volatile nature, all of the carbon dioxide is quickly expired through the respiratory system as it is formed.

Non-volatile acids

A more serious problem is the formation of strong nonvolatile sulfuric acid from sulfur-containing amino acids, such as methionine and cysteine. On average, 60 mEq of sulfuric acid is formed for every 100 g of protein metabolized. Much of the 100 mEq of hydrogen ions mentioned above consists of this acid. Such strong acids have only a fleeting existence in the body, for they immediately react with plasma buffers, particularly with bicarbonate, as described later in the discussion of chemical buffers. In this rapid buffer action, the weak acid of the buffer system is substituted for the strong acid. The buffer bases are depleted by this reaction, however, and must eventually be restored. This ultimately requires the excretion of an equivalent quantity of hydrogen ions by the kidneys. In addition to sulfuric acid, smaller amounts of phosphoric acid are formed in the hydrolysis of the phosphodiesters of phosphoproteins and phospholipids.

Various other compounds not normally present in the diet or formed in metabolism (e.g., ammonium chloride) can cause an acidemia when administered to an animal. Here the ammonium ion is acidic, yielding in solution a hydrogen ion and ammonia. After absorption into the body fluids, the ammonia is rapidly removed for the synthesis of urea in the liver. The hydrogen ions remaining, electrically balanced by chloride ions, cause an acidemia. Reaction with buffer base occurs, and the overall effect is identical to the addition of a strong acid to the body fluids. Ultimately hydrogen ions must be excreted by the kidneys in order to restore the buffer base.

Formation of excess base

During the metabolism of feeds of plant origin, large amounts of base are formed and appear in the bloodstream as bicarbonate. For example, grasses contain salts of malic, aconitic, and citric acids, apparently in the form of potassium, calcium, and magnesium salts or complexes. These organic salts are completely metabolized to carbon dioxide and water in the mammalian body, but they enter the metabolic cycle (i.e., citric acid cycle) in the form of undissociated organic acids. The ultimate source of hydrogen ions for the conversion of such organic salts to their acid form is the carbonic acid derived from hydration of carbon dioxide:

$$CO_2 + H_2O \leftrightharpoons H_2CO_3 \leftrightharpoons H^+ + HCO_3^-.$$

Thus as the anions of malic, aconitic, and citric acids are oxidized, hydrogen ions are removed and bicarbonate ions accumulate. The bicarbonate ions are electrically balanced by potassium and other cations. The excess bicarbonate raises the bicarbonate/carbonic acid ratio, and plasma pH rises. This tendency toward metabolic alkalosis is corrected by the excretion of bicarbonate in the urine, rendering the urine alkaline. Typically, the urine of herbivores is also high in potassium.

The normal balance of acids and bases

The opposing tendencies of the metabolic processes to produce both acids and bases cancel one another to a certain degree. However, the high protein rations of some animals, largely derived from meat products, produce a predominance of acidic products, while the diets of other animals, derived from plant materials, produce a predominance of basic products. Dogs, cats, and other carnivores, as well as omnivores eating a high-protein diet (most remarkably the human) and animals that are not eating (in which case body proteins are being metabolized for energy production), have to contend with an excess of acid and excrete an acidic urine. Ruminants, equids, and other herbivores have an excess of base and excrete an alkaline urine high in bicarbonate.

Ammonia, ureogenesis, and acid/base balance

The traditional view is that when proteins and amino acids are metabolized the primary nitrogenous end product is ammonia. Nearly all the ammonia immediately reacts with carbonic acid yielding ammonium and bicarbonate ions; that is, the equilibrium at body fluid pH is far to the right:

$$NH_3 + H_2CO_3 \leftrightharpoons NH_4^+ + HCO_3^-.$$

Most of the ammonium ions are used in the hepatic synthesis of urea:

$$2NH_4^+ + CO_2 \rightarrow 2H^+ + \text{urea} + H_2O.$$

The hydrogen ions formed react with the bicarbonate to reform carbonic acid, and overall there is no effect on acid-base balance. However, some ammonium ions are also taken up in the hepatic formation of glutamine. As far as this portion of the metabolic ammonia goes, an equivalent amount of hydrogen ion is not formed because it is not used in urea synthesis. In effect, the glutamine serves to carry excess hydrogen ions to the kidney, where the ions are excreted in the form of ammonium (NH_4^+). This will be discussed further in the section on hydrogen ion excretion by the kidney.

Chemical buffers of the extracellular fluid

A buffer system consists of a mixture of a weak acid and its conjugate base. An example is a solution of carbonic acid and bicarbonate ion. When a buffer system is present, the addition of an acid or a base will result in a much smaller shift of pH than would occur if no buffers were present. If a strong acid is added to the solution, the added hydrogen ions are bound by the buffer base, forming more of the weak acid. For example, if sulfuric acid were added to the bicarbonate buffer system, the reaction would be

$$2H^+ + SO_4^{2-} + 2HCO_3^- \rightarrow 2H_2CO_3 + SO_4^{2-}$$

In effect, the added strong acid has been replaced by the weak acid of the buffer system.

The relationship between pH and the mixture of a weak acid and its conjugate base is given by the Henderson-Hasselbalch equation:

$$pH = pK + \log \frac{(\text{base})}{(\text{acid})}$$

The dissociation constant of the weak acid is represented by K, and pK is the negative logarithm of K. In this context, pK can be defined as the pH at which the acid and base of the buffer system are in equal concentrations, (i.e., the pH at which the ratio of base to acid is 1). Thus the Henderson-Hasselbalch equation shows that the pH of a solution containing such a buffer system is determined by the ratio of the base to the acid. The effectiveness of most buffer systems is greatest at a pH equal to the pK of its weak acid and over a range extending one pH unit above and one pH unit below the pK value.

When an acid is added to the buffer system, a shift of pH is resisted, but the ratio of base to acid decreases, and the pH is somewhat depressed. If more acid were added, a further decrease of the base/acid ratio would occur because the base would be used up in reaction with the added hydrogen ions. Thus the protective function of buffer systems is limited and, unless the favorable ratio of base to acid is restored, the buffers will become exhausted with repeated addition of acid and acidemia will result. The restoration of buffer base ultimately requires the formation and secretion of hydrogen ions by the kidney tubules. If, instead, a strong base were added to the body fluids, it would react with the acid of the buffer and thus form more buffer base. This ultimately must be corrected by renal excretion of base and retention of hydrogen ions.

The principal buffer systems of the blood are the bicarbonate, plasma protein, phosphate, and hemoglobin buffers. Of these, the most important are bicarbonate and hemoglobin. If a strong acid is added to blood in vitro, 53 percent of the buffer action is due to bicarbonate, 35 percent to hemoglobin, 7 percent to plasma protein, and 5 percent to phosphates. The total buffering capacity of the blood is considerable and is adequate to prevent a pH shift beyond the vital limit, even if the entire daily metabolic output of nonvolatile acid were suddenly added. In reality, however, the blood alone is never required to buffer all acid products at one time. The buffers in the interstitial fluid (mostly bicarbonate) rapidly assume part of the load, and in time intracellular buffers also participate. Finally, excretion of acid by the lungs and kidneys begins immediately to reduce the total load.

The bicarbonate buffer system

The bicarbonate buffer system is the principal buffer of the blood and of the ECF. Chemically, the weak acid component of the bicarbonate buffer system is carbonic acid, H_2CO_3, and the Henderson-Hasselbalch equation is

$$\mathrm{pH} = \mathrm{pK} + \log \frac{[\mathrm{HCO_3}^-]}{[\mathrm{H_2CO_3}]}$$

where K is the dissociation constant for H_2CO_3. However, only about one of every 800 carbon dioxide molecules dissolved in body fluids is hydrated to form one carbonic acid molecule. In fact, measurement of true carbonic acid concentration is difficult and usually impractical. Instead, the total concentration of dissolved CO_2, which includes and is proportional to true $[H_2CO_3]$, is used as the concentration of the acid component in the Henderson-Hasselbalch equation. The concentration of dissolved carbon dioxide can easily be calculated as the product of carbon dioxide tension in the fluid and the solubility coefficient, s, for carbon dioxide. The value of s under body conditions is 0.03 mMol/mm Hg. For example, normal P_{CO_2} in arterial blood is 40 mm Hg, and thus $s \cdot P_{CO_2} = 1.2$ mMol CO_2 dissolved per liter of blood. The dissociation constant K in the Henderson-Hasselbalch equation is for the dissociation of the weak acid component. When $s \cdot P_{CO_2}$ is substituted for $[H_2CO_3]$, the dissociation constant becomes an apparent dissociation constant, indicated by the use of a prime sign (K′). The useful form of the Henderson-Hasselbalch equation is then

$$\mathrm{pH} = \mathrm{pK}' + \log \frac{[\mathrm{HCO_3}^-]}{[s \cdot P_{CO_2}]}$$

where pK′ = 6.1. If pH and P_{CO_2} are measured, $[HCO_3^-]$ can be calculated. The ratio of bicarbonate to dissolved carbon dioxide is normally about 20, far from the ideal buffer ratio of 1. Despite this, the bicarbonate system is very effective, partly because carbon dioxide is in plentiful supply in the body and thus P_{CO_2} can be maintained or varied rapidly by changes in the rate at which carbon dioxide is removed by pulmonary ventilation. In fact, if the lungs are normal, arterial P_{CO_2} will be held constant near 40 mm Hg even when considerable amounts of carbon dioxide are being produced by reaction with acids.

The hemoglobin buffer system

Hemoglobin is the second most important blood buffer. At normal blood pH, the hemoglobin molecules are present in part in the form of proteinate ions (Hb^-). These basic ions, with their weak acids (HHb), form a buffer pair. When acid is added to the blood, the reaction

$$H^+ + Hb^- \leftrightharpoons HHb$$

shifts to the right and the ratio of base to acid is decreased. The buffer reactions of reduced and oxygenated hemoglobin are similar, but the reduced hemoglobin ion is a stronger base.

Other buffer systems

The plasma proteins also exist to a certain extent as proteinate ions at body pH and bind hydrogen ions in a manner similar to hemoglobin. The components of the phosphate buffers at blood pH are HPO_4^{2-} (the base) and $H_2PO_4^-$ (the weak acid). This buffer system plays a minor role in the blood.

The cells of the body also contain large amounts of buffering compounds that, in the aggregate, could be more important than the blood buffers. These are assumed to be mainly intracellular proteinate ions and their weak acidic forms and the intracellular phosphates. The phosphate buffers are important intracellular buffers because of their greater intracellular concentration and also because their pK of 6.8 is closer to intracellular fluid pH than it is to extracellular fluid pH. In addition a type of buffering is effected by exchange of hydrogen ions for cations loosely bound to the vast surface of crystallites in the skeleton. These buffering actions develop slowly, and it is believed that they operate primarily in chronic acidotic states.

The isohydric principle

Although the reactions of the various buffer systems have been considered as though each were the only buffer present, all of the buffer systems in the ECF react in unison. When hydrogen ions are added to the ECF, each base of each buffer pair will bind hydrogen ions; hence all buffers share the imposed acid load. Since the pH involved is the same for all buffers in a solution, the buffers are interrelated through their common hydrogen ion concentration as illustrated in Fig. 32.1. Each pK is that characteristic of the weak acid of each buffer pair. This interrelationship is often referred to as the isohydric principle. As a result of this principle, addition of an acid or base to a solution containing several buffers will result in a change in the ratios of all the buffer pairs.

Respiratory adjustment of Pco_2

Blood Pco_2 can be varied extensively because the partial pressure of carbon dioxide in the lung alveoli generally determines the amount of carbon dioxide dissolved in the blood. This respiratory mechanism depends on the exquisite sensitivity of the respiratory control systems to changes in blood Pco_2 and pH (see Chap 13). A small increase in Pco_2 or decrease in pH stimulates pulmonary ventilation so that the rate of carbon dioxide expiration increases. If acid has been added to the body fluids, the first reaction is a purely chemical buffering that results in the formation of additional carbonic acid and a depletion of bicarbonate:

$$H^+ + HCO_3^- \rightarrow H_2CO_3 \rightarrow CO_2 + H_2O.$$

As a result, the $[HCO_3^-]/(s{\cdot}Pco_2)$ ratio falls, and consequently pH falls. However, the increase in carbon dioxide and decrease in pH stimulate breathing, causing first a rapid expiration of the extra carbon dioxide and then, because pH is still below normal, slow expiration of additional carbon dioxide so that over a period of hours Pco_2 in arterial blood

$$\log\frac{[\text{Proteinate}^-]}{[\text{H Proteinate}]} + pK_d \qquad pK_a' + \log\frac{[HCO_3^-]}{s \cdot P_{CO_2}}$$

$$\searrow \quad \swarrow$$

$$pH$$

$$\nearrow \quad \nwarrow$$

$$\log\frac{[HPO_4^{--}]}{[H_2PO_4^-]} + pK_c \qquad pK_b + \log\frac{[Hb^-]}{[HHb]}$$

Figure 32.1. The isohydric principle illustrated for some of the buffers of the blood.

decreases to below a normal level. As a result, the $[HCO_3^-]/(s{\cdot}Pco_2)$ ratio is returned to nearly its normal value, and pH is also nearly back to 7.4. However, although the ratio of base to acid is nearly normal, the amounts of each are subnormal. This adjustment of Pco_2 by the respiratory system is compensatory; full correction of the acid-base abnormality can be effected only by renal excretion of hydrogen ions and production of bicarbonate. When an alkali is added to the blood, a similar but opposite respiratory response occurs and additional carbon dioxide is retained in ECF. This increases Pco_2 to balance the increase in $[HCO_3^-]$ that results from the reaction of the added alkali with carbonic acid. These respiratory adjustments of Pco_2 during an acid or base disturbance begin to be effective within minutes, but several hours may be required before the adjustments are maximal.

Excretion of hydrogen and bicarbonate ions by the kidney

When acids or bases are added to the body fluids, chemical buffers remove the immediate threat to the body from altered $[H^+]$, but a depletion of buffer bases or acids occurs. For example, if sulfuric acid is added, a reaction with bicarbonate ions results in the formation of carbonic acid, which can be removed largely by expiration of carbon dioxide. Excretion of the sulfate ion in the urine would not correct the deficit of bicarbonate ions and would, in addition, cause the loss of some strong cations, such as sodium ions, that would be necessary for electrical balance in the urine. In effect, the problem is solved within the kidney by formation of hydrogen ions through a mechanism that forms one bicarbonate ion for every hydrogen ion formed. The hydrogen ions are secreted into the tubular fluid in exchange for cation, while the bicarbonate ions move into the plasma. In addition, hydrogen ions are captured in the form of NH_4^+ in the liver and transported as glutamine from the liver to the kidney, where the NH_4^+ is secreted into the tubular fluid. By these means, hydrogen ions, equivalent in amount to those added as sulfuric acid, are excreted and the amount of bicarbonate in plasma is restored to its normal level.

Mechanism of hydrogen ion secretion

The basic mechanism of hydrogen ion secretion is outlined in Fig. 32.2. In this scheme a hydrogen ion is derived within the tubule cell from carbonic acid formed from carbon dioxide. The carbonic anhydrase ensures a sufficiently rapid formation of carbonic acid. As carbonic acid dissociates, both hydrogen ions and bicarbonate ions are formed. The hydrogen ions are secreted into the tubular fluid, while the bicarbonate ions move to the blood. Electrical balance is maintained by a simultaneous movement of tubular sodium ions into the cells in exchange for hydrogen ions and further movement of sodium into the blood with bicarbonate ions.

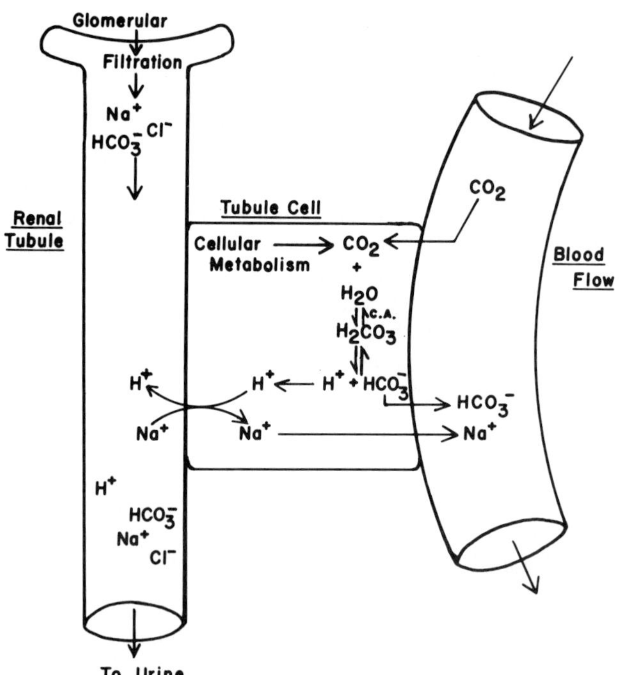

Figure 32.2. Secretion of H^+ by renal tubule cell with restoration of blood bicarbonate and conservation of filtered Na^+. C.A. is carbonic anhydrase.

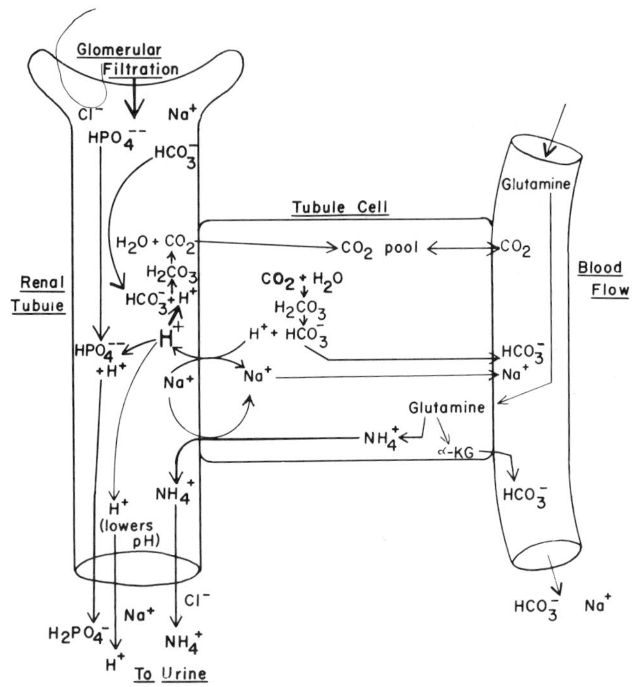

Figure 32.3. Excretion of H^+ in urine under conditions in which the rate of H^+ secretion into the tubule exceeds the rate of bicarbonate filtration. The H^+s in excess of those needed to bring about absorption of all bicarbonate appear in the urine, and they lower urinary pH. However, only a small fraction of the H^+s to be excreted from the body are in simple solution in urine. Many H^+s secreted by renal tubules or collecting ducts are bound to filtered HPO_4^{2-}. In addition, a large amount of H^+ in prolonged acidic conditions is in the form of NH_4^+ derived from glutamine where, for each NH_4^+ secreted into the urine, a HCO_3^- is restored to the plasma from the metabolism of α-ketoglutarate. (In the figure α-KG = α-ketoglutarate.)

Large amounts of hydrogen ion are secreted into the proximal tubules, but most of these react with filtered bicarbonate, and pH falls little. If all the bicarbonate is absorbed by this process in the proximal tubules, then in the distal tubules secreted hydrogen ions cause the pH to fall. Although some acidification may occur in the proximal tubules, the hydrogen ion concentration gradient that can be developed there is small. In the distal tubules and collecting ducts, however, the active transport of hydrogen ions can operate against a high hydrogen ion concentration gradient and can depress pH in the urine to pH 4 to 5. The ion-for-ion exchange with tubular sodium ions means that not only is the urine acidified but sodium ions are restored to the body fluids.

This simple hypothetical scheme may have to be modified, for recent evidence indicates that the actual source of hydrogen ions is not carbonic acid but, rather, a metabolic process that yields a hydroxyl ion for each hydrogen ion secreted. The strongly basic hydroxyl ion would then be neutralized by a hydrogen ion from carbonic acid. The overall result, however, is identical: hydrogen ions are secreted into the urine and bicarbonate ions in equivalent amounts are added to the blood. The further reactions of the secreted hydrogen ions with bicarbonate and other compounds derived from the glomerular filtrate are not shown in Fig. 32.2 but, rather, are considered below and in Fig. 32.3.

The rate of hydrogen ion secretion by renal tubule cells is largely determined by their intracellular pH. A high pH depresses hydrogen ion secretion into the tubular lumen while a low intracellular pH increases the rate. Generally, intracellular pH changes as blood pH or P_{CO_2} changes; thus acidemia and hypercapnia result in increased hydrogen ion secretion, and alkalemia and hypocapnia result in decreased hydrogen ion secretion. Intracellular [K^+] also has an important effect on acid secretion. A high [K^+] results in an increase in intracellular pH and hence a decrease in hydrogen ion secretion into the urine. A low intracellular [K^+] conversely results in increased acid secretion into the urine. The cause of this effect of potassium on intracellular pH is not well understood, but one explanation is that as potassium ions enter the cells, they displace hydrogen ions as the balancing cations for anionic sites on protein and other organic molecules. The hydrogen ions leave the cells and intracellular pH rises. Since most of the cells of the body would be involved in this process, the release of hydrogen ions by cells may be sufficient to cause a fall in pH of the ECF. There may then exist the paradoxical situation in which hydrogen ion secretion into the urine is depressed by the high intracellular pH, while at the same time there is an extracellular acidemia. Potassium-deficient states result in low intracellular [K^+], high [H^+], and enhanced hydrogen ion secretion into the urine. The secretion of hydrogen ions involves addition of bicarbonate ions to the ECF, and this can occur despite an existing alkalemia.

Bicarbonate reabsorption

The principal base of the plasma, bicarbonate ion, is present in the glomerular filtrate, and the amount filtered each day into the renal tubule is many times the total amount present in the body. Obviously, most of this bicarbonate must be reabsorbed from the tubular fluid under all circumstances. The mechanism of bicarbonate reabsorption is linked to the mechanism of hydrogen ion secretion into the tubular fluid (see Fig. 32.3). When bicarbonate ions are present in the tubular fluid, secreted hydrogen ions react with them:

$$H^+ + HCO_3^- \rightarrow H_2CO_3 \rightarrow CO_2 + H_2O.$$

The carbon dioxide thus formed in the tubule readily equilibrates with the general body pool of carbon dioxide. When the hydrogen ions are formed and secreted, however, bicarbonate ions are also formed, and for each hydrogen ion secreted one bicarbonate ion is added to the plasma. Thus, for every bicarbonate ion removed from the tubular fluid by reaction with a hydrogen ion, a bicarbonate ion is added to the blood. In effect, bicarbonate is reabsorbed from the tubular fluid and restored to the blood.

Bicarbonate excretion

Whether or not all of the filtered bicarbonate ions will be reabsorbed depends on the rate of hydrogen ion secretion into the tubular fluid and the rate of bicarbonate ion filtration. If the hydrogen ion secretion rate exceeds the bicarbonate ion filtration rate, nearly all bicarbonate ions will be reabsorbed and none will appear in the urine (Fig. 32.3). If the hydrogen ion secretion rate is less than the bicarbonate ion filtration rate, some bicarbonate ions will escape reabsorption and will appear in the urine (Fig. 32.4). Generally, under an acid stress, the hydrogen ion secretion rate rises, causing reabsorption of all bicarbonate and acidification of the urine by the excess hydrogen ions. If the acid stress involves strong acids that react with and depress plasma bicarbonate, the amount of bicarbonate filtered also falls and even greater acidification of the urine occurs. Under an acute base stress there is usually a marked increase in plasma bicarbonate that results in a corresponding increase in glomerular filtration of bicarbonate into the tubule. This great increase in filtered bicarbonate ion overwhelms tubular reabsorption processes, and a much larger fraction of the filtered bicarbonate ion escapes into and alkalinizes the urine (Fig. 32.4). Under those circumstances, changes in hydrogen ion secretion and consequently in bicarbonate reabsorption are relatively unimportant. Under more moderate, long-lasting base stress, however, reduced secretion of hydrogen ion with a corresponding decrease in bicarbonate ion (and sodium ion) reabsorption will effectively favor removal of excess base from the body.

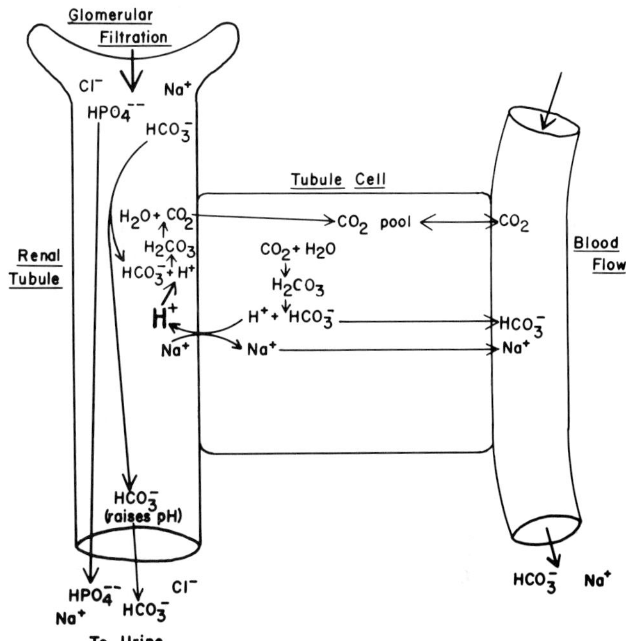

Figure 32.4. Excretion of bicarbonate under conditions where the rate of HCO_3^- filtration exceeds the rate of H^+ secretion into the tubules. All of the secreted H^+ reacts with filtered HCO_3^-, and the bicarbonate that escapes reaction with H^+ appears in the alkaline urine.

Urinary excretion of hydrogen ions

The secretion of excess hydrogen ions into the urine results in an acid urine, but the quantity of acid that can be excreted as free hydrogen ions is limited. Urine can be acidified only to a pH of about 4.5. This means that most of the hydrogen ions to be excreted must be bound by bases and are not in free solution. The most important of these bases is HPO_4^{2-} and ammonia. Phosphate is present at pH 7.4 in the glomerular filtrate, mostly in the form of HPO_4^{2-}. As the tubular fluid is acidified by hydrogen ion secretion, the basic HPO_4^{2-} takes up and binds hydrogen ions to form predominantly $H_2PO_4^-$. Part of the cation that electrically balances HPO_4^{2-} in the glomerular filtrate (mostly sodium ions) is exchanged with the secreted hydrogen ion and thus is returned to the blood. These processes are illustrated in Fig. 32.3.

In addition, a large fraction of excess H^+ is excreted in the urine in the form of NH_4^+. Until recently, the major source of NH_4^+ in the urine was believed to be the release of ammonia (NH_3) within renal tubule cells by the action of renal glutaminase on glutamine and other plasma amino acids. This NH_3 diffuses into the tubular fluid, and if excess hydrogen ions are being secreted the NH_3 binds them to form NH_4^+. The NH_4^+ is excreted in the urine, carrying with it the bound hydrogen ions, without a further depression of urinary pH.

Recently, however, a new concept of the pathway of NH_4^+ in bringing about the excretion of acid, which probably accounts for most urinary NH_4^+, has been formulated. This pathway begins in the liver with the metabolic NH_4^+ that is an end product of protein metabolism. Some of this NH_4^+ is diverted from urea synthesis to the formation of glutamine. The glutamine is carried by the circulation to the tubular epithelium of the kidney. There the metabolism of glutamine to α-ketoglutarate releases the NH_4^+s, which are then secreted into the urine. The further metabolism of α-ketoglutarate yields bicarbonate, which is added to the blood. When there is a need to excrete more hydrogen ions, the production of glutamine in the liver rises, greatly increasing the amount of NH_4^+ excreted in the urine. Overall, excess hydrogen ions have been excreted and an equivalent amount of bicarbonate returned to the blood. These processes are schematically shown in Fig. 32.3.

If, instead of excess acid there is an excess of base being released in body metabolism, this will result in a decrease in H^+ secretion by renal tubules and collecting ducts, an increase in bicarbonate excretion, and an alkaline urine. In this case, much less glutamine is formed and virtually no ammonium ions appear in the urine. As shown in Fig. 32.4, much bicarbonate will be excreted in an alkaline urine.

ACID-BASE BALANCE DISTURBANCES

The pH of the ECF is determined by the ratio of conjugate bases to their weak acids, as expressed for each buffer pair in the Henderson-Hasselbalch equation. The total amount of base in whole blood, including bicarbonate, hemoglobin, and the other bases of lesser importance, is called buffer base. Buffer base characteristically has a normal value of about 48 mEq/L of blood, but this varies somewhat with hemoglobin concentration. These bases constitute the metabolic component that determines blood pH, and acid-base disturbances that involve primarily an abnormal decrease or increase of these bases are known as *metabolic acidosis* or *metabolic alkalosis*, respectively. The weak acids in the blood, taken together, are usually measured in terms of dissolved carbon dioxide (i.e., s·P_{CO_2}, or simply P_{CO_2}). According to the isohydric principle, all other weak acids of the buffer pairs (mostly the acid form of hemoglobin) follow carbon dioxide changes. Acid-base disturbances that involve primarily abnormal increase or decrease of P_{CO_2}, which will usually be due to some problem of the respiratory system, are called *respiratory acidosis* or *respiratory alkalosis*, respectively.

When an acid-base disturbance occurs with the development of one of these four processes, the first and immediate response is amelioration of the effect on pH by reaction with buffers in the blood and interstitial fluid. A second response is compensation in which the component not primarily affected by the initial disturbance is adjusted so as to bring blood pH back toward normal. Thus, if abnormal pulmonary ventilation is the primary defect, compensation by renal action on excretion of hydrogen and bicarbonate ions will develop. Such compensation is called incomplete if pH is not returned to the normal range and complete if pH is returned to the normal range. Even if compensation is complete, the quantities of the metabolic or respiratory component primarily affected will not have been restored to normal. A final response to the primary disturbance is one that acts to restore the acid-base component primarily affected; this is called *correction*. Complete correction of the disturbance has been brought about when blood pH and concentration of all acid-base components have been restored to normal.

Metabolic acidosis

The addition of strong acid to or the loss of base (bicarbonate) from the ECF is known as metabolic acidosis. Characteristically, there is present an acidemia which, if severe, threatens life. Typical disease conditions that cause metabolic acidosis include ketosis and diabetes mellitus in which β-hydroxybutyric acid and acetoacetic acid are produced, renal acidosis in which there is a failure of bicarbonate reabsorption and it is lost in the urine, capture myopathy after intense exercise in which metabolic acids of uncertain origin are produced, and diarrhea in which pancreatic juice containing bicarbonate is not reabsorbed and is lost. In all these cases, $[HCO_3^-]$ falls either as a result of reaction with the added acid or because of direct loss from ECF, and pH falls. By the isohydric principle, a fall in $[HCO_3^-]$ will result in a fall in all buffer bases of the ECF and red cells. This condition of low blood concentration of buffer bases is called hypobasemia.

It might be expected that plasma P_{CO_2} would rise as a result of the production of carbon dioxide, as acid reacts with bicarbonate. The respiratory control systems are very sensitive to changes in P_{CO_2}, however, and will rapidly correct any deviation from the normal of 40 mm Hg. Usually no change in plasma P_{CO_2} as a result of buffer action will be detected. The fall in pH persists, however, and will act as a stimulus to the respiratory control system, resulting in an increase in alveolar ventilation and a fall in P_{CO_2}. This respiratory adjustment of plasma P_{CO_2} will begin within a few minutes but will not be maximally developed for up to 24 hours. Conversely, if the deficit of bicarbonate is suddenly corrected by therapeutic injection of bicarbonate, the respiratory compensation (i.e., low P_{CO_2}) will persist for some hours (overcompensation).

Compensation by decreasing P_{CO_2} will bring the ratio of conjugate base to weak acid back toward the normal value, but the hypobasemia will persist until the lost bicarbonate is replaced. This requires renal corrective action: excretion of hydrogen ions and restoration of plasma [HCO_3^-]. The acidemia acts as a stimulus to the secretion of hydrogen ions by the renal tubule cells into the tubular fluid. This first ensures that all bicarbonate in the glomerular filtrate will be reabsorbed. Then excess hydrogen ions beyond those required to effect reabsorption of all bicarbonate ions will begin to acidify the urine. Most of those excess hydrogen ions will be excreted from the body combined with urinary buffer bases. For each hydrogen ion excreted, one bicarbonate ion will be restored to the plasma. This will continue as long as the acidemia persists.

In some cases renal action may be adequate to correct the hypobasemia completely. This would be the outcome of a short-term stress; for example, after the injection of a small quantity of strong acid, the acid would be excreted by the kidney and bicarbonate would be restored. In mild continuing acid-base disturbance (for example, preclinical ketosis), renal action may also be sufficient to restore plasma bicarbonate as rapidly as it is destroyed by the continuous release of organic acids within the body. In many severe diseases, however, renal action will not be sufficient to keep up with the release of acid products within the body, and a serious acidemia will develop. Here complete correction will be attained either when the disease has been terminated or as the result of vigorous acid-base therapeutic action.

Metabolic alkalosis

The gain of base (hydroxyl or bicarbonate ions) or loss of strong acid by the ECF results in the process called metabolic alkalosis. Typically, an alkalemia is present. Some common conditions that usually result in metabolic alkalosis are persistent vomiting in which gastric acid is lost from the body, potassium deficiency in which renal tubule cells secrete inappropriate amounts of hydrogen ion into the urine, oxidation of ingested or injected salts of organic acids such as lactate or citrate, and injection of bicarbonate solutions. In all of these conditions there is an increase of [HCO_3^-] in the ECF, which then secondarily results in an upward adjustment of all buffer bases, which is known as hyperbasemia. Most of the responses of the body are corresponding but opposite to those found in metabolic acidosis. The hyperbasemia is accompanied by alkalemia. The rise in pH will depress pulmonary ventilation, and P_{CO_2} will rise. This respiratory compensation will bring pH back down toward the normal level, but the hyperbasemia persists. Renal correction consists of decreased secretion of hydrogen ions and hence increased excretion of bicarbonate, which will continue until the alkalemia is abolished.

Respiratory acidosis

If excretion of carbon dioxide by the lungs falls below the rate of carbon dioxide production in the body, respiratory acidosis develops. Here the primary change will be an increase in blood P_{CO_2} (hypercapnia), and the primary defect will be the inability of the lungs to expire carbon dioxide at a normal rate. This may be because of depression of the respiratory centers in the central nervous system, some abnormality of the chest wall or respiratory muscles that impedes the bellows action of the thorax, or obstructions to gas movement or diffusion within the lung. Either ventilation of the lung alveoli is diminished or diffusion between alveoli and capillary blood is impeded. The rise in P_{CO_2} represents a rise in carbonic acid, and buffer reactions occur with the nonbicarbonate bases. Hemoglobin is the most important of these bases, and the reaction with it will be

$$H_2CO_3 + Hb^- \leftrightharpoons HCO_3^- + HHb$$

This interaction between blood buffers results in an appreciable rise of plasma [HCO3−]. The buffer action ameliorates the fall in pH caused by the rise in carbonic acid. Within a few hours renal compensation becomes evident: the low pH stimulates increased secretion of hydrogen ions into the urine with a concomitant increase in plasma [HCO_3^-]. This renal compensation may require several days for maximal effect; it may be complete if pH is moved back into the normal range or partial if significant acidemia persists. Complete correction of respiratory acidosis will not be possible until recovery from the pulmonary disease occurs.

Respiratory alkalosis

When alveolar hyperventilation occurs, the expiration of carbon dioxide may exceed the rate of its production within the body, and respiratory alkalosis may develop. This is characterized by low plasma P_{CO_2} (hypocapnia) and alkalemia. Usually the hyperventilation is caused by some abnormal stimulus to the respiratory centers, either directly as in ammonia toxicity or indirectly as when hypoxemia acts reflexly via the peripheral chemoreceptors. Initially, plasma [HCO_3^-] is unchanged by the fall of P_{CO_2}, but buffer reactions with the nonbicarbonate buffers occur immediately. Using the reaction with hemoglobin as the example,

$$\begin{array}{l} HHb + HCO_3^- \rightarrow Hb^- + H_2CO_3 \\ \qquad\qquad\qquad\qquad\qquad\quad \downarrow \\ \qquad\qquad\qquad\qquad\qquad CO_2 \text{ (removed)} \end{array}$$

Thus [HCO_3^-] falls somewhat and Hb^- rises by an equivalent amount. Renal compensation begins in a few hours and reaches its maximal capacity after several days; alkalemia depresses the rate of hydrogen ion secretion by renal tubules and excretion of filtered bicarbonate rises. This results in a further fall of plasma [HCO_3^-], and the [HCO_3^-]/($s \cdot P_{CO_2}$) ratio moves back toward its normal value, as does blood pH. However, final correction of the primary change in P_{CO_2} can be brought about only by recovery from the cause of the hyperventilation.

EVALUATION OF ACID-BASE STATUS

The blood or plasma variables involved in assessment of acid-base disturbances are pH, P_{CO_2}, plasma $[HCO_3^-]$ or whole blood buffer base, and hemoglobin concentration. Two systems of clinical evaluation that differ in the value used as the metabolic component are frequently used: One is based on plasma $[HCO_3^-]$ and the other on the concept of "base excess." Both systems use P_{CO_2} as the respiratory component. The first system uses the pH-bicarbonate diagram (see Fig. 32.5) on which are plotted values taken from plasma separated from oxygenated whole blood. The diagram then includes the influence of hemoglobin as a blood buffer. The other system uses whole blood values that can be plotted on the Siggaard-Andersen alignment nomogram (see Fig. 32.6).

The pH-bicarbonate diagram

The assessment of an acid-base disturbance is aided by the pH-bicarbonate diagram, which expresses the relationship between P_{CO_2}, $[HCO_3^-]$, and pH of the plasma (Fig. 32.5). This diagram, based on the Henderson-Hasselbalch equation, is for plasma that was exposed to the particular P_{CO_2} before being separated from the erythrocytes of fully oxygenated blood. Therefore any buffering effect includes that of the erythrocytes and their hemoglobin. The diagram is constructed by substitution of values for pH into the equation while P_{CO_2} is held constant and then solving for $[HCO_3^-]$. The average normal values for plasma bicarbonate (24 mmol/L), for pH (7.40), and for P_{CO_2} (40 mm Hg) determine the "normal point" shown in the figure. If P_{CO_2} is held constant, the plot of pH values against $[HCO_3^-]$ will form a slightly curved line called a carbon dioxide isobar.

If normal whole blood is exposed to various pressures of carbon dioxide and then the pH and $[HCO_3^-]$ of separated plasma are measured, a "normal buffer line" results. This is, in effect, a titration of the blood with carbon dioxide and represents the changes that occur in uncompensated respiratory acidosis and alkalosis (points A and B, respectively). One should bear in mind that the slope of the normal buffer line will vary with hemoglobin concentration; here a normal, average hemoglobin level is assumed. If metabolic base is added to the blood, the concentration of bicarbonate ions will increase, either as a result of reaction of the base (e.g., hydroxyl ions) with carbonic acid or if bicarbonate is itself the base added. The carbon dioxide titration curve will then parallel the normal buffer line but will lie above it because of the additional bicarbonate ions present. After addition of metabolic acid, a similar shift occurs, but it will be downward because bicarbonate ions are used up in reaction with the added acid. A shift along the 40 mm Hg carbon dioxide isobar from the normal point upward as excess base is added represents uncompensated metabolic alkalosis (D). A downward shift along this isobar as excess acid is added represents uncompensated metabolic acidosis (C). Note that although these reactions will cause the release or removal of carbon dioxide, initially P_{CO_2} does not change much as metabolic acidosis or alkalosis develops. This is because the respiratory system rapidly adjusts blood P_{CO_2} through changes in pulmonary ventilation, keeping P_{CO_2} close to its normal value at first. Despite the initial constant

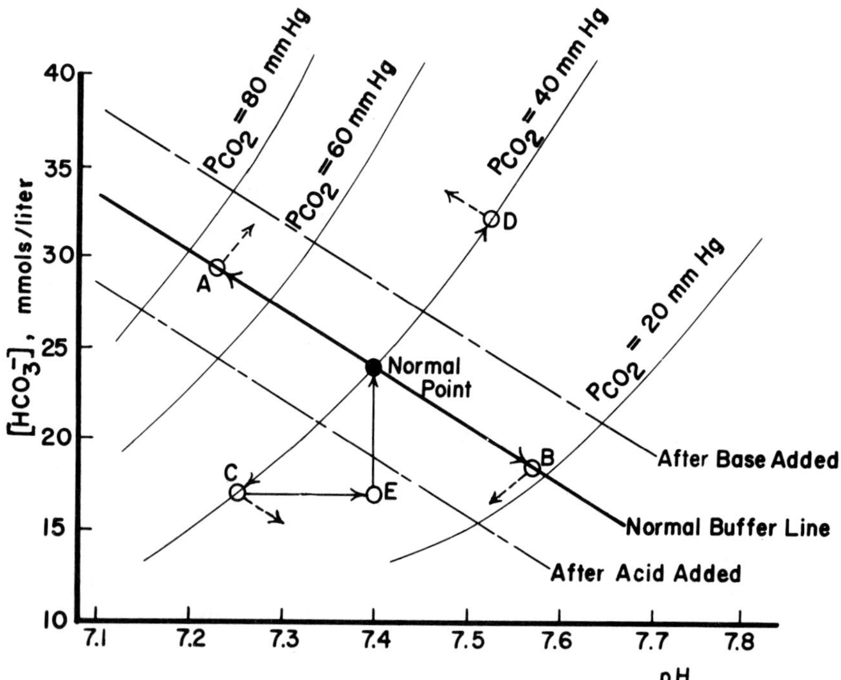

Figure 32.5. The pH-bicarbonate diagram for oxygenated human blood equilibrated with CO_2 before separation of plasma from erythrocytes.

P_{CO_2}, however, plasma pH deviates from normal during these metabolic acid-base disturbances. The shift in pH will influence pulmonary ventilation, and consequently P_{CO_2} changes. For example, when added acid reacts with bicarbonate to form more carbon dioxide, the excess carbon dioxide is quickly blown off but pH will remain slightly depressed. The depressed pH then causes a further exhalation of carbon dioxide, and P_{CO_2} falls slowly to a level below normal.

The shifts of pH and $[HCO_3^-]$ in these uncompensated acid-base disturbances are the result of reaction of the added acid or base with the chemical buffers. According to the isohydric principle, the changes in all the buffers are reflected by these changes in $[HCO_3^-]$ and pH. In the animal, however, respiratory and renal compensation would soon become effective. In Fig. 32.5 a short broken line points in the direction of the initial respiratory or renal compensation. For a respiratory acidosis (point A in the figure, short broken line and arrow), the renal compensation consists of increased tubular secretion of hydrogen ion with equivalent amounts of bicarbonate ion added to the plasma. This increases bicarbonate concentration and moves plasma pH toward the normal value. A renal compensatory response also occurs in respiratory alkalosis (point B, broken line), resulting however in increased excretion of bicarbonate and a shift of pH toward the normal value.

Compensation for metabolic disturbances is brought about by respiratory adjustment of plasma P_{CO_2}. Metabolic acidosis is represented by point C in Fig. 32.5, and the respiratory compensatory response depresses plasma P_{CO_2} and bicarbonate slightly. The result is a shift of pH toward the normal value (broken line). A corresponding compensatory response occurs in metabolic alkalosis (point D), where decreased lung ventilation raises P_{CO_2}, and bicarbonate slightly, with a consequent shift of pH toward the normal value (broken line).

In metabolic acidosis and alkalosis, respiratory compensation will usually be supported by renal adjustment of plasma bicarbonate. For example, point C represents uncompensated metabolic acidosis in which $[HCO_3^-]$ has decreased whereas P_{CO_2} is little changed. The decreased pH would soon cause an increase in respiratory ventilation and a lower P_{CO_2} (the short broken line). Renal attempts to restore bicarbonate will have already begun, however, and as a result the pathway of changes will more nearly follow the solid line to point E. The combined action of respiratory and renal processes can bring pH back to the normal range. However, plasma bicarbonate would still be depressed. Renal excretion of acid and restoration of bicarbonate would bring the status back toward normal (along the line from E to the normal point), but complete correction of the acidosis would require recovery from the diseased condition. If the primary problem were kidney disease, the renal adjustments of bicarbonate might be seriously impaired, rendering the condition more serious. In any case, the acid-base disturbance would not be completely corrected until the normal point was reached.

In respiratory acidosis and alkalosis, renal compensation ameliorates the condition. If the primary problem is respiratory disease, however, correction will await recovery from the disease. In many severe or prolonged diseases the acid-base balance disturbance would likely be only partially compensated. Furthermore, complex combinations of acidosis and alkalosis may result from separate disease processes occurring simultaneously in the animal.

Base excess and the Siggaard-Andersen nomogram

The objective of the Siggaard-Andersen nomogram is to determine the deviation from the normal value of the total quantity of buffer bases (i.e., "buffer base" or BB) of a particular blood sample. This deviation, called *base excess* (BE), can be defined most specifically as the amount of strong acid or base that must be added to a liter of oxygenated whole blood to bring its pH to 7.40. It follows that normal [BB] = actual [BB] − [BE]. If actual [BB] is abnormally high, [BE] will be positive; if actual [BB] is abnormally low, [BE] will be negative. Sometimes the term *base deficit* is used to indicate the negative condition. In an animal without acid-base disturbance, normal [BB] is approximately 48 mEq/L of whole blood. This value will vary with the amount of hemoglobin present, and nomograms include a correction for variations in hemoglobin concentration. Accurate calculation of whole blood acid-base values is difficult; instead, nomograms must be used that have been developed from data derived from direct determination of such blood values in vitro when titrated with strong acid or base.

Arterial or free-flowing (arterialized) capillary blood samples are obtained with special precautions to prevent loss of blood gases, and pH and P_{CO_2} are measured under carefully controlled conditions at 37° C. Hemoglobin concentration is also determined. The Siggaard-Andersen alignment nomogram (Fig. 32.6) is the simplest method of applying these data. A line is drawn from the point on the P_{CO_2} scale determined by the measured value through the corresponding point on the pH scale and then extended to the bicarbonate and base excess scales. Plasma $[HCO_3^-]$ can be read directly. Base excess will vary with hemoglobin concentration; the intersection of the line drawn with the appropriate hemoglobin concentration line is also an intersection with a BE line, which indicates the deviation of BB from normal. As an example, data from a dog with an acid-base disturbance are plotted on Fig. 32.6. Points A and B are the measured values for P_{CO_2} (65 mm Hg) and pH (7.13). These values in themselves suggest the presence of a respiratory acidosis. Point C gives a plasma $[HCO_3^-]$ of 21.2 mEq/L and, since in this case [Hb] was found to be 15 g/dl, point D leads to the BE value of −10 mEq/L, indicating the further complication of metabolic acidosis.

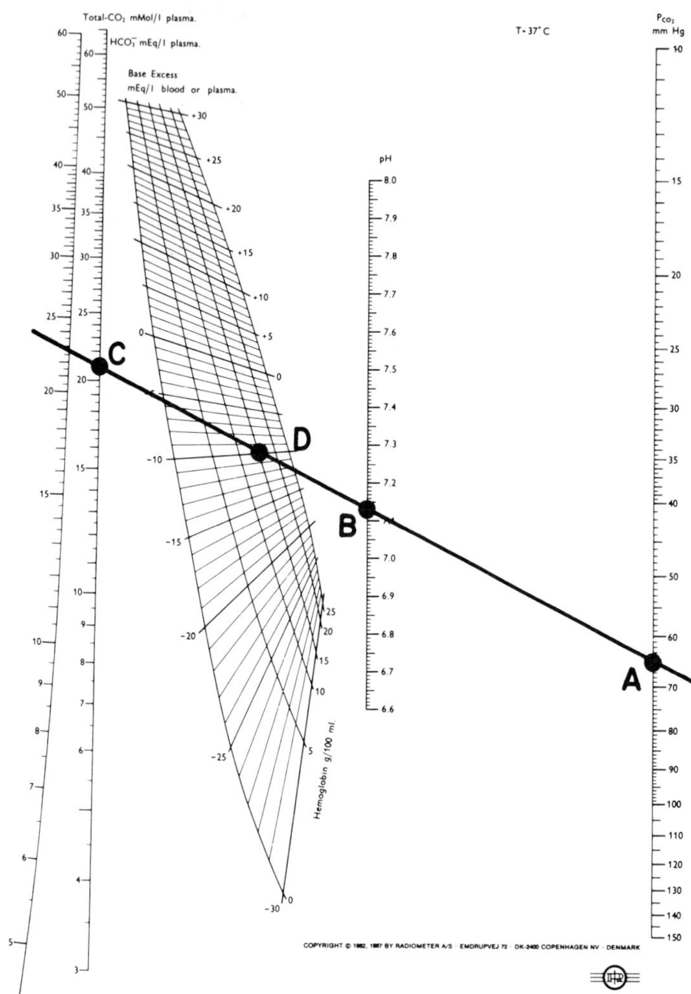

Figure 32.6. Siggaard-Andersen alignment nomogram with values plotted for a whole blood sample at A and B.

The Siggaard-Andersen alignment nomogram can also be used for the determination of plasma values with use of the scales for pH, P_{CO_2}, plasma bicarbonate, and total plasma carbon dioxide content when any two are known. Total carbon dioxide is the carbon dioxide present after strong acid is added to a sample of plasma, converting all bicarbonate to carbon dioxide. Advanced texts should be consulted for information about other forms of such nomograms that have been developed for clinical use.

It should be noted that full oxygenation of the blood used in the evaluation of acid-base status described in the procedures above is assumed. If the condition of the patient suggests that even arterial blood may not be fully oxygenated, or if venous blood must be used, the results must be corrected for the difference in buffering capacity between oxygenated and reduced hemoglobin.

The Siggaard-Andersen nomograms were developed for use with human blood; hence normal [BB] and [BE] (48 and 0 mEq/L, respectively) are specifically for average oxygenated human blood at pH = 7.40, P_{CO_2} = 40 mm Hg, and 37° C. There are slight variations from these human values among domestic mammals because of differences in hemoglobin buffering capacity, plasma [HCO_3^-], and plasma protein concentration. These variations from the human are relatively small, and the nomograms can be used to determine approximate BE for most domestic mammals. For example, the blood of normal dogs and ruminants has acid-base characteristics very similar to those of human blood. Normal young pigs, however, may show a consistent positive deviation of [BE] of about 6 to 8 mEq/L. The nomograms are still suitable for use with pigs, but the positive deviate value for normal [BE] would have to be considered. The application of the Siggaard-Andersen nomograms to other species should be done judiciously.

Use of anion gap to evaluate acid-base status

The anion-gap method does not involve precise measurements of pH or P_{CO_2}, and it has been found to be useful in some clinical situations. If concentrations of plasma sodium, potassium, chloride, and bicarbonate ions are measured, then the sum of the cation concentrations will usually exceed the sum of the anions. This is the anion gap. Unmeasured anions include sulfates, phosphates, proteinate ions, and anions of organic acids. There are also small amounts of unmeasured cations: calcium and magnesium. The method is most useful in evaluation of metabolic acidosis. In ketosis, for example, bicarbonate will decrease as it reacts with the ketonic acids, whose anions acetoacetate and β-hydroxybutyrate will accumulate (but are not measured). The anion gap will then increase far beyond its normal level. However, if the cause of the metabolic acidosis is the loss of both sodium and bicarbonate ions, there may be no change in the anion gap. This can occur in diarrhea. Also, if the loss of bicarbonate ions is exactly balanced by a gain of chloride ions, no anion gap will be evident. This can occur in renal disease. Clearly, the anion gap method must be used with caution.

REFERENCES

Atkinson, D.E., and Bourke, E. 1987. Metabolic aspects of the regulation of systemic pH. *Am. J. Physiol.* 252:F947–56.

Blatherwick, N.R. 1920. Neutrality regulation in cattle. *J. Biol. Chem.* 42:517–39.

Cornelius, L.M., and Rawlings, C.A. 1981. Arterial blood gas and acid-base values in dogs with various diseases and signs of disease. *J. Am. Vet. Med. Assoc.* 178:992–95.

Dale, H.E., Goberdhan, C.K., and Brody, S. 1954. A comparison of the effects of starvation and thermal stress on the acid-base balance of dairy cattle. *Am. J. Vet. Res.* 15:197–201.

Davenport, H.W. 1974. *The ABC of Acid-Base Chemistry.* 6th ed. University of Chicago Press, Chicago.

Dobson, A. 1980. Acid-base balance in animals. In A.T. Phillipson, L.W. Hall, and W.R. Pritchard, eds. *Scientific Foundations of Veterinary Medicine*. Heineman, London. Pp. 112–25.

Feigl, E.O., and D'Alecy, L.G. 1972. Normal arterial blood pH, oxygen, and carbon dioxide tensions in unanesthetized dogs. *J. Appl. Physiol.* 32:152–53.

Feldman, B.F., and Rosenberg, D.P. 1981. Clinical use of anion and osmolal gaps in veterinary medicine. *J. Am. Vet. Med. Assoc.* 178:396–98.

Good, D.W. 1989. New concepts in renal ammonium excretion. In D.W. Seldin and G. Giebisch, eds. *The Regulation of Acid-Base Balance*. Raven Press, New York. Pp. 169–83.

Harthoorn, A.M. 1975. A relationship between acid-base balance and capture myopathy in zebra (*Equus burchelli*) and an apparent therapy. *Vet. Rec.* 95:337–42.

Orsini, J.A. 1989. Pathophysiology, diagnosis, and treatment of clinical acid-base disorders. *Compendium: Small Animal* 11:593–604.

Phillips, G.D. 1970. The assessment of blood acid-base parameters in ruminants. *Br. Vet. J.* 126:325–31.

Pickrell, J.A. 1973. The rapid processing of canine blood gas tension and pH measurements. *Am. J. Vet. Res.* 34:95–100.

Prior, R.L., Grunes, D.L., Patterson, R.P., Smith, F.W., Mayland, H.F., and Visek, W.J. 1973. Partition chromatography for quantitating effects of fertilization on plant acids. *J. Agric. Food Chem.* 21:73–77.

Rodkey, W.G., Hannon, J.P., Dramise, J.G., White, R.D., Welsh, D.C., and Persky, B.N. 1978. Arterialized capillary blood used to determine the acid-base and blood gas status of dogs. *Am. J. Vet. Res.* 39:459–64.

Sampson, J., and Hayden, C.E. 1935. The acid-base balance in cows and ewes during and after pregnancy, with special reference to milk fever and acetonemia. *J. Am. Vet. Med. Assoc.* 39:13–23.

Scott, D., and McIntosh, G.H. 1975. Changes in blood composition and in urinary mineral excretion in the pig in response to acute acid-base disturbance. *Q. J. Exp. Physiol.* 60:131–40.

Seldin, D.W., and Giebisch, G., eds. 1989. *The Regulation of Acid-Base Balance*. Raven Press, New York.

Siggaard-Andersen, O. 1974. *The Acid-Base Status of the Blood*. 4th ed. Williams & Wilkins, Baltimore.

Stewart, P.A. 1981. *How to Understand Acid-Base*. Elsevier, New York. P.144.

Swan, R.C., Pitts, R.F., and Madisso, H. 1955. Neutralization of infused acid by nephrectomized dogs. *J. Clin. Invest.* 34:205–12.

Walser, M. 1986. Roles of urea production, ammonium excretion, and amino acid oxidation in acid-base balance. *Am. J. Physiol.* 250:F181–88.

Winters, R.W., Engel, K., and Dell, R.B. 1969. *Acid Base Physiology in Medicine*. 2d ed. London Co., Cleveland.

Wise, W.C. 1973. Normal arterial blood gases and chemical components in the unanesthetized dog. *J. App. Physiol.* 35:427–29.

CHAPTER 33

The Skin* | by Harpal S. Bal

GENERAL ANATOMY

Skin is the largest organ in the body, not in surface area but in bulk. It protects the animal organism from desiccation and from the environment while maintaining communication with the outside. Figure 33.1 shows the anatomical structures of the skin. Two of the main components of the skin are the epidermis, which consists of keratinized stratified squamous epithelium, and the dermis (corium), which is made up of intricately woven collagenous, elastic, and reticular fibers with cellular elements, smooth muscle fibers, and the amorphous ground substance (now designated as glycosaminoglycans). These two skin components are mutually dependent. Epidermis with its keratin is affected by cellular and humoral dermal factors. Hair growth is dependent on the dermal papillae, and their integrity is essential for the continued existence of the hair follicle. A follicle can regenerate its papillary cells.

The structure and thickness of the skin of domestic animals vary according to breed, age, and sex in certain species. Average skin thickness of general body areas is 2.7 mm in adult sheep, 6 mm in cattle, and 2.9 mm in goats. The dog's skin is 1 mm or more in thickness in the head and neck regions, where it is the thickest. The horse's skin varies in thickness from 1 to 5 mm and is thickest on the dorsal surface of the tail and at the attachment of the mane.

The skin of the domestic animal becomes more uniform in structure, smoother, tighter, and more dense after castration.

*Part of this chapter has been taken from the chapter in the eighth edition written by Milton Orkin and Robert M. Schwartzman.

Epidermis

The epidermis consists of an upper horny layer of dead keratinized cells (stratum corneum) and a lower viable layer of cells (stratum basale). The cells of the viable epidermis, which are produced by proliferation of basal cells, are called keratinocytes.

Epidermis is further subdivided into the stratum basale or germinativum, the stratum spinosum (prickle-cell layer), and the stratum granulosum. The stratum basale (basal layer) is a layer one or two cells thick. It is in contact with the basement membrane of the dermis below and with the stratum spinosum (prickle-cell layer) of variable thickness above. These basal cells are low columnar or cuboidal with their long axis aligned vertical to the skin surface. Cell division, which is necessary for the replacement of the superficial cells, occurs in this layer only when the animal is sleeping, unlike that of the hair follicle, which continues 24 hours a day.

The stratum spinosum or prickle-cell layer was so named because the cell junctions of this layer look like spines, which were first described as intercellular bridges. Seen with the light microscope, these spines are artifacts of tissue preparation. The plasma membrane between the cell junctions shrinks as a result of dehydration caused by the tissues when immersed in alcohol. The cell junctions, which remain intact, appear to project as spines from the surface of the cells. These spines do not exist in the living animal. They are now called desmosomes or maculae adherentes.

In the cells of the stratum spinosum, cysteine (sulfhydryl groups), lysosomal hydrolases, and protein-bound phospholipids accumulate after mitotic divisions. In the cells of upper layers near the skin surface, disulfide groups increase because of the formation of cystine and the oxidation of

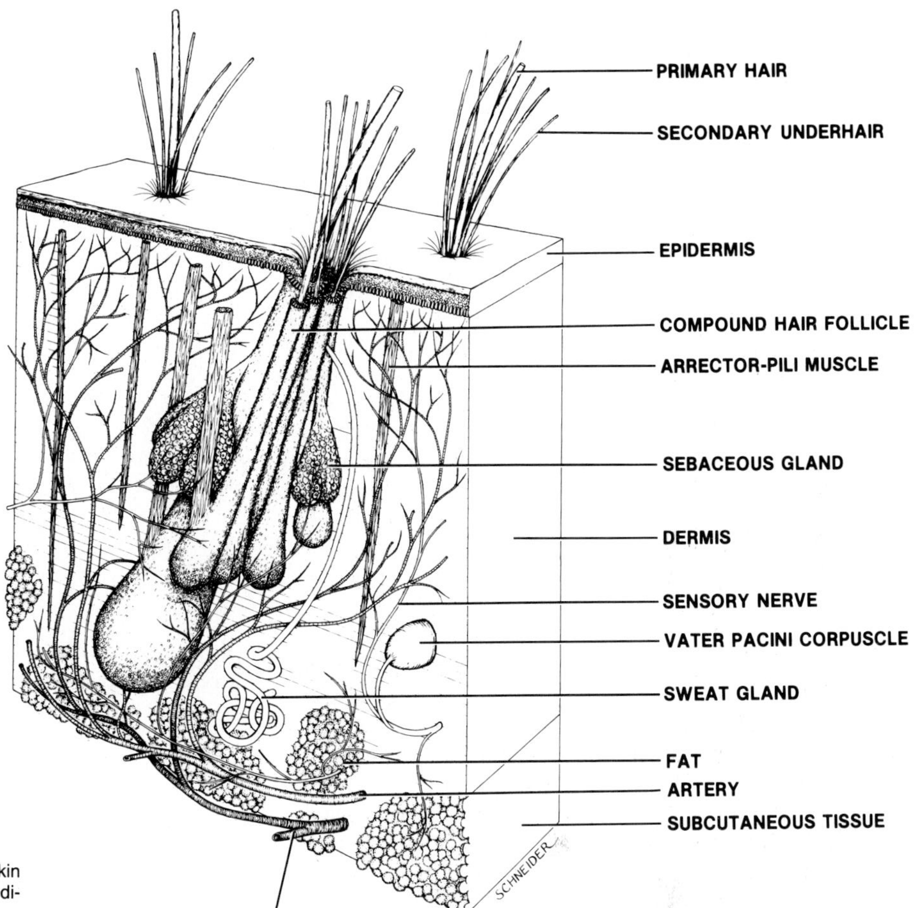

Figure 33.1. Composite drawing of dog skin showing anatomical structures in three dimensions.

adjacent sulfhydryl moieties. In malignant and proliferative conditions of the epidermis, the cells of this layer also divide by mitosis.

The stratum granulosum or granular layer is a transitional zone between the viable epidermal cells below and the dead keratinized material above. Its nuclei are absent or abnormal, and keratohyaline granules appear in the cell cytoplasm. Absence of the keratohyaline granules in this layer is associated with the production of parakeratotic keratin in psoriasis and exfoliative dermatitis, when the cells of the stratum corneum retain their nuclei and appear as scales.

In cattle, the stratum granulosum is found only in the perianal region and occasionally over the extremities. In dogs, the stratum in these areas has about 15 layers of cells and consists of a single layer in the ventral region of the neck, the abdominal, sternal, axillary, and shoulder regions, and the flank, tail, and back. It is absent in the mandibular, temporal, and dorsal portions of the head and the outer covering of the ear. In swine, one to five layers of flat polygonal cells constitute this stratum in the thicker skin regions, but there is only a single layer or the cells are sporadic in thin skin. In goats, this stratum is represented by five layers of diamond-shaped cells in some body areas and is rarely noticeable in others.

Cytoplasmic contents of the cells of the stratum granulosum are hydrolyzed before formation of the keratin layer. Basophilia of this layer is due to mineralization, predominantly of calcium and magnesium, as well as to the mordant action of the metallic ions. Many metallic ions are attached to the keratohyaline granules.

The stratum lucidum (a thin hyaline layer above the stratum granulosum) is generally absent in the skin of the domestic animals except in specialized areas such as the perianal region, the hoof margins, the teat, and over the Achilles tendon insertion in cattle, in the ovine lip and muzzle, and in the planum nasale of the dog and cat.

The cellular stratification is the reflection of various stages through which the basal cells pass in their gradual conversion to the horny material of the stratum corneum.

Stratum corneum is the most superficial keratinized layer above the stratum lucidum (when present) and the stratum granulosum. This layer is the epidermal water barrier and is formed of broad lamellar sheets of lipids consisting of 40 percent ceramides (naturally occurring sphingolipids as cerebrocide, galactocyl), 25 percent cholesterol, 10 percent cholesteryl sulfate, and 25 percent free fatty acids. These lipids are also synthesized in the epidermis of the pig and remain until they are lost by desquamation. Small amounts of triglycerides in the pig stratum corneum may be environmental contaminants.

In the horse, the mean cell-renewal time of the epidermis is approximately 17 days. In the dog, altered epidermal keratinization leads to seborrhea.

Melanocytes

The melanocytes differentiate from the neural crest cells of neuroectodermal origin. They are recognized by the presence of the pigment melanin (melanosomes) in their cytoplasm; they can bear many dendritic processes, appear as bipolar cells, or even be amorphous, depending on their location and functional state. Keratinocytes acquire melanin by phagocytosis of the dendritic processes of the melanocytes laden with melanosomes (Table 33.1).

In the human skin, it is established that a single basal melanocyte transfers melanin to 36 keratinocytes. With advancing age, the number of melanocytes in the skin declines. More melanocytes are observed in areas of the skin that are exposed to the sun. Melanin in the epidermis protects the skin from damage by ultraviolet light.

According to the recent concept, melanogenesis and melanocyte proliferation are regulated by keratinocytes and Langerhans cells. Arachidonic acid and its metabolites, leukotrienes, and prostaglandins secreted by keratinocytes and Langerhans cells regulate melanogenesis locally. Ultraviolet light and inflammation increase production of melanin. Androgens, estrogens, glucocorticoid, and thyroid hormones also modulate melanogenesis. The mechanisms are poorly understood.

Mast cells

Increased pigmentation of the skin occurs in urticaria pigmentosa and in mast cell tumors of dogs. Mast cells also have a positive reaction to dopa, which provides intermediates in the metabolism of phenylalanine and tyrosine and the production of norepinephrine, epinephrine, and melanin.

On degranulation, the mast cells release heparin, histamine, and serotonin (Table 33.1).

Langerhans cells

Langerhans cells are present in the epidermis. It has recently been demonstrated that they are involved in the immune response of the skin. Therefore renewed interest has been focused on the structure and distribution of these cells in different species. Langerhans cells are well recognized in the dog, more than in other species of domestic animals. Langerhans cells in the dog lack the specific granules (Bir-

Table 33.1. Table of skin function

	Secretion/production	Function
Cells of epidermis		
Keratinocyte	Keratin of horny layer	Effective barrier to water absorption and loss; protection from physical, chemical, and foreign bodies as bacteria, viruses, ectoparasites, etc.
	Hair	General protection; insulation from excessive cold environment, temperature, cuts, abrasions, thermal radiation, injury and chemical irritation
	Claws, horn, hoof	Self-defense, locomotion, protection, and hunting for food (claws)
	Cytokines-interleukins (IL-1, IL-3, IL-6), and other factors	Stimulation of immune response, as activation of T lymphocytes, mast cell growth, thymocyte maturation, and stimulation of hematopoiesis, macrophages, neutrophils, and killer T cell activity
Langerhans cell	Release of lymphokines	Take up antigens; present antigens to antigen primed T cells; activate T cells
Melanocyte	Melanin pigment	Transfers pigment to keratinocytes; protects keratinocyte from ultraviolet rays of sun; provides color to hair, wool, and skin
Cells of dermis		
Fibroblast	Secretion of intercellular substance, collagenous, reticular, and elastic fibers	Furnishes strength, texture, and elasticity and protection to subcutaneous tissue
Mast cell	Heparin, histamine, and serotonin	Anticoagulation and stimulation of local inflammatory reaction to dispose of foreign bodies (antigens)
Macrophage	Lysozymes, hydrogen peroxide, interleukins, superoxide (O_3)	Phagocytosis of foreign bodies, cytocidal effect on cancer cells, and active in immune reaction in stimulating B and T lymphocytes
Lymphocytes	Lymphokines	Involved in all types of immune reaction
Pericytes around blood capillaries of dermis		An undifferentiated cell that can differentiate in some other connective tissue cells such as fibroblasts; the potential property of this cell helps during granulation or healing process of the dermis

Lymphokines are soluble lymphocyte-derived mediators. Monokines represent a subset of lymphokines. Interleukins are partially composed of lymphokines and monokines. Interleukins are biologically active mediators that transmit growth and differentiation signals among leukocytes.

beck) seen in the cells of humans. These cells are present in skin, lymph nodes, spleen, and thymus. Their lineage is from the mononuclear phagocytic system. They express major histocompatibility complex class II products and serve as antigen-presenting cells. Langerhans cells have receptors for complement and immunoglobulin G fragment monomer. Langerhans cells are also capable of producing interleukin type I (IL-1). IL-1 acts as (1) a lymphocyte blastogenic factor, (2) an antibody production-enhancing factor, (3) an endogenous pyrogen, and (4) a fibroblast-stimulating factor. IL-1 increases collagen type IV production by murine mammary epithelial cells. Langerhans cells have been observed in domestic animals, especially ruminants. Cattle of the holstein and Brahman breeds exhibit an immune-mediated resistance to ticks. Langerhans cells also synthesize and express gene-associated antigens. Ultraviolet light and systemic glucocorticoids depress their numbers and function.

Merkel cells

Merkel cells are found in epidermis with hairy surfaces, in nail matrix, in palms, and in subepidermal mesenchyme. They are considered to be sensory receptors or transducers because of their close association with nerve terminals.

Some dermatologists refer to the cells of the epidermis other than the keratinocytes as dendritic cells. Under pathological conditions, however, the epidermis may be invaded by a variety of dermal cells.

Basement membrane

The basal surface of epithelial cells rests on an extracellular linear matrix known as the *basement membrane*. It consists of a basal lamina secreted by the basal cells of the epidermis and a reticular lamina synthesized by connective tissue. It has been estimated that 40 to 50 proteins form the basement membrane. The fibrous component of the basement membrane is made up of type IV collagen, which has bonding sites for laminin, fibronectin, and heparin sulfate proteoglycans. These constituents of the basement membrane mediate the cell-substrate adhesion. If the integrity of the basement membrane is disrupted, it permits the malignant tumors to invade the distant sites. Metastasis of cancer cells is facilitated if the continuity of the basement membrane breaks down. The basement membrane maintains the epidermis in a productive differentiated state, stabilizes epithelial cell architecture, and facilitates the movement of nutrients, oxygen, and useful cells of the dermis across this interface into the epidermis.

Dermis

Dermis is the fibrous connective tissue of skin (Fig. 33.2). Epidermis and the cutaneous appendages grow upon and within it and sustain their nourishment from it. Collagen makes up the bulk of connective tissue; elastic and reticular fibers constitute relatively small segments. The dermis may be divided into a superficial *papillary layer* and a thick, *deep reticular layer*. Aside from the hooves, lips, and snout of the ox, pig, and other animals, however, it is only in humans that the dermis of the general body surface is clearly definable into two segments.

The major part of the dermis of the pig consists of a massive three-dimensional network of collagen fibers and bundles that cross each other in two main directions. Several smaller fiber bundles pass through the network in various other directions and form a dense interwoven pattern. Structural differences exist in different regions of the body.

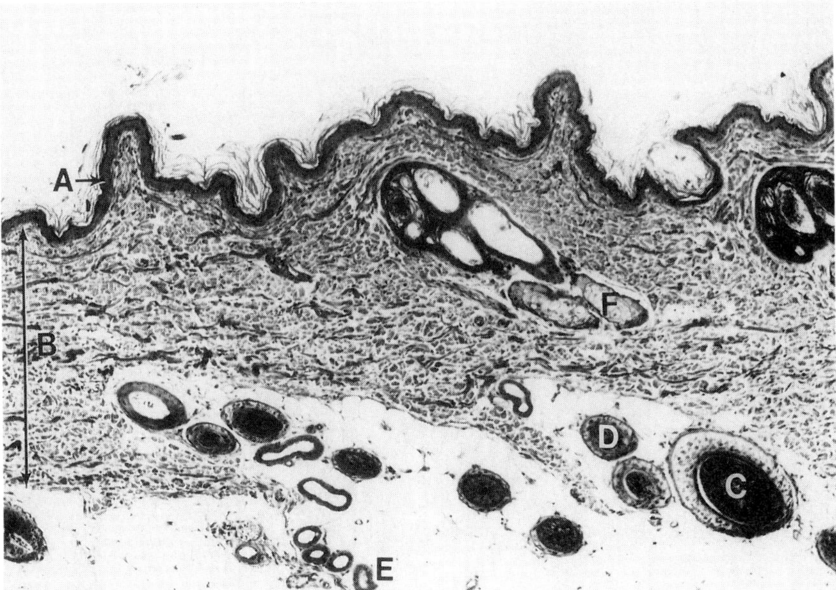

Figure 33.2. Microscopic section of the dog skin. ×90. Hematoxylin-eosin stain. Epidermis (A); dermis (B), thickness indicated by double-pointed arrow; primary hair follicle (C); secondary hair follicle (D); sweat glands (E); sebaceous gland (F).

The intercellular substances of the dermis, designated *glycosaminoglycans*, are mucopolysaccharides. Metabolism of cells, control of electrolytes and water in the extracellular fluids, calcification, and lubrication are the important functions of the glycosaminoglycans.

Hypodermis

The layer known as the hypodermis consists of loose fibrous connective tissue infiltrated with fat or adipose tissue and connects the skin to the underlying structures of the body, such as the muscles and bones. The hypodermis is the subcutaneous tissue shown in Fig. 33.1. The distribution of fat in the hypodermis is influenced by estrogenic hormones. Large masses of fat that make up a cushion or pad are called panniculus adiposus. Such masses are found in bacon and pork fatback and in footpads and digital cushions, where they serve as shock absorbers. Fat that is stored in the hypodermis insulates the body while maintaining its contour. Hypodermic injections of medicinal agents may be deposited in this layer.

GENERAL PHYSIOLOGY

Mechanical protection

Hair, hooves, nails, feathers, and the horny layer of the epidermis afford mechanical protection to underlying parts. The horny layer is thickest where chances of injury by external factors are greatest.

Hair

Because of its fibrous and bulky nature, hair affords great protection against cuts, abrasions, thermal and radiation injury, and chemical irritants. Hair is also an efficient filter and insulator. Few substances actually contact the skin of hairy animals. Physical traumas are usually blunted before they reach the cutaneous surface.

Tactile hair

The thick hair shafts growing above the lips and close to the nose in cats, dogs, and horses are very sensitive to touch. Therefore they may be used for sensory perception. The tactile hair follicle has an outer dermal sheath and an inner dermal sheath. These dermal sheaths are interconnected by bands of connective tissue or trabeculae. Spaces between the trabeculae are lined with endothelium and filled with blood and are called *blood sinuses*. Therefore these hairs have also been referred to as sinus hairs. Some voluntary control and movement of tactile hairs are facilitated by skeletal muscle fibers that attach to the outerdermal sheath. Sensitivity of the tactile hair is due to significant innervation of dermal sheaths, trabeculae, and the pressure exerted by the engorged blood in the sinuses on dermal sheaths of the hair follicle (Fig. 33.3).

Stratum corneum

From a phylogenetic point of view, keratinization came about when the vertebrates attempted to adapt themselves to life on land. In larval forms of amphibia there is a tegument, which is similar to that of fishes and has cilia on the surface. Adult amphibia develop a kind of keratinizing epidermis. The epidermis of reptiles develops an impressive horny layer. Mammals and birds have very similar epidermal shedding processes.

In many mammals there is an inverse relationship between the thickness of the epidermis and hairiness. An extreme example is the sheep, whose epidermis is about three cells thick and whose stratum corneum is trivial.

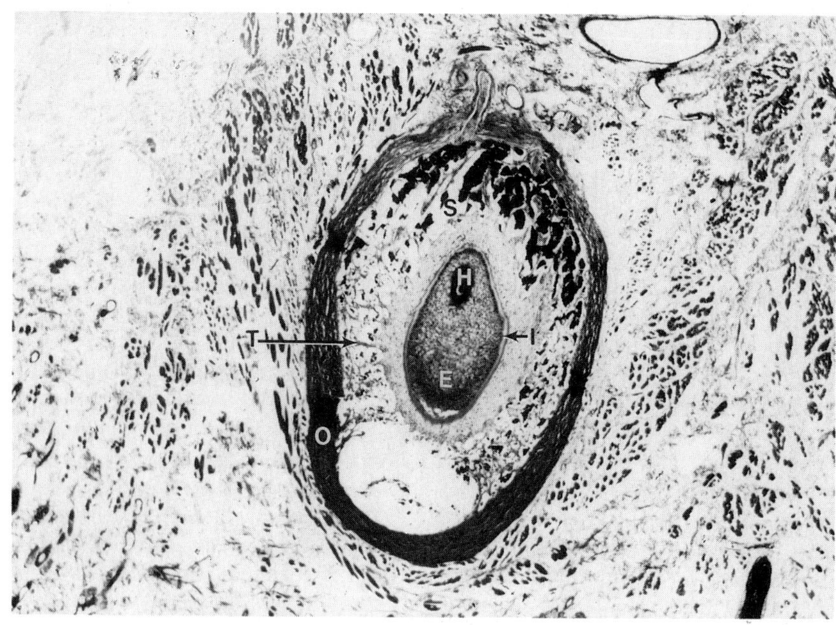

Figure 33.3. Section of the tactile hair follicle. ×90. Hematoxylin-eosin stain. Outer dermal sheath (O); connective tissue trabeculae (T); blood sinuses (S); inner dermal sheath (I); external root sheath of hair (E); hair (H).

Wherever fur is dense and thick, as in the rabbit, mouse, dog, and cat, the stratum corneum is minute. In many animals, such as deer, cattle, horses, and rabbits, it is so fragile that it cannot be separated into a sheet.

Having lost most of its hair, human skin is exposed to many noxious environmental influences. Thus the epidermis has become much thicker; it has become tough and durable, and yet it is flexible and plastic. It is remarkably efficient as a chemical- and waterproofing membrane. The exclusive function of the epidermis is to afford protection by virtue of its end product, the horny layer.

The major portion of hair, horn, hoof, feather, nail, and the stratum corneum of the skin is composed of albuminoid proteins.

Permeability

The epidermis is an effective barrier to the penetration of a wide variety of substances, the absorption of which depends on their properties as well as on the state of the skin. In general the skin has a higher order of impermeability than do other biological membranes. Overall cutaneous permeability is largely determined by the least penetrable layer (i.e., the stratum corneum).

Passage of materials into mammalian skin occurs through two main pathways: transepidermal and transappendageal (essentially through the pilosebaceous apparatus). Transepidermal absorption is thought to be limited by a superficial barrier between the stratum corneum and the uppermost layers of living epidermis. This barrier is particularly effective in preventing the passage of water and some water-soluble substances such as electrolytes. Substances unable to penetrate the superficial barrier may be absorbed in varying quantities through the more permeable cells of the sebaceous gland, the sebaceous gland duct, and the follicular epithelium. Once a substance has passed through the superficial barrier, there is apparently no significant impediment to its penetration into the remaining layers of the epidermis and the corium, after which there is ready entry into capillaries and lymph vessels and then into the general circulation.

Membrane permeability is thought to be determined largely by the lipid-protein structure of cellular membranes. This theory proposes that materials that are lipid soluble (alcohols, ketones, and so forth) penetrate the cell wall because of its lipid content, while uptake of water by cell membrane protein provides entry for water-soluble substances. Substances that are soluble in both lipids and water penetrate most rapidly of all. Permeability rates are generally lower at anatomical sites where the stratum corneum is thickest. The skin-surface lipid film probably plays a relatively small role in opposing percutaneous (through unbroken skin) absorption.

Factors that promote physiological absorption include the following: Increasing temperature, short of producing cellular damage, tends to increase penetration. Increased blood flow or hyperemia is an important factor in facilitating percutaneous absorption, particularly via the transepidermal route. It is probably most significant for gases and vapors, to which skin, like most other tissues, is highly permeable. With gases there is definite evidence that increasing concentration will yield increasing penetration.

Factors that promote absorption by barrier injury include the following: Mechanical trauma sufficient to produce breaks in barrier continuity increases permeability. Injurious agents such as mustard gas, acids, and alkalies damage the barrier membrane, thus increasing permeability. Absorption of either predominantly lipid- or water-soluble compounds may be aided by prior application of organic solvents such as benzene or chloroform. Absorption is also facilitated by inflammatory changes that impair barrier permeability and are accompanied by hyperemia. Finally, cell permeability is increased after persistent hydration of the stratum corneum.

Specific substances

1. *Water*. There is evidence to suggest the transepidermal inward movement of water. The continuous outward movement of water through the epidermis is well known.

2. *Electrolytes*. In animals there is evidence of percutaneous penetration of electrolytes, but in humans this is debatable.

3. *Lipid-soluble substances*. Lipid-soluble substances are absorbed rapidly and completely through the skin. Compounds that are soluble in both lipids and water penetrate so rapidly that the rate of absorption approaches that of gastrointestinal or even parenteral absorption (e.g., subcutaneous injections). This rapidity suggests that the route of absorption is transepidermal.

(a) The rapidly absorbed lipid-soluble substances are salicylic acid, carbolic acid (phenol), fat-soluble vitamins (A, D, and K), and sex hormones (estrogens, testosterone, and progesterone).

(b) *Heavy metals*. Mercury has received a great deal of attention because of its historical significance in the treatment of syphilis by cutaneous inunction. Metallic mercury incorporated in ointments penetrates the intact skin through hair follicles and sebaceous glands. It can then be found in tissues, body fluids, and excreta. Lead penetrates the skin to a much lesser degree. The percutaneous absorption of arsenic, as well as certain other heavy metals (e.g., mercury, tin, copper, bismuth, and antimony), depends on the transformation of the original lipid-insoluble compound into a lipid-soluble metal oleate. This may occur in or on the horny layer by combination of the salt of the heavy metal with fatty acids of sebum or outside the body when incorporated in ointment bases containing fatty acids.

4. *Gases*. All gases and many vaporized and volatile substances easily penetrate the skin, with the remarkable exception of carbon monoxide. The process appears to be one of simple diffusion across the entire skin, which be-

haves like an inert membrane. Ease of percutaneous absorption has been demonstrated for oxygen, nitrogen, helium, carbon dioxide, hydrogen sulfide, hydrogen cyanide, and vapors of ammonia, nitrobenzene, dinitrotoluene, and volatile aromatic oils.

Actinic irradiation

Sunlight may be divided arbitrarily into ultraviolet, visible, and infrared spectral regions. The intensity and spectral distribution of sunlight vary greatly with season, latitude, time of day, and changes in the earth's atmosphere.

The main sites of biological action of light rays are the skin and superficial tissues. Infrared rays are absorbed in the upper layers of the skin, where they can have a marked thermal effect; action at greater depth is insignificant. Visible light penetrates to a much greater extent than infrared. Intense irradiation with visible light can raise tissue temperature by several degrees to a depth of centimeters, while the surface of the skin is relatively little affected. Increased blood flow and enhanced sweat gland activity can follow. Ultraviolet rays differ significantly from other rays in their ability to produce chemical changes in superficial tissues.

Effects of sunlight

The formation of vitamin D and the resultant antirachitic action are the most clear-cut effects produced by sunlight.

Sunburn appears to be the result of direct injury of the cells of the epidermis by ultraviolet irradiation, with the subsequent elaboration from these cells of substances that bring about the specific physiological response. This may account for the long latent period between exposure and the development of clinical features. Ultraviolet light may exert its injurious action by altering proteins and/or nucleic acids. Sunburn is much less common in animals than in humans because animal skin is better protected by hair and pigment.

There is a wealth of convincing evidence that sunlight is one of the major causes of cancer of the skin in humans. The major lines of evidence are that cancer of the skin (1) occurs principally on the parts of the body most exposed to sunlight; (2) is more common among outdoor workers than among indoor workers; (3) is much more common in southern regions of the United States than in northern regions; (4) is much less prevalent in blacks than in whites, presumably because the skin of the former is more resistant to the harmful effects of sunlight; and (5) can be induced in laboratory animals (mice and rats) on exposure to ultraviolet irradiation.

Photosensitization may be produced in humans or in animals by toxic or allergic mechanisms, with or without the intervention of photosensitizing agents. These agents may be chemicals, such as drugs or coal-tar derivatives, or plant products. They may reach the skin by contact, ingestion, or injection. Endogenous substances, such as abnormal metabolites or toxins or other products absorbed from infection, also may act as photosensitizers. Photosensitivity occurs in erythropoietic porphyria in cattle and in humans and in certain types of hepatic porphyrias in humans. Liver damage may be associated with other forms of light sensitivity in animals.

Protective mechanisms

There are five pigments that play a role in the origin of skin color: melanin, melanoid (degradation product of melanin), oxyhemoglobin, reduced hemoglobin, and carotene. Of these five, melanin is the most important. It is a yellow to black pigment produced in the cytoplasm of melanocytes, which forms a horizontal network at the dermoepidermal junction. In mammals the amino acid tyrosine is the starting point for the production of melanin; the copper-containing enzyme tyrosinase catalyzes the entire sequence in which tyrosine is converted to melanin.

One of the direct or indirect targets of ultraviolet exposure of the skin is the melanocyte. Ultraviolet radiant energy is a highly effective agent for stimulating melanin formation.

In the domesticated water buffalo of India, the dorsal and lateral regions of the skin that are more exposed to sunlight exhibit greater pigmentation by melanin than the ventral or less exposed regions. This phenomenon appears to occur in all breeds of water buffalo, whether in temperate, subtropical, or tropical zones.

As with mechanical protection, hair and stratum corneum, particularly when thick, also are effective biological ultraviolet filters. Albino or vitiliginous skin of humans can develop increased resistance to ultraviolet irradiation by graded exposures, presumably by thickening of the stratum corneum.

Sweat glands

Two types of sweat gland have been described: *apocrine* and *eccrine* (merocrine). It was accepted that the apocrine glands shed part of their cytoplasm as a part of their secretion. Electron micrographs have revealed that the mode of secretion in these glands is apical decapitation and is, therefore, apocrine in nature. These so-called apocrine glands in humans rarely respond to thermal stimulation but elaborate their secretions slowly and sparsely.

Among the domestic animals, apocrine sweat glands are found in cattle, sheep, horses, swine, goats, dogs, and cats. Horses and cows rely partially on apocrine sweat glands for dissipation of body heat. In the dog, cat, goat, and pig, the apocrine glands are not well developed and have limited function in loss of body heat.

Structure

The detailed structure of the apocrine sweat glands has been described in human subjects. In other animal species, the structure of these glands is likely to vary because of their diverse mechanism of secretion. In humans, the apocrine glands have a secretory coil embedded in the dermis and a duct that conveys the secretory product to the pilosebaceous canal. The secretory coil of these glands is lined with epithelial cells of varying shapes, depending on the secretory activity. Myoepithelial cells, which are functionally contractile, surround the secretory cells. A basal lamina is found outside the myoepithelial cells. Secretory cells may have single, large, rounded nuclei, or they may be binucleated. Fine basophilic granules are seen at the base of the secretory cells when stained with basic stains. The terminal part of the duct is funnel shaped, with cells becoming multilayered. The ductal cells are surrounded by the myoepithelial cells. The dilation of some segments of sweat glands is seen in children and young adults and is not necessarily a phenomenon of old age.

There are large coiled glands in the region of the scrotum, interdigital pouch, infraorbital pouch, prepuce, and inguinal area of sheep. The glands of the scrotum produce more sweat per unit of area than glands of other skin regions. The goat has compound tubular sweat glands in the planum nasale. In cattle, the sweat glands are saccular, and noncoiled in general body areas, saccular and coiled around natural openings and skin margin areas. The ducts of the apocrine sweat glands open into the upper regions of the hair follicles after penetrating the epidermal cells of the follicle (Fig. 33.1). The number of sweat glands varies from 600/cm^2 in Shorthorn cattle to 1600/cm^2 in Zebu cattle. It is suggested that the greater number of sweat glands in the Zebu cattle is linked with their ability to regulate the body temperature in hot conditions. The sweat glands of the Zebu cattle and banteng are simple sacs. The yak has convoluted sweat glands. The sweat glands in the water buffalo from India, Pakistan, Iraq, Turkey, and Egypt are much less convoluted than those in the skin of Southeast Asian breeds. The multilobular sweat glands of the wisent are the largest among bovidae and the mammals.

The eccrine (merocrine) sweat glands are located in the planum nasale of the ox and pig, the footpads of the dog and cat, the carpal region in the swine (carpal glands), and the frog of the hoof in ungulates. These are coiled simple tubular glands. Two types of cell have been described in the secretory portion of these glands; a dark cell containing ribosomes exhibits a basophilic property when stained with hematoxylin and eosin stain, and a lighter-staining cell is probably involved in fluid transport. Similar to the apocrine secretory cells, these cells of the eccrine sweat glands are also surrounded by the myoepithelial cells. The shape of the secretory cells consists of simple cuboidal epithelium. The ducts of these glands have a two-layered epithelium supported by a basal lamina. Unlike the apocrine glands, the ducts of these glands open on the surface of the skin epidermis. In the footpads of the dog, the sweat glands are embedded in the adipose tissue.

Functions

The major function of the apocrine sweat glands is thermoregulation. After vigorous exercise, horses sweat profusely, and heat loss from body surface occurs as a result of evaporation of sweat. Similar heat loss also occurs in donkeys, camels, and cattle. The heat tolerance of the desert donkey is due to its sweat output. Evaporation of sweat is not impeded in animals with fur. Body heat of the dog is lost through panting and evaporation (see Chap. 13), although sweat glands are present all over the body. Evaporation from the surfaces of the mucous membrane of the large mouth and tongue of the dog controls the body temperature quite effectively.

A number of species of small-mouthed mammals, however, have no sweat glands and do not pant. In some of these animals saliva substitutes for sweat. In hot weather the body of the mouse is entirely wet; salivation is profuse. The mouse first wets the frontal portion of its chest and abdomen, then rubs saliva all over the body with its legs. The evaporation of the saliva removes heat. During heat stress, cattle are known to salivate continually.

During panting the increase of salivation is significant, and large amounts of water are evaporated. Panting and salivation are the two most important processes for controlling body temperatures in animals that have limited numbers of sweat glands. An increase in body temperature in hot weather is a common phenomenon in animals, while the body temperature of humans is kept normal by a superbly developed sweat mechanism.

The elephant has an enormous body and a small mouth. It appears to show neither panting nor intense salivation; no sweat glands can be detected. Elephants frequently suck water into their trunks and spray it over their heads, backs, and sides. If water is not available, they appear to attain temperature control by inserting their trunks into their mouths and using saliva in much the same way.

In thermoregulatory sweating, general sweat outbreak is effected in two ways: First, warmed blood from the periphery, arriving at the brain, stimulates the hypothalamic thermoregulatory centers. Second, afferent nerve impulses from the periphery stimulate the same centers via a reflex mechanism.

Perspiration on the palms and soles, in contrast to the general body surface, is not increased at all by ordinary thermal stimuli but is easily stimulated by mental or sensory agents. Insensible perspiration at these sites is very large. In animals, mental stress is almost always accompanied by muscular work, such as that involved in self-defense and in the battle for food. It is therefore of great advantage to animals for the pads of their feet to become wet when they are excited, since this provides an adhesive surface to facilitate physical work. In human beings mental stress is not necessarily accompanied by muscular activity; however, this may still be an atavistic trait.

Because of the qualities of its constituents, sweat has been considered similar to urine. Sweat, however, is the most dilute animal fluid; most of its solid constituents are exceedingly small in quantity, and therefore it would seem unlikely that sweating plays a significant role in excretion.

One of the recently recognized functions of the sweat

glands is the secretion of pheromones. Pheromones are substances that emit a specific odor when secreted on the surface of the body of an animal. This odor stimulates the olfactory senses of an animal of the same species, which then responds with a specific behavior. The glands secreting pheromones are also called *scent glands*. The scent glands, which secrete very actively in both sexes during the breeding season, elaborate a scanty viscous secretion containing volatile substances and mucopolysaccharides and are most developed in species with a strong olfactory sense. The function of scent glands is to enable males and females to locate one another during the breeding season, a matter of particular importance in normally solitary animals. The volatile scent can be detected by other members of a species over long distances.

Scent glands are not confined to the urogenital skin. Elephants have musth glands behind their eyes. Glands in the belly of the male musk deer secrete musk, which is used in the manufacture of all high-quality perfume. Scent glands of the goat, however, are sebaceous. Scent glands also play a significant and subtle role in communication between microsmatic animals (animals with a feeble sense of smell), a significance they may once have had in human communications. The apocrine glands seem to develop under the influence of gonadal hormones, but, once developed, they function independently.

The nature of secretions varies according to the gland and the region of the body: apocrine glands in the axillary region of the human body elaborate a malodorous substance; the secretion of the ceruminous glands mixes with the sebum secreted by the sebaceous glands of the external ear canal to form cerumen; a venomous poison is secreted from the skin glands of the duckbill platypus through an opening in the spine in each hindfoot.

Innervation

Sweat glands in the dog and horse have dual autonomic innervation; that is, the sweat glands may respond to intradermal epinephrine and acetylcholine. Eccrine glands of the paws of the cat and the footpads of the dog are anatomically and pharmacologically cholinergic. Adrenergic sweating occurs when adrenergic agents stimulate myoepithelium of the sweat glands pressing out preformed sweat droplets.

Sebaceous glands

Generally the sebaceous glands in the domestic animals are associated with the hair follicles and open via the pilosebaceous canal into the upper part of the follicle. They secrete sebum, a fatty lubricant.

The perianal or circumanal glands of the dog are modified sebaceous glands that exist as solid alveolar masses. The alveoli consist of small darkly staining peripheral cells and large cytoplasm-rich central cells; they are devoid of ducts and resemble endocrine glands. They are present in both sexes at birth but are best developed after puberty, forming a ring around the anus. Their function is not clear, but their involvement in steroid metabolism is suggested. Tumors of the circumanal glands, seen exclusively in the males, may occur anywhere around the anus or above it, at the base of the tail, or at the side of the prepuce as a result of metastasis. Perianal or circumanal glands are one and the same thing.

Sebaceous glands of dogs appear to be similar to the human glands. In the cat, the sebaceous gland complexes are dispersed in the connective tissue of the wall of the anal sac at fairly regular intervals. In newborn pigs the sebaceous glands are rudimentary but may still contain functional cells. In sheep the sebaceous glands are associated with the upper third of the wool or the hair follicle. Glandular epithelium is lobulated and the lobules are separated by connective tissue trabeculae. In cattle the size of the sebaceous glands is inversely proportional to the hair density. They are more highly developed in the perianal region and at the horn, hoof, and muzzle margins but absent in the hairless areas. In the goat, the sebaceous glands open independently of the hair follicles in the perianal region and on the eyelids. At the junctions of the hoof with the skin, the base of the horn, the base of ear, and in the perianal region the sebaceous glands appear as large branched alveolar glands.

The scent glands of the goat, which are modified sebaceous glands, are located around the caudomedial aspect of the base of the horn. Found in both sexes, they are usually smaller in castrated males and pregnant females. During breeding season, they become hypertrophied and very odorous in the male, and the odor is attributed to the presence of capric or caproic acids secreted by the glands. As the activity of these glands is dependent on the mating season, it can be correlated with gonadal function.

Some mammals, such as whales and porpoises, are relatively free of sebaceous glands. In laboratory animals aggregates of glands, such as the preputial and inguinal glands in rats, mice, rabbits, and gerbils, become encapsulated to form specialized organs. Sebaceous glands can also differentiate or form in other organs. They are often found in the parotid and submaxillary glands of humans. The occurrence of sebaceous metaplasia in the salivary glands is surprising because it happens so often. Sebaceous metaplasia has been found in the cervix uteri, larynx, and esophagus.

Secretion of sebum

A number of factors contribute to the secretion of sebum. The contraction of the arrectores pilorum muscles may have some effect. The viscosity of the sebum and its spread on the skin and hair may be affected by the skin temperature. Growth and differentiation of the sebaceous glands are not affected by the complete denervation of the skin areas. The flow of sebum from the sebaceous glands is a continuous process. The quantity of sebum released in a given time per unit area is proportional to the total glandular volume. This function is attributed to the entire mass of differentiated secretory cells.

Hormonal effects

Hormones regulate the size and rate of maturation of the sebaceous glands. At birth the sebaceous glands are large; they become smaller in infancy and childhood and grow larger at puberty and adulthood; sebum production in women drops after menopause. Testosterone has a direct effect on the sebaceous glands, which, after a week's interval, respond with enlarged growth in areas where the hormone is locally injected. Eunuchs normally produce very little sebum, and its production is increased by testosterone administration.

Large doses of progesterone injected into laboratory animals cause glandular enlargement, but physiological doses of progesterone (50 mg per day) administered intramuscularly to women produced no response in the sebaceous glands. There is no increase in sebum production during the luteal phase of the menstrual cycle, which is too short to stimulate sebaceous glands.

Estrogens administered in large doses over a prolonged period suppress sebum production, although, unlike testosterone, injections of estrogens have no local effect on the growth or enlargement of the sebaceous glands. Regardless of the amounts of estrogens administered locally, sebum production can be reactivated by androgen.

Adrenalectomy decreases sebum production in male rats. Glucocorticoids, on the other hand, do not stimulate sebum secretion. Adrenal androgens may play a significant role in the pituitary-adrenal and androgen-sebaceous gland stimulatory cycle. In male animals and in men, testicular testosterone is the controlling factor, whereas in female animals and in women it is the ovarian and adrenal androgens. The specific tropic hormone that stimulates the secretion of sebum is dihydrotestosterone, which is produced by the catalytic action of the enzyme α-reductase in its conversion from testosterone and other androgens.

Characteristic odors in ranting boars emanate from the preputial glands. The agent responsible for the body odor is lipophilic and probably a muscone (an oily cyclic ketone that is the chief odoriferous constituent of musk and is used in perfumes). Preputial glands dependent on the male sex hormone for secretory activity produce a fat-diffusible material that is responsible for sexual odor in boar carcasses. Odors of these glands cause an immobilization reflex in estrus sows during mating.

Functions of sebum

In domestic animals sebum provides luster to the hair coat and acts as an emollient to the keratinized superficial layer of the skin. Sebum may also act as a bacteriostatic and fungistatic agent.

Sebum also seems to function as a pheromone or olfactant signal. Sebums secreted by the different glands of various animal species have characteristic odors. Sometimes olfactory perceptions in birds are manifested in changes in breathing rate, blood pressure, heartbeat, and widening of pupils. Ability to produce scent signals varies with species and season, depending on sex, social status, age, density of population, and other factors.

SKIN GRAFTING

The past two decades have seen several useful developments in the science and techniques of skin grafting. In human medicine and surgery, skin grafting is a useful tool for the replacement of large skin surfaces that have been lost as a result of severe burning or accidental wounds. The pig has been used for skin research because the pattern of circulation in porcine skin somewhat resembles that in human skin. Among all the laboratory animal skins investigated for research, the skin of the pig appears to have closest anatomical similarities to that of humans.

Two types of grafting are in practice: split-thickness grafting and full-thickness grafting. Split-thickness grafting is an economical procedure in which part of the skin is shaved off for grafting. A split-thickness skin graft includes the epidermis and a variable section of the dermis. A full-thickness graft includes the epidermis along with the entire dermis and the appendages.

Split-thickness skin grafts

Split-thickness skin grafts are placed on areas where the superficial parts of the skin (epidermis) are damaged or lost. The graft is kept viable by the tissue fluid nutrients derived from the capillaries of the tissue on which the graft is planted. New fibroblasts develop from pericytes of the capillaries of the bed (underlying tissue) and synthesize the ground substance (glycosaminoglycans), which anchors the grafted tissue. The damaged skin then has a new epidermis from the graft. The capillaries from the bed on which the graft is placed grow into the graft to revascularize it.

The site from which the split-thickness graft is shaved off has reserve epidermal cells in the external root sheaths of the hair follicles and sweat glands. Epidermis is, therefore, rejuvenated from the external root sheaths especially and resurfaces the skin. The new epidermal growth, especially in the pig's skin, is from the external root sheaths; in humans it is from the sweat glands as well.

Full-thickness skin grafts

The full-thickness graft is planted on the surfaces of clean, uncontaminated wounds. A split-thickness graft may be used initially on traumatic and burn wounds and later replaced by full-thickness grafts.

Full-thickness grafts require full vascularization. In experimental studies of the pig skin, it was observed that the capillaries of the bed and the graft anastomose and that blood flows in the larger vessels of the graft in about 7 days.

Later, in addition to the existing vessels, new vessels grow into the graft and anastomose with the new capillaries proliferated from the bed. In veterinary medicine skin grafting has been attempted with some degree of success in the horse and in small animals. The pig is used extensively as a research animal for skin grafting for the reasons mentioned above.

In small animals, especially the dog, *pedicle grafting* of the skin is done. In this method, skin is stretched from the adjacent part to the damaged part of the skin in need of the graft without disrupting the blood supply. One edge of the skin remains connected with the original blood supply while the other is attached to the new bed. Cats have thin skin; therefore full-thickness skin grafting is more convenient.

IMMUNE PROPERTIES OF SKIN

Skin is the largest organ of the body. It protects the body against the effects of environmental toxins, pathogenic organisms, and many other substances that cause irritation and allergic reactions. In hairy as well as in thickly keratinized skin, toxins and allergens can enter through openings of the sweat gland ducts and hair follicles. The properties of Langerhans cells and their antigen-presenting abilities have been discussed. During the decade of the 1980s the skin-associated lymphoid tissues (SALTs) and their importance came to light. The following observations support the concept of the functional immunological relationship of the skin with the immune system.

1. A group of nonactivated T lymphocytes have a tendency to migrate into the epidermis of the skin from the lymph nodes adjacent to the skin.
2. Skin has antigen-presenting cells that originate from the lymphatic or hematopoietic tissue (Langerhans cells). These cells take in the antigen, process it, and present it to the reacting lymphocytes.
3. Recognition of some antigens can be facilitated by means of T lymphocytes.
4. In the absence or deficiency of antigen-presenting cells, activated lymphocytes are unable to produce a specific response.

REFERENCES

Abraham, W., Wertz, P.W., Landmann, L., and Downing, D.T. 1987. Stratum corneum lipid liposomes: Calcium-induced transformation into lamellar sheets. *J. Invest. Dermatol.* 88:212–14.

Adloph, E.F., and Dill, D.B. 1938. Observations on water metabolism in the desert. *Am. J. Physiol.* 123:369–78.

Allington, H.V. 1956. Eczematous and polymorphous hypersensitivity to light. In R.B. Baer, ed., *Allergic Dermatoses due to Physical Agents*. J.B. Lippincott, Philadelphia. Pp. 25–47.

Andrew, W. 1952. A comparison of age changes in salivary glands of man and the rat. *J. Gerontol.* 7:178–90.

Aoki, T. 1962. Stimulation of human axillary sweat glands by cholinergic agents. *J. Invest. Dermatol.* 38:41–4.

Aoki, T., and Wada, M. 1951. Functional activity of the sweat glands in the hairy skin of the dog. *Science* 114:123–24.

Baker, B.B., and Stannard, A.A. 1988. Epidermal cell renewal in the horse. *Am. J. Vet. Res.* 49:520–521.

Bal, H.S., and Ghoshal, N.G. 1976. The "scent glands" of the goat (*Capra hircus*). *Zentralbl. Veterinaermed.*, ser. C, 5:104.

Becker, A.B., Chung, K.F., McDonald, D.M., Lazarus, S.C., Frick, D.L., and Gold, W.M. 1985. Mast cell heterogeneity in dog skin. *Anat. Rec.* 213:477–80.

Biedermann, W. 1926. Vergleichende Physiologie des integumentes der Wirbeltiere. *Ergeb. Biol.* 1:120–36.

Billingham, R.E., and Medawar, P.B. 1953. A study of the branched cells of the mammalian epidermis with special references to the fate of their division products. *Phil. Trans. Roy. Soc.* 237:151–69.

Blum, H.F. 1945. The physiologic effects of sunlight on man. *Physiol. Rev.* 25:483–530.

Breathnach, A.S., and Robins, E.J. 1970. Ultrastructural observations on Merkel cells in human fetal skin. *J. Anat.* 106:4110.

Breathnach, A.S., Silver, W.K., Smith, T., and Heyner, S. 1968. Langerhans cells in mouse skin experimentally deprived of its neural crest component. *J. Invest. Dermatol.* 50:147–60.

Calhoun, M.L., and Stinson, A.W. 1976. Skin. In H.-D. Dellmann and E.M. Brown, eds., *Textbook of Veterinary Histology*. Lea & Febiger, Philadelphia. P. 463.

Calvery, H.D., Draize, J.H., and Laug, E.P. 1946. The metabolism and permeability of normal skin. *Physiol. Rev.* 26:510–40.

Davson, H., and Danielli, J.F. 1952. *The Permeability of Natural Membranes*. Cambridge Univ. Press, London, New York.

Donnelly, G.H., and Navidi, S. 1950. Sebaceous glands in the cervix uteri. *J. Pathol. Bacteriol.* 62:453–54.

Doupe, J., and Sharp, M.E. 1943. Studies in denervation: (G)-Sebaceous secretion. *J. Neurol. Psychiatry* 6:133–35.

Dutt, R.H., Simpson, E.C., Christian, J.C., and Barnhart, C.E. 1959. Identification of preputial glands as the site of production of sexual odour in the boar. *J. Anim. Sci.* 13:1557.

Edwards, E.A., and Duntley, S.R. 1939. The pigments and color of living human skin. *Am. J. Anat.* 65:1–33.

Ferguson, K.A., and Dowling, D.F. 1955. The function of cattle sweat glands. *Aust. J. Agric. Res.* 6:640–4.

FitzGerald, M.J.T. 1968. The innervation of the epidermis. In D.R. Kenshalo, ed., *The Skin Senses*. Charles C Thomas, Springfield, Ill. Pp. 61–83.

Fitzpatrick, T.B., and Szabo, G. 1957. The melanocyte: Cytology and cytochemistry. *J. Invest. Dermatol.* 32:197–209.

Forrest, J.W., Fleet, M.R., and Rogers, G.E. 1985. Characterization of melanocytes in wool bearing skin of merino sheep. *Aust. J. Biol. Sci.* 38:245–57.

Frey, J., Chamson, A., and Jean-Marie, G. 1989. Collagen and lipid biosynthesis in a case of epitheliogenesis imperfecta in cattle. *J. Invest. Dermatol.* 93:83–86.

Geipel, P. 1949. Talgdruse im Kehlkopf. *Zentralbl. Allg. Pathol. Pathol. Anat.* 83:69–71.

Goldberg, A. 1965. The hepatic porphyrias. In A. Rook and G.S. Walton, eds., *Comparative Physiology of the Skin*. Blackwell Scientific, Oxford. Pp. 345–50.

Goldsberry, S., and Calhoun, M.L. 1959. The comparative histology of the skin of Hereford and Aberdeen Angus cattle. *Am. J. Vet. Res.* 20:61–68.

Goodall, McC. 1970. Innervation and inhibition of eccrine and apocrine sweating. *J. Clin. Pharmacol.* 10:235–46.

Greer, B., and Calhoun, M.L. 1966. Anal sacs of the cat (*Felis domesticus*). *Am. J. Vet. Res.* 27:773–81.

Ham, A.W., and Cormack, D.H. 1979. *Histology*. J.B. Lippincott, Philadelphia. Pp. 637–39.

Hamilton, J.B. 1941. Male hormone substance: A prime factor in acne. *J. Clin. Endocrinol.* 1:570–92.

Hamperl, H. 1931. Beitrage zur normalen pathologischen histologie menschlicher Speicheldrusen. *Z. Mikrosk. Anat. Forsch.* 27:1–55.

Hartz, P.H. 1946. Development of sebaceous glands from intralobular ducts of the parotid gland. *Arch. Pathol.* 41:651–54.

Hashimoto, K. 1972. Fine structure of Merkel cells in human mucosa. *J. Invest. Dermatol.* 58:381–7.

Hedberg, C.L., Wertz, P.W., and Downing, D.T. 1988. The nonpolar lipids of pig epidermis. *J. Invest. Dermatol.* 90:225–29.

Hurley, J.H., and W.B. Shelley. 1960. *The Human Apocrine Sweat Gland in Health and Disease*. Charles C Thomas, Springfield, Ill. Pp. 23–26, 51–55.

Jarret, A. 1973. *The Physiology and Pathophysiology of the Skin*. Academic, New York. Vol. 1, pp. 3–44.

Jenkinson, D.M. 1969. Sweat gland function in domestic animals. In S.Y. Botelho, F.B. Brooks, and W.B. Shelley, eds., *Exocrine Glands*. Proc. Internat. Cong. Physiol. Sci. 14th Satellite Symposium, University of Pennsylvania Press, Philadelphia. Pp. 201–16.

Jenkinson, D.M., and Nay, T. 1975. The sweat glands and hair follicles of different species of bovidae. *Aust. J. Biol. Sci.* 28:55–68.

Jorgenson, S.K., and With, T.K. 1965. Congenital porphyria in animals other than man. In A. Rook and G.S. Walton, eds., *Comparative Physiology and Pathology of the Skin*. Blackwell Scientific, Oxford. Pp. 317–31.

Kligman, A.M. 1964. The biology of the stratum corneum. In W. Montagna and W.C. Lobitz, Jr., eds., *The Epidermis*. Academic, New York. Pp. 387–430.

Kligman, A.M., and Shelley, W.B. 1958. An investigation of the biology of the human sebaceous gland. *J. Invest. Dermatol.* 30:99–125.

Kovacs, R. 1950. *Light Therapy*. Charles C Thomas, Springfield, Ill. Pp. 14–17.

Kozlowski, G.P., and Calhoun, M.L. 1969. Microscopic anatomy of the integument of sheep. *Am. J. Vet. Res.* 30:1267–79.

Kral, F., and Schwartzman, R.M. 1964. *Veterinary and Comparative Dermatology*. J.B. Lippincott, Philadelphia. Pp. 8,122–29.

Kuno, U. 1956. *Human Perspiration*. Charles C Thomas, Springfield, Ill.

Lovatt Evans, C., and Smith, D.F.G. 1956. Sweating responses in horses. *Proc. R. Soc.*, ser. B 145:61–83.

Lovell, J.E., and Getty, R. 1957. The hair follicle, epidermis, dermis, and skin glands of the dog. *Am. J. Vet. Res.* 38:873–85.

Maldi, A.H., and Khamas, W.A. 1986. Light microscopic study of the vasculature of the skin of one humped camel. *Indian J. Anim. Sci.* 56:669–73.

Malkinson, F.D. 1964. Permeability of the stratum corneum. In W. Montagna and W.C. Lobitz, Jr., eds., *The Epidermis*. Academic, New York. Pp. 435–48.

Maloiy, G.M.O. 1971. Temperature regulation in the donkey (*Equus asimis*). *Biochem. Physiol.* 39A:403–12.

Marcarian, H.Q., and Calhoun, M.L. 1966. Microscopic anatomy of the integument of adult swine. *Am. J. Vet. Res.* 27:765–72.

Masson, P. 1951. My conception of cellular naevi. *Cancer* 4:9–38.

Medawar, P.B. 1953. The micro-anatomy of the mammalian epidermis. *Q. J. Microsc. Sci.* 94:481–503.

Meyer, W., Neurand, K., and Radke, B. 1982. Collagen fibre arrangement in the skin of the pig. *J. Anat.* 134, 1:139–48.

Meza Chavez, L. 1949. Sebaceous glands in normal and neoplastic parotid glands: Possible significance of sebaceous glands in respect to the origin of tumors of the salivary glands. *Am. J. Pathol.* 25:627–45.

Milewich, L., and Sontheimer, R.D. 1989. Steroid hormone metabolism by human epidermal keratinocytes. *J. Invest. Dermatol.* 93:292.

Montagna, W. 1963. Comparative aspects of sebaceous glands. In W. Montagna, R.A. Ellis, and A.F. Silver, eds., *Advances in Biology of Skin*. Vol. 4, *Sebaceous Glands*. Pergamon, New York. Pp. 32–45.

Montagna, W., and Ford, D.M. 1969. Histology and cytochemistry of human skin. XXXIII. The eyelid. *Arch. Dermatol.* 100:328–35.

Montagna, W., and Parakkal, P.F. 1974. *The Structure and Function of Skin*. 3d ed. Academic, New York. Pp. 75–95, 280–331, 332–59, 371–406.

Montes, L.F., Baker, B.L.,and Curtis, A.C. 1960. The cytology and the large axillary sweat glands in man. *J. Invest. Dermatol.* 35:273–91.

Moore, P.E., and Mariassy, A.T. 1986. Dendritic (Langerhans) cells in canine epidermis; ultrastructure and distribution (Abstract). *Anat. Histol. Embryol.* 15:178–79.

Mottag, J.H., and Zelickson, A.S. 1967. Melanin transfer: A possible phagocytic process. *J. Invest. Dermatol.* 49:605–10.

Munnel, J.F. 1986. Langerhans cells in domestic animals (Abstract). *Anat. Histol. Embryol.* 15:179.

Mykytowycz, R. 1970. The role of skin glands in mammalian communication. In J.W. Johnson, D.G. Moulton, and A. Turk, eds., *Advances in Chemoreception*. Appleton-Century-Crofts, New York. Vol. 1, pp. 327–60.

Okun, M.R. 1965. Histogenesis of melanocytes. *J. Invest. Dermatol.* 44:285–99.

Okun, M.R., and Zook, B.C. 1967. Histological parallels between mastocytoma and melanoma. *Arch. Dermatol.* 95:275–86.

Oliver, R.F. 1966. Regeneration of dermal papilla in rat vibrissae. *J. Invest. Dermatol.* 47:496–97.

Ota, R. 1950. Zytologische und histologische Untersuchungen der apokrinen Schweissdrusen in den normalen, keinen Achselgeruch (Osmidrosis axillae) gebenden Achselhauten von Japanern. *Arch. Anat. Jap.* 1:285–308.

Overton, E. 1924. *Studien uber die Narkose*. Fischer, Jena.

Piepkorn, M., Fleckman, P., Carney, H., and Linker, A. 1987. Glycosaminoglycan synthesis by proliferating and differentiated keratinocytes. *J. Invest. Dermatol.* 88:215–19.

Pontein, B. 1960. Grafted skin: Observations on innervation and other qualities. *Acta Chir. Scand.* 257(suppl.):1–78.

Rothman, S. 1943. The principles of percutaneous absorption. *J. Lab. Clin. Med.* 28:1305–21.

Rothman, S. 1954. *Physiology and Biochemistry of the Skin*. University of Chicago Press, Chicago.

Rothman, S. 1964. Keratinization in historical perspective. In W. Montagna and W.C. Lobitz, Jr., eds., *The Epidermis*. Academic, New York. Pp. 172.

Rudolph, R., Fisher, J.C., and Ninnemann, J.L. 1979. *Skin Grafting*. Little, Brown, Boston. Pp. 167–75.

Ryder, M.L. 1973. *Hair*. Edward Arnold, London. P. 1.

Sar, M., and Calhoun, M.L. 1966. The microscopic anatomy of the integument of the common American goat. *Am. J. Vet. Res.* 27:444–56.

Schiefferdecker, P. 1922. Die Hautdrusen des Menschen und des Saugetieres, ihre Bedeutung sowie die Muscularis sexualis. *Zoologica* 72:1–154.

Schmidt-Nielsen, K. 1975. *Animal Physiology: Adaptation and Environment*. University Press, Cambridge, England.

Schmidt-Nielsen, K., Schmidt-Nielsen, B., Jarnum, S.A., and Houpt, T.R. 1957. Temperature of the camel and its relation to water economy. *Am. J. Physiol.* 188:103–12.

Singh, A. 1962. Skin pigmentation in buffalo calves. *Can. Vet. J.* 3:343–46.

Sisson, S. 1975. Common integument. In R. Getty, ed., *Sisson and Grossman's The Anatomy of the Domestic Animals*. W.B. Saunders, Philadelphia. Vol. 1, pp. 728–35.

Spearman, R.I.C. 1973. *The Integument*. Cambridge Univ. Press, Cambridge. Pp. 134–38.

Straus, J.S., Kligman, A.M., and Pochi, E.E. 1962. The effect of androgens and estrogens on human sebaceous glands. *J. Invest. Dermatol.* 39:139–55.

Takayasu, S., and Adachi, K. 1970. Hormonal control of metabolism in hamster costovertebral glands. *J. Invest. Dermatol.* 55:13–9.

Thody, A.J., and Shuster, S. 1971a. Sebotrophic activity of β-lipotrophin. *J. Endocrinol.* 50:533–34.

Thody, A.J., and Shuster, S. 1971b. The effect of hypophysectomy on the response of the sebaceous gland to testosterone propionate. *J. Endocrinol.* 49:329–33.

Thody, A.J., and Shuster, S. 1971c. Effect of adrenalectomy and adrenocorticotrophic hormone on sebum secretion in the rat. *J. Endocrinol.* 49:325–28.

Trautman, A., and Febiger, J. 1957. *Fundamentals of the Histology of Domestic Animals*. 9th ed. McGraw-Hill, New York. Pp. 346–57.

Webb, A.J., and Calhoun, M.L. 1954. The microscopic anatomy of the skin of mongrel dogs. *Am. J. Vet. Res.* 15:274–80.

Wenzel, B.M. 1967. Olfactory perception in birds. In T. Hayashi, ed., *Proceedings of the Second International Symposium on Olfaction and Taste*. Pergamon, Tokyo, London. Pp. 203–17.

Wilson, J.A. 1941. *Modern Practice in Leather Manufacture*. Reinhold, New York.

PART **VI** | # ENDOCRINOLOGY, REPRODUCTION, AND LACTATION

CHAPTER **34**

Endocrine Glands | by William M. Dickson

INTRODUCTION

The various functions of the body must be able to respond, in a coordinated and appropriate manner, to diverse physical and chemical changes arising from both within and outside the body. Such perturbations may act directly upon a responding cell or upon a sensing cell, which then transmits the information to effector or target cells. In the nervous system, information is gathered, transported, integrated and disseminated by electric nerve impulses via the central and peripheral nerve networks. Alternatively, information may be transmitted from sensor to effector cells by means of chemical messengers traveling in the body fluids. These messengers adjust and correlate metabolic functions by acting on their target cells in various ways, including (1) activation of intracellular enzymes, (2) influencing the movement of substances or ions between intracellular compartments, (3) inducing enzyme synthesis, and (4) changing the permeability of the plasma membrane, thereby affecting transport to and from the extracellular space. This type of control is particularly important for the maintenance of homeostasis and the regulation of growth and reproduction.

There are three basic ways in which cells communicate:

1. They form gap junctions between adjacent cells, directly joining the cytoplasm of the two cells. This allows small molecules to pass, which couples the cells electrically and metabolically.
2. They display plasma membrane-bound signaling molecules in the extracellular matrix, which influence neighboring cells.

3. They secrete chemicals that communicate with cells some distance away. This type is subdivided as follows:
   a. Paracrine transmission—diffusion of the messenger through the interstitial fluid. Sometimes the messenger affects the cell which secretes it; this has been termed *autocrine*.
   b. Neurocrine transmission. The messenger travels a short distance from neuron to neuron or from neuron to a target cell. Release of the neurotransmitter occurs as a result of an electrical signal.
   c. Endocrine transmission. The messenger, termed a *hormone*, is secreted directly into and transported by the circulating blood.
   d. Exocrine transmission—whenever the agent is secreted to the exterior of the body. Certain gastrointestinal hormones are secreted into the lumen of the gastrointestinal tract and exert a regulatory effect on distal cells lining the tract. Another type of exocrine regulation occurs when a chemical substance from one individual exerts its effect upon another individual of the same species. Such substances, called *pheromones*, are either secreted from an exocrine gland or are found in an excretory product such as urine. These regulatory agents are most important in insects, but there are several examples of mammalian pheromones that affect reproductive function.

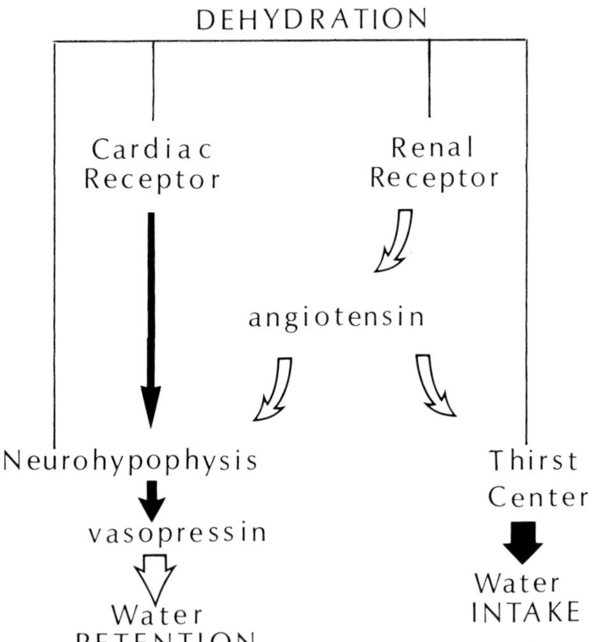

Figure 34.1. Simplified example of a multiple neural and humoral control. Open arrows represent humoral transport; closed arrows represent neural pathways.

There are close interrelationships between the various regulatory components. The nervous system is basically concerned with rapid activities and with behavior, whereas humoral control is dominant for homeostasis and slow, sustained adaptations such as growth and reproduction; it is common to find a mixture of control modes and pathways for any given function or perturbation (Fig. 34.1). In addition, a single control pathway may use a mixture of delivery systems. Nervous stimulation may affect he synthesis, release, or effect of a hormone or paracrine agent, and humoral regulators have been shown to stimulate or modulate nerve impulses. The endocrine cells of the adrenal medulla secrete their hormones in response to neural stimulation from preganglionic neurons of the autonomic nervous system. Certain neurons in the hypothalamus have evolved into neuroendocrine cells in which hormone is synthesized in the cell body, transported within the axon, and released into the bloodstream after nervous stimulation.

Another unifying link between neural and humoral control lies in the fact that the two systems share transmitters. Many biologically active amines (epinephrine, serotonin, dopamine, histamine) and peptides (somatostatin, enkephalin, thyroid-regulating hormone) have been found in both neural and endocrine tissue.

A hormone is classically defined as a compound that is synthesized and secreted by a specialized group of cells (often organized into a discrete organ—the endocrine gland), is transported via the bloodstream, and exerts it regulatory effect of a distant group of effector or target cells. As our knowledge of humoral transmission has expanded, this definition has proved to be too restrictive. Substances generally considered to be hormones (e.g., prostaglandins, somatomedins, angiotensin) are not synthesized or secreted by specialized cells or tissues. In other instances (somatostatin, glucagon, epinephrine), secretion may occur from either endocrine or nonendocrine tissue. Renin, most often regarded as a hormone, is an enzyme that exerts its effect within the bloodstream. In this chapter, regulatory agents that are transported via the circulation will be termed hormones.

Hormone chemistry, receptors, and mechanism of action

Hormones can be roughly divided into two classes according to solubility, target cell receptors, and mechanism of action (Table 34.1). The protein, polypeptide, and amine hormones are water-soluble, bind with receptors in the plasma membrane of the target cell, and frequently exert their effect by activation of intracellular enzymes or by alteration of membrane permeability. The relatively water-insoluble steroids and iodinated amino acids interact with nuclear and, perhaps, mitochondrial or cytosolic receptors and affect protein synthesis through stimulation of messenger ribonucleic acid (RNA). Because of their solubility characteristics, these two classes differ in their form of blood

Table 34.1. Chemistry and source of principal hormones

Hormone	Abbreviation or synonym	Number of amino acids (molecular wt.)	Sources
Amines			
Epinephrine*	Catecholamine (collective term)		Adrenal medulla, central nervous system (CNS)
Norepinephrine*			Adrenal medulla, CNS, sympathetic nerves
Dopamine*			CNS, sympathetic nerves
Polypeptides and simple proteins			
Thyrotropin-releasing hormone*	TRH	3	Hypothalamus, CNS, gastrointestinal (GI) tract
Enkephalins		5	CNS, GI tract
Vasopressin*	ADH	8	Neurohypophysis, CNS
Oxytocin	OT	8	Neurohypophysis, CNS, corpus luteum
Angiotensin II		8	Circulating blood
Gonadotropin-releasing hormone*	GnRH, LH/FSH RH	10	Hypothalamus, CNS, autonomic nerves
Somatotropin-release-inhibiting hormone	SRIF, Somatostatin	14	Hypothalamus, CNS, pancreas, GI tract
Gastrin		17	GI tract
Secretin		27	GI tract
Glucagon*		29	Pancreas, GI tract
β-endorphin		31	CNS, hypothalamus, GI tract
Calcitonin*	CT	32	Thyroid gland
Cholecystokinin	CCK	33	GI tract
Adrenocorticotropin*	ACTH	39	Adenohypophysis
Insulin		51	Pancreas
Parathyroid hormone	PTH	84	Parathyroid gland
β-lipotropin	B-LPH	91	Adenohypophysis
Growth hormone	STH, somatotropin	(21,500)	Adenohypophysis
Prolactin	PRL	(22,000)	Adenohypophysis
Glycoproteins			
Thyroid-stimulating hormone*	TSH	(28,000)	Adenohypophysis
Luteinizing hormone*	LH, ICSH	(28,000)	Adenohypophysis
Follicle-stimulating hormone*	FSH	(36,000)	Adenohypophysis
Iodinated amino acids			
Thyroxine	T_4		Thyroid gland
Triiodothyronine	T_3		Thyroid gland
Steroids			
Cortisol	Hydrocortisone		Adrenal cortex
Estradiol			Ovary, testes, placenta
Testosterone			Testes, ovary, adrenal cortex
Progesterone			Ovary, placenta, adrenal cortex
Aldosterone	Electrocortin		Adrenal cortex
Dihydroxycholecalciferol	Dihydroxy-vitamin D		Kidney

*Activates adenylate cyclase.

transport; those of the first class are transported as free hormones, whereas the insoluble hormone are bound to blood plasma proteins. Free hormones generally have a much shorter half-life in the circulation than those that are protein bound (Table 34.2).

Another possible basis for distinguishing among hormones is found in the embryologic origin of the secreting cells. Current evidence favors the concept that virtually all cells that secrete protein, polypeptide, and amine hormones originate from a specialized region of the ectoblast. Cells that secrete steroids and iodinated amino acids are derived from mesoderm and endoderm, respectively. Many cells that secrete water-soluble hormones have such similar morphological and biochemical characteristics that they have been collectively termed APUD cells, a name reflecting their ability to take up and decarboxylate aromatic-amine precursors. Clinical relevance of this idea is demonstrated by the occurrence of protein-, polypeptide-, and amine-secreting tumors found in both endocrine (medullary carcinoma of the thyroid) and nonendocrine (carcinoma of the lung) tissues. Such tumors may be multiple in the same individual, may occur in association with nonendocrine tumors of neural crest tissue, and occasionally may secrete more than one hormone. Considering that the endocrine glands that secrete steroids and iodinated amino acids are

Table 34.2. Circulatory half-lives of certain representative hormones

Hormone	Chemical type	Approximate half-life
Epinephrine	Amine	20–40 seconds
Vasopressin	Peptide	10–15 minutes
ACTH	Peptide	7–12 minutes
Insulin	Peptide	6–10 minutes
Growth hormone	Peptide	20–25 minutes
TSH	Glycoprotein	75–80 minutes
LH	Glycoprotein	20–50 minutes
FSH	Glycoprotein	3–4 hours
Aldosterone	Steroid	15–30 minutes
Cortisol	Steroid	80–120 minutes
1,25-DHCC	Steroid	15 hours
T_3	Iodinated amino acid	1–2 days
T_4	Iodinated amino acid	1 week

Data from Felig et al., 1987.

themselves regulated by protein hormones from the adenohypophysis, it is possible that virtually all body functions are controlled by cells with a similar embryological origin.

Hormone receptors

Hormone receptors play three important and linked roles in hormone function:

1. Receptors are relatively hormone specific. Thus, whereas the nervous system achieves anatomically specific impulses to discrete groups of cells, all cells are exposed to hormones in the bloodstream. Through binding with the specific receptors found only in certain cells, the endocrine system is able to elicit biochemically specific responses from cells throughout the body as well as organ- or tissue-specific responses. In instances where two hormones are chemically related, however, the receptor for one may bind the other with markedly less affinity; this is called *specificity spillover*.

2. The number and affinity of the receptors affect the magnitude of the target cell response. Often an increased concentration of circulating hormone results in decreased receptor numbers in the target cells. This has been termed *downregulation* and results from both occupancy of receptor sites and loss of unoccupied receptor sites. Sometimes increased circulating hormone (e.g., prolactin, angiotensin), stimulates receptor numbers. It is also possible to find hormone regulation of receptor numbers for other hormones; for example, estrogens increase the number of oxytocin receptors. Although less common, receptor affinity may also be affected. This is particularly true for receptors that are capable of binding several hormone molecules; binding of the first molecule changes the conformation of the receptor so that the affinity of the remaining sites is changed. Decreased affinity is known as *negative cooperativity.*

3. Hormone receptors are essential in the transfer of information from hormone to target cell. As far as is known, all receptors are proteins that contain a site or sites to which to hormone is bound. Binding changes the conformation of the receptor, initiating certain intracellular or membrane changes that constitute the response of the cell. The essentiality of the receptor is illustrated by the fact that an antibody to the receptor can often, on binding to the receptor, initiate the same response as the hormone.

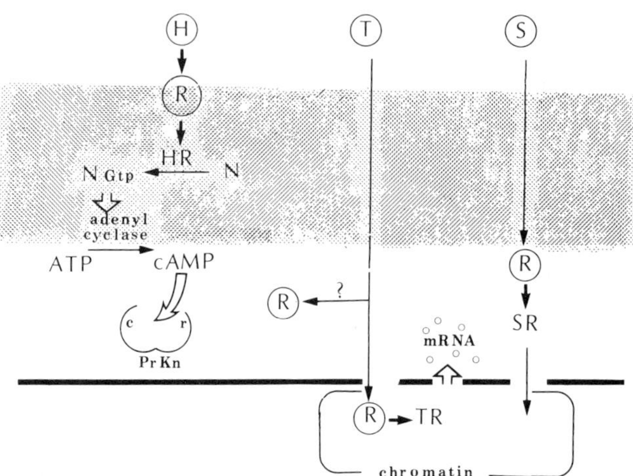

Figure 34.2. Diagram illustrating hormone-receptor interaction of protein hormone (H), thyroid hormone (T), steroid hormone (S), receptor (R), regulator protein (N), and protein kinase (PrKn). (c, catalytic subunit; r, regulatory subunit; Gtp, guanine triphosphate.) Shaded area indicates the plasma membrane, and heavy solid line indicates the nuclear membrane.

Mechanism of action of plasma membrane receptors

The binding of water-soluble hormones to their plasma membrane receptors results in the generation of one or more "second messengers" and in changes in the membrane itself. These "second messengers" then regulate the intracellular events that constitute the target cell response.

The best-defined and most common second messenger system involves cyclic adenosine monophosphate (cAMP). A membrane protein, known as guanine nucleotide regulatory protein, is affected by the hormone-receptor complex in such a way that it binds guanosine triphosphate. The resultant protein-GTP activates the enzyme adenylate cyclase, which, in turn, catalyzes the formation of cAMP from adenosine triphosphate (ATP). This cyclic nucleotide then activates cAMP-dependent protein kinase. There are also examples wherein the hormone-receptor complex inhibits the adenylate cyclase (fig. 34.2). Another cyclic nucleotide, cyclic guanosine monophosphate, has also been shown to act as a "second messenger."

Movement of calcium ions into the cell cytosol is a common cellular response to external stimuli. This calcium is derived either from the extracellular fluid or from calcium stores in the mitochondria, microsomes, or plasma membrane. Increased cytosolic calcium is very important in the cellular response to hormonal stimulation. Although the calcium ion itself may activate certain enzymes, the biological actions of calcium are usually mediated by an interaction with calcium-binding proteins such as calmodulin. Calcium-calmodulin activates certain metabolic enzymes, affects adenylate cyclase, guanylate cyclase, and phosphodiesterase, and participates in the control of membrane permeability.

Membrane phospholipids and their metabolic products play an important role in the target cell response to peptide hormone-receptor binding.

1. Increased membrane fluidity with consequent changes in receptor mobility results from methylation of phosphatidylethanolamine to phosphatidylcholine.

2. Arachidonic acid precursors for the synthesis of prostaglandins and related compounds are generated.

3. There is increased formation of polyphosphoinositides, which function within the cell to activate certain metabolic enzymes and to mobilize calcium from intracellular stores.

Mechanism of action of nuclear receptors

Steroid hormones pass freely through the plasma membrane and bind to intracellular receptors. Until recently, it was thought that the receptors were located in the cytoplasm; however, it is now thought that most, if not all, are found within the nucleus. In any case, the receptor-hormone complex is then activated and binds with high affinity to sites in the nucleus. This binding results in changes in the transcription of genes, which initiate the synthesis of specific messenger RNA (mRNA) and proteins. The mRNA response is variable, depending on the steroid and the target organ; that is, there may be either a decrease or an increase, and the magnitude can be modest to very high. While these transcriptional changes appear to involve binding to regulatory deoxyribonucleic acid sequences, the exact molecular mechanisms are not known.

Changes in mRNA levels effect a change in the rates of synthesis of the various proteins translated. For example, 1,25-dihydroxycholecalciferol increases synthesis of calcium-binding protein in the cytoplasm of the intestinal epithelium, and adrenal glucocorticoids increase the concentration of amino transferases in liver cells. The effect of steroid hormones is usually an increase in the rate of mRNA synthesis, but occasionally specific gene transcription is decreased; this may be particularly important for the feedback effects of steroids on their respective tropic hormones.

The binding sites for the iodinated amino acid hormones secreted by the thyroid gland appear to be both nuclear and cytoplasmic; however, the receptor affinity of the latter is much lower and their binding to thyroid hormone shows less correlation with the cellular response. The mechanism of action is probably much the same as with steroids, since thyroid hormones cause increased α-glycerol phosphate dehydrogenase levels and can restore certain enzymes that were decreased after thyroidectomy. Some proteins are altered by both steroids and thyroid hormones, some are affected by one or the other, and some require both; this latter situation may account for the "permissive" interaction between glucocorticoids and thyroid hormone.

Regulation of hormone secretion and activity

Diverse humoral and neural means are employed in the regulation of hormone secretion. Some hormones are secreted in response to the concentration of chemical compounds or ions in the extracellular fluid, others response to neural stimuli, and still others are controlled by hormones from another endocrine gland. Individual pathways will be discussed for specific hormones or glands in the following pages.

Virtually all control system are regulated, at least in part, by feedback. In *negative feedback*, which is the most common, the target cell response inhibits the regulating signal. For example, adrenocorticotropic hormone (ACTH) stimulates the secretion of cortisol, and the increased blood concentration of free cortisol inhibits the adenohypophyseal secretion of ACTH, either directly or by diminishing hypothalamic corticotropin-releasing hormone. *Positive feedback* is generally regarded as a "runaway" process in that the target cell response stimulates the regulating signal, which in turn stimulates more target cell response. However, at least one good example of positive feedback has been described: Luteinizing hormone from the adenohypophysis stimulates increased estradiol secretion by the ovary which, probably through the action of hypothalamic gonadotropin-regulating hormone, increases the secretion of luteinizing hormone. Termination of positive feedback may occur through an inability of the involved cells to respond further because of substrate exhaustion or receptor downgrading.

Another relatively general feature of hormone synthesis, secretion, and activity that may constitute a regulatory step is the existence of hormone precursors. These are inactive molecules, usually of greater molecular weight, which are converted into the active form just before or during secretion (insulin, parathormone, ACTH), during circulation through other organs (angiotensin II, 1,25-dihydroxycholecalciferol), or even after entry into the target cell (triiodothyronine, dihydrotestosterone).

The activity of a hormone is greatly influenced by its interaction with one or more other hormones involved in the regulation of the same or related functions. It is common, particularly in the regulation of homeostasis, to find two hormones acting antagonistically. For example, increased insulin secretion results in hypoglycemia, while increased glucagon secretion will cause hyperglycemia. In some instances, the secretion of two antagonists may increase following the same stimulus. Amino acid absorption from the intestine stimulates both insulin and glucagon; this glucagon-induced increase in blood sugar concentration serves to prevent a transient intense hypoglycemia resulting from insulin. Another type of interaction is seen when two hormones, acting together, have a greater total effect than the sum of their individual effects; this is known as *synergism*. The toxicity of catecholamines is markedly increased in animals given thyroxine, and beta-adrenergic blocking agents are used to treat acute hyperthyroidism. Whenever one hormone is required for another hormone to exert its response, it is termed a *permissive* effect. This type of interaction is exemplified by the need for a small amount of adrenal glucocorticoid to be present for catecholamines to exert their calorigenic and lipolytic effects. Commonly, in the control of general body function (i.e., growth, development, reproduction, fuel metabolism, response to stress), multiple humoral agents interacting in various ways are used to "fine tune" the eventual response.

Diagnosis of endocrine dysfunction

The detection and diagnosis of endocrine dysfunction are based on both physical signs of hormone deficiency or excess and laboratory assay of hormone concentration or of the concentration of compounds regulated by the hormone involved. Although often empirical, the physical signs are

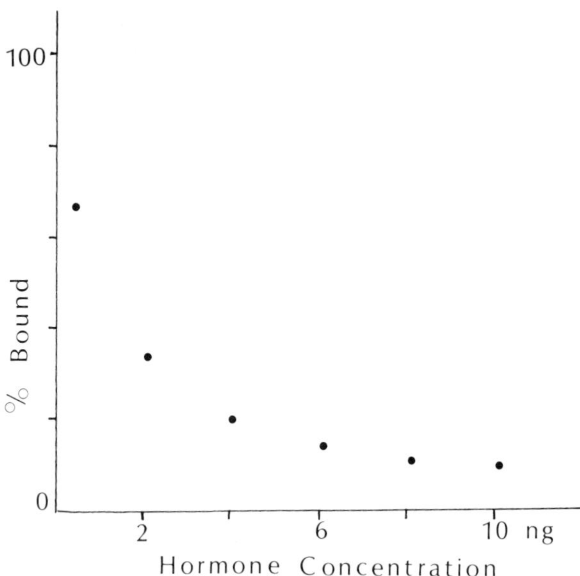

Figure 34.3. Effect of hormone concentration on protein binding in a competitive-protein-binding assay.

usually similar to those observed in experimental animals deprived of a certain gland, given hormone antagonists or inhibitors, or administered exogenous hormone. Laboratory verification of the diagnosis is important in that the dysfunction may arise from abnormal secretion, an abnormality of regulation, receptor defects, or inability of the target cell to respond.

The concentration of hormones in body fluids is measured, in virtually all cases, by some form of competitive-protein-binding assay. In such assays, a small known amount of labeled hormone is reacted with the binding protein and the sample that contains unlabeled hormone. The hormone-protein complex is separated, and the amount of bound labeled hormone is measured. The percent of labeled hormone that was bound is then compared with a standard curve (prepared with known amounts of unlabeled hormone) to ascertain the concentration of hormone in the sample. Since there is competition between labeled and unlabeled hormone for binding sites, the percent of labeled hormone that is bound will decrease with increasing concentrations of unlabeled hormone (Fig. 34.3). Blood transport proteins were initially used in these assays and purified specific receptor protein is gaining popularity, but the most common binding protein used in these assays consists of hormone antibody. These antibodies are generated by injection of pure hormone or hormone complexed to a specific protein into experimental animals. Similar assays are also used to estimate receptor numbers and affinity.

Protein hormone antibodies are also important clinically in that patients on long-term hormone replacement therapy may become refractory to treatment because of endogenous antibody production against hormones derived from another species.

Since hormones respond to and(or) initiate changes, rates of hormone secretion and, subsequently, hormone concentration in the bloodstream fluctuate. Hormone concentrations can vary widely in periods as short as a minute or two. For this reason, it is especially useful to apply procedures in which the gland is manipulated and the hormone secretory response is measured. If a deficiency is suspected, concentrations of hormones should be measured after some stimulus known to increase hormone secretion. Tentative diagnosis of overactivity would be confirmed by application of an inhibitory procedure.

HYPOPHYSIS CEREBRI AND HYPOTHALAMUS

The hypophysis cerebri (or pituitary gland) and the hypothalamus are intimately related morphologically and functionally. The hypothalamus, through the hypophysis, regulates many important peripheral endocrine glands and is the center of a large number of the complex autonomic neural control pathways.

Morphology and nomenclature

The pituitary gland is formed early in embryonic life from the fusion of two ectodermal processes. An evagination from the roof of the embryonic buccal area (Rathke's pouch) extends upward toward the brain and is met by an outpouching of the floor of the third ventricle. This outpouching becomes the neurohypophysis, and the region derived from oral epithelium becomes the adenohypophysis.

Hypothalamus and neurohypophysis

The hypothalamus is that part of the diencephalon that lies ventral to the thalamus and forms the floor of the third ventricle. Usually the hypothalamus is considered to include the optic chiasma, the tuber cinereum, the mamillary bodies, the median eminence, the infundibulum, and the neurohypophysis. The latter two parts are also included in descriptions of pituitary morphology; however, since the infundibulum and the neurohypophysis constitute ventral projections of the neural tissue of the hypothalamus, they are logically included with this structure.

Hypothalamic and neurohypophyseal tissue is composed of connective tissue, nonmedullated axons, and neuroglia (pituicytes). Between the median eminence and the neurohypophysis proper, the axons run more or less parallel to one another, and most of them pass through the neural stalk to end in the neurohypophysis. For the most part, axons arise from two nuclei in the hypothalamus: the supraoptic and the paraventricular. Neurosecretory material within the axons is visible in electron micrographs as numerous spherical bodies (Herring bodies), 100 to 180 nm in diameter, with the typical appearance of the secretory granules seen in the pancreas or in the adenohypophyseal cells.

Adenohypophysis

The adenohypophysis lies anterior to the neurohypophysis and is divided into three parts: the pars intermedia, the pars tuberalis, and the pars distalis. The pars intermedia is formed by a layer of cells contiguous to the neurohypophysis, and the pars tuberalis consists of a layer of cells surrounding the neural stalk. The pars distalis comprises the bulk of the adenohypophysis and consists of branching cords of cells separated by sinusoids. On the basis of older histological techniques, adenohypophyseal cells were classified as acidophil, basophil, or chromophobe, depending on the presence of absence of granules with an affinity for certain dyes. Modern techniques of electron microscopy and immunochemistry have enabled cytologists to identify five types of secretory cells in the adenohypophysis: *somatotrops*, which secrete growth hormone; *corticotrops*, which secrete ACTH and beta-lipotropin (β-LPH); *mammotrops*, which secrete prolactin; *thyrotrops*, which secrete thyroid-stimulating hormone (TSH); *gonadotrops*, which secrete follicle-stimulating hormone (FSH) and luteinizing hormone (LH). Chromophobes probably represent degranulated secretory cells.

Hypophyseal-portal system

Arterial blood enters the pituitary gland through the dorsal and ventral hypophyseal arteries, which carry nutrients and oxygen to the adenohypophysis and neurohypophysis, respectively. The dorsal hypophyseal artery ends in capillary plexuses in the median eminence and pituitary stalk.

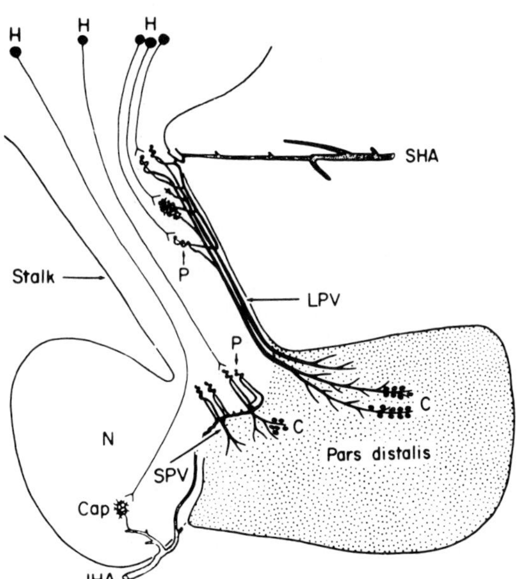

Figure 34.4. Some of the possible neurovascular connections between hypothalamic nuclei and the pituitary gland: nerve cells (H), parenchymal cells (C), primary capillary bed (P), long portal vessels (LPV), short portal vessels (SPV), posterior lobe (N), posterior lobe capillary bed (Cap), dorsal (superior) hypophyseal artery (SHA), ventral (inferior) hypophyseal artery (IHA). (From Hume-Adams, Daniel, and Prichard 1964, *Endocrinology* 75:120–26.)

Venous blood draining these plexuses is collected in two series of parallel veins running down the anterior surface of the stalk and draining into sinusoidal capillaries in the pars distalis. The ventral and central part of the pars distalis receives blood from "long" portal vessels, whereas the "short" portal vessels drain into capillaries in the more dorsal and peripheral regions (Fig. 34.4). This constitutes the hypophyseal-portal system, which is the route by which the hypothalamic regulating hormones enter and control the secretion of adenohypophyseal hormones.

Hormones of the neurohypophysis

Neurohypophyseal hormonal activity was first demonstrated by Oliver and Schafer in 1895. They found that the intravenous injection of whole pituitary extracts produced a prolonged rise in blood pressure. Soon afterward, this effect was shown to be identifiable with the pars nervosa. Subsequent studies, culminating in the work of DuVigneaud and his collaborators, have resulted in the isolation, purification, and synthesis of the neurohypophyseal hormones.

Chemistry

The compounds isolated from the pars nervosa are nonpeptides consisting of a 20-carbon hexapeptide ring with a tripeptide tail. Several nonpeptides that have biological activity have been studied, but only four occur naturally: oxytocin (Fig. 34.5), arginine vasopressin, lysine vasopressin, and arginine vasotocin. Vasopressins differ from oxytocin in that phenylalanine is substituted for isoleucine and either arginine or lysine occupies the position of leucine. Arginine vasotocin is intermediate in that arginine substitutes for leucine but isoleucine is present as in oxytocin.

Secretion

Two nuclei in the hypothalamus, the supraoptic and the parventricular, synthesize both vasopressin and oxytocin. The two hormones are complexed with neurophysin, a 95 amino acid polypeptide, and are transported within the axons to terminals in the neurohypophysis. There appears to be a specific neurophysin for each hormone. On stimulation of the cell body, the complex is dissociated and the hormone and its neurophysin are released into the bloodstream from the neurohypophysis. Thus the axons serve as both humoral and neural transport cells.

Vasopressin

If hypertonic saline solution is injected into the carotid artery, a greater concentration of the urine and a decreased urine volume are observed. If an animal is water-loaded, an increased volume of dilute urine is excreted. This latter effect can be obliterated by the injection of a small amount of posterior pituitary extract. Purification and fractionation led to the term *antidiuretic hormone* for the fraction which

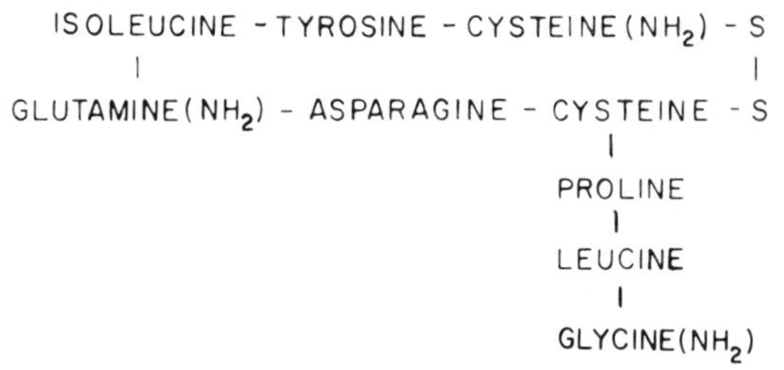

```
ISOLEUCINE - TYROSINE - CYSTEINE(NH2) - S
    |                                   |
GLUTAMINE(NH2) - ASPARAGINE - CYSTEINE - S
                                  |
                               PROLINE
                                  |
                               LEUCINE
                                  |
                               GLYCINE(NH2)
```

Figure 34.5. The amino acid arrangement in the oxytocin molecule.

exhibited this activity. Further research established that antidiuretic hormone and vasopressin were identical. The natural hormone in most mammals is arginine vasopressin, but the domestic pig and some related species utilize lysine vasopressin. In birds, arginine vasotocin exerts the diuretic effect.

Control of vasopressin secretion. Secretion of vasopressin is stimulated by increased osmolarity of the circulating blood, decreased blood volume, hypotension, angiotensin II, or acute hypoglycemia. Hypertonicity of the blood circulating in the hypothalamus is sensed by osmoreceptor cells, whereas reduced blood volume or pressure results in secretion of vasopressin through afferent nerves from the low-pressure and high-pressure stretch receptors in the vascular system and by the generation of angiotensin II (discussed later). In humans, nausea, trauma, pain, and anxiety will cause increased release of vasopressin. Environmental temperature also influences secretion of vasopressin. Exposure to cold depresses plasma vasopressin, whereas a hot environment has the opposite effect.

Function of vasopressin. The target organ for vasopressin is the kidney. As the glomerular filtrate passes through the proximal tubule, sodium, chloride, and water pass into the bloodstream simultaneously. Thus the filtrate remains iso-osmotic. In the loop of Henle, a countercurrent multiplier mechanism enables the reabsorption of large quantities of sodium chloride in excess of water, and the urine entering the distal tubule is hypotonic. In the absence of vasopressin, the distal tubule and collecting duct are impermeable to water; in the presence of vasopressin, however, about 85 percent of the water is reabsorbed. Current evidence suggests that vasopressin, through cAMP, binds to serosal surface receptors and increases the water permeability on the mucosal surface of renal cells.

Hemorrhage, with drastic reduction in blood volume, is the only situation in which sufficient vasopressin is released to give a pressor response. In dogs, the dose required to give a pressor effect is 10 times the amount needed to achieve maximal effects on the kidney. Further, arginine vasotocin is a vasodepressor in birds.

Oxytocin

Oxytocin exerts its functional activity entirely on reproduction. Cannulation of the teat canal of a lactating cow or goat results in the collection of only a minor portion of the total amount of milk in the gland. Gaines postulated in 1915 that the action of posterior pituitary extract on the mammary gland resulted in a constriction of the alveoli and subsequent milk ejection. In 1941 Ely and Peterson observed milk ejection in a denervated mammary gland perfused with blood to which posterior pituitary extract had been added.

Control of oxytocin secretion. Increased oxytocin secretion from the neurohypophysis occurs after suckling and during copulation or parturition. These are excellent examples of neuroendocrine reflexes. The afferent stimulus, suckling or cervical stimulation, is neural in nature, travels to the hypothalamic nuclei, and causes increased oxytocin release from the neurohypophysis.

Function of oxytocin. Milk ejection or "letdown" results from the contraction, stimulated by oxytocin, of the myoepithelial cells surrounding the alveoli.

It is generally agreed that oxytocin exerts a stimulatory effect upon the myometrium, provided the myometrium is under estrogen dominance; this occurs during the follicular phase of the estrous cycle and during the latter part of pregnancy. During the follicular phase of the cycle, mating results in release of oxytocin, which may aid sperm transport through increased uterine contractions. In late pregnancy, oxytocin-stimulated contractions of the uterus are useful in parturition. The assumption that oxytocin participates in the process of labor is supported by evidence that stretching the cervix induces a release of oxytocin and that the oxytocin activity of the blood of some mammals increases substantially during parturition. The uterus of the pregnant ewe or bitch, however, does not respond to this hormone unless labor has commenced. In the laying hen, arginine vasotocin causes an increase in intrauterine pressure and may be functionally involved in oviposition.

Extrapituitary oxytocin. In addition to secretion from the neurohypophysis, oxytocin is also synthesized and secreted by cells in the corpus luteum of the estrous cycle. In concert with estrogen and prostaglandin, this oxytocin is apparently involved in the dissolution of the corpus luteum after a cycle in which pregnancy did not occur. This will be discussed in Chapter 36.

Hormones of the adenohypophysis

Seven well-established hormones are secreted from the pars distalis of the adenohypophysis: FSH, LH, TSH, somatotropic hormone (growth hormone, STH), prolactin, ACTH, and beta-lipotropin. The secretion of the pars intermedia is less certain. Extracts of this area contain melanocyte-stimulating hormone (alpha and beta-MSH) and corticotropinlike intermediate peptide (CLIP), which are biologically active in suitable assay systems; It is unclear, however, whether these agents are secreted from the mammalian hypophysis.

Regulation of adenohypophyseal secretion

The afferent input that regulates the hormone output from the adenohypophysis is both humoral and neural and, like the neurohypophysis, is centered in the hypothalamus. Adenohypophyseal control, however, is mediated by the hypothalamic regulatory hormones. These hormones are synthesized in hypothalamic nuclei, transported to the median eminence by axon transport, and released into the primary capillary plexus; they reach the adenohypophysis via the long and short hypophyseal portal veins and stimulate or inhibit the secretion of the adenohypophyseal hormones. The hormone-secreting neurons of the hypothalamus are influenced by multiple neural inputs and, in most cases, are also affected by humoral stimuli. Many of these hypothalamic hormones have been found throughout the brain and in extraneural sites, such as the gastrointestinal tract and the pancreas; this has led to the suggestion that they should be termed *hypophysiotropic hormones*.

Hypothalamic hormones

Six hypothalamic regulatory hormones have been characterized:

1. Gonadotropin-releasing hormone (GnRH) is a decapeptide, pGlu-His-Trp-Ser-Tyr-Gly-Leu-Arg-Pro-Gly-NH_2, which stimulates the secretion of both FSH and LH. Evidence has been presented that differential secretion of FSH and LH is achieved by variations in the frequency and amplitude of GnRH pulses.

2. Thyrotropin-releasing hormone is a tripeptide, pGlu-His-Pro-NH_2, which stimulates the release of TSH. When injected, this hormone also stimulates the release of prolactin, but the physiological importance of this effect is unknown.

3. Dopamine, the catecholamine precursor of norepinephrine, has been established as the hypothalamic regulatory hormone that inhibits prolactin secretion. Dopamine also inhibits the secretion of TSH.

4. Somatostatin is a tetradecapeptide that contains a disulfide bridge and has the amino acid sequence Ala-Gly-Cys-Lys-Asn-Phe-Phe-Trp-Lys-Thr-Phe-Thr-Ser-Cys. Somatostatin inhibits STH secretion. This hormone is also found in the pancreas and gastrointestinal tract, where it exerts widespread inhibitory effects.

5. Growth hormone-releasing hormone is a 44 amino acid polypeptide that stimulates STH secretion.

6. Corticotropin-releasing hormone is a 41 amino acid polypeptide that stimulates release of all the peptide components from proopiomelanocortin. The adenohypophyseal response to corticotropin-releasing hormone is potentiated by both vasopressin and catecholamines.

Various substances have been reported to cause increased prolactin release. Of these, vasoactive intestinal peptide, a 28 amino acid polypeptide, best fulfils the role of a physiological prolactin-releasing hormone. Both stimulatory and inhibitory substances that affect MSH (MSH-RF and MSH-IF) have been found; both appear to be derivatives of oxytocin.

When the hypophyseal portal delivery of regulatory hormones is interrupted, either by section of the pituitary stalk or by transplantation of the hypophysis, there is a decrease in the secretion of all the adenohypophyseal hormones except prolactin, which, in mammals, is increased. In birds, the predominant hypothalamic regulation of prolactin appears to be stimulatory.

Humoral input

The best examples of relatively uncomplicated feedback in the control of efferent hypophyseal secretion are found in the secretions of the thyroid gland and the adrenal cortex. Suppression of the thyroid gland or adrenal cortex, either by chemical means or by removal, leads to an increased output of TSH and ACTH, respectively. Conversely, the administration of thyroid hormone or cortisol leads to a decreased secretion of these tropic hormones. One manifestation of feedback is the phenomenon of *compensatory hypertrophy*, which is exemplified by growth of the thyroid gland in response to a simple iodine deficiency. In such a case, the gland is unable to manufacture thyroid hormone, the pituitary gland is uninhibited, and increased TSH is secreted. As a result, the gland continues to undergo hypertrophy and hyperplasia, and the condition known as "goiter" results. The opposite effects can be demonstrated by sustained thyroxine administration, which results in inhibition of pituitary TSH and atrophy of the thyroid gland.

With respect to the gonadotropins, feedback is not so clear-cut. The striking elevation of blood gonadotropin concentration after castration has long been established, and it is well known that injection of sex hormones will depress pituitary gonadotropin output. The most active sex steroids in this regard are estrogens. Estrogen can act as a positive feedback agent as well as a negative one; during the proestrus phase of the estrous cycle, the progressive increase in estrogen secretion by the developing follicle stimulates increased GnRH secretion and sensitizes the adenohypophysis to the action of GnRH. The result is a sudden and massive increase in LH secretion, which culminates in ovulation. There is little doubt that progesterone is a potent inhibitor of ovulation during the luteal and gravid phases of the reproductive cycle. Exogenous administration of progesterone will inhibit ovulation in rats, guinea pigs, sheep, and cattle. In the male, castration results in increased secretion of both FSH and LH, but subsequent administration of testosterone lowers only the LH secretion. *Inhibin*, a water-soluble protein secreted by the Sertoli cells in the testis, is the FSH inhibitor.

The site at which target gland hormones feed back to regulate adenohypophyseal secretion is somewhat variable. It appears that thyroid hormones act primarily on the adenohypophysis itself, adrenal cortical hormones mostly inhibit through the hypothalamic hormones, and, as noted, gonadal hormones exert their action in both areas.

STH secretion is also regulated by hormonal afferents, but in this case the feedback agents are not hormones from specific target endocrine glands. In humans, hypoglycemia, prolonged fasting, exercise, and increased blood amino acid concentration will stimulate STH secretion. However, reports on the use of these stimuli to provide STH secretion in the dog have been conflicting. Somatomedins or insulinlike growth factors, peptides whose generation is STH-dependent, inhibit STH secretion at both the hypothalamic and adenohypophyseal levels.

Neural inputs

There are diverse neural inputs to the hypothalamic nuclei, which affect adenohypophyseal function. In the case of ACTH, circadian rhythm and stimuli reflecting stress to the animal override the cortisol feedback noted above. The circadian rhythm appears to be correlated with the activity of the animal; in animals that are active during the daylight hours, ACTH release begins to increase before awakening and reaches a peak during midmorning. The diurnal variation in ACTH and cortisol concentrations is not as evident in domestic animals as in humans and is obliterated by stressor stimuli such as restraint, pain, fear, or apprehension. STH secretion is also affected by sleep and stress; STH concentrations increase during the early hours of sleep and, as with ACTH, are increased by stress.

The increase in thyroid activity associated with exposure to cold and the decrease associated with high environmental temperatures are dependent on the hypothalamic-hypophyseal pathway but are mediated through neural afferents from the temperature-sensing center in the brain.

Neural stimuli are also well known in the control of reproduction. In animals such as the cat, rabbit, camel, and llama, stimulation of the cervix during copulation results in the LH surge that precedes ovulation. Seasonal reproductive cycles are initiated and terminated by neural pathways that sense light duration. Pheromones exert their effect on reproduction through afferents from the olfactory area. Prolactin secretion is increased after stimulation of the mammary nipples during suckling.

Chemistry of adenohypophyseal hormones

On the basis of chemical similarities, the hormones of the adenohypophysis can be divided into three groups: (1) the glycoproteins, (2) STH and prolactin, and (3) ACTH, β-LPH, and MSH.

The structure of the glycoproteins, FSH, LH, and TSH, involves a noncovalent bonding of two subunits. The alpha subunit is identical for the three glycoproteins and is inactive, whereas the beta subunits differ and contain the biological activity. When separated, administration of the beta subunit alone exhibits weak biological activity compared with the intact hormone. The alpha subunit of ovine LH consists of 96 amino acids with 5 disulfide bonds and 2 oligosaccharide units. The beta subunit includes 119 amino acids, 6 disulfide bonds, and 1 oligosaccharide unit.

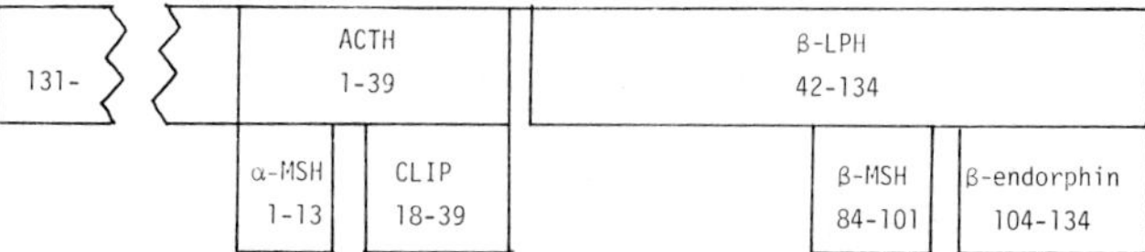

Figure 34.6. Diagram of the structure of pro-opiocortin showing the amino acid sequences of ACTH, β-LPH, α-MSH, CLIP, β-MSH, and β-endorphin. Met-enkephalin sequence occupies the positions 104–108. Numbering proceeds from approximately the center of the molecule, and the hormone-containing portion lies to the right, while the signal peptide is to the left.

STH and prolactin are large simple proteins with a molecular weight of about 22,000 and 190 amino acids with 1 or 2 disulfide bridges. There is considerable chemical similarity between STH and prolactin within a species but significant differences among species. Animals not only respond best to the homologous hormone but may produce antibodies against STH or prolactin from another species.

The corticotropes of the pars distalis and the cells of the pars intermedia synthesize a large precursor protein that is enzymatically degraded into several hormones and biologically active peptides. The precursor protein, *proopiocortin* (Fig. 34.6) is hydrolyzed in the pars distalis to ACTH and β-LPH, whereas in the pars intermedia the products a α-MSH and CLIP. The amino acid sequences of the endogenous opiates, β-endorphin and met-enkephalin, are found within β-LPH.

Role in reproduction

Prolactin and the pituitary gonadotropins, FSH and LH, exert their effects entirely on reproduction. Prolactin functions in the initiation and maintenance of lactation and, in some mammals, has a tropic effect on the corpus luteum. FSH and LH regulate the production of sex gametes and the secretion of hormones from the gonads. The specific effects of these hormones are discussed in Chapters 35 to 38.

Function of adrenocorticotropic hormone

The administration of ACTH to normal animals or animals subjected to hypophysectomy results in increased adrenocortical activity. There is an increased secretion of adrenocortical steroids into the adrenal vein, a loss of lipid from the adrenocortical cells, decreased adrenal cholesterol and ascorbic acid concentrations, adrenal hypertrophy and hyperplasia, and an increase in adrenal blood flow. Prolonged pituitary insufficiency leads to decreased adrenocortical responsiveness to ACTH, and repeated ACTH administration is necessary to elicit increased glucocorticoid secretion. The fact that hypertrophy and hyperplasia after ACTH administration are limited to the zona reticularis and zona fasciculata and that the increased steroid secretion consists of cortisol and corticosterone leads to the conclusion that ACTH is of no importance in the control of aldosterone secretion from the zona glomerulosa. ACTH will stimulate the production of aldosterone, however, and there is evidence that aldosterone secretion is initiated by ACTH after acute blood loss or a similar severe stress. Injected ACTH is more effective in stimulating aldosterone output if the dietary content of sodium has been low. ACTH acts, through adenylate cyclase, to increase cholesterol conversion to pregnenolone and stimulates the 17-hydroxylation of progesterone.

It is probable that the effects of ACTH are not limited to the adrenal gland. The following changes have been observed when ACTH has been administered to animals after adrenalectomy: mobilization of nonesterified fatty acids and neutral fats from the fat depots, enhanced ketogenesis, increased muscle glycogen, hypoglycemia, and decreased plasma amino acid concentration. ACTH also prolongs the biological half-life of cortisol injected in animals after adrenalectomy. These effects and those of STH are interrelated in the so-called "diabetogenic" action of crude pituitary extracts.

Function of thyroid-stimulating hormone

When TSH is administered to experimental animals, both morphological and functional changes are seen in the thyroid gland. The height of the alveolar epithelium is increased, and the stored colloid becomes vacuolated and depleted. After hypophysectomy, there is a decrease in all the functional aspects of thyroid physiology, including the accumulation of iodine, the organic binding of iodine, the formation of thyroid hormones, and the release of thyroid hormones into the circulation. Administration of TSH reverses these effects. While TSH affects all aspects of thyroid hormone synthesis and release, its principal action appears to be on colloid endocytosis and hormone release. There is no convincing evidence of normal extrathyroidal activity of TSH.

Function of growth hormone

Anabolic effects

A variety of endocrine and paracrine agents are involved in the control of growth. Of these, STH is primary during the period from birth to maturity. In the intact animal, pituitary hormones join with other endocrine and paracrine secretions to achieve coordinated body growth. After hypophysectomy, however, STH is the most potent agent in increasing the reduced growth rate in the animal in which adrenal, thyroid, and gonadal function is markedly impaired. Furthermore, STH is the only hormone capable of stimulating increased and abnormally rapid growth in the intact animal. The effects of STH are observed particularly in bone, cartilage, muscle, kidney, and liver. The epiphyseal disks of long bones are very sensitive to STH. In fact, the best bioassay method for growth hormone involves measurement of an increase in the width of the epiphyseal disk of the rat tibia. Mitotic activity is stimulated in growing bones, and elevated osteoblastic activity can be observed. Most of the anabolic actions of STH are effected through peripheral peptides, the somatomedins. Two principal somatomedins, A and C, have been identified; both bear a structural resemblance to insulin and are sometimes called insulinlike growth factors II and I. The liver appears to be an important source of somatomedin synthesis. These rather small peptides (molecular weight of about 7500) circulate in the plasma bound to a large plasma protein; dissociation occurs at sites of elevated hydrogen ion concentration. Circulating somatomedin concentrations can be decreased by the administration of estrogens and certain other synthetic steroids. Because of the diminished negative feedback, this may account for the excessive STH secretion in dogs given medroxyprogesterone.

In addition to these two somatomedians, several peripheral growth factors have been described. These include nerve growth factor, ovarian growth factor, platelet-derived growth factor, epidermal growth factor, and fibroblast growth factor.

Cellular effects of growth hormone deficiency and administration are readily observed in the liver cells. Hypophysectomy causes a decrease in cell size, nuclear and cytoplasmic RNA, and nuclear and cytoplasmic protein. STH reverses these changes. A direct anabolic effect of STH is indicated by the increased uptake of radioactively labeled amino acids when STH is added to an in vitro diaphragm preparation.

In the normal animal, if one kidney is removed, there is a compensatory hypertrophy of the other kidney; this will not occur in the absence of STH. In addition, STH appears to affect the kidney in a manner not entirely related to growth alone. Hypophysectomy causes a decreased glomerular filtration rate, a diminished renal blood flow, and reduced tubular secretion. These defects are corrected by the administration of STH and thyroid hormone but not by thyroid hormone alone.

Growth in the central nervous system appears to be relatively independent of growth hormone, as is the growth of the thyroid, adrenals, and gonads.

Studies in the lactating cow reveal an interesting galactopoietic effect after the injection of STH. A highly significant and linear relationship has been demonstrated between the *logarithm of the dose* of STH and an increase in milk yield. This effect is probably due to growth of the mammary gland. The availability of commercial synthetic bovine growth hormone, through recombinant DNA technology, may prove to be important in both dairy and beef production.

Catabolic effects

In muscle and adipose tissue, growth hormone acts as an antagonist to insulin; animals that have undergone hypophysectomy are quite sensitive to insulin administration.

This antagonism assumes increased importance in view of the possibility that hypoglycemia stimulates STH secretion. Growth hormone, in the presence of cortisol, has the ability to mobilize fat from adipose tissue and increase the blood level of the so-called "ketone bodies." These diabetogenic properties are similar to changes seen in fasting and may be an adaptation to reduced food intake. In the dog and cat, excessive growth hormone results in damage to the insulin-secreting cells of the pancreatic islets, which further enhances ketogenesis through insulin deprivation.

Function of melanocyte-stimulating hormone and beta-lipotropin

Many species of reptiles, amphibians, and fish show a marked color change in response to changes in illumination, temperature, or humidity. This color change results from the dispersion or concentration of pigment granules in the melanophores. This phenomenon is at least partially due to a hormone secreted by the pars intermedia of the adenohypophysis and named *intermedin* or *melanocyte-stimulating hormone* (MSH). Many of these observations resulted from studies using mammalian pars intermedia, but no function has been established for this hormone in warm-blooded animals.

In the pars intermedia, α-MSH and β-MSH are cleaved from ACTH and β-LPH, respectively. Cleavage of ACTH also produces CLIP (Fig. 34.6), a fragment with corticotropinlike activity. Increased circulating concentrations of this fragment may be responsible for the signs of adrenocortical hyperfunction that have been observed in horses with tumors of the pars intermedia.

Although the physiological role of β-LPH is as yet unknown, the occurrence of the amino acid sequences of β-endorphin and met-enkephalin within β-LPH and the discovery of opiate receptors in the central nervous system suggest that this hormone may act as a prohormone for the endogenous opiates. Since ACTH and β-LPH are released in response to the same stimuli, it is possible that these opiates effect a neural response to stress.

PINEAL GLAND

Although the existence of the pineal body (epiphysis cerebri) has been known since the second century AD, its function has remained obscure. In the frog, it appears to be a photoreceptor, and bovine pineal glands contain a factor that blanches pigment cells in tadpoles. This skin factor, *melatonin* (N-acetyl-5-methoxytryptamine), has been isolated and identified, and only the pineal gland has the enzyme necessary for melatonin synthesis.

The delayed sexual development associated with pineal tumors in children led to the speculation that the pineal gland was inhibitory to the gonads. Evidence that supports this concept has accumulated. The increased ovarian weight and shortened estrous cycles that result when rats are exposed to continuous illumination can be duplicated by pinealectomy whereas, conversely, the injection of pineal extracts or melatonin results in decreased ovarian weight and lengthened cycles. Further, sectioning of the sympathetic nerves to the pineal counters the effect of constant lighting. On the basis of these findings and experiments in which the pineal was studied under different lighting schedules, it has been suggested that light impinging on the retina causes a change in the sympathetic output of the anterior cervical ganglion, which then inhibits pineal melatonin synthesis and release. There has been demonstrated a daily rhythmic activity in melatonin synthesis, which is entirely dependent on environmental lighting. However, melatonin secretion occurs during the dark in both daylight-activity animals and nocturnal animals; thus the pineal gland acts, basically, to relay light-dark information to the hypothalamus or adenohypophysis, whatever the activity or reproductive pattern.

THYROID GLAND

The thyroid gland is unique among endocrine glands in that its secretion, the thyroid hormones, include in their structure a specific chemical element, *iodine*. The function of the thyroid gland involves the concentration of iodide and the synthesis, storage, and secretion of the thyroid hormone. Although salivary and mammary glands accumulate iodine, the amount accumulated is of little significance compared with that which is trapped by the thyroid gland. More than 90 percent of administered iodine can be accounted for by thyroid uptake and urinary excretion.

Morphology

The thyroid gland is one of the first endocrine glands to appear in the developing individual. In the human, pig, and rabbit, the embryonic thyroid gland is functional at approximately midterm. In the chick, function begins on the seventh to ninth day of incubation. In most mammals, the thyroid lies just caudal to the larynx on the first or second tracheal ring and consists of two lateral lobes connected by a narrow isthmus. In birds, the thyroid consists of two lobes lying on either side of the trachea at the level of the clavicle.

Microscopically, the thyroid gland contains numerous closely packed small sacs filled with a clear, viscous fluid. The sacs or follicles are lined simple epithelium that varies from squamous in inactive glands to tall columnar in more active thyroids. On fixation and staining with hematoxylin and eosin, the material with the follicle is seen as a noncellular, homogeneous, acidophilic mass, which is sometimes vacuolated. Cytological features are sometimes used as criteria of the functional state of the gland. In active glands the colloid is nonuniform, may be somewhat basophilic, and usually contains numerous vacuoles; the height of the lining epithelium increases, and the number of secretory droplets in the follicular cells is increased. Electron microscopy has revealed numerous filamentous villi projecting from the

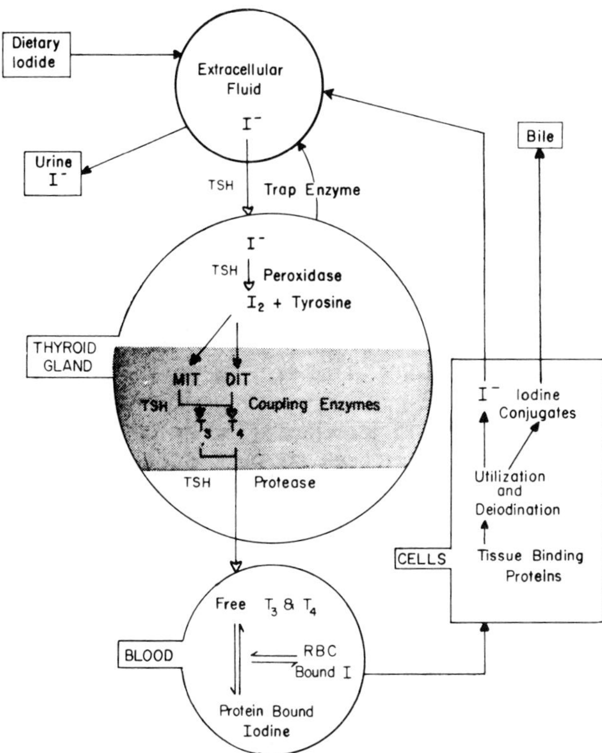

Figure 34.7. Major pathways of iodine metabolism (shaded area indicates thyroglobulin).

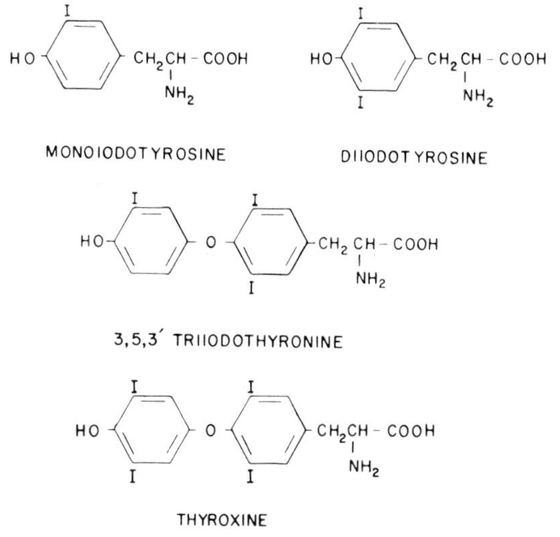

MONOIODOTYROSINE

DIIODOTYROSINE

3,5,3′ TRIIODOTHYRONINE

THYROXINE

Figure 34.8. Structural formulas of the iodinated amino acids in the thyroid gland.

follicular cells into the lumen. These microvilli afford a great increase in the inner surface area of the follicles.

Metabolism of iodine

Iodide trap

Iodine occurs throughout the animal body, but a very high percentage of the total amount is concentrated in the thyroid gland (Fig. 34.7) despite the fact that this gland constitutes only 0.2 percent of the body weight. Iodine is present in animal tissue in two forms: inorganic iodide and organically bound iodine. Iodide occurs in extremely low concentration, around 1 to 2 μg/dl of blood serum, except in the dog, in which the serum contains 5 to 10 μg/dl. The levels of organically bound iodine vary greatly and may reach 500 mg/100 g in the desiccated thyroid gland. Many forms of organically bound iodine are found, including monoiodotyrosine (MIT), diiodotyrosine (DIT), triiodothyronine (T_3), reverse triiodothyronine (rT_3), and thyroxine (T_4) (Fig. 34.8).

Iodide accumulation in the thyroid gland is expressed in terms of the thyroid uptake (the percentage of administered iodine accumulating within the gland) or by the T/S ratio, which is the ratio of concentration of iodide in the thyroid to that in the blood serum. Thyroid accumulation of iodine is measured by the administration of radioactive iodine and subsequent counting of radioactivity over the thyroid area. Results with this technique are somewhat variable and depend on the time that has elapsed since administration and on the counting equipment. The normal T/S ratio is about 25 and may increase to 500 when the gland is being stimulated by TSH. The ratio may decrease to 1 if thyroid inhibitors are administered.

Previous administration or ingestion of iodine-containing compounds greatly affects both thyroid uptake and T:S ratio.

Certain chemical radicals, thiocyanate, perchlorate, or nitrate inhibit the operation of the thyroid iodide trap. Since this inhibition can be reversed by large doses of iodide, it is thought that these radicals compete with iodide for some component of the trapping mechanism.

Synthesis of thyroid hormones

After the iodide is accumulated in the thyroid gland, it is oxidized to iodine in a reaction that is probably mediated by a peroxidase enzyme. The iodine is then transported to the lumen of the thyroid follicle, where it iodinates tyrosine molecules located on the surface of the luminal colloid. The luminal colloid consists of a glycoprotein called thyroglobulin, which has a molecular weight of 660,000. Tyrosine is iodinated to form MIT and DIT. The coupling of the iodotyrosines to form iodothyronines has two possible routes—the combination of two DIT molecules to form T_4 or the combination of one DIT with one MIT to form T_3 (3,5,3′ triiodothyronine) or rT_3 (3,3,5′ triiodothyronine). The likelihood that these reactions are enzymatically controlled is indicated by the fact that cell-free supernatant fluid of centrifuged homogenized thyroid tissue is unable to promote protein iodination beyond the MIT stage; the enzyme involved appears to be a thyroid peroxidase.

The organic binding of iodine into compounds that have

thyroid hormone activity is also inhibited by certain chemical agents. These will be described later.

Release and transport of thyroid hormone

Secretion of thyroid hormones is initiated by endocytosis of colloid near the inner surface of the thyroid cell. The ingested droplets of colloid are then degraded by lysosomal enzymes releasing the iodinated amino acids.

Two of the iodinated amino acids, T_3 and T_4, are secreted into the bloodstream. The two iodotyrosines are deiodinated within the gland by an enzyme that has been termed deiodinase. This cycle, which is intrathyroidal, reclaims the iodine from tyrosine. In the canine, intrathyroidal "scavenging" of iodide from the iodotyrosines is much less apparent than in the human. Of the two iodinated thyronines, thyroxine is predominant in all animals; approximately 33 percent of the total iodine in the gland is in the form of T_4, and usually less than 10 percent is in the form of T_3.

If radioactive iodine is injected into an animal and a blood sample is assayed for iodine activity after a suitable period of time, this activity is found to reside for the most part in the blood proteins. There is considerable species variation in the specific binding proteins and in the binding affinity for T_3 and T_4. In humans, thyroid hormones are primarily bound to a globulin called thyroid-binding globulin (TBG) with secondary binding onto albumin and a prealbumin fraction. Binding proteins are similar in sheep, goat, and cattle plasma. In the horse and dog, in addition to albumin binding, there are multiple globulins that bind T_3 and T_4. In the human, a very low percentage of hormone circulates unbound (about 0.03 percent of T_4 and 0.3 percent of T_3). In canine plasma, the binding proteins have 100 to 200 times less affinity; thus, though most of the circulating hormone is bound, free hormone concentrations in the dog exceed those in humans.

Most of the circulating T_3 is derived from peripheral deiodination of T_4 by the enzyme 5′-deiodinase. The inhibition of this enzyme by fasting, illness, or the administration of glucocorticoids or propylthiouracil, an antithyroid drug, will increase the T_4/T_3 ratio. Low circulating T_3 is also found in fetal or umbilical cord plasma. In such cases, the deiodination of T_4 increases but the product becomes rT_3, a biologically inactive triiodothyronine. The converse, decreased T_4/T_3 ratios, is common with iodine deficiency; in this case, however, the increased T_3 arises from preferential thyroid gland secretion of T_3 as opposed to T_4. Further, in hyperthyroidism, T_3 secretion may increase to a greater extent than T_4.

The in vivo potency of T_3 is about 3 times that of T_4. This and the lesser binding affinity of blood proteins for T_3 have led to the suggestion that T_4 is a prohormone. There is, evidence, however, that T_4 has intrinsic biological activity that is not dependent on conversion to T_3.

Table 34.3 lists total T_4 concentrations and T_4/T_3 ratios in the plasma of euthyroid animals for seven domestic species and for humans. It should be emphasized that in the diagnosis of thyroid dysfunction, measurement of total T_4 or T_3 concentration must be interpreted with caution. There is considerable variability with age, breed, environmental temperature, nutritional status, and health as well as a wide range of "normal" values. Further, total measurements do not reflect the free hormone concentration, which is the element of importance to the target cells.

Table 34.3. Total serum thyroxine and T_4/T_3 ratio in domestic animals

Animal	N	T_4 (μg/dl + SD)	Source	T_4/T_3*
Dog	20	1.12 + 0.14	Kelley and Oehme 1974	16
Cat	40	0.95 + 0.50	Ling et al 1974	34
Horse	157	1.57 + 0.62	Thomas and Adams 1978	21
Pig	10	3.32 + 0.80	Reap et al 1978	37
Goat	10	3.45 + 0.47	Reap et al 1978	24
Sheep	12	3.70 + 0.60	Sutherland and Irvine 1973	44
Cattle	19	4.28 + 0.17	Kelley and Oehme 1974	67
Human	1141	6.2 + 1.7	Murphy 1969	67

*Data from Reap et al. 1978.

Distribution and fate of thyroid hormones

Thyroxine and triiodothyronine have been detected in almost every tissue of the body. Skeletal muscle and liver represent the major extravascular extrathyroidal stores. Intracellular metabolic conversions of T_3 and T_4 include (1) deiodination by 5′-deiodinase and 5-deiodinase, (2) deamination, alone or in conjunction with oxidation or decarboxylation, and (3) glucuronide or sulfate conjugation. Not all of these transformations occur in all tissues; for example, skeletal muscle can only deiodinate, whereas all the conversions listed take place in the liver. Glucuronide and sulfate conjugations are regarded as detoxifying mechanisms and take place principally in the liver. These esters are excreted in the bile. Subsequent intestinal degradation of the esters and reabsorption of iodide into the bloodstream is termed the *enterohepatic cycle*. As with the intrathyroidal recovery of iodide from MIT and DIT, this process is much more efficient in the human than in the dog.

Effects of thyroid hormones

Thyroid hormones influence virtually every organ in the body. The effects of these hormones can be roughly divided into two sections: (1) growth and development and (2) metabolic.

Effects on growth and development

Growth and differentiation. One of the most striking effects of thyroid hormones is their effect on metamorphosis in amphibian larvae. If thyroxine is administered to tadpoles, they will become miniature frogs, whereas thyroidectomy will produce giant tadpoles. While thyroid-induced metamorphosis is restricted to amphibians, thyroid hormones will cause maturational changes in other vertebrates. In young birds and mammals, removal of the thyroid gland is followed by slowing or stoppage of growth, and the administration of thyroxine counteracts this effect. If growth hormone is given to thyroidectomized animals, there is an increased growth rate, largely through stimulation of the epiphyseal cartilage, but little differentiation occurs. If, however, thyroxine is given to an animal that was deprived of its pituitary gland at an early age, there will be rapid differentiation and ossification of the epiphyses with no appreciable effect on length. Although the effects of thyroid hormone are primarily on differentiation, it should be pointed out again that the maximum growth rate of animals after hypophysectomy is obtained with the injection of both STH and thyroxine rather than STH alone. The growth and eruption of the teeth are also under thyroid control, as are the horns of sheep and the antlers of deer. Hypothyroidism severely retards the eruption of permanent teeth.

Feathers, skin, and hair. Thyroidectomy will usually inhibit the molting of feathers, whereas thyroxine injection favors it. It appears as if, insofar ar this function is concerned, the thyroid operates in conjunction with the sex steroids. The regeneration of feathers after the molt is again stimulated by thyroxine in conjunction with steroid hormones. It is possible that the two hormones act in sequence, so that one causes the feather germ cell to be receptive to the action of the other ("permissive action"). Another example of cooperation between sex steroids and the thyroid is seen in the rooster, in which thyroidectomy results regressive changes in the comb that cannot be repaired by the administration of testosterone.

In mammals, both skin and hair are affected by thyroid changes. After thyroidectomy cattle and sheep have thinner hair, and the individual hairs are coarse and brittle. It appears that the normal development of the wool-producing follicles of sheep requires thyroxine in excess of that needed for growth; thus a thyroid deficiency in the growing lamb may severely impair the quality of the adult fleece. In humans and dogs, the subcutaneous edema of mucopolysaccharide-rich material is responsible for the name *myxedema* which has been used in hypothyroid individuals. Myxedema and alopecia have also been observed in calves and pigs born to iodine-deficient mothers.

Reproduction. The relationship between the thyroid and the gonads in both male and female animals is of particular interest. Reproductive failure is often a major sign of deficiency, and the birth of excessive numbers of weak or dead young has been noted in goitrous areas (iodine-deficient soils) for many years. Abortion, stillbirth, and the live birth of weak young are major results of hypothyroidism. Less severe deficiencies will result in delayed puberty, irregular estrus, and anestrus in females. It has been reported, however, that hypothyroid females ovulate and are fertile if bred at the proper time. In the male, thyroidectomy results in decreased testicular growth, impaired spermatogenesis, and lowered libido. In rams, a seasonal reduction in semen quality has been associated with hypothyroidism.

An accessory reproductive gland that appears to be sensitive to the effect of the thyroid hormones is the mammary gland. Thyroxine has been thought to be a powerful galactopoietic agent, and thyromimetic compounds have been used to increase milk production. Artificially iodinated casein (equivalent to 0.5 percent crystalline thyroxine) has been fed to dairy cattle at a rate of 1 to 1.5 g per 45 kg of body weight daily, resulting in an increase in milk production of 10 to 30 percent. To achieve this, addition of thyroactive substances must be accompanied by an increase of approximately 20 percent in the daily energy intake. Despite this additional intake, decreases in body weight have been noted when thyroprotein was fed. Control cows fed at 125 percent TDN (total digestible nutrients) achieved lactation levels as high as those given thyroprotein. A disadvantage of feeding thyroprotein in an effort to increase milk production is the increased susceptibility of these animals to high environmental temperature; instances of severe heat exhaustion have been reported in such situations.

Nervous system. The nervous system is particularly affected by a severe alteration in thyroid function. Hypothyroidism is prenatal animals results in defective brainstem-cortical connections, deficient axonal dendritic branching, delayed myelinization, reduced central nervous system (CNS), enzymes, retention of the immature external granular zone of the cerebellum, and decreased brain weight. It has been shown that thyroid hormones are instrumental in the generation of nerve growth factor; this may explain some of the neural changes that result from prenatal hypothyroidism.

Metabolic effects

Thermogenesis and increased oxygen consumption. The best-known function of thyroid hormones in the mammal is their ability to increase the rate of oxygen consumption. This and the increased thyroid activity that follows low environmental temperature support the hypothesis that the thyroid hormones are involved in thermoregulation by increasing internal heat production. Oxygen consumption is low in tissues removed from hypothyroid animals but high in those from hyperthyroid animals.

Stimulation of metabolic rate by thyroid hormones can be explained, to a great extent, by increased production of Na^+-K^+ ATPase. Increased oxygen consumption is correlated closely with increased sodium transport and inhibition of Na^+-K^+ ATPase by ouabain abolishes this response by thyroid hormone. As a result of increased ATP hydrolysis, there is increased mitochondrial oxidative metabolism; there is also evidence of a direct effect of thyroid hormone on the mitochondria.

The calorigenic effect is generally correlated with the number of nuclear T_3 receptors, but in the brain in which such receptors are present no thermogenic response is seen. Retina and testis are also unresponsive to thyroid hormone.

Nerve and muscle. Nerve function at all levels is influenced by the thyroid. Injection of thyroxine causes increased spontaneous electrical activity in the brain, a decreased threshold of sensitivity to a variety of stimuli, decreased reflex time, and increased neuromuscular irritability.

Both hypothyroidism and hyperthyroidism are characterized by disturbances in muscle tissue. In hyperthyroidism, a negative nitrogen balance and creatinuria suggest a rapid metabolism of muscle protein and an impairment of creatinine production from creatine. The "energy" of the hyperthyroid animal is apparent rather than real, and these animals require twice the usual amount of oxygen and nutrients to accomplish a given amount of muscle work. Muscular hypotonus is characteristic of low thyroid activity.

Interaction with catecholamines. There is a very important relationship between thyroid hormones and the catecholamines, epinephrine and norepinephrine. The lipolytic effect of epinephrine is markedly potentiated by the administration of thyroid hormones, and thyrotoxic animals cannot tolerate normal doses of epinephrine. Pharmacological blockade of the adrenergic nerves inhibits the calorigenic action of thyroid hormone and, *propranolol*, a beta-adrenergic blocking agent, has been used in the treatment of hyperthyroidism. The catecholamine-thyroid interaction can be explained in part by thyroid hormone inhibition of monoamineoxidase and by increased numbers of beta-adrenergic receptors stimulated by T_3 or T_4.

Effects on metabolic enzymes. Thyroid hormones stimulate or activate certain key enzymes. In addition to Na^+-K^+ ATPase, already noted, these include α-glycerol phosphate dehydrogenase, hexokinase, malic enzyme (a decarboxylase), citric cleavage enzyme, diphosphoglycerate mutase, and cytochromes b and c. In hypothyroid birds, inhibition of trimethylamine oxidation is thought to be responsible for "tainted" eggs. The conversion of carotene to vitamin A also requires adequate thyroid secretion.

It has been suggested that thyroid hormones stimulate catabolic pathways and inhibit anabolic pathways. These hormones stimulate hepatic glycolysis, increase glucogenesis and gluconeogenesis, enhance lipolysis, and decrease sensitivity to the actions of the antilipolytic action of insulin. Further, T_3 and T_4 appear to stimulate growth hormone secretion and there is evidence that glucagon lipolysis is decreased in hypothyroid animals.

The administration of thyroxine in high doses for a sustained period of time will accelerate protein catabolism and result in a negative nitrogen balance accompanied by diuresis. Since this diuresis occurs together with increased urinary potassium, it is probably secondary to the protein catabolism. In the hypothyroid, myxedematous individual, the administration of thyroxine results in increased protein synthesis and marked diuresis; this apparently results from the mobilization of the extracellular myxedema fluid.

Mechanism of action

The most accessible and most studied indicator of thyroid function is the effect of thyroid hormones on tissue oxygen consumption. For many years, it was thought that thyroid hormones exerted their effect by uncoupling oxidation and phosphorylation. The swelling of the mitochondria after the addition of thyroxine perhaps altered the internal spatial relationships of the mitochondria and impeded phosphorylation. However, the uncoupling effect could be produced only by high concentrations of thyroid hormones in vitro or after the administration of toxic doses to the animal (1 to 2 percent thyroid powder in the diet); no uncoupling, loss of respiratory control, or mitochondrial swelling could be produced when hypermetabolism was induced with small amounts of hormone. As previously noted, there is evidence of direct thyroid hormone action on mitochondria. It is now thought that the calorigenic effects result from increased nuclear transcription of mRNA coding for Na^+-K^+ ATPase.

Antithyroid compounds

Enlargement of the thyroid, known as "goiter," can be associated with hypothyroidism, euthyroidism, or hyperthyroidism (Fig. 34.9). Simple iodine-deficient goiter, formerly the leading type of goiter in farm animals, has been virtually eliminated through the use of iodized salt. However, certain foodstuffs contain substances that inhibit thyroid activity. The cruciferous plants (cabbage, kale, rutabaga, turnip, rapeseed) contain a compound, progoitrin, that is converted in the gastrointestinal tract to a potent antithyroid compound, goitrin (Fig. 34.10). In addition, many of these plants contain other goitrogens such as thiocyanate. In some parts of the world (e.g., Australia and Finland) plant goitrogens are of importance in animal goiters and, because of their secretion into milk, are also of interest with respect to the human goiter that is endemic to these areas. Certainly, the ingestion of goitrogenic material increases the iodine requirement.

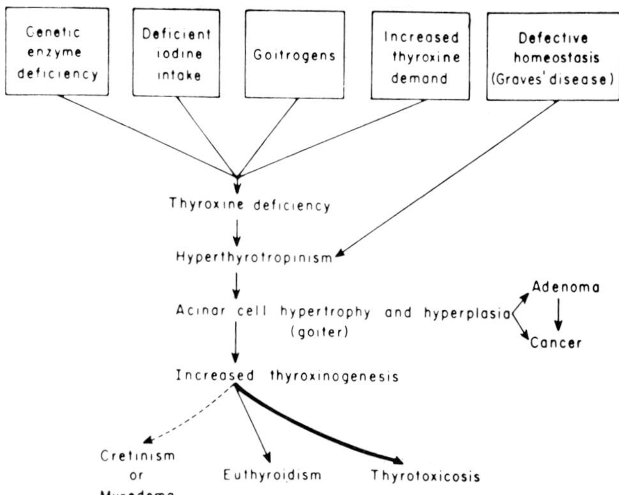

Figure 34.9. Mechanism of goitrogenesis. (From Williams and Bakke 1962, in Williams, ed., *Textbook of Endocrinology,* 3d ed., W.B. Saunders, Philadelphia.)

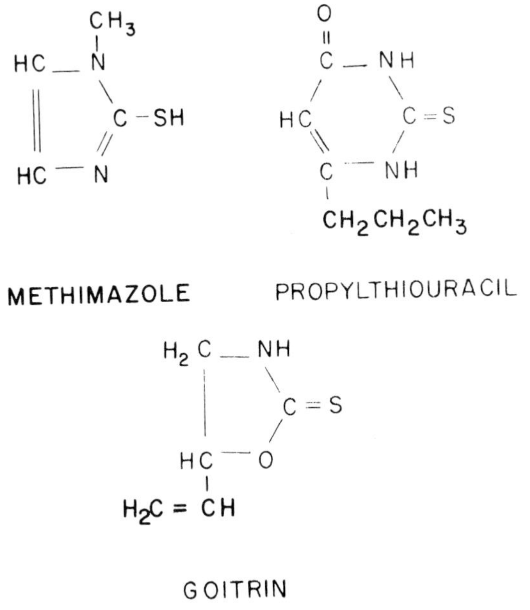

METHIMAZOLE

PROPYLTHIOURACIL

GOITRIN

Figure 34.10. Chemical structure of two commonly used antithyroid agents (methimazole and propylthiouracil) and that of the most important natural goitrogen (goitrin).

Since thiocyanate and other chemical radicals interfere with the trapping of iodide (Fig. 34.7) by the thyroid gland, the goitrogenicity of these radicals can be overcome by the feeding of excess iodide. It is more difficult to overcome the effect of goitrin and related compounds, however, since they interfere with the organic binding of iodine but not with the iodine trap. An important outcome of studies of antithyroid activities in plants has been the development of a series of potent antithyroid drugs with therapeutic value in the treatment of hyperthyroidism. The compounds that exert the most potent antithyroid activity are the thiocarbamides (Fig. 34.10). These thiourea and thiouracil compounds all inhibit the conversion of iodide to iodine, the organic binding of molecular iodine with tyrosine, and the conversion of T_4 to T_3. Other antithyroid drugs include the sulfonamides, *p*-aminosalicylic acid, amphenone, phenylbutazone, and chlorpromazine.

Thyroid dysfunction

Thyroid dysfunction is relatively uncommon in sheep, cattle, and swine. Occasionally a severe iodine deficiency or the excessive ingestion of goitrogenic foodstuffs during gestation results in the birth of dead or weak young, but thyroid disease in the adult is seldom diagnosed. Subclinical hypothyroidism has been suggested as a factor in decreased libido in the male and silent estrus in the female.

In the horse, neoplasia of the thyroid is relatively common in older animals but is not usually accompanied by clinical signs. On the basis of seasonal occurrence, breed incidence, and clinical signs, chronic laminitis in horses feeding on lush green pasture has been related to hypothyroidism, and the administration of thyroid extract in such cases has been recommended.

Table 34.4. Clinical signs of thyroid dysfunction in the dog

Hyperthyroidism	Hypothyroidism
Polyuria	Alopecia
Polyphagia	Dry, dull, coarse hair
Weight loss	Hyperpigmentation
Weakness and fatigue	Lethargy
Heat sensitivity	Cold sensitivity
Nervousness	Myxedema (facial primarily)
Tachycardia	Anemia (normocytic, normochromic)
Heart murmurs	Hypercholesterolemia
	Galactorrhea*

*Probably occurs because of excess TRH, which stimulates prolactin.

The clinical signs of hypothyroidism and hyperthyroidism in the dog are listed in Table 34.4. Hypothyroidism in this species is not uncommon but is rarely due to iodine deficiency. Although the cause is not known, circulating antibodies to thyroglobulin have been found. Hyperthyroidism appears to result from functional thyroid tumors; clinical signs are usually relatively mild.

Hyperthyroidism is said to be the most common endocrine disorder in old cats. The signs are similar to those in the dog and include hyperactivity, weight loss, polydipsia, and tachycardia. Hypothyroidism in this species is less common and is difficult to detect.

One of the major metabolic results of thyroid deficiency is an increase in the serum cholesterol level. This finding has been used by clinicians as a "suggestive" indicator of hypothyroidism; however, cholesterol synthesis is increased in thyroxine excess and reduced in thyroxine deficiency. These contradictory observations have been attributed to decreased biliary excretion of cholesterol in hypothyroid animals, causing increased blood cholesterol despite reduced synthesis.

Obesity and hypothyroidism

The total fat content of the body is eventually decreased in animals that have a marked thyroid deficiency, and there is little evidence to support the concept of thyroid obesity. In fact, weight loss in obese animals is accompanied by decreased plasma T_3, whereas overfeeding increases T_3. The relationship of the thyroid to fat deposition has been of interest to livestock producers in their search for a means of improving meat quality and increasing the efficiency of weight gain. Feeding trials after partial thyroidectomy or the administration of thyroid inhibitors have not resulted in sufficient improvement to justify these practices.

HORMONES ASSOCIATED WITH CALCIUM AND SKELETAL METABOLISM

The movement of calcium in and out of the skeleton and the maintenance of proper calcium concentration in the extracellular and intracellular fluid are essential for many critical body functions. The regulation of calcium concentration and dynamic bone remodeling is the responsibility of three hormones: *parathyroid hormone* (also called parathormone or PTH) from the parathyroid gland, *calcitonin* (CT) from the parafollicular cells within the thyroid gland, and 1,25-*dihydroxycholecalciferol* (1,25-DHCC) which is a derivative of vitamin D.

PARATHYROID GLAND

The parathyroid glands were first adequately described in 1880 by Sandstrom, and in 1891 Gley proved that a complete thyroidectomy was not fatal if the parathyroids were left intact. In 1909 MacCallum and Voegtlin related the parathyroid to calcium metabolism by alleviating the signs of thyroparathyroidectomy with the administration of calcium salts.

Morphology

In domestic animals, parathyroid glands consist of one or two pairs of beanlike organs located within or near the thyroid gland. In dogs, cats, and ruminants the caudal pair of glands are located just within the thyroid gland at the medial surface, and in the horse this pair of glands lie near the bifurcation of the carotid trunk. The cranial pair of glands lie anterior to the thyroid in the ruminants and the horse, and they are found at the craniolateral pole of the thyroid gland in the dog and cat. The pig has a single pair of parathyroid glands lying just anterior to the thyroid.

Microscopically, the epithelial cells of the parathyroid have been divided into various types. In general, however, in most species there are two cell types; chief cells and oxyphil cells. Other cell types are thought to represent differing degrees of secretory activity of the chief cell. It appears that chief cells are the source of parathormone and parathyroid secretory protein. The function of the oxyphil cells is not known.

Chemistry of parathyroid hormone

PTH is a simple straight-chain polypeptide of 84 amino acids and has a molecular weight of 9500. It is initially synthesized by chief cell ribosomes as the 115–amino acid precursor, preproPTH. Proteolytic cleavage of the NH_2-terminal 25 amino acids converts preproPTH to proPTH, which moves through the endoplasmic reticulum to the Golgi apparatus, where it is enzymatically degraded to PTH by removal of the NH_2-terminal hexapeptide. Active PTH may be secreted directly or packaged into secretory granules. The secretory granules also contain a large protein, parathyroid secretory protein, which is analogous to the neurophysins secreted by the pars nervosa in that it is secreted in concert with PTH.

Regulation of parathyroid secretion

The parathyroid glands, together with the pancreatic islets, exemplify direct humoral control of endocrine activity by a specific blood constituent. Low-calcium diets lead to hypertrophy and hyperplasia of the parathyroid glands, and perfusion of the parathyroids with calcium-free blood results in the appearance of PTH in the glandular effluent. Hypercalcemia, on the other hand, inhibits PTH secretion. Although ionized calcium is the main regulatory agent, PTH secretion is also stimulated by low magnesium levels and by sympathetic neural discharge or epinephrine.

Effect of parathyroid hormone on bone

If a fragment of bone is placed immediately adjacent to a parathyroid gland, the part of the bone next to the gland dissolves after several weeks and the part away from the gland proliferates. Tissues other than parathyroid do not produce this effect. If an animal is injected with radioactive calcium during a rapid growth period and given PTH after the calcium has stabilized into bone, considerable radioactivity is released into the blood. This experiment clearly indicates that PTH is able to mobilize calcium from bone. The increase in proline and hydroxyproline in the blood after PTH treatment suggests that PTH affects the ground substance of bone as well as the mineral components.

In vitro histological changes that occur in bone growth in tissue culture next to parathyroid tissue include (1) disappearance of typical osteoblasts, (2) formation of multinuclear osteoclasts, (3) dissolusion of bone matrix, and (4) proliferation of connective tissue on the side of the bone opposite the parathyroid tissue. These changes are similar to those observed in vivo in *osteitis fibrosa cystica*, which often results from a functional parathyroid adenoma.

The action of PTH on bone can be divided into two stages. One of these stages, *osteocytic osteolysis*, occurs within the Haversian system and is concerned primarily with *mineral homeostasis*; calcium released by this process travels via the minicirculation of bone to the endosteal surface and then to the extracellular fluid and the circulation. In this process, which is rapid, PTH stimulates the activity of resorptive osteocytes, and calcium is released into the body fluids without extensive bone remodeling. The other stage, *osteoclastic bone resorption*, is the process that accomplishes bone remodeling and is primary to *skeletal homeostasis*. PTH stimulates the conversion of osteoprogenitor cells (possibly macrophages) to osteoclasts, sustains osteoclastic activity, and inhibits osteoblastic activity. This is a relatively slow response, and this action of PTH appears to depend on a localized increase in ionized calcium, which is attained by osteocytic osteolysis. (Chapter 30 should be consulted for details of bone remodeling.)

Both cAMP and calcium messenger systems appear to be operative in the effect of PTH on bone cells. It has been suggested that the osteoclastic action of PTH is mediated through an osteoblastic paracrine factor; osteoblasts have specific PTH receptors, and PTH stimulates cAMP formation much more readily in osteoblasts than in osteoclasts. Osteoclastic bone resorption is a complex process involving monocytes, prostaglandins, and an osteocyte-activating

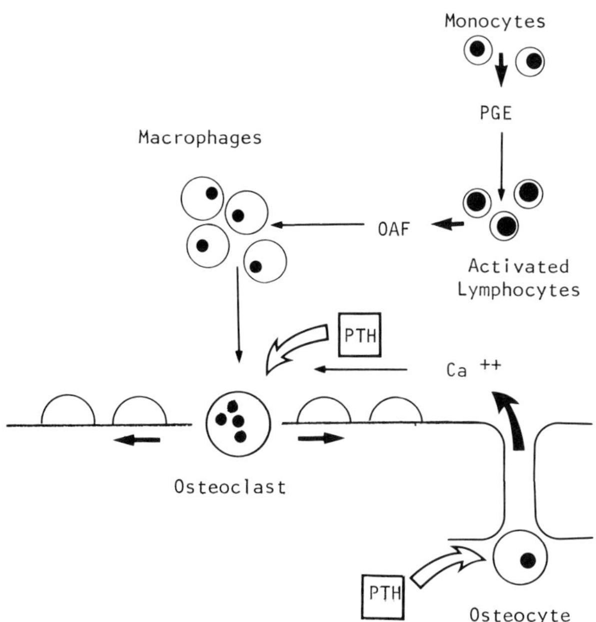

Figure 34.11. Schematic of osteoclastic and osteocytic osteolysis depicting sites of PTH action. Half-circles of bone surface represent osteoblasts contracting away from the resorption area. OAF, osteoclast activating factor; PGE, prostaglandin E.

factor from activated lymphocytes as well as PTH, calcium, and 1,25-DHCC (Fig. 34.11). The detailed interaction among the various humoral agents is still not completely understood.

Effect of parathyroid hormone on the kidney

The injection of PTH results in increased phosphate excretion, which may reach levels as much as 20 times the normal rate. Since ionic calcium and phosphate in the blood and extracellular fluid (ECF) behave in a reciprocal manner ($Ca \times PO_4$ = a constant), an increased diuresis of phosphate lowers the plasma phosphate level and allows an increased calcium concentration. PTH also enhances the renal retention of calcium. PTH inhibits the resorption of phosphate through receptors in the proximal convoluted tubules of the kidney, and phosphate diuresis is accompanied by increased excretion of sodium and bicarbonate. The PTH-stimulated increase in calcium resorption takes place through the distal convoluted tubules and the collecting ducts. In addition, PTH is the primary agent that stimulates 1-hydroxylase to effect the renal conversion of 25-hydroxycholecalciferol to 1,25-dihydroxycholecalciferol.

Other effects

If PTH is injected into a rat after parathyroidectomy and an intestinal loop is isolated, an increased transport of calcium from the loop can be demonstrated. Decreased calcium absorption has also been observed from Thiry-Vella fistulas constructed in dogs subjected to parathyroidectomy. (A Thiry-Vella fistula is an exposure of both ends of a section of intestine to the exterior with the mesenteric attachment preserved and the cut ends of the intestine anastomosed.) Absorption could be returned to normal with the injection of parathyroid extract; however, PTH stimulation of absorption is not seen in vitamin D–deficient animals.

When lactating rats are injected with PTH, there is a decrease in the calcium concentration in the milk, and yet PTH has been shown to stimulate the secretion of prolactin. Since this latter effect is found on systemic administration but not after intraventricular injection, it may result from increased circulating calcium levels.

CALCITONIN

Hypercalcemic perfusion of the thyroid/parathyroid glands of the dog leads to a fall in systemic calcium levels that is greater and more rapid than can be attributed to a simple inhibition of PTH secretion. If a similar experiment is conducted in the goat, in which the external parathyroid can be perfused without thyroid participation, systemic calcium does not decrease to the same extent. These and other studies led to the discovery of CT, a hormone of thyroid origin that works with PTH in a dual control of blood calcium concentration.

Origin and chemistry of calcitonin

In mammals, CT is secreted by the parafollicular or C cells that are found in the interstitial tissue between the follicles of the thyroid gland. These cells represent ultimobranchial gland tissue that is incorporated within the thyroid during embryonic development. In fish, amphibia, reptiles, and birds, in which the thyroid and ultimobranchial glands are separated, no CT can be extracted from the thyroid, whereas the ultimobranchial tissue contains 100 times the hormone content of a similar weight of porcine thyroid. CT-secreting cells are derived from cells of the neural crest that have migrated into and become incorporated within the ultimobranchial pharyngeal pouch of the embryo.

CT is a 32–amino acid peptide with 1 disulfide bridge and a molecular weight of 3000. While there is considerable species variation, the NH_2 terminal that contains the 1–7 disulfide bridge is similar in those species that have been characterized.

Regulation and function of calcitonin

Hypercalcemia and, to a lesser extent, increased levels of blood magnesium will stimulate the output of CT, and the opposite changes in the concentration of these ions will inhibit CT secretion. In addition, it has been shown that gastrointestinal hormones (either gastrin or cholecystokinin) stimulated by the presence of food in the stomach and intestine are CT secretagogues. CT, in turn, inhibits gastrin secretion. The gastrin-CT regulatory pathway may be of importance in conserving calcium after a calcium-rich meal, particularly in pregnant, lactating, or suckling animals.

The major role of CT is the inhibition of osteoclastic bone resorption through depression of osteoclastic activity and prevention of osteoclast formation. Since bone resorption almost always precedes bone formation, this leads to a general decrease in bone remodeling. CT also inhibits osteocytic osteolysis. In contrast to CT-PTH antagonism on bone, CT is similar to PTH in its effects on renal phosphate resorption. CT, however, not only inhibits phosphate resorption but enhances calcium diuresis, whereas PTH stimulates calcium retention. There is doubt as to the physiological importance of the CT renal effects inasmuch as high doses must be employed to achieve them.

The role of CT in the hydroxylation of 25-hydroxycholecalciferol and in the intestinal absorption of calcium is less certain. In both cases, inhibition by CT has been reported but may be indirect.

1,25-DIHYDROXYCHOLECALCIFEROL

It has been known for many years that an adequate supply of vitamin D is necessary for normal bone structure and function. Vitamin D may be ingested in the diet as irradiated ergosterol (D_2) or cholecalciferol (D_3), or it may be synthesized in the epidermis from 7-dehydrocholesterol. Epidermal synthesis occurs through rapid ultraviolet irradiation to previtamin D and a heat-mediated conversion of previtamin D to vitamin D. The latter reaction is much slower (50 percent conversion in 24 hours at body temperature) and allows a sustained release into the circulation.

Formation of 1,25-dihydroxycholecalciferol

It is now well established that vitamin D must undergo hydroxylations within the body to become biologically active. After absorption or synthesis, vitamin D is transported in the bloodstream bound to a specific blood globulin. The first activation step consists of 25-hydroxylation (see Fig. 30.23) in the liver. This initial hydroxyl derivative has weak biological activity but has the highest affinity for the binding globulin. The second hydroxylation takes place in the kidney and can occur at one of two positions, depending on the calcium need. Renal 1-hydroxylase activation produces 1,25-dihydroxycholecalciferol (1,25-DHCC), which is the most potent and physiologically effective metabolite. This enzyme step is stimulated by PTH, low serum calcium concentration, low serum phosphate concentration, prolactin, and estrogens and is inhibited by high serum calcium concentration, high serum phosphate concentration, and possibly CT. Of the agents that stimulate 1-hydroxylation, PTH appears to be the most important. There is a reciprocal relationship between 1,25-DHCC and the renal hydroxylases; 1,25-DHCC inhibits the synthesis of 1-hydroxylase and stimulates the synthesis of 24-hydroxylase. Whenever 1,25-DHCC formation is depressed, 24,25-DHCC is formed. In animals with normal blood calcium levels, the latter dihydroxyl derivative is found in greater concentration in the circulation than 1,25-DHCC.

Function of 1,25-dihydroxylcholecalciferol

The major function of 1,25-DHCC is to stimulate intestinal calcium absorption through the enhancement of calcium-binding protein and calcium-ATPase within the cells lining the intestine. This hormone also stimulates the absorption of phosphate. In addition to its effect on absorption, 1,25-DHCC is necessary for the growth and mineralization of cartilage and for osteoclastic bone resorption and osteocytic osteolysis. There is a permissive interaction between 1,25-DHCC and PTH in that small amounts of 1,25-DHCC are necessary for PTH activity; however, high concentrations of 1,25-DHCC are capable of stimulating osteoclastic bone resorption without PTH interaction. There is evidence that 1,25-DHCC acts on the parathyroid gland to inhibit the secretion of PTH. The other hydroxyl derivative, 24,25-DHCC, has very weak biological activity.

Whether 1,25-DHCC has a direct effect on bone forma-

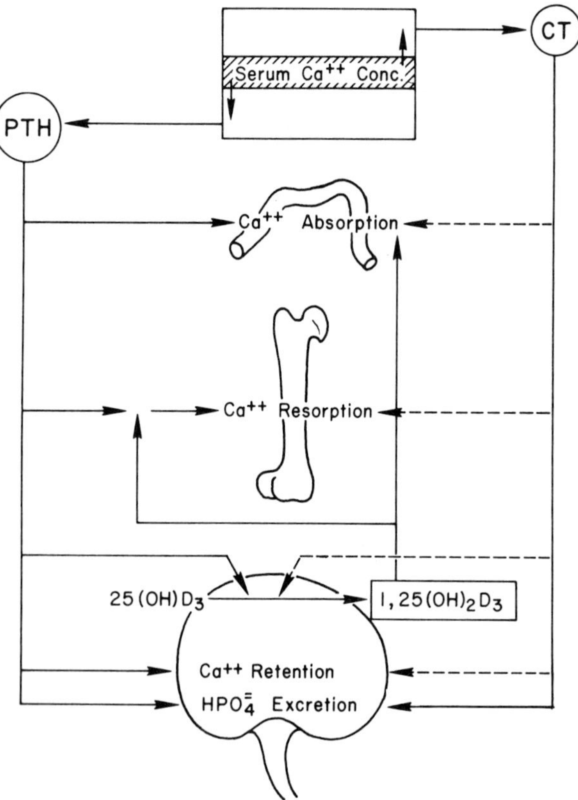

Figure 34.12. Parathyroid hormone (PTH), calcitonin (CT), 1,25-dihydroxycholecalciferol [$1,25(OH)_2D_3$], and calcium homeostasis. Solid line indicates stimulation; broken line shows inhibition.

tion and mineralization is controversial; some investigators have suggested that a metabolite of vitamin D, other than either 1,25-DHCC or 24,25-DHCC, is involved.

Figure 34.12 summarizes the effects of PTH, CT, and 1,25-DHCC on calcium homeostasis.

DISORDERS OF HORMONES THAT AFFECT CALCIUM HOMEOSTASIS

Hypocalcemia

In the dog, complete extirpation of the parathyroid glands is followed within 24 hours by severe neuromuscular dysfunction that eventually terminates in death. There are increased involuntary muscle spasms and periodic contractions of large groups of muscles, constituting what is known as *tetany*. These signs can be alleviated by the administration of calcium, and an acute decrease in ionic calcium in the body fluids results in a similar syndrome. Acute hypocalcemia from PTH deficiency is very uncommon in domestic animals.

A more common acute hypocalcemia occurs in the cow and the bitch at or near parturition. This probably results from the sudden demand on calcium reserves imposed by lactation. The condition does not result from decreased secretion of PTH; nor can it be attributed to a sudden increase in CT. There is evidence, however, that refractory or unresponsive PTH receptors may be involved. Further, it is possible that the feeding of high-calcium rations during gestation may result in "sluggishness" of parathyroid response; thus, in the cow, low-calcium rations have been employed during the last 2 weeks of gestation to prevent this condition.

Chronic hypocalcemia from dietary cause (calcium deficiency, vitamin D deficiency, excess phosphate absorption) or from kidney disease is much more frequent in domestic animals. In these conditions, the hypocalcemia is seldom severe enough to cause tetany, but the resulting hyperparathyroidism leads to skeletal demineralization (i.e., *rubber jaw syndrome* in dogs) or excess bone resorption (i.e., *renal osteitis fibrosa cystica*). Nutritional *secondary* hyperparathyroidism usually occurs in carnivores as a result of an all-meat diet. In the horse, this condition results from a diet that is high in phosphate relative to calcium. Kidney disease causes hypocalcemia because of increased calcium diuresis, phosphate retention, or an inability to form 1,25-DHCC.

Hypercalcemia

Primary hyperparathyroidism is associated with a functional adenoma of the parathyroid gland from which PTH is secreted in increased amounts despite hypercalcemia. The signs associated with this condition include renal calculi, excessive bone resorption, joint and skeletal pain, weakness, anorexia, vomiting, and polyuria. Occasionally, PTH or a PTH-like peptide is secreted in excessive quantities from a tumor that is not of parathyroid gland origin; this is referred to as *pseudohyperparathyroidism*.

Calcitonin dysfunction

There is no evidence of a clinical syndrome resulting from decreased secretion of CT, but hypersecretion, from a medullary carcinoma of the thyroid, has been observed in bulls and in humans. In this syndrome, clinical signs are few; osteosclerosis has been noted, but calcium and phosphate levels are usually just below normal.

ENDOCRINE SECRETIONS OF THE PANCREAS

In 1788 Cawley associated *diabetes* with the pancreas, and in 1869 Langerhans described islets of specialized glandular tissue dispersed among the pancreatic acini. Twenty years later, von Mehring and Minkowski found that pancreatectomy in the dog was followed by glycosuria. Finally, in 1921, Banting and Best were able to isolate insulin from the pancreatic islets. Since then, the importance of the endocrine secretions of the pancreas in the control of metabolism has been well established. Four main humoral regulators are found in pancreatic islet cells: insulin, glucagon, somatostatin, and pancreatic polypeptide.

Morphology

The pancreas is a V-shaped organ lying along the duodenum. It is composed primarily of pancreatic acini, which secrete the pancreatic enzymes that are important in digestion. These enzymes constitute the exocrine part of the pancreas and are liberated into the intestinal lumen by way of the pancreatic duct system. Scattered throughout the pancreas are small (about 0.3 mm in diameter) islets of cells that are structurally different from those in the acini. Islet tissue is arranged with branching irregular cords of cells among a rich capillary plexus. Four major cell types are found in the islets: the glucagon-producing alpha cells, the insulin-producing beta cells, the somatostatin-producing delta cells, and the F cells, in which pancreatic polypeptide is found.

Although the endocrine secretions of the islet cells affect target tissue throughout the body, it is important to note that pancreatic venous effluent passes through the liver before it reaches the main circulation. Thus the liver, because of the increased concentrations of pancreatic hormones passing through it, becomes the major target organ.

Chemistry

The determination of the exact structure of insulin by Sanger and his associates in 1955 stands as a landmark in protein biochemistry. The chemical structure of cattle insulin is depicted in Fig. 34.13. The insulin molecule contains two amino acid chains joined by two disulfide bridges with a third disulfide bridge in the A chain. There are 51 amino acids, and the molecular weight is approximately 5700.

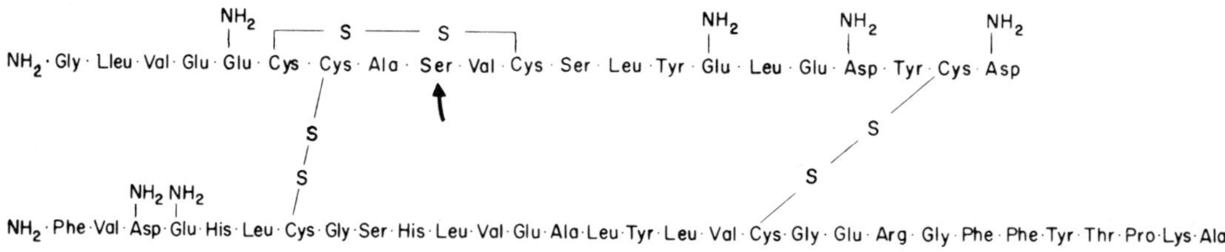

Figure 34.13. Amino acid sequence of ox insulin. (Arrow points to position No. 9 of the A chain.)

The insulin molecule is initially synthesized as a single chain, preproinsulin. The removal of a 23–amino acid signal peptide from the C terminal and the formation of disulfide bridges results in proinsulin. Except upon prolonged secretion, a 31–amino acid peptide (C peptide) is removed before secretion resulting in the two-chain insulin molecule. The C peptide is found within the secretory granules, together with insulin, and is secreted concurrently; assays of its concentration have been used to assess endogenous insulin production in patients undergoing insulin therapy.

Insulin from the ox, sheep, horse, pig, dog, and whale differs only in positions 8, 9, and 10 of the A chain, but there are more extreme differences in other animals. For example, rat insulin differs from bovine at four points in the A chain and at three points in the B chain. Insulin from one species is mildly antigenic when injected into another; occasionally, humans with diabetes have to use porcine insulin when they become refractory to bovine insulin.

Glucagon is a straight-chain polypeptide with a molecular weight of about 3500 and 29 amino acids. Similar to insulin and PTH, glucagon is initially synthesized as a larger molecule and degraded to the active form before secretion.

The chemistry of somatostatin has been described previously. Pancreatic polypeptide is a linear peptide with 36 amino acids.

Function of insulin

In insulin-sensitive tissues, except for the liver, the principal effect of insulin on carbohydrate metabolism is that it allows the transport of glucose across the cell membrane. Muscle and fat cells depend on facilitated diffusion for glucose entry and are relatively impermeable to glucose in the absence of insulin. In the liver, which is freely permeable to glucose entry, insulin stimulates glucose uptake by increasing the activity of enzymes that are responsible for glycogenesis and lipogenesis and inhibiting those that catalyze glycogenolysis.

Insulin has equally important effects on fat and protein metabolism. Insulin increases the transport of most amino acids into muscle, stimulates protein synthesis, and inhibits protein catabolism. In adipose tissue, insulin induces the synthesis of lipoprotein lipase, inhibits intracellular lipase, and enhances fatty acid esterification. Further, insulin stimulates the hepatic synthesis of fatty acids. Thus, insulin is a hormone that promotes anabolism and is the main regulatory for the disposition of nutrients; insulin has been termed the hormone of the "fed state."

Insulin also protects the body against hyperkalemia by stimulating the entry of potassium into muscle and fat cells. The specific effects of insulin are summarized in Table 34.5.

There is considerable variation in the response of different tissues to insulin. Brain, kidney, intestines, and erythrocytes show little response to insulin in comparison to liver, muscle, adipose tissue, and leukocytes.

Effect of insulin deficiency

In insulin deficiency, the ability of the peripheral tissues to use glucose either for oxidation or, in the case of the liver or muscle, for the synthesis of glycogen is greatly impaired. This leads to hyperglycemia from increased glycogenolysis and increased gluconeogenesis, and, as a result, sugar is excreted in the urine. Since the loss of glucose through the urine necessarily involves the loss of water and electrolytes, polyuria, dehydration, and hemoconcentration result. The marked dehydration, hemoconcentration, and reduced circulating blood volume result in shock, and eventually anuria ensues because of the marked decrease in kidney blood flow. In the dog whose pancreas has been

Table 34.5. Principal effects of insulin

Liver	
Glucokinase	+
Glycogen synthetase	+
Phosphofructokinase	+
Gluconeogenesis	−
Phosphorylase	−
Ketogenesis	−
Protein synthesis	+
Fat synthesis	+
Fatty acid synthesis	+
Muscle	
Glucose entry	+
Phosphofructokinase	+
Amino acid uptake	+
Ketone uptake	+
Protein catabolism	−
Potassium uptake	+
Adipose tissue	
Glucose entry	+
Triglyceride synthesis	+
Lipoprotein lipase	+
Hormone-sensitive lipase	−
Potassium entry	+

removed, the blood sugar concentration rises from a normal of 80 to 120 mg/dl to 300 to 500 mg/dl, glycosuria and polyuria occur, and the animal becomes dehydrated, then comatose, and dies within a few days.

Insulin deficiency has a marked effect on fat metabolism. Fat is used by the normal animal as a means of storing food energy; the liver and adipose tissue convert carbohydrate into fat for storage. In the insulin-deprived animal, glucose utilization is depressed and the animal is forced to mobilize fat from the storage depots to provide energy for cellular function. Adipose tissue is catabolized and the resultant fatty acids are oxidized, primarily in the liver, to the two-carbon acetyl coenzyme A (CoA). The accumulating acetyl CoA is converted to acetoacetic or beta-hydroxybutyric acid. These compound together with acetone constitute the *ketone bodies*. The resultant ketonemia and ketonuria deplete the body of fixed base, causing acidosis, and contribute to urinary sodium loss, which enhances the dehydration.

Decreased glucose utilization resulting from insulin deficiency leads to a marked increase in gluconeogenesis, which must, in turn, involve an increase in protein catabolism. The increase in protein catabolism is further increased by intracellular dehydration and is accompanied by hyperkalemia and potassium diuresis. also, insulin appears to depress the formation of the enzymes necessary for gluconeogenesis; thus the deficiency of this hormone contributes directly to the increased gluconeogenesis.

Insulin deprivation also results in various enzyme defects (e.g., liver glucokinase, pyruvate dehydrogenase, and acetyl CoA carboxylase). The metabolic sequelae of insulin deprivation are summarized in Fig. 34.14.

In many omnivorous and herbivorous animals, pancreatectomy or the injection of a beta-cell toxicant (alloxan) induces a relatively mild condition that is easily controlled with small doses of insulin. Pancreatectomy induces hyperglycemia and glycosuria in carnivorous birds, but in many herbivorous bird species, particularly the duck, this operation is followed by hypoglycemia. The difference has been attributed to the predominance of alpha cells in the pancreas of the duck.

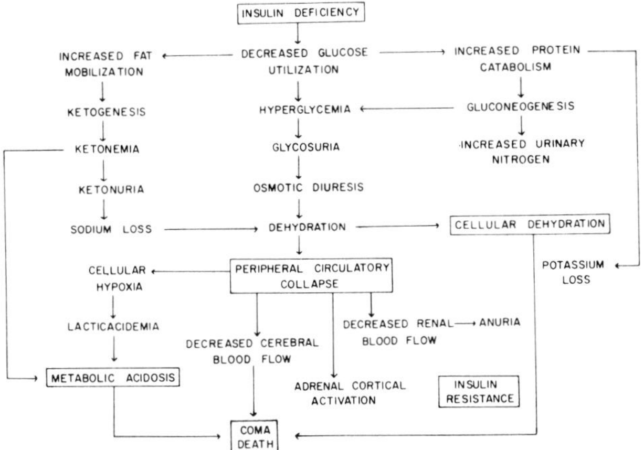

Figure 34.14. Metabolic and physiological sequelae to pancreatectomy.

Mechanism of action of insulin

The use of glucose by the cell involves the diffusion of glucose from the capillary onto the cell surface, the transport of glucose through the cell membrane, and the intracellular phosphorylation of glucose. Although extracellular glucose concentrations are high in comparison with the concentration within the cell, the membrane transport system appears to be distinct from simple diffusion and probably involves a membrane carrier system.

It is now generally agreed that in muscle and fat it is this membrane transport system that is influenced by insulin. It has been suggested that a glucose barrier in muscle cells is maintained by the constant application of energy; insulin is thought to interfere with this barrier. This hypothesis is supported by the fact that anoxia and various metabolic poisons enhance the entry of glucose from the ECF into the cell. The enzymes involved in the various metabolic reactions of insulin occur in the cell in sufficiently great amounts to handle large quantities of glucose. It is probable that the membrane transport system is rate limiting and the action of insulin on this site is of more importance than any effect it may have on phosphorylation.

In the liver, however, the plasma membrane is freely permeable to glucose and insulin exerts its effect on phosphorylation. The initial step in glucose metabolism, phosphorylation, is accomplished by the enzymes, hexokinase and glucokinase. The former, found in muscle and fat as well as liver, is not hormonally dependent and is saturated at physiological concentrations of blood glucose. Glucokinase, found only in liver, is induced by insulin and is only half-saturated at 180 mg/dl. Insulin also stimulates glucose metabolism and glycogen synthesis by facilitating the phosphorylation of fructose-6-phosphate and by inhibiting both glycogenolysis and gluconeogenesis.

Function of glucagon

Glucagon is much more effective if injected into a hepatic portal vessel than into a systemic vessel, and in the latter instance this hormone is virtually ineffective if the hepatic portal vessels are blocked. The isolated perfused liver is extremely susceptible to the glycogenolytic action of glucagon. The addition of glucagon to the perfusing fluid also results in an enhancement of protein catabolism.

Glucagon activates adenylate cyclase in liver cells, which stimulates phosphorylase and results in increased breakdown of glycogen. Glucagon also increases gluconeogenesis, elevates the metabolic rate, and inhibits hepatic lipogenesis. The increased metabolic rate is thought to result from increased hepatic deamination of amino acids. Inhibition of lipogenesis results in enhanced fatty acid oxidation and ketogenesis. A further action of glucagon is the stimulation of insulin and somatostatin secretion.

The predominance of glucagon in the pancreas in some species of birds indicates that the hormone may be physiologically more important in this vertebrate class than in the mammal; however, these animals are not nearly as dependent on glucagon as most animals are on insulin.

Function of somatostatin and pancreatic polypeptide

Somatostatin is a ubiquitous humoral regulatory agent that has been found in the CNS, pancreas, and cells lining the gastrointestinal tract. As a hypothalamic hormone, somatostatin inhibits the secretion of growth hormone and, possibly, thyroid-stimulating hormone. It is found in the retina and in the substantia gelatinosa of the spinal cord and may act as a neurotransmitter or modulator in these areas. Pancreatic somatostatin is secreted by the delta cells of the islets of Langerhans and is thought to affect neighboring alpha and beta cells through paracrine transmission or, perhaps, by passage through gap junctions. Somatostatin inhibits the secretion of both glucagon and insulin. Secreted by the gastric D cells into the lumen of the gastrointestinal tract, somatostatin inhibits the secretion of gastrin, secretin, and cholecystokinin (CCK), pancreatic exocrine secretion, gastric acid secretion, gastrointestinal motility, and the absorption of glucose. Thus, this compound appears to be a general inhibitory agent, which slows the influx of nutrients into the circulation and moderates the metabolic effects of insulin, glucagon, and growth hormone.

The secretion of pancreatic polypeptide is stimulated by the ingestion of protein or by exercise or fasting and is inhibited by somatostatin. Pancreatic polypeptide has been isolated from the pancreas and measured in the blood, but no definite function has been established.

Control of insulin and glucagon

In view of the many and diverse pathways of glucose utilization and the number of humoral agents that influence glucose metabolism, the variation in systemic blood glucose concentration is remarkably small. Among the endocrine organs that influence glucose concentration, the internal secretions of the pancreas are of primary importance inasmuch as their secretion is directly controlled by the blood glucose level. Cross-circulation experiments have been used to demonstrate this control. If pancreatic venous blood from a hypoglycemic animal is cross-circulated into a second, normal animal, the blood glucose of the recipient will increase. Conversely, if the donor has been given glucose, the blood sugar of the recipient will be reduced. These observations are attributed to increased secretion of glucagon or insulin, respectively, by the donor in response to its altered blood glucose concentration.

Of the various stimuli that stimulate the secretion of insulin, glucose is the most important. It appears that glucose metabolism within the beta cell produces the stimulus and that some glucose metabolite is responsible; metabolic inhibitors such as 2-deoxyglucose or mannoheptulose inhibit insulin secretion. An increase in intracellular calcium is believed to be the final triggering step in the release of insulin from the islet cell. Depressed insulin secretion has been observed in hypocalcemic cows and pigs.

Factors other than hyperglycemia have been shown to increase insulin secretion. Protein ingestion or the intravenous injection of amino acids will stimulate insulin secretion, even when agents (epinephrine, benzthiazide) that inhibit glucose-stimulated secretion are given. In the sheep, a species in which short-chain fatty acids are important as an energy source, butyrate and propionate cause release of insulin and long-chain fatty acids stimulate insulin release in the dog.

An important stimulatory effect on insulin secretion is exerted by the gastrointestinal hormones, gastrin, secretin, CCK, and others. Such hormones, stimulated by food ingestion, cause insulin to be released before glucose or amino acid absorption—an *anticipatory control*. Insulin secretion is also stimulated by either pancreatic glucagon or the glucagon that is secreted by intestinal cells (enteric glucagon). Finally, there is a possible CNS control of insulin secretion. Cholinergic fibers are seen surrounding the islet cells, and vagus nerve stimulation of insulin secretion has been demonstrated. Conversely, the adrenergic neurotransmitters, epinephrine and norepinephrine, inhibit glucose-stimulated insulin release. This autonomic nervous system regulation is particularly reflected in the hypoinsulinemia that accompanies exercise or stress-induced hyperglycemia.

Glucagon secretion is stimulated by hypoglycemia, amino acid absorption or infusion, gastrin, CCK, and exercise or stress. Glucagon is inhibited by glucose, free fatty acids, secretin, insulin, and somatostatin. The increased glucagon secretion after protein ingestion serves to prevent the hypoglycemia that might result from the concurrent stimulation of insulin secretion. Glucagon secretion reaches a peak during the first part of a period of fasting and declines thereafter; thus gluconeogenesis is promoted while the body is adjusting to the use of fatty acids and ketones as principal sources of energy. Pancreatic somatostatin release is enhanced by virtually every stimulus that increases insulin secretion.

ADRENAL GLAND

With the possible exception of pituitary secretions, the secretions of the adrenal glands are the most diverse in their effects. In mammals, the adrenal glands are embryologically, morphologically, and functionally separable into two distinct organs: the adrenal cortex and the adrenal medulla. Cortical hormones are steroids and exert their primary activity on carbohydrate and electrolyte metabolism, while those secreted from the medulla are amines with effects similar to those of postganglionic sympathetic neurotransmitters. Both parts of the gland appear to be important in the adaptation of the animal to adverse environmental influences.

Morphology

In birds and mammals, the adrenal glands consist of two bilaterally symmetrical, small, ellipsoid organs found at the anterior poles of the kidneys. The distance from the kidney and the proximity to the posterior vena cava vary from species to species and from right gland to left gland. On cross section, the mammalian adrenal is seen to be separated into an external cortex surrounding internal medullary tissue. In birds, the medullary tissue is scattered throughout the cortical tissue.

Adrenal medulla

In 1865 Henle observed that a brownish coloration resulted when adrenal medullary tissue was subjected to potassium bichromate. This reaction led to the name *chromaffin cells* for cells containing catecholamines. Critical review of this and similar reactions (green color with ferric chloride, blue color with ferric ferricyanide, blackening with osmium tetroxide) has not confirmed the early confidence in the specificity of these methods for the catecholamines. Adrenal medullary tissue is relatively homogeneous, contains secretory granules, and is often arranged in lobules. Two different medullary cells have been identified: epinephrine-secreting cells and norepinephrine-secreting cells. In cattle, the epinephrine cells are concentrated in the outer part of the medulla.

This part of the adrenal gland arises from the neural crest, and the chromaffin cells differentiate from neuroblasts. For this reason, and because the nerve supply to the adrenal medulla consists of preganglionic sympathetic neurons, the cells of the adrenal medulla are regarded as modified postganglionic sympathetic neurons.

Adrenal cortex

The adrenal cortex is derived from the mesodermal coelomic epithelium. This part of the gland is thus embryologically associated with the other important steroidogenic endocrine glands, the gonads. The mammalian adrenal cortex is typically divided into three zones: zona reticularis, zona fasciculata, and zona glomerulosa. The inner zona reticularis lies adjacent to the medulla and consists of randomly arranged cells with densely staining cytoplasm and a high percentage of pyknotic nuclei. In the middle zona fasciculata the cells are arranged in columns, and in the outer zona glomerulosa there is a looped or whorled arrangement resulting in an acinar appearance.

The histological appearance of the adrenocortical cells in the two outer zones varies with the stage of activity of the gland because of the depletion of certain substances during secretion. The cells of the inactive gland are vacuolated and have a foamy appearance because of the presence of large amounts of lipid. Increased secretory activity results in the depletion of lipid, cholesterol, and ascorbic acid, resulting in a more compact cell.

The zonation of the adrenal cortex varies somewhat among species. In the cow and sheep, the zona fasciculata is divided into an inner and an outer portion, and an intermediate zone can be distinguished between the zona fasciculata and the zona glomerulosa. In the juvenile mouse and rabbit, there is an inner cortical zone, consisting of healthy cells with large vesicular nuclei. This is called the X zone and is replaced by the zona reticularis at puberty in the male mouse or during the first pregnancy in the female.

After hypophysectomy, the zona fasciculata undergoes degeneration, whereas the zona glomerulosa remains virtually unchanged. In addition, there is considerable evidence that the injection of ACTH results in more marked lipid depletion of the zona fasciculata.

Chemistry and metabolism of the adrenal medullary hormones

The hormones of the adrenal medulla consist of two amines derived from tyrosine, which differ only in the presence or absence of a terminal methyl group (Fig. 34.15). The amino acid tyrosine is converted to dihydroxyphenylalanine (dopa), which is then converted to dopamine by a decarboxylase. Beta hydroxylation of dopamine results in norepinephrine, and the terminal methylation of norepinephrine results in epinephrine. Although epinephrine has been found in the CNS, the medulla is the primary source of this hormone. Norepinephrine is secreted both by the medulla and by postganglionic sympathetic neurons.

The ratio of epinephrine to norepinephrine secreted by the adrenal medulla varies considerably among species (Table 34.6) and with age. Epinephrine usually predominates over norepinephrine in the secretion from the adult mammalian gland, and in rabbits and guinea pigs norepinephrine

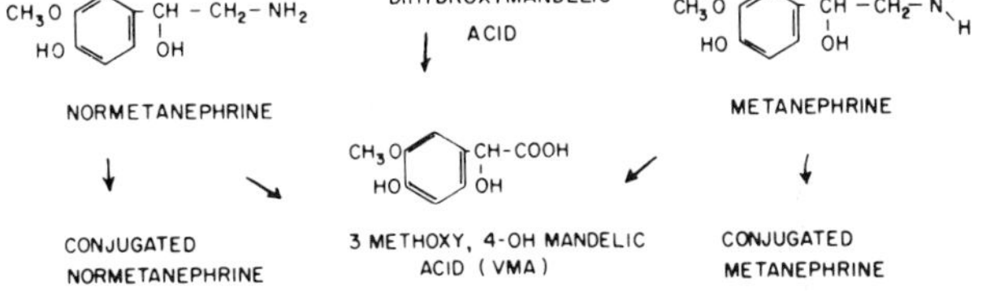

Figure 34.15. Biosynthesis and metabolism of the catecholamines.

Table 34.6. Catecholamines in adrenal glands from various adult mammalian species

Species	Norepinephrine (%)	Total catecholamines (mg/g whole gland)
Rabbit	2	0.48
Human	17	0.6
Sheep	33	0.75
Horse	20	0.84
Cat	41	1
Dog	27	1.5
Cow	29	1.8
Pig	49	2.24

Modified from West 1955, *Q. Rev. Biol.* 30:116–37.

is a minor constituent. In contrast, the adrenal medullary output of the whale and of chickens is about 80 percent norepinephrine. Fetal adrenal tissue appears to contain predominantly norepinephrine in all species. At birth, the rabbit adrenal medulla contains approximately 70 percent norepinephrine compared with a 2 percent concentration in adult tissue.

There is considerable speculation and no real agreement about the differential release of the two amines in response to varying physiological demand. The ratio of epinephrine to norepinephrine in the secretion from the canine medulla is not varied by any of various stimuli, but differential release has been observed in the human, cat, rabbit, and rat. The glucocorticoids of the adrenal cortex stimulate the conversion of norepinephrine to epinephrine by inducing the enzyme phenylethanolamine-N-methyltransferase.

Enzymatic degradation of the adrenal medullary hormones occurs through O-methylation brought about by the enzyme catechol-O-methyltransferase and by oxidative deamination through monoamine oxidase (Fig. 34.15). After administration of labeled epinephrine, 45 percent of the radioactivity appearing in the urine was found in 3-methoxy,4-hydroxymandelic acid, whereas 34 percent was found in free or conjugated metanephrine. Metanephrine and normetanephrine appear in the urine, either as free compounds or as sulfates or glucuronides. Inactivation of the catecholamines is rapid as evidenced by the half-life of epinephrine, which has been estimated at 20 to 40 seconds.

Function and control of the adrenal medulla

The chromaffin cell hormones are not essential for life, as removal of the adrenal medulla does not result in marked physiological change. This is at least partially due to the fact that the sympathetic nervous system remains intact after this operation and the function of the adrenal medulla appears to be, largely, reinforcement of this system.

Historically, there have been two contrasting theories regarding the general function of adrenal medullary secretion. The first of these, the *emergency theory*, was articulated by Cannon (1932) and is commonly referred to as the "fight-or-flight" hypothesis. Advocates of the opposing view held that the target cells were maintained in a constant state of responsiveness to epinephrine and/or norepinephrine. This theory became known as the *tonus theory*. As is often the case in such controversies, there is increasing realization that both points of view may be correct. It appears that adrenal medullary secretion is a continuous process that increases to a striking degree during an emergency.

Adrenergic receptors

The diverse and similar effects of epinephrine and norepinephrine are in large part explained by the hypothesis of two adrenergic receptors. The alpha receptors are stimulatory, with the exception of those in the intestinal smooth muscle, whereas the beta receptors are inhibitory, with the exception of those in cardiac muscle. Epinephrine and norepinephrine react with both receptors, but the alpha effect of norepinephrine is more potent than that of epinephrine, whereas epinephrine has a more potent beta action.

Specific effects

Small to moderate doses of epinephrine decrease total peripheral circulatory resistance because of vasodilation of blood vessels in the skeletal muscle (beta inhibitory receptors); epinephrine, however, constricts cutaneous vessels and those of the hepatic, mesenteric, and uterine vasculature. Thus, this hormone redistributes blood flow to that area, which is important for "fight or flight." Norepinephrine, on the other hand, increases peripheral resistance and is a generalized vasoconstrictor, with the exception of the coronary vessels. These catecholamines accelerate the rate of depolarization and enhance transmission in the cardiac muscle and cardiac transmission fibers, increasing the speed and force of contraction and hastening relaxation in cardiac muscle; thus heart rate increases (*chronotropic effect*) and the force of contraction is enhanced (*inotropic effect*). A combination of the cardiac and peripheral vasculature effects results in a difference in their action on blood pressure; epinephrine causes increased systolic blood pressure and decreased diastolic pressure, with little effect on mean blood pressure, while norepinephrine increases systolic, diastolic, and mean pressures.

Both amines produce bronchiolar dilatation and an increased rate and depth of respiration. An adequate supply of tissue oxygen is further guaranteed by the epinephrine-induced contraction of the spleen, increasing the peripheral concentration of erythroctes.

The ciliary muscle of the eye, bronchial musculature, esophageal muscle, stomach wall muscle, and bladder detrusor muscle are relaxed by the catecholamines through the beta receptors, whereas the smooth muscles of the radial iris muscle in the eye, the pylorus of the stomach, the intestinal sphincters, and the trigone and sphincter muscles of the bladder are constricted through the alpha receptors.

The smooth muscle of the intestine is also inhibited but apparently contains both alpha and beta receptors.

There is some species variation in the bladder response and species variation as well as reproductive state is apparent in the effects of the catecholamines on the reproductive organs. In the nonpregnant cat, epinephrine generally inhibits uterine motility, but in the pregnant cat its injection is followed by contraction. In the rabbit epinephrine causes uterine contraction, whereas in the dog the uterus first contracts and then relaxes.

Catecholamines have pronounced metabolic effects: hyperglycemia, increased calorigenesis, lipolysis, elevated blood lactate, and increased serum potassium. Hyperglycemia results from enhanced liver glycogenolysis, while increased blood lactate ensues from stimulation of muscle glycogenolysis. The calorigenic effect of the catecholamines probably results from cutaneous vasoconstriction, increased muscle metabolism, and a rise in lactic acid oxidation in the liver. Increased activity of the sympathetic nervous system and the adrenal medulla may be the most important physiological stimulus for the mobilization of fatty acids from adipose tissue and their subsequent release into the bloodstream.

In experiments in which the time of reaction to a stimulus is measured, the transmission of information in and out of the CNS appears to be facilitated by the catecholamines. The question of the importance of adrenergic pathways in the CNS has aroused considerable interest, particularly since such pathways appear to be important to the secretion of hypothalamic regulating hormones.

Control

As previously implied, the sympathetic nervous system and the adrenal medulla are stimulated to increased activity by situations that pose a threat to the animal. However,a feedback mechanism appears to operate through increased blood pressure and its effects on the carotid sinus and vasomotor center to limit the maximum secretion rate of these hormones. In the cat, a maximum secretion rate of 10 μg/min has been observed; this corresponds to a dose of 0.02 ml of a 1:1000 solution of epinephrine.

Glycogenolytic action of epinephrine

The second messenger concept of hormonal action was essentially initiated by studies concerned with the effect of epinephrine on glycogenolysis. Epinephrine, acting via beta-adrenergic receptors, activates adenylate cyclase, resulting in increased intracellular cAMP. cAMP activates the enzyme phosphorylase kinase; this then converts inactive phosphorylase to active phosphorylase, which catalyzes the breakdown of glycogen. The catecholamines also increase glycogenolysis, through alpha-adrenergic receptors, by promoting an increase in intracellular calcium.

Table 34.7. Naturally occurring adrenal cortical steroids

Common names	Functional name
Cortisol, 17-hydroxycorticosterone, hydrocortisone, compound F*	Glucocorticoid
Corticosterone, compound B†	Glucocorticoid
Cortisone, 17-hydroxy-11-dehydrocorticosterone, compound E	Glucocorticoid
11-Dehydrocorticosterone, compound A	Glucocorticoid
Deoxycorticosterone	Mineralocorticoid
17-Hydroxy-11-deoxycorticosterone, compound S	Mineralocorticoid
Aldosterone, electrocortin*	Mineralocorticoid

*Principal secretory product in most species.
†Chemical name = 4-pregnene-11 beta,21-diol-3,20-dione.
For details of steroid chemistry, see Dorfman and Ungar 1953, Klyne 1957.

Chemistry of the adrenocortical hormones

A large number of biologically active and inactive steroids have been isolated from mammalian adrenocortical tissue; however, most of these represent intermediates or metabolites rather than true adrenocortical hormones. The adrenocortical hormones are derivatives of the 21-carbon pregnane nuclei, and the true secretions have a double bond between C-4 and C-5. There are seven generally recognized adrenocortical hormones, which differ in structure in only three positions: C-11, C-13, and C-17. (These corticosteroids are listed in Table 34.7.)

Structure and relationship to function

Six of these hormones can be considered modifications of corticosterone (4-pregnene-11B,21-diol-3,20-dione). The seventh hormone, aldosterone, is unique in that the angular methyl group on C-13 is replaced by an aldehyde; this aldehyde group is in equilibrium with a hemiacetal ring structure between C-11 and C-13 (Fig. 34.16).

Soon after the chemical structure of the corticosteroids was established, it was noted that corticoids with a hydroxyl or ketone group on C-11 had greater physiological activity with respect to carbohydrate metabolism than corticoids with no substituents at this position; such steroids, exemplified by cortisol, cortisone, and ll-dehydrocorticosterone are termed *glucocorticoids*. Adrenocortical steroids with no substituents at C-11 have a greater effect on electrolyte metabolism than the glucocorticoids and are termed *mineralocorticoids*; 11-deoxycorticosterone and 17-hydroxy-11-deoxycorticosterone are examples of this category. Aldosterone, the most potent mineralocorticoid, proved to be the exception to this pattern. The glucocorticoid activity of 11-hydroxy and 11-carbonyl hormones is further enhanced by 17-hydroxylation. In most animals, cortisol is the principal glucocorticoid secreted and aldosterone is the principal mineralocorticoid.

Synthesis, blood transport, and metabolism

The biosynthesis of the adrenocortical steroids is a process that involves many steps (an abbreviated version is

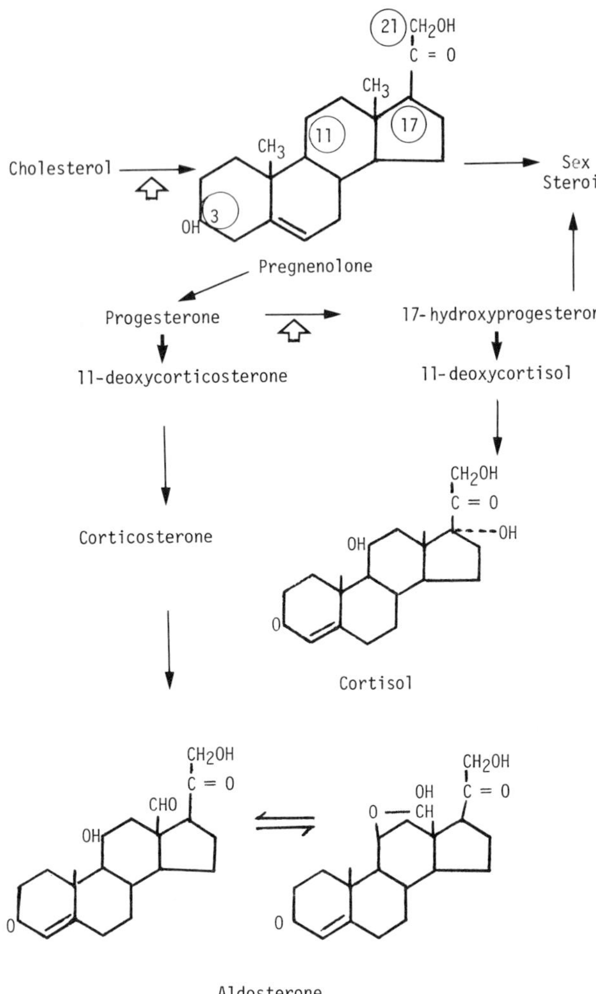

Figure 34.16. Adrenal cortical steroid biosynthesis. Circled numbers indicate sites of important enzymatic transformations; open arrow indicates site of ACTH action.

given in Fig. 34.16). Although cholesterol is probably the basic substrate for steroid synthesis within the adrenal gland, the synthesis of cholesterol from two-carbon acetyl fragments occurs and may be important in situations of great demand on the secretory capacity of the adrenal. On stimulation of the adrenal gland with ACTH, adrenocortical cholesterol and ascorbic acid in the zona fasciculata are quickly depleted and the adrenal venous steroid concentration is increased. While the cholesterol depletion of the adrenal cortex has obvious purpose, the ascorbic acid depletion is less well understood. ACTH promotes adrenocortical steroidogenesis through the activation of phosphorylase and is important in the conversion of cholesterol to pregnenolone and in 17-hydroxylation.

Adrenal hormones are secreted into the bloodstream as free steroids but are transported bound to plasma proteins. About 90 to 97 percent of the blood cortisol is bound, whereas blood aldosterone is about 60 percent bound. Also, the binding affinity is much less for aldosterone than for cortisol.

Steroid hormones are catabolized and inactivated principally in the liver, the kidney, and the target organs themselves. The liver is most important because of its well-developed ability to form sulfates by esterification and glucuronides by conjugation; these compounds are biologically inactive, and their water solubility facilitates their elimination in the bile or urine. In humans, 60 to 70 percent of the metabolites appear in the urine as glucuronides. In the dog, the principal metabolites of cortisol are cortol, 3-epiallocortol, and cortolone, all of which have a trihydroxy side chain; the dihydroxy, 20-ketone compounds, tetrahydrocortisol and tetrahydrocortisone are excreted in lesser quantities. About 10 percent of the metabolites are 19-carbon rather than 21-carbon compounds. Only about 1 percent of the secreted cortisol escapes inactivation.

Function and control of aldosterone

One of the most striking physiological changes observed after the removal of both adrenal glands in mammals and birds is marked sodium diuresis. Electrolyte changes in the blood after adrenalectomy include decreases in blood sodium, chloride, and bicarbonate levels and a rise in blood potassium concentration. Continued sodium and fluid losses lead to dehydration, hypotension, reduced renal blood flow, and increased blood levels of nonprotein nitrogen and phosphate. In many species, death can be delayed or completely averted by a high dietary sodium intake. In adrenal insufficiency, the injection of aldosterone and other mineralocorticoids enhances sodium retention and reduces elevated blood potassium (hyperkalemia).

Specific effect of mineralocorticoids

The kidney is the primary site of sodium retention after the release of aldosterone into the circulation. In this organ, the effect of aldosterone appears to be on active reabsorption of sodium and secretion of potassium in the cortical collecting tubules and on hydrogen ion secretion in the medullary collecting ducts. Aldosterone also has a permissive effect on the response of the renal collecting ducts to vasopressin.

In common with other steroids, aldosterone acts by increasing intracellular mRNA and protein synthesis. Whether aldosterone-induced proteins increase cell permeability, increase the activity of the energy-dependent sodium pump, or simply provide energy through substrate oxidation is not certain. The kaliuretic effect of aldosterone is not nearly as apparent when sodium intake is restricted.

Although aldosterone can have glucocorticoidlike effects, its concentration in the blood (0.08 μg/dl of whole blood in humans) indicates that the hormone is secreted in amounts too small to contribute to this aspect of adrenal cortical function. Although their mineralocorticoid action is very small compared with that of aldosterone, the relatively large amounts of cortisol and/or corticosterone that are secreted into the bloodstream become a factor in sodium retention and potassium diuresis.

Excess mineralocorticoid activity, whether from an aldosterone-secreting tumor, excess corticoid therapy, or enzyme deficiency leading to accumulation of deoxycortisol, gives rise to an increased plasma sodium concentration, a fall in plasma potassium concentration, hypochloremic alkalosis, and excess ECF volume. When the ECF expansion reaches a certain point, however, "escape" occurs and sodium excretion increases; thus edema is not a common feature of excess aldosterone. This "escape" may be due to direct or indirect stimulation of a hormone from the heart, which has been termed the *atrial natriuretic factor* (ANF).

The mineralocorticoids also enhance sodium retention in extrarenal tissues; these include sweat glands, salivary glands, intestinal mucosa, and sodium exchange between intracellular and extracellular fluid.

Control of aldosterone secretion

At present, evidence favors the concept that aldosterone secretion is controlled by three pathways.

1. In 1960 it was discovered that the kidney was the source of a potent aldosterone-stimulating factor and that removal of the kidneys in dogs after hypophysectomy was followed by a 50 percent reduction in the rate of aldosterone secretion. In addition, acute hemorrhage, a potent stimulus for aldosterone production, did not augment the secretion of this hormone in dogs that had undergone nephrectomy and hypophysectomy. Since then, fractionation studies with kidney extracts have indicated that the only fraction with aldosterone-stimulating activity was that containing renin. Further, intravenous infusions of renin or angiotensin II stimulate the secretion of aldosterone. A decrease in ECF volume or blood volume results in a decrease in renal perfusion and the release of renin from the juxtaglomerular apparatus. *Renin* is an enzyme that acts upon a circulating blood globulin, angiotensinogen or renal substrate, to form angiotensin I, which is further split, principally in the lung, by *converting enzyme* to angiotensin II. Angiotensin II stimulates the secretion of aldosterone.

2. It has been known for some time that hypophysectomy decreases the rate of secretion of aldosterone and that ACTH can prevent the depressing effect of hypophysectomy on secondary hyperaldosteronism. On the other hand, maximal aldosterone secretion has been observed in dogs with low plasma levels of ACTH and a low output of glucocorticoids. From these findings, it appears that in some instances of severe stress ACTH initiates aldosterone secretion, whereas in other instances, such as severe hemorrhage, ACTH augments the secretion that has been initiated by angiotensin II.

Increased aldosterone secretion can be caused by a variety of stimuli: laparotomy, hemorrhage, vena caval constriction, and congestive heart failure. The effects of these stimuli can be explained on the basis of decreased renal blood flow or increased ACTH output.

3. A small (1 mEq/L) increase in plasma potassium ion concentration will stimulate an increased secretion of aldosterone without an increase in angiotensin. Similarly, a decreased sodium concentration in the blood will stimulate aldosterone, but the magnitude of change necessary is greater. It has been shown that the angiotensin receptors in the zona glomerulosa have increased affinity when the sodium ion concentration in the blood is decreased.

Increases in potassium or angiotensin stimulate aldosterone secretion by increasing the conversion of cholesterol to pregnenolone and by stimulating the conversion of corticosterone to aldosterone.

Function of the glucocorticoids

The metabolic consequences of a complete loss of adrenocortical activity are far reaching and include almost every organ, system, and tissue in the body. When the minerolocorticoid deoxycorticosterone became available for experimental use, it was recognized that, while this hormone could reverse many of these changes, many metabolic defects continued to be present. In all species in which complete removal of the adrenal cortex has been effected (dog, human, rat, sheep, cow, pig, and horse), the results of this operation include weakness, easy fatigability, hypotension, marked intolerance to fasting, exaggerated response to insulin, and decreased ability to withstand stresses.

Although it is difficult to distinguish between effects resulting from a deficiency in mineralocorticoids and those resulting from a deficiency in glucocorticoids, replacement therapy in animals that have undergone adrenalectomy has clearly indicated that a deficiency in glucocorticoid function has serious and widespread results in general body metabolism. For example, after adrenalectomy the animal shows a striking inability to excrete a large water intake, and this defect is present even after the administration of the mineralocorticoid, deoxycorticosterone. Cortisol, on the other hand, will correct this deficiency in water metabolism and, if administered in large enough amounts, has sufficient salt-retentive activity to maintain life in animals after adrenalectomy.

Effect on carbohydrate metabolism

The primary effects of the glucocorticoids on carbohydrate metabolism are enhancement of gluconeogenesis and peripheral antagonism to the effects of insulin. The typical hypoglycemia and liver glycogen depletion that follow adrenalectomy are corrected with the administration of a potent glucocorticoid such as cortisol. Even in this regard, glucocorticoids are primarily operative in the stressed animal; these hormones are required for gluconeogenesis in animals with insulin deficiency or in fasted animals but not for basal gluconeogenesis in the fed state. Cortisol exerts a permissive effect in that glucagon and epinephrine require it to exert their gluconeogenic and glycogenolytic actions.

Glucocorticoids exert a significant effect on carbohydrate metabolism by inhibiting glucose uptake and metabolism in peripheral tissues, particularly muscle and fat cells—the so-called *anti-insulin effects*. Animals with glucocorticoid deficiency are very sensitive to insulin. With respect to liver glycogen, howver, the effects of cortisol and insulin are similar; cortisol stimulates increased liver glycogen deposition by inhibiting the formation of inactive phosphorylase and by stimulating glycogen synthetase. This effect is perceived as a response to stress and is designed to protect against long-term food deprivation.

Because of the insulin antagonism exhibited by cortisol and the hyperglycemia produced by large doses of this compound, chronic overdosage can lead to a metabolic syndrome known as steroid diabetes. It is possible that pregnancy toxemia in sheep is a diabetes-like syndrome resulting from adrenocortical hyperfunction coupled with severe undernutrition. In this disease, the typical diabetic hyperglycemia is only potential; the ewe is hypoglycemic as a result of high fetal demand for glucose.

Effect on fat metabolism

Chronic administration of glucocorticoid hormones leads to hyperlipemia and hypercholesterolemia and to a centripetal redistribution of body fat. There is lipolysis and increased plasma free fatty acids. It is not known why fat is lost in some areas (limbs) and gained in others (head and trunk).

Effect on protein metabolism

Glucocorticoids inhibit the synthesis and stimulate the breakdown of protein and RNA in muscle, skin, adipose tissue, lymphoid tissue, and connective tissue but have little effect in this respect on brain or cardiac tissue, and actually stimulate protein synthesis in the liver. Again, the effect is protective; recruitment of glucose substrates from the less immediately essential tissues and sparing of the more critical tissues.

Chronic overdosage with cortisol leads to a decrease in muscle protein and fibrosis of muscle tissue; after adrenalectomy, animals suffer from extreme muscle weakness that can be reversed only with the administration of a glucocorticoid.

The protein-mobilizing or catabolic effect of cortisol is quite apparent in its effect on bone metabolism. In glucocorticoid excess, there is decreased development of cartilage, interruption of growth, and an inhibition of the formation of new bone. There is also a direct effect in that cortisol inhibits the secretion of growth hormone from the adenohypophysis.

Effect on lymphoid tissue

Glucocorticoids cause lysis of lymphoid tissue and a reduction in circulating lymphocytes and eosinophils. After the injection of either ACTH or cortisol, the decrease in peripheral blood lymphocytes and eosinophils may amount to as much as 45 to 50 percent for the former and up to 90 percent for the latter. In humans, dogs, horses, and pigs this decrease will reach a peak in about 4 hours; in the cow, however, the maximum decrease is seen between 8 and 10 hours after the injection. The physiological role of this process is not well understood.

Effect on water excretion

As previously indicated, the glucocorticoid hormones enhance water diuresis. Although glucocorticoids inhibit vasopressin secretion and appear to antagonize the effect of vasopressin on the distal nephron of the kidney, it is probable that the enhancement of water excretion results from their ability to increase the glomerular filtration rate. Although cortisol and other glucocorticoids have considerable sodium-retentive activity, the aforementioned diuretic effect may result in an actual loss of sodium from the body after the administration of glucocorticoids. Furthermore, glucocorticoids may stimulate the secretion of ANF.

Effects on inflammation and immunity

Of all the diverse ways in which the glucocorticoids have been exploited in clinical practice, they have been used to the greatest extent for the inhibition of inflammation. When tissue is injured, the typical inflammatory response includes extravasation of fluid into the tissue spaces, leukocytic infiltration, hyperemia, and connective tissue synthesis. After the administration of cortisol or another glucocorticoid, there is a decrease in hyperemia, diminished cellular response, a decrease in exudation, and an inhibition of fibroblast formation. Many of the local anti-inflammatory effects of cortisol may be due to stabilization of lysosomal membranes preventing the release of proteolytic and other enzymes.

In all phases of glucocorticoid activity, it is difficult to separate physiological effects from responses to the exogenous administration of large doses. For example, the administration of reasonably normal doses of cortisol does not reduce the circulating antibody level, whereas large doses eventually reduce both production and release of antibodies. Early in cortisol therapy there may be an increase in circulating antibodies in the blood as a result of lysis of fixed plasma cells and lymphocytes. Increased cortisol levels during stress may help prevent autoimmune responses to antigens released after cell damage.

The anti-inflammatory action of the glucocorticoids may also account for their ability to diminish an allergic response, as these hormones do not interfere with histamine effects but will prevent histamine release. Glucocorticoids

Table 34.8. Relative potencies of selected natural and synthetic adrenal corticoids

	Sodium retention	Anti-inflammatory	Carbohydrate activity
Cortisol	Slight	1	1
Cortisone	Slight	0.8	0.8
Deoxycorticosterone	1	0*	Minimal
Aldosterone	30	0.3	0.3
Prednisolone	Minimal	4	3
Dexamethasone	0	25	Minimal
2-Methyl,9-fluorocortisol	100	10	10

*Usually classified as pro-inflammatory.
Data from Forsham 1962, in Williams, ed., *Textbook of Endocrinology,* W.B. Saunders, Philadelphia; Prunty 1958, in Gardiner-Hill, ed., *Modern Trends in Endocrinology,* Hoeber, New York.

also inhibit the action of phosphorylase A_2, a plasma membrane enzyme that initiates the conversion of arachidonic acid to inflammatory agents such as prostaglandins, thromboxanes, leukotrienes, and other eicosanoids.

The clinical usefulness of certain glucocorticoid effects has led to the development of a large number of steroids in which various structural alterations have been made in the molecule to enhance certain of the physiological actions while diminishing others. As an example, one of the more popular anti-inflammatory agents, dexamethasone, has 25 times the anti-inflammatory potency of cortisol and very little effect on sodium retention. Table 34.8 compares the potencies of several of the normal and synthetic steroids.

Effect on the nervous system

In adrenal insufficiency, electroencephalography reveals a slowing of the electrical discharges of the CNS whereas cortisol injection lowers the brain threshold for electrical excitation. Some steroids, given in very large doses, act as anesthetics. Adrenal insufficiency also results in increased sensitivity of the gustatory and olfactory receptors. In humans, glucocorticoid administration commonly effects a feeling of well-being (euphoria), but patients with hyperadrenocorticism are usually depressed.

One of the most important and little understood functions of cortisol has been described as a "permissive effect." Many cells that are responsive to a variety of stimuli will respond to these stimuli only if they are exposed to a certain baseline concentration of adrenocortical steroids. This permissive action is demonstrated by the lack of response of the arterioles to the pressor effect of norepinephrine in animals subjected to adrenalectomy. The calorigenic action of both glucagon and the catecholamines also requires glucocorticoids. As previously noted, the conversion of norepinephrine to epinephrine in the adrenal medulla is dependent on the glucocorticoids.

Effects on gastrointestinal absorption

In animals that have undergone adrenalectomy there is a diminished absorption of glucose and calcium from the gastrointestinal tract. Thus the oral glucose tolerance test can be easily misinterpreted in the adrenal-deficient animal. It is possible that adrenocorticoids are equally important in the transport of glucose across other membranes such as the placenta. This would explain the observation that the blood glucose concentration of fasted pregnant ewes that have had a adrenalectomy does not fall as rapidly as that of intact fasted pregnant controls. Glucocorticoids also increase fat absorption and stimulate gastric acid and pepsin secretion. Thus it has been suggested that, in humans, continuous stress contributes to the formation of peptic ulcers.

Effect of fetal cortisol

The importance of the fetal hypothalamus and pituitary in initiating parturition has been suspected for many years. It is now certain that, in many species, cortisol from the fetal adrenal cortex acts upon the placenta to reduce progesterone and increase estrogen secretion. Reduced progesterone and elevated estrogen concentrations promote the synthesis and release of prostaglandin $F_{2\alpha}$ ($PGF_{2\alpha}$), and uterine contractions are stimulated. Injection of cortisol or a highly potent steroid such as dexamethasone near the end of gestation will often induce labor.

Elevated fetal cortisol appears to be of importance in preparing the fetus for extrauterine existence. Increased cortisol before birth induces the production of lung surfactant, hepatic enzymes, digestive enzymes, and epidermal protein.

Control of glucocorticoid secretion

The secretion of adrenal glucocorticoids from the zona fasciculata of the adrenal cortex is controlled by ACTH. In the absence of ACTH, the production of glucocorticoids falls to very low levels and the adrenal cortex undergoes atrophy. Adrenal atrophy will also result from the continued exogenous administration of glucocorticoids since ACTH secretion can be inhibited by the increased cortisol concentration. Thus, ACTH and the adrenal glucocorticoids are reciprocally related in a negative-feedback mechanism. It should be emphasized that, in common with the other effects of cortisol, it is the "free" cortisol level that inhibits ACTH. Alterations in the concentration of plasma corticoid–binding protein may affect total concentration of blood cortisol without altering the "free" or effective concentration.

Many stimuli are capable of eliciting the release of ACTH from the anterior pituitary, even when the plasma cortisol levels are elevated. Included in this category are many types of noxious agents or stimuli that require an adaptation of the organism to meet a potential danger. In animals not subjected to stress, there is a definite diurnal variation in ACTH release and blood corticoid concentration. This diurnal cycle is related to the activity pattern of the species; in the mouse maximal corticoid secretion occurs during the night, when the animal is active, whereas in species that are active in the daylight hours the maximal secretion occurs early in the day.

Adrenal cortex and adaptation

One of the most striking results of adrenalectomy is the inability of the animal to resist adverse conditions that require reintegration of the internal metabolism of the organism for defense against injury. In 1936 Selye published the first of a long series of observations on the stereotyped response of the organism to a variety of noxious stimuli. Selye termed this response the *general adaptation syndrome* and divided it into three phases: the alarm reaction, the stage of resistance, and the stage of exhaustion. According to his hypothesis, adverse stimuli or "stressors" have nonspecific as well as specific damaging effects on the organism, and the organism responds in nonspecific as well as specific ways. Although the nervous system, kidney, and many endocrine glands are involved in the various body responses that are termed nonspecific, the adrenal cortex is assigned the leading role in this body adaptation. In a sense, the role of the adrenal cortex in adaptation represents an extension and reinforcement of what Cannon originally termed the "fight-or-flight" response of the adrenal medulla. For example, the organism's need for glucose is satisfied through glycogenolysis and gluconeogenesis resulting from increased secretion of epinephrine, while at the same time the glucocorticoids enhance these processes, promote hepatic glycogenesis, and recruit glyconeogenetic substrate from peripheral tissues. This hypothesis stimulated a considerable amount of research, and it has been considerably modified since 1946, when it was first formulated in detail. The permissive action of the corticoid hormones in adaptation was demonstrated by Engel (1957), who observed the triphasic response in rats provided with exogenous corticoids after adrenalectomy. While there is substantial evidence of the importance of the adrenal cortex to the adaptation of the organism to adverse stimuli, adaptation is a complex process with many facets, and various response patterns result from different combinations of general reactions and specific responses. Figure 34.17 diagrams some of the reactions that occur in response to hypotension resulting from hemorrhage.

Many examples of animal adaptation involving adrenal participation have been described. Domestic chickens subjected to overcrowding exhibit adrenal hypertrophy and increased adrenal weights of wild mammals appear to be a reasonably accurate measure of overpopulation. It has been speculated that these overactive adrenals may reflect part of a mechanism to limit and delay reproduction. Excess glucocorticoids have been shown to inhibit LH release in both males and females and to enhance the ability of the sex steroids to suppress gonadotropin secretion through negative feedback. The latter effect may account for the ability of glucocorticoids to delay the onset of puberty.

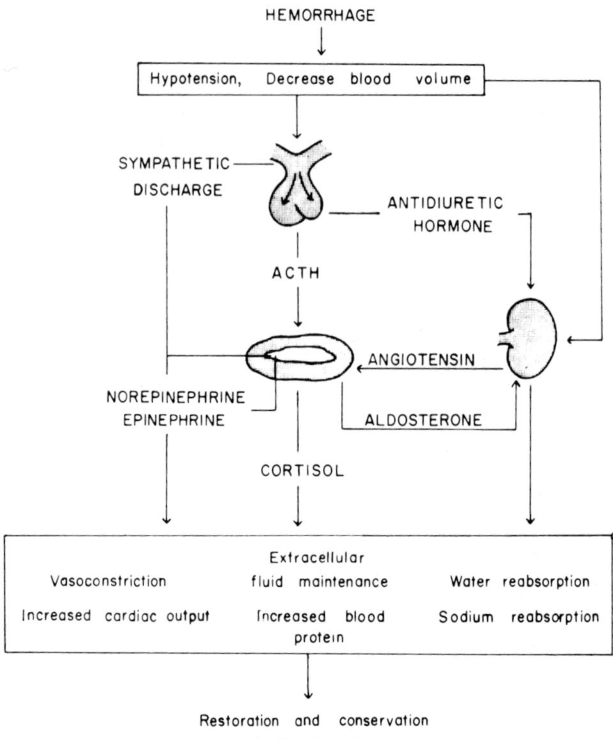

Figure 34.17. Endocrine responses to hemorrhage.

Adrenocortical dysfunction

Both hypofunction and hyperfunction of the adrenal cortex have been observed in domestic animals, and adrenocortical dysfunction constitutes one of the more commonly diagnosed endocrinopathies in the dog. The signs of adrenocortical dysfunction in this species are listed in Table 34.9. Hypofunction of the adrenal cortex varies greatly in severity; often the condition may be detected when an animal cannot respond normally to a stressful situation. The

Table 34.9. Signs of adrenocortical dysfunction in the dog

Hypofunction	Hyperfunction
Loss of weight	Thin, rough haircoat
Depression, lethargy	Thin epidermis
Fatigability	Keratin accumulation in skin
Gastrointestinal disturbances	Hyperpigmentation*
Dehydration	Cutaneous mineralization
Hyperpigmentation*	Centripetal fat distribution
Muscle weakness	Hepatomegaly
Hypotension	Muscle weakness
Hemoconcentration	Polyuria†
Moderate hypoglycemia	Polydipsia†
Plasma Na : K ratio of less than 25	Lymphopenia
Plasma cortisol less than 1.5 μg/dl (small increase 1 hour after administration of ACTH)	Eosinopenia
	Mild hyperglycemia
	Exaggerated response to ACTH (greater than 25 μg/dl)

*Due to excess ACTH.
†Results from pressure of tumor on ADH neurons.

disease results more commonly from primary adrenocortical insufficiency rather than from adenohypophyseal dysfunction. On the other hand, hyperfunction of the adrenal cortex in the dog or horse may be due to a functional tumor of the pars distalis or pars intermedia. In some cases, as in humans, the pars distalis appears to be insensitive to cortisol feedback. Autonomous functional tumors of the cortex are rare.

Laboratory diagnosis of adrenocortical dysfunction should not be based on a single plasma cortisol assay. Plasma cortisol concentrations vary widely, and the variation can occur within a very short time. Stress of any kind (transport, handling, presence of strangers, blood sampling, etc.) will markedly increase the cortisol concentration. Furthermore, although there is some uncertainty as to the occurrence and magnitude of diurnal variation in domestic animals, fivefold increases in cortisol concentration have been reported for morning samples as opposed to those taken in the afternoon. Perturbation tests, such as stimulation with ACTH or suppression with dexamethasone, are very helpful in detecting dysfunction and determining the site of the dysfunction.

Whenever adrenocortical steroids are administered in relatively high doses and for extended periods of time, the adrenal cortex of the patient becomes unresponsive to endogenous ACTH stimulation and the pituitary shows a sluggish response to stressful stimuli. If the corticoid therapy is then suddenly withdrawn, the resulting adrenocortical hypofunction can have dangerous consequences. This can be avoided by administering the steroid on alternate days so that the pituitary gland is not constantly depressed and the cortex retains some endogenous secretion.

The marked protein catabolism that occurs during high-dose, long-term corticosteroid therapy may lead to delayed wound healing, osteopenia, muscle weakness, and decreased antibody response. In addition, care must be exercised in the administration of high doses of corticoids to animals with localized infections; the anti-inflammatory effect of the steroid may result in systemic dissemination of the infection.

Adrenocortical sex steroids

In normal animals, the adrenal cortex secretes small amounts of androgenic and estrogenic steroids. The contribution, if any, of these steroids to normal function is not known; however, certain adrenal tumors produce sex steroids in excessive quantity and cause clinical signs. Masculinizing adrenocortical hyperplasia has been reported in a female mink, and it has been suggested that excessive adrenal androgens are sometimes responsible for anestrus in the cow.

A deficiency of the hydroxylating enzymes necessary in the synthesis of cortisol removes the negative feedback on ACTH and results in hyperstimulation of the adrenal cortex. The biosynthetic pathway is then directed toward synthesis of certain intermediates and the sex steroids. Such enzyme deficiencies are usually found in the newborn and are characterized by signs of androgen excess and sometimes by salt retention caused by excessive deoxycorticosterone. If the enzyme block is severe and occurs early in the biosynthetic pathway, death results. Enzyme deficiencies of this kind have not been reported in domestic animals.

PROSTAGLANDINS

In 1934 von Euler found that seminal fluid contained lipid-soluble material that lowered arterial blood pressure and stimulated isolated intestinal and smooth muscle. Assuming the origin to be the prostate gland, he named these substances *prostaglandins* (PGs); subsequent work has shown that they originate from the seminal vesicles. In 1960 Bergstrom purified and isolated the active principles, and in the late 1970s the biosynthesis of PGs, thromboxanes, and leukotrienes from arachidonic acid was described. The leukotrienes are generated through the action of the enzyme 5-lipooxygenase on arachidonic acid and are primarily involved in inflammatory processes. The thromboxanes and PGs result from the action of cyclooxygenase (Fig. 34.18) on arachidonic acid and exert various effects throughout the body. Two of these products, thromboxane and prostacyclin, are very short lived and probably do not appear in the circulation; prostacyclin, produced in the lung and endothelium of blood vessels, inhibits platelet aggregation whereas thromboxane is proaggregatory. The so-called "classic" prostaglandins, PGE and PGF, have been detected in circulating blood but are almost completely degraded on one passage through the lung and liver. Prostaglandins are named according to the structure of the five-membered ring with a subscript indicating the degree of unsaturation of the side chains.

The prostaglandins, even when administered in small quantity, have marked and diverse effects on many systems. Closely related prostaglandins often exert opposite effects. PGEs are generally vasodilators, and $PGF_{2\alpha}$ is a potent vasoconstrictor. PGE is thought to be involved in the shunting of renal blood flow from the cortex to the juxtaglomerular nephrons during renal hemodynamic stress.

Prostaglandins are, for the most part, proinflammatory and cause fever when injected into the third ventricle; the antipyretic and analgesic effects of aspirin and other drugs are due to their ability to inhibit the synthesis of prostaglandins from arachidonic acid. The anti-inflammatory action of the steroids is partly attributable to an interference in prostaglandin synthesis.

Prostaglandins enhance the motility and secretion of the small intestine (an important side effect of PG administration is diarrhea) but PGE_2 has been shown to inhibit gastric acid secretion and to prevent gastric and intestinal mucosal lesions induced by aspirin.

Inhalation of $PGF_{2\alpha}$ causes bronchospasm while PGE_2

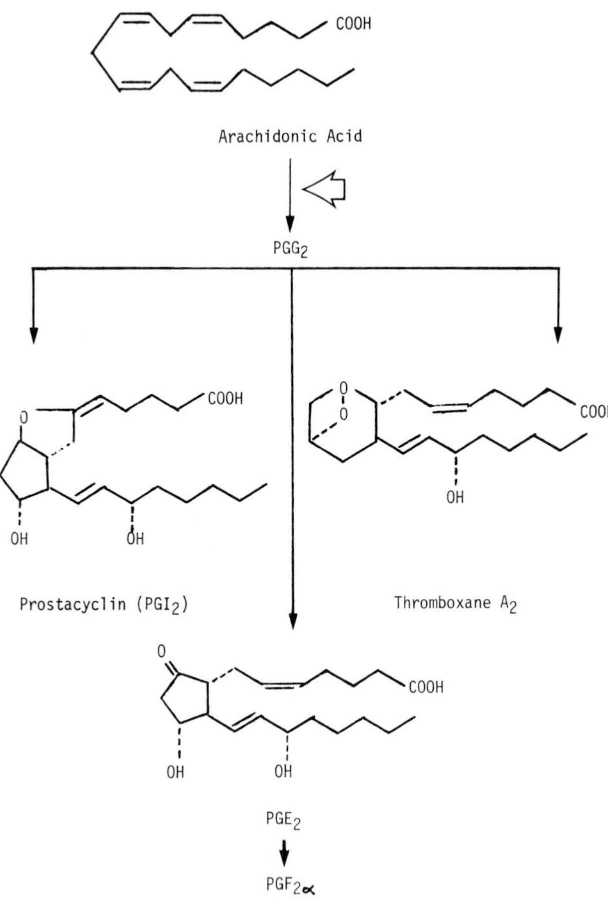

Figure 34.18. Three major pathways of prostaglandin synthesis. Open arrow indicates site of aspirin inhibition.

causes bronchodilation; asthmatic humans are extremely sensitive to the bronchoconstricting effect of $PGF_{2\alpha}$.

The role of PGs in reproduction has generated considerable attention, and in veterinary medicine reproduction is certainly the area where therapeutic application of these compounds has been most applied. The specific effects of the PGs in reproduction will be discussed in the chapters dealing with reproduction.

HORMONES FROM OTHER ORGANS

A number of humoral regulatory compounds are secreted from cells in organs not generally considered to be endocrine glands. These include renin and erythropoietin from the kidney, ANFs from the heart, the hormones secreted by gastric and intestinal mucosa, and the thymus gland secretions.

Renin-angiotensin system

The juxtaglomerular apparatus of the kidney consists of the juxtaglomerular cells, which are epithelioid cells in the media of the afferent arteriole to the glomerulus, and the macula densa, which is a region of modified kidney distal tubule cells lying in close proximity to the glomerulus and its arterioles. The juxtaglomerular cells contain and secrete renin in response to low pressure in the afferent arteriole or to decreased sodium and chloride flux in the macula densa. Renin secretion is also stimulated by prostaglandins and sympathetic nerve discharge and inhibited by vasopressin and angiotensin II.

Renin is a proteolytic glycoprotein enzyme with a molecular weight of about 40,000. Renin acts upon angiotensinogen (renin substrate), which is a circulating glycoprotein of hepatic origin, to liberate the decapeptide angiotensin I. This biologically inactive peptide is then degraded to the octapeptide angiotensin II by an enzyme termed *converting enzyme*. While much of this conversion takes place in the lung, converting enzyme is present in all endothelial cells, and angiotensin II generation occurs throughout the body. Angiotensin II stimulates aldosterone secretion from the adrenal cortex and is a potent systemic vasoconstrictor. The efferent glomerular arteriole seems to be very sensitive to angiotensin; this efferent arteriolar constriction tends to increase the glomerular filtration rate, which aids in the excretion of toxic metabolites even during systemic hypotension.

In sodium-depleted animals the pressor receptors for angiotensin II are less sensitive, whereas those in the adrenal cortex show increased sensitivity. Thus the predominant effect of angiotensin II can be adjusted somewhat according to the situation.

Angiotensin II also stimulates the thirst center in the hypothalamus to increase water intake, stimulates increased vasopressin secretion, and appears to act directly on the distal tubule to increase sodium and water retention. It has also been shown to stimulate salt and water absorption in the jejunum and colon and to induce formation of blood vessels.

Angiotensin II is metabolized to angiotensin III, a heptapeptide with much less vasopressor activity but with virtually equal activity on the adrenal gland. Further degradation leads to various inactive metabolites. The half-life of angiotensin II is very short, but renin activity persists for longer periods, leading to a reasonably sustained effect.

Atrial natriuretic factor

In 1956 Kisch reported the presence of secretory granules in cardiac atrial cells, and it was later shown that atrial extracts have vasodilatory and natriuretic activity. The existence of an atrial hormone, termed *atrial natriuretic factor* (ANF), is now well established.

The predominant form of the hormone, which is stored in the heart, is the 126 amino acid proANF; on secretion, this is cleaved, generating the 28 amino acid, biologically active hormone, ANF. The secretion of ANF is stimulated whenever atrial pressure is increased, either by pressor stimulants or by an increase in atrial stretch volume.

The effects of ANF on the kidney are natriuretic and diuretic; ANF stimulates an increase in glomerular filtration rate and the renal excretion of water, sodium, chloride, magnesium, calcium and phosphate. The increased glomerular filtration rate does not account for the increased urinary solute concentration; in fact, the urinary sodium concentration commonly exceeds the plasma sodium concentration after ANF injection.

Atrial natriuretic factor blocks the secretion of vasopressin from the neurohypophysis and the angiotensin II, potassium, or ACTH-stimulated release of aldosterone from the adrenal cortex.

The effects of ANF on the vasculature are somewhat conflicting and vary with the experimental preparation. In vitro, ANF has vasodilatory actions and opposes the vasopressor actions of catecholamines or angiotensin II. In vivo, the injection of ANF in rats increases blood flow to the kidney, gastrointestinal tract, heart, testes, lung, and spleen with no change in cardiac output, but in the dog the blood flow increase is confined to the kidney. In general, ANF causes a decrease in blood pressure in both normal and hypertensive animals; whether this results from fluid loss, decreased cardiac output, or peripheral vasodilation is not clear.

In summary, ANF appears to be a hormone that protects the animal against fluid volume overload and elevated blood pressure.

Erythropoietin

Adjustments in red blood cell production and release are mediated by *erythropoietin*, a circulating glycoprotein with a molecular weight of about 23,000. Erythropoietin, a substance produced by the kidney in response to hypoxia, stimulates certain stem cells in bone marrow to differentiate into proerythroblasts.

Gastrointestinal hormones

Various humoral agents are secreted by mucosal cells in the stomach and intestine and are carried by the circulation or within the intestinal lumen to influence the functions of the stomach, intestine, pancreas, and gallbladder. Table 34.10 summarizes these compounds. The major gastrointestinal hormones have been discussed in Chapter 16.

A number of humoral regulators have been detected in both gastrointestinal tissue and the CNS. Substance P, neurotensin, somatostatin, and serotonin have been isolated from both areas. Immunoreactive sites have been found in the CNS for CCK, vasoactive intestinal polypeptide, motilin, and bombesin, whereas such sites have been reported in the gastrointestinal tract for enkephalin, endorphin, and thyrotropin-releasing hormone. The significance of these observations is unclear.

Serotonin is found in certain special silver-staining cells that are particularly common in the mucosa of the gastrointestinal tract and in association with the bile ducts. These cells represent the *enterochromaffin tissue*. Serotonin is also found in high concentration in certain parts of the CNS and in the blood platelets. The latter represent a storage or transport site and can accumulate large quantities of this substance. Serotonin exerts diverse and interesting effects, including contraction of intestinal smooth muscle, dilatation of the coronary vascular bed, constriction of the afferent glomerular arterioles, and depression of activity in the CNS. Serotonin has a complicated effect on blood pressure; depending on the dose and the species, its effects may be either hypertensive or hypotensive.

Table 34.10. Gastrointestinal peptides

	Major secretory source	Gastrointestinal or metabolic effect	
Gastrin	Stomach	Gastric secretion	+
		Glucagon	+
		Insulin	+
		Calcitonin	+
Gastric inhibitory peptide (GIP)	Duodenum	Gastric secretion	−
		Gastric motility	−
		Insulin	+
Motilin	Duodenum	Gastric secretion	+
Cholecystokinin (CCK)	Duodenum	Gallbladder contraction	+
		Pancreatic enzymes	+
		Glucagon	+
		Gastric motility	−
Secretin	Duodenum, jejunum	Pancreatic juice volume and HCO_3	+
Vasoactive intestinal peptide (VIP)	Ileum	Intestinal juice volume and electrolyte	+
		Gastric acid secretion	−
Substance P	Gastrointestinal tract	Intestinal motility	+
Bombesin	Stomach	Gastric secretion	+
		Intestinal motility	+
		Gastrin, VIP, GIP, secretin, motilin	−
Somatostatin	Stomach	Pancreatic secretion	−
		Gastric secretion	−
		Gastric motility	−
		Gallbladder contraction	−
		Insulin	−
		Glucagon	−

+, increase; −, decrease.

Thymus gland

The thymus gland is a unique organ in that it is large and active in the newborn, reaches the apex of its activity at puberty, and declines in activity slowly but steadily thereafter. The thymus is particularly sensitive to the lympholytic action of adrenal glucocorticoids.

Various experiments have demonstrated that the thymus is essential for the normal development and maintenance of immunological competence. Mice that have been subjected to thymectomy at birth develop a condition called *wasting disease*, which can be prevented by an implant of thymus tissue; this is the case, even when the implant is enclosed in a diffusion compartment that excludes the exit of cells. It has been proposed that, normally, a thymic hormone reacts with the lymphoid cells in the thymus and other lymphoid tissues to produce cells that are capable of recognizing and reacting with antigens. Whenever one of these competent but uncommitted lymphoid cells encounters and reacts with an antigen, it begins to multiply and gives rise to plasma cells, which synthesize the appropriate antibodies.

Various protein substances varying in molecular weight from less than 1000 to 200,000 have been isolated from the thymus and proposed as thymic hormones. Wasting disease can be prevented by injections of homeostatic thymic hormone, thymosin, or thymic humoral factor. Homeostatic thymic hormone or lymphocyte-stimulating hormone is capable of increasing the lymphocyte/polymorphonuclear cell ratio, and either thymosin or thymic humoral factor can stimulate cell-mediated immunity.

Actions not directly related to the immune response and the lymphoid system have been ascribed to thymic extracts. A neuromuscular blocking agent, *thymin*, is thought to be released in excess in autoimmune thymitis and causes depression of neuromuscular transmission.

REFERENCES

Dorfman, R.I., and Ungar, F. 1953. *Metabolism of Steroid Hormones*. Burgess, Philadelphia.

Felig, P., Baxter, J.D., Broadus, A.E., and Frohman, L.A. 1987. *Endocrinology and Metabolism*. 2d ed. McGraw-Hill, New York.

Gardiner-Hill, H., ed. 1958. *Modern Trends in Endocrinology*. Hoeber, New York.

Hume-Adams, J., Daniel, P.M., and Prichard, M.L. 1964. Distribution of hypophyseal portal blood in the anterior lobe of the pituitary gland. *Endocrinology* 75:120–26.

Kelley, S.T., and Oehme, F.W. 1974. Circulating thyroid levels in dogs, horses, and cattle. *Vet. Small Anim. Clinician* 69:1531–33.

Klyne, W. 1957. *The Chemistry of the Steroids*. Methuen, London.

Ling, G.V., Lowenstine, L.K., and Kaneko, J.J. 1974. Serum thyroxine and triiodothyronine uptake values in normal adult cats. *Am. J. Vet. Res.* 35:1247–49.

Murphy, B.E.P. 1969. Distribution of values for serum T_4 concentration in euthyroid, hypothyroid, and hyperthyroid patients. *Recent Prog. Horm. Res.* 25:563–610.

Reap, M., Cass, C., and Hightower, D. 1978. Thyroxine and triiodothyronine levels in ten species of animals. *Southwestern Vet.* 31:31–34.

Sutherland, R.L., and Irvine, C.H.G. 1973. Total plasma thyroxine concentration in horses, pigs, cattle, and sheep: Anion exchange resin chromatography and ceric arsenite colorimetry. *Am. J. Vet. Res.* 34:1261–70.

Thomas, C.L., and Adams, J.C. 1978. Thyroxine levels in horses. *Am. J. Vet. Res.* 39:1239.

West, G.B. 1955. The comparative pharmacology of the suprarenal medulla. *Q. Rev. Biol.* 30:116–37.

Williams, R.H. 1974. *Textbook of Endocrinology*. 5th ed. W.B. Saunders, Philadelphia.

CHAPTER 35

Male Reproductive Processes | by George H. Stabenfeldt and Lars-Eric Edqvist

The male gonad, the testis, has two major functions: first, to produce germ cells called spermatzoa that transmit the male genes to the offspring and, second, to produce androgens, which give the individual male characteristics including the drive and the means to deliver germ cells to the female. The spermatozoa are produced within the seminiferous tubules of the testes by the process called spermatogenesis. During spermatogenesis, the number of chromosomes characteristic of each species is halved, so that each new individual receives one-half of its genes as a random sample from its sire and a similar contribution from its dam. The Leydig cell, found in the interstitium of the testis, and the Sertoli cell, located within the seminiferous tubule, support the production of germ cells. The spermatozoa pass from the seminiferous tubules into the epididymides, where they mature until they are ejaculated. The secretions of the accessory glands (seminal vesicles, bulbourethral glands, and prostate) provide nutrients to spermatozoa at the time of ejaculation.

ANATOMICAL ASPECTS

The main functional parts of the male genital system of domestic animals are the penis, scrotum and testes, rete tubules, efferent tubules, epididymides, vasa deferentia, accessory glands including the ampulla, prostate, seminal vesicles, and bulbourethral glands (Fig. 35.1).

The reproductive organs of male domestic animals have several unique features. In the ram, the penis is characterized by a filiform appendage containing the urethra. The large size of the accessory glands (seminal vesicles and bulbourethral glands) of the boar contribute to the remarkably large volume of semen produced by this species. The boar also has the largest testes per unit of body weight of the domestic animals. The preputial diverticulum of the boar is well developed and usually contains degenerating epithelial cells and urine. The penis of the stallion is vascular and has a urethra that protrudes several centimeters from the surface of the glans penis of the stallion. The penis of the bull, ram, and boar contains a sigmoid flexure that is straightened during erection and extension of the penis.

The most remarkable features of the reproductive tract of the male dog are the os penis and the absence of all accessory glands except the prostate and ampullae. The penis of the cat is distinguished by the presence of spines and by its posterior orientation. The cat, dog, and pig have posterior presentations of their scrotal testes while the bull, buck, ram, and stallion have ventral presentations.

SPERMATOGENESIS

The spermatogonium

The term *spermatogenesis* indicates the entire developmental process involved in the transformation of the stem cell, or *spermatogonium*, into a *spermatozoon*. The process begins at the wall of the seminiferous tubule, which is lined with spermatogonia, and ends with the release of mature spermatozoa in the lumen of the seminiferous tubule. Sper-

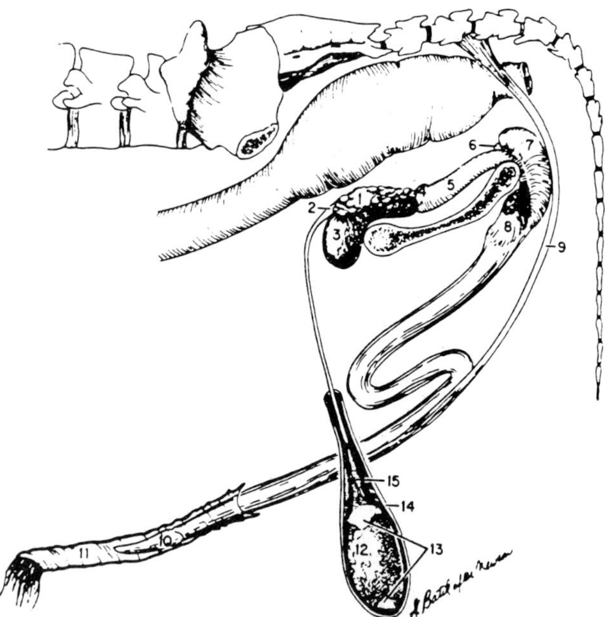

Figure 35.1. Reproductive organs of the bull: 1, seminal vesicle; 2, ampulla; 3, urinary bladder; 4, prostate; 5, urethral muscle surrounding the pelvic urethra; 6, bulbourethral gland; 7, bulbocavernosus muscle; 8, ischiocavernosus muscle; 9, retractor penis muscle; 10, glans penis; 11, preputial membrane and cavity; 12, testis; 13, epididymis; 14, scrotum; 15, spermatic cord.

matogenesis involves mitotic proliferation, meiotic division, and differentiation of the haploid spermatid.

Spermatogenesis is initiated when spermatogonia undergo mitosis. One spermatogonium formed by the initial mitotic division does not divide and differentiate further but remains in a basal state of differentiation; in essence, it replaces the parental cell. The other spermatogonium undergoes mitosis. The basic function of mitosis is to ensure the production of large numbers of germ cells. The process of germ cell production differs in the male and female in that (1) the supply of germ cells is replenished (maintained) in the male, whereas germ cells continue to decrease throughout the reproductive life of the female, and (2) germ cell numbers are greatly increased during spermatogenesis by mitosis in the male, whereas mitosis ceases at birth in the female and oogenesis involves the development of a limited number of preformed germ cells.

Mitosis

The first major phase of spermatogenesis, *mitosis*, has a species-specific number of divisions. For example, after the initial mitotic division, there are three divisions in man, four in the bull, buck (rabbit) and ram, and five divisions in the rat. At the end of the final mitotic division in the bull, for example, 16 cells would have been formed; these are known as *primary spermatocytes* (see Fig. 35.2). From a quantitative standpoint, the greater the number of mitotic divisions, the greater the number of spermatozoa produced per unit weight of testis. At the end of the mitotic phase, the germ cells that are now primary spermatocytes enter the first prophase of meiosis, where development is arrested for a variable period of time.

Deoxyribonucleic acid is synthesized during and throughout the last mitotic division. There is some evidence that autosomal chromosomes continue to code for messenger ribonucleic acid during meiosis and the first part of spermiogenesis. If so, this suggests that the haploid gene complement may have some influence on the development of genetic material within the finished male germ cell.

Meiosis

Meiosis, the second major step in spermatogenesis, has as its function the reduction of the chromosome number of the germ cell to the haploid state. This is essential to allow the union of haploid spermatozoa and oocytes to form new individuals with the correct number of chromosomes. The first stage of meiosis is completed with cell division and a 50 percent reduction in the chromosome number. The resultant cell is a *secondary spermatocyte*. Although the cells are technically haploid at this stage, a further division is required because the chromosomes replicate at the beginning of meiosis. After the second cell division of meiosis, the cells are called *spermatids*.

Spermiogenesis

The third and final step in spermatogenesis involves the maturation of spermatids into spermatozoa, a process called *spermiogenesis*. Maturation involves (1) formation of a tail to aid movement within the female reproductive tract, (2) development of mitochondria to furnish energy during movement in the female tract, and (3) development of an organelle, the acrosome that allows penetration of the oocyte. A considerable amount of cytoplasm is extruded from the cell during spermatogenesis. Remnants of cytoplasm are sometimes observed attached to the spermatozoon and are referred to as cytoplasmic droplets. The presence of cytoplasmic droplets is sometimes interpreted as an indication that the maturation process is not complete. Cytoplasmic bridges that have held developing clones of spermatozoa together during development disappear at the end of spermiogenesis. Spermiogenesis starts in the seminiferous tubules and finishes in the epididymis.

As previously indicated, 16 primary spermatocytes could arise in the bull from the mitotic divisions of one spermatogonium. This number would be further expanded to 64 because of the two cell divisions that occur during meiosis. Cell loss, however, occurs at all points of the multiplication process and the total number of mature spermatozoa produced is almost always less than the theoretical number.

The process of spermatogenesis involves the cloning of a large number of spermatogonia. Cells within a clone are not identical, however, because of meiotic chiasma formation.

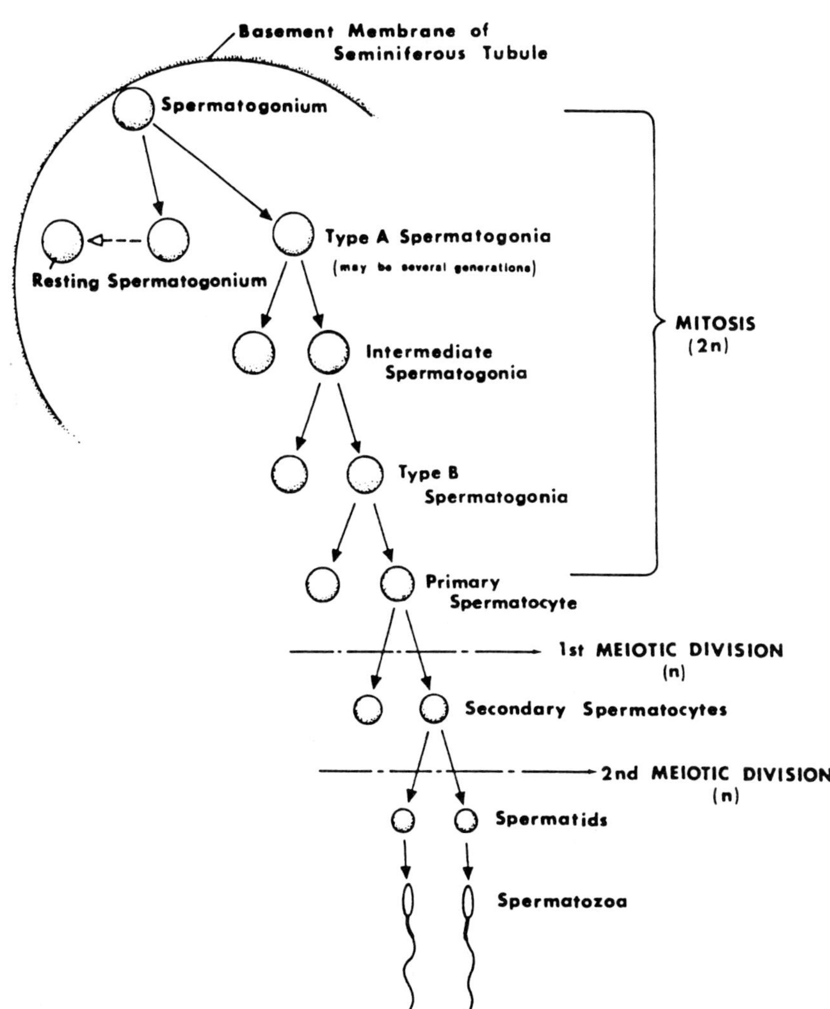

Figure 35.2. Diagrammatic representation of spermatogenesis, which involves transformation of spermatogonia into spermatozoa. The initial mitotic division of a spermatogonium produces one cell that replaces the original spermatogonium and one cell that continues to divide (type A). The type A spermatogonium divides progressively to form other generations of type A (e.g., type A2, A3, A4), the number of generations being a function of the species. Most type A spermatogonia divide to form intermediate spermatogonia, which in turn divide to form type B spermatogonia. Primary spermatocytes are formed at the last mitotic division. A reduction in chromosome number occurs during meiosis, with secondary spermatocytes being produced by the first meiotic division and spermatids by the second meiotic division. The differentiation process to this point is called spermatocytogenesis. Spermatids then differentiate into spermatozoa by the process of spermiogenesis. (From McDonald, 1989, *Veterinary Endocrinology and Reproduction*, 4th ed., Lea & Febiger, Philadelphia. Reprinted with permission.)

This process increases the genetic variability of germ cells in spite of a common ancestral source (within a clone).

Spermatogenic cycle

Spermatogenesis is initiated at the same cell site at regular intervals (Fig. 35.3), the interval being designated a *spermatogenic cycle*. Each spermatogonium that replaces the parental cell begins to divide at a time interval that is characteristic of each species. The spermatogenic cycle for various species is as follows: pig, 8 days; sheep, 10 days; rat, 12 day; cattle, 14 days; and human, 16 days.

There is a fairly precise relationship between the duration of the spermatogenic cycle and spermatogenesis, i.e., spermatogenesis is approximately four times the duration of the spermatogenic cycle. For example, in the bull with a spermatogenic cycle of 14 days, mitotic proliferation requires about one cycle (14 days) and meiotic division requires two cycles (28 days). Spermiogenesis requires 22 to 23 days before sperm are released into the lumen of the seminiferous tubule. Thus the process of spermatogenesis in the bull requires 4.6 spermatogenic cycles:

$$\frac{(14 + 28 + 22)}{14}$$

Although the period of spermiogenesis does not precisely equal one spermatogenic cycle, initiation of the mitotic division of a spermatogonium of a certain cell line coincides with the beginning of meiosis of related cells and the beginning of spermiogenesis of another population of related cells. Because of this relationship, characteristic cell associations occur within a cloning area of the seminiferous tubule (Fig. 35.3).

Spermatogenic wave

Spermatogenesis is coordinated as to areas (lengthwise) of the seminiferous tubule, a phenomenon called the *sper-*

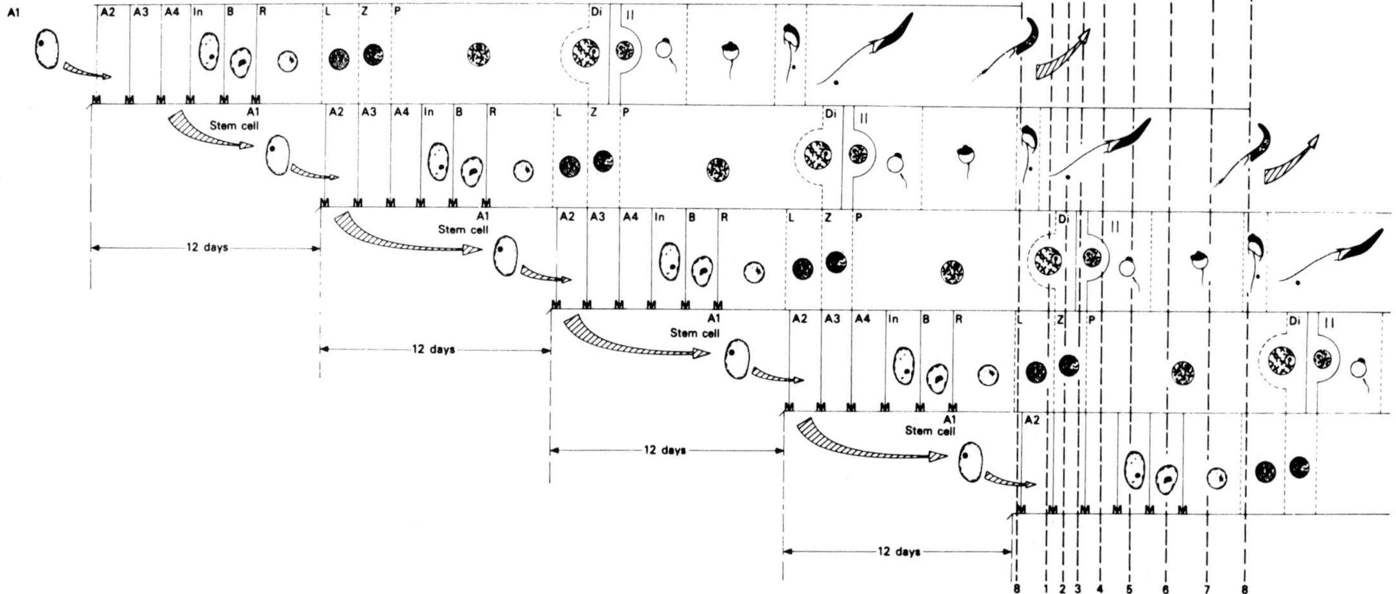

Figure 35.3. The top panel illustrates the passage of one rat spermatozoon through the spermatogenic process. The length of the blocks interconnecting each cellular stage illustrated is proportional to the amount of time it takes to progress through the different stages. Note that where new cell types arise by mitosis (M), solid bars interconnect adjacent blocks. During meiotic prophase and spermiogenesis, however, cells change morphology by steady and progressive differentiation, not by quantum jumps. For these cells, the broken bars interconnecting adjacent boxes indicate that the cells illustrated are samples chosen from a continuum of change. Progressively developing spermatogonia are indicated by A, In, and B; resting (R), leptotene (L), zygotene (Z), pachytene (P), and diplotene (Di) are the primary spermatocytes; II, secondary spermatocytes. Each of the lower panels shows the history of other spermatozoa that commenced development by cyclic reentry of the same stem-cell population into spermatogenesis at progressively later time intervals. The length of one spermatogenic cycle is indicated. Note that four cycles elapse before the upper spermatozoon, and its cohorts in the clone, complete development and are released. Thus several different cell types will be present at the same point in the tubule at the same time, although at different points along a radial axis through the tubule. (Slightly modified from Johnson and Everitt 1980, *Essential Reproduction,* Blackwell Scientific Publications, Oxford.)

matogenic wave (Fig. 35.4). There is evidence in the rat that the most central area of the seminiferous tubule is activated first at puberty (i.e., all spermatognia within a certain limited longitudinal area of the tubule are programmed to begin dividing at the same time). Areas adjacent to this area are observed to have progressively earlier stages of spermatogenesis. In other animals (e.g., humans) the area of cell coordination can be relatively small and occupy only one portion of the seminiferous tubule on a longitudinal basis.

Spermatogenesis, once initiated, is a process in which spermatozoa are produced continuously as a result of regional coordination of sperm production because of the spermatogenic wave phenomenon. Interruptions occur normally in some species (i.e., seasonal breeders). In these animals, spermatogenesis is initiated and terminated each year.

The Sertoli cell

The other major cell type within the seminiferous tubule is the *Sertoli cell* (Fig. 35.5). The Sertoli cell is important for controlling the development of germ cells with respect to both nutritive and regulatory function. The Sertoli cells are large, have prominent nucleoli, and are basally situated within the tubule. These cells have long processes that sur-

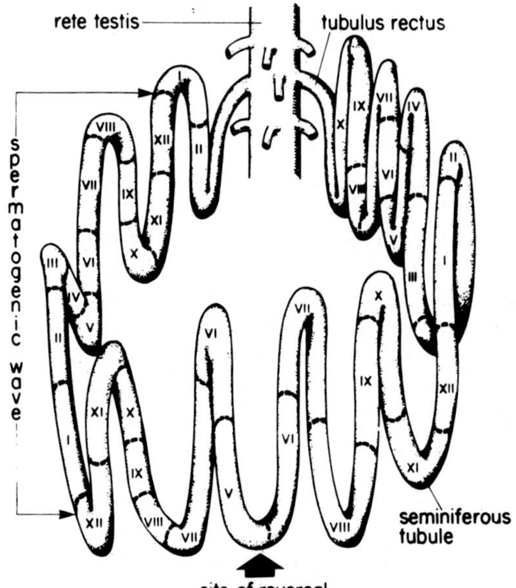

Figure 35.4. Diagrammatic representation of the spermatogenic wave. In this phenomenon, all spermatogonia within a certain area of the seminiferous tubule are programmed to begin dividing at the same time. Successive stages of development, designated I to XII, are adjacent to each other. This process allows for the continuous supply of mature spermatozoa. (From Hafez 1987, *Reproduction in Farm Animals*, 5th ed., Lea & Febiger, Philadelphia. Reprinted with permission.)

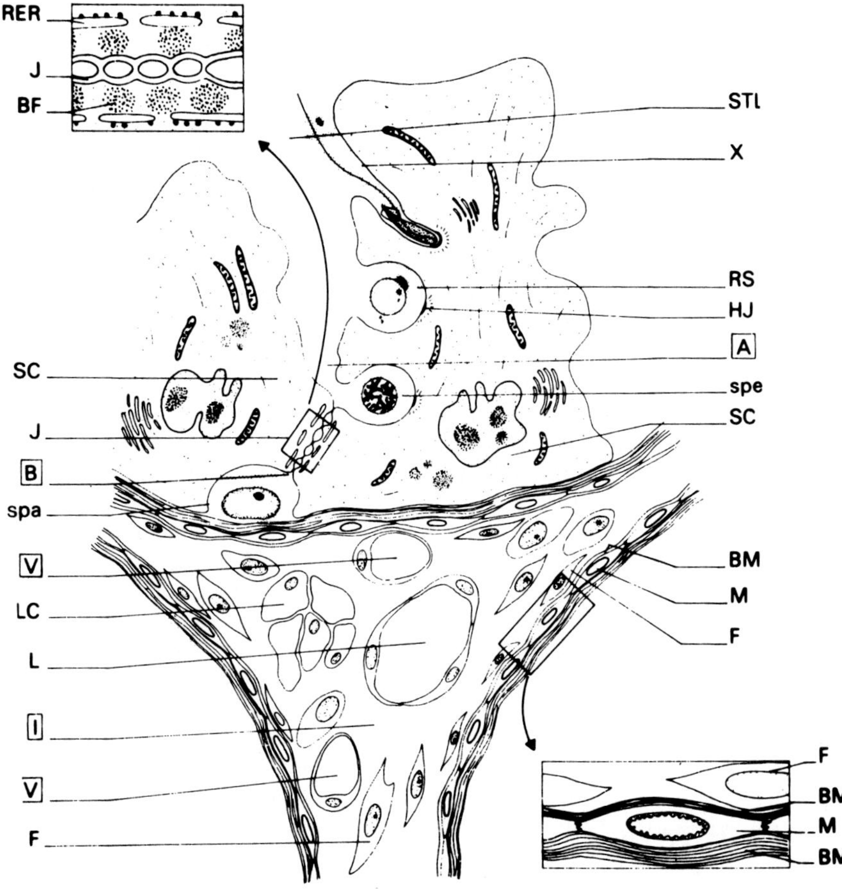

Figure 35.5. Cross section through part of an adult testis. There are four compartments in the testis: the vascular (V); interstitial (I), including the lymphatic vessels (L) and containing the Leydig cells (LC); basal (B); and adluminal (A) compartments. The basal and adluminal compartments lie within the seminiferous tubules. An acellular basement membrane (BM) containing myoid cells (M) and invested with a loose coat of interstitial fibrocytes (F) separates the interstitial and basal compartments. Myoid cells are linked to each other by punctate junctions. The basal and adluminal compartments are separated by rows of zonular junctional complexes (J) linking together adjacent Sertoli cells (SC) around the complete circumference of the seminiferous tubule. Beneath the region of junctional complexes are bundles of filaments (BF) running parallel to the surface around the "waist" of the Sertoli cells, and beneath the filaments are cisternae of rough endoplasmic reticulum (RER). Within the basal compartment are the spermatogonia (spa), whereas spermatocytes (spe), round spermatids (RS), and spermatozoa (X) are shown in the adluminal compartment (STL, seminiferous tubule lumen) and in intimate contact with the Sertoli cells, which form anchoring "hemi junctions" (HJ) with the elongating spermatids. (From Johnson and Everitt 1980, *Essential Reproduction*, Blackwell Scientific Publications, Oxford.)

round the spermatocytes and spermatids and provide an intimate interaction with germ cells throughout their development. During the process of maturation, spermatocytes that originate from spermatogonia in the basal compartment of the tubule move through the tight junctions formed between Sertoli cells and finish their development in the adluminal (central) compartment of the tubule.

On maturation, the spermatozoa are released from the Sertoli cell and become free in the lumen of the seminiferous tubule. The Sertoli cell is thought to be the main source of fluid that is secreted into the lumen of the tubule. The number of Sertoli cells remains constant during spermatogenesis.

HORMONAL CONTROL OF SPERMATOGENESIS

Two cell types are responsible for hormone production within the testis: the Leydig cell and the Sertoli cell. The Leydig cell is located outside the seminiferous tubule in the interstitium (also called *interstitial cell*) (Fig. 35.5). The hormonal control of these cells is presented in Fig. 35.6.

The Leydig cell

The main function of the Leydig cell is production of testosterone, which is important for the development and maintenance of spermatogenesis and male characteristics.

Leydig cell production of testosterone is controlled by the gonadotropin, luteinizing hormone (LH) (earlier called interstitial cell-stimulating hormone). LH binds specifically to Leydig cell membranes and activates cyclic adenosine monophosphate. This process initiates the activation of protein kinases, which catalyze the phosphorylation of intracellular proteins and the mobilization of steroid precursors, mainly through the conversion of cholesterol to pregnenolone. The main biosynthetic pathways from pregnenolone involve either Δ5-intermediates (pregnenolone, 17α-hydroxypregnenolone, dehydroepiandrosterone, and 5-androstenediol), or Δ4-intermediates (progesterone, 17α-hydroxyprogesterone, and 4-androstenedione) (see Fig. 36.1). There is considerable variability among species as to pathways that are utilized.

LH also has a tropic effect on the Leydig cells, stimulating them to undergo hypertrophy. Removal of LH leads to

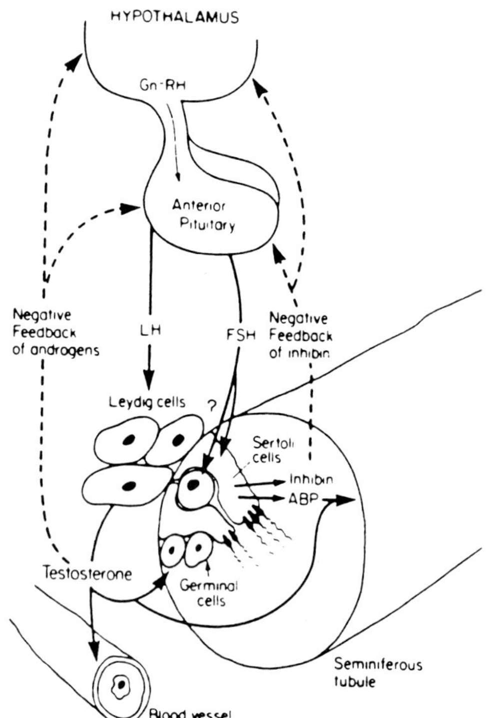

Figure 35.6. Diagrammatic representation of the endocrine control of the testis. The hypothalamus secretes gonadotropin-releasing hormone (GnRH) that stimulates secretion of LH and FSH from the anterior pituitary. LH stimulates Leydig cells to produce testosterone, which in turn suppresses GnRH and gonadotropin secretion by negative-feedback inhibition. FSH stimulates Sertoli cell activity, including the secretion of androgen-binding protein (ABP), the conversion of androgens to estrogens, and the secretion of inhibin. Inhibin has a negative-feedback effect on FSH secretion. (From Hafez 1987, *Reproduction in Farm Animals*, 5th ed., Lea & Febiger, Philadelphia. Reprinted with permission.)

cessation of testosterone production and a great reduction in the size of the Leydig cells.

A sensitive negative-feedback system operates between LH and testosterone secretion. Increases in LH secretion are followed within 30 to 60 minutes by increased levels of testosterone, which last from 1 to several hours. Negative-feedback inhibition of LH secretion by testosterone is followed by a resultant decline in testosterone synthesis.

Testosterone produced by the Leydig cells moves into the seminiferous tubule by either simple or facilitated diffusion. High intratesticular concentrations of testosterone are required for spermatogenesis and especially for the process of meiosis. Testosterone also moves readily into the blood vascular system, where it is important for the development and maintenance of libido, secretory activity of the male accessory organs, and development of general body features associated with the male phenotype, such as increased muscle mass.

Boar testes secrete considerable amounts of C-16 unsaturated androgens. Plasma concentrations of 5α-androstenone, the major C-16 unsaturated androgen, is usually higher than the testosterone concentration. These steroids are partly excreted in the saliva, where they act as pheromones, facilitating the expression of the rigidity reflex, or copulatory stance, of the sow in estrus. The C-16 unsaturated androgens are an important component of the odor of boar urine and are responsible for the undesirable flavor of boar meat, the so-called *boar taint*.

The Sertoli cell

The secretory activity of the Sertoli cell is controlled by follicle-stimulating hormone (FSH) (Fig. 35.6). Membrane receptors for FSH and cytoplasmic and nuclear receptors for androgens are present in Sertoli cells. The Sertoli cell converts testosterone produced by the Leydig cell into estrogens. This situation is analogous to that in the female in which testosterone is produced by cells outside the basement membrane (theca) and subsequently is converted into estrogens by the cells inside the basement membrane (granulosa). Estrogens move into both the adluminal and the basal compartments of the testis. From the latter compartment, estrogens can move into the blood vascular system where large amounts of estrogens are found in the blood of some species, particularly the stallion. The function of estrogens in spermatogenesis is not known.

The Sertoli cell converts testosterone into dihydrotestosterone, an androgen of greater biological potency than testosterone; testosterone also moves through the Sertoli cell into the adluminal compartment without being transformed. The Sertoli cell synthesizes a protein, *androgen-binding protein* (ABP), which binds androgens within the adluminal compartment. The function of this protein is not known, although it may serve as a means of stabilizing the concentration of androgens in the seminiferous tubules for use in both spermatogenesis and Sertoli cell function.

The Sertoli cell is also a source of *inhibin*, a protein molecule that suppresses FSH secretion at the level of the pituitary gland (gonadotropes). Inhibin has subunits that are linked by disulfide bonds: an α-subunit with a molecular weight of about 18,000 that is common to both forms of inhibin (A and B) and a β-subunit that varies in molecular weight (13,800 to 14,700) and gives inhibin its biological identity. In the presence of high spermatogenic and, therefore, high Sertoli cell activity, FSH concentrations tend to be low because of the production of inhibin by the Sertoli cell. One of the signs that the spermatogenic process is depressed, at least as concerns Sertoli cell activity, is a high FSH value in a male.

The gonadotropins

LH is required for spermatogenesis because of its role in testosterone production. Testosterone alone, however, is not adequate for the continuation of spermatogenesis, with a block to spermatogenesis occurring at meiosis in the absence of gonadotropins other than LH (demonstrated in hypophysectomy studies in rats). FSH is important for the completion of meiosis of germ cells through its influence on Sertoli cell activity. There is some evidence that a third gonadotropin is important for spermatogenesis (i.e., prolactin which facilitates the interaction of LH with its receptors located on the Leydig cells).

COMPARTMENTS OF THE TESTIS

There are four compartments within the testis. They are the vascular and interstitial compartments, which are external to the seminiferous tubule, and the basal and adluminal compartments, which are internal to the seminiferous tubule (see Fig. 35.5). The undifferentiated spermatogonia are in the basal compartment, with the differentiating germ cells located in the adluminal part of the seminiferous tubule. The intertubular and intratubular cell populations are separated by a barrier composed of the basement membrane, which contains myoid cells and fibrocytes. Within the tubules, the tight junctional complexes of the Sertoli cells act as a barrier between luminal and adluminal spaces. The Sertoli cell complex controls both the passage of molecules and developing germ cells. The barrier, formed mainly by the Sertoli cells, is known as the *blood-testis barrier*.

Blood-testis barrier

The blood-testis barrier has two main functions. First, it allows the creation of an adluminal environment in which the metabolism of spermatozoa is controlled. For example, potassium ions, selectively secreted into the adluminal space, are important for maintaining spermatozoa in a quiescent state. Second, the blood-testis barrier protects against the movement of spermatozoa into the interstitium of the testis. Because the spermatozoon becomes haploid during its formation as a secondary spermatocyte, it is not recognized as "self" by the general defense mechanisms of the body. The leakage of spermatozoa into the interstitium results in the development of a severe inflammatory reaction involving mainly monocytic type cells. The inflammatory response to spermatozoa can result in the obliteration of areas of the testis. These types of reaction are more often observed in the epididymis, suggesting that the barrier may not be as effective in the epididymis as within the seminiferous tubules of the testis.

The epididymis

The epididymis is important for both maturation and storage of spermatozoa (Fig. 35.7). Spermatozoa do not gain the ability to move and penetrate an oocyte until they have passed through the epididymis. The presence of a *forward-motility protein* in the epididymis allows the spermatozoon to become motile. Further maturation of the acrosome occurs within the epididymis, which allows the sperm to penetrate the oocyte.

The metabolism of spermatozoa in the epididymis is low. Two factors that contribute to this are (1) the small amount of oxidizable substrate present (except for lactic acid) and (2) high concentrations of potassium which are inhibitory to motility.

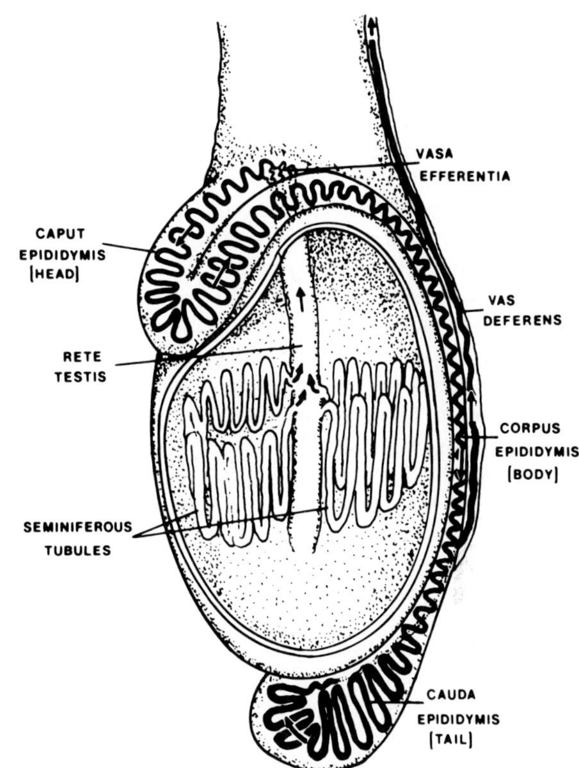

Figure 35.7. Diagrammatic representation of the duct system by which spermatozoa leave the testis (seminiferous tubules, rete testis, and vasa efferentia) and the excurrent duct system which stores (epididymis) and transports (vas deferens) spermatozoa. (From Hafez 1987, *Reproduction in Farm Animals*, 5th ed., Lea & Febiger, Philadelphia. Reprinted with permission.)

Epididymal function is dependent on the presence of adluminal testosterone. The absence of testosterone in the epididymis, caused by ligation of the efferent ductules, results in degeneration of the epididymis. The epididymis has some capacity for degrading and absorbing ABP.

The head of the epididymis absorbs considerable amounts of fluid that originates in the seminiferous tubule. This absorption results in a high concentration of spermatozoa in the tail of the epididymis, with the tail storing about 80 percent of the mature germ cells. In the absence of ejaculation, the main fate of spermatozoa is spontaneous discharge into the urethra and out in the urine. Resorption of spermatozoa by the epididymis does not occur.

Obstructive lesions in the epididymis affect the testicle differently, depending on the site of obstruction. If the lesion is in the head, degeneration of the testis occurs through the accumulation of fluid and the development of pressure within the seminiferous tubules. If the lesion is in the tail, the testicle may appear normal because fluid can still be absorbed by the head of the epididymis. Obviously, both conditions result in infertility of the affected animal.

MALE ACCESSORY ORGANS

Physical characteristics

In addition to the testes, epididymides, and the system of ducts that transport spermatozoa to the exterior of the animal, the male genital system consists of various glands that add their secretions to the spermatozoa at the time of ejaculation. These include the ampullae, seminal vesicles, prostate, and bulbourethral glands (see Fig. 35.1).

The size and location of the accessory sex glands vary considerably among the domestic animals. The prostate, for example, is disseminated in the ram and the goat, whereas in the boar and the bull the gland is both disseminated and discrete. The prostate is a compact gland in the dog. Distinct dorsal, ventral, and lateral lobes are present in some species. The prostate is a compound tubuloalveolar gland in all domestic animals.

The ampulla is an enlargement that arises at the distal end of the ductus deferens. It is most prominent in the dog and horse. The seminal vesicles are elongated glands with complex internal villous projections; they are relatively large in domestic animals, especially in the boar. The bulbourethral glands, also compound tubuloalveolar glands, are the most caudally located accessory organs and are found just anterior to the bulbocavernosus muscle. They are remarkably large, cylindrical structures in the boar.

Chemical composition and function of seminal plasma

The secretion of the male accessory sex organs is known collectively as seminal plasma. This fluid, released at the time of ejaculation, provides an ionically balanced and nutritive environment that is conducive to the survival of sperm within the female reproductive tract.

Fructose is the major source of energy for spermatozoa in seminal plasma of the bull, ram, goat, and rabbit. It is derived mainly from the seminal vesicles and is metabolized to lactic acid by spermatozoa. Sorbitol, a sugar alcohol that is present in the semen and accessory glands of several domestic species, is readily reduced to fructose. The seminal vesicles also produce inositol, a nonreducing carbohydrate, in large amounts in the boar and in smaller amounts in the bull, ram, and stallion. Inositol has also been found in ampullary secretions of the stallion. The physiologic significance of this substance is not known, except that it could serve as a source of carbohydrate through conversion to fructose.

Boar seminal vesicles secrete a large quantity of ergothioneine, a sulfur-containing base thought to protect the spermatozoa from the toxic effects of oxidizing agents. Ampullary secretions of the stallion also contain ergothioneine. This is important because both boar and stallion semen has characteristics, such as large volume, low sperm concentration, and low amounts of glycolyzable sugars, that make it particularly vulnerable to oxidizing agents. Ascorbic acid, produced by the seminal vesicles of most other species, is also a strong reducing substance. Seminal vesicle secretions contain many other substances, such as citric acid, amino acids, proteins, sodium, potassium, lipids, and phosphorylcholine. Choline is produced from phosphorylcholine by the action of acid phosphatase as well as numerous proteolytic enzymes.

Prostaglandins (E_1, E_2, E_3, $F_{1\alpha}$, $F_{2\alpha}$) are another group of compounds found in seminal plasma. Von Euler first discovered these compounds and, because he believed them to be of prostatic origin, named them for the prostate. In men they originate mainly from the seminal vesicles, whereas in the ram prostaglandins originate from both the prostate and the seminal vesicles. The prostaglandins F series cause smooth muscle contraction, which may aid the passage of spermatozoa through the female reproductive tract. Ram seminal vesicles are particularly rich sources of the enzymes needed to convert the long-chain, highly unsaturated fatty acids, dihomo-α-linolenic and arachidonic, to prostaglandins.

The dorsolateral lobe of the prostate has a remarkably high content of zinc. Zinc is an integral part of the enzyme carbonic anhydrase; although it is also associated with lactic dehydrogenase in the semen, its exact role in prostatic secretions is not known. Prostatic secretions also contain fructose, citric acid, cholesterol, numerous proteins, and, in some species, free amino acids. Enzymes that occur in seminal plasma, including acid and alkaline phophatases, proteolytic enzymes, glycosidases, and aspartate aminotransferase, probably originate in the prostate.

The nitrogenous base, spermine, which is produced by the human prostate, is absent in the semen of domestic animals. A conjugated protein called sperm antiagglutinin, which prevents head-to-head agglutination of sperm, is also produced by the prostate.

The secretory activity of the accessory organs is hormonally dependent. Castration abolishes the secretion of the accessory organs, with function being restored by the administration of testosterone.

TESTOSTERONE IN THE PERIPHERAL SYSTEM

Control of testosterone secretion

The secretion of testosterone by Leydig cells is under the control of LH. LH secretion, in turn, is controlled by episodic release of gonadotropin hormone-releasing hormone (GnRH). The number of episodic LH releases varies from 4 to 5 per 24 hours in the bull to up to 12 per 24 hours in the ram. The episodic LH release pattern of a certain minimal frequency is essential for the secretion of testosterone.

Testosterone moves from the interstitium, which surrounds the Leydig cell, into three areas: blood vessel, lymphatic vessel, or seminiferous tubule. The largest amount of testosterone is transported from the Leydig cell via the blood vascular system. The presence of various plasma proteins, including *sex hormone–binding* globulin, is important not only for transport but also for secretion of testosterone. In the absence or reduction of testosterone-binding proteins, production of testosterone declines. This suggests that increased concentrations of testosterone in the interstitium (in the absence of ABP) inhibit testosterone production.

Attempts to control testosterone secretion and spermatogenesis have produced interesting results with respect to the importance of local production of testosterone in the maintenance of spermatogenesis. Spermatogenesis decreases after the administration of testosterone sufficient to effect negative-feedback inhibition of LH secretion. Spermatogenesis is inhibited by this procedure because levels of testosterone barely above physiologic amounts can inhibit LH release (and inhibit testosterone synthesis); yet the exogenously derived testosterone does not reach the interstitium in amounts sufficient to maintain spermatogenesis. The high intratesticular concentration of testosterone provided by the Leydig cell is essential for spermatogenesis.

The episodic secretion of testosterone makes it difficult to make an accurate assessment of Leydig cell function by measurement of only one blood sample. An assessment of normalcy as concerns testosterone production by the testis is made if the particular testosterone value is at least equal to values observed at the nadir of the episodic cycle (i.e., about 1 ng per milliliter of plasma). Values of testosterone can be as high as 10 ng per milliliter of plasma.

Functions

The peripheral functions of testosterone include the development and maintenance of (1) libido, (2) secretory activity of the accessory organs, and (3) general body features that are associated with the male.

Testosterone is essential for libido, and castration is usually effective in eliminating male sex drive. Castration, however, does not invariably dampen male libido, as evidenced by the fact that castrated male horses are sometimes presented as being potentially cryptorchid because of the expression of normal libido. It appears that sexual drive can be maintained in some castrated animals by low concentrations of testosterone, probably of adrenal origin.

Testosterone is important for the development and maintenance of the secretory epithelium of the accessory sex organs. The route of transfer from the Leydig cell is via the general circulation and not via the seminiferous tubule, as occurs for maintenance of the epididymis. The discovery by Huggins and coworkers at the University of Chicago of the importance of testosterone in secretions from the canine prostate led to one of the first attempts to treat neoplasia on a physiologic basis. The finding that testosterone-dependent prostatic secretions could be inhibited by the administration of a synthetic estrogen, diethylstilbestrol, led to Huggins' being awarded a Nobel prize in physiology and medicine.

Testosterone is also important for the development of various general body characteristics. Structural and (or) functional changes that are characteristic of the male include (1) a myotropic (or anabolic) effect that involves an increase in muscle mass through the retention of nitrogen (the thickening of the muscles of the vocal cords of the larynx, which decreases the pitch of the male voice, represents a myotropic effect); (2) hair growth patterns (in humans, testosterone has a positive effect on the face, a negative effect on the head); and (3) calcification of antlers in seasonal breeders that shed horns on a yearly basis.

Some behavioral changes influenced by testosterone include (1) urinary patterns of male dogs, which involve the raising of a hind limb as a prelude to urination; (2) aggressiveness that may be more of a characteristic of the male than of the female; and (3) the marking of a territory by substances known as pheromones, which can be produced by the kidney under the influence of testosterone.

TESTICULAR FUNCTION

Puberty

Most of the information available on factors that influence puberty in the male comes from sheep. As presented in Chap. 36, a *change in photoperiod* following a minimal exposure to a long photoperiod is the factor that is critical to the initiation of puberty in the female lamb. A change in photoperiod does not appear to be as critical for the onset of puberty in the male lamb in that changes associated with the initiation of spermatogenesis are often under way by, or before, the occurrence of the summer solstice. Reduced sensitivity to steroid feedback inhibition of gonadotropin secretion in the male lamb is important for the onset of spermatogenesis, but this change in sensitivity does not appear to be highly related to photoperiod in the male.

Changes that lead to the onset of puberty begin as early as 15 weeks of age. Because spermatogenesis and subsequent maturation of sperm require at least 2 months, the male lamb does not enter puberty, defined as the ability to release mature germ cells, until the age of about 30 weeks. This age is similar to the age at onset of puberty in the female lamb. In general, onset of puberty in male sheep is more gradual than the more abrupt process that occurs in the female.

Photoperiod

Both sheep and goats undergo major periods of testicular regression and activation as a result of photoperiod changes. Testicular activity in adults of both species is adversely affected by increasing photoperiod and restored by decreasing photoperiod. The resultant effect on fertility depends on the breed of sheep. In the Soay ram, spermatogenesis is terminated from November to July (in the northern hemisphere). In the other extreme, it is not uncommon for successful breedings to occur during the spring, even though fertility is reduced for most breeds during this time.

Decreasing light causes a reduction in spermatogenic and endocrine functions of the gonads of the stallion, although fertility is only reduced, not abolished. Slight reductions in fertility are sometimes noted in cattle and swine during the winter.

A major contributor to our knowledge of the effect of photoperiod on male sheep has been G.A. Lincoln of Edinburgh, Scotland. Reproductive activity is increased in the ram in response to decreasing light via its effect on the hypothalamus and pineal gland, the result being the increased secretion of gonadotropins from the anterior pituitary gland. An increase in the frequency of release of GnRH from the hypothalamus, and thus release of LH from the anterior pituitary, is central to the establishment of testicular function in pubertal animals or reestablishment in mature animals. In one study, the number of episodic releases of LH averaged one episode per 24 hours during testicular quiescence, five episodes per 24 hours during activation, and 12 episodes per 24 hours during normal testicular activity.

Testicular production of testosterone also varies as a function of season in response to LH release. Although the episodic release of LH, which occurs in the off-season, is of high amplitude, testosterone production by the Leydig cell is minimal because the frequency of LH release is low and the Leydig cell is relatively unresponsive to LH (Fig. 35.8). During the physiologic breeding season, LH release of much smaller amplitude but longer duration elicits the release of a relatively large amount of testosterone. Basal concentrations of both LH and testosterone are higher at this time than in animals with inactive testes.

Although baseline concentrations of FSH are greatly increased during testicular activation, values decline to relatively low ones when activation is complete. Both the frequency and the amplitude of episodic LH release increase during the activation process, but only increased frequency is maintained after the testes are fully activated. Baseline concentrations of LH change very little during the entire process. Sustained release of testosterone in response to LH pulses does not occur until 30 to 50 days after the photoperiod change. Prolactin concentrations also change (decrease) in response to decreasing light in sheep whose basal levels are reached about 5 weeks after the light change. The significance of this pattern of prolactin is not known. The testis requires upward of 60 days before the seminiferous tubules become sufficiently developed to have an impact on testicular size.

The long-day photoperiod in adult male sheep is inhibitory to GnRH synthesis and release, and even small amounts of testosterone can enhance the inhibition. Under short-day photoperiod, the inhibition of GnRH synthesis is removed and testosterone is less effective in inhibiting GnRH synthesis. This situation is comparable to that observed in the ewe with increased sensitivity to negative-feedback inhibition of gonadotropin secretion by estrogen observed during the anestrum and decreased sensitivity during the breeding season (see Chap. 36).

The pineal gland mediates the effect of photoperiod in the ram (see Fig. 36.12). Removal of the superior cervical ganglia renders the pineal gland inactive as judged by its enzymatic activity. This mode of pineal inhibition blocks the negative photoperiod response in the ram, which allows the testes to remain in an active state without regard to the photoperiod.

Melatonin is released daily in the ram during the dark period (as in other species). It has been shown in experimental studies that melatonin release occurs in rams at the same time (2400 hours), whether they have been exposed to

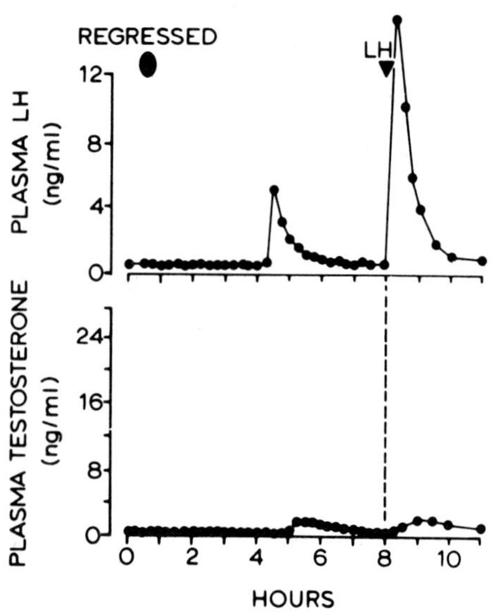

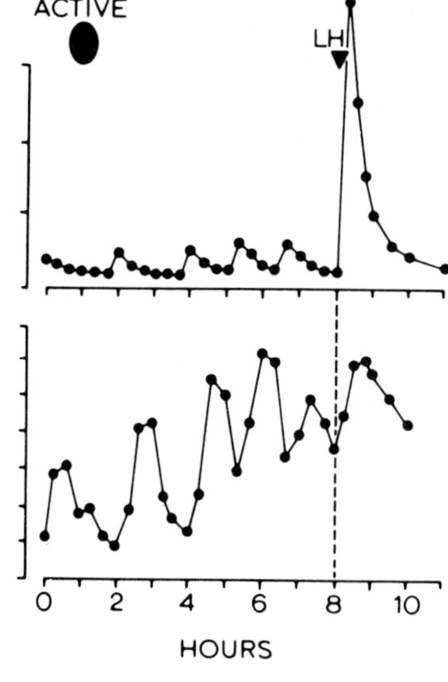

Figure 35.8. Short-term changes in the concentration of luteinizing hormone (LH) and testosterone in the blood plasma of one adult Soay ram sampled at 15- to 30-minute intervals for 11 hours at two stages of the sexual cycle, namely, when the testes were fully regressed and when they were fully enlarged (active). Toward the end of the sampling period the animals were given an intravenous injection of 40 μg of LH. (From Lincoln and Short 1980, *Recent Prog. Horm. Res.* 36:1–52.)

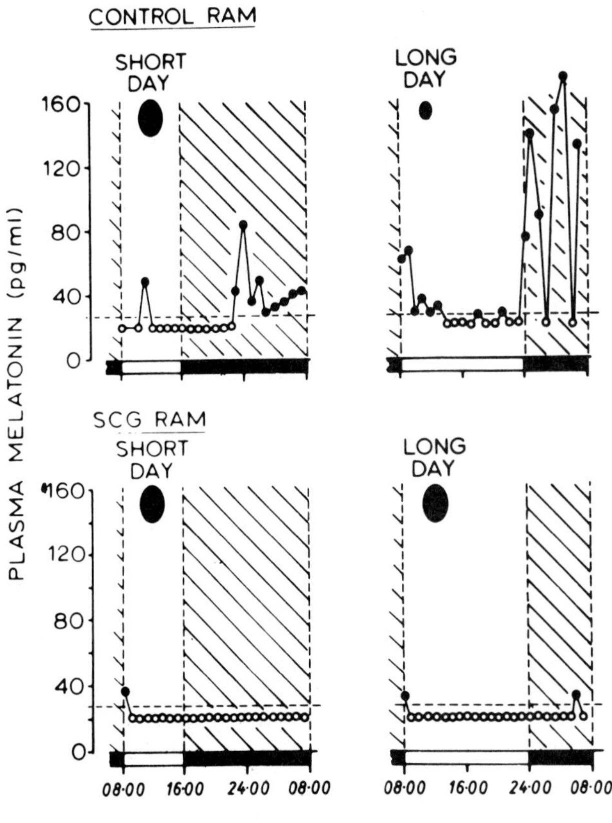

Figure 35.9. Changes in the concentration of melatonin in the blood plasma of one control Soay ram (*top*) and one Soay ram after superior cervical ganglionectomy (*bottom*) sampled at hourly intervals for 24 hours in week 7 during a 16-week period of short days (8 hours light; 16 hours dark) and for a similar time in week 9 during a subsequent 16-week period of long days (16 hours light; 8 hours dark). Note that regression of the testes (indicated by solid oval) occurred in the control ram on exposure to long days, but no such regression occurred in the ram that had undergone ganglionectomy. Note also that melatonin secretion began at about 2400 hours in the control ram, regardless of whether the onset of darkness was 1600 or 2400 hours. (From Lincoln and Short 1980, *Recent Prog. Horm. Res.* 36:1–52.)

darkness beginning at 1600 hours (16 hours of darkness, short day), or 2400 hours (8 hours of darkness, long day) (Fig. 35.9). The release of melatonin is much greater in the long-day rams, even though darkness is of shorter duration. It is perhaps surprising that more melatonin is released in a shorter dark period than in a longer dark period. Melatonin synthesis occurs on a circadian basis (daily rhythm), and the timing of the onset of darkness appears to be critically important to the response.

The phenomenon of *photorefractoriness* has been observed in some seasonal-breeding males. This phenomenon is present in many of the autumn-breeding species of deer in which testicular activity is present for only a limited time. Soay rams, a primitive breed, begin to undergo testicular regression in early November in Edinburgh 4 to 6 weeks before the time of light reversal (December 21). Thus, for some seasonal-breeding males, a change to an unfavorable photoperiod is not required for the cessation of active testicular function; the hypothalamus becomes unresponsive as concerns the release of GnRH in a pulsatile manner of sufficient frequency to maintain the testis.

In seasonal breeders such as sheep, the male has a longer sexual season than the female. The male enters the fertile state earlier and remains fertile longer than the female. This ensures that females at all stages of the breeding season have an opportunity to become pregnant.

Location of testes

All of the common domestic animals have testes that are located in scrotal sacs exterior to the abdominal cavity. Other animals (elephant, dolphin, whale, armadillo) have intra-abdominal testes. While a scrotal location, which provides for a lower testicular temperature, is essential for spermatogenesis in domestic animals, there is no information that would indicate that the scrotal testes of domestic animals are superior to the abdominally located testes in other species.

The scrotum regulates testicular temperature by two specialized mechanisms. First, prior to its entry into the testicle, arterial blood is cooled by a countercurrent heat exchange with venous blood in the pampiniform plexus located outside the testis in the spermatic cord. The extensive convolutions of the arterial and venous vessels allow heat to be transferred from the arterial side to the cooler venous side that drains the testicle. Second, activity of the external cremaster and tunica dartos muscles allows the testicles to be drawn close to the body as the temperature decreases (via contraction) and to move farther away as the temperature increases (via relaxation).

The temperature-regulatory mechanisms maintain the internal temperature of the testis at about 4 to 7°C below rectal temperature when the environmental temperature ranges from 5 to 21°C. Increases in environmental temperature to 35 to 40°C can reduce the temperature differential that can be attained to 2 to 3°C. Fertility is lower in both cattle and swine inseminated with semen collected during the summer, which suggests a deleterious effect of heat on spermatogenesis in these species. Sperm production is also lower in the ram during the summer months because of increased scrotal temperature.

The abnormal retention of testes in the abdominal cavity of domestic animals is known as *cryptorchidism*. The retained testicle can be found anywhere along the fetal migration path from the caudal pole of the kidney to the inguinal ring. The condition can be either unilateral or bilateral. In the latter case, the animal is sterile because body temperature is incompatible with spermatogenesis. Testosterone production by the Leydig cells continues, although at concentrations that are 50 percent, or less, of normal. These levels of testosterone, although reduced, are sufficient to

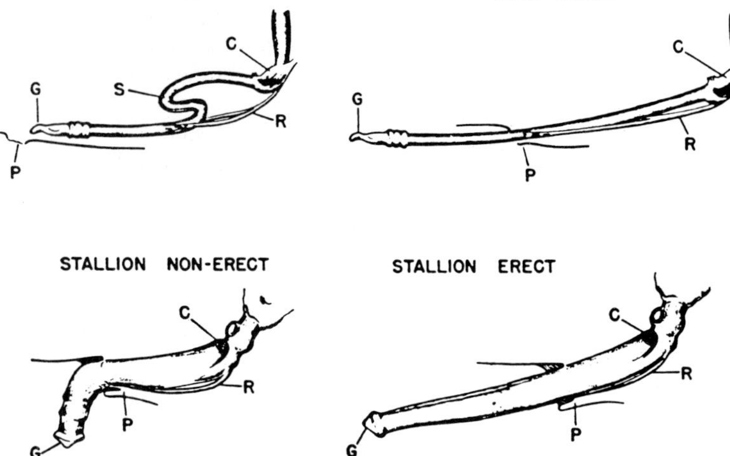

Figure 35.10. Diagrammatic representation of the erection process in the bull and stallion. The fibroelastic nature of the penis of the bull does not allow for much engorgement, and erection of the penis occurs because of the relaxation of the retractor penis muscle which allows the sigmoid flexure to be straightened. The stallion has a large cavernous body, and erection of the penis occurs through enlargement due to filling of the corpus cavernosum and spongiosum. C, cavernous muscle; G, glans; P, prepuce; R, retractor penile muscle; S, sigmoid flexure. (From Hafez 1987, *Reproduction in Farm Animals*, 5th ed., Lea & Febiger, Philadelphia. Reprinted with permission.)

maintain libido. One problem of veterinary practitioners involves the differentiation of the cryptorchid from the castrated horse. As mentioned previously, this situation occurs because some castrated horses maintain libido in the presence of very low testosterone concentrations. The determination of plasma testosterone concentrations is useful when one needs to differentiate the cryptorchid from the castrate. Cryptorchid testes also present problems, as in the dog, because of the increased incidence of neoplasia observed in this species.

ERECTION AND EJACULATION

Erection of the penis is under control of the autonomic nervous system. Erection is accomplished by the synergy of two mechanisms. First, during sexual excitement the corpus cavernosum and corpus spongiosum of the penis become engorged as a result of arteriolar dilation. Simultaneously, the venules contract, trapping the blood in the penis. Second, the ischiocavernosus and bulbospongiosus muscles increase their tone and occlude venous return by pressing the dorsal vein of the penis against the ischial arch. The process of venous engorgement results in the development of extremely high pressures within the vascular system; for example, pressures in the corpus cavernosum may exceed 15,000 mm Hg.

The extent to which the penis expands during erection depends on the capacity of the cavernous body. Ruminants and boars have fibroelastic organs that restrict the amount of enlargement possible in these species (Fig. 35.10). Protrusion of the penis in these species is due to relaxation of the retractor penis muscle, which allows the sigmoid flexure to be straightened. The penis of the stallion is highly vascular and has a large cavernous body, which accounts for the increase in size that occurs during erection (Fig. 35.10). Protrusion of the penis in the horse occurs through enlargement due to filling of the corpus cavernosum and spongiosum.

In the dog, final distention of the penis does not occur until after intromission. The presence of a bony structure, the os penis, in the dog (and cat) facilitates intromission. In the cat, the presence of spines on the glans penis may be important for vaginal stimulation, a prerequisite for ovulation.

Ejaculation, defined as the ejection of semen via the

Table 35.1. Information on accessory glands, penile type, and ejaculation in domestic animals

	Accessory glands					Volume of ejaculate			
Species	Seminal vesicles	Prostate gland	Bulbourethral gland	Ampulla	Type of penis	Mean (ml)	Range (ml)	Time of ejaculation	Site of semen deposition
Bull	+	+	+	+	Fibroelastic	6	2–10	Approximately 1 sec	Vagina
Ram	+	+	+	+	Fibroelastic	1	0.7–2	Approximately 1 sec	Vagina
Boar	+	+	+	+	Fibroelastic	225*	150–500	10–20 min	Uterus
Stallion	+	+	+	+	Vascular	60*	20–250	10–15 sec	Uterus
Dog	–	+	–	+	Vascular (os penis)	9	2–16	30–40 min	Vagina
Cat	–	+	+	+	Vascular (os penis)	0.05	0.01–0.2	Approximately 1 sec	Vagina

*Represents gel-free portion.

excretory ducts, is initiated through the stimulation of sensory nerves located in the glans penis. This stimulation, in turn, triggers a series of peristaltic contractions of the muscular walls in the epididymis, vas deferens, and urethra. These contractions move spermatozoa from the epididymis and vas deferens and fluids from the accessory glands through the ducts leading to the external urethral orifice. In the bull and the ram, spermatozoa are mixed almost instantaneously with fluids from the accessory glands in the urethra before emission of the semen. In the stallion, boar, and dog, the spermatozoa are mixed sequentially with fluids from the accessory glands; sequential ejaculates are sperm-free, sperm-rich and, finally, sperm-poor (See Table 35.1 for details concerning accessory glands and ejaculation.)

REFERENCES

Austin, C.R., and Short, R.V., eds. 1972–1980. *Reproduction in Mammals*. Vols. 1 though 8. Cambridge Univ. Press, Cambridge. (See Chap. 36 for titles.)

Austin, C.R., and Short, R.V., eds. 1982–1986. *Reproduction in Mammals*. 2d ed. Vols. 1 through 5. Cambridge Univ. Press, Cambridge. (See Chap. 36 for titles.)

Burger, H., and deKretser, D., eds. 1981. *Comprehensive Endocrinology: The Testis*. Raven Press, New York.

Cupps, P.T., ed. 1991. *Reproduction in Domestic Animals*. 4th ed. Academic Press, San Diego.

Hafez, E.S.E., ed. 1987. *Reproduction in Farm Animals*. 5th ed. Lea & Febiger, Philadelphia.

Johnson, M., and Everitt, B. 1988. *Essential Reproduction*. 3d ed. Blackwell Scientific Publications, Oxford.

Knobil, E., and Neill, J.D., eds. 1988. *The Physiology of Reproduction*. Raven Press, New York.

Lincoln, G.A., and Short, R.V. 1980. Seasonal breeding: Nature's contraceptive. *Recent Prog. Horm. Res*. 36:1–52.

McDonald, L.E., and Pineda, M.H. eds. 1989. *Veterinary Endocrinology and Reproduction*. Lea & Febiger, Philadelphia.

Setchell, B.P. 1978. *The Mammalian Testis*. Cornell Univ. Press, Ithaca.

CHAPTER 36

Female Reproductive Processes | by George H. Stabenfeldt and Lars-Eric Edqvist

REPRODUCTIVE HORMONES

Gonadal hormones

Types

The major types of steroid hormone involved in female reproductive processes are pregnanes and estranes. The most important pregnane is progesterone, which is produced by the corpus luteum (CL), placenta, and adrenal cortex. Progesterone synthesis by the CL is controlled by luteinizing hormone (LH) in the nonpregnant animal; prolactin (PRL) also supports the CL (luteotropic effect) in some species, particularly the rat, mouse, and ewe. Estradiol-17β and estrone are the primary estranes in domestic nonpregnant and pregnant animals, respectively. Estriol, another important estrogen, is found only in primates during pregnancy. The sites of estrogen production are the ovary (granulosa cells of ovarian follicles), the fetoplacental unit, and the adrenal cortex. Ovarian estrogen synthesis is controlled by follicle-stimulating hormone (FSH), which has an effect on the granulosa cells. LH also plays a vital role in estrogen synthesis in that it controls production of the essential precursor molecule (testosterone) by the theca interna cells.

Figure 36.1 shows that all steroids are derived by common biosynthetic pathways.

Transport

Steroid hormones are lipid-soluble and therefore have limited solubility in water. To compensate for this, for transport, steroids are bound to plasma proteins, some of which have high specificity for steroids. Sex hormone–binding globulin, for example, has a high binding affinity

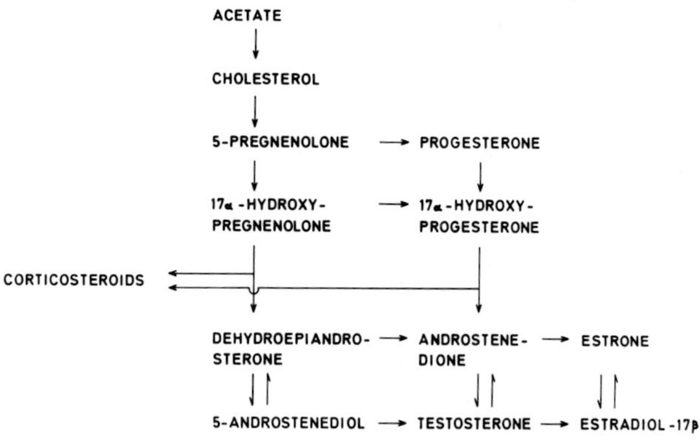

Figure 36.1. Pathway for the synthesis of biologically active steroids from acetate. The steroids secreted from the gonads and the adrenal cortex are formed from acetate and cholesterol. (From Edqvist and Stabenfeldt 1980, in Kaneko, ed., *Clinical Biochemistry of Domestic Animals,* Academic Press, New York.)

for estrogens. Cortisol-binding globulin, which has a high affinity for cortisol and corticosterone, also is important for progesterone transport. The proteins that bind steroids with high affinity have low capacity. Albumin, on the other hand, which is a protein with low binding affinity for steroids, is an important transport vehicle because of its high concentration and, therefore, high capacity in plasma. The largest portion of a steroid hormone present in blood is bound to proteins with less than 5 percent of the hormone unbound or free.

Function

Although the steroids are lipid-soluble and capable of permeating all cells of the body, certain cells are able to concentrate and use steroids through the synthesis of specific cytoplasmic receptors. Cells that selectively bind specific steroids are called target cells for the hormone in question. The steroid-cytoplasmic receptor complex is transferred to the nucleus wherein the complex binds to specific sites on the chromatin. The synthesis of ribonucleic acid (RNA) polymerase follows and, as a result, messenger RNA is synthesized. Protein synthetic capabilities of a cell are turned on for a specific purpose, often within 30 minutes after the initial steroid–cytoplasmic-receptor interaction.

Estrogen causes several important tissue responses. (1) It stimulates growth of endometrial glands, necessary for the maintenance of the zygote before implantation; (2) it stimulates ductal growth in the mammary gland; (3) it causes secretory activity in the oviduct, which enhances survival of oocyte and spermatozoon; (4) it initiates sexual receptivity; (5) it regulates gonadotropin secretion, including the ovulatory release of LH from the anterior pituitary; (6) it may be responsible for the release of prostaglandin $F_{2\alpha}$ ($PGF_{2\alpha}$) from both the nongravid uterus and the gravid uterus at parturition (in both cases to cause regression of the CL); (7) it stops growth of long bones by initiating closure of the epiphyseal growth plate; (8) it promotes protein anabolism; and (9) it is epitheliotropic.

The important tissue responses caused by progesterone include (1) promotion of endometrial gland growth; (2) promotion of lobuloalveolar growth in the mammary gland; (3) promotion of secretory activity of the oviduct and endometrial glands to provide nutrients for the developing zygote before its implantation; (4) promotion of estrus in some species (ewe and bitch) in coordination with estrogen; (5) prevention of contractility of the uterus during pregnancy; and (6) regulation of secretion of gonadotropins. It is important to recognize that the actions of progesterone often occur in synergism with estrogen and often require estrogen priming.

Synthesis and clearance

The concentrations of steroid hormones in blood depend mainly on rates of synthesis and rates of degradation. The amount of steroid synthesized can be relatively stable (as with progesterone from the mature CL), can increase steadily across a sustained interval of time (as with estrogen from developing follicle), or, as in the case of the male (Chap. 35), can fluctuate rapidly over a few hours (testosterone produced by Leydig cells). Production rates can also change rapidly as steroid hormone–producing cells undergo change. For example, estrogen production by granulosa cells declines rapidly (to basal concentrations within 24 hours) in concert with the preovulatory surge of LH. Similarly, progesterone declines steadily over a period of 36 hours after the initiation of luteolysis.

The metabolic clearance rate of steroids is rapid, with a turnover rate of 20 to 30 minutes or less for most steroids. Steroids are conjugated with glucuronic acid and (or) sulfates by the liver, which renders them water-soluble in both bile and urine. Steroids are also rendered inactive by metabolism to compounds that have greatly reduced biologic activity. In most situations, the clearance rate of steroids is relatively constant, so that blood concentrations are a good measure of changes in production rates.

Interconversion of steroids

Some steroids can be metabolized to other biologically active compounds. In primates, for example, both estradiol-17β and androstenedione can be converted into estrone. Although the liver is the main site of conversion, this process also occurs in peripheral tissues. In women, the major portion of estrone comes from metabolism of the hormone by various tissues, and only a minor portion of the hormone in the plasma is derived by synthesis and release from the primary source, the ovary.

Intracellular conversion of steroids can also be important for the biological activity of the compound. The enzyme 5α-reductase is present in many tissues that are targets for androgens. In these tissues, testosterone is converted to 5α-dihydrotestosterone, a compound with more biologic activity than testosterone. In the young animal, the absence of this enzyme is protective in that this prevents premature androgenization in response to the presence of testosterone. In the male rat, testosterone is converted to estradiol-17β within the hypothalamus. In this instance, estradiol-17β is essential for the development and maintenance of male behavior.

Anterior pituitary hormones

Structure and function

Three hormones produced by the anterior pituitary are important for reproductive processes in the female: FSH, LH, and PRL. Both FSH and LH have carbohydrate moieties which, together with thyrotropic hormone, form a group of pituitary hormones classified as glycoprotein. The glycoprotein hormones have two subunits that are noncovalently linked. Within a species, the α-subunits for all of the glycoprotein hormones are identical. The β-subunits are different as to both amino acid and carbohydrate content, which confers the specificity of action of the hormone.

The main function of FSH is to promote the growth of follicles. LH is important for the ovulatory process and the luteinization of the granulosa, which results in the formation of the CL. The actions of FSH and LH are synergistic.

PRL has an ancestral commonality with growth hormone. Both are simple, single-chain, globular proteins of similar molecular weight (22,000 to 24,000) and amino acid residues (190 to 200 amino acids). PRL is characterized as containing three disulfide bridges and two tryptophan molecules. In mammals the most important functions of PRL concern the development of secretory tissue in the mammary gland and the maintenance of lactation. PRL is luteotropic in some species, such as the rat and mouse, and probably sheep. The biphasic daily release of PRL is essential for the establishment of sustained luteal activity in mice and rats as compared with the one-day duration of luteal activity observed in normally cycling rodents (in the absence of PRL).

Mechanism of action

Protein hormones bind to specific receptors located on the surface of target cells. This contrasts with the cytoplasmic binding of steroid hormones. The cell-surface receptor is integrated with a cell-membrane receptor. On binding of the protein hormone to the receptor, the enzyme adenyl cyclase is activated to convert adenosine triphosphate (ATP) to the nucleotide adenosine monophosphate (3,5-AMP) cyclic AMP (cAMP) (the second messenger) activates intracellular protein kinases. These kinases activate enzyme systems that allow the physiological effect of the hormone to be achieved. LH, for example, causes the synthesis of an inducer protein and, as a result, the production of progesterone by mitochondria.

Control of secretion

Hypothalamic control of the anterior pituitary is carried out by small peptide hormones that are released in the median eminence and transported to the anterior pituitary by a portal system of capillaries. Figure 36.2 depicts the interaction of the hypothalamus, hypophysis, and ovary as concerns the development of ovarian follicles. The release of FSH and LH is controlled by a 10–amino acid peptide originally called luteinizing hormone-releasing factor, then luteinizing hormone-releasing hormone, and now known as gonadotropin-releasing hormone (GnRH). There is still question as to whether GnRH controls both LH and FSH, because LH synthesis and release are much more responsive to GnRH than are FSH synthesis and release.

There are basically two ways in which the secretion of gonadotropins is influenced. One is to vary the frequency or amplitude of the pulse release of GnRH. It has been conclusively shown that pulsatile release of GnRH is essential for the maintenance of LH and FSH secretion by the anterior pituitary. Another way to influence FSH and LH secretion is to change the sensitivity of the anterior pituitary to the pulses of GnRH through the modulatory effects of estrogen and progesterone. In general, increasing concentrations of estrogen cause an increase in sensitivity to GnRH and result in an increased release of gonadotropins; progesterone has an opposite effect.

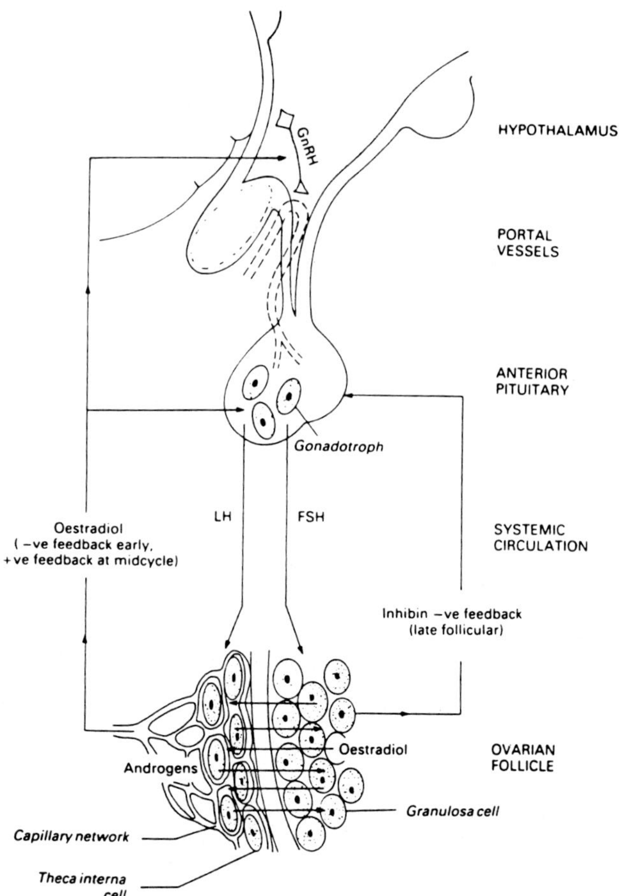

Figure 36.2. Diagrammatic presentation of the interactions of the hypothalamus, pituitary, and ovary in control of ovarian follicle development. –ve, negative; +ve, positive. (From Johnson and Everitt, *Essential Reproduction*, 3d ed., Blackwell Scientific Publications, Oxford.)

The fundamental emphasis of the control of PRL secretion concerns inhibition of secretion by hypothalamic factors (Fig. 36.3). This concept comes from studies in which transection of the pituitary stalk results in greatly increased concentrations of PRL. One prolactin inhibitory factor is thought to be dopamine, a catecholamine. Dopamine is released from neurons in the median eminence and is carried by the hypophyseal portal system to the anterior pituitary, with decreased dopamine synthesis leading to increased PRL release. The prohormone for GnRH, GnRH-associated protein, and gamma amino butyric acid, also inhibit PRL secretion. Like the gonadotropins, PRL is re-

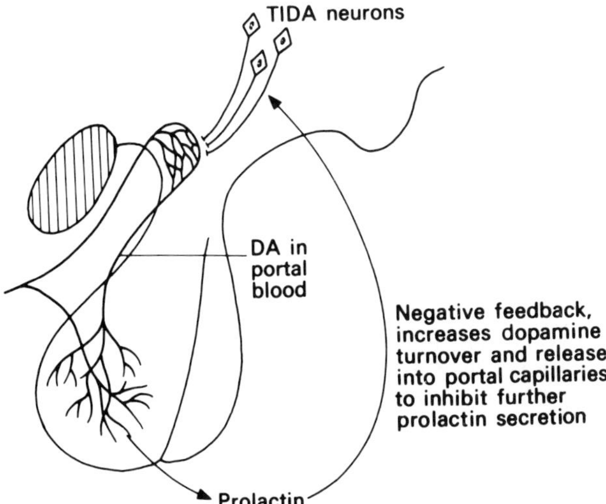

Figure 36.3. Diagrammatic presentation of negative-feedback control of prolactin secretion. Prolactin, secreted by lactotrophs in the anterior pituitary, blocks further prolactin secretion by increasing the turnover of dopamine (DA) in tuberoinfundibular dopamine (TIDA) neurons located in the arcuate nucleus. Dopamine reaches the lactotrophs via the portal capillaries wherein prolactin secretion is inhibited. (From Johnson and Everitt, *Essential Reproduction*, 3d ed., Blackwell Scientific Publications, Oxford.)

leased in a pulsatile fashion, possibly because of a waxing and waning of inhibitory factor synthesis. PRL is released by the administration of thyrotropin-releasing hormone, the biologic significance of which is not known. Also, stress causes the release of PRL.

The ways in which steroids, particularly estrogens, affect the release of gonadotropins are both interesting and contrasting. Estradiol-17β can have a suppressive effect on gonadotropin release, a phenomenon called negative feedback. A second, and contrasting, phenomenon known as positive feedback occurs when a surge release of gonadotropins occurs in response to gradually increasing concentrations of estrogens. This latter phenomenon requires exposure of the hypothalamus and pituitary to sustained elevations of estrogen; both time and concentration are important. Negative feedback, on the other hand, requires a short duration of exposure to basal or minimal concentrations. The sexual cycle of the male lacks an abrupt cyclical phenomenon such as the gonadotropin surge required for ovulation in the female. Thus the male does not have a positive-feedback system, and gonadotropin secretion is under negative-feedback control.

OVARIAN FUNCTION

Folliculogenesis

The establishment of cyclic ovarian activity at puberty is important for the formation and release of gametes as well as for the establishment of mature sexual capabilities. In the female, the hypothalamopituitary system develops in the absence of hormonal stimuli.

Gamete production proceeds in the embryonic ovary through mitotic division of the primordial germ cells. Mitosis ceases at birth, with the maximal number of oocytes that a female will ever have being present at this time; if destruction of the gametes occurs, the animal will become infertile. Meiosis is soon initiated by factors from the rete ovarii but is arrested at the dictyotene (resting) stage, with resumption of meiosis not occurring until the onset of puberty. In primates, the interval from the initiation of meiosis to its resumption in the last oocyte to be developed can be as long as 50 to 55 years!

The control of the reestablishment of growth and development of the primordial follicle is not understood except that it is independent of gonadotropin influence. During the initial *hormone-independent* phase of follicle development, the oocyte increases in size and activity, which includes the production of RNA and ribosomes. The *follicular cells*, which initially formed around the oocyte, begin to grow and divide during this period and become *granulosa cells*. These cells produce a glycoproteinaceous substance that forms a layer immediately around the oocyte called the *zona pellucida*. Granulosa cells maintain contact with oocytes by cytoplasmic processes that form gap junctions with the oocyte. Gap junctions, also formed between the granulosa cells, are important for communication among these cells, which lack a direct blood supply. Spindle-shaped cells that organize around the exterior of the basement membrane are called *theca cells*. Nutrients are supplied to the granulosa cells and oocyte from the vascularized theca.

The follicle at the end of the hormone-independent stage is still preantral. The synthesis of receptors for FSH and estrogen in the granulosa and of LH receptors in the theca is required for follicles to enter the *hormone-dependent* stage. FSH influences estrogen production by causing the granulosa cells to convert androgens, produced in the theca under the influence of LH, to estrogens. The association of the theca and the granulosa is shown in Fig. 36.2.

FSH also induces its own receptors; this allows the follicle to become increasingly responsive to a relatively steady amount of FSH in the plasma. Estrogens are mitogenic and cause growth and division of the granulosa. They also induce additional FSH receptors in the granulosa. As the granulosa develops under the influence of FSH and estrogen, it begins to synthesize and release secretions that cause cell separation, resulting in the formation of a space called an *antrum*. The developmental sequence of an oocyte and its investments is shown in Fig. 36.4.

Substances, probably of granulosa cell origin, that are capable of inhibiting maturation of the follicle appear in follicular fluid. These inhibitors control the growth of the follicle, which consists of both oocyte and surrounding supporting cells, so that oocyte and follicular cell maturation is coordinated. A factor known as the *oocyte–maturation inhibiting factor* prevents the resumption of meiosis. A *luteinization-inhibiting factor* prevents the gran-

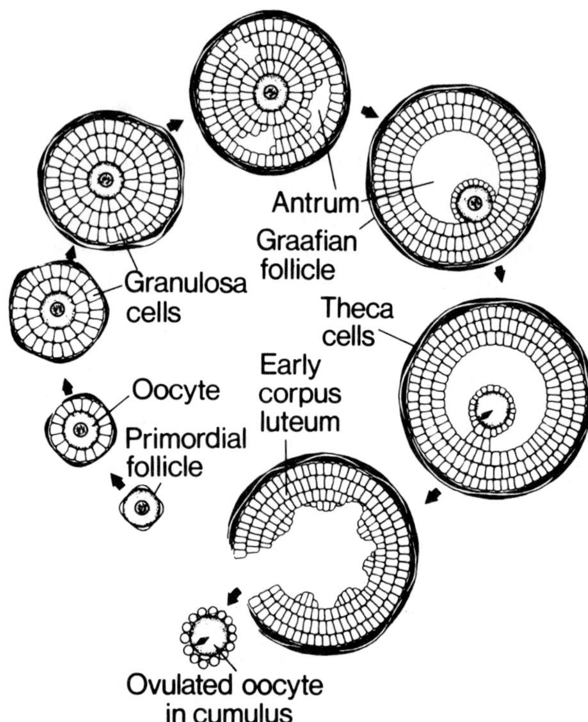

Figure 36.4. Diagrammatic representation of follicular growth. (From Baker 1972, in Austin and Short, eds., *Reproduction in Mammals,* No. 1, Cambridge Univ. Press, Cambridge.)

ulosa from being luteinized prematurely. *Folliculostatin*, or *inhibin*, produced by the granulosa is a protein hormone that inhibits follicle growth. Inhibin causes a progressive negative-feedback inhibition of FSH synthesis and release, especially during the latter part of folliculogenesis, just before ovulation.

FSH, besides inducing additional receptors for FSH, also induces receptors for LH in the granulosa. LH, on the other hand, decreases the number of FSH receptors on the granulosa, especially during the preovulatory surge of LH. These receptor changes are important for the conversion of the granulosa from estrogen secretion in the follicular phase to progesterone secretion in the luteal phase of the estrous cycle.

Ovulation

Selection of the ovulatory follicle

A few follicles leave the primordial state each day and begin to develop. Follicular development results in either atresia and destruction or ovulation. An obvious question presents itself: What determines which follicles will be ovulated and which will undergo atresia? It is important to recognize that follicles continue to grow and develop in domestic animals during all phases of the estrous cycle, including the luteal phase. As shown by ultrasonographic studies in cattle, several dominant follicles develop during the luteal phase of the cycle at about 10-day intervals. Either the second or the third dominant follicle that develops during the luteal phase goes on to be the ovulatory follicle. The selection of the second or third follicle as the ovulatory follicle depends on the timing of initiation of regression of the CL. If CL regression occurs earlier, the second dominant follicle continues to develop through ovulation; if later, the third dominant follicle becomes the ovulatory follicle.

Events interior to the follicle

As a result of the preovulatory LH surge (Fig. 36.5), three important changes occur within the antral follicle within the 24 hours preceding ovulation. These changes are as follows:

1. The preovulatory LH surge affects the maturation of the oocyte. LH blocks the synthesis of oocyte-inhibiting factors (produced by the granulosa), which allows meiosis, held in abeyance since entering prophase months or even years before, to resume approximately 24 hours before ovulation. Meiosis I is completed before ovulation in most species (first polar body formed), but meiosis does not continue until the occurrence of fertilization.

2. The endocrine nature of the follicle is also changed by the LH surge. As indicated previously, FSH induces the formation of LH receptors in the granulosa cells. With the surge release of LH, the granulosa becomes responsive to LH and begins to secrete progesterone (instead of converting androgens to estrogens under the influence of FSH). The granulosa thus begins its conversion to a luteal type of structure even before ovulation. In some species (e.g., primates) the luteinization process is under way before ovulation, and the resulting production of progesterone enhances the ability of estrogen to cause LH release. In the dog, preovulatory luteinization and the resultant progesterone synthesis are important for keying the onset of sexual receptivity.

3. The LH surge also influences the ovulatory process per se through stimulation of the production of intrafollicular substances (again, probably of granulosa origin), which promote the rupture of the follicle. For example, prostaglandins such as $PGF_{2\alpha}$ and PGE appear in follicular fluid during the last few hours before ovulation. Concomitant with prostaglandin synthesis is the increased formation of multivesicular bodies, which form as outpockets of fibroblasts that are a part of the exposed follicle wall. Multivesicular bodies appear to secrete proteolytic enzymes, which cause dissolution of the ground substance surrounding the fibroblasts. The result is dissolution of an area of the protruding follicular capsule, which allows the oocyte to escape.

Relaxin concentrations also have been shown to increase in follicular fluid before ovulation. Relaxin is noted for its ability to cause disorganization of connective tissue fibers

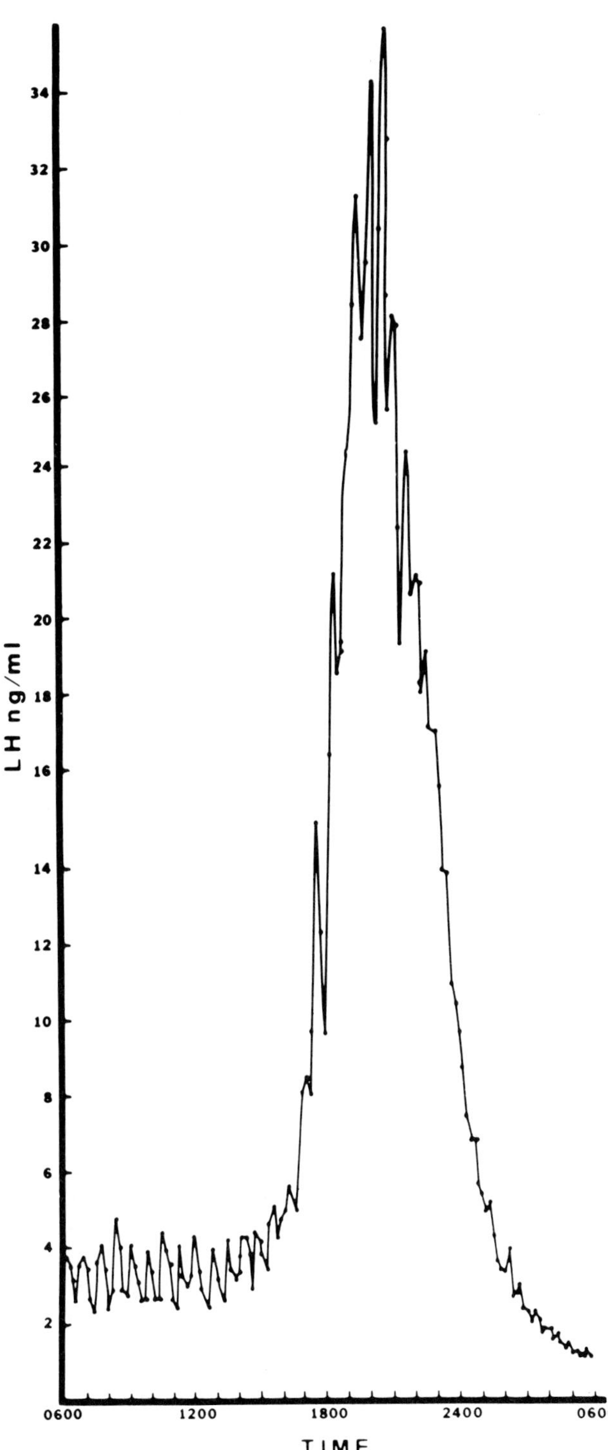

Figure 36.5. Preovulatory surge of plasma luteinizing hormone (LH) in the cow. (From Rahe et al. 1980, *Endocrinology* 107:498. © 1980 The Endocrine Society.)

of the cervix and pelvic ligaments, resulting in loss of cellular continuity and increased tissue pliability at parturition. Relaxin may have a similar effect on connective tissue of the follicular wall, which may lead to actual disruption of the wall.

Events exterior to the follicle

An interplay occurs between the ovary, hypothalamus, and anterior pituitary and allows the ovary to communicate that a follicle(s) is ready for rupture (ovulation). The ovarian signal is estrogen produced by the ripening ovarian follicle. Increasing maturity of the follicle is indicated by its secretion of increasing amounts of estrogen. The response of the hypothalamus and anterior pituitary is to release gonadotropins in increasing frequency, which results in the preovulatory surge in gonadotropins.

Two aspects of estrogen synthesis and (or) concentration appear to be important for the surge release of gonadotropins. First, there is a time requirement for exposure of the hypothalamus and pituitary to estrogen and, second, certain concentrations of estrogens are required for LH to be released in a surge fashion. The interval from reaching certain critical concentrations of estrogen to the release of LH is relatively short; for example, the injection of estradiol into anestrous ewes in amounts as small as 10 μg has been shown to effect LH release within 12 hours.

Estrogen effects LH release through an action on both the hypothalamus and the anterior pituitary. The means by which estrogen effects release of GnRH within the hypothalamus involves stimulation of catecholaminergic neurons involving the synthesis and release of both dopamine and norepinephrine. The catecholaminergic neurons, in turn, influence GnRH-secreting neurons. The effect of estrogen at the level of the anterior pituitary is to increase the sensitivity of the pituitary gonadotropes to GnRH. The release of GnRH is also modulated by the opioid peptide β-endorphin. This peptide is a derivative of a larger molecule, pro-opiomelanocortin, which is produced by the intermediate lobe of the pituitary. The pharmacologic administration of endorphin suppresses both the amplitude and the frequency of pulsatile release of gonadotropins. This finding has led to a suggestion that endorphins mediate the negative-feedback effects of progesterone on pulsatile gonadotropin secretion during the luteal phase. Nevertheless, the importance of endorphins as physiologic modulators of gonadotropin secretion remains to be shown.

Recently, an approach has been developed that allows monitoring of GnRH secretion by the equine hypothalamus with a cannula placed via the facial vein into the intercavernal sinus; the sinus receives blood directly from the pituitary. Pulsatile secretion of GnRH is responsible for the pulsatile release of LH from the anterior pituitary. The continuous infusion of large doses of GnRH can result in downregulation of GnRH-binding sites on gonadotropes, thus decreasing the responsiveness of the anterior pituitary as concerns LH release and blocking ovulation. On the other

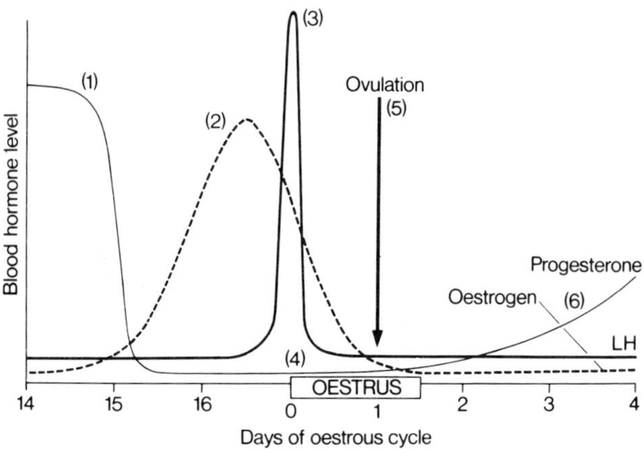

Figure 36.6. Periovulatory endocrine events in the ewe. (1) Regression of the corpus luteum (CL) (progesterone declines); (2) growth of follicles (estrogen increases); (3) surge release of luteinizing hormone (LH) from anterior pituitary; (4) onset of estrus; (5) ovulation; (6) development of the new CL. (From Short 1972, in Austin and Short, eds., *Reproduction in Mammals,* No. 3, Cambridge Univ. Press, Cambridge.)

hand, continuous infusion of low doses of GnRH can cause folliculogenesis and ovulation.

A large surge release of LH is essential for the initiation of ovulation. The release of LH is accompanied by a smaller FSH surge that may be synergistic with LH as concerns ovulation. The duration of the ovulatory surge of LH is relatively short in most animals (e.g., 4 to 5 hours in rabbits, 4 to 12 hours in cats, 6 to 12 hours in cattle, sheep, and goats, and 24 hours in dogs and pigs). The one exception is the horse, which has a broad LH surge occurring over a period of up to 7 days. This exception is partially explained by the high carbohydrate (sialic acid) content of equine LH, which protects it from degradation.

The interval from beginning LH release to ovulation is relatively precise for most species: 12 hours in rabbits, 24 to 32 hours in cats, cattle, and sheep, and 36 hours in pigs. The relationship between estrogen, progesterone, LH release, and ovulation in the ewe is shown in Fig. 36.6.

The surge release of LH initiates and coordinates the events of ovulation and sexual receptivity through increased GnRH synthesis. This is manifested through the hypothalamus, which controls LH release as well as estrous activity.

Spontaneity of ovulation

In many species, ovulation occurs spontaneously after normal follicle growth during the estrous or menstrual cycle. This means that a secretory pattern of estrogen associated with a developing dominant follicle(s) is almost always able to elicit a surge release of LH that results in ovulation. Examples of spontaneous ovulators include the bitch, cow, doe (goat), mare, sow, primates, and some laboratory species, including the mouse, rat, and guinea pig. (In this chapter, *doe* will always refer to the goat unless otherwise specified.)

Induced ovulators are animals that do not ovulate spontaneously, even in association with normal follicle development. These species, which include the cat, rabbit, ferret, mink, and members of the Camelidae family, require copulation for ovulation to be induced. Within minutes of vaginal stimulation, copulation initiates the ovulatory release of LH through sensory pathways in the spinal cord. Estrogen priming of the hypothalamus and anterior pituitary in induced ovulators is an essential prerequisite for copulation to induce GnRH and LH release leading to ovulation.

The main cause of ovulatory failure in animals is an inability to grow follicles. As discussed below, environmental and physiologic influences, such as unfavorable photoperiod, lactation, or inadequate nutrition, are the main indirect causes of ovulatory failure. Ovulatory failure, per se, is rare among spontaneous ovulators. It is generally considered that animals with the capability to grow follicles almost always are able to release LH in response to the estrogen stimulus.

Corpus luteum

Formation, function, maintenance

Formation of the CL begins with the conversion of the granulosa from estrogen to progesterone secretion, called *luteinization* of the granulosa, by the preovulatory LH surge. In some species, the theca also makes a contribution to the cellular composition of the CL. A fibrin clot that forms in the cavity of the ruptured follicle serves as the framework upon which luteal cells develop. The membrane separating granulosa and theca is disrupted, and this allows blood vessels to grow into the interior of the follicle and to vascularize fingers of tissues that contain granulosa and theca cells. In many animals, the preovulatory LH surge is the driving force for both formation and initial maintenance of the CL, with basal circulating concentrations of LH sufficient for continued maintenance of the CL.

Prolactin (in addition to LH) may be important for maintenance of the CL in a few animals, such as sheep, dogs, mice, and rats. Luteal function in the bitch requires the presence of both LH and PRL for the secretion of progesterone throughout pregnancy or pseudopregnancy. In rodent species, such as the rat and mouse, copulation is necessary for initiation of the daily biphasic release of PRL that is essential for CL maintenance. In the absence of copulation in the rat and mouse, the luteal phase is short (about 1 day), which gives the animal the reproductive advantage of returning to a potentially fertile state within a few days.

Regression of the corpus luteum

In 1925 it was shown that hysterectomy of the guinea pig during the luteal phase of the estrous cycle resulted in prolongation of the life of the CL. Since then it has been

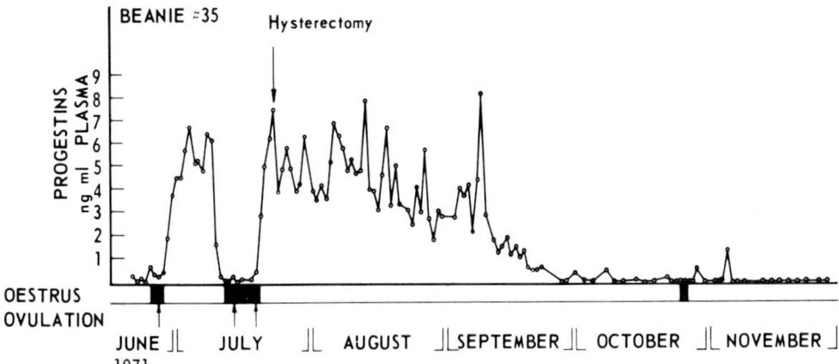

Figure 36.7. The effect of hysterectomy on luteal activity in the mare. Note the prolongation of luteal activity after hysterectomy. Horizontal bars indicate sexual receptivity; up arrows indicate ovulation. (From Stabenfeldt et al. 1974, *J. Reprod. Fert.* 37:343.)

established that the uterus plays a major role in controlling the life span of the CL in nonpregnant animals, especially the large domestic species (cow, doe, ewe, mare, sow). The importance of the uterus with respect to CL life span in the mare is demonstrated in Fig. 36.7, in which hysterectomy is shown to have prolonged the luteal phase. Species in which the uterus appears not to play a role in CL regression include the dog, cat, and primates.

$PGF_{2\alpha}$ is the substance that initiates regression of the CL in the large domestic species. $PGF_{2\alpha}$ is synthesized and released in a pulsatile mode beginning approximately 14 days after ovulation. In the cow, for example, individual $PGF_{2\alpha}$ surges average 5 to 6 hours in duration, with about the same interval intervening between surges. Functional luteolysis, which involves a decline in progesterone secretion, usually begins 3 to 6 hours after the initiation of $PGF_{2\alpha}$ release. Regression of the CL is usually complete within 24 to 48 hours in the large domestic species. $PGF_{2\alpha}$ release patterns for the goat are shown in Fig. 36.8.

The sow has a somewhat different pattern of $PGF_{2\alpha}$ release in that increased secretion of $PGF_{2\alpha}$ occurs several days before the initiation of functional luteolysis. This is consistent with the fact that porcine CL is very unresponsive to exogenously administered $PGF_{2\alpha}$ until relatively late in the luteal phase of the estrous cycle. As a result, the use of $PGF_{2\alpha}$ for the manipulation of the estrous cycle of the pig is somewhat limited in scope.

There is some evidence that the uterus requires a minimal priming time by progesterone before $PGF_{2\alpha}$ can be synthesized and released. The synthesis and release of $PGF_{2\alpha}$ usually begin about 14 days after ovulation. There are indications from utero-ovarian transplant experiments in the ewe that estrogens may play a key role in initiating $PGF_{2\alpha}$ synthesis. The source of estrogen is likely the antral follicle that develops late in the luteal phase of the estrous cycle. Even though follicles often can and do grow during all parts of the luteal phase, only estrogen from late luteal phase antral follicles effects $PGF_{2\alpha}$ synthesis and release. It appears that uterine subcellular components involved in the synthesis of $PGF_{2\alpha}$ require time (i.e., about 2 weeks after ovulation) before enzyme systems for $PGF_{2\alpha}$ synthesis can be activated under physiologic conditions.

Enhancement of $PGF_{2\alpha}$ synthesis and release appears to occur during regression of the CL. This suggests that declining progesterone concentrations facilitate release of $PGF_{2\alpha}$. The enhanced release of $PGF_{2\alpha}$ serves to ensure regression of the CL. Cessation of $PGF_{2\alpha}$ synthesis, on the other hand, occurs within hours after progesterone concentrations are reduced to basal values.

In sheep, a role for oxytocin has been established in stimulation of uterine $PGF_{2\alpha}$ synthesis and release. The ovine CL synthesizes and stores oxytocin during the estrous cycle. A pulse of $PGF_{2\alpha}$ causes both decreased progesterone synthesis and the release of oxytocin from the luteal tissue. Oxytocin then causes subsequent synthesis and release of $PGF_{2\alpha}$ by the uterus. The interaction between the uterus and the ovary is akin to dance partners in a tango, with first one leading and then the other. A prerequisite for uterine response to oxytocin, the oxytocin receptor, is induced by estrogen produced by developing antral follicles. It is likely that $PGF_{2\alpha}$ synthesis and release, induced by estrogens from antral follicles, start the process. There are occasional false starts in which pulsatile $PGF_{2\alpha}$ synthesis and release do not elicit either a decrease in progesterone or the release of oxytocin. Usually, though, the process of luteolysis is under way by the second or third pulse of $PGF_{2\alpha}$.

Mechanisms of luteal regression

Corpora lutea are richly vascularized and are very susceptible to changes in blood flow. Since $PGF_{2\alpha}$ causes contraction of smooth muscle, a reduction of blood supply to the CL by constriction of the arterial system is one mechanism by which luteolysis is effected. Another means of initiating regression is through a disturbance of cellular synthetic pathways. Specific binding sites for $PGF_{2\alpha}$ develop on the plasma membrane of luteal cells, and $PGF_{2\alpha}$ binding may either prevent or interfere with LH binding. It is also possible that the binding of $PGF_{2\alpha}$ initiates intracellular changes that interfere with steroidogenesis.

Transport of $PGF_{2\alpha}$

The source of $PGF_{2\alpha}$ that controls the life span of the CL is the uterus. Since there are no arteriole-venule shunts

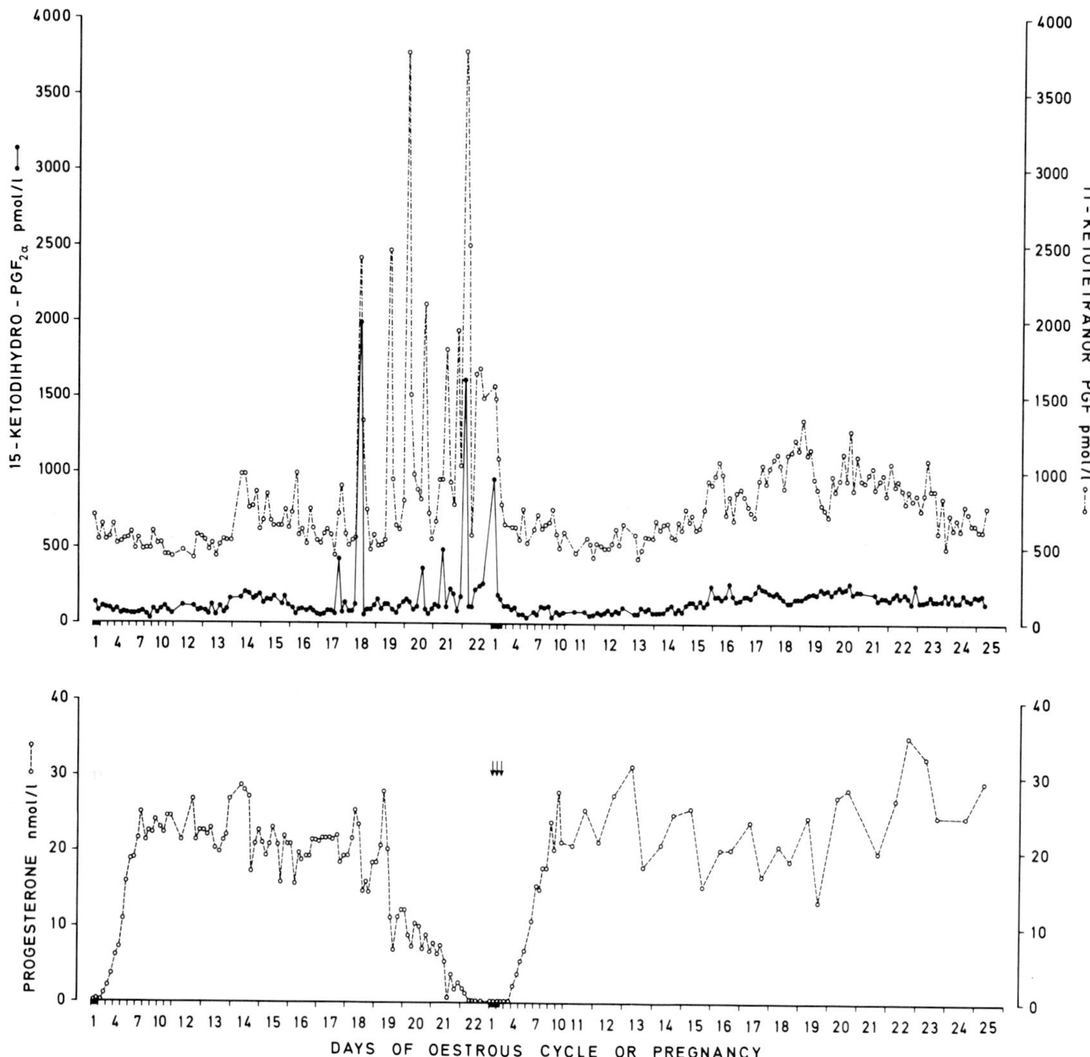

Figure 36.8. The release of prostaglandin $F_{2\alpha}$ ($PGF_{2\alpha}$) as reflected by concentrations of its main metabolite 15-keto-13–14-dihydro-$PGF_{2\alpha}$ (● - - - ●) and the more degraded 11-ketotetranor PGF metabolites (○ - · - · - ○) and luteal activity as indicated by progesterone concentrations (○ - - ○) during an estrous cycle and early pregnancy in a goat. Note the release of $PGF_{2\alpha}$ (as indicated by metabolite concentrations) in association with luteolysis and the absence of release at the comparable time in early pregnancy. Arrows indicate the time of mating. (From Fredriksson, Kindahl, and Edqvist 1984, *Anim. Reprod. Sci.* 7:537.)

between the ovarian artery and the utero-ovarian vein, $PGF_{2\alpha}$ must either pass via the general circulation (*general transfer*) to reach the ovary or be transferred from the utero-ovarian vein to the ovarian artery by *local transfer* mechanisms. Local transfer involves the movement of $PGF_{2\alpha}$ from an area of high concentration (utero-ovarian vein) to an area of lower concentration (ovarian artery) via a countercurrent type of exchange mechanism (Fig. 36.9). This route of transfer has functional merit because a high percentage of $PGF_{2\alpha}$ (more than 90 percent) is metabolized to biologically inactive compounds such as 15-keto-13,14-dihydroprostaglandin $F_{2\alpha}$, by one passage through the lungs. Local transfer thus allows the conservation of the biologically active molecule.

The local route of transfer of $PGF_{2\alpha}$ is particularly important in the cow and ewe for controlling luteal activity. In this situation only the uterine horn adjacent to the ovary containing the CL can influence regression of the CL.

In pigs and horses, $PGF_{2\alpha}$ is transferred effectively through the general circulation. Two conditions must exist for this to occur: higher production rates of $PGF_{2\alpha}$ and a lower rate of $PGF_{2\alpha}$ degradation in the lungs. The transport

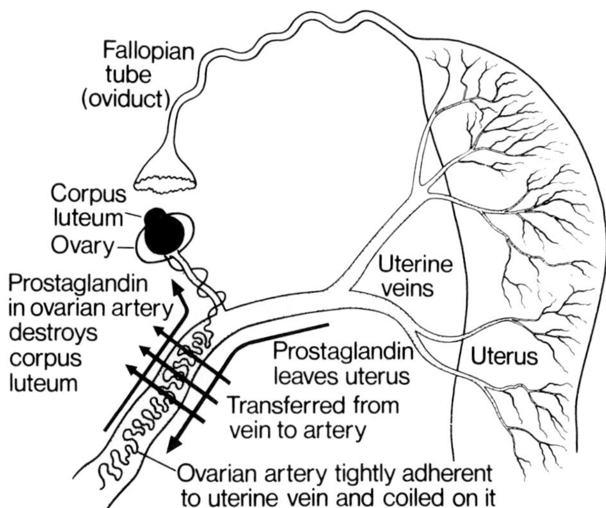

Figure 36.9. The route of transfer proposed for the movement of $PGF_{2\alpha}$ from the uteroovarian vein to the ovarian artery to effect luteolysis. (From Short 1972, in Austin and Short, eds., *Reproduction in Mammals,* No. 3, Cambridge Univ. Press, Cambridge.)

of the biologically active form of $PGF_{2\alpha}$ by the general transfer route means that each uterine horn can influence the life span of the CL on the contralateral ovary.

Control of luteal activity in other species

The reason for the demise of the CL in the nonpregnant dog or (pseudopregnant) cat is not known. Luteal activity is generally prolonged in both species (75 days for the dog; 35 days for the cat). In both species, peak luteal activity is achieved in about 20 to 25 days, followed by a 15-day decline in activity in the cat and a 50-day decline in the dog. The gradual decline in luteal activity suggests the occurrence of a slow "wearing-out" process instead of the acute lytic process that occurs in large domestic animal species.

In primates, peak luteal activity is achieved about 8 days after ovulation and is followed by a gradual decline in luteal activity over a similar time span. As indicated previously, the uterus does not appear to control the life span of the CL in primates. For women, this means that cyclic ovarian activity continues after removal of the uterus.

Abnormalities in control of the CL

Spontaneous prolongation of luteal activity occurs in large domestic animals. The basic cause is a failure of the endometrium to synthesize $PGF_{2\alpha}$ at the proper time (about 14 days after ovulation). The result is prolonged luteal activity that can range in duration from 1 to 5 months. Although the incidence in various species is not precisely known, horses have an incidence of 15 to 20 percent while sheep and cattle probably have an incidence of less than 5 percent. Mares appear to have a species predilection to the development of persistent CL. There are at least two possible explanations for the persistent luteal phase: (1) synthesizing enzymes are not formed and (or) substrates for $PGF_{2\alpha}$ synthesis are not available on a subcellular basis and (2) the signal for initiation of $PGF_{2\alpha}$ synthesis and release is inadequate.

Uterine abnormalities can result in prolongation of CL activity. In cows and ewes, *uterus unicornis* (one uterine horn present because of a developmental abnormality) results in the prolongation of CL activity if ovulation (and CL formation) occurs on the side contralateral to the intact uterine horn. In pigs, a uterine anomaly involving an isolated uterine horn (constriction due to segmental aplasia) is incompatible with pregnancy because the isolated horn is not influenced by the pregnancy. The synthesis and release of $PGF_{2\alpha}$ occur at the usual time for nonpregnant animals and result in the regression of both sets of CL (swine ovulate in both ovaries) and loss of the pregnancy.

Inflammatory processes can initiate the synthesis of $PGF_{2\alpha}$. The elicitation of acute inflammatory responses within the endometrium can cause synthesis of $PGF_{2\alpha}$ in nonpregnant animals before postovulation day 14, resulting in premature regression of the CL and shortening of the estrous cycle. The endometrium must have had a minimum of 4 to 5 days of progesterone priming (5 to 6 days after ovulation) before the inflammatory process can elicit the release of $PGF_{2\alpha}$. Endogenous $PGF_{2\alpha}$ synthesis and release also occur after acidic saline infusion in utero in the mare or iodine infusion in utero in the cow during the luteal phase. In the mare, $PGF_{2\alpha}$ synthesis begins within minutes of infusion, and regression of the CL is usually under way within 6 to 9 hours. In the cow, iodine solution causes destruction of the endometrial epithelium, and it is only on reestablishment of the epithelium and stromal elements of the uterus 3 to 5 days later that the regenerating tissues spontaneously release $PGF_{2\alpha}$. In both situations, the normal CL life span is usually shortened.

Chronic inflammatory processes of the uterus in the mare can result in destruction of the endometrium and loss of ability to synthesize $PGF_{2\alpha}$; the end result is often pyometra. In the mare luteal activity may be prolonged in the mare for months in cases of severe obliterative endometritis because this is incompatible with the synthesis and release of $PGF_{2\alpha}$. The presence of pyometra in the cow also results in a loss of ability of the endometrium to synthesize $PGF_{2\alpha}$; most cows with pyometra have a persistent CL. The presence of pyometra in the cow, however, does not cause a poor prognosis for fertility, because tissue damage is much less extensive than in the horse. Goats have persistent luteal phases in conjunction with the accumulation of uterine fluid, a condition known as "starburst" because of the amount of fluid released once regression of the CL occurs. The accumulation of fluid in the uterus in the ewe and the cow may also result from prolonged luteal phases.

In general, abnormalities in estrous cycle lengths are almost always related to uterine dysfunction in large domestic animals.

SEXUAL RECEPTIVITY

Hormonal changes that drive sexual attractiveness are relatively subtle, or of low magnitude. In the cat, for example, an increase in estradiol-17β concentrations in plasma from 10 pg/ml to 20 pg/ml results in sexual receptivity. The concept of synergism is also important in that often several hormones combine to produce sexual receptivity. The sequence in which the hormones appear is important for their synergistic action, and there are basic differences in hormone requirements for sexual receptivity among species.

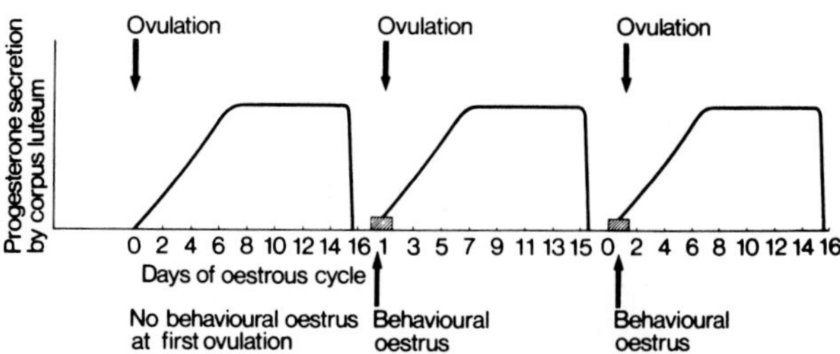

Figure 36.10. The estrous cycle of the ewe. Note the short interval between regression of the corpus luteum (CL) and the subsequent ovulation that allows progesterone priming of the hypothalamus to be effective (with estrogen) in eliciting sexual receptivity. Also note that the first ovulation of the season is not accompanied by estrus. (From Short 1972, in Austin and Short, eds., *Reproduction in Mammals,* No. 3, Cambridge Univ. Press, Cambridge.)

Steroids

Estrogen derived from developing antral follicles is required by all domestic animals for the initiation of sexual receptivity. Progesterone derived from either the preovulatory follicle or the CL is also often important for the manifestation of sexual receptivity.

Progesterone plays an obligatory role in estrous manifestation in the ewe and bitch. In the ewe, priming of the hypothalamus with progesterone before the production of estrogen by the developing dominant follicle is essential for the expression of estrus. This requirement is shown by the fact that sheep do not show estrus in conjunction with the first ovulation of the breeding season. At this time, most sheep have been exposed to very low levels of progesterone for a number of months. The sexual centers of the hypothalamus become primed once a CL forms after the first ovulation, and estrus occurs in conjunction with the next growth wave of an antral follicle. Progestational imprinting of the sexual centers of the hypothalamus is retained for a short period in the absence of progesterone in that progesterone values are low for about 24 hours between the end of luteolysis and the onset of estrus in sheep (Fig. 36.10).

The bitch requires progesterone for the manifestation of estrus, but in a different sequence than in the ewe. In the dog, a long period of sexual attractiveness (proestrus) occurs in response to estrogen produced during preovulatory follicle development. A small increase in progesterone concentrations, which occurs during the preovulatory LH surge, is important for the initiation of sexual receptivity. The granulosa cells of the preovulatory follicles that are undergoing preovulatory luteinization are the source of progesterone. Progesterone is also important for the maintenance of estrus because the bitch remains in estrus for a number of days in concert with the initial development of corpora lutea and the associated increase in progesterone secretion.

There is evidence that progesterone is important for the expression of sexual receptivity in cows and sows. In one study in which cows were monitored continuously with a camera in the postpartum period, only 50 percent of the animals were sexually receptive in conjunction with the first postpartum ovulation. Most dairy cows have at least a 15- to 20-day interval from calving to first ovulation, during which time progesterone concentrations are low. In a study in pigs, it was shown that 32 percent of a group of sows failed to show estrus with the first ovulation after lactation. Pigs have low progesterone concentrations for the first 40 to 50 postpartum days (lactational anestrus) before the first ovulation. It is likely that both situations represent conditions in which the prolonged absence of progesterone has decreased the sexual sensitivity of animals to the increase in estrogen associated with development of the first ovulatory follicle(s).

In the cat, goat, and horse there is no evidence that progesterone plays any synergistic role with estrogen in eliciting sexual receptivity. All three species show estrus with the first follicular activity of the season (all are seasonal breeders) after months of low progesterone concentrations. Goats are thus different from sheep with respect to their progesterone requirement for the expression of estrus. This is advantageous for the goat because it can be bred in conjunction with the first ovulation of the breeding season.

One additional steroid hormone, testosterone, deserves mention for its role in the maintenance of libido in primates. Each month a number of antral follicles are formed, although usually only one is ovulated. The theca interna of the follicles undergoing atresia forms an active tissue of the ovary, which secretes androgens, both testosterone and androstenedione. This androgenic contribution of the primate ovary (and possibly of the adrenal cortex) is important for libido in primates.

Protein hormones

There is both circumstantial and experimental evidence to suggest that GnRH has a role in sexual receptivity. The experimental evidence comes from the lordotic responses of ovariectomized rats and the sexual receptivity of prepubertal gilts, which occur within 24 hours of treatment with GnRH. In gilts, sexual receptivity in association with

GnRH treatment occurs without a concomitant increase in estrogen.

The circumstantial evidence that GnRH has a role in estrous manifestation comes from the close correlation of the onset of sexual receptivity and the initiation of the preovulatory LH release. There is evidence to show that the onset of sexual receptivity begins in conjunction with the initiation of the LH surge. The response of the sexual centers could be the result of either an increase in GnRH secretion or increased responsiveness to GnRH because of estrogen priming. The action is presumed to be mediated within the central nervous system (i.e., within the sexual centers of the hypothalamus).

REPRODUCTIVE CYCLES

Puberty

The term *puberty* is used to define the onset of reproductive life and, for the female, the initiation of cyclic ovarian activity. In the female, puberty is usually associated with the first appearance of estrus; puberty also includes the events that immediately precede the onset of ovarian activity.

The mechanism of pubertal onset has been studied extensively in sheep. From birth until the age of about 7 to 8 months, hypothalamic secretion of gonadotropins is very sensitive to negative-feedback inhibition by estrogen. During this time, small amounts of estrogen are sufficient to inhibit gonadotropin synthesis and release. Under these physiologic conditions, follicles are not able to develop to any significant extent. At about the seventh to the eighth month of life in ewe lambs, two events occur that allow the establishment of ovarian cyclicity. First, there is a decrease in the sensitivity of the hypothalamus to estrogen feedback. In this situation, the frequency of GnRH pulsatile release from the hypothalamus increases and gonadotropins begin to be secreted in significant amounts. The higher frequency of GnRH pulsatile release stimulates follicle development to the point of antrum formation and final follicle development. Second, the increased secretion of estrogen results in positive-feedback stimulation of the hypothalamus and anterior pituitary with a resultant discharge of gonadotropins. This gonadotropin surge does not cause ovulation, but it does cause significant production of progesterone, probably from luteinized ovarian follicles. The progesterone phase is short lived and is followed in a few days by another surge of LH, which leads to ovulation. The role of FSH in the onset of puberty is somewhat unclear in that female lambs at 10 to 12 weeks of age have FSH concentrations that are similar to those of adult animals. Figure 36.11 summarizes the endocrine events associated with puberty in sheep.

The establishment of sexual maturity or ovulatory cycles in primates, in contrast to that in domestic animal species, takes a longer period of time. Menstrual cycle intervals are irregular for the first few months to several years after the onset of menstruation. Photoperiod has been shown to influence the onset of puberty in macaque monkeys, with about 20 percent of females entering puberty during the autumn (favorable photoperiod of decreasing light) when they are about 30 months of age; the rest enter puberty 1 year later at about 42 months of age. The onset of puberty is defined as the first appearance of menstruation, or *menarche*.

It has been suggested that adult animals, such as sheep, that are influenced by the photoperiod revert to the prepubertal state during anestrum. This is based on the fact that the hypothalamus is sensitive to estrogen negative feedback during anestrum, gradually becoming less sensitive during the transition to the breeding season. The other similarity is that adult animals undergo the same endocrine pattern in initiating ovarian cyclicity at the beginning of the breeding season (i.e., a double LH surge separated by a small surge of progesterone). There is a critical difference, though, between pubertal and adult sheep in that adult ewes do not

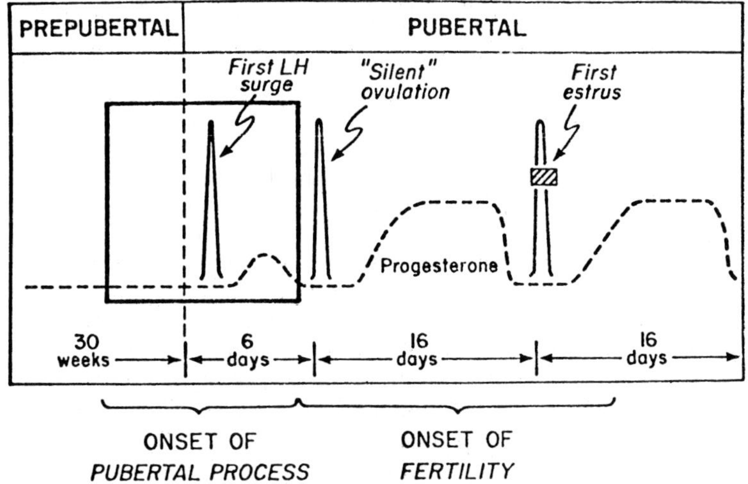

Figure 36.11. A diagrammatic representation of the prepubertal and pubertal endocrine events in sheep. Note that the first major LH release (enclosed in box) does not result in ovulation. LH, luteinizing hormone. (Slightly modified from Foster and Ryan 1979, *Ann. Biol. Anim. Biochim. Biophys.* 19:1369.)

need decreasing light as a cue for the onset of ovarian activity; they simply become refractory to the long photoperiod of spring and summer.

Finally, the attainment of a "critical" body size is essential to the onset of puberty. In sheep, for example, the size required for onset of puberty is about 40 kg. For all species of livestock, a high level of energy intake allows puberty to occur at the earliest time possible. Onset of puberty is usually delayed in undernourished animals. The onset of pulsatile secretion of gonadotropins is delayed in these animals, probably because of the absence of growth factors, which is monitored by the hypothalamus.

Estrous and menstrual cycles

Generally, two types of reproductive cycle are recognized: *estrual* and *menstrual*. The term *estrous cycle* refers to the rhythmic phenomenon observed in all mammals (except some primates) in which there are regular but limited periods of sexual receptivity (called *estrus*), which occur at intervals that are characteristic for a species. One cycle interval is defined as the time from the onset of one period of sexual receptivity to the next or as the interval between successive ovulations.

The name *estrus* is derived from the Greek word *oistros* meaning "gadfly" and was used to describe the behavior of cows when attacked by such flies. The British spelling of the word, *oestrus*, reflects its Greek origin.

Estrous cycle terminology was originally developed to describe the distinct stages of the cycle observed in such animals as the guinea pig, rat, and mouse. In some instances, the adaptation of the terminology to domestic animals seems contrived. The classic terminology is as follows:

Estrus is the time of sexual receptivity, with ovulation usually occurring at about the end of estrus. The word *heat* is a colloquial term that is often substituted for estrus.

Metestrus is the period of early CL development (at least in large domestic species); the onset is usually defined as beginning with the end of estrus; duration is a few days.

Diestrus is the period of mature luteal activity that begins about 4 days after ovulation and ends with the regression of the CL.

Proestrus is the period of rapid follicle growth that precedes the onset of estrus. In large domestic species, this phase occurs after the regression of the CL.

It should be noted that the classic terminology includes descriptions of behavioral (estrus) and ovarian (metestrus, diestrus, proestrus) changes. Terminologies restricted to either behavioral or ovarian changes are commonly substituted. The terms *estrus–sexually receptive* and *diestrus–sexually nonreceptive* describe behavioral changes. In behavioral terminology, diestrus encompasses the classic stages of metestrus, diestrus, and proestrus, at least in large domestic species. *Proestrus* is used in the dog and cat to indicate increased sexual interest, but with lack of acceptance of the male as concerns copulation. The terms *follicular* (which encompasses the classic stages of proestrus and estrus) and *luteal* (which includes the classic stages of metestrus and diestrus) are descriptive of ovarian activity.

In contrast to the estrous cycle terminology that focuses on cyclic sexual activity, *menstrual cycle* terminology is based on changes that occur within the uterus (endometrium) as a result of cyclic ovarian activity. Most primate species, including most monkeys, the great apes, and humans, have menstrual cycles.

In primates, as in domestic animals, development of the endometrium is under the control of estrogen and progesterone. A unique aspect of the proliferation of the primate endometrium concerns the development of a spiral arterial blood supply. With regression of the CL and withdrawal of progesterone, the elongated and coiled arteries of the endometrium collapse with a resultant sloughing of an extensive amount of the endometrium. The process involves some hemorrhage, and the discharge of red-tinged fluids is called *menstruation*.

Listed below are some of the differences that exist between estrous and menstrual cycles:

1. The numbering of the menstrual cycle begins with the onset of menstruation and represents the end of the luteal phase; the numbering of the estrous cycle begins with the onset of sexual receptivity and represents the late follicular phase. (It should be noted that the luteal phase ended for domestic animals before onset of the cycle.)

2. Significant follicular growth does not occur during the luteal phase in primates, and thus the 12- to 13-day follicle growth phase begins after luteal regression. As a result, ovulation does not occur until about the midpoint of an average 28- to 30-day menstrual cycle. Ovulation in animals with estrous cycles usually occurs shortly after the onset of the cycle (estrus).

3. Sexual receptivity is not limited to a certain time of the menstrual cycle, as is the case in animals that have estrous cycles. Certain peaks in sexual activity in primates are noted, including the time before ovulation and before menstruation.

4. The amount of endometrial tissue lost is greater in animals with menstrual cycles than in those with estrous cycles. There is sloughing of tissues below the level of the epithelium in primates. In domestic animals, the analogous situation involves the sloughing of an epithelial layer of cells at the end of the luteal phase (not usually observed). The sanguineous discharge observed in the bitch during proestrus and in the cow after ovulation is not equivalent to menstruation.

Factors influencing reproductive cycles

The basic system for control of ovarian activity includes pulsatile release of GnRH and gonadotropins by the hypothalamus and anterior pituitary, respectively. The system is held under control by the gonadal steroids, estrogen and

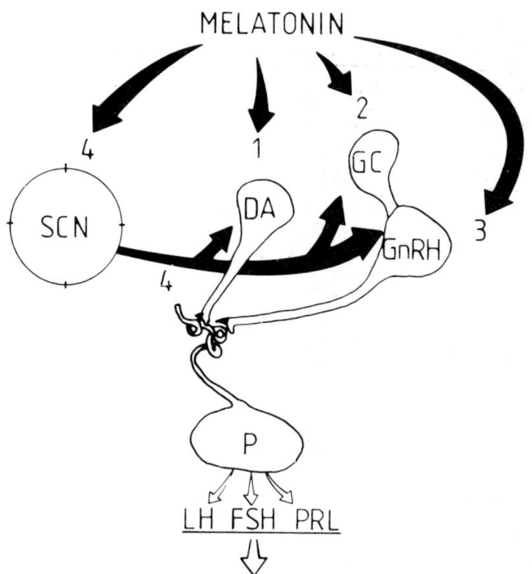

Figure 36.12. Pathways by which melatonin could act to regulate seasonal reproduction: (1) increase the activity of dopaminergic neurons thought to inhibit prolactin secretion; (2) regulate the activity of neurons that control gonadotropin releasing hormone (GnRH); (3) act directly on, or modulate, the sensitivity of the GnRH-producing neurons to sex steroids; (4) regulate the activity of the photoperiodic timer (suprachiasmatic nucleus, SCN), which acts on neurons producing dopamine, neurons controlling GnRH-producing neurons, and/or neurons directly producing GnRH. DA, dopaminergic neurons; FSH, follicle stimulating hormone; GC, neurons controlling GnRH secretion; LH, luteinizing hormone; P, pituitary; PRL, prolactin. (From Forsberg 1990, PhD Thesis, Report 8, Dept. of Clinical Chemistry, College of Veterinary Medicine, Swedish University of Agricultural Sciences, Uppsala, Sweden.)

testosterone. Superimposed on this control system are external factors that can modify normal reproductive activity. Such factors include photoperiod, temperature, nutrition, and social factors, which are conveyed by the olfactory, auditory, visual, and sensory systems. Information regarding these various factors is transmitted through the central nervous system and modified in the hypothalamus to eventually affect gonadotropin secretion by the anterior pituitary.

Photoperiod

Light is the most potent environmental factor affecting reproductive cycles in seasonal breeders. Of the domestic species, the queen, doe (goat), ewe, and mare are affected by photoperiod. Unlike many other climatic variables, changes in day length follow a predictable pattern from one year to the next, and therefore changes in photoperiod are reliable for predicting changes in reproductive activity. The pineal gland is involved in relaying changes that occur in the photoperiod. Photic information is transmitted from the retinal cells of the eye, via the optic nerves, to the suprachiasmatic nuclei, which are located in the anterior hypothalamus. Output from this nucleus is transmitted via the paraventricular nucleus to the superior cervical ganglia via autonomic nervous system tracts and then finally to the pineal gland (epiphysis cerebri). The signal released by the pineal gland is the hormone melatonin, which plays a critical role in subsequently modifying hypothalamic-pituitary-gonadal activity (Fig. 36.12). Melatonin signals the duration of the photoperiod, with the resultant response by the reproductive system varying according to the species and the particular nature of their seasonal breeding strategy.

Different responses to photoperiod are observed in animals. Both the queen and the mare become anestrus late in the autumn because of decreasing light, and ovarian cycles are reestablished by increasing light. The reverse situation occurs in ewes and does; that is, ovarian activity ceases with increasing light and is reestablished with decreasing light (Fig.36.13).

There is evidence to suggest that the ease of reestablishing ovarian cyclicity in pigs after lactation is dependent on photoperiod. In one Norwegian study, 93.5 percent of the sows and gilts resumed ovarian activity within 10 days of weaning during the months of January through June; 66.7 percent resumed ovarian activity within the same post-weaning interval during July through December. Although the queen and the mare respond similarly to photoperiod, the cat enters anestrum earlier than the mare (October instead of November) and resumes cyclic ovarian activity earlier (mid-January instead of late February to March) in the California setting of latitude 38.5° north. The turn-off response time for gonadal activity for the cat and horse (decreasing photoperiod) is longer than the turn-on response time (increasing photoperiod) (Fig. 36.13).

The dog is moderately affected by the photoperiod, even though estrous cycles begin at all months of the year. Although the difference is small, a significantly greater percentage of dogs show estrus during the increasing photo-

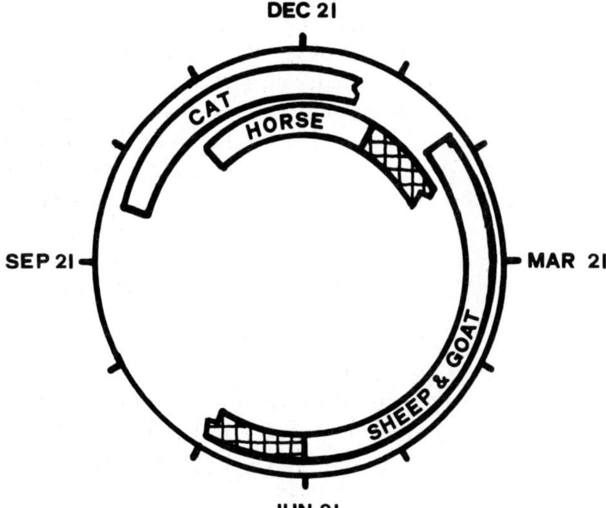

Figure 36.13. A diagrammatic representation of the effect of photoperiod on ovarian activity in the cat, horse, sheep, and goat. The bars represent periods of ovarian inactivity (anestrum). The transitional period for the horse, sheep, and goat is shown by the hatched portion of the bar.

period (spring) than during the decreasing (autumn) photoperiod.

In addition to differences in photoperiod responses between species, there are also genetic differences within species, as shown by the photoperiod response in sheep. For example, the Rambouillet breed begins ovarian cyclicity in July, whereas the Finnish Landrace breed begins reproductive cycles closer to September 1. The Finnish Landrace ewes, on the other hand, are more resistant than some breeds to the inhibitory effects of increasing photoperiod; they often have ovarian cycles through March. The Mediterranean breeds are noted for their prolonged breeding seasons. Ovarian cyclicity in these breeds can begin in the spring (before the summer solstice), which suggests the presence of an endogenous regulator.

Changing photoperiod by artificial means is the most effective way to manipulate those animals that are influenced by photoperiod, especially on an individual animal basis. For animals that respond to increasing light for the reestablishment of ovarian activity (queen, mare), increased light beginning about 1 month before the expected onset of anestrum should result in continuous ovarian activity. If one wants to reestablish ovarian cyclicity (e.g., in a winter anestrum mare), a minimum of 2 months' exposure to the appropriate photoperiod is required.

For animals that initiate ovarian activity in response to decreasing light, the problem of photoperiod manipulation is difficult in the absence of light-controlled barns. One solution is to put the animals in an environment in which light is suddenly extended and, after a period of time, suddenly decreased. A change in light (in this case, a decrease) is important for stimulation of ovarian activity and can be done in a photoperiod time frame that is usually suppressive of ovarian activity. Recently melatonin implants in sheep have been used to advance (make earlier) the breeding time of sheep as well as to increase the ovulatory rate (to midseason form) as compared with that usually observed at the beginning of the breeding season. Although the mechanism is not known, it may be that chronic exposure of ewes to melatonin disrupts the suppressive effects of circadian timing of melatonin release observed under increasing light.

When one is attempting to manipulate animals by changing the photoperiod (or by other means), it is useful to know that varying degrees of hypothalamic suppression occur during the anestrum. The *deep anestrum*, attained shortly after the cessation of ovarian activity, lasts for a number of months, depending on the particular species or breed. *Transitional anestrum*, the period between deep anestrum and cyclic ovarian activity, lasts for about a month (Fig. 36.13). During this period, the hypothalamus and pituitary begin to increase gonadotropin secretion, and some follicle growth occurs. It is during this period of time that photoperiod-sensitive animals are most easily manipulated.

Temperature

Temperature plays a very minor role in affecting the reproductive cycles of domestic animals. Warmer than normal summer temperatures advance the breeding season of sheep. High temperatures adversely affect reproductive cycles only under extreme conditions, including conditions under which cows are unable to get rid of their heat load at night. In this situation, embryonic mortality (especially before implantation) is the main effect noted, with reproductive cycles remaining normal.

Nutrition

The two main areas in which nutrition can affect reproductive patterns in domestic animals are (1) the onset of puberty and (or) the breeding season (for seasonal breeders) and (2) the reestablishment of ovarian activity after parturition. A drought, especially in areas that have been overgrazed, can cause a delay in the onset of puberty or the breeding season because of malnutrition.

The deleterious effect of low nutrition on reproductive cycles of sexually mature animals represents a major problem in domestic animals, particularly in cattle. Most beef cattle, for example, are fed a limited ration in the winter season and can be in a negative metabolic balance at parturition. Because of the importance of 12-month calving intervals, and because gestation lasts 280 days in cattle, animals must be successfully impregnated within 85 days after delivery to maintain a 12-month calving interval. As it often takes 45 to 60 days after calving to re-establish ovarian cyclicity in beef cattle under optimal feed conditions, conception must occur within a 25- to 40-day period after cycling begins if the 12-month interval is to be maintained. Beef cows that conceive late in the breeding season and deliver late calves as a result are usually culled.

The reestablishment of regular ovarian cyclicity can be a problem in the heavily producing dairy cow because of a negative metabolic balance for the first 60 to 90 days of lactation, even though the animal may be fed ad libitum. There is little that one can do in this situation except wait for the reestablishment of metabolic balance and accept the fact that heavily producing cows may not be able to calve at 12-month intervals.

A technique called *flushing* can be used to increase the number of ova shed, particularly in animals with multiple births (e.g., ewes and sows). This involves a sudden shift in feed from suboptimal to optimal for animals that have established cyclic ovarian activity. In one experiment, the ovulatory rate was increased from 133 ovulations per 100 ewes to 217 ovulations per 100 ewes with an increase in the level of nutrition.

Pheromones

Chemicals that allow communication between animals of the same species are called *pheromones* (*sex pheromones* if sexual activity is affected). Pheromones are important for modifying the behavior of both males and females. Males are attracted to females by odors emanating from vaginal secretions. One compound, methyl-*p*-hydroxybenzoate, has been isolated from the vaginal secretions of dogs in proestrus and estrus and shown to elicit intense anogenital interest by males when applied to females (see Chap. 49). Females are also influenced by odors of the male. Sows in estrus, for example, will assume a breeding stance (hind legs braced, or "rigidity reflex") if exposed to the urine of a boar. Note that in this situation the sow's perception of odor changes because of her changing physiologic state and not because of changes in the boar's urine. The androgen, 5α-androstenone, may contribute to the male odor (also called the *boar taint*).

Two classic phenomena involving pheromones have been reported in mice. The *Whitten effect* involves the synchronization of estrous cycles by the introduction of a male into a group of females. Female mice tend to have erratic cycling patterns, or no ovarian activity, when housed in large numbers without a male. The introduction of a male causes females to resume ovarian cyclicity in a highly synchronized manner (a significant number of females are in estrus the third day after introduction of the male). The effect of the male is to initiate gonadotropin synthesis and release.

The *Bruce effect* involves the manipulation of pregnancy by pheromones. If a recently bred female mouse is placed in a cage with a strange male, the pregnancy fails. This is due to blockage of PRL secretion and, with a decline in PRL secretion, CL regresses and the pregnancy fails. The effect is thought to be pheromonal in origin because loss of pregnancy can occur if the pregnant animal is placed in a cage previously inhabited by a strange male.

A practical use of pheromones (a *Whitten type of effect*) is made through the introduction of a ram into a breeding flock of sheep during the transitional period between deep anestrum and the breeding season. The so-called *ram effect* tends to both (1) advance the time of onset of the breeding season and (2) synchronize estrus. The physiologic mechanism involves the acceleration of gonadotropin release with final development of antral follicles and ovulation. A similar effect has been observed in swine with the introduction of boars into pens of prepubertal gilts (daily for short periods), which advances the onset of puberty.

Sound

Sounds from the male have been demonstrated to elicit behavioral responses (sexual) in the female. In pigs, about 50 percent of estrous sows exhibit the *rigidity reflex* if pressure is put on their backs. The response is increased to 75 percent if animals are exposed to sounds of the male.

In cats, the male often makes characteristic chirping sounds in the presence of estrous females. Females can be influenced by the chirp, even to the point of stopping in midstride to assume a lordotic posture.

Vision

Visual cues can also affect reproductive behavioral patterns. There are a number of species of birds in which displays by the male, including both the presentation of colored plumage and characteristic movements influence reproductive behavior of the female. In subhuman primates, females that are sexually receptive alert the male through particular body movements as well as by the development of changes in skin color associated with the perineal region. The absence of movement by the female (e.g., the cow or ewe) when approached by the male can be used as a cue that the female may be receptive.

Physical contact

Physical contact of a female with a male causes the female to become immobile (i.e., exhibit the so-called *rigidity reflex*). Ewes in estrus move freely in a pen of ewes but often cease movement on the first contact with a male. The ewes' desire for physical contact with the male can be used to detect females in estrus. If a male is placed in a pen adjacent to a group of ewes, ewes that are in estrus will place themselves immediately adjacent to the male. (In Britain this is called *tupping*.)

Reproductive senescence

The end of cyclic ovarian activity in primates, a well-defined phenomenon called *menopause*, occurs at about 45 to 50 years of age in the human female. The basic physiologic change in primates is a gradual lack of responsiveness of the ovary to gonadotropins. It is not clear whether follicles fail to leave their primordial state or are not responsive to gonadotropins once follicle growth begins. With a gradual decline in ovarian secretion of estrogen, gonadotropin synthesis and release increase because the hypothalamus has been relieved of negative-feedback inhibition. One of the commercial products of this phenomenon is *human menopausal gonadotropin*, a substance with FSH and LH activity, which is extracted from the urine of postmenopausal women.

The phenomenon of reproductive *senescence* is not recognized in domestic animals. This may be due, in part, to the fact that many domestic animals have lives that are shortened for economic or humane reasons. One effect of age has been noted in dogs in that estrous cycle intervals tend to increase from the norm of 7.5 months to 12- to 15-month intervals with advancing age.

Cat

Puberty

Most cats born in the spring and summer months enter puberty at the start of the next breeding season (mid-

January in the northern hemisphere). The age at onset of puberty in female cats averages between 8 and 10 months; the range is 4 to 20 months. The wide age range at puberty is likely due to failure of the kitten to develop at a normal rate, coupled with the intervention of a subsequent negative photoperiod. Males have spermatozoa present in seminiferous tubules by the age of 6 to 8 months and ejaculate by 7 to 9 months.

Estrous cycle

The cat is unique among the domestic species in that ovulation is induced by copulation. If female cats do not have contact with a male, they have estrous cycle intervals of about 16 days. These estrous cycles can be continuous throughout the breeding season (January to October). This type of cycle involves 7- to 8-day follicular phases in which follicles grow and regress (Fig. 36.14) followed by about 8 to 9 days of ovarian inactivity. Another type of cycle is observed in nonpregnant cats that copulate but fail to conceive. These animals have a minimum interval of 42 days between estrus states, which involves a luteal phase of 35 days and a subsequent minimal interval of 7 days before the onset of subsequent follicle development. These animals are referred to as being *pseudopregnant*.

The onset of estrus in cats usually occurs 1 to 3 days after the onset of follicle growth and extends for a day longer than the follicular phase; the duration of estrus is about 6 to 7 days.

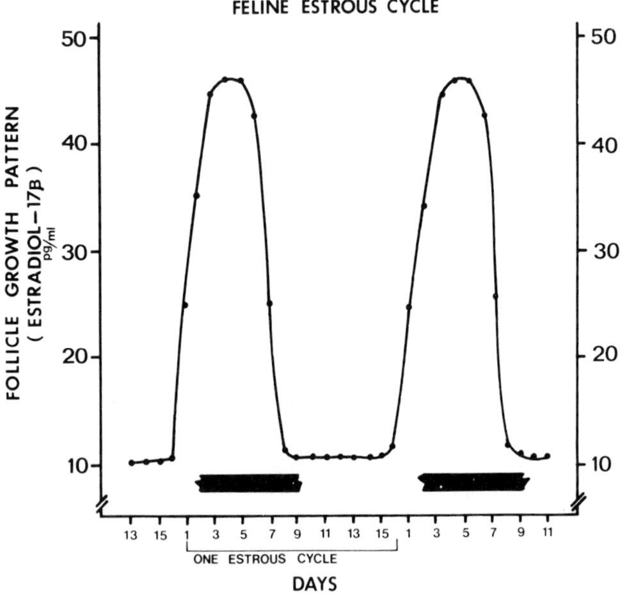

Figure 36.14. A diagrammatic representation of follicle dynamics in the cat. Cohorts of follicles grow and regress over 8-day periods in the absence of coitus; approximately the same interval of time occurs between follicle development. Estrus (horizontal black bars) begins slightly after the start of follicle growth and extends slightly beyond the end of follicle growth. (Adapted from Shille, Lundström, and Stabenfeldt 1979, *Biol. Reprod.* 21:953.)

There is considerable variability in the expression of estrus by the cat. Some cats do not manifest estrus, even though cyclic follicular activity can be demonstrated by changes in blood estrogen values. Other animals show continuous estrous activity including the period between follicular phases when estrogen concentrations are low. Others with continuous estrus have overlapping follicle waves, much the same as occurs in the rabbit.

The behavior of cats in estrus is striking. With the onset of estrus there is an increase in the affection shown to almost any object (e.g., table legs, doorjambs, humans, etc.). Behavior during estrus includes crawling with the chest against floor, rolling, and vocalizing sounds that are lower than usual in pitch.

Mating behavior of the male involves mounting, grasping the back of the neck (for stability), and paddling the hind legs against the sides of the female. The latter action causes the female to present the perineal region dorsally so that intromission can be accomplished. This orientation is important because the penis of the male is oriented in a posterior manner. Ejaculation is usually completed within 10 to 15 seconds of mounting. The male dismounts rapidly after ejaculation because the female immediately becomes sexually and aggressively nonreceptive. After an initial refractory period of about 10 minutes, copulation usually occurs again. As many as four or five intromissions and ejaculations can occur in the first hour of contact. The number of copulations observed over a 4-hour period has ranged from 8 to 12. The refractory period of the female tends to increase with each copulation.

Cats show partner preference, with some males being acceptable to a large number of females and others acceptable to only some females.

Ovulation and luteal activity

Intromission by the male initiates a surge release of LH (within minutes) in the queen that has a duration of 4 to 16 hours (Fig. 36.15); ovulation occurs 24 to 32 hours later. If pregnancy does not occur after breeding (and ovulation) a luteal phase of 35 to 40 days occurs (Fig. 36.16).

Dog

Puberty

Dogs usually attain puberty 2 to 3 months after they reach adult body size, usually between 6 and 12 months of age, and generally without regard to the time of year. Smaller breeds reach puberty before large breeds because they reach adult size earlier.

Estrous cycle

The estrous cycle interval in dogs is exceptional because of its length, averaging approximately 7.5 months. Estrous cycle intervals are affected by breed; for example, German shepherds have estrous cycle intervals of about 150 days, whereas boxers and Boston terriers have intervals of 240

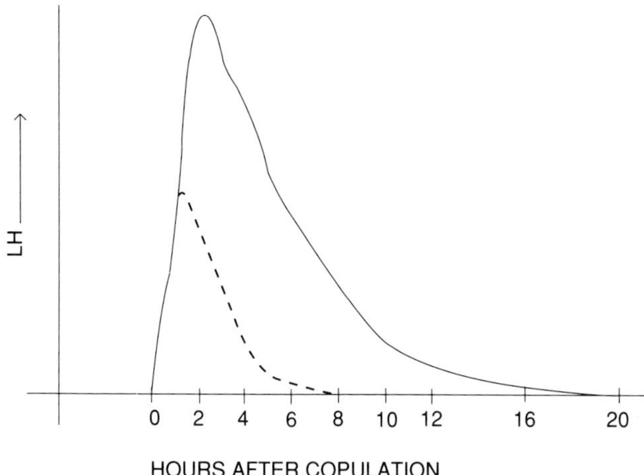

Figure 36.15. Luteinizing hormone (LH) release in cats after copulation. Ovulation occurred in conjunction with both patterns of LH release. (Adapted from Shille et al. 1983, *J. Reprod. Fert.* 68:29.)

days. Pregnancy also affects the duration of the estrous cycle with intervals tending to increase in conjunction with pregnancy. Estrous cycles begin at all times of the year, although there is a small but significant increase in the incidence of estrus in the late winter and spring months.

The estrous cycle of the dog is characterized by the long duration of its component parts. Proestrus (animals are sexually attractive, but not receptive) is 7 to 10 days, estrus is 7 to 10 days, and diestrus is 75 to 80 days. The dog is also unusual in having an anestrous period of 75 to 175 days. As indicated previously, the dog can have estrous cycles any time of the year, although there is a small, but significant, increase in incidence from January through June.

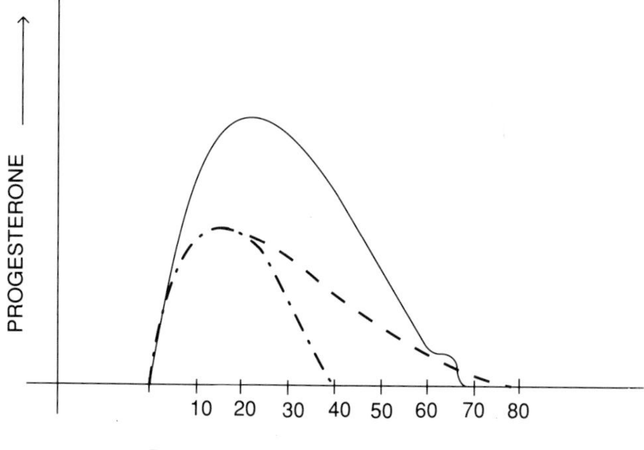

Figure 36.16. Luteal activity (progesterone patterns) in nonpregnant dogs (*broken line*), pregnant dogs (*solid line*), and pseudopregnant cats (*broken line with dots*). (Dog data adapted from Smith and McDonald 1974, *Endocrinology* 94:404, copyright the Endocrine Society. Cat data adapted from Shille and Stabenfeldt 1979, *Biol. Reprod.* 21:1217.)

Ovulation

Ovulation occurs within 24 to 48 hours after the LH surge, which terminates proestrus and initiates estrus. The time of ovulation can be approximated through an examination of cytological changes observed in vaginal fluids, and all changes are based on the increasing estrogen concentrations that characterize proestrus. The vaginal epithelium is stimulated by estrogens to undergo mitosis. Cell division occurs at the basal lamina, with cells being progressively pushed away from the basal lamina toward the lumen of the vagina. Cells begin to undergo degeneration as they are displaced from their nutritive supply. Four epithelial cell types are generally recognized: (1) parabasal, (2) intermediate, (3) superficial, and (4) anuclear. The first two cell types have been classified as *noncornified* and the last two as *cornified*. Full cornification (all anuclear and superficial cells present) is usually achieved within a day or two after the end of the follicular phase. Because LH is released at the end of the follicular phase, and because ovulation occurs a day later, the day that full cornification is reached and the day that ovulation occurs are often as close as 1 or 2 days.

White blood cells disappear from the vaginal smear within a few days after the onset of proestrus. This is because the main route for their appearance, the vaginal epithelial wall, increases in thickness, thus blocking the entrance of white blood cells into the vagina. Red blood cells that appear in vaginal smears during proestrus originate from the developing blood vascular system of the endometrium under estrogen stimulation.

In the dog, oocytes are ovulated before the meiotic formation of the first polar body. The first polar body is formed in the oviduct between 48 and 60 hours after ovulation. Fertilization is delayed for this period of time because sperm penetration does not occur until after formation of the first polar body. The delay in fertilization, however, does not cause fertility problems because of the 4- to 5-day longevity of dog semen. Also, canine oocytes have an unusually long life span for fertilization after formation of the first polar body (i.e., about 48 hours).

Luteal activity

As mentioned previously, the nonpregnant dog has a luteal phase of about 75 days (Fig. 36.16). Luteal activity reaches a peak about 25 days after ovulation and then slowly declines. Luteal activity is longer in the nonpregnant dog than in the pregnant dog because luteal activity is terminated in the pregnant dog at about 63 to 65 days of gestation (24 hours before delivery).

The glandular elements of the endometrium develop (as in all animals) under progesterone influence during the luteal phase. The time required to return the endometrium to a basal (normal) state of proliferation after regression of the CL is long (i.e., at least 30 days after CL regression in the nonpregnant animal and at least 60 days after parturition). The prolonged periods of progesterone exposure, together with the responsiveness of the endometrium, eventually result in cystic endometrial hyperplasia. Such a change in the endometrium is the basis for the relatively high incidence of pyometra in the dog.

Cattle

Puberty

In cattle, both breed and nutrition play a role in the onset of puberty. A high level of energy intake allows the earliest possible initiation of puberty with both the size and the age of an animal being important in determining the onset of puberty. Smaller breeds attain puberty earlier, as follows: Jersey (8 months), Guernsey (11 months), Holstein (11 months), and Ayrshire (13 months).

Estrous cycle

The length of the estrous cycle is 21 days (range, 18 to 24). Estrous cycle lengths are more consistent within individual animals than among animals. The duration of estrus is about 18 hours for *Bos taurus*. One of the important tropical beef cattle breeds, the Brahman (*Bos indicus*),has periods of estrus as short as 2 to 14 hours. The duration of estrus is increased if more than one animal is in estrus at the same time. Also, detection of estrus is usually easiest when animals are being moved (e.g., to the milking parlor).

Knowledge of behavioral changes associated with estrus is important for effective heat detection. These changes include restlessness, increased alertness, increased interest in other animals, mounting other animals, standing for others to mount, decreased appetite, and a more placid temperament. Important physical changes include decreased milk production, relaxation of the vulva, increased redness of the vulva, and vulvar discharge of clear, stringy mucus.

Ovulation

The preovulatory gonadotropin surge begins in concert with the onset of sexual receptivity, peaks within 6 hours, and is usually complete in 10 to 12 hours (see Fig. 36.5). Ovulation occurs about 30 to 32 hours after the onset of estrus. The cow is the only domestic species that ovulates after the cessation of estrus (i.e., about 12 to 14 hours after). This information has been important for development of the optimal time for the artificial insemination of cattle (i.e., about 12 hours after the animal is first detected in estrus) (Fig. 36.17).

Luteal activity

Luteal activity lasts about 16 days in the cow, which is about 2 days longer than for other large domestic species. $PGF_{2\alpha}$ release begins on about day 18 of a 21- to 22-day cycle. Regression of the CL is usually complete by day 20, with rapid follicle growth leading to the expression of estrus within 2 days of luteolysis. It is common for the first postpartum estrous cycle in dairy cows to be shortened to as little as 10 days in duration. It is believed that the shortened cycle is due to regression of the CL caused by premature $PGF_{2\alpha}$ synthesis and release from a uterus that is still undergoing involution.

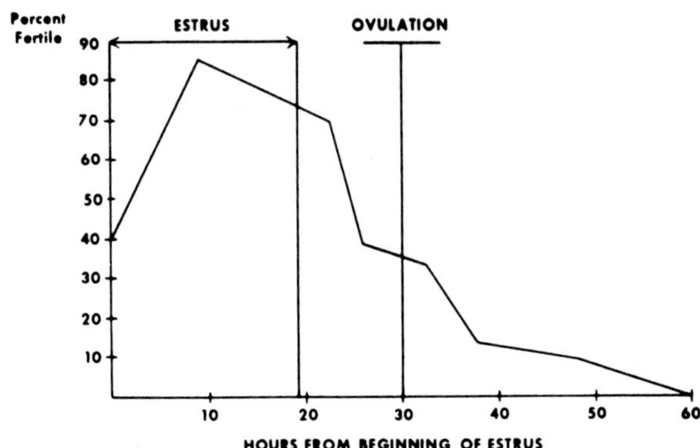

Figure 36.17. The effect of time of insemination on conception rate in cattle. (Adapted from Trimberger 1948, *Nebr. Agric. Exp. St. Res. Bull.* 153.)

Ovarian pathophysiology

Follicular cysts. Follicular cysts are thin-walled follicles, sometimes called thecal cysts, with no evidence of luteinization of the granulosa. The incidence is highest in the immediate postpartum period of the mature, heavily producing cow. In most cases the cystic structures are not accompanied by signs of sexual receptivity or aggressiveness and are usually spontaneously resolved by postpartum day 60. The basic cause is thought to be a malfunction of the hypothalamopituitary system with insufficient release of LH.

The endocrine driving force for sexual behavior is not associated with the enlarged (cystic) follicle because the follicle, although retaining its structural form, degenerates within a few days after reaching its optimal preovulatory size if it is not ovulated. When nymphomania occurs in conjunction with the syndrome, the adrenal cortex is thought to be involved and, in fact, adrenal hyperplasia has been recognized in some animals with cystic follicles. The adrenal cortex not only converts progesterone to corticoids, but it also forms testosterone and estrogen. A malfunction in the adrenal cortex could divert the system toward estrogen and testosterone production, causing continual overt sexual behavior. This concept is supported by the fact that a number of cows with this syndrome assume male behavioral attitudes. This particular syndrome is self-perpetuating in that the adrenal cortex is driven by ACTH, but estrogen and testosterone produced by the adrenal cortex do not effect negative feedback inhibition of ACTH release.

Luteal cysts. Luteal cysts are follicular structures that have undergone partial luteinization without the occurrence of ovulation. The end result is a follicular type of structure that contains a thin outer ring of luteal tissue. The structure can produce small amounts of progesterone and prevent cyclic ovarian activity.

From a clinical standpoint, it is probably not important to be able to differentiate luteal from follicular cysts in cattle inasmuch as the treatment of both conditions is the same. Treatment involves the use of luteotropic substances, such as LH, human chorionic gonadotropin (hCG), or GnRH, with the aim being the production of a luteal structure comparable to a normal CL. Exposure of the hypothalamus to progesterone (endogenous in this case) for a period approximately equal to the normal luteal phase often allows the hypothalamus to reestablish normal synthesis and release of gonadotropins. With removal of the CL (by endogenous release, or exogenous administration of $PGF_{2\alpha}$), the estrous cycle can be reestablished with the growth of new follicles. The manual rupture of follicular cysts is usually not an effective treatment because the ruptured cyst does not luteinize and the follicular cysts often recur.

Cystic corpus luteum. Many corpora lutea have central cavities of up to 25 percent of the CL volume without affecting CL activity. Most cystic corpora lutea are able to produce progesterone in amounts compatible with normal physiological functioning of the reproductive system.

Persistent corpus luteum. The incidence of spontaneous persistence of the luteal phase in cattle in the postpartum period is probably less than 5 percent in animals that have normal genitalia. Some of the conditions or situations in which persistent corpora lutea are found include (1) distention of the uterus with fluid of the noninflammatory (mucometra or hydrometra) type, (2) distention of the uterus with fluid of the inflammatory (pyometra) type, and (3) mummification of the fetus.

Horse

Puberty

The onset of puberty for the filly usually occurs at between 12 and 18 months, or during the season that follows birth of the foal.

Estrous cycle

The estrous cycle of the mare averages 22 days, with a range of 19 to 25 days. Estrous cycle lengths can be erratic during the transitional period from winter anestrum to the physiologic breeding season. This is because mares grow follicles in the transitional period without being able to ovulate them. Mares often develop a series of overlapping dominant follicles during transition, with only short periods between follicles, and intervals between estrus states can be very short as a result. These short estrus intervals do not represent estrous cycles, in the true sense, because ovulation and subsequent luteal activity are absent. Usually two or three dominant follicles develop before ovulation in mares during the transitional period.

Estrous cycles become stable in length as soon as the first ovulation of the season occurs. Cycles tend to become lengthened in the autumn because of a delay in the initiation of folliculogenesis after luteolysis. This is due to the inhibitory effect of the decreasing photoperiod. Estrous cycle activity stops abruptly at the end of the physiologic breeding season.

Estrus

The duration of estrus in the mare is 5 to 6 days. Prolonged periods of estrus are observed in the transition period, as indicated, in conjunction with overlapping follicle waves and in the absence of ovulation. The occurrence of normal diestrous intervals (15 to 16 days) in mares after estrus strongly suggests that the mare has ovulated. Prolongation of estrus, once normal estrous cycles have been established, is a strong indication that ovulation has been delayed.

Estrus can be determined in mares by teasing with a stallion. The typical response for a mare in estrus is to squat and urinate, elevate the tail, stand with the hind legs apart, and rhythmically evert the clitoris. Some animals, including those with foals at their side, may not show estrus, even though they have normal cyclic ovarian activity. Estrogen production is often normal in these cases, suggesting sources of malfunction (e.g., the hypothalamus) other than the ovary.

Ovulation

Ovulation occurs about 24 hours before the end of estrus in the mare. Estrus ends because ovulation occurs; therefore the cessation of estrus in mares during the physiologic breeding season is indicative of the occurrence of ovulation. The interval from the onset of estrus to ovulation can be variable because of differences in follicle dynamics; therefore it is difficult to predict the time of ovulation from the onset of estrus. The usual alternative is to anticipate ovulation through palpation of the ovaries through the rectum.

The mare is unique in the prolonged elevation of LH observed during the estrous cycle. A progressive increase in LH concentration begins at the completion of CL regression and continues for 4 to 5 days, with ovulation occurring around the third day of this rise; the return to baseline may require another 4 or 5 days.

The mare is unique among domestic animals in that ovulation may occur during the luteal phase of the estrous cycle. (One estimate is that this occurs in about 5 percent of the cycles.) Estrous cycle lengths usually are not changed in this situation because the CL formed during the luteal phase is usually of sufficient age to be responsive to the lytic effects of $PGF_{2\alpha}$, which is released 14 days from the time of formation of the original CL.

The mare is also unusual in that she ovulates through a restricted area of the ovary, the ovulation fossa. It is located on the ventral surface of the ovary and is bounded by the attachment of the fimbria on one side and the utero-ovarian ligament on the other. This site of ovulation is the result of the migration of cortical ovarian tissue and its invagination on the ventral surface of the ovary during fetal development.

Approximately 25 percent of the estrous cycles of the mare have more than one ovulation. This is surprising in light of the fact that uterine capacity is generally limited to one fetus. Twin foals surviving to term represent about 1 percent of total foalings.

Luteal activity

Luteal activity lasts about 14 days in the nonpregnant mare. Functional regression of the CL begins within 6 hours after endogenous release of $PGF_{2\alpha}$ and is complete within 36 hours. The mare is usually in estrus within 24 hours after regression of the CL. As previously indicated, spontaneous prolongation of the CL occurs in the mare and is probably the most important breeding problem of normal animals (incidence, 15 to 20%). The persistent luteal phase occurs because of a failure to synthesize and release $PGF_{2\alpha}$ in amounts adequate to cause regression of the CL (Fig. 36.18). The luteal phase also can be prolonged if the endometrium has undergone chronic destruction of tissue elements, or it can be shortened if the endometrium is subjected to acute inflammatory processes.

Sheep

Puberty

In the northern hemisphere, most lambs are born between December and March. Almost all lambs will enter puberty the next fall at the age of 8 to 9 months. In one study at the University of California, Davis, 95 percent of the ewe lambs manifested estrus during the autumn after their birth; 100 percent had cyclic ovarian activity as determined by endocrine analysis. Ewe lambs often do not express estrus until the third (or more) ovulation after the onset of puberty. The ewe lamb thus appears to need more endocrine priming for manifesting the first estrus of puberty than do adult ewes entering the breeding season.

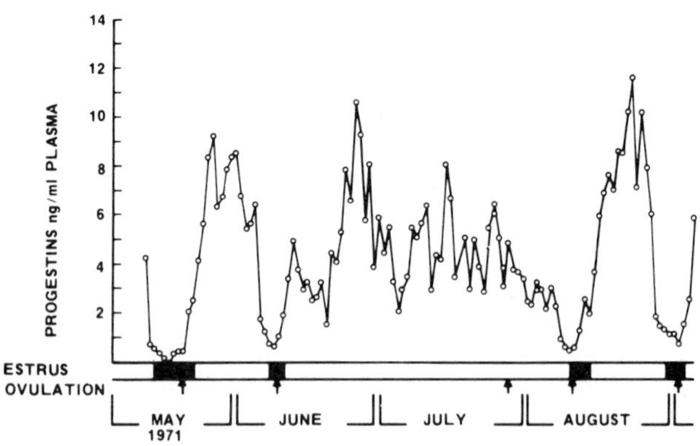

Figure 36.18. Progestin (progesterone) concentrations in the blood of a nonpregnant mare with a persistent corpus luteum (luteal phase from about June 10 to August 10). Notice the regular estrous cycles before and after the period of persistent corpus luteum. Also notice that ovulation occurred late in July during the persistent luteal phase. Arrows indicate ovulation; horizontal bars indicate estrus. (Slightly modified from Stabenfeldt et al. 1974, *Equine Vet. J.* 6:158.)

Estrous cycle

The length of the estrous cycle is 17 days. The estrous cycle is shorter in sheep than in cows, sows, and does because the antral follicle is further advanced at the time of regression of the CL. The interval from CL regression to the onset of estrus is usually only 24 hours.

The ewe is seasonally polyestrus; she has repeated estrous cycles within a physiologic breeding season that lasts about 6 to 7 months.

The duration of estrus in sheep averages 36 hours. Breeds with higher ovulation rates tend to have longer periods of sexual receptivity than breeds with lower ovulation rates.

The following points are important for understanding sexual behavior in the ewe. (1) Prior exposure to progesterone (from CL) for 1 to several days is necessary for sexual receptivity. (2) Homosexual activity can occur in a flock, although it is not certain that the riding activity is directed at animals that are sexually receptive. (3) If females in estrus are separated from males by a barrier, they will tend to place themselves in close proximity to the males. (4) Ewes that have copulatory contact with a male tend to lose their attractiveness to other males. This point has important implications as concerns the use of an infertile ram in a flock of range-managed ewes. (5) Fluttering of the tail is a prominent sign of estrus.

Ovulation

LH is released in conjunction with the start of estrus, and ovulation occurs approximately 30 to 32 hours later. LH release tends to be delayed in ewes that have higher ovulation rates. Preovulatory gonadotropin release terminates active follicle growth, and a delay in gonadotropin release in animals with high ovulation rates presumably allows additional follicles to mature and develop to the point of ovulation. Luteal production of progesterone, as reflected in the plasma, is the same regardless of the natural ovulatory rate within a breed. It is only when corpora lutea are increased beyond the normal number that increased concentrations of progesterone in the blood are observed.

Luteal activity lasts about 14 days in the nonpregnant ewe. Spontaneous persistence of the corpus luteum occurs in the ewe at an incidence rate of 2 to 3 percent.

Pig

Puberty

Puberty is usually attained by the age of 6 to 7 months. The first ovulation of puberty is accompanied by sexual receptivity. Puberty can be delayed for several months in pigs held under conditions of intensive management. Various schemes have been used to bring these animals into puberty, including the daily introduction of males, hormone treatment with equine chorionic gonadotropin (eCG) followed by hCG or GnRH, and (or) transportation of animals from one site to another.

The pig is usually bred at the third estrus of puberty because ovulatory rates tend to increase through the third ovulation. If pigs are bred at the onset of puberty, or the first estrus, special attention must be paid to nutrition because the animals will be both growing and nurturing fetuses during their first gestation.

Estrous cycle

The length of the estrous cycle is 21 days. The average duration of estrus is 2 days. The most prominent physical change during estrus involves swelling of the vulva to the point that it tends to gap open.

Behavioral changes associated with estrus in pigs include restlessness, decreased appetite, and decreased pitch of vocal sounds. Estrus can be detected by elicitation of the rigidity reflex via the application of back pressure.

Ovulation

LH release and the onset of estrus are closely related, as in other animals. Ovulation occurs about 36 to 42 hours after the onset of estrus, or about 6 hours before the end of estrus. Breeding tends to shorten the estrus-to-ovulation interval.

Ovulation almost always occurs in both ovaries. The ovulatory rate is usually greater (16 to 17) than uterine capacity (about 12). Because the fertilization rate is high, a reduction of embryo numbers usually occurs by day 30 of gestation.

Luteal activity

Luteal activity lasts about 14 days in the sow. The sow has a long interval (5 to 6 days) from CL regression to estrus. Developing follicles produce estrogen during this 5- to 6-day interval; animals do not show signs of estrus during this time. This is further indication of the importance of the increased pulsatility of GnRH (which drives the preovulatory gonadotropin surge) for initiating the onset of sexual receptivity in the pig.

Main breeding problems

Anatomical defects that isolate uterine segments can be deleterious to fertility in swine. As indicated previously, a "blind" horn produces $PGF_{2\alpha}$, even when fetuses are present in the adjacent horn. This results in regression of both sets of CL and the loss of the pregnancy. The recurrence of estrous cycles on a regular basis in spite of breeding is suggestive of the presence of an isolated uterine horn.

Another problem of the reproductive system of pigs involves the development of follicular cysts. In this syndrome, large numbers of thin-walled cysts are observed on both ovaries (usually after the animals are sent to the packing plant).

One of the important syndromes in pigs involves failure to initiate lactation in the immediate postpartum period. The syndrome is known by the acronym MMA, which stands for the presence of mastitis, metritis, and agalactia. Prolactin is significantly less in pigs with the syndrome than in normal animals. The concept of endocrine malfunction is supported by the fact that pigs with gestation periods 2 to 3 days longer than normal have a higher incidence of this disease. Animals in herds with a predisposition to the disease have a reduced incidence of the disease if induced to deliver at the normal time of 113 days.

Goat

Puberty

Goats usually enter puberty the autumn after their birth. Goats are similar to sheep with respect to age at first estrus (7 to 8 months) because breeding season and gestation lengths are similar; puberty can occur as early as 4 to 5 months. Most goats are bred during the second breeding season after their birth at an average age of 17 to 18 months. Estrus is manifested with the first ovulation at the start of puberty.

Estrous cycle

The estrous cycle averages 21 days in duration (range, 19 to 22 days). Both the follicular and luteal phases of the cycle are longer than in the ewe.

The duration of estrus, not as well documented as in other species, is about 30 to 36 hours. Does are particularly active and vocal during estrus. The tail is maintained in an erect position and is vigorously wagged during estrus. The tendency for animals in estrus to present themselves in close approximation to the male is highly characteristic of the estrous doe. Copulation occurs rapidly, with intromission and ejaculation completed within a few seconds.

The ovulatory surge of LH is relatively short in duration (i.e., about 9 hours). The surge is closely related to the onset of sexual receptivity. The precise time of ovulation is still not well documented, although one report indicates its occurrence at 33 hours after the onset of estrus.

In the goat, the phenomenon of pseudopregnancy exists, with the animal appearing to be pregnant and even overdue. The udder may be enlarged and the uterus filled with fluid, although no fetuses are present. Progesterone concentrations are usually elevated, suggesting the possibility that prolonged luteal activity is a factor in the development of the syndrome. Regression of the CL induced by $PGF_{2\alpha}$ results in discharge of the uterine fluid.

Data on the duration of various aspects of the estrous cycle are presented in Table 36.1.

POSTPARTUM OVARIAN ACTIVITY

Domestic animls vary in the ease with which they establish cyclic ovarian activity after parturition. In the follow-

Table 36.1. Average lengths of various parts of the reproductive cycles of domestic animals

Species	Length of estrous cycle (days)	Length of estrus	Time of ovulation	Time fertilized ova enter uterus (after conception) (days)	Time of implantation (after conception) (days)	Type of placenta	Length of pregnancy (days)
Cow	21	18 h	12 h after end of estrus	3–4	30–35	Epitheliochorial	280
Ewe*	17	36 h	30 h after beginning of estrus	3–4	15–18	Syndesmochorial	147
Sow	21	45 h	36–40 h after beginning of estrus	3–4	14–20	Epitheliochorial	113
Mare*	21	5–6 days	Last day of estrus	3–4	30–35	Epitheliochorial	345
Doe* (goat)	20	40 h	30–36 h after beginning of estrus	4	20–25	Syndesmochorial	147
Bitch	In estrus at 7- to 8-month intervals depending on breed	Proestrus, 9 days; estrus, 7–9 days	First or second day of estrus	5–6	15	Endotheliochorial	64
Queen*	16 (nonbred) (pseudopregnancy lasts 36 days)	5–6 days	Induced 24–32 h after coitus	4	13	Endotheliochorial	65

*Seasonally polyestrous.
Modified from Hansel and McEntee 1977, in Swenson, ed., *Dukes' Physiology of Domestic Animals,* 9th ed., Cornell Univ. Press, Ithaca, N.Y.

ing section, animals will be presented in the order of ease with which the postpartum ovarian activity is established.

The mare begins to grow follicles within hours of delivery. This occurs because the mare has high concentrations of FSH during the last part of gestation, which initiates follicle growth; ovulation occurs about 11 to 12 days after parturition (so-called foal heat). Lactation is not suppressive of ovarian function in the mare, although some mares may not express estrus when suckling a foal. Conception is possible at the postpartum estrus because the microvillus type of placentation of the mare allows for rapid involution of the uterus.

Follicular development in the cow is influenced by the method of milk removal. Suckling has a more suppressive effect than mechanical milking. Dairy cattle will often ovulate between postpartum days 15 and 20. The minimum period for uterine involution is 25 to 30 days, so the earliest possible time of conception would be at the second ovulation (assuming the first ovulation at day 15 to 20). The time interval for beef cattle is longer, the first ovulation usually not occurring until at least 45 days after parturition.

The ewe and the doe often deliver during the time of year in which the increased photoperiod is beginning to turn off cyclic ovarian activity. Therefore, the interval from parturition to the first postpartum ovulation is usually a matter of 5 to 6 months. Ewes that lamb during the autumn breeding season, however, have been observed in estrus as early as 38 days after parturition. Progesterone studies indicate that the first ovulation (sexually unexpressed) occurred as early as 3 weeks after parturition. Thus lactation per se is not strongly suppressive of ovarian activity in sheep.

Lactation is usually suppressive of follicle growth in the queen in that follicle growth usually does not begin until 7 to 10 days after weaning; cats occasionally manifest estrus and conceive during lactation. Involution of the uterus is rapid in the cat, and conception is possible at the first postpartum estrus.

In the sow lactation suppresses follicle growth, and animals usually do not ovulate until at least 7 to 10 days after weaning (weaning usually occurs between 4 and 6 weeks after parturition). Conception is possible at this time because the uterus is fully involuted. The reason for lactational suppression of ovarian follicle activity is not fully known, but a process that stimulates PRL release (via dopamine inhibition) may interfere with gonadotropin release. In addition, piglets tend to suckle frequently (i.e., every hour), and this could promote continual inhibition of gonadotropin secretion.

The bitch has the longest postpartum interval of any of the domestic species before ovarian activity recurs. Ovarian activity usually does not resume for 3 to 5 months after weaning, an interval that tends to negate any influence of lactation on the resumption of folliculogenesis. The reason(s) for this long period of ovarian inactivity is not known; nor do we understand the mechanisms that initiate gonadotropin secretion leading to the onset of the next estrous cycle.

PREGNANCY

The period of pregnancy (gestation) starts with fertilization and ends with parturition. The average lengths of gestation for some species are given in Table 36.1. It should be noted that both breed and sex differences exist (e.g., the average gestation period is 278 days for Ayrshire and Holstein-Friesian cows and 292 days for Brown Swiss cows). Gestation periods are slightly longer when cows or mares have a male rather than a female fetus. In sheep, the sex of the fetus does not appear to affect the length of gestation. In general, the larger the litter, the earlier the delivery.

Ovum transport

At the time of ovulation the fimbriae of the oviducts are engorged with blood and are in close contact with the surface of the ovary. The contractile activity of the fimbriae sweeps the ovulated oocyte(s) into the funnel-shaped abdominal opening of the oviduct called the infundibulum. The oocyte is then transported to the ampullary part of the oviduct through contraction of the oviductal musculature and through movement of mucosal cilia that beat toward the uterus. This allows the oocyte(s) to move against the flow of oviductal fluid.

Transport of spermatozoa

Rapid phase

Semen that is deposited in the cervical canal or into the uterine lumen is rapidly distributed along the uterine horns and oviducts. The rapid phase of transport results in spermatozoa being present in the oviducts within minutes after insemination. Although the mechanisms by which this transport occurs are imperfectly understood, it is obvious that the motility of the spermatozoa is of little significance. Two factors are important: (1) negative uterine pressure and (2) contraction of the uterus and oviduct(s). The latter may be aided by substances in seminal plasma, such as prostaglandins, which promote smooth muscle contraction. Oxytocin, released in the female because of copulatory stimulation, also causes increased tone and contractility of the uterus and oviducts.

Prolonged phase

The spermatozoa that are rapidly transported are not those involved in fertilization inasmuch as rapid transport causes structural damage to the cells. Also, capacitation of spermatozoa, which is necessary for fertilization, does not occur.

Spermatozoa destined to be involved in fertilization are transported slowly and appear to be stored in parts of the tubular genitalia in so-called sperm reservoirs. In animals that deposit semen in the vagina (e.g., ruminants), the cervix appears to have an important role as a sperm reservoir from which spermatozoa are transported to the uterus and oviducts over a period of hours. Other sperm reservoirs are located in the oviducts near the uterotubal junction. This sperm reservoir, formed between 6 and 12 hours after deposition of semen, remains relatively unchanged for about 24 hours before sperm numbers begin to decline. During the same period, spermatozoa disappear from other areas of the genital tract because of phagocytosis by leukocytes. The environment created within the uterotubal junction is favorable for increasing the longevity of spermatozoa, perhaps through a decrease in metabolism as occurs within the epididymis. Spermatozoa pass from the oviductal storage areas into the oviducts, where their numbers are maintained at relatively constant levels, dependent on the size of the sperm reservoir.

Spermatozoa retain their fertilizing capacity in the female tract for 24 to 48 hours in the cow, ewe, and sow, for as long as 90 hours in the bitch, and for 5 days in the mare. Motility is not a sign of fertilizing capability per se, because spermatozoa usually retain their motility in the female genital tract twice as long as their fertilizing capacity. Sperm transport in the female genital tract can be summarized as occurring in three stages: initial rapid transport, establishment of reservoirs, and slow release from the reservoirs.

The duration of estrus is such that ovulation often occurs 24 hours or more after the onset of estrus, allowing for insemination of the female before ovulation. There are two main points to be emphasized: (1) The fertilizing life span of spermatozoa is, on the average, at least twice as long as that of ova, and (2) spermatozoa require a few hours in the female tract to gain the ability to fertilize. Thus spermatozoa are waiting in large numbers to ensure the fertilization of ova or an ovum immediately after ovulation.

Capacitation

Spermatozoa must undergo some changes after they are deposited in the female reproductive tract in order to acquire the ability to penetrate the zona pellucida and fertilize the ova. This process, referred to as *capacitation*, requires several hours. During capacitation, glycoproteins originating from seminal plasma or epididymal fluid are removed from the sperm surfaces and hydrolytic enzymes are activated in the acrosome. The actual process that capacitation allows is the *acrosome reaction*. This reaction involves the fusion and vesiculation of the plasma and outer acrosome membranes (see Chap. 35) to form ports through which the acrosome enzymes hyaluronidase and the trypsinlike acrosin escape. The acrosomal reaction occurs only in capacitated spermatozoa and is considered by some to be a part of the process of capacitation.

Fertilization

In most domestic animals, oocytes remain viable for up to 18 hours after ovulation. In the cow, ewe, and sow, the first polar body has been formed and metaphase of the second maturational division initiated at the time of ovulation. The second maturational division is not completed until fertilization occurs. In the horse, dog, and fox, oocytes are ovulated before formation of the first polar body. In the dog, formation of the first polar body is not complete until 48 to 60 hours after ovulation.

The process of fertilization can be defined as the fusion of the male and the female gametes to form one single cell called the *zygote*. The first step of fertilization involves the passage of the spermatozoon through the zona pellucida. The spermatozoon penetrates the zona pellucida with the aid of the enzymes hyaluronidase and acrosin. The motility of the sperm is also important for the penetration of the zona; once contact with the plasma membrane of the ovum occurs, spermatozoon motility ceases.

At the time of fertilization, the ovum consists of a nucleus surrounded by a plasma (vitelline) membrane (Fig. 36.19). The ovum is invested with a mucoprotein coat called the *zona pellucida*. The special granulosa cells (*cumulus oophorus)* that surround the zona pellucida are usually lost soon after ovulation.

When the spermatozoon penetrates the zona pellucida, the *zona reaction* occurs. This protective reaction prevents penetration of the vitelline membrane by other spermatozoa. This is important since polyspermy is deleterious to the development of a normal *zygote*. The incidence of polyspermic zygotes in most mammalian species is only about 1 to 2 percent. Once the spermatozoon penetrates the ovum, its head enlarges and converts into the male pronucleus. Both male and female pronuclei enlarge many times before they move toward each other through the cytoplasm. The gamete membranes come in contact and eventually fuse, incorporating sperm and egg nuclei into a single cell. This process, known as *syngamy*, signals the completion of fertilization and the formation of the zygote.

Embryo cleavage, transport and uterine accommodation

After the first cleavage of the zygote, the second cleavage usually occurs first in the larger of the two blastomeres before formation of the four-cell zygote (Fig. 36.19). By the 16- to 32-cell stage, the cells form a circular, slightly lobulated structure called a *morula*. When the zygote is 6 to 8 days old, a cavitation is formed within the embryo, and the entire structure is then known as a *blastocyst*. The term *embryo* is used for the blastocyst stage until there is a differentiation of the organ systems and the placenta. After this stage the conceptus is referred to as a *fetus*.

For the first few days after ovulation, uterine conditions, which had been favorable for the transport of spermatozoa, become unfavorable for the survival of zygotes. Retention

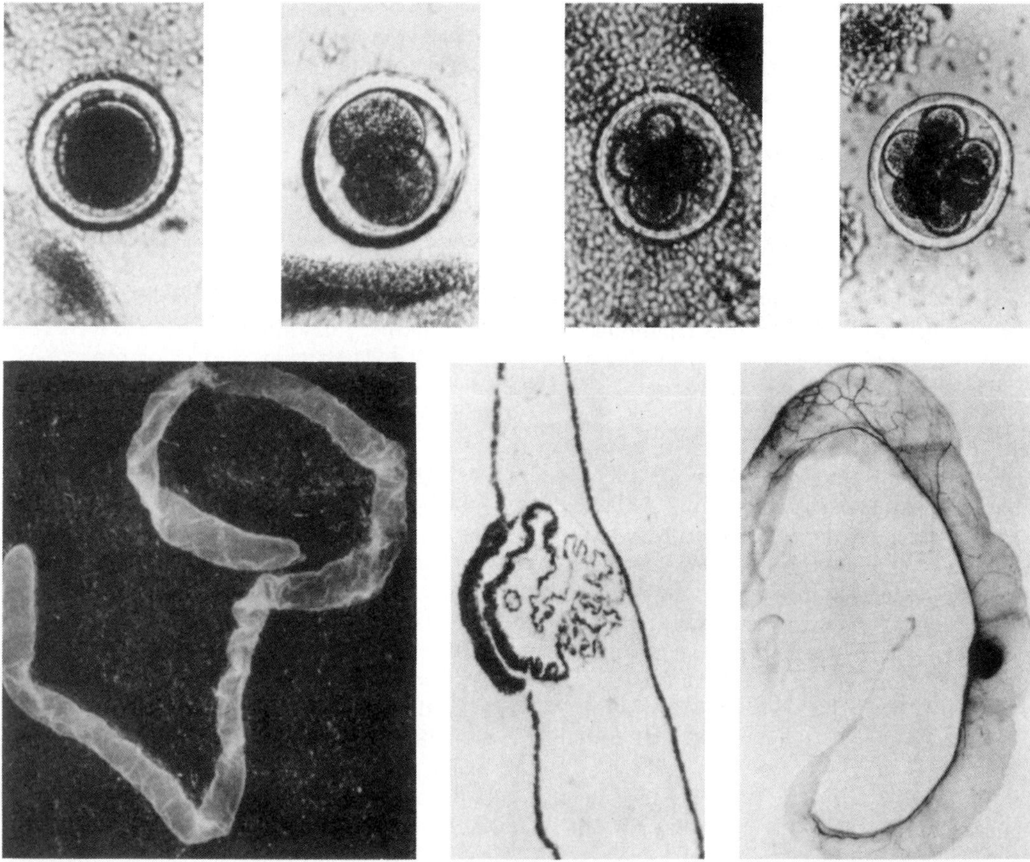

Figure 36.19. Development of cow embryo. (*top, left to right*) Unfertilized ovum and two-, six-, and eight-cell embryos removed from oviduct 2 to 3 days after estrus. Note the zone pellucida, vitellus, and vitelline membrane. Outside diameters range from 146 to 165 μm. (*bottom left*) Fourteen-day embryo, overall length 70 mm. (*bottom center*) Section through the embryonic disk of the 14-day embryo. Note beginning mesoderm formation. The embryo disk is 0.58 mm in diameter. (*bottom right*) Thirty-five-day embryo removed at the beginning of implantation. The embryo is 12 mm long; the entire vesicle (dilated) is 45 cm in length. (From Hansel and McEntee 1977, in Swenson, ed., *Dukes' Physiology of Domestic Animals,* 9th ed., Cornell Univ. Press, Ithaca, N.Y.)

of zygotes in the oviducts allows development to proceed at the same time the uterus is cleaning up the remnant of spermatozoa that were left behind and preparing to nurture the zygotes. Zygotes usually remain in the oviduct for 3 to 5 days before being transferred into the uterus. Data from the mare indicate that differentiation occurs between zygotes and oocytes; oocytes are retained in the oviduct (to degenerate slowly), whereas zygotes are passed into the uterus. Estrogen influences the motility of the oviducts and thus the passage of zygotes from the oviducts into the uterus.

Before the passage of embryos into the uterus, progesterone from the developing CL has been preparing the uterus to retain and nurture the embryos. Progesterone decreases the muscular activity and tonicity of the uterus and promotes the development of a glandular epithelium, which is responsible for producing *uterine milk*.

The nutritive requirements of the embryo are supplied by yolk material and secretions of the oviducts and uterus (uterine milk). Implantation begins 2 to 5 weeks after conception in domestic animal species, and thus the "free living" state of the embryo is longer in these animals than in primate species in which an intimate relationship (interstitial implantation) begins 1 week after ovulation.

In litter-bearing animals, spacing of zygotes in the uterus is important for high rates of implantation and subsequent normal fetal development. The distribution of embryos is effected by contraction of the uterine musculature in response to the presence of embryos. A local phenomenon occurs in the immediate vicinity of the implanting zygote, which prevents the overlapping of implantation by other zygotes. Transuterine migration of zygotes is important for the proper spacing of zygotes in species that have multiple young. Even though spacing appears to be evenly applied in litter-bearing animals, embryos develop best if they are either toward the tip or the body of the uterine horn. This phenomenon is probably correlated with the vascular architecture of the uteroplacental unit.

Maternal recognition of pregnancy

For pregnancy to be established in large domestic animals, the presence of an embryo in utero must be recognized in the dam and translated into prolongation of the life span of the CL and its continual secretion of progesterone. If corpora lutea are not maintained during early pregnancy, abortion will occur in all domestic animals. As has been pointed out previously, uterine-derived $PGF_{2\alpha}$ is the luteolysin in large domestic animals. One absolute prerequisite for the maintenance of pregnancy in these animals is inhibition of the secretion of $PGF_{2\alpha}$ in a pulsatile form.

As the fetal-maternal attachment in large domestic species occurs at a time that is longer than the normal CL life span, the process of implantation cannot serve as a signal for ensuring the rescue of the CL. It appears important that embryos interact with a large area of the endometrium as a prerequisite for the establishment of pregnancy. In litter-bearing animals, spacing of blastocysts between the two uterine horns allows contact with the endometrial surface to be made throughout the length of the uterine horns. In animals that have one fetus (e.g., the mare) the interaction of the embryo and the endometrium occurs by movement of the embryo throughout both uterine horns. The interaction between the blastocysts and the endometrium results in signals from the embryo(s) or the endometrium, which result in maintenance, or at least prevents regression, of the CL. This process is best known in the pig.

Sow

The 12-day-old preimplantation blastocyst of the pig has the capacity to synthesize estrogens (mainly estrone) from available precursors. This synthesis begins at days 12 to 13, which is before the time of permanent fetal-maternal attachment. Elevated concentrations of estrone sulfate (main conjugate) are present in the maternal circulation as early as day 16 of pregnancy. The initial synthesis of estrogen begins at a time when the blastocysts are undergoing rapid growth. The day 10 blastocyst is about 2 mm in diameter, on day 11 it has changed into a flaccid sac about 5 mm in diameter, and by day 14 a considerable elongation that reaches 1 m in length has occurred.

Spacing of blastocysts between the two uterine horns allows contact with the endometrial surface to be made over most of the length of the uterine horns. Failure to establish this contact leads to pregnancy failure. A minimal number of blastocysts (4 or 5) must be present in utero to ensure sufficient endometrial contact for gestation to be maintained. Concomitant with the rapid elongation of the blastocyst and its ability to synthesize estrogens is a marked reduction in the capacity of the uterus to synthesize $PGF_{2\alpha}$ in a pulsatile manner that passively prevents luteolysis, allowing the CL to continue to be functional. The importance of estrogen secretion from the blastocyst for CL maintenance is suggested by the fact that estrogen administration to nonpregnant pigs during the luteal phase prolongs the CL life span.

Cow, Ewe, and Doe

In the cow, ewe, and doe the preimplantation blastocyst also undergoes a considerable elongation at the time the CL life span needs to be extended (Fig. 36.19). The synthesis and release of $PGF_{2\alpha}$ in a pulsatile fashion are abolished (Fig. 36.8).

In the cow, the existence of a luteotropic factor of embryonic origin has been suggested on the basis of the high concentrations of progesterone that have been observed in pregnant as compared with nonpregnant heifers. Also, a protein (protein B) of placental origin has been identified in cattle, beginning at about day 20 of gestation. The role of this protein in the establishment of pregnancy of cattle is, as yet, unknown.

Another possible fetal signal for pregnancy maintenance

is a protein called trophoblastin, which has been found in both sheep and cattle. The possibility that this molecule plays an immunologic role in the establishment of pregnancy is based on its close structural homology with interferon.

Mare

In the mare, the blastocyst does not undergo elongation as occurs in the sow and the domestic ruminant species. The embryo does move, though, throughout both uterine horns before its fixation in the base of one horn at day 16 of gestation. This movement of the embryo is probably important for the blockage of pulsatile $PGF_{2\alpha}$ synthesis and release.

The mare produces a gonadotropin called equine chorionic gonadotropin (eCG) (orginally called pregnant mares' serum gonadotropin, PMSG, by its discoverer, Professor Harold Cole). Its synthesis does not begin, however, until about day 35 of gestation; therefore eCG cannot play a role in the early maternal recognition of pregnancy in the mare.

Bitch and Queen

In both the dog and the cat, implantation occurs well before the time that luteal demise would occur if the animal were not pregnant (Fig. 36.16). The luteal life span in the nonpregnant dog is longer, in fact, than in the pregnant bitch, so rescue of the CL is not essential, in one sense, in the dog. The enhancement of progesterone secretion observed between days 20 and 30 of gestation suggests the presence of a placental luteotropin in the dog.

In the cat, ovulation without conception results in a luteal life span that lasts for about 35 to 40 days (Fig. 36.16). Because implantation begins about 13 days after ovulation (conception), the cat does not need a signal of blastocyst origin to maintain CL function. Later, however, a luteotropin from the placenta (as yet unidentified) influences the CL to continue progesterone secretion until the processes associated with parturition terminate luteal activity.

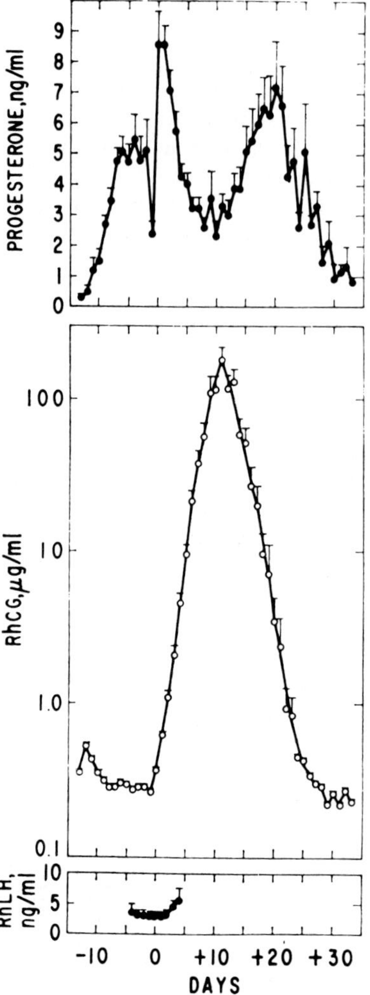

Figure 36.20. The rescue of the corpus luteum in early pregnancy in the rhesus monkey. Note the sharp increase in progesterone concentrations in blood after the initial appearance of MCG (RhCG) (0, day of CL rescue). Rescue of the CL occurs between days 10 and 12 after conception. (From Knobil 1973, *Biol. Reprod.* 8:246.)

Primates

Primates use an active process for bridging the gap between the nonpregnant and pregnant states. Implantation begins 6 to 8 days after fertilization; therefore the process of implantation can serve as a signal for prolongation of the life span of the CL. The form of implantation (i.e., interstitial) is important because it allows the trophoblastic cells to begin to secrete CG (hCG in humans and mCG in monkeys) within 1 or 2 days after implantation. Chorionic gonadotropin is luteotropic, and CL activity is almost immediately enhanced and extended. Human CG can be detected in the maternal peripheral blood as early as days 8 to 10 after ovulation. There is little room for error in primates for the rescue of the CL at the onset of pregnancy in that the luteal phase is only 14 days in duration, and rescue of the CL must begin at least 3 or 4 days before the end of the luteal phase. Determination of hCG in urine is used as a pregnancy test in humans. The hormonal changes associated with maintenance of the CL during early pregnancy of the rhesus monkey are shown in Fig. 36.20.

Implantation

The embryo is considered to be implanted when it becomes fixed in position and forms both physical and functional contact with the uterus. The time of implantation is easy to define for species in which the embryo becomes buried in the wall of the uterus. In primates, for example, the blastocyst passes through the uterine epithelium into the interstitium so that it is effectively separated from the uterine cavity by about day 7 after ovulation.

In domestic animals, the time of implantation is more

difficult to define. This is because the areas of attachment between the trophoblastic cells of the placenta and the epithelial surface of the uterus develop slowly over a period of days, making the precise time of implantation difficult to determine. As the implantation process is gradual, ranges of time are usually presented during which the embryo makes a definitive union with the endometrium. The following are times (days) for the initiation of implantation in various species after ovulation: humans, 6 to 8; rabbits, 7; cats, 13; sheep, 15 to 18; swine, 14 to 20; horses, 30 to 35; cattle, 30 to 35 (see Table 36.1).

Embryonic mortality

For an interaction to occur between the embryo and the endometrium, the development of the uterus must be in synchrony with the development of the embryo. It is well established in large domestic animals that fertilization rates are high (i.e., about 90 percent). The most significant time of early embryonic mortality in these species is when the fetal-maternal attachment is being established. Delayed passage or development of embryos within the oviduct or impaired development of the endometrium can contribute to asynchrony between the uterus and the embryo, with reproductive failure being the result.

It has been suggested that the fertilization of oocytes at the end of their fertilizable period results in the development of abnormal embryos and embryonic loss. This may be one explanation for the most common identifiable cause of embryonic mortality in animals (i.e., chromosomal abnormalities). The usual situation in domestic animals is that in the majority of embryonic losses the cause is neither identified nor diagnosed. The advent of ultrasonography has been important for the study of embryonic mortality in that embryonic development can be followed as early as 12 to 13 days (in horses and cats).

Immunology of pregnancy

The fetus inherits transplantation antigens from its sire, which brings forth the question how the dam tolerates and even nourishes foreign tissue without rejection, as would occur with a skin graft that had the same transplantation antigens.

One important factor appears to be the complete separation of maternal and fetal circulation that exists so that the mother is not sensitized to fetal antigens. In some species, it appears that the isolation of the fetus is accomplished by a fibrinoid layer that surrounds the trophoblast, particularly in species with deciduate implantation. This layer may prevent the passage of fetal antigens into the dam. Animals with epitheliochorial placentae do not have this protection (see Table 36.1). The recent finding that a protein produced by the fetus (trophoblast) is structurally related to interferon suggests the possibility of the embryo producing substances that modify the immunologic response of the dam.

The placenta

The trophoblastic cells of the embryo participate in formation of the placenta. In the chorioallantoic placenta that is characteristic of domestic animals, the outer layer of the allantois is fused to the chorion. The fetal umbilical vessels penetrate the amnion and then are distributed over the surface of the placenta in the connective tissue layer between the allantois and chorion.

The chorionic placentae of mammals are usually classified according to the number of distinct tissues that separate maternal and fetal blood. In less developed species, more barriers are interposed between the two circulatory systems. Fewer barriers are present in species that are more complex, so that the placenta becomes more permeable to the passage of nutrients.

Endocrinology of gestation

Sources of endocrine support for pregnancy

Progesterone is essential for the maintenance of pregnancy; the source is either the CL, the placenta, or both. In animals in which placental production of progesterone is low (e.g., the sow and doe), corpora lutea are essential throughout pregnancy. In other animals, the placenta varies in its capability for synthesizing progesterone. Placental production of progesterone occurs in the cow, but pregnancy continues in only a few animals that are subjected to ovariectomy on about day 225 of gestation. Placental production of progesterone is therefore marginal in the cow and occurs only in the latter part of gestation. In the bitch, the same situation exists as for the cow, in that ovariectomy on days 50 to 55 results in only a few animals going to term; placental production of progesterone is marginal in the dog. Placental production of progesterone is sufficiently established in the cat by day 40 that ovariectomy does not disrupt pregnancy. In sheep, placental production of progesterone is established by about day 50, so that ovariectomy after this time does not adversely affect the outcome of the pregnancy. Progesterone production by the placenta in the mare is established by day 70 of pregnancy, so that ovariectomy at this time usually does not result in abortion. In primates, placental production of progesterone is probably adequate to maintain pregnancy by as early as 3 to 4 weeks after implantation.

In species such as sheep and primates, luteal production of progesterone continues throughout pregnancy, even though placental production is dominant. In the mare, on the other hand, with CL regression midway during gestation, placental progesterone is solely responsible for pregnancy maintenance by about day 150 of gestation.

Hormones of fetoplacental origin

In addition to progesterone, the major steroid produced by the placenta is estrogen. In domestic animals the major estrogen produced during pregnancy is estrone, and in primates it is estriol. In contrast to the production of progesterone, which is by the placenta only, the synthesis of estrogen requires an interaction between the placenta and the fetus. This fetoplacental interaction has been best described by Diczfalusy, a Hungarian immigrant to Sweden, who showed that the placenta of the primate was unable to produce estrogen from progesterone, even though these steroids were closely associated in the steroid biochemical pathway. This inability was due to the absence of appropriate enzyme systems. In primates, the key fetal organ is the fetal zone of the adrenal cortex, which converts pregnenolone (supplied by the placenta) to an androgen, dehydroepiandrosterone. This androgen is returned to the placenta, which converts it to an estrogen. A similar system exists in the horse, except that the fetal gonads serve as the intermediary organ for the conversion of pregnenolone to estrogen. The use of the fetal gonad in the horse as the endocrine intermediary explains the large size of the fetal gonads during pregnancy (peak size achieved at about 7 months), with the gonads being larger at times than those of the dam.

Estrogen concentrations are useful for determining the status of the fetus in that the fetus participates in the synthesis of estrogens. Estriol values are used in humans to assess the activity of the fetus (in conjunction with ultrasonography). Estrone conjugate concentrations in blood or urine are useful in the mare for determination of pregnancy beginning at about day 40 of gestation. The initial increase in estrogen concentrations is thought to be due to stimulation of the ovaries by eCG. By about day 70, estrogen concentrations almost entirely reflect production by the fetoplacental unit and the beginning presence of free estrone; in addition to estrone conjugates, estrone concentrations can then be used to assess the viability of the fetus throughout the rest of pregnancy. Estrone concentrations tend to increase relatively late in gestation in other domestic animals (bitch, cow, doe, ewe, and queen) and, as such, have little practical application for either determination of pregnancy or the assessment of fetal well-being.

The assay of estrogen conjugate concentrations in urine (or plasma) has been useful for the assessment of estrogen secretion in both humans and horses. The number of conjugates that are formed during estrogen metabolism (of a variety of estrogens) is relatively small. As a result, estrogen values tend to be amplified when conjugate concentrations are measured, making the assessment of estrogen dynamics much easier, particularly in domestic animals wherein concentrations of unconjugated estrogens in plasma are low in comparison to primates. Useful information can be obtained from urine obtained from the soil, for the conjugates of estrogen are very stable.

The protein hormones produced during pregnancy tend to be of placental origin. One of these hormones, *relaxin*, is produced by the placenta of the cat, dog, and horse begin-

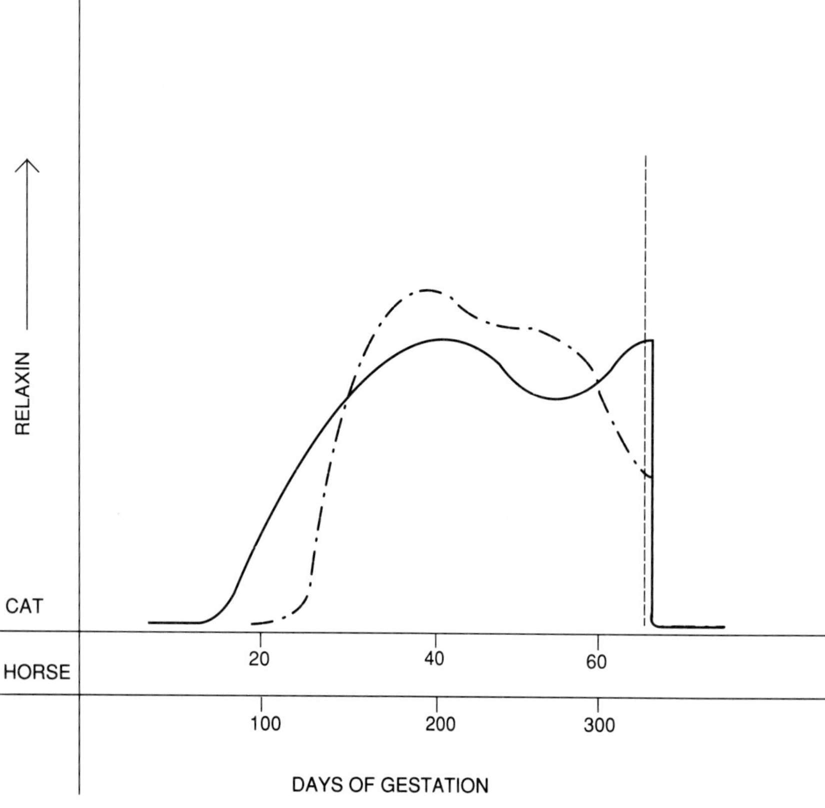

Figure 36.21. Plasma relaxin activity during pregnancy in horses (*solid line*) and cats (*broken line*). Dashed vertical line indicates the times of parturition. (Horse data adapted from Stewart and Stabenfeldt 1981, *Biol. Reprod.* 25:281. Cat data adapted from Stewart and Stabenfeldt 1985, *Biol. Reprod.* 32:848.)

ning at about days 20, 20 and 70 of pregnancy, respectively (Fig. 36.21). One of the suggested functions of relaxin during pregnancy is maintenance of the quiescent uterus (in conjunction with progesterone). In exception to the general rule of protein hormone production by the placenta, relaxin is produced in the CL of pigs, cattle, and primates during pregnancy.

Placental lactogen (PL), a protein hormone produced during pregnancy, has been identified in primates (also called *chorionic somatomammotropin* in humans), goats, sheep, and cattle. In addition to its lactogenic properties (prolactinlike), it has somatomammotropic biological activity similar to insulin and growth hormone in that it increases protein synthesis, increases lipolysis, and decreases gluconeogenesis. There is some evidence that PL in dairy cattle affects alveolar development that occurs in association with the subsequent lactation.

As mentioned previously, gonadotropic hormones produced by the trophoblast, and called chorionic gonadotropins (CG), have been identified in both primates and horses. The structure and action of these hormones are similar to the gonadotropins produced by the anterior pituitary. In primates, CG stimulates and extends the activity of the CL (progesterone production) during the early establishment of pregnancy. In mares, CG is produced by specialized trophoblastic (chorionic girdle) cells that invade the endometrium at about day 35 of gestation and form discrete tissue bodies called *endometrial cups*. The initial effect of eCG is to stimulate the ovary to produce estrogens. The source of the estrogen appears to be the primary CL of pregnancy in that ovariectomy, or luteolysis induced by prostaglandin treatment (pregnancy supported by exogenous progesterone administration), prevents the estrogen rise at days 35 to 40. Equine chorionic gonadotropin also is probably responsible for the development of additional (secondary) CL from the standpoint of both production of follicles and luteinization or ovulation of the follicles. Interestingly, groups of follicles (destined to be secondary CL) can begin their development as late as 3 weeks after the onset of eCG production. The importance of secondary CL in the mare is unknown inasmuch as progesterone production by the primary CL is adequate to maintain pregnancy until the takeover by the placenta at about day 70 of gestation (see Fig. 36.22).

There is circumstantial evidence in cats and dogs that the placentae of these species produce a luteotropic hormone. In cats, the luteal phase is extended from the usual 35 to 40 days observed in the nonpregnant (pseudopregnant) animal. In dogs, the presence of a luteotropin is suggested by the enhancement of progesterone production observed by days 20 to 30 of pregnancy.

Two hormones of importance in pregnancy that are not of fetoplacental origin are $PGF_{2\alpha}$ and PRL. Although the source of $PGF_{2\alpha}$ synthesis is not known for certain, it is likely to be the endometrium. In the mare, for example, $PGF_{2\alpha}$ concentrations increase 100-fold from early pregnancy to term. This increased synthetic capacity is important because a massive release of $PGF_{2\alpha}$ controls the onset of delivery in the mare.

PRL, an important hormone of pregnancy, originates from the anterior pituitary, with increased secretion during pregnancy due to the effects of estrogen on the lactotropes. PRL is important for the initiation (and subsequent maintenance) of lactation.

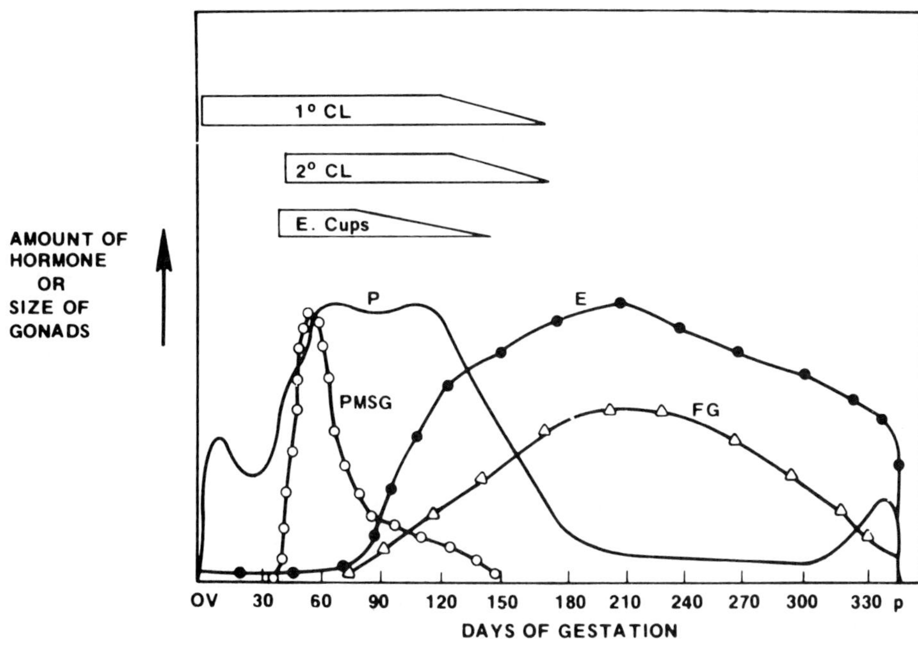

Figure 36.22. The endocrinology of pregnancy in the mare. PMSG, pregnant mare's serum gonadotropin; P, progesterone; E, estrogen; FG, fetal gonads; 1° CL, primary corpus luteum; 2° CL, secondary corpus luteum; E. cups, endometrial cups. (From Stabenfeldt and Hughes 1977, in Cole and Cupps, eds., *Reproduction in Domestic Animals,* 3d ed., Academic Press, New York.)

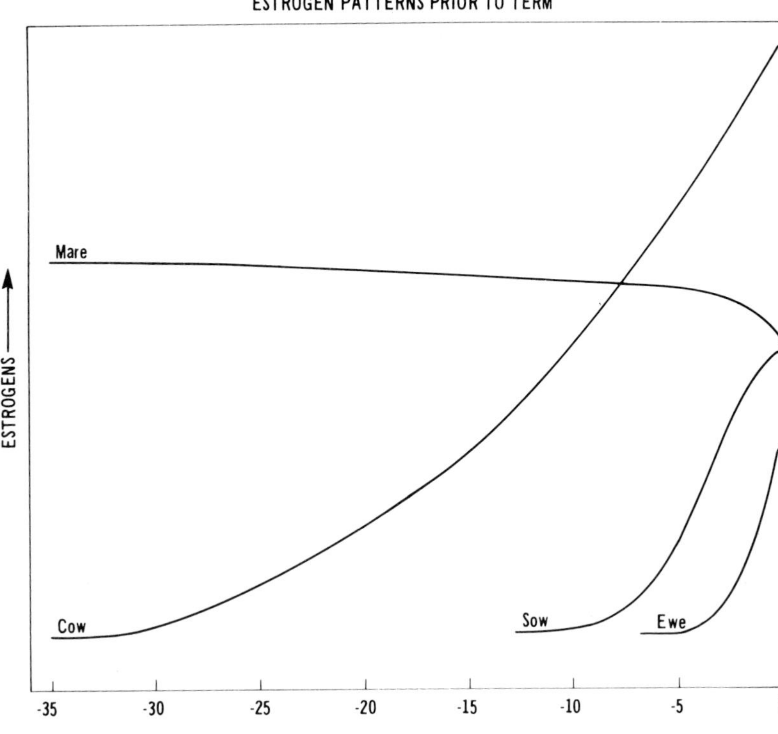

Figure 36.23. Estrogen patterns in the mare, cow, sow, and ewe before parturition (O). (From Edqvist and Stabenfeldt 1980, in Kaneko, ed., *Clinical Biochemistry of Domestic Animals,* Academic Press, New York.)

PARTURITION

For delivery of the fetus(es), it is necessary that the uterine myometrium be converted from a quiescent (essential for pregnancy maintenance) to an actively contracting organ. In the following discussion, data from both the cow and the ewe are used to develop the endocrine basis of parturition.

Sequence of preparturient endocrine events

Progesterone is responsible (perhaps in conjunction with relaxin) for the maintenance of a quiescent myometrium and a contracted cervix. One of the initial preparturient events observed in the dam is a changeover from progesterone to estrogen production, which begins at 3 to 4 weeks before parturition in the cow and at less than 5 days in the ewe (Fig. 36.23). Increased estrogen production is important for the synthesis of contractile proteins of the myometrium and the formation of gap junctions between myometrial cells. The former allows for the development of forceful uterine contractions and the latter allows for coordination of contractions in association with the delivery process.

The critical question, then, is what initiates the changeover from progesterone to estrogen synthesis in the immediate prepartum period. The answer lies within the adrenal cortex of the fetus. In sheep, it has been shown that fetal cortisol production results in the induction of enzymes that are important for the movement of steroids down the biosynthetic pathway from progesterone to estrogen, specifically, 17_{α}-hydroxylase and C17–20 lyase. The maturation of the fetus and particularly the fetal adrenal cortex is the key factor in the initial movement toward parturition.

As can be seen from the estrogen data for the cow, the changes that are initiated by the fetus occur weeks before the delivery process itself. The question: What initiates the final acute phase of the parturitional process? In domestic animals and primates, greatly accelerated synthesis and release of $PGF_{2\alpha}$ are the factors that initiate the final delivery process. Estrogens are probably important for the initiation of the $PGF_{2\alpha}$ surge in some species, whereas oxytocin may be the initiating factor in others. In mares, for example, small amounts of oxytocin (as little as 5 to 10 IU) administered intravenously near term result in a massive release of $PGF_{2\alpha}$ within a few minutes and the initiation of delivery.

In general, $PGF_{2\alpha}$ synthesis and release occur 24 to 36 hours before term in domestic animals. $PGF_{2\alpha}$ initiates regression of the CL, which results in progesterone withdrawal, much in the same manner as occurs during the termination of the luteal phase in the estrous cycle of large domestic species. Prepartum luteolysis passively allows the myometrium to become more contractile. In addition, $PGF_{2\alpha}$ exerts a direct effect on uterine musculature by increasing its contractile state. This is effected, in part, by its ability to decrease sarcoplasmic binding of calcium ions, thus freeing them to interact in the contractile process. This initial increase in contractility of the uterine musculature is important for the start of the first stage of labor (i.e., the presentation of the fetus at the internal os of the cervix in the so-called diver's position). $PGF_{2\alpha}$ also has an indirect effect on uterine contractility by making the uterine musculature more sensitive to oxytocin. Finally, there is some evidence that $PGF_{2\alpha}$ is involved in relaxation of the cervix, possibly through the dissolution of ground substance that binds fibroblasts and fibrocytes together (again, in a manner similar to that observed with the rupture of the follicle, i.e., ovulation).

It is likely that relaxin also plays an important role in parturition through its effect on relaxation of the cervix. Relaxin is also important for the softening of the tissues that surround the pelvic canal, which in turn allows the fetus to have maximal space for its passage through the pelvis. The release of relaxin in the immediate prepartum period occurs in the sow and cow through the effect of $PGF_{2\alpha}$ on the CL, the source of relaxin in these animals. The positioning of the fetus and the dilation of the cervix constitute stage 1 of parturition.

The release of oxytocin is initiated by engagement of the fetus in the pelvic canal, which initiates impulses to travel through the spinal cord to the hypothalamus (Ferguson's reflex). Oxytocin enhances the rhythmic contraction of the uterine musculature (in concert with $PGF_{2\alpha}$) during the delivery process. The stage of expulsion of the fetus is referred to as the second stage of parturition.

In the mare, $PGF_{2\alpha}$ synthesis and release result in a precipitous onset of parturition, with dilation of the cervix occurring within 15 to 20 minutes and delivery usually occurring within 60 minutes of the initial rise in $PGF_{2\alpha}$. In this species corpora lutea are not present, and progesterone withdrawal does not occur before delivery. The placenta must carry on all functions, including progestational and nutritive support for the fetus, up to the time of delivery. In this situation, it is not possible for the placenta to stop certain functions (progestational support of pregnancy) and carry on others (nutritive and gas exchange). The massive release of $PGF_{2\alpha}$ overrides the progesterone support of pregnancy in this instance. There is a similar relationship to $PGF_{2\alpha}$ release and absence of progesterone withdrawal with respect in primates. Figure 36.24 summarizes the endocrine events that lead to parturition.

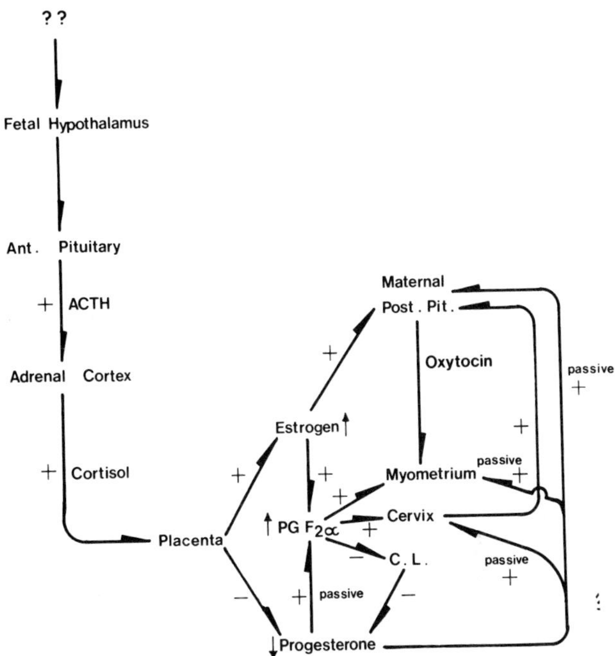

Figure 36.24. Relationship of endocrine events that lead to parturition in the ewe. +, stimulation; −, inhibition. (Adapted from Liggins et al. 1973, *Rec. Progr. Horm. Res.* 29:111.)

Importance of the fetus

As indicated previously, the fetus plays a pivotal role in initiation of the delivery process. In the 1960s, experimental studies by Liggins and Kenneday showed the importance of the fetal anterior pituitary, and studies by Drost showed the importance of fetal adrenals in initiation of the delivery process. Destruction of most of the fetal anterior pituitary by electrocautery or removal of the fetal adrenals resulted in prolonged gestation in sheep. The concept arose that the fetal hypophyseal-adrenal system was essential in sheep, and possibly all domestic species, for the delivery of the fetus(es).

Abnormalities in development of the anterior pituitary and the adrenals have led to prolonged gestation in both Holstein and Guernsey cattle. Both syndromes have a genetic basis that has an autosomal recessive basis. In Guernseys, the anterior pituitary does not develop and the neonatal calf ceases to grow after 7 months of age (because of the absence of tropic growth factors). In Holsteins the pituitary gland is present, but there is an absence of cells that produce ACTH. The fetus continues to grow past term, with fetal death usually the result of an inadequate nutrient supply. In both syndromes, the adrenal cortices are present but usually have some degree of abnormal organization. These syndromes occur only if the homozygous condition is present with the defect being lethal. Carriers of these diseases are obviously heterozygous for the condition.

Abnormalities in gestation length can occur as a result of the ingestion of alkaloidal agents during the early formative stages of the embryo. For example, ingestion of the plant *Veratrum californicum* by sheep during the period of early organogenesis, particularly days 10 to 15 of gestation, can cause a disruption in the formation of the hypothalamus and anterior pituitary. Gestation is prolonged because of the absence of a normal hypothalamohypophyseal-adrenocortical axis. The lambs often have a cyclopean appearance because the eyes are organized at the same time as the hypothalamus and anterior pituitary. The disease is usually limited to animals bred early in the breeding season because the plant grows at high elevations and is killed by cold temperatures in the early autumn. Dystocia is a common end result of the disease.

Microorganisms, such as the bluetongue virus, also cause a disruption of organogenesis if present at the critical time of development. In particular, sheep that contract this disease will have prolonged pregnancies involving cyclopean lambs similar to those caused by the ingestion of *Veratrum californicum*.

Prolongation of gestation can also occur as the result of the ingestion of substances that inhibit physiologic hypothalamo-pituitary activity. The ingestion by sheep of plant leaves from a shrub called *Salsola tuberculata* in southwest Africa causes prolonged gestation. Drought conditions force the ewes to graze the leaves from this shrub, and prolongation of gestation occurs when the shrub is ingested in the latter third of gestation. Gross abnormalities of the fetus do not occur in this syndrome.

Finally, premature delivery appears to occur because of a defect in Angora goats, a defect that involves the premature development of fetal adrenal glands.

REFERENCES

Austin, C.R., and Short, R.V., eds. 1976. *Reproduction in Mammals*. No. 6. *The Evolution of Reproduction*. Cambridge Univ. Press, Cambridge.

Austin, C.R., and Short, R.V., eds. 1979. *Reproduction in Mammals*. No. 7. *Mechanisms of Hormone Action*. Cambridge Univ. Press, Cambridge.

Austin, C.R., and Short, R.V., eds. 1980. *Reproduction in Mammals*. No. 8 *Human Sexuality*. Cambridge Univ. Press, Cambridge.

Austin, C.R., and Short, R.V., eds. 1982. *Reproduction in Mammals*. No. 1. *Germ Cells and Fertilization*. 2d ed. Cambridge Univ. Press, Cambridge.

Austin, C.R., and Short, R.V., eds. 1982. *Reproduction in Mammals*. No. 2. *Embryonic and Fetal Development*. 2d ed. Cambridge Univ. Press, Cambridge.

Austin, C.R., and Short, R.V., eds. 1984. *Reproduction in Mammals*. No. 3. *Hormonal Control of Reproduction*. 2d ed. Cambridge Univ. Press, Cambridge.

Austin, C.R., and Short, R.V., eds. 1984. *Reproduction in Mammals*. No. 4. *Reproductive Fitness*. 2d ed. Cambridge Univ. Press, Cambridge.

Austin, C.R., and Short, R.V., eds. 1986. *Reproduction in Mammals*. No. 5. *Manipulating Reproduction*. 2d ed. Cambridge Univ. Press, Cambridge.

Cole, H.H., and Cupps, P.T., eds. 1977. *Reproduction in Domestic Animals*. 3d ed. Academic Press, New York.

Concannon, P.W., Morton, D.B., and Weir, Barbara J., eds. 1989. *Dog and cat reproduction, contraception and artificial insemination. J. Reprod. Fert.* 39 (suppl.).

Cupps, P.T., ed. 1991. *Reproduction in Domestic Animals*. 4th ed. Academic Press, San Diego.

Edqvist, L.-E., and Kindahl, H., eds. 1981. Prostaglandins in animal reproduction. *I. Acta Vet. Scand.* 77 (suppl.).

Edqvist, L-E., and Kindahl, H., eds. 1984. *Prostaglandins in Animal Reproduction. II. Animal Reprod. Science, vol. 7.*

Feldman, E.C., and Nelson, R.W. 1987. *Canine and Feline Endocrinology and Reproduction*. W.B. Saunders, Philadelphia.

Hafez, E.S.E., ed. 1987. *Reproduction in Farm Animals*. 5th ed. Lea & Febiger, Philadelphia.

Johnson, M., and Everitt, B. 1988. *Essential Reproduction*. 3rd ed. Blackwell Scientific Publications, Oxford.

Knobil, E., and Neill, J.D., eds. 1988. *The Physiology of Reproduction*. Raven Press, New York.

McDonald, L.E., and Pineda, M.H., eds. 1989. *Veterinary Endocrinology and Reproduction*. 4th ed. Lea & Febiger, Philadelphia.

CHAPTER 37

The Mammary Gland and Lactation | by Chung S. Park and Norman L. Jacobson

The mammary gland, like sebaceous and sweat glands, is a cutaneous gland. Histologically, in the more advanced mammals it is a compound tubuloalveolar type that originates from the ectoderm. Although the mammary gland is basically similar in all mammals, there are wide species variations in the appearance of the gland and in the relative amounts of the components secreted.

The most primitive of present-day mammals is the egg-laying monotreme, of which one representative is the duck-billed platypus. The primary difference between the mammary gland of the platypus and that of higher mammals is the absence of a nipple. The milk is expressed from 100 or more ducts (or glands) located in two lines lateral to the ventral midline of the animal. The milk accumulates on the abdominal fur, which is licked by the young.

A somewhat more advanced type of mammal is the marsupial, whose young are born in a very immature state. The newborn marsupial, if it is to survive, must find its way quickly to a nipple, which in most marsupials is located in a pouch. If there are more young than nipples, the latecomers perish.

The most advanced mammals are those with true placentas. About 95 percent of the mammals existing today belong to this group.

FUNCTIONAL ANATOMY OF THE MAMMARY GLAND

External

The mammary glands of cattle, sheep, goats, horses, and whales are located in the inguinal region; those of primates and elephants in the thoracic region; and those of pigs, rodents, and carnivores along the ventral surface of both the thorax and abdomen.

Normally, cattle have four functional teats and glands, whereas sheep and goats have two; each teat has one streak canal and drains a separate gland. The glands and teats of domestic animals are known collectively as the udder. Pigs and horses usually have two streak canals per teat, with each canal serving a separate secretory area. In rodents, carnivores, and primates the number of streak canals per teat ranges up to 10 or 20.

Because more is known about bovine mammary glands than about those of other mammals, more attention will be given here to that species. A cow's udder is composed of two halves, each of which has two teats, and each teat drains a separate gland (quarter). The quarters are separated by connective tissue, and each has a separate milk-collecting system (Fig. 37.1).

In addition to the four normal teats, there may be supernumerary teats associated either with a small gland, with a normal gland, or with no secretory area. About 40 percent of all cows have supernumerary teats. These teats are usually oriented similarly to normal teats and may be caudad to (most common), between, or fused with the normal teats. Supernumerary teats are also found in sheep, goats, pigs, and horses. In these species, with the exception of the horse, rudimentary teats are usually found in the male.

The empty weight of the lactating udder of dairy cows is usually 14 to 32 kg. Capacity is not necessarily closely correlated with empty udder weight since the ratio of par-

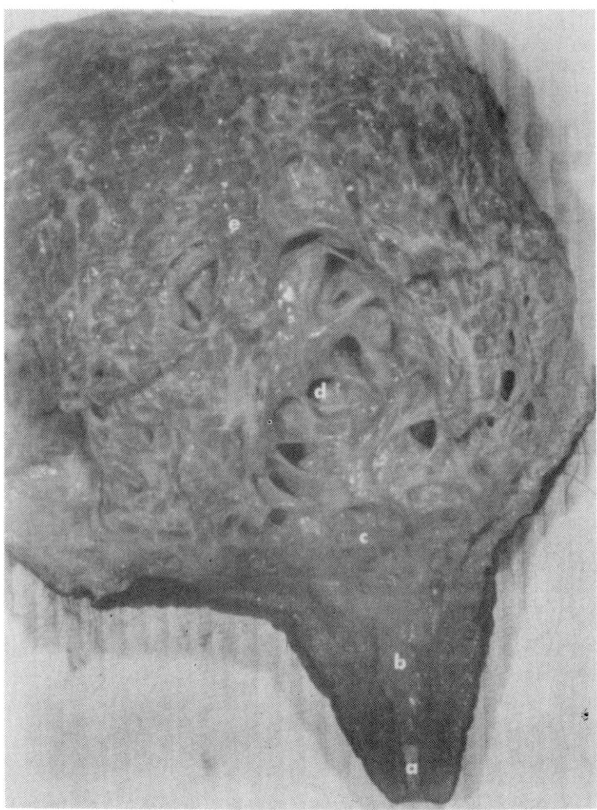

Figure 37.1. Vertical section through one quarter of a bovine udder: a, streak canal; b, teat cistern; c, gland cistern; d, large duct at point of entry into gland cistern; and e, secretory tissue.

enchyma (secretory tissue) to stroma (connective tissue) also varies widely. The weight and capacity of the udder usually increase until the cow reaches maturity at about 6 years of age.

Internal

Supporting structure

The two halves of the bovine udder are separated by the median suspensory ligament, which is formed by two lamellae of elastic connective tissue originating from the abdominal tunic (Fig. 37.2). The posterior extremity of this ligament is attached to the prepubic tendon. The lateral suspensory ligaments are composed largely of fibrous, nonelastic strands giving rise to numerous lamellae that penetrate the gland and become continuous with the interstitial tissue of the udder. The lateral suspensory ligaments are attached to the prepubic and subpubic tendons, which in turn are attached to the pelvic symphysis. The lateral and median suspensory ligaments are the primary structures supporting the bovine udder. On the ventral surface of the udder, the lamellae of the median suspensory ligament and the lateral suspensory ligaments provide a saclike support for the mammary gland. The skin offers little mechanical support but does protect the udder.

Milk-collecting system

The bovine teat has a small cistern terminating at its distal extremity in the streak canal, which is the opening to the exterior of the teat (Figs. 37.1 and 37.3). Radiating upward from the streak canal into the teat is a structure known as Fürstenberg's rosette, which is composed of about seven or eight loose folds of double-layered epithelium and underlying connective tissue; each fold has a number of secondary folds. In cattle, the primary structure responsible for retention of milk is a sphincter muscle surrounding the streak canal. In the pig, which usually has two streak canals per teat (each canal draining a separate gland area), the streak canal is tightly closed by longitudinal folds originating in the teat cistern. Each streak canal also has a circular elastic connective tissue band. Only a few muscle fiber bundles are found. Large ducts empty into a gland cistern located above each teat (Figs. 37.1 and 37.3). These ducts branch profusely, ultimately ending in secretory units called alveoli or acini (Figs. 37.3 and 37.4).

The epithelium of the skin and the lining of the streak canal are of the stratified squamous type; the teat, gland cisterns, and ducts are lined with a two-layer epithelium—a layer of cuboidal cells overlaid with high cylindrical cells. There is a gradual change in the epithelial lining of the ducts to the single layer of epithelium characteristic of the alveoli.

Alveoli are generally recognized as the basic functional units of the lactating mammary gland (Figs. 37.3, 37.4, and 37.5). Milk is formed in the epithelial cells of the alveolus. The alveolus, when filled with milk, is approximately 100 to 300 μm in diameter. The size of the alveolus is affected by many factors, particularly the amount of milk in the lumen.

The alveoli are grouped together in units known as lobules, each of which is surrounded by a distinct connective tissue septum. The lobule in the bovine is less than 1 mm^3 in volume. Lobules, in turn, are grouped together into larger units called lobes, which are surrounded by more extensive connective tissue septa (Fig. 37.3).

The alveoli are surrounded by contractile myoepithelial cells that are involved in the milk-ejection (or milk-letdown) reflex (Figs. 37.4 and 37.5). Myoepithelial cells also are located along the ducts. Apparently these cells are widely distributed among mammals, since they have been identified in the cat, dog, goat, pig, rabbit, rat, sheep, and human.

Blood supply

The main route followed by blood in passing from the heart to mammary glands in the inguinal region is by way of the caudal aorta, the right and left common iliac arteries (from this point the route continues to be bilateral), the

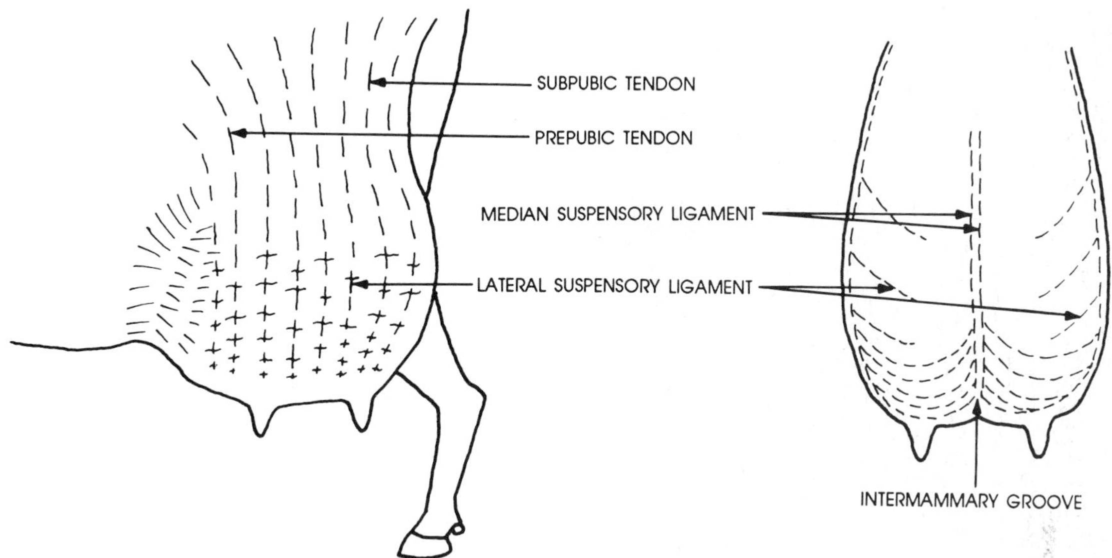

Figure 37.2. Suspensory apparatus of the bovine udder. (Redrawn from Smith 1959, *Physiology of Lactation*, 5th ed., Iowa State University Press, Ames.)

external iliac arteries, and the external pudic arteries. The mammary arteries that originate from the external pudic arteries form cranial and caudal branches, which supply the cranial and caudal portions of the udder, respectively. Numerous branches from these vessels provide blood to all parts of the mammary gland.

A major route for the return of blood from the udder to the heart is via veins traversing much the same route as the arteries just described. The blood passes through the external pudic veins, the external iliac veins, and the caudal vena cava. The subcutaneous abdominal veins (caudal and cranial superficial epigastric veins) provide a potential route for passage of blood from the udder to the heart by way of the

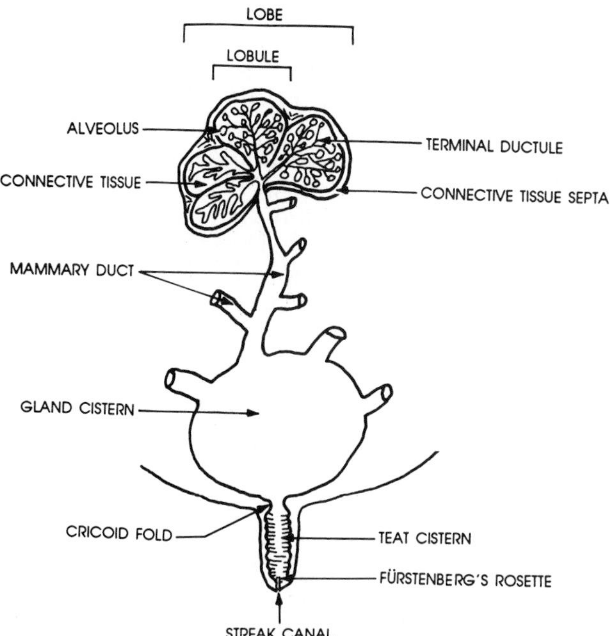

Figure 37.3. Duct and lobuloalveolar systems of the bovine mammary gland. (Redrawn from Bath et al. 1985, *Dairy Cattle: Principles, Practices, Problems, Profits,* 3d ed., Lea & Febiger, Philadelphia. Reproduced with permission.)

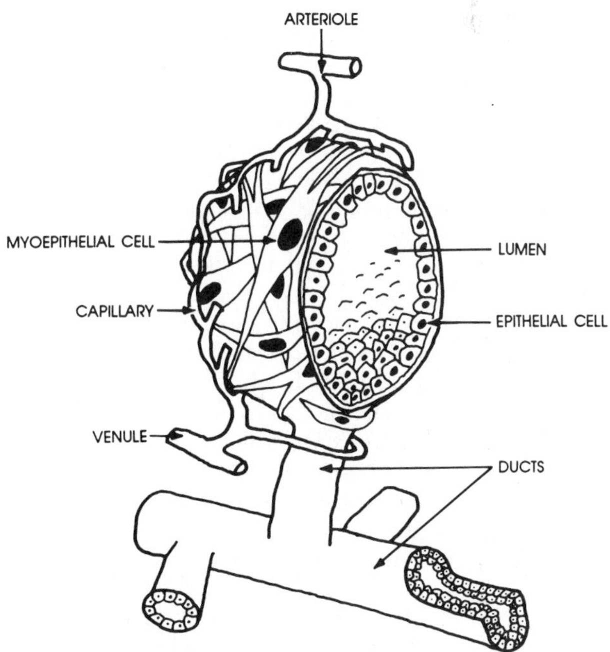

Figure 37.4. An alveolus surrounded by blood vessels and myoepithelial cells in the mammary gland. (Drawn by C.B. Choi.)

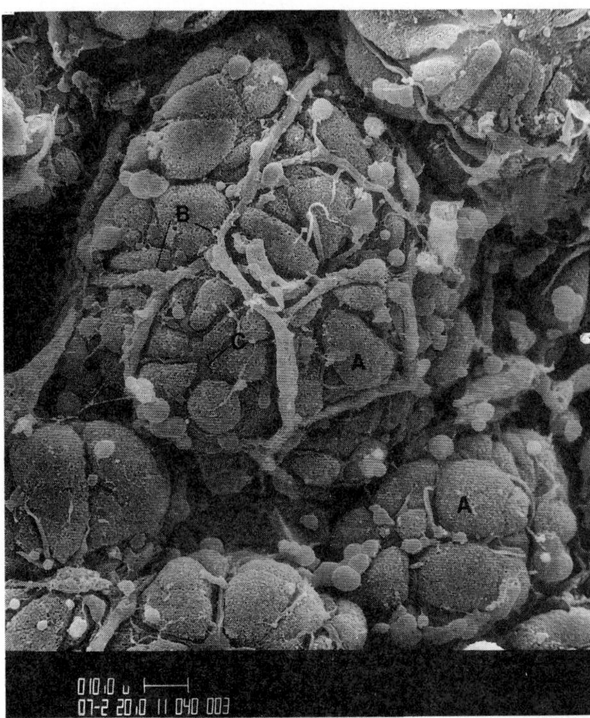

Figure 37.5. Scanning electron micrograph of lactating murine mammary tissue incubated in collagenase and hyaluronidase to digest extraneous tissues. An alveolus is shown with individual secretory cells (A), surrounded by an encircling blood vessel (B) and myoepithelial cells (C). (From Caruolo 1980, *J. Dairy Sci.* 63:1987–98.)

cranial vena cava. The valve structure in male and virgin female cattle, sheep, and goats is such that most of the blood caudal to the umbilical region is directed toward the udder. As the animal ages, the valves become ineffective and blood may flow either way. In the lactating animal an appreciable amount of blood is removed from the udder through the subcutaneous abdominal veins. In addition, a portion of blood is drained from the mammary glands by the perineal veins via the internal pudic veins. The relative amount of blood passing through this route compared with that returning to the heart via the external pudic veins depends in part on the position of the animal. When the animal is lying down, blood flow through one of the subcutaneous abdominal veins might easily be obstructed. A less common return route, which is not always present, is from the lateral surface of the udder to the medial surface of the thigh and through to the saphenous vein. Extensive anastomosing of veins within the udder allows for alternative venous routes in any particular region.

Blood supply differs according to mammary gland location. In the sow, for example, the caudal glands receive blood from the caudal aorta as described for the cow, and the cranial glands receive blood by way of the internal and external thoracic arteries.

The ratio of volume of blood circulating through the mammary gland to volume of milk produced has been the subject of many studies. In the dairy cow producing at a moderate level the ratio is about 670:1.

Lymph

Body fluids and solutes are continuously being exchanged between the blood plasma and the interstitial fluid, the lymph. Mammary glands have an extensive network of lymphatic vessels, which in the cow leave the udder by way of the supramammary lymph nodes. The efferent vessels from the supramammary lymph nodes pass through the inguinal canal to the external iliac (or deep inguinal) lymph nodes. By way of the lumbar trunks, lymph passes through the cisterna chyli and thoracic duct into the venous system near the origin of the cranial vena cava.

The flow of lymph from the mammary ducts is much greater in animals that are lactating than in those that are not. Lymph is moved by a pressure differential caused by breathing, the pressure in the blood capillaries, and the contraction of the muscles. When an excessive amount of lymph accumulates between the skin and the secretory tissue of the udder, edema develops. This is most serious in first-calf heifers and in older cows with pendulous udders at the time of parturition.

Nerve supply

The bovine udder is supplied with sensory (afferent) and motor (efferent) nerves. The afferent nerves consist of ventral branches of the first and second lumbar nerves; the inguinal nerve, consisting of ventral branches of the second, third, and fourth lumbar nerves; and the superficial perineal nerve, which is a branch of the pudic nerve (Fig. 37.6).

The ventral branches of the first and second lumbar nerves supply a small area of the cranial part of the udder, principally the skin. The inguinal nerve is located anterior to the external iliac blood vessels as they descend through the internal inguinal ring, where the inguinal nerve divides into cranial and caudal nerves. The cranial inguinal nerve innervates the fold of the flank and the cranial part of the forequarter and foreteat (including the apex). The cranial branch of the caudal inguinal nerve (or branches) supplies the skin of the lateral part of the forequarter and the caudal portion of the foreteat and, to a lesser degree, the glandular tissue. The caudal branch of the caudal inguinal nerve innervates the lymph node area, the glandular tissue of the rear quarter, and the caudal part of the forequarter, the rear teat, and the skin of the rear quarter except the caudal portion above the base of the teat. The skin of the caudal part of the udder above the teat is innervated by the superficial perineal nerve. These afferent nerves are significant in the milk-ejection process; however, neither secretion nor ejection of milk in the bovine requires efferent nerve fibers.

The efferent fibers of the bovine udder originate from the lumbar sympathetic plexus, pass through the inguinal can-

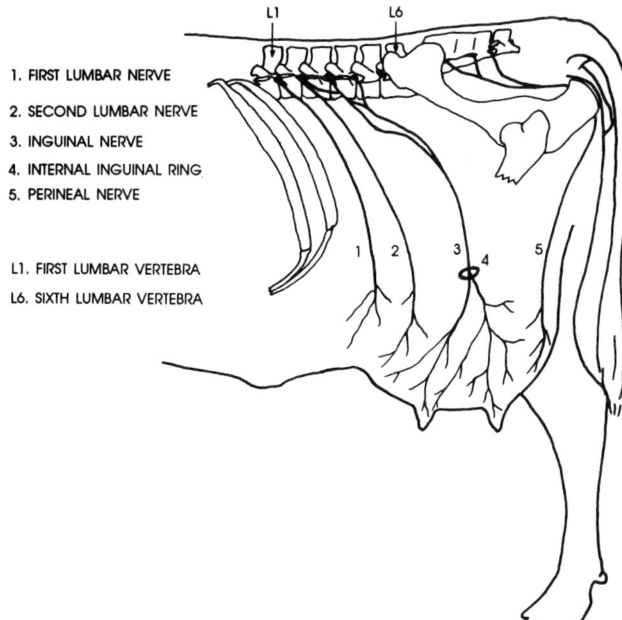

Figure 37.6. Innervation of the udder. (Drawn by C.B. Choi.)

al, and induce vasoconstriction. The mammary gland apparently is not innervated by parasympathetic fibers, which would be expected because of its cutaneous origin. The nerves of the mammary gland are located in connective tissue and are not in direct contact with the alveolar cells. Moreover, they apparently have no direct effect on rate of milk secretion or on milk composition.

MAMMARY GROWTH, DIFFERENTIATION, AND LACTATION

Milk secretion involves both intracellular synthesis of milk and subsequent passage of milk from the cytoplasm of the epithelial cells into the alveolar lumen. Milk removal includes the passive withdrawal of milk from the cisterns and the active ejection of milk from the alveolar lumina. *Lactation* refers to the combined processes of milk secretion and removal. *Mammogenesis* describes the development of the mammary gland; *lactogenesis* is the initiation of milk secretion; and *galactopoiesis* is used in a general sense to refer to the maintenance of milk secretion and/or the enhancement of established lactation.

Hormones regulate normal growth, development, and differentiation of the mammary gland and subsequent lactation. The endocrine glands most intimately associated with mammary function are the pituitary, hypothalamus, ovaries, and placenta, but other glands indirectly influence lactation (Table 37.1, also see Chap. 34).

Mammogenesis

At peak development during lactation the mammary gland consists of ductular and secretory alveolar epithelial cells (parenchyma) embraced in a heterogeneous matrix of cells, including myoepithelial cells, adipocytes, and fibroblasts. These latter three cell types make up the stroma. In addition, leukocytes, cells associated with the vascular system, and neurons are found in the mammary gland. Mammary growth is the major determinant of bovine milk yield capacity; the number of mammary alveolar cells directly influences milk yield. Estimates of the correlation between milk yield and mammary alveolar epithelial cell numbers range between 0.50 and 0.85. Conversely, increased proportions of fibroblasts and adipocytes in the

Table 37.1. Major hormones affecting mammary function

Endocrine gland	Hormone secreted	Major function associated with mammary gland
Anterior pituitary	Follicle-stimulating hormone (FSH)	Estrogen secretion from ovarian follicles
	Luteinizing hormone (LH)	Progesterone secretion from corpus luteum
	Prolactin (PRL)	Mammary growth; initiation and maintenance of lactation
	Growth hormone (GH)	Stimulates milk production
	Thyroid-stimulating hormone (TSH)	Stimulates thyroid gland to secrete thyroxine, triiodothyronine
	Adrenocorticotropic hormone (ACTH)	Stimulates adrenal gland to secrete glucocorticoids
Posterior pituitary	Oxytocin	Milk ejection
Hypothalamus	Growth hormone-releasing hormone	Stimulates GH release
	Somatostatin	Inhibits GH release
	Thyrotropin-releasing hormone (TRH)	Stimulates TSH (also prolactin and GH) release
	Corticotropin-releasing factor	Stimulates ACTH release
	Prolactin-inhibiting factor (dopamine)	Inhibits prolactin release
Thyroid	Thyroxine; triiodothyronine	Stimulates oxygen consumption, protein synthesis, and milk yield
	Thyrocalcitonin	Calcium and phosphorus metabolism
Parathyroid	Parathyroid hormone	Calcium and phosphorus metabolism
Pancreas	Insulin	Glucose metabolism
Adrenal cortex	Glucocorticoids (cortisol, corticosterone)	Initiation and maintenance of lactation
	Mineralocorticoids (aldosterone)	Electrolyte and mineral metabolism
Adrenal medulla	Epinephrine and norepinephrine	Inhibition of milk ejection
Ovary	Estradiol	Mammary duct growth
	Progesterone	Mammary lobule-alveolar growth; inhibition of lactogenesis
Placenta	Estradiol	See ovary
	Progesterone (species dependent)	See ovary
	Placental lactogen	Mammary growth

Adapted from Tucker 1985, in Larson, ed., *Lactation,* Iowa University Press, Ames, Iowa.

mammary gland are associated with reduced milk yield in cows.

Growth of the mammary gland takes place during various reproductive epochs beginning prenatal to early lactation. Mammary development during fetal and prepubertal stages is not necessarily under hormonal control. During puberty, pregnancy, and nursing, however, growth and development are largely under the influence of hormonal changes. The bulk of mammary growth takes place during pregnancy, and then the mammary glands regress after peak lactation. This cycle repeats itself with each pregnancy and lactation.

Mammary development in the fetus

When the bovine embryo is about 35 days old, a mammary line forms from the stratum germinativum (in the malpighian layer) on either side of and parallel to the ventral midline. At approximately 60 days, the mammary bud sinks deeper into the dermis and the teat begins to form. Up to this point development in the male and female is similar, although teat development proceeds somewhat more slowly in the male. The proliferating ectoderm moves deeper into the mesenchyme, forming what is known as a primary sprout. At about 100 days, formation of canals begins at the proximal end of the sprout and proceeds gradually toward the distal end, eventually producing an opening to the exterior. Secondary sprouts develop from the proximal end of the primary sprout, and canalization begins at the end adjacent to the primary sprout. The cavity within the primary sprout eventually develops into the gland and teat cisterns, and the cavities in the secondary sprouts develop into the major ducts.

Mammary growth from birth to conception

At birth the bovine udder has distinct teat and gland cisterns, but the major ducts are developed to only a limited extent. The difference between male and female is relatively small. The vascular and lymphatic systems are organized essentially as they will be in the mature udder. Adipose and other connective tissues are also well organized. A large fatty pad makes up a large part of the udder. Development of the mammary glands in other species with some modifications proceeds in a similar manner. Mammary apparatus from birth to puberty undergoes relatively little development. Mammary growth rate is consistent with body growth rate (isometric growth) until onset of ovarian activity preceding puberty. Size increase is largely due to an increase in connective tissue and fat.

Beginning just before the first estrous cycle (puberty), bovine mammary parenchyma begins to grow at a rate faster than whole body growth. This growth rate is referred to as allometric growth. This rapid mammary growth continues for several estrous cycles and then returns to an isometric pattern until conception. Allometric growth begins again at conception and continues, in most species, after parturition for variable periods of time. During each recurring estrous cycle, the mammary gland is stimulated by estrogen from the ovary and prolactin and somatotropin from the adenohypophysis (anterior pituitary) gland. The growth mainly involves lengthening and branching of the ducts. In species that experience long estrous cycles with a functional luteal phase (cattle, goats, pigs, horses, and humans), progesterone is produced by the corpus luteum and is available to synergize with estrogen, prolactin, and somatotropin to stimulate growth and differentiation of mammary ducts into a lobuloalveolar system.

Mammary development after conception

Most mammary growth occurs during pregnancy. The rate of growth remains exponential throughout gestation. Increase in cell numbers continues into early lactation in most species, although the extent of lactational mammary growth varies from less than 10% in ruminants to as much as 50% in rats. After 3 to 4 months of gestation in cows, mammary ducts elongate further and alveoli form and begin to replace stroma (adipocytes) in the supramammary fat pad. Lobuloalveolar development is extensive by the end of the sixth month. In the sow, lobuloalveolar development is essentially completed by midpregnancy (second month).

Mammary epithelial cells complete differentiation during pregnancy. A marked increase in gene expression takes place during pregnancy with increasing concentrations of messenger ribonucleic acid (mRNA) and increasing rates of synthesis of milk components. Some milk constituents even appear in blood (alpha-lactalbumin and caseins) and spill over into urine (lactose). These events can be considered the onset of lactogenesis stage I (see "Lactogenesis" section), with the accumulation of precolostrum in the mammary gland. There is variation among species in the onset of this phase and, within a given species, initiation of the synthesis of different milk components is not necessarily coincidental.

Accelerated mammary growth during pregnancy is due most likely to increased and synchronous secretion of estrogen and progesterone. Achievement of growth in response to estrogen and progesterone requires coincidental secretion of prolactin and perhaps somatotropin. Placental lactogen secretion increases during pregnancy and probably stimulates substantial mammary growth (synergistic with estrogen and progesterone) in those species in which the hormone enters the maternal circulation.

Mammary involution

In most species, the cessation of suckling or milking rapidly brings about mammary involution, which is characterized by a decrease in number of mammary epithelial cells and also in secretory activity per cell. Lysosomal enzymes are released, and many epithelial cells are lysed. Myoepithelial cells remain in the gland during involution and maintain the structure of the remaining epithelial cells. The space previously occupied by the degenerating alveoli is replaced with adipose cells. The extent to which alveoli degenerate varies with species and is governed by the ability of estrous cycle hormones to maintain lobuloalveolar structures. If an animal enters the dry period (period of nonlactation) in advanced stages of pregnancy, the decrease in cell number is much less than if the animal enters the dry period in early stages of pregnancy. As many as 50 percent of the mammary epithelial cells may be carried over from one lactation to the next. This may explain why milk production of dairy cows is associated more closely with successive pregnancies than with age. Dry periods that are too short (i.e., less than 6 weeks) reduce the increase in mammary cell numbers that occur during early phases of the subsequent lactation of the dairy cows.

Nutrition

Nutritional status plays an important role in mammary development, differentiation, and subsequent lactation. Mammary growth that occurs during critical hormone-dependent stages of development, including prepubertal to late gestation periods, is sensitive to the plane of nutrition. Changes in feeding intensity (nutrient density) can alter the secretion of one or more hormones, such as somatotropin and corticoids, that regulate mammary growth and differentiation. In growing dairy heifers, either overfeeding or severely restricting nutrient intake inhibits normal development of the mammary gland, especially the degree of parenchymal cell proliferation. Although the extent of pubertal mammary development is relatively small, the interaction of hormones and nutritional status during this period of development is of great importance for continual and full development of the mammary gland during gestation. The nutritional status of dairy heifers, especially 2 to 3 months before parturition, is also critical to maximal mammary proliferation and subsequent lactational performance. After a period of diet restriction, an increase in nutrient density (both protein and energy) during the late stage of gestation results in an increase in mammary growth and milk yields in the bovine, the rat, and the pig.

Lactogenesis

Lactogenesis is a process of differentiation whereby the mammary alveolar cells acquire the ability to secrete milk; it is conveniently defined as a two-stage (I and II) mechanism. The first stage of lactogenesis consists of partial enzymatic and cytologic differentiation of the alveolar cells and coincides with limited milk secretion before parturition. The second stage begins with the copious secretion of all milk components shortly before parturition and extends throughout several days postpartum in most species.

The onset of copious milk secretion at parturition to meet the nutritional requirements of relatively well-developed neonates is a feature of lactation in all placental mammals. The two main theories to account for this phenomenon are (1) that there is an increased positive stimulus from lactogenic hormones, especially prolactin and glucocorticoids, and (2) that secretion is released from inhibition by progesterone. Many species will initiate substantial milk secretion during pregnancy in response to exogenous glucocorticoids. Exogenous prolactin is effective only in rabbits. Placental lactogen, a polypeptide hormone of placental origin, may be of importance in the lactogenic process of some species, although its role in bovine mammary function is not established. If prolactin secretion is blocked by the dopamine agonist bromocriptine, normal onset of lactogenesis (stage II) is prevented in rats, rabbits, and pigs. In ruminants prolactin inhibition at parturition delays, but does not totally prevent, lactogenesis stage II when milking is continued.

Withdrawal of progesterone triggers lactogenesis in the presence of prolactin and glucocorticoids. Progesterone inhibits prolactin stimulation of its own receptor and also inhibits many other actions of prolactin, including transcription, stabilization, and translation of mRNAs for milk proteins. Progesterone decreases the ability of prolactin to induce secretion of α-lactalbumin, an enzyme moiety of lactose synthase (formerly lactose synthetase). Moreover, progesterone significantly reduces the synergism between estrogen and prolactin. The progesterone block on lactogenesis is not, however, absolute. If it were absolute, then simultaneous pregnancy and lactation would be impossible.

Prepartum milking generally initiates lactation in pregnant animals. Transmission of neural impulses from the teat to the hypothalamus probably results in the release of prolactin and ACTH, which in turn induces mammary cell secretion. However, neural components of the milking stimulus are not required to stimulate lactogenesis because the alveoli will be distended with milk, even if milking is not permitted before or immediately after parturition.

Galactopoiesis

Maintenance of lactation requires maintenance of alveolar cell numbers, synthetic activity per cell, and efficacy of the milk-ejection reflex. After parturition, there is a marked increase in milk yield in cows, which reaches a maximum in 2 to 8 weeks and then gradually declines (lactation curve). During this decline the rate of mammary cell loss presumably exceeds the rate of cell division. This loss of secretory cells lowers milk yield as lactation advances. In some species such as cattle and horses, conception may occur during lactation. Early stages of gestation have little effect on milk production and mammary cell numbers, but milk yield and mammary cell number decrease after the fifth month of concurrent gestation compared with nonpregnant cows.

A hormonal complex controls lactation, but unless milk is removed frequently from the mammary gland, synthesis of milk will not persist despite an adequate hormonal status.

Conversely, maintenance of intense suckling or milking to provide adequate milk removal will not maintain lactation indefinitely. Oxytocin is required for milk removal, whereas several other hormones are essential for maintenance of intense milk synthesis and secretion. Although there are species variations, growth hormone, ACTH (or glucocorticoids), thyroid-stimulating hormone, insulin, and parathyroid hormone are required for maintenance of lactation. Thyroid hormones influence milk synthesis as well as the intensity and duration of milk secretion. Administration of parathyroid hormone stimulates milk yield and increases concentration of plasma calcium. Interaction between the parathyroid and vitamin D metabolites also is important for maintaining lactation. Insulin concentrations are negatively correlated with milk yield. In rodents at least, mammary uptake of insulin associated with uptake of glucose is maintained throughout and is essential for maintenance of lactation. ACTH plays a direct role in maintaining lactation by exerting its effects on maintenance of mammary cell numbers and metabolic activity.

Exogenous prolactin has very little galactopoietic effect in lactating cows, but it causes a slight increase in milk yield of goats in late lactation. Prolactin injection into lactating rabbits increases milk production and the concentration of lactose in milk. Large doses of ACTH or of adrenal glucocorticoids inhibit lactation in rats and ruminants. The galactopoietic effects of thyroprotein (iodinated casein) usually last only 2 to 4 months; however, no net benefit over the entire lactation results. The feeding of thyroprotein causes an increased need for nutrients, a loss of body weight, and increases in heart rate, respiration rate, and body temperature.

It has been known for many years that growth hormone has a dose-dependent effect on stimulation of milk yield in dairy cows. Growth hormone does not produce its effects by direct stimulation of the mammary gland in ruminants. Rather, growth hormone appears to exert its galactopoietic effect by partitioning available nutrients from body tissues and toward milk synthesis. Commercial exploitation of such an effect was not practical until the advent of recombinant deoxyribonucleic acid (DNA) procedures that have allowed the synthesis of bovine growth hormone (also called bovine somatotropin) economically in the laboratory. The increased milk yield from exogenous somatotropin (pituitary-derived or recombinantly derived) persists in lactating cows. Whether or not growth hormone will have long-term beneficial effects on milk production and efficiency is yet to be determined.

There is no evidence that nerves directly affect maintenance of secretory activity of the mammary alveolar epithelium. However, stimulation of the mammary afferent nerves via the hypothalamus causes a variety of hormonal responses. Feed intake and water consumption markedly affect rates of milk secretion, and both of these processes are regulated by the hypothalamus. The role of the nervous system in lactation associated with the milk-ejection reflex is discussed in the subsequent "Milk Removal" section. For example, if milking is stopped, milk synthesis stops, and the secretory cells of the udder are rapidly lost.

MILK SYNTHESIS AND SECRETION

Mammary gland metabolism

Metabolic change associated with lactation

A striking feature of metabolic adaptation related to the onset of lactation is the considerable increase in food and water intake accompanied by hypertrophy of the intestinal tract to allow for more rapid absorption of the nutrients. There is also hypertrophy of the mammary gland, liver, and heart. Numerous tissues are involved in absorbing and mobilizing nutrients to meet the metabolic requirements of lactation (Table 37.2). Peripheral tissue requirements are reduced to ensure adequate nutrient availability for milk synthesis. This metabolic balance between mammary gland and body nutrients is largely regulated by the central nervous system via hormones, neuropeptides, and neurotransmitters (see Chap. 36).

Epithelial cell structure and function

Lactating mammary epithelial cells are highly differentiated and easily discernible from nonlactating cells at the ultrastructural level (Fig. 37.7). Precursors from blood are taken into the cells through the basal and lateral membranes, and milk is discharged through the apical membrane into the lumen. Mammary epithelial cells are typical secretory cells that have a well-developed endoplasmic reticulum (ER) and Golgi apparatus. Export proteins, synthesized in the rough endoplasmic reticulum (RER), are modified in the Golgi apparatus, where most of the nonfat milk constituents are also added. Secretory vesicles originate in

Table 37.2. Partial list of metabolic adaptations associated with onset of lactation

Function	Metabolic change	Tissues involved
Milk synthesis	Increased use of nutrients	Mammary gland
Intake and digestion	Increased food and water consumption	Central nervous system
	Hypertrophy of digestive tract	All segments of digestive tract
	Increased capacity for nutrient absorption	
Lipid metabolism	Increased lipolysis	Adipose tissue
	Decreased lipogenesis	
Glucose metabolism	Increased gluconeogenesis, increased glycogenolysis	Liver
	Utilization of acetate for energy (ruminants)	Mammary gland
Protein metabolism	Mobilization of protein reserves	Muscle and other body tissues
Mineral metabolism	Increased absorption and mobilization of reserves	Gut, bone, kidney, liver
Water metabolism	Increased absorption and expansion of plasma volume	Gut, kidney, central nervous system

Adapted from Collier 1985, in Larson, ed., *Lactation,* Iowa University Press, Ames.

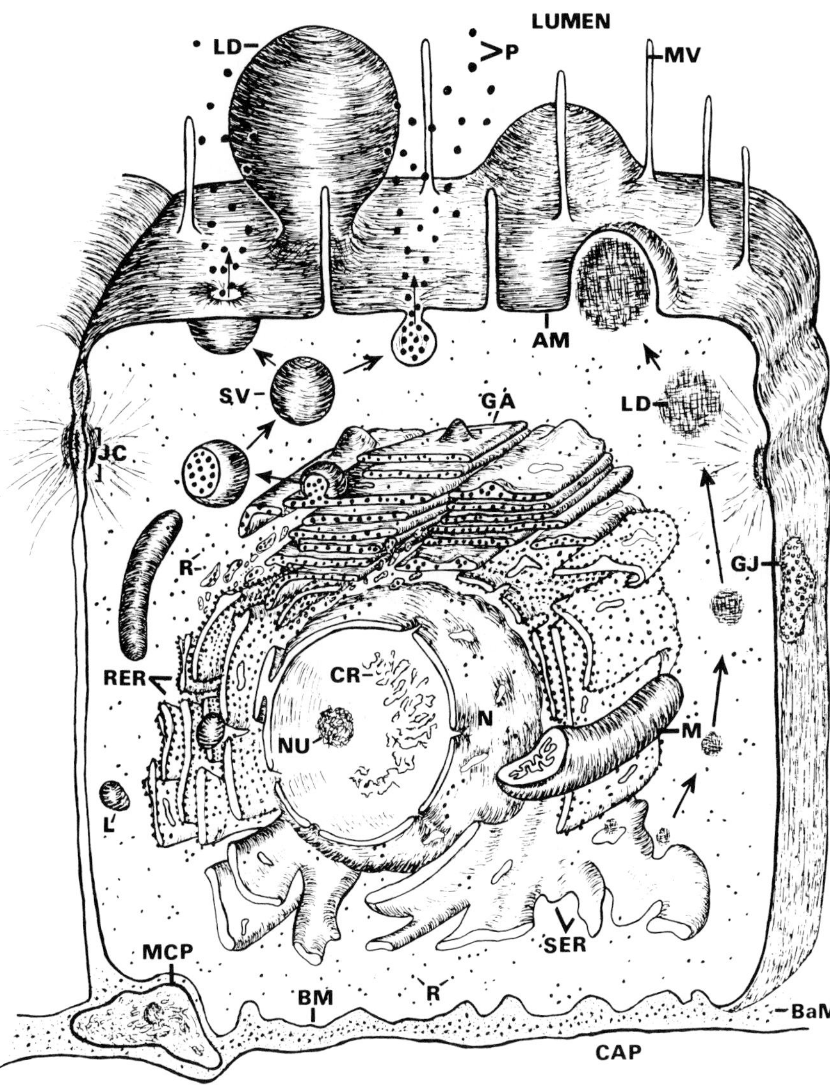

Figure 37.7. Diagrammatic representation of a secretory cell in the alveolar epithelium of the lactating mammary gland. AM, apical plasma membrane; BM, basal plasma membrane; BaM, basement membrane; CAP, capillary; CR, chromosomes; GA, Golgi apparatus; GJ, gap junction; JC, junctional complex; L, lysosome; LD, lipid droplet (globule); M, mitochondrion; MCP, myoepithelial cell process; MV, microvillus; N, nucleus; NU, nucleolus; P, protein (casein micelle); R, ribosomes (free and bound); RER, rough endoplasmic reticulum; SER, smooth endoplasmic reticulum; SV, secretory vesicle. Precursors from the bloodstream capillary (CAP) enter the cell and exit into the lumen as milk constituents. (From Larson 1985, in Larson, ed., *Lactation*, Iowa State University Press, Ames. Reprinted by permission © 1985 by Iowa State University Press, Ames, Iowa 50010.)

the Golgi apparatus to carry milk components to the surface of the cell. Glycolysis, fatty acid synthesis, and amino acid activation occur in the cytosol. Energy transfer from oxidizable substrates to adenosine triphosphate takes place in the mitochondria. Citrate and compounds used in nonessential amino acid synthesis are also synthesized in the mitochondria. Lysosomes contain hydrolytic enzymes and play a major role in cell destruction during involution at the end of lactation.

Energy metabolism

Glucose is the primary energy substrate in the nonruminant, whereas glucose (propionate) and acetate are the main energy sources in ruminant animals (Fig. 37.8, Chaps. 21 and 24). Because of their availability and high rate of uptake by the lactating mammary gland, acetate and, to a lesser extent, β-hydroxybutyric acid are considered the most important energy metabolites in mammary gland metabolism of ruminants. Two of the most significant functions of acetate are to supply carbon for de novo synthesis of fatty acids and to generate adenosine triphosphate through the tricarboxylic acid cycle and electron transport system. Glucose plays a central role in the metabolism of the mammary gland. Glucose can be used in one of three ways: (1) conversion to the galactose moiety of lactose; (2) formation of triose phosphate via the glycolytic pathway; and (3) conversion to 6-phosphogluconate via the pentose phosphate pathway. These pathways generate immediate precursors and cofactors for the synthesis of milk components (protein, fat, and lipid).

Blood glucose concentrations in cattle and sheep are lower (40 to 80 mg/dl) than blood glucose concentrations in

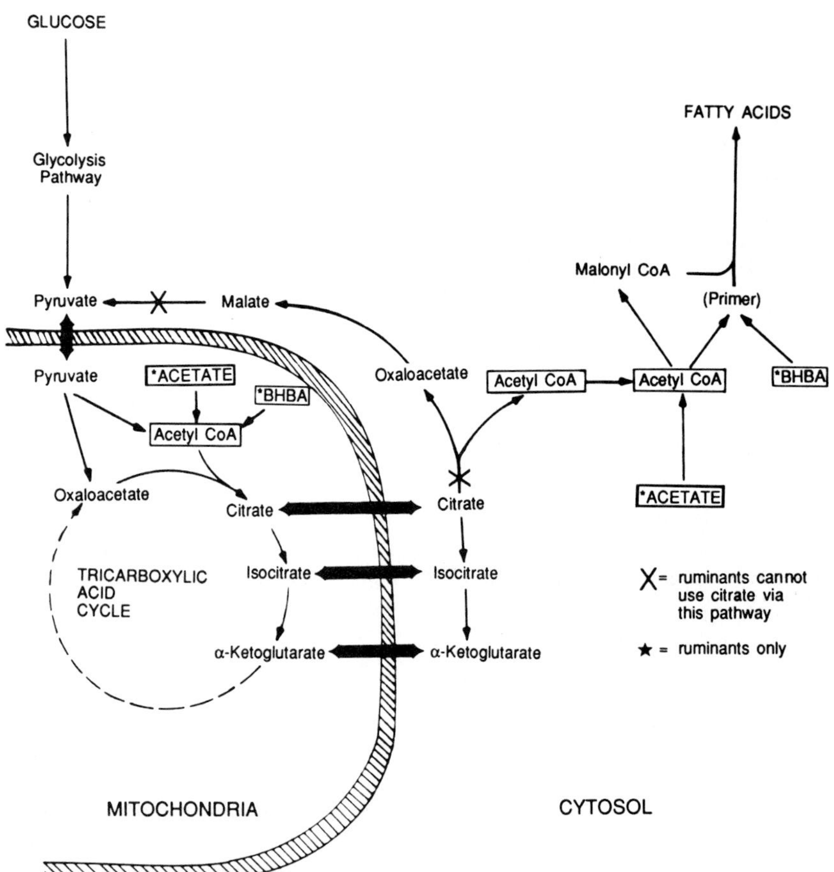

Figure 37.8. Energy and fatty acid metabolism in lactating mammary cells. (Redrawn from Bauman and Davis 1974, in Larson and Smith, eds., *Lactation: A Comprehensive Treatise*, Academic Press, New York.)

nonruminants (80 to 120 mg/dl). Because of low blood glucose levels and high availability of acetate for energy production, ruminants have developed glucose-sparing mechanisms in several tissues, most noticeably in the mammary gland, to prevent hypoglycemia under conditions of great metabolic demand, such as lactation. Glucose restriction ensures that glucose carbon is not used in synthetic and oxidative reactions where other substrates, such as acetate, could be used as effectively. The most noteworthy example of such restriction is the exclusion of glucose as a carbon source in fatty acid synthesis in ruminant tissue by a lack of the citrate cleavage enzyme essential for the generation of cytoplasmic acetyl-coenzyme A (CoA) from glucose in the nonruminants (Fig. 37.8).

Biosynthesis of milk components

Milk fat

Fats in bovine milk are characterized as mixed triglycerides with a large proportion of short-chain fatty acids (C_4–C_{16}). The fatty acids, glycerol, and other related intermediates are synthesized in the cytosol, and biosynthesis of triglycerols takes place in or near the endoplasmic reticulum of the mammary epithelial cells.

There are three major sources of fatty acids. The first, and one of prime importance in ruminants, is synthesis of fatty acids in the mammary gland from acetate and β-hydroxybutyric acid transported from the rumen. Acetate, via the malonyl CoA pathway, contributes to all short-chain (C_4–C_{14}) fatty acids and to a portion of the C_{16} acids in ruminants. The reduced nicotinamide adenine dinucleotide phosphate required for reductive steps is from the pentose phosphate pathway and the citric acid cycle (cytoplasmic isocitrate dehydrogenase). Ruminants cannot cycle acetyl CoA derived from glucose in the mitochondria, but glucose is a major source of acetyl CoA in nonruminants (Fig. 37.8). The second source of fatty acids is triglycerides present in circulating chylomicrons and low-density lipoproteins. These fatty acids, more than 14 carbons in length, are of either dietary or rumen microbial origin and are mainly C_{16} (palmitic) and C_{18} (stearic, oleic, and linoleic) acids. More than half of the fatty acids in cow's milk are derived directly from the blood; one-third are C_{16} acids, and most are C_{18} acids. The third source is cytoplasmic acetyl CoA from glucose through glycolysis and the citric acid cycle.

The primary source of glycerol for triglycerides in most

species is glycerol-3-phosphate, derived either from the glycolytic pathway or from the lipolysis of triglycerides during fatty acid uptake by the mammary gland. Two major pathways for the synthesis of triglycerides are known. The α-glycerol phosphate pathway, in which phosphatidic acids are formed, predominates in mammary tissue. On removal of the phosphate molecule from phosphatidic acid, a third long-chain acyl CoA molecule is attached to a 1, 2-diglyceride to form the triglyceride. The monoglyceride pathway, a second route, involves the formation of a 1, 2-diglyceride from the acylation of 2-monoglyceride.

Milk protein

The major milk proteins synthesized for export in bovine mammary epithelial cells are the casein proteins, (α_s-, β-, and κ-casein), β-lactoglobulin, and α-lactalbumin. The caseins constitute the greater part of bovine milk proteins with α_s-casein predominating. Proteins analogous to most of these are found in varying amounts in the milks of most species (see Table 37.4). Lactoferrin and lysosomal enzymes are quantitatively important proteins in milk. Immunoglobulins and blood serum albumin enter the mammary cell as preformed proteins from the blood.

Mechanisms of protein synthesis in the mammary gland appear to be comparable to those found in most other protein-synthesizing cells. Milk protein synthesis is controlled by hormonal regulation of gene transcription, the stability of mRNA, and the rate of mRNA translation. Milk proteins for export are synthesized from free amino acid according to predetermined plans encoded in the genes. Each cell has a complete genome in its nucleus. In the presence of DNA-dependent RNA polymerase and appropriate nucleotide precursors, DNA is transcribed to mRNA. The mRNA carries the encoded message from the nucleus to the cytoplasmic ribosomes located on RER, where the mRNA is translated into specific amino acid sequences of milk proteins. As with other secreted proteins, milk proteins are synthesized with an N-terminal sequence, which enables them to traverse the membrane of the ER. After synthesis in the RER, the proteins are transported to the Golgi complex, where posttranslational modifications of milk proteins, such as chain folding and phosphorylation of caseins, occur. Several genetic variants of the major milk proteins, derived from mutations, are known. The genetic polymorphs of milk proteins can serve as useful indices of an animal's history as well as of physical properties of the milk proteins from different animals.

Lactose

Lactose, a disaccharide composed of glucose and galactose, is the predominant carbohydrate found almost exclusively in milks and in the mammary glands of many species. Glucose is the only precursor of lactose. Two molecules of glucose must enter the mammary epithelial cell for each molecule of lactose formed. One glucose unit is converted to galactose. Lactose synthase catalyzes the reaction of glucose and galactose to form lactose in the Golgi apparatus. This enzyme is composed of two subunits: (1) galactosyl transferase, found both in mammary cells and in cells of other tissues, and (2) α-lactalbumin, a whey protein component of milk. Glucose is a poor acceptor of galactosyl residues, but in the presence of α-lactalbumin the galactosyl transferase is so altered that glucose becomes an effective acceptor for galactose at physiological glucose concentrations. Progesterone appears to repress the synthesis of α-lactalbumin during pregnancy. After the decline of plasma progesterone and enhanced secretion of prolactin at parturition, α-lactalbumin increases resulting in formation of active lactose synthase, thereby allowing the initiation of lactose synthesis. Thus α-lactalbumin may be the rate-limiting enzyme in the initiation of lactation.

Other components

Calcium, phosphorus, potassium, chloride, sodium, and magnesium are the primary minerals in milk. Although minerals in milk are derived from the blood, it is not known conclusively whether they are absorbed in proportion to their concentration in blood or whether there are mechanisms that allow selective uptake. There is evidence that the mammary epithelial cell can discharge minerals back into blood as well as into milk, which would suggest some type of active transport mechanism.

Lactose, sodium, and potassium concentrations are usually constant in milk. These components plus chloride maintain osmotic equilibrium in milk. Water moves into milk to maintain osmotic equilibrium with that of blood; consequently, the secretion of lactose, potassium, sodium, and chloride into milk determines the volume of milk produced.

Vitamins cannot be synthesized by the mammary gland. They are synthesized by bacteria in the rumen; converted from precursors in the liver, small intestine, and the skin; or derived directly from feed sources. Generally, the vitamin content of milk can be increased by increasing the vitamin concentration in the blood that supplies the mammary gland.

Secretion of Milk

Cellular secretion

Milk proteins synthesized in the RER move to the Golgi complex where phosphorylation of threonine and serine residues of casein as well as glycosylation of certain other milk proteins occur. Nonfat milk constituents (lactose, proteins, and salts) are then incorporated into Golgi vesicles. These secretory vesicles, containing essentially nonfat constituents, travel toward the apical surface of the mammary epithelial cells and fuse with the plasma membrane, where the vesicular contents are discharged into the lumen (exocytosis). Cytoplasmic lipid particles coalesce to form larger droplets as they migrate from the ER toward the apical membrane. These lipid droplets traverse to the membrane and bud off as globules encased in an envelope of apical plasma membrane. The movement of milk constituents occurs in a sequential manner in the mammary cell. It is believed that all of the membranes, starting with the nuclear envelope, ER, Golgi apparatus, secretory vesicles, and plasma membranes, are functionally connected. Basal and lateral membranes of the cell also are likely derived from Golgi vesicles. The role of microtubules in milk synthesis is not clear since inhibitors of microtubular function, such as colchicine, inhibit cellular secretion but not milk synthesis. However, microtubules are probably important in differentiation of the secretory cells during the second stage of lactogenesis.

The transport of blood immunoglobulins (Igs) into the lacteal secretion occurs by a specific mammary epithelial intracellular transport mechanism. Leukocytes cross the mammary barrier, either by passing between the epithelial cells through the tight junctional complex or by pushing a secretory cell out of the epithelial layer into the lumen. Tight junctions exist between epithelial cells of the alveoli. Some transport (transudation) of ions and lactose across leaky junctional complexes probably occurs after oxytocin injections and in late lactation. Increased concentrations of milk components in blood also are associated with increased migration of leukocytes into milk (i.e., increased milk somatic cell counts correlate with increased serum α-lactalbumin).

Regulation of mammary gene expression

The opportunity to study mammary tissue–specific and hormone-regulated milk protein gene expression has been enhanced by the recent development of recombinant DNA techniques. Emphasis has been placed on identification of control elements in mammary genes and use of them to target the expression of foreign genes in the mammary gland. Three basic strategies have been used to study the expression of milk protein genes on a molecular level. Cloned genes may be (1) transfected into mammary-derived cell lines, (2) analyzed in vitro, or (3) integrated into the germ line of transgenic animals. These studies indicate that the production of milk with enhanced nutritional value as well as large-scale synthesis of medically important proteins in transgenic lactating animals may be attainable.

PHYSIOLOGY OF MILKING

Milk secretion rate

Milk secretion is a continuous process, although its secretion rate is not constant. Moreover, the mammary gland is freed of its accumulated secretion only periodically. This unique physiology indicates that secretions already produced may influence further secretory processes. The capacity of the mammary gland to store and secrete milk determines the rate of milk secretion and the productivity of the mammary gland.

Milk-secretion rate depends in part on the pressure that accumulates within the mammary gland and, perhaps more important, on feedback regulation by specific milk components. Low intra-alveolar pressure and reduced negative feedback characteristic of the period immediately after milking or nursing probably facilitate the transport of newly synthesized milk into the alveolar lumen. As secretion continues between milkings, pressure increases and concentration of milk components increases. The buildup of newly synthesized milk inhibits the uptake of milk precursors by chemical feedback mechanisms, physical factors, or both. Physical factors are a result of the distended alveoli partially displacing all other intramammary compartments, including the blood vessels. The intramammary pressure in a dairy cow's udder before milking ranges between 0 and 8 mm Hg. Washing the udder, which stimulates milk letdown (see "Milk-Ejection Reflex" section), results in markedly higher intramammary pressure (35 to 55 mm Hg). The increased pressure resulting from milk letdown slowly declines, even if no milk is removed from the gland. Within approximately 1 hour after the last milking, the udder pressure rapidly increases to about 8 mm Hg; this increase is believed to be caused by the residual (or complementary) milk that is left in the udder after a normal milking. Thereafter, a gradual increase in pressure is experienced and is followed by an accelerated pressure increase that represents overfilling of alveoli, ducts, and gland cistern.

Frequent removal of milk is conducive to increased milk-secretion rates and decreased intramammary pressures. An inverse relationship between milk secretion rate and udder pressure has been recognized. Moreover, there is evidence that increased frequency of milking enhances milk yield and reduces loss of mammary secretory cells, which are under local control (i.e., autocrine mechanisms) within the mammary gland. The possibility also exists that specific components in milk may act within the mammary cell to inhibit their own secretion independent of intramammary pressure. For instance, elevated intramammary pressure does not appear to inhibit milk fat synthesis to the extent that it inhibits the synthesis of other milk components. Nonetheless, these mechanisms serve to adjust rate of milk secretion to rate of milk removal by nursing offspring.

Milk removal

Milk-ejection reflex

The removal of milk from the mammary gland of most species is dependent on a neurohormonal reflex that results in milk ejection. This process involves activation of neural receptors in the skin of the teat. Mechanical stimulation of the teats, such as milking or suckling, initiates the neural reflex, which travels from the teats to the spinal cord, to the paraventricular and supraoptic nuclei of the hypothalamus, and then to the neurohypophysis (posterior pituitary) gland, where oxytocin is discharged into the blood. It is also apparent that oxytocin release can be induced by higher brain centers via conditioned responses (e.g., a mother's milk letdown in response to the cry of her infant) or external stimuli (e.g., audiovisual and olfactory cues). Oxytocin binds to receptors on and thereby causes contraction of the myoepithelial cells, thus completing the circuit and evoking ejection (letdown) of milk. The number of oxytocin receptors on the myoepithelial cells reaches a maximum during the first lactation and then probably persists for the lifetime of the myoepithelial cell.

The milk-ejection reflex is inhibited by various stressful stimuli (pain, fright, and emotional disturbances). Stress increases discharge of epinephrine and norepinephrine. These catecholamines then cause contraction of smooth muscles, thereby partially occluding the mammary ducts and blood vessels, preventing oxytocin from reaching the myoepithelial cells. Epinephrine can also block oxytocin binding to the myoepithelial cells. The most common cause of failure of milk ejection, seen particularly in primiparous cows, is associated with the stress of milking during the early postpartum period. Reactions to stress may also prevent milk ejection by blocking release of oxytocin.

Mechanical milking

Pulsation rate (number of cycles of alternating negative and atmospheric pressure), pulsation ratio, vacuum level, and cluster weight affect the rate of peak milk flow or stripping milk yield. Pulsation ratio is the ratio of time that a vacuum is applied to the pulsation chamber to the time atmospheric air is admitted to the chamber. Each interacts with the other, such that there is no equation to describe the ideal combination. Recommended settings for milking equipment should be pulsation rates of 50 to 80 cycles per minute, favoring the lower of these rates; pulsation ratios of 50:50 to 70:30; vacuum levels of 43 to 50 kPa, depending on the amount and distance milk must be lifted; and cluster weights of 1.4 to 3.6 kg. Vacuum level should be adequate to prevent cluster falloff but low enough to allow milking at a reasonable speed without injury to teat ends and internal teat walls. Air slips and machine stripping should be minimized. Teat dipping with an approved product after milking should be practiced to prevent intramammary infections.

BIOLOGICAL FUNCTION OF MILK

Nutritive value and colostrum

Milk is essential for the growth and development of young mammals. Milk provides energy in the form of lactose and fat and amino acids in the form of protein. It is also a source of antibodies, vitamins, and minerals. Because of wide variation in composition, it is difficult to discern the relationship between milk composition and nutritive requirements of the young. In general, species that nurse their young on demand tend to furnish milk of lower solids and caloric content than those that nurse at scheduled intervals.

Milk of cows can serve as the sole or major component in the diet of human infants. In comparison with human milk, bovine milk contains more calcium, phosphorus, thiamine, riboflavin, and protein but less carbohydrate. Lactose promotes absorption of calcium from the gut and may reduce the incidence of diarrhea in the newborn. Lactose intolerance in humans is not uncommon, however.

Table 37.3. Composition of bovine colostrum and normal whole milk

Constituent	Colostrum (%)	Whole milk (%)
Total solids	23.9	12.9
Lactose	2.7	5.0
Fat	6.7	4.0
Protein	14.3	3.2
Casein	5.2	2.6
Albumin	1.5	.47
Immunoglobulin	6.0	.09
Ash	1.1	.7
Vitamin A (ng/dl)	295.0	34.0
Specific gravity (g/ml)	1.056	1.032

Modified from Roy 1969, in Cuthbertson, ed., *Nutrition of Animals of Agricultural Importance,* Part 2, Pergamon, Oxford; Parrish, Wise, Hughes, and Atkenson 1950, *J. Dairy Sci.* 33:457.

Colostrum, which is formed in the mammary glands before parturition, is the first milk secreted after parturition. Colostrum is of primary significance to the neonate. It is highly nutritious and in some species contains components essential for survival during the neonatal period. High levels of vitamin A are important in correcting the low vitamin A reserves common in newborn calves and pigs. Total solids, protein, and ash are considerably greater in colostrum than in normal milk (Table 37.3). Lactose content, however, is much lower. The remarkably high protein content in colostrum is due largely to an increase in casein and globulin, especially immunoglobulins. The predominant immunoglobulin in bovine colostrum is IgG. On ingestion, IgG imparts systemic immunity to the neonate. This is especially important for neonates of domestic species (cow, sheep, pig), since these species have epitheliochorial placentas, which do not allow transfer of Ig from the maternal to the fetal systems. In the human and rabbit, IgG is transported across the placenta to the developing embryo; therefore, in these species, Ig concentration in colostrum is much lower and is composed chiefly of IgA and IgM. Transfer of Ig in dogs, cats, and rodents occurs via both routes.

Species variation

Gross milk composition of 30 species, including at least one species of each of 17 orders, is given in Table 37.4. Composition varies greatly among species: protein varies from less than 1 to 14 percent, fat from a trace to more than 50 percent, lactose from a trace to 7 percent, mineral (as ash) from 0.2 to 2 percent, and calculated energy from 40 to 330 kcal/100 g. In general, milk of marine mammals has a high fat and, therefore, high energy content. Many rapidly growing species, such as rabbit and rat, have a high protein content, although the relationship between rate of attainment of maturity and level of protein is not consistent. The marked differences and the multitudes of nutritive compo-

Table 37.4. Composition of milks of various animals

Animal	Genus and species	Percentage by weight							Energy (kcal/100 g)
				Protein					
		Water	Fat	Casein	Whey	Total	Lactose	Ash	
Aardvark	*Orycteropus afer*	68.5	12.1	9.5	4.8	14.3	4.6	1.4	184
Bat, fringed	*Myotis thysanodes*	59.5	17.9	ND*	ND*	12.1	3.4	1.6	223
Bear, black	*Ursus americanus*	55.5	24.5	8.8	5.7	14.5	0.4	1.8	280
Buffalo, water	*Bubalis bubalis*	82.8	7.4	3.2	0.6	3.8	4.8	0.8	101
Camel	*Camelus dromedarius*	86.5	4.0	2.7	0.9	3.6	5.0	0.8	70
Cow	*Bos taurus*	87.3	3.9	2.6	0.6	3.2	4.6	0.7	66
Dog	*Canis familiaris*	76.4	10.7	5.1	2.3	7.4	3.3	1.2	139
Dolphin	*Tursiops truncatus*	58.3	33.0	3.9	2.9	6.8	1.1	0.7	329
Donkey	*Equus asinus*	88.3	1.4	1.0	1.0	2.0	7.4	0.5	44
Echidna	*Tachyglossus aculeatus*	ND*	19.6	8.4	2.9	11.3	2.8	0.8	233
Elephant, Indian	*Elephas maximus*	78.1	11.6	1.9	3.0	4.9	4.7	0.7	143
Goat	*Capra hircus*	86.7	4.5	2.6	0.6	3.2	4.3	0.8	70
Guinea pig	*Cavia porcellus*	83.6	3.9	6.6	1.5	8.1	3.0	0.8	80
Hedgehog	*Erinaceus europaeus*	79.4	10.1	ND*	ND*	7.2	2.0	2.3	100
Horse	*Equus caballus*	88.8	1.9	1.3	1.2	2.5	6.2	0.5	52
Human	*Homo sapiens*	87.1	4.5	0.4	0.5	0.9	7.1	0.2	72
Kangaroo, red	*Macropus rufus*	80.0	3.4	2.3	2.3	4.6	6.7	1.4	76
Manatee	*Trichechus manatus*	87.0	6.9	ND*	ND*	6.3	0.3	1.0	88
Opossum	*Didelphis virginiana*	76.8	11.3	ND*	ND*	8.4	1.6	1.7	142
Pig	*Sus scrofa*	81.2	6.8	2.8	2.0	4.8	5.5	1.0	102
Rabbit	*Oryctolagus cuniculus*	67.2	15.3	9.3	4.6	13.9	2.1	1.8	202
Rat	*Rattus norvegicus*	79.0	10.3	6.4	2.0	8.4	2.6	1.3	137
Reindeer	*Rangifer tarandus*	66.7	18.0	8.6	1.5	10.1	2.8	1.5	214
Seal, fur	*Callorhinus ursinus*	34.6	53.3	4.6	4.3	8.9	0.1	0.5	516
Sheep	*Ovis aries*	82.0	7.2	3.9	0.7	4.6	4.8	0.9	102
Shrew, tree	*Tupaia belangeri*	59.6	25.6	ND*	ND*	10.4	1.5	ND*	278
Sloth	*Bradypus variegatus*	83.1	2.7	ND*	ND*	6.5	2.8	0.9	62
Squirrel, gray	*Sciurus carolinensis*	60.4	24.7	5.0	2.4	7.4	3.7	1.0	267
Yak	*Bos grunniens*	82.7	6.5	ND*	ND*	5.8	4.6	0.9	100
Zebu	*Bos indicus*	86.5	4.7	2.6	0.6	3.2	4.7	0.7	74

*ND, not determined.
Modified from Jenness 1986, *J. Dairy Sci.* 69:869–85.

nents of milk of various species perhaps result from processes of selection and breeding. The ability of caseins to form micelles carrying large amounts of casein and phosphate appears to constitute a distinct selective advantage, especially for species whose young grow rapidly. There are major differences in milk composition, even among and within breeds of cattle; these differences can be accentuated by genetic selection.

Lactation is the final phase of reproduction and is essential for breeding success. Lactation plays a variable role in the overall reproductive strategies, which include wide ranges in litter size, growth rate, length of gestation, length of lactation, and kind and extent of parental care provided to the young. The fraction of total growth supplied by milk and the state of development during which milk contributes to growth vary greatly. This contribution to total growth is minimal in such species as guinea pigs but very high in some marsupials and primates. Although the overall daily capacity for energy transfer via milk is rather constant in many species (125 kcal/$kg^{0.75}$ body weight), the nutritive composition of milk differs greatly among species and may vary during lactation. The lactation capacity of a species involves an interaction of several factors: physiological status and growth rate of the nursling, genetic pattern, environmental stress, nursing habits, and availability of food and water to the mother.

FACTORS AFFECTING LACTATION

Nutritional, physiological, and environmental factors

Essential nutrients required for optimum growth and lactation are carbohydrates (as the primary energy source), lipids, protein, minerals, vitamins, and water. The nutrient requirements of domestic animals, including needs during lactation, have been studied and summarized in a series of publications by the National Research Council. Although all nutrients are of immense importance, energy is considered the most limiting factor because it is necessary for proper metabolism of all remaining nutrients. In lactation, energy is important from the standpoint of timing as well as amount. Inadequate energy at the beginning of lactation, when demands are greatest, will decrease milk production to a far greater extent than inadequate energy in the latter part of lactation. Cows at peak lactation are in negative energy balance, which is desirable from the standpoint of efficient milk production because body fat reserves are used to meet energy requirements.

Alteration of protein intake has a slight effect on the milk composition, especially milk protein, although a drastic reduction in protein intake will lower the milk yield significantly. Increasing protein content of the diet of the lactating cow above the National Research Council requirements (varying from 15 to 19 percent in the diet dry matter, depending on the level of milk production) has no effect on yield and causes only a slight increase in the nonprotein nitrogen content of the milk.

Milk fat content, strongly influenced by heredity in the cow, is by far the most variable constituent of milk. Diets can also influence composition and yield of milk fat. In general, diets that result in a low ruminal acetate/propionate ratio (high concentrate diets) lead to decreased milk fat synthesis, occasionally accompanied by a modest increase in milk protein. Fat in the diet of the cow has relatively little effect on the fat content of the milk. Inclusion of minimum concentrations of fiber (19 percent as acid detergent fiber) in diets of lactating cattle is essential for optimum rumen fermentation to maintain the fat level in milk. Milk fats of ruminants are highly saturated because of extensive hydrogenation of dietary unsaturated fatty acids in the rumen. For an increase in the polyunsaturated fatty acid content of milk fat, unsaturated fatty acids (vegetable oils) have been treated and fed to cows in ways that prevent hydrogenation by the ruminal bacteria.

Stage of lactation also influences the composition and yield of milk. At parturition milk production commences at a relatively high rate, and the amount secreted continues to increase for about 4 to 8 weeks in cows. After the peak is attained, milk production gradually declines. The rate of decline is commonly referred to as persistency. Fat, protein, and lactose contents in milk tend to rise slightly as lactation progresses.

Pregnancy reduces the milk yield of the cow; by the eighth month of gestation, milk yield may be reduced by 20 percent. The recommended ideal dry period for cows is 6 to 8 weeks. Either shorter or longer dry periods will reduce subsequent milk production. Milk yield increases at a decreasing rate until about the eighth year of age, depending on the breed of cattle, and then decreases at an increasing rate. In general, larger cows produce more milk than smaller ones, but milk yield does not vary in direct proportion to body weight. Rather, it varies approximately by the metabolic body size (kg$^{0.75}$ of body weight).

Milking twice daily yields at least 40 percent more milk than milking once daily; milking three times a day may yield a 5 to 20 percent increase over twice-a-day milking; and milking four times a day may yield an additional 5 to 10 percent. Thus, the response to more frequent milking diminishes with increasing frequency. Physiological factors that contribute to increased production with frequent milking are (1) less intramammary pressure, (2) increased stimulation by hormones (e.g., prolactin), and (3) less negative feedback on the cellular synthesis as a result of buildup of milk components.

Animals exposed to environmental stress will undergo metabolic adaptations to alleviate the effects of stress. These include alterations in basal metabolism, acid-base balance, water and electrolyte metabolism, change in rumen fermentation, and endocrine function. The environmental temperature directly alters both milk yield and composition by affecting basal metabolism, food intake, rate of passage of digesta, and nutrient requirements for maintenance (Fig. 37.9). However, this effect is strongly dependent on the species of the animal. Tropical cattle (*Bos indicus*) tolerate heat much better than *Bos taurus*, although

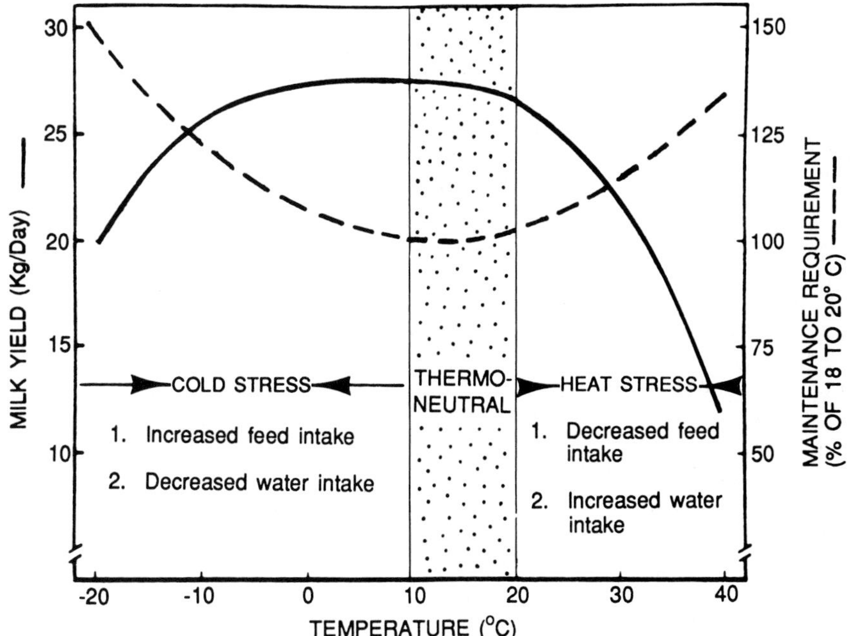

Figure 37.9. Effect of ambient temperature on maintenance requirements and milk yield in 600 kg cattle. (Slightly modified from Collier 1985, in Larson, ed., *Lactation*, Iowa State University Press, Ames. Reprinted by permission © 1985 by Iowa State University Press, Ames, Iowa 50010.)

milk yields from tropical species typically are lower. Holsteins and larger breeds are somewhat more tolerant of lower temperatures, whereas smaller breeds, especially the jersey, are more tolerant of higher temperatures. Within a relative humidity range of 60 to 80 percent, milk yield is unaffected by temperature changes between 10° and 20° C. This temperature range is referred to as the thermoneutral zone. An animal exposed to this temperature can maintain constant body temperature without changing its basal metabolism. Heat stress reduces feed intake and increases water intake, causing a rapid decline in milk yield as maintenance requirements increase and nutrient intake decreases. Above 40° C, feed consumption and milk production decline (Fig. 37.9). Cold stress increases feed intake, which prevents a decline in milk yield until temperatures go below −5° C. Decrease in milk yield during cold stress is due primarily to increased body-maintenance requirements.

There also are pronounced seasonal variations in bovine milk composition. Milk fat, total solids and protein, and solids-not-fat are greatest during the cold months. Fat and protein are generally less during hot months. These variations are compounded in part by seasonal changes in forage type and availability.

Mastitis and metabolic disturbances

Mastitis

Mastitis is an inflammatory reaction of the mammary gland to bacterial, chemical, thermal, or mechanical injury. Inflammation is characterized by gross swelling, heat, redness, pain, and disturbed function and will result in a decrease in milk production and a change in milk composition.

It is estimated that 5 to 10 percent of all cows produce abnormal milk at any given time, and 40 percent of the cows in the United States are infected with pathogenic bacteria in two or more quarters. The most common mastitis-causing pathogens are staphylococci and streptococci, although coliforms may be acutely important as causative agents in some herds. Yeasts such as *Candida albicans* may also cause severe and chronic mastitis.

The mammary gland is protected by a complex system of primary and secondary defense mechanisms. The primary defense mechanisms are those that prevent entry of pathogens into the mammary gland and are associated with the streak canal. The secondary defense mechanisms include chemical, cellular, and immunological components located within the mammary gland. Most screening tests for inflammation measure the number of leukocytes and mammary cell numbers in milk. The most common cow-side tests for leukocyte numbers present in milk are the strip cup and the California mastitis test. Other tests, such as the Wisconsin mastitis test or somatic (mammary epithelial) cell count, are usually conducted in a laboratory.

Many factors predispose an animal to an invading organism or allow a preexisting low-grade infection to become more active. Prevention is the key in development of mastitis-control programs. A control program should emphasize those managerial and environmental factors that affect susceptibility to mastitis.

Metabolic disturbances

In dairy cows metabolic disturbances such as milk fever, ketosis, grass tetany, udder edema, fat cow syndrome, and retained placenta may be directly or indirectly related to nutrition. Most of these disorders occur at or shortly after parturition and represent a failure of the cow to adjust to the rapid onset and stress of high milk production.

Milk fever (parturient paresis) is one of the most common disorders associated with lactation in dairy cows. It occurs at or soon after parturition and the beginning of lactation. It is characterized by a generalized paresis, circulatory collapse, and a gradual loss of consciousness. When the disease is not treated, death often results. Blood calcium and inorganic phosphorus levels drop sharply. In most cases prompt recovery will follow after the administration of calcium into the blood (e.g., infusion of calcium borogluconate). However, relapses requiring repeat treatment are rather common. This syndrome seldom occurs at first parturition and is most common in high-producing animals. Limiting calcium intake during the dry period (late gestation) but increasing it at calving time reduces the incidence of milk fever. Other preventive practices include incomplete milking during the first 3 days after calving and administration of vitamin D 3 to 5 days before calving.

Fat cow syndrome is the presence of excessive obesity in the dry cow. The syndrome is characterized by inappetence, reduced milk yield, and extensive loss of body condition. The extent of organ (especially liver) fat deposition is determined by various predisposing factors, such as the presence of certain diseases or stressful complications during calving, which lead to tissue mobilization. The incidence may be reduced by avoidance of the overconditioning of cows during late lactation and dry period and by formulation of diets that maximize feed intake after calving.

Grass tetany, a magnesium-deficiency disease that is aggravated by high levels of milk production, is discussed in Chapter 29. *Ketosis*, a metabolic disease associated with lactation in dairy cows as well as with pregnancy in ewes, is discussed in Chapter 27.

REFERENCES

Bauman, D.E., and Davis, C.L. 1974. Biosynthesis of milk fat. In B.L. Larson and V.R. Smith, eds., *Lactation: A Comprehensive Treatise*, vol. II. Academic Press, New York. Pp. 31–75.

Caruolo, E.V. 1980. Scanning electron microscope visualization of the mammary gland secretory unit and of myoepithelial cells. *J. Dairy Sci.* 63:1987–98.

Collier, R.J. 1985. Nutritional, metabolic, and environmental aspects of lactation. In B.L. Larson, ed., *Lactation*. Iowa State University Press, Ames. Pp. 80–128.

Jenness, R. 1986. Lactational performance of various mammalian species. *J. Dairy Sci.* 69:869–85.

Larson, B.L. 1985. Biosynthesis and cellular secretion of milk. In B.L. Larson, ed., *Lactation*. Iowa State University Press, Ames. Pp. 129–63.

Parrish, D.B., Wise, G.H., Hughes, J.S., and Atkeson, F.W. 1950. Properties of the colostrum of dairy cow. V. Yield, specific gravity and concentrations of total solids and its various components of colostrum and early milk. *J. Dairy Sci*. 33:457–65.

Roy, J.H. 1969. The nutrition of dairy calf. In D. Cuthbertson, ed., *Nutrition of Animals of Agricultural Importance*. Pergamon Press, New York. Part 2.

Schmidt, G.H. 1971. *Biology of Lactation*. W.H. Freeman & Company, San Francisco. P. 11.

Smith, V.R. 1959. *Physiology of Lactation*, 5th ed. Iowa State University Press, Ames.

Tucker, H.A. 1985. Endocrine and neural control of the mammary gland. In B.L. Larson, ed., *Lactation*. Iowa State University Press, Ames. Pp. 39–79.

CHAPTER 38

Avian Reproduction | by William H. Burke

This chapter will deal primarily with the domestic chicken (*Gallus domesticus*) and to a lesser degree with the domestic turkey (*Meleagris gallopavo*). Because of their economic importance, these two species have been subjected to heavy selection for increased reproductive potential. The Japanese quail (*Coturnix coturnix japonica*) has been domesticated and used for egg production in Japan and other Asian countries. It begins to lay at the age of 6 to 8 weeks, is very responsive to photoperiod manipulation, amenable to experimental manipulation, and is inexpensive to maintain. It has been widely used in research in avian reproduction and endocrinology with the often unstated assumption that it represents a "model" animal and that studies with it are applicable to chickens and turkeys. Therefore frequent mention will be made of it in this chapter. It should be kept in mind that the reproductive characteristics of these species do not reflect the wide variety of reproductive habits of the thousands of wild avian species adapted to diverse environments. Many of the anatomical and physiological characteristics described here are found to greater or lesser degrees in many wild birds, but details of reproductive characteristics vary greatly among species. In most cases, the offspring of poultry are quite mature and precocial when hatched, whereas the young of most birds hatch in a very immature state. Most species of poultry are polygamous, whereas the vast majority of wild birds are monogamous. These very differences may explain why domestic poultry were amenable to domestication.

Reproduction in birds is characterized by ovoviviparity. In this mode of reproduction the potential offspring leaves the mother's body after a very short period of embryonic development and undergoes the major portion of its development outside her body. Although this mode of reproduction is found in several mammals and many reptiles, it is found universally in birds. To meet the needs imposed by ovoviviparity, the avian egg, at the time it is laid, must be able to support embryonic and fetal growth. It contains nutrient materials in the yolk, albumin, and shell. It contains water and protective membranes, and it is surrounded by a protective shell. At the time a fertilized egg is laid, the embryo has already developed to the gastrula stage.

Table 38.1. Reproductive hormones, their site of origin, their actions, and their regulation in poultry

Hormones	Site of origin	Action	Regulation
Luteinizing hormone	Anterior pituitary	Induces ovulation, stimulates steriodogenesis	Hypothalamic GnRH
Follicle-stimulating hormone	Anterior pituitary	Stimulates sertoli cell development in males; stimulates ovarian function but precise role is unclear	Hypothalamic GnRH
Prolactin	Anterior pituitary	Induces incubation and the accompanying ovarian regression	Hypothalamic factors such as VIP and serotonin are most strongly implicated
Arginine vasotocin	Posterior pituitary	Causes oviposition	Ill defined
Testosterone	Leydig cells of the testes; granulosa and theca cells of the ovary	Growth of accessory sex organs in males; growth of head furnishings in both sexes; male sexual behavior; oviduct growth and differentiation; albumin secretion	Luteinizing hormone
Estradiol	Theca cells of the ovary	Oviduct growth and differentiation; albumin secretion; vitellogenesis; increased calcium metabolism; female feather pattern; female sexual behavior	Luteinizing hormone; follicle-stimulating hormone?
Progesterone	Granulosa cells of mature follicles	Oviduct growth and differentiation; albumin secretion; evokes preovulatory luteinizing hormone surge	Luteinizing hormone; follicle-stimulating hormone?

REPRODUCTIVE ENDOCRINOLOGY

Anterior pituitary hormones

The avian anterior pituitary secretes the same complement of hormones as the mammalian pituitary gland (Table 38.1). Luteinizing hormone (LH), follicle-stimulating hormone (FSH), thyroid-stimulating hormone, prolactin (PRL), somatotropic (growth) hormone (STH), and adrenocorticotropic hormone (ACTH) have each been isolated and purified from pituitary glands of one or more avian species. Although the anterior pituitary hormones of birds, mammals, and other tetrapod vertebrates show some common properties, there are also distinct differences in their biological activities and chemical properties. Generally, antibodies raised against mammalian pituitary hormones show limited cross-reaction with avian hormones and vice versa. This means that immunological tests for measuring levels of pituitary hormones in the general circulation have had to be developed to study avian endocrinology. This has been accomplished for chicken and turkey LH, PRL, STH; chicken FSH; and turkey ACTH. The availability of these techniques has led to rapid advances in our understanding of avian reproductive endocrinology, but there are still many gaps in our knowledge.

Release of avian gonadotropins from the anterior pituitary is regulated by one or more hypothalamic factors. The pure decapeptide that is known to be the regulator of gonadotropin release in mammals is also a potent releaser of avian gonadotropins. Although this substance causes LH and FSH release in birds, the chicken's own gonadotropin-releasing hormones (GnRHs) differ from that of mammals. Two active GnRHs have been isolated from the chicken's hypothalamus, characterized, and chemically synthesized. Chicken GnRH I (cGnRH I) has a glutamine residue at position 8 rather than the arginine found in mammalian GnRH. Chicken GnRH II differs from cGNRH I and from mammalian GnRH in 3 of the 10 amino acid residues. Both cGnRHs are biologically active. However, anatomical evidence suggests that neurons that secrete cGnRH I (but not cGnRH II) terminate in the median eminence and are therefore positioned to elicit responses from the anterior pituitary. The physiological role of cGnRH II is uncertain at this time.

Prolactin release from the avian pituitary is under stimulatory control of the hypothalamus rather than the chronic inhibition characteristic of mammals. A number of peptides, including vasoactive intestinal polypeptide, thyrotropin releasing hormone, arginine vasotocin, and neurotensin, evoke the release of prolactin from the avian anterior pituitary. There is increasing evidence that vasoactive intestinal polypeptide is the prolactin releaser responsible for the hyperprolactinemia associated with incubation. Several neurotransmitters evoke the release of prolactin from the avian pituitary. Among these, serotonin appears to be the most important. Dopamine probably plays a minor role in the regulation of prolactin secretion in birds. Its effect is inhibitory as in mammals. The interactions of these central nervous system (CNS) elements in the regulation of prolactin secretion in different physiological conditions remain to be elucidated.

Posterior pituitary hormones

The neurohypophyseal hormones of birds have antidiuretic, oxytocic, and vasoactive actions. Although these hormones have much in common throughout the vertebrates, there are distinct and important differences in their amino acid composition. The active principles released from the avian posterior pituitary are arginine vasotocin (AVT) and mesotocin (MT). AVT is the normal antidiuretic hormone in birds and also is more active than MT in inducing uterine contractions. Thus this single molecule appears to serve two separate physiological roles. Whereas arginine vasopressin (AVP) is a potent vasoconstrictor in mammals, posterior pituitary hormones have mixed effects in birds. They cause relaxation of some vascular smooth muscle and

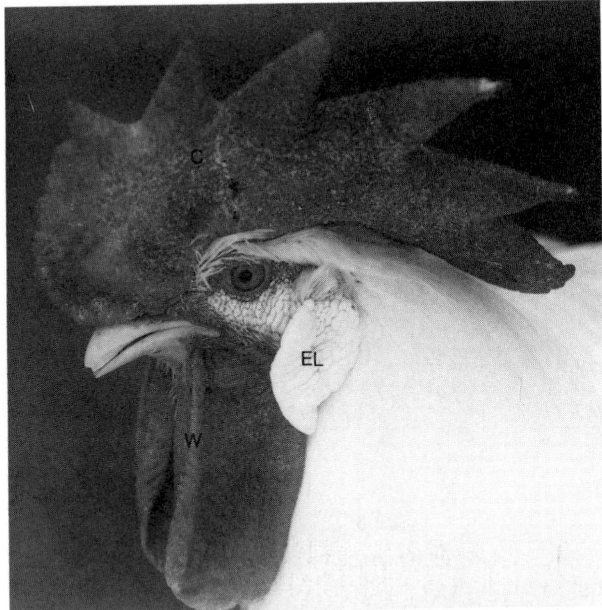

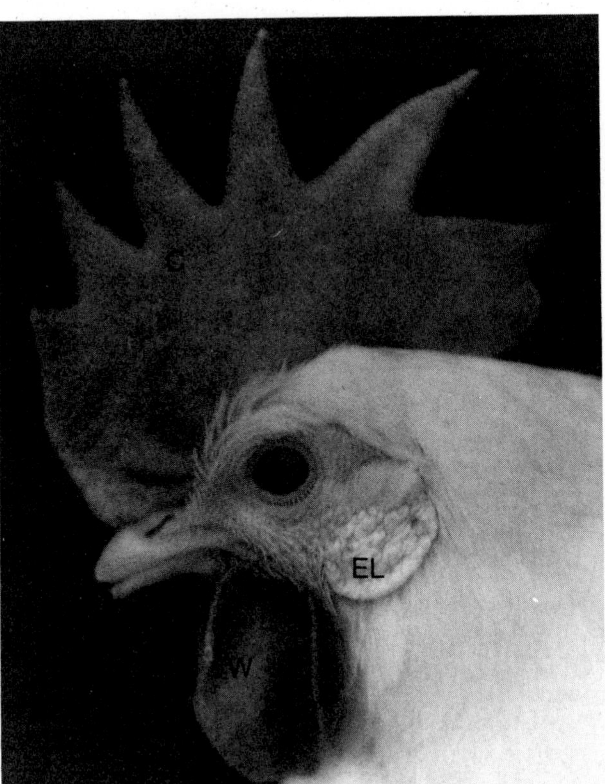

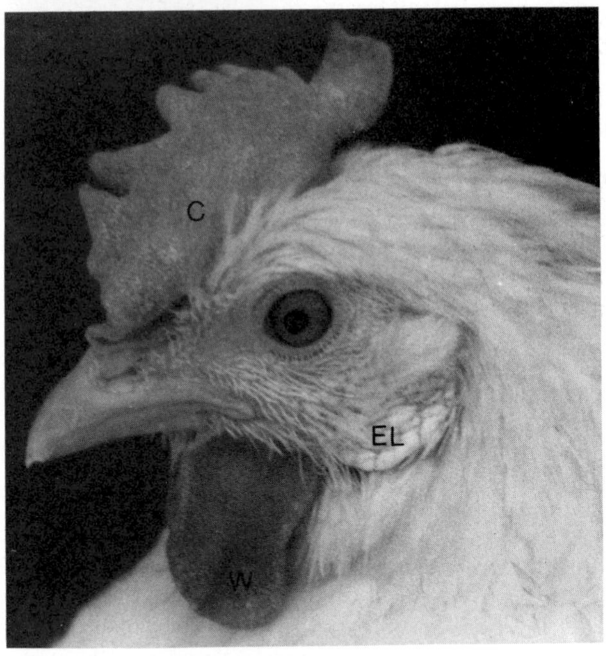

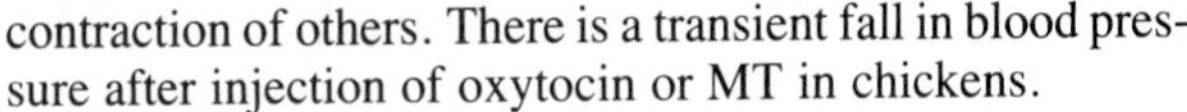

Figure 38.1. Head furnishings of chickens: (*Upper left*) sexually active male; (*upper right*) sexually active laying female; (*lower*) previously laying female who has stopped laying and undergone ovarian regression. C, comb; W, wattles; EL, earlobes. These structures are developed in response to androgenic hormones. The large, well-developed head furnishings of the sexually mature male and laying female are indicative of androgen secretion by gonads of these birds. The shrunken comb of the nonlaying female shows the effects of androgen deficiency resulting from ovarian regression and marked reduction in ovarian steroidogenesis.

contraction of others. There is a transient fall in blood pressure after injection of oxytocin or MT in chickens.

Gonadal hormones

Avian gonads produce steroid hormones that act throughout the body, affecting development of the reproductive duct systems, head furnishings such as comb and wattles (Fig. 38.1), feathers, voice, blood composition, nutrient absorption, and behavior. The predominant testicular steroid is testosterone, while the ovary secretes estrogens, progesterone, and testosterone.

PHOTOPERIODISM

Reproductive activity in many avian species is controlled by environmental stimuli that synchronize breeding seasons with the optimum time of year for survival of offspring. Day length regulates breeding seasons of many wild and domestic species; sexual activity increases with longer days and decreases with shorter ones.

Photosensitivity

The length of photoperiod that stimulates the gonads under natural conditions differs among species. A light period of approximately 12 hours out of each 24 hours stimulates the gonads in many species. The total time of light exposure is not the critical factor; many experiments have shown that short, correctly spaced intervals of light are fully capable of stimulating gonadal growth even with far less than 12 total hours of light. It appears that there is a circadian rhythm in the brain's sensitivity to light, and the rhythm is synchronized by dawn. When the brain is exposed to additional light 12 or more hours after dawn, it acts on as yet unknown biochemical mechanisms to cause the hypothalamus to release increased amounts of GnRH. Circulating levels of LH and FSH are increased with just 1 day of exposure to "long" photoperiods.

Chickens and turkeys are responsive to light stimulation, and artificial light regulation is a common tool used to retard or stimulate reproduction. Even though these species are responsive to light stimulation, they will eventually become sexually mature on short photoperiods, and chickens will lay when kept in total darkness. Some wild birds, however, remain sexually immature indefinitely unless they are exposed to an appropriate photoperiod.

Nonretinal photoreception

Removal of the eyes does not interfere with photosexual responsiveness. This suggests that light acts via some nonvisual pathway to stimulate the gonads. More than 50 years ago, a French physiologist, Jacques Benoit, showed that light directed onto the empty orbits of eyeless ducks stimulated testis growth. Similar experiments have verified the presence of nonretinal photoreceptors in a number of avian species. Elegant experiments have demonstrated that the nonretinal photoreceptors regulating the photosexual response are located in discrete areas of the hypothalamus, as are GnRH neurons. Neurons containing the visual pigment *opsin* have been identified in close proximity to GnRH-secreting cell bodies. Thus a picture of an independent hypothalamic complex totally responsible for photoperiodically induced gonadal growth is developing. In support of this concept are the findings in several species of birds that not only are eyes not required for light-induced gonadal growth but they play no role whatsoever. The gonads of eyeless Japanese quail develop normally in response to long photoperiods but fail to regress when the birds are switched to short photoperiods. Thus, in this species and perhaps in others, the eyes may be an essential part of the mechanisms regulating seasonal gonadal regression. Poultry producers tend to regard light as the primary environmental regulator of reproduction. While photoperiod strongly regulates reproductive cycles of many wild species, they are also regulated by species-specific factors such as mate choice, water levels, and nest site availability. The biochemical and anatomical mechanisms by which these factors are integrated with photoperiod to regulate GnRH secretion are not known.

Photorefractoriness

Another interesting facet of the photosexual response is the phenomenon of light refractoriness (Fig. 38.2). Many

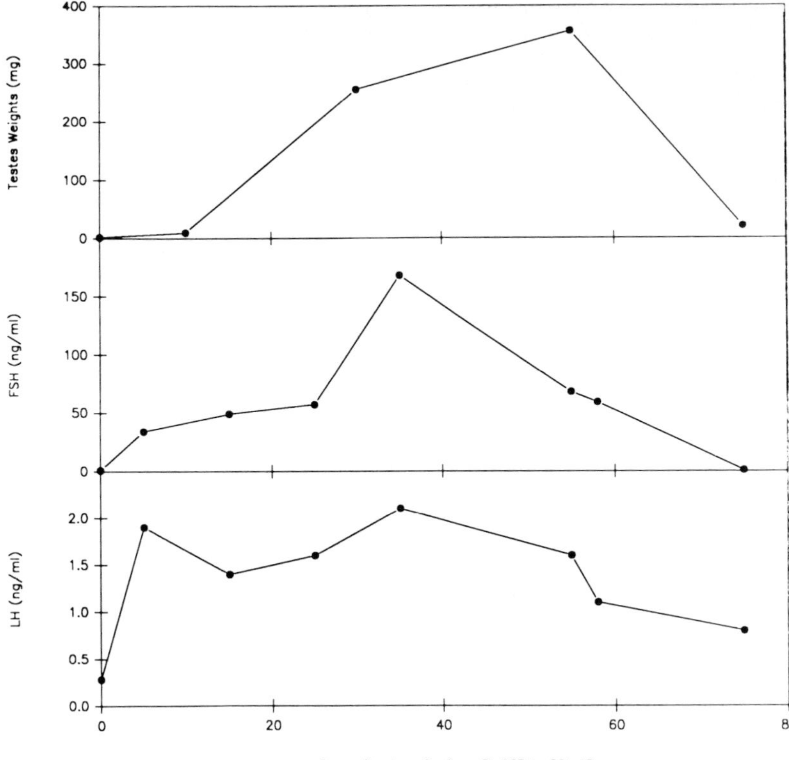

Figure 38.2. Changes in testes weights and plasma gonadotropin levels of the White Crowned Sparrow after the shift from a photoperiod of 8L:16D to a photoperiod of 20L:4D. Even though the birds continue to be exposed to the gonad-stimulating photoperiod, gonadotropin levels fall and the gonads regress. The birds have become photorefractory. Photorefractoriness occurs in many temperate-zone wild species during early summer, even though the natural day length exceeds that required to elicit gonad growth in photosensitive individuals. (Data adapted from Wingfield et al. 1980, *Gen. Comp. Endocrinol.* 42:464–740.)

avian species require prepubertal exposure to a non-gonad-stimulatory light regimen before they are able to respond to stimulatory photoperiods. A nonstimulatory light regimen of short days (real or simulated winter) must follow each reproductively active period if a second period of reproductive activity is to occur. Photorefractoriness also terminates the breeding season in many species. In these species plasma levels of FSH and LH decline and the gonads regress, even though the photoperiod is still long. The photoreceptive mechanisms have become refractory to further photostimulation. In some wild species annual rhythms of gonadal activity occur even if they are continuously experimentally exposed to long days (Fig. 38.2). In these species annual changes in day length may synchronize reproductive cycles but are not absolutely required for them. As flocks of chickens and turkeys lay, an increasing number of individuals undergo gonadal regression. This occurs earlier in turkeys than in broiler breeder hens and earlier in them than in commercial egg-laying hens. It also occurs in males. There are many possible reasons for this gonadal regression, including illness, injury, and social stresses. In some individuals this may be an expression of photorefractoriness. Turkeys are generally believed to express photorefractoriness to a greater degree than chickens.

The physiological basis of photorefractoriness is unknown. The phenomenon may provide a mechanism to prevent egg laying at times of the year when offspring would have little chance of reaching maturity before migration time or of surviving a winter in nonmigratory species. There is increasing evidence in some migratory species that photorefractoriness is caused by an interaction of thyroid hormones and prolactin. This regulatory mechanism appears not to operate in turkeys, even though photorefractoriness occurs in this species.

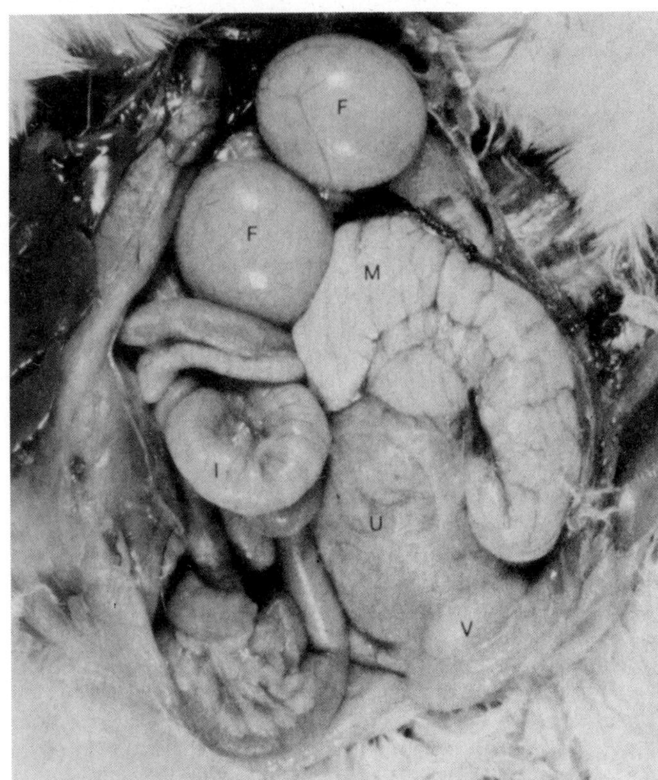

Figure 38.3. Reproductive tract in the body cavity of a hen, showing coiling of the long (80 cm) oviduct, the large amount of space devoted to these organs, and the proximity of the ovary and oviduct. F, large ovarian follicles; M, magnum; U, uterus containing a developing egg; V, coiled vagina tightly bound to the uterus by connective tissue; I, intestine.

ANATOMY OF THE OVARY

In all domestic species of birds only the left ovary and oviduct are normally functional (Fig. 38.3), although occasional individuals are found with left and right functional ovaries or oviducts. The functional left ovary is tightly attached to the dorsal body wall just anterior to the left kidney and posterior to the left lung and adheres closely to the posterior vena cava.

Follicular hierarchy

The mature, functional ovaries of birds are relatively large. For example, the ovary of a 2 kg chicken may weigh 40 to 50 g. The largest three to five follicles account for all but about 6 g. This group of follicles, with the most mature called the F1, the next most mature F2, and so on down to about F5, is often termed the follicular hierarchy (Fig. 38.4). Each differs from the adjacent one by about 1 day's growth.

In addition to the relatively few rapidly developing follicles that are readily visible, the ovary contains many intermediate-sized follicles and many more that are microscopic (Fig. 38.4). Estimates of the total number of follicles in the chicken ovary vary. Early workers counted 2500 with the naked eye and 12,000 with the microscope. In the life of an individual, only a small fraction of these will develop to the point of ovulation.

Follicular structure

The immature avian follicle consists of an oocyte surrounded by follicular cells. The oocyte contains the nucleus and cellular organelles and has a limiting membrane typical of cells throughout the body. The mature follicle differs markedly from the oocyte. It has grown to gigantic proportions by the addition of yolk material. The yolky material is surrounded by a proteinaceous membrane, variously termed the perivitelline or vitelline membrane, which is probably secreted by the surrounding follicular cells (Figs. 38.5 and 38.6). The nucleus of the ovum lies beneath the perivitelline layer and above the surface of the yolk. Surrounding the perivitelline layer is a layer of granulosa cells which have processes that penetrate it and are in contact with the underlying yolk.

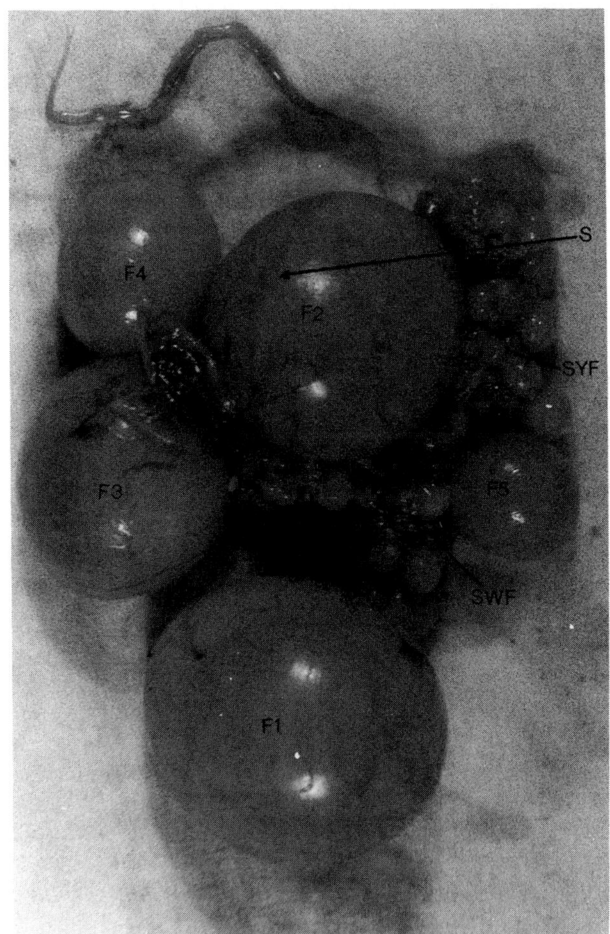

Figure 38.4. Ovary of a sexually mature hen showing five large follicles comprising the follicular hierarchy (F1-F5), small yellow follicles (SYF) that have entered the intermediate growth phase of yellow yolk deposition, and small white follicles (SWF) in which no yellow yolk has yet been deposited. The remnants of the wall from a postovulatory follicle (POF) that released the egg seen in the shell gland in Fig. 38.3 can be seen. The avascular stigma (S), along which rupture of the F2 follicle would have occurred, is apparent.

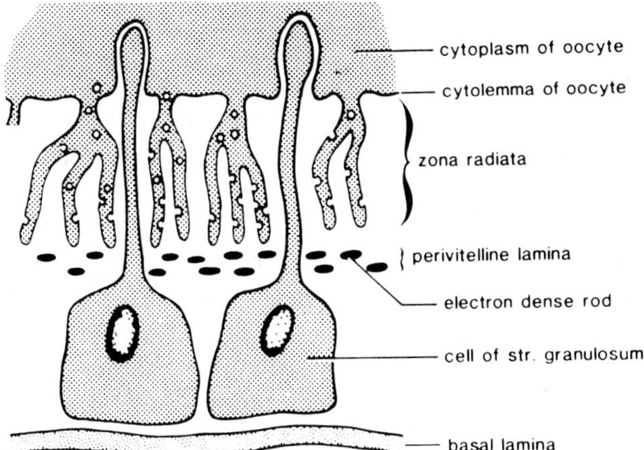

Figure 38.6. An enlarged section of the junction between the inner follicular wall and the yolk. Fingerlike projections of the oocyte cytolemma and the granulosa cells allow transfer of materials from blood into the yolk. Some materials are presumably transferred through the granulosa cells while others are picked up by pinocytotic activity of the cytolemma. The perivitelline lamina consists of a network of long intermeshed fibers secreted by cells of the granulosa layer. This meshwork, then called the perivitelline or vitelline membrane, remains around the yolk at the time of ovulation and provides the mechanical strength necessary to contain the yolk's contents. (From King and McClelland 1984, *Birds: Their Structure and Function*, Bailliere Tindall, London.)

The granulosa layer is surrounded by thecal layers, which are well vascularized and innervated. The granulosa layer and components of the theca interna are active in steroidogenesis.

A complex vascular system exists in the rapidly growing follicles with a particularly extensive venous component. Prominent veins are readily discernible over most of the follicular surface. A relatively avascular band, the stigma (Fig. 38.4), is present on each follicle, and it is along this band that follicular rupture occurs when the oocyte is released.

Figure 38.5. Diagrammatic section through the wall of a mature follicle. The walls of the mature and nearly mature follicles are highly vascular. In the living bird many large blood vessels are visible on follicle walls. These vessels can still be seen in Figs. 38.3 and 38.4, even though the hen was dead. A single arterial supply, the intramural artery, courses through the superficial tunic of the follicle wall and sends branches to terminate in capillary beds just outside the granulosa cells. Several large venous systems—the internal, middle, and external intramural veins—are present in the follicular wall. It has been suggested that the sluggish nature of blood flow in these large veins allows for the massive flow of yolk materials from the blood into the growing yolk. The theca interna and granulosa layers are active steroidogenic tissues. The small boxed segment of the inner follicular wall is shown in more detail in Fig. 38.6. (From King and McClelland 1984, *Birds: Their Structure and Function*, Bailliere Tindall, London.)

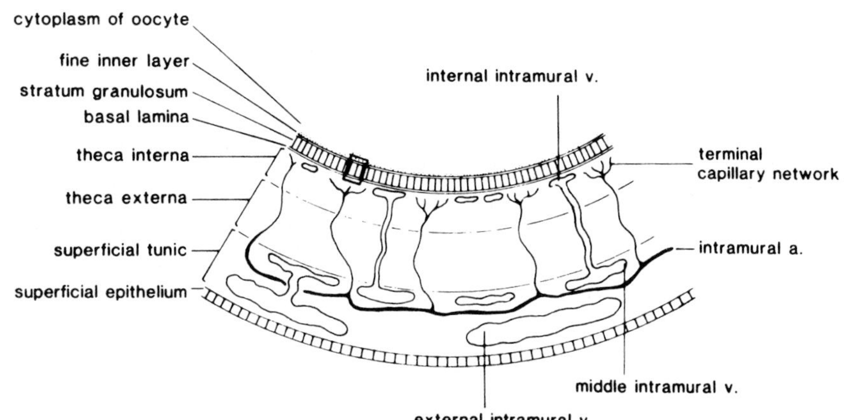

In addition to follicles in many stages of development, the ovary of actively ovulating birds contains the remnants of follicles that have ruptured (Fig. 38.4). These structures, which appear much like grape skins after the contents have been squeezed out, regress rapidly, but they appear to function for a short time in regulating ova transport through the oviduct. The details of this regulatory mechanism remain unclear, but removal of the ruptured follicle causes delayed oviposition of the ovum released from it. No structure analogous to the corpus luteum of mammals forms in these postovulatory follicles.

Ovarian medulla

All of the ovarian structures described to this point make up the cortex of the ovary. Beneath the cortex is a region rich in vascular, neural, and connective tissue termed the medulla. In addition to nerves associated with the ovarian vasculature, the maturing follicles receive sympathetic innervation. Interruption of these nerves by pharmacological means blocks ovulation.

OOGENESIS

It has often been stated that all of the potential ova that a female bird will ever have are present in her ovary by the time she is hatched, but recent work has shown that oogenesis persists for 2 to 3 days thereafter. As the ovary matures and individual follicles begin to grow, a small round, white disk is seen on the surface of each follicle, under the vitelline membrane. This disk, the blastodisk, contains the chromosomal material of the ovum. The disk sits atop a column of white yolk, the latebra, which extends to the center of the oocyte. Before ovulation the oocyte completes the first meiotic division, but meiosis is not completed until the blastodisk is penetrated by a spermatozoon. After fertilization the blastodisk is termed a blastoderm, and by the time the egg is laid the blastoderm is, in fact, an embryo and can be identified as such with the naked eye in most eggs opened for examination.

FOLLICULAR GROWTH

The smallest visible follicles appear white, while intermediate-sized follicles are yellow, indicating that yolk deposition has begun (Fig. 38.4). Studies of the chicken show that the initial phase of yellow yolk deposition is relatively slow, occurring over a period of some 60 days. During this time follicles achieve a diameter of about 6 mm. Some individual follicles then undergo a rapid growth phase during which they grow to 30 to 40 mm in 9 to 11 days. The mechanism that selects individual follicles to undergo the rapid growth phase, which may culminate in ovulation or occasionally in atresia and regression, is unknown.

Yellow egg yolk is a complex mixture of water, lipid, protein, and numerous other microcomponents, including vitamins and minerals. Most of the lipid exists in lipoprotein form, and these compounds are often complexed with Ca or Fe. Phospholipids such as lecithin and cephalin are also found in substantial quantities in yolk. Yolk proteins and lipoproteins are formed in the liver under the influence of estrogens, transported to the ovary, and deposited in developing follicles. Total plasma lipids are markedly increased in estrogenized birds (i.e., laying females, females just before sexual maturity, immature estrogen-treated females, and estrogen-treated males); as a consequence their plasmas often appear white or creamy.

Yolk is not a physically homogeneous substance but consists of granular fractions suspended in a continuous phase. The composition of egg yolk has been extensively studied, and various names have been given to its fractions. Much of the free protein in yolk is clearly identical to blood proteins and probably is derived from them. For example, the water-soluble proteins in egg yolk, called livetins, contain serum albumin, serum γ-globulin, and transferrins.

The yellow color typical of egg yolk is due to xanthophyll pigments in the diet. Diets low in xanthophyll result in light yellow or white egg yolks.

OVARIAN STEROIDOGENESIS

Steroid hormones are secreted by follicular granulosa and thecal cells (Figs. 38.5 and 38.6) and by nonfollicular interstitial cells of the hen's ovary. In the weeks before the first ovulation, growth of the oviduct gives evidence of ovarian estrogen secretion, and growth of the comb and wattles attest to the secretion of androgens. At this time many small white follicles are present on the ovary, but there are no yolk-filled large yellow follicles. These observations and much information from in vitro studies point to the small follicles as the main source of estrogens. In fact, it has been calculated that they are responsible for as much as 97 percent of the ovarian estrogen output in the laying hen. The probable source of estradiol and androgens in the small follicles is the theca cell. The δ-5 pathway whereby pregnenolone is converted to dihydroepiandrosterone, thence to androstenedione, and finally to estradiol is active in these follicles. Quite a different picture of steroidogenesis has emerged from studies of the follicular hierarchy (i.e., follicles F5 to F1). Granulosa cells of these follicles are the source of ovarian progesterone, with increasing amounts being produced as the follicles progress toward maturity (Fig. 38.10). This progesterone is released into the bloodstream. It also diffuses to nearby theca cells, where it is converted into androstenedione and some of it is further metabolized to estradiol. The ability of the theca cells to convert progesterone to androstenedione is diminished or lost as the most mature follicle approaches ovulation. Thus increasing amounts of progesterone are released from the F1 follicle into the blood in the hours preceding ovulation. The elevation of plasma progesterone stimulates LH release from the pituitary gland, and it is a key factor in events leading up to ovulation. (See "Regulation of the Ovulatory Cycle" below.)

It is clear that LH can stimulate granulosa cell and thecal

cell steroidogenesis in follicles at all stages of maturity. A role for FSH in steroidogenesis is more problematical. FSH receptors are present on granulosa cells of large follicles, and their adenyl cyclase activity is stimulated by FSH. FSH receptor numbers and FSH stimulated progesterone synthesis of large follicles have been reported to diminish in the days preceding ovulation of a given follicle. It should be noted that some researchers report no effects of FSH on steroidogenesis of follicles at any stage. Final clarification of this issue awaits the preparation of larger amounts of pure, potent avian FSH. Prolactin may inhibit ovarian steroidogenesis. Although earlier work suggested that it inhibited synthesis of progesterone and estradiol, more recent in vitro studies support an effect on estradiol biosynthesis alone.

ANATOMY OF THE OVIDUCT

In avian anatomy the term *oviduct* is used to describe the complete tubular genitalia of the female. It is large, weighing about 60 g in a sexually mature chicken and extending from the ovary to the cloaca. The oviduct is highly coiled (Fig. 38.3), but when removed from the bird it can be straightened out to a length of 70 to 80 cm (Fig. 38.7). The oviduct presents the typical hollow tubular organ structure, that is, a mucosal layer surrounded by a tunica muscularis that is bounded by serosa. The muscularis layer contains inner circular and outer longitudinal fibers. The oviduct can be subdivided into five functional regions. From the ovarian end, they are the infundibulum, magnum, isthmus, uterus (shell gland), and vagina. Some anatomists subdivide the shell gland into a tubular portion and a pouchlike portion. The vagina attaches to the cloaca, a region through which pass digestive wastes, kidney wastes, and genital tract products. Each of the five regions is easily identified by gross appearance and microscopic structure, and each has specific functions.

At its funnel-shaped anterior extremity, the infundibulum is a thin membranous tissue with scanty smooth muscle. In the posterior tubular region it becomes more heavily muscled and glandular. There is a gradual transition from posterior infundibulum to anterior magnum. The infundibulum is aglandular except in its posterior regions, where a gradual transition to glands characteristic of the magnum occurs. Visual observation and motion pictures have shown the infundibulum to be very motile as the time of ovulation approaches. It has been observed to engulf a follicle before ovulation and to be well around it by the time the ovum is released. Thus the concept of an ovum dropping from the ovary and then being picked up after ovulation is not necessarily accurate. The infundibulum is the site of fertilization, and it is often assumed that sperm cannot penetrate the ovum after it begins to be covered by albumin.

Secretion of albumin (egg white) is the function of the magnum (Table 38.2). As the name implies, this segment of the oviduct is the longest, and it has thickened, whitish walls. The mucosa of the magnum is densely packed with

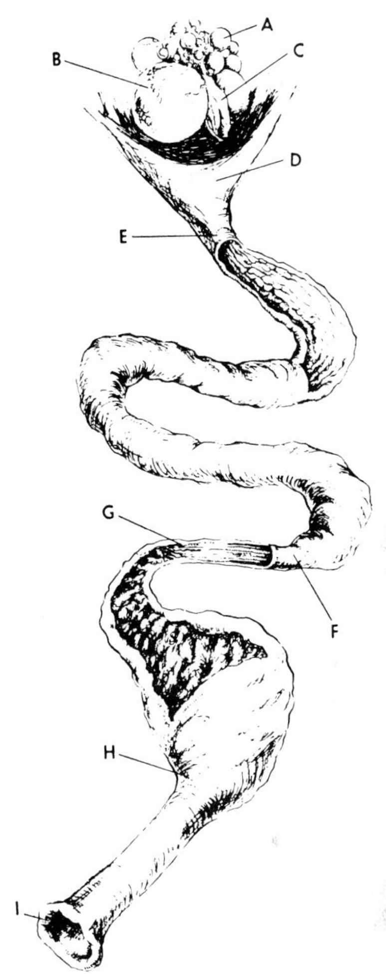

Figure 38.7. Reproductive tract of the laying hen. A, immature ovum of ovary; B, mature ovum; C, ruptured ovarian follicle; D, infundibulum or funnel of oviduct; E, beginning of albumin-secreting region or magnum; F, end of magnum and beginning of isthmus; G, end of isthmus and beginning of uterus; H, end of uterus and beginning of vagina; I, opening of oviduct into cloaca. (From Sturkie 1970, in Swenson, ed., *Dukes' Physiology of Domestic Animals*, 8th ed., Cornell Univ. Press, Ithaca, N.Y.)

Table 38.2. Formation of the hen's egg

Oviduct segment	Length* (cm)	Function	Time spent
Infundibulum	8	Pick up of ovulated ova Site of fertilization	15 min
Magnum	33	Secretion of albumin	3 h
Isthmus	10	Secretion of shell membranes	1½ h
Shell gland	12	Addition of fluid to egg (plumping) Stratification of albumin Shell production Secretion of shell pigments (if present)	20 h
Vagina	12	Sperm storage Egg transport	1 min

*Length of the segments differs with size of the hen and changes greatly, depending on relaxation or contraction of the muscular walls.

tubular glands that open onto its surface. The epithelial cells consist of ciliated cells and nonciliated goblet cells. Albumin is made up of many protein components in varying proportions. Specific biological properties can be attributed to certain of these proteins when they are tested in vitro, but whether they actually serve any more specific role than that of providing a protein reserve for embryonic growth is not clear. The regulation of magnal secretion involves estrogenic, androgenic, and progestogenic hormones. Growth of the oviduct and development of secretory tissue are undoubtedly dependent on estrogens, but estrogens alone will not bring the magnum to a fully functional state. Epithelial goblet cells, which secrete the biotin-binding protein avidin, are dependent on progesterone for their function. Under certain experimental conditions, testosterone synergizes with estrogen in causing magnal development, while progesterone is sometimes antagonistic. Other work has shown that progesterone can either synergize with or antagonize estrogenic stimulation, depending on the dose. Progesterone antagonizes estrogen-induced cytodifferentiation of magnal cells, but it synergizes with estrogen to evoke secretion from previously differentiated secretory glands. The relative importance and dynamic interactions of these three hormones in normal laying females have not been clarified; they are obviously complex.

The isthmus is separated from the magnum by a narrow (1 mm) nonglandular band that is clearly distinguishable to the eye. It secretes the two keratinous, fibrous shell membranes that form an enclosing sac that hold in the egg contents and serve as a support upon which the hard shell is deposited.

The shell gland serves to add fluid to the developing egg, secretes the hard shell, adds a proteinaceous cuticle over the hard shell, and in some birds secretes shell pigments. The part connecting to the isthmus is termed the tubular shell gland. It enlarges and becomes more pouchlike as it approaches its junction with the vagina. This thick-walled muscular organ has long narrow mucosal folds covered with ciliated and nonciliated epithelial cells. A dense layer of tubular glands underlies the epithelium.

The uterus is separated from the vagina by a constricting muscle sometimes called the uterovaginal sphincter. Just beyond this in the vagina are tubular glands capable of prolonged storage of spermatozoa. The vaginal mucosa contains few glands other than these. The vagina is the terminal part of the oviduct and is attached to the cloaca. Its function appears to be the transport and storage of sperm and the transport of eggs; it adds nothing to the eggs that move through it.

EGG FORMATION

Time required

A schematic diagram of a complete egg is shown in Fig. 38.8. Approximately 25 to 26 hours elapse from the time an oocyte is released from the ovary until the finished product, an egg, is released from the body. It is the function of the oviduct to store and transport sperm, to pick up ova, to provide a site for fertilization and early embryonic growth, and to add nutritive and protective layers around the embryo. The time spent in each segment of the oviduct and the functions of these segments are shown in Table 38.2.

Fertilization; albumin and membrane secretion

The infundibulum has not generally been considered to play a role in egg formation, other than that of transport and serving as the site of fertilization.

The magnum secretes and stores albumin before egg formation and releases the proteinaceous material as the ovum passes. The stimulus for release of this material has often been assumed to be mechanical distention due to the passage of a yolk. Distention by a yolk is not absolutely necessary, however, since small eggs that have no yolk at all are sometimes laid and small foreign objects placed in the infundibulum can pass down the oviduct and become coated with albumin, shell membranes, and shell. The volume of

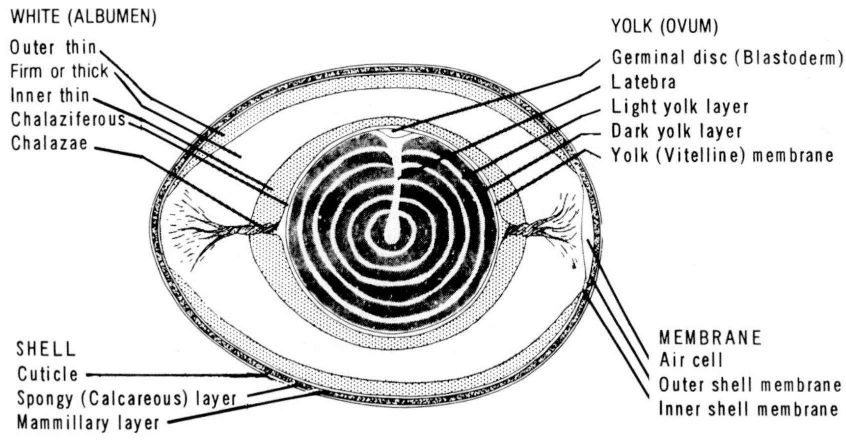

Figure 38.8. Diagram of a cross section of the hen's egg. The parts, their origin, and their functions are described in the text. The yolk materials are continuously transported from the blood into the yolk, once rapid follicular growth begins. The concentric circles, if they are seen, are due to intermittent transfer of pigments. During the night, when hens are not eating, blood carotinoid levels fall and their transfer into yolk is decreased. These rings are not prominent in eggs from modern egg-laying hens, housed under long photoperiods with continuous access to feed. The latebra consists of a column of white yolk material atop which the chromosomal material rests. Fertilization takes place at this site, and early embryonic growth begins here. (Taken from USDA Agricultural Handbook 75, *Egg Grading Manual*.)

albumin surrounding an ovum as it leaves the magnum is only about one-half of that in a finished egg. At this time the albumin is thicker and more viscous than in a finished egg, and it is not separated into layers. Fluids added later increase albumin volume.

Two shell membranes are laid down around the albumin as it passes through the isthmus. These layers are closely apposed except at the blunt end of the egg, where they usually separate, forming an air cell after the egg is laid. Since surgical extirpation of portions of the isthmus results in deformed eggs, it seems that the characteristic egg shape is due to factors in the isthmus. Although deposition of the bulk of the eggshell undoubtedly occurs in the uterus, initial calcification of specific sites on the shell membrane occurs in the isthmus.

Shell formation

During the first 5 hours that the developing egg spends in the shell gland, fluid is added to the albumin, approximately doubling its volume. This added fluid and the mechanical effects of turning result in stratification of the egg white into four recognizable regions. Extending out from the yolk toward both ends of the egg are white, twisted strands of protein called the chalazae. The inner albumin layer extends around the yolk, and the chalazae represent extensions of this layer. Just outside this layer is a watery white layer, then a viscous white layer, and then another less viscous white layer. The formation of such a highly organized structure suggests that it has some importance in embryonic development. It is often suggested that the chalazae serve to hold the yolk and developing embryo in the center of the egg to prevent embryonic adhesion to the shell membranes. Eggs with poor albumin quality (i.e., albumin that is thin and watery) tend to hatch more poorly than those with albumin of good quality.

Shell is secreted most actively during the last 15 hours that the egg spends in the uterus. It is made up of calcium carbonate (98 percent) and a glycoprotein matrix (2 percent). The crystalline part of the shell consists of columns of material embedded in the outer shell membrane. These columns are separated by pores that extend from the outside of the egg to the shell membranes and allow gas exchange by the embryo. Outside the shell is a thin proteinaceous layer, the cuticle, which may block the entrance of bacteria.

Many birds lay uniformly colored or patterned eggs. The uniformly colored eggs, whether brown, blue, or green, are colored by pigments derived from the red blood cells. The porphyrin pigments are distributed throughout the shell but are more concentrated in its outer layer. Eggs that are speckled or have a colored pattern contain pigments in the cuticular layer. These pigments are also derived from porphyrins. On a freshly laid wet egg, the cuticle and cuticular pigments can easily be rubbed off. It is interesting to note that eggs from particular birds often have a uniform pattern day after day.

The source of calcium for shell formation is a subject of much interest. Of course the origin of the hen's calcium is dietary, but female birds have mechanisms for making large amounts of calcium available over a relatively short time. The hen deposits about 2 g of calcium on the egg in 15 hours. This is equivalent to removing the total amount of circulating calcium every 15 minutes during shell formation. As puberty approaches, ovarian estrogen secretion brings about marked changes in calcium handling in birds. Under the influence of this hormone, circulating calcium levels rise from about 10 mg per deciliter of plasma to about 25 mg, the rise being in the protein-bound (nondiffusible) fraction. In addition, estrogen stimulates the deposition of 4 to 5 g of calcium in the hollow medullary region of bones; with the onset of reproductive activity, calcium-binding proteins are increased in the gut mucosa, and calcium absorption becomes much more efficient. All of the calcium secreted into the uterine lumen during shell formation is derived from the blood, and the blood calcium is obtained from feed and from the bones. In the laying hen, medullary bone is in a dynamic state, continuously being deposited and broken down. A sizable fraction of each shell's calcium is derived from this source. Actual shell formation involves the secretion of calcium into the shell gland lumen by uterine epithelial cells, the secretion of a carbonate (bicarbonate ions) source by the subepithelial tubular glands, and the interaction of these components to form calcium carbonate. Insufficient calcium can lead to faulty shell formation, as can inhibition of carbonic anhydrase, an enzyme that catalyzes the conversion of CO_2 and H_2O to H_2CO_3. Hot environments, associated with panting and low blood CO_2, can result in thin eggshells.

Major changes in uterine fluid composition occur during the ovulatory cycle. Experimentally, significant changes in uterine fluid composition have resulted from administration of the adrenal steroids, corticosterone, and aldosterone. Furthermore, an aldosterone antagonist, spironolactone, can affect the composition of this fluid. These findings suggest an involvement of mineralocorticoid hormones in the regulation of uterine fluid composition.

FEMALE REPRODUCTIVE CYCLES

Ovulatory cycle

The ovulatory cycle of the domestic hen is about 24 to 26 hours long, and cycles may occur for many days without interruption. The eggs laid day after day without interruption are commonly called a clutch, although some reserve this term for the group of eggs that wild birds incubate at one time. Eventually, a series of ovulatory days is interrupted by one or more anovulatory days, after which ovulation is resumed. When hens are young and laying at a very high rate, the interval between ovulations and the time required to form an egg may approximate 24 hours. Very long clutches are possible at this time. As hens age, the interovulatory intervals within a clutch approach 25 to 26 hours

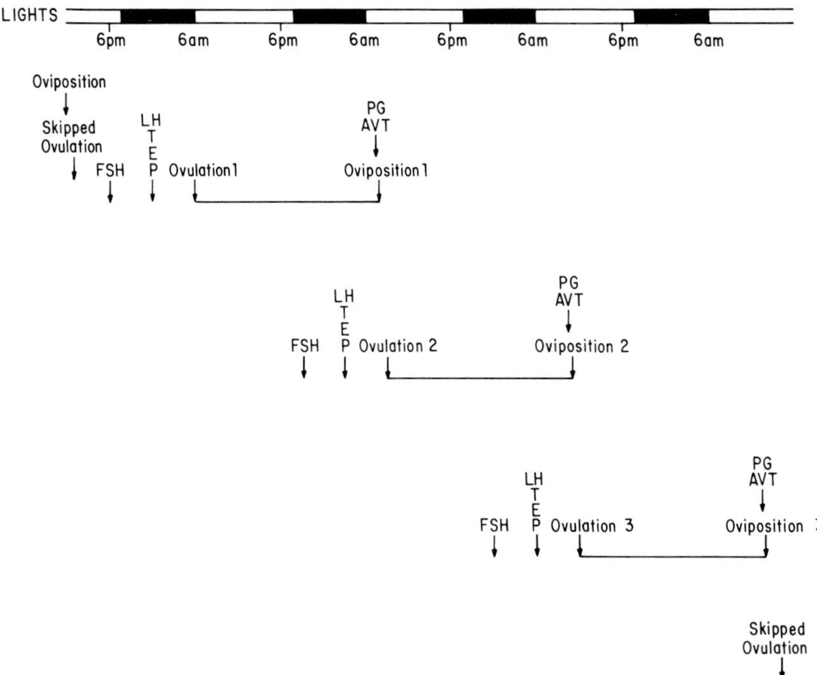

Figure 38.9. Time relations among hormonal events, ovulation, and oviposition in a hypothetical three-egg clutch. Lights were on from 6 AM to 8 PM each day. One clutch ended when ovulation did not closely follow an oviposition ("skipped ovulation" in upper left-hand region of diagram). The hormonal events responsible for initiating the next clutch occurred during the following dark period. The ovulation resulting from this LH surge took place about 6 AM and the first egg of the clutch was laid about 26 hours later. This oviposition was quickly followed by ovulation of the second ovum of the clutch. The increases in FSH, LH, estradiol (E), progesterone (P), and testosterone (T) are not abrupt but, rather, occur over a few hours, peaking approximately at the times shown. The increased blood levels of arginine vasotocin (AVT) and prostaglandin (PG) that are associated with oviposition occur rather abruptly shortly before oviposition. After ovulation 3 days in a row, with each ovulation occurring later in the day, the hormonal events responsible for ovulation again failed and the clutch ended.

and shorter clutches result. The time relations between events in the ovulatory cycle of the hen have been extensively studied and described (Figs. 38.9, 38.10, and 38.11), but the internal regulatory mechanisms are not understood.

Chicken clutches range from 1 to 30 or more eggs. While clutch size is based on ovarian activity, the most obvious manifestation of this activity is the production of a complete egg. Ovulation and oviposition (the act of laying) are not absolutely related, but those events are usually very highly correlated. As many as 11 to 20 percent of the ovulated ova are released into the abdominal cavity; since they do not enter the oviduct, no eggs result. This tendency is more pronounced in hens at the onset of ovarian activity, but some individuals are permanent "internal layers." This condition can often be attributed to some oviducal abnormality. Large fast-growing breeds of chickens and turkeys are often poor egg producers, but recent work has indicated that they may actually produce more yolks than better layers. This apparent contradiction might be due to lower rates of oviducal capture of ovulated ova in the large breeds, or greater atresia rates of partially developed follicles. Ova that do not get picked up by the oviduct are reabsorbed, but eggs that escape from the oviduct after the shell membrane or shell is formed tend to be retained, and many may accumulate in the abdominal cavity. Hens with an accumulation of eggs in the abdominal cavity can often be recognized by gross abdominal distention and by their penguinlike posture.

Oviposition patterns

In the past, much attention has been paid to the time relationships between ovipositions within a sequence. The term *lag* was introduced to describe the time greater than 24 hours that elapsed between eggs within a sequence. In hens laying short and middle-length sequences, interesting pat-

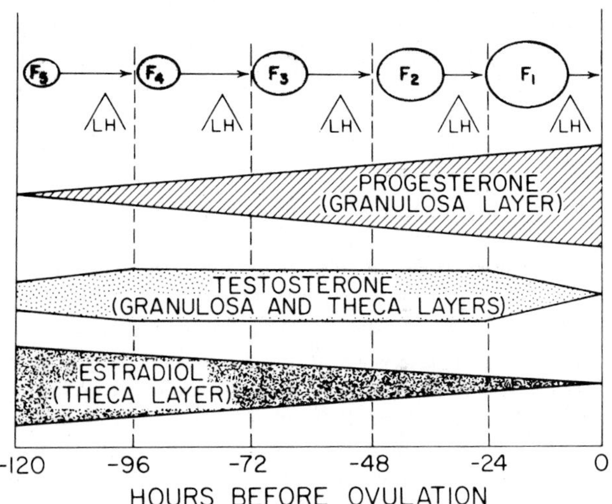

Figure 38.10. The pattern of steroidogenesis changes as follicles mature from the F_5 to the most mature F_1. As a follicle matures, progressively less progesterone is converted to androgens and estrogens; consequently more progesterone is released into the blood. (From Bahr et al. 1980, *Biol. Reprod.* 29:326–334.)

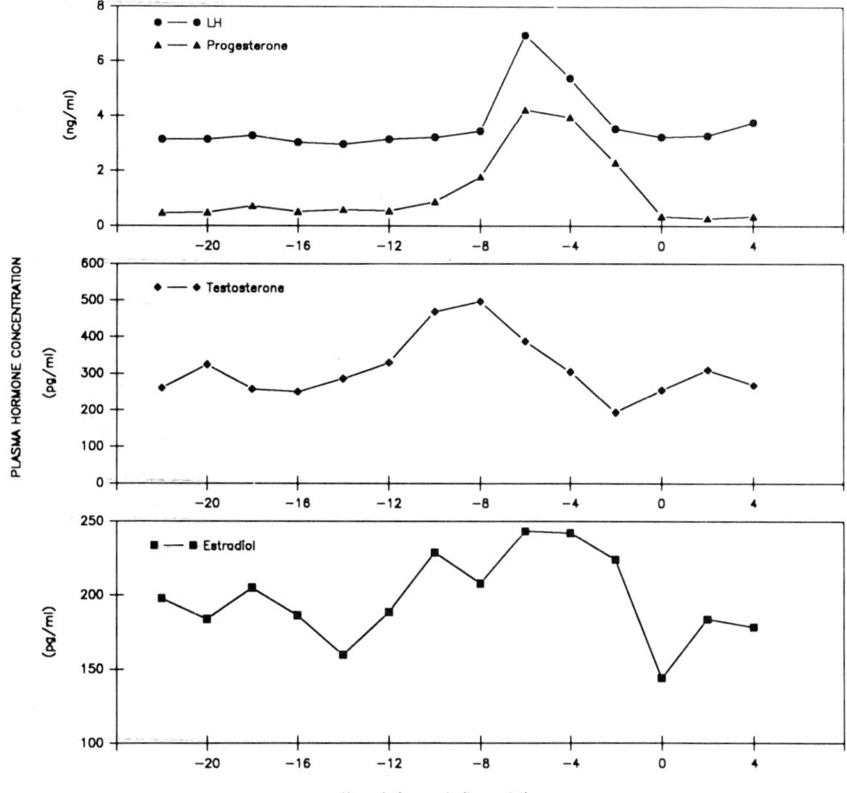

Figure 38.11. Plasma levels of LH and progesterone increase simultaneously about 4 to 8 hours before ovulation. The LH surge is responsible for setting in motion the biochemical events that lead to ovulation. These two hormones are involved in a positive feedback loop, each stimulating release of the other. At high levels, progesterone inhibits LH release and thus may be responsible for termination of its surge. An elevation in plasma prolactin levels (not shown) occurs during the descending phase of the LH-progesterone surge. It may terminate the surge by interfering with progesterone synthesis. In this figure plasma testosterone levels are shown to be elevated before LH and progesterone while estradiol levels increase at the same time. Some investigators find both the estradiol and testosterone peaks to precede those of LH and progesterone. Other investigators find the testosterone peak to occur at the same time as those of progesterone and LH. The magnitude of the ovulatory cycle peaks in birds is much less than the magnitude of those measured in domestic mammals. (Data adapted from Johnson and van Tienhoven 1980, *Biol. Reprod.* 23:386–93.)

terns of lag could be described. In modern-day commercial egg layers in which 92 to 95 percent of the hens may lay every day during the peak periods of production, these patterns are less apparent. The first egg of a sequence is generally laid early in the morning, at just about the time the lights come on. Subsequent eggs in the sequence are laid later and later in the day until the last egg in a sequence is laid in late afternoon. Chickens rarely lay in the dark part of the photoperiod. The oviposition pattern described is simply a reflection of the pattern of release of LH, the ovulation-inducing hormone. LH release occurs about 32 hours before oviposition of the egg whose ovulation it induced. Thus, in chickens, virtually all LH releases are restricted to the dark phase of the photoperiod. Species differ in oviposition time patterns and, by implication, in LH release patterns. The maximum number of eggs is oviposited in midmorning in chickens, about midday in turkeys, late afternoon to early evening in *Coturnix* quail, and from midnight to early morning in ducks.

Usually, but not invariably, an oviducal egg will be laid before the next ovulation occurs (Fig. 38.9). Within a clutch, the interval from oviposition to the following ovulation averages about 35 minutes, with a range of 15 to 75 minutes.

Egg production

The productivity of female poultry is determined by the length of their egg-laying life, the length of sequences, and the intervals between sequences. Commercial egg-laying hens are perhaps the most productive type of poultry, although they are rivaled by some breeds of ducks. Egg production of commercial egg layers is greatly influenced by management decisions as well as reproductive biology. Some flocks will begin to lay at about 22 weeks of age and lay continuously for about a year. Other flocks will lay for about 45 weeks, be forced into a period of reproductive inactivity, and then be stimulated to lay for an additional 35 weeks. In the first case an average production of 260 eggs per hen is typical. In the second case each hen might well lay nearly 500 eggs in her productive lifetime. Breeds of chicken selected for meat production rather than egg production lay far fewer eggs. Typically they lay about 160 eggs in a 40-week period, then are marketed for meat. Turkey hens lay about 110 eggs in a 28-week laying period and are then marketed for meat.

REGULATION OF THE OVULATORY CYCLE

The mechanisms responsible for ovulation and for its failure, which leads to skipped days in the ovulatory cycle, have intrigued investigators for decades. The development of radioimmunoassays for avian reproductive hormones has led to a great increase in knowledge in this area (Figs. 38.10 and 38.11).

LH is a key in the hen's ovulatory cycle (Fig. 38.11). It is the hormone directly responsible for the induction of ovulation. Blood levels of LH increase some 4 to 8 hours before each ovulation, and in chickens housed in usual photoperiods (i.e., 15 hours light; 9 hours dark)) the LH surges occur only during the dark period. With ovulatory cycles being some 25 to 26 hours in length, the LH surges occur progressively later in the dark period with each subsequent egg in a clutch. Eventually the LH surge would fall into the lighted portion of the day, but the release mechanism then fails and no LH release occurs. The restriction of LH surges to the dark portion of the photoperiod is not strictly adhered to by turkeys, and, in fact, chickens will release LH during lighted hours if they are housed under continuous light. Thus the LH release mechanism is not dependent on dark, but release normally occurs during this period. If LH release is elicited, premature ovulations occur; if normal LH release is blocked, ovulation fails. All evidence supports the role of LH as the only ovulation-inducing hormone.

Progesterone is the other key hormone in the hen's ovulatory cycle. Progesterone and LH are involved in a positive-feedback loop. As the most mature follicle approaches ovulation, its pattern of steroid synthesis changes, leading to the production of more progesterone (Fig. 38.10). The release of increasing amounts of progesterone into the blood stimulates the release of more LH from the pituitary into the blood. The LH, in turn, stimulates more progesterone synthesis and release. This mutually stimulatory positive-feedback system functions for several hours until peak levels of both hormones are attained in the 4 to 8-hour period before ovulation (Fig. 38.11). Plasma levels of both hormones then fall. Interference with synthesis or release of either of these hormones into the hen's blood blocks preovulatory peaking of the other. It should be noted that this relationship between LH and progesterone is quite different from the relationship in many mammals. In most mammals elevated levels of plasma progesterone, such as those in the luteal phase of the cycle or during pregnancy, block the release of LH from the pituitary. High levels of progesterone can also block LH release in the hen. Thus low but rising levels of progesterone may serve to initiate and elicit the preovulatory LH peak, whereas peak levels of progesterone may serve to terminate it.

Changes in plasma levels of other ovarian hormones also occur during the ovulatory cycle (Fig. 38.11). Plasma testosterone levels rise just before or concurrent with the rise in LH and progesterone. Testosterone, like progesterone, can stimulate LH release at certain levels and suppress it at high levels. Plasma estradiol levels change, although information is mixed regarding the time of its rise. Some evidence suggests that its rise precedes that of LH, progesterone, and testosterone, whereas other evidence suggests a concurrent rise. The preovulatory rise in estradiol is small, and it does not stimulate the ovulatory surge of LH as does the greater rise in many mammals. Thus it seems not to play a role in the regulation of the ovulatory cycle. The magnitude of the ovulatory cycle changes in these hormones is on the order of a few fold, much less than changes during the mammalian ovulatory cycle.

Information on FSH levels in the hen's ovulatory cycle is sparse, primarily because of difficulty in establishing specific assay methods capable of measuring FSH in the blood. Earlier bioassay studies, based on the use of large pools of blood from many hens, suggested that two peaks of circulating FSH occur during each ovulatory cycle, one 25 hours before ovulation and the other 11 hours before. The limited data based on radioimmunoassay of plasma from individual hens show a single small peak 11 to 14 hours before ovulation. The precise role of FSH in the ovulatory cycle has not yet been defined.

PRL levels increase during the period in the ovulatory cycle when LH, progesterone, testosterone, and estradiol levels are decreasing. This information, coupled with other studies showing that exogenously administered PRL (of mammalian origin) blocks LH-induced ovulation in the hen and LH- and FSH-induced steroidogenesis in the turkey, suggests a possible role of PRL in the ovulatory cycle. According to this hypothesis, PRL levels rise and serve as a turn-off mechanism for the preovulatory LH-steroid hormone cascade.

Much remains to be learned about the precise hormonal mechanisms that regulate ovarian function and the ovulatory cycle of birds. Figure 38.9 shows a composite picture of hormonal events, ovulation, and oviposition in a hypothetical three-egg clutch.

BROODINESS

Incubation behavior

Broodiness, that is, the incubation behavior of birds, has virtually disappeared from chickens selected for egg production, but it is common in chickens used for meat, in turkeys, and in other domestic species of birds. Turkeys, particularly the modern broad-breasted strains selected for meat production, retain much of their ancestors' reproductive patterns, even in confinement. After a few weeks of laying eggs, many turkeys exhibit a desire to incubate them. Although this trait is indispensable for the survival of most species of wild birds, it is undesirable in modern poultry operations. This situation arises because of an apparent incompatibility between ovarian activity and incubation. When hens become broody, their ovaries regress and egg production ceases. Since it is more efficient to incubate eggs artificially than to allow the hens to do it, broodiness is undesirable.

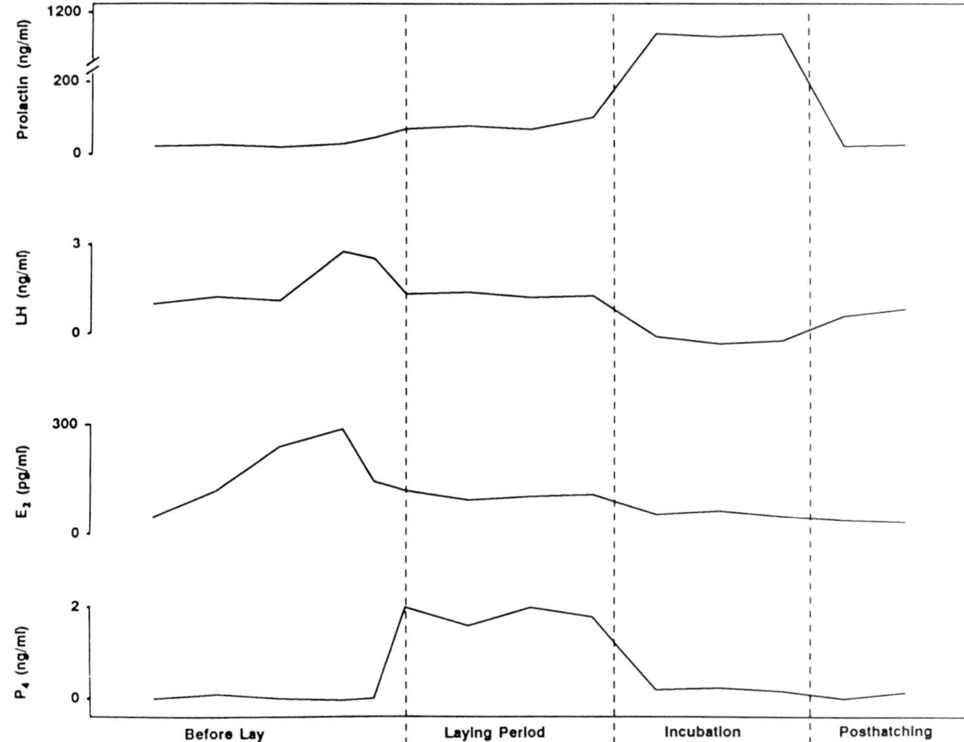

Figure 38.12. Diagrammatic scheme of plasma hormone levels during the reproductive life cycle of a typical gallinaceous female. Some weeks before the first egg is laid, plasma LH and estradiol levels begin to increase. Androgen levels (not shown) increase during this same time. The increased levels of estrogens cause growth of the oviduct and radical changes in calcium metabolism. As the first ovulation approaches, plasma levels of progesterone increase markedly. Prolactin levels increase slightly before lay and continue to increase in the early laying period. Plasma LH, progesterone, and estradiol fall to intermediate levels during the laying period, with periodic surges associated with ovulation. If the female incubates eggs, there is a dramatic increase in plasma prolactin levels at the onset of this period. Levels of the other hormones then fall very low. On hatching of the young, plasma prolactin levels fall sharply whereas LH levels increase slightly.

Prevention of broodiness

Many management techniques are used to prevent or discourage broodiness, but basically they all involve placing the hen in strange, uncomfortable surroundings. This may be done by removing nests or nesting material (e.g., using a wire floor), adding intense 24-hour lights, shifting from one pen into a new pen or barn, or shifting from an inside pen to an outside pasture. Several pharmacological treatments have been shown to influence broodiness. For example, treatment of turkey hens with pimozide, a dopamine receptor blocking agent, at the first sign of broodiness is partially effective in preventing it. Oral administration of parachlorophenylalanine, a serotonin synthesis inhibitor, suppresses plasma PRL levels and interrupts broodiness in turkeys but not in chickens. Neither of these compounds is approved for commercial use in poultry. All these techniques may work to some degree, but the key to success is early recognition of incipient broodiness and early treatment. Increased levels of serum PRL and decreased serum LH, estradiol, and progesterone levels precede the behavioral signs of broodiness by some days (Fig. 38.12), indicating that pituitary and ovarian functions are changing before broodiness is apparent. Since the behavioral signs of broodiness follow the changes in internal function, it is not possible to prevent the endocrine changes with current broody control techniques, but it is possible to reverse them after they are well under way. Invariably this results in some loss in egg production, even when the best-known broody treatments are used. If broodiness is allowed to persist for some days before treatment begins, ovarian regression will have set in and several weeks may elapse before ovulation resumes. If no treatment is given, hens will persist indefinitely in their broody behavior.

Prolactin's role in broodiness

For many years, indirect studies suggested that PRL is a causal factor in the behavioral and ovarian changes that are associated with broodiness. Injections of mammalian PRL sometimes induced incubation behavior, sometimes caused ovarian regression, and interfered with LH- and FSH-induced steroidogenesis. It is now clear that increased circulating levels of PRL precede broodiness and that PRL levels fall dramatically when management techniques to treat broodiness are applied (Fig. 38.12). PRL levels in turkeys rise when hens are confined to nests with eggs, a procedure that induces broodiness.

The studies cited above support the involvement of PRL in broodiness and the associated ovarian regression. Earlier in the chapter the effects of various neuropeptides and neurotransmitters on plasma PRL were discussed. Even though much detailed information is now at hand, the causal link between the hen's environment, hyperprolactinemia, and broodiness remain unknown. It is known that nocturnal nesting increases night by night in the period just before behavioral broodiness in chickens. Denervation of the so-called brood patch area on the ventral surface of the turkey's breast decreases nesting time, decreases plasma prolactin levels, and blocks broodiness. Plasma prolactin levels fall rapidly if incubating hens are deprived of the opportunity to nest and rise rapidly when these hens are again given access to the nest. On the basis of these observations, it might be proposed that tactile sensory input from brood patch receptors alters neurotransmitter and neurohormonal activity in the hypothalamus in a manner to elicit prolactin release. Elevated prolactin levels could then act to cause gonadal regression and cessation of laying. Either the changes in CNS activity or the elevated prolactin levels might be responsible for the marked anorexia of incubation. The elevated prolactin levels, alone or in combination with ovarian steroids, would elicit brood patch hyperemia and perhaps increased brood patch sensitivity to tactile stimuli.

In many other species similar relationships exist between prolactin, incubation, and gonadal regression. In some species the relationships are very different. For example, pigeons and doves lay two eggs and then begin to incubate. In these species prolactin does not initiate incubation. In fact, prolactin levels rise only during the latter half of incubation and stimulate proliferation of the crop-sac mucosa in preparation for crop milk production. Crop milk, as the sloughed mucosal cell slurry is known, is fed to the squabs after hatching. In some species, such as cockatiels and parakeets, females begin to incubate soon after laying the first of many eggs. As a result, there is an extremely asynchronous hatch, with chicks emerging over several weeks. The role of prolactin in incubation of these birds has not been investigated.

OVIPOSITION

Egg expulsion

The act of oviposition (laying of the egg) involves the coordinated interaction of a number of body systems. The smooth muscles of the shell gland contract, and those separating the shell gland and vagina relax. Feathers in the vent and abdominal region relax while abdominal skeletal muscles contract (the bearing-down reflex). As these coordinated muscular activities expel the egg, respiratory rate increases and the hen's comb blanches.

Regulation of oviposition

The precise factor that triggers oviposition when the egg is ready to be laid is not known. There is strong evidence supporting the involvement of posterior pituitary hormones, prostaglandins, and a factor(s) from the ruptured ovarian follicle in oviposition. Injection of AVT, oxytocin, or AVP will induce oviposition within minutes. The posterior pituitary content of AVT drops before oviposition, while levels in the blood increase markedly. In addition AVT is a potent stimulator of uterine smooth muscle contractions in vitro. These lines of evidence clearly show an involvement of this hormone in oviposition. Similar statements can be made about prostaglandins. Prostaglandins of the E and F series (PGEs and PGFs) stimulate contraction of uterine muscle in vitro. PGE_1 is a potent inducer of oviposition. While $PGF_{2\alpha}$ can also induce oviposition, much higher doses are needed. Blood levels of 15-keto-13,14-dihydro-$PGF_{2\alpha}$, the stable metabolite of $PGF_{2\alpha}$, increase five- or sixfold in the hour preceding oviposition. Thus there is good support for an important role of prostaglandins as regulators of oviposition.

A third major factor to be considered as a regulator of the oviposition of a particular egg is the follicle from which it was released. Surgical removal of the ruptured follicle, or its granulosa cell layer, delays oviposition of the egg that was released from that follicle. In some cases the egg is held for days. Prostaglandin levels in the wall of the ruptured follicle increase dramatically before oviposition. Prostaglandins may be the factor by which the ruptured follicle affects oviposition.

An understanding of the control of oviposition must seek to integrate the actions of neurohypophyseal hormones, prostaglandins, the ruptured follicle, and other factors. Other factors can induce or prevent oviposition. For example, electrical or mechanical stimulation of the preoptic region of the hypothalamus causes premature oviposition, as does general anesthesia with sodium pentobarbital. Ephedrine or epinephrine causes relaxation of uterine muscle and retards oviposition, while acetylcholine stimulates it. Thus oviposition in birds, like parturition in mammals, is influenced by multiple control systems, the details of which remain to be unraveled.

NESTING

Floor eggs

Accumulation of eggs in a nest is obviously a prerequisite for incubation; a group of eggs must be gathered in one spot so the female can sit on all of them simultaneously. Domestic birds still retain strong nesting behavior and the urge to deposit eggs in a nest. Nonetheless, oviposition of eggs on the floor rather than in nests is a serious management problem. Floor-laid eggs are generally dirty, contaminated, and unfit for eating or hatching. The incidence of floor eggs may be affected by environmental factors during the growing period and during the laying period. For example, hens allowed to roost during the growing period lay fewer floor eggs. More eggs are laid in nests if houses are uniformly well lighted with no dark corners. Both chickens and turkeys can be trained to lay in nests if repeatedly placed in them early in the laying period.

Control of nesting

The assumption might be made that a hen nests when it has an egg ready to be laid, but this is not necessarily so.

The stimulus for nesting appears to be related to the ovulation that occurred about 24 to 25 hours earlier, rather than to the actual presence of an egg in the uterus. Usually both nesting and a nearly complete egg coincide 24 to 25 hours after ovulation. If these events are separated by stopping engulfment of the ovum or transplantation of the ovary to another site in the body, nesting behavior still proceeds at the expected time after ovulation. At least 95 percent of nestings are associated with a prior ovulation, and nesting is a much better indicator of prior ovulation than is oviposition. The ovarian signal that evokes nesting behavior cannot be neural, since normal nesting is observed in hens whose ovaries have been severed from normal nervous connections. Thus an unknown hormonal mechanism may be responsible.

ANATOMY OF THE MALE REPRODUCTIVE TRACT

Testes

The following description of male anatomy is based primarily on the rooster. Males of all avian species have internally placed rather than scrotal testes. In domestic birds they are located just anterior to the kidneys and are attached to the dorsal body wall (Fig. 38.13). The testes of birds are larger, relative to body weight, than those of mammals, and in many species there is bilateral asymmetry, with the left gonad larger than the right. Whether the mechanisms that are responsible for testicular asymmetry are the same as those that cause the marked ovarian asymmetry in birds is unknown. The testes are often whitish, although functional black, partial black, or olive green testes are normal in some breeds or species of birds. The testes are soft and lack the connective tissue septa commonly found in mammals. The great mass of testicular tissue is composed of seminiferous tubules, with relatively few Leydig cells visible in microscopic sections. As a consequence of their intra-abdominal location, avian testes function at body temperature (about 41 to 42°C for domestic species), a feat that would be impossible for most mammals. It has been suggested that the testes are cooled by airflow in the abdominal air sacs. This hypothesis is unsupported by experimental evidence and is almost certainly untrue.

Accessory organs

The accessory tubular organs associated with the testes are relatively undeveloped in birds; birds have no seminal vesicles, bulbourethral glands, or prostate glands. Tightly apposed to each testis is a small structure that has often been termed an epididymis (Fig. 38.14). The epididymal region consists of efferent tubules that carry sperm from the testis to a single epididymal duct, which is apparent on the epididymal surface. This duct is short (about 2 to 4 cm) and is quite unlike the mammalian structure of the same name. Leading from each epididymis is a coiled tube, the vas or ductus deferens (see Figs. 38.13, 38.14, and 38.15), which traverses posteriorly, is attached to the dorsal body wall, and terminates at a small papilla in the cloaca. Just before its termination the vas deferens becomes enlarged and serves as a storage site for spermatozoa, as does the entire duct. Each vas deferens penetrates a small papilla and ejects the semen through it into the cloaca. At the time of sexual excitation several small folds in the ventral cloaca become

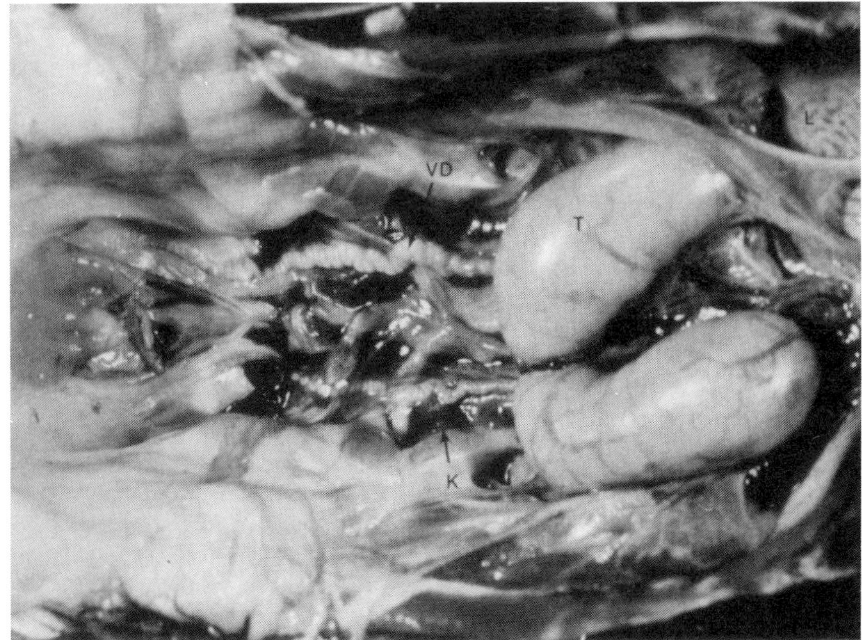

Figure 38.13. Internal reproductive organs of the rooster, showing the testes (T) and coiled vas deferens (VD), which carries sperm to the ejaculatory apparatus in the cloaca. The proximity of the gonads to the lungs (L) and kidneys (K) can be noted. The epididymal region is not apparent.

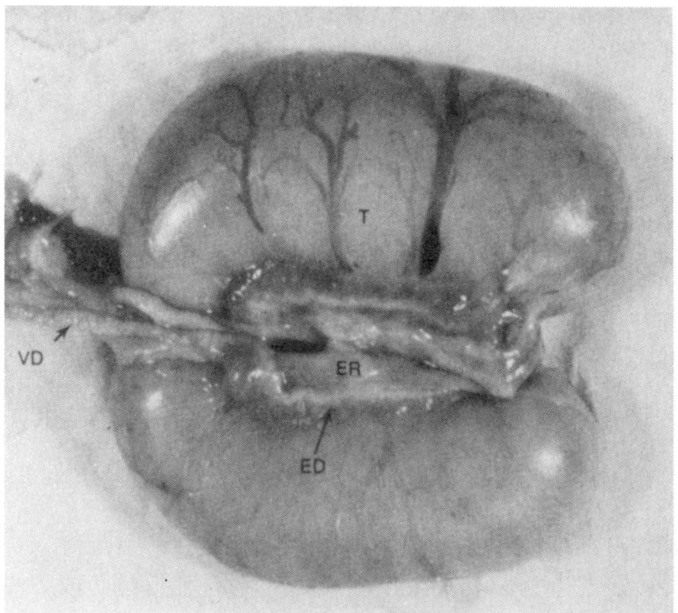

Figure 38.14. Rooster testes (T) removed from the body and viewed from the dorsal aspect. The whitish ductus epididymis (DE) in the small epididymal region (ER) collects sperm leaving the testis and joins with the vas deferens (VD). Sperm taken from this region of the vas deferens (*upper third*) are already capable of fertilization.

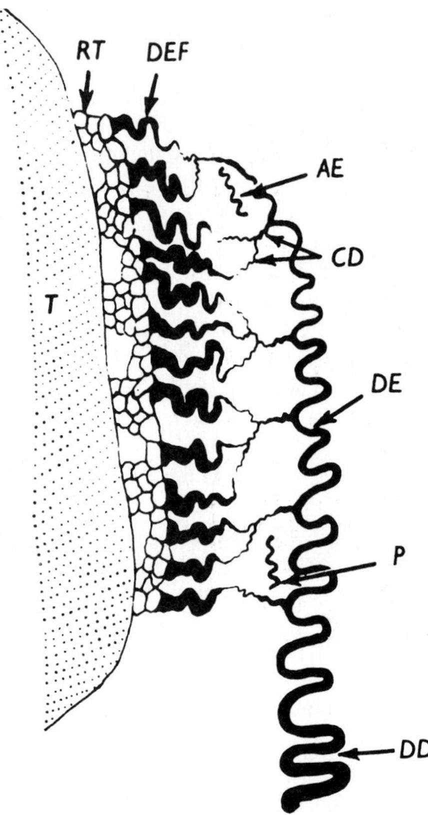

Figure 38.15. Schematic diagram of the excurrent duct system in the epididymal region. The seminiferous tubules of the testis (T), which are not shown, terminate in a network of rete testes (RT). The large efferent ducts (DEF) arise from the RT and terminate in collecting ducts (CD). AE is appendix epididymis. The relatively few CD terminate on the ductus epididymis (DE), which, as it leaves the region of the testes, becomes the enlarged coiled ductus deferens (DD, same as vas deferens). P is paradidymis. The right and left DD course caudally on the ventral surface of the respective kidney. The terminal part of each DD is dilated into a sperm-storing receptacle just before it penetrates the lateral cloacal wall and terminates in a papillae (From Tingari 1971, *J. Anat.* 109:423–435.)

engorged with lymphatic fluid and protrude, forming a troughlike structure to direct the flow of semen (Figs. 38.16 and 38.17). The phalluses of the rooster, the tom, and many other birds are small and do not function as intromittent organs. Semen is transferred to the female by touching the rudimentary phallus to the everted vagina. Ducks and geese, however, have sizable penises (Fig. 38.18), and mating is accomplished by intromission. The vasa deferentia and cloacal ejaculatory apparatus probably receive both sympathetic and parasympathetic innervation. External stroking of the base of the tail causes protrusion of the genitalia and often forceful expulsion of semen from the rooster. Similar stimulation elicits phallic eversion in the tom, but the viscous semen is generally released only after pressure is applied to the terminal storage depots in the vasa deferentia. In the female the same sort of manipulation evokes vaginal eversion, an event that also occurs during natural mating while the male treads on the female's back. Neural pathways underlying these responses have not been described. It seems likely that stimulation of this region by treading or by manual means activates a reflex arc involving touch or pressure receptors, sensory neurons, and the autonomic nervous system.

Sperm transport and maturation

The physiological role that the various juxtatesticular structures play in maturation of spermatozoa is relatively unstudied in birds. Applying names used for mammalian tissues to structures in the avian tract may cause misleading conclusions regarding functional similarities. The mammalian epididymis is clearly a site of great importance in sperm maturation, but the importance of the avian epididymis in sperm maturation is not clear. It is relatively minuscule compared with that of the mammal, and transit time through it is on the order of a day or so. In fact, estimates of total transit time from the testes to the terminal region of the vasa deferentia range from 1 to 4 days. Early studies indicated that sperm taken from the testis or epididymis of the cock were capable of producing fertility, but at a very low level. More recently it has been shown that cock spermatozoa taken from the testes produce very high levels of fertility if insemination takes place high up in the oviduct. These recent findings suggest that cock sperm, unlike those of mammals, are functionally mature before they leave the testes. Sperm from upper, middle, and lower

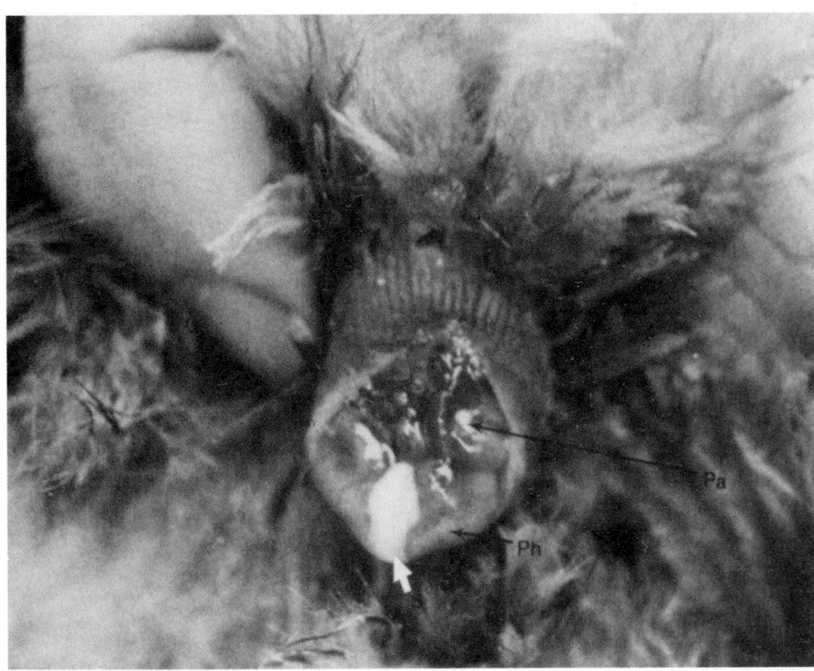

Figure 38.16. The small phallic region (P) of a rooster everted for semen collection by manual stroking of the abdominal and tail head regions. After eversion is obtained, the fingers are moved to the cloacal region to maintain the eversion and squeeze semen from the terminal segment of the vas deferens. Semen (S) can be seen running from the troughlike structures formed by engorgement of cloacal tissues with lymphatic fluid during sexual excitation. Semen can be seen emanating high up on the cloacal wall, where one of the bilateral papillae (V) is visible. Each vas deferens terminates in one of these papillae.

regions of the vas deferens of the cock have about equal fertilizing ability. It has also been shown that the vasa deferentia of the cock have the ability to preserve sperm trapped in them.

ENDOCRINE REGULATION OF THE TESTIS

The general pattern of dual gonadotropic influence on testicular function appears to hold in birds. Testicular growth is stimulated by either LH or FSH, but the gonadotropins have different target cells. LH acts on Leydig cells to promote their development and testosterone production. FSH acts on Sertoli cells. Full testicular function is brought about by the combined action of FSH and testosterone. With the onset of a photostimulatory photoperiod, there are rapid increases in blood levels of LH and FSH. Within days after the levels of these hormones increase, they again decrease, as the negative feedback influence of testicular products exert themselves. Levels of LH decline when testosterone levels are increasing. Testosterone undoubtedly is the major feedback regulator of LH secretion. Levels of FSH decline more slowly than those of LH and do so as the testes are approaching full size. By the time the testes have reached full size, FSH levels are only about one-fourth the peak levels attained several weeks earlier. The different time courses of the rise and decline of LH and FSH suggest that they are not being influenced by the same regulatory factor. The testes of birds may elaborate a nonsteroidal regulator of FSH secretion, as do the testes of mammals.

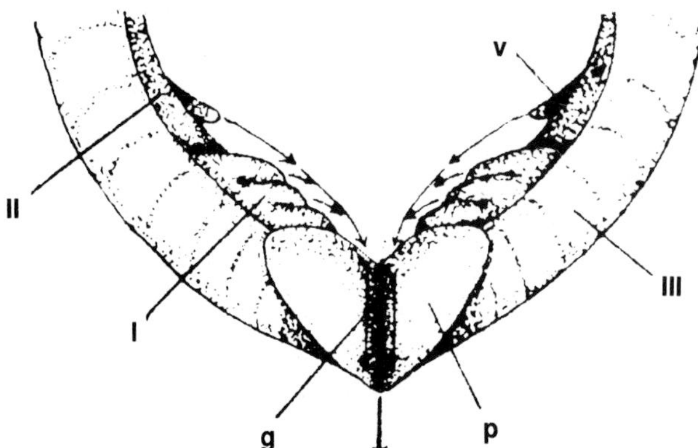

Figure 38.17. Diagram showing the ejaculatory process in the cock. Semen is released from the papillary process of the vas deferens (v) (identified as DD, a ductus deferens in the previous figure). Arrows show the flow of semen across the swollen lymphatic fold (I) and through the groove (g) of the erect phallus (p). Transparent lymphatic fluid can be released from the lymphatic fold and mix with semen. The addition of large amounts of lymphatic fluid to semen often occurs when semen is forcefully expressed during manual ejaculation. It is considered an undesirable adulterant. The second (II) and third (III) folds of the cloaca are evident. (From Nishiyama 1955, *J. Fac. Agric. Kyushu Univ.* 10:277–306).

SEMEN

Semen is a mixture of sperm cells and carrying fluids. In domestic birds the ejaculate is characteristically highly concentrated and of low volume. Artificial collection of semen from chickens and turkeys is widely practiced and relatively simple. Nearly all of the information available regarding physical and chemical characteristics of avian semen have been obtained from semen collected in this

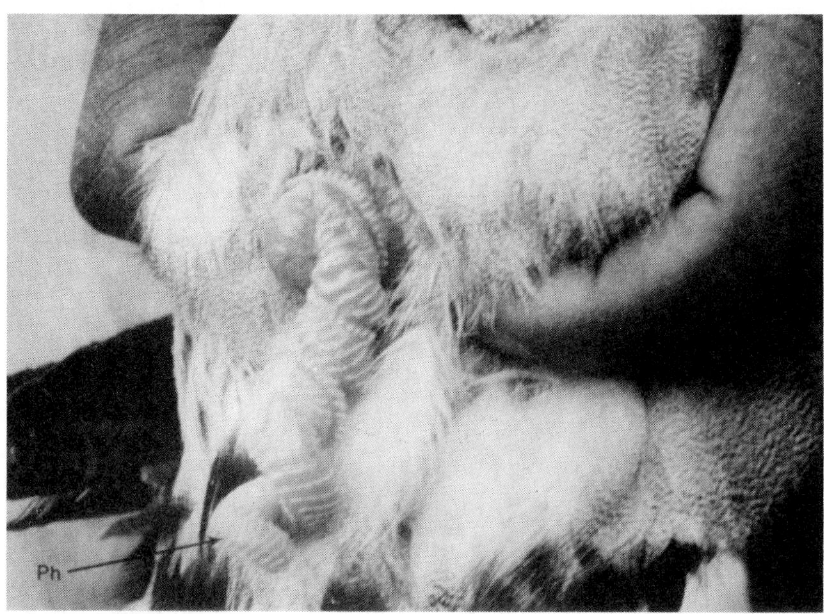

Figure 38.18. Long coiled phallus (Ph) of a mallard drake. This structure, about 7 to 8 cm long, coils into the cloaca when the duck is not sexually aroused. To evert the phallus for semen collection, the duck was held with its abdominal region up and digital pressure was applied around the cloaca. This type of penis is found in both ducks and geese.

manner. The composition of semen thus obtained is quite variable, the sperm cells being mixed with secretory fluids from the engorged phallic apparatus and with digestive and urinary tract wastes. The contributions of these factors are not easily controlled, and consequently considerable variation in semen composition has been reported. The average volume of cock ejaculate is about 0.5 ml, but amounts considerably above and below this are commonly obtained. The sperm cell concentration of such an ejaculate averages around 4 billion per milliliter of semen. Semen volume of turkey toms tends to average around 0.25 to 0.35 ml, with concentrations of 8 to 12 billion sperm per milliliter. Thus the number of sperm released at each ejaculation in these two species does not differ markedly, both being in the

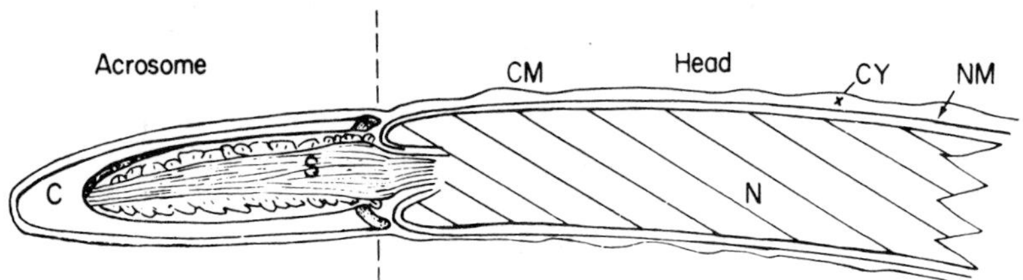

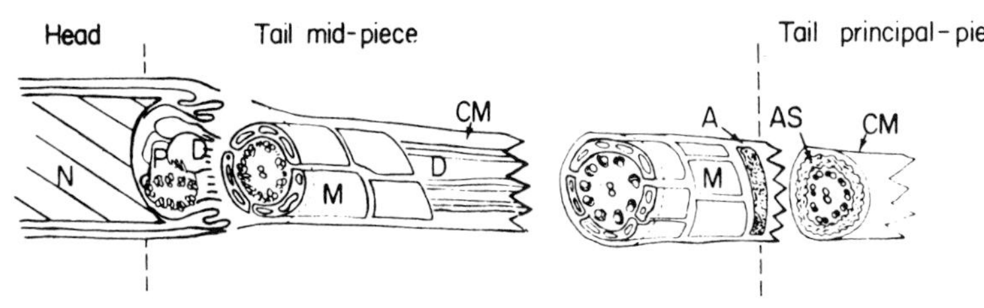

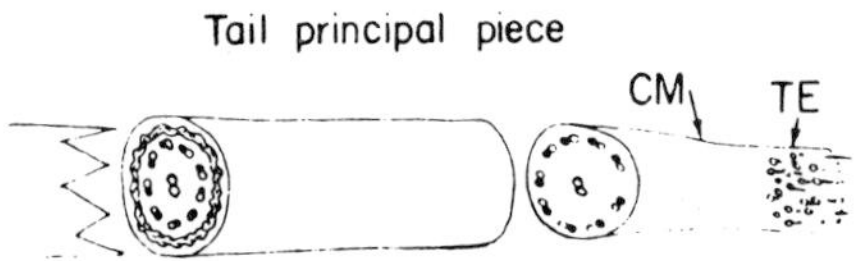

Figure 38.19. Semidiagrammatic drawing of fowl spermatozoa showing the principal ultrastructural components. The acrosome cap is cut away to show the underlying spine. C, acrosome cap; S, acrosome spine; N, nuclear material of the head; CM, cytoplasmic membrane; CY, cytoplasmic remnants; NM, nuclear membrane; P, proximal centriole; D, distal centriole; M, mitochondrion; A, annulus; AS, amorphous sheath; TE, tail end where the 9 + 2 fibril structure breaks down. (From Lake 1971, in Bell and Freeman, eds., *Physiology and Biochemistry of the Domestic Fowl*, vol. 3, Academic Press, London.)

range of 2 to 4 billion cells. There are striking differences in the chemical composition of seminal fluids of birds and mammals (and, indeed, among mammals), the physiological meanings of which remain obscure.

Spermatozoa of the chicken and turkey are similar in shape, but differ from mammalian sperm. In these avian species the sperm head is narrow and long (0.5 × 12.5 μm) with a small acrosome overlying the apical end of the nucleus (Fig. 38.19). The middle piece and the main piece of the tail together are about 94 μm long, for a total sperm length of about 110 μm. The diameter of the tail is about 0.5 μm or slightly less, giving the sperm an overall filiform shape.

SPERM STORAGE IN VIVO

Females of many avian species can store sperm in specialized oviducal glands for prolonged periods and can produce fertile eggs for days, weeks, or even months after a single mating or artificial insemination. Early studies suggested that sperm were stored in mucosal crypts of the infundibulum. Although these structures do have the ability to store sperm, the most important normal sperm-storage tissue is probably located in the vagina, very near its junction with the uterus. Sperm are found in these uterovaginal sperm-storage glands shortly after mating or artificial insemination and persist there for the fertile period of the female. Sperm are seldom found in the infundibular storage sites unless semen is introduced into oviduct in such a manner that it bypasses the uterovaginal glands. There is evidence that sperm move from the uterovaginal area to the infundibulum after oviposition and there await the arrival of the next ovulated ovum, which may take place within minutes. Other work has shown that the passage of an egg through the uterovaginal area is not essential for sperm release, but the mechanism that does bring about their release is not known. It may well be that the uterovaginal and infundibular storage areas act in concert. The biochemical basis for the ability of these glands to store sperm is not known. It is often hypothesized that they provide a microenvironment that nourishes the sperm or that they induce reversible sperm quiescence; they may function in both ways.

ARTIFICIAL INSEMINATION

Commercial artificial insemination of poultry

All commercial breeding turkey hens are bred by artificial insemination (AI). The widespread use of AI came not from a desire to spread the genes of outstanding males but from low fertility levels achieved by natural mating. Broad-breasted turkey toms have resulted from generations of intense selection for size and conformation. Along with extreme development of the pectoral muscles have come a diminished libido and a reduced ability to mate. Modern toms lack the coordination and dexterity to complete sufficient matings to assure high fertility. In addition, partial completion of the mating act, even without transfer of semen to the female, can result in variable periods of sexual refractoriness during which hens will not remate.

Commercial use of AI in chickens is not widely practiced in the United States since natural matings generally result in satisfactory fertility levels. Artificial insemination of broiler breeder hens with semen from select sires might well lead to more rapid genetic improvement in growth and other production characteristics of broilers. Conversion from natural mating to artificial insemination would require availability of skilled labor and major investments in new types of housing. The broiler industry has not found the cost-benefit relationship attractive. Some limited commercial AI of chickens, guinea fowl, and ducks is practiced in other countries. These species all have shorter fertile periods than the turkey after AI or natural mating. This necessitates AI at least every 7 days to maintain peak levels of fertility. Approximately 100 million sperm per AI are required for optimum fertility in chickens.

Artificial insemination, as it is practiced commercially in the turkey industry, proceeds as follows. Semen from many toms is collected in a common pool and mixed. The semen is protected from temperature extremes. This pool of semen from unidentified toms is used to inseminate an indeterminant group of unidentified hens, with no attention to individual matings or parentage of resulting offspring. Each hen is inseminated with about 0.025 ml of semen dispensed from a short plastic straw. To accomplish this, one worker causes the vagina to protrude or evert by placing pressure around the cloacal and abdominal region. When the vagina is everted, a second worker inserts the inseminating straw 5 to 7 cm into the vagina. Abdominal pressure is relaxed, and the semen, containing about 200 million sperm, is expelled into the vagina. Most studies show that placement of the semen close to the uterovaginal storage glands, but not beyond them in the uterus, results in maximum fertility. Although turkey hens will produce fertile eggs 40 or more days after a single AI, it is common practice to inseminate them at intervals of 7 to 14 days to assure maximum fertility. Although lower fertility does result from inseminations carried out when hens are carrying hard-shelled eggs (i.e., near the time of oviposition), turkey hens are inseminated commercially without regard to ovulatory stage.

Fertility patterns

The fertility of a flock of hens depends in large part on unknown factors within the females. Some flocks have excellent fertility with infrequent insemination; others require more frequent AI to attain and maintain moderate fertility levels. A general recommendation for insemination of commercial flocks is therefore hard to make. With the use of AI in turkeys, it is common to obtain 85 percent fertile eggs from a flock during their 25- to 28-week laying season. Other flocks will average only 60 percent fertile eggs. The reasons for such differences are not fully known. Poor results are sometimes attributable to poor insemination technique, but at other times some hens are simply incapable of producing fertile eggs. The causes of the latter condition are not known.

Semen diluents

Many diluents for avian semen have been developed, and some of these have been widely used with turkeys and other species. The composition of successfully used diluents differs greatly, precluding generalizations about the composition of an ideal poultry semen extender. The simplest diluent, used with some success, has been a 1 percent sodium chloride solution. Most of the diluents used for poultry semen are buffered mixtures of different salts, which may or may not contain a nutrient source. Dilution rates used with poultry semen tend to be low. One part of semen may be mixed with 1 to 4 parts of diluent. When insemination is practiced, the volume of diluted semen used must be adjusted to assure that the female receives an adequate number of sperm.

Traditionally, it has been recommended that chicken and turkey semen be used within 30 to 45 minutes after collection. With recent advances in semen diluents and semen-handling techniques, excellent fertility can be obtained from chicken and turkey semen stored unfrozen for 6, 12, 18, or even 24 hours. Storage conditions and diluents have differed markedly. With most diluents, avian sperm survive best when kept cool (5 to 15°C) and well oxygenated. Some diluents, however, allow preservation of chicken spermatozoa at 41°C for 24 hours. These advances make possible rather dramatic changes in turkey AI. Turkey toms have generally been housed near the hens for whom they provide semen. This often leads to inefficient utilization of the males' reproductive capacity. Some large turkey-breeding farms, with many flocks of hens, are now using central stud farms. Semen from a stud farm is collected, diluted, and handled to maximize its longevity. Semen can then be distributed to hen farms located several hours away. Maximum utilization of the sperm-producing capacity of rigorously chosen elite males allows greater investment in their housing. In turn, males housed in ideal conditions live longer, are healthier, and produce high-quality semen over a long period.

Frozen semen

Efforts toward long-term preservation of chicken and turkey semen are being made. Fertility levels of 90 percent or more have been obtained after AI of chicken semen that had been frozen in liquid nitrogen. In contrast, fertility levels of more than 10 percent are only rarely obtained with frozen turkey semen. The freezing of chicken semen is a multistepped and labor-intense procedure. In addition, only a small number of hens can be bred with an ejaculate of frozen chicken semen. These considerations make widespread commercial use of frozen chicken semen impractical. This technology can be used, however, to conserve selected valuable germ plasm.

EMBRYO DEVELOPMENT

Early development

At the time it is laid the fertile egg is already carrying an embryo at the gastrula stage of development. Fertilization has occurred some 24 to 26 hours earlier, and the nuclear region of the fertilized egg has undergone repeated division. After oviposition, embryonic development can be arrested by cooling of the egg. In fact, development can be arrested, started again by heating, rearrested by cooling, and later reinitiated and carried to completion by proper incubation. The percentage of embryos that live through the incubation period and hatch decreases with the length of time the eggs have been stored. Prolonged storage of sperm in the female tract also tends to decrease the viability of embryos that result from such sperm. Often the last several fertile eggs laid in a hen's fertile period die early in incubation, presumably because the sperm have grown stale or weak.

Synchronization of hatching

Under normal or optimal conditions of artificial incubation, the chicken embryo will hatch after 21 days and the turkey after 28 days. These are average figures; considerable variation in emergence time exists between individuals. In several species, such as the bobwhite quail and the *Coturnix* quail, which show only a few hours' variance in hatching time, the rate of embryonic development is influenced by signals transmitted from egg to egg. This communication synchronizes hatching time, a feature that might be of considerable survival value in the wild. In *Coturnix* quail, with an incubation period of about 17.5 days, and in bobwhite quail, with an incubation period of about 23 days, embryo development can be accelerated by a full day and the young will still hatch fully mature.

Incubation conditions

Many factors influence the development of avian embryos. Some are environmental, and others are associated with characteristics of the egg itself. The environmental factors most often considered are temperature, humidity, concentration of oxygen and carbon dioxide, and turning of the eggs. While there are rather wide ranges of these factors within which some eggs will hatch, the ranges over which maximum hatches can be obtained under artificial conditions are much narrower. Recommendations for these factors vary somewhat with the age of the embryo, the type of equipment, and the species. Incubation temperatures of about 37.5°C and relative humidity of about 60 percent have generally been considered satisfactory for most of the incubation period in chickens and turkeys. Incubation temperature is often reduced about 0.5°C and humidity increased to about 65 to 68 percent after chicken eggs have been incubated for 18 days and turkey eggs for 25 days. In these last few days of incubation the embryo's beak pierces the air cell and lung ventilation begins. The embryo then breaks through the shell and emerges. Much mortality can occur during these critical events if humidity is low and embryos become dry and stick to the shell membranes.

In the past these general incubation recommendations were considered adequate. With continued striving to obtain maximum reproductive efficiency, more critical appraisals of incubation conditions are being made. Eggs lose water throughout incubation. The amount of water lost is affected by the number of pores in the shell, pore diameter, pore length, and moisture level in the incubator. Shell characteristics vary a great deal from hen to hen, between strains of hens, and with the length of time hens have been laying. An 11.5 to 12.0 percent weight loss during the first 19 days of incubation in chickens or the first 25 days in turkeys is considered optimum. Uniform weight loss cannot be achieved if eggs that differ greatly in shell characteristics are incubated under the same relative humidity. Improved hatchability can be achieved if incubator moisture levels are altered on the basis of shell conductance of eggs being incubated. It may be impractical to do this in modern hatcheries, where many thousands of eggs from different flocks are incubated in the same incubators.

During the first 18 to 19 days of incubation in chickens and the first 25 to 26 days in turkeys, the exchange of oxygen and carbon dioxide between embryos and the atmosphere takes place via chorioallantoic blood vessels underlying the shell. Before lung ventilation the exchange of these gases depends on shell pore characteristics, as described above, and on partial pressure differences between the embryo's blood gases and the atmosphere. Traditionally, atmospheric oxygen levels have been considered adequate for eggs incubated at low altitudes, whereas the addition of oxygen to incubators at an altitude above 1500 meters is beneficial. Incubator carbon dioxide levels above 1 percent should be avoided.

Embryo mortality

Embryo mortality in chicken and turkey eggs tends to follow a well-defined pattern. The first peak in embryo mortality is noted at about 3 to 4 days of incubation, and the second occurs at about the time lung ventilation begins. The early mortality peak, which represents about 2 percent of broiler chicken eggs, is often attributed to chromosomal abnormalities. The late peak, which represents about 2.5 to 3.0 percent of broiler chicken eggs, may be due to failure of critical organ systems to mature synchronously at this important time in the embryo's life. These peaks are somewhat smaller in embryos of commercial egg-laying chickens and somewhat larger in turkeys. Mortality between these peaks is generally very low, totaling less than 0.5 percent of the fertile eggs. Nutrient deficiencies in the mother's diet can increase mortality during this time. Many specific genes that produce gross physical abnormalities and cause death of chicken and turkey embryos have been identified. Genetic selection for improved hatchability has eliminated most of these from commercial strains of poultry.

PARTHENOGENESIS

Parthenogenesis, the development of unfertilized eggs, is a well-documented phenomenon in turkeys. By genetic selection, the incidence of parthenogenesis has been increased to more than 40 percent in eggs of experimental flocks. Most of the parthenogenetic embryos die, but about 1 percent of them complete development and hatch. All of these have been diploid males, but testis weights are low and only 20 percent of them produce semen.

REFERENCES

Aiken, R.N.C. 1971. The oviduct. In D.J. Bell and B.M. Freeman, eds., *Physiology and Biochemistry of the Domestic Fowl*, vol. 3, Academic Press, London. Pp. 1237–89.

Cunningham, F.J., Wilson, S.C., Knight, P.G., and Gladwell, R.T. 1984. Chicken ovulation cycle. *J. Exp. Zool.* 232:485–94.

El Halawani, M.E., Fehrer, S., Hargis, B.M., and Porter, T.E. 1988. Incubation behavior in the domestic turkey: Physiological correlates. *CRC Crit. Rev. Poult. Biol.* 1:285–314.

Follett, B.K., and Robinson, J.E. 1980. Photoperiod and gonadotropin secretion in birds. *Prog. Reprod. Biol.* 5:39–61.

George, J.C. 1980. Structure and physiology of posterior lobe hormones. In A. Epple and M.H. Stetson, eds., *Avian Endocrinology.* Academic Press, New York. Pp. 85–115.

Gilbert, A.E. 1979. Female genital organs. In A.S. King and J. McLelland, eds., *Form and Function in Birds*, vol. 1, Academic Press, London. Pp. 237–360.

Goldsmith, A.R., and Follett, B.K. 1980. Pituitary hormones. In A. Epple and M.H. Stetson, eds., *Avian Endocrinology.* Academic Press, New York. Pp. 147–65.

Howarth, B. 1984. Maturation of spermatozoa and mechanism of fertilization. In F.J. Cunningham, P.E. Lake, and D. Hewitt, eds., *Reproductive Biology of Poultry.* Longman Group Ltd., Essex. Pp. 161–74.

Lake, P.E. 1971. The male in reproduction. In D.J. Bell and B.M. Freeman, eds., *Physiology and Biochemistry of the Domestic Fowl*, vol. 3. Academic Press, London. Pp. 1411–47.

Lake, P.E. 1984. The male in reproduction. In B.M. Freeman, ed., *Physiology and Biochemistry of the Fowl*, vol. 5, Academic Press, London. Pp. 381–405.

Lake, P.E. 1986. The history and future of cryopreservation of germ plasm. *Poultry Sci.* 65:1–15.

Lake, P.E., and Stewart, J.M. 1978. *Artificial Insemination in Poultry.* Bulletin 213, Ministry of Agriculture, Fisheries and Food, Her Majesty's Stationary Office, London.

Nicholls, T.J., Goldsmith, A.R., and Dawson, A. 1984. Photorefractoriness in European starlings: Associated hypothalamic changes and the involvement of thyroid hormones and prolactin. *J. Exp. Zool.* 232:567–72.

Robinson, F.E., Etches, R.J., Anderson-Langmuir, C.E., Burke, W.H., Cheng, K.W., Cunningham, F.J., Ishii, S., and Talbot, R.T. 1987. Steroidogenic relationships of gonadotropic hormones in the ovary of the hen (*Gallus domesticus*). *Gen. Comp. Endocrinol.* 69:455–66.

Scanes, C.G. 1984. Hypothalmic, pituitary and gonadal cycles. In F.J. Cunningham, P.E. Lake, and D. Hewitt, eds., *Reproductive Biology of Poultry.* Longman Group Ltd., Essex. Pp. 1–14.

Scanes, C.G., Stockell-Hartree, A., and Cunningham, F.J. 1984. The pituitary gland. In B.M. Freeman, ed., *Physiology and Biochemistry of the Fowl*, vol. 5, Academic Press, London. Pp. 40–84.

Sharp, P.J. 1980. Female reproduction. In A. Epple and M.H. Stetson, eds., *Avian Endocrinology.* Academic Press, New York. Pp. 435–54.

Solomon, S.E. 1983. Oviduct. In B.M. Freeman, ed., *Physiology and Biochemistry of the Fowl*, vol. 4, Academic Press, London. Pp. 379–417.

Wilson, S.C., and Cunningham, F.J. 1984. Endocrine control of the ovulation cycle. In F.J. Cunningham, P.E. Lake, and D. Hewitt, eds., *Reproductive Biology of Poultry.* Longman Group Ltd., Essex. Pp. 29–49.

PART **VII** | **NERVOUS SYSTEM, SPECIAL SENSES, SKELETAL MUSCLE, AND TEMPERATURE REGULATION**

CHAPTER **39**

Design and Basic Function of the Nervous System | by W. R. Klemm

GENERAL FUNCTION

Input information from sensory receptors into the nervous system results in output instructions to muscles and glands. The processing of input data often requires reference to memory and conscious evaluation before leading to decisions to alter behavior appropriate to the sensory input (Fig. 39.1).

Input information for the central nervous system (CNS) originates in the external environment as well as within the body (Chap. 41). This information is received by peripheral sensory organs such as the eye, ear, and nose. Other sensory receptors, such as those for pain, touch, pressure, and temperature are actual processes of nerve cells, either bare endings or highly specialized structures.

Changes in physical environment are transduced (converted to another form) by sensory receptors, and this transduction must be coded. The initial coding is achieved by a relatively slow change in voltage across the membrane of the receptor; the relation between stimulus intensity and magnitude of change in receptor voltage is often logarithmic.

For most sensory receptors the next stage of coding occurs as the slow receptor voltage change triggers the discharge of impulses—brief (about 1 millisecond) transmembrane voltage changes—that move from the receptor via the attached neuronal process into the CNS. Impulses code information in various ways: by latency between stimulus and impulse discharge, by the number of impulses in a burst, by the interval between and among impulses in a burst, or by rate of change in impulse frequency.

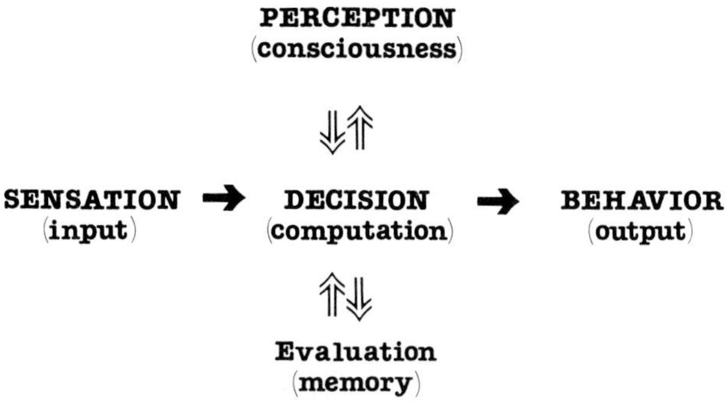

PERCEPTION (**consciousness**)

⇓⇑

SENSATION (**input**) ➔ **DECISION** (**computation**) ➔ **BEHAVIOR** (**output**)

⇑⇓

Evaluation (**memory**)

Figure 39.1. Sensory input (sensation) provides the basic information about an animal's environment to which it may need to respond. Then the nervous system engages in a group of processing reactions designed ultimately to arrive at a decision about the appropriate response. Decision making requires computation of the properties of the stimulus; this processing may or may not be conducted at the level of conscious perception. In addition, the stimulus is evaluated in terms of its biological significance, which typically requires reference to memory of past learned experiences; these, in turn, are evaluated in the current working memory. Once the appropriate response is determined, the nervous system issues its output in the form of patterns of glandular secretions and muscle contraction (behavior).

The next stage of information transfer, or processing, occurs when the impulses from receptors reach other neurons (Chap. 40). The message transfer begins with the release of chemical secretions (neurotransmitters) that diffuse across the intercellular gap (the synapse) to react with the membrane of the neuron that contacts the receptor. The neurotransmitter then causes a relatively slow change in transmembrane voltage, somewhat analogous to the change that stimuli induce in sensory receptor organs. Finally, this slow voltage change, if of the right polarity, may trigger the neuron to discharge impulses to the next neurons in line or to the effector organs (glands and muscles). The slow voltage change must reach a certain magnitude, or threshold, before impulses can be triggered. This scheme allows a great deal of processing to occur at this level. Because a given neuron receives information from as many as a thousand other neurons, the slow voltage changes contributed by each can interact, adding or subtracting to determine whether threshold for impulse discharge is reached.

Input information may lead almost directly to output instructions; such simple function is usually confined to simple reflexes in the spinal cord, such as the knee jerk, in which the neuron carrying sensory input connects directly to the output (or motor) neuron (Chap. 40). Even at this level, however, processing still occurs in the sensory receptor's membrane voltage, in the chemical release in the synapse, in the membrane voltage of the motoneuron, and even at the neuromuscular junction.

More commonly, many nerve cells must process input signals before they generate output signals. For example, the routing of sensory impulses is regulated by inherited functional pathways for such signals and their complex interconnections. Also, the brain compares incoming information with stored information of previous experiences, called memory, before processing and generating output signals; often this process occurs consciously (Chap. 48).

ORGANIZATIONAL PRINCIPLES

Basic modes of operation

Nerve cells can have only two main actions on other nerve cells: excitatory or inhibitory. Because neurons are organized into networks, excitatory and inhibitory effects can be orchestrated into complex patterns of information flow and processing and flow. Spinal reflexes have the simplest organization (see Chap. 40). A reflex is a specific, usually stereotyped response to stimulation. Most reflexes are genetically determined by the anatomical organization of neurons that mediate the reflex. For example, in the withdrawal reflex in which a dog withdraws its foot in response to toe pinch, each activated sensory neuron sends input into the spinal cord that automatically relays excitation back into nerves that excite muscles of that leg. Some reflexes may also have inhibitory components. In the flexion reflex, for example, sensory input excites some neurons in the cord that inhibit the antagonists (extensors) of the flexor muscles of that limb. This organization of neurons, called *reciprocal innervation,* is found in many kinds of reflexes.

Another basic mode of nervous system operation is mutual regulation, where two pools of neurons reciprocally affect the same function or behavior. In a sense, this organization provides checks and balances that regulate functions within reasonable limits. Some of the functions and behaviors that are regulated in this way are respiration, blood pressure, heart rate, various visceral secretions and movements, temperature control, eating, drinking, sleep, and approach and avoidance drives. Paired control centers are often reciprocally inhibitory, but in some cases, such as sleep and approach-avoidance centers, the mutual regulation may be more complex.

In a neural network, excitation, inhibition, reflex action, and mutual regulation all operate to control a behavioral act (Fig. 39.2).

Mechanisms of information processing

While there are many elegant and mathematical ways of explaining information processing, at the neuronal level it consists of the specific chemical and physical transformations that occur when the nervous system detects, analyzes, and responds to changes in environment. That analysis may involve filtering or averaging of information so that some is lost. Information may be transformed or erased, especially when contrasted and compared with the stored information that is called *memory*. Ultimately, information may be added to existing memory or may emerge from the analysis process in the form of output for appropriate operation of glands and muscles.

Processing reactions take place at all levels of the nervous system, from the coding in sensory receptors, to synaptic reactions and associated patterns of impulse generation, to the routing through neuronal networks, to profuse interactions of widespread neuronal subsystems.

Many interesting analogies can be drawn between certain principles of computer and engineering technology and information-processing phenomena in the nervous system. Such properties as triggering, gating, switching, and synchronizing occur in the nervous system. Also observable are amplitude discrimination, filtering, amplification, linear-to-logarithmic signal transformation, complex waveform generation, and frequency modulation. Such basic operations occur as counting, averaging, integration, differentiation, sign inversion, correlation, coincidence detection, delay, phase, shift, and interval measurement.

Coding of sensory input

A sense organ generally codes the quantity of information that it receives in terms of the magnitude of the change in its membrane potential (generator potential); this change in potential is, in turn, associated with a corresponding change in impulse discharge rate (Chap. 41). With continued stimulation, most sense organs tend to adapt or habituate; that is, their stimulus-induced change in impulse rate tends to decrease with time.

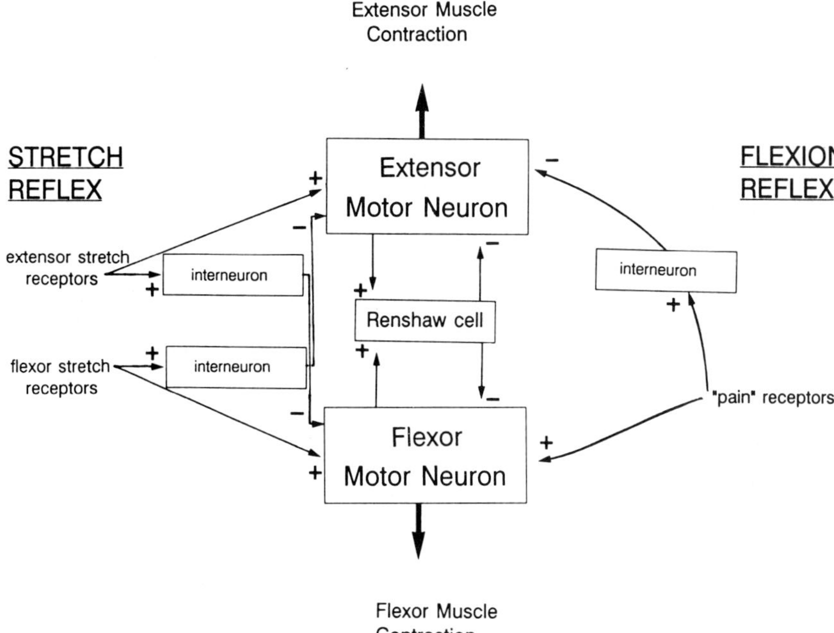

Figure 39.2. Example of mutual regulation in neuronal networks by the basic processes of excitation and inhibition. Examples are taken from the mechanisms of the stretch reflex (where a muscle reflexly contracts when it is stretched) and the flexion reflex (where a muscle reflexly contracts in response to painful stimuli). When stretch receptors in an extensor muscle are excited by stretch (see Chaps. 40 and 41), the appropriate extensor motor neuron causes contraction of that extensor muscle. Then, via inhibitory interneurons, the antagonistic flexor muscle is inhibited so that a limb, for example, achieves extension. Also, concurrently, an interneuron pool of Renshaw cells, is excited, which in turn inhibits and shuts off the activity of the extensor motor neuron, so that extension is not excessive. Comparable phenomena occur when stretch receptors in flexor muscles are activated by stretch. In flexion reflex phenomena, painful stimuli cause a withdrawal of the affected body region. In limbs, for example, flexors are directly excited to contract, while at the same time, via an inhibitory interneuronal pool, the extensors are inhibited.

Action-potential patterns

Many neurons discharge impulses continually, and information is carried in some incompletely understood way by changes in the rate of discharge and/or the distribution of patterns of intervals between and among impulses.

Other neurons, particularly if they are sensory or motor, may have some rather specific response patterns to an input stimulus: (1) *phasic-tonic*, in which an initial high rate decreases as accommodation develops to continued stimulation, (2) *on*, in which the initial response stops abruptly in response to a simultaneously induced inhibitory processes, (3) *off*, in which presence of the stimulus first causes inhibition, followed by a delayed or rebound excitation, and (4) *serial on*, in which recurrent inhibition can develop oscillatory discharge.

Relation of unit activity to population (ensemble) activity

Discharge of impulses in any given neuron cannot possibly, by itself, convey much meaningful information. For example, the subjective impression of a visual scene is not derived from the discharge pattern of a single visual cortex neuron, especially since that neuron probably discharges in the perception of various other scenes or even in the absence of a scene. In other words, neuronal ensembles have gestalt properties (properties of the whole that do not exist in and cannot be summed from the parts). This gestalt principle probably also applies to the operations of systems of several other kinds of neuronal ensemble. For example, sleep may be explained by a gestalt view of the function of several populations of neurons that are critical to sleep but are widely scattered in different parts of the brain (Chap. 48).

Synaptic processing

Once information about stimuli enters the CNS, chemical and electrical changes in the synapses provide enormous capacity for processing that information as it passes from neuron to neuron. Release of the chemical transmitter can produce a graded change in the membrane voltage of the postsynaptic neuron. If the polarity of that potential is in the right direction, the cell becomes excited and begins to discharge impulses; this change is called an excitatory postsynaptic potential (EPSP) (see Chap. 40). Cells are inhibited if the voltage change is of the opposite polarity, a so-called inhibitory postsynaptic potential (IPSP). Because the discharge threshold across a synapse is a function of the presynaptic volleys that act upon it, and because a given neuron may receive branches from many axons, the passage of impulses in a network of such synapses can be highly varied. The subsequent change in stimulation threshold of the postsynaptic membrane can be enhanced or inhibited, depending on the transmitter chemical involved and the ion permeabilities. Thus the synapse acts as a decision point at which information converges, and is modified by algebraic processing of EPSPs and IPSPs (Fig. 39.3). In addition to the IPSP inhibitory mechanism, there is a presynaptic kind of inhibition that involves either a hyperpolarization of the inhibited axon or a persistent depolarization; whether it is the former or the latter depends on the specific neurons involved.

When inhibition occurs at specific points in an interac-

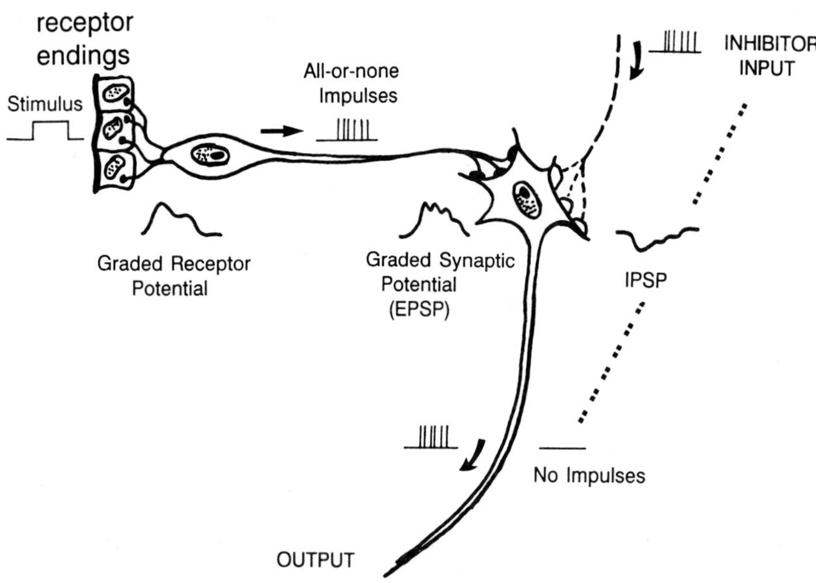

Figure 39.3. Illustration of how processing occurs in the synapse, compared with processing in sensory receptors. Excitatory environmental stimuli produce a graded change in membrane potential of sensory organs, which, if large enough, triggers the discharge of all-or-none impulses that are conducted into the central nervous system. At synaptic junctions, postsynaptic neurons develop graded changes in membrane potential; if the shift is depolarizing (EPSP), it may reach the threshold required for discharging impulses. At the same time there may be other inhibitory influences (IPSP) that hyperpolarize the postsynaptic cell, algebraically antagonizing the excitatory influence.

tive circuit of neurons (Fig. 39.4), it can act as a gate to route information flow. In circuits where the inhibition is fed back into the input neurons, a synchronization of the activity of many neurons can occur; this process is believed to underlie the production of large, rhythmic, electroencephalographic (EEG) waves, such as alpha waves (8 to 12/s) from the visual cortex of humans and θ waves (4 to 7/s) from the hippocampus of mammals.

Coding for the quality of a stimulus depends largely on how neurons are organized into networks of the pathways through which nerve impulses are propagated. Some of these paths are "hard-wired," built-in under genetic control during embryonic development. The simplest network is the spinal reflex arc (one kind was illustrated in Fig. 39.2). Information arising from sensory receptors in the skin flows directly back to contract muscles from that area. In a flexion reflex, for example, strong stimulation causes withdrawal of the stimulated limb, and information is usually interpreted as pain at that limb because of the hard-wired circuitry. Similarly, animals see because axons from the retina propagate impulses to a specific zone of neurons in the cortex at the back of the brain. Sound is not seen, for example, because auditory receptors do not send impulses to the visual receiving areas of the brain.

At least four basic types of circuit are found in the CNS of

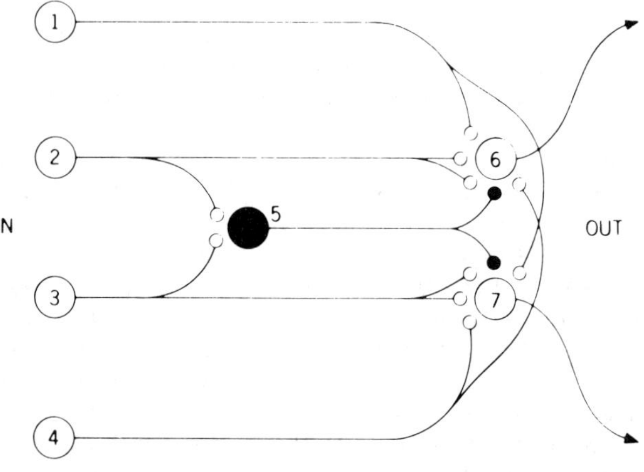

INPUT NEURONS ACTIVATED	OUTPUT NEURONS ACTIVATED			
	NONE	6 ONLY	7 ONLY	6 AND 7
1	X			
1&2		X		
1&3			X	
1&4				X
2		X		
2&3	X			
2&4		X		
3			X	
3&4			X	
4	X			

Figure 39.4. (*Top*) Pool of excitatory neurons and an inhibitory neuron (solid circle), illustrating the effect of circuit design and threshold for excitation on routing of information. Assume that impulses begin in the four input neurons on the left and that a net of at least two excitatory terminals must be active to release enough transmitter chemical to reach the threshold for exciting subsequent neurons. Input from neuron 2, for instance, would excite neuron 6 because two axon terminals are active. Input from 2 and 3, however, would not have an output because the inhibitory neuron would also be activated, and its inhibitory transmitter would cancel part of the effect of the two active excitatory terminals at 6 and 7. Note from the summary table (*bottom*) that many output possibilities exist. Still further complexity could be achieved, as it is in brain circuits, by drawing in branches that feed back excitatory or inhibitory effect on other neurons in the circuit. (From W.R. Klemm, *Science, The Brain, and Our Future*, Bobbs-Merrill, Indianapolis; copyright 1972 by the Regents of the University of Colorado.)

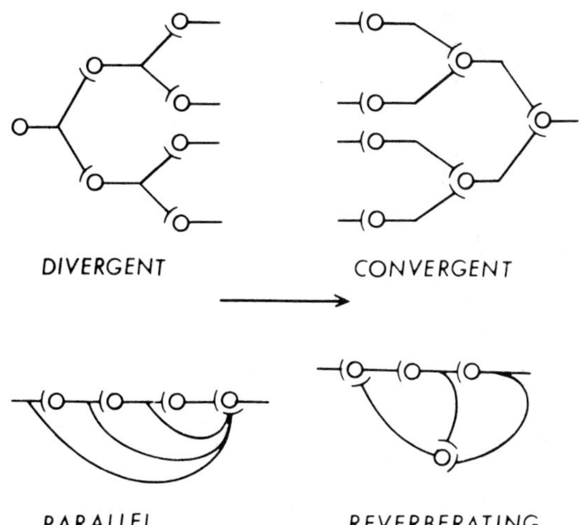

Figure 39.5. Common types of circuits in the nervous system. Arrow indicates direction of impulse propagation. (Modified from Guyton 1964, *Function of the Human Body*, 2d ed., W.B. Saunders, Philadelphia.)

mammals: divergent, convergent, parallel, and reverberating (Fig. 39.5).

In a divergent circuit, one neuron ultimately affects many neurons. A typical example of such circuitry is found in certain nerves in the cortex that initiate voluntary motor activity. Connections of a given cortical cell fan out so that an initial impulse in the brain results in many impulses reaching many muscle fiber units.

A convergent circuit has the reverse arrangement: impulses from many nerves ultimately impinge on a single neuron. This enables a neuron to receive information from a wide range of receptors. The spinal cord provides an example: a neuron may receive sensory input from the skin and from viscera (see Chap. 41).

The parallel circuit provides for special functions that are not obtainable in the first two circuits: a single impulse can initiate a series of impulses in other neurons. Those impulses that must cross synapses before reaching the target are delayed because synaptic transmission is slower than axonal transmission. Thus the arrival of impulses at the target is protracted but not self-perpetuating.

The fourth type of circuit not only provides for the protracted receipt of impulses at the target but also is self-perpetuating, and electrical disturbances in the circuit can be continuous. One input impulse can drive an oscillatory network in which impulses continually circulate around the circuit. Two obvious examples of this type of circuit are in the nervous control of respiration (see Chap. 13) and in the cycling of impulses between the cerebral cortex and certain subcortical centers.

Very sophisticated discrimination and evaluation of stimulus information can occur when networks are engaged that are not hard-wired but, rather, can change their functional organization in response to inputs.

Processing in the cerebral cortex

Beyond the cell level, mechanisms of information processing are poorly understood. Perhaps most is known about processing in the visual system (Chap. 42). Two rules seem evident: (1) processing becomes more sophisticated as the sensory input is passed from the periphery to the visual cortex and (2) neurons in different cortical levels are responsive to different attributes of visual stimuli. As examples, neurons in the retina function mainly to detect patterns of light, with comparatively minor capability to discriminate orientation of light stimulus. But progressive capability to detect orientation of light patterns occurs in the lateral geniculate body of the thalamus and visual cortex; here a given cell may respond to only one orientation of light stimulus. Within the cortex, there is further specialization, in that some cells respond to various colors while others respond to moving light patterns.

Studies of neuronal responses to visual stimuli have indicated that the visual cortex is functionally organized into adjacent columns of about 1 to 2 mm^2 each. How these individual processing units are orchestrated to produce integrated analysis of a visual scene is not known, but the units must be coupled in some way.

The visual system contains different kinds of feature-detector neurons. In the retina there are some neurons that respond if the edge of an object is lighter or darker than the background; some retinal cells will discharge to a moving edge, while others discharge in response to a general reduction in brightness.

Similar divisions of labor exist among neurons in the visual cortex. In the primary visual cortex of cats, many neurons respond to simple line stimuli such as light slits, dark bars, and edges. The selectivity of the responses varies with the depth from the cortical surface. The orientation of the line stimuli greatly influences which neurons will discharge.

A popular alternative explanation of these bar- and edge-responsive cells is that they merely indicate that the brain is breaking down a complex visual scene into its individual spatial frequencies (spatial frequency is analogous to temporal frequency). It does seem that the low spatial-frequency content (i.e., broad or wide parts of the scene) carries information about the basic nature of objects, while high spatial-frequency content conveys the details.

The modern theory for the processing of visual information is that separate operations, called channels, process a given restricted range of spatial frequencies. Describing a visual scene in terms of spatial-frequency content is convenient because one can mathematically decompose and reconstruct the image. The image of a dog, for example, consists of a mixture of a few low spatial frequencies that make up the gross outline and many high spatial frequencies that create the detail of small parts of the body. Implications of this concept of vision include the idea that the spatial-frequency channels of the visual cortex actually function as filters for distinguishing components of an object and for separating one object from another in the "mind's eye" (see Fig. 49.2).

Relative localization of function

There are many examples of specific functions being governed by an anatomically defined pool of neurons (centers). Examples include specific reflexes, arousal, sleep, dreaming, reward and aversive responses, regulation of viscera, and specific sensory and motor functions of the neocortex.

As long ago as 1870, stimulation of certain cortical areas was known to cause contractions of certain muscles. The location for visual recognition was shown in 1881 to be in the occipital cortex. Various studies in humans have revealed that higher cerebral functions (speech, music, mathematics, and so on) are segregated into one hemisphere or the other. Such asymmetrical function in animals is generally not looked for, but recent studies in monkeys show that they process photographs of monkey faces most effectively in the right hemisphere, while the left hemisphere operates best on tilted lines.

Various other functions are also localized: respiratory and cardiovascular reflex control (brain stem); pituitary control (hypothalamus); control of various homeostatic functions such as body temperature, thirst, hunger, and water balance (hypothalamus); memory consolidation (hippocampus); and motor coordination (cerebellum). Even single neurons can have very specific functions: there are visual cortex cells so specialized that they only "look at" edges or at corners, and then only at certain angles.

Computational maps

Some neural computations occur in maps—arrays of neurons in which the tuning of neighboring neurons for a particular parameter value varies predictably. Each such array is tuned somewhat differently, and they operate on inputs in parallel. The information represented in such maps is transformed almost instantly into a place-coded (topographic) probability distribution. Among the map systems that have been discovered are those for visual line orientation and direction of motion, auditory maps of amplitude and time interval, and motor maps of movements.

The tuning of individual neurons for mapped parameter values is broad relative to the range of the map. Thus, any given stimulus of the right type tends to activate neurons throughout the map, but the locations of peak activity code the precise information about the mapped parameter.

The antilocalization view

Despite these many demonstrations of localized function, an antilocalization view can also be argued. This view holds that the brain has interdependent parts. There is, for example, a certain amount of plasticity in the nervous system; damage to one part may be at least partially compensated for by other parts. Moreover, some functions are not clearly localized; for example, attempts to disrupt memory of learned tasks in rats with lesions of various parts of the cortex revealed that the critical factor was how much cortex was destroyed, not where the lesion was.

One reason for the confusion about localization versus distributed processing is that the brain parts are so highly interconnected. The brain stem and subcortical structures in the telencephalon have extensive projections to the cerebral cortex. In general, there are reciprocal projections back to subcortical structures, but two major neurotransmitter systems, using norepinephrine and acetylcholine, supply input without receiving projections back from the cortex. The significance of such connections may be that where the connections are reciprocal, the cortex has feedback control over its sources of input, whereas those inputs without reciprocal connections can modulate cortical function more independently.

Damage to brain tissue creates an imbalance in a variety of functions, some of which may be reflected in functions that are not normally attributable to the damaged area. In some cases, the postlesion deficit is partially due to abrupt imposition of inhibitory influences, and these influences can be removed by judicious placement of other lesions. Although these ideas have potential relevance for veterinary medicine, no specific procedures have been developed for creating therapeutic lesions.

The best understanding of the brain comes from reconciliation of the apparent contradictions between the localization and antilocalization viewpoints. There is truth to both positions, and they are not mutually exclusive. These issues obviously have implications for clinical management of animals with brain lesions. If one holds too strongly to the localization view, therapeutic options become very limited. The antilocalization view could stimulate research into experimental evaluation of admixtures of special training exercises and judicious application of deliberate, multistage creation of lesions.

Hierarchical control and interdependence

Invertebrates such as lobsters, gastropods, and crayfish have specific groupings of neurons that reflexly elicit escape swimming. These circuits have identifiable sensory neurons, interneurons, and motoneurons, as well as "command" neurons that activate the entire network's output and achieve a stereotyped and relatively complete repertoire of behavior.

The extent to which such "preprogrammed" command-neuron circuitry exists in mammals is not known, but such circuitry probably does exist in masked form because of the extensive interaction with other, less stereotypically organized neurons and circuits. The best-known examples of such command circuits in mammals involve systems that regulate hand and eye movements.

When considering the gross organization of more advanced nervous systems, one is tempted to view them as a hierarchy of subsystems that the cerebral cortex "supervises." In humans, for instance, neurons in the spinal cord can carry out mundane control functions for their respective body segment while the cortical neurons are "free to think higher thoughts." However, the assignment of rank order to the spinal cord and subsystems in the brain is not as obvious as it may seem. Although the part of the brain that provides intelligence, the neocortex, ranks above the reflex systems in the brain stem and spinal cord, there are practical limits on the degree of control exerted by the neocortex. If control were absolute, for example, animals would not succumb to the dizziness and ataxia associated with motion sickness and the vestibular system of the brain stem. Animals would be able to suppress the pain that is mediated in the thalamus. They could stave off sleep indefinitely by keeping the reticular activating system active.

It thus seems more reasonable to regard the nervous system as a hierarchy of semiautonomous subsystems whose rank order is variable; any subsystem may take part in many types of interrelationship. Whichever subsystem happens to dominate a situation, each subsystem is independent only to a certain extent, being subordinate to the unit above it and modulated by the inputs from its own subordinate subsystems. This design feature of the mammalian nervous system provides maximum flexibility and is probably the basis for the brain's marvelous effectiveness.

Interaction with hormonal systems

The nervous system is the body's chief coordinating agency, exerting control over almost all functions; for example, the endocrine system, which regulates metabolism and growth, is not only controlled by the nervous system but also is, to a large extent, part of it. One part of the brain, the hypothalamus, releases secretions that regulate the master endocrine gland, the pituitary. The fact that hormones from the endocrine system also act upon the nervous system suggests that it is a control system with feedback not only from the impulse-conducting nerve pathways but also from hormones. The interrelations of neural and hormonal systems are summarized in Fig. 39.6.

Hormone-feedback effects are often mediated in the hypothalamus by circulating hormones. Hormones have specific receptor-binding sites in the hypothalamus, and such binding produces both physiological and behavioral consequences. For example, injection of estrogen directly into the hypothalamus of a cat whose ovaries have been removed can restore sexual behavior and even induce nymphomania. (Because this treatment does not immediately affect the ovary or uterus, it indicates a direct central effect.) Another principle that this example illustrates is that the level of hormone may alter the probability and intensity of the associated behavior but does not alter its *form*.

Besides affecting pituitary and adrenal function, glucocorticoids have important direct effects on neural processes that affect behavior. Treatment of sick animals with glucocorticoids often makes them seem to feel better. Adrenocorticotropic hormone (ACTH), glucocorticoids, and even certain peptide fragments of ACTH that have no endocrine function have distinct but poorly understood influences on learning and various behaviors.

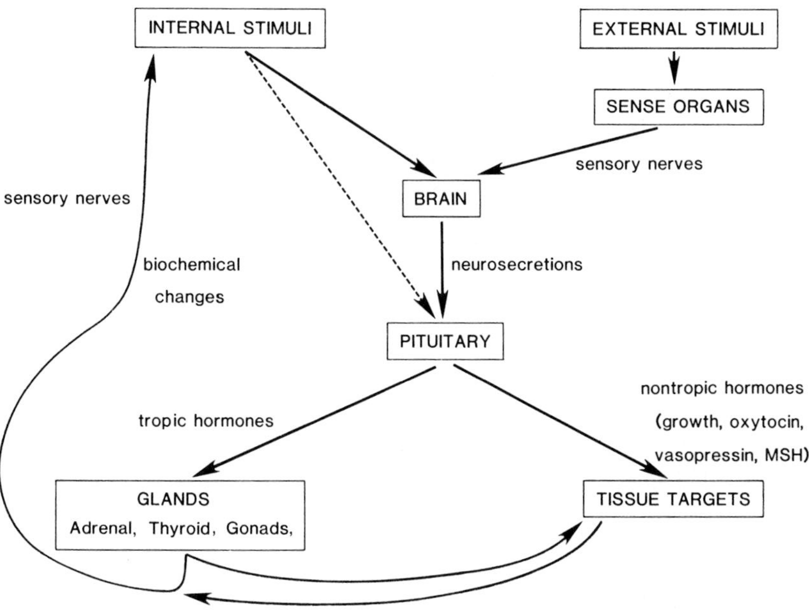

Figure 39.6. Diagram of the interrelations among various endocrine organs and the nervous system. The brain, particularly the hypothalamus and associated limbic system structures, integrates both internal and external stimuli and regulates the pituitary, which in turn governs function of other major endocrine glands via tropic hormones and which has direct actions governing such functions as growth and fluid balance. Feedback information from glands and target tissues is received in the form of biochemical and neuronal messages: these messages provide the internal stimuli that influence the brain and the hypothalamus in their regulatory control. MSH, melanocyte-stimulating hormone.

CELLS OF THE NERVOUS SYSTEM

Neurons

The neuron, the basic unit of the nervous system, consists of a cell body with a nucleus and the usual organelles, and often with a long process called an axon (Fig. 39.7).

Although neurons appear in many forms (Fig. 39.7), and many atypical forms occur, they are classified by the number and arrangement of their processes.

Unipolar cells, having a single process, are rare in higher animals. They are somewhat more common in lower vertebrates and invertebrates. The physiological relation of the single process to the cell body is not clear.

Bipolar cells have two processes, one axon and one dendrite. In vertebrates these cells are well exemplified in the retina by sensory cells with a short axon and dendrite. Similar cells occur elsewhere. In higher vertebrates the nerve cells in spinal nerve ganglia are embryologically bipolar. The two processes later fuse near the cell body into one process with a T-shaped appearance. One branch becomes an axis cylinder of a peripheral afferent nerve fiber; the other branch passes into the CNS by way of the dorsal root of a spinal nerve. Although both branches are anatomically axons, the peripheral branch is physiologically a dendrite that conducts impulses centrally.

Multipolar cells have numerous branching dendrites and an axon, which may be long or short. Typical multipolar cells with long axons are the motor nerve cells (motoneurons) in the ventral gray column of the spinal cord. The axons of these neurons emerge from the CNS in spinal nerves to become peripheral motor nerve fibers. The axons of other multipolar cells, instead of leaving the gray matter, are very short and break up into numerous branches in the vicinity of the cell body. By means of these cells, an afferent neuron may be placed into relation with a great many motor neurons. They are designated as internuncial neurons or interneurons.

Neuron organelles function similarly to those of any cell: chromosomes carry "ancestral wisdom," mitochondria regulate energy supply, microsomal particles control biochemical synthesis, and cell membranes surround the cytoplasm and regulate transport of solutes. Mature neurons are unusual also in that they normally do not divide. Why mature neurons do not divide is unknown, but the reason may be related to one or more of the other unusual features of neurons: (1) they express a higher fraction of the genome than other cells, (2) the ribonucleic acid is clustered as "Nissl substance" on endoplasmic reticulum, (3) they are closely invested by supporting cells (glia), (4) they continuously exhibit pulsatile membrane voltage changes and associated ionic fluxes, and (5) they have an extensive cytoskeleton of tubules and filaments for transporting chemicals throughout an extensive proliferation of protoplasmic processes. Finally, a special pigment, lipofuscin, accumulates in the cytoplasm as the neuron ages or if its mitochondria or lysosomes are damaged.

Axons terminate in branches that interact with branches of other neurons. These *synaptic* contacts permit impulse transmission between neurons, typically from the axonal

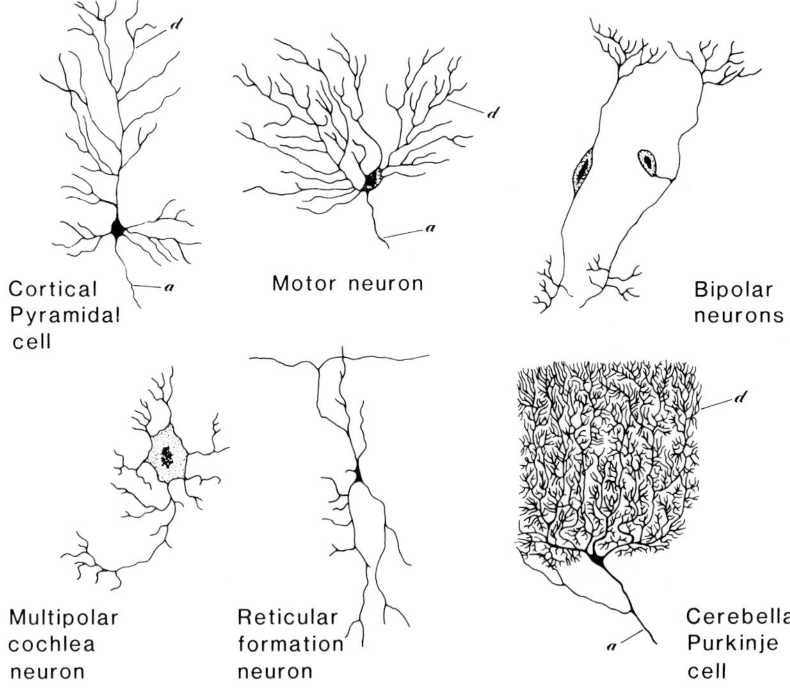

Figure 39.7. Different structural types of neurons. Despite their differences in shape and function, all neurons have in common dendrite (d) branches, which receive input from other neurons, and an axon (a), which carries impulse output away from the cell body. The axon of many neurons is enclosed in a sheath of membranes (myelin) of glia cells (not shown). Axons of some neurons may project for much longer distances than indicated (e.g., the full length of a leg).

branches of one neuron to the short dendrites of an adjacent neuron body. The active region of a synaptic membrane is presumed to be the isolated dark patches near the membrane, which are seen in electron micrographs (see Chap. 40).

The cell synthesizes many chemicals that are constantly transported to the periphery, as was initially demonstrated in experiments in which ligation of an axon caused bulging on the side nearest the cell body. Simple diffusion and hydrostatic gradients alone cannot account for this transport; time-lapse photographs have indicated that peristaltic motions of axons may assist in propelling material down the axon. The rate of transport depends on the nature of transported materials. Some chemicals move slowly, about 1 to 6 mm/day, perhaps being oriented in their direction of flow along the 10 nm (diameter) neurofibrils that are parallel to the long axis of the axon. Also in the same axis are the neurotubules of about 24 nm, which are considered transport ducts for the chemicals that have been observed to move at such very fast rates as 100 to 1000 mm/day.

The term *nerve* signifies a group of fibers made up of the processes of many neurons, closely enveloped in tough connective tissue, which connects the brain with the periphery. Nerve cell bodies that are grouped in clusters in the brain and spinal cord are sometimes called *nuclei*. Some nuclei also occur outside the brain and spinal cord; these have connective tissue sheaths and are called *ganglia*.

Neuronal number

The total number of neurons in the nervous system ranges from a few hundred in primitive invertebrates to about 30 million in advanced invertebrates, such as the octopus, to well over 200 billion for large mammals, such as whales and elephants. Estimates for the human brain are on the order of 85 billion, and each neuron may have as many as 1000 synaptic contacts. Number alone does not determine intellect, unless one is willing to concede that elephants and whales are smarter than humans. Whales and elephants also do not have the extensive motor capabilities and behavioral repertoire of humans, or even of domestic animals such as dogs and cats.

Brain weight is proportional to body weight, but the relationship is a power function of body weight that ranges widely, from 0.1 to 0.8. It is generally true, however, that phyla whose members have larger brains and more neurons respond to environmental change with a greater range and versatility of behavior.

Special neuronal functions

Generation of electricity

The nervous system's electrical activity is the most conspicuous aspect of nervous tissue function. Electrical activity arises from the fact that ions distribute differentially on either side of the cell membrane. Flow of ions across neuronal membrane is regulated by so-called ion channels, which are proteins that undergo conformational changes to open and close a pathway selectively for a specific ion to flow down its electrochemical gradient (see Chap. 41).

Electrophysiological data are usually expressed as voltage, or the potential force generated by the separation of electrically charged ions. The most fundamental biological potential is the steady cell voltage that exists between the inside and the outside of the resting or unstimulated neuron (see Chap. 40).

Activity in adjacent neurons alters the direction and magnitude of this polarization of postsynaptic neurons. If the membrane polarity tends to reverse to the extent of achieving a critical threshold level of depolarization, a nerve impulse is discharged. Such membrane potential changes are called postsynaptic potentials. A neuron receives not only excitatory postsynaptic input but often also inhibitory (hyperpolarizing) input, which can be added to determine the net level of polarization and excitability.

Electrodes placed in the brain or on the scalp record a composite sum of the voltages caused by extracellular currents near the electrodes, compounded from postsynaptic voltages, impulses, and even glial cell depolarizations. This sum of electrical activity is the EEG, which has been a useful diagnostic tool in human medicine for years and is also being used in veterinary medicine. The EEG is useful in the diagnosis and prognosis of animal patients with brain damage; the diagnostic capabilities, however, are usually not pathognomonic.

Secretion of chemicals

The electrical impulse current usually is unable to influence the postsynaptic neuron directly. The electrical disturbance releases a chemical transmitter from the presynaptic neuron, which diffuses across the synapse, reacts with molecular receptors on the postsynaptic membrane, and initiates a new electrical disturbance in the neuron (or target muscle or gland). This neurochemical transducer system includes means for synthesizing, storing, and releasing the transmitter. Moreover, the system can destroy the released transmitter, thus ensuring only transient activation of postsynaptic membranes. Some neurons, instead of releasing an excitatory transmitter, release a substance that actually *inhibits* postsynaptic activation. Some neurosecretions are hormones (i.e., transported in the blood)—for example, epinephrine, which is released from modified neurons in the adrenal medulla (see Chaps. 34 and 46).

Growth

Neurons stop dividing shortly after birth, but their axons and dendrites grow extensively during the period before adulthood. Some scientists believe that some growth occurs also in the adult animal. Maturation of behavior parallels proliferation of neuronal processes; presumably this growth creates new contact areas among neurons and new information-processing networks.

One aspect of growth has particular medical importance. Since the brain grows at a much faster rate than the body, its growth depends critically on a proper supply of nutrients; deficiencies during the growing stage can cause permanent damage. Animal experiments also indicate that sensory and learning experiences help stimulate neuronal and glial growth.

Growth of axonal processes is especially important in regenerating cut nerves (Chap. 40). When regeneration occurs, the original innervation sites are preferentially reinnervated; some believe that this is evidence of some kind of chemical cuing that is provided by the target sites to guide the direction of regrowth. Commonly, however, regeneration of nerves is thwarted because the axonal sprouts fail to align with the original glial sheaths (Chap. 40).

There is no reliable therapy for promoting reinnervation in the brain, although systemically injected gangliosides reportedly promote reinnervation (see "Biochemistry," this chapter). Present therapy must rely on the use of highly structured and intensive learning situations. To a limited degree, the brain can reorganize itself so that the new circuits are used to compensate for damage. The extent to which recovery from damage can occur varies with the locus of the damage and the extent of topographic mapping involved. More recovery can be expected if the neuronal damage occurred in gradual and successive stages than if it occurred all at once.

One of the more interesting features of embryogenesis is the death of certain structures that are genetically programmed (e.g., regression of the tail in amphibian metamorphosis). In addition, restrictive conditions at the target area for axonal growth cause a sporadic scattering of dying neurons as well as more localized areas of dying neuron clusters. Sometimes, in places where many neurons are "competing" to innervate a given restricted target, as many as 50 percent of the neurons will die. It is not clear what these cells are competing for, because sometimes there is sufficient space. One idea is that the competition is for finite amounts of a trophic chemical. One chemical that has been isolated from nerve tissue is a protein known as *nerve growth factor* (NGF), because it promotes growth and functional differentiation of neurons. NGF can also reduce or prevent normal cell death during embryogenesis.

Exogenous administration of NGF seems to inhibit naturally occurring cell death and to promote survival of neurons with cut axons. The active component of NGF consists of two similar 118–amino acid polypeptides with a sequence that has some similarities to insulin. The NGF gene has recently been mapped in humans and some other species. Cloning of the gene will make possible medical use of NGF.

Neurons may die when deprived of their afferent input, and some systemic degenerative disease of the nervous system may reflect this process. The mechanism is not known, but one recent study has shown that this secondary cell death in cells that no longer receive inputs from their normal neurotransmitter (gamma-aminobutyric acid, GABA) can be prevented if the tissue is externally supplied with GABA.

Functional differences among neurons

Even among neurons that are anatomically similar, functional differences exist. Chemicals have different effects on different parts of the nervous system. Carbon disulfide exerts its greatest effect in destroying a portion of the brain involved in motor functions (the caudate nucleus). Vitamin deficiencies initiate degenerations in specific portions of the nervous system. Some neurons are especially sensitive to such factors as the osmotic balance in surrounding fluid, others to carbon dioxide concentrations, others to blood glucose, and still others to hormones.

Differences among nerve cells are illustrated by the different chemical neurohumors released by various neurons. Another, more subtle, indication of chemical differences among neurons is in the specificities exhibited during development and regeneration of cut nerves. During embryonic growth, neuronal processes grow and somehow "recognize" their appropriate targets so that a final, appropriate connection is made and growth stops.

Glia cells

The connective tissue cells of the brain are called *glia cells*, or *neuroglia*. Depending on the counting technique used, they outnumber neurons as much as tenfold. The dense packing of so many neurons and the even more numerous glia causes nervous tissue to have less extracellular space than other tissue. Neuroglia are considered to interact with neurons in a supportive and symbiotic way. Like neurons, glia are metabolically quite active.

Glia form loose ensheathments around neurons, except when myelin is formed by the systematic spiralization and compaction of glial cytoplasmic processes (Fig. 39.8). Cells that form myelin in peripheral nerves are called *Schwann cells*. The myelin-forming cells in the CNS are called *oligodendrocytes*. The cytoplasm and membrane of both these cells wrap around neuronal processes; the junctions between adjacent glia cells form the nodes of Ranvier, which are relatively uninsulated patches of neuronal membrane (Fig. 39.9). Because nerve impulses can skip from node to node, impulse conduction is much faster in myelinated nerves (see Chap. 40). Another consequence of glial ensheathment is that the extremely sensitive neuronal membranes are more or less shielded from straying neurotransmitters, neurohumors, and toxins.

Another very common type of glia cell is the astrocyte, which has cytoplasmic processes, many of which attach to blood vessels to help form the so-called blood-brain barrier. Astrocytes differ also from oligodendrocytes in having a more lucent cytoplasm, fewer organelles, and microfilaments gathered into bundles.

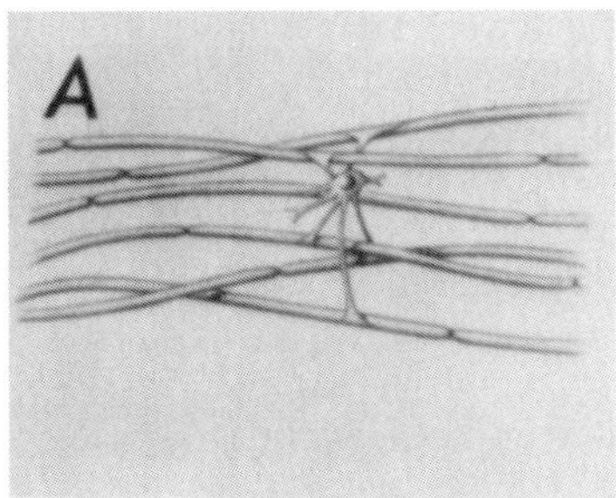

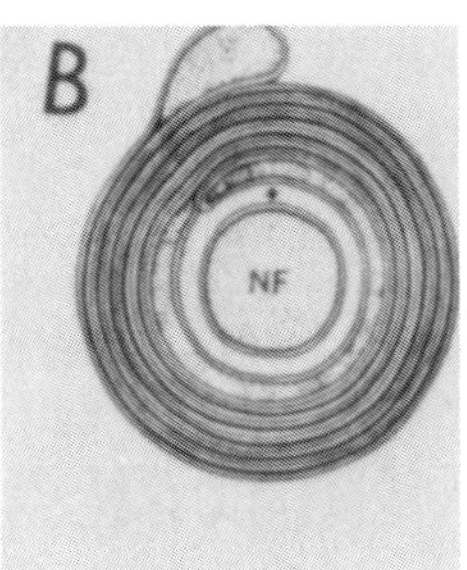

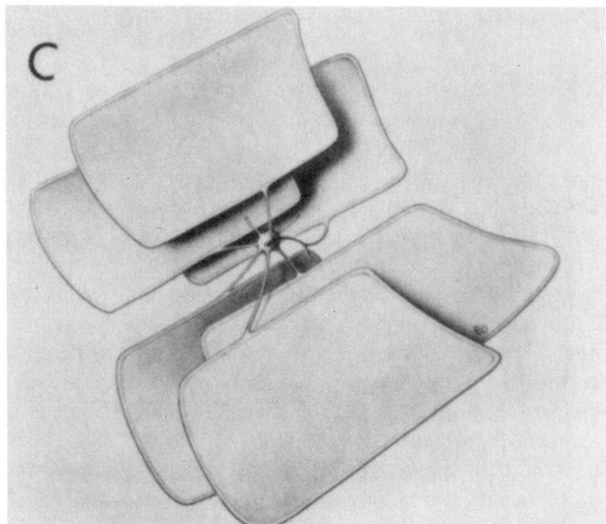

Figure 39.8. Central nervous system glial cell body. (*A*) With its cytoplasmic extensions wrapped around several axons. (*B*) Cross section of a wrapped nerve fiber (NF). (*C*) The cell with the cytoplasmic extensions unwrapped. (From Bunge 1970, in Schmitt, ed., *The Neurosciences: Second Study Program*, Rockefeller Univ. Press, New York.)

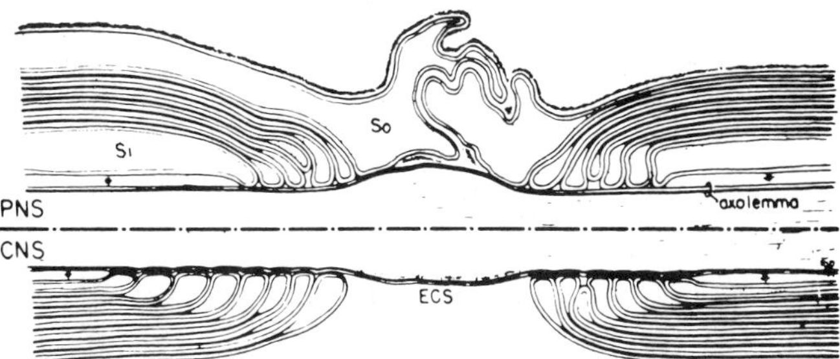

Figure 39.9. Node formed by junction of two glial cells of a myelinated nerve fiber, showing the contrast in structure in the peripheral nervous system (PNS, above) and in the central nervous system (CNS, below). In the PNS, the Schwann type of glial cell provides an internal collar (Si) and an outer collar (So) of cytoplasm for the compact myelin. Contact with extracellular space (ECS) is more intimate in the CNS nodes. (From Bunge 1970, in Schmitt, ed., *The Neurosciences: Second Study Program*, Rockefeller Univ. Press, New York).

A third kind of cell, the microglia, is sometimes misleadingly referred to as a glial type. These are ameboid, phagocytic cells that invade the nervous system from the blood; they originate from leukocytes. Microglia are very small, with dark nuclei, sparse cytoplasm, and irregular, short processes. Microglia are important in the degeneration reactions that accompany CNS damage. They invade damaged areas and phagocytize debris; later they may transform into macrophages. Other glial reactions to damage include reactive hyperplasia of astrocytes and of oligodendrocytes. Such increases have been observed in many diseases and even as a response to increased sensory stimulation and motor activity.

Other cell types that are sometimes called glia include the ependymal cells, which line the ventricles and spinal canal, pituicytes in the neural part of the pituitary, and the satellite cells in sympathetic and spinal ganglia.

Membrane potentials of glia cells have been recorded with microelectrodes. Impulse discharge in adjacent nerve fibers can depolarize nearby glia; the excitation results from K^+ release from the neuron. The glia cell response is long lasting and graded; it can summate to very large voltage shifts (up to 48 mV), provided neuron discharges are rapid. There is also a reciprocal relationship wherein neurons discharge in response to depolarization of nearby glia.

Certain glia act as a "sink" for transmitters that have been released. High-affinity uptake has been demonstrated in glia cells for glutamate, GABA, serotonin, and the catecholamines. Some neurotransmitters that are taken up may be destroyed in the glia; for example, glia have high levels of catechol-O-methyltransferase, which is an enzyme that destroys catecholamines. Recent experiments show that there is a glial-neuronal-glial communication system in which glia can transfer certain chemicals to neurons, whereupon the chemicals are transported down the length of axons and released, and some of the molecules are recovered by glia.

Glia cells are involved in epilepsy, a disorder of animals and humans in which there are uncontrollable spasms of muscles and paroxysms of massive neuronal discharge. Epilepsy often originates in localized areas of the brain; in these areas astrocytes proliferate and form so-called glial scars. These scars may develop in response to the increased release of K^+ associated with hyperactive neurons. The gliosis also tends to produce a positive-feedback effect wherein neuronal hyperactivity increases. By reducing the extracellular space, gliosis tends to increase the concentration of extracellular K^+, which in turn promotes hyperactivity of neurons in that area.

BIOCHEMISTRY

Chemical composition

The nervous system, like all tissues, is composed mostly of water (82 percent of the gray matter, 72 percent of the white matter). Most of this water (85 percent) is intracellular. Much of the water is not freely moving but rather is constrained by hydrogen bonding to membranes and organelles. The solutes, such as glucose, electrolytes, and amino acids, constitute only about 1 percent of the total mass in cerebrospinal fluid (CSF) and about 2 percent in intracellular compartments.

Most nervous system solids (40 to 65 percent) are complex lipids. These lipids are usually quite different from lipids in other body regions. Their composition is conspicuously altered in such genetic diseases as cerebral lipidoses. Neutral fat is not present in normal brain.

There are two dominant "families" of lipids: glycerolipids, made from a glycerol backbone, and sphingolipids, made from sphingosine, a C18 amino alcohol.

Phosphorylated glycerolipids form the bulk of the lipid bilayer of cell membranes in which apolar acyl chains face each other in the membrane interior, whereas polar phosphate head groups associate with surface water (see Fig. 40.16). The best-known glycerolipids include phosphatidylcholine, phosphatidylinositol, and phosphatidylserine. Another group, the phosphatidylinositides, are important "second messengers" in signal transduction (see Chap. 40).

Sphingolipids commonly are derivatives of ceramide, which is sphingosine that contains two aliphatic chains attached at the amino group ("N-acylated"). The ceramide backbone is then used to synthesize such compounds as sphingomyelin, cerebrosides, and gangliosides. Not much is known about the function of sphingomyelin or cerebrosides, but gangliosides, which contain sugars and sialic (neuraminic) acid moieties attached to the ceramide, appear to influence axonal growth and synaptic transmission (Chap. 40).

Proteins in the nervous system generally occur in complexes with lipids. Lipoproteins are proteins that contain lipid. Proteolipids behave as lipids but contain protein; they are especially concentrated in myelin. These lipid-protein complexes constitute the vast bulk of total CNS lipid; they differ from related complexes in plasma in that they are not soluble in water.

Radioactive isotope studies show that proteins of the nervous system have extensive and even rapid turnover, comparable to secreting glandular tissue. Most of the synthesis occurs in Nissl granules. The immunological properties of nervous system proteins are poorly understood, but they may be factors in autoimmune allergic encephalitides and also in memory processes.

An important class of neural proteins is the glycoproteins. These compounds are complex sugar–containing proteins that are embedded in neuronal membranes, where they participate in receptor reactions with hormones, transmitters, and neurotoxins.

Membrane transport

Transmembrane ion gradients are a major source of potential energy that is fundamental to the ionic current generation that is characteristic of neurons (Chap. 40). Active transport protein systems in the cell membrane create these gradients. Transport proteins form highly specific complexes with their substrates; during the transport, proteins typically undergo conformational and binding affinity changes as they load the ion on one face of the membrane and release it on the other side. The relationship of transport rate to ion concentration can be described in the same way as enzyme kinetics.

The known transport systems involve cations: H^+, Ca^{2+}, Na^+, and K^+. The transport of Na^+ and K^+ is coupled; that is, Na^+ is extruded at the same time that K^+ is brought into the cell. The process requires adenosine triphosphate, which is produced by a membrane-bound enzyme, Na^+-K^+ ATPase. Operation of this transport system is thought to account for 25 to 40 percent of all the oxygen consumed by the brain.

Oxidative metabolism

Nerve tissue generates considerable metabolic activity to sustain impulse conduction and to synthesize, store, and release its secretions (see also Chap. 40). Stasis of brain circulation for 8 minutes in dogs causes severe and permanent damage, including loss of function of the cerebral cortex, of auditory reflexes, of the ability to stand and walk, and of emotional reactions and vocalization. The respiratory and cardiovascular regulatory centers are more resistant and can be revived after complete interruption of their blood supply for as long as 30 minutes.

Since hypoxia causes such rapid loss of cerebral functions, the brain evidently derives the bulk of its energy from aerobic sources. The newborn is much more tolerant to hypoxia than the adult is because the metabolic rate of the newborn's brain is low and more energy can be derived anaerobically. Newborn puppies and kittens tolerate an exposure of about 24 minutes to an oxygen-free atmosphere.

The importance of glucose as a fuel for the brain is indicated by the loss of about 20 mg glucose per 100 ml of blood as blood passes through the brain. The brain does not require insulin for the oxidation of carbohydrate, which suggests that the cell barriers to glucose presented by most cells are not present in most nerve cells. Although the brain normally uses only glucose as an energy substrate, it can use ketone bodies during certain disease states, such as starvation. Transport of glucose into the brain from both blood and CSF results from a membrane transport system that facilitates diffusion independent of energy and leads to equilibration of glucose across the membrane, mediating equally a rapid flux in and out of the cell.

The amount of oxygen consumed by nervous tissue is especially large during periods of hyperactivity, such as muscular convulsions. Even in the resting brain of the dog, for example, about 50 percent of the oxygen supplied to the head is used by the brain; the brain, which weighs only 1 percent of the body, accounts for about 8 percent of the total oxygen consumption of the body at rest. Regional differences in oxygen consumption can be visualized by a radiographic technique, called positron emission tomography, that uses isotopic glucose. Blood flow to various parts of the nervous system varies widely, with only slight circulation to white areas and marked circulation to gray areas such as the cortex. During depression of neural functions, the blood flow in nervous tissue is reduced.

Local changes in oxygen and carbon dioxide content regulate the brain's blood supply, which is carried by carotid and vertebral arteries. The CSF supplies little nutrition to the brain, having as its main function the mechanical cushioning of the CNS.

Neurosecretions

Neurons secrete, and are responsive to, a wide variety of chemicals: "neurotransmitters" that allow one neuron to excite or inhibit another neuron at the synapses, and "neuromodulator" chemicals that fine-tune various neurotransmitter functions by adjusting the sensitivity of those systems. Synaptic transmission is ultimately associated with altered conductance across the membrane of specific ions. The conformational changes and channel opening are regulated by membrane potential changes in some ion channel systems (Na^+, K^+, and Ca^{2+}) and by specific neurotransmitter-receptor interactions in other systems (acetylcholine and GABA, for example).

Neurotransmitters affect virtually all physiological processes in the brain and all behaviors, and any given process or behavior is generally influenced by more than one neurotransmitter or neuromodulator.

The standard criteria for deciding which neurochemicals actually have a transmitter function are that the candidate transmitter must be normally present, synthesized, stored, released, reacted with postsynaptic membranes to alter polarization, and destroyed or otherwise removed from the site of action (see Fig. 39.10). There are now more than 50 recognized neurotransmitters. The reason for the variety of these transmitters is not at all clear, but such communication systems certainly provide an enormous amount of highly specific synaptic messages.

Neurotransmitters affect postsynaptic membranes by binding reversibly with certain sites or receptors, which they "recognize" on the basis of compatible size, three-dimensional shape, and electric-charge distribution. Similar to the "lock-and-key" reactions of enzymes and substrates, the transmitter is thought to react only with receptors, destructive enzymes, and drugs that have compatible physical and electrochemical characteristics of the binding site of the molecule.

Many transmitters have multiple receptors and multiple functions. Dopamine, for example, has at least two receptors with such diverse actions as the following: (1) inhibition of neurons in the caudate nucleus of the brain, (2) inhibition of postganglionic neurons in the superior cervical ganglion, (3) activation of adenylate cyclase in postsynaptic neurons, (4) stimulation of parathyroid hormone release, (5) inhibition of prolactin release from the anterior pituitary, and (6) regulation of β-endorphin release from the intermediate pituitary.

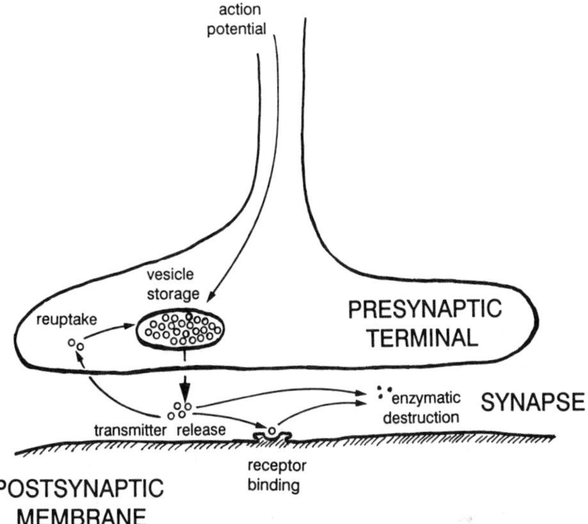

Figure 39.10. Diagram of the basic principles of neurochemical transmission in the nervous system. As action potentials move into presynaptic terminals, stored neurotransmitter is released into the synapse. Released transmitter participates in three reactions: (1) binding to stereospecific receptors on postsynaptic membrane, (2) enzymatic binding and destruction, and (3) reuptake into the presynaptic terminal. Each of the three reactions is vulnerable to drug treatment, and many neuropharmacological drugs exist to exploit these mechanisms.

For many decades a central doctrine of neurophysiology was that a given neuron contained only one kind of neurotransmitter, but that is not true for many neurons. For example, the "classic" neurotransmitters (GABA, acetylcholine, dopamine, norepinephrine, and serotonin) coexist in certain neurons with a peptide (commonly cholecystokinin, enkephalin, endorphin, substance P, neuropeptide Y, or somatostatin). The functional significance of dual transmitters seems to be that one member of a pair modulates the postsynaptic effect of the other or its presynaptic release.

Historically, as the list of neurotransmitters grew, concepts of transmitter actions expanded to include a variety of second messenger systems that regulate both active and passive ionic conductances across membranes (Chap. 40). Current research thrusts focus on elucidation of how transmitters interact to regulate common synaptic targets.

Drug and chemical barriers

Although the brain has very high blood flow (about 10 ml/g/min, which is 10 times the rate for resting muscle), many drugs and chemicals have difficulty entering the brain. This barrier is created by endothelial cells, which in the CNS have tight intercellular junctions, rather than the leaky junctions that are characteristic of endothelial cells elsewhere in the body. The tightness of junctions in the CNS seems to be imposed by some unknown secretion from the astrocytes that surround the endothelial cells.

Some brain areas, however, seem to lack a blood-brain barrier; these areas include the pineal gland, the posterior lobe of the pituitary, and the area postrema (a small region in the roof of the fourth ventricle). Also, in the rest of the brain, there is no barrier for many drugs that have a high lipid affinity.

ANATOMICAL DIVISION

Sensory receptors

A receptor cell initiates sensory input into the nervous system by responding to a change in energy in its environment, inducing appropriate patterns of nerve impulses in its axons. Receptors vary greatly in structure and functions, being highly specialized and usually modality specific (see Chaps. 41 to 43).

Peripheral nerves

In the peripheral system many fibers are grouped into trunks that connect with the CNS. The connecting fibers course in spinal and cranial nerves, many of which contain both afferent (input) and efferent (output) fibers.

At various places outside the CNS are collections of neurons called ganglia. Axons or nerves that send impulses into ganglia are called presynaptic or preganglionic; those that send impulses out of a ganglion are called postsynaptic or postganglionic. The peripheral ganglia, together with their presynaptic and postsynaptic nerves, are a major part of the autonomic nervous system, which functions to maintain homeostasis of viscera, glands, and cardiac and smooth muscle (see Chap. 46).

Spinal cord

The spinal cord contains many nerve tracts that connect the brain stem and higher centers with the spinal nerves. To a large degree, sensory and motor tracts are segregated in the cord. For example, proprioceptive impulses arising from the periphery ascend in the dorsal cord (fasciculus cuneatus and fasciculus gracilis) and in the lateral cord (spinocerebellar tract). Other sensory impulses, such as those for pain, temperature, and touch, ascend in various tracts located in lateral and ventral portions of the cord (see Chap. 41). Descending motor tracts, such as the corticospinal, rubrospinal, and tectospinal, occur in the lateral cord; the vestibulospinal tract and another branch of the corticospinal tract occur in the ventral cord (see Chap. 44). In addition to communicating with higher centers, the cord also has many neurons that process reflexes locally, so that higher centers are only slightly involved. The consequences of spinal cord lesions thus depend on what part of the cord is damaged.

Brain

Fiber tracts

The white matter of the cerebral hemispheres consists of three types of myelinated nerve fiber: association, commissural, and projection fibers. Association fibers connect different cortical regions. Commissural fibers form the connecting links between the two cerebral hemispheres. Projection fibers, motor and sensory, connect the cerebral cortex with the brain stem and spinal cord.

Specific structures

The brain (Fig. 39.11) is composed of a stem that contains fiber tracts and many neuronal centers for regulating, automatically and without volition, many visceral functions, particularly emesis, coughing, respiration, blood pressure, and heart rate. These centers are located in that portion of the brain stem that is continuous with the spinal cord—the medulla oblongata.

The medulla connects rostrally with the pons, which lies directly under the cerebellum and contains many relays with motor systems. The cerebellum functions in regulating body posture and movement (see Chap. 44).

Emerging from the various portions of the brain stem are the cranial nerves. All of the cranial nerves except the first two (olfactory and optic) connect with the brain stem (Table 39.1).

Rostral to the pons is the midbrain or mesencephalon. Dorsally, there are four rounded prominences called colliculi. These function as visual and auditory reflex centers. Ventrally, the midbrain contains motor centers (red nucleus and substantia nigra), nuclei of cranial nerves III and IV, and fiber bundles from the cerebral cortex (cerebral peduncles).

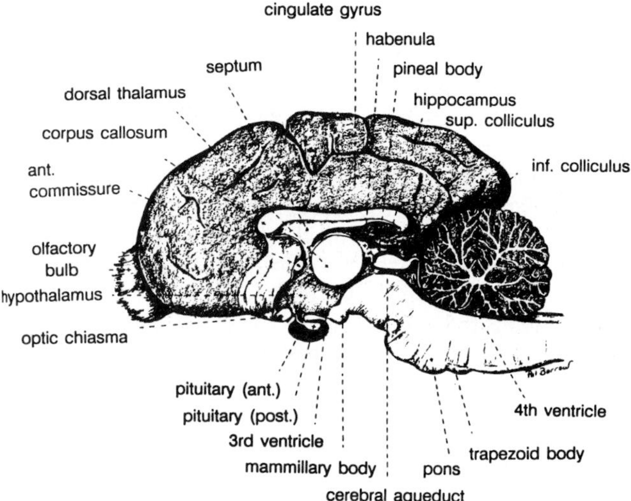

Figure 39.11. Midsagittal section of a dog brain. (Modified from Miller 1952, *Guide to the Dissection of the Dog*, 3d ed., Edwards, Ann Arbor, Mich.)

Table 39.1. Cranial nerves

Number	Name	Function	Location
I	Olfactory	Sensory	Bulb at anterior end
II	Optic	Sensory	Anterior to pituitary
III	Oculomotor	Motor	Posterior to pituitary
IV	Trochlear	Motor	Posterior to colliculi
V	Trigeminal	Mixed	Ventral pons
VI	Abducens	Motor	Posteroventral pons
VII	Facial	Mixed	Posteroventral pons
VIII	Acoustic	Sensory	Posteroventral pons
IX	Glossopharyngeal	Mixed	Lateral medulla
X	Vagus	Mixed	Lateral medulla
XI	Spinal accessory	Motor	Lateral medulla
XII	Hypoglossal	Motor	Lateral medulla

The reticular formation extends within the central core of the brain stem from the medulla, through the pons and midbrain, to the anterior end of the thalamus. Although superficially homogeneous, the reticular formation contains assorted nuclear aggregates. In the caudal portion are the well-known centers for control of respiration and cardiac activity. Some centers in the reticular formation tend to promote sleep whereas other reticular centers promote wakefulness (Chap. 48). Many regions of the reticular formation facilitate motor activity, and at least one zone contains a major inhibitory system (see Chap. 44).

The midbrain leads directly to the diencephalon, or interbrain, which consists, from the bottom up, of the pituitary gland, the hypothalamus, the subthalamus, the thalamus, and the epithalamus. A CSF-filled third ventricle separates the thalamus into two symmetrical portions.

The pituitary, or hypophysis, is an endocrine gland (see Chap. 34). The hypothalamus integrates functions carried out through the autonomic nervous system. In the hypothalamus are other areas that regulate such functions as temperature, hunger, thirst, and sexual drive (see Chap. 49).

The subthalamus is a small area that functions in the regulation of motor activity.

The thalamus, the largest component of the diencephalon, consists of a great number of nuclei that project sensory input to the cortex. Other thalamic nuclei participate in affective behavior (Chap. 49) or in sleep and arousal (Chap. 48).

The epithalamus contains the habenula, which is an olfactory center, and the pineal gland, which is a neurosecretory organ that regulates gonadal hormones and certain daily rhythms.

The thalamus and the rest of the brain rostral to it are paired. The major portion of the paired systems is the telencephalon, the most conspicuous components of which are the cerebral hemispheres. Each cerebral hemisphere contains a mantle of cells, the cerebral cortex. The cortex of primitive animals has mainly olfactory and emotional functions. A later development in reptiles, birds, and mammals added the neocortex, which displaced more primitive cortex medially. Neocortex development is best developed in primates and humans. Certain discrete portions of the neocortex control precise sensory and motor activities. The large amount of remaining cortex functions less specifically in sensory-motor regulation and in memory and problem solving (Fig. 39.12).

Under the cortex of the telencephalon and anterolateral to the thalamus are the basal ganglia—clusters of nerve cells and the fiber tracts involved in motor activity (see Chap. 44).

The CSF in the ventricles bathes and cushions inner structures of the brain and surrounds the whole outer surface of the brain.

Specific neurotransmitter pathways

For certain transmitters, the neurons that make the transmitters are scattered widely throughout the brain. Very often the neurons associated with a given transmitter are gathered together to form distinct pathways and well-defined points of axonal termination.

Noradrenergic pathways. The cells that make norepinephrine as a transmitter have cell bodies that are concentrated in a few regions of the pons and medulla. A major

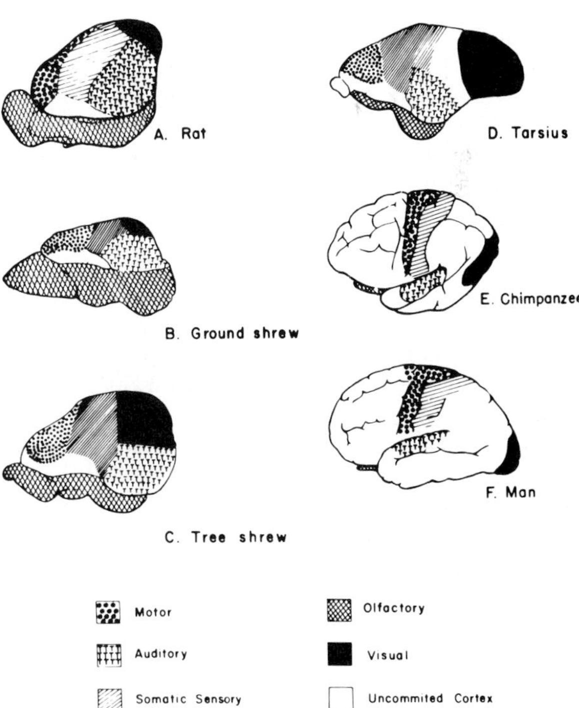

Figure 39.12. Diagram of the cerebral cortex of various species to illustrate the primary functions of various parts of the cortex. Note that the amount of uncommitted (nonspecific) cortex shows a relative increase in the higher primates. (Modified from Penfield 1966, in Eccles, ed., *Brain and Conscious Experience,* Springer-Verlag, New York.)

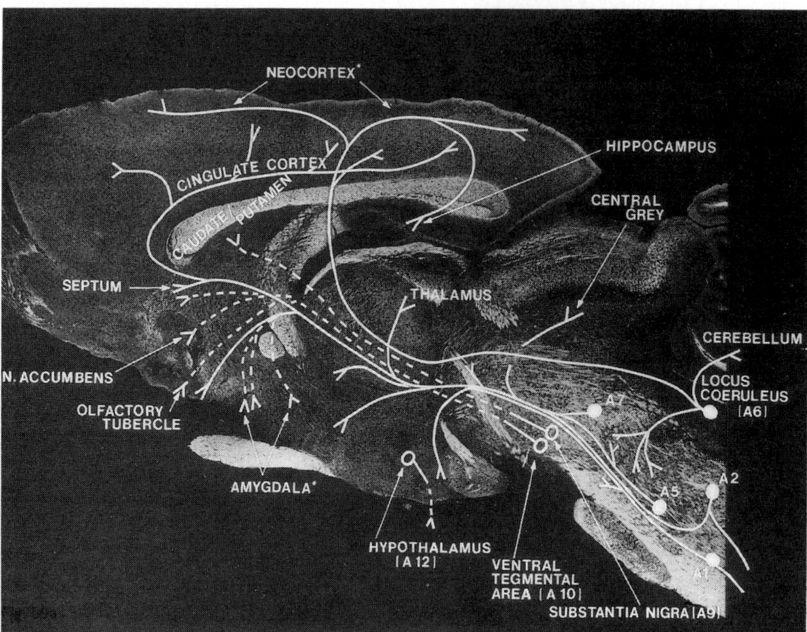

Figure 39.13. Histological section of the rat brain near the midline, showing diagrammatically the pathways for two major neurotransmitter systems. Dopaminergic pathways are indicated as open circles and broken lines, whereas noradrenergic pathways are indicated by closed circles and solid lines. Both systems also send descending projections into the spinal cord. (An asterisk indicates lateral to the plane shown.) (Reprinted with permission from *Prog. Neuro-Psychopharmacol.* 5:1–33, W.R. Klemm, Opiate mechanisms: Evaluation of research involving neuronal action potentials. Copyright 1981, Pergamon Press, Ltd.)

group is in the locus ceruleus. The axons from these cell bodies project widely in both ascending and descending directions (Fig. 39.13). Norepinephrine innervation is sparse in most parts of the brain (only about 1 percent of the total brain terminals contain norepinephrine), but particularly rich innervation occurs in such places as the Purkinje cell layer of the cerebellar cortex, the hypothalamus, and several other parts of the limbic system (see Fig. 39.15 and Chap. 49). Descending projections also terminate widely in the spinal cord.

Dopaminergic pathways. Cell bodies that contain dopamine are gathered together in several places; one grouping occurs in a deeply pigmented area of the brain stem known as the substantia nigra. The axons of these cells project to the caudate nucleus and putamen. Another major dopamine system, called the mesolimbic system, originates from the ventral tegmental area of the mesencephalon and projects to various structures of the limbic system (Fig. 39.13).

A final pathway is a system involving dopaminergic cell bodies in the tuberal swelling area of the hypothalamus that innervate the pituitary stalk in the area of the median eminence (A12 cells, Fig. 39.13).

Serotonergic pathways. The cell bodies that contain serotonin are located mostly along the midline of the brain stem in so-called raphe nuclei. Axons from these cells spread widely and have terminals in the cortex, basal ganglia, and many parts of the limbic system. There are also projections into the cerebellum and descending projections to many levels of the spinal cord.

Cholinergic pathways. Cell bodies that contain acetylcholine occur in many scattered areas. Certain areas of special concentration, however, exist in the septum, which supplies input into the limbic system, and in the "basal nucleus of Meynert," which supplies the neocortex. There is also a major projection system arising in the brain-stem reticular formation and terminating widely in the colliculi, thalamus, hypothalamus, and various components of the limbic system.

Endogenous opiate (endorphin) pathways. Two naturally occurring endorphins, both of which are pentapeptides, are concentrated mostly in the neurohypophysis, hypothalamus, striatum, and septum. A similar distribution occurs with β-endorphin, except that it does not occur in the striatum. β-endorphin cell bodies are located mainly in the basal hypothalamus, and the fibers are distributed to the midline areas of the hypothalamus and pons. Endorphin fibers are most prominent in the basal ganglia, amygdala, and parts of the spinal cord.

"Local circuit" transmitter systems. Some transmitter systems do not involve distinct projection pathways. This is particularly true of the inhibitory transmitter, glycine, which occurs in innumerable small interneurons in the gray matter of the spinal cord. The major inhibitory transmitter of the brain, GABA, occurs in interneurons (basket cells) of the hippocampus, cerebellar cortex, and elsewhere. Of the few GABAergic cells that have long projections, the most notable are the Purkinje cells of the cerebellar cortex, which inhibit cells of the deep nuclei of the cerebellum. There is also GABAergic projection from the basal ganglia to the substantia nigra.

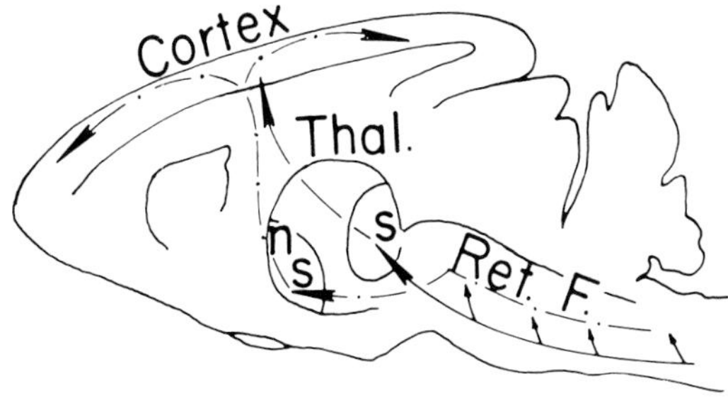

Figure 39.14. The major sensory pathways in the brain: s, specific thalamic sensory nuclei; ns, nonspecific thalamic sensory nuclei. Spinothalamic afferents enter specific thalamic nuclei, whereas nonspecific thalamic areas receive indirect innervation from polysynaptic pathways in the reticular formation. Thal., thalamus; Ret. F., reticular formation.

MAJOR FUNCTIONAL SYSTEMS

Sensory

The primary sensory pathway, in an oversimplified view, contains a chain of three neurons (Fig. 39.14). The first neuron conveys impulses from the periphery into the spinal cord or cranial nerve nuclei. The second neuron projects to cells in lateral and posterior areas of the thalamus; some second neurons terminate on motor neurons in the spinal cord and thus form a basis for spinal reflexes (see Chap. 41). The thalamic third neuron projects to sensory portions of the cerebral cortex. Excitability of neurons in this chain is partially regulated by the sensory cortex, which exerts excitation and inhibition on ascending paths.

Proprioceptive impulses are a special case in that some first-order neurons terminate in the nucleus gracilis and nucleus cuneatus in the medulla. The second neuron passes to the thalamus, and the third from the thalamus to the cortex; additional paths exist where the second neuron relays in the brain stem, from which third neurons pass to the cerebellum.

The second sensory route is via the reticular formation of the brain stem, which receives collateral innervation from ascending primary paths (see Chap. 41). At the same time that impulses are arriving over primary pathways, branches from those pathways feed into the highly synaptic reticular region of the brain stem, where the impulses propagate rostrally to medial and anteroventral regions of the thalamus, and then to widespread regions of the cortex. The apparent function of this secondary sensory system is to cause a generalized activation of the cortex rather than to preserve information about the quality of a specific sensation (Chap. 48).

Consciousness

The brain's function can be described as a continuum of states ranging from alert wakefulness to sleep. The brain-stem reticular formation regulates the spectrum of states of consciousness (see Chap. 48).

When the brain-stem reticular formation is active, it provides a tonic excitatory drive for the whole cortex. In a sense, the reticular formation can be said to "arouse" cortical cells to be more receptive to sensory information arriving over the primary pathways. These events are accomplished by behavioral alertness. Conversely, depression of reticular activity leads to behavioral sedation. Destruction of the reticular formation causes permanent unconsciousness and coma.

Depression of the brain-stem reticular formation facilitates sleep, but sleep is more than a passive phenomenon. Sleep also appears to be promoted by activity in such areas as the preoptic region of the hypothalamus and the solitary tract region of the medulla. The dream stages of sleep appear to be produced actively by regions in the pontine reticular formation (see Chap. 48).

Emotion

Many factors govern animal motivation to behave in certain ways. One of these factors is the interaction with the sensory environment, wherein an animal assesses the "value" of a desired stimulus. These interactions reflect the reinforcing or rewarding properties of stimuli as opposed to their aversive or painful properties. The reward or punishment decisions made by the brain are made mainly in the brain stem and the so-called "limbic system" (Fig. 39.15) (see also Chap. 49).

In the more primitive animals, the olfactory sense dominates behavior. The olfactory portions of the brains of such animals are relatively large and constitute a major portion of the limbic system. In higher animals the components of the limbic system (such as the septum, hippocampus, amygdala, and cingulate portion of the cortex) regulate many aspects of emotion and behavior. In fact, it was the viral disease rabies, which damages the hippocampus and results in profound emotional disorders, that originally suggested the role of the limbic system in emotional behavior.

Although many details of the limbic system's function are lacking, much research effort has revealed that this system controls such drives as sex, appetite, and thirst and such emotions as euphoria, depression, rage, and fear. Moreover, the limbic system exerts control over hypothalamic autonomic centers.

Study of self-stimulation phenomenon, where animals operate levers to deliver electric current through electrodes implanted in certain limbic areas, shows that animals will work to the point of exhaustion to provide stimulation of these areas. The limbic system also appears to have a crucial role in the consolidation of temporary memories into permanent form.

Motor

Motor systems can be classified into two types: (1) from the pyramidal system or (2) from the extrapyramidal system

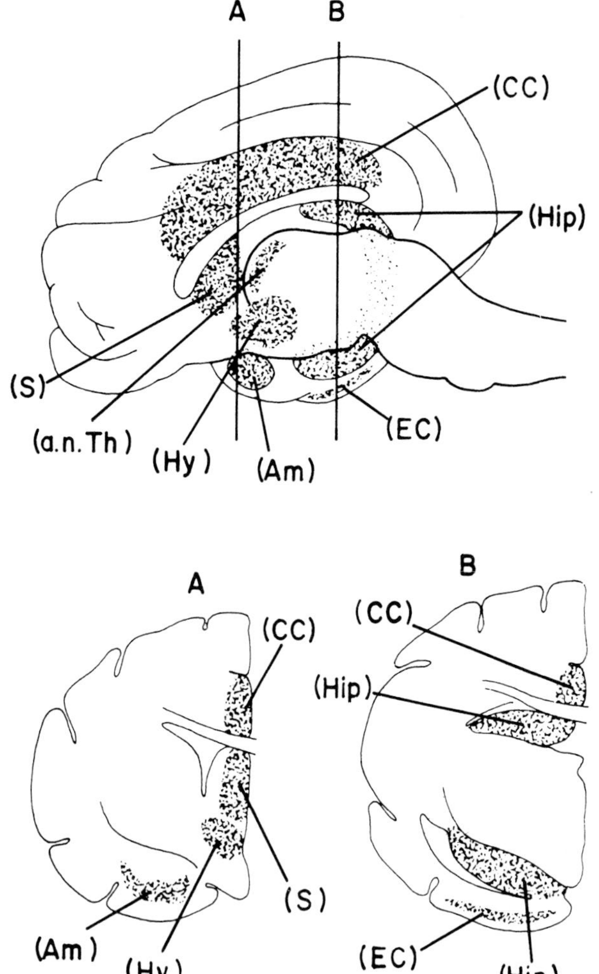

Figure 39.15. Major components of the limbic system and their relative positions. (*Top*) Vertical slice through midline of the brain. (*Bottom*) Cross sections at two different anteroposterior levels. Am, amygdala; a.n. Th., anterior nucleus of thalamus; CC, cingulate cortex; EC, entorhinal cortex; Hip, hippocampus; Hy, hypothalamus; S, septum. (From Lane, ed., 1976, *Life, The Individual, The Species*, C.V. Mosby, St. Louis.)

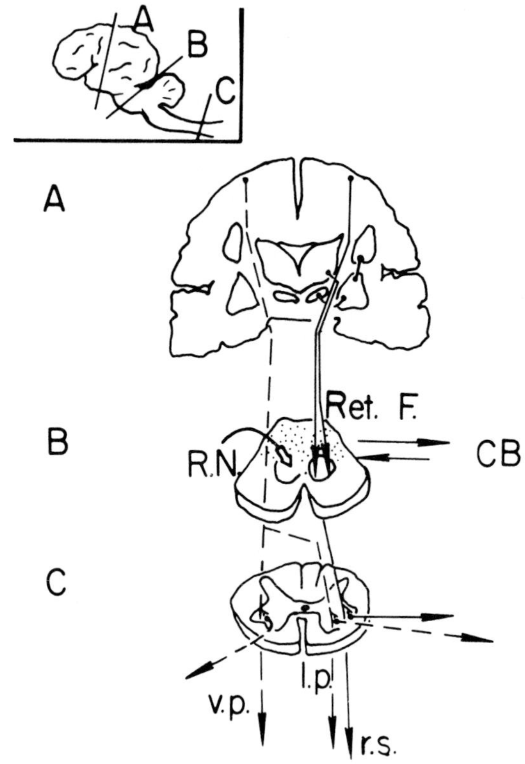

Figure 39.16. Major motor pathways in the central nervous system (CNS), showing one-half of the bilaterally symmetrical pyramidal and extrapyramidal systems. Insert (*top*) locates A, B, and C sections. The pyramidal system (*left*) arises in layer V of the cortex (not shown) and is composed of fiber tracts in the spinal cord (ventral and lateral pyramidal tracts; v.p. and l.p.) that make contact with lower motoneurons in the cord. The extrapyramidal system (*right*) has fibers in the cortex that act on subcortical areas, especially the reticular formation (Ret. F.) and the red nucleus (R.N.). Thalamic and basal ganglia influences are also exerted. The cerebellum (CB) exerts its servomechanism functions primarily by way of the brainstem structures. The inhibitory and facilitatory functions of the motor portions of the reticular formation are mediated by way of the reticulospinal tract (r.s.).

(Fig. 39.16, see also Chap. 44). The pyramidal system consists of pyramid-shaped cells in the cortex and their efferent pathways to skeletal muscles. Impulses arising from other areas of the cortex and subcortex initiate discharge of these pyramidal cells, which then send impulses down a long bundle of nerve fibers (pyramidal tract or corticospinal tract). At the level of the pons the tract splits into a ventral and a lateral bundle that course in the spinal cord. Along various points in the ventral horn of the spinal cord, synaptic junctions are made with neurons that go to muscles. Motor activity of this pyramidal system is voluntary and, because of the high degree of localized function in the motor cortex, can be very precise and discrete.

The extrapyramidal system includes all motor portions of the CNS that are not in the pyramidal system. Most important are the basal ganglia (caudate nucleus, putamen, globus pallidus, subthalamus, red nucleus, substantia nigra, brain-stem reticular formation) and some portions of the thalamus and cortex. These brain nuclei play the dominant role of motor regulation in lower animals such as birds, which have a poorly developed motor cortex. Even in the cat and the dog, these brain areas dominate motor activity, as shown by studies in which removal of the motor cortex does not have major effects on motor ability. Indeed, rudimentary locomotion reflexes are generated by central pattern generators in the brain stem and spinal cord below the level of consciousness. The so-called "mesencephalic locomotor region" is a major source of locomotor drive. There is also a group of cells in the medial medulla that cause global inhibition of movement.

The cerebellum monitors various states of inertia and momentum of muscles through a feedback mechanism by which signals go to the cerebral cortex to make necessary adjustments. The cerebellum receives impulses from receptors in joints and muscles that signal the physical state of the muscles and joints. It also receives stimuli from the equilibrium apparatus in the inner ear. Finally, the cerebellum receives impulses from the motor cortex. The efferent signals of the cerebellum go primarily to motor centers in the brain stem and to the motor cortex.

To summarize motor function, one can say that the extrapyramidal system maintains an organized background of muscle tone, posture, and gross movements upon which the pyramidal system can direct discrete and precise movements.

Visceral control

A major subsystem of the brain regulates visceral functions, such as the activity of the cardiovascular, gastrointestinal, and urogenital systems (Fig. 39.17). These functions are monitored and modulated by the autonomic nervous system (see Chap. 46). This system has dual components, one enhancing organ function and the other opposing it. Activation of the sympathetic portion of this system results in a fast heart rate and increased blood pressure; activation of the parasympathetic portion has the opposite effects. The dual innervation of the various organs also arises from rather ill-defined dual centers in the hypothalamus, which in turn are influenced by the action of other brain areas. For example, in the posterior portion of the hypothalamus are centers that control emergency sympathetic responses that prepare the animal for "fight or flight." Other centers in the anterior hypothalamus and in the septal area apparently control parasympathetic functions such as rest, recovery, digestion, and elimination.

At least in animals, autonomic functions generally have been considered to be automatic and not subject to voluntary control.

The autonomic nervous system is a primary outlet for the processing and "decisions" of the limbic system. Emotional stress in animals is most clearly manifest in changes in heart rate, blood pressure, and other indicators of visceral function. Recordings of such autonomic effects from dogs have shown that the degree of the response to stress depends on two major factors: (1) the value of the actual need (drive) and (2) the brain's estimation of the probability that the drive can be satisfied. The brain's comparison of these two factors activates the mechanisms that produce emotions and associated autonomic responses.

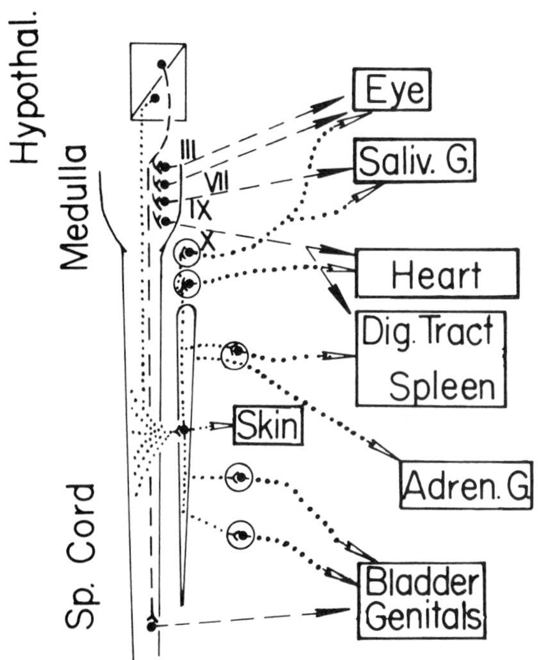

Figure 39.17. Simplified diagram of the autonomic nervous system. Dotted lines, sympathetic division; broken lines, parasympathetic division. Sympathetic fibers are shown emerging from the thoracolumbar regions of the spinal cord and making synaptic junctions in the sympathetic trunk or in cervical, coeliac, or mesenteric ganglia (exception: innervation of the adrenal medulla). Parasympathetic fibers are shown emerging from the cranial and sacral nerves and making synaptic junctions in the target organs. Sp, spinal; Hypothal., hypothalamus; Saliv. G., salivary gland; Dig., digestive; Adren. G., adrenal gland.

REFERENCES

Adelman, G., ed. 1987. *Encyclopedia of Neuroscience*. Birkhaeuser, Boston.

Berkley, K.J., and Contos, N. 1987. A glial-neuronal-glia communication system in the mammalian central nervous system. *Brain Res.* 414:49–67.

Bloom, F.E. 1988. Neurotransmitters: Past, present, and future directions. *FASEB J.* 2:32–41.

Chagas, C., Gattass, R., and Gross, C. 1985. *Pattern Recognition Mechanisms*. Springer-Verlag, New York.

Cooper, J.R., Bloom, F.E., and Roth, R.H. 1986. *The Biochemical Basis of Neuropharmacology*, 5th ed. Oxford Univ. Press, New York.

Garcia-Rill, E., and Skinner, R. D. 1987. The mesencephalic locomotor region. I. Activation of a medullary projection site. *Brain Res.* 411:1–12.

Grillner, S., and Wallen, P. 1985. Central pattern generators for locomotion, with special reference to vertebrates. *Annu. Rev. Neurosci.* 8:233–61.

Hamilton, C.R., and Vermeire, B.A. 1988. Complementary hemispheric specialization in monkeys. *Science* 242:1691–94.

Janzer, R.C., and Raff, M.C. 1987. Astrocytes induce blood- brain barrier properties in endothelial cells. *Nature* 325:253–57.

Kandel, E.R., and Schwartz, J.H. 1985. *Principles of Neural Science*. 2d ed. Elsevier, New York.

Klemm, W.R., and Sherry, C.J. 1982. Do neurons process information by relative intervals in spike trains? *Neurosci. Biobehav. Rev.* 6:429–37.

Knudsen, E.I., duLac, S., and Esterly, S.D. 1987. Computational maps in the brain. *Annu. Rev. Neurosci.* 10:41–65.

Kromer, L.F. 1987. Nerve growth factor treatment after brain injury prevents neuronal death. *Science* 235:214–16.

Kuffler, S.W., Nicholls, J.G., and Martin, A.R. 1984. *From Neuron to Brain*, 2d ed. Sinauer Associates, Sunderland, Mass.

Levi-Montalcini, R., ed. 1986. *Molecular Aspects of Neurobiology*, Springer-Verlag, New York.

Matthews, G.G. 1986. *Cellular Physiology of Nerve and Muscle*. Blackwell, Palo Alto, Calif.

McGeer, P.L., Eccles, J.C., and McGeer, E.G. 1987. *Molecular Neurobiology of the Mammalian Brain*, 2d ed. Plenum Press, New York.

Mesulam, M.-Marsel. 1987. Asymmetry of neural feedback in the organization of behavioral states. *Science* 237:537–38.

Millhorn, D.E., and Hokfelt, T. 1988. Chemical messengers and their coexistence in individual neurons. *News Physiol. Sci.* 3:1–4.

Saji, M., and Reis, D.J. 1987. Delayed transneuronal death of substantia nigra neurons prevented by gamma-aminobutyric acid agonist. *Science*. 235:66–69.

Shepherd, G.M. 1988. *Neurobiology*. Oxford Univ. Press, New York.

Siegel, G., Agranoff, B., Albers, R.W., and Molinoff, P. eds. 1989. *Basic Neurochemistry*, Raven Press, N.Y.

Williams, R. W., and Herrup, K. 1988. The control of neuron number. *Annu. Rev. Neurosci.* 11: 423–53.

Worden, F.G., Swazey, J.P., and Adelman, G. 1975. *The Neurosciences: Paths of Discovery*. MIT Press, Cambridge, Mass.

CHAPTER 40

Nerves, Junctions, and Reflexes | by Ainsley Iggo and W. R. Klemm

IONIC BASIS FOR NEURONAL ACTIVITY

Ionic composition

The ionic composition inside neurons and their fibers is quite different from that of the extracellular fluids. Four ions are of particular importance to neuronal function (Table 40.1); note that all but potassium have much higher extracellular concentrations under resting conditions. Thus there is a concentration gradient that influences the flow of ions when membrane permeability changes, as it does when neurons discharge impulses.

There is also an electrostatic gradient arising because these ions are electrically charged and the resting neuron is electronegative on the inside relative to the outside. If a microelectrode is placed inside a neuron and another electrode is placed outside, an oscilloscope display will reveal that the magnitude of this charge differential in an inactive neuron is on the order of 70 mV (Fig. 40.1). This degree of

Table 40.1. Representative ionic concentrations of mammalian neurons under resting, unstimulated conditions

	Ionic concentrations (mM/L)	
	Intracellular	Extracellular
Sodium	10	140
Potassium	140	5
Chloride	4	100
Calcium	0.01	10

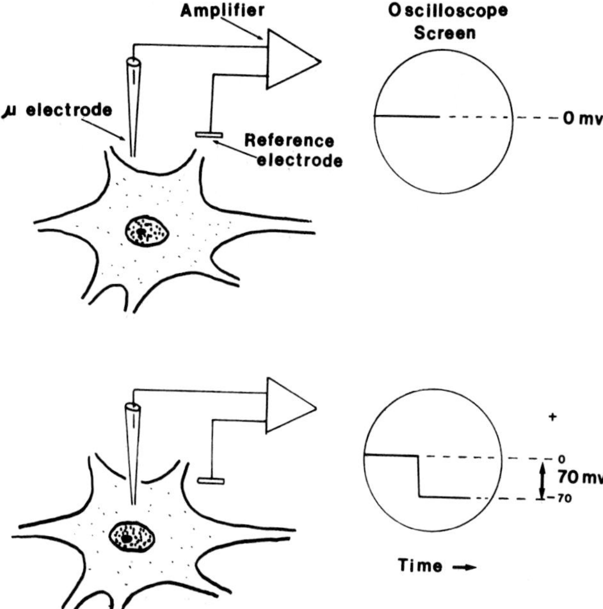

Figure 40.1. Demonstration of the steady electrostatic gradient that exists in resting nerve cells. (*Top*) When a "differential amplifier" that senses the voltage *difference* between two electrodes is used, no voltage gradient is seen between two points on the extracellular medium. However, when one electrode is placed inside the cell (*bottom*), a steady voltage gradient of about −70 mV is detected.

charge separation is quite large when expressed in terms of square meters of membrane thickness. The charge differential arises because there is an asymmetrical distribution of ions inside and outside the cell; there are more negatively charged ions (and fewer positive ions) inside the cell than there are outside.

The asymmetrical ion distribution arises because the neuronal membrane is a barrier, particularly for cellular proteins, which carry a net electronegative charge.

Active ion transport

A major factor affecting ionic distribution is the presence of an active transport system ("pump") for sodium and potassium. The pumping action, transporting sodium ions outward while moving potassium ions inward, is achieved by a large membrane-bound protein and its associated lipids, Na^+-K^+ ATPase. Metabolic energy is needed to maintain this asymmetrical distribution, as is readily demonstrated by use of poisons that prevent the formation of ATP. Sodium, for example, is normally "pumped out" of the neuron by a transport system dependent on adenosine triphosphate (ATP), but this efflux is abolished when poisons are used to prevent the formation of ATP (Fig. 40.2). In the absence of active transport, sodium, being electropositive, is attracted to stay inside the cell, which is electronegative.

There are also transport systems for Ca^{2+}, one of which is a different type of ATPase. A specific protein, known as calmodulin, is an intracellular binder of Ca^{2+} and acts as a reservoir while limiting the amount of free Ca^{2+}. Ca^{2+} tends to be bound at the membrane surface by electronegative sialic acid moieties of glycoproteins and glycolipids (gangliosides).

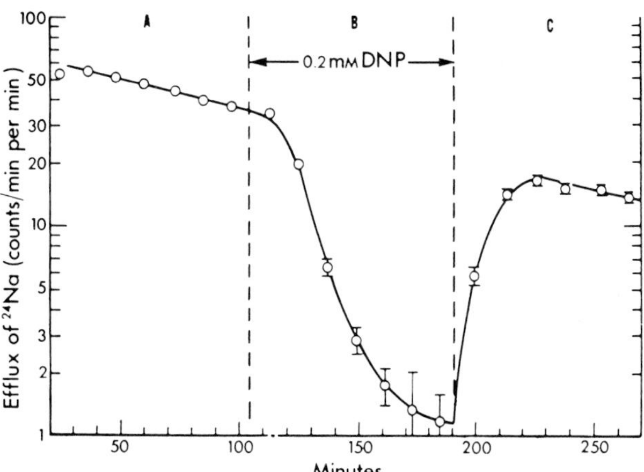

Figure 40.2. Demonstration of the dependence of sodium efflux from the cell on oxidative phosphorylation. The amount of radioactive sodium moving out of a Sepia axon that was bathed in artificial sea water is shown in (A) and (C). At time = 100 minutes, dinitrophenol (DNP) was added to the bath to poison the ATP system, and this arrested the sodium efflux. (From Hodgkin and Keynes 1955, *J. Physiol.* 128:28–60.)

BIOELECTRICITY

Membrane potentials

With the sodium-potassium pump at equilibrium, the membrane voltage remains essentially constant. Although seemingly "at rest," the neuron is poised for "explosive" action because of two important kinds of gradient. One is a concentration gradient wherein passive diffusion forces would, if the membrane permeability should change, erase the high concentration of sodium on the outside and the high concentration of potassium on the inside. The other is the electrostatic gradient, wherein the inside negativity would, if the membrane permeability should change, electrically attract the positively charged sodium ions to come inside the neuron.

The basis for the resting membrane potential can be quantified by the so-called Goldman equation:

$$\text{Em} = \text{RT/F} \log_e \frac{\text{Pk}[\text{K}^+]_o + \text{PNa}[\text{Na}^+]_o + \text{PCl}[\text{Cl}^-]_i}{\text{Pk}[\text{K}^+]_i + \text{PNa}[\text{Na}^+]_i + \text{PCl}[\text{Cl}^-]_o}$$

where Em is the membrane potential, R is the gas constant, T is the absolute temperature, F is the Faraday constant, P is the permeability constant for each of the key ions, and the ion concentrations inside and outside the cell. The absolute value of Em varies among neurons but is generally on the order of 70 mV.

Action potentials ("impulses")

Should anything disturb the resting membrane permeability to ionic flow, then sodium would diffuse down its concentration and electrostatic gradients to enter the neuron, resulting in a temporary reversal of the membrane potential (Fig. 40.3). Likewise, potassium would diffuse down its concentration gradient to leave the neuron. This is exactly what happens when a neuronal receptor organ is excited by its environmental stimulus (see Chap. 41) or when a neuron is excited by electrical stimulation or by chemicals released from other neurons (see "Junctional Transmission" below). Sodium enters neurons via pores ("channels") in specific receptor proteins that traverse the plasma membrane. As sodium enters the cell, the positive charge that it carries cancels the internal negativity and, in fact, actually reverses the neuron's polarity so that the membrane voltage temporarily becomes about 60 mv, inside positive. This change is sudden and is the most conspicuous sign of activity; it therefore is called an *action potential*.

The process is also called "depolarization" because the electrical polarization of the resting membrane is reversed. The amplitude of the action potential is limited by both concentration and electrical gradients. As sodium diffuses inward, it changes both the concentration and the electrical gradients that enable the influx. At about 60 mv positive an "equilibrium potential" is reached where the forces compelling influx are offset by the forces that develop to stop influx. For a given axon, the amplitude of the action poten-

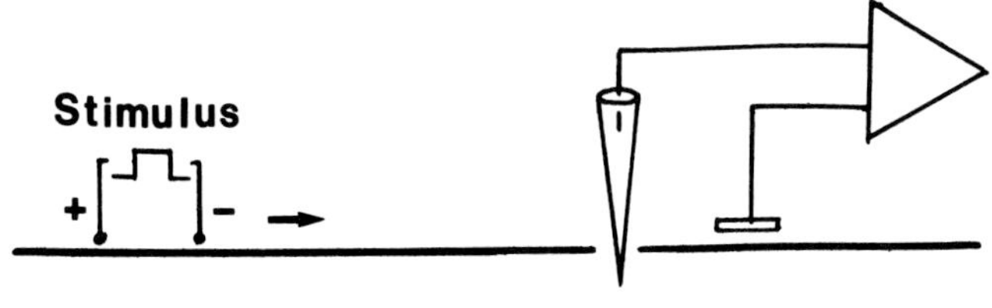

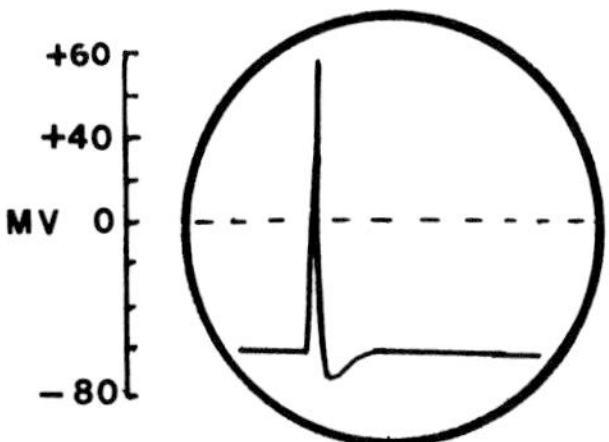

Figure 40.3. (*Top*) Diagram of experimental setup to record an axon's response to an applied excitatory stimulus (on the left). An intracellular microelectrode is coupled or "referenced" to an extracellular macroelectrode. (*Bottom*) Oscilloscope display of the action potential, as it would appear when the propagating depolarization reaches the microelectrode.

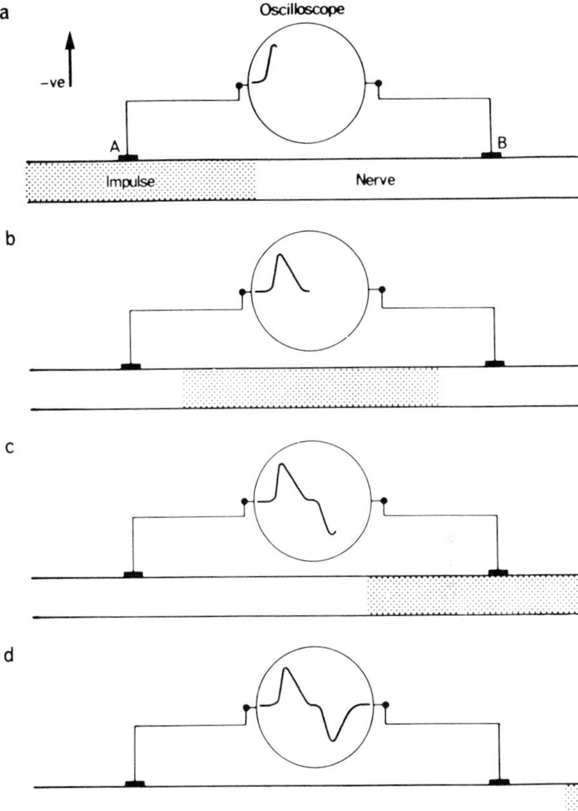

Figure 40.4. Display of the action potential waveform recorded from two extracellular electrodes, as is commonly done in student laboratories. These recordings are commonly made with the oscilloscope amplifiers in a "differential" mode, wherein the voltage amplified is the difference between the potential at electrode A and electrode B. If the scope is set so that a negative potential at A causes the beam to deflect upward, then as an action potential propagates under electrode A, there will be an upward spike. Oscilloscope input B in this case would display a negative potential downward, and when the action potential spreads under electrode B the waveform will be upside down, assuming that the two electrodes are far enough apart that algebraic interactions do not occur between points A and B. In a typical experiment with frog sciatic nerve, for example, it is not possible to get the two electrodes far enough apart to show the biphasic character as two separate "spikes." This same action potential takes on different values but retains a similar shape, if microelectrode recordings are used. In this case, the magnitude of the potential is much greater because the ionic current is passing through the very high resistance of the membrane (recall Ohm's law). Also, this kind of recording allows the display of the absolute resting (direct current) membrane potential of about −60 to −70 mV. Note that in this case, the action potential present at the microelectrode is being "referenced" to the other electrode that is extracellular, and thus there is no opportunity to see any biphasic nature of the action potential. With microelectrode recording, the oscilloscope shows the action potential to consist of a reversed polarization, with the inside positive.

tial is generally the same each time it is generated. This is the so-called "all-or-none" principle; a neuron discharges either an action potential of full amplitude or none at all. The amplitude is generally constant, irrespective of the strength of the excitatory stimulus and, usually, the frequency of generation. However, a few neuronal types that fire in rapid bursts may produce action potentials in the burst that show a progressive decrease in amplitude.

The all-or-none principle does not apply to action potentials as they are recorded from a peripheral nerve, which contains axons of many different neurons and thus produce a compound or composite action potential (see "Activity in Nerve Trunks" below).

Appearance of the action potential

The action potential is described as a plot of volts versus time. As could be expected, the waveform features a rapid rise and fall in potential. The absolute values obtained depend on the recording environment. For example, if two extracellular electrodes are placed outside an axon, the peak depolarization will be a only few millivolts, seen as an upward deflection of an oscilloscope beam when the action potential is directly under one electrode and seen as a downward deflection when the action potential has moved to under the second electrode (Fig. 40.4).

The point is that sodium influx accounts for the action potential. What is the significance of the potassium efflux? It also continues until its equilibrium potential is reached, which occurs somewhat later than is the case for sodium influx. Since potassium is leaving the neuron, it carries electropositivity with it; that is, the efflux tends to make the inside of the neuron electronegative, thus tending to cancel the electropositivity that was created by sodium influx. In short, potassium efflux terminates the action potential.

These offsetting tendencies were first demonstrated on observation of the flux of radiolabeled sodium and potassium in nerves that were repeatedly excited by electrical stimulation. It was not possible, however, to determine the simultaneous relations of ionic flux during a single action potential until the so-called voltage clamp technique was discovered. This procedure employs electronic feedback circuitry in an electrical stimulator so that the membrane voltage can be clamped or held constant. If, for example, the neuron is clamped in a depolarized state and the extracellular sodium and potassium currents are monitored, it can be seen that there is an initial inward sodium current followed by an outward potassium current (Fig. 40.5). If potassium efflux is insufficient to restore the overall membrane potential to the resting normal state, a second electrical stimulus may not be able to reexcite sodium conductance. This process is responsible for refractory-period phenomena (see below).

Only a few number of ions have to move to create the voltage change, on the order of only 4 pmol/cm^2, as measured in invertebrate neurons. For this reason, neurons can sustain a high rate of impulse activity, even for brief periods of anoxia. At some point, however, enough sodium ions have entered the cell and enough potassium ions have left that active transport processes are essential to restore ion concentrations back to their resting levels.

The restoration of normal ionic equilibrium is often manifest in the aftermath of the action potential in the form of small and long-lasting "after potentials." As might be expected, they are highly vulnerable to metabolic influences.

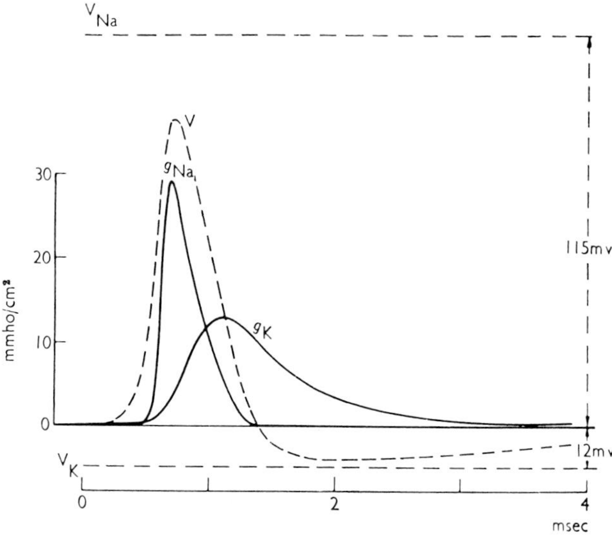

Figure 40.5. Concurrent relations between membrane voltage (V) (*broken lines*) and sodium and potassium currents (gNa and gK), as determined in classic voltage clamp studies on giant squid axon. Note that sodium conductance is rapidly inactivated, whereas potassium conductance is delayed and prolonged. V_{Na}, sodium equilibrium potential. V_K, potassium equilibrium potential. (From Hodgkin and Huxley 1952, *J. Physiol.* 117:500–44.)

Electrical response properties of neurons

Threshold phenomena

When an axon is excited electrically, the stimulus has to reach a certain magnitude, or threshold, in order to open the sodium channels and trigger an action potential. A stronger stimulus may cause the action potential to occur more quickly but will not otherwise change it. In many excitable neurons with a resting potential of 50 to 90 mV (inside negative), the depolarization magnitude required is 10 to 20 mV.

Subthreshold stimuli do "sensitize" sodium channels for a time that decays exponentially when the stimulating current is withdrawn. Delivery of a second stimulus during the decay from the first may trigger an action potential at a lower than usual stimulus intensity.

Accommodation

A decline in axonal excitability can occur if a stimulus has a very slow time course. Such accommodation occurs because prolonged subthreshold currents prevent regenerative increase in sodium permeability. As a result, the axon passes into a refractory state.

A similar kind of refractoriness can occur with certain muscle-relaxant drugs, such as succinylcholine and decamethonium, that produce a sustained degree of depolarization and thus prevent the regenerative increase in sodium permeability needed to generate new action potentials. Local anesthetics generally do not cause depolarization block but apparently block conduction by a direct inactivation of sodium channels.

Refractoriness

When an action potential is triggered, there is a brief subsequent period of depressed excitability during which the axon is refractory to the genesis of another impulse. Immediately after an impulse, the axon is absolutely refractory; that is, another impulse cannot be triggered, no matter how intense the stimulus. This period is followed by another, longer, period in which the refractoriness is relative; that is, a second impulse may be triggered, but the stimulus intensity required for doing so will be higher (Fig. 40.6).

Propagation of action potentials

Once an action potential is triggered, for whatever reason, it propagates or spreads throughout the various contiguous regions of neuronal membrane. This spread is most evident as a rapid conduction of the impulse of electrical discharge along an axon. In an axon, one can think of a localized "spot" of depolarization as acting as an electrical stimulus to adjacent spots of membrane, thus triggering them into depolarization and conduction of the action potential (Fig. 40.7).

Propagation occurs because any localized point of depolarization can serve as an electrical stimulus for depolarizing an adjacent point. The voltage change at a point of

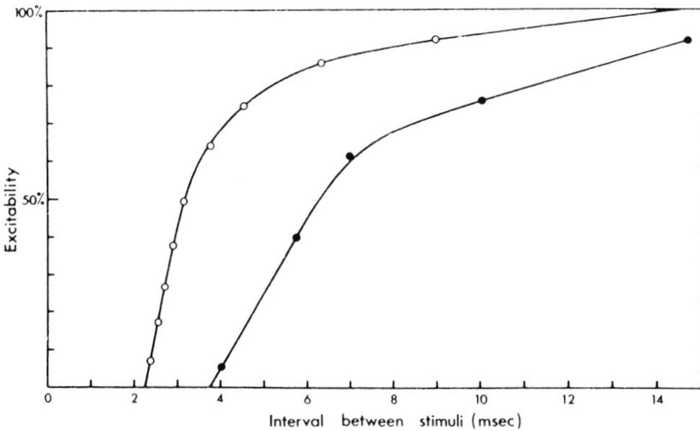

Figure 40.6. Curves to illustrate the recovery of excitability after an initial impulse; experiment was conducted with paired stimuli, delivered at various intervals. In both sciatic nerve (*open circles*) and sartorius muscle (*closed circles*) of frog, full excitability is not restored until about 14 ms has elapsed since the initial impulse. For about 2 to 4 ms after the initial stimulus, the tissue is absolutely refractory, followed by a gradual return to normal (relative refractory period). (Modified from Adrian 1921, *J. Physiol.* 55:193–225.)

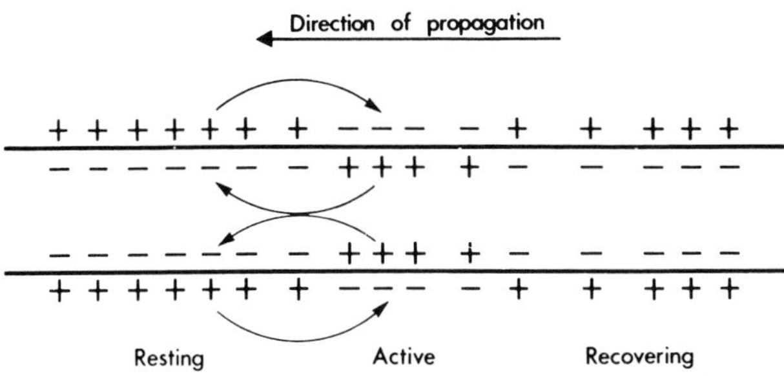

Figure 40.7. Distribution of the electrical charges across a neuronal membrane at rest (outside positive, inside negative) and during the genesis of an action potential (outside negative, inside positive). Arrows indicate the flow of ionic current through the membrane, which depolarizes adjacent membrane ahead of the "spot" of depolarization and which repolarizes adjacent membrane in the wake of the propagated action potential.

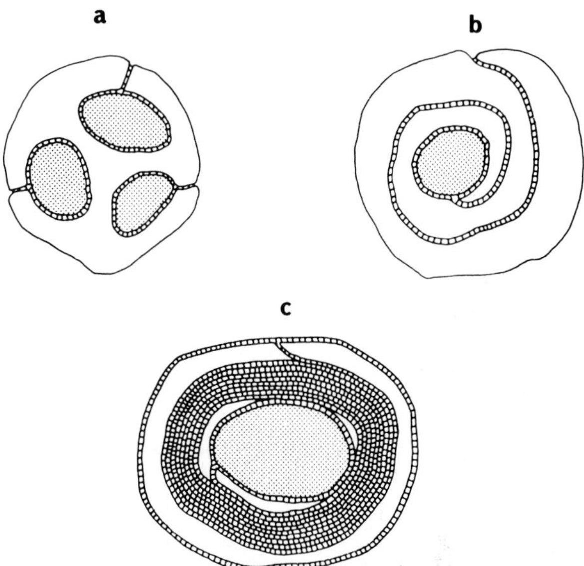

Figure 40.8. Illustration of different ways that glial cells can form a coating of myelin around axons. (*a*) Membrane of a peripheral glia cell (Schwann cell) that is adjacent to three axons, but does not actually form a myelin coat; (*b*) early stage of myelin formation in which a few turns of glial membrane engulf the axon; (*c*) fully developed myelination in which cytoplasm is largely extruded and a tight wrapping of membrane surrounds the axon. In vertebrates, very small-diameter axons (<1 μm) are often unmyelinated. Conduction in these axons is relatively slow, not only because of the small diameter but also because there is no myelin.

depolarization actually changes the conformation of proteinaceous channels in adjacent membrane so that sodium ions can penetrate and diffuse down their concentration and electrostatic gradients. These channels are more properly called voltage-gaited sodium channels (see below). The speed at which propagation occurs is governed by the size (diameter) of the axon, with larger axons conducting impulses faster.

The role of myelin

Myelin is a covering around axons that is produced by glia cells that wrap their cell membranes around and around a segment of axon (Fig. 40.8; see also Chap. 39).

Role of myelin in conduction velocity. A long myelinated axon is coated with the membranes of many adjacent glia cells. At the axial junction between the membrane wrappings of adjacent glial cells there is a gap, or node (node of Ranvier). Each node is a region where ion flux is essentially the same as in an unmyelinated axon, whereas obviously ions cannot flow across the numerous layers of glial membrane in the internodal regions. Thus, when an action potential propagates down a myelinated axon, the sodium/potassium fluxes can occur only at the nodes. Because myelin is a very effective electrical insulator, voltage-gaited sodium channels in the axon can be activated only at the nodes. Current flow of an action potential can seem to "leap" or skip from node to node and does not depend on successive depolarization of the entire surface of an axon (Fig. 40.9).

To illustrate the functional importance of myelination, let us consider that an unmyelinated squid axon with a conduction speed of 20 m/s is 500 μm in diameter. That same speed can be achieved in a myelinated frog axon that is only 20 μm in diameter. In mammals, because of the higher body temperature, a myelinated fiber 20 μm in diameter conducts at 120 m/s. Myelination, because it achieves high transmission rates with smaller fibers, allows peripheral nerves to remain quite small, although they contain many thousands of separate information paths, each of which conducting at high speed.

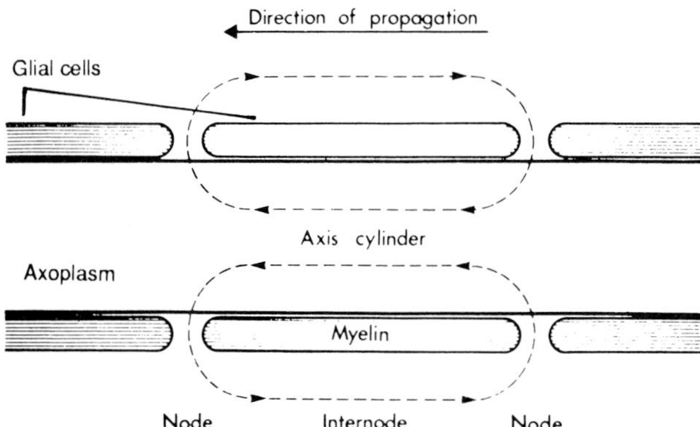

Figure 40.9. Propagation of action potential in myelinated axon. The continuous axon is surrounded by the membranes of glial cells (three shown here), and current flow occurs at the junctions (nodes of Ranvier) between the glial cells.

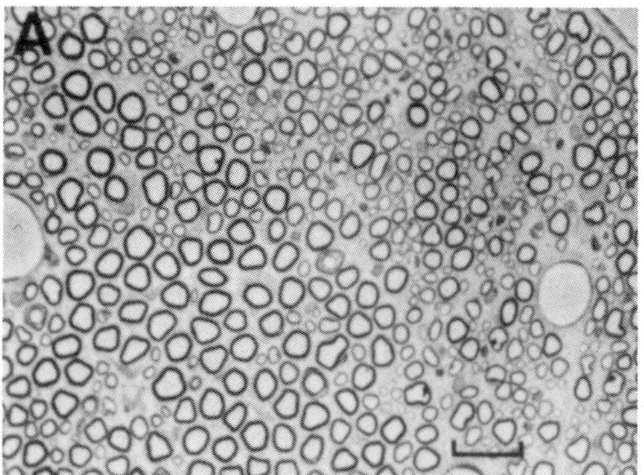

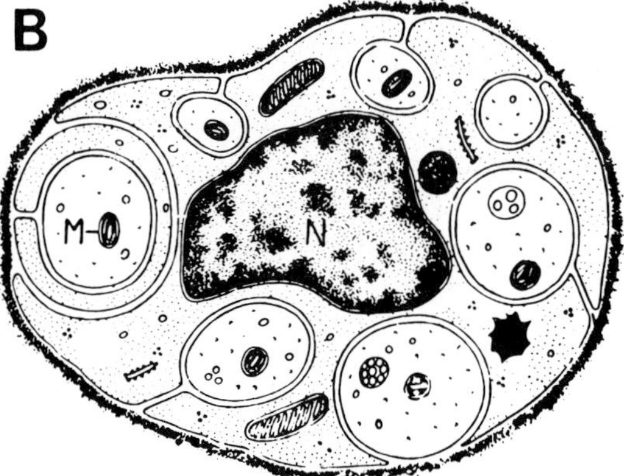

Figure 40.10. Histological cross section of a nerve (*A*) and diagram (*B*) of component parts. In (*A*) a rat sciatic nerve (×365) contains many myelinated axons (1 to 10 μm)(dark circles), which in turn are gathered together within a connective sheath (upper right-hand corner). (From Webster and Collins 1964, *J. Neuropath. Exp. Neurol.* 23:109–26.) In (*B*) an electron micrograph-based drawing of a single Schwann cell shows the cell to engulf seven non-myelinated axons. N, nucleus of Schwann cell; M, mitochondrion inside an axon. (From Elfvin 1958, *J. Ultrastruct. Res.* 1:428- 54.)

ACTIVITY IN NERVE TRUNKS

Peripheral nerves link the CNS and the periphery. When action potentials are initiated, they spread via these peripheral nerves and their axons, either into the CNS or outward from the CNS.

Composition of peripheral nerves

Peripheral nerves are formed from the axons of many neurons that have their cell bodies located in (a) dorsal root ganglia and cranial nerve ganglia (these are *afferent,* sensory neurons), (b) the ventral horn of the spinal cord or corresponding cranial nerve nuclei in the brain stem (these are *efferent,* or motor, axons), and (c) autonomic nuclei of the brain stem and spinal cord or the peripheral ganglia of the autonomic system (which give rise to the efferent fibers of the autonomic nervous system).

The nerves that connect the brain and spinal cord to peripheral structures are formed from many individual axons—often thousands, or even millions, as in the case of the optic nerve. Individual axons are always surrounded and supported by Schwann cells, and many axons will have a fully developed myelin sheath. These elements, in turn, are surrounded and supported by connective tissue sheaths, which are permeated by blood vessels and lymphatics (Fig. 40.10).

All spinal nerves contain both afferent and efferent components that originate from the dorsal and ventral roots, respectively, of the spinal cord. The sciatic nerve, for example, contains about equal numbers of each kind, but the muscular and cutaneous branches contain a predominance of efferent and afferent axons, respectively.

The visceral nerves, such as the vagus and splanchnic nerves, are also mixed nerves.

Classification of axons in nerves

The axons within nerves have been classified in one of two complementary ways, on the basis of either conduction velocity or fiber diameter. The conduction velocity scheme includes an A group, subdivided into alpha, beta, gamma, and delta according to descending order of conduction speed. All the myelinated axons of spinal nerves are in this group; in the cat, representative conduction speeds are 40 to 120 m/s for alpha and 4 to 25 m/s for delta. There is also a B group of fibers, which are, by definition, preganglionic autonomic efferents with conduction velocities of 3 to 16 m/s. C fibers are very slow-conducting unmyelinated fibers, less than 1 μm in diameter, which are mostly postganglionic sympathetic fibers.

The relative proportions of different groups of axons in nerves vary with species. In rats and rabbits, for example, there are proportionately more C fibers, whereas ruminants have relatively few.

Electrical properties of nerves

Because nerves contain fibers of varying diameter, and because the excitation thresholds are more or less directly proportional to fiber diameter, the electrical activity that is commonly recorded in laboratory demonstrations of nerve activity is more complex than is the action potential from a single axon. The all-or-none principle applies only to the individual axons contained therein. A weak electrical stimulus, for example, may be at discharge threshold for A fibers of a nerve without exciting any C fibers. Thus such a weak stimulus would produce a summed action potential of all the A fibers in the nerve, as seen from a pair of extracellular electrodes placed on the nerve. Higher-intensity stimulation would activate all contained fibers and thus produce a "compound" action potential that is summed from all the unitary action potentials.

Conduction velocity of the various component fibers also affects the waveform of the compound action potential. Not all fibers conduct at the same speed, and thus the contribution to the total nerve action potential from fibers that have different conduction speed will produce delayed small bumps on the oscillographic tracing. At the locus of a given recording electrode, the action potentials from the fastest conducting fibers will arrive first, followed by delayed voltage changes that re being produced by the more slowly conducting fibers. In a typical nerve, the most conspicuous part of the compound action potential will be contributed by A alpha fibers, followed in turn by the contribution of A delta fibers; depending on the nerve, there may also be evident smaller contributions from B and C fibers (Fig. 40.11).

Responses of nerves to damage

Although mature neurons have lost the ability to divide (see Chap. 39), damage to neuronal processes such as axons can often be repaired. When a nerve is transected, for example, the region distal to the cut degenerates in a few days, but the proximal portion remains viable and able to conduct impulses. The cell body does show some initial liquification of chromatin, and RNA metabolism is stimulated after cutting of the axon. The distal portion dies rapidly because it depends on descending transport processes from the neuronal soma. Even the distal myelin eventually disappears, suggesting that Schwann cells also depend on a viable axon. What survives is the connective tissue neurilemma, containing new glia cells as they proliferate, which provides a substrate and conduit that directs regrowth of the axonal process from the proximal end of the transection. Optimal regeneration occurs only if the severed stumps are surgically rejoined, a procedure that is commonly employed in human neurosurgery with varying degrees of success. The time required for regeneration of the nerve fiber depends on the distance between the severed ends as well as the distance to the target muscle or gland. If reinnervation does not take place, the neuron and its axonal stump may atrophy and die, or the stump may continue to grow into a benign tumor; such neuromas are a problem, especially in horses, and may require neurectomies to be performed.

Commonly a denervated target organ becomes supersensitive to its normal neurotransmitter. For example, a neuromuscular junction that has lost its innervation becomes supersensitive to exogenously applied acetylcholine.

In the case of afferent fibers, the receptor end-organs of cut fibers degenerate along with the fiber. If the receptor achieves reinnervation of its target, in the spinal cord for example, then the normal selective sensitive and function may return.

Central nervous system

Repair of damaged fiber tracts in the CNS is usually poorly achieved. The generally accepted explanation is that glia "scars" form and block the proper regrowth of axonal processes. Experimentally, repair of damage has been pro-

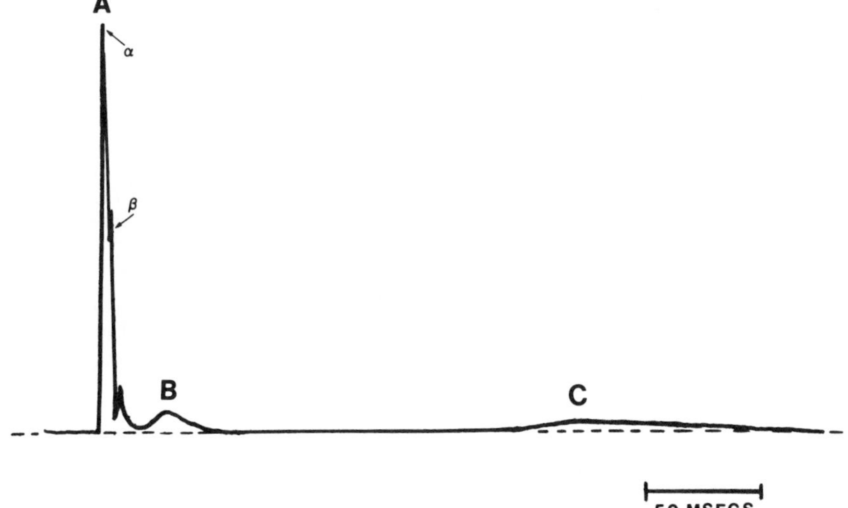

Figure 40.11. Illustration of a compound-action potential from a mixed-fiber nerve, showing the relative amplitudes and time relationships of the various components. Because of the short duration of the A-fiber component, it is usually not feasible to see the entire complex clearly in a single sweep of an oscilloscope beam.

moted by localized application of growth factors, such as nerve growth factor. Even more promising are the growth-promoting effects that have been reported for the systemic administration of gangliosides, which can cross the blood-brain barrier and which are potent stimulants of neuronal growth. Results are probably best when lesions are in nuclear groups, where regeneration does not require the reformation of major fiber tracts. Medical applications of these findings have not been exploited.

JUNCTIONAL TRANSMISSION

A central issue of the neuron doctrine, that each neuron is a distinct functional unit, is the question of how neurons "communicate" with each other. There are only two possibilities: electrical and chemical communication. For many years the prevailing view was that of electrical ("electrotonic" or "ephaptic") communication, wherein an impulse in one neuron, for example, acted as an electrical stimulus to trigger the genesis of an action potential in a target neuron. In some tissues, electrical conduction is clearly the mechanism of communication. This is known because the transfer of activity from one cell to an adjacent cell occurs almost instantly, far to quickly to have been accomplished by chemical means. Cells in which this kind of transmission occurs have very close or tight contacts (about 3nm) between their adjacent membranes—so-called "gap junctions." These junctions have a special topography (Fig. 40.12) in which structural elements extend across each of the apposed cell membranes and allow a continuous connection of the cytoplasm and a direct physical "conduit" for ionic flux between the apposed cells. In addition to electric charge carriers, other larger molecules can be exchanged through these gap junctions.

Electrical coupling

Gap junctions are rather common in certain epithelial tissues, and some have also been seen in neural tissues. The over-all functional role in neurophysiology is not clear, because the preponderance of evidence favors chemical transmission as the predominant communication mechanism in vertebrate nervous systems (see below).

It is also theoretically possible, and much experimental evidence supports the view, that voltage fields of nervous activity act remotely as "electrical stimulators" upon neuronal tissue. This is an extension of the idea that impulse conduction in myelinated axons skips from node to node because the impulse voltage at one node excites the adjacent node. Indeed, one has to wonder about the possibility of "cross-talk" in a nerve that contains hundreds and thousands of myelinated axons. If impulses at one node in a

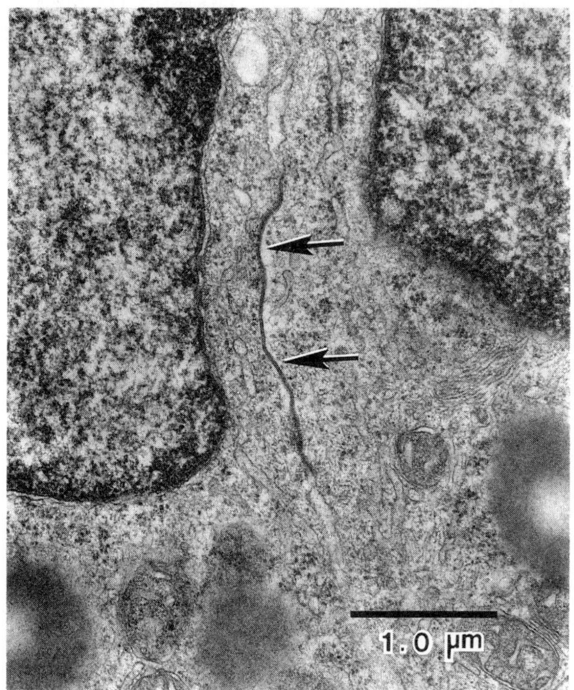

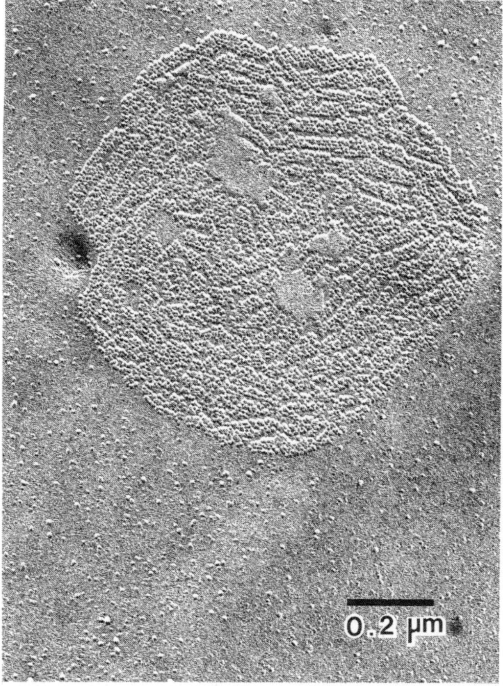

Figure 40.12. Transmission electron micrographs of gap junctions. (*Left*) A large gap junction (*arrows*) connecting two ovarian granulosa cells can be seen in thin sections as regions of closely apposed membranes separated by a 2 nm gap. (*Right*) Freeze-fractured and platinum shadow–cast replica of the plasma membrane from the same cell type reveals the ordered organization of connecting channel-forming particles (connexons). Each channel comprises two annular units that are paired identical units in the adjacent cells. Each connexon consists of six identical protein subunits (connexins). The aqueous channel measures about 1.5 nm in diameter. (Photographs courtesy of Dr. Robert Burghardt, Dept. Vet. Anatomy and Public Health, Texas A & M University.)

given axon excite activity in the next node of that axon, why can they not excite activity in a nearby node of another axon? Also, in cortical tissues that exhibit coherent electrical activity, as reflected in large electroencephalographic rhythms, there is convincing evidence that the ionic currents underlying those rhythms are large enough to cause an electrotonic influence on the excitability of the neurons that are participating in those rhythms. For example, the large "theta waves" seen in the hippocampus of domestic animals have been shown to regulate the flow of input from the entorhinal cortex through the hippocampus. Although this idea of electrical communication is subject to much current debate, there is no question that chemical communication is a dominant factor in the operation of nervous systems.

Chemical coupling

The basic idea of chemical communication is quite simple: When an axon discharges an impulse, the electrical change causes the release of certain "transmitter" chemicals contained in the axon terminal. These transmitters then diffuse across the space (synapse) (about 25 nm) that separates it from the adjacent cell, whereupon the transmitter interacts stereospecifically with a molecular receptor on the postsynaptic membrane. The transmitter-receptor interaction triggers a cascade of postsynaptic and intracellular events that either excite or inhibit the postsynaptic cell.

Synaptic (and neuromuscular) junctions are anatomically and physiologically specialized for chemical communication. The consequence of chemical transmission varies with the type of junction; in neuromuscular junctions, for example, the action is always excitatory, whereas the action may be either excitatory or inhibitory in junctions with smooth muscle or in interneuronal synapses.

Transmission from axons to skeletal muscle

When an impulse in a motor axon supplying a skeletal muscle arrives at the neuromuscular junction, it normally evokes a membrane potential depolarization and action potential in the target muscle. One of the first clues that this transmission process did not involve direct electrical coupling came from the observation that neuromuscular transmission could be blocked by curare (a plant extract used by South American Indians on the tips of the blowpipe arrows they use to capture monkeys and other prey). We now know that neuromuscular transmission depends on release of acetylcholine from an axon terminal, which reacts with a specific class of receptors (nicotinic) on the postjunctional membrane of muscle cells; curare is a specific blocker of nicotinic receptors (the commonly used muscle relaxant, d-tubocurarine, is a purified form of curare).

The junction between an axon terminal and a muscle is structurally highly specialized to provide a storage mechanism for acetylcholine and to provide physical proximity between the sites of acetylcholine release and the membrane receptor region of muscle (Fig. 40.13).

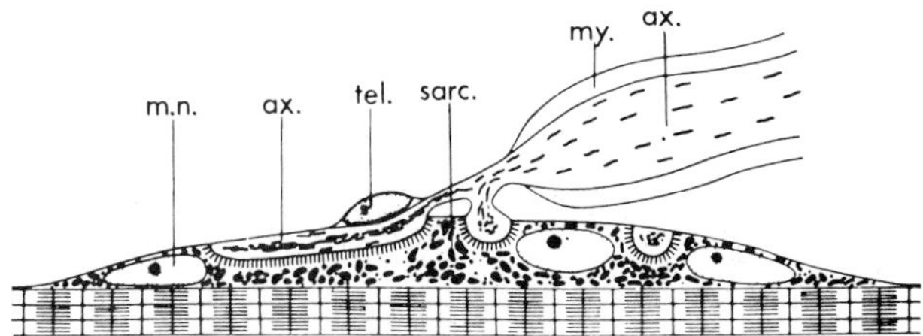

Figure 40.13. Schematic diagram of frog neuromuscular junction. The axon (ax.) sheds its myelin (my.), divides near the muscle, and ends in several grooves in the membrane of the muscle cell (two shown here). The membrane of the muscle cell. (From Couteaux 1960, in Bourne, ed., *The Structure and Function of Muscle*, Academic Press, New York.)

Acetylcholine transmitter

Acetylcholine release from axon terminals occurs in response to an action potential and an associated influx of Ca^{2+}. The influx of Ca^{2+} triggers the release of stored acetylcholine, which is released in small packets, or "quanta," of 1000 to 10,000 molecules. Released acetylcholine diffuses across the junction and binds to the nicotinic receptors on muscle membrane. This, in turn, depolarizes muscle membrane and allows sodium to rush in down its concentration and electrostatic gradient, and thus produce an action potential in the muscle, which in turn causes the muscle cell to contract (see Chap. 45). Some drugs duplicate acetylcholine action, either by mimicking the action on nicotinic receptors (carbamylcholine) or by enhancing the amount of acetylcholine in the junction by preventing its enzymatic destruction after release (physostigmine, certain organophosphorous pesticides, and "nerve gases" used in warfare). The depolarizing action of acetylcholine normally lasts only a few milliseconds because it is rapidly destroyed by the enzyme acetylcholinesterase. Drug inhibition of this enzyme can markedly prolong the size and duration of the end-plate potential (Fig. 40.14). Such drugs are highly dangerous because they not only impair respira-

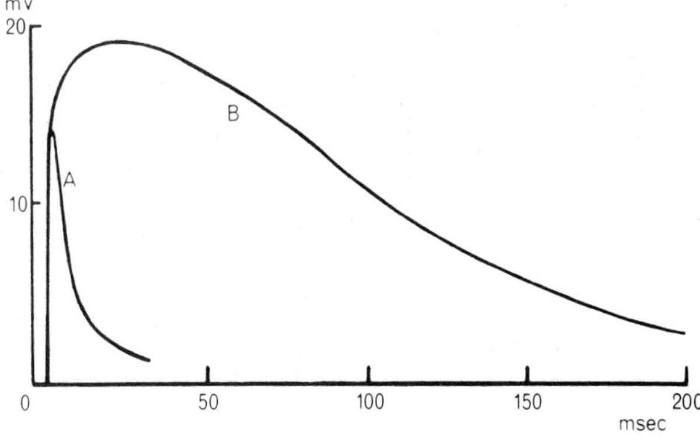

Figure 40.14. Effect of an anticholinesterase (prostigmine) on the size and duration of the motor end-plate potential. The normal potential (A) was larger and lasted much longer when the cholinesterase was inhibited (B). (From Fatt and Katz 1951, *J. Physiol.* 115:320–70.)

tion but also potentiate acetylcholine action in viscera at parasympathetic terminals (see Chap. 46) and in autonomic ganglia, which are also cholinergic (see below).

Clinical implications of calcium ion

Extracellular calcium ions must have a concentration of at least 10^{-4}M for acetylcholine to be released. Impaired transmitter release often occurs clinically in high-producing dairy cows, which lose too much calcium to their milk. Such cows become paralyzed, but symptoms can be relieved dramatically by intravenous infusion of calcium ions in a suitable form, such as calcium gluconate.

Transmission from axons to smooth muscle

The basic principles of chemical transmission are the same for smooth muscles as for skeletal muscles. However, smooth muscles do not have such specialized neuromuscular junctions as skeletal muscles. Also, the transmitter action may be either excitatory or inhibitory and, in either case, will probably persist much longer than the effect in skeletal muscle. In part this is because the enzymatic inactivation systems are not as prominent in smooth muscle junctions. The physiological consequence is that autonomic effects (Chap. 46) last long after the stimuli that triggered them.

The common transmitters released from postganglionic autonomic neurons are acetylcholine in parasymapathetic neurons and noradrenalin in sympathetic neurons. Details concerning these transmitters and their various receptor subtypes are presented in the Chap. on the autonomic nervous system (Chap. 46).

Synaptic (interneuronal) transmission

Synaptic regions have morphological specialization of both presynaptic and postsynaptic membranes. Several kinds of such junctions are known: axosomatic, between axons and soma or cell body (for example, between axons and cell bodies in autonomic ganglia); axoaxonic, between two axons (for example, the junction between axons of spinal interneurons and primary afferent fibers); axodendritic, between axons and dendrites (for example, in the dorsal horn of the spinal cord); and dendrodendritic, between dendrites (for example, in cerebellar cortex).

Regardless of type, there is no continuity of cytoplasm, as with gap junctions, across the synapse; electron micrographs clearly show a gap of about 20 to 30 nm. Both presynaptic and postsynaptic membranes are thickened and modified (Fig. 40.15). The presynaptic terminal contains more than the usual density of mitochondria, and there are also numerous storage vesicles for neurotransmitter. The presynapatic terminal is specialized for storage and release of neurotransmitter, which diffuses across the synaptic gap to bind with specific postsynaptic receptor proteins. The binding is transient, so that transmitter in the gap can also be destroyed enzymatically, can be taken back up into the presynaptic terminal, or may sometimes even bind to presynaptic "autoreceptors." Postsynaptically, neural membranes are modified by the incorporation into the lipid bilayer of specific receptor proteins and their associated complex lipids, called gangliosides (Fig. 40.16).

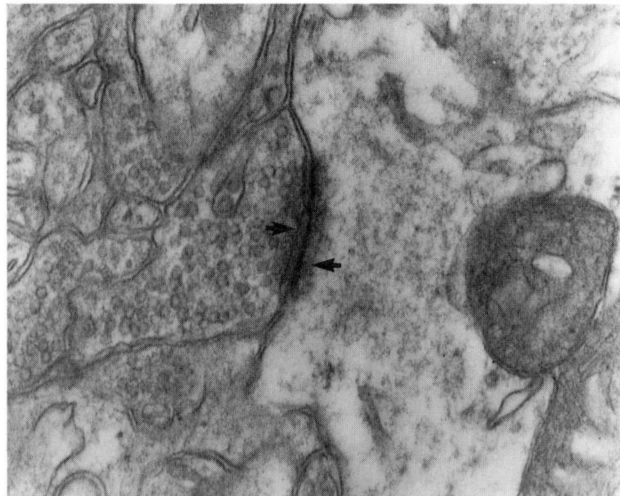

Figure 40.15. Transmission electron micrograph of several axon terminals (*near center of photograph*), indicated by the inclusion of numerous circular vesicles. Region of an active synapse is indicated by thickened darker membrane (*arrows*). Magnification: ×30,500. (Photograph courtesy of Drs. Evelyn Tiffany-Castiglioni and Oscar Illanes, Dept. Vet. Anatomy and Public Health, Texas A & M University.)

The density of synaptic junctions is extraordinary. As much as 65 percent of the surface of a neuron's soma and dendrites may be covered with synapses from afferent terminals. The neurotransmitter-receptor interactions may either depolarize or hyperpolarize the postsynaptic target (Fig. 40.17).

Ion channels

Postsynaptic activity is ultimately governed by the flow of ions through specialized ion channels. These are of two types: (1) voltage-gated (i.e. regulated by membrane voltage per se, as is seen in axonal propagation of impulses) and (2) chemically gated (i.e., regulated by neurotransmitter). These two types of channel are differentially affected by poisons; tetrodotoxin, for example, blocks voltage-gated but not chemically gated Na^+ channels, while cobra venom does just the opposite.

Microelectrode techniques ("patch clamp") that involve recording of current flow through only one or a few ion channels reveal that the channels open in an all-or-none fashion. The graded over-all changes in postsynaptic potentials arise because the channels of the whole neuron open in staggered sequence.

Excitatory neurotransmission

Such systems cause sodium channels to open and allow sodium ions to enter the cell. The net response is graded: a small depolarization occurs if a few channels open, while a

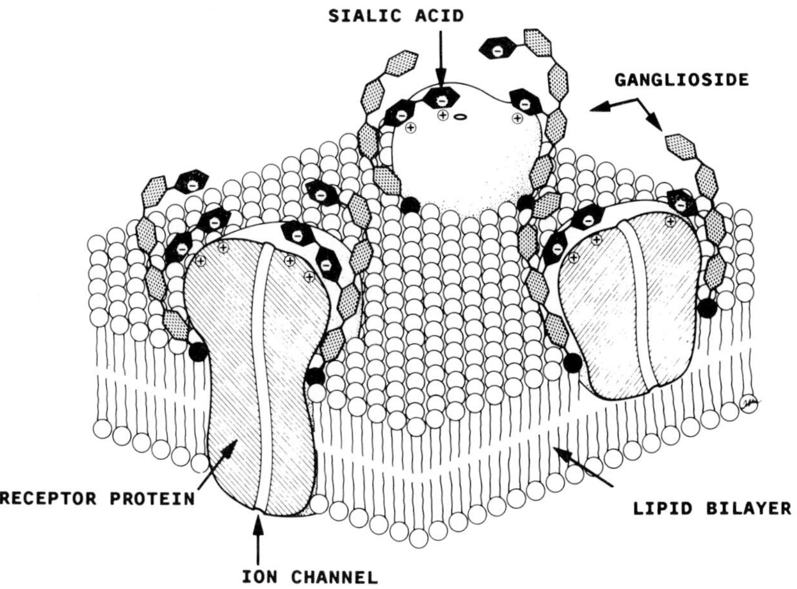

Figure 40.16. Modification of the conventional diagram of plasma membrane to reflect the molecular composition in the synapse. Shown are the presence of specific receptor proteins, their channels through which ions can flow, and the surrounding ganglioside lipids, with their extracellularly projecting sugar and sialic acid moieties. (Reprinted from *Alcohol*, volume 7, W. R. Klemm, Dehydration: A new alcohol theory, pp. 49–59, copyright 1990, with permission from Pergamon Press Ltd, Headington Hill Hall, Oxford 0X3 0BW, UK.)

large depolarization and impulse discharge occurs if many channels are open (see discussion on ion channels, below). The potential change is called an "excitatory postsynaptic potential", or EPSP. The associated ion flow gradually declines to zero, as it runs down the electrochemical gradient; the duration is usually on the order of several milliseconds. Another key feature of chemical neurotransmission is that as long as the membrane potentials are below threshold for firing impulses, the membrane potential can

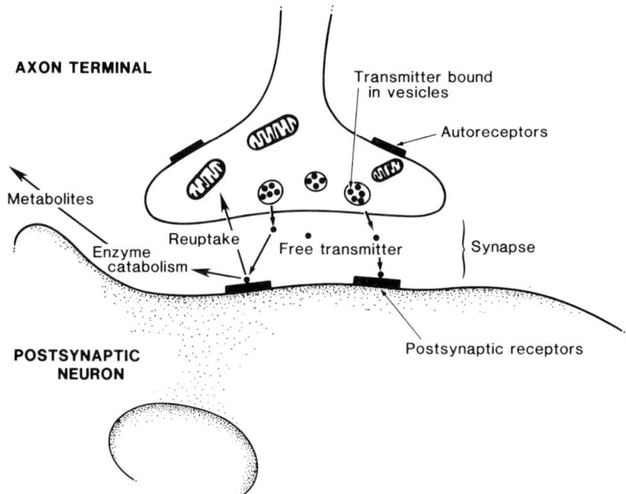

Figure 40.17. Diagram of presynaptic and postsynaptic elements and associated neurotransmission mechanisms. Presynaptic terminals synthesize and store neurotransmitter chemicals. When the terminal is depolarized, transmitter is released into the synaptic gap, whereupon it temporarily can bind to specialized postsynaptic receptor proteins. Transmitter can also be destroyed enzymatically or may even bind temporarily to presynaptic autoreceptors, which in turn regulate release of transmitter.

summate inputs. That is, if a neurotransmitter at one synapse causes a small depolarization, a simultaneous release of that transmitter at another synapse located elsewhere on the same soma will summate to cause a larger depolarization. This so-called spatial summation mechanism (Fig. 40.18) is complemented by temporal summation, wherein successive releases of transmitter from one synapse will cause progressive increase in depolarization as long as the presynaptic changes occur faster than the decay rate of the membrane potential changes in the postsynaptic neuron. Neurotransmitter effects last several times longer than presynaptic impulses and thereby allow summation of effect. Thus the EPSP differs from action potentials in a fundamental way, it summates inputs and expresses a graded response, as opposed to the all-or-none response of impulse discharge. The summation process is an integral feature of the nervous system's ability to process information (see Chap. 39).

At the same time that a given postsynaptic neuron is receiving and summating excitatory neurotransmitter, it may also be receiving "conflicting" messages that are telling it to shut down firing. These inhibitory influences are mediated by inhibitory neurotransmitter systems that cause postsynaptic membranes to hyperpolarize. Such effects are generally attributed to the opening of selective ion channels that either allow intracellular potassium to leave the postsynaptic cell or allow extracellular chloride to enter. In either case, the net effect is to add to the intracellular negativity and move the membrane potential farther away from the threshold for generating impulses.

When EPSPs and inhibiting postsynaptic potentials (IPSPs) are generated simultaneously in the same cell, the output response will be determined by the relative strengths of the excitatory and inhibitory inputs. Output "instructions," in

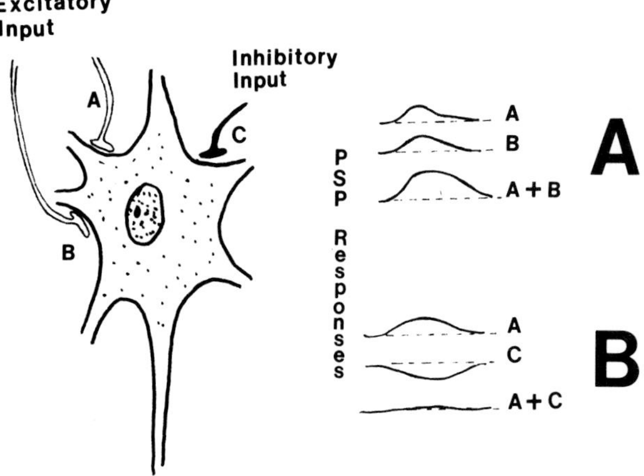

Figure 40.18. Schematic diagram of the summation of changes in postsynaptic membrane that can occur in excitatory neurotransmitter systems. (*A*) When excitatory inputs are received simultaneously at several synapses on the same neuron, the postsynaptic potentials summate ("spatial summation"), bringing the membrane potential closer to the threshold for firing an action potential. (*B*) When inhibitory input is received at a synapse, it tends to cancel the effect of a simultaneous excitatory input.

the form of impulse generation, are thus determined by this algebraic processing of information.

Major neurotransmitters

More than 100 neurotransmitters and neuronal chemicals that modulate transmitter action have been discovered. The best known transmitters include acetylcholine, dopamine, norepinephrine, and serotonin. In recent years the greatest research activity has involved neuropeptides. Research has shown that it is common for more than one transmitter to coexist in the same neuron—a violation of the old "Dale's principle," which held that a given neuron makes only one transmitter.

Receptors

Each transmitter has its own receptor molecule. Three receptors have been particularly well studied: the receptors for acetylcholine, for γ-aminobutyric acid (GABA) (a major inhibitory transmitter), and for glycine/glutamate (major excitatory transmitters acting on the so-called N-methyl-*d*-aspartate [NMDA] receptor). The last two types of receptors are particularly interesting because they have multiple sites, including receptor sites where primary neurotransmitter effects occur and other "recognition sites" at which binding creates allosteric effects on the receptor sites.

A high degree of structural homology is exhibited by one group of receptors: the "muscarinic" acetylcholine receptor and several subtypes of receptors for norepinephrine. These feature a short string of amino acids that projects extracellularly while continuing in the membrane as a sequence of seven coils; these, in turn, continue in the cytosol as a series of three loose loops.

Presynaptic inhibition

A presynaptic inhibitory mechanism has been discovered. Here, the inhibition is produced by depression of excitatory presynaptic terminals, and thus the inhibition does not depend on the genesis of postsynaptic IPSPs. Presynaptic terminals release less of their excitatory transmitter when they are excited in the normal way, and the EPSPs normally generated are smaller than usual. Thus inhibition of output results even though IPSPs are never produced. One very important feature of presynaptic inhibition is that it has a very long time course, on the order of 100 or more milliseconds.

Presynaptic autoregulation

Axon terminals can act as receptive structures as well as being transmissive. Their own transmitters may be among the chemical signals that they detect, translating that binding into a modulation of transmitter release.

Second messengers

Neurotransmitters and their receptors often do more than just alter ion channels.

The transduction of input, whether it be at sensory receptors or at synapses, typically involves the gating of ion channels (Fig. 40.19). In some cases this involves a direct action of postsynaptic depolarization, and in others it involves an indirect action between the extracellular ligand and the molecules (receptors) of the ion gate. A good example of transmitter action is the nicotinic acetylcholine system, in which the receptor and the ion channel are part of the same glycoprotein complex; such systems are fast but exhibit little capability for amplification.

In other cases, the ion gate actions are amplified indirectly by a chain of biochemical events, a cascade of biochemical reactions that serve to amplify the input. The cascade begins with an initial formation of second messenger molecules, such as cyclic adenosine monophosphate (cAMP), cyclic guanosine monophosphate (cGMP), or phosphoinositides. These are commonly coupled to a series of postsynaptic biochemical reactions that act in cascade fashion to produce activated, phosphorylated proteins that cause the ultimate change in cellular activity (Fig. 40.19, bottom). The addition of charged phosphate groups to protein can alter conformation and thereby change the function of an enzyme, a regulatory protein, or an ion channel subunit.

Although there are several distinct second messenger systems, all seem to share common principles. In particular, high-energy phosphate bonds are formed on proteins and activate them to catalyze cellular responses. Finally, phosphatases cleave the activated phosphate groups, terminate the second messenger action, and thus allow regeneration of the system.

Cyclic AMP

Adenosine triphosphate (ATP), in the presence of the enzyme adenylate cyclase becomes converted into cAMP,

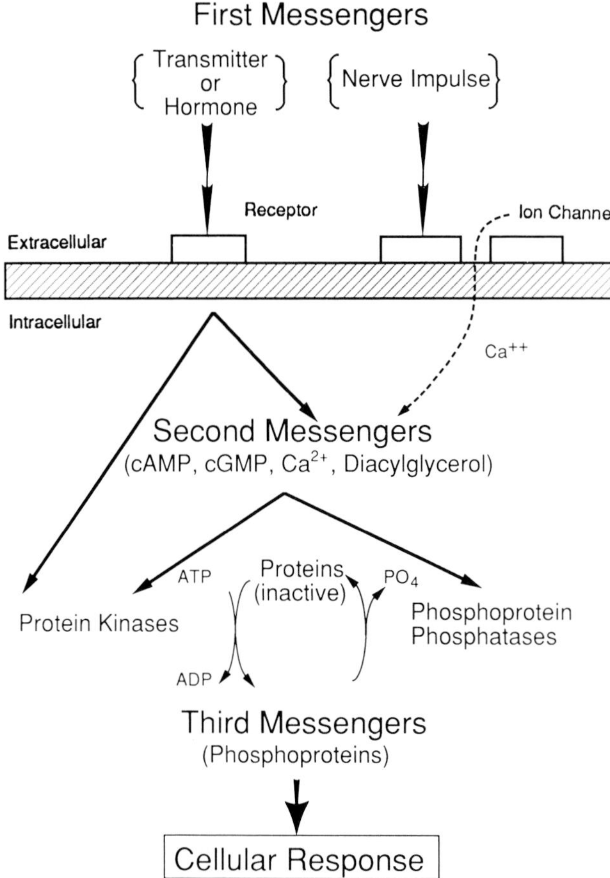

Figure 40.19. Diagram of the principles of synaptic transduction. In some synaptic systems a presynaptic nerve impulse opens voltage-gated ion channels (*top right*), whereas in others a transmitter-receptor interaction is involved (*top left*). In both cases, "second messenger" chemicals may emerge; these activate protein kinases that produce an ATP-dependent phosphorylation of specific "third messenger" proteins, which provide the proximate influence on cellular activity.

yielding two phosphate groups and hydrogen ion in the process. Cyclic AMP has three primary actions in the neuron: functioning of microtubules, synthesis of neurotransmitter, and synthesis of a second messenger for neurotransmitter-receptor reactions. Among the transmitters that are known to activate this system are norepinephrine, dopamine, serotonin, histamine, adenosine, and various peptides, as well as some prostaglandins.

The transmitter-receptor actions produce a cascade of biochemical reactions that ultimately produce the cellular response (Fig. 40.20).

The actual cascade of reactions is quite complicated. It appears to include the following steps: (1) binding of transmitter to receptor, (2) displacement of guanine diphosphate (GDP) from its bonding to a "G" protein, which may be either excitatory or inhibitory, (3) replacement of the GDP on the G protein by guanine triphosphate (GTP), (4) activation of adenylate cyclase by Ca^{2+}-calmodulin action on the G protein, (5) formation of cAMP, (6) coupling of cAMP to

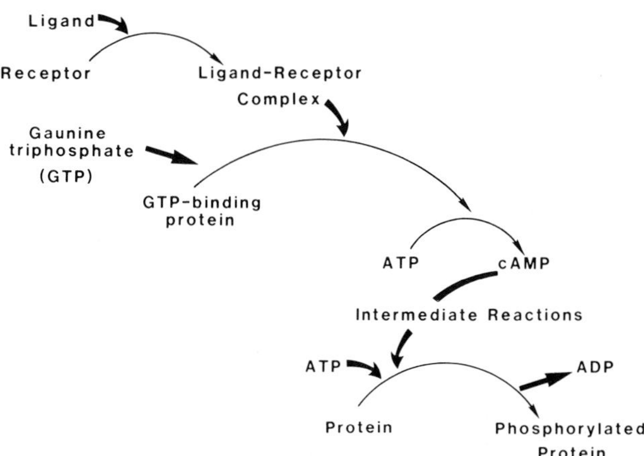

Figure 40.20. Illustration of the cascade of biochemical reactions associated with the cyclic AMP second messenger system. When neurotransmitter or drug ligand binds with the membrane receptor (*upper left*), the complex initiates binding of GTP to a specific protein, which in turn triggers the formation of cyclic AMP. Cyclic AMP in turn initiates a series of reactions that ultimately lead to formation of the phosphorylated proteins that are the proximate cause of the cellular response.

a regulatory subunit of a protein kinase, (7) phosphorylation of protein by protein kinase, (8) intracellular actions produced by the phosphorylated protein, (9) termination of G protein action by hydrolysis of GTP to GDP, and (10) termination of cAMP action by phosphodiesterase.

In the case of inhibitory transmitters, the coupling between the G protein and adenylate cyclase inhibits the formation of cAMP, thus inhibiting subsequent steps in the cascade.

There is also a parallel cascade second messenger system involving cGMP, wherein GTP is converted into cGMP. This system seems to be most conspicuous in the cerebellum and may be involved in the action of acetylcholine.

Phosphatidylinositol

In some synapses, the transmitter-receptor interaction cleaves membrane phosphatidylinositol, which yields a diacylglycerol residue and inositol triphosphate (ITP). ITP has second messenger properties. When ITP breaks down, it gives rise to two second messengers that act synergistically to activate a protein kinase that phosphorylates certain proteins that permit release of bound calcium inside the cell. The amplification steps occur because one molecule of catalyst can regulate the reactions of many substrate molecules. Known agonists of ITP breakdown include substance P, neurotensin, acetylcholine, norepinephrine, serotonin, histamine, glutamate, and vasopressin.

Calcium

Calcium is a vital component in a variety of presynaptic and postsynaptic reactions. Ca^{2+} has its own voltage-dependent ion channel through membranes, its own ATP-linked pump, specialized binding proteins, and specialized protein kinases. Extracellularly, much of the Ca^{2+} is probably sequestered by the sialic acid residues of membrane-bound glycolipids (gangliosides) and glycoproteins. There is both an electrostatic and a concentration gradient for calcium entry into the neuron. When a neuron is depolarized, Ca^{2+} enters the presynaptic membrane via a specific calcium channel. Once inside, Ca^{2+} again becomes sequestered by virtually every presynaptic protein. One of particular importance is known as calmodulin; calmodulin becomes activated when bound to Ca^{2+}, and it can then initiate a series of important presynaptic actions. The best known action is the adhesion of presynaptic vesicles to the cell membrane, where exocytosis of neurotransmitter occurs. Neurotransmitters that are known to be releasable by this mechanism include norepinephrine, dopamine, and acetylcholine. In recent years a whole class of Ca^{2+}-channel–binding drugs (verapamil, nifedipine, diltiazem) has been developed; in humans these are used for angina, hypertension, and various kinds of cardiac arrhythmia.

Pharmacological consequences of neurotransmission

Because neurotransmitter systems require biochemical mechanisms for synthesis, storage, release, and receptor binding, the nervous system provides numerous opportunities for pharmacological intervention and for the treatment of neural disorders. Numerous drugs are in wide use for alteration of neurotransmitter functions, and the list of new drugs under development grows steadily. A particularly unexploited area of therapeutic opportunity is the development of drugs that act at various stages in the second messenger systems.

REFLEX ACTION

Principles

Reflexes are relatively simple involuntary, stereotyped, reactions to peripheral stimulation. Several specific reflexes are routinely used in clinical neurological examinations. The neural circuitry for reflexes is commonly referred to as a "reflex arc," primarily because the reflex circuits in the spinal cord have an arclike anatomy; it should be noted, however, that there are also cranial reflexes. Five neural elements commonly make up a reflex arc: (1) a receptor organ, (2) an afferent neuron, (3) interneurons in the cord or brain, (4) efferent neurons, and (5) an effector organ, which may be a skeletal muscle, a smooth muscle, or a gland. In some of the simpler (monosynaptic) reflexes, the interneuron may not be required.

Many aspects of animal behavior (see Chap. 49) include a very complex series of muscle and gland responses that are also involuntary and stereotyped; these could be called complex or compound reflexes, but many people prefer to use other terminology, such as *reaction* or *response*.

Spinal cord reflexes

Spinal cord reflexes have a great deal of clinical value, because defects in these reflexes are very useful in determination of the location and magnitude of damage to the spinal cord. In dogs, the most common cause of such damage is a "slipped disk" (protrusion of the intervertebral disk).

Flexion (withdrawal) reflex

If a noxious stimulus, such as a toe pinch, is applied to a limb, the animal will withdraw the limb automatically. This can occur in animals with spinal lesion or transection, as long as the spinal damage does not involve the circuitry of the reflex itself. The reflex arcs that produce this withdrawal involve many synapses, which excite those muscle groups that will produce withdrawal by contraction of flexors. At the same time, extensors are inhibited (Fig. 40.21).

This reflex is very useful clinically. If it is intact, it reveals that the associated region of spinal cord, muscles, and nerves is intact. Furthermore, associated behavioral signs can give evidence of the integrity of ascending paths to the brain. It is also a measure of anesthesia, although it can still be present under light stages of anesthesia where the animal is unconscious (see Chap. 48).

Crossed extensor reflex

The basics of the crossed extensor reflex are best illustrated in humans. On stepping on a tack or a piece of glass,

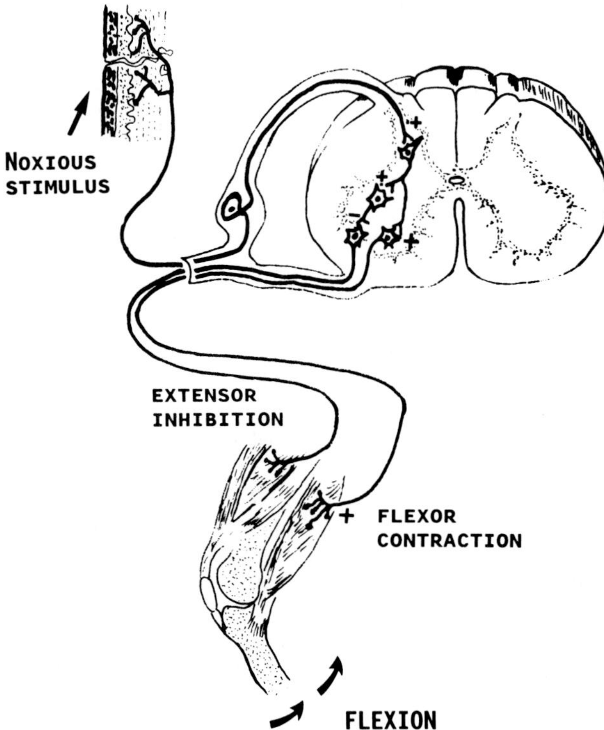

Figure 40.21. Illustration of the spinal pathways involved in mediating the flexor reflex. Noxious stimulation of a limb, for example, initiates an excitatory spike train that activates alpha motoneurons that supply flexor muscles of that same limb. Concurrently, inhibitory interneurons in the cord are activated to inhibit the alpha motoneurons that supply the extensors of that same limb.

one reflexly withdraws the affected limb and simultaneously extends the opposite limb. This reflex includes the same neurons as the withdrawal reflex but, in addition, recruits the neurons that control extension of the opposite limb. If a flexor reflex is induced in a recumbent animal, the crossed extensor reflex is usually not seen, except when it has been released from inhibition by a lesion in the brain.

Myotatic (stretch) reflex

The myotatic reflex occurs in response to sudden stretching of muscle, such as can be produced by sudden tapping of a tendon. The sense organ is the muscle spindle (see Chap. 41); when it is activated by stretch of the muscle, the annulospiral ending part of the spindle generates a discharge of impulses, carried in so-called Ia afferent fibers and routed through the spinal cord via the dorsal horn onto motoneurons (alpha motoneurons) in the ventral horn of the same spinal segment. The alpha motoneurons that are "wired" in this circuit are connected to the same muscles that contained the activated spindle. At the same time, the circuitry is so connected that the Ia discharge inhibits the alpha motoneurons of muscles that are antagonists of the stretched muscle. For example, if a flexor muscle is stretched, the myotatic reflex causes it to contract while the corresponding extensor muscle is inhibited. Thus the consequence of muscle stretch is to contract the stretched muscle, thus opposing the stretch and shutting off afferent discharge. This is the basis for the knee-jerk or ankle-jerk reflex that is routinely used in clinical neurology to assess the integrity of the spinal cord at various levels. The purpose of this reflex system is thus to expedite movements in response to prior movements. It also serves to promote muscle tone; that is, there is a low level of continuous contraction of skeletal muscle.

Muscle tone is regulated by other motoneurons that activate the small muscle fibers of the spindle itself, the so-called intrafusal fibers (see Chap. 41). This provides another way that extrafusal muscle fibers can be made to contract. Small motoneurons, called gamma motoneurons (also called gamma efferents), in the ventral horn of the cord supply excitatory drive to the intrafusal muscle fibers of the spindle. When gamma motoneurons are activated, they cause contraction of intrafusal fibers, which in turn stretches the spindle and triggers the myotatic reflexes. When there is a sustained low level of gamma efferent activity, there will be sustained muscle tonus. Normally, gamma efferent activity is under control of descending influences from the brain (see Chap. 44).

Alpha motoneurons may be excited directly to produce somatic movement with simultaneous coactivation of gamma motor neurons, or gamma motor neurons may be excited to initiate the myotatic reflexes that produce somatic movement. Locomotion seems to involve both mechanisms. In voluntary motor activity, alpha and gamma motor neurons are excited simultaneously so that as extrafusal muscle fibers shorten, intrafusal fibers also shorten in order that myotatic reflexes can be maintained in a muscle of shorter length.

Inverse myotatic reflex

The Golgi tendon organ mediates an inverse myotatic reflex. As discussed in Chapter 41, these receptors are relatively insensitive to stretch of an extrafusal muscle fiber but are easily excited by extrafusal muscle contraction, which puts stretch on the tendon. Thus the Golgi tendon organ is a sensor of muscle contraction. Afferents from Golgi organs, so-called Ib afferents, contribute to multipsynaptic reflex arcs in the cord that inhibit alpha motoneurons and relax the muscle that contains the tendon organ, while at the same time activating contraction of the antagonists to that muscle.

Thus this reflex acts as a brake on excessive contraction of muscles and prevents damage. Human weight lifters, for example, will experience sudden collapse if they try to lift too much; their Golgi tendon organs protect them from damaging their muscles. In animals this reflex is best demonstrated under decerebrate or brain damage conditions; in such situations, strong passive flexion of a limb will produce passive stretch on the spindle, producing contraction of the muscle, but the Golgi tendon organ reflex may then become dominant, causing a "clasp-knife" reflex, wherein the muscle tension abruptly melts away after an initial strong resistance.

Scratch reflex

Dogs scratch a lot. There is a simple reflex basis for this action, although it typically has a voluntary component. The reflex nature can be demonstrated, at least in some dogs, by moving the fingers rapidly back and forth over the skin of the dorsolateral parts of the thorax, the ventral abdomen, or the caudal part of the ear. The reflex can even be produced in animals with lesions in the cervical cord, thus indicating that the arc is resident in the cord.

Micturition reflex

When animals undergo major spinal cord damage, there is an initial period when urination reflexes stop. As several days elapse, however, reflex urination may return. This reflex is initiated by bladder afferents that are stimulated as the bladder fills and is stretched. The reflex system, located in the lumbosacral enlargement, includes the pelvic nerve and the hypogastric nerves as afferent inputs and efferent fibers to the bladder in the pelvic nerve and to the external urethral sphincter in the pudendal nerve.

The micturition reflex is facilitated by cutaneous afferents from the perineal region. This is best illustrated in intact cows, where tickling the skin of the perineum may reflexly trigger urination.

In intact animals, the micturition reflex centers in the cord are modulated by centers within the brain-stem reticular formation.

There are many other reflex actions that involve the spinal cord, including defecation, eructation, erection, and ejaculation. Some of these are discussed in the chapters dealing with other systems.

REFERENCES

Augustine, G.J., Charlton, M.P., and Smith, S.J. 1987. Calcium action in synaptic transmitter release. *Annu. Rev. Neurosci.* 10:633–94.

Bawin, S.M., Sheppard, A.R., Mahoney, M.D., and Adey, W.R. 1984. Influences of sinusoidal fields on excitability in the rat hippocampal slice. *Brain Res.* 323: 227–37.

Bloom, F.E. 1986. Molecular diversity and neuronal function. In R. Levi Montalcini, P. Calissano, E.R. Kandel, and A. Maggi, eds., *Molecular Aspects of Neurobiology*. Springer-Verlag, Berlin. Pp. 188–92.

Changeaux, J.P., Davillers-Thiery, A., and Chemouilli, P. 1984. Acetylcholine receptor: An allosteric protein. *Science* 225:1335–45.

Cockroft, S., and Gomperts, B.D. 1985. Role of guanine nucleotide binding protein in the activation of polyphosphoinosotide phosphodiesterase. *Nature* 314:534–36.

Cotman, C.W., Monaghan, D.T., and Ganong, A.H. 1988. Excitatory amino acid neurotransmission: NMDA receptors and Hebb-type synaptic plasticity. *Annu. Rev. Neurosci.* 11:61–80.

DeLahunta, A. 1983. *Veterinary Neuroanatomy and Clinical Neurology*. W.B. Saunders, Philadelphia.

DeMello, W.C. 1987. *Cell-to-Cell Communication*. Plenum Press, New York.

Eccles, J.C. 1982. The synapse: From electrical to chemical transmission. *Annu. Rev. Neurosci.* 6:325–39.

Gorio, A., and Haber, B. 1985. *Neurobiology of Gangliosides*. A.R. Liss, Inc., New York.

Hertzberg, E.L., and Johnson, R.G. 1988. *Gap Junctions*. A.R. Liss, Inc., New York.

Kennedy, M.B. 1983. Experimental approaches to understanding the role of protein phosphorylation in the regulation of neuronal function. *Annu. Rev. Neurosci.* 6:527–46.

Krueger, B.K. 1989. Toward an understanding of structure and function of ion channels. *FASEB J.* 3:1906–14.

Levitan, I.B. 1988. Modulation of ion channels in neurons and other cells. *Annu. Rev. Neuroscience*. Annual Reviews, Palo Alto, Ca. Pp. 119–36.

Lichtstein, D., and Rodbard, D. 1987. A second look at the second messenger hypothesis. *Life Sci.* 40:2041–51.

Millhorn, D.E., and Hokfelt, T. 1988. Chemical messengers and their coexistence in individual neurons. *News Physiol. Sci.* 3:1–5.

Pace, U., and Lancet, D. 1987. Molecular mechanisms of vertebrate olfaction: Implications for pheromone biochemistry. In G.D. Prestwich and G.J. Blomquist, eds. *Pheromone Biochemistry*. Academic Press, New York. Pp. 529–46.

Putney, J.W., Jr., ed. 1986. *Phosphoinositides and Receptor Mechanisms*. Vol. 7. *Receptor Biochemistry and Methodology*. A.R. Liss, New York.

Reuter, H. 1987. Modulation of ion channels by phosphorylation and second messengers. *News Physiol. Sci.* 2:168–71.

Starke, K. 1989. Presynaptic autoregulation: Does it play a role? *News Physiol. Sci.* 4:1–4.

Tallman, J.F., and Gallager, D.W. 1985. The GABA-ergic system: A locus of benzodiazepine action. *Annu. Rev. Neurosci.* 8:21–44.

Venter, J.C., Fraser, C.M., Kerlavage, A.R., and Buck, M.A. 1989. Molecular biology of adrenergic and muscarinic cholineregic receptors. *Biochem. Pharmacol.* 38:1197–1208.

Zucker, R.S., and Haydon, P.G. 1988. Membrane potential has no direct role in evoking neurotransmitter release. *Nature* 335:360–62.

CHAPTER 41

Somesthetic Sensory Mechanisms | by Ainsley Iggo and W. R. Klemm

This chapter describes some basic principles of sensory function and some of the features of whole-body sensory functions ("somesthesia"). Functions of some special senses are explained elsewhere: vision in Chapter 42 and hearing, taste, and smell in Chapter 43.

PRINCIPLES OF AFFERENT ACTIVITY

The central nervous system (CNS) must have "information" for processing and action. The input of this information comes from specialized nerve endings and organs that convert (transduce) the physical nature of the environment, both external and internal, into a nerve impulse code that can be "read" by the CNS. This kind of input is called CNS afferent, meaning "coming into or toward" the CNS.

Organizational plan

Afferent activity is conveyed as action potentials (Chap. 40) via nerves into the dorsal roots of spinal nerves or into cranial nerve nuclei of the brain stem. The axons in these peripheral nerves are functionally the same as dendrites in that they bring impulse input into the cell body, even though the length of many of these fibers makes them seem like axons.

The excitation is typically conveyed via a peripheral or cranial nerve fiber to a first-order neuronal cell body, located either in the dorsal root ganglion of spinal nerves or in a cranial nerve ganglion. From here, the cell's output fiber synapses with a second neuron in the spinal cord or brain stem, respectively, that relays the output to a third neuronal cell body located in the thalamus. Axons of the third neurons project sensory input to the final destination in the cerebral cortex (i.e., sensory cortex) (Fig. 41.1).

In addition to this trisynaptic path, which typically mediates conscious sensations, stimuli can be routed to motoneurons directly or indirectly via interneurons to activate reflexes (see Chap. 40).

All sensory receptors have at least three common properties: they (1) have a defined receptive field on or in the body, (2) are activated by select kinds of stimuli, and (3) have a distinct rate of adaptation to the presence of continuous stimulus.

Receptive field

The body area from which a response can be aroused is called a receptive field, and the size of that field varies with the amount of innervation that is present. For example, a dog's ears are quite sensitive to pulling and pressure, because there are many nerve fibers there; the receptive fields are quite small, in that stimulation of a very small point of skin is likely to elicit a response. Conversely, receptive fields over the back are relatively larger, requiring that more surface of the back be stimulated to evoke a response. Individual afferent fibers also have a receptive field, responding to stimuli applied to any place within it.

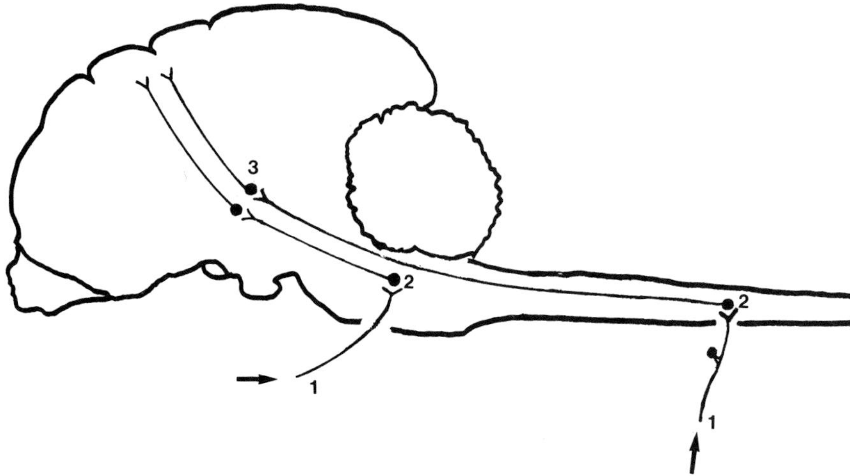

Figure 41.1. General anatomical plan for sensory pathways. Peripheral input enters via a fiber of a first-order neuron, whose cell body is in a cranial nerve ganglion for stimuli involving the head or in the dorsal root ganglion of spinal nerves, in the case of stimuli involving the trunk or limbs. Second-order neurons in the dorsal horn (or in the brain stem in the case of proprioceptive stimuli and certain cranial nerve inputs) relay the input to the thalamus, wherein third-order neurons project the input to the sensory cortex.

In spinal nerves, each dorsal root receives input from a defined region of the body, called a *dermatome*. Adjacent dermatomes have overlapping receptive fields.

Selective sensitivity

Sensory receptors, which are specialized nerve endings or organs, belong to one of two main physiological groups: (1) exteroceptors, which detect stimuli that arise external to the body, and (2) interoceptors, which detect stimuli that originate within the body.

Exteroceptors include the special senses for vision and hearing (see Chap. 42), as well as such senses as the vomeronasal sense (Chap. 49), olfaction, and taste (Chap. 43). Exteroceptor functions that are discussed in this chapter are those that affect the outer surface of the body, such as touch, pressure, warmth, and cold. Interoceptors include sensory units in the viscera, equilibrium sensors in the inner ear, and a special class of receptors devoted to detecting position of limbs and muscle tone (so-called proprioceptors).

Each of these kinds of receptor is selective for its type of stimulus. The selectivity is manifest in especially low thresholds for activation of a particular kind of stimulus. Thermal receptors are particularly sensitive to temperature change, and chemoreceptors are especially sensitive to chemical changes. Most receptors can respond to stimuli for which they are not specialized, but the thresholds are much higher. For example, the retina of the eye has a very low threshold for responding to light, but it can respond to pressure at a much higher threshold.

Sensitivity of receptors is commonly quantified in terms of plots of response versus a stimulus parameter. For example, the output of thermal receptors has a maximum at temperatures that are specific to the receptor type (Fig. 41.2). Such curves define the effective range of stimuli.

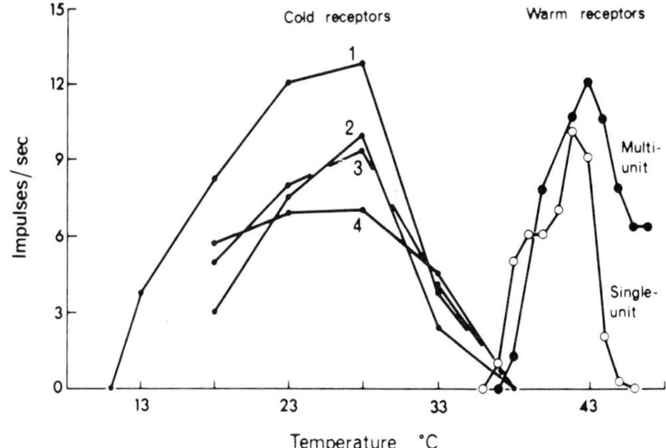

Figure 41.2. Temperature sensitivity curves for four cold receptors and two warm receptors in the scrotal skin of the rat. Each data point is the mean impulse discharge rate after the skin had been held at the given temperature for at least 3 minutes. (From Iggo 1969, *J. Physiol.* 200:403–30.)

Adaptation

Most sensory receptors are tuned to respond to change. That is, the receptor responds by generating impulses whenever it suddenly receives an applied stimulus or the nature of that stimulus changes. If the stimulus continues, however, there is a tendency for the receptor to habituate or adapt and stop responding (Fig. 41.3). Some receptors adapt rapidly, others adapt slowly, and some never adapt. There is a biological advantage to having different receptors that adapt at different rates. Those afferent units that adapt rapidly are well suited to signaling sudden changes in stimulus, and this is useful for such stimuli as sights, sounds, and touch. On the other hand, slowly adapting receptors can keep the CNS informed of long-lasting stimuli, and they are useful for stimuli that are harmful and cause pain.

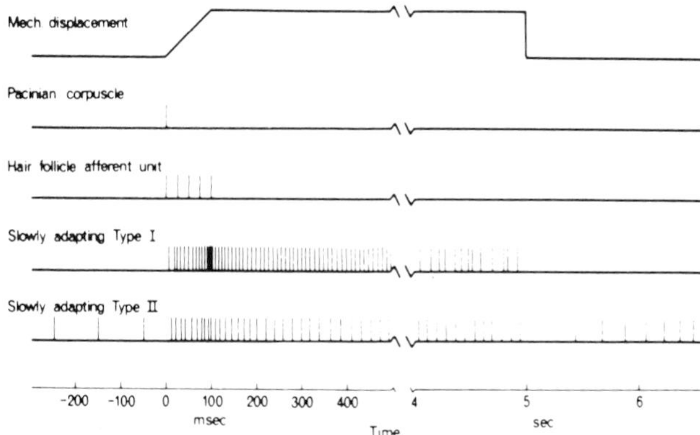

Figure 41.3. Differences in the rate of adaptation in different kinds of skin receptors. A mechanical probe, upper tracing, is shown displacing the skin. Pacinian corpuscles and hair follicle stimuli are very rapidly adapting, producing only a few initial impulses. Slowly adapting units, with or without resting discharge, show sustained levels of impulse activity as long as the stimulus persists.

Adaptation is not the same as fatigue. A fatigued receptor cannot be excited by withdrawal and reapplication of the stimulus.

Mechanisms by which receptors adapt

Mechanisms vary with the kind of receptor involved. For example, in some mechanoreceptors physical structure contributes in large measure to the adaptation. In visual receptors (rods and cones), the adaptation involves changes in chemical composition.

Poorly adapting ("static") receptors

Receptors that do not adapt readily keep the brain informed of the presence of stimulus. This is biologically useful for certain kinds of stimuli; for example, the brain ought to be apprised of the location of joints and limbs in space at all times, so that responses to other stimuli that require movement will occur rapidly and correctly. Other examples of static receptors include baroreceptors for blood pressure, chemoreceptors for blood gases, sound receptors in the ear, receptors in the vestibular apparatus, and pain receptors; in each case a continuous discharge is biologically useful.

Rapidly adapting receptors

Rapidly adapting receptors react strongly only when a change in stimulus is taking place. Because the number of impulses generated by such receptors is directly related to the rate at which the change takes place, these receptors can be considered stimulus-rate receptors. Thus the Pacinian corpuscles that transduce skin pressure stimuli are able to signal to the brain the rate at which pressure changes on the skin are occurring.

Specific modalities

Each type of sensation to which an animal responds is called a modality of sensation (sight, sound, touch, temperature). For each modality, there are usually specialized sensory cells, or receptors, that are sensitive to that modality and that transduce the stimulus into nerve impulses.

Even within a given modality, there can be much sensory selectivity (Fig. 41.4).

Coding mechanisms

Place and stimulus-quality coding

All sensory modalities are converted into nerve impulses. How, then, does the nervous system know what the original sense modality was? A major part of the answer is that each sense modality tends to have its own pathways and circuits in the spinal cord and brain. For instance, if a dog's toe is pinched, the sense modalities of pressure and pain are correctly interpreted in the spinal cord because there is a genetically determined reflex pathway that couples the incoming impulses to spinal motoneurons, which in turn deliver impulses to the correct muscles to produce a withdrawal response. At the same time, there are alternate ascending pathways that allow the sensory impulses to be sent to the brain, so that the brain can be consciously aware of the stimulus (i.e., perceive it).

For a given modality, the ascending pathways have their own topography. For example, a dog does not see odor or smell sights because each stimulus is detected and processed in its own anatomical pathway. Moreover, stimulation of a given receptor, by whatever means, elicits the

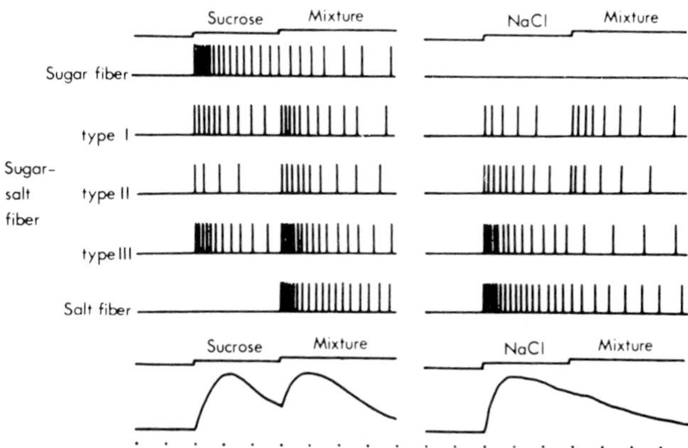

Figure 41.4. Diagram of the impulse discharge in taste cells recorded from isolated nerve fibers in the chorda tympani of dogs. Three types of unit are tested by three solutions: sugar (0.5M sucrose), salt (0.5M NaCl), and a sugar-salt mixture. Note that the fiber of the sugar cell (*top tracing*) responds only to sugar and a mixture that contains sugar. A fiber of a salt cell (*bottom tracing*) responds only to salt or to a mixture that contains salt. Fibers of dual-responsive cells (types I to III) are excited in varying degrees by both sugar and salt. (From Funakoshi and Zotterman 1963, *Acta Physiol. Scand.* 57:193–200.)

same sensation; for example, electrical stimulation of the optic nerve elicits sensations of light.

Spatial discrimination is a function of receptor density.

Intensity coding

In most sensory systems, the more intense the stimulus, the higher the rate of impulse discharge along the respective pathways (Fig. 41.5). The dynamic range is so large that it has to be expressed on a logarithmic or power scale. Also, the more intense the stimulus, the more likely it is to activate a large ensemble of receptors.

Frequency "tuning"

Certain neurons, such as those organized in columns perpendicular to the surface of auditory and visual neocortex, are tuned to respond best at certain stimulus frequencies, temporal frequencies of sound stimuli, and spatial frequencies of visual stimuli. The receptive fields are mapped topographically in the cortex. For certain features, the cortical maps are computed in other topographically located cortical regions, and the response projects into another new locus. In bats, for example, cells in one part of the auditory cortex are coded specifically for such calculated parameters of sound as target size and distance and others are mapped for varying velocity.

Distributed processing

Sensations that are perceived in the consciousness are processed in the neocortex. However, a basic principle of mammalian sensory systems is that the processing is distributed to other CNS and even peripheral levels. Much processing goes on subconsciously in the thalamus and in the dorsal horn gray matter of the cord. In the case of stimuli from the head, a major nuclear group, the sensory nucleus of cranial nerve V, traverses most of the entire length of the brain stem. Preprocessing even occurs peripherally, most notably in the retina, the cochlea, and the olfactory bulb.

The processing is reflected in the changes in temporal order of spike trains in CNS locations. Interspike intervals are generally stereotyped in sensory receptor discharge, but complex serial dependencies in spike-train intervals can be seen from CNS neurons.

The sensory receptor cells themselves produce some processing of the features that are extracted from a stimulus. Habituation is a clear example. Even more complex processing can occur. With some unmyelinated nociceptors, for example, high-frequency stimulation will sensitize the receptor so that it responds more vigorously to a stimulus than it would if it were preexposed to stimuli delivered at a slower rate.

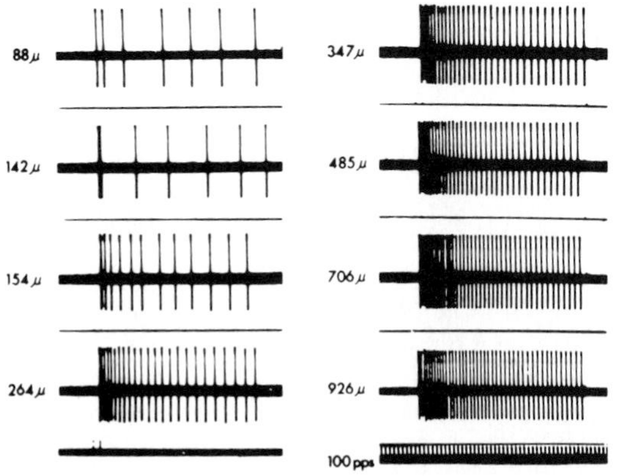

Figure 41.5. Impulse discharge in the afferent fiber of a single cutaneous mechanoreceptor in the hairy skin of a cat in response to mechanical pressure pulses of various intensities. Values shown indicate the distance of skin displacement. Up to a point, there is a conspicuous increase in impulse frequency with increases in stimulus intensity. This receptor also shows a gradual, adaptive slowing of discharge as the stimulus is sustained. (From Werner and Mountcastle 1965, *J. Neurophysiol.* 28:359–97.)

Descending control of spinal afferents

Descending impulses from more cranial parts of the CNS can inhibit or facilitate discharge of second-order cells in the dorsal horn. Thus the brain can "fine tune" the sensitivity of peripheral sensation. Such actions may be involved in the mechanism of focused attention (see Chap. 48). In addition, there may be local actions involving recurrent excitation or inhibition wherein a neuron can regulate its own discharge by feedback from collaterals of its own axon. Descending influences are thought to be particularly important in the perception of pain (see below and also Chap. 48).

SOMATIC SENSORY SYSTEMS

Somatic sensations

Somatic sensations are those that come from the body ("soma"). For convenience of discussion, these are distinct from special senses that deal with visual, auditory, taste, smell, and vestibular (equilibrium) senses. There are three types of somatic sensation: (1) mechanoreceptive senses, which detect mechanical displacement of some bodily tissue, (2) thermoreceptive senses, which detect changes in temperature, and (3) pain or nociceptive senses.

Types of sensory receptor

Receptors are classified according to the origin of stimuli to which they respond. *Exteroceptors* respond to stimuli outside the body, such as light, sound, skin sensation, and some chemical sensations. *Proprioceptors* respond to stimuli originating in muscles and tendons that convey information about the relative position of body parts and the position of the body in space. *Interoceptors* respond to stimuli associated with internal bodily conditions, such as blood pressure and glucose concentration of blood.

Histologically, many of the specific receptors have their own unique structure, as may be described in a textbook of histology. Functionally, the sensory receptors are classified into several categories:

Mechanoreceptors	Skin tactile sensations
	Deep touch receptors
	Sound receptors
	Equilibrium receptors
	Arterial pressure receptors
Thermoreceptors	Cold and warmth
Electromagnetic receptors	Vision
Electroreceptors	Voltage fields (fish, monotremes)
Chemoreceptors	Smell
	Taste
	Vomeronasal sensations
	Arterial oxygen
	Osmolality
	Blood CO_2
	Hormone receptors
Nociceptors	Painful sensations

Cutaneous mechanoreceptors

At least ten kinds of afferent receptor have been described in the hairy skin of mammals. The central connection of the afferent fibers determines the kind of sensation perceived. Studies in humans provide good evidence that there are separate sensory pathways for touch, pressure, temperature, and pain.

Most of the receptors in the skin are associated with hair follicles and are responsive to movement of skin hair. These units adapt rapidly.

Slowly adapting mechanoreceptors are scattered among the hairs and have small receptive fields. These discharge lasting 5 to 10 minutes or longer after stimulus onset. There are also rapidly adapting mechanoreceptors and high-threshold mechanoreceptors. Some mechanoreceptors in the skin have high thresholds, and firm pressure on the skin is needed to excite them.

All of the skin mechanoreceptors are thermally responsive, although they are not especially sensitive to temperature change.

Cutaneous thermoreceptors

There are two types: cold receptors, which discharge with a fall in skin temperature, and warm receptors, which have an opposite response. Both types discharge steadily at a particular constant temperature, and discharge increases when the temperature changes appropriately (Fig. 41.6). Both types have small receptive fields, and they are relatively insensitive to mechanical stimulation.

Cold and warm receptors have maximal sensitivities at different temperatures, about 15°C apart (see Fig. 41.2).

Cutaneous nociceptors

Nociceptors respond only to intense or noxious stimuli. When an animal is conscious, such stimulation can be perceived as pain (see Chap. 48).

One common feature of all the skin nociceptors is that they become less responsive if the stimulus is repeated at frequent intervals (for example, less than 30 seconds). Some of these receptors are excited by bradykinin, a polypeptide that is produced in tissues during inflammation.

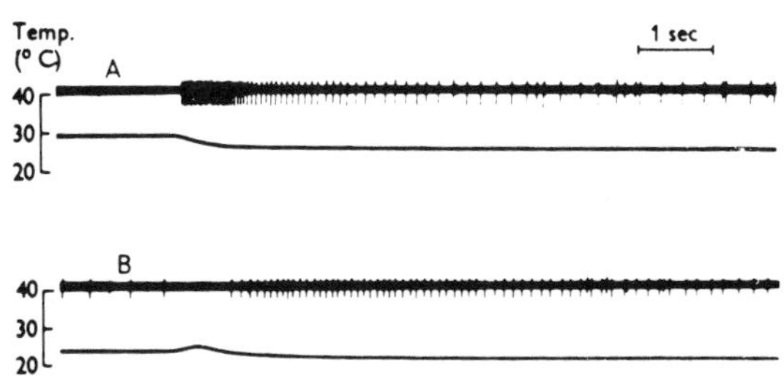

Figure 41.6. Impulse discharge in cutaneous cold receptor in the hairy skin of the cat. In (*A*) the initial steady temperature of 29°C was decreased to 25°C, producing a brisk discharge that adapted slowly. In (*B*), at a steady temperature of 22°C, there was a steady background discharge that was increased when the temperature fell to 20.5°C. (From Hensel et al. 1960, *J. Physiol.* 153:113–26.)

Equilibrium (vestibular) receptors

Vestibular receptors detect the position and motion of the head and body. The receptors, located in the inner ear on both sides of the head, provide sensory information that helps to regulate a variety of subconscious reflexes associated with posture and eye movement.

The vestibular sense organs are contained along with the auditory sense organs within the bony labyrinth, which is a series of cavities within the petrous part of the temporal bone. Inside the bone is a membranous labyrinth, which contains both vestibular and auditory sense organs. Both organs are filled with a fluid called endolymph (see Chap. 43). One portion of the vestibular apparatus, the saccule, communicates freely with the cochlea. Although housed together (Fig. 41.7), vestibular and hearing sense organs function quite independently.

The vestibular organ has two parts: (1) the so-called otolith organs containing the utricle and the saccule, which detect the position of the head in a gravitational field and also detect linear acceleration forces on the head, and (2) the so-called semicircular canals, which lie in three different planes. These planes are perpendicular to each other and are thus sensitive to acceleration and changes in acceleration in each of the three planes.

Both the otolith organs and the semicircular canals contain specialized receptor hair cells, whose surface microvilli are suspended in the endolymph (Fig. 41.7). These microvilli are specialized, consisting of about 40 to 70 stereocilia and one kinocilium per cell. Hair cells respond to movements of the microvilli as endolymph moves in response to head movements and to any gravitational changes. If the stereocilia are bent toward the kinocilium, the hair cell depolarizes, which in turn causes impulse discharge in the afferent fibers of the eighth cranial nerve. If

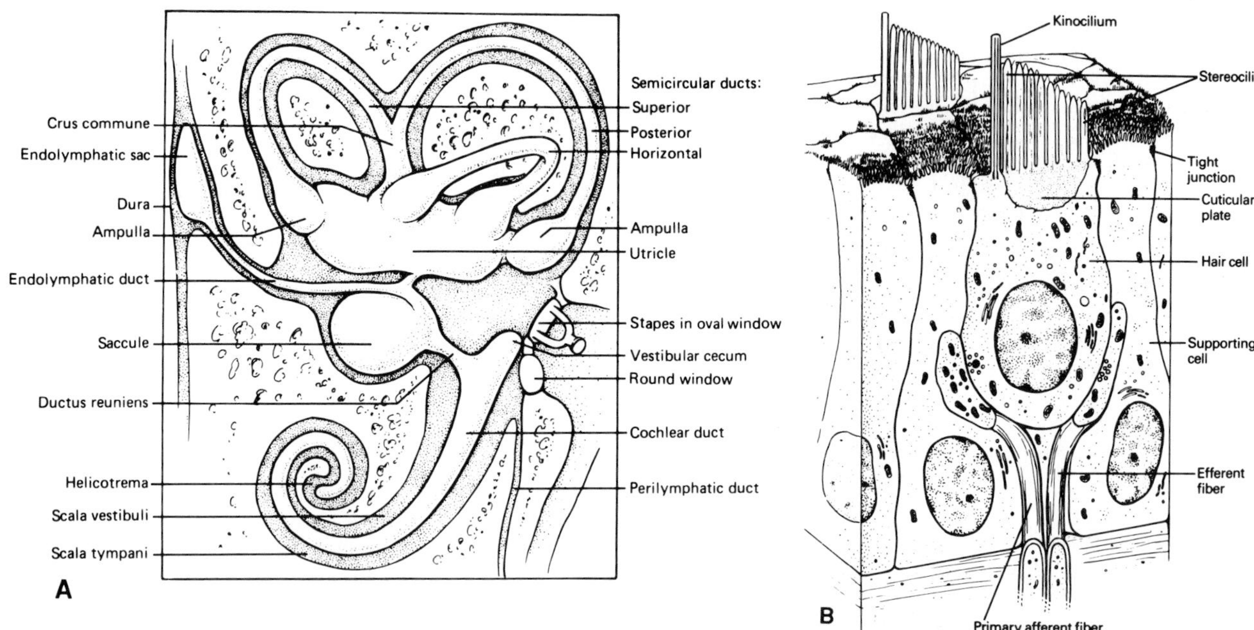

Figure 41.7. (*A*) Arrangement of the membranous labyrinth containing auditory structures (cochlear duct) and vestibular structures (utricle, saccule, and two of the three semicircular canals). (*B*) Hair cells of the vestibular sensory epithelium, which are surrounded by supporting cells, to which they are joined at the apical surfaces by gap junctions. The surface of the hair cell that is exposed to endolymph movements (*top*) contains microvilli that move in response to endolymph movement. When a hair cell is depolarized, it initiates impulse discharge in the primary afferent (called afferent because it sends input via the vestibular nerve to vestibular nuclei in the brain stem). The efferent fiber comes from cells in the brain stem that provide a pathway for the brain to regulate activity of vestibular receptor cells. (From Kelly, 1985, in Kandel and Schwartz, eds., *Principles of Neuroscience*, 2d ed., Elsevier, New York, pp. 584–96.)

stereocilia are bent in the other direction, hair cells hyperpolarize, and discharge in afferent fibers is arrested.

Impulse output from the hair cells is conveyed via the vestibular nerve to bipolar cell bodies in the vestibular ganglion, which in turn projects into vestibular nuclei in the brain stem. There are four vestibular nuclei in the brain stem, each of which has distinctive connections with the spinal cord, oculomotor nuclei (cranial nerves III, IV, and VI), and the cerebellum.

This system is very important clinically; vestibular disorders can produce nausea, abnormal eye movements (particularly strabismus and nystagmus), loss of balance and ataxia, abnormal posture, and altered tonic head and neck reflexes.

Visceral receptors

Numerous interoceptors occur in the walls of the alimentary tract. The receptors in the mucosa are sensitive to pH. For example, in the stomach mucosa some receptors respond to acidic solutions (pH 3 or lower) whereas other receptors respond to pH 8 or higher. Both types adapt slowly. These receptors also can respond to mild touch, so they may normally be involved in peristaltic reflexes.

In ruminants, there are receptors that respond to the acetate ion, which triggers reflex inhibition of rumen contraction. Other receptors can initiate or inhibit eructation.

One group of visceral receptors responds to distention. These receptors are crucial in peristalsis, because when distention occurs their impulses stimulate peristalsis. Paradoxically, these same receptors discharge during contraction (Fig. 41.8). With both kinds of stimulus, the rate of impulse discharge is slowly adapting and more or less proportional to the intraluminal pressure change. Frequency of discharge during a contraction overlaps discharge during

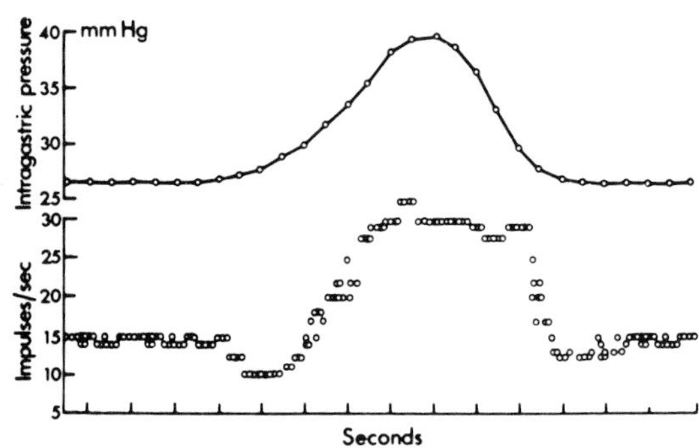

Figure 41.8. Illustration of the relationship between intraluminal pressure change (*upper tracing*) and rate of impulse discharge from the distention receptors (*lower tracing*). Data taken from a slowly adapting tension receptor in the wall of the esophageal groove in a goat. Similar receptors are found all along the alimentary canal and in the urinary bladder. (From Iggo and Leek 1966, *Acta Neuroveg.* 28:353–59.)

distention, so that the CNS apparently cannot distinguish between the two types of stimulus.

Ruminants have distention receptors that can distinguish between gaseous and fluid distention. Gaseous distention of a region around the cardia can evoke eructation, whereas fluid distention of this same region abolishes reflex opening of the cardia.

Sensory mechanisms

Flow receptors. Some visceral organs have flow receptors. For example, some pudendal nerve fibers fire bursts of impulses when fluid flows rapidly through the urethra, and the rate of discharge is proportional to the rate of flow. This discharge initiates reflex contraction of the bladder and relaxation of the urethra.

Mesenteric receptors. Pacinian corpuscle mechanoreceptors are located in mesentery near blood vessels. There are also some other less rapidly adapting mechanoreceptors located around mesenteric arteries. The significance of these receptors is not known.

Proprioceptors

The major proprioceptors are divided into those that signal the CNS about the state of muscle tone and those that signal the tension on tendons in the joints.

Muscle receptors. These receptors have a highly distinctive, fusiform structure (Fig. 41.9) called a muscle spindle, which is embedded among the large contractile muscle fibers in skeletal muscles. Spindles contain internal structures that respond to stretch: (1) primary endings wind around the fibers (intrafusal fibers) in the equatorial region of the spindle and (2) secondary endings surround or end on the intrafusal muscle fibers located toward the poles of the spindle. Primary endings continue in spinal nerves as the largest-diameter components, so-called group Ia fibers that are 12 to 20 μm in diameter).

Both primary and secondary endings respond to stretch of the extrafusal muscle, and they adapt very slowly to steady muscle stretch. A similar effect can occur when intrafusal muscle fibers contract, because that also stretches the sensory endings. When extrafusal fibers contract, the

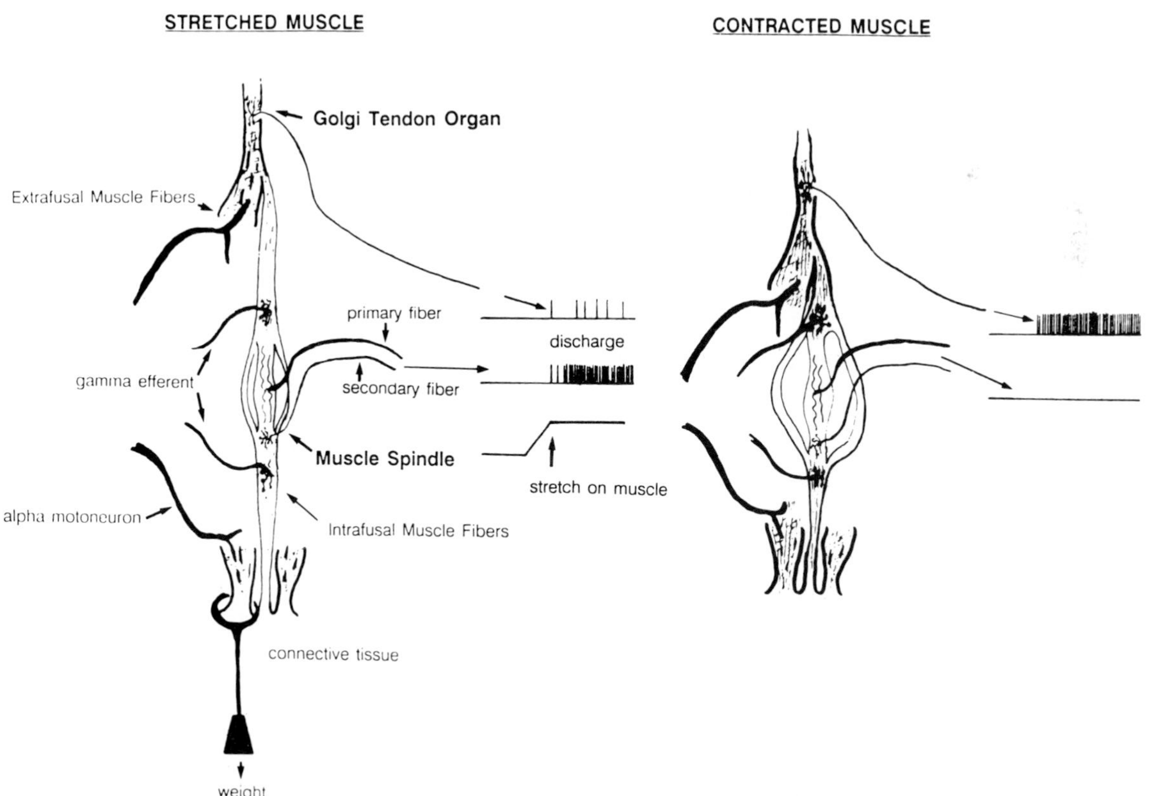

Figure 41.9. Effect of muscle stretch and active muscle contraction on the impulse output of muscle spindles and Golgi tendon organs. When the main muscle (extrafusal fibers) is passively loaded, both primary and secondary spindle afferents discharge a burst of impulses, while the Golgi endings produce little or no response. The equivalent effect is achieved if there is excitation of the intrafusal fibers of the spindle, which selectively stretches the spindle apparatus. When the extrafusal muscle is made to contract by alpha motoneuron input, extra tension is put on the Golgi organ, which discharges vigorously, while spindle efferents are silent because the spindle apparatus is relaxed and not stretched.

spindle shortens, and this tends to stop its discharge. There are many important physiological and clinical consequences of the reflexes associated with this mechanism (see Chap. 44).

Golgi tendon organs. Golgi tendon organs are receptors that are found in the tendons, where they are arranged in series with extrafusal muscle fibers, rather than parallel as in the case of spindles (Fig. 41.9). They respond with a slowly adapting discharge when the muscle is stretched, but the discharge increases further if the muscle contracts. The threshold at which tension initiates impulse discharge is higher than that for spindles. Because Golgi discharge inhibits contraction of extrafusal fibers, this enables Golgi tendon organs to operate as a "fail safe" system that can shut off contraction if the muscle tension gets so high that physical damage to the muscle and tendons is about to occur.

Joint receptors. Individual slowly adapting afferent units in the joints are sensitive to the position or angle of the joint. For each given fiber, there is an optimum angle at which discharge rate is highest. Many of the receptors are maximally active at extremes of joint movement. There are also similar rapidly adapting joint receptors that have larger-diameter fibers.

TRANSDUCTION OF SENSORY STIMULI INTO NERVE IMPULSES

Generator potentials in receptors

The common property of sensory receptors, irrespective of the physical nature of the stimulus, is that stimulation induces a localized flow of ionic current that, in turn, can trigger a train of action potentials in the receptor's nerve fiber. Whether or not impulses discharge depends on the magnitude of the generator potential.

Like action potentials (Chap. 40), generator potentials develop with the opening of membrane channels for Na^+ and K^+. Unlike action potentials, generator potentials are graded, and they summate algebraically in response to repeated stimulation. In fact, many receptors have been experimentally characterized in terms of the relationship of stimulus strength to size of generator potential.

Stimulus-response relations

One important characteristic of many receptor types is that they operate over a wide range of stimulus intensity (Fig. 41.10). A dog can feel the weight of a flea and the weight of a strong toe pinch. In humans, experiments have determined that the range for somatic sensations can be as large as 100,000 to 1. Such responses are typically proportional to the logarithm of the stimulus intensity. Stimulus intensity can be quantified in terms of the minimal detectable change. Studies performed in this way obey the so-called Weber-Fechner law, which holds that the ratio of a change in stimulus strength required for perception of a change is a constant. For example, a person who could detect a 5 g change while holding a 50 g reference weight

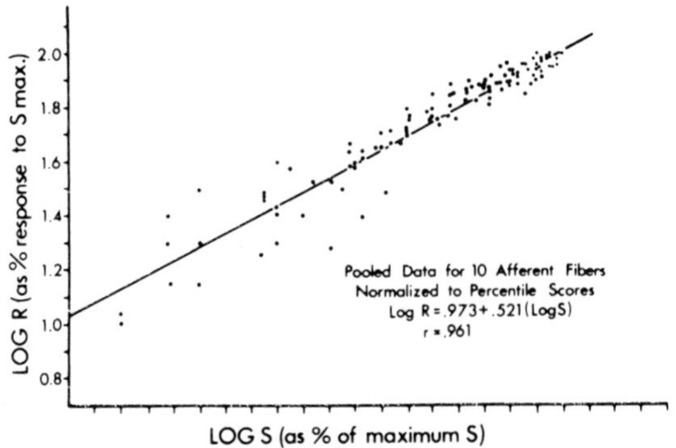

Figure 41.10. Log-log plot of neural impulse discharge rate (R) in receptors of cat skin, plotted as a function of the magnitude of mechanical stimulation. (From Werner and Mountcastle 1965, *J. Neurophysiol.* 28:359–97.)

would be able to detect a 50 g change if the reference weight were 500 g. A more direct way to study perception of stimulus intensity is to perform experiments in humans and ask them to assign relative scores of perceived intensity as stimulus intensity is changed. Experiments of this kind demonstrate the Stevens power law, which holds that perceived intensity is equal to the actual stimulus intensity, raised to a specified power (the value of the power parameter varies with type of sensory receptor).

TRANSMISSION OF SENSORY INPUTS

Sensory inputs generate impulses that are conducted in nerve fibers of varying diameters. The diameter of the fiber roughly governs the speed at which the impulses spread into the central nervous system. In the case of spinal nerves, for example, fibers are classified into types A, B, and C, with each type further subdivided according to fiber diameter. The large-diameter A fibers are myelinated, and they conduct at the fastest speeds (70 to 120 m/s). Type C fibers are the smallest in diameter and the slowest conducting. They constitute all of the postganglionic autonomic fibers (see Chap. 46) and more than half of all sensory fibers. Because C fibers are small, they can convey much sensory information to the central nervous system without creating the need for giant-sized nerves. The trade-off is in the slow speed of conduction, on the order of 0.5 m/s; for most sensory information, however, that is more than adequate. For the few instances in which much faster input is needed (as, for example, with proprioceptive and touch stimuli), the input is routed in the fast-conducting A fibers. In the case of pain stimuli, some are conducted in A fibers (sharp pain), while others are conducted in C fibers (dull, burning, or aching pain).

Tactile inputs

The specialized tactile receptors transmit their signals in rapidly conducting beta type A fibers, which have conduction velocities on the order of 30 to 60 m/s. Cruder types of pressure signals, as detected by free nerve endings, conduct at slow rates of 1 to 8 m/s in small axons.

Kinesthetic inputs

Kinesthetic sensations are those that allow recognition of the orientation of the different parts of the body with respect to each other as well as of the rates of movement of the different body parts. This information is typically transduced in the sensory endings in joint capsules and ligaments. It is transmitted at high speeds in A fibers. The appropriate sequencing of motor commands to extensors and flexors in a dog chasing a rabbit (and in the fleeing rabbit), for example, could not occur at high speed without a continuous high-speed updating of the CNS on the succession of changes in body parts during the running.

Thermal inputs

So far, no specialized skin receptors for heat or cold have been identified. Bare nerve endings can be responsive to temperature changes. However, a given bare nerve ending seems to respond to either cold or warmth but not both. Thermal receptors are somewhat unusual in that they can respond to sudden changes in temperature as well as to sustained temperatures. For example, the impulse rate in a cold receptor rapidly becomes quite high after a sudden lowering of temperature; as that temperature is maintained, the impulse rate declines to a steady plateau that is higher than the firing rate at the original temperature.

The number of cold and warm receptors is relatively small, and thus there must be a great deal of spatial summation before an animal becomes consciously aware of cold or heat. Small, highly localized cold or warm stimuli may not be felt intensely.

Thermal sensations are conducted in very small, myelinated, second-order fibers that travel in the lateral spinothalamic tract. Thus lesions of this part of the cord would disrupt perception of thermal as well as nociceptive stimuli.

Ascending projection pathways

Impulses in spinal nerves arrive in the dorsal gray matter (dorsal horn) of the spinal cord, whereupon they are fed into long axons that project in the white matter of the cord to the brain. Some first-order afferent neurons send collaterals into the dorsal columns directly and others project via the dorsal horn where they end on second-order neurons that project via the lateral white matter to the thalamus.

Dorsal column projections

The sensations carried in first-order neurons in the dorsal columns include touch and pressure sensations that require high resolution of the location of the origin on the body, proprioceptive senses of muscle contraction and tendon stretching, and phasic sensations such as vibration. In the cord the neurons are heavily myelinated, and this system is thus a high-speed projection pathway. The impulses reach their first synaptic junction in two relay nuclei in the brain stem (the cuneate and gracilis nuclei). From here, the second-order neurons in the chain project impulses into posterior and ventral parts of the thalamus, where another synaptic junction occurs. The third-order neurons in the chain then project impulses into specific regions of the neocortex, mainly to the postcentral gyrus regions but also to nearby cortical regions.

Throughout this three-step projection pathway, the sensory information is topographically organized; that is, the body is mapped in the neural tissue. For example, in the dorsal spinal column, fibers from lower parts of the body are clustered toward the center area; fibers from anterior (rostral) parts of the body collect as successive layers on the lateral sides of the dorsal columns. In the thalamus, the tail end of the body is represented by the most lateral parts of the thalamus, while rostral body parts are located more medially.

Dorsal column projections involve divergent circuitry (Chap. 39). This can be demonstrated by a record of the impulse-firing activity at each level of the projection chain in response to a peripheral stimulus. For example, a weak touch stimulus will evoke activity in a few neurons in the brain-stem relay nuclei, and a stronger stimulus will evoke activity in many more second-order neurons. This divergence continues to develop in the thalamic and neocortical receptive areas.

Because the projection goes to the neocortex, it is not surprising that the sensations can be consciously perceived (see Chap. 48). Thus animals with lesions along this pathway, such as spinal disk protrusions that compress this part of the cord, may not "know" where their limbs are.

Lateral column projections

The lateral column conveys tactile, pressure, nociceptive, joint afferent, muscle spindle, and Golgi tendon organ stimuli. The central targets include the thalamus, the brainstem reticulum, and the cerebellum.

Tactile and pressure sensations, as well as pain sensations arising from overstimulation of pressure sensors or thermal receptors, propagate in a spinocervical tract in the lateral column. This tract is well developed in nonprimates. Fibers in this tract conduct very rapidly, with conduction velocities greater than 100 m/s.

The spinothalamic system, which is dominant in primates but less so in nonprimates, is also found in the lateral column. It ascends as two tracts, the more lateral one conveying nociceptive and thermal sensations and the ventral one conveying tactile and joint angle afferents. Afferents entering the dorsal root synapse with second-order neurons, and their axons cross over and ascend to the thalamus on the other side.

Several sense modalities ascend in spinoreticular tracts. One group of muscle and high-threshold joint afferents, along with some cutaneous afferents, project into the lateral reticular nucleus, whereupon there is a relay to the cerebellum. Other afferents end on second-order neurons whose axons cross over in the cord and ascend to various levels of the brain-stem reticular formation, which in turn provides both ascending reticulothalamic and descending reticulospinal tracts.

Muscle afferents are also conveyed in a spinovestibular tract to the lateral vestibular nucleus, which helps to regulate posture and locomotion.

Muscle spindle and Golgi tendon organ afferents synapse on second-order neurons, fibers of which ascend in a dorsal spinocerebellar tract to the anterior lobe and paramedian and pyramis lobes of the cerebellum. There is also a ventral spinocerebellar tract that ascends, mostly contralaterally, to convey afferents from muscle spindles, Golgi tendon organs, and flexor reflex afferents. As these afferents enter to synapse on second-order neurons in the dorsal horn, they are strongly affected by descending tracts from the cortex and red nucleus, which determine whether information from flexor reflex or spindle afferents are relayed to the cerebellum.

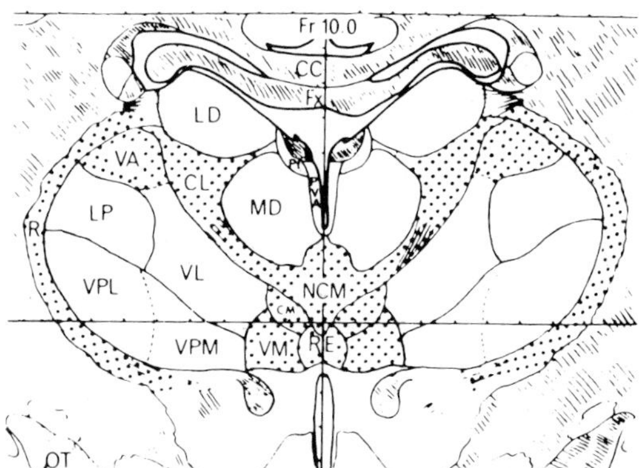

Figure 41.11. Cross section near the middle of the thalamus of a cat to show the various nuclei. Nonspecific nuclei (*stippled*) include the medial (RE) and intralaminar complexes (CL, NCM) and nucleus reticularis (R). Specific nuclei include a ventral group (ventrolateral, ventroposteromedial, ventroposterolateral, VL, VPM, VPL) and a dorsal group (medial and lateral dorsal, MD, LD). Other structures: CC, corpus callosum; Fx, fornix; OT, optic tract. (From Jasper 1960, in *Handbook of Physiology*, sec. 1, Magoun, ed., *Neurophysiology*, Am. Physiol. Soc., Washington, D.C., vol. 2, pp. 1307–21.

THALAMIC RELAYS

The thalamus is the great sensory ganglion of the brain stem, being interposed in the pathway from peripheral receptors and the cerebral cortex, where conscious perception of afferent activity occurs. The thalamus contains many distinct clusters (nuclei) of cell bodies that are topographically organized to receive input from selected parts of the body and to relay output to selected parts of the cerebral cortex. Not all of these nuclei have specific sensory functions, but many do. For example, in the dorsal group of thalamic nuclei (Fig. 41.11), the lateral geniculate nucleus receives fibers from the optic tract and projects visual information to the posterior part of the cortex (visual cortex). The medial geniculate receives inputs that are relayed from the cochlea and projects output to the lateral part of the cortex (auditory cortex). The ventrobasal complex (VPL and VPM in Fig. 41.11) receives input from the spinothalamic tract and the trigeminal tract and projects to the somatosensory region of the cortex (sensory cortex). The ventrolateral (VL) nuclei receive information from the cerebellum and relay it to the part of the cerebral cortex that initiates movements (motor cortex, see Chap. 44).

Specific projection pathways

The specific projection pathways include sensory nuclei that constitute a specific projection system, in that specific afferent input from the periphery is processed in the thalamus and then relayed to precise regions within the cortex for conscious perception. For example, the ventrobasal complex has a very precise point-to-point relationship both with its receptive fields and with somatic sensory areas of the cerebral cortex. Tactile and kinesthetic activity from the contralateral side of the body projects via this region to the somatic sensory area of the cortex. The representation of the body in the ventrobasal complex is proportional to the innervation density of the various parts. As a result, the body image is distorted. Animals such as the rabbit have a relative dominance of trigeminal representation, while the cat has a more balanced spinal and trigeminal projection and a corresponding enlargement of the VPL nucleus to accommodate the projection from the trunk and limbs. In the monkey, the hands and feet have a very rich afferent innervation and are more highly developed as tactile and prehensile organs; these structures have a larger share of the representation, with a correspondingly greater enlargement of the ventrolateral part of the ventrobasal complex.

There is another group of nuclei in the dorsal and anterior thalamus that are not specific sensory processing and relay nuclei (Fig. 41.11, stippled regions). These include some nuclei that are part of the limbic system (see Chap. 49), and some medial nuclei (RE, NCM, and CL in Fig. 41.11) that are part of a nonspecific sensory projection to the cortex (see below). Also, part of this nonspecific system is the reticular nucleus that surrounds the rest of the thalamic nuclei and extends the full length of the thalamus.

Nonspecific projection system

The stippled nuclei in Fig. 41.11 form a system of projection to the cortex that is not point to point, as is the specific projection system. Interesting phenomena, the recruiting response and a similar augmenting response, occur when these areas are electrically stimulated at continuous slow frequencies (4 to 10 per second). The electroencephalogram (EEG) over the cerebral cortex during such stimulation exhibits stimulus-bound large waves that tend to wax and wane in amplitude. This projection system is thought to be involved in the genesis of relaxed states and sleep (see Chap. 49).

SENSORY (SOMESTHETIC) CORTEX

The outer cerebral cortex of mammals is called neocortex. The neocortex is of two types. One has neurons that are connected in point-to-point fashion with either muscles (see Chap. 44) or specific sensory projection pathways. The other, sometimes called the association cortex, interacts with the motor and sensory cortex in performing the higher cognitive functions of the brain.

All vertebrates have a paleocortex, which processes information subconsciously and dominates in amphibians, reptiles, and birds. In mammals, this remnant persists, usually folded beneath the neocortex, and functions primarily as part of the limbic system (see Chap. 49).

The relay paths of specific sensory systems (visual, auditory, etc.) through the different thalamic nuclei retain their separation in the projection to the neocortex. The projections into the sensory cortex are generally from the opposite side of the body, except in sheep and goats. Each kind of afferent fiber goes to a different region of the cortex. The tongue and the face are represented at the most medial end of the sensory cortex, whereas the hind leg is represented on the lateral convexity of its surface. The precise location and extent of the sensory areas depend on the degree of development of the cerebral cortex, which is most profound in primates and least developed in such domesticated species as ruminants. Even in ruminants, however, the cerebral cortex is impressively developed, especially in comparison with many nondomestic mammalian species, such as rodents. The surface area devoted to a given part of the body is generally proportional to the adaptational importance of the body part in question. Pigs, for example, have a large representation for the snout, horses for the mouth and lips, and monkeys for the hands.

The consequence of damage to the sensory cortex depends on the extent to which that sensation is represented in the cortex. A related, very practical application of this knowledge is that the amount of pain and distress evoked by a peripheral injury depends on how extensively the body part is represented in the sensory cortex. In ruminants, for example, very little of the body's trunk is represented in the sensory cortex, and that explains why these animals can be quite indifferent to the surgical insertion of a ruminal cannula through a wound in the flank. On the other hand, injuries to the face are more distressing, especially in dogs, cats, and monkeys.

There are additional so-called secondary sensory areas that are less well organized topographically and that receive bilateral inputs. Ablation experiments in dogs, cats, and monkeys have established that tactile discrimination is impaired when the primary somatic sensory area is removed, but recovery will take place. More severe deficits occur when there is bilateral removal of both the primary and the secondary sensory cortex. This sensory loss was not recovered in the experiments that have been reported.

The gustatory, or taste, area of the cortex receives ipsilateral projections of the ventrobasal part of the thalamus. The taste area of the cortex is located at the medial end of the facial area. In rats, bilateral removal of the taste area abolishes their ability to discriminate tastes.

SPECIFIC SENSORY PERCEPTIONS

As mentioned, for sensory input of whatever kind to be registered as a perception, the animal must be conscious (see Chap. 48). From the human perspective, it may not usually matter much whether a domestic animal responds consciously or unconsciously to a given stimulus. In the case of pain, however, there are esthetic and humane-treatment considerations that are important. The latter are covered in more detail in Chap. 48, because the whole question of whether a given stimulus is inhumane hinges on whether or not the animal is conscious. People interested in animal welfare have a special need to understand the physiological principles involved here.

Appetite

Hunger is a conscious sensation that in part is caused by contractions of the empty stomach. This relationship does not hold in the same way for ruminants, in which rumen and reticulum contractions actually increase after eating.

Gastrointestinal fibers in the vagus nerve may have a role in satiety. The ingestion of food by a sham-fed dog (that is, a dog with an esophagostomy) may be reduced if a balloon, inserted through a gastric fistula, is inflated in the stomach, while the animal is feeding. This effect is different from the chemical influences associated with absorption after eating.

The chemical regulation of appetite is extremely complex and, to this day, is still not well understood despite decades of intense research. One thing seems clear: There are groups of neurons in the hypothalamus that regulate appetite. Lesion and electrical stimulation studies in several species have shown that there is some kind of satiety center in the medial hypothalamus and a feeding center in the lateral hypothalamus. (Thirst may also be regulated by reciprocally acting centers in the hypothalamus.) (See Chap. 49 for more discussion of appetitive behavior.)

Somatic sensations

Touch sensations

Touch stimulation of the hairless skin activates Meissner corpuscles, whereas vibration activates Pacinian corpuscles. These receptors are the terminals of large myelinated fibers, which enter uninterruptedly in the dorsal column of the spinal cord to relay with second-order neurons (Fig.

40.1) in the medulla; these neurons send crossed projections to ventral and posterior parts of the thalamus. Touch stimulation of the face and head projects centrally via the trigeminal nerve.

Thermal sensations

Psychophysical experiments in humans show that temperature sensation from the skin arises from small spots. A small probe above skin temperature elicits a sensation of warmth, and the opposite arises from a probe lower than skin temperature. The quality of the sensation depends on both initial temperature of the skin and rate of change of temperature. This is because the thermoreceptors adapt to the prevailing temperature. When the temperature is changed, they discharge at frequencies that depend on both the initial temperature and the rate of temperature change.

Thermal stimulation of certain areas of the body surface in the cat, dog, rat, and rabbit evokes powerful thermoregulatory reflexes. The extent to which these are associated with conscious sensations is not always clear. Heating the scrotal skin of a ram or the udder of a ewe to 40°C causes breathing to become rapid and shallow, and the animal pants. Similar heating of an equivalent area of the shorn skin of the flank does not have this effect.

Tickle and itch

Common experience with dogs shows that they itch. There is no way to know whether animals can perceive tickle sensation. It is known that the sham scratching that one can elicit in dogs by light stroking of the skin on the side of the belly and flank is a spinal reflex that does not require control from the brain. Presumably, cats experience a tickle-related kind of sensation when they stroke and rub their whiskers.

Conscious proprioception

Unlike the proprioceptive inputs that go to the cerebellum via tracts in the lateral cord, certain inputs that ascend in the dorsal cord project to the neocortex, where they are consciously perceived. Certain movement abnormalities, such as foot dragging or knuckling, occur because the animal does not know about the abnormal movement. However, animal neurological tests do not readily discriminate between spinocerebellar and spinocerebral proprioceptive lesions.

Visceral sensations

Viscera do not give rise to a wide range of sensations. Much of the sensory activity in viscera controls visceral reflexes, and it is not processed consciously. For example, abdominal and thoracic viscera can be handled in conscious human subjects without producing any sensation. Also, conscious ruminants give no behavioral sign of sensation on manual probing of a fistulated reticulum and rumen, even when the manipulations are strong enough to elicit reflex gastric movements.

In humans the range of visceral sensations includes fullness or distention and thermal sensations. Normal propulsive movements are not perceived; if contractions become intense, however, then they may be felt as pain. Casual observations of animals indicate that they seem to register bladder and rectal fullness consciously. A housetrained dog intentionally seeks to be let outdoors when it needs to urinate or defecate. Many major visceral reflexes, such as the carotid sinus reflex and local vascular pool reflexes, are never perceived by humans, nor presumably by animals.

Three cranial nerves (facial, glossopharyngeal, and vagus) contain general visceral afferents. These pass into the solitary tract, a prominent structure in the lateral medulla, and then relay with second-order neurons in the nucleus of the solitary tract, which in turn projects to the thalamus and then to the neocortex. Some special visceral afferents include those that mediate the senses of taste, olfaction, and vomeronasal function.

Visceral pain

The most sensitive parts of the viscera for producing pain are the peritoneal linings; inflammation of the peritoneum (peritonitis) can be extremely painful. Severe distention of hollow viscera can also cause pain; so can severe contractions, as in intestinal colic. Other sources of visceral pain include the passing of solid objects such as urinary calculi, high levels of hydrogen ion concentration, or inflammation. Inflammation may also lower the pain threshold for other sources of pain, such as distention or extreme contraction.

Most of the nociceptive stimuli from viscera enter the sympathetic division of the autonomic nervous system (see Chap. 46).

Nociceptive sensations

The afferent fibers that transmit pain-producting stimuli are small in diameter. Those that are myelinated probably account for sharp, rapidly produced pain, while the unmyelinated (C) fibers probably account for the slow-onset, long-lasting (aching) kind of pain.

These small fibers project via dorsal horn neurons into tracts in the ventrolateral quadrants of the spinal cord. From there, the pathway goes to specific thalamic nuclei that, in turn, project fibers into the cerebral cortex. In addition, many of these small fibers relay in the brain-stem reticular formation and other thalamic areas.

Various kinds of stimuli excite impulse activity in the ventrolateral fibers, but discharge becomes more vigorous if noxious stimuli are used. Thus alleviation of pain could be accomplished by drugs or other input stimuli that attenuate the impulse discharge in ventrolateral pathways. Descending neural influences from the cortex might have that effect.

Once the impulses enter the CNS, they become subject to a great deal of modification, either by drugs or by interaction with the influences of other kinds of stimuli. This interaction can occur at all levels of the CNS and may be especially important in those parts that do not have topographical representation of the body or stereotypical relay functions. Such areas include the so-called substantia gelatinosa of the spinal cord, the reticular formation and central gray area of the brain stem, the nonspecific thalamic nuclei, and many areas of the cerebral cortex.

Pain pathways

Painful stimuli trigger impulses in four major ascending systems (Fig. 41.12). These inputs ascend to the thalamus, where they then relay to the sensory cortex for conscious awareness.

Gate control theory of pain

Before an animal can perceive nociceptive stimuli as pain, the impulse trains must arrive in the brain. The substantia gelatinosa of the cord is a key relay point where nociceptive input either propagates to the brain or is interrupted. The substantia gelatinosa may contain a gate control circuit that can close off the flow of nociceptive input. The proposed details for how this gate works have not been experimentally confirmed, although there is clinical evidence that activity in the large myelinated and rapidly adapting touch fibers that enter the dorsal columns can shut off pain perception. Direct or even transcutaneous stimulation of dorsal column sensory inputs can alleviate pain. Also, the gate control theory posits a role for inhibition descending from the brain, for which there is good evidence.

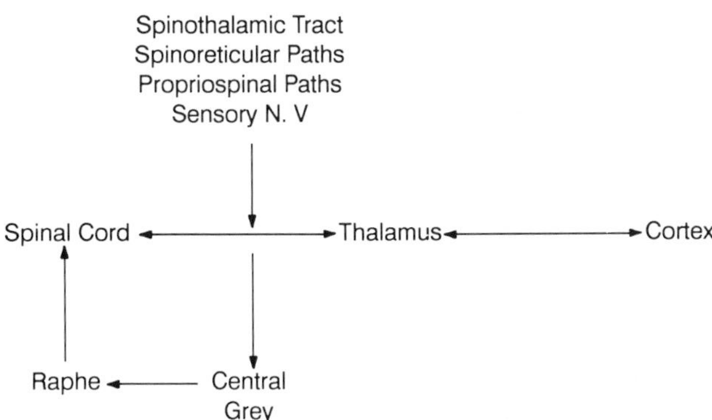

Figure 41.12. Nociceptive inputs are shown entering the CNS via three major spinal cord tracts and the sensory nucleus of the trigeminal nerve. Rostral projections go to the thalamus and neocortex. There are also descending influences from neocortex and thalamus, as well as brain-stem connections linking the central gray and raphe nuclei.

Brain-stem modulation of nociceptive inputs

Descending inhibitory influences on pain-producing stimuli are anatomically and neurochemically diverse. Several brain-stem nuclei seem to be important (particularly the periaqueductal gray matter and the raphe magnus nucleus). Coactivation of spinal serotonergic and noradrenergic systems is a general finding, and endogenous opioids play a major role. In addition to noxious stimuli, cardiopulmonary vagal afferents also can engage the endogenous systems of pain control.

Although pain occurs in the conscious mind, the brain stem is a primary locus for processing and mediation of nociceptive input, as well as the behaviors that develop from such input. Particularly well known are the opiatergic systems in the central (periaqueductal) gray matter of the brain stem, the serotonergic raphe magnus nucleus, and the adjacent medullary reticular formation areas. Some reticular formation areas convey nociceptive input into the central gray matter, whereas other reticular areas provide descending inhibitory influences to the dorsal horn region of the cord.

Behavioral expression of pain

Animals express the presence of pain in a variety of ways. The obvious signs are vocalization, growling, hissing, snarling, biting, and withdrawal of the affected part. Less obvious signs would include increases in respiration, blood pressure, and heart rate, pupillary dilation, and perhaps, in chronic pain, behavioral depression. Experience, skill, and judgment are needed to interpret the presence of pain as well as to judge how effectively the pain is relieved by treatment.

A wide range of damaging stimuli can cause pain. As long as the stimulus is intense, pain can be perceived from a wide range of thermal, chemical, and mechanical stimuli.

Psychophysical studies of pain in humans reveal that there are several qualities of painful sensation. Superficial or cutaneous pain is highly localized and is sharp and pricking in quality. One kind of surface pain is of short latency, is mediated by myelinated (group III) fibers, and has a "bright" quality. A second kind has a longer latency and is mediated by nonmyelinated fibers; it is more diffuse and has an aching, throbbing quality.

"Psychic" dimensions to pain

Because pain operates in the conscious domain, it is not surprising that altered states of consciousness and neocortical function can affect the perception of pain. These principles are easier to demonstrate in humans, but they seem to apply also to animals. Pain is less intense if an animal is sedated. Distraction by other kinds of stimuli can reduce pain. The affective (emotional) state of an animal can influence pain. To some extent, pain can be lessened by cortical decisions to evoke behaviors that conflict with impulse "traffic" associated with pain. For example, dogs in a fight often do not exhibit signs of pain until the fight is over.

Humane treatment issues

Pain is discussed at some length in Chapter 49, because the issue of consciousness is central to whether or not nociceptive stimuli are perceived as noxious. The peripheral disturbances that evoke pain can continue to persist in the absence of brain function. For example, toe pinch withdrawal reflexes can still occur when the spinal cord is severed or when the brain is made unconscious by light levels of anesthetic.

A stimulus that is ordinarily painful will not be painful if the conduction pathway to the cortex is interrupted, as by spinal cord lesions, or if neocortical function is disrupted, as by anesthetics. During anesthesia, for example, sensory information is still *received* in the brain, as indicated by evoked response recording, but it is not *perceived*. Medically, this is an important distinction.

Knowledge about pain in animals in inevitably inferential, usually based on analogy with human experience. It is inferred that stimuli are noxious and strong enough to cause animals to perceive pain if those same stimuli cause pain in humans, if they approximate the tissue damage caused in humans, and if they produce appropriate behaviors in animals.

In a conscious animal, signs of pain perception can become apparent: crying out, escape/avoidance behavior, "favoring" certain unusual limb positions, facial grimaces (especially in primates), or vocalizations (especially ultrasonic alarm cries in rodents and certain other species). However, in an animal that cannot exhibit much behavior (as, for example, an animal paralyzed with muscle relaxants or dissociative anesthetics such as ketamine), signs of pain perception would be more subtle: increased heart and respiratory rates, pupil dilation, and EEG activation. Under anesthesia, which dilates the pupils for reasons other than pain, it can be assumed that pain is not perceived as long as the other signs are not present. Presence of spinal and cranial reflexes is not a reliable indicator of pain because these reflexes operate at a subconscious level; the toe pinch reflex, for example, is mediated solely in the cord. Pain, therefore, is probably not felt, even during light anesthesia, because cardiovascular and respiratory functions are suppressed and the EEG is deactivated.

Referred Pain

Nociceptive input from viscera can sometimes be referred to the body surface; that is, visceral pain cannot be perceived with great accuracy. Often, the referred pain seems to originate from body surface areas that are in the same embryological dermatome as the visceral organ that is producing the pain. This is the kind of pain that commonly accompanies heart attack in humans. The pain is felt in the left arm and over the chest surface, whereas the nociceptive discharges are actually initiated in the heart.

The explanation for this confusion is that the visceral nerve fibers synapse in the dorsal horn of the cord on some of the same neurons that receive skin nerve fibers. Thus the brain knows only that the first-order neurons in the cord were activated; it does not know whether they were activated by visceral or somatic stimuli.

Referred pain can be very misleading in veterinary situations. For example, there is a case report of a bitch with a denuded tail, due to her having gnawed at it, that was not helped by surgical removal of the offending part of the tail. Relief followed only the discovery and treatment of a subcutaneous cyst on the thigh.

The convergence of sensory inputs that underlie referred pain also provide therapeutic opportunities wherein cutaneous stimulation can modify the pain (see below).

SENSORY DYSFUNCTION—MEDICAL IMPLICATIONS

Hypoesthesia and hyperesthesia

Loss of sensation typically accompanies damage to sensory nerves or their conducting pathways. Above-normal sensation is most commonly seen in overactive spinal reflexes, such as the muscle stretch reflex that occurs when the spinal cord is damaged rostral to the cord segments that contain the reflex circuitry. The cause is actually a release of motoneurons from tonic descending inhibition.

Itching/tickling

The sensations of itching and tickling are poorly understood; they probably involve simultaneous activation of several types of sensory receptors. Scratching, particularly in dogs, can become excessive to the point of self-inflicted damage. Treatment must be aimed at reducing the intensity of peripheral stimulation. CNS factors are also involved, as can be seen when a dog stops scratching as soon as his attention is distracted toward something else.

Self-mutilation

The bizarre behavior of self-mutilation often involves chewing and destruction of extremities that are irritated. It may result from an extreme form of itching, but little is known about the causes. One form is genetically transmitted as an autosomal recessive.

Spinal cord trauma

Lesions of the cord that affect the sensory conducting pathways in the lateral and ventral parts of the cord will disrupt normal sensation. Cord lesions most commonly arise from trauma or rupture of intervertebral disks. These lesions are diagnosed by certain neurological examination procedures. For example, if simple spinal reflexes are normal, one can assume that the primary sensory and motor nerve fibers are normal. Certain postural reactions and behavioral responses to pain assess the integrity of ascending sensory conducting pathways.

Alleviation of pain

Obviously, anything that can reduce the nociceptive discharge from sensory receptors can alleviate pain. Local anesthetics work because they block the conduction of impulses in afferent fibers. A more permanent treatment requires removal of the source of irritation at the receptor site.

Neurophysiological bases for counterirritation, acupuncture, and related methods for alleviating pain

The mechanisms of pain relief afforded by counterirritation procedures are not completely understood, but they probably involve suppression of activity in nociceptive pathways arising in the dorsal horn (substantia gelatinosa) of the spinal cord.

Suppression of nociceptive projection can be achieved by generation of spike discharge from mechanoreceptor afferent units, whether they are triggered by electrical stimulation of nerve trunks or by chemical or mechanical stimulation of the skin. One of the first things a veterinarian learns about giving injections is techniques to reduce pain and the associated "startle" response. An example is the technique used with cattle whereby one holds the injection needle between the thumb and forefinger, while pounding on the leg with the base of the hand; after two or three rhythmic pounds, the hand is then turned so that the next pounding by the hand also thrusts in the needle. This works, in part, because the cow is consciously aware of the heavy pressure stimuli from the pounding, and this masks the conscious awareness of the simultaneous nociceptive stimulus. This effect might also be explained in terms of the gate control theory.

The gate control theory might also explain counterirritation therapy, which is a medical procedure in which one applies a continuous stimulus that is different from the nociceptive stimulus, which it masks. Likewise, acupuncture might be explained in similar ways.

Electrical stimulation of brain

Analgesia can be induced in animals and humans by electrical stimulation of medial brain-stem structures, such as the raphe nuclei and the central, periaqueductal gray matter. These sites also have high levels of endogenous opiate peptides. These neural systems, which are coupled to higher brain centers, provide the means whereby analgesia can be produced by such factors as emotional state, expectation, attention, volition, blood pressure, stress, counterirritation, and certain drugs.

Whole-head electrical stimulation, so-called "electrical anesthesia" (see Chap. 48), can also produce what appears to be anesthesia, accompanied by analgesia.

Analgesics

In the case of aspirin, a substantial part of the analgesic effect is peripheral; aspirin's suppression of prostaglandin production reduces the irritation produced by bradykinin. Currently, a very active field of research is the study of mechanisms of action of aspirinlike compounds.

Opiates act directly on brain-stem opiate receptor systems that disrupt the rostral projection of nociceptive stimuli. Apparently, the reason that the brain has membrane receptors for opiates is that the brain's own opiatergic peptide neurotransmitters developed as an adaptive mechanism for minimizing excessive pain.

Anesthesia

The most commonly used injectable agents are barbiturates; the most commonly used inhalant anesthetics are methoxyflurane and halothane. Local anesthetics, such as procaine and lidocaine, block the ion conductance channels that are responsible for action potential generation. General anesthetics are effective in concentrations that have little effect on peripheral nerves; they act with greatest potency at the synapses, particularly in reticular formation and neocortex (see Chap. 48).

Numerous theories have been advanced to explain the molecular basis for anesthesia. These range from nonspecific effects such as "fluidizing" of the lipid components of the membrane to more specific action on such biochemicals as Na^+-K^+ ATPase, various neurotransmitter systems, enzymes associated with cellular oxidation, and Ca^{2+} transport and binding systems. Distinguishing of primary from secondary effects is difficult, but it is tempting to regard transmitter effects as secondary to other more basic actions on or within the membranes. Fluidization of membrane lipid certainly must have a profound effect on the conformation of membrane-bound proteins. The newest theory is that anesthetics displace and perturb surface-bound water, thus altering conformation of membrane proteins. Perhaps those proteins that normally serve to open the sodium conductance channels no longer have the proper conformation during anesthesia. Gangliosides, which are concentrated around receptor proteins of synapses, may also be involved in mediating anesthetic action.

REFERENCES

Akil, H., Watson, S.J., Young, E., Lewis, M.E., Khachaturian, H., and Walker, J.M. 1984. Endogenous opioids: Biology and function. *Annu. Rev. Neurosci.* 7:223–55.

Basbaum, A.I., and Fields, H.L. 1984. Endogenous pain control. *Annu. Rev. Neurosci.* 7:309–38.

Carstens, E.E. 1987. Endogenous pain suppression mechanisms. *JAVMA* 191:1203–06.

Casey, K.L., and Morrow, T.J. 1983. Supraspinal pain mechanisms in the cat, in R.L. Kitchell and H.H. Erickson, eds., *Animal Pain: Perception and Alleviation*. American Physiological Society, Bethesda, Md. Pp. 63–81.

Dennis, S.G., and Melzack, R. 1983. Perspectives on phylogenetic evolution of pain expression, in R.L. Kitchell and H.H. Erickson, eds., *Animal Pain: Perception and Alleviation*. American Physiological Society, Bethesda, Md. Pp. 151–60.

Edeline, J.-M. and Neuenschwander-El Massioui, N. 1988. Retention of CS-UCS association learned under ketamine anesthesia. *Brain Res.* 457:274–80.

Firestein, S., and Werblin, F. 1989. Odor-induced membrane currents in vertebrate-olfactory receptor neurons. *Science* 244:79–82.

Gebhart, G.F., and Randich, A. 1989. Brainstem modulation of nociception. In W. R. Klemm and R. P. Vertes, eds., *Brainstem Mechanisms of Behavior*. Wiley & Sons, New York.

Halpern, M. 1987. The organization and function of the vomeronasal system. *Annu. Rev. Neurosci.* 10:325–62.

Iggo, A. 1982. Cutaneous sensory mechanisms. In H.B. Barlow and J.D. Mollon, eds., *The Senses*. Cambridge Univ. Press, Cambridge.

Iggo, A., and Andres, K.H. 1982. Morphology of cutaneous receptors. *Annu. Rev. Neurosci.* 5:1–31.

Imig, T.J., and Morel, A. 1984. Organization of the thalamocortical auditory system in the cat. *Annu. Rev. Neurosci.* 6:95–120.

Jacobs, V.L., Sis, R.F., Chenoweth, P.J., Klemm, W.R., and Sherry, C.J. 1981. Structures of the bovine vomeronasal complex and its relationships to the palate: Tongue manipulation. *Acta Anat.* 110:48–58.

Johnson, K.O., and Hsiao. 1992. Neural mechanisms of tactural form and texture perception. *Annu. Rev. Neurosci.* 15:227–50.

Klemm, W.R., and Sherry, C.J. 1982. Do neurons process information by relative intervals in spike trains? *Neurosci. Biobehav. Rev.* 6:429–37.

Lineberry, C.G. 1981. Laboratory animals in pain research, in W.I. Gay, ed., *Methods of Animal Experimentation*, Vol. 6. Academic Press, New York. Pp. 237–311.

Spray, D.C., 1986a. Cutaneous temperature receptors. *Annu. Rev. Physiol.* 48:625–38.

Spray, D.C. 1986b. Symposium on visceral sensation. *Prog. Brain Res.* Vol. 67. Elsevier, New York.

Spray, D.C. 1992. Sensory transduction. *Society of General Physiologists 45th Annual Symposium,* Rockefeller Univ. Press, New York.

CHAPTER 42

Special Senses I: Vision | by Dwight B. Coulter and Gretchen M. Schmidt

ANATOMY

The eye is composed of the eyeball or globe, the optic nerve, and the accessory structures—eyelids, conjunctivae, lacrimal apparatus, and extraocular muscles. The eyeball contains the aqueous humor, iris, lens, and vitreous humor and is enclosed by three tunics or coats (Fig. 42.1). The extraocular muscles, found covering the eyeball posterior to the limbal attachment of the conjunctiva, are in turn covered with a capsule, the fascia bulbi (Tenon's capsule).

The fibrous tunic or external coat of the eyeball consists of an anterior part, the transparent cornea, and a posterior part, the opaque sclera. The vascular tunic (uveal tract) or middle coat is composed of the choroid, ciliary body, and iris. The nerve tunic (retina) or inner coat is transparent and sensitive to light. Embryologically, the retina is a part of the brain; the optic nerve is a cerebral tract.

The transparent lens is suspended from a ring of tissue, the ciliary body, in the transparent aqueous humor ante-

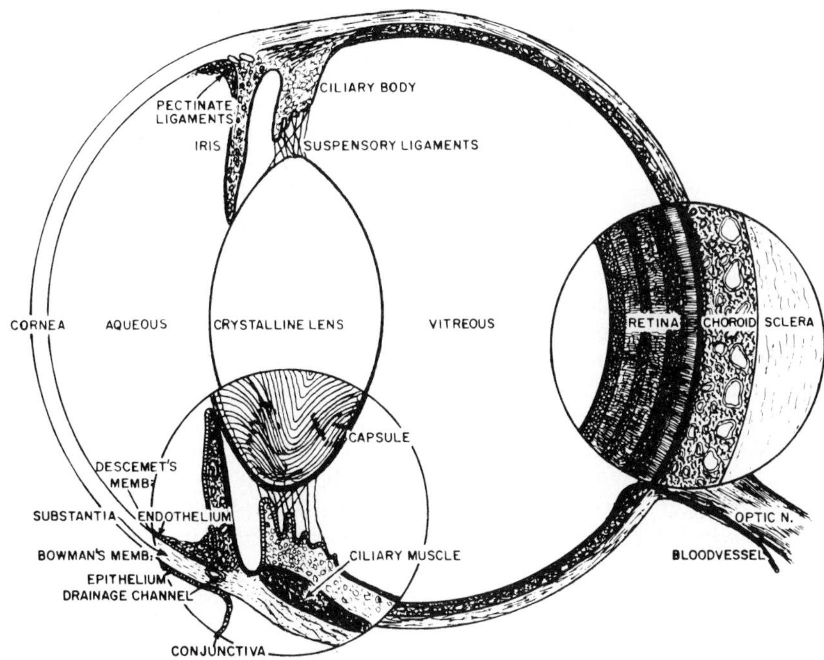

Figure 42.1. Section of the eye of a cat. The two circles enclose magnified sections of the macroscopic drawing. Not to scale.

riorly and the transparent vitreous humor posteriorly. The iris is a diaphragm that divides the aqueous humor into anterior and posterior chambers. Its central opening is the pupil. Morphological changes in the living eye are evaluated by means of gross visual inspection, the ophthalmoscope, radiographs, ultrasonograms, computerized tomograms, and magnetic resonance images.

EYELIDS AND LACRIMAL SYSTEM

Puppies, kittens, rats, rabbits, and mice are born with their eyelids closed. The eyes open at the age of 1 to 2 weeks, but both eyes do not always open on the same day. Horses, ruminants, pigs, and guinea pigs are born with their eyes open. Precocious birds, such as chickens, are hatched with their eyes open, whereas altricial birds, such as parrots, are hatched with their eyes closed.

The frequency of blinking varies among domestic animals. Cats tend to blink the least. In domestic mammals the upper eyelid is most movable; in domestic birds the lower lid is more movable. Normal blinking maintains the tear film over the corneal surface, helps to remove debris, and assists in the drainage of tears into the lacrimal apparatus.

The *menace reaction*, a blink in response to a menacing gesture, cannot be elicited from an otherwise intact animal if sufficient damage has occurred to the contralateral cerebral cortex. The menace reaction should be differentiated from the *palpebral reflex*, a blink in response to stimulation of skin receptors of the lid or conjunctiva. Some of the sensory innervation of the conjunctiva is contained in the oculomotor nerve and is a subsidiary pathway of the trigeminal (fifth) cranial nerve. The *corneal reflex* is a blink in response to touching of the cornea.

The nictitating membrane or third eyelid, found in the medial canthus of domestic animals, aids in protection of the cornea, and its gland produces tears. It is larger and more mobile in domestic birds than in domestic mammals. The multiunit smooth muscle that draws the feline nictitating membrane into the medial canthus is innervated by postganglionic adrenergic sympathetic nerve axons with cell bodies located in the anterior cervical ganglion. Although the receptors are adrenergic (alpha 1), the muscle responds to administration of acetylcholine or histamine. Protrusion of the nictitating membrane over the eyeball, an early sign of tetanus, follows contraction of the retractor bulbi muscle. Paralysis of cervical sympathetic nerves to the eye, as in Horner's syndrome, also results in protrusion of the nictitating membrane.

Closure of the lids or suturing of the lids closed does not completely deprive the eye of light stimuli. Both eyelids and the nictitating membrane transmit some of the longer wavelengths of light; the amount transmitted depends on lid pigmentation.

The precorneal tear film is divided into three layers. The outer layer is a thin, oily layer produced by the sebaceous glands of the eyelids. This layer prevents evaporation of the underlying layers and overflow of the tear film onto the eyelids. The middle aqueous layer is secreted by the lacrimal gland, the gland of the nictitating membrane, and accessory lacrimal glands in the conjunctiva. Compared with primates, domestic animals have very low levels of lysozyme in their tears, but the immunoglobulins are similar to those of primates. Irritation increases the lysozyme concentration. Compared with plasma, tears are slightly alkaline and higher in potassium, and they have a lower but correlating concentration of glucose. Lacrimation is increased by stimulation of the ophthalmic branch of the trigeminal nerve. The harderian gland is one of several lacrimal glands found in a variety of animals, including amphibians, reptiles, birds, and mammals, but not terrestrial carnivores and nonhuman primates. The lipid-rich secretion of the harderian gland may contain a pheromone in some species, and in the chicken it contains a large number of antibody-producing plasma cells. The inner layer of the tear film is produced by the conjunctival goblet cells and sometimes by the deep gland of the nictitating membrane. With the aid of blinking, mucin is absorbed by the hydrophobic corneal epithelium and provides a hydrophilic surface for the aqueous tear fluid. The lacrimal secretions either pass through the lacrimal puncta and canaliculi into the nasal cavity and are swallowed or they flow out through the nostrils. Blinking, facial muscle movement, and breathing facilitate the excretion. Epiphora (overflow of tears) occurs if the punctum or the canaliculus (lacrimal duct) of an eye is nonpatent (blocked).

CORNEA

The cornea is the strongest optical portion of the eye because of the air-to-tissue interface. The optical power of the eye is reduced under water when water interfaces with the cornea. In birds the cornea may play a role in accommodation. To function as a refracting medium, the cornea must be transparent. Its transparency depends on the absence of blood vessels, the state of relative deturgescence, and the arrangement of the stromal collagen fibrils. The aqueous humor, limbal capillaries, and tears enable the cornea to maintain the metabolism necessary for corneal deturgescence. If corneal metabolism is decreased, the cornea becomes overhydrated (edematous) and loses its transparency. Corneal stromal deturgescence is a function of the hydrophobic epithelial and endothelial cell layers.

Drugs that have both polar (water-soluble) and nonpolar (lipid- soluble) forms can penetrate the cornea. The appearance of blood vessels in the cornea indicates a pathologic process. The ophthalmic branch of the trigeminal (fifth) cranial nerve is the cornea's source of sensory (touch and pain) innervation. The sensory fibers of the cornea have an axon reflex that, when stimulated, results in miosis, hyperemia, ocular hypertension, and increased protein in the aqueous humor. Substance P, the neurotransmitter of axons conducting the modality of pain, has been found in aqueous humor of the rabbit after intracranial stimulation of the trigeminal nerve.

AQUEOUS HUMOR

Aqueous humor, the transparent fluid that fills the anterior and posterior chambers between the cornea and the lens, is formed in the posterior chamber by filtration across the fenestrated capillaries in the ciliary processes and by secretion of solutes accompanied by water across the ciliary epithelium. The aqueous humor is formed at about 15 ± 10 μl per minute. In birds, the pecten, a highly vascular structure projecting from the fundus at the base of the optic nerve into the vitreous humor, may play a role in aqueous humor production. As waste products are discharged from surrounding tissues into the aqueous humor, the aqueous humor changes in composition while flowing from the posterior chamber, where it is formed, to the anterior chamber, where it drains into uveal venous blood. The aqueous humor contains far less protein and urea than plasma but more ascorbic acid. Normal aqueous humor, like secreted cerebral spinal fluid and synovial fluids, does not clot. When pathological processes break down the blood–aqueous humor barrier, protein leaks in, as evidenced by clotting. Carbonic anhydrase inhibitors slow the rate of entry of bicarbonate into the aqueous humor. Cats and rabbits have relatively high bicarbonate levels with low chloride concentrations; in ruminants, horses, and primates bicarbonate levels are low and chloride concentrations are high. Potassium ion concentrations are higher in dogs than in cats and rabbits. In other words, there is a fair amount of variation in ion concentrations among species. Beta-adrenergic blocking agents can decrease aqueous humor formation, and it is suspected that centers in the brain affect aqueous humor formation. Aqueous humor circulation in the anterior chamber results from convection (temperature differences) within the eye. When the eyelids are closed, however, temperature within the eye is fairly uniform.

The outflow of aqueous humor through the spaces of Fontana of the trabecular meshwork at the angle between the cornea and the iris can be affected by the condition of the endothelium, tension of the iris, and tension of the ciliary muscle. Aqueous humor outflow, if blocked, can be facilitated by drug-induced miosis. Contraction of the ciliary muscle increases the outflow. Some literature suggests that Schlemm's canal in the primate eye is uniquely instrumental in aqueous humor drainage. Although the aqueous humor plexus of the dog is grossly different from Schlemm's canal, ultrastructurally the two are the same. The aqueous humor plexus of the eye of a nonprimate mammal or a bird may not have the simple canal-like appearance, as it is an extremely plexiform conformation in the deep tissues of the anterior scleral segment, but functionally the aqueous humor plexus and Schlemm's canal are analogues. Ruminants may have both an intrascleral venous plexus and a canal of Schlemm. The intrascleral venous plexus and the posterior or uveoscleral pathway apparently serve as intrascleral conduits for exiting aqueous humor and uveal venous blood, which eventually mix. The primate eye lacks the numerous interconnections between the aqueous humor and uveal vessels. This lack may account for the greater incidence of breakdowns in primate ocular homeostatic mechanisms. Because of the direct removal of aqueous humor into the venous system, a lymphatic drainage system for the eye is not found.

Intraocular pressure varies from about 10 to 25 mm Hg, depending on the animal and also on the method of determination. Tonometers for measuring intraocular pressure vary from simple instruments consisting of a footplate, a plunger, and a recording scale to pneumatonographs, which flatten or indent the cornea with a silicone sensor membrane driven by compressed gas. Extraocular muscle contraction, especially of the retractor bulbi, can temporarily elevate the intraocular pressure. Intraocular pressure also varies with fluctuations in aqueous production and drainage, venous and arterial pressures, and respiration.

IRIS AND PUPIL

The pupil is the opening in the iris through which light is transmitted. The irides of the young are often a different color than those of the adult. Bird irides contain pigmented connective tissue cells and lipids. The lipid colors are affected by diet; for example, a corn diet promotes a yellow coloring. Heterochromic irides (e.g., one blue and one brown eye) occur in domestic mammals. Blue irides, associated with deafness and white fur, occur in dogs, cats, mink, rabbits, and mice. The incidence of deafness associated with heterochromic irides in cattle and horses has not been documented. Eyes with a blue iris often lack a tapetum and/or choroidal pigment. (The tapetum, a structure in the back of the eye or fundus that reflects light, is discussed under "Retina" below.)

Pupils are dark or pink in ambient room light. An eye with a dark pupil may or may not have a tapetum, but a pink pupil indicates a lack of tapetum. If a light beam in a dark environment is directed through the pupil, a fundic reflection will be colored (e.g., blue, green, orange, or yellow) if a tapetum is present or pink to red if there is no tapetum. The pink or red color is from the hemoglobin in the choroidal vessels. Complete albinos have pink irides; incomplete albinos, such as Siamese cats, may have blue irides. Albinos have pigment cells that are defective in pigment production, but other syndromes involve a lack of pigment cells caused by a lack of cell migration during embryological development.

Pupil shape varies in animals. The pupil may be round or may have the shape of a horizontal ellipse, a vertical ellipse, or a vertical slit. The primary function of irides is to provide an optimal amount of light for the retina by varying pupil size. When light elicits miosis in one eye, miosis occurs in the other eye, even if it is in the dark (Fig. 42.2).

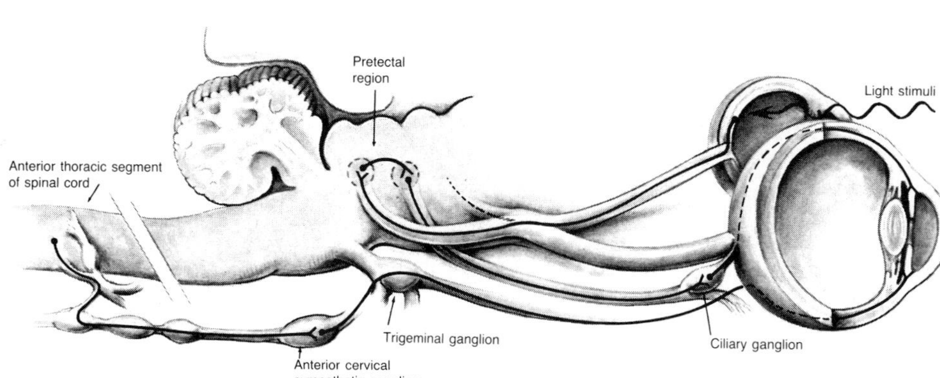

Figure 42.2. A scheme of the neural circuit for the pupillary light reflex. Sensory impulses from the retina affect the pretectal nuclei. The motor impulses travel down the oculomotor cranial nerve (III) via the ciliary ganglion to the constrictor iris muscle. Light in one eye affects the nonstimulated eye (as shown) as well as the stimulated eye (motor innervation of stimulated eye not shown). When light stimulates one eye and produces a reflex response in the opposite pupil, this is called the consensual light reflex. Also shown is the sympathetic innervation to the dilator muscle of the iris, which is not involved in the pupillary light reflex. The dilator muscle is also affected by circulating catecholamines from the adrenal medulla.

Another function of irides is the maintenance of clarity of aqueous humor. The surface epithelial cells phagocytize debris. The function of black masses (corpora nigra, umbraculum, or granula iridis) on the edges of the irides of horses and ruminants is not known. The iris may also help keep light in focus on the retina. When the pupils decrease in size, optical aberration is decreased. *Aberration* refers to the condition in which light rays striking the periphery of a lens are refracted differently from those striking the central portion. However, the irides of certain animals, such as horses and ruminants, do not contract to the extent of those of dogs, cats, and chickens, and therefore the blocking of aberrantly refracted rays by the iris may not be important in animals with large pupils and lenses.

The muscles of mammal irides are of the smooth muscle type. In birds, however, the iris muscles are striated and have cholinergic nicotinic receptors. In mammals the constrictor or sphincter muscle fibers have cholinergic muscarinic receptors innervated by the oculomotor nerve (parasympathetic portion), and the dilator muscle fibers have alpha$_1$-adrenergic receptors innervated by sympathetic nerves that follow the long ciliary nerve (part of the ophthalmic branch of the trigeminal nerve). Most, but not all, parasympathetic nerves synapse in the ciliary ganglia. Practically all the cells in the ciliary ganglia innervate the intrinsic muscles of the eye, with the vast majority innervating the ciliary muscle. Pupil size is determined mainly by iris muscles but may also be affected by turgescence and detumescence of the iris blood vessels. Injury to the eyeball often results in iridal hyperemia and miosis as well as increased protein in the aqueous and increased intraocular pressure. Axonal reflexes may be involved in these reactions.

Hippus is a tremor of the iris muscle. Respiratory hippus can occur occasionally in normal cats and is analogous to respiratory cardiac sinus arrhythmia in dogs. That is to say, there may be a variation in a cat's parasympathetic tone that correlates with respiration.

Some other factors that affect iridal dynamics are known. Morphine acts on the brain oculomotor nucleus to cause miosis in the dog, whereas morphine causes mydriasis in the cat because catecholamines are released from the adrenal glands. The iris-dilator muscle becomes hypersensitive to catecholamines after the muscle has been denervated. Hypersensitivity is greater in postganglionic denervation than in preganglionic denervation. Paralysis of cervical sympathetic nerves to the eye, such as would occur after unilateral denervation of cervical sympathetic nerves (Horner's syndrome), results in a paralysis of the iris-dilator muscle of the denervated eye and a unilateral miosis. This sign of Horner's syndrome in which the two pupils are not of equal size (anisocoria) is seen best in subdued light.

LENS

The crystalline lens focuses entering light on the retina. Keeping the image of visual stimuli on the retina by the lens is a dynamic form of accommodation. (A discussion of accommodation appears under "Optics and Ocular Movement" below.) The lens, surrounded by a capsule, is suspended from the ciliary processes by zonules. When the ciliary muscle contracts and tension on the zonules decreases, the lens becomes thick (more convex), especially the anterior surface. As the lens thickens, it may even push the iris anteriorly, as shown in Fig. 42.8C. The ciliary muscle is innervated by parasympathetic neurons. Most neurons in the ciliary ganglia innervate the ciliary muscles. The cholinergic muscarinic receptors can be blocked by atropine. Beta $_2$-adrenergic receptors, when stimulated, inhibit the ciliary muscle. Thus when an animal becomes excited and sympathetic tone increases, the lens becomes less convex, and the eye is accommodated for viewing distant objects.

The lens, when normal, is transparent because of a lack of blood vessels, the arrangement of its cells, and a high concentration of special proteins called crystallins. The lens is called crystalline because of its transparent appearance, not because of any crystalline arrangement of its molecules. The protein concentration of the fiber cells averages about 35 percent of the wet weight but may be as high as 70 percent in the inner nuclear region. There are three antigenically distinct crystallin proteins in mammals (often four in birds). The crystallins are formed early in fetal life and sequestered; therefore, if the crystallins accidentally leak out in adults, an immune response to the crystallin proteins may occur. Lens proteins are organ-specific immunologically but not species-specific. The lens proteins, once formed in the lens, persist and probably stay there for the animal's lifetime.

VITREOUS HUMOR

The vitreous humor is a clear hydrogel containing hyaluronic acid and a framework of collagen fibrils similar to those in articular cartilage. Except for the hyaluronic acid and collagen, the composition of vitreous humor is very similar to that of the aqueous humor. Nutrients slowly diffuse from the ciliary body to the retina through the vitreous humor.

Gradients of nutrients and waste products occur in both aqueous and vitreous humors; neither humor should be considered homogeneous. Changes in the blood-retinal or blood-vitreous humor barrier affect the vitreous humor, but, because of the relatively large volume, changes are usually much slower in the vitreous humor than in the aqueous humor. No barrier exists between the aqueous humor and the vitreous humor or between the vitreous humor and the retina.

In the embryo, the hyaloid artery courses from the optic disc to the posterior lens capsule. Normally it regresses within a few weeks after birth, but it may be seen with an ophthalmoscope in foals and calves. Remnants may be seen in mature animals, but usually there is only an irregular fibrous hyaloid canal.

The vitreous humor provides physical support to the lens and holds the retina against the choroid. Physicochemical change in the vitreous hydrogel is a cause of lens luxations and retinal detachments.

RETINA

Figure 42.3 shows the sequence of cells involved in sensation generally and in vision specifically. All but one layer (pigment epithelium) of the normal retina is transparent. To stimulate the photoreceptors, light must pass through the transparent retinal layers. Photoreceptors (rods and cones) are hyperpolarized by light, probably as a result of decreased membrane permeability to sodium ions. Receptors for somatic senses of an animal body are depolarized by an appropriate stimulus, and the depolarization initiates action potentials or a release of transmitter substance. It is thought that photoreceptors release most of their transmitter substance in the dark while depolarized. Most retinal cells have graded potentials; only ganglion cells have all-or-none action potentials transmitted over relatively long axons that make up the optic nerves. Thus the retinal cells integrate the

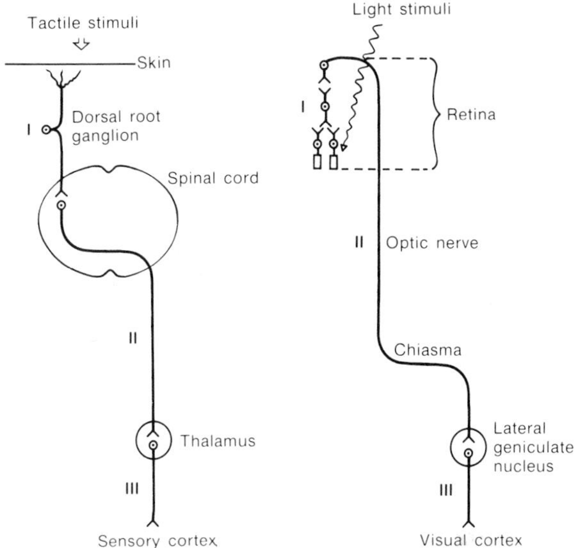

Figure 42.3. Comparison of a cutaneous sensory pathway (*left*) and the visual pathway (*right*). The first or primary neurons (I) in both pathways are bipolar cells in a three-neuron pathway to the cerebral cortex.

photoreceptor activity so that light increases ganglion cell axon action potentials. Horizontal cells, amacrine cells, and glia cells are involved in this integration. For instance, it has been found that certain roughly circular zones of the retina surrounding one type of ganglion cell will, when stimulated, increase a ganglion cell's activity. Such zones are surrounded by zones that, when stimulated, decrease the ganglion cell's activity. Conversely, still other circular zones, when stimulated, decrease another type of ganglion cell activity, and stimulation of the surrounding areas often increases the ganglion cell activity. Thus central and surrounding retinal areas are antagonistic to each other, indicating that activity of ganglion cells is affected by stimuli in other areas of the retina. Further evidence of retinal cell integration is shown by the fact that certain ganglion cells respond only to light moving in a particular direction across the retina. In birds, the brain exerts control, via centrifugal pathways, over transmission in the retina through its effects on amacrine cells.

The retinas of domestic mammals contain mostly rods, while retinas of domestic birds contain mostly cones. The number of cones of domestic mammal retinas is highest in the central region. Also, the number of photoreceptors per bipolar cell decreases toward the more sensitive central parts of the retina. When a number of cells synapse on another cell (e.g., when a number of photoreceptor cells synapse on one bipolar cell), the phenomenon is called convergence. The number of photoreceptors per bipolar cell decreases (less convergence) toward the central parts of the retina where sensitivity and visual acuity are greatest. Visual acuity is the extent to which details and forms of objects can be perceived accurately. A foveal region is an area of high visual acuity, provided the light intensity is sufficient. The foveas of primates and birds contain only cones, and in the foveal area the ratio of cones to bipolar cells is 1:1 (no convergence). Retinal structures are displaced over a fovea so that the cones are exposed to light less impeded by retinal structures. Domestic mammals lack foveas but do have more sensitive, cone-rich central areas or visual streaks shaped like the pupil. These sensitive areas or streaks cannot be seen with the ophthalmoscope. Figure 42.4 shows the fundic structures that are seen ophthalmoscopically.

The rods are extremely sensitive to light except at the red end of the spectrum and are used for night (scotopic) vision; cones function best for daylight (photopic) vision. Because there is less convergence of cones, cone vision has greater acuity; rod vision lacks resolution. This lack of resolution in rod vision is due, for the most part, to the convergence of rods on bipolar cells.

The photosensitive pigment in outer-segment disc membranes of rods is called *rhodopsin*. Light changes the molecular shape of rhodopsin from the cis to the trans form, which then splits by hydrolysis into scotopsin (a protein) and retinal (vitamin A aldehyde). Some of the retinal is enzymatically changed into retinol (vitamin A alcohol), which in turn is stored as a fatty acid ester (retinyl ester) in the pigment cells (Fig. 42.5). The cis form of the vitamin A is necessary to form rhodopsin and requires isomerases (enzymes). This *cis*-retinal joins scotopsin to form rhodopsin. This formation of rhodopsin is an exothermic reaction. The newly synthesized rhodopsin moves from the rod inner segment to the outer segment discs, which are continuously being formed. In the dark, rhodopsin accumulates in the disc membranes so that the rods become very sensitive to light. This process is called dark adaptation. It takes 20 to 40 minutes for the photoreceptors to become maximally sensitive to light. In light, the concentration of rhodopsin decreases; the rods thus become insensitive, and vision is the result of cone stimulation (light adaptation). Light adaptation is complete in about 5 minutes. Avitaminosis A causes visual abnormalities. One of the earliest signs of avitaminosis A is night blindness (nyctalopia).

When light bleaches rhodopsin, membrane permeability to sodium ions decreases because of the changes in molecular configuration affecting membrane channels. Because discs may be separated from the cell (rod) membrane, calcium ions have also been suspected of decreasing membrane permeability to sodium ions. As discs (saccules) are separated from the rods, the pigment epithelium phagocytizes and digests the discs from the outer segments. Cone discs are also shed, but mostly in darkness, whereas rods shed most of their discs in light. In most species it is difficult to separate rods from cones solely on a morphological basis. The metabolism of photopigments from cones has not been as well defined as that of rhodopsin. Iodopsin is a photolabile retinal-containing pigment (a photopsin) isolated from the cone-dominated retina of the chicken. There

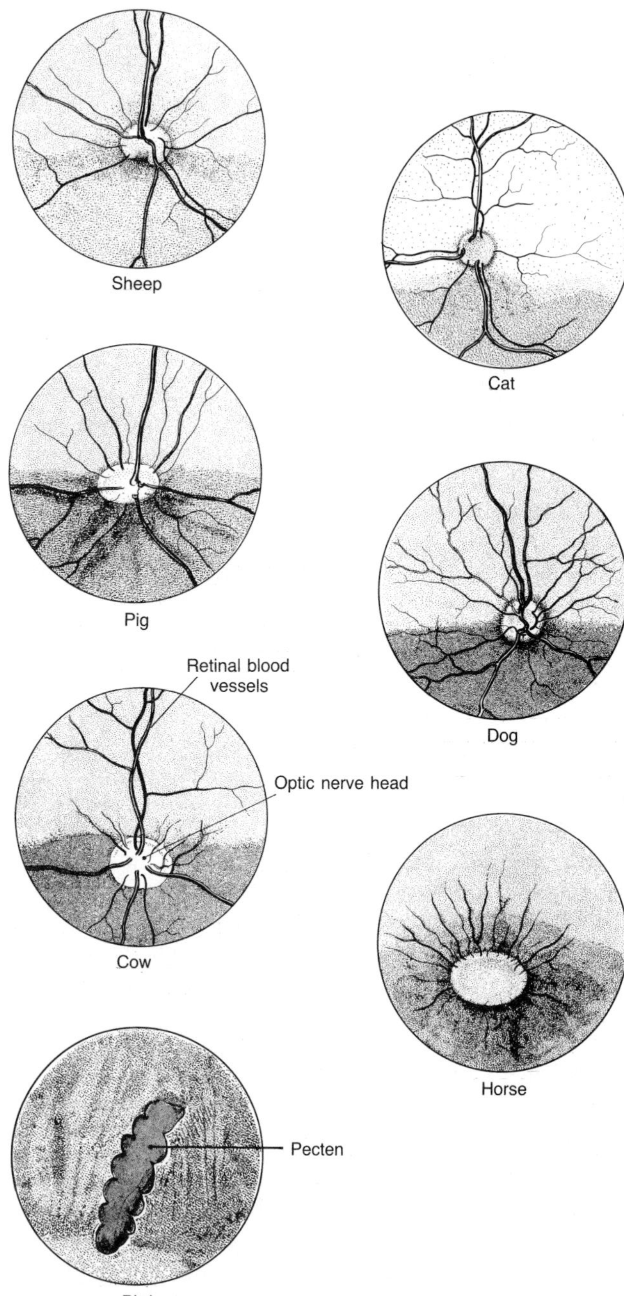

Figure 42.4. Drawings of fundi of seven domestic animals as seen by ophthalmoscopy.

are other retinal-containing pigments of cones, bleached in accordance with the color of the light, but their occurrence in domestic animals is not definite. The only difference between rod and cone pigments is within the opsin (protein) component. It is thought that vitamin A is required for normal cone function as well as for rod function. In birds, colored oil droplets found in cones may play a part in cone

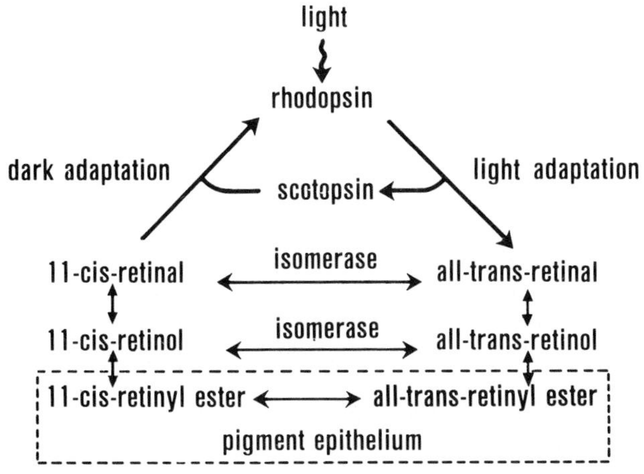

Figure 42.5. Breakdown and resynthesis of rhodopsin in the retina (in and around rod discs) and the pigment epithelium. Retinal (an aldehyde), retinol (an alcohol), and retinyl (a fatty acid ester) are forms of the vitamin A derived from carotenes.

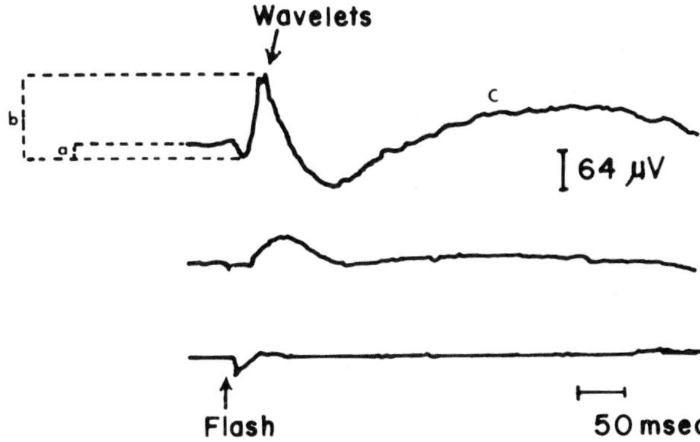

Figure 42.6. Three electroretinograms from a dog's eye. The recording electrode was on the cornea and the reference electrode on the nasion. Each of the three recordings is an average of 32 flashes (1 flash per second, < 10 μs flash duration) as computed by a signal averager. (*Top*) Bright white flashes in the dark. The wavelets superimposed on the b wave do not consistently occur unless special techniques are employed. (*Middle*) Dim blue flashes in the dark. This scotopic potential is primarily from rod activity. (*Bottom*) Bright red flashes in ambient light. This photopic potential is primarily from cone activity.

function. There is evidence of four spectral classes of cones in the retinas of a number of birds. One class of cones is responsive to short wavelengths (ultraviolet).

In the cat, the amino acid taurine is necessary for photoreceptor cell function and viability. If taurine-deficient diets—for example, certain dog foods—are fed to cats, photoreceptor abnormalities occur initially in the area centralis (region of maximal cone concentration). A decline in feline retinal taurine content is associated with changes in retinal electrical activity such as increased latencies and decreased amplitudes.

The record of gross electrical activity (potential changes) of the retina is called an electroretinogram (ERG). An ERG can be elicited from mammals (Fig. 42.6) and birds by a flash of light. The waves of an ERG elicited by a flash of light are the a, b, and c waves. The a-wave probably originates from the photoreceptors; the b wave from glia cells and perhaps horizontal, amacrine, and bipolar neurons; and the c wave from the pigment epithelium. Changes in either the eye or the stimulus will affect the ERG (Fig. 42.6). An ERG can be elicited after severance of the optic nerve (axons of ganglion cells).

Successive flashes of light elicit a separate ERG (with a, b, or c waves) for each flash, but if the frequency of flashes is increased, a point is reached at which separate ERGs cannot be differentiated; that is, fusion occurs. The frequency at which fusion occurs is called the critical frequency for flicker fusion. At low light intensity, fusion may occur at 2 to 6 flashes per second, whereas at high light intensity it may occur at 40 to 60 flashes per second.

Oscillatory potentials (wavelets) are low-amplitude oscillations superimposed on the b wave of an ERG. Oscillatory potentials are not seen to any extent with routine light flashes but can be elicited under special conditions with bright flashes. Oscillatory potentials have been recorded from cats, rabbits, guinea pigs, mice, pigeons, and primates. Their origin is not yet known. The oscillatory potentials may be selectively reduced or extinguished in some retinopathies while the amplitudes of the a and b waves remain normal.

ERGs are especially important in the evaluation of retinal function when the ocular fundus cannot be examined ophthalmoscopically, as in the case of cataracts, and in the detection of retinopathies before the retina shows ophthalmoscopic changes. It should be remembered that although an ERG may be isoelectric (flat), indicating loss of vision, a pupillary light reflex may still be present.

In addition to flash-elicited ERGs, there are pattern-elicited ERGs. The pattern is usually of checkerboard design and is displayed for viewing on a cathode-ray tube or in goggles worn by the animal. The squares reverse color without changing total light output (luminance). It is thought that pattern-elicited ERGs, unlike flash-elicited ERGs, are partially derived from optic nerve activity and that the absence of such responses may be diagnostic of loss of optic nerve function.

Some domestic mammals (cats, dogs, horses, ruminants) usually have a tapetum (Fig. 42.7), which reflects light back through the retina. In individual animals, the tapetum may be missing in one or both eyes. The tapetum increases sensitivity to light and is the source of the colored fundus (eyeground) reflection seen when a bright light is shined into an animal's eye. For example, in colored photographs taken indoors with a flash, the pupils of humans may be red and those of dogs orange or yellow if the flash is directed appropriately to elicit a fundic reflection. A discussion of pupil color appears under "Iris and Pupil," above. When a tapetum is lacking in an animal's eye, as in pigs, the fundic reflection is red because of blood in the choroid.

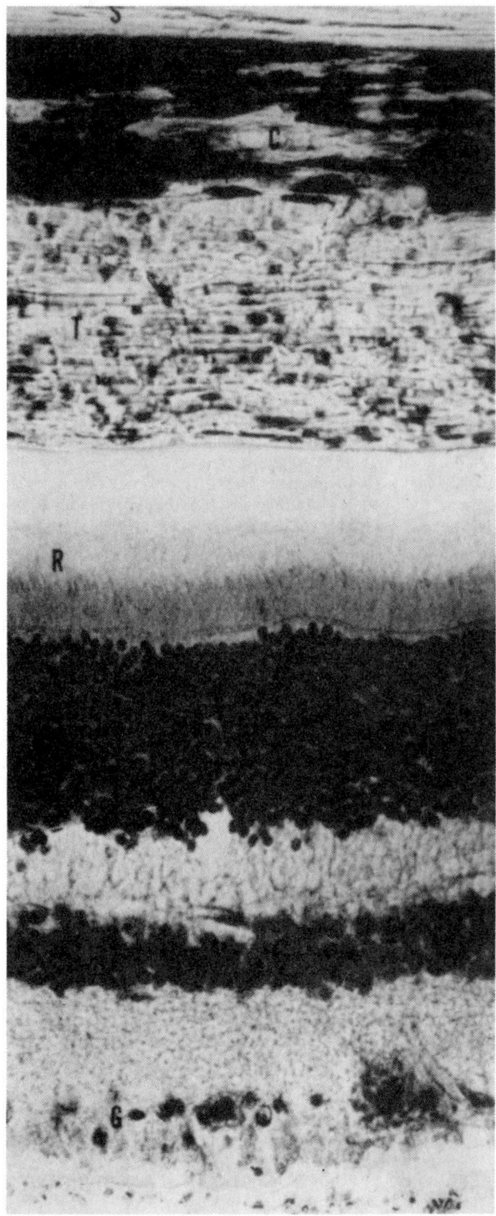

Figure 42.7. Tapetum lucidum (layer of choroid) of a cat seen as a broad band of cell layers (T) between the pigment layer of the choroid (C) and the retina. Melanin is absent from pigmented epithelium of retina (outer layer of retina) where tapetum is present. S, sclera; R, receptors; G, ganglion cells. (See Fig. 42.1, magnified section of retina, choroid, and sclera, for orientation.)

Complete degeneration of the retina results in a brighter tapetal reflection (hyperreflection).

The choroidal blood supplies most of the metabolic needs of the retina, even in those animals with retinal blood vessels. Normal retinal blood vessel growth is stimulated in the neonate by a relative oxygen deficiency. (The neonate retina receives less oxygen under atmospheric pressure than it did before birth.) If a neonate is placed in a hyperbaric oxygen environment and then returned to a normal atmospheric pressure, the relative oxygen deficiency in the normal atmosphere causes the retinal vessels to grow over the retina, resulting in blindness.

OPTICS AND OCULAR MOVEMENT

The curvature and refractive index of a lens, determine the power of a lens expressed in diopters (D). Refraction is the deflection of light as it passes from one medium into another of different optical density. The refractive index is the ratio of the velocity of light in a vacuum to the velocity of light in a medium. Table 42.1 shows the refractive index for air, water, and various parts of the eye of a horse. Because the eye contains a variety of tissues through which light must pass, refraction in the eye is complex.

Parallel light passing into a medium perpendicularly is not refracted. If parallel rays of light (collimated light) pass through one surface of a biconvex lens, they are refracted and converge to a focus or point beyond the other surface of the lens. The distance between the lens and the point of convergence is defined as the principal focal length. The reciprocal of the principal focal length in meters equals the power of the lens in diopters. As a source of light or an object reflecting light approaches a lens, the light rays become nonparallel with respect to the lens surface, and the convergence point or focus falls beyond the principal focal length (farther away from the lens). Glass lenses can be convergent (+D), bringing the focal point nearer to the lens, or divergent (−D), taking the focal point farther from the lens. If the principal focal length of the eye of a horse is 40 mm (0.04 m), the dioptic power is 25 D.

The light reflected from an object after passing through a lens is upside down and reversed. An image on the retina is upside down and reversed with reference to an object viewed by an eye. The ratio of eye lens-to-image distance to object-to-eye lens distance equals the ratio of image size to object size.

In an optical instrument an image is kept in focus by moving a lens with respect to the object, whereas in the eye the lens changes its power or D to keep the image in focus on the retina by changing its shape. This changing of shape is called accommodation. In other words, a glass lens has an unchanging principal focal length, whereas the eye lens can change its principal focal length. Figure 42.8 shows

Table 42.1. Refractive index for air, water, and parts of the eye of a horse

Medium	Refractive index
Air	Near 1.000
Water	1.333 (varies with temperature)
Cornea	1.370
Aqueous humor	1.335
Lens	1.420
Vitreous humor	1.335

From Knill, Eagleton, and Harver 1977, *Am. J. Vet. Res.* 38:735–37.

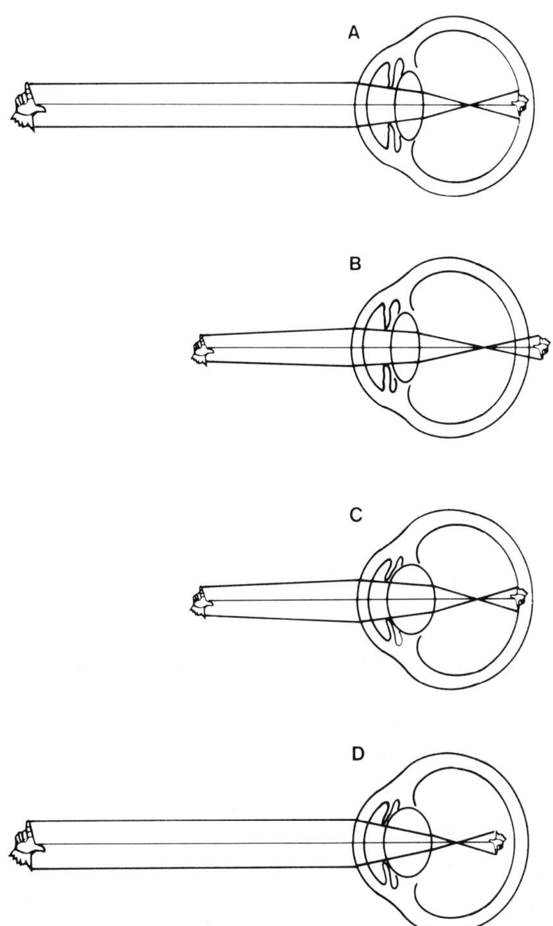

Figure 42.8. (*A*) An emmetropic eye viewing an object at a distance. Reflected light rays from a distant object are parallel, and thus the image is focused on the retina. (*B*) An unaccommodated eye viewing a close object. Reflected light rays from a close object are nonparallel. (*C*) An accommodated eye viewing a close object. Note the change in lens shape. (*D*) An ametropic eye viewing an object at a distance with too powerful a lens.

what happens to the image as the object distance and lens power vary. As an object approaches the eye, the ring of ciliary muscle contracts, lessening the tension on the zonules attached to the lens capsule. As the tension on the lens decreases, the lens thickens (Fig. 42.8C), thus increasing its dioptic power and keeping the image on the retina.

An eye is *emmetropic* if the resting eye focuses parallel light rays on the retina—in other words, if the image of a distant object is in focus on the retina. If such an image is not in focus in a resting eye, the eye is described as *ametropic*. Ametropia is the consequence of some error of refraction (e.g., too weak or too powerful a lens or too short or too long an eyeball). If parallel light rays passing through the resting eye focus in front of the retina, the ametropic eye is myopic; if the parallel rays focus in the back of the retina, the eye is hypermetropic (the state of hyperopia).

The capacity for accommodation in domestic animals varies from species to species. Predatory mammals such as dogs and cats can increase the power of their lenses more than those that are preyed upon, such as horses and ruminants. In the case of cats, accommodation can be so dynamic that the lens pushes the iris anteriorly as it becomes more convex. The capacity for accommodation probably varies with the breed, within species as well as among individuals. Most domestic mammals cannot dynamically accommodate to the extent that humans can.

Birds are good accommodators. Each eye is able to accommodate independently of the other. Chicks have an impressive range of accommodation, even on the first day of life. In birds the ability to accommodate declines with age.

In the horse, ciliary muscles are weak, and the dynamic accommodation by a change in lens shape occurs to a lesser extent than in predators. It is evident that the horse must move its head or its eye, or both, for optimal visual acuity. It may be that the horse uses a form of static accommodation, the ramp retina (Fig. 42.9). According to the ramp retina concept, light entering the eye ventrally travels farther from the lens to the retina, and light entering more dorsally travels a shorter distance from the lens to the retina. The eye is oriented so that light enters ventrally for near vision and dorsally for far vision. Whether head and eye movement indicates that the horse has a ramp retina, uses the movement to keep the image on the most sensitive parts of the retina, or both has not been resolved. In any case, the inability of the horse to accommodate rapidly probably causes many horses to shy after a sudden movement.

To keep images on the most sensitive parts of the retina, all animals use neck muscles and ocular muscles. Saccadic movements are rapid eye movements, caused by extraocular muscle contraction, which occur when an animal is

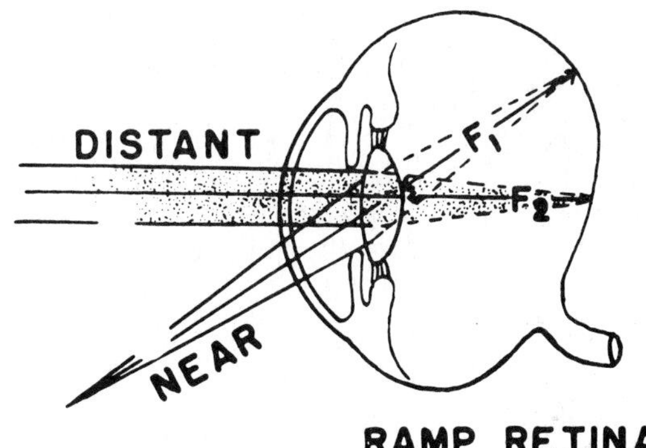

Figure 42.9. Ramp-shaped retina, which provides a longer focal length for viewing downward (F_1) than for viewing along the axis of the eye (F_2). This means that lower, nearer objects are in focus without, or with minimal, accommodation. The head and eye movement indicates that the horse may have a ramp retina. (From Prince, Diesem, Eglitis, and Ruskell 1960, *Anatomy and Histology of the Eye and Orbit in Domestic Animals*, Charles C Thomas, Springfield, Ill.)

tracking visual stimuli, in nystagmus (discussed below), and in rapid eye movement of sleep. The fixational microsaccades that occur in humans probably do not occur in domestic animals. Muscle spindles are absent from the extraocular muscles of some domestic animals (dogs, cats, rabbits, birds) and present in others (primates, ruminants, pigs). How the lack of spindles affects function is not known, but it is known that the muscle spindle population is greatest in antigravity muscles. Extraocular muscles are not antigravity muscles; therefore it is not surprising to find few or no spindles in them. Table 42.2 lists the functions of the extraocular muscles. Usually both eyes move together in what are called conjugate movements. Convergent movements bring the two pupils toward each other as attention is focused on objects near the animal. Drugs (general anesthetics, for example) that decrease skeletal muscle tone decrease extraocular muscle tone so that the eyeballs can no longer be maintained in their normal position.

Nystagmus is a rhythmical oscillation—either horizontal, rotary, or vertical—of the eyeballs. Jerk nystagmus is nystagmus in which the oscillations are faster in one direction than in the other. By convention, the direction of eye movement in jerk nystagmus is identified by the direction of the quick component (i.e., left or right, dorsal or ventral). Optokinetic nystagmus is brought on by visual stimuli, either when the visual stimuli are moving and the head is stationary or when the head and body are moving and the visual stimuli are stationary. Optokinetic nystagmus is subcortical in domestic animals; that is, it can be evoked in the absence of the cerebral hemispheres. In humans, optokinetic nystagmus cannot be elicited without the cerebral cortex. Lesions of the anterior colliculi can affect fixation on visual stimuli.

Rotatory and postrotatory nystagmus, types of vestibular (labyrinthine) nystagmus, are elicited by stimulation of the semicircular canals (Fig. 42.10). Acceleration or deceleration during rotation of the head causes inertial displacement of the endolymph in the semicircular canals, resulting in bending of the cupula. If the eyes are open during rotation, optokinetic and rotary nystagmus enhance each other. Postrotatory nystagmus lasts 20 ± 5 seconds but is reduced if the eyes open during rotation. Caloric nystagmus is elicited by placing cold (18°C) or warm water (48°C) in an ear. Cold-water stimulation usually produces nystagmus in a direction away from the stimulated ear; warm-water stimulation usually produces nystagmus toward the stimulated ear. Caloric stimulation of nystagmus is not dependable in domestic animals. This lack of dependability is probably due to variation in the distance from the ear canal to the inner ear (labyrinth). Galvanic nystagmus is elicited by direct current stimulation of the vestibular portion of the eighth cranial nerve.

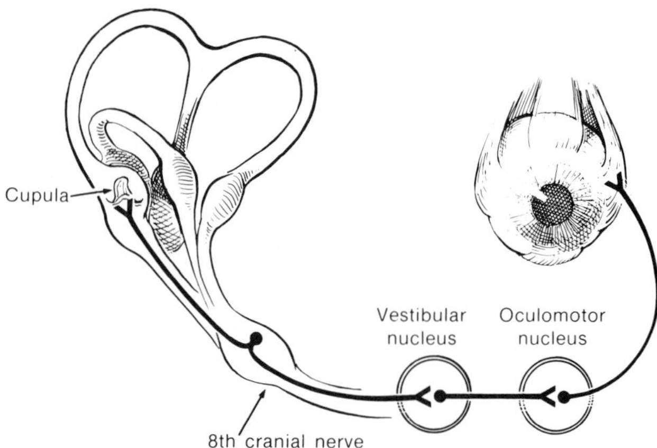

Figure 42.10. A scheme of the neural circuit from a cupula to an extraocular muscle. The cupula moves when inertial displacement of endolymph occurs in the semicircular canals during acceleration or deceleration as the head rotates. Synergistic and antagonistic muscles are appropriately innervated (not shown), and also the contralateral eye has appropriate synergistic and antagonistic innervation (not shown). When the ipsilateral eye moves temporally, the contralateral eye moves nasally.

Table 42.2. Extraocular muscles and their main function

Muscle	Main function*
Lateral rectus	Abduction
Medial rectus	Adduction
Dorsal rectus	Elevation
Ventral rectus	Depression
Ventral oblique	Outward rolling
Dorsal oblique	Inward rolling
Retractor bulbi	Retraction

*No eye movement is carried out by one extraocular muscle acting alone.

Ocular nystagmus is a wandering or searching movement of the eyes associated with congenital blindness. Anesthetics and diseases of the vestibular (labyrinth) mechanism, brain stem, or cerebellum can cause nystagmus. After unilateral or bilateral destruction of the labyrinth, cats have a spontaneous nystagmus and lose their equilibrium. These signs disappear within a few days to a week. White cats have been shown to have varying degrees of vestibular and/or optokinetic dysfunction when compared with normally pigmented cats.

Kittens are born with divergent *strabismus*, which is evident after the eyes open. Normal eye alignment, which is dependent on visual stimuli, develops at about 6 weeks of age. Convergent strabismus (crossed eyes) is commonly seen in adult Siamese cats and in other albino mammals as a result of defects in the lateral geniculate nucleus (a part of the thalamus).

An electro-oculogram is a record of difference in potential between the front and the back of the eyeball. The recording electrode is placed subcutaneously at the lateral canthus of the eye, and the reference electrode is placed subcutaneously on the neck; recording electrodes can be placed above or below the eye. The potential varies with eyeball movement; therefore eye movement can be recorded on an electro-oculogram.

Manipulation of extraocular muscles during ocular surgery often slows the heart. This slowing of the heart is called the oculocardiac reflex. In unanesthetized dogs, clinicians may apply pressure to the eyeballs and slow the heart while listening to heart sounds. The reflex involves the trigeminal (sensory) and vagal (motor) nerves. Occasionally, the heart will beat faster or arrhythmias will occur, rather than the heart beating slower, because the sympathetic output may override the parasympathetic effect of the vagi.

VISUAL PATHWAYS

The axons of the ganglion cells in the retina make up the optic nerves. Most of the ganglion cells synapse in the lateral geniculate body (thalamus), and then the cells in the lateral geniculate body project to the visual cortex (striate cortex of the occipital lobe; see Fig. 42.3). A second pathway of ganglion cell axons leads to the anterior rostral colliculus or pretectal region (Fig. 42.2).

Analysis of feline ganglion cell axon projections to the brain has shown that the nasal and temporal portions of the retina overlap along a vertical median strip. In this visual streak, an area of maximal ganglion cell density, 50 percent of the axons project to the ipsilateral lateral geniculate nucleus of the thalamus and 50 percent to the contralateral lateral geniculate nucleus. On the nasal side of the strip, 100 percent of the cells project contralaterally; temporal to it, 75 percent of the cells project ipsilaterally and 25 percent contralaterally. Animals whose eyes are positioned laterally in the skull have more ganglion cell axons projecting contralaterally than do animals whose eyes are positioned well to the front of the head.

Ganglion cells have been classified into X, Y, and W cells, depending on the electrophysiological responses of ganglion cell axons. X cells demonstrate a sustained response to stimuli and participate in high-acuity vision. Y cells respond to rearrangement of stimuli (phasic or transient response) and are important in the initial analysis of crude form. W cells project to the rostral colliculus and are involved in head and eye movement. Siamese cats have a significantly lower percentage of Y cells than X cells when compared with other breeds of cats, and an eye of a Siamese cat is primarily represented in the contralateral cerebral cortex. Siamese cats have lower critical flicker fusion than other breeds of cats because of their lower number of Y cells. The abnormal retinal projections of many albino mammals cause the strabismus that often occurs in albinos. Albino mammals usually have abnormal lateral geniculate nuclei.

Potentials recorded from the visual cortex (occipital cortex) are called *visual evoked responses* (VERs). Like ERGs, VERs are flash-elicited and pattern-elicited responses. Patterns are often a checkerboard design with the squares reversing color (pattern shift). With the flash-elicited VERs, it is difficult to differentiate retinal activity from cortical activity, especially in small animals. Bilateral disease of the visual cortex causes abnormal pattern-elicited VERs; if the lesions are extensive, the animal may be cortically blind, (i.e., cannot perceive visual stimuli).

There is a transfer of visual cortical activity from one cerebral hemisphere to the other. Experiments in cats have shown that the corpus callosum plays a part in normal binocular vision and depth perception.

VISION

What an animal actually perceives through vision is, of course, unknown. However, on the basis of behavioral, biochemical, electrophysiological, and anatomical investigations, some ideas as to how animal vision compares with human vision have been presented. It is thought that primates, birds, reptiles, amphibians, and fish perceive color to a much greater extent than do domestic mammals. For instance, feline cones are maximally sensitive to green, so cats can discriminate blue from gray or green most of the time, provided the stimuli subtend a large visual angle. Memory and learning that colors have significance are factors in an animal's ability to distinguish colors as well as the appropriate photoreceptors and retinal integration. When devising behavioral tests to quantitate an animal's ability to discriminate colors, one must take care to keep luminance

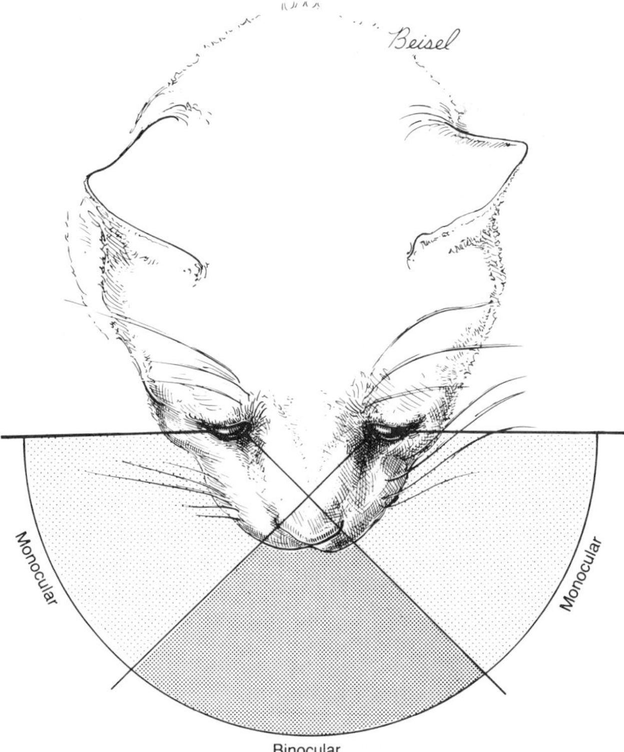

Figure 42.11. Field of vision of a cat, showing a large central binocular area resulting from the forward position of the eyes.

constant. If luminance is not constant, the animal may base behavioral responses on luminance rather than on color.

Tests have indicated that visual resolution of cats is similar to that of humans. Birds of prey with more than one fovea probably have excellent resolution with their sensitive cones strategically placed; for example, some birds have strip fovea on the dorsal part of the fundus for scanning the ground or water for prey.

The anatomical placement of the eyes in the head certainly has a great influence on what is seen (Fig. 42.11 and 42.12). The entire spatial area that can be viewed by an eye is called the field of vision. The visual fields of two eyes overlap centrally. There is a great deal of variation among breeds within species for some domestic mammals (dogs, horses). The wider-set eyes of herbivores that are preyed upon enable them to have a panoramic field of vision. The areas immediately in front of the nose and behind the hindquarters are outside the field of vision for some mammals (rabbits, horses). The rabbit even has a small binocular field behind it when it raises its head. A horse, when holding its head high or when grazing, can scan a 360-degree field of vision.

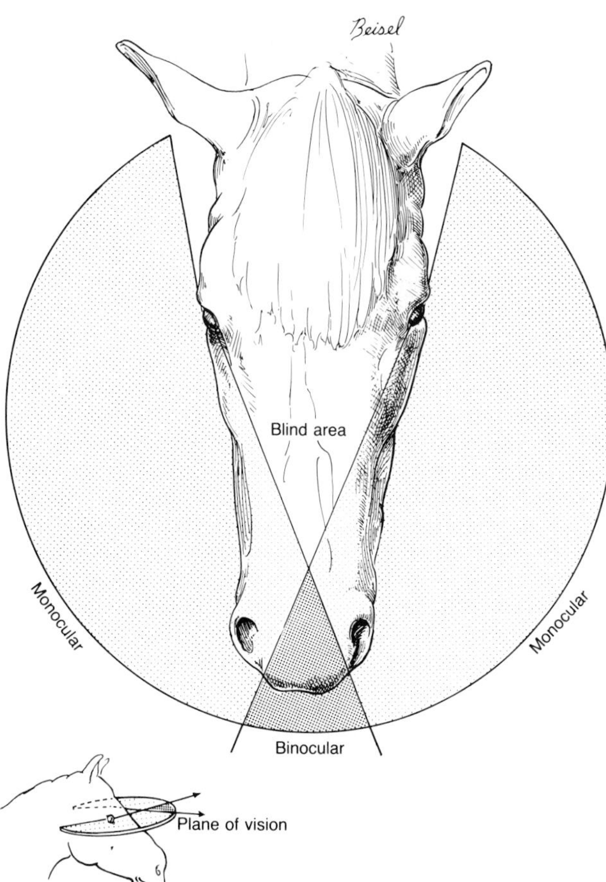

Figure 42.12. Field of vision of a horse. When the eyes are cast down (not shown), there is a blind spot in front of the nose. When the eyes are cast posteriorly at the level of the body (not shown), there is a blind spot immediately behind the horse's body.

REFERENCES

Aquirre, G.D., and Rubin, L.F. 1975. Rod-cone dysplasia (progressive retinal atrophy) in Irish Setters. *J. Am. Vet. Med. Assoc.* 166:157–64.

Apt, L., Isenberg, S., and Gaffney, W.L. 1973. The oculocardiac reflex in strabismus surgery. *Am. J. Ophth.* 76:533–36.

Bedford, P.G.C., and Grierson, I. 1986. Aqueous drainage in the dog. *Res. Vet. Sci.* 41:172–86.

Bentley, P.J. 1986. The crystalline lens of the eye: An organismal microcosm. *News Physiol. Sci.* 1:195–99.

Bergsma, D.R., and Brown, K.S. 1971. White fur, blue eyes, and deafness in the domestic cat. *J. Heredity* 62:171–85.

Blake, R., and Crawford, M.L. 1974. Development of strabismus in Siamese cats. *Brain Res.* 77:492–96.

Blakemore, C., and Cummings, R.M. 1975. Eye-opening in kittens. *Vision Res.* 15:1417–18.

Bridges, C.D., and Alvavez, R.A. 1987. The visual cycle operates via an isomerase acting on all-trans retinol in the pigment epithelium. *Science* 236:1678–80.

Chen, D.-M., and Goldsmith, T.H. 1986. Four spectral classes of cone in the retinas of birds. *J. Comp. Physiol. A* 159:473–99.

Cornwell, A.C. 1974. Electroretinographic responses following monocular visual deprivation in kittens. *Vision Res.* 14:1223–27.

Coulter, D.B., and Schmidt, G.M. 1984. The eye and vision. In M.J. Swenson, ed., *Dukes' Physiology of Domestic Animals*. 10th ed. Cornell University Press, Ithaca, New York.

Crawford, M.L., and Marc, R.E. 1976. Light transmission of cat and monkey eyelids. *Vision Res.* 16:323–24.

Cruise, L.J., and McClure, R. 1981. Posterior pathway for aqueous humor drainage in the dog. *Am. J. Vet. Res.* 42:992–95.

Guillery, R.W. 1974. Visual pathways in albinos. *Sci. Am.* 230:44–54.

Hamasaki, D.I., and Maquire, G.W. 1985. Physiological development of the kitten's retina: An ERG study. *Vision Res.* 25:1537–43.

Hammond, P. 1978. The neural basis for colour description in the domestic cat. *Vision Res.* 18:233–35.

Hayes, K.C., Carey, R.E., and Schmidt, S.Y. 1975. Retinal degeneration associated with taurine deficiency in the cat. *Science* 188:949–50.

Hill, D.W., and Houseman, J. 1980. Retinal blood flow to tapetal and pigmented fundus in the cat. *Exp. Eye Res.* 30:245–52.

Kalil, R.E., Jhaveri, S.R., and Richards, W. 1971. Anomalous retinal pathways in the Siamese cat: An inadequate substrate for normal binocular vision. *Science* 174:302–5.

Kato, I., Kawasaki, T., Aoyazi, M., Sato, Y., and Mizukoshi, K. 1979. Loss of visual suppression of caloric nystagmus in cats. *Acta Otolaryngol.* 87:499–505.

Knill, L.M., Eagleton, R.O., and Harver, E. 1977. Physical optics of the equine eye. *Am. J. Vet. Res.* 38:735–37.

Kowler, E., and Steinman, R.M. 1980. Small saccades serve no useful purpose: Reply to a letter by R.W. Ditchburn. *Vision Res.* 20:273–76.

Lee, H.K., and Wang, S.C. 1975. Mechanism of morphine-induced miosis in the dog. *J. Pharmacol. Exp. Ther.* 193:415–31.

Loop, M.S., Bruce, L.L., and Petuchowski, S. 1979. Cat color vision: The effect of stimulus size, shape and viewing distance. *Vision Res.* 19:507–13.

Loop, M.S., and Frey, T.J. 1981. Critical flicker fusion in Siamese cats. *Exp. Brain Res.* 43:65–68.

Loop, M.S., Petuchowski, S., and Smith, D.C. 1980. Critical flicker fusion in normal and binocularly deprived cats. *Vision Res.* 20:49–57.

Malnati, G.A., Marshall, A.E., and Coulter, D.B. 1981. Electroretinographic components of the canine visual evoked response. *Am. J. Vet. Res.* 42:159–63.

McFadden, S.A., and Reymond, L. 1985. A further look at the binocular visual field of the pigeon (Columba livia). *Vision Res.* 25:1741–46.

Mitchell, D.E., Griffin, F., Wilkinson, F., Anderson, P., and Smith, M.L. 1976. Visual resolution in young kittens. *Vision Res*. 16:363–66.

Moses, Robert A., ed. 1981. *Adler's Physiology of the Eye*. 7th ed. C.V. Mosby, St. Louis.

Roberts, S.R., and Erickson, O.F. 1962. Dog tear secretion and tear proteins. *J. Small Anim. Pract*. 3:1–5.

Robles, S.S., and Anderson, J.H. 1978. Compensation of vestibular deficits in the cat. *Brain Res*. 147:183–87.

Rodriguez-Peralta, L. 1975. The blood aqueous barrier in five species. *Am. J. Ophthalmol*. 80:713–25.

Saibil, H.R. 1986. From photon to receptor potential: The biochemistry of vision. *News Physiol. Sci*. 1:122–25.

Schaeffel, F., and Howland, H.C. 1987. Corneal accommodation in chick and pigeon. *Comp. Physiol. A* 160:375–84.

Schaeffel, F., Howland, H.C., and Farkas, L. 1986. Natural accommodation in the growing chickens. *Vision Res*. 26:1977–93.

Schmidt, S.Y., Berson, E.L., and Hayes, K.C. 1976. Retinal degeneration in cats fed casein. I. Taurine deficiency. *Invest. Ophthalmol*. 15:47–52.

Schwartz, B. 1964. The effect of lid closure temperature gradients in the rabbit eye. *Invest. Ophthalmol*. 3:100–106.

Sherman, S.M., Guillery, R.W., Kaas, J.H., and Sanderson, K.J. 1974. Behavioral, electrophysiological and morphological studies of binocular competition in the development of the geniculocortical pathways of cats. *J. Comp. Neurol*. 158:1–18.

Sivak, J.G., and Allen, D.B. 1975. An evaluation of the "ramp" retina of the horse eye. *Vision Res*. 15:1353–56.

Sivak, J.G., Hildebrand, T.E., Lebert, C.G., Myshak, L.M., and Ryall, L.A. 1986. Ocular accommodation in chickens: Corneal vs lenticular accommodation and effect of age. *Vision Res*. 26:1865–72.

Stone, J. 1966. The naso-temporal division of the cat's retina. *J. Comp. Neurol*. 126:585–600.

Szabuniewicz, M., McCrady, J.D., and Banknieder, A.R. 1966. Ophthalmodynamometry for clinical measurement of blood pressure in the goat. *Southwestern Vet*. 19:283–86.

Thibos, L.N., Levick, W.R., and Mortstyn, R. 1980. Ocular pigmentation in white and Siamese cats. *Invest. Ophthalmol. & Vision Sci*. 19:475–86.

Tusa, R.J., Rosenquiat, A.C., and Palmer, L.A. 1979. Retinotopic organization of areas 18 and 19 in the cat. *J. Comp. Neurol*. 185:657–78.

Vakkur, G.J., and Bishop, P.O. 1963. The schematic eye in the cat. *Vision Res*. 3:357–81.

Vakkur, G.J., Bishop, P.O., and Kozak, W. 1963. Visual optics in the cat, including posterior nodal distance and retinal landmarks. *Vision Res*. 3:289–314.

Van Buskirk, E.M. 1979. The canine eye: The vessels of aqueous drainage. *Invest. Ophthalmol. & Vision Sci*. 18:223–30.

Waldorf, R.A., Polsinelli, D.J., Knister, J.R., and Kohut, R.I. 1977. Vestibular and optokinetic responses of the white cat. *Acta Otolaryngol*. 84:72–79.

Wallenstein, M.C., and Wang, S.C. 1979. Mechanism of morphine-induced mydriasis in the cat. *Am. J. Physiol*. 236:R292–96.

Wallman, J., Gottlieb, M.D., Rajaram, V., and Fugate-Wentzek, L.A. 1987. Local retinal regions control local eye growth and myopia. *Science* 237:73–77.

Wistow, G., and Piatigorsky, J. 1987. Recruitment of enzymes as lens structural proteins. *Science* 236:1554–56.

Witzel, D.A., Riis, R.C., Rebhun, W.C., and Hillman, R.B. 1977. Night blindness in the Appaloosa: Sibling occurrence. *J. Equine Med. Surg*. 1:383–86.

CHAPTER 43

Special Senses II: Taste, Smell, and Hearing

by Morley R. Kare, Gary K. Beauchamp, and Roger R. Marsh

THE CHEMICAL SENSES

The animal body is a network of chemical receptors (chemoreceptors). All cell membranes respond to chemical stimulation. Some cells have become specialized to respond only to chemical stimuli from the external environment, whereas others, such as those in the carotid bodies, respond only to internal chemical stimuli. The former are collectively referred to as the chemical senses. This arbitrary division is bridged by the chemical receptors in the gut.

Fish have chemoreceptors distributed over the body surface. In amphibians, reactions to chemicals applied to the surface of the skin are observed; however, other specialized chemical receptors are concentrated in the oral cavity. For all air-breathing animals, chemoreception is primarily associated with the orally located taste buds or with the nasal chemoreceptors.

The chemical senses have been divided into three classes: (1) olfaction or smell, (2) gustation or taste, and (3) the common chemical sense. Olfaction is characterized by a sensitivity to volatile substances in extreme dilution. This accounts for its description as a distance receptor. The gustatory receptors usually require more gross contact with the chemical stimulant. The common chemical sense is reserved for the nonspecific stimulants, which are often irritants. The divisions among smell, taste, and the common chemical sense are arbitrary and can overlap because a single chemical may affect all three categories. Furthermore, a fourth chemical sense mediated by the terminal nerve (cranial nerve 0) has been identified. Its function and stimulators are not known, but it is speculated that it is involved in modulation of reproductive physiology.

COMMON CHEMICAL SENSE

In the higher vertebrates the common chemical sense is mediated primarily by the trigeminal nerve that innervates the nasal and oral cavities and the cornea. The major function of the common chemical sense has long been presumed to be the detection of noxious chemical stimuli and the initiation of appropriate protective reflexes, which are among the strongest reflexes in the body. Concentrations of nonnoxious compounds also stimulate trigeminal chemoreceptors, however, and the common chemical sense can interact with other chemical senses to produce an overall sensation.

TASTE

The function of taste is generally associated with the ingestion of food. Some investigators suggest that it encourages nutritional prudence; that is, taste provides the animal with a cue as to the value of a food. There is evidence that selection behavior based on taste is complementary to physiological need. For example, in a choice situation (water versus saline solution) the adrenalectomized rat will select the salt necessary to maintain life. There are a number of reports, many unsupported, that imply that taste has been developed to permit an animal to reject toxic substances and accept nutritious food or food products; wild animals, however, can be attracted to some poisonous baits, and many nutritionally useful food materials can be distasteful (e.g., alfalfa to the fowl). It is obvious that, for both wild and domestic animals, taste is not always a reliable guide to nutritional merits.

A most important function of taste is its effect on digestion and possibly metabolism. Taste and olfaction serve as gatekeepers, determining what food will enter the digestive tract. It is common knowledge that sensory information can initiate eating and stimulate salivary flow. The function and importance of saliva vary with the species, but generally saliva facilitates deglutition by its function as a lubricant.

Early in this century, Pavlov demonstrated that oral stimulation in the conscious dog increases the flow of gastric and pancreatic juices. In recent years, with the use of more sophisticated techniques, evidence has accumulated that nutrients can be metered and monitored orally. Information in the mouth can stimulate increased oxygen consumption, affect activity along the digestive tract, initiate the release of metabolic hormones, and modify biliary, gastric, and pancreatic functions. In turn, the nutritive state can feed back information that can affect the sense organs.

It is apparent that orally derived information can influence digestion and metabolism; however, there is only a modest amount of scientific information available for assessment of the nutritional contribution of the sensory qualities of food.

Taste receptors

The taste organs of mammals have their seat in the mucosa of the oral and pharyngeal cavities. The maximal concentration of receptors is in the mucosa of the tongue, particularly the dorsum.

All mammals and birds that have been studied have taste organs that are commonly referred to as taste buds (Fig. 43.1). The distribution of taste buds varies greatly among species. Taste buds are usually concentrated on the circumvallate and fungiform papillae. The taste buds in cows and sheep are generally oval in shape; their length is approximately 100 μm, and their width varies from 20 to 45 μm. The taste buds of the horse are slightly smaller and melon shaped, whereas those of goats are still smaller, irregular ovals of about 30 by 60 μm. The pig has spindle-shaped 20 by 90 μm buds. In the cat and the dog, the taste buds are circular with a diameter of approximately 30 μm. Avian taste buds have shape characteristics that are intermediate between those of fish and mammals and that resemble those of reptiles. Chicken taste receptors are approximately 30 μm wide and 70 μm long.

Although taste buds are characteristically found on the tongue, they have also been found on various structures related to the oral cavity, such as the upper margins of the gullet, epiglottis, soft palate, pharynx, and larynx.

The tip of the tongue of the cow is well supplied with taste buds; the middle has relatively few; and the back, which contains the circumvallate papillae, has by far the greatest number. There are, in fact, approximately 10 times as many taste buds on the relatively few circumvallate papillae as there are on the fungiform papillae.

In the dog, the reverse is true; the greatest concentration of taste buds is on the anterior portion of the tongue. In the chicken, there are no taste buds on the highly cornified anterior portion of the tongue; furthermore, there are few buds on the base of the tongue and on the floor of the pharynx.

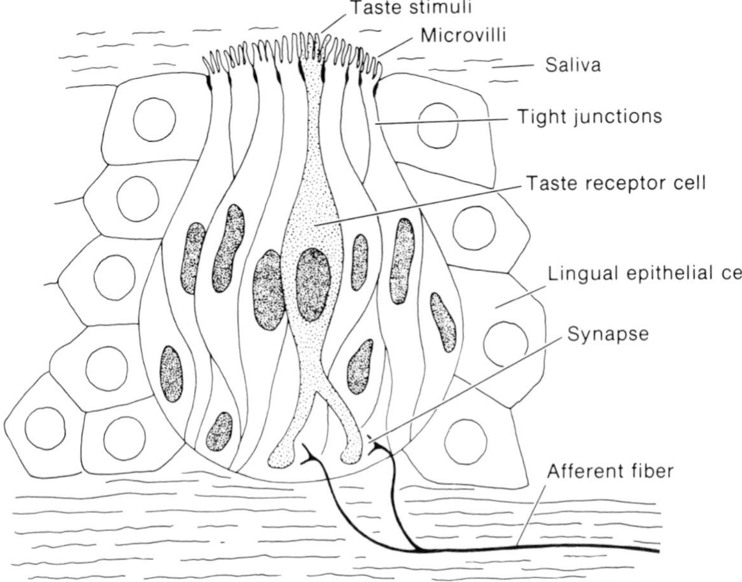

Figure 43.1. Schematic of an idealized taste bud containing taste receptor cells. Chemicals dissolved in saliva interact with the apical portion of the taste receptor cell, inducing changes in membrane conductance. These changes are communicated to the CNS through synapses with neurons at the base of the cell. Supporting cells may differentiate into taste cells. (Redrawn and modified from Kinnamon 1989, *Trends Neurosci.* 11:491–96.)

Cells in the outer layer of the taste buds are continually undergoing mitotic division. The relationship of age to number of taste buds is not uniform among species. The maximum number is in 5- to 7-month human fetuses; in contrast, no taste buds are found in the rat until the ninth postpartum day, with the maximum being reached at 12 weeks.

The taste buds degenerate when the taste nerves to them are cut. They will reappear very quickly when the nerve fibers regenerate. Taste buds transplanted to eyeless orbits in the adult newt regenerate after extensive invasion of the transplant by nerve fibers of the orbit.

Early studies provided extensive information on the size and precise distribution of taste buds on the papillae and on the number of taste receptors in the various domestic animals. However, the relationship between the total number or type of taste buds and the taste threshold or spectrum is complex. The chicken, with its relatively few taste receptors (Table 43.1), responds to chemical solutions to which the cow, with a thousand times as many buds, is unresponsive. Nonetheless, the cow responds behaviorally to many more taste stimulants than the bird.

Anatomy

In the typical mammal, taste receptors in the posterior one-third of the tongue are supplied with nerve fibers from the ninth cranial nerve (glossopharyngeal). Receptors located on the anterior two-thirds of the tongue receive nerve fibers from the chorda tympani branch of the seventh cranial nerve (facial). The tenth cranial nerve (vagus) services taste receptors in the pharynx and larynx. All three of these neural pathways, after passing through their respective cranial ganglia, terminate in the medulla or pons of the brain. At the medulla, these nerve fibers are collected through a tract (tractus solitarius) that extends to the second-order neurons of the solitary nucleus. The solitary nucleus fibers ascend and terminate in the caudal end of the pontine parabrachial nuclei. From this pontine taste area, ascending fibers travel via the ipsilateral bundle to a thalamic gustatory relay, which in turn projects to a small band of cortex. Subcortical regions that receive taste input include the central nucleus of the amygdala, lateral hypothalamus, ventrobasal thalamus, parabrachial nuclei, and red nucleus of the solitary tract.

Table 43.1. Number of taste buds in various animals

Animal	Taste buds	References
Chicken	24	Lindenmaier and Kare 1959
Pigeon	37	Moore and Elliot 1946
Starling	200	Bath 1906
Duck	200	Bath 1906
Parrot	350	Bath 1906
Kitten	473	Elliot 1937
Bat	800	Moncrieff 1951
Dog	1,706	Holliday 1940
Human	9,000	Cole 1941
Pig and goat	15,000	Moncrieff 1951
Rabbit	17,000	Moncrieff 1951
Calf	25,000	Davies et al. 1979
Catfish	100,000	Hyman 1942

There is, of course, considerable species variation in the importance of specific nerves for transmission of taste information. A unique posterior receptive field for the chorda tympani in the calf has been related to the possibility that chemoreception plays a significant role in the mechanism of rumination. In the fowl, taste buds are limited to the posterior portion of the tongue that is served by the lingual branch of the glossopharyngeal nerve.

Mechanisms of taste stimulation

The initial events in taste recognition vary according to the taste stimulus. For both acids (sour) and sodium chloride (salt), specific membrane receptors do not appear to be required. Instead, taste cell membrane conductance changes are controlled by voltage-dependent ion channels selective for Na^+, Ca^{2+}, and K^+. For example, it is now thought that salt taste occurs by passive influx of Na^+ into the taste cell through these sodium channels. Since these channels are specific to Na^+ and Li^+, few compounds other than NaCl or LiCl elicit a salty taste. This specificity to Na ions may be a consequence of the unique importance of regulating sodium in species, such as herbivores, that could be under sodium stress.

Contrasting with sour and salty tastes, it is believed that transduction of sugars (sweet), some amino acids, and bitter compounds involves specific membrane receptors. It is thought that, for sweet taste, the receptors are proteins and are responsive to certain conformations of molecules; any molecule having the appropriate conformation would be perceived as sweet. In light of the great species difference in response to substances that humans describe as sweet, it would appear likely that the structure of the receptors would also be species-specific.

After initial identification of a taste stimulus, the information is processed, perhaps with second messengers such as cyclic adenosine monophosphate, with the final common pathway being cell depolarization and influx of Ca^{2+}. Presumably, the intensity of a taste is a function of the rate of firing of the nerve.

Deficiencies of vitamins A and pyridoxine, sodium, nickel, zinc, copper, and other nutrients have been reported to affect taste and/or smell function. There is evidence to suggest that deficiencies of other micronutrients as well as macronutrients will lead directly or indirectly to altered taste or olfactory behavior. The searching behavior of malnourished animals is common knowledge and can be observed in specific hungers. In view of the relationship of the chemical senses to food acceptance by both humans and animals, it is surprising that there has been so little research in this field.

No pattern, whether chemical, physical, or nutritional, explains all the comparative results. An explanation in terms of detailed function has been sought. The chicken, which is indifferent to sugars, has a relatively high blood glucose concentration, while the ruminant, which responds so dramatically to sugar solutions, has a low circulating blood glucose concentration. A general relationship between blood glucose and sweet taste preference is challenged by observations derived from work with the cat and the armadillo, which are indifferent behaviorally to sugars but which have blood glucose concentrations similar to those found in humans.

Some food habits of animals are seasonal in nature. Perhaps taste directs or follows the abrupt feeding changes of birds that are insectivorous part of the year and granivorous the rest of the time. The diet of ruminants also changes abruptly from the high-protein diet of the suckling calf to the low-protein herbivorous diet of the adult. Taste might also take part in the intensive feeding that precedes hibernation or migration. Whether taste changes direct or follow these altered eating patterns and whether structural changes in taste receptors have occurred are unresolved questions.

Methods of study

The sense of taste in domestic animals has not been the subject of extensive scientific investigation until recently. Folklore and casual observations are the basis for many of the current opinions as to what taste sensations can be perceived.

The most commonly used method to evaluate the sense of taste in an animal is the preference test. Typical of this approach is the two-choice situation in which the material to be tested is added to one of two otherwise identical food or fluid choices, and the animal's preference and intake are then recorded. This type of testing is difficult to reproduce since the chemical and physical context in which a taste stimulant might be tested can substantially modify the taste quality. Thus, although an animal may preferentially ingest salt in solution, the same concentration of salt in feed may have no influence on intake. There is further complication because variables that modify taste reception can be different for each species.

Electrophysiological studies involve the application of substances to the tongue of the anesthetized subject and the measurement of consequent changes in electrical activity on the related taste nerve (Fig. 43.2). The results will indicate whether the chemical evoked a peripheral discharge but not whether the chemical had a taste that was appealing or offending to the animal (Figs. 43.3 and 43.4). Although there are examples of good relationships between behavioral and electrophysiological responses, there are also abrupt contradictions. For example, concentrations of sucrose solutions that will elicit avid selection and ingestion responses in calves are not detectable electrophysiologically. Furthermore, sucrose octaacetate at concentrations that evoke no behavioral response in the fowl is an effective electrophysiological stimulant. The behavioral response commonly measures preference thresholds, and the electrophysiological recordings can be related to discrimination thresholds. In current electrophysiological research consid-

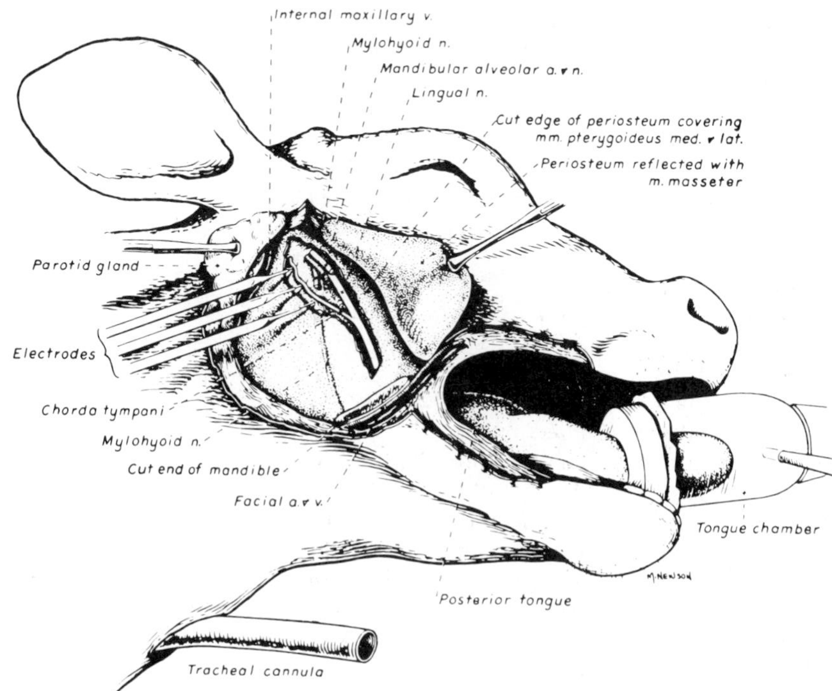

Figure 43.2. Preparation of the head of a calf for electrophysiological recording, showing anatomical landmarks, position of electrodes, and tongue chamber used for flowing the stimulating solutions over the anterior part of the tongue. The right cheek is cut open and sutured to provide access to the posterior part of the tongue. V., vein; n., nerve; a., artery; m., muscle (mm plural); med., medial; lat., lateral. (From Bernard 1964, *Am. J. Physiol.* 206:827–35.)

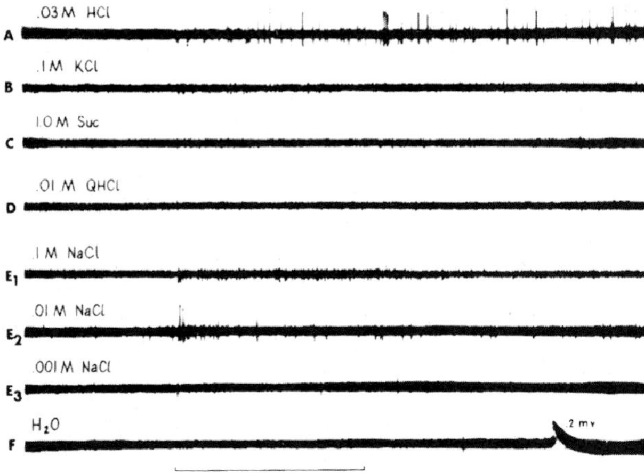

Figure 43.3. Electrophysiological responses of a single neuron in the gustatory system of a white rat, obtained in the medulla from the cell body of a neuron extending from medulla to thalamus, the second in the chain of three neurons from tongue to cortex. These responses are qualitatively similar to those of the neurons of the gustatory systems of all mammals so far investigated. The all-or-nothing principle of nerve action is seen in the similarity of the size of these voltage changes or spikes. The slight variations in spike amplitude between records are due to small displacements in electrode position relative to the neuron, while within each record some short-term "fatigue" is seen in spike height. This neuron responds to many stimuli; as is probably true of all gustatory neurons of all animals. It is quite sensitive to NaCl and HCl but not very sensitive to sucrose (Suc.) or quinine hydrochloride (QHCl); other neurons have different patterns of sensitivity, providing a basis for discrimination among stimuli. $E_1 - E_3$ show that spike frequency here, as in most sensory neurons, is a function of stimulus intensity. F shows that this neuron does not respond to water; some species (dog, cat, rabbit, chicken) have neurons that are sensitive to water. (Unpublished data of Dr. R.P. Erickson, Duke University.)

erable emphasis has been on single-fiber as opposed to whole-nerve recordings. Recent studies of taste neurophysiology have employed the patch-clamp technique. With this technique, electrical activity of individual receptor cells is beginning to be characterized.

Species variability

A common assumption is that animals share the human taste world. This is usually qualified to indicate varying degrees of taste deficiency in animals. The basis for this assumption may be the fact that so much of the behavioral taste research has been carried out on the laboratory rat, which, by chance, happens to have a sense of taste similar in many aspects to that of humans. Recent evidence, however, clearly establishes that each animal species lives in a separate taste world. It is more realistic to accept that each species has a sense of taste complementary to its own ecological needs and that similarities with humans are instances of overlapping rather than more complete development. For humans, taste sensations are classified by means of verbal reports into the categories of sweet, sour, bitter, and salty. With animals, it is often more appropriate to divide responses into pleasant, unpleasant, and indifferent. Nevertheless, comparison of the responses of various ani-

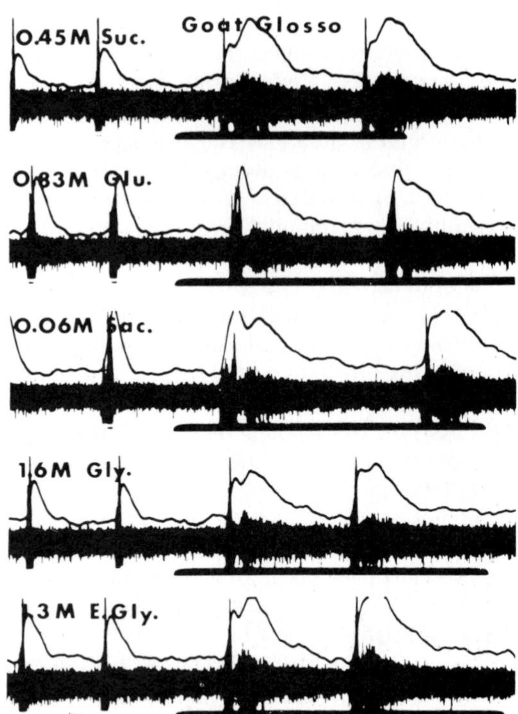

Figure 43.4. Electrophysiological records from the whole lingual branch of the glossopharyngeal nerve of a goat. Suc., sucrose; Glu., glucose; Sac., sodium saccharinate; Gly., glycerine; E. Gly., ethylene glycol. (From Bell and Kitchell 1966, *J. Physiol.* 183:145–51.)

mal species with those of humans necessitates reference to the classic divisions.

A comparison of selected species' responses to tastes is presented in Table 43.2. As can be observed, there is great variation among species in response to the classic categories.

Fowl

The chicken and many other species of birds are indifferent to the common sugars; xylose, however, is offensive

Table 43.2. Species differences in behavioral responses to human taste sensations and amino acids

	Sweet	Sour	Salty	Bitter	Amino acids
Chicken	0,–	0	–	0,–	?
Ruminants	+++[a]	–	–	–[b]	?[f]
Cats	0[c]	—	?,–	—	++[d]
Dogs	++[f]	?	0	0[e]	?
Pigs	+++[f]	?	+	–	?

Key: +++, highly preferred; ++, preferred; +, slightly preferred; 0, indifferent; –, slightly rejected; —, rejected; ?, unclear or unknown. For details and references, see Jacobs, Beauchamp, and Kare, 1978.

[a]Little response to lactose, maltose, or artificial sweeteners in cows.
[b]Whereas cows reject bitter quinine hydrochloride, goats are tolerant.
[c]Adult cats; also avoid artificial sweeteners.
[d]Casein hydrolysate as well as some individual amino acids such as proline.
[e]Sucrose octa-acetate.
[f]Saccharine not preferred.

to the chicken. The fowl exhibits indifference and then an aversion to increasingly concentrated salt solutions. This is in contrast to many mammals that prefer hypotonic salt concentrations to pure water. Fowl will not voluntarily ingest salt solutions in concentrations beyond the capacity of their elimination system. However, they exhibit unexplainable responses to some salts. For example, heavy metal compounds are relatively offensive, and yet fowl indifferently accept lithium and cadmium chlorides, which are lethal. Birds have a wide range of tolerance for acidity and alkalinity in their drinking water: chicks will accept strong mineral acid solutions over extended periods of time.

Sucrose octaacetate at a concentration that is bitter to humans is readily accepted by the fowl and by many other avian species. However, quinine sulfate, which is used extensively as a standard bitter stimulus for humans and rats, is also rejected by many species of birds. Some of the defensive secretions of insects have a uniquely offensive taste for birds. Taste apparently can be important in this predator-prey relationship, although visual cues and social context are more important.

Dimethyl anthranilate, which is used in the human food industry, is uniquely offensive to the fowl and to many other members of the class Aves in a 1:10,000 concentration. Particularly with regard to sweet and bitter tastes, human sensory judgment is thus not a reliable guide to how the bird will respond.

Ruminants

Most of the work on taste in ruminants has been carried out with calves. The work must be interpreted with caution because this species undergoes an abrupt dietary change early in life, switching from milk to a typically herbivorous diet.

Calves, when offered a choice between pure water and even a 1% sucrose solution, which is insipid to humans, will select the sucrose almost exclusively. Furthermore, this sucrose solution brings about a doubling of daily fluid intake. The calf is indifferent to lactose, and in the rat also this sugar is not greatly preferred over water (Figs. 43.5 and 43.6). In contrast, the opossum strongly prefers lactose to water. Further, the calf selects xylose, which is the only sugar reported to be offensive to the fowl. The calf is indifferent to saccharin solutions at levels that are sweet or pleasant to humans and rats. A screening of several other synthetic sweeteners used by humans failed to reveal any marked preferences. Both calves and goats exhibit pronounced preferences for glucose.

The calf has a wide pH tolerance. In contrast to the fowl, however, it shows a greater degree of acceptance on the alkaline side and less on the acid side. Further, calves are less responsive to mineral acids than they are to organic acids.

There is a substantial tolerance for sodium chloride by calves and goats. This taste response has been used in situations in which salt is added to a protein supplement for the purpose of regulating intake. Although goats are unusually tolerant of quinine hydrochloride, calves reject solutions at the 0.0001 M concentration. Dairy cows, however, are not offended by sucrose octaacetate at concentrations that are repugnant to humans.

There are species and strain differences among sheep, goats, and pigmy goats in behavioral responses to a variety of taste substances. Of particular interest were the findings

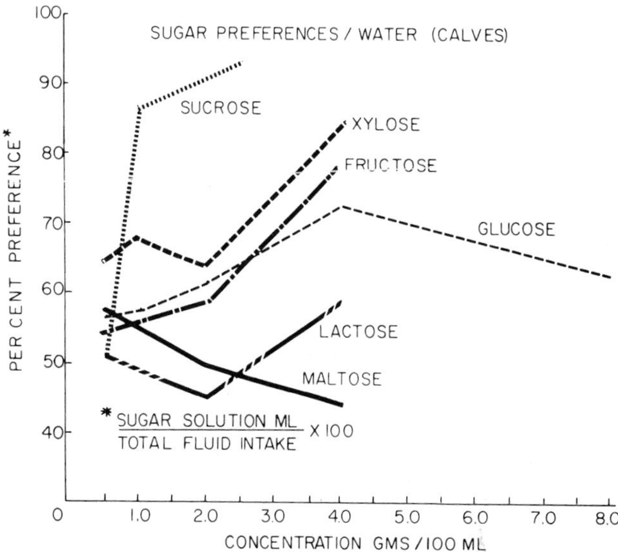

Figure 43.5. Response of the calf to various sugar solutions in a two-choice preference test (sugar versus water). With the exception of maltose and lactose, marked preferences for the sugars are indicated. (Reprinted with permission from Kare and Ficken 1963, in Zotterman, ed., *Olfaction and Taste*, Pergamon, Oxford.)

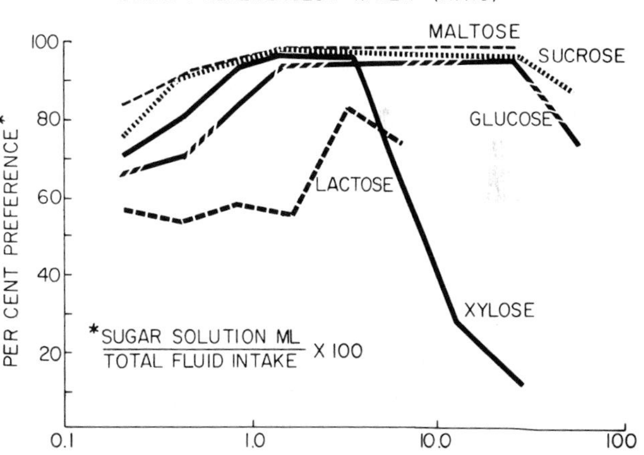

Figure 43.6. Response of the rat to various sugar solutions in a two-choice preference test (sugar versus water). (Reprinted with permission from Kare and Ficken 1963, in Zotterman, ed., *Olfaction and Taste*, Pergamon, Oxford.)

that mature sheep apparently exhibited no preference for sucrose, and goats exhibited only a very mild preference at relatively low concentrations. These responses are in marked contrast to the responses of calves (Fig. 43.5).

Cats

Mature cats on an adequate diet exhibit no preference for sucrose, lactose, maltose, fructose, glucose, or mannose. In fact, large intake of at least one sugar—sucrose—can cause vomiting, diarrhea, and even death in cats. Cats avoid saccharin and cyclamate in high concentrations. Quinine and citric acid are also avoided. The cat's response to sodium chloride in solution is unsettled; there is one report of a slight preference at one concentration. Thus cats are indifferent to or avoid most common taste substances. Both wild and domestic cats prefer solutions of hydrolyzed protein and several individual amino acids to water. Thus the flavor preference profile of this strict carnivore corresponds to the natural food preferences.

Dogs

Mature dogs were presented with glucose, fructose, sucrose, maltose, or saccharin incorporated into standard biscuits. Although there was substantial individual variation, all the sugar-containing biscuits were selected or at least tolerated indifferently. Some of the dogs were markedly offended by the saccharin. Sucrose octaacetate in concentrations offensive to rats and humans was accepted indifferently by dogs. In conscious dogs with gastric and intestinal fistulas, it has been observed that the nature and volume of pancreatic secretions are influenced by taste stimuli.

Pigs

Pigs respond to sucrose solutions. The preference for glucose and lactose is more modest. In a test with saccharin, a minority of pigs were offended at every concentration offered. A majority of pigs selected saccharin solutions, however, even at concentrations excessively sweet (2.5%) to humans. Pigs appear to show no preference for sodium cyclamate, a substance that is sweet to humans. Salt intoxication of pigs is periodically reported. Nevertheless, where pure water was available, test animals would not consume lethal quantities of salt. The pig rejects some quinine salts.

Fish

Taste in catfish, an important species in aquaculture, has been the focus of much study because of the exquisite sensitivity of this system. Catfish often feed on the bottom of bodies of very murky water, which may be why their taste sensitivity is so well developed. Taste receptor cells are located throughout the entire surface of the skin but are concentrated on the whiskers or barbels. The catfish, in addition to being able to detect differences in concentration of tastes, also has the ability to localize the source of these compounds. As would be expected for an aquatic animal that eats animal products, the catfish taste system is especially sensitive to amino acids, perhaps resembling most cats in this regard. Biochemical evidence suggests at least two distinct receptor sites, one for basic amino acids and the other for neutral amino acids.

Individual variability

Every species studied thus far has exhibited considerable individual variability. For example, in their response to the common sugars, calves varied from indifference to pronounced preference. In a litter of pigs that was tested with a wide range of concentrations of saccharin solutions, some were found to have a marked preference for the synthetic sweetener and others to reject it. Many dogs actively rejected saccharin in low concentrations in their food, but a small minority were indifferent and a few preferred it.

Individual variation has been studied in chickens and quail. In a single-stimulus procedure, several chlorides at various concentrations were tested. Different individuals had markedly different thresholds (the lowest concentration at which the intake differed significantly from that of water). No individual was found to be completely taste blind, since all birds responded if the concentration reached a sufficiently high level. The response of the individual animals was chemical-specific and concentration-dependent.

A breeding program was carried out in which birds sensitive to ferric chloride were selected and mated and those insensitive to the chemical were also mated. After five generations, there was a statistically significant difference between those with high-threshold and those with low-threshold parents. The findings suggest that the taste for ferric chloride has a genetic basis. Parallel studies with laboratory strains of mice and rats have clearly demonstrated that individual differences in taste among individuals of a species may be under genetic control.

Nutrition

The function of taste in the physiological economy of the vertebrate animal body has not been established, although it is often closely related to nutrition. The cat and the fowl on an adequate diet are both indifferent to sucrose solutions. When caloric intake in feed is restricted, a chick will select a sucrose solution and will increase fluid intake to make up the deficiency. A similarly "correct" nutritional choice was not made when the sugar was replaced with an isocaloric solution of fat or protein. In fact, the domestic fowl acutely depleted of protein will avoid a casein solution and will select only water, apparently because of the taste.

Feed that has been rendered so distasteful to the fowl that it was totally avoided in a choice situation did not influence intake when there was no alternative. The response to the taste quality was modified by hunger. In fact, the offensiveness had to be increased almost tenfold in a no-choice situation to effect a reduced intake over an extended period.

Many herbivores need extra salt to maintain sodium balance. Salt-deficient animals respond immediately, if salt is available, by ingesting quantities sufficient to make up the deficit. Taste is an important mediator of this behavior. Unlike the rat and the sheep, the dog and the cat do not appear to have a spontaneous appetite for salt. Furthermore, there is some evidence that cats, at least, cannot even detect a salt taste. Perhaps there is no mechanism to detect salt since, as carnivores, they would starve long before sodium depletion could occur.

Rats and other omnivores and herbivores seem to have a similar specific appetite for sweets inasmuch as food-deprived and insulin-treated animals respond with an increase in intake of sweet solutions. There appear to be no specific hungers for vitamins; instead, when animals are made thiamine deficient and then are presented with a choice between two differently flavored diets, one thiamine-sufficient and the other thiamine-deficient, they must learn to associate the flavor of the thiamine-sufficient diet with recovery from the deficiency. Once this association is made, they will preferentially ingest the diet containing thiamine. Similarly, in the absence of specific receptors to detect water, the thirsty animal may learn to associate the sensory characteristics of water with relief from depletion.

Aggressive and exploratory behaviors develop in animals after depletion of calcium or of other minerals. The degree to which this behavior is directed by taste has not been established. Furthermore, the overall food preference behavior of domestic animals is not a reliable guide to nutritional adequacy of a diet.

The nutritional "wisdom" of jungle fowl was compared with that of domestic chickens and that of wild Norway rats was compared with that of laboratory rats. In both instances, the wild animals were found to be more precise in their caloric regulation or correction. Further, they tended to be more responsive to the nutritional and physiological consequences of their diet than to the sensory qualities. The laboratory rat was particularly "self-indulgent." It may well be that, with domestication, acute sensory mechanisms would be disadvantageous. For this reason, experimental work with highly selected populations may be less than ideal for discerning function of the chemical senses.

Temperature

Temperature can substantially modify the reaction to taste stimulation. The domestic fowl is acutely sensitive to the temperature of water. Acceptability decreases as the temperature of water increases above ambient levels. In fact, fowl will discriminate between choices with a temperature difference of only a few degrees Celsius, rejecting the higher temperature. The chicken will suffer from acute thirst rather than drink water 5°C above its body temperature. At the other extreme, the chicken will readily accept water down to the level of freezing. A sizable minority of chickens lacks this sensitivity to temperature; when it is present, however, response to it takes precedence over the response to chemical stimulants. These findings are important when one is trying to induce animals to take medicine.

SMELL

Olfaction in animals is mediated by several distinct sensory systems. The two most important ones are the main olfactory system, with receptors in the dorsocaudal portion of the nasal cavity, and the accessory olfactory system, with receptors localized within the vomeronasal or Jacobson's organ located near the external nares. The former system is the one humans are most familiar with, as it subserves the sense of smell; the accessory olfactory system is either diffuse or lacking in adult humans and Old World monkeys and apes. Recent evidence implicates the accessory olfactory system in mediating responses to sex odors in a variety of species.

Anatomy

The olfactory system consists of paired nostrils (external nares), internal nares (choanae), nasal cavities or chambers, receptor cells, olfactory nerves, and the olfactory bulbs of the brain.

Main olfactory system

The paired nasal cavities are divided by an epithelium-covered medial septum, which is supported by partially ossified cartilage. Their lateral walls consist of turbinate bones named for the facial bones of which they are a part. It is on the ethmoid turbinate bones that the specialized olfactory epithelium is found (Fig. 43.7). In all animals the nasoturbinate bones remain fairly simple elongated structures; the maxilloturbinate bones, however, vary considerably in their complexity. In the horse, pig, sheep, and cow, the maxilloturbinate bones are similar to the nasoturbinate bones in their simplicity. By contrast, in the rabbit, numerous folds run from anterodorsal to posteroventral in the

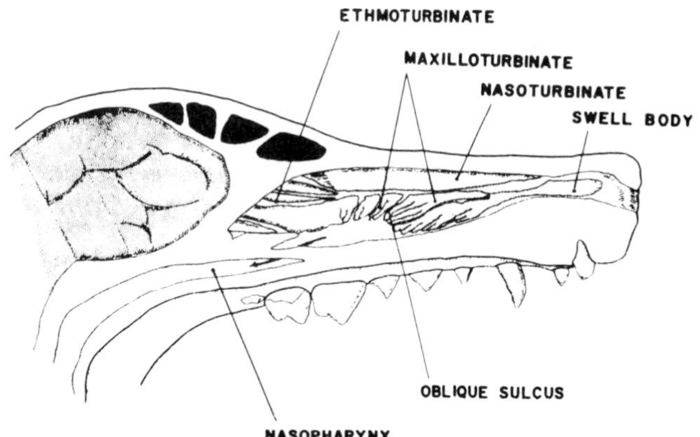

Figure 43.7. Normal anatomy of midsagittal section of a dog's head with septum removed. (From Becker and King 1957, *A.M.A. Arch. Otolaryngol.* 65:428–36.)

maxilloturbinate bones. This condition of complexity also occurs in the cat and to an even greater extent in the dog (see Fig. 43.8). The olfactory areas in keen-scented animals have been increased through a lengthening of the nose and a folding of the turbinate bones. Furthermore, this development has involved excavation of the frontal and sphenoid bones with an extension of the olfactory ethmoturbinate bones into recesses or sinuses. The respiratory epithelium is present to a proportionally larger extent than is the olfactory epithelium to provide greater filtration and warming of inspired air.

The surface area of the microvilli and cilia of the olfactory mucosa is enormous and may often exceed that of the entire body surface. The mobility of the external nares during sniffing suggests that this organ's structure is important to olfaction. Posteriorly, there exists a bony subethmoidal shelf, which is found below the ethmoidal turbinates and is so situated that it forces inspired air into the olfactory epithelium. A complete washing-out of the region on expiration does not occur by virtue of the recess created by an inspiration. The recess permits the accumulation of odor molecules that would be unrecognizable in a single sniff. Such a shelf is not seen among primates. The epiglottis forms, with the soft palate, a partition that permits those animals in which it is best developed to inspire air through the nose while eating. Thus, with the mouth open, the animal is alert for predators and also can effect an olfactory screening of its forage.

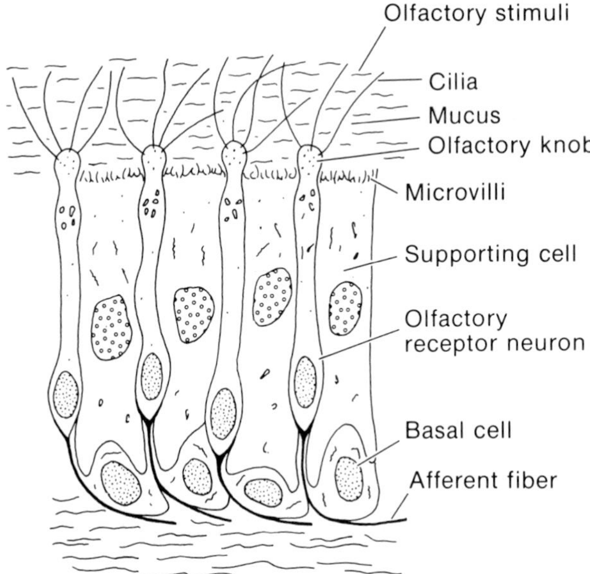

Figure 43.8. Schematic of olfactory receptor sheet. Chemicals dissolved in mucus interact with molecular receptors located on the cilia of the receptor neurons. Membrane conductance changes stimulate action potentials. Note the absence of synapses; the olfactory receptor cell synapses first in the olfactory bulb. Olfactory receptor neurons, unlike almost all other CNS neurons, regenerate periodically, possibly differentiating from the supporting cells. (Redrawn and modified from Moulton and Beidler 1967, *Physiol. Rev.* 47:1–39.)

In normal inspiration by awake dogs, air enters the vestibule and traverses through all meatuses (passages) as far back as the anterior tips of the ethmoidal turbinates. The mainstream, however, takes a downward path anterior to this to enter the nasopharynx. Expired air flows primarily through the ventral meatus, with a small flow through the middle meatus. There is no air flow in the dorsal meatus or over the ethmoid region. This observation adds some support to the hypothesized function of the ethmoid shelf. Sniffing, on the other hand, fills the entire nasal chamber.

The lining of the anterior part of the nasal cavity (the vestibule) is continuous with that of the nostrils and may contain hair, as in the horse or pig, or it may be bare, as in the cow and dog. Cilia play a role in clearing nasal passages.

The olfactory portion of the nasal mucous membrane is confined largely to the region of the ethmoidal turbinate bones and to the opposing portion of the septum. The olfactory cells (Fig. 43.8) extend throughout the whole layer of olfactory epithelium. These are bipolar nerve cells that consist of a small oval cell body that contains a nucleus and a scant amount of cytoplasm. The distal process or dendrite is termed the olfactory rod, and it projects beyond the free surface and bears olfactory cilia. The latter probably bear the receptor elements. The cilia are constantly bathed in a coating of mucus; chemicals must first dissolve in this mucus to produce odors. Comparative studies of the olfactory epithelium reveal no substantial difference among animals with a keen sense of smell and those with one that is apparently less developed.

The central processes of the bipolar olfactory cells become the olfactory nerve fibers. Each of the fibers is a direct continuation of the axon of a single olfactory receptor and remains separate, without synapse, until it reaches the olfactory bulb. The nerve fibers then form a dense external layer of olfactory nerve fibers around the olfactory bulb. From this point, they turn inward to end in the glomeruli. A glomerulus is an encapsulated group of synaptic connections of the fine terminal branches of the olfactory fibers and the dendrites of both the mitral and tufted cells whose cell bodies are located more deeply in the bulb. Olfactory cells undergo a continual turnover with a life expectancy of one to several months.

Accessory olfactory system

Receptors for the accessory olfactory system are located within the vomeronasal organ (VNO). This organ consists of paired cigar-shaped structures that are located medially, usually along the anterior portion of the nasal septum (Fig. 43.9). The VNO opens at one end and forms a blind sac at the other. The location of this opening is variable. For example, in rodents the opening is into the nasal cavity; in cats it is into the nasopalatine canal, which connects the

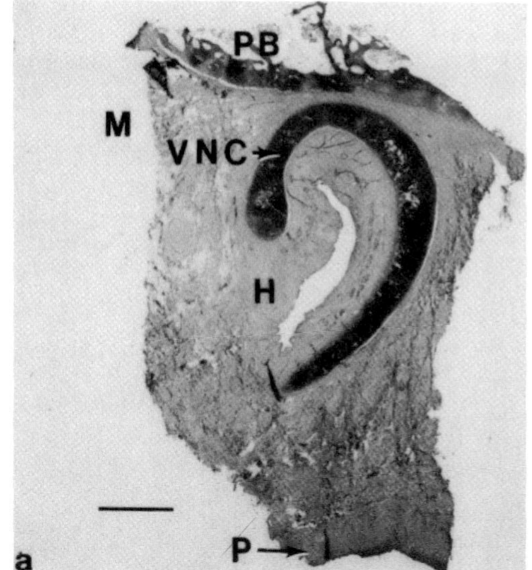

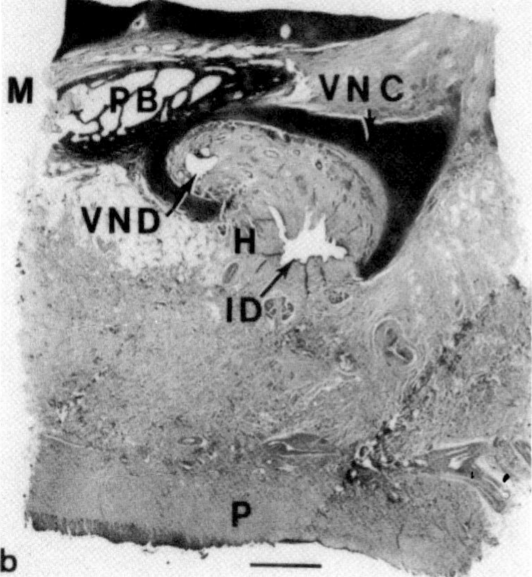

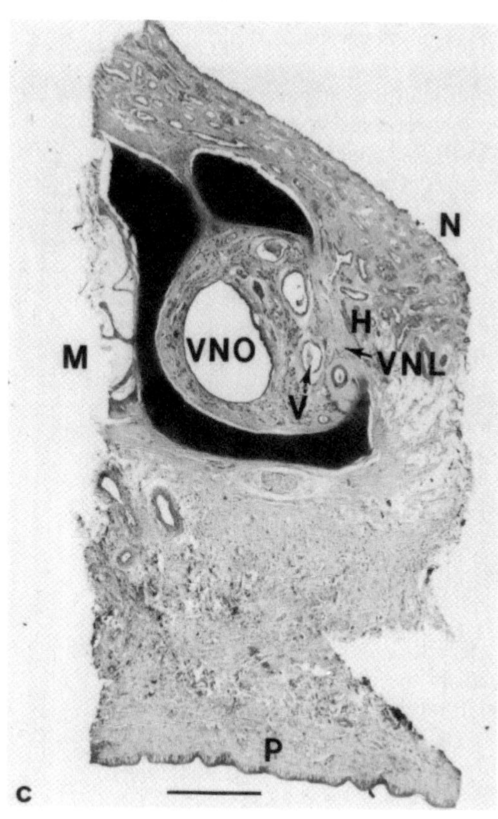

Figure 43.9. Photomicrographs of histologic sections of the cow's head in the area of the vomeronasal organ (VNO). A section near the origin of one VNO off the midline (M) is shown in (*a*). The vomeronasal cartilage (VNC) forms a comma-shaped structure ventral to the palatine bone (PB) and dorsal to the palate (P). A hilus (H) is directed vetromedially. In (*b*), taken approximately 0.5 cm caudal to (*a*), a distinct incisive duct (ID) and a vomeronasal duct (VND) along which chemostimulatory molecules travel into the VNO are evident. The VNO with numerous blood vessels lying adjacent to it and penetrating the vomeronasal ligament (VNL) is shown in (*c*). The nasal cavity (N) is now evident. Farther caudal to (*c*), the VNO ends in a blind sac. Apparently, the VNO sucks in and expels liquids containing molecules that stimulate receptors located within it. Bar = 2 mm. (From Jacobs et al. 1981, *Acta Anat.* 110:48–58 with permission of S. Karger AG, Basel.)

nasal and oral cavities; in cows it opens directly into the oral cavity.

The receptor tissue of the VNO lies generally on the medial surface of the organ with epithelium of the respiratory type on the lateral surface. The receptors are similar to those of the main olfactory system, with the exception that they lack cilia and have only microvilli instead (see Fig. 43.8). The vomeronasal receptors, like the main olfactory receptors, constantly regenerate. The locus of this organ near the exterior is partially responsible for the enduring speculation that it may be involved in perception of large, nonvolatile molecules that normally could not reach the main olfactory system. It appears that for molecules to enter the VNO they must first become dissolved in mucus. The VNO has a pumping mechanism that serves to suck molecules into the organ through the lumen and then pump them back out into the surrounding area. This mechanism is innervated by autonomic efferents in the nasopalatine nerve; if these nerves are severed, the normal functioning of the VNO is interrupted.

A variety of behavioral mechanisms are likely to be involved in transporting substances to the VNO. Flehmen, the facial grimace observed in many species, including ungulates and cats, has been postulated to function by drawing fluids, particularly urine, into the VNO. Among bulls examining estrogen-primed cows, the tongue is used to compress the hard palate, which presumably induces pressure changes in the VNO and thereby serves to draw chemical substance into the receptor area.

The receptors of the VNO, like those of the main olfactory system, are primary neurons projecting directly to the olfactory bulb (Fig. 43.8). However, there is generally an anatomically distinct portion of the olfactory bulb, the accessory olfactory bulb, that receives VNO input. The accessory olfactory bulb also has distinct glomeruli where the vomeronasal nerve synapses with other cells located within the structure.

Mechanisms of olfactory stimulation

No olfactory receptors have yet been fully characterized, so the precise details of how odorous chemicals exert their effects are not known. It is thought that the olfactory stimulus interacts with specific macromolecular receptor sites, probably protein, localized on the cilia. The number of different receptor sites is not known but may be very large in order to encompass all the varied odors that an animal can detect and discriminate.

After interaction with a receptor site, cell membrane depolarization occurs. Recent biochemical and neurophysiological studies indicate that, as in taste, depolarization is followed by intracellular activation of second messengers that are necessary to evoke an action potential, thereby sending a signal to the olfactory bulb. Complex processing of olfactory information begins in the olfactory bulb.

Although it is widely assumed that there is a similar sequence of events for vomeronasal receptors, no experimental evidence is available for this system. Since the accessory system may be responsive to large, nonvolatile molecules, such as proteins, novel transductive mechanisms are possible.

Olfaction and the central nervous system

Considerable progress has been made in describing the neuroanatomical connections. The main olfactory system and the accessory olfactory system maintain relatively separate central pathways (Fig. 43.10). Generally, the main olfactory connections involve thalamic and telencephalic cortical areas, whereas the accessory olfactory system is more involved with the diencephalon, particularly the hypothalamus. These anatomical facts suggest that it is the accessory olfactory system that mediates many of the behavioral and neuroendocrine responses to sex odors (see below).

Methods of study

Behavioral tests are difficult to design, and the results from these tests may not lend themselves to simple assessment. Part of the problem is the difficulty of quantifying stimuli and responses. In addition, an odor may be meaningful only in a specific context. The delivery of a stimulus restricted solely to the olfactory receptor can also be a major problem. To meet these and other objections, some investigators have developed specially built chambers that permit introduction of the odor isolated from auditory, visual, or pressure cues.

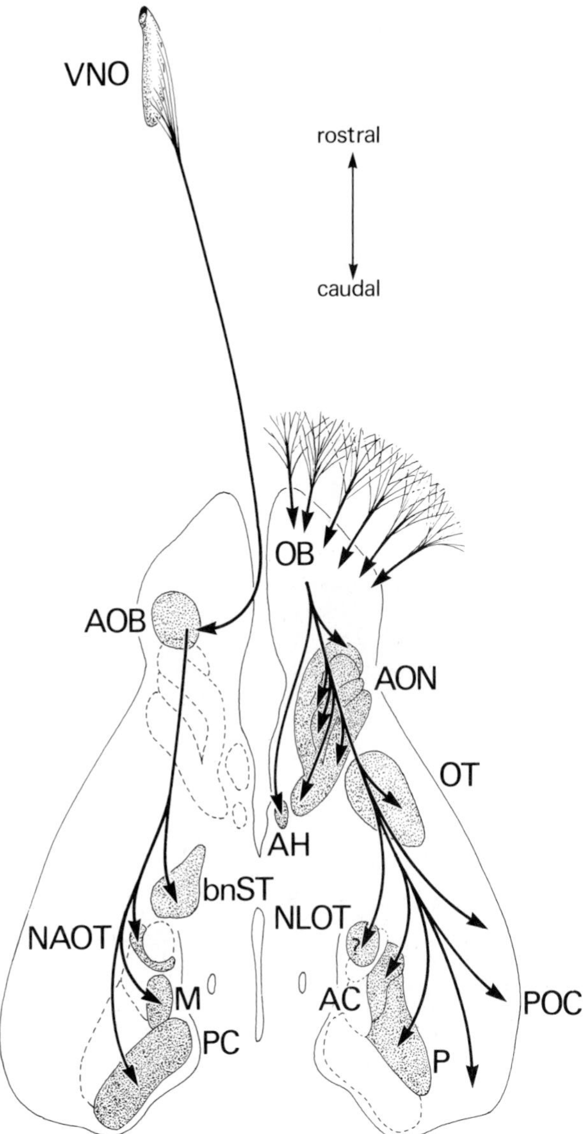

Figure 43.10. Schematic view of a horizontal section of a rat's brain comparing the independent primary and secondary projections (ipsilateral only) of the olfactory and vomeronasal systems (right and left halves, respectively). For clarity, secondary contralateral projections and many olfactory bulbar projections to rostral midline structures are not shown. AC, anterior cortical nucleus of the amygdala; AH, anterior hippocampus; AOB, accessory olfactory bulb; AON, anterior olfactory nucleus; bnST, bed nucleus of the stria terminalis; M, medial nucleus of the amygdala; NAOT, nucleus of the accessory olfactory tract; NLOT, nucleus of the lateral olfactory tract; OB, olfactory bulb; OT, olfactory tubercle; P, periamygdaloid region; PC, posterior cortical nucleus of the amygdala; POC, primary olfactory cortex; VNO, vomeronasal organ. (From Wysocki 1979, *Neurosci. Biobehav. Rev.* 3:301–41.)

A widely used experimental method is the recording of the electrical activity that follows stimulation of the olfactory system. In some cases these electrophysiological recordings are made from the olfactory epithelium, from the nerve fibers, and from the olfactory bulb.

Most of the early electrical measurements reported represent activity from a collection of receptors. Recently techniques that allow records to be made of the action potentials in a single primary olfactory receptor have been described. A further substantial advance in this area results from the use of unanesthetized and unrestrained animals that sniff the stimulant by themselves.

Little electrophysiological work has been carried out on domestic animals. This may be in part because the olfactory nerve is extremely short in mammals and in a difficult location. Furthermore, since electrophysiology does not distinguish between the pleasant and the unpleasant, the results have limited practical application.

Species variability

There are very large differences in relative size of olfactory structures and in ability to detect odors among species. The dog is reported to be able to detect odors several orders of magnitude lower in concentration than are detected by humans. Very sensitive animals, such as dogs, are labeled *macrosmatic* whereas animals that can detect odors but are much less sensitive, such as some species of birds, are termed *microsmatic*. Some animals, such as sea mammals (dolphins, whales), totally lack an olfactory apparatus, cannot smell, and are termed *anosmic*.

Although it is generally assumed that the size of the olfactory bulb in relation to the rest of the brain is a good indication of how sensitive an animal is to odors, this is not necessarily the case. Recent evidence indicates that some species of birds, such as cowbirds, that have relatively small olfactory bulbs are surprisingly sensitive to at least some odors. However, the birds with the largest olfactory bulbs, such as kiwis and some arctic birds, also appear to make the most use of odor and to be the most sensitive.

Most domestic mammals are probably quite sensitive to odors. However, few comparative studies of olfactory sensitivity have been conducted on species other than dogs, rats, and humans, so precise comparisons cannot be made.

It has not yet been possible to classify odors into any logical groupings on the basis of their quality. Although volatile chemicals with similar chemical structures may have similar odors, in other cases they may not. Similarly, structurally different chemicals may have similar odors. Moreover, there is little evidence that odors that humans judge as similar are also perceived as similar by other species. Thus, as with taste, it is likely that each species has its own olfactory world that may be very different from our own. The dog may not only be more sensitive to odors but may also perceive odors in a very different way.

Behavior

Nutrition

It is difficult to measure the extent to which the sense of smell is necessary to locate and discriminate among foods. It has been reported that the domesticated animal is less sensitive to the nutritional and toxic consequences of a food choice and more responsive to the sensory qualities of food than is its wild counterpart. This conclusion could complicate the selection of animals for a study of the function of smell.

Cats selected dry chow suffused with the odor of meat in preference to the same chow suffused with air only. Furthermore, cats that were poisoned with lithium chloride soon after eating the odor-laden dry food avoided the odor-laden chow during subsequent trials; that is, it was possible to develop a conditioned aversion to the meat odor.

Dogs that have been made anosmatic (unable to smell) by treatment of the olfactory receptor area with caustic zinc sulfate fail to distinguish among lamb, pork, beef, and horse meat. In contrast, dogs that could smell exhibited definite preferences. Apparently, dogs use smell to distinguish among meats. However, anosmatic dogs did prefer a bland diet mixed with horse meat to the bland diet alone, suggesting that taste or texture without odor is sufficient for discriminating meat from nonmeat.

Several Russian ethological studies suggest that behavioral responses to meat odors are innately determined. Dogs begin responding with salivation to meat odors at approximately the age at which weaning would normally occur, even though they have had no prior experience eating meat. One cannot eliminate the possibility that there are similar chemicals in milk to which salivation has been conditioned.

Various aromatic mixtures have been recommended for animal feeds. Typical ingredients of these mixtures are anise, fenugreek, and onion. The inference is that these odors render food more appealing and hence increase food intake. Nonetheless, there is no evidence to justify this. Furthermore, preference tests indicate that many of these flavors are actually offensive to the animal for which they are sold. Even if they were appealing, there is no evidence to indicate that long-term control of intake would be altered by these flavors.

In studies with heifers, dogs, and pigs, attempts have been made to cater to the chemical senses of these animals. Short, transitory increases in food intake were observed; however, they were approximately equal to the modest depression in intake recorded when the additive was removed. Enhancement of the smell or taste appeared to be warranted only when food intake was depressed because of abnormal circumstances (e.g., a strange environment or a substantial change in the diet). Here, a return to normal intake has been effected more rapidly by an increase in the sensory appeal.

No behavioral function of smell is apparent in the domestic fowl. However, some evidence indicates that the odors of plants may be a factor in their selection for lining the nests of some bird species. Odors clearly play a role in food selection in several species of birds, such as kiwis, vultures, and shearwaters, and there are indications that some social behaviors of ducks may be influenced by odors. Apparently birds are more responsive to odors than was earlier thought.

Social behavior

The main olfactory system and the accessory olfactory system play important roles in the regulation of reproductive and other social behavior in many mammalian species. Animals are commonly attracted to and sexually stimulated by chemical signals produced by members of the opposite sex. Individual recognition, maintenance of the mother-young dyad, elicitation of aggression, and establishment of dominance have all been demonstrated to occur via olfactory signals. In fact, the social world of many mammals is probably dominated by these chemical messages.

The sources of these chemical messages are manifold. Skin glands are found throughout the mammals. In small mammals (e.g., shrews, hamsters, guinea pigs), many of these are modified sebaceous glands that develop from the hair follicle. In large mammals, odor-producing areas usually are mixed sebaceous and sweat (apocrine) glands. The location and type of gland vary with the species, and many species have developed specific behaviors (often termed scent-marking behaviors) that serve to place the glandular material on a surface. One advantage of olfactory signals is that they remain long after the animal that deposited them has left the area. Territories and home ranges can thereby be labeled.

In addition to skin glands, urine serves as an important source of olfactory signals. Here, too, specialized behaviors have been developed for marking the environment, as is immediately evident with dogs. Other sources of odors include saliva, feces, vaginal secretions, and accessory glands in the eye (harderian glands). Control of gland size, production of the odorous material, and frequency of placement are often regulated by hormonal status. For example, skin gland size and scent-marking behavior are often sexually dimorphic; dominant male animals may have larger, more productive glands and may mark more frequently.

In pigs it has been shown that a steroid metabolite in boar saliva is capable of enhancing the lordosis response to back pressure in receptive females. Urine appears to play a role in stimulating the mounting of a dummy by young stallions, and chemical signals may play a role in the detection of estrus by bulls. In dogs, urine and vaginal secretions from estrous bitches are very attractive to intact males, provided the males have had sexual experience; inexperienced males are not as attracted. A component in vaginal secretions of estrous bitches, methyl-*p*-hydroxybenzoate, has been reported to stimulate male mounting behavior. Olfactory cues are also important in mother-young recognition in goats, sheep, and horses and probably in other domestic mammals.

In most species, chemical signals probably act in concert with visual, tactile, and auditory cues to ensure reproduction. Even when one sense is eliminated, the others may be able to ensure appropriate behavior. Furthermore, domestication may have diminished the specificity of response to precise chemical signals.

There is now a large body of research that shows that chemical signals from members of the same species may also influence reproductive physiology. For example, urine-based signals may affect the regularity of estrous cycles and even the age at which reproductive maturation occurs. Such phenomena as synchronization of estrus may in part be mediated by chemical signals.

It appears that the main olfactory system and the accessory olfactory system act together in the perception of biologically meaningful odors, but in some cases at least the accessory system is more important. Recent studies with rodents have demonstrated that when the VNO is deafferentated, behavioral and neuroendocrine responses to odors are disrupted. These findings are consistent with the neuroanatomical connections of this organ (Fig. 43.10). Among the large domestic mammals, studies on goats and bulls are also lending support to the hypothesis of a critical role for the vomeronasal–accessory olfactory system.

The ability of many mammals to identify individuals on the basis of extremely small amounts of secretions is probably the basis for the tracking ability of some species, especially dogs. Much of the information on the tracking ability of dogs is anecdotal, and olfactory thresholds are not separated from discrimination among odors or from training. It has been reported that, indoors, dogs are capable of detecting human traces for as long as 6 weeks.

HEARING

All of the domestic animals are capable of hearing sounds in their environment. Hearing in the mammal and in the bird is generally recognized to be more highly developed than in any other class of animals. Although the hearing apparatus is not identical in all domestic species (the bird's ear differs substantially from that of mammals), the basic structures and modes of functioning share a common pattern. The ear in all domestic animals efficiently converts acoustical information from the environment to nerve impulses that are transmitted to the central nervous system (CNS). The mammalian ear, especially, is sensitive to sounds of a wide range of intensities and frequencies. Humans, for example, can detect sounds whose pressures are on the order of thousandths of a microbar (a microbar is one millionth of the standard atmospheric pressure) and yet can tolerate pressures a million times as high for brief periods. The ears of many mammals are sensitive to frequencies covering a range of nearly 10 octaves.

Auditory stimuli

Sound, the stimulus for hearing, consists of patterns of pressure waves propagated through the air. In the case of a pure tone, the pattern is simple, consisting of sinusoidal waves of pressure. The number of waves per second is the frequency of the tone (*Hertz*, abbreviated Hz, has replaced *cycles per second* as the term for this unit of measurement). Pitch is the perceptual counterpart of frequency; sounds with a high frequency are perceived as being high in pitch. Few sounds in nature are as simple as this, however. Many tones, such as vowel sounds in man and sustained tones of musical instruments, consist of a complex pattern of waves. These can be resolved into a fundamental frequency, corresponding to the rate at which the pattern repeats itself, and harmonics or overtones. These are combinations of sine waves whose frequencies are multiples of the fundamental frequency. Such signals are described by their spectra, the spectrum being a representation of the relative strengths of the constituent sine waves. It is largely the harmonics that determine the character of different musical instruments and distinguish speech sounds from one another. Not all sounds can be resolved into discrete frequency components. Noise and noiselike sounds consist of more or less random pressure fluctuations. Such sounds are said to have continuous spectra, comprising energy of many frequencies within a range rather than the clearly defined harmonic frequencies that contribute to tonal stimuli.

The other major attribute of sound, besides frequency, is intensity. For a tone of a given frequency, perceived loudness depends on intensity, but loudness also varies according to frequency; the ears of any species are more sensitive to some frequencies than to others, and these sounds, at a given physical intensity, seem louder than sounds to which the animal is less sensitive.

Anatomy

The ear is made up of three divisions: the external ear, consisting of the pinna or auricle and the external auditory meatus (ear canal); the middle ear, consisting of the tympanic cavity containing the ossicles, the Eustachian tube with its diverticulum, the guttural pouch (in the Equidae); and the inner ear or labyrinth, consisting of an acoustic part, the cochlea, and a nonacoustic part, the vestibular organ (Fig. 43.11). The vestibular system contains receptors sensitive to linear acceleration and gravity and others that detect angular acceleration or rotation. These receptors are important in permitting the animal to orient itself in space, as they provide feedback during movements of the head and body. The vestibular system is described in detail in Chapter 44. The cochlea, supplied by the cochlear branch of the acoustic nerve, contains the receptor cells and associated structures that convert the mechanical energy of sound vibrations into nerve impulses. All the parts of the ear contribute to its sensitivity. The outer ear first collects sound waves and guides them to the eardrum, then the middle ear structures transmit them efficiently from the air to the much denser liquid within the inner ear. There minuscule fluid displacements are analyzed as to frequency and encoded as pulses traveling up the auditory nerve to the brain.

Auricle

The function of the auricle is to collect sound waves, which are then transmitted to the tympanic membrane by way of the external auditory meatus. The mobility of the auricle in most mammals enhances its value as a collector of sound waves by enabling it to be turned in the direction of the sound. The human pinnae contribute relatively little to the collection of sound, and pinnae are totally absent in birds.

Tympanic membrane

Completely separating the external auditory meatus of the external ear from the tympanic cavity of the middle ear is a thin septum known as the tympanic membrane or ear-

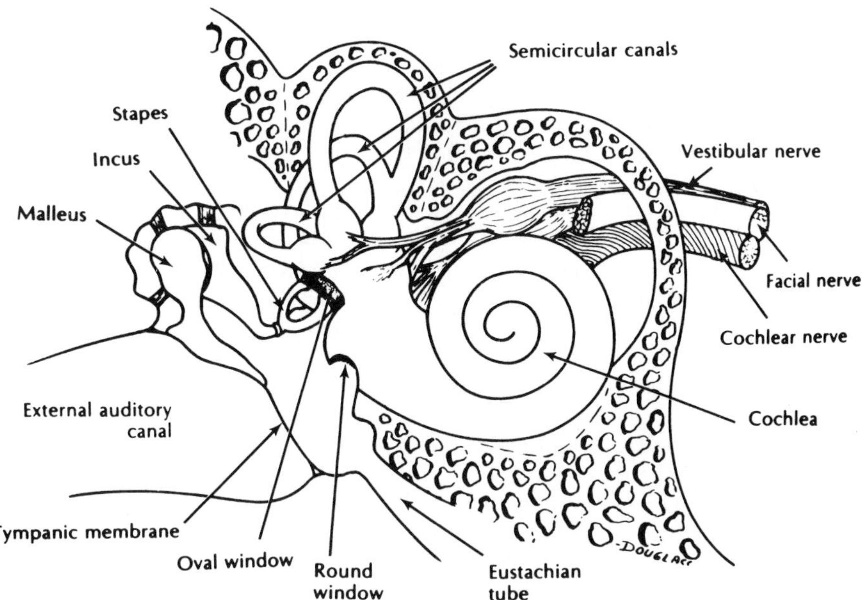

Figure 43.11. Mammalian ear. The anatomy has been altered somewhat for clarity, and the footplate of the stapes has been withdrawn from the oval window in which it is normally seated. The ossicles—the malleus, incus, and stapes—conduct sound waves from the tympanic membrane or eardrum to the cochlea, which contains the receptor cells. The semicircular canals are part of the vestibular system. The facial nerve, shown cut here, courses through the wall of the middle ear. The Eustachian tube equilibrates middle ear pressure with atmospheric pressure. (From V. Goodhill [ed.] 1979, *Ear Diseases, Deafness and Dizziness*, Harper & Row, Hagerstown, Md.)

drum. It is composed of three layers: the external layer, which is continuous with the skin lining the external auditory meatus; the middle layer, which is composed of radially and circularly arranged connective tissue fibers; and the internal layer, which is continuous with the mucous membrane of the tympanic cavity. Attached to the internal surface of the membrane is the manubrium or handle of the malleus, the first of the auditory ossicles (Fig. 43.11). Thus vibrations of the tympanic membrane are transmitted to the chain of bones and, by them, to the inner ear.

Auditory ossicles

The ossicles are three small bones (the malleus, the incus, and the stapes, popularly known as the hammer, the anvil, and the stirrup) in the mammalian tympanic cavity. They comprise a chain extending from the tympanic membrane to the oval window, which opens into the inner ear (Fig. 43.11). The ossicles, together with the tympanic membrane, greatly increase the efficiency with which sound is transmitted to the inner ear. Air is a highly compressible, low-density medium. If sound traveling through the air strikes the surface of water, with its much greater density, a large change in impedance, or opposition to movement, is encountered; the great majority of the sound energy is reflected and only 1 percent is transmitted to the water. The inner ear contains fluids composed mostly of water, through which sound must travel in order to stimulate the receptor cells. The ossicles concentrate the force of the sound striking the eardrum on the much smaller area of the oval window, with a corresponding increase in pressure. The eardrum is readily displaced by sound waves, so that little energy is reflected, and the mechanical advantage of the ossicles compensates for the greater impedance of the cochlea.

The impedance-matching function is due not just to the relative areas of the eardrum and oval window but also, to a lesser degree, to a lever action in the ossicles themselves. The malleus has a long process coupled to the eardrum and a short process at right angles (the short process is perpendicular to the plane of the page in Fig. 43.11, pointing toward the viewer, whereas the long process points down toward the bottom of the page). The incus, or anvil, is joined to the malleus by a rigid joint (ankylosed in many species). Again in Fig. 43.11, protruding back away from the viewer is the short process of the incus, which, along with the short process of the malleus, forms a pivot whose axis is nearly perpendicular to the plane of the page. Force applied to the eardrum causes rotation about this axis and displacement of the long process of the incus, which extends down to articulate with the stapes, or stirrup. Since the long process of the malleus is longer than that of the incus, there is an increase in the force applied to the stapes. The crura (the curved arms of the stapes) transmit the force to the footplate of the stapes, a plate of bone that fits into the oval window and acts as a piston to displace the fluid in the inner ear. Tendons attached to the malleus and incus maintain their position, and connective tissue holds the footplate of the stapes in place.

The middle ear structure of birds is much simpler, and transmission of sound is less efficient. A simple columella (meaning "little column") of bone is suspended in the middle ear, one end being coupled to the tympanic membrane and the other forming a piston in the oval window. This structure lacks the lever action of the mammalian ossicles and may be less efficient in other respects since the ratio of eardrum to oval window area is not as large as in mammals.

Eustachian tube and guttural pouch

Connecting the tympanic cavity with the pharynx is the Eustachian tube, which ensures that the air pressure in the tympanic cavity shall be the same as that outside the body. The pharyngeal aperture of the tube is opened during swallowing, correcting any inequality of atmospheric pressure on the two sides of the tympanic membrane.

The guttural pouch, among domestic animals found only in Equidae, is a remarkable diverticulum of the Eustachian tube. The average capacity of each pouch in the horse is said to be about 300 ml. The function of the guttural pouch is not known. Experiments show that, in the horse, air enters the guttural pouch through the relaxed aperture of the Eustachian tube during expiration and leaves mainly during the expiratory pause. During inspiration the aperture of the Eustachian tube is closed.

Cochlea

The inner ear consists of a single structure, the labyrinth, which contains specialized structures for detection of both sound and motion. The vestibular labyrinth consists of the semicircular canals, which detect rotation (Fig. 43.11), plus gravity receptors (not visible in Fig. 43.11). Their functions are described in Chapter 44. The acoustic portion of the labyrinth is the cochlea, the coiled structure shown in Fig. 43.11. As the cross section in Fig. 43.12 illustrates, the mammalian cochlea contains a fluid-filled tube wound around a central bony core, the modiolus. This tube consists of three compartments—the scala vestibuli, the scala media (also known as the cochlear duct), and the scala tympani. The scala media, which contains the receptor cells and related structures, is separated from other scalae by Reisner's membrane above and by the basilar membrane below. The scala vestibuli communicates with the oval window, through which sound vibrations are transmitted by the stapes, while the round window, in contact with the scala tympani, compensates for the pressure changes associated with sound stimuli.

Whereas the fluid in the scala tympani and vestibuli, perilymph, is similar to cerebrospinal fluid, the scala media contains endolymph, whose electrolyte concentrations are more similar to those of intracellular fluid. The existence of a separate endolymph-filled compartment is significant.

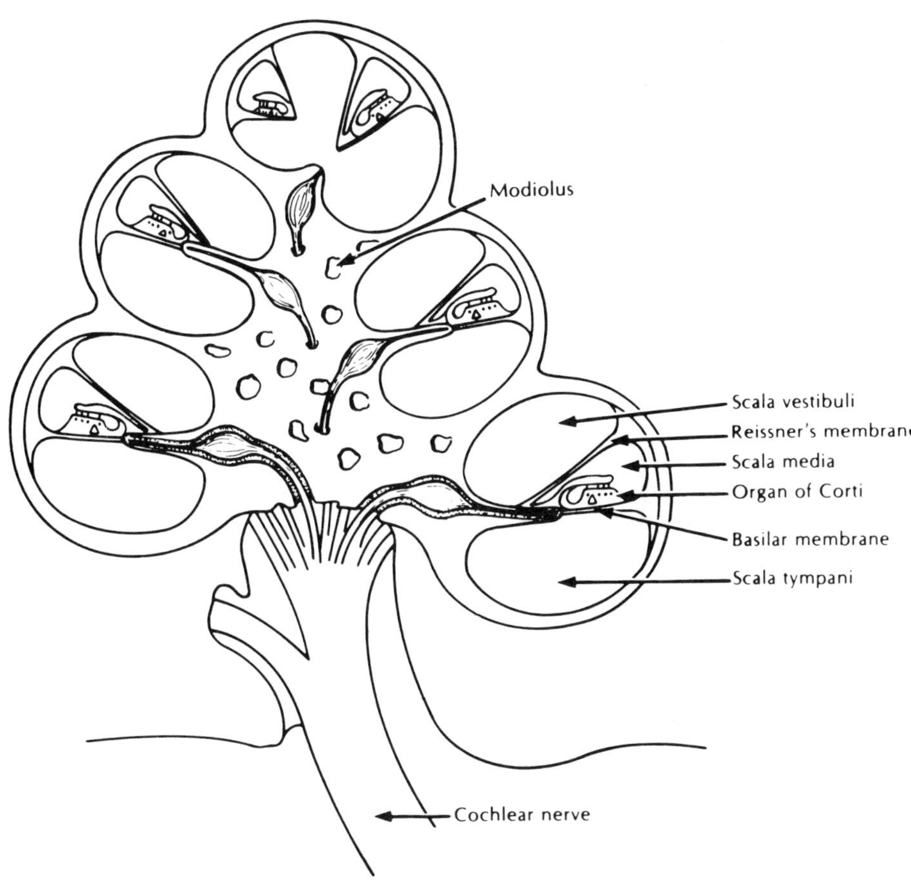

Figure 43.12. Cross section of mammalian cochlea. It has the form of a tube coiled about the modiolus from which nerve fibers radiate. The organ of Corti, shown in more detail in Fig. 43.13, contains the receptor cells and related structures. The scala vestibuli communicates with the oval window, through which sound energy is transmitted by the stapes. Acoustically, the scala media and the scala vestibuli form a single conduit; the thin Reisner's membrane serves only to prevent the fluids of the two compartments from mixing. The scala tympani provides a return path for the sound waves to the round window. (From V. Goodhill [ed.] 1979, *Ear Diseases, Deafness and Dizziness*, Harper & Row, Hagerstown, Md.)

Perilymph, in common with other extracellular fluids, contains high sodium and low potassium concentrations, whereas endolymph is low in sodium and high in potassium. The consequence of this difference in electrolytes is that there is an electrical potential, or voltage difference, on the order of 80 mV between the scala media and the scala tympani that permits depolarization by an appropriate stimulus. Depolarization of the receptor cells causes release of a neurotransmitter, which stimulates the auditory nerve.

In the auditory system the receptor cells—the cells that actually convert mechanical energy into neurotransmitter release—are known as hair cells because of the stiff stereocilia projecting from their apical surface. The hair cells are contained in the organ of Corti, along with supporting cells and the dendrites of the auditory nerve, which synapse with the hair cells at their bases (Fig. 43.13). The organ of Corti rests on the basilar membrane and, in turn, is overlaid with the tectorial membrane, a gelatinous structure. The hair cells are situated with their stereocilia near or in contact with the tectorial membrane, so that vibrations deflecting the basilar membrane result in bending of the stereocilia. This, in turn, causes an ion flux through the hair cell, resulting in release of a transmitter substance that stimulates the auditory nerve fibers.

There are two classes of hair cells in the mammalian organ of Corti. The three rows of outer hair cells (Fig. 43.13) differ from the single row of inner hair cells in a number of ways, most notably their patterns of innervation. Few afferent neurons project from the outer hair cells to the CNS—only one neuron for many hair cells. Conversely, each inner hair cell synapses with several afferent neurons. The two classes of hair cells also differ greatly in their pattern of efferent innervation—neurons presumed to have some sort of regulatory function, which carry signals out from the brain. It is now suggested by many that only the inner hair cells serve as receptors, with the outer hair cells being said to participate in increasing the sensitivity or frequency selectivity of the cochlea in some manner.

Avian cochlea

The cochlea of the bird differs considerably from that of the mammal. It is short and nearly straight, rather than coiled. The hair cells form a broad pavement rather than four individual rows.

Mechanism of hearing

Sound waves entering the external auditory ear throw the tympanic membrane into vibration. With relatively little

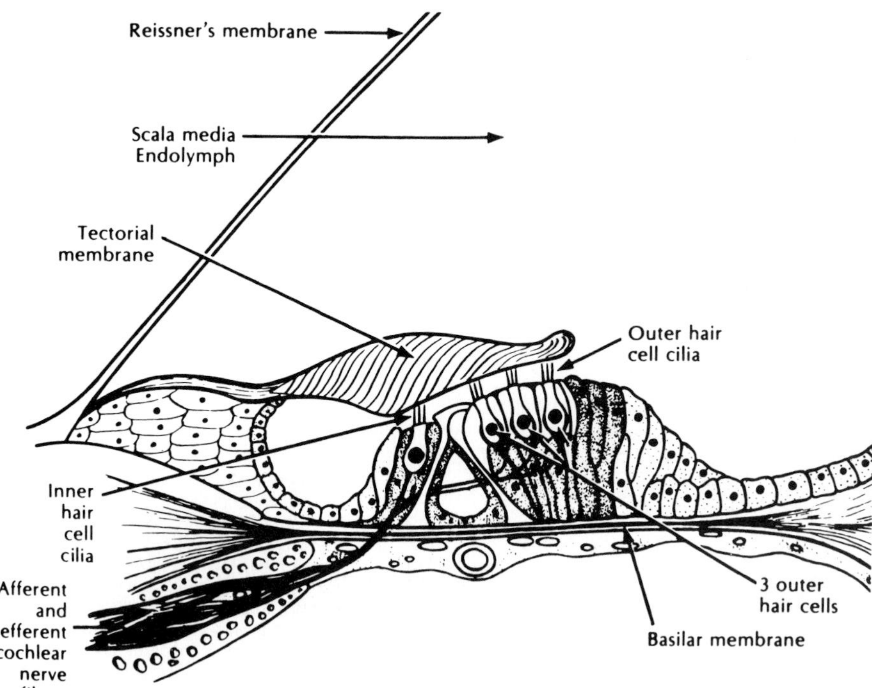

Figure 43.13. Organ of Corti. As the basilar membrane is flexed by sound waves traveling through the scalae vestibuli and media, the cilia of the hair cells are deflected by the tectorial membrane. This alters the ionic current through the hair cells, stimulating the release of neurotransmitter at their synapses with cochlear nerve fibers. The endolymph within the scala media, having a remarkably high potassium concentration, provides the voltage potential that drives the ionic current. (From V. Goodhill [ed.] 1979, *Ear Diseases, Deafness and Dizziness*, Harper & Row, Hagerstown, Md.)

energy loss, the waves thus generated are transmitted mechanically across the tympanic cavity by action of the auditory ossicles. The movements of the footplate of the stapes set up waves in the perilymph of the labyrinth, which cause the basilar membrane to vibrate. As this membrane moves up and down, the hair cells are displaced. As the basilar membrane moves up and down, the tectorial membrane moves laterally relative to the hair cells. Since the tips of the outer hair cells' stereocilia are embedded in the tectorial membrane, they are bent by this motion. The stereocilia of the inner hair cells also are bent, the motion being transmitted through the thin layer of fluid under the tectorial membrane. The bending of the cilia in some manner alters the permeability of the hair cell to ion flow; bending of the cilia in one direction increases flow, and bending in the opposite direction decreases the ionic current. This fluctuating current mimics, within limits, the acoustic signal reaching the ear; one can place an electrode on the round window and record an electrical signal, known as the cochlear microphonic potential, that reflects this current flow. The current flow through the hair cell results in the release of a neurotransmitter from the base of the hair cell where it synapses with the fibers of the auditory nerve. This neurotransmitter is the stimulus that initiates a nerve impulse to the brain.

Because the basilar membrane at the basal end of the cochlea is stiffer than at the apical end, low-frequency sound waves do not greatly deflect it at the basal end but travel instead toward the apex before reaching the point of maximal deflection of the basilar membrane and thus maximal hair cell stimulation (Fig. 43.14). High-frequency waves displace the membrane near the round window, thus losing their energy before they reach more apical regions. The result is that each region of the basilar membrane is differentially sensitive to a different frequency, and stimulation of nerve fibers from that region provides the CNS with information as to the frequency of the sound.

Range of hearing

Traditionally, hearing sensitivity in animals has been assessed by behavioral techniques. For example, the animal can be trained to obtain food by pressing a lever and then be taught that this behavior produces food only in the presence of a sound. Hearing sensitivity can be estimated by determining the intensity of sounds at various frequencies that will cause the animal to press the lever. More recently, electrophysiological methods have provided more direct evidence of auditory function. Electrical activity elicited by acoustic stimulation can be recorded from the cochlea itself, or neuronal activity can be recorded from the auditory nerve or various points in the CNS.

The range of frequencies that can be detected varies among the species. Humans can detect sounds in the range from 20 to 20,000 Hz, although sensitivity is poor at both extremes. Some animals can perceive frequencies much higher than 20,000 Hz. The upper pitch unit of dogs is generally thought to be about twice that of humans. The silent dog whistle emits some frequencies too high for humans to hear but below the upper pitch limit for dogs. The frequency most audible to the rat appears to be 40,000. Frequencies as high as 98,000 cause potential changes in

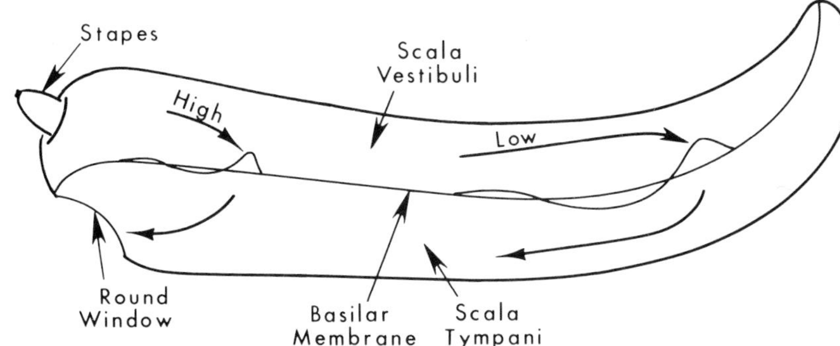

Figure 43.14. Schematic of the cochlea, shown uncoiled. The scala media, which is acoustically continuous with the scala vestibuli, is omitted. Sound waves are introduced by the stapes, then travel up the scalae to a point at which the basilar membrane has a corresponding resonance (near the base for high frequencies; near the apex for low frequencies). At this point the basilar membrane is deformed, stimulating the hair cells; thus the frequency of the signal is detected by the place along the basilar membrane that is maximally excited. In the process, the vibrations are transmitted through the basilar membrane and travel back to the round window.

the cochlea of the bat. In terms of sensitivity (the least loud sound perceivable at a given frequency), dogs and humans are about equal at low frequency, but dogs appear markedly superior at frequencies between 1000 and 8000. Studies of the range of hearing in adult birds indicate that they are approximately as sensitive as humans. The larger domestic animals—sheep, cattle, and horses—have similar ranges of hearing; the upper limit for cats may approach 100,000 Hz.

Frequency ranges appear to be determined by mechanical factors. The transmission of high frequencies into the cochlea is limited by the mass of the tympanic membrane and ossicles. Another factor, the volume of air in the middle ear, limits the low frequencies. This air must be compressed for the tympanic membrane to move in and out, and the excursion of the tympanic membrane is greatest for low-frequency sounds. Certain small animals extend their low-frequency sensitivity by having enlarged middle ear cavities; in the chinchilla, especially, the middle ear consists of a large bubblelike shell of bone, accounting for the greater part of the size of the posterior skull. Birds generally have a narrower range of hearing than mammals, probably because of similar mechanical constraints on the transmission of sound to the cochlea.

Localization of sound

Two cues aid in identifying the direction from which sounds come. The first is the relative loudness of the sound at the two ears. This cue is most effective for high-frequency sounds, since these are most attenuated for the ear turned away from the source. The second cue is the difference in time of arrival of the sound between the two ears. There are neurons within the CNS that are exquisitely sensitive to the delays between the responses from the two ears. Movements of the pinna aid in the localization of sound sources, as is evident on observing a horse or deer that has detected a strange sound.

Hearing impairment

Loss of hearing in domestic animals is of two general types. Sensorineural impairment involves disease of the cochlea or the cochlear branch of the auditory nerve; conductive loss occurs when the sound waves cannot be transmitted efficiently to the inner ear. In the latter instance the causes include occlusion of the exterior meatus, rupture of the eardrum, and malfunction of the ossicles. The most common cause of hearing impairment in humans and laboratory animals (and probably other species) is otitis media —inflammatory or infectious processes resulting in the accumulation of fluid in the middle ear, which interferes with the mobility of the eardrum.

In sensorineural loss the most common site of a lesion is the hair cell, although degeneration of supporting structures and nerve fibers is often noted. In domestic animals the major causes of sensorineural impairment are noise trauma, congenital anomalies and hereditary defects, and toxicity related to drug administration. Degeneration of the cochlea with aging has been found in the horse, cat, and other species. Hereditary impairment can be associated with albinism in cats and some other species but is not a constant finding. Hereditary deafness has been described in cocker spaniels and bull terriers, and a progressive hereditary loss (becoming worse with time) is not uncommon among dalmatians. In many cases of sensorineural impairment, a sound of moderate intensity may be inaudible but quickly becomes louder as its intensity is increased. This rapid growth in loudness is known as recruitment. In such a case, loud sounds, such as a handclap or a voice at close range, may elicit a normal response, obscuring a substantial hearing deficit.

Many of the aminoglycoside antibiotics (kanamycin and streptomycin, for example) are ototoxic at serum levels above certain limits. Hearing loss may not appear until after the drug has been discontinued. The loop diuretics (those acting in the loop of Henle; e.g., furosemide) may potentiate the toxicity of aminoglycosides.

Objective testing of hearing impairment is now feasible and, at least in auditory research, quite routine. The method involves recording of electrical activity originating from the auditory nerve and nuclei within the brain-stem auditory pathways with the use of scalp electrodes. These potentials, known collectively as brain-stem auditory evoked responses (BAERs), or by similar terms, are quite small when measured at the scalp but can be detected by a form of computer processing known as signal averaging. This involves collection of the responses to hundreds or thousands of stimulus presentations. When the responses are averaged, the pattern elicited by the sound can be detected whereas extraneous interference is reduced. Since the stimulus can be repeated very rapidly (20 times a second is common), the data collection need not take a great deal of time. Figure 43.15 illustrates a series of BAERs recorded from a dog. A high intensity is tested first, then the intensity is reduced until the response disappears. The limitations of the test are that specialized equipment costing tens of thousands of dollars is used and that the animal must be asleep to avoid interference from muscle activity.

A method of detecting middle ear problems, known as impedance audiometry, has widespread use with human infants and children and may have veterinary applications. The principle is that the normal tympanic membrane has a low acoustic impedance or resistance to the transmission of sound; sound waves striking the normal tympanic membrane are readily transmitted via the ossicles into the inner ear. If the tympanic membrane is rendered immobile by the accumulation of fluid in the middle ear, its impedance is greatly increased, with the result that sound is reflected back rather than penetrating the middle ear. The test involves introduction of a tone into the ear canal and measurement of the resultant sound pressure in the canal, which is a function of the amount of energy reflected from the tympanic membrane.

Besides detecting the fluid that accompanies otitis media, impedance audiometry can detect an excessively compliant tympanic membrane, indicative of discontinuity of the ossicles, or abnormal air pressure in the middle ear space. The latter measure is made by varying the pressure in the ear canal; only when the pressure on the outside is equal to the pressure in the middle ear will the tympanic membrane have its greatest compliance.

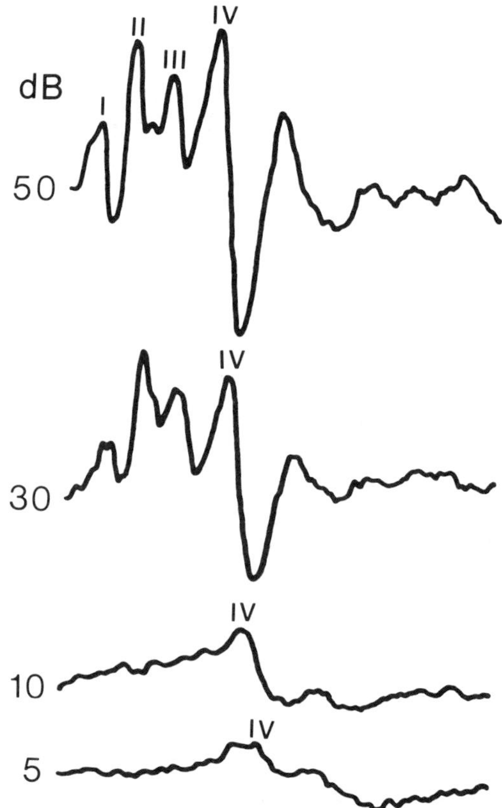

Figure 43.15. Brain-stem auditory evoked response, recorded from domestic dog. If the ear is stimulated by clicks—abrupt auditory stimuli—a characteristic pattern of waves can be recorded from scalp electrodes with the aid of computer processing. At high intensities several waves (the number varies with species, electrode placement, and recording technique) can be seen originating from the auditory nerve and various neurons within the brain-stem auditory pathways. The earlier waves become obscure at low intensities, but some activity (here wave IV) can be seen at very low intensities, confirming that the cochlea has detected the signal. The decibel (dB) scale is a relative scale of intensity of the stimulus, relative to the average threshold for eliciting the response.

Behavior

The primary behavioral functions of audition are detection of environmental sounds (including those of predator and prey) and communication with the same species. Less common behavioral functions of audition are communication with other species, as in threat signals or voice communication between humans and domestic animals, and echolocation for hunting and navigation.

Few domestic animals need to rely on sound for hunting prey or eluding predators, although the related orienting responses to novel sound are certainly evident in many species. Sound still plays an important role in intraspecific communication in domestic animals. Functions include maintenance of contact between parent and offspring, sexual communication, warning of danger and threatening of adversaries, and definition and defense of territory. Dogs, like other gregarious species of Canidae, employ a wide variety of sounds for social purposes, including greeting, play activity, establishment of hierarchy, and simply maintaining social contact over long distances, as evidenced by the group barking of domestic dogs and the howling of wolves. In pigs, sounds produced by the young appear to have a role in nursing, and the rhythmic *chant de coeur* or mating sound produced by the boar may play a role in inducing female receptivity.

Among birds, vocal communication is remarkably elaborate. The birdcalls of many species have not only innate but also learned components and complex patterns. Indeed, it is often the pattern more than the pitch of the individual components that carries the message. Birdcalls most frequently serve to announce territory and attract mates. Song is also involved in the maintenance of pair bonds—mates in a number of species engage in reciprocal calling patterns.

Many of the domestic birds are precocial, that is, the young are ambulatory and able to feed themselves at hatching. In such species, the calls of the young serve to maintain contact with the mother. Among chickens, at least, these calls are essential to the hen's recognition of her young. A chick in view of the mother elicits no recognition if the chick's distress call cannot be heard, and a deafened hen will even kill chicks approaching the nest when she fails to discriminate them from predators.

REFERENCES

Adams, M.G. 1980. Odour-producing organs of mammals. In D.M. Stoddart, ed., *Olfaction in Mammals*. Academic Press, New York: Pp. 57–86.

Albone, E.S. 1984. *Mammalian Semiochemistry*. Wiley & Sons, Chichester.

Anisko, J.J. 1976. Communication by chemical signals in Canidae. In R.L. Doty, ed., *Mammalian Olfaction, Reproductive Processes and Behavior*. Academic Press, New York. Pp. 283–93.

Bath, W. 1906. Die Greschmacksorgane der Vögel und Krokodile. *Arch. Biontol.* 1:1–47.

Brand, J.G., Naim, M., and Kare, M.R. 1981. Taste and nutrition. In M. Rechcigl, ed., *Handbook of Nutritional Requirements in a Functional Context, vol. 2*. CRC Press, Boca Ration, Fla. Pp. 255–82.

Brand, J.G., Teeter, J.H., Cagan, R.H., and Kare, M.R., eds., 1989. *Chemical Senses. Volume I. Receptor Events and Transduction in Taste and Olfaction*. Marcel Dekker, New York.

Cole, E.C. 1941. *Comparative Histology*. Blakiston, Philadelphia.

Davies, R.O., Kare, M.R., and Cagan, R.H. 1979. Distribution of taste buds on fungiform and circumvallate papillae of bovine tongue. *Anat. Rec.* 195:443–46.

Denton, D. 1984. The hunger for salt. Springer-Verlag, New York.

Donaldson, J.A., and Miller, J.M. 1980. Anatomy of the ear. In M.M. Paparella and D.A. Shumrick, eds., *Otolaryngology*, vol. I. W.B. Saunders, Philadelphia. Pp. 26–62.

Elliott, R. 1937. Total distribution of taste buds on the tongue of the kitten at birth. *J. Comp. Neurol.* 66:361–73.

Fay, R.R. 1988. *Hearing in Vertebrates: A Psychophysics Databook*. Hill-Fay Assoc., Winnetka, IL.

Holliday, J.C. 1940. Total distribution of taste buds on the tongue of the pup. *Ohio J. Sci.* 40:337–44.

Honrubia, V., and Goodhill, V. 1979. Clinical anatomy and physiology of the peripheral ear. In V. Goodhill, ed., *Ear Diseases, Deafness and Dizziness*. Harper & Row, Hagerstown, Md. Pp. 4–63.

Houpt, K.A., and Wolski, T.R. 1982. *Domestic Animal Behavior for Veterinarians and Animal Scientists*. Iowa State University Press, Ames.

Hyman, L.H. 1942. *Comparative Vertebrate Anatomy*, 2d ed. University of Chicago Press, Chicago.

Jacobs, W.W., Beauchamp, G.K., and Kare, M.R. 1978. Progress in animal flavor research. In R.W. Bullard, ed., *Animal Flavor Chemistry*. American Chemical Society, New York.

Kare, M.R. and Rogers, J.G., Jr. 1976. The special senses. In P.D. Sturkie, ed., *Avian Physiology*. Springer, Berlin.

Laing, D.G., Cain, W.S., McBride, R.L., and Ache, B., eds., 1989. *Perception of Complex Tastes and Smells*. Academic Press, Sydney.

Lawrence, M. 1991. Introduction to inner ear (fluid) physiology. In M.M. Paparella, D.A. Shumrick, J.L. Gluckman, and W.L. Meyerhoff, eds. *Otolaryngology*, 3d ed. Vol. I. W.B. Saunders, Philadelphia. Pp. 199–217.

Lerner, S.A., Matz, G.J., and Hawkins, J.E. 1981. *Aminoglycoside Ototoxicity*. Little, Brown, Boston.

Lindenmaier, P., and Kare, M.R. 1959. The taste end-organs of the chicken. *Poult. Sci.* 38:545–50.

Moncrieff, R.W. 1951. *The Chemical Senses*. Leonard Hill, London.

Moore, C.A., and Elliott, R. 1946. Numerical and regional distribution of taste buds on the tongue of the bird. *J. Comp. Neurol.* 84:119–32.

Pickles, J.O. 1988. *An Introduction to the Physiology of Hearing*. Academic Press, London.

Vandenbergh, J.G., ed., 1983. *Pheromones and Reproduction in Mammals*. Academic Press, New York.

Wysocki, C.J. 1979. Neurobehavioral evidence for the involvement of the vomeronasal system in mammalian reproduction. *Neurosci. Biobehav. Rev.* 3:301–41.

CHAPTER 44

Regulation of Motor Activity | by James E. Breazile

Somatic motor control involves a wide variety of movements, which include walking, running, backing, voluntary stepping with one or more feet, prehension, mastication, swallowing, respiration, eye movements, and control of urinary and fecal continence. Each of these types of movement requires brain controls that receive sensory input from the tissues involved, from other environmental stimuli, and from other activity that is simultaneously taking place within the central nervous system. Such control systems use a large number of brain structures for even the simplest somatic movement.

The basic units of somatic motor activity are brain-stem and spinal cord reflex arcs, which are discussed in Chapter 40. In most cases voluntary movements are carried out through the modification of activity in tonically active reflex arcs. Reflex arcs (receptor organs → afferent neurons → interneurons → motor neurons → muscle) represent *feed-forward control* in which there is limited means for modification of the motor action. Feed-forward systems are fast, but they tend to produce movements that lack stability and accuracy of motor action. In all reflex arcs, one or more central nervous system neurons are involved in the neural pathway, allowing synaptic modification by central nervous system activity.

The final common pathway of all influences on somatic motor control involves the neurons of the brain stem and the spinal cord that innervate skeletal muscle. These neurons give rise to large-diameter axons (class A alpha) and are thus called *alpha motor neurons*. Motor neurons that supply intrafusal muscle fibers give rise to class A gamma axons and are called *gamma motor neurons*. Each alpha motor neuron provides an axon that exits the ventral root and supplies one motor unit (see Chap. 45). The cell bodies of motor neurons are proportional in size to the size of the motor unit with which they are associated. Thus those that supply large motor units have large cell bodies and those that supply small motor units have small cell bodies. Motor neuron excitability is inversely related to the size of the cell body. As a skeletal muscle is stimulated through central nervous system excitation, small motor neurons are excited first; then, with increased excitatory force, larger motor units are recruited. When motor neurons are inhibited by central mechanisms, large motor neurons are the first to be inhibited. This orderly recruitment and inhibition in relation to the size of motor units is called the *size principle of motor neuronal excitability*.

Axons from alpha motor neurons branch within the gray matter of the spinal cord into one to six recurrent collaterals that synapse upon interneurons within the vicinity of the original cell bodies. One group of these interneurons (known as *Renshaw cells*) inhibits alpha motor neurons giving rise to the collaterals. This provides a short negative-feedback control to alpha motor neuron activity and tends to limit the frequency and duration of action potential production. Because large motor neurons are more easily inhibited than small motor neurons, Renshaw cell inhibition tends to contribute to the orderly recruitment of small to large motor units as somatic muscle contraction force is increased. The excitability of Renshaw cells is influenced by descending neural activity from the brain as well as by cutaneous and muscle sensory afferents. In this way, these inhibitory interneurons provide a means for other neural influences to alter reflex activity.

For an appreciation of some of the problems involved in an examination of control mechanisms of motor activity, a common, seemingly simple motor behavior in the dog will be considered. The control that is required for a dog to run, jump, and catch a tossed Frisbee is complex. It is necessary for the dog to maintain a fixed visual image of the Frisbee on the retina throughout the movement. The speed of locomotion, the timing of the jump, and the head, neck, and jaw movements must all be coordinated to place the jaws in the appropriate position to catch the Frisbee. Once the catch has been made, it is necessary that body and limb movements allow the dog to return safely to the ground and for locomotion to continue.

Accuracy and stability in somatic motor action require a number of feedback-control systems (Fig. 44.1). There are three components to a feedback control: a sensing system, a set point system, and an error-detecting and reset mechanism. Sensory receptors and afferent neurons represent the sensing system of the reflex arc and generate somatic movement. Cognitive regions of the brain serve as sensing systems for intentional, voluntary movements. Other neural structures are required for set point determination and for error detection and reset.

Set point systems predetermine the desired rate, duration, and range of movement required to accomplish an established goal. In eye movements, the set point might be the maintenance of a stable visual image on the retina. In somatic motor control, the set point may be the movement of a limb to provide appropriate postural support. In the Frisbee-catching dog, the ultimate set point is the position of the jaws to grasp the Frisbee in the air, with all motor activity preceding this point being determined by the set point. Several individual set points may have to be achieved before the complete performance of the single motor action.

In the organization of voluntary movements, set point activities occur within regions of the central nervous system that are involved with motivational activities, in which animals voluntarily determine the desired set points for movements. In many cases, however, set points are established without voluntary intervention. The latter is seen in many limb reflexes, as in Renshaw inhibitory feedback control, in which the set point is determined by the intensity and location of the activating sensory stimulation and other central neural activity that must be integrated with the reflex. It is obvious that if the set point in a reflex movement is flexion of a limb and the situation in which the animal is postured causes the animal to fall down, the set point would be detrimental to the animal. In this situation, neural activity controling the maintenance of posture intervenes in the reflex action and provides a new set point for limb movement.

Error-detection and reset systems require a great deal of information to carry out their function. Initially information from the set point device is necessary to determine whether there is an error. Error-detection and reset mechanisms must then receive information concerning the resting state of the animal before initiation of the movement and continue to receive information concerning the effect of the movement. The major error-detecting and reset system of the brain is the cerebellum.

VESTIBULO-OCULAR REFLEX

The vestibulo-ocular reflex represents a relatively simple reflex action, controlling eye movements to provide a stable visual field as the head is turned. This reflex arc provides an example of a feedback-control mechanism. Rotation of the head is sensed by the semicircular canals of the vestibular system, as described below.

The pathway diagrammed in Fig. 44.2 shows a direct projection of the vestibular nerve to the vestibulocochlear nuclei. The vestibular nuclei, in turn, project directly to the oculomotor nucleus for eye muscle control, completing the reflex arc. By itself, this pathway provides a direct control of eye movements when the head is rotated, but a great deal of instability is observed.

The purpose of the vestibulo-ocular reflex is to maintain a stable visual image on the retina during head movements. The set point in this case is the retinal activity generated by the visual image. This control system feeds back to the vestibular nuclei to modify the reflex activity and assure the desired output. The cerebellum functions as the error-detection and reset mechanism. The reflex pathways with their feedback components are indicated in Fig. 44.3. It will be noted that not only does the visual system have a controlling influence on the vestibular relay of sensory information but the vestibular input itself passes through the cerebellum to influence the vestibular relay. This type of dual control is characteristic of somatic motor controls. There is a direct feed-forward control (the reflex arc), par-

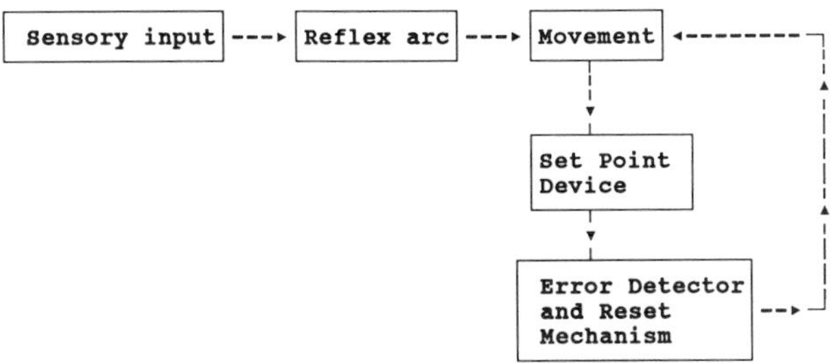

Figure 44.1. Elements of a feedback control system.

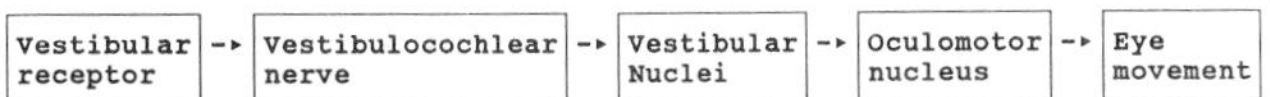

Figure 44.2. Components of vestibulo-ocular reflex arc.

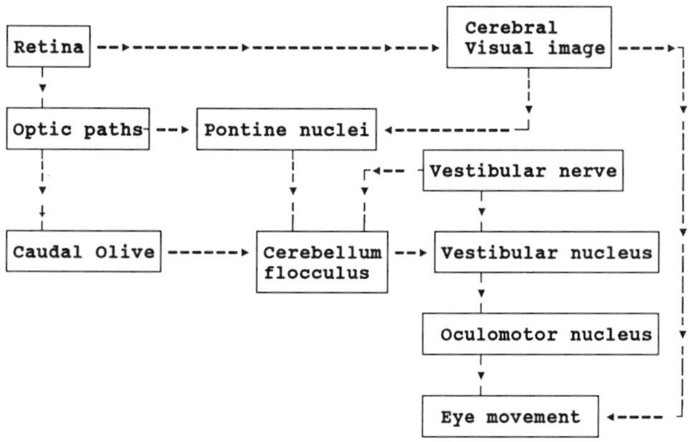

Figure 44.3. Components of vestibulo-ocular reflex pathways with feedback controls.

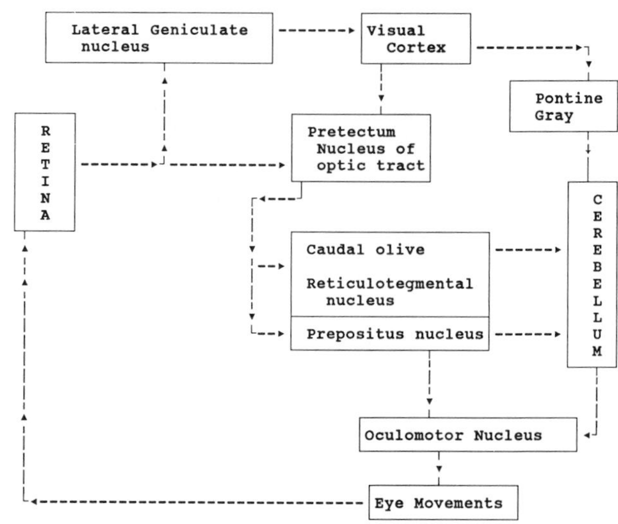

Figure 44.4. Elements of optokinetic nystagmus reflex with feedback controls

alleled by an indirect feed-forward system (vestibulo-cerebello-vestibular), coupled to a feedback controller (visual-cerebello-vestibular).

The cerebellum plays a key role as an integrator of the motor action, with a major effect of providing stability for motor activity. In the vestibulo-ocular reflex, the cerebellum receives, from the retina, input concerned with movement of the visual image. The cerebellum then modifies (resets) the reflex arc to maintain a stable retinal image.

HORIZONTAL OPTOKINETIC NYSTAGMUS

Horizontal optokinetic nystagmus is a rhythmic physiological movement of the eyes in response to a moving visual field, as when one is looking at telephone poles from a moving vehicle. This reflex involves visual input as the primary sensory regulator. The purpose of the reflex is to provide a fixed visual image on the retina during a slow movement of the eyes in the direction opposite that of body movement. Thereafter, the eyes are rapidly moved to a new position and a new visual image is maintained during another slow movement of the eyes. These alternating actions are repeated. The neural pathway for optokinetic nystagmus is illustrated in Fig. 44.4.

In this reflex movement, the shortest pathway for the control of eye movements is a feed-forward pathway from the retina, through the nucleus of the optic tract (NOT),and the prepositus nucleus (PPN) to the oculomotor nucleus (ON) (retina→NOT→PPN→ON).

A second feed-forward system consists of the pathway from the retina through the lateral geniculate (LG) to the visual cortex (VC) and then to the nucleus of the optic tract, where it converges with visual input from the retina. The latter (retina→LG→VC→NOT→PPN→ON) appears to be the dominant feed-forward influence for the reflex action, providing the set point for control of eye movement.

The convergence of visual cortex efferents, through the pontine gray and retinal input through the pretectum, caudal olive, reticulotegmental, and prepositus nuclei to the cerebellum, allows the cerebellum to serve as an *error detector*. Through its direct and indirect projections to the oculomotor nucleus, errors in eye movements are corrected and stability of visual image on the retina is produced.

It should not be concluded that the pathways illustrated for either vestibulo-ocular or optokinetic eye movements represent all the brain structures used. Even though control mechanisms for optokinetic eye movements and those for vestibulo-ocular movements vary in complexity, the same basic elements are required. In both cases the visual image provides the set point, established in the visual areas of the cerebral cortex. The cerebellum serves as the error-detection and reset mechanism, providing accuracy and stability to the reflex movement.

BRAIN CONTROL OF REFLEX LIMB MOVEMENTS

Motor controls in eye movements are relatively simple. The eye is a relatively inelastic structure of extremely small mass, in a low-viscosity, nearly frictionless medium. On the other hand, movements of the postural and limb muscles involve inertia, gravity, external loads, elasticity of ligaments and tendons, and antagonistic muscle tone. It becomes obvious that brain control of postural and limb movements must involve a greater degree of complexity of feed-forward and feedback mechanisms than is required for eye movement. Feedback controls of eye movements are primarily dependent on visual feedback to maintain stable vision or vestibular input to compensate for head movements. Because of the variable load conditions that occur in limb movements, proprioceptive feedback controls that reflect muscle stretch and degree of muscle contraction are necessary.

Inverse myotatic reflexes (Fig. 44.5) and the gamma loops of myotatic reflexes (Figs. 44.6 and 44.7), described in Chapter 40, serve as major sensory inputs to the spinal cord and the brain, contributing to the control of limb movements. As illustrated in Fig. 44.8, these reflex arcs are interactive and have extensive sensory connections with the brain. The gamma motor neuron activity of the spinal cord is established primarily through the activity of the pontine and medullary reticulospinal tracts. As described in Chapter 40, the gamma motor system activity maintains a low-level, tonic activity of skeletal muscle known as muscle tone. The inverse myotatic reflex, activated by muscle contraction, acts to dampen muscle contraction. Through Ia afferents the brain receives information concerning the activity of the gamma loops and the degree of muscle stretch, and through Ib afferents, it receives information concerning the degree of contraction of skeletal muscle. Both Ia and Ib afferents transmit information concerning activity of their reflex arcs to the cerebellum by way of the dorsal and ventral spinocerebellar tracts. Ia afferents also transmit information to the somatic motor and premotor areas of the cerebral cortex. These areas of the cerebral cortex also receive input from other areas of the cerebral hemisphere concerning the total sensory environment of the animal.

It can be seen from Figs. 44.7 and 44.8 that there is a long latency reflex arc for the myotatic reflex that passes through the cerebral cortex. It should also be noted that both reflex arcs have direct input to the cerebellum. The inhibitory limbs of the reflex arcs (reciprocal innervation) have been omitted from the figures for the sake of simplicity. It can be concluded from these illustrations that even a reflex movement of the limbs, involving the myotatic and inverse myotatic reflex arcs, is continually under control by the brain. The brain is necessary to provide a set point (the motor and

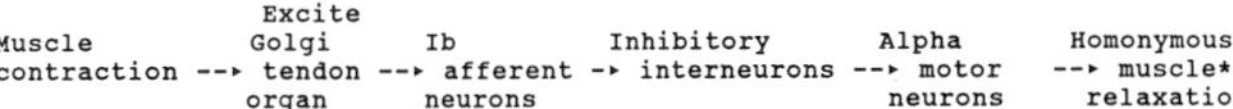

Figure 44.5. Inverse myotatic reflex arc, demonstrating the mechanism of self-inhibition of muscle contraction. * A homonomous muscle is the one that contains the receptor organ.

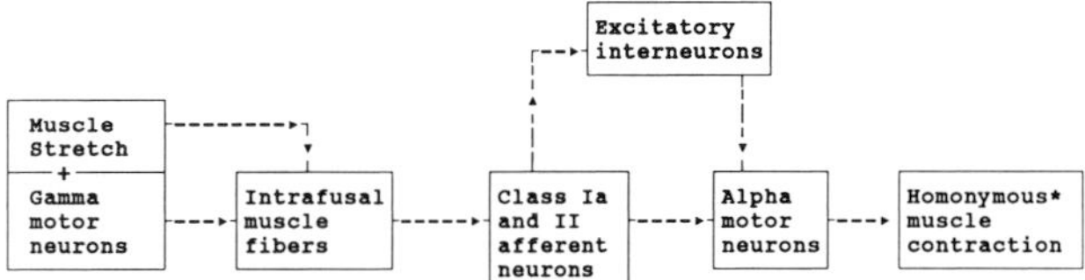

Figure 44.6. Myotatic reflex arc, demonstrating the combined effect of muscle stretch and gamma motor neuron activity.

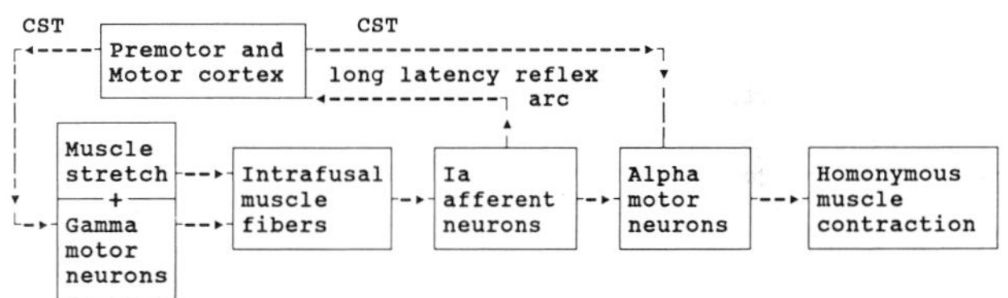

Figure 44.7. Myotatic reflex arc, demonstrating the long latency reflex arc through the premotor and motor cortex. Note that this arc produces coactivation of the alpha and gamma motor neurons. The corticospinal tract (CST) is one of several descending tracts that are involved.

premotor cortex) and for error detection (cerebellum) of these spinal cord reflexes. The feedback loops through which the cerebellum corrects errors in reflex action involving the motor and premotor cortex are discussed below. It should be noted that the motor cortex, through a number of

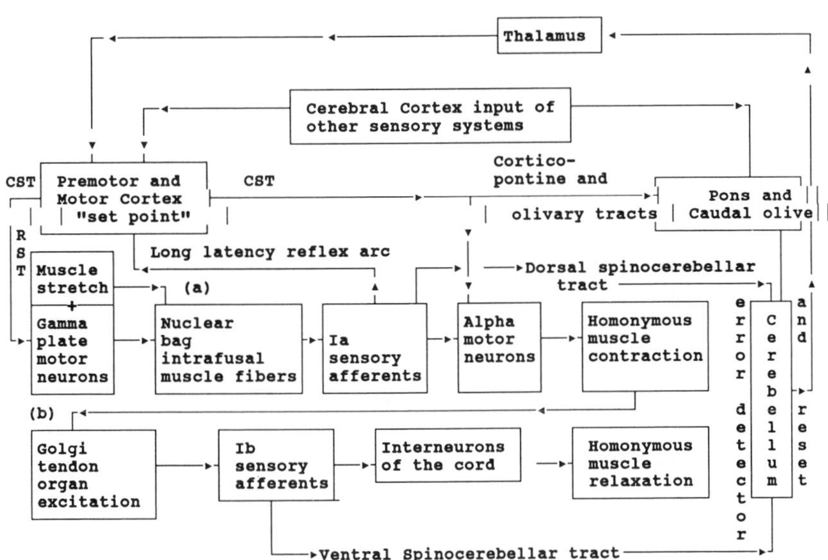

Figure 44.8. Schematic of the combined reflex and brain connections of (a) the myotatic (Fig. 44.6) and (b) the inverse myotatic reflex (Fig. 44.5) arcs of the spinal cord. Note that the premotor and motor cortices provide the set point for reflex activity and the cerebellum serves as error detector and reset of the reflex activity. CST is the corticospinal tract.

descending tracts, influences the excitability of both the alpha and the gamma motor neurons of the spinal cord.

SPINAL SHOCK

Dependence of spinal motor mechanisms on the brain is best demonstrated by the motor capacity of the spinal cord after transection of its connections with the brain stem. Transection of the spinal cord at its junction with the medulla produces death because of a failure of respiration. Transection of the cord caudal to the emergence of the phrenic nerve allows respiration to continue. Such a transection produces a period of time in which there is a total lack of spinal cord somatic and visceral reflexes caudal to the level of the transection. This state of *areflexia* is called *spinal shock*. The duration of spinal shock varies with the level of the spinal cord transection (more prolonged in caudal thoracic and lumbar transections than in cervical or cranial thoracic transections) and the age of the animal (more prolonged in mature than in immature animals) and is increased with the degree of encephalization (dependence of spinal cord mechanisms on brain control). In most domestic species, some reflexes (anal, genital, and withdrawal) return within 10 to 15 minutes. Patellar myotatic reflexes generally return within 30 minutes. Within 2 to 3 hours, withdrawal and myotatic reflexes become hyperexcitable, and they are more easily elicited than in the normal animal. This *hyperreflexia* is accompanied by a diminished resting muscle tone. Visceral reflexes generally take longer to recover from spinal shock than do somatic reflexes. Within 1 to 2 weeks, however, all visceral reflexes caudal to the transection are functional. Visceral reflexes of nonprimates, unlike somatic reflexes, do not develop post–spinal shock hyperreflexia.

The physiological basis for spinal shock resides in the removal of excitatory influences and the enhancement of inhibitory influences on motor neurons of the isolated spinal cord. The mechanisms that produce these effects are not known, but Renshaw cell hyperactivity has been implicated as playing a role in enhanced inhibition of motor neurons. Studies of partial spinal cord transection conducted in the cat have demonstrated that transection of the ventral reticulospinal and vestibulospinal tracts will produce spinal shock. In primates, however, transection of the corticospinal tract results in spinal shock that is nearly as complete as that resulting from cord transection. Transection of the corticospinal tract in cats and dogs does not produce spinal shock. It is apparent, therefore, that the removal of descending tracts to produce spinal shock in a given species depends on the importance of the individual tracts involved in controlling excitability of motor neurons.

SCHIFF-SHERRINGTON RIGIDITY

Dependence of thoracic limb motor control on caudal portions of the spinal cord and on brain mechanisms is demonstrated by transections of the mid to caudal thoracic spinal cord. Transection of the spinal cord at levels caudal to the origin of the brachial plexus and cranial to that of the lumbosacral plexus results in an antigravity rigidity of the pectoral limbs and neck. This is called *Schiff-Sherrington rigidity* in honor of the scientists who first committed it to study. Schiff-Sherrington rigidity is an *alpha rigidity*. Rigidity results from increased excitability of alpha motor neurons to extensor muscles and diminished excitability of their antagonists, the flexor muscles. The cord transection interrupts propriospinal tract axons arising from the lumbosacral spinal cord that normally inhibit alpha motor neurons to cervical and pectoral limb antigravity muscles and excite alpha motor neurons to their antagonists. The duration of Schiff-Sherrington rigidity varies among species. In the dog it can be demonstrated for several hours after cord transection, being quite severe initially and barely detectable after 24 hours.

Compensation for Schiff-Sherrington rigidity requires an increase of other inhibitory influences on cervicothoracic antigravity motor neurons. Two possible mechanisms have been described. The cerebellum exerts a tonic inhibitory influence on cervicothoracic alpha motor neurons, through its relationship with the vestibulospinal and reticulospinal tracts. The class Ia and II afferents from muscle spindles of the pectoral limbs also inhibit contralateral antigravity alpha motor neurons. The former is demonstrated in lesions of the anterior lobe of the cerebellum, which produces a marked *decerebellate alpha rigidity*. The latter is demonstrated by unilateral transection of the dorsal roots of brachial plexus spinal nerves producing an alpha antigravity rigidity in the opposite limb. The manner in which cerebellar and forelimb afferent tonic inhibition is altered to allow compensation for Schiff-Sherrington rigidity is not known.

DECEREBRATE RIGIDITY

If the brain stem is transected on a plane passing between the rostral and caudal colliculi of the midbrain and caudal to the red nucleus, a marked increase in muscle tone in antigravity (extensor) muscles results. All four limbs are markedly extended, and the head and tail are elevated. This postural response is called *decerebrate rigidity*. Decerebrate rigidity results in part from an increased activity of the medullary and pontine reticulospinal and vestibulospinal tracts. The principal effect of this activity is to produce hyperexcitability of spinal cord gamma motor neurons and their gamma loops. Because decerebrate rigidity is due primarily to increased gamma motor neuron activity, it is referred to as a *gamma rigidity*. Because of its reflex nature, the rigidity is diminished by transection of dorsal roots of spinal nerves that supply limb muscles. After such a transection, however, considerable rigidity remains in the pectoral limbs. This rigidity (called an *alpha rigidity*) is due to hyperactivity of alpha motor neurons induced by vestibulospinal tracts and afferents from neck muscles and joints. This alpha rigidity can be abolished by transection of

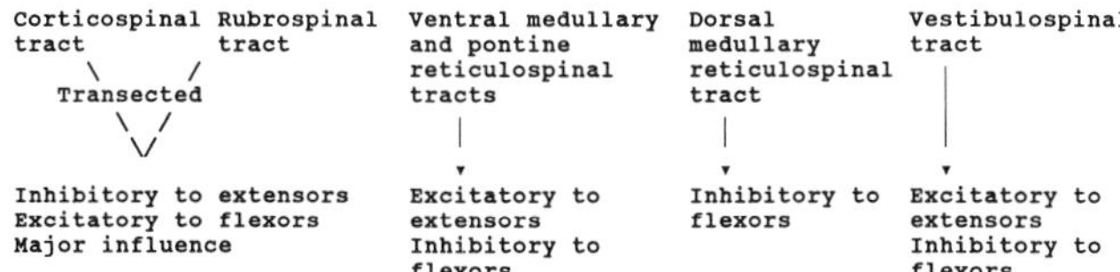

Figure 44.9. Primary influence of descending somatic motor tracts involved in the production of decerebrate rigidity.

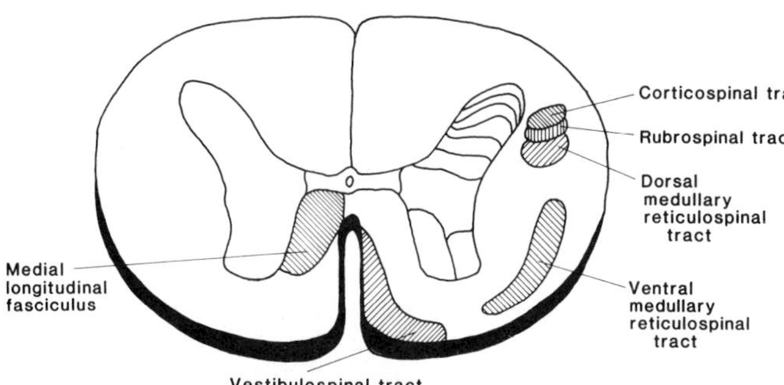

Figure 44.10. A representation of some of the descending axonal systems of the spinal cord, illustrating their relative location within the white matter. The medial longitudinal fasciculus contains a number of motor tracts, including the medial vestibulospinal tract.

the vestibular component of the eighth cranial nerve and the dorsal roots of cervical nerves. In decerebrate rigidity, although extensor muscles are hyperactive, flexor muscles are hypotonic and flexor reflexes are inhibited.

The brain-stem transection resulting in decerebrate rigidity interrupts many tracts. Two major somatic motor tracts interrupted are the corticospinal and rubrospinal tracts, both of which are excitatory to alpha and gamma motor neurons innervating flexor muscles and inhibitory to motor neurons innervating extensors (Figs. 44.9 and 44.10). The vestibulospinal tracts exert a powerful excitatory effect on extensor motor neurons. There are three descending tracts from the pontine and medullary reticular formation that exert influences on flexor and extensor motor neurons. These tracts are the dorsal and ventral medullary and the pontine reticulospinal tracts. The latter two tracts are excitatory to gamma and alpha motor neurons of extensor muscles, and the dorsal medullary reticulospinal tract exerts a tonic inhibitory effect on flexor motor neurons (Fig. 44.9).

It is clear that no single tract is responsible for the development of decerebrate rigidity. It is also clear that, although the pelvic limbs demonstrate predominantly a gamma rigidity in decerebration, the pectoral limbs exhibit a combination of both alpha and gamma effects.

CEREBELLUM IN MOTOR CONTROL

The cerebellum is a portion of the metencephalon and is attached to the pons and medulla by way of the rostral, middle, and caudal cerebellar peduncles. The peduncles contain axons that pass between the cerebellum and the brain stem and spinal cord. The surface of the cerebellum is characterized by numerous folds called *folia*, separated by *sulci*, and by larger *lobes* and *lobules*, separated by *fissures*. The cerebellar surface is characterized by two hemispheres with a central *vermis*. There are three lobes of the cerebellum; the *anterior lobe*, which lies rostral to the primary fissure, the *posterior lobe*, caudal to the primary fissure, and the *flocculonodular lobe*, separated from the caudal portion of the posterior lobe by the posterolateral fissure. On an anatomical and functional basis, the vermis and paravermal region of the cortex is organized into three functional strips that extend rostrocaudally across the cerebellum (Fig. 44.11). There is a medial vermal region, associated with the underlying fastigial nucleus and the medullary and pontine reticular formation. This medial vermal strip is concerned primarily with maintenance of muscle tone through influence on the pontine and medullary reticulospinal tracts projecting to alpha and gamma motor neurons of the spinal cord. There is a lateral vermal area associated with the lateral vestibular nucleus and concerned with maintenance of head and eye posture. The more lateral, paravermal region is associated with the underlying interpositus nucleus and is concerned with control of voluntary somatic movements.

The cerebellar cortex has a similar cytoarchitectural organization throughout and appears to use similar mechanisms in all parts for handling neural information. The cortex is composed of gray matter and is organized into three layers: an outer molecular layer, an intermediate Purkinje cell layer, and a deep granular cell layer.

The molecular layer contains the cell bodies of basket and outer stellate cells (Fig. 44.12). The Purkinje cell layer contains the Purkinje cell bodies, and the granular cell layer contains the cell bodies of the Golgi type II neurons and granular cells. Figure 44.12 demonstrates the relationship of these cells to each other and to the mossy fibers and the climbing fibers, which provide afferent inputs to the cere-

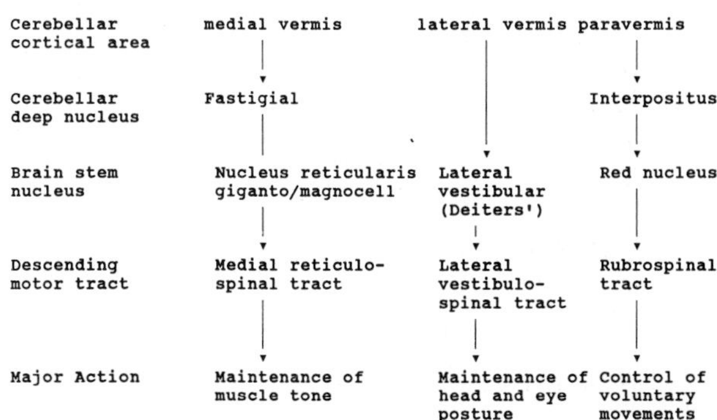

Figure 44.11. Representation of the main pathways through which the cerebellar influence is exerted on reticulospinal, lateral vestibulospinal, and rubrospinal tract.

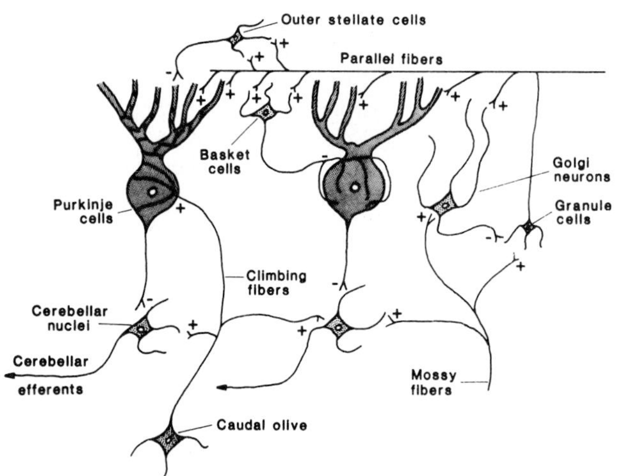

Figure 44.12. A schematic illustration of the neural elements of the cerebellar cortex. Afferents to the cortex and deep nuclei are represented by mossy fibers and climbing fibers. A plus sign indicates an excitatory synaptic influence on postsynaptic neurons, and a minus sign indicates an inhibitory synaptic influence.

bellar cortex. The pathway of information flow within the cerebellum is as follows:

1. Afferent information from all cerebellar afferent systems, with the exception of the olivocerebellar tract, enters the cerebellum through mossy fibers and excites cerebellar nuclei, Golgi type II neurons, and granular cells of the cortical granular cell layer.

2. Granular cells, through their parallel fibers, excite outer stellate cells, basket cells, and Purkinje cells and are immediately inhibited by Golgi type II neurons.

3. Purkinje cells inhibit cerebellar nuclei and neurons of the lateral vestibular nucleus and momentarily stop excitatory efferent activity passing from these nuclei to other parts of the central nervous system.

4. Purkinje cells are immediately inhibited by outer stellate cells and basket cells.

5. At the time of peak inhibition of Purkinje cells, climbing fiber activity arrives to produce an excitatory input to the cerebellar nuclei and the Purkinje cells, producing a second brief burst of action potentials from Purkinje cells.

6. Purkinje cells again momentarily inhibit cerebellar or vestibular nuclei, interrupting their excitatory efferent influence on extracerebellar structures.

The time delay between arrival of extracerebellar information over mossy fibers and climbing fibers is important in the timing of Purkinje cell inhibition of cerebellar and lateral vestibular nuclei to interrupt outflow from the cerebellum. This outflow is in all cases excitatory to the nuclei of termination of efferents from the cerebellar and lateral vestibular nuclei. This inhibition produces a brief period of removal of excitation (known as *inhibition through disfacilitation*) interrupting excitatory drive to those structures influenced by the cerebellum. It appears that the only mode through which the cerebellar cortex can operate is through inhibition of extracerebellar nuclei by disfacilitation.

In the previous examples, it has been emphasized that the cerebellum is an error-detection and reset device for somatic movements. For it to carry out this function, it is necessary that it receive input from a set point determinant. This information can then be compared with input derived from the external environment and from the muscles, tendons, and joints involved in movement and posture, degree of muscle tone, and rates of contraction and relaxation of muscles during movement. With this information, the cerebellum can compare the movement being made with the set point information and, through efferent pathways to the motor control neurons, correct errors as the movement is being carried out. The principal connections of the cerebellum involved in this process are illustrated in Fig. 44.13.

It can be seen from Fig. 44.13 that influences from the cerebral cortex involving other ongoing motor and sensory events are integrated with spinal cord input to determine the pattern of motor action that will be allowed. Afferents to the cerebellum represent, in density, about two times that of cerebellar efferents. The major afferent pathways are primarily the dorsal and ventral spinocerebellar, olivocerebellar, reticulocerebellar, vestibulocerebellar, and pontocerebellar tracts (Figs. 44.3, 44.4, 44.8, and 44.13).

The dorsal spinocerebellar tract arises from the dorsal nucleus (of Clarke), located within the dorsomedial portion of lamina VII of the spinal gray, and extends from the eighth cervical (C-8) to the third lumbar (L-3) segment of the cord. This tract projects ipsilaterally within the dorsolateral portion of the lateral funiculus to terminate in the anterior lobe

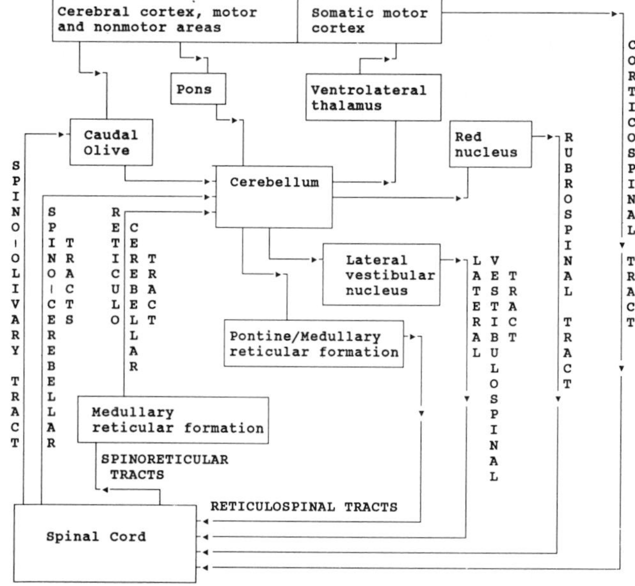

Figure 44.13. Cerebellar control for voluntary limb movements. The afferents and efferents of the cerebellum for control are illustrated.

and the paramedian and pyramis lobules of the cerebellum. The dorsal spinocerebellar tract principally contains axons that are excited by class Ia and II afferents from muscle spindles and by Ib afferents from Golgi tendon organs, as well as cutaneous, touch, and pressure axons. Afferents from thoracic, lumbar, sacral, and caudal nerves are contained within the dorsal spinocerebellar tract.

Class Ia afferents to the cervical spinal cord have descending projections that reach the dorsal nucleus of the thoracic spinal cord and therefore activate the dorsal spinocerebellar tract. These afferents, as well as Ib afferents from Golgi tendon organs of cervical muscles, joint angle, cutaneous, and pressure afferents of the neck, also project axons to the lateral cuneate nucleus, forming part of the spino-cuneato-cerebellar tract. This tract has terminations in the cerebellum that are very similar to those of the dorsal spinocerebellar tract.

The ventral spinocerebellar tract arises from neurons that occupy laminae VI and VII of the spinal gray along the entire length of the spinal cord. The ventral spinocerebellar tract axons cross to the opposite side of the spinal cord and project to the cerebellum through the rostral cerebellar peduncle. This tract is activated principally by class Ib afferents from Golgi tendon organs, although there is some activation by tactile and joint angle receptors. The ventral spinocerebellar tract terminates within the same regions of the cerebellar cortex as does the dorsal spinocerebellar tract.

Spino-reticulo-cerebellar tracts relay through the lateral reticular nucleus of the medulla and carry information derived from flexor reflex afferents entering the spinal cord. Flexor reflex afferents represent class II and III muscle afferents, cutaneous afferents, and high-threshold joint sensory afferents. At the spinal level these afferents elicit flexor reflexes. The projections to the cerebellum provide information concerning stimuli that are likely to be aversive. These tracts arise primarily from laminae VI, VII, and VIII of the spinal gray matter and project bilaterally to the brain within the ventral and lateral portions of the lateral funiculus.

The spino-olivary tract arises from laminae IV, V, and VI of the dorsal horn, crosses to the opposite side of the cord, ascends along the ventral lateral portion of the lateral funiculus, and terminates within the caudal olivary complex of the medulla oblongata. This tract is excited by cutaneous, muscle, and joint afferents. Other inputs from the cerebral hemispheres to the caudal olivary complex provide input concerning a wide variety of somatic motor and sensory activity. The olivocerebellar tract crosses within the medulla to terminate within the cerebellum as the sole source of cortical climbing fibers. As already outlined, these fibers are critical to the normal function of the cerebellum.

The pontine gray matter receives input from the entire cerebral hemisphere and transmits information to the cerebellum. This cortico-ponto-cerebellar pathway is constantly active, providing the cerebellum with neural analogues of both sensory and motor activity of the cerebrum.

When cerebellar afferents and efferents are compared, it is apparent that there are extensive reciprocal connections between the cerebellum and other central nervous system structures (Fig. 44.13). This reciprocal nature of cerebellar connections has led to the concept that the cerebellum functions as a follow-up servomechanism for correction (error detection and reset) of motor activity as it is carried out. This function has been illustrated in the previously described motor activities. In addition, the cerebellum smooths out motor irregularities produced by alterations in the environment, compares the intended motor action with the activity of muscle, joint, and cutaneous afferent activity produced by the movement, and makes adjustments so that the intended motor action is well coordinated with postural maintenance.

There are a number of closed loops in the cerebellar control pathways; for example, vestibulo-cerebello-vestibular, spino-cerebello-spinal (via rubrospinal, corticospinal, reticulospinal, and vestibulospinal tracts), and cerebro-cerebello-cerebral loops are well established in all mammals (Fig. 44.13). These loops are continually active, processing ongoing environmental information with reflex activity and intended somatic movements. The components of the cerebellum that function in such closed-loop feedback pathways occupy the most medial corticonuclear components of the cerebellum (vestibular, fastigial, and interpositus nuclei).

Another type of loop, an open loop involving nonreciprocal connections (such as cerebro-cerebellar from the sensory and association areas of the cerebral cortex) affects the spinal cord and brain-stem mechanisms through systems that do not immediately feed back to the origin of the activity for modification of ongoing activity. These latter loops involve the more laterally located corticonuclear components of the cerebellum (interpositus and dentate nuclei).

Closed feedback loops are relatively insensitive to exter-

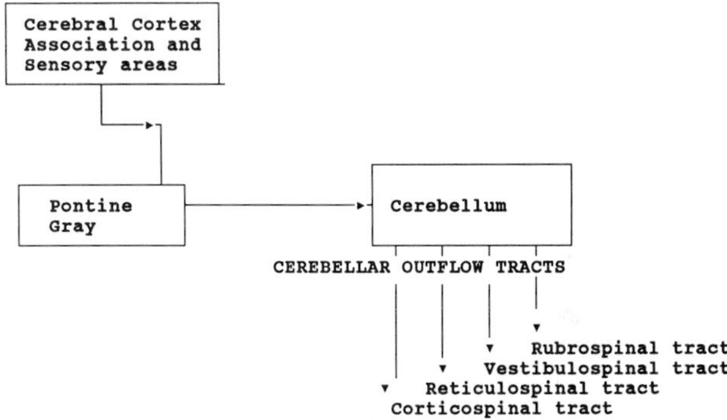

Figure 44.14. Feed-forward loops through the cerebellum for somatic motor control that do not involve tactile and vestibular input.

nal disturbances and other changes in control values and require considerable loop time for their action. A relatively uncomplicated pathway from input to output is required for a good feedback-control loop to function. In motor control, many motor activities are carried out at far too rapid a rate to allow a feedback system to operate. In these cases, feed-forward loops, with their shorter loop time, allow rapid motor action to occur. Figure 44.14 illustrates a feed-forward loop for cerebellar function in rapid motor acts.

PATTERN GENERATORS FOR RHYTHMIC MOTOR ACTIVITY

Many somatic motor actions demonstrate a rhythmicity produced by interneurons interacting in an organized fashion. These populations of interneurons are referred to as *pattern generators*. Pattern generators are composed of two reciprocating half-centers—one for excitation of a group of muscles and relaxation of their antagonists and the other for excitation of the antagonists and inhibition of the agonists. Pattern generators, with the possible exception of those that regulate respiration, do not have an inherent pacemaker function but require excitation either from the brain or from sensory input to the nervous system. The pattern generator of the respiratory system has long been recognized to determine the basic rate and rhythm of respiration. A detailed discussion of this mechanism is presented in Chapter 13. Similar pattern generators for mastication, rumination, and eructation are located within the brain stem. The basic mechanism for synchronized, sequential limb movements during locomotion resides within the locomotor pattern generators of the spinal cord.

SPINAL CORD PATTERN GENERATORS FOR LOCOMOTION

Walk, trot, and gallop (or in some cases canter) are the three basic gaits of most quadrupeds. Some animals, such as many cats and camels, do not gallop, in which case the gallop gait is replaced by a canter. In all these actions, however, each individual limb undergoes a characteristic movement called a *step cycle*. A step cycle is the period from the instant a foot leaves the ground, until it leaves the ground again during locomotion. Each step cycle is divided into two phases—a *swing phase* and a *support phase*. During the swing phase the foot is free of the supporting surface and undergoes, first, a flexion and then an extension to strike the surface. The support phase involves an extension of the limb to bear the animal's weight. The end of the support phase represents a period of extensor propulsion and provides most of the force of movement.

There are four locomotor pattern generators within the spinal cord. Each generator governs the somatic motor activity of one limb. These populations of interneurons are located deep within the dorsal horn, bordering on the intermediate gray of the spinal cord. Each generator contains a half-center for excitation and inhibition of limb-extensor muscles and another half-center for excitation and inhibition of limb-flexor muscles. The four pattern generators are interrelated in their activity through crossed and uncrossed, ascending and descending axonal systems, including the propriospinal and ventral spinocerebellar tracts of the surrounding white matter. These tracts serve to interconnect the pattern generators with each other and produce the interlimb coordination of the gaits of locomotion.

Locomotor pattern generators require a tonic excitatory input from the brain and/or through peripheral nerves to activate them. When activated, these generators can produce all phases of step cycles for walking, trotting, or galloping (or cantering). With increasing speeds of forward movement, the duration of the swing phase of the step cycle remains relatively constant. The supporting phase, however, is gradually shortened, resulting in a step cycle of shortened duration. The speed of locomotion is determined by the distance that individual limbs travel during the swing phase. This distance is proportional to the propulsive force provided by the terminal, extensor component of the support phase. The pattern of motor neuron activity, resulting in smooth, stable limb movements during the step cycle, is basically dependent on the activity of the pattern generator for the individual limbs as modified by reflex and other central influences.

The role of the other brain-stem structures and the cerebellum in activation of the spinal cord pattern generators during walking appears to be to provide and control descending tract activity for regulation of the generators and to provide postural stability. Stimulation of the mesencephalic locomotor area, discussed below, is associated with rhythmic waxing and waning of activity in the reticulospinal, rubrospinal, and vestibulospinal tracts. The reticulospinal and rubrospinal tracts show an increased activity during the swing phase of the step cycle and the vestibulospinal tracts during the support phase. Direct stimulation of these tracts, however, does not influence the sequence of muscle activity but alters the intensity of activity during the periods of the step cycle in which they ordinarily would be active. It is clear that activity of these descending tracts does not establish the rhythm of locomotion. The entire range of locomotion can be produced by stimulation of the mesencephalic locomotor area in cats in which the cerebellum has been removed. In these animals, the phasic discharge of the descending tracts does not occur and the animals lack the good coordination of limb movements observed in similar animals with the cerebellum intact. The relationship of the cerebellum to the neurons of these descending tracts is indicated in Fig. 44.13. The cerebellum, therefore, appears to be an important component of a feedback regulatory system involving the reticulospinal, vestibulospinal, and rubrospinal tracts. This system produces stability and determines the force of muscle contraction during locomotion.

The lateral vestibular (Deiters') nucleus gives rise to the

lateral vestibulospinal tract, while the red nucleus is the origin of the rubrospinal tract. Both paths provide excitatory synaptic terminals at all levels of the cat's spinal cord. The overall effect of the lateral vestibulospinal tract is to facilitate extensor (or antigravity) motor neurons, and that of the rubrospinal tract is to facilitate flexor (or orthogravity) motor neurons.

SUBTHALAMIC LOCOMOTOR AREA

An intact brain is necessary to produce normal locomotion with the maintenance of a stable posture and without disturbances in pattern, synchrony, and strength of muscle activity. In the cat, large portions of the brain may be removed with little indication of locomotor alteration. A cat in which both cerebral hemispheres, including all subcortical nuclear structures and the rostral and dorsal portions of the thalamus, have been removed, leaving intact the caudal portion of the subthalamus, can walk almost normally. Such an animal demonstrates spontaneous walking with a well-coordinated gait and normal maintenance of postural equilibrium but cannot avoid obstacles placed in its path. This decerebrate animal cannot carry out the fine motor control that is necessary to climb a ladder or to walk on a narrow ledge. If electrode stimulation is carried out within a small area of the diencephalon called the *subthalamic locomotor area*, located just dorsal and medial to the subthalamic nucleus, the animal will demonstrate an increase in speed of walking as the intensity of stimulus is increased. At a critical walking speed, the pattern of locomotion changes from a walk to a trot and, at higher speeds, to a gallop or a canter. The gait of locomotion initiated in this manner is related to speed. The speed of movement is, in turn, related to the intensity of stimulus applied to the subthalamic locomotor area of the brain.

The anatomic location of the subthalamic locomotor area has not been clearly delineated, and it is possible that it corresponds to an area of concentrated axons projecting from other motor centers of the brain toward their nuclei of termination. Therefore, it is not truly a locomotor center. The subthalamic nucleus, however, is very much an integral component of the somatic motor controls.

MESENCEPHALIC LOCOMOTOR AREA

Bilateral lesions in the subthalamic locomotor area of the brain abolish spontaneous locomotion in decerebrate animals. If, however, electrical stimulation is applied to the mesencephalic tegmentum within the pedunculopontine nucleus, walking and running with good postural maintenance can again be elicited in the decerebrate cat. This region of the midbrain is called the *mesencephalic locomotor area*. As with subthalamic locomotor area stimulation, increasing the intensity of stimulation results in increased speed of walking, followed by trotting and galloping or cantering. The synchrony of joint movements and the sequence of limb movements occur as in the intact animal.

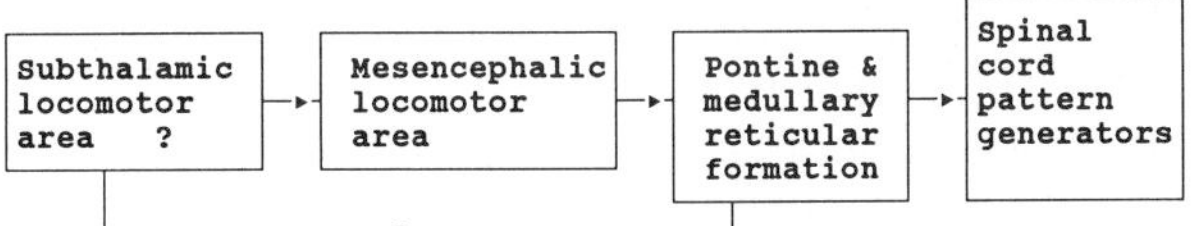

Figure 44.15. Subthalamic and mesencephalic locomotor areas and their relationships to spinal cord locomotor pattern generators.

Although lesions of the mesencephalic locomotor area do not prevent the initiation of locomotion through stimulation of the subthalamic area, it appears from anatomic and physiologic studies that the subthalamic locomotor area normally elicits its motor action through the mesencephalic locomotor area (Fig. 44.15).

In animals with intact brains, it is unlikely that the mesencephalic or subthalamic locomotor areas initiate and carry out locomotion; they probably represent focal areas through which cerebral locomotor mechanisms have their function. From anatomic and physiologic studies, it is apparent that these areas are an integral part of the general cerebral locomotor control mechanism involving the cerebral cortex and basal ganglia.

BASAL GANGLIA

The basal ganglia (Fig. 44.16) are a collection of nuclear structures within the telencephalon, midbrain, and subthalamus that are significantly involved in the organization of somatic motor activity. The components of this system include the caudate nucleus, putamen, globus pallidus, endopeduncular nucleus, subthalamic nucleus, and substantia nigra. Some authors include the amygdaloid nuclear complex of the temporal lobes of the hemispheres, which has significant olfactory and limbic system functions. Others will include the red nucleus of the mesencephalon, which serves as a somatic motor control system but is more cor-

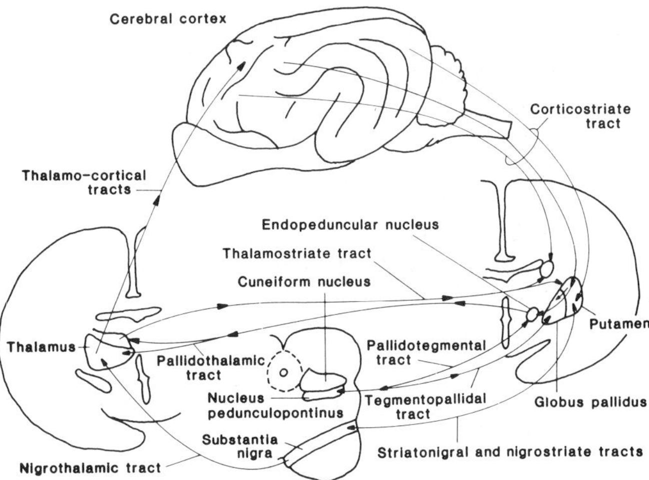

Figure 44.16. Schematic illustration of some of the feedback loops that operate in the involvement of the basal ganglia in motor control.

rectly seen as a major efferent system for the cerebral motor cortex and cerebellar control of motor activity. Classically, the basal ganglia have been thought to function as an internal loop system from most of the cerebral cortex to the striatum, to globus pallidus and substantia nigra, to the thalamus, and then to the motor cortex for carrying out somatic motor activation. The major circuitry of the basal ganglia is illustrated in Figs. 44.16 and 44.17.

The *caudate nucleus* and the *putamen* are collectively known as the *corpus striatum* (or simply the *striatum*) because they develop from a single nuclear structure and become partially separated by the internal capsule during cerebrogenesis. In this way, the caudate nucleus comes to lie dorsomedial and the putamen ventrolateral to the internal capsule. The primordial common origin is reflected by cellular bridges extending through the internal capsule connecting the two structures. The striatum receives excitatory projections from the cerebral cortex, nucleus centre medianum (one of the intralaminar nuclei of the thalamus), and substantia nigra (pars compacta). The substantia nigra provides a well-known excitatory, dopaminergic input, which shows deficiency of transmitter agent in Parkinson's disease in humans. Patients with Parkinson's disease demonstrate postural instability, tremor, and rigidy and exhibit difficulty in the initiation of movement. Treatment of monkeys with a piperidine derivative, N-methyl-4-phenyl-1-,2,5,6-tetrahydropyridine, produces a condition very similar to Parkinson's disease and is associated with deficiency of dopamine in the basal ganglia.

Bilateral lesions of the substantia nigra occur in horses poisoned with yellow star thistle. These animals demonstrate a lack of ability to prehend food with their lips (the major prehension organ of the horse). They exhibit a passivity of facial expression, somewhat reminiscent of the human patient with Parkinson's disease.

Striatal outputs terminate in the globus pallidus (which, in primates, has external and internal segments, with the endopeduncular nucleus of nonprimates representing the internal segment) and in the substantia nigra (pars reticulata). These striatonigral axons are well known as the gamma aminobutyric acid projections of the striatum.

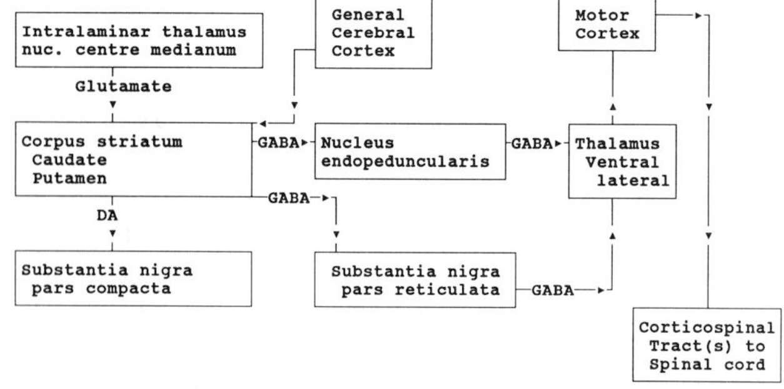

Figure 44.17. Major functional neural connections of the basal ganglia demonstrating the neurotransmitters assumed to provide transmission of either excitatory (dopamine [DA] and glutamate) or inhibitory (gamma amino butyric acid [GABA]) influences.

The major outputs of the basal ganglia arise in the endopeduncular nucleus and the substantia nigra and project to the ventral lateral thalamus for relay to the somatic motor and premotor cortex. These outputs also use gamma aminobutyric acid as a neurotransmitter and are inhibitory to the ventral lateral thalamus. It can be seen from the schematic (Fig. 44.17) that when the corpus striatum is excited, it will inhibit the endopeduncular nucleus and the substantia nigra and remove inhibition of the ventral lateral thalamus. The net result is increased excitability of the ventral lateral thalamus, with increased excitation of the motor cortex.

The basal ganglia are organized to function through a system of feedback loops (Figs. 44.16 and 44.17). These feedback loops contain a number of synaptic junctions through which other neural influences can modify the loop activity. Feedback loops require time for adjustment and function best in the generation of slowly developing activities. The basal ganglia receive input from the sensory, motor, and association areas of the cerebral cortex. They cooperate with these areas of the cerebral hemisphere in the preprogramming of somatic muscle activity in voluntary motor activation. The continual activity of the basal ganglion loop system results in a continuous excitation of the mesencephalic locomotor area (nucleus pedunculopontinus). This tonic input to the locomotor center is capable of exciting spinal cord locomotor pattern generators involved in the control of locomotion.

Few well-controlled studies have been conducted in domestic animals to determine the deficiencies that result from basal ganglion damage. Bilateral lesions in the head of the caudate nucleus in the cat result in locomotor hyperactivity, which is nearly identical to that produced by lesions in the prefrontal association area. In these animals locomotor activity is increased with increased ambient light or sound stimuli. Hyperactivity ceases in a quiet, darkened environment. Unilateral lesions of the caudate nucleus produce hyperactivity and circling in the direction of the side of the lesion.

CEREBRAL CORTEX IN MOTOR CONTROL

The neural circuitry of the cerebral cortex is designed to process spatial and temporal patterns of neural activity underlying motor functions. The functions of the somatic motor areas of the cerebral cortex are to translate goal-directed motor programs into appropriate coordinated muscle activity. Three functional areas of the cerebral cortex—the primary motor area, a premotor area, and a supplemental motor area—have been demonstrated to play a role in the processing of somatic motor activity. The primary motor cortex is located in the precruciate region of the hemisphere and serves as the origin of a major portion of the corticospinal and corticobulbar tracts for control of motor activities derived from the brain stem and spinal cord. Ablation of the primary cortex has the most severe functional consequences, and neural activity of the primary area more clearly synchronizes the final motor output. The supplemental and premotor areas of the hemisphere are adjacent to the primary area, and they demonstrate less specificity in regard to motor control and less severity of deficits when damaged.

When electrical stimulation is applied to the somatic motor areas of the cerebral cortex, muscle movement can be elicited. When a systematic study of this nature is carried out, a somatotropic organization emerges, allowing the mapping of a rough figurine of the animal's musculature on the cerebral surface. The relative degree of cortical motor control to various body parts is reflected in the area of the cerebral cortex that is involved in controlling muscles in that region of the body. In pigs and horses, the lips and nose are represented in large areas of the cortex, whereas the legs and feet have little representation. In the raccoon, on the other hand, the forepaws have a large representation, reflecting the fine digital control exhibited by these animals.

The supplemental and premotor cortical areas are involved in preprogramming of motor activity, particularly that which is dependent on sensory guidance. These areas would be quite important in the dog catching a Frisbee in that they would be responsible for the final integration of vision, speed, and distance judgment necessary to provide proper timing of the jump, posturing of the head, and jaw activity to catch the Frisbee. An important role of the premotor cortex in preprogramming of movements is establishment of the motor set, or the state of readiness to make a particular movement. To accomplish this, the premotor cortex receives input from a number of visual, auditory, and somatic sensory areas of the cerebral hemisphere as well as from the cerebellum and amygdala. In a complex movement, a number of motor sets may be required to complete the movement. In the Frisbee-catching dog, a motor set would be required for the jump, to allow collection of the limbs and a proper spring to propel the dog on its proper trajectory. Another motor set would then be required to provide a setting from which the head and neck movements could be made, and an additional motor set would be required for opening the jaws and grasping the Frisbee.

The primary motor area is interconnected with the premotor and supplemental motor areas and is involved in the integration of premotor activity into a motor act. Important in this integration is continual sensory input from muscles and skin to the somatic motor cortex (Fig. 44.18). Another important sensorimotor loop of the primary motor cortex involves the cerebellum (Fig. 44.19). This loop is integrated with input from the basal ganglia, as described above. Although these loops are reflex in nature and operate in unconscious adjustments of muscle activity, they are also functional in voluntary somatic motor movements.

The corticospinal tract is the major descending tract from the primary motor cortex (Fig. 44.10). The axons of this

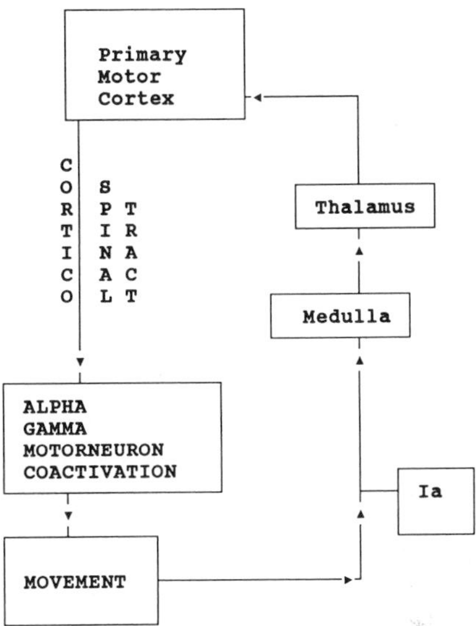

Figure 44.18. Functional loop involving the primary motor cortex, mediating voluntary motor activity. This represents the "long loop" of the myotatic reflex depicted in Fig. 44.7.

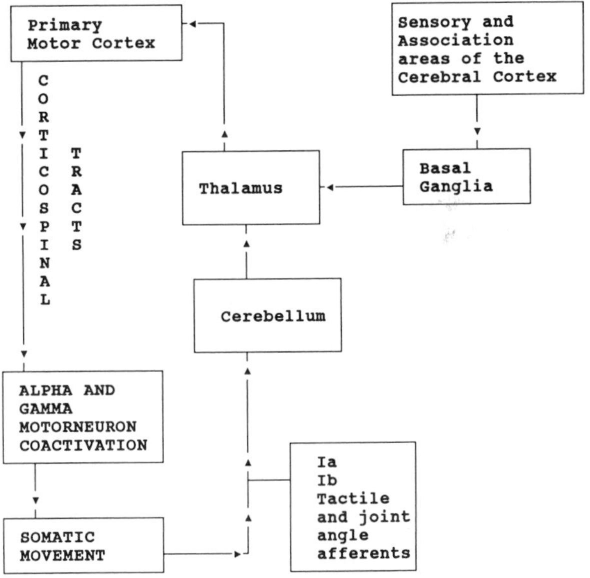

Figure 44.19. Illustration of the interaction of the basal ganglia and the cerebellum in the control of somatic motor cortex control of voluntary movement.

tract originate from pyramidal cells in layers III and V of the motor cortex. These axons pass through the internal capsule and cerebral peduncles with other axons that contribute to corticothalamic, corticopontine, and corticomedullary tracts, some of which provide motor control to striated muscles of the eye, tongue, face, mandible, pharynx, and larynx. Others terminate within the brain-stem reticular formation and sensory relay nuclei of the brain stem for sensory control functions. The corticospinal tract emerges from the caudal surface of the pons as the medullary pyramids, extending along the ventral surface of the medulla. At the spinomedullary junction, the pyramids decussate and give rise to lateral and ventral corticospinal tracts, descending within the lateral and ventral funiculi, respectively.

The function of the corticospinal tract is much more important in primates than in nonprimate mammals. Transection of the pyramid or ablation of the primary motor cortex in monkeys produces severe deficits of motor control contralateral to the side of the lesion. These deficits are characterized by paresis (weakness of motor action) and a loss of control of fine movement, with a marked deficit in coordination of limb movements during locomotion. Similar lesions in humans produce paralysis. In cats and dogs, transection produces a persistent hypermetria and loss of tactile placing and hopping reflexes in the affected limbs.

The function of the primary motor cortex in domestic nonprimates is to correlate somatic motor activity with somatic and vestibular sensory inputs. The primary motor cortex and the tracts that originate from it (the corticospinal, corticorubral and corticoreticular tracts) do not appear to function in the decision-making process of locomotion, in the timing of rapid movements, or in the generation of slow movements. Although it is generally considered that the somatic motor cortex is an important element in the voluntary motor control system, it is not necessary for the normal conduct of voluntary motor action in most domestic animals.

ASSOCIATION AREAS OF THE CEREBRAL CORTEX

The association areas of the cerebral hemispheres represent most of the cortex that is not occupied by primary or secondary sensory or motor cortex. These areas represent a large proportion of the cerebral cortex and have generally been relegated the function of associating various sensory functions into some meaningful sensory perception that relates to memory. The association cortex has also been incriminated in a large number of functions, such as the patterning of various behaviors, memory, recall, intellect, and limbic system functions associated with visceral and endocrine controls. The association cortex is involved in the organization and initiation of somatic motor activities.

A series of repeatable electroencephalographic alterations preceding specific motor acts have been well demonstrated in primates and the cat. At about 150 ms before the initiation of a voluntary motor act, a readiness potential is recorded over the frontal and parietal association cortex areas. About 90 ms before movement, a second premotion potential is recorded over the same areas. Even though the movement may involve only one limb (such as pressing a lever with the right forepaw), these potentials are recorded bilaterally. Within 50 ms before the movement, a third potential change, the motor potential, is recorded over the motor cortex opposite the side of the movement. It appears that preplanning of the movement involves the association of a variety of cortical activities before involvement of the primary motor cortex.

There are three general association areas that are topographically and anatomically separable (Fig. 44.20). The *frontal cortex* (often called the orbitofrontal area or prefrontal association area) lies rostral to the primary motor cortex and extends to the ventral and medial surface of the frontal portion of the hemisphere. The *temporal* association area occupies the nonauditory portion of the temporal lobe of the brain, and the *parietotemporo-occipital* association area lies caudal to the somatosensory cortex and lateral to the visual cortex. The three association areas are interconnected by fibers of the cerebral cortical white matter, so that each receives axons from and projects axons to the others. Although all association cortex areas may function in preprogramming of a planned or voluntary movement, it appears that locomotion programming more likely occurs, at least in its final stages, within the prefrontal association cortex.

The prefrontal association cortex is closely associated with structures of the limbic system, which is important in the organization of behavioral responses resulting in endocrine, visceral, and somatic motor activity. An influence of the prefrontal cortex on locomotor activity is demonstrated by ablation of the region in the cat or monkey. Such a lesion results in an initial period of hypoactivity, followed in a few days (in the cat) to a few weeks (in the monkey) by hyperactivity. The hyperactivity is reflected in continuous, stereotyped, aimless pacing. The pacing is diminished or may disappear in the dark and is increased with increasing ambient illumination or sound. Such hyperactivity can be diminished or stopped with administration of amphetamines or other cerebral stimulants. Lesions of the prefrontal association areas also result in learning deficits that may or may not be related to the influence on somatic motor activity.

The role of the prefrontal association cortex in the organization and initiation of somatic motor activity is made more obvious by the fact that a significant efferent pathway

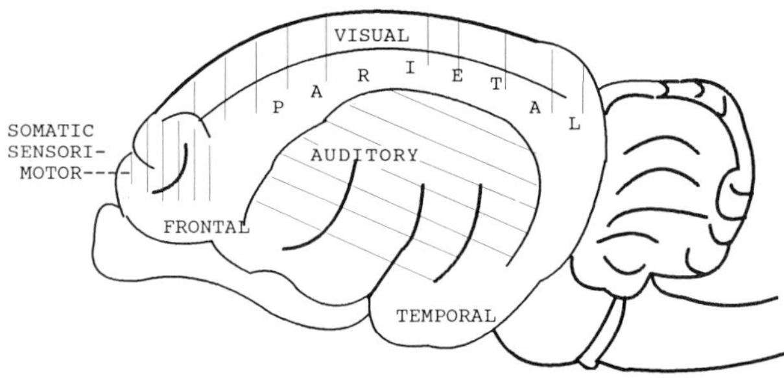

Figure 44.20. Schematic of the functional areas of the cerebral cortex, indicating the location of the frontal, parietal, and temporal association areas. The relationship of the association areas to sensory and motor areas can be seen.

from this area of the cortex projects to the head of the caudate nucleus. The caudate nucleus is a portion of the basal ganglia that has long been recognized as being an important somatic motor control system. Two distinctive efferent systems have been demonstrated to project from the prefrontal association cortex to the caudate nucleus; a ventral projection from the ventral surface of the cortex to the ventrolateral portions of the head of the caudate nucleus and a dorsal projection from the dorsolateral area of the prefrontal cortex to the rostral and dorsal portions of the head of the caudate nucleus. These projections are quite important in the preprogramming of voluntary movements.

BRAIN-STEM RETICULAR FORMATION AND MOTOR CONTROL

The brain-stem reticular formation (described in Chap. 48) plays a key role in somatic and visceral motor control. Reticulospinal tracts arising from the medullary and pontine reticular formation have long been recognized to play a significant role in somatic motor control. Reticulospinal tract neurons represent a major component of the *upper motor neurons* in veterinary clinical neurology. Damage to descending tracts in the spinal cord produces what is called an *upper motor neuron disorder*. Upper motor neuron disorders are characterized by a diminished muscle tone and hyperreflexia of somatic musculature. This combination produces an interesting condition known as *spasticity*. Spasticity is characterized by the nature of resistance to passive flexion of a joint. As a joint is flexed by manual force, there is at first no resistance to movement. This is referred to as the *free area* of the movement. The free area of passive movement results from a diminished muscle tone and, presumably, diminished gamma loop activity. As the joint flexion progresses, however, there is a gradual building of resistance to flexion. The resistance to movement represents hyperexcitability of myotatic reflex arcs.

Other functions of the medullary and pontine reticular formation and the reticulospinal tracts include respiratory control (Fig. 44.21), cardiovascular regulation (Fig. 44.22), micturition control (Fig. 44.23), emesis (Fig. 44.24), and, in ruminants, eructation and rumination, deglutition, mastication, suckling, coughing, and many other similar responses. In some cases the reticular formation serves to provide interneurons for reflex arcs carrying out these functions. In other instances, aggregates of reticular formation neurons interact to provide functional centers within which these responses are organized. These centers are referred to as centers for cardiovascular control, respiration, micturition, deglutition, emesis, and rumination. In fact, they are not separate and distinct centers but overlap considerably with each other. Neurons functioning in the control of one system lie adjacent to neurons that control other systems.

The caudal pontine and rostral medullary reticular formation can be divided into three zones based on their relationships to (1) the limbic system; (2) oculomotor, neck, ear, and trunk postural motor neurons; and (3) cranial nerve control to the trigeminal, facial, vagus, glossopharyngeal, and respiratory nerves. These zones are illustrated in Fig. 44.24. From this illustration, it can be seen that these regions of the reticular formation contain neurons that represent the last in a chain of neurons (often called *premotor neurons*) that affect a wide range of motor actions.

Optokinetic and vestibulo-ocular reflexes cause a slow movement of the eyes with a quick return. The brain mechanisms for slow movements have been described above. The rapid return to establish a new fixed image on the retina is called a *saccadic movement*. The medial medullary and pontine reticular formation are essential for the production

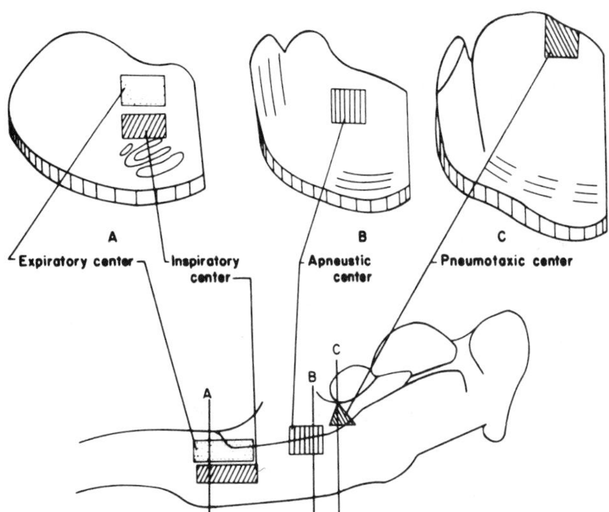

Figure 44.21. Location of respiratory centers within the reticular formtion of the brain stem.

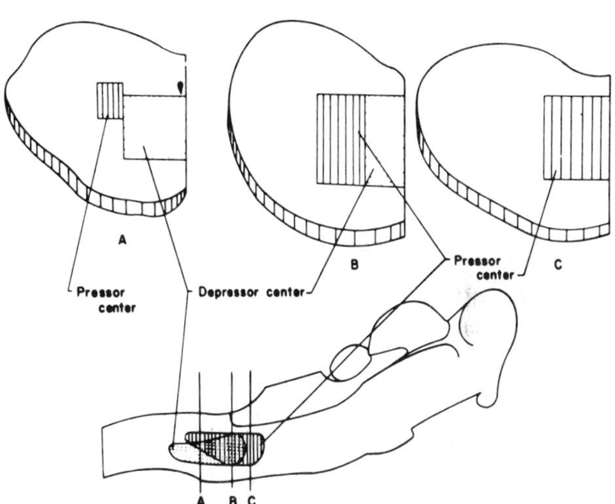

Figure 44.22. Location of the vasomotor centers within the reticular formation of the brain stem.

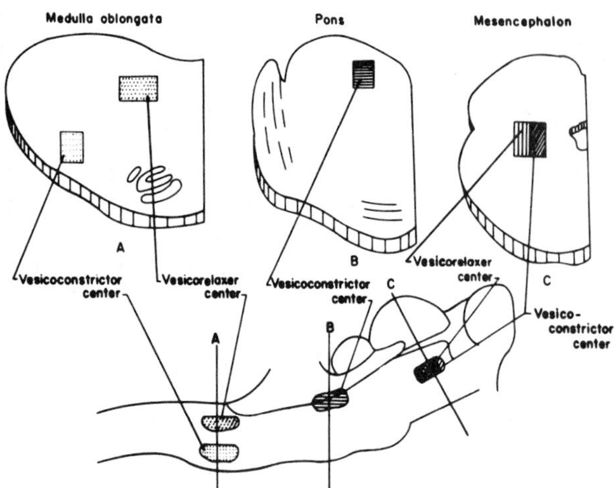

Figure 44.23. Location of micturition centers within the reticular formation of the brain stem.

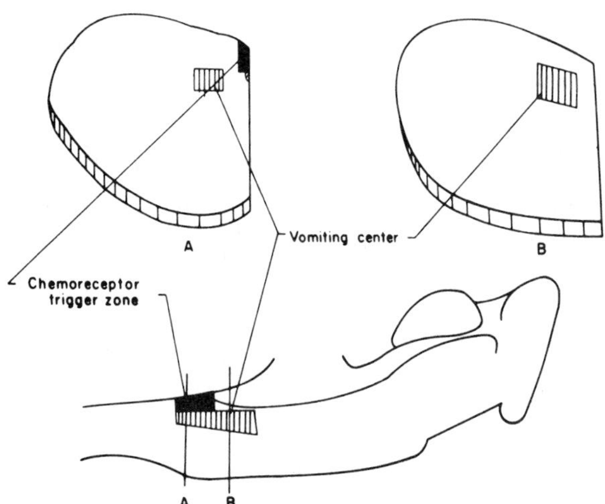

Figure 44.24. Location of the chemoreceptor trigger zone and the emetic center within the reticular formation of the brain stem.

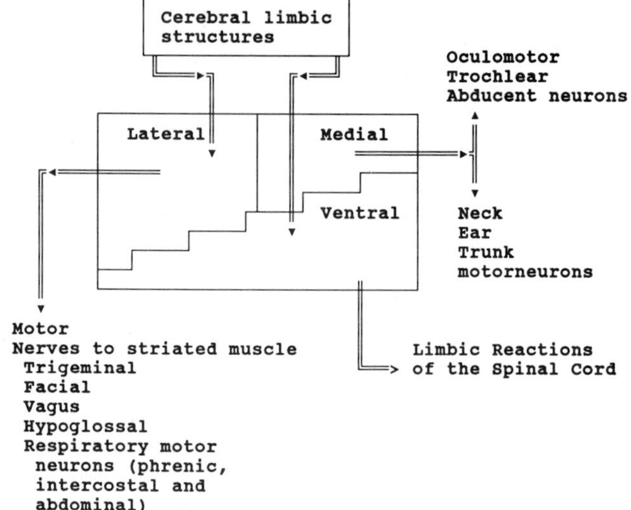

Figure 44.25. Caudal pontine and rostral medullary reticular formation can be divided into three transverse zones on the basis of anatomical and physiological properties.

of saccadic eye movements. Input to the reticular formation is derived from the visual areas of the cerebral cortex and the rostral colliculus. It appears that all the motor neuron innervation for saccadic movements come from the medial medullary and pontine reticular formation. The same regions of the reticular formation also provide descending tracts for the mediation of ear, neck, and postural trunk muscle activity (Fig. 44.25).

The ventral portion of the caudal pontine and medullary reticular formation, specifically the raphe nuclei (magnus and pallidus) and the adjacent areas, projects reticulospinal tract axons, which terminate throughout the full length of the spinal cord. The axons project to parasympathetic motor neurons of the caudal brain stem and to parasympathetic and sympathetic neurons of the spinal cord. Nucleus raphe pallidus also projects axons to cranial nerve motor neurons of the trigeminal, facial, glossopharyngeal, and hypoglossal nerves (but not to the oculomotor, trochlear, and abducent motor nuclei). Many of these neurons contain serotonin, substance P, and leu-enkephalin, which serve as neurotransmitters for somatic and autonomic responses to limbic system inputs.

Nucleus subcoeruleus and the nucleus of Kölliker-Fuse, located in the dorsolateral pontine tegmentum, are considered to be specializations of the pontine reticular formation. These nuclei project to the dorsal horn and intermediate gray and to autonomic and somatic motor nuclei throughout the length of the spinal cord. These nuclei also project axons to autonomic and somatic motor nuclei of the caudal brain stem (trigeminal, facial, vagus, and hypoglossal) but not to the motor nuclei innervating extrinsic eye muscles. Both nuclei contain norepinephrine, which serves as a neurotransmitter. Lesions of these nuclei result in a depletion of norepinephrine throughout the spinal cord.

The lateral part of the pontine and medullary reticular formation controls trigeminal, facial, vagal, and hypoglossal neurons of the brain stem and respiratory motor neurons (phrenic, intercostal, and abdominal motor neurons) of the spinal cord (Fig. 44.25). This spinal projection of the reticulospinal tracts represents the neural basis for respiration, swallowing, and vomiting. This region of the reticular formation, in addition to the ventral area, receives considerable afferent input from structures of the cerebral limbic system through which blood pressure and respiration are controlled in emotional behavior. The medial region of the pontine and medullary reticular formation does not receive limbic system afferents, which indicates that the ocular movement and postural control systems are not under such direct control in emotional behavior.

POSTURAL CONTROL

For each species of animal there is a recognized normal posture or attitude within the field of gravity. The maintenance of this posture is accomplished through the continuous activity of a complex of interacting *postural reflexes*. There are three general types of postural reflex: local static reactions, segmental static reactions, and general static reactions. The latter include tonic neck and labyrinthine reflexes.

Local static reactions of the limbs are involved in producing a fixed standing posture that prevents collapse under the force of gravity. These reactions involve simultaneous contraction of antagonistic muscle groups. The myotatic reflex, which is a major antigravity response, is not in itself sufficient to provide postural support. Cutaneous reflexes are also involved.

Local static reactions are operative in the intact animal but can best be observed in the dog from which the cerebellum has been removed. In this *decerebellate* animal there are exaggerated myotatic reflexes, and an antigravity hypertonicity is produced. A light touch to the foot pads produces a reflex in which the limb follows the finger as though it were a magnet. This response, which was at first called the "magnet response," is generally known as the "positive supporting response". It is found that the tactile pressure applied to the digital pads not only produces a cutaneous reflex response but, through spreading of the toes, also produces enhanced myotatic reflexes in the interosseous muscles. The limb is then extended against the pressure, and, once active resistance to extension is met, other muscles are stretched and their myotatic reflexes become more active, producing a postural support response by the limb.

Segmental static reactions are represented by the crossed extensor reflex produced by class Ib and class II afferents of spinal nerves. When a pectoral limb is caused to extend, either from the action of a positive supporting reaction or from a crossed extensor reflex initiated by a noxious stimulus to the contralateral pectoral limb, the contralateral pelvic limb also extends. It is often stated that crossed extensor reflexes are "abnormal or clinical" reflexes, inasmuch as they are best seen in the hyperreflexic animal, but there is no doubt that they are normal physiologic reflexes in the intact animal. These reflexes involve sensory input to a local area but elicit reflex actions over wide regions of the spinal cord. The same reflex occurs in the opposite direction. When a pelvic limb is caused to extend, the opposite forelimb similarly extends. The reflex arcs in these instances involve the propriospinal system of the spinal cord. Segmental static reactions apparently use spinal cord pathways that are functional in quadrupedal locomotion.

General static reactions include tonic neck reflexes and tonic labyrinthine reflexes. As both types of reflex produce many of the same responses and are stimulated by similar inputs, it is necessary to eliminate one in order to study the other. Tonic neck reflexes, therefore, can be studied in their pure form only when the vestibular labyrinth has been bilaterally destroyed or when the vestibular component of the eighth cranial nerve is bilaterally transected.

Tonic neck reflexes are produced by movements of the head and are initiated by stretch receptors in the joint capsules of the cervical vertebrae. If the head is rotated so that an animal is looking at something to the right without turning the body, there is an increase in extensor postural tone in both right limbs and a relaxation of extensor postural tone in both left limbs. Rotation of the head dorsally, as in a cat looking up at a bird, produces an extension of both pectoral limbs and a diminished extensor tone in the pelvic limbs. Rotation of the head ventrally, as in a cat looking under a stool, produces a flexion of the pectoral limbs and an extension of the pelvic limbs. These reflexes obviously are useful in altering the posture of animals in accord with the location of their intended visual field.

VESTIBULAR SYSTEM AND LABYRINTHINE RESPONSES

The inner ear, which lies within the petrous part of the temporal bone, is a continuous series of fluid-filled cavities, the *bony (osseous) labyrinth*, that are lined with a thin periosteum and a delicate epithelioid layer. The bony labyrinth contains *perilymph*, which resembles extracellular fluid with a high concentration of protein. Perilymph is continuous between the auditory and vestibular parts of the labyrinth. The auditory part is the *cochlea*, and the vestibular part is the *vestibulum* and the *semicircular canals*. The bony labyrinth contains a continuous series of epithelium-lined chambers and ducts known as the *membranous labyrinth*.

The vestibular component of the membranous labyrinth is composed of two widely communicating membranous sacs—the *saccule* and the *utricle*—and *three semicircular canals* (Fig. 44.26). The membranous labyrinth is filled with *endolymph*. Endolymph contains low concentrations of protein, high concentrations of potassium, and considerable quantities of mucopolysaccharides. The vestibular receptor organs represent specialized areas of neuroepithelium located within the saccule, the utricle, and each of the semicircular canals. The receptors of the saccule and utricle are called *maculae*, and those of the semicircular canals are called *cristae ampullaris*.

The maculae are called *otolithic organs* because of their structure. They are composed of a plaque of *hair cells* that serve as sensory receptor cells. Hair cells have on their luminal surface a large number of stereocilia and a single kinetocilium. These structures project from the cell surface into an overlying *statoconial membrane* that is covered with a layer of *otoliths*. The statoconial membrane is composed of mucopolysaccharides, which embed the cilia.

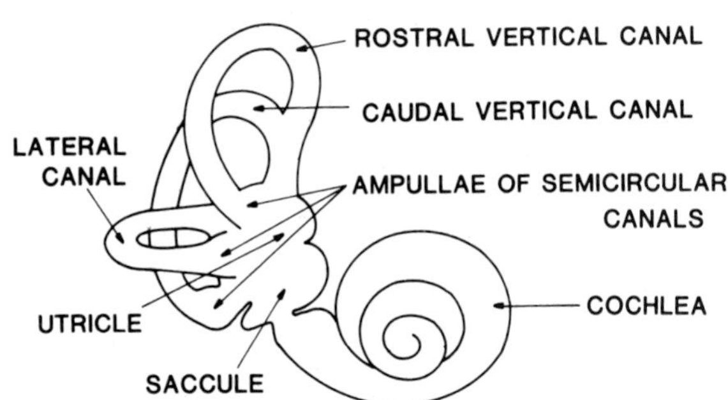

Figure 44.26. A schematic of the mammalian labyrinth, illustrating the semicircular canals and their relationship to the utriculus and sacculus and the relationship of the vestibular system to the auditory system, represented by the cochlea.

Otoliths are calcite or calcium carbonate concretions. The density of the otoliths causes them to move as the position of the head is altered within the field of gravity. As the otoliths move, the statoconial membrane causes the cilia of the hair cells to bend. Bending of the cilia serves as a means of stimulating the receptor cells and exciting afferent activity in the vestibular component of the eighth cranial nerve.

The macula of the saccule does not appear to be functional in domestic animals. The macula of the utricle, however, excites a number of postural responses aimed at maintaining the head in an upright position within a field of gravity and in maintaining a fixed retinal image through control of eye movements. The reflexes elicited to maintain a stable position of the head in space are called *labyrinthine righting reflexes*. A righting reflex can be demonstrated in the intact blindfolded cat that is held upside down and dropped. The cat rapidly turns and lands on its four feet. Although this righting reflex is initiated by the macula of the utricle, a number of other sensory inputs are involved. The first movement made by the cat is a rotation of the head (*labyrinthine righting reflex*) toward an upright posture. This rotation is followed immediately by a rotation of the upper body (*neck righting reflex*). These two reactions are then followed by a rotation of the lower body to complete the turn. This righting response can be elicited in an otherwise intact animal in which both vestibular receptors have been destroyed, but it is slower or incomplete. If, however, such a cat is blindfolded, it will fall without any attempt at righting. It is clear that visual input facilitates the righting reflexes.

The macula of the utricle is also functional in postural adjustments during linear acceleration. If an animal is accelerated in any direction, it will turn in the direction of its travel, extend its limbs, and spread its digits to contact a supporting surface. This is referred to as the *vestibular placing reflex*. This reaction is also reinforced by vision, but unilateral destruction of the macula of the utricle results in a loss of the vestibular placing reflexes on the affected side.

The cristae ampullaris lie within one end of each membranous semicircular canal. The site of the crista within each canal is represented by a dilatation of both the membranous and osseous canals, known as the *ampulla* (Fig. 44.26). Within the membranous ampulla, the crista represents a transverse ridge of connective tissue covered with hair cells, similar to those of the maculae. The cilia of these receptor cells are covered with a mucopolysaccharide *cupola* that obliterates the membranous canal. When the head is rotated, the inertia of the endolymph within the semicircular canal causes it to move in the direction opposite that of rotation. This movement of endolymph causes the cupola to be deformed. Deformation of the cupola, in turn, bends the cilia of the hair cells and serves to excite vestibular afferent activity. These receptors are well organized to detect either positive or negative rotatory acceleration. The three semicircular canals are oriented in planes approximately at right angles to each other and are termed, respectively, lateral (horizontal), anterior vertical, and caudal vertical. With this orientation, at least one of the canals will be rotating in the direction of the head when it is turned. If rotation of the head is continued at a constant velocity, the inertia of endolymph will soon be overcome and no excitatory input will result. This property of the semicircular canals causes the receptors to detect rotatory acceleration but not constant velocity of rotation.

When semicircular canals are continuously stimulated, one of the most obvious responses is *vestibular nystagmus*. Nystagmus is a rhythmic to-and-fro movement of the eyes, consisting of two components: a slow deviation in the direction opposite the rotation, followed by a rapid (saccadic) deviation in the direction of rotation. By convention, the direction of nystagmus is said to be in the direction of the fast component. If, therefore, the head is rotated to the left, the fast component will be to the left and the direction of nystagmus would be said to be to the left. The central nervous system structures involved in nystagmus include a combination of those that produce vestibulo-ocular reflexes and those responsible for saccadic eye movements, both of which are described earlier in this chapter.

Since the semicircular canal receptors can detect only acceleration, if the head rotation is continued at a constant velocity, vestibular nystagmus will be discontinued throughout the rotation, but optokinetic eye movements may be observed. When a continuous rotation is terminated, however, an inertial endolymph flow is again induced, and nystagmus will occur again. Nystagmus that occurs at the end of rotation is called *postrotational nystagmus*. The direction of postrotational nystagmus is opposite that of rotational nystagmus.

Since excitation of semicircular canal receptors depends on movement of endolymph, anything that causes endolymph to move can serve as an adequate stimulus to these receptors. Temperature differences along the canal will initiate convection currents in endolymph and serve to excite the receptors. This can be accomplished by flushing the external ear canal with hot (45°C) or cold (12°C) water.

Motion sickness is a condition that develops in animals subjected to a prolonged intermittent stimulation of either otolithic organs (linear acceleration and/or deceleration), such as swinging on a swing, or the semicircular canal receptors (rotatory acceleration or deceleration). Such stimulation is caused by moving automobiles, airplanes, or ships producing motion sickness during transportation. The syndrome of motion sickness is characterized in dogs by salivation, swallowing, a drop in blood pressure, and vomiting, all of which are characteristic of a true vomiting reflex. The vestibular nuclei of the brain stem have extensive input into the emetic center.

Ablation of the nodulus and uvula of the cerebellum renders an animal refractory to motion sickness. It is clear that the cerebellum plays a role in the production and prevention of motion sickness, but the extent of this role has not been determined.

REFERENCES

Amimia, M., and Yamaguchi, T. 1984. Fictive locomotion of the forelimb evoked by stimulation of the mesencephalic locomotor region in the decerebrate cat. *Neurosci Lett* 50:91–96.

Armstrong, D.M. 1986. Supraspinal contributions to the initiation and control of locomotion in the cat. *Prog. Neurobiol.* 26:273–361.

Armstrong, D.M. 1988. The supraspinal control of mammalian locomotion. *J. Physiol.* 405:1–37.

Armstrong, D.M., and Drew, T. 1984a. Discharges of pyramidal tract and other motor cortical neurones during locomotion in the cat. *J. Physiol.* 346:471–95.

Armstrong, D.M., and Drew, T. 1984b. Locomotor-related neuronal discharges in cat motor cortex compared with peripheral receptive fields and evoked movements. *J. Physiol.* 346:497–517.

Armstrong, D.M., and Drew, T. 1985. Forelimb electromyographic responses to motor cortex stimulation during locomotion in the cat. *J. Physiol.* 367:327–51.

Armstrong, D.M., and Edgley, S.A. 1984a. Discharges of nucleus interpositus neurones during locomotion in the cat. *J. Physiol.* 351:411–32.

Armstrong, D.M., and Edgley, S.A. 1984b. Discharges in Purkinje cells in the paravermal part of the cerebellar anterior lobe during locomotion in the cat. *J. Physiol.* 352:403–24.

Armstrong, D.M., Edgley, S.A., and Lidierth, M. 1988. Complex spikes in Purkinje cells of the paravermal part of the anterior lobe of the cat cerebellum during locomotion. *J. Physiol.* 400:405–14.

Asanuma, H., Zarzecki, P., Jankowska, E., Hongo T., and Marcus, S. 1979. Projections of individual pyramidal tract neurons to lumbar motor nuclei of the monkey. *Exp. Brain Res.* 34:73–89.

Baev, K.V., Berezovskii, V.K., Kebkalo, T.G., and Savoskina, L.A. 1985. Projections from structures of the cat forebrain to the hypothalamic locomotor region. *Neurophysiology* 17:183–89.

Barnes, C.D., Joynt, R.J., and Schottelius, B.A. 1962. Motoneuron resting potentials in spinal shock. *Am. J. Physiol.* 203: 1113–16.

Beloozerova, I.N. and M.G. Sirota, 1986a. Activity of motosensory cortex neurons in cat during natural walking on crosspieces of a horizontal ladder. *Neurophysiology* 18:543–45.

Beloozerova, I.N., and Sirota, M.G. 1986b. Activity of motosensory cortex neurons in cat during natural walking with stepping over obstacles. *Neurophysiology* 18:546–49.

Berezovskii, V.K., Kebalo, T.G., and Savoskina, L.A. 1984. Afferent brainstem projections to the hypothalamic locomotor region of the cat brain. *Neurophysiology* 16:279–86.

Burke, R.E. 1981. Motor units: Anatomy, physiology and functional organization. In V.B. Brooks, ed., *Handbook of Physiology*, Section 1, Vol II, Part 1. Americah Physiological Society, Bethesda, Md. Pp 345–422.

Buttner-Ennever, J., and Holstege, G. 1986. Anatomy of premotor centers in the reticular formation controlling oculomotor, skeletomotor and autonomic motor systems. *Prog. Brain Res.*, 64:89–98.

DeLong, M.R., Alexander, G.E., Mitchell, S.J., and Richardson, R.T. 1986. The contribution of basal ganglia to limb control. *Prog. Brain Res.* 68:161–75.

Drew, T. 1987. Discharge patterns of pyramidal tract neurones in motor cortex during a locomotion task requiring a precise control of limb trajectory. *Soc. Neurosci. Abstr.* 13:72.17.

Drew, T., Dubuc, R., and Rossignol, S. 1986. The discharge patterns of reticulospinal and other reticular neurones in chronic, unrestrained cats walking on a treadmill. *J. Neurophysiol.* 55:375–401.

Drew, T. and Rossignol, S. 1984. Phase-dependent responses evoked in limb muscles by stimulation of medullary reticular formation during locomotion in thalamic cats. *J. Neurophysiol.* 52:653–57.

Eccles, J.C. 1986. Learning in the motor system. *Prog. Brain Res.* 64:3–18.

Edwards, S.B. 1975. Autoradiographic studies of projections of the midbrain reticular formation: Descending projections of nucleus cuneiformis. *J. Comp. Neurol.* 161:341–58.

Eidelberg, E., Story, J.L., Meyer, B.L., and Nystel, J. 1980. Stepping in chronic spinal cats. *Exp. Brain Res.* 40:241–46.

Eidelberg, E., and Yu, J. 1981. Effects of corticospinal lesions upon treadmill locomotion in cats. *Exp. Brain Res.* 45:101–3.

Feldman, J.L., and Grillner, S. 1983. Control of vertebrate respiration and locomotion: A brief account. *Physiologist* 26: 310–16.

Fetz, E.E. 1984. Functional organization of motor and sensory cortex: Symmetries and parallels. In G.M. Edelman, W.E. Gall, and W.M. Cowan, eds., *Dynamic Aspects of Neocortical Function*. John Wiley & Sons, New York. Pp. 453–73.

Fetz, E.E., Cheney, P.D., and Palmer, S.S. 1986. Activity of forelimb motor units and corticomotoneuronal cells during ramp-and-hold torque responses: Comparisons with oculomotor cells. *Prog. Brain Res.* 64:133–41.

Forssberg, H., Grillner, S., and Halbertsma, J. 1980. The locomotion of the low spinal cat.I. Coordination within a limb. *Acta Physiol. Scand.* 108:269–81.

Forssberg, H., Grillner, S., Halbertsma, J., and Rossignol, S. 1980. The locomotion of the low spinal cat. 2. Interlimb coordination. *Acta Physiol. Scand.* 108:283–95.

Freund, H.J. 1983. Motor unit and muscle activity in voluntary motor control. *Physiol. Rev.* 63:387–436.

Fuchs, A.F., Kaneko, C.R.S., and Scudder, C.A. 1985. Brainstem control of saccadic eye movements. *Annu. Rev. Neurosci.* 8:307–37.

Fulton, J.F., and McCouch, G.P. 1937. The relation of the motor area of primates to the hyporeflexia ("spinal shock") of spinal transection. *J. Nerv. Ment. Dis.* 86:125–46.

Garcia-Rill, E. 1986. The basal ganglia and the locomotor regions. *Brain Res. Rev.* 11:47–63.

Garcia-Rill, E., Skinner, R.D., and Fitzgerald, J.A. 1983. Activity in the mesencephalic locomotor region during locomotion. *Exp. Neurol.* 82:609–22.

Garcia-Rill, E., Skinner, R.D., Gilmore, S.A., and Owings, R. 1983. Connections of the mesencephalic locomotor region (MLR). II. Afferents and efferents. *Brain Res. Bull.* 10:63–71.

Grillner, S. 1981. Control of locomotion in bipeds, tetrapods and fish. In V.B. Brooks, ed., *Handbook of Physiology, The Nervous System*, vol. II. *Motor Control*, part 2. American Physiological Society, Bethesda, Md. Pp. 1179–1236.

Grillner, S., and Wallen, P. 1985. Central pattern generators for locomotion, with special reference to vertebrates. *Ann. Rev. Neurosci.* 8:233–61.

Hoffmann, K.-P. 1986. Visual inputs relevant for the optokinetic nystagmus in mammals. *Prog. Brain Res.* 64:75–84.

Holstege, G., Van Neerven, J., and Evertse, F. 1984. Some anatomical observations on axonal connections from brain stem areas physiologically identified as related to respiration. *Neurosci. Lett., Suppl.* 18:S83.

Ito, M., Shiida, T., Yagi, N., and Yamamoto, M. 1974. The cerebellar modification of rabbits horizontal vestibulo-ocular reflex induced by sustained head rotation combined with visual stimulation. *Proc. Jpn. Acad. Sci.* 50:85–89.

Kebkalo, T.G., Berezovskii, V.K., and Esipenko, V.B. 1986. Efferent projections of mesencephalic locomotor neurons in the cat. *Neurophysiology* 18:96–102.

Lisberger, S.G., Morris, E.J., and Tychsen, L. 1987. Visual motion processing and sensory-motor integration for smooth pursuit eye movements. *Annu. Rev. Neurosci.* 10:97–129.

McCouch, G.P., Hughes, J., and Stewart, W.B. 1941. Crossed inhibition of the flexor reflex in the spinal mammal. *J. Neurophysiol.* 4: 547–54.

Palmer, C., Marks, W.B., and Bak, M.J. 1985. The responses of cat motor cortical units to electrical cutaneous stimulation during locomotion and during lifting, falling and landing. *Exp. Brain Res.* 58: 102–16.

Shimamura, M., and Kogure, I. 1983. Discharge patterns of reticulospinal neurons corresponding with quadripedal leg movements in thalamic cats. *Brain Res.* 230:27–34.

Steeves, J.D., and Jordan, L.M. 1984. Autoradiographic demonstration of the projections from the mesencephalic locomotor region. *Brain Res.* 307:263–76.

Steeves, J.D., Jordan, L.M., Schmidt, B., and Skovgaard, B.J. 1980. Effect of norepinephrine and 5-hydroxytryptamine depletion on locomotion in the mesencephalic cat. *Brain Res.* 185:349–62.

Udo, M., Kamei, H., Matsukawa, K., and Tanaka, K. 1982. Interlimb coordination in cat locomotion investigated with perturbation. II. Correlates in neuronal activity of Deiters' cells of decerebrate walking cats. *Exp. Brain Res.* 46:438–47.

Wiesendanger, M. 1986. Experimental evidence for the existence of a proprioceptive transcortical loop. *Prog. Brain Res.* 64:67–74.

Wise, S. P. 1985. The primate premotor cortex: Past, present and preparatory, *Annu. Rev. Neurosci.* 8:1–19.

Yu, J., and Eidelberg, E. 1983. Recovery of locomotor function in cats after localized cerebellar lesions. *Brain Res.* 273:121–31.

CHAPTER 45

Skeletal Muscle Physiology | by James E. Breazile

A great proportion of the body mass is composed of skeletal muscle. The metabolism and action of skeletal muscle are important in a wide variety of body movements and in the maintenance of body temperature. Skeletal muscle is organized to provide a wide variety of actions. Besides providing the force for somatic movements, skeletal muscle provides control of the larynx and pharynx and at least part of the esophagus in vocalization, deglutition, eructation, and regurgitation. The external anal and urethral sphincters provide urinary and fecal continence. Extrinsic eye muscles provide fixation of the eye and the maintenance of a stable image on the retina during head movement. The muscles of mastication and the muscles of the tongue are important in food prehension, mastication, and deglutition. Because of the wide variety of actions required of skeletal muscle, the anatomic organization of individual muscles demonstrates numerous variations.

Some skeletal muscles that have limited shortening in contraction and move heavy loads, such as the gluteals, are organized in a pennate structure with muscle fibers radiating from a central tendon. Muscles that demonstrate greater shortening in contraction and move relatively light loads, such as the sartorius, are composed of slender muscle fibers that extend along the length of the muscle belly. Muscles are attached at their extremities to connective tissue raphe, tendons, or aponeuroses through which movement of body parts is mediated. Each muscle is best organized to produce the type of contraction and transmission of tension to its tendon for the desired function of the muscle.

CELLULAR STRUCTURE OF SKELETAL MUSCLE

Skeletal muscles are mainly composed of multinucleated cells, called *muscle fibers* or *myocytes*. Microscopically, the fibers of skeletal muscle microscopically appear to be cross-striated when viewed perpendicular to their long axes (Fig. 45.1). Because of this property, skeletal muscle is referred to as "striated" muscle. Cardiac muscle is also striated, and much of what is known of the structure and function of cardiac muscle also applies to skeletal muscle. There are, however, some features of cardiac muscle that do not apply to skeletal muscle.

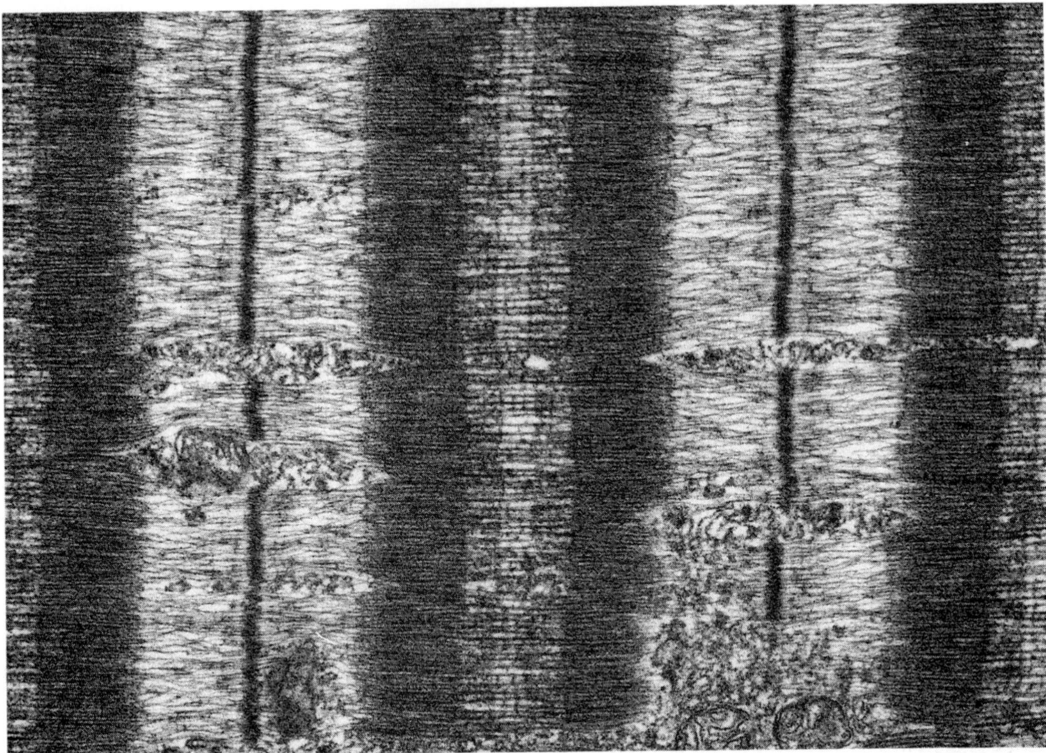

Figure 45.1. Electron micrograph of a longitudinal section through skeletal muscle, indicating the cross-striations produced by the myofilaments and identifying the bands produced.

CONNECTIVE TISSUE ELEMENTS OF SKELETAL MUSCLE

Skeletal muscle cells are bound together by connective tissue sheaths, which are independent of the individual cell membranes except through association with the basal lamina of myocytes. The basal lamina is intimately related to surrounding connective tissues (Fig. 45.2). The connective tissue sheaths of skeletal muscle are organized into three divisions—the epimysial sheath (epimysium), which surrounds the entire muscle belly; the perimysial sheath (perimysium), which surrounds 10 to 20 muscle fibers forming muscle fasciculi; and the endomysium, which surrounds individual muscle fibers. The connective tissue sheaths of the epimysium and the perimysium consist of thick connective tissue containing many collagen fibers and some elastic fibers. In a contracted muscle the perimysium and the epimysium may demonstrate some folding, but in relaxed muscle these sheaths are relatively smooth. Endomysium is composed of two types of filament. There are thick filaments approximately 50 nm in diameter, which are clearly collagen filaments, and thin filaments about 20 nm in diameter that appear to be precursor forms of collagen. The endomysium provides immediate mechanical support to individual muscle cells. Blood vessels and nerves are con-

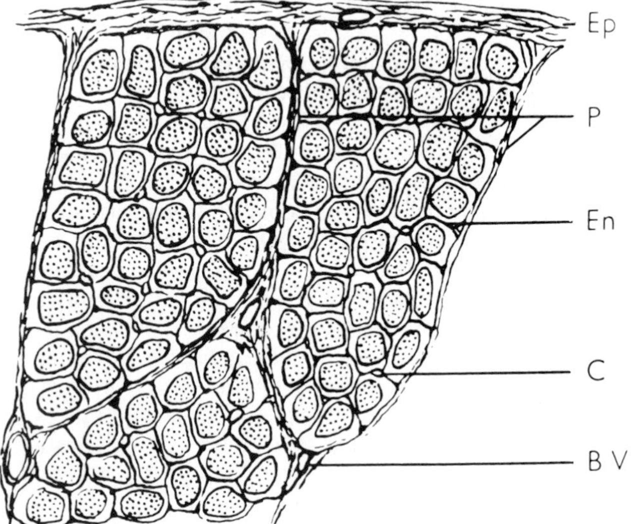

Figure 45.2. Diagram of a cross section through a portion of a muscle belly, illustrating the connective tissue sheaths. Ep, epimysium; P, perimysium; En, endomysium; BV, blood vessels; C, capillaries. (From Gould 1973, in Bourne, ed., *The Structure and Function of Muscle*, 2nd ed., vol. 2, Academic Press, New York.)

tained within the connective tissue sheaths and are supported by them as they pass to and from individual muscle fibers or muscle fasciculi. The connective tissue sheaths are important in attachment of muscle fibers to tendons, raphe, and aponeuroses. Because collagen is quite inelastic, the connective tissue sheaths contribute little to the elastic properties of skeletal muscle unless muscles are stretched beyond their normal functional lengths. The elastic properties of skeletal muscle rest primarily with the characteristics of the muscle cells themselves.

BASEMENT MEMBRANE AND MYOTENDINOUS JUNCTION

The basement membrane of muscle fibers represents a coating on the surface of the sarcolemma that is continuous with the surrounding endomysium of the muscle. The basement membrane consists of an inner basal lamina that contains the proteins laminin, fibronectin, and type IV collagen and an outer, reticular lamina composed of the proteins fibronectin, type V collagen, and another protein known as a high-salt soluble protein. The basal lamina is firmly associated with the underlying sarcolemma and cannot be mechanically removed without damage to the cell membrane. The reticular lamina is continuous with the overlying endomysial connective tissues. At the myotendinous junction, the reticular lamina and the endomysium blend with the perimysial sheath to become continuous with tendons of origin and insertion of the muscle. Satellite cells, often called *pericytes*, are located within the basal lamina and sometimes contact the surface of the sarcolemma. These cells are thought to represent precursors of muscle cells, differentiating in response to muscle damage to replace dead myocytes.

SARCOLEMMA STRUCTURE AND FUNCTION

Each skeletal muscle cell (referred to as a muscle fiber or a myocyte) is enclosed within a cell membrane, the sarcolemma. The sarcolemma not only provides mechanical support for the cell as its cell membrane and serves to attach muscle fibers through its basement membrane to connective tissue for physical movements, but it also generates and propagates action potentials in much the same fashion as the nerve cell membrane. The sarcolemma, however, has a variation that is not found in the neuronal cell membrane. The sarcolemma is continued into the interior of the cell as a transverse tubular system, providing a very large surface area of cell membrane in the vicinity of the contractile elements of muscle.

NEUROMUSCULAR RELATIONSHIPS AND ACTION POTENTIALS

Skeletal muscle innervation

Action potentials do not occur spontaneously in skeletal muscle. Rather, they are produced in response to action potentials in motor neuron axons. A single alpha motor neuron axon, through branching, may innervate a large number of skeletal muscle fibers. A single motor neuron axon with all of its branches and the muscle fibers that it innervates are together defined as a *motor unit*. The ratio of motor axons to the number of muscle fibers innervated in a given skeletal muscle is an indication of the size of the motor units and is called the *innervation ratio*. Innervation ratios vary among skeletal muscles, depending on the degree of motor control required. The extrinsic eye muscles, for example, in which a high degree of motor control is necessary to maintain steady vision, have an innervation ratio of 1:2 to 1:4, whereas those of some large somatic muscles have ratios of 1:800 or more.

NEUROMUSCULAR JUNCTION

Motor axons terminate at the surface of skeletal muscle fibers at sites called *neuromuscular junctions*. At neuromuscular junctions the sarcolemma is modified to form a *motor end plate*. The motor end plate represents a circumscribed area, usually near the middle of the muscle fiber, in which there are numerous surface folds that indent the surface of the muscle fiber. Motor neuron axon terminals lie within the folds, where they release acetylcholine from the numerous transmitter vesicles contained within the nerve terminals. Acetylcholine vesicles are released in response to depolarization-induced calcium influx into the nerve terminals as a result of action potentials in the motor axons. Calcium influx into the axon terminal occurs through voltage-dependent calcium channels. These channels can be at least partially blocked by magnesium and other divalent cations, which may account for the means by which $MgSO_4$ produces a reduction in neuromuscular transmission. The means by which a rise in intracellular calcium concentration induces neurotransmitter release is not known. One of the mechanisms that has been suggested involves the formation of a calcium-calmodulin complex that directly functions to initiate exocytosis of synaptic vesicles.

The toxin of *Clostridium botulinum* attaches to axon terminals and prevents the release of acetylcholine. The condition produced is called *botulism*, and it can result in profound skeletal muscle paralysis to the point of respiratory failure and death. Alpha latrotoxin, a polypeptide neurotoxin of the venom of the black widow spider (*Latrodectus mactans tredecimguttatus*), stimulates the release of acetylcholine from motor nerve terminals. These actions result in depletion of acetylcholine within the nerve terminals and produce skeletal muscle paralysis.

The sarcolemma surface within the motor end plate contains complexes of intrinsic proteins, which serve as receptor molecules for acetylcholine. The released acetylcholine diffuses across the 50 to 100 nm space between the nerve terminals and the motor end-plate membrane and attaches to the acetylcholine receptors. On the attachment of acetylcholine to a receptor, a transducer action is initiated through an increase in membrane permeability to small ions (Na^+, K^+, and Cl^-). The increased diffusion rate of these ions depolarizes the motor end-plate membrane.

The depolarization of the motor end-plate membrane induced by acetylcholine interacting with the membrane-bound receptors is called a *motor end-plate potential*. The motor end-plate region of the sarcolemma is electrically inexcitable; therefore, although it does depolarize, it does not generate an action potential. The surrounding sarcolemma is electrically excitable, however, and can generate action potentials. The depolarization of the motor end-plate membrane electrotonically depolarizes the surrounding sarcolemma to a threshold membrane potential and produces an action potential, which is then conducted over the surface of the muscle fiber. The sarcolemma of the motor end-plate contains, in addition to acetylcholine receptor complexes, an intrinsic protein complex that serves as an acetylcholine esterase. This enzyme rapidly degrades acetylcholine (within 1 to 2 ms) to acetate and choline, resulting in the rapid inactivation of the acetylcholine-receptor complex. Neuromuscular junction activity is therefore a very brief event, with the duration of the end-plate potential varying from 15 to 20 ms.

The acetylcholine content of individual transmitter vesicles of motor nerve endings (between 4,000 and 10,000 molecules) is known as a quantum. Each quantum of transmitter, activating a population of receptor proteins, produces a miniature end-plate potential. Because there is a continuous low level of spontaneous release of acetylcholine vesicles in the resting state, resulting in activation of acetylcholine receptors, miniature end-plate potentials can be recorded from innervated muscle cells. The production of end-plate potentials for muscle contraction results from the temporal and spatial summation of thousands of individual miniature end-plate potentials.

ACETYLCHOLINE RECEPTORS

Acetylcholine receptors of skeletal muscle are classed as *phasic receptors*. Their response to the attachment of acetylcholine or other activating agents is limited to 1 to 2 ms, even if acetylcholine is not degraded and the transmitter-receptor complex is maintained. This time represents the duration of change in sarcolemma permeability to small ions. If the acetylcholine is not degraded by acetylcholine esterase, even though acetylcholine remains attached to the receptor, the transducer mechanism producing the end-plate potentials is not reactivated and a neuromuscular block occurs, resulting in skeletal muscle paralysis. Acetylcholine receptors of the motor end-plate can also be activated by other choline derivatives, such as succinylcholine, and by nicotine to produce a transient excitation of skeletal muscle. Since there are no local enzymes present to rapidly hydrolyze these agents, they continue to occupy the receptor sites until they are metabolized and block the attachment of acetylcholine. This effect also results in a neuromuscular paralysis. Curare can attach to the acetylcholine receptors but does not initiate changes in ion permeability or end-plate potentials. Curare, however, blocks the attachment of acetylcholine and prevents neuromuscular transmission, leading to skeletal muscle paralysis.

Acetylcholine receptors are pentamers containing four types of protein subunits, known respectively as alpha (two units), beta, gamma (or epsilon), and delta (Fig. 45.3). As skeletal muscle cells mature, gamma proteins are replaced by epsilon proteins to provide the properties of the adult neuromuscular junction. In the embryo, acetylcholine receptors are present on skeletal muscle cell precursors before innervation with motor axons. These cells (myoblasts and fused myoblasts forming myotubes) have 100 to 500 functional acetylcholine receptors per square micrometer of cell membrane. The receptors have a short half-life of 17 to 22 hours and are distributed over the entire surface of the cells. Embryonic receptors have an activation time of 3 to 10 ms in response to acetylcholine. When the myotube is contacted during development or reinnervation by an axon, acetylcholine receptors become clustered under the nerve terminal with a density of 1000 to 2000/μm^2 of cell membrane and with a sharp decline in numbers of extrajunctional receptors. The junctional receptors have a half-life of about 11 days, and the duration of their activation is shortened to 1 to 2 ms. After birth, during muscle membrane maturation, the number of receptor molecules within the motor end-plate membrane continues to increase by 15 to 20 times.

When mature skeletal muscle is denervated, there is a return to an embryonic state in regard to receptor distribution on the muscle cells as evidenced by a proliferation of acetylcholine receptors over the entire sarcolemma. A simi-

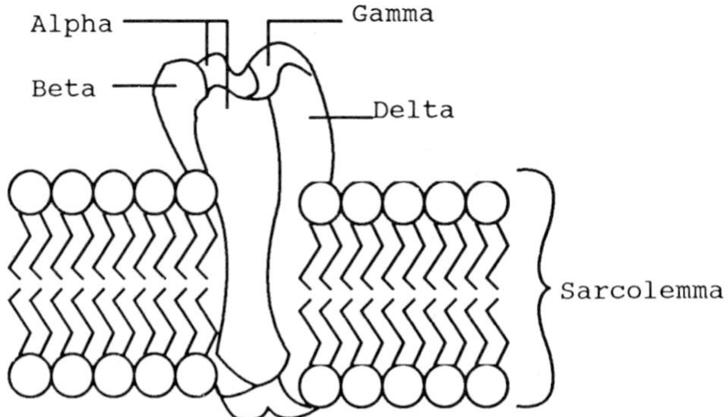

Figure 45.3. Model of the acetylcholine receptor protein complex of the sarcolemma of skeletal muscle. The relationships of the alpha, beta, gamma, and delta proteins are illustrated.

lar increase in numbers and distribution of acetylcholine receptors occurs when neuromuscular transmission is blocked, either by blocking of action potential production in innervating nerves or by blocking of the acetylcholine receptors with curare. It appears, therefore, that electrical activity of the sarcolemma is important in determining the distribution of acetylcholine receptors within the sarcolemma. Indeed, direct electrical stimulation of the muscle prevents or reverses the increase in extrajunctional acetylcholine receptors in denervated muscle.

The newly formed receptors of denervated muscle cells are sensitive to circulating levels of acetylcholine and are capable of activation of skeletal muscle. This activity can be recorded as action potentials of individual muscle cells. In electromyographic recording, this activity is known as *denervation* (or fibrillation) *potential*.

The mechanism of regulation of the number and distribution of acetylcholine receptors of skeletal muscle is not known but, as indicated above, appears to involve electrical activity of the sarcolemma. This activity has been related to the intracellular concentration of Ca^{2+}. Chronically increased levels of intracellular Ca^{2+} result in a decrease in production of acetylcholine receptors. It appears that the local increase in acetylcholine receptors within the motor end-plate, with a diminished number in the extrajunctional sarcolemma, involves a peptide containing 37 amino acids. This peptide, called calcitonin gene-related peptide (CGRP), is contained within the axon terminals of spinal motor neurons within the vesicles that contain acetylcholine. CGRP is cosecreted with acetylcholine and is responsible for activation of protein production by a group of muscle cell nuclei that are clustered beneath the motor end-plate membrane. These nuclei, described by Ranvier in 1875, as "fundamental nuclei," appear to be specialized to generate acetylcholine receptor proteins. In this model, the corelease of CGRP with acetylcholine locally increases the production of receptor proteins through a cyclic adenosine monophosphate second-messenger mechanism.

Myasthenia gravis is a neuromuscular disorder in which autoantibodies are produced against acetylcholine receptors. Many of the receptors undergo degeneration as a result of complement activation or they function abnormally because of combination with antibodies. Reduced receptor numbers, with normal amounts of acetylcholine released, lead to exercise-induced paralysis through blockade of neuromuscular transmission. Treatment with a drug, such as edrophonium HCl, that blocks the action of acetylcholinesterase immediately reverses the paralysis. Myasthenia gravis has occasionally been associated with failure of the thymus to undergo its normal atrophy at puberty. The relationship between the thymus and acetylcholine receptors appears to involve a common antigen. Antibodies to the antigen formed on thymocytes also attach to acetylcholine receptors.

MEMBRANE POTENTIALS OF SKELETAL MUSCLE

The sarcolemma separates intracellular and extracellular fluids, which have markedly different ionic compositions. The intracellular fluid contains a high concentration of K^+ (about 145 mEq/L) and of organic anions, such as proteins, adenosine triphosphate (ATP), and adenosine diphosphate (ADP), and low concentrations of Na^+ and Cl^- (about 5 mEq/L of each). The extracellular fluid contains high concentrations of Na^+ (145 mEq/L) and Cl^- (100 mEq/L) and a low concentration of K^+ (2.4 mEq/L) ions. There are few or no large organic anions in the extracellular fluid. Organic anions cannot diffuse through the sarcolemma. The sarcolemma is quite permeable to potassium ions, so that potassium ions diffuse out of the cell, leaving behind the large impermeable organic anions, producing a membrane potential (Em) that is positive extracellular relative to intracellular fluid. If K^+ were the only diffusible ion, the membrane potential would reach a level at which the force of the K^+ concentration gradient would be equaled by the opposing force of the membrane potential. The membrane potential at this level is called the K^+ equilibrium potential (E_K+). There is a slight inward diffusion of Na^+, however, which slightly diminishes this K^+ diffusion potential so that the resulting membrane potential of skeletal muscle is about 90 mV in magnitude. The Na^+-K^+ pump of the sarcolemma contributes slightly to the resting membrane potential, because approximately three sodium ions are transported out for every two potassium ions transported into the cell. The potential, however, is determined primarily by the relative diffusion rates of Na^+ and K^+ ions.

ACTION POTENTIALS OF SKELETAL MUSCLE

Action potentials of skeletal muscle are produced in the same manner as those of nerve cells. After an initial depolarization of the electrically excitable sarcolemma to a threshold membrane potential, produced by the action of acetylcholine and acetylcholine receptors, there is a spontaneous, all-or-none, time limited increase in permeability of the sarcolemma to Na^+. The all-or-none property of change in permeability to Na^+ indicates a maximal change that cannot be increased or decreased after a threshold membrane potential is reached. The resulting increase in diffusion rate of Na^+ causes the membrane potential to move toward the equilibrium potential for Na^+ (about +65 mV, in the intracellular fluid relative to the extracellular fluid). Because of the simultaneous diffusion of K^+, however, the membrane potential reaches only about 10 mV, positive intracellular, producing a small overshoot. Immediately after this increase in Na^+ permeability, there is a voltage-sensitive, time-limited increase in permeability to K^+ as Na^+ permeability returns to normal levels. The membrane potential therefore returns rapidly toward the equilibrium potential for K^+, resulting in repolarization of the sarcolemma. When K+ permeability returns to resting levels, the membrane potential is restored. The sarcolemmal depolarization, resulting from the action potential amplitude of about 100 mV from resting levels, serves to depolarize adjacent sarcolemma to threshold and the action potential is conducted along the membrane.

In cardiac muscle, calcium ion diffusion from the extracellular to the intracellular fluid is an important contribution to the action potential and contributes to the calcium available for initiation of muscle contraction. In skeletal muscle, although there is a slight inward diffusion of calcium ions during the action potential, it does not appear to contribute significantly to action potential production or to skeletal muscle contraction mechanisms.

TRANSVERSE TUBULE SYSTEM

The transverse tubule system (T tubules) of mammalian skeletal muscle extends deep into the muscle cell at the level of junction of the A and I bands (Fig. 45.1). In frog twitch-muscle cells, T tubules enter the muscle cells at the Z lines (Fig. 45.4). T tubules serve to provide an avenue for the depolarization resulting from the action potential of the sarcolemma to pass into the cell. The density of T tubules within myocytes varies between cells with different physiological properties so that in muscle cells with fast-twitch properties it is about twice as extensive as in slow-twitch myocytes (described below). About 80 percent of the T tubule membrane (T membrane) surface makes contact with the surface of the sarcoplasmic reticulum (SR) membranes of the cell. At these specialized T-SR junctions, two cisternae of the sarcoplasmic reticulum contact one T tubule to form a skeletal muscle triad of tubular structures (Figs. 45.4 and 45.5).

SARCOPLASMIC RETICULUM

The SR is an elaborately branched, anastomosing, membranous, tubular network within the muscle cell, extensively overlying bundles of myofibrils (Fig.45.4). The tubules extend throughout the sarcomere and have dilated extremities known as terminal cisternae. Two terminal cisternae of the SR contact the transverse tubule membranes to form the triad of skeletal muscle (Fig. 45.5). The SR mem-

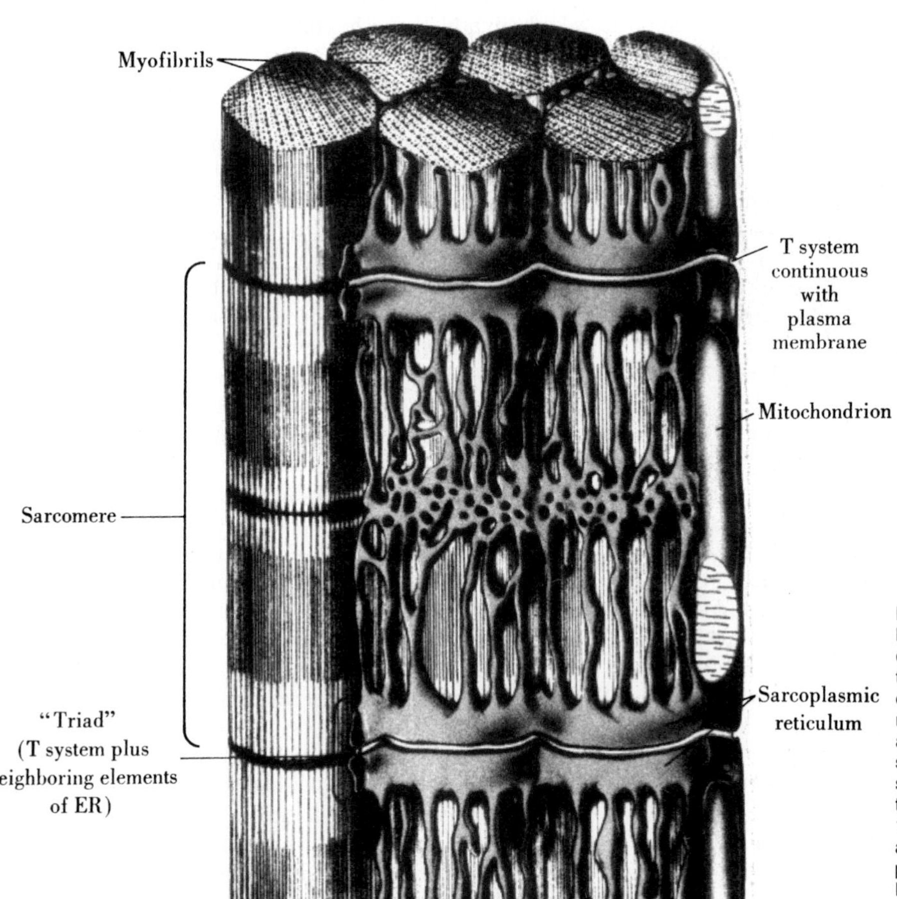

Figure 45.4. Diagram of the transverse tubular system and the sarcoplasmic reticulum of frog skeletal muscle. Transverse tubules (T tubules) are shown at the level of each Z band, and the sarcoplasmic reticular membranes form an extensive network around each myofibril. The cisternae of the sarcoplasmic reticulum and their relationship to the transverse tubules are illustrated. (From A.B. Novikoff and E. Holtzman 1970, *Cells and Organelles*, Holt, Rinehart and Winston, New York. Reproduced by permission of Holt, Rinehart and Winston, Inc., and L.D. Peachey and D.W. Fawcett. Modified from *J. Cell. Biol.*, vol. 25, no. 3, pt. 2, pp. 209–31, 1965.)

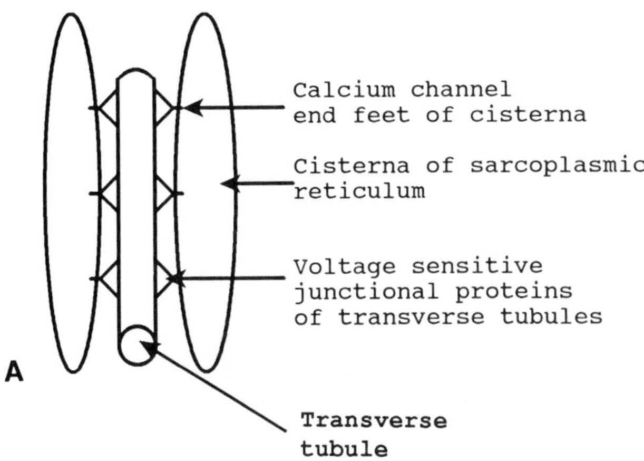

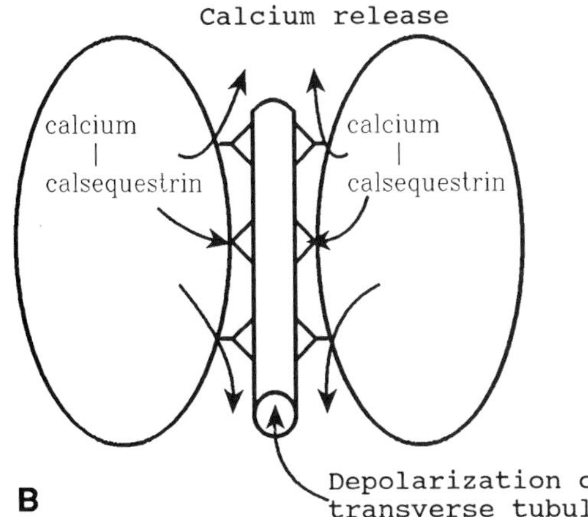

Figure 45.5. (*A*) Schematic of the sites of interaction between the transverse tubules and the sarcoplasmic reticulum, forming the triad of skeletal muscle. (*B*) Sites of calcium release from the cisternae of the sarcoplasmic reticulum in response to depolarization of the transverse tubules are illustrated.

brane, but not the membrane involved in the formation of triads, contains large numbers of calcium pump proteins, with Ca^{2+} sensitive ATPase activity. These proteins are functional in actively transporting Ca^{2+} ions from the cytoplasm into the cisternae of the reticulum. The lumen of the SR contains about 98 percent of the total calcium of the cell. Within the SR, calcium is bound to calsequestrin, a protein with a high affinity for calcium. Calsequestrin, when saturated, can bind up to 43 moles of calcium per mole of protein. This calcium is released into the cytoplasm in response to the influence of the depolarized transverse tubules on the SR at the triads (Fig. 45.5).

In humans and in pigs, there is a hereditary disorder called *malignant hyperthermia* in which defective activation of calcium channels of the SR takes place. The activation of calcium channels can be triggered by the general anesthetic halothane and results in extremely strong muscle contractions and heat production. Halothane-induced calcium channel activation can be reversed by the drug dantrolene, a direct-acting muscle relaxant that reduces Ca^{2+} release from the SR.

Within the triad, SR membranes are separated from the transverse tubule membranes by about 12 nm. *End-feet*, 12 to 25 nm wide and spaced 28.5 nm apart, bridge the space between the two membranes and appear to be the structural basis for functional interaction. The end-feet represent proteins of the SR membranes (foot proteins), which span the gap between the membranes and contact a junctional protein of the T membranes (Fig. 45.5). These T membrane junctional proteins characteristically bind the chemical dihydropyridine, which also binds to and serves as a marker for calcium channels of other membranes. The molecules in the T membranes of skeletal muscle appear to serve as voltage sensors rather than as calcium channels. When the membrane potential of the T membrane is diminished from resting levels to between 40 and 60 mV, the voltage-sensitive T membrane proteins activate phospholipase C, which acts on T membrane phosphatidylinositol 4,5-bisphosphate to produce inositol 1,4,5-trisphosphate ($INSP_3$) and diacylglycerol. The $INSP_3$ acts on the SR membrane foot proteins to activate the release of calcium into the cytoplasm. The foot proteins of the SR membrane apparently serve as calcium channels, developing high permeability to calcium on activation. $INSP_3$ has a short half-life and is rapidly degraded by inositol triphosphatase. The time required for this chemical mediation of calcium release (estimated to be 0.5 ms) contributes to the total time delay (latency time) of excitation contraction coupling.

When the transverse tubules are maintained in a depolarized state for 100 to 200 ms, as occurs with repetitive action potential production at high frequency or accumulation of K^+ in the extracellular fluid, there is a marked decline in the rate of release of calcium from transverse tubules. This inactivation of calcium release results from released calcium binding to a high-affinity calcium receptor on the release channel, producing a conformational change in the channel and diminishing its permeability. In this way, maintained depolarization of the sarcolemma leads to inactivation of muscle cell contraction.

Within the cytoplasm, the calcium is mostly bound to a cytosolic protein called *calmodulin*. Calmodulin transports cytoplasmic calcium to its sites of action. Calcium release from the SR and its cytosolic transport by calmodulin play a critical role in the initiation of skeletal muscle contraction.

MYOFIBRILS AND MYOFILAMENTS

The cytoplasm of skeletal muscle cells contains a large number of 1 to 2 μm, cylindrical, longitudinally arranged bundles known as myofibrils (muscle fibrils in Fig. 45.6). Cross-striations, the dominant microscopic characteristic

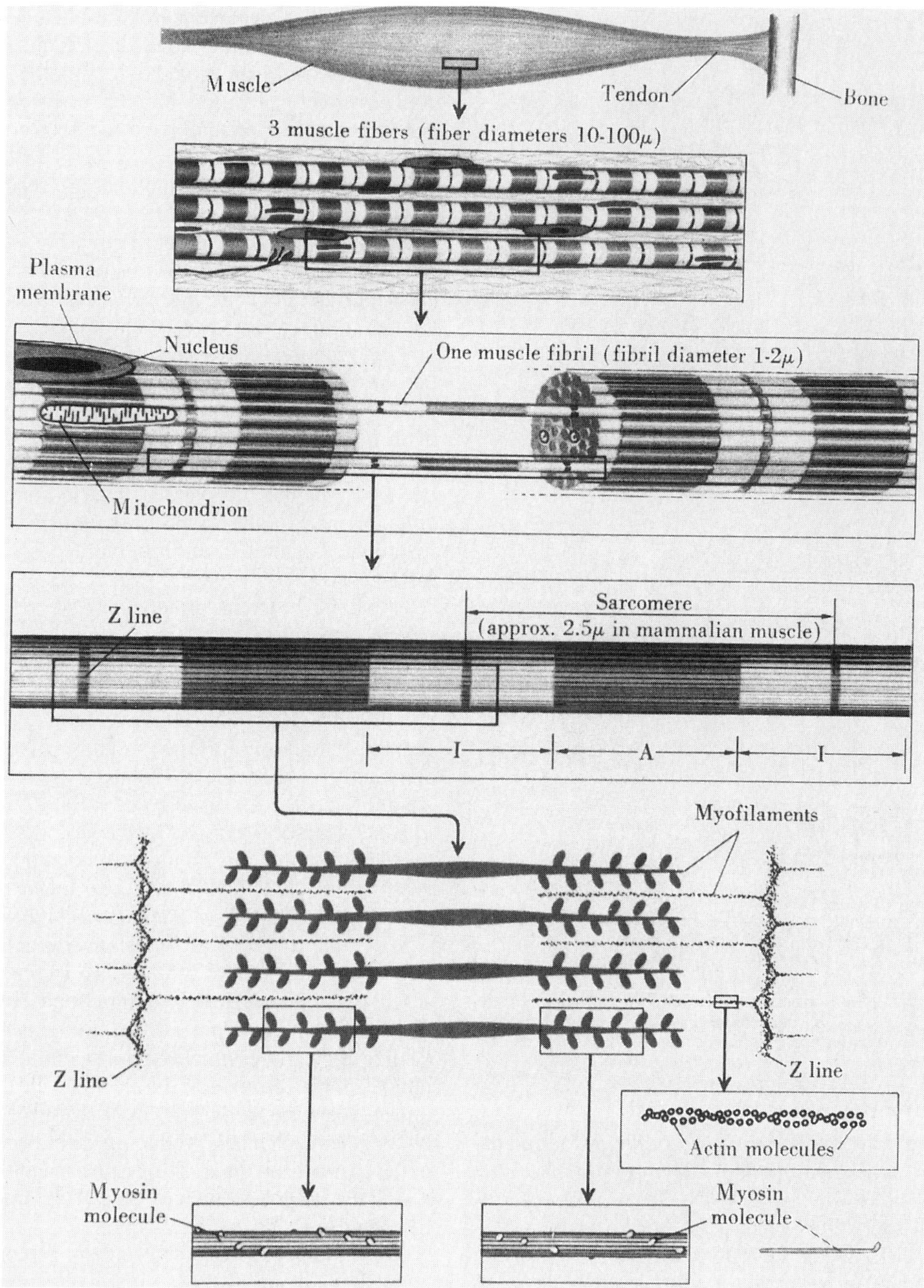

Figure 45.6. Diagram of the components of a vertebrate skeletal muscle illustrating various levels of organization from the gross muscle to the molecular components. (See text for a description.)

of skeletal muscle, are produced by an orderly arrangement of the contractile proteins within the myofibrils forming the myofilaments of the muscle cells. Cross-striations are produced by alternate thick and thin bands extending across the cytoplasm of each cell. Bands composed mainly of isotropic proteins (actin, tropomyosin, and troponin) form I bands, which are interrupted by bands composed primarily of anisotropic proteins (myosin) forming A bands. Each of the I bands is divided into two equal parts by an intervening dark band, the Z line. The interval between adjacent Z lines is called a sarcomere and represents the functional and structural unit of skeletal muscle. Each sarcomere of a muscle cell is identical to all other sarcomeres of a given muscle cell. The length of individual sarcomeres varies between 1.5 μm when the muscle is contracted and 3.6 μm when the relaxed muscle is stretched. As an individual sarcomere contracts, adjacent Z lines approach each other. The contraction of many sarcomeres produces the overall muscle contraction.

Electron microscopic and histochemical examinations of skeletal muscle cells demonstrate two basic types of myofilament within the sarcomere. These are known, respectively, as thick and thin myo-filaments. Thin myofilaments are composed of actin, troponin, and tropomyosin. Thick myofilaments are composed of myosin. It is the organization of the myofilaments within the myofibrils that produces the cross-striated appearance of skeletal muscle. Thick myofilaments are about 12 nm in diameter and 1.6 μm long, and the thin myofilaments are about 8 nm in diameter and 1 μm in length. Thin myofilaments are continuous with the Z lines and extend into the sarcomere but do not, except in strong muscle contraction, reach the sarcomere center. Thick myofilaments lie within the center of the sarcomere, overlapping on each end with the thin myofilaments. Thin myofilaments are arranged in a hexagonal array around each thick filament, allowing for extensive interaction between the thick and thin myofilaments in muscle contraction.

STRUCTURE AND FUNCTION OF THICK MYOFILAMENTS

Thick myofilaments comprise aggregations of myosin molecules. Myosin is a protein with a molecular weight of about 470,000, consisting of a dimer with an elongated tail (about 160 nm in length). The myosin tail contains two polypeptide chains (called light meromyosin, with a molecular weight of about 160,000) united to two heavier chains (called heavy meromyosin, with a molecular weight of about 360,000), which combine to form an alpha helix (Fig. 45.7). At one end of each heavy meromyosin chain there is a globular component (called the globular head) to which are covalently bound four light myosin polypeptides (called light myosin chains) with molecular weights ranging from 15,000 to 16,000. The myosin light chains are classified on the basis of chemical differences as L1, L2, or L3 chains. The globular heads of myosin are often referred to as cross-bridges as they attach and detach from the thin myofilaments in muscle contraction (Fig. 45.8).

The junction of the globular head of myosin with the remainder of the heavy meromyosin molecule functions as a hinge, producing a site of bending of the myosin molecule after its interaction with actin. This hinge is thought to contribute a major portion of the force of muscle contraction. When the globular head bends at the hinge, the force of this action simultaneously stretches the heavy meromyosin molecule. The elasticity of the heavy meromyosin contributes to the expenditure of energy in muscle contraction.

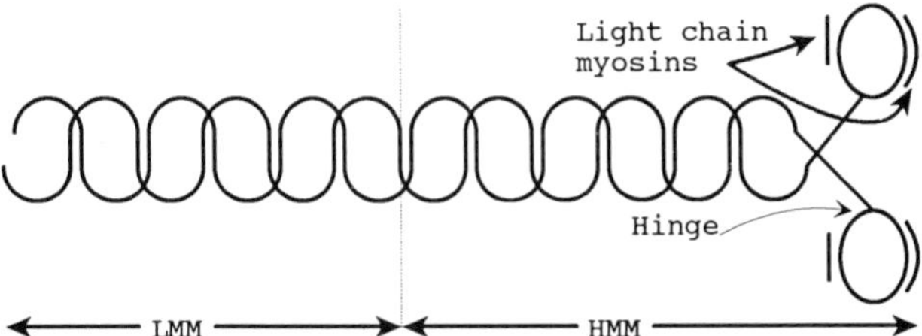

Figure 45.7. Schematic of a myosin molecule, illustrating the alpha helix organization, junction between light and heavy meromysins, the two globular heads, and location of the hinge and of light chain myosins. LMM, light meromysin; HMM, heavy meromysin

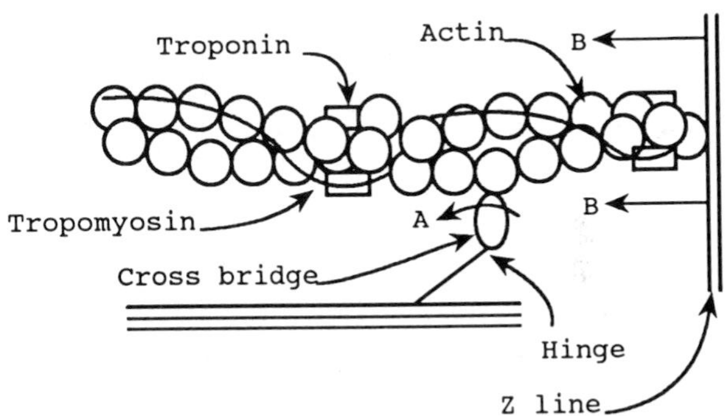

Figure 45.8. Schematic of the interaction of myosin cross-bridges with the actin of the thin myofilaments. During muscle contraction, thousands of such interactions occur to pull the Z lines toward each other, shortening the sarcomere. Also illustrated are the components of thin myofilaments and their relationships. The letters A and B represent movements of the globular heads of myosin and of the Z lines in muscle shortening.

The globular head of the myosin molecule contains actin-induced ATPase activity (which appears to be a property of the light-chain myosin molecules) that interacts chemically with the actin proteins of the thin filaments. Myosin molecules are classified on the basis of the rate at which they hydrolyze ATP, into *slow, fast*, and *superfast* myosin ATPase activities. Within the thick myofilament, all myosin molecules have the same polarity of relationship to the thick myofilament, with myosin tails oriented toward the center of the sarcomere and myosin heads toward the Z line. Because of this arrangement, there are no globular heads near the middle of the thick myofilament. This region corresponds to the H line seen with the light microscope.

Globular heads of myosin attach to adjacent actin molecules of thin myofilaments during muscle contraction. Bending of the myosin molecule at the hinge pulls the actin and the associated thin filament and Z lines toward the center of the sarcomere, resulting in sarcomere shortening.

STRUCTURE AND FUNCTION OF THIN MYOFILAMENTS

Thin myofilaments are composed of actin, tropomyosin, and troponin in a ratio of 7 actin to 1 tropomyosin and 1 troponin molecule (Fig. 45.9). Actin is a globular protein

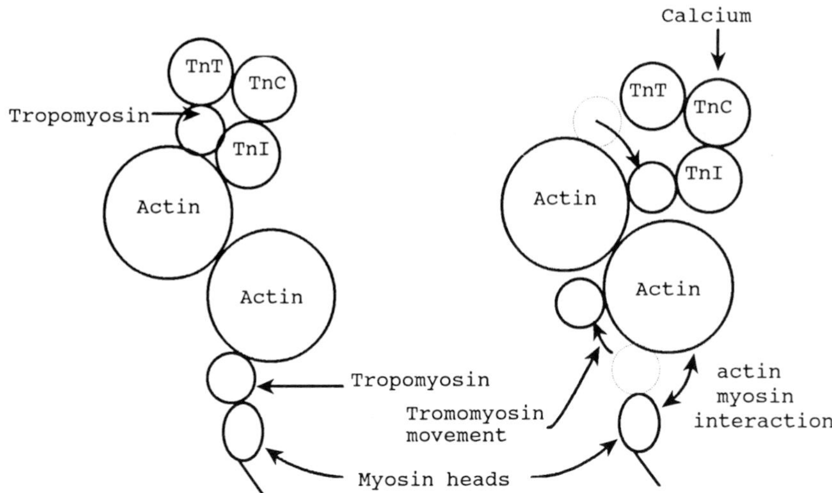

Figure 45.9. A schematic of a cross section of a thin myofilament, illustrating topographic relationships between its components. These relationships are illustrated in the state of muscle relaxation (*left*) and in contraction (*right*) in which tropomyosin movement, allowing interaction between actin and myosin, is demonstrated. TnT, TnC, and TnI are troponin (Tn) proteins based on amino acid sequence.

(known as G-actin) with a molecular weight of about 42,000. In the presence of cytoplasmic ATP, actin molecules form a fibrous polymer (known as fibrous or F-actin) consisting of about 300 G-actin units.

Tropomyosin is an elongated protein, about 40 nm in length with a molecular weight of about 35,000, consisting of a double alpha helix. Two helices of tropomyosin lie at 180 degrees from each other, within the grooves formed by the actin polymer (Fig. 45.9). At resting concentrations of cytoplasmic calcium (about 10^{-8} M), tropomyosin in this position blocks interaction between myosin globular heads and actin molecules and serves to inhibit muscle contraction. Since the inhibition of myosin and actin interaction results from the topographic relationship of tropomyosin to these two molecules, the inhibition is called *steric hindrance*.

Troponin is a complex of three proteins: troponin-T (Tn-T), troponin-I(Tn-I), and troponin-C (Tn-C). Troponin-T binds the troponin complex to tropomyosin at each end of the tropomyosin units (an interval of about 42 nm). Troponin I binds to both actin and tropomyosin and, in the resting muscle cell, maintains the steric hindrance of tropomyosin on actin and myosin interaction. Troponin-C has a high affinity for calcium ions. The binding of cytoplasmic calcium to Tn-C is a critical stage in the mechanism of muscle contraction. When cytoplasmic calcium ion concentrations rise to a sufficient level (about 10^{-6} to 10^{-5} molar), calcium binding to Tn-C affects Tn-I, causing tropomyosin to move closer to the groove of the two-strand actin helix. This movement results in the removal of steric hindrance of actin interaction with myosin, allowing muscle contraction (Fig. 45.9).

Although there are other proteins within the thick and thin myofilaments, they represent only a small portion of the protein of muscle and their function in contraction is not known.

EXCITATION CONTRACTION COUPLING

Excitation contraction coupling is the series of activities involved in translation of an action potential on the sarcolemma into a muscle contraction. The mechanisms of excitation contraction coupling are described above as they involve each element of excitation and contraction. In summary, the sequential events of skeletal muscle contraction are as follows:

1. An action potential of the sarcolemma depolarizes the transverse tubule system of the muscle cell.
2. Depolarization of the transverse tubules induces the release of calcium from the SR.
3. The released calcium binds to Tn-C, initiating alterations in Tn-I.
4. Alterations in Tn-I result in a movement of tropomyosin relative to actin and myosin and remove steric hindrance to their interaction.
5. Actin and myosin interact to form an actin-myosin complex that activates the myosin ATPase, releasing energy for muscle contraction and inducing a bending of the myosin molecules at the hinge region of the heavy meromyosin.
6. This action pulls the thin myofilaments and their associated Z lines toward the center of the sarcomere, resulting in muscle shortening.

This representation of muscle contraction is referred to as the *sliding filament model* and explains most of the physical and chemical events of skeletal muscle contraction. For significant muscle shortening (from a stretched sarcomere length of 3.6 μm to a contracted length of 1.5 μm), it is necessary that the myosin molecules release from the initial actin molecule, restore it to its original position, and reattach to another actin. This action is repeated many times. Each of the thousands of myosin heads within a thick myofilament acts independently of the others. As some myosin heads detach from actin and are restored to their original shape, others are attached and bending, so that there is a continuous recycling of actin and myosin interactions to produce a smooth muscle contraction.

ROLE OF ATP IN MUSCLE CONTRACTION AND RELAXATION

During the cyclic attachment and detachment of myosin globular heads, ATP is hydrolyzed to provide energy for the muscle contraction. Although ATP is the immediate source of energy for muscle contraction, there is no change in ATP concentration within muscle cells during moderate muscle activity. The ATP used in muscle contraction is readily replaced through phosphorylation of ADP from creatine phosphate, which represents a major store of energy for skeletal muscle. The concentration of ATP in muscle cells at rest is about 5 μmol/g of tissue, whereas that of creatine phosphate is about five times greater. Creatine phosphate interacts with a cytoplasmic enzyme, *creatine kinase*, to form ATP from ADP. In this way, ATP and ADP are continually recycled during muscle contraction to provide a continual source of energy.

ATP and creatine phosphate in resting muscle cells represent stores of energy that are available for muscle contraction. These stores are maintained through the continued generation of ATP from glycolysis and through the oxidation of acetyl coenzyme A derived from pyruvic acid through oxidative metabolism involving the citric acid cycle. The regeneration of creatine phosphate is a slower process than that of ATP, so that in repeated muscle contraction the creatine phosphate store is diminished while the ATP concentration is maintained. Creatine phosphate concentrations are then restored after muscle relaxation has occurred. Creatine phosphate is restored through the metabolism of glycogen in anaerobic metabolism (glycolysis) or through the metabolism of glucose or fatty acids in aerobic metabolism (oxidation). The regeneration of creatine phosphate ultimately requires oxygen, either to metabolize glucose and fatty acids to creatine phosphate or to restore the glycogen used during an anaerobic period of muscle contraction. The oxygen required in this restoration is referred to as the oxygen debt of skeletal muscle.

The hydrolysis of ATP and its regeneration are critical events in skeletal muscle contraction. In the absence of ATP, actin and myosin bind firmly to each other, forming *rigor complexes*. Such a condition occurs in rigor mortis after the consumption of energy sources and ATP from dying muscle cells. A number of steps involving ATP and its hydrolysis occur in muscle contraction. Cytosolic ATP attaches to the myosin component of an actin-myosin complex and causes the rigor complex to dissociate into actin and ATP-myosin. This action, with the steric hindrance of actin and myosin interaction provided by tropomyosin, maintains a relaxed state in the muscle. When intracellular calcium is increased and the action of Tn-I on the structural relationship of tropomyosin to actin and myosin is exerted, steric hindrance of myosin and actin interaction is removed. On exposure to actin, the myosin ATPase hydrolyzes ATP to ADP, and the energy released is stored. Actin and myosin complexes are formed and the stored energy is released to provide energy for the bending of the myosin molecule at the hinge at the junction of the globular head. Bending of the hinge pulls the thin filament toward the center of the sarcomere. Another molecule of ATP then attaches to the myosin molecule, causes it to detach from actin, and restores it to its original position, restarting the cycle.

MUSCLE RELAXATION

Muscle relaxation is essentially a reversal of the mechanisms of contraction. After the depolarization of the sarcolemma and the transverse tubule system is terminated, calcium pumps of the sarcoplasmic reticulum actively transport calcium ions from the cytoplasm into the tubules of the sarcoplasmic reticulum, where it is rebound to calsequestrin. The removal of calcium from the cytoplasm results in a release of calcium from Tn-C–calcium complexes. Both Tn-C and Tn-I are altered, and they cause tropomyosin to move out of the groove between the actin molecules. This action reestablishes steric hindrance of actin and myosin interaction, and muscle relaxation takes place.

Myotonia is a condition in which skeletal muscle continues to be excited after voluntary effort or stimulation has been terminated. The muscle cells appear to remain depolarized because of an altered chloride permeability within the transverse tubular membranes, and contraction continues. Animals affected with myotonia demonstrate an increase in muscle size (hypertrophy) but have a normal resting muscle tone. Normal resting muscle tone in the face of continued sarcoplasmic depolarization results from an inhibition of calcium release from the sarcoplasmic reticulum as described on page 861.

SKELETAL MUSCLE FIBER TYPES

It has long been recognized that skeletal muscle could be classified, on the basis of myoglobin content and rate of contraction, as *white, red, fast,* and *slow*. Types of skeletal muscle fiber have been identified on the basis of physiological, ultrastructural, histochemical, biochemical, and immunological examination findings. On the basis of primary energy source (oxidative or aerobic versus glycolytic or anaerobic) and rate of fiber contraction, mammalian skeletal muscle fibers are classified as slow-twitch (type I), oxidative, and fast-twitch (type II) glycolytic fibers. Although there is a range in oxidative energy dependence between them, type I fibers are always oxidative. Type II fibers display a range of dependency on oxidative or glycolytic energy. The use of histochemical techniques that demonstrate the relative concentrations and pH stability of myosin ATPase content of muscle fibers allows the separation of fibers into type I and type II and the subclassification of type II fibers as types IIA, IIB, IIC, and IIM.

Table 45.1. Skeletal muscle fiber types

Fiber type and contraction velocity	Fatigue resistance	Glycolytic or oxidative	ATPase type
Red slow type I	High	Oxidative	Slow
Red fast type IIA	High or intermediate	Oxidative	Fast
White fast type IIB	Low	Glycolytic	Fast
Intermediate type IIC	Intermediate	Oxidative	Fast and slow
Superfast type IIM	Unknown	Glycolytic and oxidative	Superfast*

*Superfast myosin has been isolated from the superfast contracting jaw muscle of the cat. This myosin differs from both slow and fast myosin and has an ATPase activity three times that of fast myosin.

With the use of a combination of parameters, including shortening velocity, fatigue resistance, metabolism, and myosin ATPase characteristics, skeletal muscle fibers can then be classified into the following types: red, slow, type I; red, fast, type IIA; white, fast, type IIB; intermediate, type IIC; and superfast, type IIM fibers (Table 45.1). These classifications indicate that skeletal muscle is composed of a heterogenous population of muscle fibers that are organized to best accomplish the function of the muscle in which they are contained.

Deficiencies of specific muscle fiber types have been described in clinical disorders in animals. A type II muscle fiber deficiency of Labrador retrievers appears to be associated with a simple autosomal recessive genetic transmission. Affected animals exhibit extreme fatigue with exercise but quickly recover after rest. Plasma creatine levels are elevated in these animals. Creatine is normally formed in the liver and is converted to creatinine in type II skeletal muscle cells. The absence of these cells results in the excretion of up to 30 times the normal levels of creatine in the urine.

Irish terrier and golden retriever dogs exhibit a sex-linked myopathy that results in degeneration of all muscle fiber types. Signs of muscle degeneration appear at about 8 weeks of age and are progressive.

PLASTICITY OF SKELETAL MUSCLE

Plasticity of skeletal muscle refers to the capacity of myofilament proteins to undergo extensive changes in response to functional demands involving hormonal influences and exercise, both during neonatal development and in adulthood. Skeletal muscles that are rendered inactive, either through immobilization or through denervation, lose mass (atrophy) and have a marked decrease in muscle cell protein content. There are extensive data demonstrating that different types of physical training can alter both the size and the composition of skeletal muscle. These changes are reflected in quantitative and qualitative changes in specific structural proteins of the myofilaments and of the metabolic enzymes. Since these alterations involve the synthesis of new proteins, genetic expression mechanisms are involved.

Immunohistochemical studies with myosin-specific antibodies have demonstrated a high degree of control of the relative proportions of different (fast versus slow) myosin heavy-chain and light-chain isoforms during muscle growth. Fast and slow types of myosin heavy-chain isoforms are interconvertible in a given muscle and influence the functional properties of the muscle. It is clear that prolonged endurance exercise increases the level of mitochondrial proteins, increasing the oxidative capacity of the muscle, without affecting the muscle size. Weight training, on the other hand, increases muscle size but slightly decreases the density of mitochondrial proteins. Cross-innervation experiments, in which nerves to slow-twitch muscles are replaced with nerves that normally innervate fast-twitch muscles, result in a change in myosin ATPase from the slow to the fast form. Stimulation of a slow muscle through chronic direct stimulation, without neural activation, results in similar changes. When slow skeletal muscle is denervated or immobilized, the same transformation occurs. This suggests that the endogenous genetic nature of skeletal muscle is to produce fast myofilaments and that the expression of slow isoforms is dependent on motor nerve activity. Although these observations indicate that plasticity of muscle proteins depends on the degree and type of activity exhibited by the muscle, the mechanisms through which activity is translated into genetic alterations are not known.

MECHANICAL CHARACTERISTICS OF MUSCLE CONTRACTIONS

When a single stimulus is applied to a muscle, a short, brisk contraction followed by relaxation to resting tension or length results. This type of muscle contraction is known as a *muscle twitch* (Fig. 45.10). If the muscle is fixed at both ends so that it cannot shorten but the tension developed by

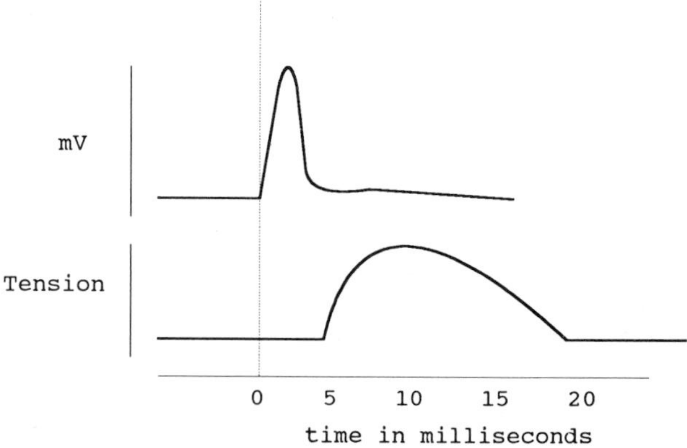

Figure 45.10. Schematic of the time relationships between an action potential (*top*) and the tension developed in a muscle twitch (*bottom*).

the muscle twitch can be measured at one of the tendons, the contraction is called an *isometric contraction* (Fig. 45.11). If the muscle is not fixed in length and bears a constant, movable load, the muscle will shorten and the contraction produced is called an *isotonic contraction*. If a muscle contracts against an elastic load, so that the load increases as the muscle shortens, the contraction is called an *auxotonic contraction*. Often skeletal muscle undergoes contraction while it is being lengthened by the load it bears; such a contraction is called a *lengthening* (or *eccentric*) *contraction*.

When skeletal muscle is activated to produce an isotonic contraction while stretched by a moderate load, there is a 2 to 3 ms interval between the stimulus and the initiation of tension development (Fig. 45.10). This interval is called the *latent period*. The latent period represents the time required for spread of the action potential over the sarcolemma and activation of excitation contraction mechanisms. In stretched muscle, there is a very brief period of latency relaxation immediately before the development of tension

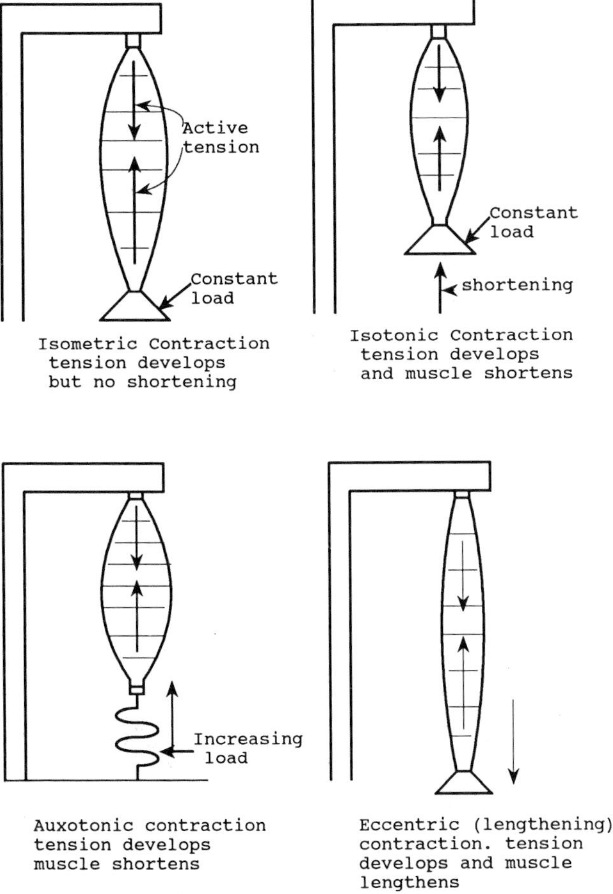

Figure 45.11. Schematic of isometric, isotonic, auxotonic, and eccentric muscle contractions.

by the muscle. The cellular mechanisms that produce the diminished tension are not known. Latency relaxation is not observed in muscles that are stimulated at lengths substantially below their normal in situ resting length.

Two types of isometric and isotonic contraction can be observed in skeletal muscle. If a load is applied and allowed to stretch the muscle before the initiation of contraction, the contraction is called a *preloaded contraction*. The tension developed by the muscle must exceed the preload before overall shortening of the muscle occurs. If the load is applied after the muscle has begun its shortening, the contraction is called an *afterloaded* contraction. The difference in response between these two types of contraction lies within the elastic components of the muscle belly. These elastic elements are viewed as comprising two components—one in series with the muscle contraction and one in parallel with it. The series elastic element resides in the myosin molecules of the thick myofilaments; the parallel elastic element is the sarcolemma. In a preloaded contraction, the elastic components are stretched before the muscle contraction occurs, and the dynamics of muscle shortening are a better measure of the actual muscle fiber–shortening dynamics. In an afterloaded contraction, the applied load will stretch the elastic elements after muscle fiber shortening has been initiated.

LENGTH-TENSION RELATIONSHIPS

When skeletal muscle is stretched, the elasticity of the myosin molecules and the sarcolemma resist stretching as elastic forces and passive tension develop in the muscle (Fig. 45.12). When the stretching force is removed, the muscle returns to its resting length. Stretch of more than 30 to 40 percent of the resting muscle length usually results in damage to muscle cells and, when released, the muscle does not return to its original length.

When muscle is stretched, the contractile properties vary in a characteristic fashion. If muscle resting lengths are plotted against the tension developed when stimulated, the resulting plot is a *length–tension curve* (Fig. 45.12). When the lengths of individual sarcomeres are compared with both the stretch of a skeletal muscle belly and the tension developed in a single contraction, a good correlation is demonstrated among the three variables. Maximum contraction strength develops at sarcomere lengths of between 2.0 and 2.25 μm (Fig. 45.13), which allow for maximum exposure of myosin heads to actin of thin myofilaments without overlapping of the opposing thin myofilaments. There is a possibility that stretching the sarcomere has the effect of increasing Tn affinity for cytosolic Ca^{2+}, thus forming more calcium Tn-C complexes and enhancing muscle contractile force. Such a mechanism has been demonstrated to operate in cardiac muscle cells and probably operates in skeletal muscle cells as well. The length of the muscle belly at which maximal contractile force develops is called the *optimal length* (Fig. 45.12). When the muscle is

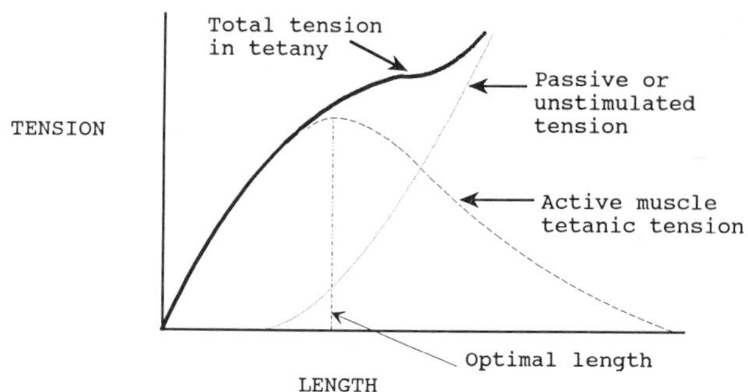

Figure 45.12. Illustration of the relationships between passive and active tension in a skeletal muscle at various lengths.

shortened or lengthened before contraction, so that sarcomere length increases or decreases from the optimal length, the tension developed in a single muscle twitch is diminished. At sarcomere lengths beyond 3.65 μm, there is no overlap of thick and thin filaments and no muscle contraction can occur (Fig. 45.13). At sarcomere lengths below 1.27 μm, there is no contraction because the thick filaments abut against the Z lines and are partially compressed.

FORCE-VELOCITY RELATIONSHIPS

The velocity of muscle shortening in isotonic contractions is determined by the load against which it contracts (Fig. 45.14). With no external load or with only a light load, there is a rapid rate of shortening. As the external load is increased, the velocity of muscle shortening diminishes. A.V. Hill developed empirical formulas to describe the relationships between velocity of shortening and external load in the sartorius muscle of the frog. Hill's equations state that $(P + a)(V + b) = K$, where P is the load applied to the muscle, V is the velocity of shortening, a is a constant of force dimensions, b is a constant with dimensions of velocity, and K is a constant. This equation indicates that force developed in the muscle is inversely related to velocity of shortening. When the load P is equal to the maximum isometric force that the muscle can develop, the load is referred to as Po. At a load of Po, V is also zero. The constants a and b are both sensitive to temperature, with a Q_{10}

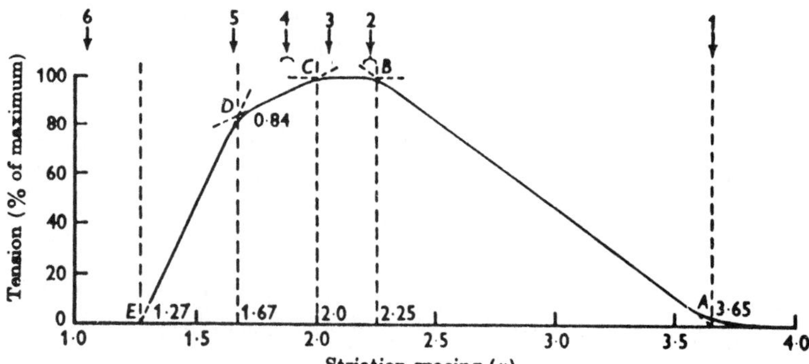

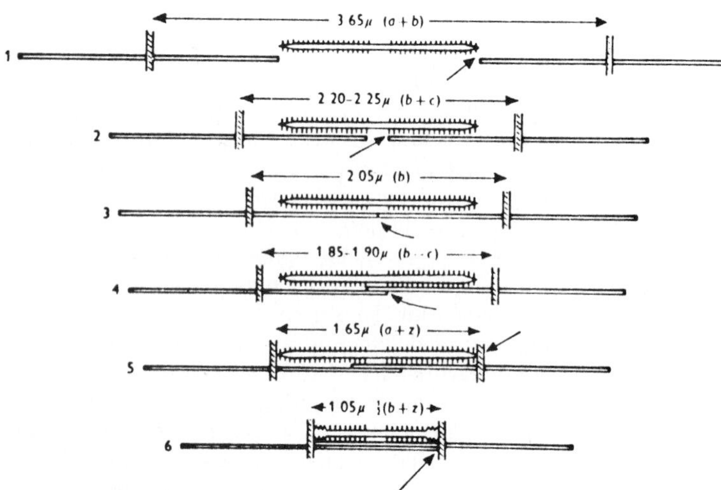

Figure 45.13. Illustration of the effects of sarcomere length on isometric tension development during a tetanic muscle contraction. Each of the schematics in the lower part demonstrates the topographic relationships of the thick and thin myofilaments at each length. The letter a refers to the length of the thick myofilaments, b to the length of the thin myofilaments and the z lines and c to the H line, in which there are no cross-bridges on the thick myofilaments. (From Gordon, Huxley, and Julian 1966, *J. Physiol.* 184:170–92).

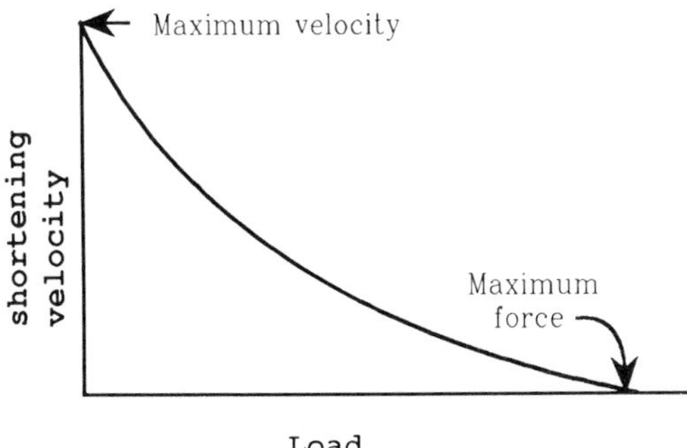

Figure 45.14. Illustration of the relationship between velocity of shortening and the maximum load against which isotonic contractions can occur.

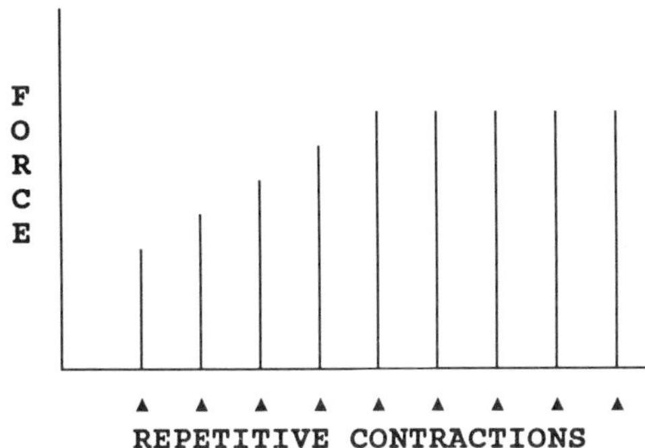

Figure 45.15. Staircase effect (treppe). Repeated maximal stimuli applied to a muscle produce a sequential increase in the force of muscle contraction until a maximum is obtained for that rate of stimulation.

from 1.5 to 2, and are thought to represent biochemical activities in the muscle fibers. The constant a is related to the heat of shortening, and constant b is related to the chemical interactions taking place within the myofilaments during contraction. One can obtain the constants a and b by plotting the value (Po-P)/V against P, which provides a straight line. The slope of the line is 1/b, and the y intercept (the Po-P/V value) is equal to a/b. Hill's equation becomes useful in determining the maximum velocity of muscle contraction, which occurs with zero load (V_{max}). Since it is impossible to obtain a true zero load in muscle, V_{max} can be calculated by the equation $V_{max} = Po(b/a)$, or from the plot of velocity of shortening against tension development and extrapolation of the plot to zero tension (load). V_{max} has often been used as a measure of the ability of muscle to do work.

REPETITIVE MUSCLE ACTION AND RECRUITMENT

The intensity of tension development by individual muscle fibers during contraction is proportional to the number of calcium Tn-C complexes formed during excitation contraction coupling. When skeletal muscles are stimulated to contract while still undergoing relaxation or during a period immediately after relaxation, a second muscle twitch is produced and develops a greater tension than the initial contraction. This effect is called *temporal summation of muscle contraction*. Temporal summation is best observed when muscle is repetitively stimulated to produce a series of contractions. Each subsequent contraction demonstrates an increase in tension over the previous contraction, until a plateau of maximum tension characteristic of the rate of activation is attained (Fig. 45.15). This effect, also called *treppe* or *ascending staircase effect*, is produced by an increasing quantity of cytosolic calcium remaining from the previous contractions. Thus each subsequent stimulus activates increasing quantities of Tn-C. If the muscle is stimulated at a sufficiently high rate to prevent relaxation between contractions, a continuous contracted state known as *tetany* results. Tetany occurs because the calcium pumps of the sarcoplasmic reticulum membranes cannot remove the cytoplasmic calcium as fast as it is released by the action potentials, so that the cytoplasmic concentration of calcium is maintained above threshold levels for muscle contraction. The maximum tension developed in tetany exceeds that developed in any individual muscle twitch and represents the maximum tension possible for the muscle. When muscle tetany is maintained for a period of time, tension begins to decrease, even though stimulation is continued. This is often called *muscle fatigue*, but it is not the fatigue that is seen in intact animals. It is rare, however, that skeletal muscles are physiologically stimulated at rates sufficient to produce tetany.

When muscle contraction force is increased through voluntary effort by the animal, increased force is the result of recruitment of additional active motor units. This condition is known as *spatial summation of muscle contraction*. Because of the properties of motor neurons that innervate skeletal muscle, recruitment of small motor units occurs initially; as force increases, larger motor units are recruited. This is known as the *size principle of motor neuron activation*.

SKELETAL MUSCLE ENERGETICS AND METABOLISM

When skeletal muscle contracts, there is a marked increase in ATP hydrolysis, representing energy utilization. According to the law of conservation of energy, the chemical energy used must equal the sum of mechanical energy and heat production by the muscle.

The energy utilization of skeletal muscle in performing work represents only 40 to 50 percent of the total energy generated from ATP. The remaining 50 to 60 percent forms heat. This heat is referred to as *initial heat*, even though it is generated both at the initiation and during the course of muscle contraction. It would appear that work accomplished by muscle contraction represents a 40 to 50 percent efficiency of energy utilization. When the total energy used, however, is compared with the heat generated and the work accomplished, the mechanical efficiency of skeletal muscle is only about 20 to 30 percent. This apparent inefficiency of muscle contraction results from the energy required to pump calcium ions out of the cytoplasm into the sarcoplasmic reticulum to maintain the sodium and potassium ion pumps and to restore the ATP used during contraction. These mechanisms use significant energy and generate additional heat, which is known as the *recovery heat* of muscle contraction.

When a muscle is stimulated to contract, to produce either a twitch or a tetany, there is an initial rapid production of heat, called *activation heat*, that is independent of the tension developed. Activation heat is determined by measurement of the heat produced and the force developed at varying muscle lengths. The plot of these values is then extrapolated to zero to obtain the theoretical heat produced at zero force development. Activation heat is thought to be the net result of Ca^{2+} transport associated with the initiation of muscle contraction. If no physical work is done by the muscle, as in an isometric contraction, there is a continual generation of heat. Muscle heat generated in this situation is called *maintenance heat*. Maintenance heat is proportional to the duration and tension of the muscle contraction. When a muscle lifts a load and does external work, the heat produced is called *shortening heat* and is proportional to the work done. Shortening heat is produced in addition to maintenance heat in an isometric contraction, even though no external work is done, and represents an enhanced interaction of actin and myosin. The proportionality between work done and shortening heat is known as the *Fenn effect*.

SKELETAL MUSCLE ENERGY METABOLISM AND THE LACTATE SHUTTLE

During rest or mild muscle activity, ATP is continuously generated through oxidative or aerobic mechanisms to the degree that oxygen is available. Because of the large density of capillaries in muscle tissues, it has been generally assumed that the oxygen supply to skeletal muscle cells is high. The blood of large arteries of mammals contains about 20 ml oxygen per 100 ml and has an oxygen tension, or Po_2, of 100 mm Hg. At rest the blood in large veins contains about 15 ml oxygen per 100 ml and has a Po_2 of about 40 mm Hg. Microelectrode measurements of tissue oxygen tension of skeletal muscles, however, indicate that the resting Po_2 is only 15 to 19 mm Hg. It is obvious, therefore, that skeletal muscle functions at all times with a limited oxygen supply when compared with most other tissues. It is proposed that the low-oxygen environment of skeletal muscle is related to the anatomic arrangement of blood vessels supplying muscle. In skeletal muscle, large and small arterioles and venules are adjacent and parallel to each other, being separated only about 40 to 80 μm. This arrangement allows a *countercurrent oxygen exchange* between the inflowing and outflowing blood. Thus oxygen is removed from the arterial blood by diffusion into the venous blood providing a low Po_2 to the tissue cells. With this arrangement of blood vessels, it would seem that there must also be a countercurrent accumulation of carbon dioxide in muscle tissue, although that has not been demonstrated at this time.

Low oxygen concentration in skeletal muscle results in anaerobic metabolism and the production of lactic acid. In the gracilis muscle of the dog, however, lactic acid production has been shown to occur when there is an apparently adequate supply of oxygen. Similarly, lactic acid production is enhanced in resting muscle after feeding. The production of lactate in these conditions represents the operation of a *lactate shuttle*. The lactate shuttle operates as a postprandial glucose-conservation mechanism by allowing absorbed plasma glucose to be converted to lactate by skeletal muscle. The muscle-generated lactate may be used by the muscle to form glycogen, or it may enter the venous blood and pass to the liver for hepatic glycogen synthesis.

The lactate shuttle operates in sustained exercise to release lactate from muscle fibers that have high rates of glycogenolysis and glycolysis. Most of this lactate is used by muscle fibers with high aerobic capacities. It is apparent that this shuttled lactate may provide a significant supply of energy to exercising muscle when compared with that provided by blood glucose.

In anaerobic metabolism of skeletal muscle, as in continued exercise, there is increased glycolysis to the point that mitochondria cannot use pyruvate or provide sufficient oxygen to cytochrome oxidase for reduction of cytosolic nicotinamide-adenine dinucleotide to prevent lactic acid accumulation in the cytosol. The formation of lactic acid has the effect of assisting in the maintenance of ATP through its effect on the phosphorylation ratio ([ATP]/[ADP]) of skeletal muscle cells. The interrelationship between ATP, ADP, creatine (Cr), and creatine phosphate (PCr^{2-}) in muscle cells is important because the hydrolysis of ATP to ADP and inorganic phosphate (Pi) is thermodynamically irreversible. ATP is generated through the mediation of creatine and creatine phosphate as indicated in the reaction: $H^+ + ADP^- + PCr^{2-} \rightarrow ATP^{2-} + Cr$. It can be seen that as the $[H^+]$ rises from the formation of lactic acid, the reaction will shift to the right and maintain the phosphorylation ratio at a higher level than normal.

Since lactic acid is relatively strong as an organic acid (pK = 3.9)and is almost completely ionized at physiological pH, it must be immediately titrated by tissue buffers to a salt in order to limit changes in cellular pH . This titration is accomplished primarily by $NaHCO_3$ of the extracellular fluid. As intracellular lactate is produced, bicarbonate ions (HCO_3^-) , derived from $NaHCO_3$ in the extracellular fluid, diffuse into the cell where they form $KHCO_3$. $KHCO_3$ reacts with lactic acid to form potassium lactate, H_2O, and CO_2. The generated CO_2 equilibrates with extracellular CO_2, and lactate ions leave the cell to associate with the Na^+ to form sodium lactate. Through this mechanism, each milliequivalent of lactate produced generates 22 ml of additional CO_2 to the extracellular fluid. The loss of $NaHCO_3$ from the extracellular fluid represents a metabolic acidosis. This mechanism alters the ratio of O_2 uptake and CO_2 generation (the respiratory quotient) by the muscle cells and produces a decreased exercise tolerance or muscle fatigue.

Muscle fatigue results from the inability to use inorganic phosphate that is formed in the hydrolysis of ATP to ADP for the restoration of ATP. Inorganic phosphate, in the form of KH_2PO_4, accumulates in the cytoplasm. KH_2PO_4 being acidic, acts directly on the contractile proteins, diminishing their ability to develop tension within sarcomeres.

SKELETAL MUSCLE ACTIVITY AND SYSTEMIC POTASSIUM EQUILIBRIUM

Skeletal muscle contains the largest single pool of K^+ in the body, representing about 75 percent of the total body K^+. During exercise, K^+ loss from human skeletal muscle may increase the plasma levels of K^+ by as much as 3 mM per minute. This represents a net loss of K^+ from skeletal muscle of about 40 mM/min. The maximum capacity for active transport of K^+ is about 125 mM/min. The magnitude of these K^+ movements allows muscle to produce large changes in extracellular K^+ during short periods. Alterations in extracellular and intracellular K^+ concentrations interfere with excitability of nerve and muscle cells, contractility of muscle cells, and systemic metabolism. There are, therefore, tight controls on the activity of Na^+-K^+ transport for the maintenance of optimum muscle function. These controls involve regulation of the basal activity and concentration of Na^+-K^+ ATPase proteins (the Na^+-K^+ pump) in muscle cell membranes.

Insulin, thyroid hormones, epinephrine, and norepinephrine influence the basal activity of the Na^+-K^+ ATPase of skeletal muscle. These ongoing controls play a significant role in systemic metabolism as well as in the gain or loss of K^+ in skeletal muscle cells.

The effect of insulin in enhancing the uptake of extracellular K^+ is well recognized. This action appears to be mediated through an enhancement of the basal activity of Na^+-K^+ ATPase, independent of the effect of insulin on glucose transport. A second messenger, or mediator, of this action on ATPase activity has not been demonstrated but is assumed to exist. The insulin effect on inward K^+ transport is accompanied by a hyperpolarization of muscle cells, indicating an increase in the K^+ concentration gradient across muscle cell membranes. The fact that increasing plasma K^+ concentrations by 1 mM stimulates insulin secretion in dogs indicates a feedback control against severe hyperkalemia involving insulin-stimulated Na^+-K^+ pumping. Minor alterations in plasma K^+ concentrations (below 1 mM) are adjusted through other regulatory mechanisms involving the liver and the kidney.

Abnormal distribution of potassium between intracellular and extracellular fluid results in clinical conditions in animals that are characterized by skeletal muscle weakness (often to the point of physical collapse and paralysis) and spontaneous, uncoordinated muscle contractions called *muscle fasciculation*. These conditions are seen in hyperkalemic periodic paralysis or weakness in horses and dogs and in hypokalemic periodic weakness or paralysis in dogs. In addition to these conditions, the cause of which is not known, decreased extracellular potassium ion concentrations may occur after intense and prolonged vomiting, excess urinary loss of potassium, or insulin administration or in fluid therapy in which potassium balance is not controlled.

Epinephrine- and norepinephrine-enhanced basal activity of skeletal muscle Na^+-K^+ pumping in the dog has been recognized for more than 50 years. Epinephrine demonstrates a potency in this action that is at least one order of magnitude greater than that of norepinephrine. The effects of epinephrine have been demonstrated to occur at plasma levels obtained during exercise. The activity is mediated through beta$_2$-adrenergic receptors of skeletal muscle cells, resulting in increased cytoplasmic cyclic adenosine monophosphate concentrations. Other beta$_2$ agonists, such as terbutaline, demonstrate the same property. The influences of epinephrine and norepinephrine are additive to the effect of insulin on basal pump activity.

Beta-adrenergic receptor activation promotes a marked increase in skeletal muscle mass (associated with a reduction in body fat content). This action, through the use of beta-agonists to increase the lean body weight of animals, could have dramatic effects in meat production. Lambs fed cimaterol (a beta-agonist) for a period of about 2 months showed a 25 to 30 percent increase in muscle weight, compared with lambs fed a control diet. This induced increase in muscle weight is accompanied by the production of additional muscle cells through mitosis of satellite cells.

Long-term controls of Na^+-K^+ pump proteins involving the concentration of these proteins in muscle cell membranes is exerted by muscle activity, thyroid hormones, and the availability of K^+. Training in dogs leads to a diminished loss of K^+ during exercise and an increase in resting membrane potentials of skeletal muscle cells. This effect appears to be mediated through elevated extracellular K^+ concentrations. Elevation of extracellular K^+ concentration, as occurs in unconditioned animals, results in an upregulation of Na^+-K^+ ATPase in muscle cell membranes as a protective mechanism against excessive loss of K^+ in working animals. When extracellular K^+ is depleted below normal levels, there is a consequent downregulation of transport proteins. The functional significance of this response is not known, but a reduction in the capacity for clearing K^+ from the extracellular fluid may assist in avoidance of severe hypokalemia and paralysis during K^+ deficiency.

The influence of thyroid hormones on basal metabolic rate has long been recognized. The means by which thyroid hormones exert this effect has been determined to be primarily through an upregulation of Na^+-K^+ ATPase concentration in cell membranes. Thyroid hormones, therefore, favor the clearance of K^+ from the extracellular fluid and, with an increase in the use of ATP, a major part of the thermogenic action of thyroid hormones and the maintenance of body temperature take place. It is estimated that up to 85 percent of thyroid hormone–mediated thermogenesis is due to enhanced Na^+-K^+ pump activity in body cells.

ACTIVITY-INDUCED MUSCLE INJURY

Activity-induced injury of skeletal muscle often occurs when muscles are active after a period of inactivity or when muscles are exposed to extraordinary conditions. The most familiar situation is muscle soreness that occurs 1 to 3 days after strenuous or unaccustomed exercise. In some cases activity-induced injury results in increased plasma levels of intracellular enzymes such as creatine kinase or lysosomal enzymes, with or without structural evidence of muscle damage. Muscle injury is generally accompanied by decreased ability to develop normal levels of force in contraction that cannot be attributed to fatigue. There is no correlation between muscle fatigue and the extent or degree of activity-induced muscle soreness. Mechanical disruption and increases in muscle hydrogen ion and lactate concentrations have been suggested as causes of this type of muscle injury.

A more severe exertional myopathy is observed in horses and working greyhounds, although it may occur in other canine breeds after strenuous exercise in poorly conditioned animals. The initiating cause is not known, but considerable muscle damage may occur. It appears that ischemia develops, resulting in muscle cramping and the release of myoglobin. Since myoglobin is readily excreted in the urine, a myoglobinuria results. In the era when draft horses were used for farm power, the condition was known as Monday morning sickness, as it would occur after a weekend of rest and heavy work on Monday.

Although it is often stated that skeletal muscle has limited regenerative power, it has been well demonstrated that muscle fiber regeneration occurs in all animal species in which it has been investigated. After either minced muscle implants or free muscle grafts, in which there is no blood or nerve supply, muscle demonstrates a remarkable ability to regenerate, vascularize, and be reinnervated. Such muscles attach to existing tendon stumps of the recipient animal so that, on regeneration, these muscles are functional.

REFERENCES

Asano, Y., Liberman, U.A., and Edelman, I.S. 1976. Thyroid thermogenesis: Relationships between Na^+-dependent respiration and Na^+K^{-+}-adenosine triphosphatase activity in rat skeletal muscle. *J. Clin. Invest.* 57:368–79.

Augustine, G.J., Charlton, M.P., and Smith, S.J. 1987. Calcium action in synaptic release. *Annu. Rev. Neurosci.* 10:633–93.

Averill, D.R. 1980. Diseases of muscle. *Vet. Clin. North Am.* 10:233–55.

Babij P., and Booth F.W. 1988. Sculpturing new muscle phenotypes, *News Physiol. Sci.* 3:100–102.

Bandman, E. 1985. Myosin isoenzyme transitions in muscle development, maturation and disease. *Int. Rev. Cytol.* 97:97–131.

Brooke, M.H., and Kaiser, K.K. 1970. Three myosin adenosine triphosphatase systems: The nature of their pH lability and sulfhydryl dependence. *J. Histochem. Cytochem.* 18:670–72.

Brooks, G.A. 1986. Lactate production under fully aerobic conditions: The lactate shuttle during rest and exercise. *Federation Proc.* 45:2924–29.

Buckingham, M.E. 1985. Actin and myosin multigene families: Their expression during the formation of skeletal muscle. *Essays Biochem.* 20:77–109.

Carlson, B.M. 1986. Regeneration of entire skeletal muscles. *Federation Proc.* 45:1456–60.

Cattaneo, A., and Grasso, A. 1989. A functional domain on the alpha-latrotoxin molecule, distinct from the binding site, involved in catecholamine secretion from PC12 cells: Identification with monoclonal antibodies, *Biochemistry* 25:2730–36.

Clausen, T. 1986. Regulation of active Na^+ -K^+ transport in skeletal muscle. *Physiol. Rev.* 66:542–80.

Drachman, D.G. 1981. The biology of myasthenia gravis. *Annu. Rev. Neurosci.* 4:195–225.

Gorczynski, R.J., and Duling, B.R. 1978. Role of oxygen in artriolar functional vasodilation in hamster striated muscle. *Am. J. Physiol.* 235 (5):H505-H515.

Harris, P.D. 1986. Movement of oxygen in skeletal muscle. *News Physiol. Sci.* 1:147–49.

Hermansen, L., Orheim, A., and Sejersted, O.M. 1984. Metabolic acidosis and changes in water and electrolyte balance in relation to fatigue during maximal exercise of short duration. *Int. J. Sport Med. Suppl.* 5:110–15.

Holloszy, J.O., and Booth, F.W. 1976. Biochemical adaptations to exercise in muscle. *Annu. Rev. Physiol.* 38:272–91.

Huang, C.L.-H. 1988. Intramembrane charge movements in skeletal muscle. *Physiol. Rev.* 68:1197–1247.

Idstrom, J.P., Harihara, S.V., Chance, B., Schersten, T., and Bylund-Felenius, A.C. 1985. Oxygen dependence of energy metabolism in contracting and recovering rat skeletal muscle. *Am. J. Physiol.* 248:17:H40–H48.

Katz, J., and McGarry, J.D. 1984. The glucose paradox: Is glucose a substrate for liver metabolism? *J. Clin. Invest.* 74:1901–09.

Kjeldsen, K., Norgaard, A., Gotzsche, C.O., Thomassen, A., and Clausen, T. 1984. Effect of thyroid function on the number of Na-K pumps in human skeletal muscle. *Lancet* 2:8–10.

Knockel, J.P., Blanchley, J.D., Johnson, J.H., and Carter, N.W. 1985. Muscle cell electrical hyperpolarization and reduced exercise hyperkalemia in physically conditioned dogs. *J. Clin. Invest.* 75:740–45.

Kramer, J.W., Hegreberg, G.A., and Hamilton, M.J. 1981. Inheritance of a neuromuscular disorder of Laborador retriever dogs. *J. Am. Vet. Med. Assoc.* 179:380–82.

Kushmerick, M. J. 1983. Energetics of muscle contraction. In L.D. Peachey, R.H. Adrian, and S.R. Geiger, eds., *Skeletal Muscle; Handbook of Physiology*, Section 10. Am. Physiol. Soc., Bethesda, Md. 189–236.

Laufer, R., Fontaine, B., Klarsfeld, A., Cartaud, J., and Changeux, J-P. 1989. Regulation of acetylcholine receptor biosynthesis during motor endplate morphogenesis. *News Physiol. Sci.* 4:5–9.

Lemos, J.R., Nordmann, J.J., Cooke, I.M., and Stuenkel, E.L. 1986. Single channels and ionic currents in peptidergic nerve terminals. *Nature* 319:410–12.

Lomo, T., and Westgaard, R.H. 1975. Control of ACh sensitivity in rat muscle fibers. *Cold Spring Harbor Symp. Quant. Biol.* 40:263–74.

Mauro, A. 1961. Satellite cells of skeletal muscle fibers. *J. Biophys. Biochem. Cytol.* 9:493–95.

Mallart, A., and Haimann, C. 1985. Differential effects of alpha-latrotoxin on mouse nerve endings and fibers. *Muscle Nerve* 8:151–57.

Newham, D.J., Jones, D.A., and Edwards, R.H.T. 1983. Large delayed plasma creatine kinase charges after stepping exercise. *Muscle Nerve* 6:380–85.

Newham, D.J., Mills, K.R., Quigley, B.M., and Edwards, R.H.T. 1983. Pain and fatigue after concentric and eccentric contractions. *Clin. Sci.* 64:55–62.

Pette, D., and Spamer, C. 1986. Metabolic properties of muscle fibers. *Federation Proc.* 45:2910–14.

Ruegg, J.C. 1987. Dependence of cardiac contractility on myofibrillar calcium sensitivity. *News Physiol. Sci.* 2:179–82.

Samaha, F.J., Guth, L., and Albers, R.W. 1970. Phenotypic differences between the actomyosin ATPase of the three fiber types of mammalian skeletal muscle. *Exp. Neurol.* 26:120–25.

Schuetze, S.M. 1987. Developmental regulation of nicotinic acetylcholine receptors. *Annu. Rev. Neurosci.* 10:403–57.

Schneider, M.F., and Simon, B.J. 1988. Inactivation of calcium release from the sarcoplasmic reticulum of frog skeletal muscle. *J. Physiol.* 405:727–45.

Swynghedauw, B. 1986. Developmental and functional adaptation of contractile proteins in cardiac and skeletal muscles. *Physiol. Rev.* 66:710–71.

Vergara, J., and Asotra, K. 1987. The chemical transmission mechanism of excitation-contraction coupling in skeletal muscle. *News Physiol. Sci.* 2:182–86.

Vergara, J., Asotra, K., and Delay, M. 1987. A chemical link in excitation-contraction coupling in skeletal muscle. In L. Mandel and D.C. Eaton, eds., *Cell Calcium and Control of Membrane Transport*. Rockefeller Univ. Press, New York. Pp. 133–51.

Wasserman, K. 1986. Anaerobiosis, lactate and gas exchange during exercise: The issues. *Federation Proc.* 45:2904–9.

Whalen, W.J., Nair, P., and Ganfield, R.A. 1973. Measurements of oxygen tension in tissues with a micro oxygen electrode. *Microvasc. Res.* 5:254–62.

Wilkie, D.R. 1986. Muscular fatigue: Effects of hydrogen ions and inorganic phosphate. *Federation Proc.* 45:2921–23.

Yang, Y.T., and McElligott, M.A. 1989. Multiple actions of β-adrenergic agonists on skeletal muscle and adipose tissue. *Biochem. J.* 261:1–10.

CHAPTER 46

Visceromotor (Autonomic) Control | by David Robertshaw

The autonomic nervous system is responsible for the visceral (or vegetative) control of the animal's body, and traditionally it has been thought to provide motor innervation to glands, to the heart, and to organs that have smooth muscle. However, the overall function of the autonomic system is to maintain the internal environment of the body within carefully defined limits. This internal control function is called *homeostasis* or, more descriptively, *homeokinesis*, a term that more accurately reflects the fact that the equilibrium is achieved by dynamic and not static processes. The term incorporates many dynamic processes, the equilibrium of which is so highly controlled that under normal circumstances they appear to be static. As a mechanism for control, the autonomic nervous system must be considered to include not only the visceral motor neurons but peripheral afferent neurons as well. The latter are nerve cells that conduct impulses to the central nervous sytem (CNS) and provide the information on which the system acts. The integrating centers use this information and activate the appropriate visceral motor neurons. The classic autonomic "system," the peripheral motor portion, is in reality merely the branch of the total autonomic program that executes its functions and, as such, is efferent in nature; that is, it conducts impulses away from the CNS.

The peripheral motor projections of the central autonomic areas are the parasympathetic (craniosacral) and sympathetic (thoracolumbar) efferent systems. Their combined activity is a modified reciprocal innervation, and in those structures that have a dual innervation the final activity of the structure represents the net balance between the opposing actions of the two parts of the efferent autonomic nervous system. The detection of changes and the conduction of information to the central integrative stations are as essential to the total mechanism as the integration itself and the subsequent peripheral execution. This basic principle of interdependence must be kept in mind in the study of the autonomic nervous system, since the division of the system into constituent parts, which is necessary for the sake of clarity, is quite artificial.

Many drugs, when administered, mimic activity of either the sympathetic or the parasympathetic nervous system; they are called *sympathomimetic* and *parasympathomimetic*, respectively. In most cases they act by direct action on the effector area by either acting in the same way as the transmitter substance or preventing its degradation and prolonging its action. Other drugs may have a central stimulating effect.

ANATOMICAL DIVISIONS

Central division

The core of the central portion of the autonomic system is the hypothalamus. This area receives specific afferent input and, through appropriate connections, exercises motor functions that produce modifications necessary for maintenance of the homeokinetic state. Superimposed upon the visceral functions of the hypothalamus is the influence of the other parts of the brain, particularly the cerebrum. The outflow from the hypothalamus affects other centers subserving visceral functions that are located in the lower brain stem. For example, respiration is controlled in the medullary region of the brain. The information associated with evaporative heat loss by panting is relayed from the temperature-regulating centers of the hypothalamus to the respiratory neurons of the medulla; the pattern of breathing is then changed so that evaporative heat loss may stabilize the internal body temperature. Evidence of cerebral involvement in visceral function is obtained from the effect of various psychic states, in both humans and animals, on blood pressure. Gastric and colonic ulcerations are all manifestations of altered autonomic function.

Peripheral efferent division

The peripheral efferent portions of the autonomic nervous system, those fibers that lead impulses away from the CNS, are classified as either *sympathetic* or *parasympathetic*. Initially, this separation was based on pharmacological evidence. When anatomical studies supported the separation, the synonyms *thoracolumbar* for the sympathetic and *craniosacral* for the parasympathetic systems were introduced. The organization of the efferent system is presented in Fig. 46.1 and may be referred to throughout the discussion of the efferent system.

The basic anatomical scheme underlying the efferent autonomic system is a two-neuron pathway with the cell bodies of the first leg of the pathway located in the CNS. The axons of these neurons leave the brain stem or spinal cord to terminate on ganglionic neurons located at varying distances from the CNS. The ganglionic neurons of the sympathetic system tend to be concentrated in grossly visible aggregates called *paravertebral ganglia*, whereas the ganglionic neurons of the parasympathetic system are more likely to be dispersed in the wall of the innervated organ. Thus the postganglionic axons of the parasympathetic nervous system are much shorter than those of the sympathetic nervous system. Since the ganglion cell is a point of anatomical reference for the pathway, the neuron leading from the CNS to the ganglion is called a *preganglionic neuron* and its fiber is called a *preganglionic fiber*. In the ganglionic synapse, the presynaptic terminal is actually the termination of the preganglionic neuron, and the postsynaptic membrane is the dendritic zone of the ganglionic neuron.

One exception to the two-neuron pattern has been found. The glandular cells that compose the medullary portion of the adrenal gland are, in reality, modified postganglionic neurons without an axon. Autonomic innervation of the adrenal medulla, then, is from preganglionic fibers only.

Craniosacral (parasympathetic) division

Cranial division. The cranial efferent division is composed of axons within cranial nerves III (oculomotor), VII (facial), and IX (glossopharyngeal), which innervate structures of the head, and cranial nerve X (vagus), whose projections supply parasympathetic innervation to the thoracic and abdominal viscera.

The autonomic preganglionic elements of the oculomotor nerve (III) leave the brain to contact ganglionic neurons in the ciliary ganglion or in the episcleral ganglia of the eye. Parasympathetic innervation supplies the pupillary constrictor muscles and is thus involved in the reflexes both for reducing light entering the eye and for accommodation to near vision. Numerous inputs affect the autonomic oculomotor responses, including both pupillary constriction and accommodation for near vision.

Parasympathetic contributions to the facial nerve (VII) are distributed in three pathways. Some pass to the sphen-

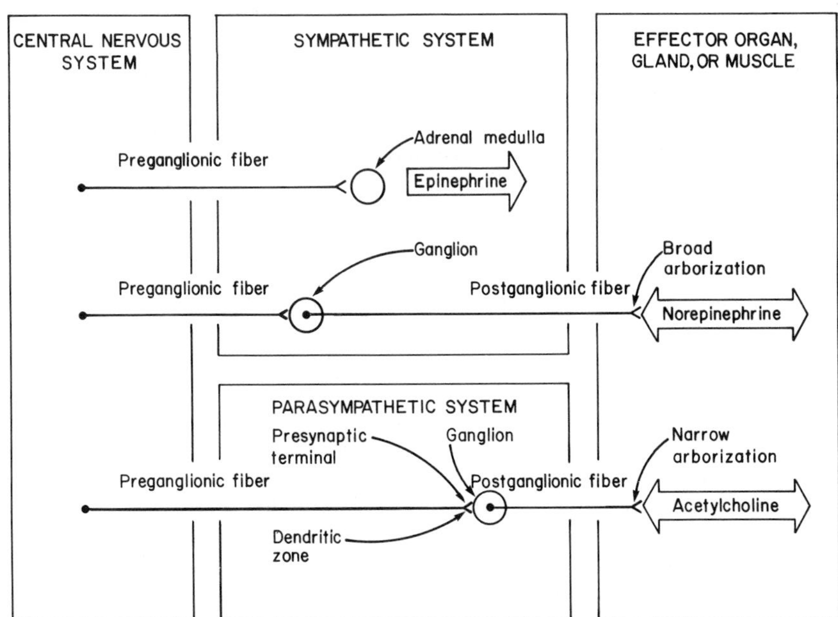

Figure 46.1. Organization of the efferent (motor) system. The boxes indicate division of the system's constituents; this artificial division is made for clarity only. Note relative lengths of preganglionic and postganglionic fibers. Most effector organs (*right box*) receive innervation from both sympathetic and para-sympathetic systems. Thus both driving force and braking mechanism are provided for effector organs that are so innervated.

opalatine (pterygopalatine) ganglion, from which postganglionic fibers innervate the lacrimal glands, the nasal and oral glands, and their associated smooth muscle. A second fiber distribution is with the chorda tympani to provide vasodilatory and secretory innervation for the submandibular and sublingual salivary glands. The third group of preganglionic fibers passes directly to the sublingual and submandibular salivary glands and ganglionic neurons in the surface of the glands.

The preganglionic neurons of the glossopharyngeal nerve (IX) pass to the otic ganglion or the tympanic plexus, from which the postganglionic fibers project secretory and vasodilatory fibers to the parotid and orbital salivary glands.

Afferent fibers from taste buds in the anterior portions of the tongue provide some of the important nervous stimuli that influence the activity of these salivary glands.

Afferent fibers to the salivatory nuclei originate in visceral afferent contributions from cranial nerves VII, IX, and X. These pathways provide the autonomic centers with gustatory impulses and are closely allied with the gagging and vomiting reflexes.

The principal parasympathetic origin of the vagus nerve (X) is the dorsal efferent nucleus of the medulla oblongata (dorsal nucleus of the vagus nerve in the dog). The fibers emerge as the parasympathetic cardiac and respiratory visceral efferents and the abdominal visceral efferents. The preganglionic fibers leave the medulla together in the vagus nerve, which provides parasympathetic innervation to all visceral structures from the caudal pharyngeal region to the upper portions of the colon. In the cervical region of several species—notably the dog, horse, and ox—the vagus runs in direct contact with the cervical sympathetic trunk, the fibers of the two structures being intermingled. Preganglionic fibers generally terminate in neurons distributed in the walls of the organs to be innervated. Before terminating, the preganglionic fibers may ramify on the surface of organs to form plexuses. (These assume the name of the organ, e.g., the cardiac plexus or the aortic plexus.)

Afferent connections to the nuclei of origin of the vagus include fibers from the hypothalamus and projections from bulbar and medullary visceral control centers (e.g., respiratory centers, cardiac centers).

Sacral division. The sacral parasympathetic efferents leave the spinal cord with the ventral roots of the sacral nerves. These preganglionic parasympathetic fibers leave the spinal cord and, with the sympathetic hypogastric nerves, form the pelvic plexus, where some of the fibers contact postganglionic neurons whereas others apparently pass on through to make ganglionic contacts in the walls of pelvic organs. The preganglionic and postganglionic fibers are distributed by way of various subsidiary plexuses and nerves to the specific organs (e.g., urethral plexus, nervus erigens). The connections to the sacral preganglionic neurons from the higher centers are provided by fibers in the ventral portions of the spinal cord. The segmental afferent (dorsal root) fibers also distribute to the preganglionic neurons of the sacral division. Pelvic innervation is apparently well interconnected, and in experimental preparations a single sacral root can provide sufficient innervation to maintain normal parasympathetic function in such reflex activities as micturition, defecation, and sexual function.

Thoracolumbar (sympathetic) division

In the thoracolumbar efferent division, the two-neuron pathway also appears with the preganglionic neurons located in the intermediolateral gray column of the thoracic and lumbar spinal cord. The preganglionic axon, which is generally myelinated, leaves the cord substance and subseuently the spinal canal with the ventral root of the segmental spinal nerve. A short distance from the canal the preganglionic fibers leave the spinal nerve to enter the paravertebral sympathetic trunk via the rami communicantes. This collection of nerve fibers and ganglionic neurons is located bilaterally on the ventral surface of the vertebrae. Although the sympathetic trunk extends from the upper cervical region to the base of the tail, it receives preganglionic fibers only from the thoracic and upper lumbar spinal cord segments. The number of preganglionic axon bundles (rami communicantes) entering the trunk varies with the species and depends on the number of vertebrae in each region. The number of thoracic rami depends on the number of thoracic vertebrae, which ranges from 18 in the horse to 13 in the dog. In the lumbar region, where the upper segments are the main source of preganglionic fibers, species variation also occurs. In humans only the first two or three lumbar segments provide preganglionic fibers, whereas in the dog, horse, and cow there are four to six lumbar contributions.

In domestic animals the sympathetic trunk extends from the cervical region to the lower sacral or first coccygeal vertebra. The cervical trunk receives its preganglionic fibers from the upper thoracic spinal cord. The preganglionic fibers terminate in the caudal, middle, or cranial cervical ganglia; the last named is the largest and most frequently present. In domestic animals more obviously than in humans, the caudal cervical ganglion and the first few thoracic ganglia combine to form the stellate ganglion. Since, as mentioned, the efferent fibers in the vagosympathetic trunk are intermingled, it is apparent that the transmission of impulses is in opposite directions; the sympathetic outflow is directed toward structures in the head, whereas vagal efferents supply structures in the thorax and abdomen. Sectioning of the vagosympathetic trunk will therefore produce evidence of denervation at quite different anatomical sites.

The sacral and coccygeal ganglia receive their preganglionic fibers from lower thoracic and lumbar segments. The ganglia themselves vary greatly in number and location among species and among individuals of the same species.

Ganglionic neurons are also located in prevertebral ganglia, which are entities separate from the sympathetic trunk. For the most part, the prevertebral ganglia are found associated with the autonomic innervation to the abdominal and pelvic viscera.

A given preganglionic fiber emerging from the thoracic or lumbar cord follows one of several possible courses (Fig. 46.2). All preganglionic fibers leave their respective spinal nerve roots as *rami communicantes* to enter and form the sympathetic trunk. From this point, the course of the fiber depends on the location of its ganglionic termination. The simplest course is for the preganglionic fiber to terminate on ganglionic neurons at the same level at which it entered. More commonly, however, the preganglionic fiber or a branch of the fiber ascends or descends some distance in the trunk before terminating on ganglion cells at other segmental levels. This course is taken by those fibers that provide preganglionic innervation to the cervical, sacral, and coccygeal ganglia. As a final alternative, the preganglionic axon may join the sympathetic trunk, pass through the trunk, often after ascending or descending a few segments, and contact a ganglion cell in one of the prevertebral ganglia.

Each preganglionic neuron exercises control over many ganglionic neurons by virtue of the terminal branching of its axon. The branches not only terminate on neurons in one ganglion but, in following an ascending or descending path, may contact neurons in several ganglia along the way. The terminal ramifications of these preganglionic fibers often number 25 or 30, thereby providing for divergence of the impulse.

The postganglionic neurons extend their axons, which are predominantly unmyelinated, directly to the organ to be innervated. The course of the postganglionic fibers varies with the location of the effector organ. From the neurons in the sympathetic trunk, the postganglionic sympathetic fibers to be distributed to cutaneous structures return in segmental bundles to the somatic spinal nerves and pass with the respective cutaneous branches to the smooth muscles of cutaneous vessels, to hair follicles, and to the cutaneous glands. In addition, sympathetic fibers accompany somatic nerves to skeletal muscle, where they provide innervation to the blood vessels. As mentioned above, the axon bundles that connect the sympathetic trunk with the somatic spinal nerve are called rami communicantes. In humans, the myelinated preganglionic bundles and the unmyelinated postganglionic bundles enter and leave the sympathetic trunk as discrete bundles and are called, respectively, white and gray rami communicantes. The rami of domestic animals are generally mixed, containing both myelinated and unmyelinated fibers, and the white and gray designations are significant only to the extent that they imply preganglionic or postganglionic function.

Postganglionic sympathetic fibers to other visceral structures generally run together as specific visceral nerves, or

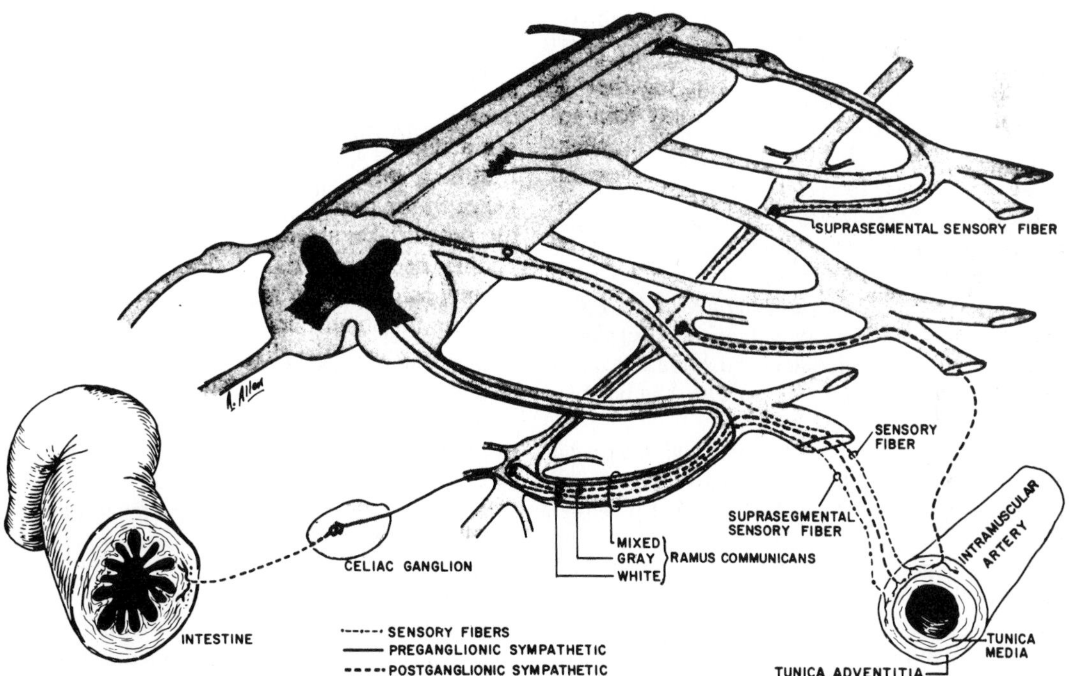

Figure 46.2. Typical sympathetic spinal reflex pathways. The afferent (sensory) limb is shown as a visceral sensory fiber. The several possibilities for efferent outflow are shown. In general, preganglionic fibers that provide central innervation to vessels of the skin and skeletal muscles terminate in the chain ganglia, and preganglionic fibers that provide central innervation to peritoneal structures pass through the chain ganglia and terminate in prevertebral ganglia.

they may join somatic nerves and run with them to the effector organs. Examples of specific visceral nerves are the splanchnic nerves, which provide sympathetic innervation to the abdominal viscera, and the hypogastric nerves, which carry sympathetic influence to the pelvic organs. Postganglionic axons from the cervical ganglion join the trigeminal (V), facial (VII), glossopharyngeal (IX), vagus (X), accessory (XI), and hypoglossal (XII) cranial nerves and often contribute to the first, second, and third cervical nerves. In addition, each spinal (segmental) nerve carries a complement of sympathetic fibers.

Central pathways to the preganglionic sympathetic neurons in the spinal cord are of two types: (1) Fibers from the brain descend in the reticulospinal tracts to the thoracic and lumbar gray matter, and (2) sensory fibers enter the dorsal roots of the spinal nerves and, through interneurons, contact the preganglionic sympathetic neurons. The sensory axons from the dorsal root ganglia also ascend the cord, providing the central integrating centers with both somatic and visceral information.

FUNCTIONS

General function

Autonomic reflex arc

The autonomic reflex arc consists, as does its somatic counterpart, of an afferent (sensory) limb and an efferent (motor) limb (see Fig. 46.2). Visceral and somatic sensory fibers entering the dorsal root send branches ascending in spinal sensory columns and also send synaptic terminals to nearby interneurons. The interneurons transmit impulses to the preganglionic neurons in the cord or brain stem. Preganglionic axons make up the efferent limb and carry the visceral motor stimuli to ganglion cells, from which postganglionic axons innervate visceral effectors. In the parasympathetic efferent system, it is more common to find long preganglionic fibers serving a relatively few ganglionic neurons in the wall of a specific organ. The degree of divergence in the parasympathetic system is limited by the diffuse arrangement of the postganglionic neurons and the degree to which a given postganglionic axon can arborize at its effector terminal. Such limited distribution is compatible with the discrete action attributed to the parasympathetic system (see Fig. 46.1).

In the sympathetic system, on the other hand, the preganglionic axon most frequently contacts relatively large numbers of ganglionic neurons located close to the preganglionic cells of origin. The chain arrangement of ganglia permits an entering preganglionic axon to contact not only a large number of neurons in a given ganglion but also, through its ascending or descending path in the chain, a large number of neurons in other ganglia. The result is a marked divergence of sympathetic motor impulses. Therefore a given axon may provide innervation to 25 to 30 ganglion cells, some of which serve more than one type of effector organ. This architectural arrangement promotes the broader action that is characteristic of the sympathetic division (see Fig. 46.1).

At the cranial level, simple multisynaptic reflex arcs may exist, and although the same basic pattern prevails as in the spinal area, the specific internal pathways are considerably more diverse and complex.

Ganglia as entities serve several functions. They act as distribution terminals for preganglionic-to-postganglionic divergence and convergence of impulses. As a result, a degree of overlap occurs so that a given postganglionic neuron may receive axon terminals from more than one preganglionic neuron. In addition, a given preganglionic neuron will contact many postganglionic neurons in the same or in different ganglia; that is, impulse divergence occurs. Interestingly, the degrees of divergence of the various ganglia are appropriate for the postganglionic innervation provided. There is minimal divergence of impulses in the cranial cervical ganglion, which provides rather discrete innervation to specific structures of the head; the celiac and mesenteric ganglia, on the other hand, provide a more generalized output to the gastrointestinal tract, and in these ganglia the divergence of impulses is maximal.

The convergence of several preganglionic fibers on a given ganglionic neuron provides the structural basis for spatial and temporal summation. It is apparent, then, that the neuron relationships in autonomic ganglia have some of the properties of CNS neurons—and, as such, exercise a degree of integrative power on the flow of impulses—and that they modify the nerve impulses to provide optimal stimulus conditions for the effector organs supplied by the postganglionic fibers.

Neurotransmitters and synaptic function

The first description of chemical transmission of neuron synapses was offered in 1921 by Loewi, who gave the name *vagusstoff* to a chemical released into the surrounding fluid as a result of vagal stimulation of the perfused heart. In the same year, Cannon and Uridil described the release of sympathin after stimulation of the nerves of the sympathetic system. It had been shown previously that injected epinephrine produced effects similar to stimulation of the sympathetic nerves. Subsequently, Dale and Feldberg gave the names *cholinergic* and *adrenergic* to synapses at which *acetylcholine* and *epinephrine* (adrenaline), respectively, were released as chemical mediators. For some time it was generally accepted that either epinephrine or sympathin was the sympathetic mediator. It was noted that sympathetic stimulation or epinephrine administration could produce either (1) relaxation of smooth muscle (e.g., intestineal and bronchiolar muscle) or (2) contraction (e.g., vascular smooth muscle and ureter). This led to a proposal that there were two types of transmitter: sympathin I associated with inhibitory functions and sympathin E subserving excitatory transmission.

In 1946 von Euler defined the adrenergic neurotransmitter as noradrenaline (*norepinephrine*), and in 1948 Ahlquist identified receptor sites in adrenergically innervated tissue as being either excitatory (alpha) or inhibitory (beta). Subsequently these two types of receptor were subdivided into $alpha_1$, $alpha_2$, $beta_1$, and $beta_2$, with the classification being based on the development of specific pharmacological antagonists. In addition, other transmitter substances were proposed to explain observations that neural stimulation could not be identified as causing the release of either acetylcholine or norepinephrine. It was suggested by Burnstock that these nonadrenergic, noncholinergic nerves released the purine nucleotide adenosine triphosphate as their transmitter substance. Although other putative autonomic transmitters (mainly in relation to enteric neurons) have been proposed, their definitive existence as transmitters has not been established. Thus 5-hydroxytryptamine (5-HT or serotonin) and γ-aminobutyric acid appear to satisfy many of the criteria as transmitter substances, possibly at interneurons in the gut. In addition, immunohistochemical studies have demonstrated that various biologically active polypeptides are localized within enteric neurons of the gastrointestinal tract and urogenital system. They are substance P, vasoactive intestinal polypeptide, neurotensin, somatostatin, bombesin, cholecystokinin, and bradykinin. Some of these substances may be modulators rather than transmitters in the traditional sense. It is possible that some of the peptides may coexist in the same terminal. They may be released only at high levels of stimulation. Thus, neuropeptide Y released from some noradrenergic neurons at high stimulation intensities may potentiate the action of norepinephrine postsynaptically. The peptides may act in many other ways; for example, substance P overrides the negative-feedback control of 5 HT release, thereby enhancing transmitter release. In other cases, the peptides may be inhibitory. In relation to the main or definitive transmitter, the action of peptides tends to be prolonged and may have a significant long-term tropic effect. Thus, in mammalian sympathetic ganglia, dopamine induces a long-term enhancement of the response to acetylcholine.

In summary, with the exceptions noted above, it is generally accepted that acetylcholine is the neurotransmitter released by nerve terminals at parasympathetic postganglionic effector junctions and that norepinephrine is the transmitter at sympathetic postganglionic effector junctions. Acetylcholine is considered to be the transmitter at ganglionic synapses in both the parasympathetic and sympathetic systems.

Cholinergic synapses

Classically, the synaptic junctions for which acetylcholine is the transmitting agent (cholinergic synapses) are described as functionally related to nicotinic activity or muscarinic activity. These designations were made at the time the neurological activity of acetylcholine was being described, and they stem from comparisons made to drug actions that were then well known. The action of the alkaloid muscarine (from the fly mushrooms) was known to involve excitement of terminals of the postganglionic fibers of the parasympathetic nervous system; consequently, these neuroeffector junctions were described as *muscarinic*. Also, the synapses at the ganglion cells of the entire autonomic nervous system, as well as the somatic myoneural junctions, were known to be excited by nicotine; hence these junctions were referred to as *nicotinic*. It is now known that the difference between the synapses resides at the postsynaptic receptor area; thus there are muscarinic and nicotinic receptors. In terms of inhibition, these two sets of receptors are also differentiable. The muscarinic receptors are blocked by the drug atropine, whereas the nicotinic receptors are not susceptible to atropine but are blocked by large doses of nicotine or by the curare drugs. The curare drugs and high doses of nicotine do not block the muscarinic receptors. These conditions are summarized in Table 46.1.

The release of acetylcholine at autonomic cholinergic sites is, so far as is known, identical to its release by the nerve terminals at skeletal muscle. Degradation of the transmitter occurs for the most part in immediate proximity to the site of transmitter release. In ganglia the active enzymes are released from storage sites primarily in the presynaptic terminal, whereas in myoneural junctions the acetylcholinesterase appears concentrated in the effector membrane. Furthermore, the nonspecific acetylcholinesterase activity in the blood is sufficiently high that excess transmitter overflowing into the circulatory system will be immediately hydrolyzed. Reuptake of acetylcholine into the nerve terminals does not occur; rather, choline produced as a result of acetylcholine hydrolysis is actively taken up and used in the synthesis of new transmitter.

Adrenergic synapses

When von Euler defined the transmitting agent at adrenergic nerve endings as norepinephrine (noradrenaline), epinephrine was relegated to the role of a humoral transmit-

Table 46.1 Classification of Cholinergic Receptors of the body

Neuronal junctions	Receptor type	Blocking agents
Smooth muscle Cardiac muscle Exocrine glands	Muscarinic	Atropine Other belladonna alkaloids
Autonomic ganglia Skeletal muscle	Nicotinic	Nicotine* (high concentrations depolarize ganglia cells principally) Bis-quaternary compounds (block ganglia) Curare (blocks skeletal muscle primarily)

*Nicotine acts in low concentrations as a stimulator, depolarizing the postsynaptic or effector membrane. In higher concentrations it blocks the same sites by preventing repolarization.

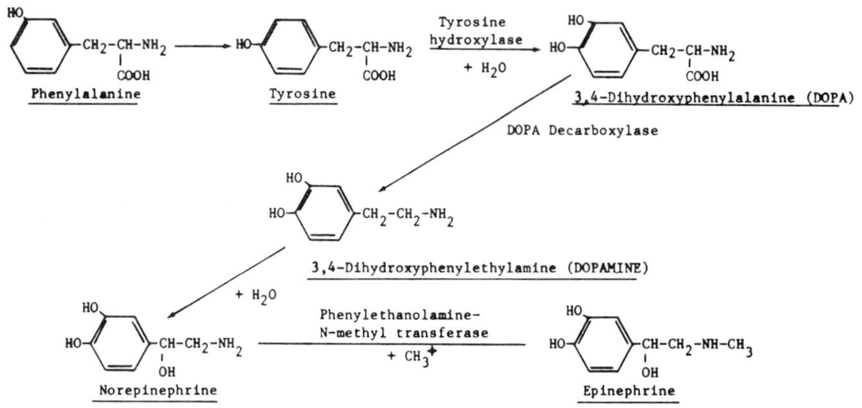

Figure 46.3. Major synthetic pathways for dopamine, norepinephrine, and epinephrine.

ter in the sympathetic nervous system. The currently accepted view is that norepinephrine is the primary secretion of adrenergic nerve cells in the peripheral autonomic system, whereas epinephrine is the primary secretion of chromaffin cells in the mammalian adrenal medulla.

The synthetic pathways of the catecholamines (dopamine, norepinephrine, and epinephrine) are described by the equations shown in Fig. 46.3. Primary raw materials are the amino acids phenylalanine and tyrosine. Intermediate steps involve the formation of 3,4-dihydroxyphenylalanine (dopa), which seems to have some primary adrenergic activity in the CNS. Generally speaking, however, the active products of this metabolic scheme are epinephrine and norepinephrine, although dopamine is being recognized as being significant in some autonomically innervated structures.

The conversion from phenylalanine or tyrosine to dopa is mediated by tyrosine hydroxylase, and the next step from the amino acid dopa to dopamine is mediated by dopa decarboxylase. These enzymes are in the cytoplasm of adrenergic neurons and adrenal medulla chromaffin cells. The accumulation of dopamine in the cytoplasm is limited by intracellular monoamine oxidase (MAO), which converts catecholamines to inactive compounds; however, dopamine can be taken up by an active process into storage vesicles and converted to norepinephrine by the action of dopamine-β-hydroxylase. Thus in adrenergic nerve terminals norepinephrine is finally synthesized at the site in which it is stored.

The rate-limiting step in the biosynthesis of norepinephrine is the tyrosine-hydroxylase reaction. The feedback inhibition of this step by the catecholamines that are produced may be an important regulatory mechanism in the formation of these compounds.

Epinephrine is formed in the mammalian adrenal medulla by phenylethanolamine-*N*-methyltransferase (PNMT). The enzyme is activated by the very high levels of glucocorticoids present in an intra-adrenal portal vascular system. The adrenal medulla normally receives the undiluted venous effluent from the adrenal cortex (as well as its own arteries), in which the concentration of glucocorticoids is 100 times the levels in systemic arterial blood. Evidence of the role of glucocorticoids as a cofactor in the methylation of norepinephrine to epinephrine by PNMT was obtained from experiments on rats that, after hypophysectomy, were unable to synthesize epinephrine or cortisol. Replacement doses of glucocorticoids failed to restore PNMT activity, but adrenocorticotropin administration was successful, thereby implicating adrenocortical cortisol synthesis as the requisite function.

As the frequency of impulses arriving at a nerve terminal (which, in the autonomic nervous system, is a nerve varicosity) increases, so does the amount of released transmitter; that is, the amount per pulse remains constant. In both the adrenal medulla and the noradrenergic nerves, the transmitter is stored in vesicles, the contents of which are discharged by a process of exocytosis. There is good evidence that only a small portion of the norepinephrine in a single vesicle is released by a nerve impulse. Thus modulation of the amount of transmitter entering the synapse may be the result not only of variations in action potential frequency but also of alterations in the amount released per action potential. This latter point is speculative because the manner by which the quantity of vesicle release may be altered is unknown, although the neuropeptides may be effective in this respect. Some of the transmitter stored in nerve endings is synthesized de novo, but some of it is norepinephrine that has been released and then taken up again for further use. This reuptake mechanism is an active process and is a way of terminating the action of released transmitter as well as reducing the need for new transmitter synthesis. Adrenergically innervated structures show the phenomenon of denervation supersensitivity; after denervation, the nerve endings degenerate and the denervated structure shows enhanced responsiveness to administered transmitter. Part of this phenomenon is explained by loss of the reuptake mechanism leaving more of the norepinephrine available to stimulate the postsynaptic effector. Some of the norepinephrine that is taken up by the nerve ending is metabolized by MAO, an enzyme present in the cytoplasm of the nerve ending. The MAO deaminates the side chain to 3,4-dihydroxymandelic acid, a physiologically inactive compound. The transmitter that escapes reuptake may diffuse into the extracellular fluid and enter the circulation. Another enzyme, catechol-*O*-methyltransferase (COMT), is located in the vicinity of the effector and inactivates part of the released transmitter by methylation of the *ortho*-OH group on the ring. Circulating epinephrine and norepinephrine are inactivated by COMT mainly in the liver and kidney.

The response to stimulation of adrenergic nerves or to elevated levels of circulating catecholamines will depend on the type of receptor affected. It has been suggested that, although most receptors are located in close proximity to the varicosities, there may be some in the walls of blood vessels that respond only to circulating catecholamines and are therefore noninnervated. The $beta_2$ receptors in the blood vessels of skeletal muscle may be an example of noninnervated receptors. Likewise, there may be alpha receptors that are more sensitive to circulating catecholamines than to neurally released transmitter, and evidence is accumulating that there are two distinct populations of receptors—innervated and noninnervated.

The concept of two types of adrenergic receptor arose out of the observation that epinephrine, norepinephrine, and the synthetic catecholamine isopropyl norepinephrine (isoproterenol) had differing relative potencies at various sites. Thus the term *alpha receptor* was applied to receptors that are highly sensitive to epinephrine and norepinephrine but less so to isoproterenol, whereas the term *beta receptor* was applied to receptors that responded most to isoproterenol, less to epinephrine, and least to norepinephrine. This classification was substantiated pharmacologically when specific alpha and beta receptor agonist and antagonist drugs were developed. It was then discovered that beta receptor activity involves stimulation of adenyl cyclase activity, leading to an increase in intracellular cyclic adenosine monophosphate (cAMP). There is evidence that the way in which $alpha_1$ and $alpha_2$ effects are mediated is quite distinct. $Alpha_2$ receptor responses are effected by inhibition of adenyl cyclase activity and thus a decrease in intracellular cAMP, whereas $alpha_1$ receptor function is mediated via activation of the phospho-inositol pathway.

A further subdivision of beta receptors was then proposed on the basis of the relative potencies of epinephrine and norepinephrine at certain sites. Thus it was noted that norepinephrine was equal to, or stronger than, epinephrine in stimulating the cardiac muscle and in mobilizing free fatty acids from adipose tissue, and such receptors were classed as $beta_1$ receptors. In the other instance, such as bronchodilation or vasodilation of skeletal muscle blood vessels, epinephrine was more potent than norepinephrine, and the receptors were designated $beta_2$ receptors. The classification has gained acceptance because of the synthesis of a number of selective $beta_1$ and $beta_2$-receptor agonists and antagonists. Isoproterenol is a general beta receptor agonist and propranolol a general beta receptor antagonist.

As indicated, it is now apparent that alpha receptors can be clearly subdivided and that the classic postsynaptic alpha receptor is of the $alpha_1$ variety, whereas the central nervous receptors and the presynaptic adrenergic receptors are $alpha_2$ receptors. However, some postsynaptic $alpha_2$ receptors that have actions in the vascular resistance vessels comparable to those of $alpha_1$ stimulation have been proposed. Presynaptic $alpha_2$ receptors are responsible for reducing transmitter release in response to neural stimulation. In fact, $alpha_2$ receptors may be responsible for inhibition of the smooth muscle of the intestine by prevention of the release of norepinephrine rather than prevention of its action. Presynaptic inhibition of transmitter release is distinct from the reuptake mechanism and may assist in economizing transmitter release or possibly may help to equalize norepinephrine concentrations in densely innervated tissue.

In addition to presynaptic inhibition of transmitter release, there is evidence of presynaptic enhancement of transmitter release via a presynaptic beta receptor. There is little information on the type of beta receptor involved; whereas presynaptic alpha receptors are present on all adrenergic nerves, the facilitatory beta receptors are not universally present. They have been demonstrated pharmacologically, and their physiological role has yet to be determined. Presumably they are more likely to be activated by elevated levels of circulating epinephrine and thus may potentiate concurrent neural stimulation under conditions of massive and general sympathetic discharge (e.g., during hemorrhage).

Presynaptic modulation of transmitter release by adrenergic receptors may not be the only method of adrenergic modulation; in many structures receiving a dual innervation, cholinergic and adrenergic fibers have been shown to run in the same nerve bundle and, within the effector tissue, may be in the same Schwann cell sheath. It has been shown that, in cardiac tissue, cutaneous arterioles, and the spleen, acetylcholine may have an inhibitory effect on the release of norepinephrine by activation of muscarinic receptors. Similarly, norepinephrine, by acting on presynaptic alpha receptors, can reduce the amount of acetylcholine released by cholinergic nerves. The receptors appear to be located at both preganglionic and postganglionic parasympathetic nerve terminals. Whether the alpha receptor is of the $alpha_1$ or $alpha_2$ type is unclear. Thus, in tissues innervated by both cholinergic parasympathetic and noradrenergic sympathetic nerves, the transmitters may interact by having opposite effects not only on the postsynaptic sites but also on transmitter release, resulting in a prejunctional antagonism.

EFFECTS ON SPECIFIC STRUCTURES

The autonomic nervous system innervates smooth muscle, cardiac muscle, and gland cells, inducing two effector reactions: excitation and inhibition. Generally, when a given organ is innervated by both sympathetic and parasympathetic fibers, the effects are reciprocal; that is, if the sympathetic excites, the parasympathetic inhibits. Sympathetic innervation alone, however, may provide reciprocal innervation through alpha-receptor (generally excitatory) and beta-receptor (generally inhibitory) nerve endings. The net result in such circumstances is determined largely by the relative density of each type of receptor and the degree of adrenomedullary stimulation; release of epinephrine from the adrenal medulla into the blood will activate both alpha and beta receptors. For example, if the receptors are mainly of the $beta_2$ type and if there is a significant number of them, elevated circulating catecholamines will result in a predominantly beta-receptor effect. Thus in the blood vessels of skeletal muscle, neural stimulation of sympathetic nerves (there being virtually no parasympathetic fibers) causes vasoconstriction, whereas an increase in circulating epinephrine will cause vasodilation through $beta_2$-receptor stimulation. This may be of physiological significance in the emergency reaction in which blood flow to skeletal muscle must be increased. An exception is the smooth muscle of the intestinal tract, which has alpha and beta sympathetic endings, both of which are inhibitory.

Following is a brief description of the autonomic effects on specific structures. It must be remembered that innervation and function vary from species to species. Some of the more important exceptions will be noted, but good comparative work is lacking for many of the species and for many of the organs. A summary of the innervations described appears in Fig. 46.4 and Table 46.2.

Some features of the innervation of specific structures are described below.

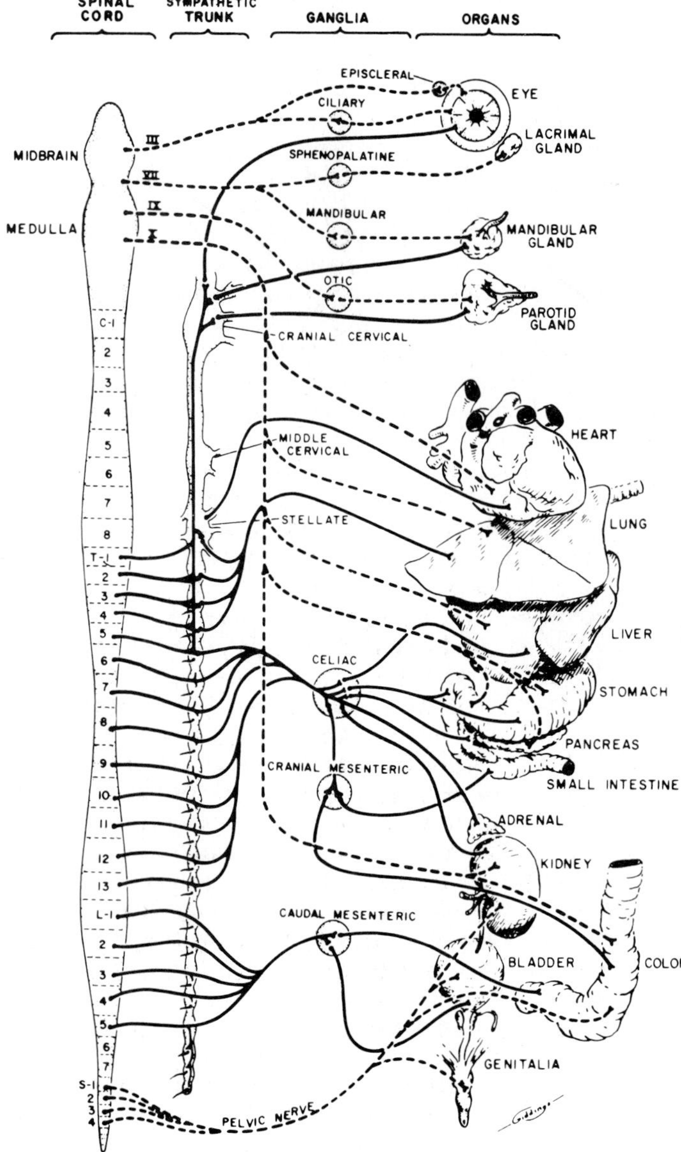

Figure 46.4. Generalized diagram of the efferent autonomic nervous system of a domestic animal. The spinal cord segmentation is characteristic of the dog, but the lumbar and sacral contributions incorporate the possibilities found in cattle and horses. The lines showing sympathetic flow are solid; parasympathetic, broken.

Structures of the head

Lacrimal glands

Parasympathetic fiber stimulation causes vasodilatation and secretion from the gland cells. Sympathetic fiber stimulation causes vasoconstriction; it has little secretory effect, but it may cause an increase in the mucous content of the secretion.

Iris musculature

Parasympathetic activity causes pupillary constriction (myosis), and sympathetic activity causes pupillary dilatation (mydriasis).

Ciliary muscle

Parasympathetic stimulation causes contraction of the ciliary muscle and thus accommodation of the lens for near vision. The evidence of sympathetic innervation is somewhat doubtful.

Nictitating membrane

Parasympathetic innervation has not been demonstrated. Sympathetic stimulation causes the membrane to be retracted.

Eyelid (Miller's or tarsal muscle)

Sympathetic nerve stimulation aids in raising the eyelid.

Submandibular and sublingual salivary glands

Parasympathetic stimulation produces vasodilatation and causes secretion of comparatively large volumes of saliva. Sympathetic fibers conduct impulses that will decrease a previously augmented circulation. It may be inferred that observed increases in basal secretion rates caused by sym-

Table 46.2. Functions of the autonomic nervous system

	Parasympathetic	Sympathetic	
Organ	Effects	Effects	Receptor types
Heart	Decreased activity	Chronotropic and inotropic effects	β
Blood vessels			
Skin and mucosa		Constriction	α
Skeletal muscle		Dilatation	α < β
Coronary		Constriction or dilatation	α < β
Abdominal		Constriction	α > β
Pulmonary		Constriction or dilatation	α = β
Eye			
Iris muscle	Constriction	Relaxation (far vision)	α
Ciliary muscle	Contraction (near vision)		β
Nictitating membrane		Retraction	α
Bronchiole	Constriction	Dilatation	β
Glands			
Sweat		Secretion	α (Ox), β (Horse)
Salivary	Secretion and vasodilatation	Constriction of myoepithelial cells and vasoconstriction	
Lacrimal gland	Secretion	Vasoconstriction	
Gastric	Secretion	Inhibition	
Pancreas	Secretion		
Liver		Glycogenolysis	
Adrenal cortex		Secretion	
Mammary		No known secretory effect	
Smooth muscle			
Skin (pilomotor)		Contraction	
Stomach and intestines			
Lumen	Increased tone and motility	Decreased tone and motility	α, β
Sphincters	Relaxation	Contraction	α
Uterus (cat and dog)			
Pregnant		Contraction (epinephrine)	
Nonpregnant		Inhibition (epinephrine)	
Milk letdown		Inhibition	
Urinary bladder	Contraction	Relaxation	β
Sphincter	Relaxation	Contraction	α
Gallbladder	Contraction	Relaxation	β
Spleen		Contraction	α
Blood coagulation		Increased rate	
Sex organs	Erection	Ejaculation	Neurogenic
Blood glucose		Increased	

pathetic stimulation are the result of myoepithelial contraction and expulsion of saliva rather than true secretion.

Parotid salivary gland

Parasympathetic innervation causes vasodilatation and augmented secretion. In ruminants the parotid gland secretes continually; although it is possible that the parasympathetic nerves provide secretory tone to the gland, basal secretion continues in spite of both parasympathetic and sympathetic neurotomy.

Sympathetic stimulation causes vasoconstriction and, in the dog, a marked increase in the organic matter of the saliva. Observations of increased saliva flow after sympathetic stimulation can be attributed to expulsion of saliva because of myoepithelial contraction.

Brain

Innervation is exclusively vasomotor. The function of the autonomic vasomotor nerves is minimal, since other vascular beds in the body act to keep the blood pressure remarkably constant, thereby assuring an equally constant rate of perfusion to the head and brain.

Thoracic viscera

Heart

Parasympathetic nerves originate in the dorsal motor nucleus of the vagus nerve (cranial nerve X) and pass with the nerve to the cardiac plexus, then to muscles of the atria, the vessels, the sinoatrial and atrioventricular nodes, and the conducting tissue. Parasympathetic stimulation has its main effects, therefore, on the atria and the conducting system where it slows down the heart rate (i.e., a negative chronotropic effect); there is virtually no effect on ventricular function. Parasympathetic innervation to the coronary blood vessels is so slight that parasympathetic stimulation has a negligible effect on coronary blood flow.

Sympathetic nerves originate in the first to fifth thoracic cord segments and enter the chain and stellate ganglia. Postganglionic fibers then reach the heart in the cardiac plexus to terminate in the sinoatrial node, the vessel walls, and the atrial and ventricular muscle. The sympathetic nerves to the heart have both positive chronotropic and inotropic effects. Their effects on coronary blood flow are difficult to evaluate since the major determinant of coronary blood flow is the local activity of the heart. Sympathetic stimulation will, therefore, indirectly increase coronary blood flow. In addition, however, the extensive sympathetic innervation to the coronary blood vessels is associated with constrictor alpha receptors and dilator $beta_2$ receptors, the former being associated with the epicardial arteries and the latter with the intramuscular vessels. Their physiological role, particularly that of the alpha receptors, is difficult to evaluate.

Lung

Respiratory movements are controlled by somatic nerves to the skeletal respiratory muscles.

The structures in the lung that are innervated by the autonomic nervous system include the smooth muscle of the airways, especially in the trachea, bronchi, and bronchioles, the smooth muscle of the pulmonary arteries and veins, and the goblet cells of the bronchial epithelium.

The parasympathetic nerves produce bronchoconstriction

and stimulation of bronchial mucous secretion. Cholinergic-blocking drugs such as atropine, therefore, may be useful in the relief of bronchospasm and the reduction of bronchial and bronchiolar secretion of mucus. Thus, the use of atropine as preanesthetic medication not only reduces salivary flow but also will prevent the accumulation of mucus in the airways. The sympathetic innervation to the smooth muscle of the airways causes relaxation and bronchial dilation. The response is mediated by $beta_2$ receptors, and thus $beta_2$ agonist drugs can be used in the emergency therapy of severe bronchospasm. It is thought that the secretion of the bronchial and bronchiolar mucous cells can be inhibited by the sympathetic innervation.

The functional role of the autonomic nerve supply to the smooth muscle of the pulmonary blood vessels is not clear. Stimulation of the vagus causes a mild pulmonary vasodilation, and sympathetic stimulation causes pulmonary vasoconstriction. The profound pulmonary vasoconstriction associated with hypoxia is independent of the sympathetic nerves or circulating catecholamines but is initiated by the low oxygen tension in the airways. The use of sympathetic blocking drugs is, therefore, ineffective in relieving the symptoms of high mountain disease in cattle (See chaps. 12 and 13).

Esophagus

The autonomic nervous system innervates only smooth muscle, not striated muscle. The type of muscle in the esophagus varies greatly among species. In the dog and in ruminants, the esophageal musculature is entirely striated; in the pig there is only a short section of smooth muscle near the gastric cardia; and in the cat and horse the caudal one-third of the esophagus has a smooth muscle coat.

Parasympathetic nerves produce smooth muscle contraction and peristalsis.

Sympathetic function is poorly defined, but presumably it is inhibitory for esophageal smooth muscle.

Abdominal and pelvic viscera

Parasympathetic stimulation produces the following effects: Smooth muscle of the walls of the gastrointestinal tract, including the rumen and gallbladder, is stimulated to contract. The smooth muscle of the sphincters of the gastrointestinal tract is affected, the manner depending to some extent on the species. In the dog and cat, the pyloric sphincter is stimulated; in the cow, parasympathetic nerves inhibit the pyloric sphincter and the reticulo-omasal sphincter. In the liver, the smooth muscle of the sphincter of the bile duct is relaxed. Glandular secretion is stimulated. Smooth muscle of the bladder is contracted. Anal sphincter and smooth muscle of the sphincter of the urinary bladder are relaxed.

Sympathetic stimulation produces the following effects: Constriction occurs in abdominal blood vessels. There is inhibition of the smooth muscle in the walls of the gastrointestinal tract, including the rumen, and the gallbladder of the dog and cat. The inhibitory effects on motility are neither adrenergic nor cholinergic and are probably mediated by purinergic transmitters. Smooth muscle contracts in the trabeculae, capsules, and blood vessels of the spleen as well as the pyloric and anal sphincters and the sphincter of the bile duct. In the cow, the reticulo-omasal sphincters are also contracted. Glycogenolysis in the liver is stimulated. Secretions of the stomach and the intestinal tract in general are inhibited by sympathetic stimulation.

In the genitalia, parasympathetic stimulation causes vasodilatation and erection of the penis and clitoris. Sympathetic nerves are responsible for ejaculation.

Cutaneous vessels, smooth muscle, and glands

There is no parasympathetic innervation to the cutaneous blood vessels of the skin; a possible exception involves the blood vessels of the human face, which dilate when stimulated, with resultant blushing. Sympathetic nerves cause cutaneous vasoconstriction. The piloerector muscles elevate hair and increase insulation. These muscles are controlled by sympathetic nerves, and the transmitter (norepinephrine) acts on alpha receptors.

The sweat glands on the general body surface of humans and some other primate species are of the eccrine type and are controlled by sympathetic cholinergic fibers. In this respect, they are similar to the sweat glands on the footpads of the dog and cat and represent an exception to the general rule that all sympathetic nerves are adrenergic. The sweat glands on the general body surface of cattle, sheep, goats, dogs, and horses, however, are of the apocrine type and are similar to the axillary glands of humans. They are controlled by adrenergic sympathetic nerves; in the case of cattle, sheep, goats, and dogs, the receptors are of the alpha type, but in horses the receptors are of the $beta_2$ variety. The receptors on the apocrine sweat glands of humans are not known.

EMERGENCY REACTION

The mobilization of the systems of the body to combat a life-threatening condition has been called the emergency or fight-or-flight reaction. It is the coordinated result of increased output of adrenal medullary secretions and of increased activity of the sympathetic nervous system. The reaction establishes in the body the optimal condition for defense of the animal's life, whether to stand and fight or to run away. There occurs a constriction of the vessels of the skin and of the intestinal tract but a dilatation of the vessels of skeletal muscle, the effect being mediated in part by circulating epinephrine as well as a possible neural component. A sympathetic cholinergic neural vasodilator pathway to skeletal muscle blood vessels has been described.

Thus neural vasodilatation probably precedes that brought about by circulating catecholamines in the early phase of the emergency reaction.

The combination of vasoconstriction and vasodilatation shifts the blood volume into a compartment somewhat smaller than the blood vascular space at rest. The volume shift is accompanied by an increased cardiac rate and output and by coronary vascular dilatation. As a consequence, there is an overall improvement in circulatory efficiency. Other notable changes include an elevated blood sugar level and metabolic rate, mydriasis and upper eyelid retraction, decreased gastrointestinal motility but contraction of the gastrointestinal and urinary sphincters, expulsion of red cells from the spleen, bronchodilatation, piloerection, decreased coagulation time, and an increased pain threshold. The utility of each of these changes when combat is imminent or when escape from combat is necessary is apparent.

Bronchodilatation and the increase in numbers of red cells provide for a more highly efficient respiratory function. Mydriasis and upper eyelid retraction improve visual acuity. Peripheral vasoconstriction, decreased coagulation time, and an increased pain threshold are all modifications that help prevent wounding or offset the psychic effects of wounds, which may detract from the need of the animal to focus on its objective. Piloerection, most notable in the dog and cat, may help to distract an adversary by causing an apparent increase in size. Decreased gastrointestinal motility and contraction of the sphincters prevent loss of the contents of the gastrointestinal tract and bladder at inconvenient times. Finally, the most important aspect of the sympathoadrenal response to fight, flight, or fright may be the mobilization of substrate by stimulation of glycogenolysis and lipolysis to provide energy.

REFERENCES

Axelrod, J. 1974. Neurotransmitters. *Sci. Am.* 230:58.

Birks, R.I., and MacIntosh, F.C. 1957. Acetylcholine metabolism at nerve-endings. *Br. Med. Bull.* 13:157–61.

Brooks, C.M., et al. 1979. *Integrative Functions of the Autonomic Nervous System.* University of Tokyo Press, Tokyo.

Burnstock, G. 1981. Neurotransmitters and trophic factors in the autonomic nervous system. *J. Physiol. (Lond.)* 313:1–35.

Donald, D.E., and Shepherd, J.T. 1980. Autonomic regulation of the pheripheral circulation. *Annu. Rev. Physiol.* 42:429.

Iversen, L.L. 1967. *The Uptake and Storage of Noradrenaline in Sympathetic Nerves.* Cambridge University Press, London.

Kunos, G. 1978. Adrenoceptors. *Annu. Rev. Pharmacol. Toxicol.* 18:291.

Landsberg, L., and Young, J.B. 1980. Catecholamine and the adrenal medulla. In P.K. Bondy and L.E. Rosenberg, eds. *Metabolic Control and Disease.* 8th ed. W. B. Saunders Co., Philadelphia. Pp. 1621.

Langer, S.Z. 1980. Presynaptic regulation of the release of catecholaminess. *Pharmacol. Rev.* 32:337–62.

Starke, K. 1981. Presynaptic receptors. *Annu. Rev. Pharmacol. Toxicol.* 21:7–30.

Su, C. 1983. Purinergic neruotransmission and neuromodulation. *Annu. Rev. Pharmacol. Toxicol.* 23:397–411.

Wurtman, R.J., Pohorecky, L.A., and Baliga, B.S. 1972. Adrenocortical control of the biosynthesis of epinephrine and proteins in the adrenal meddula. *Pharmacol. Rev.* 24:411–26.

Ungar, A., and Phillips, J.H. 1983. Regulation of the adrenal medulla. *Physiol. Rev.* 63:787–843.

CHAPTER 47

Temperature Regulation and Environmental Physiology | by Bengt E. Andersson and Hallgrímur Jónasson

POIKILOTHERMISM AND HOMEOTHERMISM

Organic life depends on reactions by which chemical energy is transformed into heat. The rate of these reactions is affected by temperature, so that heat production of living cells will increase two to three times if the temperature is raised by 10°C. The degree of acceleration with rising temperature, however, varies with different chemical reactions. A change in temperature, therefore, also changes the character of more complicated biological processes. This makes a relatively constant temperature a necessity for the efficient functioning of the complex brains of mammals and birds. These animals have developed a heat-regulating device that enables them to maintain, under ordinary conditions, a constant deep body temperature, regardless of the temperature of the surroundings. These *homeotherm*, or warm-blooded, animals can carry on their usual activities under a wide range of external temperature, whereas *poikilotherm*, or cold-blooded, animals, whose temperature varies directly with that of the environment, are dependent on the external temperature. In the cold they pass into a state of sleeplike inactivity, and in hot weather they may have to burrow into the mud to avoid disastrous overheating.

The increase in chemical activity that is achieved at the higher temperature may be the reason the deep body temperature of homeotherms is set so high (within the range of 36°C for the elephant to 41°C for birds). This high temperature also means that heat production must be continuously at a high level in a cold environment, which demands that the animals consume more food and spend more time obtaining it.

HIBERNATION

Some small mammals maintain a high body temperature, mainly under conditions of favorable environmental temperature, but abandon homeothermy in the cold. The temperature of these hibernators shows great variations, even in the warm-blooded state, and is quite dependent on the activity of the animal. During winter sleep it falls to and remains at a level only slightly above the environmental temperature. These animals show also a marked reduction in metabolism, breathing rate, and heart rate. There is, however, a protective mechanism against profound cooling. If the body temperature falls to levels near freezing, the animal wakes up and rapidly rewarms. Most hibernators arouse periodically in a rhythmic manner, and each brief arousal involves considerable energy expenditure. To meet these energy demands, some animals, such as ground squirrels and woodchucks, greatly increase their bodily fat stores during the weeks preceding hibernation. Chipmunks and hamsters, on the other hand, do not lay down depot fat but, instead, hoard food and increase their water consumption until hibernation ensues; they then eat copiously while awake. Other small hibernators include the European marmot, the American groundhog, the dormouse, and the hedgehog. Bears can hibernate without arousing for 3 to 5 months (in extreme cases, up to 7 months). Unlike other hibernators, their body temperature decreases only slightly, by about 6°C. Because of the great body mass, several days would be required for a bear to rewarm if its core temperature were reduced to the same degree as that of the smaller animals. This would be clearly disadvantageous in a time of emergency. In other aspects, bears show typical physiological adaptations to winter dormancy (e.g., a sharp reduction in heart rate and a lowered metabolic rate). The ability of all mammalian hibernators to awake from hibernation, using only heat from their own sources, is apparently due to the prominence of brown fat in mammalian hibernators. Brown fat differs from white fat in color and in metabolic properties, namely, the presence of fat-metabolizing enzyme systems. The cells of brown fat tissue are sympathetically innervated and are rich in mitochondria and cytochrome. When stimulated, these cells oxidize the fat and produce heat at a very high rate. Because the tissue is extensively vascularized, the heat is quickly distributed to other parts of the body. During arousal from hibernation, the temperature of brown fat tissue, located mainly between the shoulder blades, is among the highest in any part of the body. Fundamental differences apparently exist between the biochemical processes during hibernation and in the warm-blooded state. The blood sugar concentration in some hibernators is considerably lower during winter sleep, and in all hibernators studied the serum magnesium concentration is markedly elevated during hibernation. No single endocrine factor, however, has so far been shown to be directly involved in the control of hibernation.

BODY TEMPERATURE

Many conditions are capable of causing normal variations in the body temperature of homeotherms. Among these are age, sex, season, time of day, environmental temperature, exercise, eating, digestion, and drinking of water. Further, there are temperature differences to be found between different parts of the body, and these differences may vary considerably.

Gradients of temperature

In humans and animals there are gradients of temperature in the blood, tissues, and rectum, with the lower temperatures being toward the exterior of the body. There are also considerable variations in the different parts of the deep core. The temperature of the liver may be 1 to 2°C higher than the rectal temperature, and the brain temperature is usually somewhat higher than that of the carotid blood. These regions are thus cooled rather than warmed by arterial blood. In ruminants the intraruminal temperature is higher than the rectal temperature because of extra heat produced by the ruminant microorganisms. In a cold environment the temperature of peripheral parts of the body, such as the limbs, may be 10°C or more below core temperature.

Rectal temperature

An index of deep body temperature is most easily obtained in animals by insertion of a thermometer into the rectum. Although rectal temperature does not always represent an average of deep body temperature, it is better to measure the temperature at this selected site than to measure the temperature at various sites and call it body temperature. Further, because rectal temperature reaches equilibrium more slowly than temperatures in many other internal sites (e.g., central vessels), it is a good index of a true steady state. Since a temperature gradient exists in the rectum, it is important to insert the thermometer to a constant depth in each species or breed of animal. Table 47.1 shows the normal rectal temperatures of certain domestic animals.

Diurnal variations

The thermoregulatory mechanisms are probably linked to the mechanisms that control sleep and wakening. In animals that are active during the daytime, maximum temperatures are usually found in early afternoon and minimum temperatures early in the morning, whereas animals that are active at night have a reversed temperature rhythm. Variations related to the time of day are designated as diurnal variations. The extent of such temperature changes varies in different species. In the cow, the rectal temperature is regularly higher in the afternoon than in the morning, with a difference of about 0.5°C. Radiotelemetric recordings of deep body temperature in sheep over long periods and under field conditions have demonstrated diurnal variations of about 1°C with no discernible seasonal trends in its extent. During the shortest and longest days, the duration of the rising and falling phases of body temperature appeared to be proportional to the hours of daylight and darkness, respectively. Studies of diurnal temperature variations in the camel are of particular interest. The rectal temperature of the dehydrated camel at rest during summer may vary from 34°C to more than 40°C, whereas the diurnal variation in the winter is usually in the order of 2°C. When camels in the

Table 47.1. Rectal temperatures

	Average		Range	
Animal	°C	°F	°C	°F
Stallion	37.6	99.7	37.2–38.1	99.0–100.6
Mare	37.8	100	37.3–38.2	99.1–100.8
Donkey	37.4	99.3	36.4–38.4	97.5–101.1
Camel	37.5	99.5	34.2–40.7	93.6–105.3
Beef cow	38.3	101	36.7–39.1	98.0–102.4
Dairy cow	38.6	101.5	38.0–39.3	100.4–102.8
Sheep	39.1	102.3	38.3–39.9	100.9–103.8
Goat	39.1	102.3	38.5–39.7	101.3–103.5
Pig	39.2	102.5	38.7–39.8	101.6–103.6
Dog	38.9	102	37.9–39.9	100.2–103.8
Cat	38.6	101.5	38.1–39.2	100.5–102.5
Rabbit	39.5	103.1	38.6–40.1	101.5–104.2
Chicken (daylight)	41.7	107.1	40.6–43.0	105.0–109.4

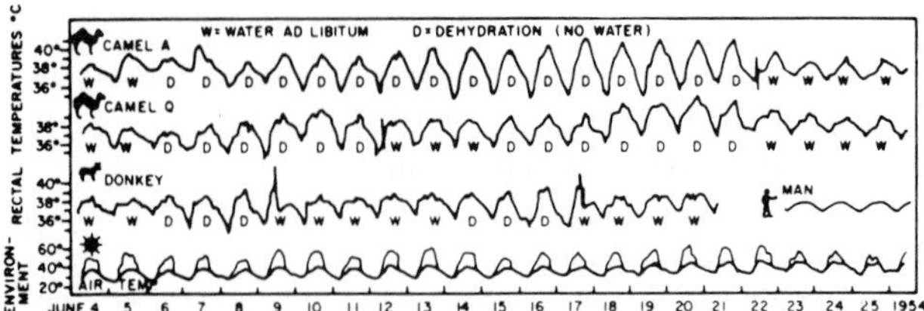

Figure 47.1. Diurnal variations in rectal temperature in two camels and one donkey for a 3-week period. Note the increase in diurnal fluctuations during dehydration. Air temperature corresponds closely to standard meteorological observations. The fine line above the heavy line refers to the integrated temperature of the environment. (From Schmidt-Nielsen, Schmidt-Nielsen, Jarnum, and Houpt 1957, *Am. J. Physiol.* 188:103–12.)

hot summer are permitted to drink ad libitum once a day, the daily variations in rectal temperature do not exceed those found during the winter months. The usual diurnal temperature variation in the donkey during the summer was found to be between 34.6 and 38.4°C (Fig. 47.1). The observations on the rectal temperature of the camel show that a very high rectal temperature, found under conditions of heat stress and water deprivation, is not necessarily a sign of failure of heat regulation. Rather, it is a manifestation of the animal's ability to preserve water that otherwise would have to be evaporated to prevent the considerable daytime rise in body temperature.

HEAT BALANCE

A thermal steady state exists only when the net effect of heat gain is balanced by the net effect of heat loss.

Heat is produced in the body by metabolic activities but may also enter from the exterior by means of radiation, conduction, and convection. In some organs, such as the liver and the heart, heat production is normally relatively constant. Skeletal muscle, on the other hand, makes a variable contribution to heat production: during muscular work more than 80 percent of the heat of the body is produced in skeletal muscle; during rest the figure is much lower.

Heat is lost from the body by radiation, conduction, and convection, evaporation of water from skin and respiratory passages, and excretion of feces and urine.

In homeotherms the various thermoregulatory mechanisms consist of a series of physiological adjustments that serve to establish a thermal steady state at the level of normal body temperature and that consequently struggle to maintain equality in heat gain and heat loss. The extent to which such adjustments are required is highly dependent on the external temperature. In general it can be stated that there exists a thermoneutral zone of constant metabolism in which variable insulation (mainly due to circulatory adjustments) is sufficient to maintain a thermal steady state. Above and below this thermoneutral zone, circulatory adjustments are no longer enough for the maintenance of heat balance. In high temperatures they must be supplemented by an increase of evaporative heat loss (sweating and panting), and in cold temperatures by increased metabolism.

PHYSIOLOGICAL RESPONSES TO HEAT

Circulatory adjustments

Cutaneous vasodilatation causes a rise in skin temperature, which steepens the thermal exchange gradient for environmental temperatures below skin temperature. This increases heat loss. The cutaneous vasomotor reactions in response to thermal changes are mediated mainly by sympathetic vasoconstrictor nerves. Peripheral vasodilatation is therefore obtained by an inhibition of sympathetic vasoconstrictor tone. Warmth may decrease vasoconstrictor tone either via a rise in central nervous system (CNS) temperature or reflexly by the mediation of thermoreceptors in the skin and other parts of the body. Local skin vasodilatation may also occur as a direct result of warmth on the blood vessels, or it may be due to the presence in the skin of bradykinin, a powerful vasodilator substance that is released from activated sweat glands.

Above an environmental temperature of about 31°C, skin vasodilatation no longer increases heat dissipation, and a rise in body temperature will result unless heat loss can be augmented by other means.

Evaporative heat loss

Evaporation of water is an effective way of cooling the body. Whereas only 1 calorie is needed to elevate the temperature of 1 g of water by 1°C, it takes almost 600 calories to evaporate the same amount of water from the body. At ordinary temperature and humidity, about 25 percent of the heat produced in resting mammals is lost by evaporation of water from the skin and respiratory passages. This insensible water loss, cutaneous and respiratory, is rather constant under basal conditions. An increased flow of blood through the skin causes it to increase somewhat, but the mechanisms of sweating and panting offer much more efficient ways to increase the evaporative heat loss.

Sweating

There are two kinds of sweat glands: eccrine glands, which are supplied by cholinergic fibers present in sympathetic nerves, and apocrine glands, which develop from hair follicles. The latter glands are generally considered not to be supplied by secretory nerves and are sensitive to epinephrine carried in the bloodstream. In humans the eccrine sweat glands alone are responsible for thermal sweating, but in many domestic animals apocrine sweat glands are important for evaporative heat loss.

Thermoregulatory sweating is elicited in two ways: (1) by a rise of the CNS temperature and (2) reflexly, by stimulation of warmth receptors in the skin and other parts of the body outside the CNS. Although reflex sweating may occur in the absence of an increased central temperature, a high skin temperature cannot elicit full-scale sweating without simultaneous CNS facilitation. The horse and other equines were once regarded as exceptions from this generalization. Earlier it was thought that equine sweat glands had no direct innervation and that sweat gland activity was controlled solely by epinephrine from the adrenal medulla. Later work shows that adrenomedullary denervation, which stops the physiological release of epinephrine by the adrenal medulla, does not alter heat-induced sweating in equines. If a skin area is sympathetically denervated, heat-induced sweating no longer takes place in that area. It can be concluded, therefore, that in equines sweating in response to heat is controlled by sympathetic nerves with epinephrine as the transmitter substance.

The relative importance of sweating as a heat-dissipation mechanism varies among species. In the dog sweating is insignificant in heat regulation, whereas panting is all the more important. In cows maximum evaporation from the skin surface amounts to about 150 $g/m^2/h$ at an external temperature of 40°C. The respiratory evaporation under the same condition is only about one-third of that amount (Fig. 47.2). Sweat secretion in the sheep is less important than in the cow. Maximum sweat secretion in shorn sheep during heat stress is 32 $g/m^2/h$, which means that a sheep may dissipate about 20 kcal per hour by sweating. Consequently, evaporative heat loss via the respiratory passages is more important in the sheep than in the cow. When the camel is exposed to the full heat load of the desert, the increase in respiratory frequency is insignificant but sweating is considerable. One characteristic of sweating in the camel in the dry desert is that there is no copious flow of sweat or conspicuous wetting of the fur. This may explain earlier erroneous reports that the camel does not sweat.

In general, the function of sweat glands in domestic animals falls short of the remarkable activity of the human sweat glands. In humans, heat loss from sweating may be as high as 1000 kcal per hour.

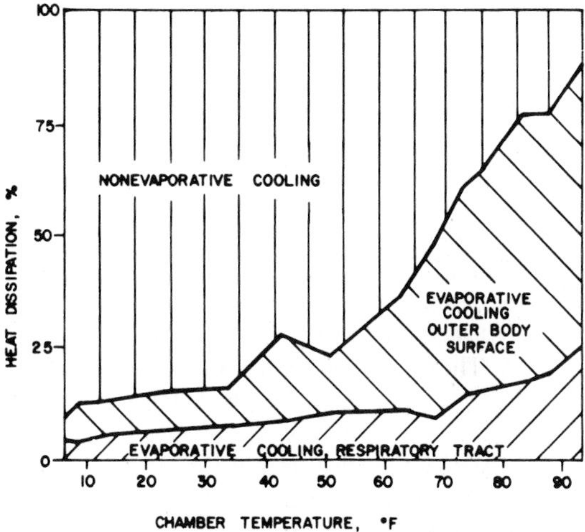

Figure 47.2. Percentages of total heat loss (averaged for jersey and holstein cows) by evaporation from the respiratory tract, evaporation from the body surface, and nonevaporative means (radiation, conduction, and convection) at different environmental temperatures in a climatic chamber. The respiratory evaporation rises slowly with rising ambient temperature, accounting for 4 to 30 percent of the total heat loss. Between ambient temperature of 5°F and approximately 50°F (−15 and +10°C), the skin evaporation is about the same as that from the respiratory tract, but from 50°F (10°C) on, surface evaporation rises markedly. The sharper rise in skin evaporation between 65 and 80°F (18 and 27°C) may correspond to the breaking out in sweat of humans at 80 to 90°F (27 to 32°C). (From Kibler and Brody, 1950, *Univ. Mo. Ag. Exp. Sta. Res. Bull.* 461.)

Panting

A heat load will, in many species, evoke polypnea (rapid breathing) and, in some, polypneic panting, that is, breathing at a frequency of between 200 and 400 breaths per minute with an open mouth. Panting is usually accompanied by increased salivary secretion and may cause a considerable increase in respiratory evaporative cooling if the humidity of the inspired air is not too high. Studies of the panting mechanism in cattle have shown that evaporative cooling occurs in the upper respiratory passages and not from cooling in the lungs. It is equally clear that in the calf and in the sheep, panting in response to a raised environmental temperature may start before there is an increase in the temperature of the blood supplying the brain. But panting may also be induced at a constant external temperature by a rise in body temperature or by local warming of the anterior hypothalamus. This shows that the panting mechanism, like sweating, may be stimulated both reflexly and centrally. Birds, which have no sweat glands, increase evaporation not only by panting but also by a mechanism named *gular flutter*. It consists of rapid oscillations of the thin floor of the mouth and the upper part of the throat.

PHYSIOLOGICAL RESPONSES TO COLD

When the environmental temperature falls, some means must be used by the homeotherm animal to prevent a drop in its body temperature. This regulation against cooling is primarily brought about by a reduction of heat loss and is known as *physical regulation*. If physical regulation is not sufficient to maintain body temperature, heat production has to be increased as a second line of defense, and this is known as *chemical regulation*.

Reduction of heat loss

Behavioral responses and increased fur insulation

A reduction of heat loss can be accomplished by the adoption of a posture that minimizes the surface area exposed to cold, such as the curled-up position of animals. During acute exposure, animals may further increase the effective insulation of the fur by piloerection. Increased fur growth and subcutaneous fat deposition are other means.

Circulatory adjustments

Vasoconstriction, mediated by vasoconstrictor nerves, occurs in the skin and superficial tissues of homeotherms exposed to cold. This accomplishes two main reductions in heat loss: (1) The decreased peripheral blood flow causes a drop in skin temperature, reducing the temperature gradient between the skin and the environment. (2) The functional insulation of the skin increases because of a reduction in the convected heat loss of perfusing blood. An increased peripheral vasoconstrictor tone may be elicited reflexly by the simulation of skin cold receptors or centrally by a lowered CNS temperature.

A very important improvement in heat economy is gained by the arrangement of deep arteries and veins running close together. Cold venous blood is transported centrally adjacent to warm arterial blood coursing peripherally. By continuous heat exchange, the returning venous blood is warmed whereas the arterial blood is cooled, which effectively minimizes heat losses in a cold environment. This countercurrent heat-exchange system permits adequate blood supply to the limbs in spite of large temperature gradients. In a cold environment the temperature of radial artery blood in a human may be about 20°C without the person feeling unendurably cold and with the rectal temperature remaining at the normal 37°C. Countercurrent heat exchange also helps to keep the temperature of the testes at the lower level necessary for spermatogenesis. Because of skin vasoconstriction in the cold, there is a shift of returning venous blood from superficial to deep channels and this increases the efficiency of the countercurrent heat-exchange system. During skin vasodilatation in a hot environment, the shift goes in the opposite direction.

Increase of heat production

The external temperature at which the heat-retaining mechanisms are no longer adequate to maintain a constant body temperature and at which heat production has to be increased is known as the lower critical temperature (t_c). This varies a great deal in different animals. Among farm animals, cattle and sheep have the lowest critical temperature and are therefore most able to withstand the cold. Since so much of the heat of the body is produced in the skeletal muscles, these structures are of primary importance for the increased metabolic rate that occurs below the critical temperature. The principal way in which the enhancement of metabolism is brought about is by shivering, which consists of rhythmic muscular contractions. An increase in heat production in animals exposed to cold may also occur in the absence of detectable muscular activity (so-called nonshivering thermogenesis).

Shivering

During sudden exposure to cold, shivering is the major contributor to the enhanced heat production. It may increase oxygen consumption by 400 percent, whereas the contribution of nonshivering thermogenesis is far less. Shivering is an involuntary function of the body and consists of a muscular tremor with a frequency of about 10 per second. The muscle oscillations are usually preceded by an increased muscular tone. The circuit consisting of gamma motoneurons, muscle spindles, and muscle afferent fibers is apparently of great importance in the control of shivering. From the thermodynamic standpoint, shivering is much more effective than voluntary muscle contractions.

Like other thermoregulatory mechanisms, shivering may be initiated and influenced by peripheral and central temperatures. Peripheral cooling may induce shivering with no change in brain temperature, and local cooling of the anterior hypothalamus or the spinal cord may elicit shivering at an external temperature that remains constant. The termination of peripherally elicited shivering by brain warming and that of centrally induced shivering by skin warming demonstrate the close association between the two mechanisms.

Nonshivering thermogenesis

There also exists a cold-stimulated thermogenesis without shivering. For instance, cold-acclimated animals, in which muscular activity is blocked by curare, may double their heat production during cold exposure. This nonshivering thermogenesis is due predominantly to the calorigenic effect of epinephrine and norepinephrine, which are both released in increased amounts in the cold. Thyroxine secretion is also stimulated by cold. The fact that thyroxine potentiates the calorigenic action of epinephrine indicates that there exists a complex and modulated interplay between various endocrine factors in the bodily defense against cold. Adrenocortical hormones may also be of importance. Particularly in newborn mammals (including human infants) and in hibernating mammals, brown fat is an important site of nonshivering thermogenesis. Cold-induced sympathetic stimulation of the brown fat markedly increases lipid metabolism and hence heat production. Brown fat tissue has probably the highest thermogenic capacity of any mammalian tissue (see "Hibernation," above). Repeated cold exposure may increase the stores of brown fat that contribute to cold acclimation.

TEMPERATURE PERCEPTION

Temperature perception is mediated by peripheral thermoreceptors and thermosensitive units in the CNS. Their joint action seems to be necessary to obtain the maximal temperature regulation against heat or cold.

Peripheral thermoreceptors

The sensations of warmth and cold in humans originate from thermoreceptors in the skin and certain mucous membranes. It is not known for sure that animals experience peripheral warmth or cold in the same manner. Nevertheless, most of the knowledge about the properties of the thermoreceptors is derived from electrophysiological studies in animals. There are two kinds of thermoreceptors: warmth receptors and cold receptors. At constant temperatures they show a steady discharge (a static response), the frequency of which is dependent on the absolute temperature (Fig. 47.3). When there is a sudden temperature rise, the warmth receptors react with a transient increase in frequency (a phasic response) but soon adapt to a new static discharge rate. The cold receptors behave in the opposite way, showing a transient increase in discharge when there is a sudden temperature drop. Certain areas of the skin seem to be of greater importance than others in the peripheral control of body temperature. For example, local warming of the scrotal skin in the ram elicits polypnea much more readily than heating of any other skin area. Recent studies involving cooling or warming of restricted parts of the body in experimental animals imply that thermosensitive elements of importance in temperature regulation also are present in deep body tissues outside the CNS.

Central nervous system thermosensitivity

CNS thermosensitivity obviously plays an important role in temperature regulation. The local warming of the anterior hypothalamus (the preoptic region) in conscious mammals activates all available physiological and behavioral heat-loss mechanisms, and local cooling of the same part of the brain stem evokes the thermoregulatory responses for heat gain. Similar thermoregulatory responses are elicited by alterations of spinal cord temperature in both mammals (Fig. 47.4) and birds. In mammals, the preoptic thermosensitivity is of greater importance for temperature regulation than spinal thermosensitivity, whereas spinal thermosensitivity seems to play a dominant role in birds.

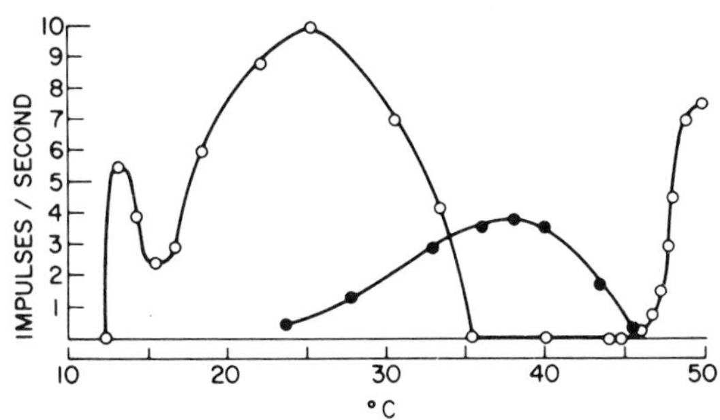

Figure 47.3. Frequency of the steady discharge of a single cold fiber (*open circles*) and of a single warm fiber (*solid circles*) when the temperature receptors of the cat's tongue are exposed to constant temperatures within the range of 10 to 50°C. (From Zotterman 1953, *Ann. Rev. Physiol.* 15:357–72.)

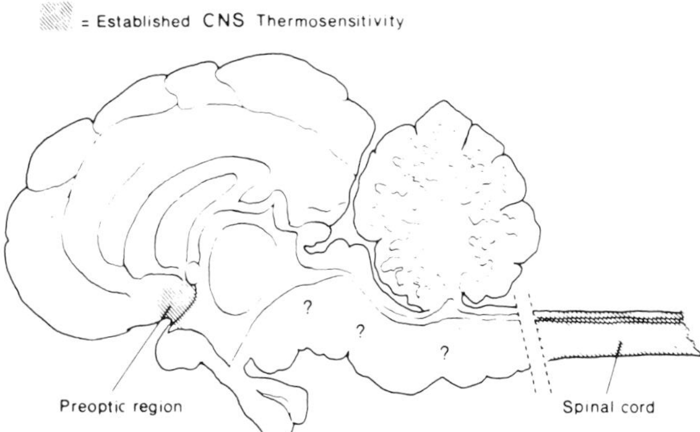

Figure 47.4. Parts of the central nervous system shown to contain temperature sensors important for mammalian temperature regulation. Sensors of that kind may also be present within the parts of the brain stem indicated with question marks.

REGULATION OF BODY TEMPERATURE

Peripheral versus central factors

A much debated problem is the relative importance of peripheral, spinal, and hypothalamic thermoreceptors for determining the set-point of the body thermostat. In general, central heat counteracts the effect of peripheral cold, and vice versa. This is indicated by the effects of local cooling and warming of the anterior hypothalamus at different external temperatures. Local cooling of the anterior hypothalamus causes marked peripheral vasoconstriction and may further cause shivering, even in a thermally neutral environment. This leads to an elevation of core temperature. The shivering response, however, is highly dependent on the external temperature. It is strong in a cold environment and weak or absent in a warm one. Local warming of the hypothalamic thermoregulatory center has the reverse effect. It inhibits the cold-defense mechanisms and activates the heat-loss mechanisms. However, the heat-loss response to central warming is highly dependent on the external temperature. It is strong in the warmth and weak in the cold. Nevertheless, by blocking the cold defense, prolonged local warming of the anterior hypothalamus may cause almost a 10°C drop in rectal temperature of goats placed in the cold.

Interaction between neural and hormonal mechanisms

As epinephrine, norepinephrine, and thyroxine are of major importance in cold-stimulated, nonshivering thermogenesis, an increased secretion of these hormones occurs in mammals during cold stress. The anterior hypothalamus participates in the control of these hormonal cold-defense mechanisms. Local warming of this part of the brain inhibits the activation of the sympathicoadrenomedullary system and the thyroid activation that normally occurs during a general cold stress. Local cooling of the anterior hypothalamus, on the other hand, causes sympathicoadrenomedullary activation and increased secretion of thyroxine (Fig. 47.5). The latter response is mediated by the release of thyrotropic hormone (TSH) from the anterior pituitary. It is therefore evident that changes in deep body temperature influence both neural and hormonal thermoregulatory mechanisms by altering the activity of thermosensitive cells in the anterior hypothalamus.

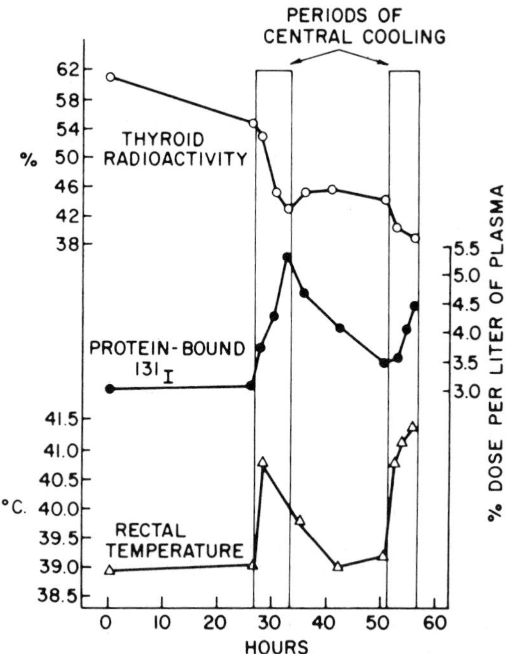

Figure 47.5. Thyroid activation elicited by local cooling of the hypothalamic thermoregulatory center of a goat (central cooling). The animal had been given 40 μc of ^{131}I as KI 3 day before the experiment. The increased release of thyroxine from the thyroid gland during central cooling is evidenced by a rapid fall in thyroid radioactivity and a steep rise of protein-bound radioiodine (PB^{131}I) in the blood plasma. Note the rise in rectal temperature during local cooling of the anterior hypothalamus. (From Andersson, Ekman, Gale, and Sundsten 1962, *Acta Physiol. Scand.* 54:191–92.)

REACTION TO EXTREME ENVIRONMENTAL TEMPERATURES

Heat tolerance

Many experimental studies have established the ability of various domestic animals to withstand external heat. The remarkable ability of the camel has been mentioned. In the sheep, the rectal temperature starts to rise above normal at an air temperature of 32°C, and open-mouth panting begins at a rectal temperature of 41°C. Unless the relative humidity is high (above 65 percent), the sheep is able to withstand for hours an external temperature as high as 43°C. Both sweating and panting are important heat-regulatory devices in this species. The same applies to cattle. In the cow, sweat gland activity increases in relation to the rise in temperature, and polypnea often occurs at rectal temperatures above 40°C.

Because of underdeveloped sweat glands and the absence of a panting mechanism, the pig has a lower heat tolerance than most other domestic animals. Its rectal temperature begins to rise above normal at an environmental temperature of 30 to 32°C. If the relative humidity is 65 percent or more, the pig cannot tolerate a prolonged exposure to a temperature of 35°C. At 40°C the pig is unable to stand an atmosphere of any humidity. A rectal temperature of 41°C. is near the danger point, and collapse easily occurs.

The rectal temperature of the dog tends to rise above normal at a room temperature of 27 to 30°C. As the environmental temperature rises, the rate of breathing increases, but the depth of breathing (tidal volume) is markedly reduced. This helps to protect the carbon dioxide content of the blood against reduction. At a rectal temperature of 41°C the dog is in danger of a breakdown in its thermal equilibrium, and at a rectal temperature of 42.5°C severe nervous symptoms develop, with danger of immediate collapse.

The rectal temperature of the cat begins to be elevated at an air temperature of 32°C, and at a relative humidity above 65 percent the cat is unable to withstand prolonged exposure to an environment temperature of 40°C. As in the dog, polypnea and panting are the main ways to increase heat loss during heat stress. In addition, a cat may increase its evaporative heat loss by spreading saliva on its coat.

In birds, evaporation that occurs as air passes through the air sacs has a cooling effect. When body temperature rises, birds pant and drink more water. At external temperatures above 27°C, the hen begins to show a rise in rectal temperature and respiratory rate. Prolonged exposure of a hen to an air temperature of 38°C is unsafe unless the relative humidity is below 75 percent. A rectal temperature of 45°C appears to be the upper limit of safety in the hen.

Adjustments during prolonged cold exposure

The lower critical temperature (t_c) varies among species but may also vary considerably among individuals of the same species dependent on climatically induced changes in body insulation. Increased insulation causes a lowering of t_c, and decreased insulation has the reverse effect.

The physiological adjustments to prolonged cold exposure can be separated into three categories: (1) changes that occur during cold exposure for a few weeks when other environmental factors remain unchanged (cold acclimation), (2) modifications that develop during the slow seasonal change from summer to winter (cold acclimatization), and (3) genetic alterations over several generations as a result of natural selection of the individuals best suited for survival in the cold climate (climatic adaptation). The principal difference between the first two is that animals acclimated to cold show persistent elevation of metabolism as a result of enzyme reactions but usually no significant lowering of t_c, whereas cold-acclimatized animals generally show no increase in metabolism but have a markedly lower t_c as the result of improved insulation.

Cold acclimation

The phenomenon of cold acclimation has been studied mainly in small animals under laboratory conditions. It involves primarily a shift from shivering to nonshivering thermogenesis occurring during the first 2 to 3 weeks of cold exposure. The increase in nonshivering thermogenesis enables the animals to survive longer than nonacclimated animals in severe cold. The nature of the physiological adjustments in the cold-acclimated animal is still largely unknown. However, definite changes in carbohydrate and fat metabolism occur, the stores of brown fat may increase, and the calorigenic effect of epinephrine and norepinephrine is potentiated during cold acclimation. Maintenance of the increased nonshivering metabolism requires the presence of the thyroid and the adrenal glands. The effect of cold acclimation is lost when the animals are placed in an environmental temperature of 30°C for 4 days.

Cold acclimatization

For animals living in a cold climate, compensation by increased heat production similar to that occurring during cold acclimation would be highly uneconomical. Mammals living under winter conditions maintain a normal body temperature mainly by adjustments that involve improved insulation. Consequently, they have a lower t_c than animals of the same species that are not acclimatized to cold. Measurements of the insulative value of the fur show marked increases in winter over summer values. Vasomotor adaptations may also be of great importance. Heat production, on the other hand, is usually not elevated in cold-acclimatized animals. In many arctic animals the metabolism in the winter is actually lower than it is during summer when measured at a given external temperature.

Climatic adaptation

The body temperature of homeotherms does not show adaptive changes. Thus the rectal temperature does not vary significantly between tropic and arctic mammals, although the latter have to live in the extreme cold. Arctic animals maintain their body temperature at a high level because of a most efficient insulation, and they do not increase their metabolism until the environmental temperature is very low. The lower critical environmental temperature is −10°C for the Eskimo dog and −30°C for the Arctic fox, whereas humans and large tropical animals have lower critical temperatures as high as 25 to 27°C. The extreme temperature gradients that exist between peripheral and central parts of the body in arctic animals do necessitate certain chemical changes in the tissues. The melting point of the marrow fat of the phalanges of the Eskimo dog, for example, has been found to be 30°C lower than that of the upper part of the femur.

HYPOTHERMIA

Hypothermia is a reduction of deep body temperature below normal in nonhibernating homeotherms. In nature hypothermia usually develops because of an exhaustion of the metabolic cold defense mechanisms. Shivering may persist for a long time, causing a depletion of the skeletal muscle and liver glycogen reserves and also a fall in the glycogen content of cardiac muscle. Concomitant with the fall in deep body temperature there is gradual slowing of the heart and a hemoconcentration as the result of a fluid shift from the blood to the tissues. The lethal low level of body temperature varies among species and among individuals of the same species. In humans and in dogs, cardiac arrest followed by respiratory depression and death may occur at a rectal temperature of about 25°C. Considerably lower levels of rectal temperature, however, have sometimes been observed in surviving humans and dogs. Because of reduced brain metabolism, mental effects are detected in humans when the rectal temperature has fallen to about 35°C, and in dogs and cats consciousness is lost at a rectal temperature of about 26°C.

To facilitate cardiac and brain surgery in humans, the use of artificially induced hypothermia has become common. Concomitantly, much experimental work has been performed on the effect of deliberate lowering of the body temperature in animals. A rapid body cooling is facilitated by initial use of anesthesia, which is no longer necessary when the rectal temperature falls below 25°C. Since cardiac arrhythmias and cardiac arrest are likely to occur at this rectal temperature, the usual level of surgical hypothermia is in the range of 25 to 30°C. (so-called moderate hypothermia). Much experimental work in both large and small animals has been performed, however, in the range of 15 to 25°C. With the information obtained from these studies, it has been possible to perform cardiac surgery in humans during deep hypothermia (i.e., at body temperatures near 15°C). Under such circumstances a certain degree of circulation is maintained by the use of an artificial heart-lung pump, and the heart may be arrested for periods of as much as 1 hour. With similar precautions taken, a dog survived 1 hour of cardiac arrest when the rectal temperature was reduced to 0°C.

FEVER AND HYPERTHERMIA

In contrast to other forms of hyperthermia, fever is a regulated rise of body temperature that is reversed to normal by treatment with antipyretics (aspirin and aspirinlike drugs). During the development of fever, the heat balance is positive because of a reduction in heat loss (skin vasoconstriction) and because of increased heat production. Later, when the body temperature reaches a certain height, the balance between heat loss and heat production is restored, and the temperature is again precisely regulated at the new high level. With termination of fever, various heat-loss mechanisms are activated and body temperature returns to its normal level.

The cause and the mechanisms underlying fever have been extensively studied in recent years. Bacteria and other microorganisms contain and produce lipopolysaccharides and other substances that have a febrile action. These *exogenous pyrogens* elicit fever indirectly through the mediation of *endogenous pyrogen(s),* which are of a protein nature and are released from monocytes and fixed tissue–

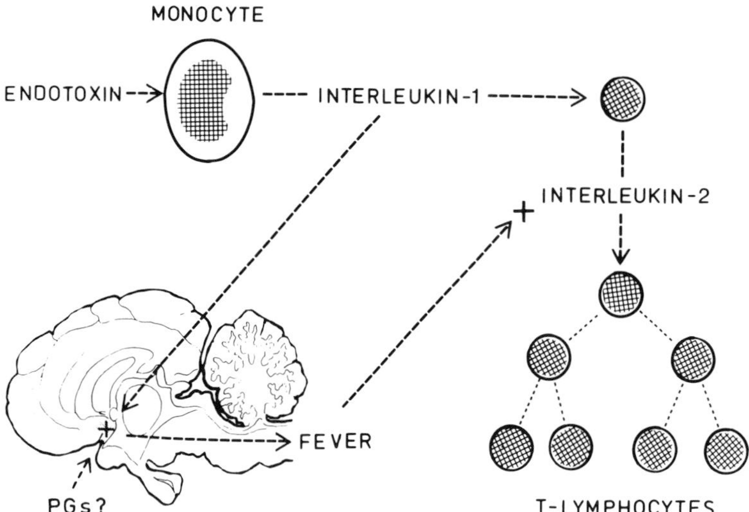

Figure 47.6. Simplified schematic illustration of the combined action of interleukin-1 as an endogenous pyrogen and a stimulator of T-lymphocyte proliferation. The proliferation is further accentuated by the fever elevation of body temperature. PGs, prostaglandins. (From Jónasson 1987, Studies on endotoxin-induced fever—associated with endocrine, renal and ophthalmic events, Doctoral thesis, Karolinska Institute, Stockholm.)

macrophages. So far, several endogenous pyrogens have been identified, of which *interleukin-1* is the most potent and the best studied. Endogenous pyrogen acts on CNS thermoregulatory mechanisms (predominantly in the preoptic region, Fig. 47.6) to facilitate cold-defense reactions and inhibit heat-dissipation reactions. The net result is an elevation of the set-point of the bodily "thermostat" and a body temperature regulated at a higher-than-normal level. There is some evidence that the thermoregulatory effect of endogenous pyrogen is secondary to stimulation of CNS prostaglandin synthesis. Speaking in favor of this is the fact that aspirin and other antipyretics are effective inhibitors of prostaglandin synthesis. Endogenous pyrogen may also be liberated from phagocytes under certain noninfectious conditions (e.g., in surgical fever).

If not complicated by cerebral damage that impairs temperature regulation, fever is generally self-limiting, with maximum body temperature of about 41°C in mammals. There is much evidence that fever is of benefit for fighting infection. The elevated body temperature in disease stimulates the formation of interferons, proteins that have antiviral and antibacterial properties. Interleukin-1 exerts many effects of importance for defense against infectious agents. Among these is the activation of T-lymphocytes, the cells primarily responsible for cell-mediated immunity. Proliferation of the T cells is enhanced by fever. Another effect of interleukin-1 is to lower the plasma iron concentration. The resulting hypoferremia reduces bacterial growth rate, since iron is essential for normal growth and division of these microorganisms. Furthermore, many laboratory studies have shown higher survival rates for infected animals with fever than for those given antipyretic drugs.

The hyperthermia characteristic of heat stroke develops when the heat production exceeds the evaporative capacity of the environment, or when the evaporative mechanisms become impaired because of great loss of body fluid and reduced blood volume. Here antipyretics are ineffective, and a reversal of body temperature can be achieved only by whole-body cooling. *Nonfebrile hyperthermia* may also develop in response to drugs that impair the heat-dissipation mechanisms and/or drastically increase the metabolic rate. A strange example is the genetically determined *malignant hyperthermia* observed in swine and humans. The malignant hyperthermia can be triggered by inhalation anesthetics and muscle relaxants that induce an inappropriate elevation of myoplasmic calcium concentration followed by a dramatic rise in muscle metabolism and heat production. Once developed, the malignant hyperthermia is lethal unless intense body cooling is initiated.

REFERENCES

Andersson, B. 1970. Central nervous and hormonal interaction in temperature regulation of the goat. In J.D. Hardy, A.P. Gagge, J.A.J. Stolwijk, eds., *Psychological and Behavioral Temperature Regulation*. Thomas, Springfield, Ill. Pp. 634–47.

Andersson, B., Ekman, L., Gale, C.C., and Sundsten, J.W. 1962. Activation of the thyroid gland by cooling of the preoptic area in the goat. *Acta Physiol. Scand.* 54:191–92.

Bligh, J., Ingram, D.L., Keynes, R.D., and Robinson, S.G. 1965. The deep body temperature of an unrestrained Welsh mountain sheep recorded by a radiotelemetric technique during a 12-month period. *J. Physiol.* 176:136–44.

Britt, B.A. 1979. Etiology and pathophysiology of malignant hyperthermia. *Fed. Proc.* 38:44–48.

Dinarello, C.A. 1988. Endogenous pyrogens. *Methods Enzymol.* 163: 495–510.

Folk, G.E., Jr. 1979. Protein and fat metabolism during mammalian hypophagia and hibernation: Introduction. *Fed. Proc.* 39:2953–54.

Folk, G.E., Jr., Larson, A., and Folk, M.A.: Physiology of hibernating bears. In Proceedings of the Third International Conference on Bear Research and Management, June 1974. *Bears—Their Biology and Management*. Edited by M.R. Pelton, J.W. Lentfer, and G.E. Folk. Morges, Switzerland, International Union for Conservation of Nature and Natural Resources, 1976, pp. 373–80.

Gale, C.C. 1973. Neuroendocrine aspects of thermoregulation. *Annu. Rev. Physiol.* 35:391–430.

Gollan, F. 1964. Cardiac arrest of one hour duration in dogs during hypothermia of 0°C followed by survival. *Fed. Proc.* 13:57.

Hensel, H. 1974. Thermoreceptors. *Annu. Rev. Physiol.* 36:233–49.

Jónasson, H. 1987. Studies on endotoxin-induced fever—Association with endocrine, renal and ophthalmic events. Doctoral thesis, Karolinska Institute, Stockholm.

Kibler, H.H., and Brody, S. 1950. Environmental physiology with special reference to domestic animals. X. Influence of temperature, 5° to 95°F, on evaporative cooling from the respiratory and exterior body surfaces in Jersey and Holstein cows. *Univ. Mo. Ag. Exp. Sta. Res. Bull.* 461.

Kluger, M.J. 1986. Is fever beneficial? *Yale J. Biol. Med.* 59:89–95.

Robertshaw, D., and Taylor, C.R. 1968. The control of sweat gland function in equines. *Proc. Internat. Union Physiol. Sci.* XXIV Internat. Cong., Washington. Vol. 7, p. 370.

Schmidt-Nielsen, K. 1979. *Animal Physiology: Adaptation and environment.* Cambridge Univ. Press, Cambridge.

Schmidt-Nielsen, K., Schmidt-Nielsen, B., Jarnum, S.A., and Houpt, T.R. 1957. Body temperature of the camel and its relation to water economy. *Am. J. Physiol.* 188:103–12.

Zotterman, Y. 1953. Special senses: Thermal receptors. *Annu. Rev. Physiol.* 15:357–72.

CHAPTER 48

Neurophysiology of Consciousness | by W. R. Klemm

ANIMAL CONSCIOUSNESS

Certain behavioral states, such as alertness and sleep, are commonly called "states of consciousness." However, since consciousness, like beauty, is in the mind of the beholder, it is semantically awkward to talk about the physiology of such an abstraction. Some philosophers distinguish between awareness and consciousness. Awareness, which all higher animals have, is a form of perception, whereas consciousness sometimes is defined as a special kind of *self*-awareness. Perhaps a more physiological definition of consciousness is that it is present if an animal has mental images (not necessarily visual) that it uses to represent the sensory world and to make choices that govern its behavior.

Humans are tempted on philosophical grounds to deny animals a consciousness. Despite the long-held "behaviorist" view that animal behavior can be explained without attributing consciousness to animals, there is growing evidence that animals, at least the higher mammals and primates, do think. Even in typical operant conditioning studies, animal subjects sometimes exhibit innovative behaviors that could not have been predicted from the design of the experiment and the behavioral "shaping" procedures.

Animals can pay attention to stimuli and do so selectively, paying special attention to those stimuli that are most biologically important at the time. Animals evidently can hold some kind of mental image of environmental situations, as has been demonstrated in experiments in which animals must delay a response to a stimulus. Animals have long-term and short-term memories. Maze studies show that they even have "working" memories that they use in problem solving. For example, an eight-arm radial maze, with all arms identical and baited with food, has been used to show that a rat can remember which of the arms he has already visited to retrieve the food reward; some workers interpret these data as indicating that the rat has created a "cognitive map" (not necessarily conscious).

Animals have a mental clock of sorts that allows them to track time. Their behaviors are often serially ordered, and the choice of sequences in a behavior can be under their voluntary control. Particularly in the wild state, animals often make choices that optimize decision making, as in diet selection and foraging strategies, for example.

Animals communicate with each other, quite sophisticatedly in some species. Higher primates can learn the rudiments of language.

Common observation of animals causes us to think of the various consciousness states as being on a continuous scale that ranges from sleep to hyperexcitability. Yet the position along such a continuum is not at all clear for such states as dreaming, tranquility, pain, hibernation, and various immobility responses.

There are two major medical implications of consciousness. One is the assessment of neurological disorders; disorders of consciousness typically indicate brain-stem lesions, which are serious and difficult to treat. The other implication is in humane animal care, particularly as it relates to pain. "Pain" is felt only in a conscious state (see also Chaps. 39 and 41). Thus a clear idea is needed of what consciousness is and how to recognize changes in it.

OBJECTIVE MEASURES OF CONSCIOUS STATES

Behavior

Various states are commonly defined in terms of observed behavior. For example, a hunting dog is *alert* when, on detecting the scent of birds, it stops, becomes tense, perks its ears, and points its tail. It is *asleep* when it lies down, curls up, closes its eyes, and does not move for a time.

Electrographic correlates

Electrical activity from various body organs can reflect the behavioral state by providing information on such functions as heart rate, muscle tone, and neuron activity. Such measures not only provide a more precise definition of behavioral states but, more important, they enable us to learn about the mechanisms that cause the various states.

Information on electrical activity of the brain is usually derived from electrodes placed on the head or within the brain and is usually displayed by pen-and-ink recorders; the written record thus obtained is called the *electroencephalogram* or *EEG*. The EEG is actually a plot of voltage changes as a function of time. The waveform of the EEG is irregular because the waves have been compounded from a mixture of different voltages and frequencies that were generated by different neuronal generators.

Most evidence suggests that the EEG comes from algebraic summation of slow membrane potential changes in the excitatory postsynaptic potential (EPSP) and inhibitory postsynaptic potential (IPSP) of individual neurons (Chap. 40). It is also possible that some of the EEG comes from membrane potential fluctuations of glia cells and from compounding of nearly synchronous impulses.

In an oversimplified way, the EEG can be said to appear in one of two forms: (1) *low voltage, fast activity (LVFA)*, in which most waves are of low voltage and short duration; and (2) *high voltage, slow activity (HVSA)*, in which most waves are of high voltage and long duration.

Usually electrical activity of the brain correlates with behavior over a wide range of normal phenomena. LVFA is usually associated with alert states, and HVSA is associated with sedated states such as sleep and anesthesia. These correlations do not always apply in certain disease or drug states.

A prominent correlate of an activated or aroused brain of dogs, cats, and other nonprimates is a rhythmic hippocampal electrical discharge (5 to 12 waves per second) known as theta rhythm. The hippocampus, a major part of the limbic system (see Chap. 49), is most noted as a site of infection for rabies virus and for its role in consolidating temporary memories into permanent form. The rhythm seems to be driven from activated neurons in the pontine reticular formation; these, in turn, activate an oscillatory pacemaker system in the septum, which supplies a major cholinergic input to the hippocampus. Theta rhythm is strongly correlated with movement and locomotion, but it also occurs any time an animal becomes aroused and has enhanced postural tone, even if immobile.

ALERTNESS

Behavioral correlates

An animal's basic response to biologically meaningful stimuli involves a succession of stages. First, there is attention or startle, depending on stimulus intensity. Then there is orientation, followed by either approach, withdrawal, or habituation.

A significant stimulus causes animals to interrupt motion and to turn eyes, ears, and nose toward the stimulus. This reflex focusing of attention and sensory investigation is called the orienting reflex.

The initial arousing and orienting responses are more reflexive than later stages. In all stages there is usually a conspicuous activation of the EEG (LVFA)(Fig. 48.1). Initial responses are triggered by a major *change* in sensation; for example, sudden cessation of continuous stimulation can be just as arousing as can sudden stimulation during continuous absence of stimulation.

With experience, the brain can learn to discriminate against certain stimuli that are of no consequence to the animal. This habituation or accommodation is indicated in the EEG by failure of the stimulus to elicit LVFA. The chief feature of arousing stimuli is their strangeness to the animal. Arousal habituation is quite relevant to the study of sleep, because it means that uniform stimulation is associated with the brain sites that cause HVSA.

One can think of arousal as a *readiness response* (Fig. 48.2). When the animal is aroused by sensory input, all relevant systems are excited by reflex action. Behavioral readiness is a state of preparedness for making appropriate behavioral responses to environmental contingencies. It has long been accepted that the brain stem, particularly its reticular formation, mediates such components of readiness as "arousal" and "orienting." The brain stem also mediates most of the other components of readiness by generating a global mobilization that includes enhanced capability for selective attention, cognition, affect, learning and memory, defense, flight, attack, pain control, sensory perception, autonomic "fight or flight," neuroendocrine stress responses, visuomotor and vestibular reflexes, muscle and postural tone, and locomotion.

The cerebral cortex is excited, enhancing consciousness and arousal level. Concurrently, muscle tone is enhanced, preparing the body for forthcoming movement instructions. Simultaneously, the limbic system is activated and allows

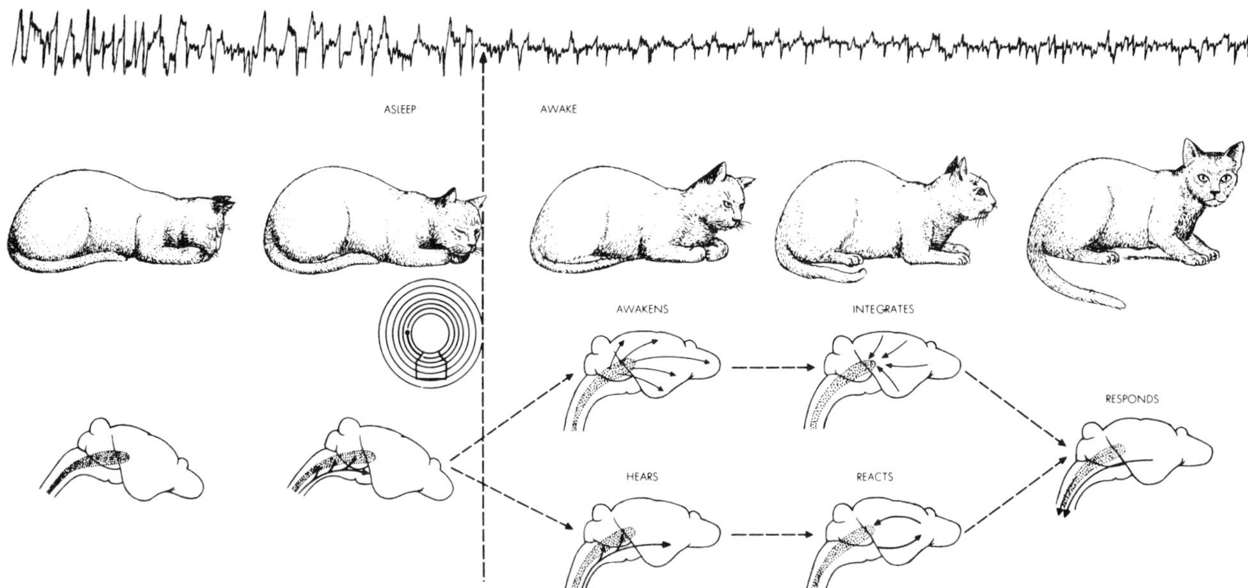

Figure 48.1. Electroencephalogram (EEG) and behavioral effects of an auditory stimulus on the reticular activating system (RAS). The brain diagram illustrates sound stimuli (*incoming solid arrows*) reaching the brain-stem reticular formation (*stippled area*) by way of collateral branches of the axons that lead to the auditory cortex (Chap. 49). At this stage, the animal has received the sensory information and thus hears without necessarily processing the information. The RAS then "awakens" the cortex diffusely so that it integrates and processes the auditory input. Associated with the RAS effect is a behavioral arousal and a desynchronization of the EEG. Interactions of RAS and cortical activity then prepare the cat to make an appropriate motor response to the sound stimulus. (From French 1957, *The Reticular Formation*.)

new stimuli to be evaluated in the context of memories. Also, at the same time, neurons of the hypothalamus and the autonomic nervous system mobilize the heart and other visceral organs for the so-called fight-or-flight situations. This constellation of responses makes an animal *ready* to respond rapidly and vigorously to biologically significant stimuli. These multiple reflexlike responses are, for the most part, very obvious during *startle reactions* of either animals or humans. Less intense stimuli may not evoke a complete readiness reflex because the brain can quickly determine that a response of great intensity is not appropriate to the stimuli.

Neurophysiological bases

Brain-stem reticular activating system

All readiness response components seem to be triggered from the brain-stem reticular formation (BSRF), the central core of the brain stem.

The following facts suggest that the reticular activating system (RAS) performs an important function in readiness: (1) Humans with lesions in the RAS area are lethargic or even comatose. (2) In experimental animals surgical isolation of the forebrain causes the cortex to generate an EEG that consists solely of HVSA. (3) Direct electrical stimulation of the RAS has unique abilities to awaken sleeping animals and to cause hyperarousal in awake animals. (4) RAS neurons develop a sustained increase in discharge just *before* behavioral and EEG signs of arousal.

The BSRF cells receive collateral sensory input from all levels of the spinal cord, including such diverse sources as cutaneous receptors of the body and head, Golgi tendon organs, aortic and carotid sinuses, several cranial nerves associated with vestibular sensors, eyes, and ears, in addition to extensive inputs from other areas of the brain stem, the cerebellum, and the cerebral cortex.

When RAS neurons are stimulated by sensory input of any kind, they relay excitation through numerous reticular synapses and finally activate widespread zones of the cerebral cortex. In contrast, sensory information that arrives in the cortex by way of the main sensory paths passes through relatively few synapses and arrives at specific and very discrete zones of the cortex (see Chap. 41).

The RAS responds in the same way to any sensory stimulus, whether from the skin, eyes, or ears, to "awaken" the cerebral cortex so that it can respond to and process stimuli.

The role of the RAS in these arousing responses can be demonstrated by direct electrical stimulation at many points within the brain-stem reticulum. Such stimulation activates the neocortex (indicated by LVFA in the EEG), the limbic system (rhythmic theta activity in the hippocampus), and postural tone (increased electromyographic activity of muscles) (Fig. 48.3). In addition, many visceral activities are activated via spread of RAS excitation into the hypothalamus.

While the obvious conclusion is that the reticular formation creates arousal by direct excitation of higher centers,

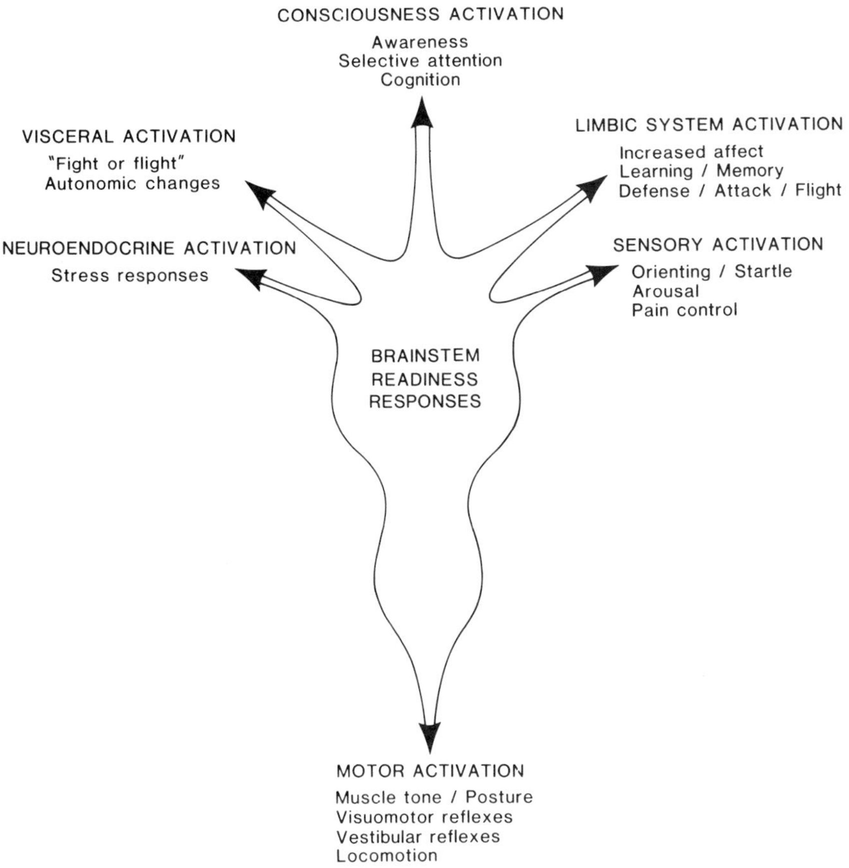

CONSCIOUSNESS ACTIVATION
Awareness
Selective attention
Cognition

VISCERAL ACTIVATION
"Fight or flight"
Autonomic changes

LIMBIC SYSTEM ACTIVATION
Increased affect
Learning / Memory
Defense / Attack / Flight

NEUROENDOCRINE ACTIVATION
Stress responses

SENSORY ACTIVATION
Orienting / Startle
Arousal
Pain control

BRAINSTEM
READINESS
RESPONSES

MOTOR ACTIVATION
Muscle tone / Posture
Visuomotor reflexes
Vestibular reflexes
Locomotion

Figure 48.2. Model of the brain stem's role in mediating behavioral "readiness" to respond to biologically meaningful stimuli. Activation of the brain stem, particularly the reticular formation and periaqueductal gray, is seen to engage a constellation of sensory, integrative, and motor responses for adaptive response to novel or intense stimuli.

one cannot yet rule out the possibility that the excitation is indirect and results from a release from inhibition.

The RAS gets extensive input from various brain regions, particularly the neocortex and limbic system, and such input can be a major factor in causing certain behavioral states. For example, the cortical and limbic system activities that are associated with the distress of a newly weaned puppy probably supply a continuous barrage of impulses to the RAS, which in turn continually excites the cortex to keep the puppy awake and howling all night.

The general view of wakefulness is that it exists whenever the tonic flow of impulses of the RAS is above the critical level for sustaining consciousness. There is a strong correlation between the impulse discharge rate in the BSRF and the level of behavioral arousal. Reduction of RAS activity, either normal or abnormal (by barbiturates, tranquilizers, experimental injury, or disease), can lead to various degrees of sedation, sleeplike states, and coma.

Selective attention

Besides nonspecific arousal effects, the RAS also seems to have a role in selective attention to specific stimuli. The RAS controls activity in the thalamic extension of the RAS,

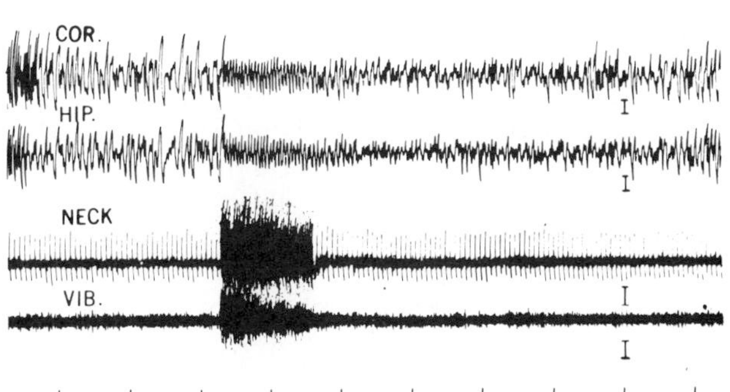

Figure 48.3. Stimulation of areas in the rat brain-stem reticular formation, showing the widespread nature of the reticular activating system. A focal point of the reticular formation was stimulated mildly (2.8 volts, 300 pulses per second), as indicated by thickened portion of the 1-second time line at the bottom. Both cortex (COR) and hippocampus (HIP) were activated, as indicated by the initial theta rhythm followed by low-voltage, fast activity in the EEG. Simultaneously, there was activation of both ascending and descending muscle activities, as revealed in the electromyogram of vibrissae (VIB) and nuchal muscles (NECK, contaminated with electrocardiographic signals). The spinal cord was transected cervically to restrict feedback variables and to achieve substantial deafferentation (note deactivated EEG before stimulation). (From Klemm 1972, *Brain Res.* 41:331–44.)

and this portion of the thalamus has powerful inhibitory effects on thalamic sensory relay nuclei. The reticular thalamus is under control of several other brain areas that seem to control sensory input to the extent that they activate the reticular thalamus to produce its inhibition. Note the similarity in principle of this so-called gate-inhibitory scheme to that which seems to operate in the spinal cord for pain (see "Pain" in this chapter).

Selective attention is particularly under the influence of certain areas in the thalamus and neocortex. Recordings of action potentials in the cortex of trained monkeys show that cells in certain areas act as "attention filters" to impair perception of stimulus features that have less biological significance. Other neurons respond better and more selectively when the monkeys are attentive to the task.

RAS and movements

The role of the RAS in general body movements has become clearer in recent years with the demonstration of correlations of neuronal discharge with locomotion and other movements. In cats, circumscribed zones within the brain-stem reticulum have been identified; stimulation of these zones causes rhythmic stepping movements in decerebrate cats and increased speed of locomotion in intact cats.

Reticular neurons alter their discharge patterns in association with a variety of functions, and it seems clear that a given neuron may participate in one or more phenomena, such as arousal, movement, activated sleep, reward, fear, conditioning, habituation, pain, and so on. This may, however, simply reflect the possibility that a given neuron controls activity of a small set of muscles that provide the behavioral manifestation of arousal, fear, pain, and other responses.

Limbic system

The limbic system (see Chap. 49), has many functions, including an influence on activated behavioral states. For example, activation of the BSRF, in turn, excites the hypothalamus to generate the fight-or-flight visceral activities of the autonomic nervous system. Memory functions best in aroused states. Other probable influences involving affective behavior are less well understood.

Cerebral cortex

The cerebral cortex receives many of the stimuli that cause changes in behavioral state. Neural activity within the cortex, moreover, often determines the state and degree of response to stimuli. If one ablates a specific sensory portion of the cortex (for example, the cells that receive sound input), then the appropriate stimulus (sound in this case) will fail to change behavior.

Although the cortex is necessary for some behavioral states, it cannot be the sole determinant because of the profound influences of subcortical areas.

The cortex helps to regulate those subcortical structures that affect it. For example, electrical stimulation at many points on the cortex can evoke neural responses in the RAS, which in turn stimulates the cortex into awareness and responsiveness.

The activation of the cerebral cortex that results from RAS activity is cholinergic. During behavioral arousal in cats, release of acetylcholine by cortical cells is greatly increased. Systemic injection of the acetylcholine blocker, atropine, prevents excitation of cortical cells by the release of acetylcholine.

Conscious direction of behavior

Intent to act arises in consciousness, presumably via complex cortical processing. The neurophysiology of such processes is difficult to study. However, one example of how to study such processes is recent work based on recording of extracellular impulses from cortical neurons that participate in complex voluntary movements. Some cells in the cortex of monkeys have firing rates that, if combined vectorially, will predict the direction of arm movement. It is known that in the cord, the neural circuits do not relate to muscles or joints in a one-to-one manner but, rather, there is much convergence of input from many parts of the limb and much divergence of output that seems to address the limb as a whole.

SLEEP

Sleep occupies much of an animal's life: up to 42 percent of ordinary ("deactivated") sleep, plus 16 percent of dream-stage ("activated") sleep in cats under laboratory conditions.

What is the purpose of sleep? It is not clear. *Rest* can be achieved without sleep. No one has been able to associate sleep with any specific life-maintaining function related to measurable physiological variables. Human experiments seem to suggest that sleep is needed for restitution of the brain but not of the body.

Sleep is necessary for good health, and animals deprived of sleep will eventually become ill. Forcing animals to stay awake can make them irritable and cause them to engage in vicious fights. Sleep deprivation apparently alters certain immune functions and does so independently of the cortisol circadian rhythm.

One purpose of sleep may be to enable the activated phase of sleep, for which some purposes seem to have been identified (see below).

Deactivated sleep

General characteristics

Sleep is recognized most obviously as a reversible unconsciousness and relative immobility of an animal. Behavior during sleep is characterized by (1) reduced ability to analyze changes in the environment, (2) increased threshold to sensory stimulation, and (3) relative muscular inactivity. The environmental influences that usually modify behavior are relatively ineffective. Likewise, in all animals except birds, the tonic proprioceptive, labyrinthine, and visual reflexes that are responsible for righting the body and maintaining normal posture do not operate during sleep.

Since one of the primary characteristics of sleep is a synchronized, HVSA type of EEG, typical sleep is sometimes called slow-wave sleep. Also conspicuous are cortical EEG spindles. By themselves, however, these electrical correlates are not specific indicators of sleep, for they can also occur in certain drug sedation states, during natural drowsiness, during anesthesia, and in certain disease conditions.

The typical stage of sleep can be referred to as *deactivated sleep (DS)* to contrast it from another, qualitatively different, stage of sleep (activated sleep) that will be discussed later.

Absence of movement is conspicuous during DS; spinal reflexes are also depressed. Muscle tone is generally reduced.

During DS, visceral functions are usually depressed because of dominance of the parasympathetic nervous system. The heart rate is slower and blood pressure is lower. Pupils constrict (subtle changes in pupil size can be monitored as an index of the degree of drowsiness). Breathing movements are slower, alveolar CO_2 levels drop, blood pH becomes slightly more acid, total metabolic rate decreases, and body temperature drops. However, no parallel signs of metabolic depression in the brain occur. Cerebral blood flow can even increase during sleep. Moreover, some neurons become more active during DS than during wakefulness.

Mechanisms of deactivated sleep

Many theories have been proposed to explain sleep, but no one theory seems sufficient by itself. Some insight is provided by the normal requirements for inducing sleep.

Sleep is best induced by limitation of movement and by restriction of excessive sensory stimulation, and it can be aided by a continuous monotonous sound. Reduction of the proprioceptive drive with muscle relaxants is also known to promote sleep. Under natural conditions, fatigue of postural tonus markedly decreases the number of proprioceptive impulses. The highest cerebral centers, thus partly isolated from afferent stimulation, are able to lapse into inactivity, and sleep results. Although fatigue is the usual cause of muscle relaxation, it is not necessary for sleep. Many times sleep and wakefulness cycles are largely controlled by conditioned responses.

There are several humoral theories of sleep. They all share the premise that certain body chemicals, usually metabolic end products, accumulate and excite the neurons that cause sleep. This possibility has prompted testing of dialysates and extracts of fluids from sleep-deprived subjects. Such studies reveal the existence of several naturally occurring peptides that promote DS.

Immunological mechanisms may be involved in the genesis of sleep. The leukocytic interleukin I, which also occurs in astrocytes, is somnogenic.

Several lines of evidence suggest that serotonin is involved in sleep control: (1) brain levels of serotonin are high in sleep and low during behavioral activity, (2) intracarotid or intravertebral injections of serotonin induce EEG and ocular signs of sleep, as does topical application of serotonin to an area on the floor of the fourth ventricle; (3) depletion of serotonin interferes with sleep; (4) in serotonin-depleted animals, injection of the serotonin precursor (5-hydroxytryptophan) tends to restore normal sleep; and (5) lesions of the serotonergic neurons in the raphe system of the brain stem interfere with sleep.

Another possibility, not mutually exclusive of serotonin mechanisms, is the possible role of acetylcholine. Cholinergic substances injected in parts of the limbic system, the preoptic region, the diffuse thalamic projection system, and the pontine reticular formation also can induce sleep.

The parasympathetic nervous system is dominant during DS. This, however, does not prove a parasympathetic cause of sleep. For example, during extreme alertness, there is activation of the sympathetic system but sympathetic activity is a consequence and not a cause of the alertness.

Since decorticate animals sleep, the basic sleep-wakefulness mechanisms must be subcortical. These subcortical mechanisms include the activating role of the RAS and the deactivating role of diencephalic and medullary structures. Diminution of RAS activity is an important predisposing cause of sleep. The basic question of why RAS activity diminishes naturally has not been satisfactorily answered.

Most evidence favors an active inhibitory process in specific hypnogenic systems as the cause of sleep.

Deactivating systems

Sleep appears to be regulated by several apparently redundant systems that cannot independently account for sleep.

Thalamic reticular areas antagonize certain activities of the RAS. These thalamic areas, known collectively as the diffuse thalamic projection system (DTPS), are separate and largely independent of the topographically specific thalamic relay nuclei (Chap. 41). The projection of the DTPS is, as the name implies, quite diffuse, projecting ascendingly to the cortex and descendingly to the midbrain reticular formation.

The DTPS is a pacemaker that can regulate cortical activity. When electrically stimulated, it produces rhythmically recurrent potentials, primarily in the frontal and parietal association cortex, which are termed *recruiting* and *augmenting* potentials (Fig. 48.4). One intriguing aspect of the interpretation of recruiting is the similarity in both morphology and topography of recruiting potentials to the spontaneous "spindles" of drowsy animals. Among the other facts that suggest a close relationship is that spindles can be triggered by a single stimulation of the DTPS. During spontaneous cortical spindling or during evoked recruiting, the pacemaker thalamic cells owe their timing to unusually large IPSPs that alternate regularly with EPSPs.

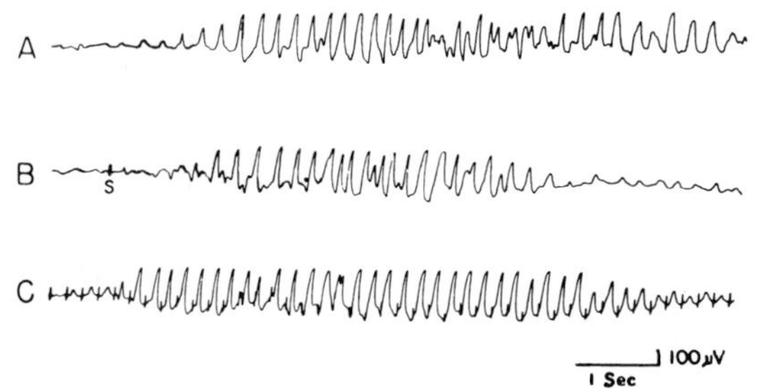

Figure 48.4. Effects of diffuse thalamic projection system stimulation in the medial thalamus of the cat on electrical activity in the cortex. The cat was under light pentobarbital anesthesia. (*A*) Spontaneous spindle burst; (*B*) a single 1 ms shock (S) triggering a spindle burst; (*C*) repetitive stimulation at 5 per second showing waxing and waning of recruiting response. (From Jasper 1960, in *Handbook of Physiology*, sec. 1, Magoun, ed., *Neurophysiology*, American Physiological Society, Washington, D.C., vol. 2).

Several other parts of the brain are antagonistic to the RAS and actually function as sleep-inducing centers.

Low-frequency stimulation of the caudate nucleus can produce spindling, HVSA, and sleep. Similar results have been reported for stimulation of the anterior preoptic regions of the hypothalamus. The preoptic region seems particularly important for the genesis of sleep.

When the brain stem of the cat is transected between the colliculi, the cat sleeps continuously, because the RAS is completely separated from the forebrain. If such a transection is made through the middle of the pons, the cat shows EEG signs of being constantly alert because of disconnection of sleep-inducing systems that are located in the lower medulla (i.e., the RAS action on the forebrain becomes virtually unopposed). Several areas in the caudal pons and rostral medulla, on appropriate stimulation, promote electrographic and behavioral signs of sleep. These areas include the pontine reticular formation, the solitary nucleus, and the ventral nucleus of the medulla.

The solitary tract nucleus is of special interest because most of its neurons increase discharge during but not before sleep; such increases do not occur in nearby neurons.

In addition, many investigators suspect that another sleep center is the *raphe*, a small group of serotonergic cells in the midline of the brain stem. However, the role of raphe nuclei is suspect, because when rats with raphe lesions are observed several weeks after creation of the lesions, there is no interference with DS. However, long-term changes in DS occur after lesions are produced in the lateral part of the periaqueductal gray matter. Perhaps the role of the raphe serotonergic cells is to trigger DS by modulating the activity of true sleep centers.

One can only speculate on the mechanisms that initiate sleep center activity. Discharge patterns in afferent proprioceptive and autonomic nerves may trigger sleep centers directly, or indirectly by release of excitatory drive. Chemical action—at the area postrema, for example—remains an important possibility.

Activated sleep

General characteristics

In 1957, EEG studies in humans revealed that during sleep there were alternating periods of EEG activity in which the waves were not synchronized but were actually desynchronized and associated with stereotyped rapid eye movements. When subjects were awakened in the midst of these episodes, they usually remembered a dream that was interrupted. Subsequently, these same physiological changes were observed to occur periodically during the sleep of animals.

This stage of sleep is qualitatively different from DS. The physiological changes are such that *activated sleep (AS)* is an appropriate name, except that the activation is not expressed behaviorally. Inhibition of motor activity during AS is one of the cardinal features. One of the paradoxes of this state is that as the RAS activity increases, there is a corresponding increase in activity of motor inhibitory systems.

In AS, there is activation of the cortical EEG, hippocampal theta rhythm, spikelike EEG waves in several vision-related brain areas (pons, lateral geniculate nuclei, and occipital cortex), bursts of rapid eye movement, and postural muscle atonia with superimposed phasic twitching.

The various aspects of muscle activity during AS may seem confusing; nuchal activity declines at the same time that face and eye muscles are phasically activated. Moreover, phasic myoclonic jerks occur in many hind limb muscles during AS; between these twitches there are periods of inactivity. The twitches contrast sharply with the tonic inhibition of nuchal and limb muscles. These twitches result from phasic barrages of nerve impulses arriving at spinal motoneurons from supraspinal levels that overwhelm the tonic inhibitory influences of other supraspinal centers. During AS, both monosynaptic and polysynaptic reflexes are markedly depressed, except for those periods when phasic twitching occurs.

The tonic depression of muscle activity probably arises in the brain-stem reticulum. A dramatic phenomenon of AS without such depressed motor activity can be demonstrated by the production of small bilateral lesions in the dorsolateral part of the pontine reticular formation. When sleeping cats with such lesions enter the AS stage, they raise their heads, make body-righting movements, alternately move their limbs, and even try to stand. Although these cats do not respond to stimuli, they act as though they are startled or searching, and sometimes they even attack nearby objects. During alert wakefulness these cats behave almost normally.

Another unusual feature is that AS is a *deep* stage of sleep, and the threshold for arousing stimuli is greater than during DS. AS does not occur in fish or amphibians, and it is poorly developed in reptiles, birds, and lower mammals. In 1-week-old kittens, typical DS seldom occurs; AS constitutes 90 percent of the total sleep time. During the second week, more variability appears in the EEG, with some arousal during wakefulness and some spindles during DS. At 3 weeks the EEG resembles that of the adult.

Since AS is associated with dreaming in humans, the question of whether a similar association exists in animals arises. Much anecdotal evidence seems to indicate that animals do dream. Sleeping dogs, for example, often pedal their feet, twitch their lips and nose, and even bark.

Mechanisms of activated sleep

The brain area that seems to be most concerned with producing AS is the pons. Neither surgical removal of the cerebellum nor complete transection of the brain stem at the midbrain level prevents the peripheral physiological signs of AS. Similarly, transection of the brain stem caudal to the pons fails to prevent EEG signs of AS. AS is abolished by lesions in the pons of intact animals, and low-level electrical stimulation of the midbrain or pontine reticular formation during DS can trigger AS. High-level stimulation during DS causes awakening.

"Executive" structures for AS are located in the pontine reticular formation. The system causing postural atonia is located in the medial part of the locus ceruleus and its immediate vicinity. These neurons have a descending pathway to the nucleus magnocellularis in the medulla, which is a zone that ultimately depresses muscle tone at the spinal level. Gigantocellular field units fire in correlation with movements, both in AS and in the awake state. They are thus not critical to the AS state and cannot be AS "executive neurons." The executive neurons appear to be located in the mediodorsal part of the pons, near the locus ceruleus, and the ventromedial part of the caudal pons and rostral medulla. In both regions, tonically activated neurons can be located during AS. What activates these neurons during AS? One possibility is input from noradrenergic and serotonergic neurons that are located nearby and that cease firing during AS (releasing the executive neurons from inhibition).

Lesion studies indicate that only the activity of certain neurons in the dorsolateral pons is crucial for the generation of AS. Total brain-stem transections at the pontomedullary junction reveal that neither the pontine reticulum nor the medullary reticulum was sufficient for generating the indices of AS; both zones need to have functional interaction to coordinate the various activities associated with AS.

At present there is much interest in the neurochemical transmitter functions that might cause and sustain AS. Many drugs and hormones alter AS, usually reducing the normal incidence. Neuropharmacological studies implicate acetylcholine, norepinephrine, and serotonin, but the mechanisms are not clearly understood.

Some insight into AS mechanisms can be gleaned from the demonstration of a biological need for AS. This has been shown in cats, for example, that were awakened every time they exhibited physiological signs of AS (but not DS). On successive days of deprivation, an increasing number of awakenings was needed. On the first day of recovery after deprivation, when sleep was not interrupted, the AS phase increased to 53 percent of the total sleep time.

It is not known why AS is necessary, but there is evidence to support several possibilities, namely, that AS (1) serves as an endogenous source of stimulation to promote maturation, (2) is needed to establish neuronal pathways serving binocular vision, (3) is an internal reward mechanism, (4) promotes consolidation of memories for recently learned events, (5) is essential for maintaining emotional stability, and (6) is required for sustaining norepinephrine and dopamine neurotransmitter systems. All of these are consistent with another possibility, namely, that AS enables "readiness rehearsal" for the forthcoming day's awake situations and experiences; it may be detrimental for the brain to sustain long periods of depression, as in DS. Accordingly, one would expect that AS deprivation would make animals less ready to respond appropriately to biologically meaningful stimuli and situations during their periods of wakefulness. This view is consistent with observations that such deprived animals show decreased reaction times, lessened orienting, decreased adrenal stress responses, lessened EEG activation responses to stimuli, and decreased performance on various conditioning paradigms. Also rehearsal for readiness during the next wakefulness period is supported by the fact that most AS occurs just before awakening.

Comparison of sleep in domestic species

There are conspicuous species differences in activity cycles. Monophasic animals, generally adults of higher species, tend to have a long rest period each day, usually at night. Many domestic animals tend to be monophasic, being most active during daylight. Most birds, which are largely responsive to optical stimuli, are also monophasic. Primates have a distinct diurnal cycle, being more active during daylight. Polyphasic animals show several alternating periods of rest and activity in a 24-hour period. Many wild mammals and the young of domestic animals are of this type.

Horses, cows, and sheep seem to sleep mostly at night, whereas pigs also sleep a lot during the day. All these species have polyphasic DS and AS, with pigs showing the most episodes of sleep. Horses have the least amount of drowsiness. A given DS episode averages about $\frac{1}{2}$ hour except in the pig, in which it is longer. Duration of the average AS period is about 10 minutes or less, except in pigs in which it is about $\frac{1}{2}$ hour.

The amount of time that animals spend sleeping seems to be a species-specific function of the animal's life-style, phylogenetic rank, and age. Many conditions can interfere with sleep; new surroundings, lack of security, quality and quantity of food, weather changes, and so on. The amount of sleep can be changed enormously by adjustment of the environment to allow complete habituation.

Cats experimentally kept in the dark remain quiescent for 18 to 20 hours out of 24. In another study, in which time cues were eliminated by constant lighting, cats slept about 57 percent of the time, mostly during the day. A troop of monkeys has been observed to sleep 8.5 hours per night in the summer and 14.5 hours in the winter. Other environmental changes, such as food scarcity, endocrine arousal of mating instincts, and danger situations, also can modify the usual sleep-wakefulness cycles.

Predator species usually sleep more than nonpredators, presumably because natural selective forces discriminate against long-sleeping prey species (Table 48.1). For example, cats sleep a great deal, and they have a high incidence of AS. Prey species, such as ruminants, rabbits, and guinea pigs, sleep very little; they also have little AS, which, because it is a deep stage of sleep, would reduce the ability of a prey animal to awaken and escape capture by a predator.

The basic phylogenetic relationship is that sleep occurs in higher species only. EEG signs of sleep, for example, do not occur in the amphibians that have been tested. There are conflicting reports on sleep in reptiles, but in birds there are EEG signs of both DS and AS. Among primitive mammals, it seems that most species exhibit signs of both DS and AS, except for the most primitive species, the anteater, which exhibits DS only. Primitive mammals also tend to have incompletely developed AS, in that some of the usual physiological correlates may be absent.

The basic age relationship is that young animals sleep more than do older ones of the same species. Moreover, most of the sleep time of the young is spent in AS, and the amount of AS time gradually decreases with maturation. The high incidence of AS in the young probably begins in the fetal stage. Fetal calves within 30 days of parturition have almost half of their total sleep time in AS; EEG signs of nonsleeping were present only about 15 percent of the time.

Table 48.1. Wakefulness and sleep times (percent of each 24 hours)

Species	Wakefulness	Deactivated sleep	Activated sleep
Fox	38.9	51.1	10
Cat	44.9	41.7	13.4
Pig	46.3	46.4	7.3
Rat	48	45	7
Cow	52.3	44.5	3.1
Sheep	66.5	31.1	2.4
Rabbit	71.3	25.5	3.1
Guinea pig	71.6	24.5	3.9
Horse	80	16.7	3.3

Animals can sleep in various positions. Among livestock species, horses are the most likely to sleep standing up, an ability that is due to the bracing support of sesamoidean ligaments. However, the horse cannot cycle through all the stages of sleep, particularly AS, unless it lies down. Pigs are the most likely to lie down. Ruminants lie down in sternal recumbency, which prevents aspiration of regurgitated rumen contents. Cattle also can exhibit DS during standing, and birds exhibit both DS and AS while perching.

The most species-related visceral effect is on the rumen-reticulum activity of ruminants (Fig. 48.5). Rumination does not usually occur during AS, and contraction rates and strength are decreased in both DS and AS. No causal relations between sleep and rumen activity have been found; in goats, tranquilization promotes sleep without a major effect on contraction rate, and atropine blocks contraction without preventing DS or AS.

The depth of sleep varies greatly with species. Cats are notoriously deep sleepers, but cattle are easily aroused from sleep.

In most species, sleep deprivation is followed by a compensatory rebound increase in sleeping when the opportunity becomes available. Not all stages of sleep are equally affected. The deepest stage of DS is made up for first, followed by a compensatory increase in amount of time

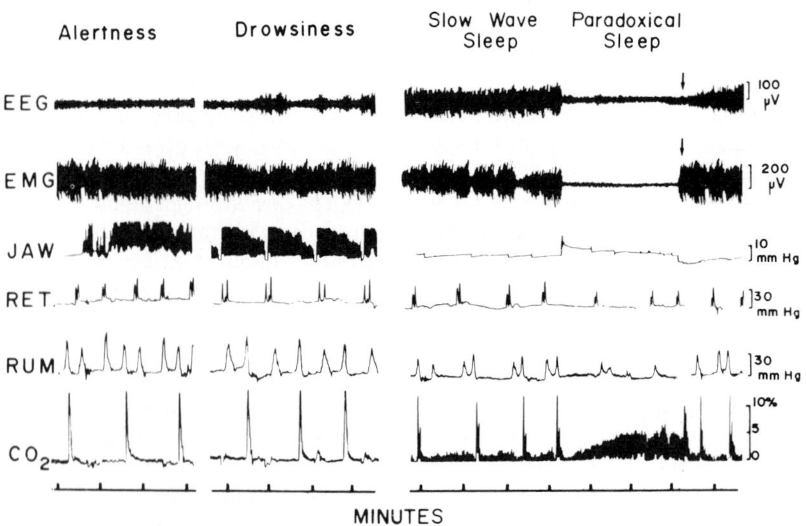

Figure 48.5. Electrographic correlates of various stages of sleep and wakefulness in cattle. As cow becomes drowsy, the EEG deactivates, muscle tone (EMG) and chewing (JAW) decrease, and some slowing of reticular (RET) and ruminal (RUM) contractions occurs. These changes progress in DS (slow-wave sleep). During AS, ending at the right-hand arrows, the EEG becomes activated, nuchal muscle tone (EMG) is abolished, and RET and RUM rate and strength of contraction decrease further, with rumination being arrested (peaks of CO_2 trace reflect eructation). (From Ruckebusch 1975, in McDonald and Warner, eds., *Digestion and Metabolism in the Ruminant* New England Pub. Unit., Armidale, Australia.)

spent in AS. Cattle, however, and perhaps other ruminants, can be deprived of AS if they are not allowed to lie down. They tend to show DS more readily while standing, and, although both DS and AS increase in the early postdeprivation period, cattle are more tolerant of AS deprivation than other species.

Narcolepsy

Sleep disorders in domestic animals are relatively rare. Only one sleep disorder, narcolepsy, has been identified in animals, and that has been seen only in dogs. Narcolepsy is a sudden "attack" of AS occurring directly from alert wakefulness without a preceding DS. Canine narcolepsy is caused by an autosomal recessive gene and is characterized by excessive daytime drowsiness and sudden attacks of AS. In affected dogs, narcolepsy is triggered by the excitement of approaching a goal, such as food, a play object, or a companion.

The sudden loss of muscle tone in narcolepsy may be caused by hyperactivity of the well-known inhibitory cells in the medial medullary reticular formation. Cholinergic stimulation of the dorsolateral pons, which projects to this medial medullary area, induces atonia, and cholinomimetic drugs aggravate clinical signs. Norepinephrine- and serotonin-uptake blockers reduce symptoms.

TRANQUILITY

Tranquility is a drug-induced state of relative depression of emotionality without corresponding sedation. Compared to sedative drugs, tranquilizers produce less dulling of senses, ataxia, soporific action, and addictiveness. Tranquilizers alter limbic system functions in ways that are not yet understood.

The selective behavioral effects of these drugs suggest a certain degree of localized function within the brain, but our understanding is incomplete. Some depression of the

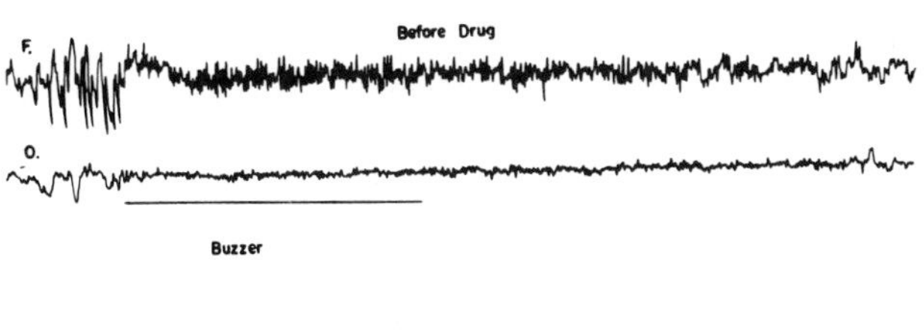

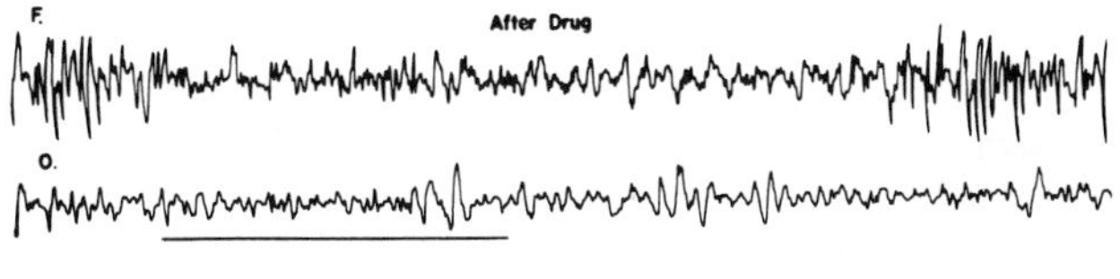

Figure 48.6. EEGs (F., frontal; O., occipital) from a rabbit illustrating a normal arousal response to a sound stimulus. After treatment (bottom) with a tranquilizing drug (chlorpromazine), the usual arousal response is not elicited.

RAS and neocortex is suggested by the observation that these drugs tend to block the EEG arousal response (Fig. 48.6) and presumably other features of the readiness response. In some species, such as cats and horses, certain tranquilizers can cause a paradoxical hyperreactivity, presumably because of disinhibitory phenomena.

PAIN

Analgesia

Pain is a conscious perception. Besides the requirement of consciousness, whether a given pattern of sensory input is perceived as painful depends on many variables. First, the sensory receptors that supply the impulses are important. The receptors that are responsible for pain are not clearly identified; some of them are probably free nerve endings. Moreover, intensity of stimulation is important; many "nonpain" receptors will mediate pain if the stimulus is very great.

Pain can be attenuated pharmacologically in one of two ways, either (1) by interfering with the propagation of the nerve impulses that carry nociceptive (pain-causing) information along specific sensory pathways or (2) by depressing consciousness and thus perception of nociceptive signals. Anesthetics and large doses of alcohol or tranquilizers probably act by depressing conscious perception, whereas "pure" analgesics, such as narcotics, act on the nociceptive pathways. Some analgesics, such as aspirin and ibuprofen, also act at the level of sensory receptors.

Anesthesia

Anesthetics abolish pain by eliminating consciousness. Impulse patterns that are normally perceived as painful are generally unimpaired or even augmented in their propagation during anesthesia, but associated evoked responses in the RAS are greatly attenuated during anesthesia. Thus, during anesthesia nociceptive input can be *received* in the neocortex but cannot be *perceived* as pain.

Animals do not have the means to express consciousness as readily as humans, and it is therefore wise to understand the actions of various drugs that are used as anesthetics. A few such agents, such as the commonly used veterinary drug, ketamine, do not really cause unconsciousness; they give that appearance simply because the animals are paralyzed and behaviorally unresponsive. Under ketamine, however, animals are mentally responsive. The drug does not alter dorsal horn neuronal responses to noxious stimuli or, apparently, their rostral projection. Noxious stimuli still evoke blood pressure increases in ketamine-treated animals, and such animals also can develop classic conditioning responses to noxious stimuli.

A common clinical experience with anesthetics is that during injection there is a transient excitement stage in which the animal seems very excited and is difficult to restrain. Sometimes anesthetics even trigger transient epileptiform seizures in diseased animals. Since anesthetics are definitely depressants, this seeming paradox has been explained as indicating disinhibition. Evidence of preferential anesthetic action on inhibitory neurons of the reticulospinal system has been presented.

Anesthetics, although they are distributed widely and uniformly throughout the brain, probably exert their most profound effect on the RAS and neocortex, presumably because they act at synaptic junctions and because these areas have so many synapses. Anesthetics fluidize membrane lipids and probably have allosteric effects on receptor proteins in the membrane because of the displacement of hydrogen-bonded water.

Anesthetics produce profound unconsciousness by selective depression of the RAS in the central core of the brain stem, rather than by deafferentiation of the more lateral spinothalamic sensory paths. As might be expected, the consequence of this RAS blocking is decreased function of many other parts of the brain. With both volatile and injectable anesthetics, HVSA dominates the EEG during a surgical plane of anesthesia. Some exceptions to this rule should be noted, however. During the early state of ether anesthesia, the EEG may be activated.

In all situations of very deep anesthesia, there is a progressive slowing and decrease in EEG activity and finally complete absence of brain waves. This absence of EEG activity is a cardinal sign that death is imminent or has already occurred.

Electrical anesthesia

Electroanesthesia is an anestheticlike state induced by the application of very large amounts of pulsating or alternating current across the head.

Electroanesthesia differs from electrosleep in several important ways. For one, much higher current densities are employed with electroanesthesia (10 to 40 mA). The stimulus frequencies are high (several hundred to thousands of cycles per second).

The question then arises as to whether animals feel pain but just cannot respond to it. The answer is not known.

There are several problems with electroanesthesia that limit its usefulness. These generally involve severe induction reactions, and there have been some side effects after anesthesia. The side effects include poor muscle relaxation, sustained contraction of respiratory muscles, laryngospasm and cyanosis, cardiac arrhythmias, and skin burns at the electrode sites.

HIBERNATION

Hibernation is a state of dormancy and fasting in mammals wherein core temperature drops but is capable of rewarming to normal via metabolic mechanisms. Unlike prolonged sleep, hibernation is a more profound biological adjustment that enables some homeothermal animals to survive a season of cold and of food scarcity by setting their thermostatic controls at very low levels and by practically abolishing activity. Presumably, species with this ability have unique thermoregulatory functions in the portion of the hypothalamus that controls body temperature by adjustments of the autonomic nervous system.

Hibernating animals become like temporary poikilotherms, with body temperatures in some species dropping to near that of the environment in cold weather. Unlike genuine poikilotherms, hibernating animals recover their ability to regulate high body temperatures in favorable environments and during periods of activity. During periods of hibernation, the most characteristic physiological changes include a marked depression of eating and metabolism, heart and respiratory rates, blood pressure, and brain electrical activity.

Hibernation is an adaptational advantage in that it permits an animal to conserve food. Those hibernators that have greatly lowered body temperature avoid freezing to death by awaking and generating body heat when their body temperature approaches freezing. Commonly, there are periodic awakenings during hibernation, even when freezing is not imminent.

The common domestic animals do not hibernate. Those species that do include the dormouse, gopher, ground squirrel, pocket mouse, hamster, hedgehog, marmot, squirrel, woodchuck, bat, and several species of birds. The bear, which was once thought only to exhibit prolonged sleep, does hibernate and experience a temperature drop of about 6.8°C, from 38.0 to 31.2°C (100.4 to 89.2°F) accompanied by lowered metabolism and lowered heart rate (see Chap. 47).

The hypothalamus and other components of the limbic system seem to be critical for hibernation. If the hypothalamus in a hibernator is damaged, there is a precipitous rather than gradual drop in body temperature during cold weather. Also, such an animal cannot protect itself by arousal when environmental temperature falls dangerously low.

Hibernation is entered through the typical stages of sleep. As the body temperature falls the incidence of AS decreases, and when temperature falls to a certain level the brain enters uninterrupted DS, until still colder temperatures produce an apparent absence of cortical electrical activity.

Hypothermia, as distinguished from true hibernation, can be induced in the nonhibernating species of domestic animals. It is entirely safe, provided certain techniques are employed, and is a useful aid in experimental surgery (see Chap. 47).

IMMOBILITY RESPONSES

An immobility response (IR) is a unique state of profound immobility and relative unresponsiveness that can be triggered by several kinds of stimulation. The best-known kinds of IR are "animal hypnosis" and drug-induced catalepsy. The most conspicuous feature is an immobility that seems to be a reflex because it is a specific, stereotyped, involuntary, and unconditioned response to specific stimuli. The state is reversible, terminating either spontaneously or on sensory stimulation.

Certain drugs, particularly dopamine-receptor blockers, can promote catalepsy in which upright, awkward postures are maintained. Animals in the "hypnosis" form of IR may seem to be unconscious, but they are not. The EEG is typically activated, and conditioned reflexes can be learned better than when the animal is not in this state. Physiological indices, such as heart and respiratory rate, during IR range from decrease to increase. The variation may be related to whether or not an animal was excited during induction.

The usual induction methods involve either fixation of vision or manual restraint. Immobilization usually requires that all animal movements be prohibited for a few seconds.

Species differences in susceptibility to the hypnosis form of IR can be quite marked, and even within a species susceptibility varies. Most of this research has been conducted in guinea pigs, rabbits, and chickens, because they are especially susceptible. Chickens can be immobilized by the commonly known technique of drawing a line in front of the beak and briefly enforcing immobility. Goats and sheep have been immobilized by manual restraint methods. Cats, although not usually considered good subjects, have been immobilized by an optic fixation method. Dogs are not good subjects, although puppies can be immobilized on their side between the ages of 4 to 7 days and 20 to 30 days. The "pointing" of adult bird dogs may be a related kind of IR.

"Animal hypnosis" is qualitatively different from DS in that it (1) is enhanced by manipulation, (2) occurs less frequently in advanced species with development, and (3) can be associated with EEG desynchrony. It differs from AS in that it has (1) no REM, (2) no persistent phasic limb twitches, (3) no absence of nuchal muscle tone, (4) periods of EEG synchrony, (5) increased incidence with tranquilizing drugs and with manipulation, and (6) decreased incidence with phylogenetically advanced species.

The relationship of "animal hypnosis" to human hypnosis is obscure, primarily because so little is known about the physiology of human hypnosis. The two states do share certain physiological features: relative analgesia, a lack of specific EEG correlates, little change in visceral function, and, most important, reduced patterned motor activity. The relationship of animal hypnosis to drug-induced catalepsy is likewise unclear. These two states have the same cardinal sign of immobility and maintenance of unusual and awkward postures; it is not known whether endogenous dopamine receptor blockade underlies the hypnosis for IR.

A working hypothesis for the mechanism of IR might assume that manipulation stimuli trigger a simultaneous descending mixture of excitation and inhibition of lower motor neurons. It should be noted that in IR there is a high state of muscle tone but no movement. Flexor reflexes seem to be inhibited during IR. The animal hypnosis form of IR can be promoted by neural systems in the brain stem, because it can be demonstrated with transections of brain just rostral to the midbrain. Thus one part of the mechanism would seem to be an activation of descending motor inhibition, known to arise from the medial medullary reticular formation. If this were the only influence, however, animals in IR would not be able to sustain awkward postures. Descending excitation of extensors is operative during IR, presumably from vestibular nuclei and reticular extensor excitatory zones in the medulla and pons. Lack of movement may arise because of inhibition of the brain-stem locomotor centers (see Chap. 44).

REFERENCES

Campbell, S.S., and Tobler, I. 1984. Animal sleep: A review of sleep duration across phylogeny. *Neurosci. Biobehav. Rev.* 8:269–300.

Folk, G.E., Jr. 1979. Protein and fat metabolism during mammalian hypophagia and hibernation. *Fed. Proc.* 39:2953–54.

Georgopoulos, A.P., Schwartz, A.B., and Kettner, R.E. 1987. Neuronal coding and robotics (a response). *Science* 237:301.

Griffin, D.R. 1984. Animal thinking. *Am. Sci.* 72:456–64.

Hobson, J.A. 1988. *The Dreaming Brain*. Basic Books, New York.

Jones, B.E. 1985. Neuroanatomical and neurochemical substrates of mechanisms underlying paradoxical sleep, p. 139–153. In D. J. McGinty, ed., *Brain Mechanisms of Sleep*. Raven Press, New York.

Katayama, Y., Dewitt, D.S., Becker, D.P., and Hayes, R.L. 1984. Behavioral evidence for a cholinoceptive pontine inhibitory area: Descending control of spinal motor output and sensory input. *Brain Res.* 296:241–62.

Kilduff, T.S., Bowersox, S.S., Kaitin, K.I., Baker, T.L., Ciaranello, R.D., and Dement, W.C. 1986. Muscarinic cholinergic receptors and the canine model of narcolepsy. *Sleep* 9:102–6.

Klemm, W.R. 1987. Resolving the controversy over humaneness of decapitation sacrifice of laboratory animals. *Lab. Anim. Sci.* 37:148–51.

Klemm, W.R. 1989. Drug effects on active immobility responses: What they tell us about neurotransmitter systems and motor functions. *Prog. Neurobiol.* 32:403–22.

Klemm, W.R., and Vertes, R., eds. 1989. *Brainstem Mechanisms of Behavior*. John Wiley & Sons, New York.

Koella, W.P. 1984. The organization and regulation of sleep. *Experientia*. 40:309–38.

McGinty, D., ed. 1985. *Brain Mechanisms of Sleep*. Raven Press, New York.

Mitler, M.M., Dement, W.C., Guilleminault, C., and Foutz, A.S. 1980. Canine narcolepsy, In *Animal Models of Neurological Disease*. Pitman Medical Ltd. Kent, England. Pp. 226–38.

Popper, K.P., and Eccles, J.C. 1977. *The Self and Its Brain*. Springer, New York.

Roitblat, H.L. 1987. *Introduction to Comparative Cognition*. W.H. Freeman & Co., New York.

Spitzer, H., Desimone, R., and Moran, J. 1988. Increased attention enhances both behavioral and neuronal performance. *Science* 240:338–40.

Waquier, A. 1985. *Sleep: Neurotransmitters and Neuromodulators*. Raven Press, New York.

CHAPTER 49

Behavioral Physiology | by W. R. Klemm

A PHYSIOLOGICAL CONCEPT OF BEHAVIOR

Behavior is an emergent property of nervous system function, and it cannot be readily explained on the basis of the properties of individual neurons or even selected neuronal populations. Behavior is the expressed sum of individual muscle contractions and hormonal secretions. The order, timing, and relative amount of muscle contractions and secretions determine what kind of behavior will occur. One can start analysis of the concept of behavior with the "final common pathway" of motoneurons (and glands) through which most of the behavioral patterns are initiated and made overt (Fig. 49.1). The interaction of sensory input and central nervous system (CNS)–initiated input to muscle and gland output neurons causes behavior to be displayed against the backdrop of the existing state of muscle tone, of primitive spinal reflexes, and of current glandular activity. Feedback modulation of behavior occurs directly on the CNS, on neurohumoral secretory cells and proprioceptors, and indirectly by the behavior itself, which may well alter both the external situation and the internal state. Accordingly, behavior is the result of the way the various nervous subsystems interact with each other and with the internal and external world.

Important to the concept of behavior is not only what behavior *is* but also what behavior *does*. Because behavior alters an animal's relationship to its external world, one of the principal consequences of behavior is adjustment of the sensory input.

Certain behaviors are relatively inflexible (stereotyped), and these consist of subunits of so-called fixed-action patterns that occur in a predictable sequence. The stimulus that initiates the sequence of subunits acts only as a trigger and exerts little or no effect on the behavior, once it is under way. Generally such patterns are genetically programmed and species-specific. Simple spinal reflexes are examples of fixed-action patterns. Another example might be the way that bulls, when presented with estrous pheromone in vitro, respond with a complex chain of specific, linked behaviors that involve attraction to and sampling of the pheromone, followed by a series of sexual preparation behaviors (see "Courtship and Mating"). However, most fixed-action patterns in domestic animals are not as fixed as they seem.

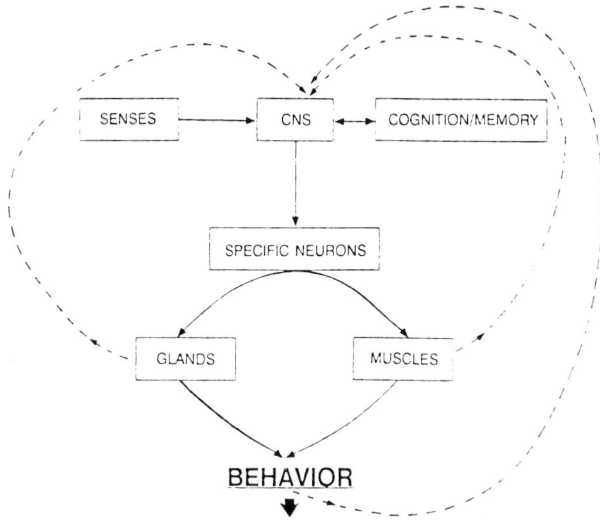

Figure 49.1. Diagram of a physiological concept of behavior. Behavior emerges from the specific pattern of motoneuron and muscle activity, which in turn is governed by sensory and other inputs, including feedback information from the muscular activity and the behavior itself. Note that behavior can be either self-initiated or driven from a variety of external or internal contingencies. CNS, central nervous system.

Most chains of reflex actions are modifiable by other stimuli and assorted CNS influences.

Most obvious animal behaviors result from serially ordered patterns of motor acts. Although the sequence is not always predictable, many types of behavior, particularly in response to a specific stimulus, are probabilistically organized; that is, one can predict the probability that a given subset of behavior will occur. This is dictated by the neuronal "wiring diagram" for inputs and outputs and by the past learning experiences of the animal.

Many complex behaviors are triggered centrally rather than as peripherally induced reflexes. In the cat, for instance, various forms of sensory deprivation have no effect on the motor discharge that underlies purring. All domestic animals have central pattern generators for locomotion. Several regions of the brain and spinal cord, when electrically or chemically stimulated, will elicit near-normal locomotor activity. The movements are stereotyped and undirected, thus suggesting that the stimulation activates a command circuit for locomotion rather than activating some motivational or drive mechanism.

CIRCADIAN RHYTHMS AND BEHAVIOR

Many physiological functions and behaviors have daily (circadian) rhythms. Times of sleep and times of activity (see Chap. 48) are the most obvious behavioral rhythms. Cattle, for example, do not sleep much, but even they have a distinct quiescent period between midnight and dawn.

Many species live in places where their activity is linked to certain rhythmic events, such as tidal actions or sunset. Such species have internal behavioral regulating rhythms that ensure that the animals perform the right behaviors at the right times. Such rhythms will persist for a time after environmental cues have changed, but eventually the "internal clock" can be reset to the new timing of the cues.

Some of the best-studied clock mechanisms involve light cycles and their influence on behavior via cyclic changes in body temperature, cortisol secretion, and hormonal responses in the pineal gland (see also Chap. 34).

In both mammals and birds, the physiological mechanisms of the pineal gland involve neural inputs from the retina to certain regions of the hypothalamus, particularly the suprachiasmatic nucleus (SCN), which in turn innervates the pineal gland. The SCN is metabolically and electrically most active in the daytime. The SCN supplies neural input to the pineal gland, whose hormone product, melatonin, has feedback influences on the SCN. Exogenously administered melatonin can entrain circadian rhythms.

Melatonin inhibits gonadal function, and since light inhibits melatonin production, long days promote reproduction in most species. One practical application is the use of long days to promote egg laying in chickens (see Chap. 38). Through these interactions, the SCN somehow modulates the amount of motor activity; that is hard to explain, because the SCN's neural output seems to be confined to the limbic system. However, experiments unrelated to circadian rhythms have implicated one limbic structure, the hippocampus, in compulsive motor activity.

Light has many interesting effects on other limbic system functions. For example, exposure of clinically depressed humans to early morning light reportedly shifts the circadian rhythm of melatonin production and alleviates the depression. The potential for influencing domestic animal behavior has not been investigated.

INGESTIVE BEHAVIOR

Modes of feeding

Filter feeding

The use of small particles as feedstuffs is usually restricted to aquatic forms; among mammals, whales are the most common example. Flexible and moving flagella or cilia direct the flow of feed-bearing liquid into "traps" of mucus-laden, threadlike tissues.

Tearing and chewing

The tearing and chewing mode of eating, common to most domestic animals, requires special mouth structures, such as the horny beaks of birds and the specialized teeth of mammals. Incisor teeth are used for cutting and gnawing, canines for tearing or piercing, and molars for crushing and grinding.

Feeding behavior

Various species chew their food in different ways. Rabbits and other rodents nibble their feed with sharp incisor teeth, while ungulates use tongue, lips, and teeth in feeding. Horses grasp forage with their teeth and tear it off, while cattle depend mostly on the tongue to encircle grass and pull it into the mouth. Sheep graze much closer to the ground than cattle because of the flexibility of their cleft upper lip. Carnivores do not have grinding molar teeth to permit lateral grinding movements; they spend very little time in eating but "wolf down" their food in large gulps.

Special feeding patterns characterize certain species. Pigs root and turn over the soil. Certain cattle breeds eat soil. Rabbits are coprophagous. Dogs bury bones or carry food from one place to another.

Social influences also affect feeding. Group-fed animals tend to eat more. Dominance relationships often develop around food sources, eventually causing dominant animals to eat more than subordinate animals.

Grazing behavior

Patterns

Cattle and sheep graze mostly in daylight, beginning around sunrise and ending about sundown; if daytime temperatures are high, cattle will graze more at night. Grazing species, especially cattle, generally function as a social unit in which every member engages in grazing, exploring, idling, or ruminating at the same time.

Goats are browsers, and because they have no taste receptors that correspond to the human bitter taste sensation, they enjoy a wide variety of plants that are distasteful to other species. Cattle prefer Bermuda grass to many other kinds of forage. When forage is scarce, cattle may eat poisonous weeds that they otherwise would ignore.

Grazing patterns affect the transmission of parasites. Cattle usually avoid herbage near manure piles, and thus the intake of parasite eggs is reduced if there is enough total forage to permit them to be selective. In pastures with mixed grass and clover, parasite eggs are concentrated on clover, and sheep are particularly prone to large infestations because they selectively graze the clover.

Distance traveled and intake

Grazing distance varies with climate, topography, availability of forage, and species. On the average, cattle graze about 3 miles per day; Brahman cattle graze longer and travel farther than European breeds. Sheep travel about 3 to 8 miles per day.

Rumination behavior

Diet affects the age at which a young animal begins rumination; nursing calves will begin rumination as soon as they begin eating grass or hay in addition to nursing.

Rumination behavior is characterized by regurgitation of rumen contents and remastication with lateral grinding movements of the jaw (Chap. 21). Rumination can occur during standing or walking but is most prominent when animals lie down specifically for that purpose. Ruminants apparently do not ruminate while asleep, but rumen contractions will persist at about the same rate as during wakefulness (Chap. 48).

The cause of regurgitation is similar to the cause of vomiting: negative esophageal pressure develops as a deep inspiration occurs with a closed glottis. Touch receptors in the reticulum are stimulated by coarse forage, thus activating a medullary reflex that controls rumination. Rumination can be interrupted temporarily by many circumstances, such as hunger, fear, pain, curiosity, or intense social interactions.

Chemoreception and feeding

Smell and taste have a great effect on the palatability and consumption of feedstuffs. Much remains to be learned about the interaction of the chemical senses in determining food intake, and the practical applications for domestic animals remain largely unexploited.

Birds have olfactory capabilities, but their food intake seems to be governed mostly by vision.

Role of early experience

Young animals often imitate the food-selection behavior of their parents. Baby calves, for example, often mimic adult grazing behavior.

Young animals are much more likely than adults to learn to accept new foods. One practical consequence is that puppies can learn to like commercial dry food and continue to like it as adults; dogs that are first exposed to it as adults often do not find it appetizing.

Dietary selection of nutrients

Physiological regulation

Of domestic animals, the pig is probably the most likely to self-select a nutritionally adequate diet if given cafeteria-style choices. Although these capabilities are poorly developed in most animals, the fact that they exist at all suggests that some physiological feedback controls operate to alter food preferences. Intake of sodium, however, is well regulated in most species. Adrenalectomy, which leads to excessive sodium loss, results in a marked appetite for sodium. Cattle are well known for their self-regulation of salt intake if they have salt-mineral blocks to lick. Sometimes animals will develop deviant food preferences if they are nutritionally deficient. Cattle grazing on phosphorus-poor land may eat bones of dead animals.

Learned taste aversions

The best-known example of such aversions is "bait shyness" of rats. Rats that survive the eating of a poisoned bait often will refuse to eat that bait again. This is a main reason that it is very difficult to exterminate colonies of rats by poisoning. The bait shyness principle has also been demonstrated in other mammals, such as coyotes and wolves.

Social influences

Social effects on ingestion run the gamut from competition to cooperation. Dogs may hunt as a pack and then fight over a bone. Cattle and sheep graze as a social activity. Feeding is even more clearly a social activity for certain species of monkeys.

THERMOREGULATORY BEHAVIOR

Thermoregulatory behavioral changes are controlled by the CNS, particularly the hypothalamus (see Chap. 47).

Hot weather adjustments

Animals seek out comfortable environments. Grazing cattle seek out shade, pigs look for mud holes, and camels alter body position to minimize sun exposure.

Metabolic heat can be reduced by decreasing food intake, and animals generally eat less when the temperature is hot.

Cold weather adjustments

Conservation of body heat is a particular problem in newborn animals because their neural thermoregulatory mechanisms are not yet mature and because they have a greater body surface-to-mass ratio. Therefore in many mammalian species the young will huddle against each other and against the mother. Such behavior quickly leads to social attachments. Moreover, the touch and odor stimuli produced by such body contact seem to be necessary for normal behavioral development, as has been shown in monkeys raised in isolation or with surrogate (artificial) mothers (see also "Maternal Behavior," below).

COMMUNICATIVE BEHAVIOR

Special communication "systems" that transmit information between and among animals include visual, auditory, and chemical cues. The detection of pertinent features of a given set of sensory cues will, of course, vary with the physiological capabilities of the species. For example, the human sensory world tends to be dominated by visual information, and humans extract this kind of information exceptionally well. A dog, on the other hand, probably gets more useful information from its sense of smell. The behaviors that are triggered by communicative signals vary, depending on whether the signal is only received or is fully perceived. Receipt of input may involve only simple reflexes, but perception of information usually involves consciousness and higher-order levels of integration that take into account the situational context, memory of past experiences, and other factors (Chap. 48).

Visual communication

Some behavioral responses to visual stimuli are genetically programmed; for example, hens in a barnyard crouch in "fear" when they see an overhead pattern that resembles a hawk. Other kinds of visual response are learned. A hungry pig will scurry to his trough if it appears that you are taking food to it. More subtle discernments depend on species differences in visual acuity. Color vision opens many new communication channels. Common examples include the sexual attraction of female birds to the colorful plumage of males and the herding and leading of female baboons by males who turn away to reveal their bright red rumps.

Visual information is communicated in terms of the contrast edges or boundaries between areas in the visual field that have different contrasts. As described elsewhere (Chaps. 39 and 41), the location and orientation of these line stimuli are detected by selectively sensitive cells in the visual cortex. Also important is the distance (i.e., "spatial frequency") across a uniform-contrast zone of a portion of the visual field. Most visual information is communicated by the low-spatial frequencies (i.e., the broader spans of visual target) rather than the high-spatial frequencies (fine details) that are not seen by all species or are not seen when there is impairment of vision (Fig. 49.2).

Some birds have exceptional capability to resolve changes in contrast, orientation, and spatial frequencies at very high speed. What other species, for example, has the adeptness of a hawk catching a field mouse that is running in the camouflage of a dry pasture? Also impressive is the visual efficiency displayed by purple martins in their high-speed aerial chases of mosquitoes.

Even in animals that are good form discriminators, such as birds and mammals, the details of the visual structure are often relatively unimportant as triggers of specific behavioral acts. One can, for example, get a bull to mount an artificial cow made of 2 × 4 inch framing lumber and covered with colored canvas, as long as estrous urine is placed on the "rear end" of the artificial cow.

In higher mammals, visual detail becomes more important. Facial expressions, particularly in primates, accomplish a great deal of communication.

Auditory communication

Certain special advantages are offered by auditory communication. Sound can go around corners. Specific sounds can be embedded in a background of noise and still be readily detected. Sound is easily "decontaminated" by the emitting animal because that animal can easily replace a given sound with another. Complex acoustic signals are most conspicuous in the communication of humans and birds.

Directionality of auditory information is enhanced because there is a hearing organ on each side of the head. In humans, for example, the wavelength of sound used in language is about equal to the distance between the ears, and the head acts as a barrier to sound propagation. At the right ear, the head creates a "shadow" of sound propagating from a source at the left (Fig. 49.3), and vice versa. The brain locates the origin by analyzing the difference in sound intensity at both ears. In animals with smaller head sizes, the wavelengths used in communication tend to be correspondingly shorter; very small animals may vocalize ultrasonically. This is because the shadow effect is magnified for very short wavelengths that are less than the width of the head.

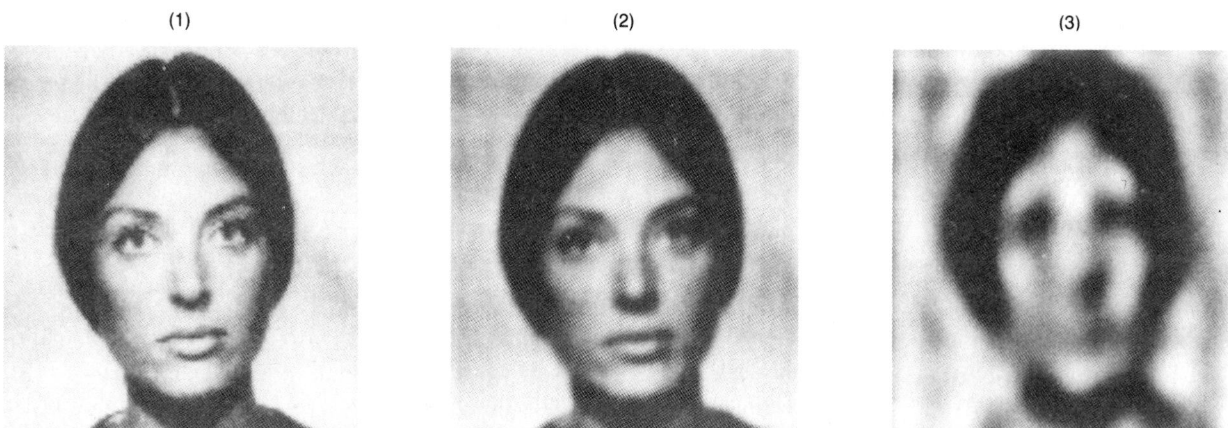

Figure 49.2. Illustration of how an animal pet, for example, might perceive its owner. The visual system conducts two-dimensional spatial frequency filtering, with the degree of fidelity varying with species. In these computer-processed photographs, the original continuous-tone portrait (*1*) was digitized, and the spatial-frequency spectra were computed by Fourier transform and attenuated by a digital filter, with a mathematical function based on visual sensitivity to contrast (*2*). This visual information was manipulated further by a low-frequency passband digital filter, and the result (*3*) approximated the low-spatial frequency information processed by a single visual "channel" (i.e., a neural system that is tuned to respond best to that spatial frequency). The filtered portraits were then reconstructed by an inverse Fourier transform. (From Ginsburg 1978, *Visual Information Processing Based on Spatial Filters Constrained by Biological Data,* AMRL-TR-78–129, National Technical Information Service, Springfield, Va.)

Birds, which communicate with wavelengths that are much longer than head dimensions, use a pressure-gradient mechanism. These animals have air cavities in the skull that connect the inner surfaces of the tympanic membranes of each ear. Movement of the right tympanum, for example, transmits sound to the inner surface of the left tympanum while sound passes around the head to the outer surface of the left tympanum. The gradient of sound intensity on the inside and outside of the tympanum determines how much it moves.

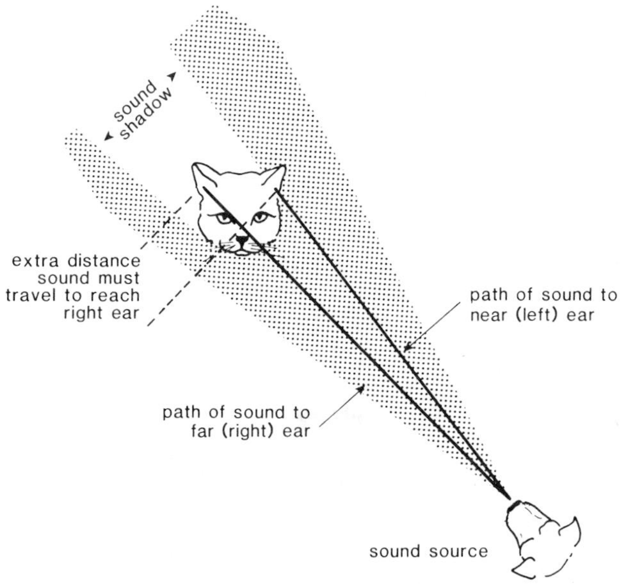

sound shadow
extra distance sound must travel to reach right ear
path of sound to near (left) ear
path of sound to far (right) ear
sound source

Figure 49.3. Localization of the origin of a sound source because of differing loudness at the two ears. The sound shadow produced by the head position relative to the direction of sound creates less sound intensity at the cat's right ear.

Chemical communication

Olfaction

Olfaction is a kind of chemical communication that has several advantages for an organism. The stimuli go around corners, can be sent over long distances, and are not affected by visual or auditory conditions. The message conveyed by such stimuli can be highly specific. The importance of olfactian is implied in the following facetious definition of a dog: "A dog is an animal that smells like a dog to another dog."

The olfactory bulb plays a role in smell communication that is similar to the role of the retina in visual communication. Similar relations exist between taste buds and the sense of taste. The senses of smell and taste are covered elsewhere (Chap. 43).

Pheromones

If a chemical that is secreted by one animal influences the behavior of another, the chemical is called a *pheromone*. In insects, many pheromones have been chemically identified, but there has been little success in identifying mammalian pheromones, probably because the behavioral assays are so complex. That is, the "fixed-action response patterns" in mammals are much more variable and distractible than those in insects.

Much of the territorial marking behavior of ungulates and of certain other mammals depends on pheromones deposited via urine or glands. Many mammals, such as dogs, label territorial boundaries with urine. One well-known mammalian pheromone is the n-butylmercaptan of the skunk.

Pheromones commonly modulate sexual behavior; the attraction of male dogs to bitches in estrus is perhaps the most commonly observed example. In rodents, male sex pheromone in the urine can accelerate the onset of puberty in young females. Adult female urine may have a similar effect of the maturation of young males. Odors from cervicovaginal secretions of cows in estrus can synchronize estrus in group-housed females. The bovine estrous pheromone also seems to be present in serum and in secretions from certain vaginal mucocutaneous glands.

Pheromones probably regulate some maternal behaviors; mothers will sometimes reject their newborn, seemingly because they "smell wrong." Similar rejection can occur if a new mother is given a newborn from another mother or even if its own newborn becomes contaminated with odors from human handling.

The mechanisms by which pheromones are detected are often assumed to be olfactory because, for example, the attraction of male dogs to bitches in estrus can occur over long distances and without visual cues.

However, not all pheromonic communication occurs via the olfactory mucosa. Experiments in which the olfactory mucosa was destroyed revealed that male hamsters could still identify bodily secretions from females that were in estrus. Presumably the vomeronasal organ (VNO) achieved this detection, because deafferentation of the VNO greatly interfered with the males' attraction to the secretions. Bull sexual responses to estrous pheromone are typically incomplete unless the bull can "taste" the sample through what appears to be VNO sampling.

The morphology of the VNO and its ducts precludes any easy access to the receptor cells. The basic arrangement is illustrated by that in cattle, in which the sensory epithelium of the VNO is found in two blind-ended sacs that are filled with mucus and that lie on either side of the base of the nasal septum (Fig. 49.4). Two bilaterally symmetrical ducts lead to these sacs; one opens into the nasal cavity, and the other opens into a pit in the midline area of the roof of the mouth near the incisor teeth.

A behavior that is associated with delivery of odorants to the VNO is a species-typical curling of the upper lip, known as *flehmen*. Extension of the neck and raising of the head are also usually observed (Fig. 49.5). This behavior occurs in most species of the cat family and in most ungulates. It occurs most often in males, particularly in association with investigation of the anogenital area of females.

In bulls the lip and tongue movements during flehmen have been studied with time-lapse photography. This re-

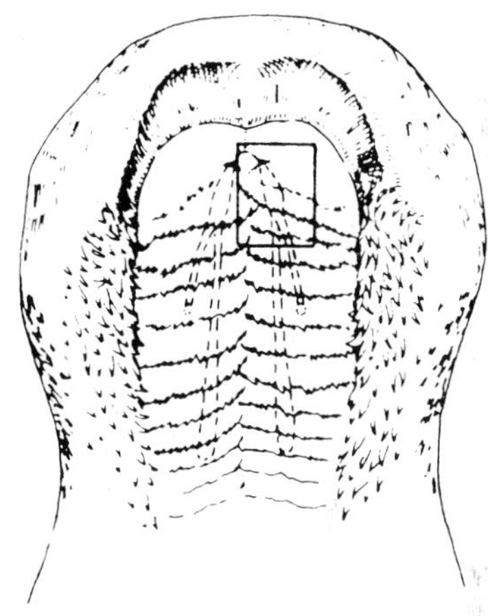

Figure 49.4. Drawing of roof of bovine mouth, superimposed on a diagram of the vomeronasal organs (parallel to the midline and coursing caudally) and the associated ducts (the lateral open-ended ducts are incisive ducts opening into the nasal cavity). (From Klemm, Sherry, Sis, Schake, and Waksman 1983, *Appl. Anim. Ethology,* 12:53–62.)

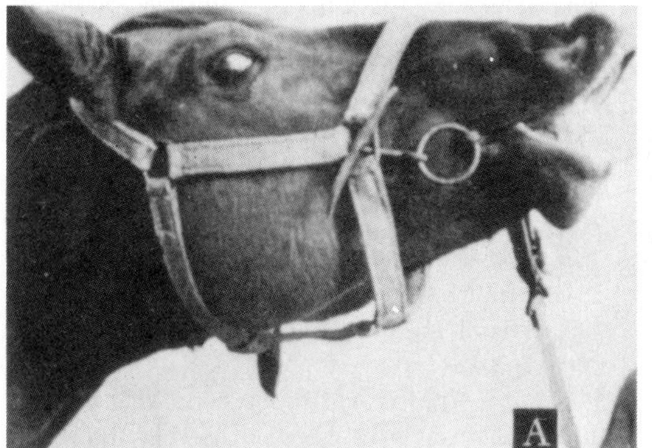

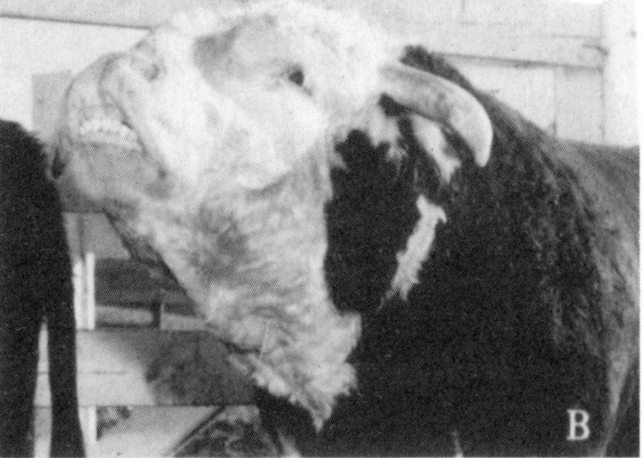

Figure 49.5. Lip-and-nose curl, known as "flehmen," in a stallion (*A*) and in a bull (*B*). (Photo A from Wierzbowski 1959, *Roczn. Nauk Roin.,* ser B., 73:753; photo B from Hafez and Schein 1969, in Hafez, ed., *Behavior of Domestic Animals,* 2nd ed., Bailliere, Tindall and Cassell, London.)

vealed that the bull places the tip of the tongue on the roof of his mouth and everts the tongue so that the ventral surface protrudes forward; a series of forward-stroking movements of the roof of the mouth seems to be associated with "sampling" of the urine for pheromone content. The bull then exhibits one or more flehmen behaviors, perhaps designed to enhance the sampling efficiency.

VNO function seems to require close proximity to the pheromone, and the chemical may even have to be delivered in solution to the VNO.

In goats application of a fluorescent dye and estrous urine to the mouth resulted in the presence of the dye in the VNO; in controls that did not show flehmen, the dye did not get far enough back into the VNO to reach the sensory epithelium. Because cavernous vascular tissue surrounds the VNO, it seems that some kind of autonomic regulation of blood flow can create a pumping action on the VNO.

The VNO efferent pathways lead to the accessory olfactory bulb, with a relay from there to the amygdala; these pathways are anatomically distinct from the olfactory mucosal pathways in all species studied thus far. The amygdala output projects into that part of the hypothalamus that participates in the cyclic preovulatory surge of gonadotropins.

SEXUAL BEHAVIOR

Courtship and mating

In primitive animals, courtship rituals commonly involve a "chained" or linked sequence of stereotyped behaviors. Even in mammals such chaining of behavioral reflexes can be evident. For example, the mating behavior of a bull often begins with his approaching the genital area of a female (probably in response to seeing the cow being mounted by others, by detection of a pheromone, or both). Then he "nuzzles" the vulva and underside of the tail; this often elicits a reflex urination by the cow, followed by the bull's licking of the vulva and underside of the tail. He then will often go through one or more cycles of flehmen behavior that is interspersed with further nuzzling and licking. The cow, in response, will signal her willingness to be mounted by the degree to which she stands still. The bull's mounting behavior seems to be governed by what he senses from the sampling of the urine and by the bodily movement cues exhibited by the cow.

Influences on sexual behavior

Sexual behavior in males is influenced particularly by the social environment, sensory capacities, and sexual stimuli. Females are sexually active only during estrus; in some species estrus is seasonal—for example, in the fall for most breeds of sheep and in the spring for horses. The cyclic behavior in females is accompanied by cyclic changes in endocrine glands and in the reproductive tract (see Chap. 36). The cyclic changes are initiated mainly through neural stimuli, such as day length (sunlight) in seasonally cyclic species, which ultimately act on the hypothalamus to regulate the release of gonadotropic hormone-releasing factors.

Behavioral signs of estrus in females often include an increase in general motor activity. In horses, cattle, and swine there are often associated changes in external genitalia, generally seen as swelling of the tissues and vaginal discharge. Estrous sows and cattle can be seen mounting other females, and they often attempt to urinate when approached by a male. Cattle are notorious for having "silent" heat, wherein cows ovulate but show no signs of estrus.

Castration and ovariectomy can greatly reduce sexual behavior, but that reduction depends largely on the animal's age and prior sexual experience; castration of sexually experienced males does not necessarily reduce mating behavior. The "buller syndrome" among castrated cattle is a significant behavioral problem in large commercial feedlots.

Also included among the stimuli that promote sexual behavior is social facilitation. Members of the opposite sex stimulate each other hormonally. For example, female sheep come into estrus sooner if rams are present in the flocks. The presence of males can also accelerate the onset of female puberty. In monkeys and hamsters, female presence accelerates onset of seasonal breeding in males. The mere presence of a female can elicit a surge in testosterone release, as has been noted in bulls, rams, boars, and laboratory animals. Puberty can be inhibited by rearing young with their family groups or by overcrowding.

In theory, any hormone that is under the control of hypothalamic releasing factors can be influenced by the sensory environment. For example, the milk letdown hormone, oxytocin, is under reflex control and subject to many conditioned influences. The mere sight or sound of a farmer moving milk cans or in other ways preparing for milking will frequently trigger milk letdown before the udder is touched. Other stimuli that are stressful will hinder oxytocin release.

Spinal reflexes dominate many sexual behaviors, as can be demonstrated in spinally transected animals. The sexual behavior of many female mammals includes a species-typical receptive posture and certain movements that are particularly noticeable during estrus. Estrogenic hormones sensitize the reflexes that underlie the movement. Stroking the skin of the vulvar area in a spinally transected dog will evoke a lateral curvature of the hindquarters and deviation of the tail to one side (such responses occur in spinally intact bitches in estrus); estrogen priming will magnify this reflex. In the spinally transected female cat, stimulation of the perineal region evokes a dorsal flexion of the pelvis, treading or stepping of the back legs, and lateral deviation of the tail (the typical movements of an intact female in estrus). Estrogen treatment magnifies the reflexes.

Higher brain functions

The role of higher brain centers in sexual behavior relates to motivation under limbic system control (see below) and environmental and contextual evaluation under cerebral cortex control. For example, removal of the cerebral cortex in males may cause them to be unresponsive to females in estrus. Similar operations in females do not necessarily abolish their sexual behaviors. This difference in cortical function also may help to explain why males are generally easily inhibited or distracted in strange surroundings. Males also are more likely to develop subtle conditioned associations between sexual contexts and neutral stimuli; the normally neutral stimuli become positively reinforcing in a sexual context.

In subcortical areas, the structure that is most obviously related to sexual behavior is the hypothalamus. The hypothalamic nuclei regulate the interactions of sex hormones and pituitary tropic factors (see Chaps. 34 and 36). In addition, the hypothalamus regulates autonomic nervous system functions that control such relevant visceral functions as penile erection, ejaculation, genital tract secretions, and so on. No doubt the motivational aspects of neural processing in other limbic areas that are closely linked to the hypothalamus contribute to the readout from the hypothalamus of glandular and smooth muscle activities that are associated with sex. Bilateral lesions of the amygdala, for example, produce a marked hypersexuality in cats.

Males and females are born with sexually undifferentiated brains, but the secretion of immature gonads quickly confers the male or female identity upon the brain. Injection of the opposite-sex hormone in a young rat only a few days old can cause it to display the sexual behaviors of the opposite sex for the rest of its life.

SOCIAL BEHAVIOR

Maternal behavior

Maternal behavior at parturition

In most domestic species, the postpartum mother licks herself, the neonate, and the placental fluid. The licking of the neonate can be quite vigorous; besides helping dry the newborn, the licking stimulates general body activity, including urination and defecation. Commonly, the placenta will be eaten. The mother generally positions herself and the neonate to facilitate nursing.

Mother-young interactions

Beyond this level (licking) of communication there are visual, tactile, taste, and olfactory communications that serve to link the pair. Once mother and offspring learn to identify each other, they also often have species-specific means of communicating. For example, baby chicks in distress will release a "fret call," which usually elicits a rapid approach by the mother. Calves and their mothers often communicate by means of individually recognizable calls. Such calling may even exist when humans cannot hear it, as with ultrasonic signals among rodents.

Bonding between mother and offspring occurs quickly. In monkeys, the principal stimulus for this bonding is tactile (touch), and this may occur to a lesser degree in other mammalian species.

Domestic animal mothers usually stay near their young; cows will call their calves if they stray too far. Mothers of most species will fight to protect their young.

The fostering behavior of the mother varies with species but is generally pronounced. Protection is afforded in many ways: cattle will hide newborn calves in tall grass; dogs will attack if they perceive danger to the young; mothers of many species require the young to stay nearby.

Mother cats teach their young to hunt mice and other small prey.

The suckling behavior of the young animal is critical to its survival, and the initial learning stages are times of great vulnerability. The sucking action is a tactile stimulus that causes release of oxytocin from the mother's neurohypophysis, which in turn promotes the letdown of milk. The lip and tongue movements of the young during suckling can be quite vigorous; in cattle, the number of pulsations during suckling ranges from 60 to 100 per minute.

If the young is separated from the mother, lactation will soon cease, especially if the young has been nursing for some time. The mother suffers considerable discomfort for the first few days after separation as the mammary gland swells with milk.

Abnormal maternal behavior

In some carnivores, the young may be cannibalized, for reasons that are not entirely clear. In sheep, prepartum ewes may steal offspring of other mothers by physically driving the mother away from the young. In all species, some mothers will reject their newborn, particularly if there is something strange about them.

In domestic animals, little is known about the effects of maternal care on the ultimate social and sexual behavior of the young. In primates, normal adult behavior requires considerable interaction with and care given by the mother during early development.

Social stress

Many social interactions among animals are stressful and can produce the typical adrenocortical hormone stress response. Aside from the obvious stresses involved in predator-prey relations and combative encounters, there are other more subtle stresses. Overcrowding and unstable social hierarchies also create stress. The temporary debilitation that is caused by such stresses as shipment of animals or unaccustomed confinement, for example, can trigger onset of certain infectious diseases (shipping fever of cattle is a well-known example).

The physiological mediation of social stress is the same as for any other kind of stress that might be induced by disease, drugs, environmental extremes, or other factors. Specifically, the autonomic nervous system activates sympathetic responses in association with increased release of hypothalamic corticotropin-releasing factor, pituitary adrenocorticotropic hormone (ACTH), and adrenocortical hormones. Hormonal effects of environmental stresses are probably mediated via the hippocampus, which is a part of the limbic system (see below), because the adrenocortical response to stress does not occur if the neural connections are cut between the hippocampus and the hypothalamus. Decreased resistance to disease often occurs during social stress. Likewise, production of milk and eggs is often decreased (see Chap. 38).

Aggressive behaviors

Aggressive behavior includes threat, attack, and retreat. Threat gestures have the adaptive advantage that they can often prevent actual fighting and bodily damage. Among the visual cueing examples are the pawing-of-the-ground behavior of angry bulls, the baring of teeth by dogs, and the arched back and raised hair of a threatened cat.

The response to aggressive gestures or other signals will often evoke either counteraggression or appeasement signals. Appeasement signals often are visual, but they may be subtle to a human observer. For example, head and neck position of cattle in social hierarchy contests often signals whether a cow that is being challenged resists the challenge or is yielding. Dogs, and sometimes primates, will signal appeasement by rolling over and spreading the hind legs to expose the abdomen and anogenital area.

Fighting is very common in carnivores and in herbivores. In all intraspecies aggressive encounters, the fighting usually serves to establish hierarchy (e.g., in cattle) or territory (e.g., in dogs). Some fighting is sexually stimulated; bulls are notorious for having vicious fights between themselves when a nearby cow is in estrus.

The physiological basis for aggressive behavior involves limbic system structures such as the hypothalamus and the amygdala. Electrical stimulation or lesions in these structures profoundly enhance or interfere with aggressive behavior; the actual influence depends on the affected brain area.

Social organization

For many species, group cohesion (e.g., of a herd of cattle or a flock of chickens) is crucial to group welfare. Cattle herds function as a unit, and each member of the group has a special social relation to all the others. Each member knows its position in the group hierarchy, and acceptance of this rank has the advantage of reducing aggressive encounters. Considerable fighting may occur, however, before the rank order is established.

For most species and breeds, the more dominant animals tend to be older males. Introduction of an alien animal into a group creates a temporary breakdown in social structure as the new animal establishes its position in the social order. The group may reject alien animals, especially if they are older. Social rank greatly affects food consumption; during food scarcity, low-ranking animals will not get as much to eat as high-ranking animals. Since aggressiveness is an important determinant of group rankings, it is not surprising to learn that brain areas that control aggression also affect social rank. Lesions of the amygdala severely disrupt the group hierarchy; for example, amygdala lesions in high-ranking monkeys cause them to become low-ranking monkeys. Interference with VNO function also seems to disrupt social organization.

EMOTIONAL BEHAVIOR: NEUROPHYSIOLOGICAL BASES

Emotions

In the early history of experiments on the neural mechanisms of emotions, several milestones led to the idea that there is a group of intimately interconnected structures that function in concert to act as an emotive brain. These milestones included discoveries that the mere handling of a decorticate dog or cat could cause marked emotional responses and that the lesions of rabies, a disease characterized by emotional disorders, occur predominantly in the hippocampus. Other studies involving lesions or electrical stimulation of various brain areas have identified several areas, such as the hypothalamus and amygdala, that are critically involved in the genesis of emotional behavior. Such areas are closely and extensively linked by reciprocal connections into a functional system known as the *limbic system* (Fig. 49.6).

The limbic system

The limbic system includes several parts of the cortex (i.e., the primitive cortex, such as cingulate and piriform cortex, and the hippocampus), the midline structure known as the septum, a cluster of nuclei collectively known as the amygdala, and the hypothalamic nuclei.

The autonomic expression of emotions is mediated ultimately by the perifornical region of the lateral hypothalamus, which projects via several brainstem relays to the intermediolateral cells of the spinal cord (Chap. 46).

The exact way that the limbic system governs behavior is not known. Whatever the mechanisms, the behavioral consequence of limbic function generally falls into one of the following categories: (1) behavioral inhibition (i.e., failure to respond or act), (2) approach or avoidance behavior, and (3) fight or flight behavior. Specific behavioral changes that occur after electrical stimulation or lesions of limbic areas are summarized in Table 49.1.

Some limbic structures perform other functions that are not so directly related to emotional behavior. For example, formation and recall of memories seem to require the function of amygdala and the hippocampus (see below). The hippocampus, in addition, seems to allow an animal to construct a spatial map, or a three-dimensional representation of the environment.

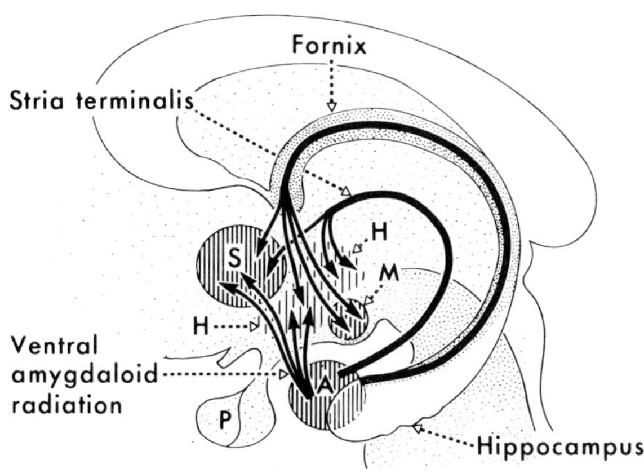

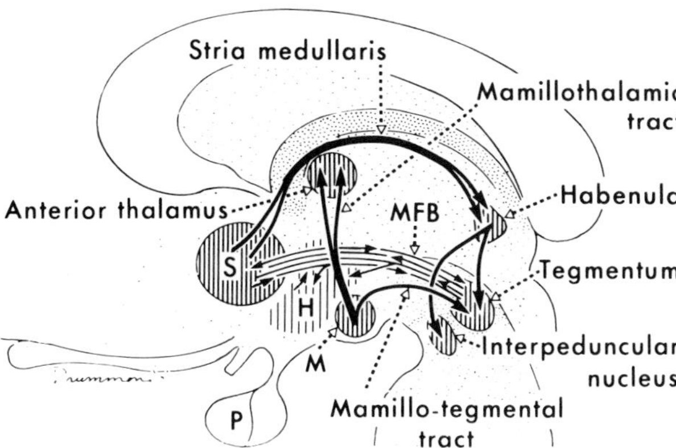

Figure 49.6. Diagrams of some of the anatomical interconnections of various parts of the limbic system. Most of the structures are midline, but the amygdala and parts of the hippocampus are lateral to the plane of the drawing. Two drawings are used for clarity of illustration. A, amygdala; H, hypothalamus; M, mammillary body; MFB, medial forebrain bundle; P, pituitary; S, septum. (From McGeer, Eccles, and McGeer 1978, *Molecular Neurobiology of the Mammalian Brain,* Plenum, New York.)

Limbic system interface between sensory input and motor output

Sensory input must be evaluated not only in terms of its exact features but also in terms of its emotional impact (i.e., the effect on drive, motivation, fear, aggressiveness, sexual desires, and so on). Thus the limbic system becomes involved in the processing of sensory input and also must be involved in producing the motor response. The relations of the hypothalamus to visceral motor control are understood reasonably well (Chap. 46). For somatic motor activity, the nucleus accumbens is particularly interesting because it is part of the limbic system but also has direct outputs to subcortical motor-control areas.

Certain motor-control areas of the brain have limbic system functions. For example, destruction or disease of the striatum (caudate nucleus and putamen) causes disorders involving autonomic homeostasis, sensorimotor integration, eating and drinking, learning and memory, and motivational and mental processes, besides expected deficits in posture and bodily movement. As another example, the dopaminergic cells in the brain stem that enhance locomotor activity via the striatum also promote motivation and euphoria.

A major challenge to our understanding of the limbic role in sensory and motor function is to explain how the emotive and cognitive functions of the brain operate together with reflex functions of the brain to initiate and maintain appropriate muscular responses.

Table 49.1. Behavioral effects of altered function in limbic areas

Brain area	Response to stimulation	Response to lesions
Cingulate gyrus	Tameness or aggression	Tameness, lack of anxiety
Septum	Defecation, micturition, tameness, hypersexuality	Irritability and attack
Amygdala	Aggression	Tameness, hypersexuality
Thalamus	Somnolence, relaxation, attack	Apathy, docility, rage
Hypothalamus	Eating, drinking, fighting, flight	Adipsia, aphagia, hyperphagia, autonomic deficits
Midbrain central gray	Fight or flight	Hyperphagia

MOTIVATION AND DRIVE

Some confusion exists in defining the difference between drives and emotions, particularly in animals. Nonetheless, to a human there are clear semantic differences between *fear*, *disappointment*, *hope*, and *anger*, on the one hand, and *hunger*, *thirst*, and *sleepiness* on the other.

Although the behavioral responses to a given stimulus may be relatively stereotyped, many variables affect the probability that such responses will occur. Often these variables relate to internal drive and motivational states. Offering food to a satiated cat, for example, is not likely to elicit eating.

The central problem with motivation is that it can be studied only by inference. Inferences about motivation can explain many behaviors, such as changes in responsiveness, goal-directed behavior, and spontaneous behavior, and can explain temporal clustering and ordering of specific behavioral patterns.

At the primitive level, motivation often arises as a "reflex" response to cues or signals that correspond, for example, to a prey, an enemy, or a social or sexual partner.

Memories of past experiences and the context created by other stimuli affect motivation. Other factors include level of arousal, level of autonomic activity, hormone levels, and emotion-producing functions within the limbic system.

Motivation usually leads to certain goal-directed behaviors. For example, if there is a drive for quenching thirst, an animal explores for water; if water is found, the goal will be approached and water will be consumed. The drive for water is thus reduced.

Many of these drives are expressions of physiological regulatory systems. In body-water regulation, a rise in osmolality, detected by osmosensitive neurons in the hypothalamus, activates water-conservation mechanisms and triggers the drive of thirst (see Chap. 31).

It is commonly assumed that there are specific functional centers for certain drive states. For example, electrical stimulation of various regions within the hypothalamus elicits, depending on the exact stimulus site, such behaviors as attack, defensive crouching, vocalization, copulation, eating, or drinking.

One should not conclude that stimulation loci are equivalent to control areas. Such stimulation could merely activate pathways that ascend or descend to a control area; alternatively, the normal balance of relations among several brain areas that mediate a given class of behaviors may be upset so that a given behavior emerges.

Convenient as the concept of brain centers is, it is an oversimplification at best. Any activity more complex than simple reflex action probably involves extensive interaction of widely separated parts of the nervous system.

Neural substrates of appetite and thirst

The physiology of appetite regulation has many practical applications in animal nutrition and veterinary medicine. Amazingly, little attention had been given this subject until recently.

Obviously, peripheral stimuli associated with taste, smell, stomach contractions, metabolic rate, and body temperature are important in the regulation of appetite and thirst. In the brain, a group of neurons in the lateral hypothalamus seems to promote the drive for eating, and a coupled group of neurons in the ventromedial hypothalamus promotes satiety; both areas are under many influences from other brain areas (Fig. 49.7). Both noradrenergic and cholinergic transmitter systems help to regulate appetite and thirst.

Utilization of glucose by hypothalamic cells is a primary influence on appetite regulation. Peptide transmitters also seem to be involved. For example, hypothalamic thyrotropin-releasing factor and cholecystokinin help to inhibit feeding. In sheep, parenteral injection of cholecystokinin inhibits feeding, and injection of cholecystokinin antibody into the cerebral ventricles stimulates feeding. Endogenous opiates interact with dopamine systems to maintain feeding. The apparent redundancy of appetite regulatory mechanisms may exist to ensure that the system is fail-safe; similar comments apply to thirst control.

It is believed that the thirst drive is affected by the octapeptide hormone, angiotensin II, acting on neurons in the anterior hypothalamus. Neurons in another nearby area, the subfornical organ, are also important in thirst regulation.

Neural substrates for aggression

Aggression seems to arise from limbic function, particularly in certain parts of the amygdala and hypothalamus. Normally, the neocortex suppresses these aggressive drives, as occurs after decortication.

The neurotransmitter systems in the limbic system are obviously important in aggression. As one example, injection of the acetylcholine mimic, carbachol, into the hypothalamus causes rats that normally do not attack mice to become killers of mice.

Under most conditions, multiple areas throughout the limbic system interact to govern aggressive behavior. Electrical stimulation or discrete lesions in various limbic areas

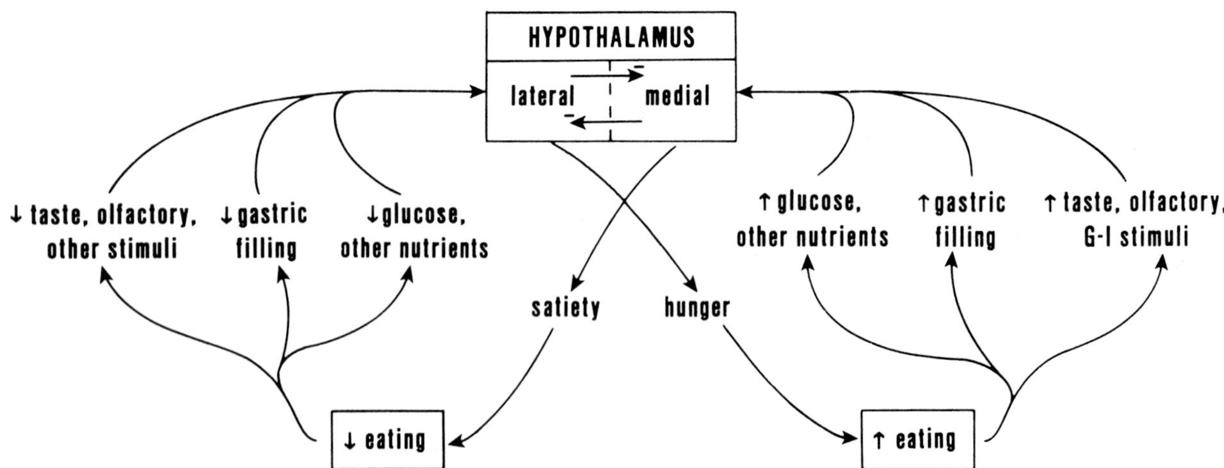

Figure 49.7. Diagram of the interrelations of various influences in the regulation of appetite. Lateral and medial parts of the hypothalamus inhibit each other, and together they form a central control for appetite regulation. Active neurons in the lateral hypothalamus initiate hunger, eating, increased blood glucose, etc. (right side of drawing), which in turn activate medial hypothalamic neurons to inhibit the lateral neurons. Opposite kinds of regulatory action appear on the left, where active medial hypothalamic neurons depress appetite and reduce taste stimuli, etc., which in turn promote activity in lateral hypothalamic neurons to promote appetite.

reveal that a variety of emotional reactions can ensue, including rage, fear, escape, "unemotional" attack, and defense (Table 49.1).

Neural substrates for reward and punishment

Certain areas of the brain mediate drives for reward or punishment (Fig. 49.8). This is shown most dramatically by experiments in which an animal is trained to press a lever that delivers (or prevents) electrical current to certain brain area via chronically implanted electrodes. Depending on the brain area implanted, an animal may press levers for hours to stimulate itself or may work vigorously at pressing levers to stop automatic delivery of current.

Positive reinforcement systems

Animals repeat behaviors that are positively reinforcing; that is, they repeat behaviors that satisfy some drive or need. The neuronal basis for such reinforcing behaviors resides in several areas of the limbic system. The effects of positive reinforcement result from electrical stimulation of such limbic areas as the lateral hypothalamus, the septum, and the medial forebrain bundle.

The neurotransmitter systems most involved in positive reinforcement seem to be catecholaminergic. It is not clear, however, whether dopamine or norepinephrine is the most important transmitter. Good arguments have been presented for both transmitters.

There may be multiple reinforcement systems. The endogenous opiate peptide system is reinforcing, and it does not seem to depend on dopamine or norepinephrine. In addition, systems that control such normally rewarding functions as eating, drinking, sexual behavior, and so on do not necessarily depend on dopamine or norepinephrine.

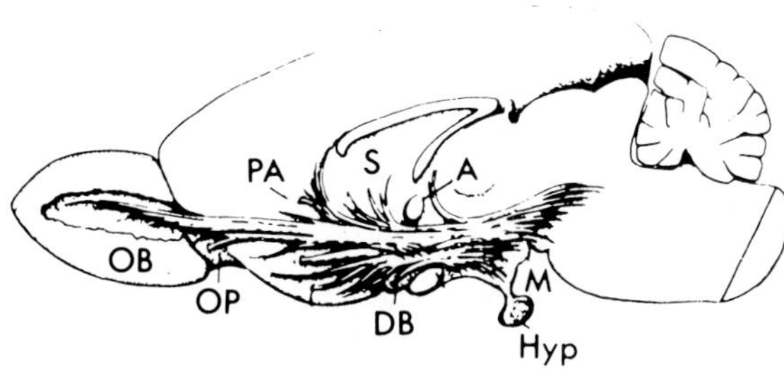

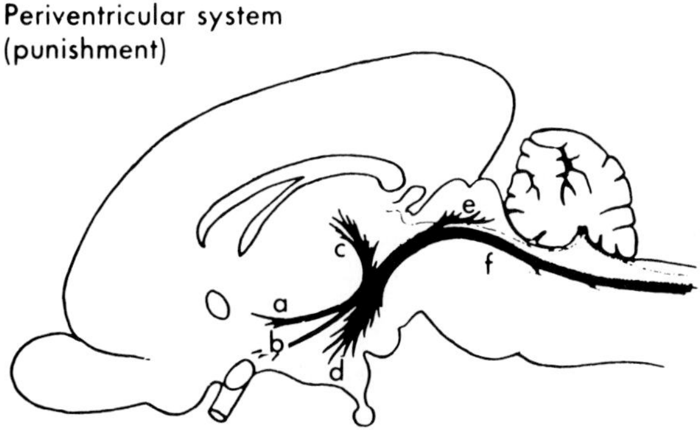

Figure 49.8. Midline views of the neural systems that regulate reward (*above*) and punishment (*below*). A, anterior commissure; DB, nucleus of the diagonal band; Hyp., hypothalamus; M, mammillary body; OB, olfactory bulb; OP, olfactory peduncle; PA, paraolfactory area; S, septum; a, periventricular nucleus; b, supraoptic nucleus; c, dorsomedial thalamus; d, posterior hypothalamus; e, tectum of midbrain; f, motor nuclei of cranial nerves. (From LeGros Clark, Beattie, Riddoch, and Dott 1938, *The Hypothalamus*, Oliver & Boyd, Ltd., Edinburgh. Used by permission of the publisher and the William Ramsay Henderson Trust.)

Negative reinforcement systems

Negatively reinforcing stimuli produce withdrawal, immobility, aversion, escape, or similar behaviors. The neural systems that mediate such behaviors occur mostly in the brain-stem reticular formation and in the periventricular and periaqueductal areas of the midbrain. The transmitter system most clearly associated with such functions is cholinergic.

LEARNING AND MEMORY

Learning and memory are coupled processes. Many aspects of these processes have great practical applications for the way one trains and manages domestic animals. The application to housebreaking of pets or the training of hunting dogs or of work animals is obvious. Other, less obvious, applications include the learned taste aversions that were mentioned earlier. The smell that is associated with the taste also can develop a conditioned association. The importance of this role of smell in formulation of pet and livestock feeds has probably been underestimated.

Kinds of learning

Imprinting

Imprinting is a kind of instantly acquired, lifelong memory that is best illustrated by the fact that baby ducks become behaviorally attached to the first living, larger animal they encounter in life (usually their mother or a chicken "setting hen"). Perhaps a similar kind of learning occurs between mammalian offspring and their mothers. The attachment of a dog to its master may involve an element of imprinting.

Conditioning (type 1)

In the simplest and classic case, an animal associates two stimuli. One stimulus produces an automatic, unlearned response, and its paired stimulus, which has no initial meaning, gradually comes to acquire meaning for the animal that learns to associate the two stimuli. In Pavlov's famous studies, for example, a hungry dog secreted stomach juices and salivated any time it saw palatable food. This response is unlearned or unconditioned and is called an unconditioned response. When a bell was rung just before the presentation of food, there was normally no response, because the dog had not yet learned its significance. With repeated presentation, however, the dog associated the bell with the food. Soon the dog started salivating as soon as it heard the bell, before it saw any food.

Conditioning (type 2)

A related kind of conditioning is known as instrumental conditioning because the animal learns a paired association by controlling the presentation of the conditioning stimulus (i.e., the animal is instrumental in controlling its own learning). One common example of such learning is so-called avoidance conditioning, wherein an animal learns to perform a certain behavior in order to prevent punishment.

Operant conditioning

Operant conditioning is a special class of instrumental conditioning that involves the animal more actively in controlling the training events. In such learning an animal must exhibit some overt behavior and is then rewarded for performing the desired behavior. A trainer can "shape" the behavior of an animal by giving suitable rewards when the animal does what the trainer wants. At first, the animal does not know what the trainer wants, but the trainer can teach that in successive, small steps. The trainer begins by rewarding the first accidental movement that comes even remotely close to the desired behavior. For example, if one wants to teach a dog to fetch a newspaper, the dog is rewarded for just approaching a newspaper. Then one successively increases the demands that must be fulfilled for reward.

Discriminative learning

In discriminative learning, a trainer rewards the animal for distinguishing one stimulus from among several by making the desired behavioral response.

Stimulus generalization

Once an animal learns to respond to a given stimulus, it may respond similarly to other similar stimuli; that is, the animal generalizes the learning situation. This process is also basic to what has been called learning-set theory, which holds that animals can learn in sets of related information. In a way, this is "learning to learn."

Habituation

After repeated stimulation without the usual association with a reward or punishment, the stimulus may soon lose its significance and the animal may stop responding. It thus learns to ignore the stimulus.

State-dependent learning

The physiological (or pharmacological) state of an animal at the time of learning or recall can affect performance. Some of the early studies of this phenomenon were done with drugs, and it was seen that an animal trained under the influence of a drug would show more complete recall if retention testing was also done while the animal was under the influence of that drug. Such observations also emphasize that the failure of recall does not necessarily suggest failure of learning. The basis for state-dependent action on storage or retrieval is not known.

Kinds of memory

Short-term memory

Short-term memories last only for the brief period immediately after learning. Recall presumably depends on and reflects the current pattern of activity in the neuronal circuits that are processing the experience. Any condition that disrupts ongoing patterns of activity can prevent the conversion, or consolidation, of short-term memories into more permanent form. The consolidation of memory also may involve an increase in the general level of arousal, as well as facilitation of specific pathways.

Factors that can interfere with consolidation include electroconvulsive shock, anesthesia, hypoxia, hypothermia, hypercapnia, and a wide variety of psychoactive drugs. In an animal's typical environment, the factor most likely to interfere with consolidation is the experience of conflicting or disruptive stimuli during or after the learning event and before enough time has elapsed for consolidation. Animal trainers are careful to construct learning environments to minimize distractions.

Long-term memory

Permanent memory is generally believed to be created by a combination of anatomical and chemical change. Learning experiences, if sufficiently intense and prolonged, can affect the proliferation and synaptic contact of axon terminals. Perhaps very subtle anatomic changes and the associated change in neuronal circuitry underlie all permanent memory. A structural basis for permanent memory has been demonstrated experimentally in a trisynaptic pathway in the hippocampus. Repeated excitatory input produces a supersensitive responsiveness in the pathway that persists, sometimes for weeks, after the stimulus. Associated physical changes include a change in the number and shape of dendritic "spines" and an increase in the number of synapses.

Principles of memory formation

The most interesting physiological aspect of memory is not the memory imprint (engram) itself but the processes whereby the stuff of memory is coded, labeled, dispatched to storage, and retrieved. The filing and coding of sensory inputs almost certainly have to involve the thalamus, because it is the principal sensory-processing system that is interposed between the environment and the cortex. Entry and recall of such labeled and coded information also involve the hippocampus and its more closely associated structures (see below).

From a variety of studies, it seems clear that memory is more of a "process" in a population than a "thing" in a place. Recent studies in cats suggest that recall of previously learned visual cues may engage between 5 million and 100 million neurons. One of the leading theories on how a learning situation is represented diffusely in the brain is that a significant sensory stimulus organizes widespread brain areas into a representational system that holds the information in a kind of buffer storage; the information in the buffer (short-term) storage can be retrieved or recodified into permanent (long-term) storage.

Less research emphasis has been placed on the neurophysiological features of two other important aspects of learning and memory: the initial encoding of stimulus features and retrieval processes. Memory mechanisms also seem to vary, depending on whether recall requires conscious attention, as in imaging or speaking, or is more subconscious, as in well-learned motor acts.

Role of the hippocampus

One part of the brain, however, that is clearly implicated in memory consolidation is the hippocampus. Lesions in this area block the ability to consolidate newly learned experiences into long-term memory.

One reason that the hippocampus is so crucial in memory processes is that it has reciprocal connections with the many cortical areas that participate in higher-order sensory processing (Fig. 49.9). It is hard for information to get processed in the brain without being routed, in part at least, through the hippocampus. Most of the input from the neo-

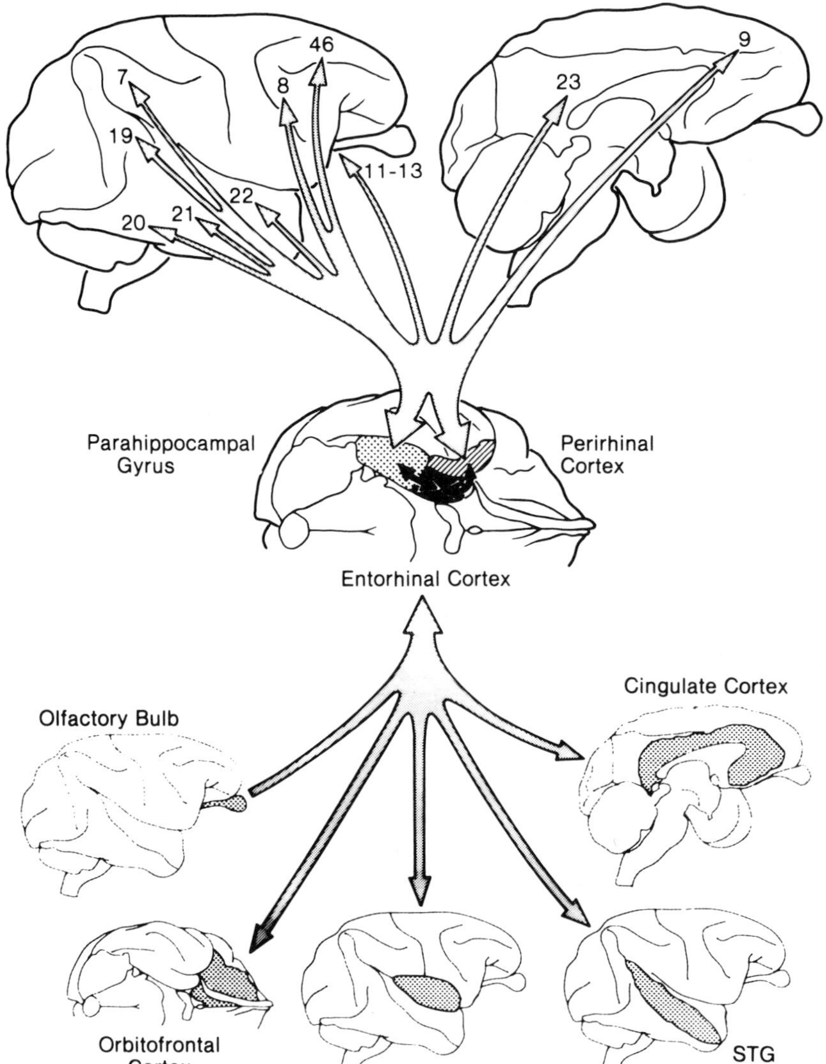

Figure 49.9. The hippocampus has a strategic location in the input and routing of inputs from many sensory sources. Reciprocal connections occur with many numbered regions of the primate neocortex, and these relay to the hippocampus (*black area*) via adjacent cortical regions (parahippocampus/perirhinal cortex—*stippled areas*). There are many other reciprocal connections that relay via the entorhinal cortex. The only pathway that is not reciprocal and that involves only one sense comes from the olfactory bulb. (From Squire, Shimamura, and Amaral 1988, in Byrne and Berry, eds., *Neural Models of Plasticity,* Academic Press, New York.)

cortex comes from several regions in the frontal, temporal, and parietal neocortex, which are relayed by cortical areas adjacent to the entorhinal cortex. The entorhinal cortex also has reciprocal connections with the hippocampus, and inputs to the hippocampus are relayed through the entorhinal cortex from many cortical regions.

Long-term postsynaptic potentiation

Memory has a representation at the cell level. For example, the responsiveness of a population of neurons can be modified by "experience," such as electrical stimulation of its inputs. If "learning" of this experience has taken place, then responsiveness at a later time when the stimulus is repeated in an enhanced response.

Chemical bases of memory

Certain biochemical changes occur during the formation of permanent memories. Because memory must be "read out" in the form of patterns of nerve impulses, the chemical storage of memory needs to be in a form that can alter the membrane permeability characteristics that govern impulse discharge. Thus the most likely place for memory-related change is in the membrane itself. Such changes may result from permanent alterations in the interior of the cell and may involve gene activation and associated ribonucleic acid (RNA) or ribosomal changes.

Turnover of both RNA and proteins is too fast to encode permanent memory. Changes in RNA and protein synthesis, however, could affect gene expression in ways that create permanent changes in synapse structure and connectivity. Many experiments have implicated protein changes in association with memory formation. Protein synthesis is involved in the formation of permanent memory because amnesia can be produced if protein synthesis in the brain is inhibited at the time of learning.

All biochemicals have a continual "turnover." This need not cause a problem for memory storage, if there is some anatomic consequence of the original chemical changes. For example, if a memory involved the formation of a new synapse, all the molecules of that synapse could be replaced, but the memory would persist as long as the synapse remained.

Drug enhancement of memory

Several drugs, in certain doses, promote the formation of certain memories. These drugs include pyrimidine bases and their precursors, corticosteroids, certain peptides such as ACTH, oxytocin, lysine vasopressin, and the stimulants pentylenetetrazol and strychnine. The vasopressin effect is particularly well documented in many animal and human studies. However, these various drug effects may be nonspecifically or indirectly related to memory. Such treatments can affect a variety of physiological states that are important to memory, states such as arousal, attentiveness, motivation, and sensitivity to rewarding or aversive features of the learning contingencies.

Most drugs either have no effect on memory or have a major impairing effect.

DEVELOPMENT OF BEHAVIOR

Functional development during embryogenesis is not as well understood as anatomical development. One generalization that seems clear is that motor functions develop earlier and more rapidly than do sensory functions. Another generalization is that neurons in many regions of the developing nervous system are initially overproduced, and their later reduction in number suggests that they compete for survival during embryogenesis and perhaps for a while after birth.

Development of behavior is particularly rapid during the early neonatal period because the brain is undergoing its most profound growth at that time. This growth is mostly due to glia cell division (neurons generally do not divide after birth) and to proliferation of dendrites and axon terminals. Dendrites develop extensive "spines" (extensions of membrane) (Fig. 49.10), which appear under electron microscopy as areas of synapse with presynaptic axon terminals.

Nerve growth factor, which is a protein containing two identical long chains of amino acids, stimulates growth of neuronal processes of some neurons. Apparently, there is also a brain-derived growth factor that has both in vivo and in vitro effects. Exogenously injected gangliosides also promote growth of neuronal processes.

One of the central ideas in modern developmental neurobiology is that neurons grow and organize their connections by use of individual chemical codes. Axons in the CNS, for example, synapse selectively with only a very limited repertoire of cell types. Muscles inactivated by denervation seem to generate some kind of unknown signal, probably chemical, for stimulation of sprouting and growth of axon terminals that can accomplish reinnervation. Cell-surface glycolipids and glycoproteins are among the probable candidates for such chemical tags.

Experience affects brain development in young animals. It is likely that even more profound environmental influences occur during embryogenesis. Embryos become motile at a very early stage of gestation, and this is clear evidence that immature neuroblasts generate impulses. This also suggests that there is ample opportunity for neural electrical activity to influence the course of tissue differentiation, but it is known from tissue-culture studies that synapse formation is not solely dependent on ongoing electrical activity.

Early experiences have profound impacts, even at the neuronal level. For example, if kittens are raised in different-structured environments where all visual input is monotonous, the responsiveness of visual cortex cells can

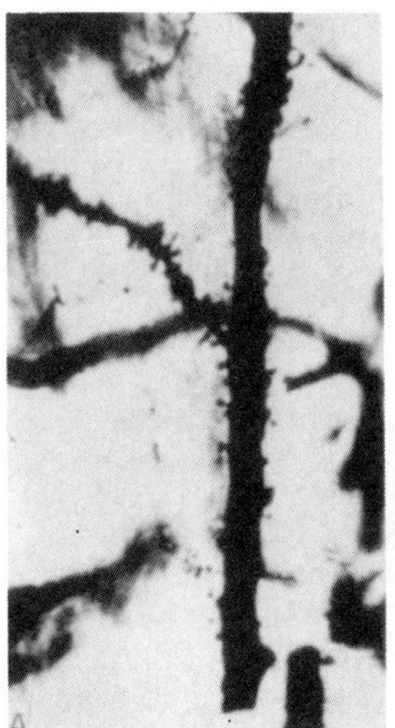

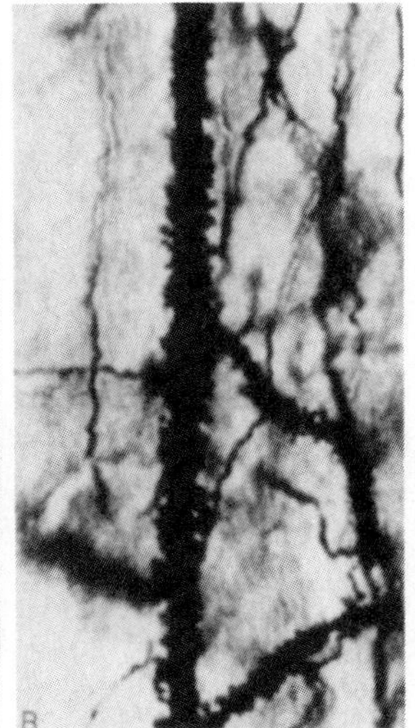

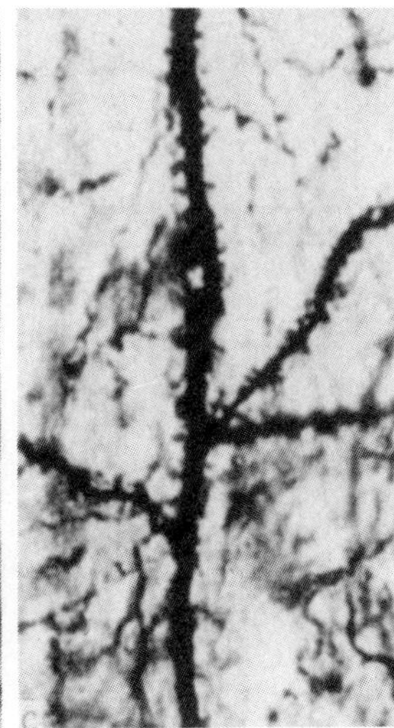

Figure 49.10. Importance of sensory input in promoting the development of synapses during development. (*A*) The loss of spines as a result of an electrolytic lesion of the geniculate, a visual relay center, given on the first day of life of a rabbit. (*B*) The spines along dendrites of pyramidal cells in the cortex of a normal 30-day-old rabbit. Note the thickness and density of the spines. (*C*) The loss of spines similar to (*A*) that occurs if the newborn rabbit has its eyes surgically removed. (From Globus 1971, in Sterman, McGinty, and Adinolfi, eds., *Brain Development and Behavior,* Academic Press, New York.)

be permanently altered. If the rearing environment contains vertically striped walls, the line-detector cells of the cortex later respond mainly to vertical stripes, whereas if the rearing environment contains horizontal stripes, the cells later respond mainly to horizontal stripes.

A more global effect of rearing environments has been demonstrated in classic experiments involving rats reared under sensorily "rich" or "poor" conditions. Rich environments include toys, running wheels, ladders, social partners, and human handling. Poor environments feature isolation and housing in a small, dim cage. Rats raised in rich environments showed significant favorable differences in cerebral cortex weight and capillary supply, number of glia cells, metabolic rate, brain acetylcholinesterase activity, and development of dendritic spines.

Gentle human handling of young animals often produces a permanent taming, or emotion-reducing, effect. Isolation or mistreatment of young animals often produces permanent behavioral disorders.

BEHAVIORAL PLASTICITY

The idea of *plasticity* is that nervous system capabilities can be changed by experiences; this is particularly demonstrable in very young animals. The idea goes beyond mere learning; the fundamental changes in the brain's anatomy and chemistry lead to changes in an animal's ability to "learn how to learn."

Plasticity presumably results when neuronal circuits change or improve connectivity. The preeminent location for the occurrence of such changes is at the synapses. Sensory input promotes synapse formation, as indicated by the degree of dendritic spines, which is greatly reduced if the sensory pathways are blocked during embryogenesis or even during early postnatal life. There is a critical period during development when the nervous system is maximally sensitive to environmental stimuli. The exact age at which this occurs, the stimuli to which it applies, and the degree of criticality vary with the species. Imprinting is a good example.

The ability to form new neuronal connections and to modify existing ones seems to decline inevitably with age (it is hard to "teach an old dog new tricks"). The first and most conspicuous sign of aging is faulty short-term memory. Older animals have little trouble performing old learned behavior but have more difficulty in consolidating new learning experiences.

The neurophysiological reasons for these effects no doubt relate to the fact that the total number of neurons in the brain decreases dramatically with age. Neurons die as aging progresses, and they are not replaced.

Development and aging can be thought of as "two sides of the same coin." Aging of the brain is manifest in a loss of neurons, reduction of neuronal branches and dendritic spines, accumulation of lipofuscin pigment, and increased glia cell proliferation. These signs can be partially delayed by three neural stimulant treatments: (1) adrenalectomy, which causes sustained increase of ACTH, (2) daily injections of ACTH fragments 4 to 9, or (3) daily injection of pentylenetetrazol.

BEHAVIORAL PATHOPHYSIOLOGY

Brain damage

A degree of recovery from brain damage can occur in mammals, particularly if the damage occurs in the young. The fact that recovery can occur argues for the principle of plasticity. If the principle is valid, it may mean that rehabilitation therapy is a very underexploited aspect of veterinary practice. The plasticity issue has been better studied in humans. Even destruction of a highly topographically organized human function such as speech can be compensated for if the lesion occurs before a child is about 10 years old. In animals, the plasticity issue is often studied by monitoring of progress after surgical creation of lesions. Such studies confirm the existence of plasticity and its age-relatedness. For example, lesions of the striate cortex are followed by eventual behavioral recovery in most mammals, provided the damage occurs at an early age. Even higher cognitive and learning functions in monkeys can be restored after lesions of the frontal cortex, if the damage occurs before the age of 5 to 12 months. Recovery rate, however, is slow and takes up to several years, and it depends on the test experiences gained during postoperative development.

The location of damage in the brain will determine the magnitude of its consequences and often determines the opportunity for later compensation. For example, damage to areas that affect appetite or to other hypothalamic areas that control vital vegetative function might so impair the general health of an animal that, without adequate nursing and supportive care, there will be no opportunity for later recovery. If learning capability is impaired by lesions in an area such as the hippocampus, then postdamage experiences may not prove helpful.

Serial ablation studies suggest a role for postdamage experience and learning in the recovery process. Sequential destruction of a brain area, as opposed to a one-step lesion, is much more likely to lead to recovery. The same principle operates even in adult animals.

Several things seem to be involved in the neurophysiological basis for recovery phenomena. One is the phenomenon known as *denervation supersensitivity;* cutting an axon, for example, makes its postsynaptic receptors supersensitive to the transmitter that is normally released by the cut axon. The response of the target tissue to that transmitter will be augmented when the transmitter is released by other axons in the vicinity. Another compensatory capability is the activation of latent synapses. Some, perhaps many, synapses in the CNS are functionally inactive or have latent capabilities. Under conditions in which they are "needed," such synapses may become functional and thus compensate for the synapses that have been lost through damage.

Another compensatory response is that of axonal regeneration and sprouting of new processes; the damaged axon may regenerate its lost fiber and reestablish the previous connection, or adjacent and undamaged axons may sprout collaterals; such changes are particularly common in an injured peripheral nerve. In the brain of mammals, the capacity for regeneration is poor, but this is not the case for certain pathways; surprisingly effective regeneration has been observed for the connections between the hypothalamus and the pituitary. If the cell bodies in an area die, that area may be partially "refilled" by proliferation of nearby axons, and this new growth creates new functional synaptic contacts.

In recent years, many studies have shown that parenteral injection of gangliosides promotes proliferation of axons and repair of neuronal damage. Also, surgically implanted fetal neurons can sometimes survive and restore some lost function.

Stress

Many stressors can cause profound and long-lasting effects on behavior. Stereotypical behaviors are common. Also common are depression and "behavioral despair," wherein the useful spontaneity of behavior is lost. These effects may result from the stress-induced release of ACTH and beta endorphin, both of which act on the brain.

In behavioral depression, there is a large decrease in brain norepinephrine. In one study involving tail-shock stress in rats, the decreased brain norepinephrine was accompanied by behavioral deficits in locomotion, rearing, and exploratory activity. Pretreatment with tyrosine prevented these effects. As in humans, animals seem to respond to social stresses with such pathological changes as hypertension, arteriosclerosis, and gastric ulcers. If the animal can alter the situation through appropriate behavior, the physiological response abates. If the animal cannot cope, behavior may become stereotyped (as may be seen in the compulsive pacing of certain zoo animals) or may be suppressed (so-called learned helplessness).

Adaptation to environmental stressors seems to involve some nervous suppressor system involving the amygdala. The hippocampus seems to be involved in the control of stress steroids.

Adverse conditions may elicit several kinds of coping effort. For example, dry sows that are confined are vigorously active initially, but then they suppress behavior or develop stereotypes. Tethered sows that have "entertaining" things to do, such as playing with a chain, may exhibit lower cortisol levels than those that do not have such opportunities.

Such observations raise new questions about the humaneness of certain commonly accepted farm practices. Physiological data are generally insufficient to permit reasoned conclusions.

Emotional stimuli also seem to affect the immune system; immune responses can be classically conditioned, for example. Lymphocytes may produce neuroendocrinelike peptide hormones. Social status seems to affect immune responsiveness; when rats live as a colony for 3 months, there is a lowering of total blood lymphocytes in subdominants but not in dominants or submissives. Neuroimmunology is an emerging new field of science that should disclose important new information about the relationships between behavior and infectious disease.

REFERENCES

Berg, D.K. 1984. New neuronal growth factors. *Annu. Rev. Neurosci.* 7: 149–70.

Bjorklund, A., and Stenevi, U. 1984. Intracerebral neural implants: Neuronal replacement and reconstruction of damaged circuitries. *Annu. Rev. Neurosci.* 7:279–308.

Brown, M.C., Holland, R.L., and Hopkins, W.G. 1981. Motor nerve sprouting. *Annu. Rev. Neurosci.* 4:17–42.

deWied, D. 1989. Neuroendocrine aspects of learning and memory processes. *News Physiol. Sci.* 4:32–6.

Dimond, S.J. 1980. *Neuropsychology*. Butterworth, London.

Freed, W.J., deMedinaceli, L., and Wyatt, R.J. 1985. Promoting functional plasticity in the damaged nervous system. *Science* 227: 1544–52.

Gorio, A., and Haber, B. 1985. *Neurobiology of Gangliosides*. A. R. Liss, New York.

Gottlieb, D.I., and Glaser, L. 1980. Cellular recognition during neural development. *Annu. Rev. Neurosci.* 3:303–18.

Greene, L.A., and Shooter, E.M. 1980. The nerve growth factor: Biochemistry, synthesis, and mechanism of action. *Annu. Rev. Neurosci.* 3:353–402.

Griffin, R.W., and Beidler, L.M. 1984. Studies in canine olfaction, taste, and feeding: A summing up and some comments on the academic-industrial relationship. *Neurosci. Biobehav. Rev.* 8:261–63.

Hafez, E.S.E., Schein, M.W., and Ewbank, R. 1969. The behavior of cattle. In E.S.E. Hafez, ed., *The Behavior of Domestic Animals*, 2nd ed. Tindall & Cassell, London. Pp. 235–95.

John, E.R. 1967. *Mechanisms of Memory.* Academic Press, New York.

John, E.R., Yang, Y., Brill, A.B., Young, R., and Ono, K. 1986. Double-labeled metabolic maps of memory. *Science* 233:1167–75.

Larson, J., Wong, D., and Lynch, G. 1986. Patterned stimulation at the theta frequency is optimal for the induction of hippocampal long-term potentiation. *Brain Res.* 368:347–50.

Lewis, D.B., and Gower, D.M. 1980. *Biology of Communication*. Halsted Press, New York.

Lewy, A.J., Sack, R.L., Miller, L.S., and Hoban, T.M. 1987. Antidepressant and circadian phase-shifting effects of light. *Science*. 235:352–54.

Lynch, G., and Larson, J. 1988. Rhythmic activity, synaptic changes, and the "how and what" of memory storage in simple cortical networks. In J.L. Davis, R.W. Newburgh, and E.J. Wegman, eds., *Brain Structure, Learning, and Memory.* Praeger, Boulder, Colo. Pp. 33–68.

Lynch, G., McGaugh, J.L., and Weinberger, N.M., eds. 1984. *Neurobiology of Learning and Memory*. Guilford Press, New York.

Mogenson, G.J., Jones, D.L., and Yim, C.Y. 1980. From motivation to action: Functional interface between the limbic system and the motor system. *Prog. Neurobiol.* 14:69–97.

Muller-Schwartze, D., and Silverstein, R.M. 1980. *Chemical Signals* Plenum Press, New York.

O'Keefe, J., and Nadel, L. 1979. The hippocampus as a cognitive map. *Behav. Brain Sci.* 2:487–533.

Overmann, S.R. 1980. Feeding behaviors. In M. R. Denny, ed., *Comparative Psychology: An Evolutionary Analysis of Animal Behavior*. John Wiley & Sons, New York. Pp. 414–35.

Purves, D., and Lichtman, J.W. 1980. Elimination of synapses in the developing nervous system. *Science* 210:153–57.

Reinis, S., and Goldman, J.M. 1980. *The Development of the Brain.* Charles C Thomas, Springfield, Ill.

Reppert, S.M., Weaver, D.R., Rivkees, S.A., and Stopa, E.G. 1988. Putative melatonin receptors in a human biological clock. *Science* 242:78–81.

Rivard, G., and Klemm, W.R. 1989. Two body fluids containing bovine estrous pheromone. *Chem. Senses* 14:273–79.

Shashoua, V.E. 1985. The role of extracellular proteins in learning and memory. *Am. Sci.* 73:364–69.

Smith, O.A., and DeVito, J.L. 1984. Central neural integration for the control of autonomic responses associated with emotion. *Annu. Rev. Neurosci.* 7:43–65.

Squire, L.R., and Butters, N., eds. 1984. *Neuropsychology of Memory*. Guilford Press, New York.

Squire, L.R., Shimamura, A.P., and Amaral, D.G. 1989. Memory and the hippocampus. In J. Byrne and W. Berry, eds., *Neural Models of Plasticity*. Academic Press. New York.

Teyler, T.J., and DiScenna, P. 1986. The hippocampal memory indexing theory. *Behav. Neurosci.* 100:147–54.

Vandenbergh, J.G. 1989. Coordination of social signals and ovarian function during sexual development. *J. Anim. Sci.* 67:1841–47.

Wiepkema, P.R., and van Adrichem, P.W.M., eds. 1987. *Biology of Stress in Farm Animals: An Integrative Approach*. M. Nijhoff Pub., distributed by Kluwer, Hingham, Mass.

Index

Page numbers followed by "f" indicate figures; those followed by "t" indicate tables.